NIEDERMEYER'S ELECTROENCEPHALOGRAPHY

DIGITAL MEDIA ACCOMPANYING THE BOOK

Individual purchasers of this book are entitled to free personal access to accompanying digital media in the online edition. Please refer to the access token card for instructions on token redemption and access.

These online ancillary materials, where available, are noted with iconography throughout the book.

🎥 Video

🔊 Audio

The corresponding media can be found on *Oxford Medicine Online*
at: www.oxfordmedicine.com/niedermeyer7e

If you are interested in access to the complete online edition, please consult with your librarian.

Access to SCORE database

Individual purchasers of this book are also entitled to free personal access to the SCORE database via URLs provided within the work.

Please refer to the unique access token card provided with the work to access **both** *Oxford Medicine Online* as well as the SCORE database.

NIEDERMEYER'S ELECTROENCEPHALOGRAPHY

Basic Principles, Clinical Applications, and Related Fields

SEVENTH EDITION

EDITED BY

Donald L. Schomer, MD

PROFESSOR, NEUROLOGY, HARVARD UNIVERSITY
DIRECTOR, LABORATORY OF CLINICAL
NEUROPHYSIOLOGY
CHIEF, COMPREHENSIVE EPILEPSY PROGRAM
DEPARTMENT OF NEUROLOGY
BETH ISRAEL DEACONESS MEDICAL CENTER
BOSTON, MA

Fernando H. Lopes da Silva, MD, PhD

EMERITUS PROFESSOR
CENTER OF NEUROSCIENCE
SWAMMERDAM INSTITUTE FOR LIFE SCIENCES
UNIVERSITY OF AMSTERDAM
AMSTERDAM, NETHERLANDS
AND
DEPARTMENT OF BIOENGINEERING
HIGH TECHNICAL INSTITUTE
UNIVERSITY OF LISBON
LISBON, PORTUGAL

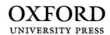

OXFORD
UNIVERSITY PRESS

OXFORD
UNIVERSITY PRESS

Oxford University Press is a department of the University of Oxford. It furthers
the University's objective of excellence in research, scholarship, and education
by publishing worldwide. Oxford is a registered trade mark of Oxford University
Press in the UK and certain other countries.

Published in the United States of America by Oxford University Press
198 Madison Avenue, New York, NY 10016, United States of America.

Library of Congress Cataloging-in-Publication Data
Names: Schomer, Donald L., editor. | Lopes da Silva, F. H., 1935– editor.
Title: Niedermeyer's electroencephalography : basic principles, clinical applications,
and related fields / edited by Donald L. Schomer, Fernando H. Lopes da Silva.
Other titles: Electroencephalography
Description: Seventh edition. | New York, NY : Oxford University Press, [2018] |
Includes bibliographical references and index.
Identifiers: LCCN 2017000250 | ISBN 9780190228484 (alk. paper)
Subjects: | MESH: Electroencephalography | Central Nervous System
Diseases—diagnosis Classification: LCC RC386.6.E43 |
NLM WL 150 | DDC 616.8/047547—dc23
LC record available at https://lccn.loc.gov/2017000250

This material is not intended to be, and should not be considered, a substitute for medical or
other professional advice. Treatment for the conditions described in this material is highly
dependent on the individual circumstances. While this material is designed to offer
accurate information with respect to the subject matter covered and to be current as of the
time it was written, research and knowledge about medical and health issues is constantly
evolving and dose schedules for medications are being revised continually, with new side effects
recognized and accounted for regularly. Readers must therefore always check the product
information and clinical procedures with the most up-to-date published product information
and data sheets provided by the manufacturers and the most recent codes of conduct and
safety regulation. The publisher and the authors make no representations or warranties to
readers, express or implied, as to the accuracy or completeness of this material. Without
limiting the foregoing, the publisher and the authors make no representations or warranties
as to the accuracy or efficacy of the drug dosages mentioned in the material. The authors and
the publisher do not accept, and expressly disclaim, any responsibility for any liability, loss or risk
that may be claimed or incurred as a consequence of the use and/or application of any of the
contents of this material.

9 8 7 6

Printed in the United States of America on acid-free paper

We would like to dedicate this book to students of clinical neurophysiology from around the world and from all the ages. We have learned so much from you and from your dedication to the better understanding of the physiological workings of the brain. We have enjoyed passing some of this great body of scientific work on to you, our students, both directly and indirectly. We now are looking forward to you, the younger members of our profession, to continue to push forward the boundaries of our field. Our heartfelt support in your endeavors.

Donald L. Schomer, MD
Fernando H. Lopes da Silva, MD, PhD

CONTENTS

PREFACE TO THE SEVENTH EDITION

We have had a challenging and fruitful last several years putting together this seventh edition of Ernst Niedermeyer's masterpiece. First, we have a new publisher, the Oxford University Press (OUP). We would like to thank Craig Panner from OUP for all of his help, support, encouragement, and counsel over the last several years as we have made this, what we believe to be, very successful transition. Also, we have partnered with the Holberg Group, the business side of the ILAE and European Consortium of Epilepsy Centers that developed the SCORE System for EEG report interpretation and reporting. They have made available to our readers a teaching module of EEG studies and reports that we hope will show us that there can be order and consistency to EEG interpretations for the international community of EEG labs.

This edition has been extensively revised from our sixth edition. We have added chapters on recording techniques related to deep brain stimulation for movement disorders and on responsive brain stimulation for epilepsy. Dr. Shils and his co-authors have included a number of audio recordings demonstrating what is actually heard in the operating room during these procedures that allows them to place their stimulating probes accurately. Drs. Thompson, Hallett, and Shibaski have combined their efforts to produce a chapter on the neurophysiological basis of myoclonus, a chapter that, for too long, has been absent from this book. Dr. Beniczky and his collaborators on the SCORE project have a new chapter providing an introduction to and the theory behind the SCORE system. Dr. Shibaski and collaborators from Japan have an intriguing chapter on how to build an automated EEG waveform interpretation system that may someday complement the SCORE system's technology. Drs. Beal and Beniczky combined their efforts in a chapter that discusses how to design and develop clinical trials through the implementation of STARD protocol designs that support and assist us in better validating our diagnostic tests and sheds considerable light on where older and sometimes classical studies may be seriously deficient. With a major ongoing push to provide meaningful EEG recording in the various ICU settings, Drs. Hirsch and Riviello and their co-authors have given us a new chapter dedicated to that subject.

The chapters dealing with basic science aspects of clinical neurophysiology have been substantially updated to reflect the huge number of studies that provide new fundamental findings regarding the biophysics, physiology, dynamics, and analysis of neuronal networks. New collaborators joined the time-honored teams of authors of these basic and analytical chapters, namely Drs. Wendling, Wadman, Congedo,

Garcia-Larrea, Palva, Hahn, and Brunner. A new chapter reflecting the clinical research area that focuses on combining EEG with other imaging techniques has been added through the significant efforts of Drs. Seeck, Spinelli, and Gotman. The burgeoning field of neurocognitive research was strengthened with the contribution of Dr. Halgren, whose life career has focused on these matters.

We have combined many chapters from the sixth edition in an attempt to bring related topics together. For example, all of the standard technical-based chapters related to the more fundamental aspects of EEG technology and recording principles have been combined into one large chapter on analog and digital technologies, polarity and electrical field determinations, and multimodal monitors such as ECG, EMG, SaO_2, and so forth. Drs. Galovic, Schmitz, and Tettenborn wrote a chapter that combines and updates the previous chapters related to EEG findings in inflammatory disorders of the brain, cerebrovascular disease, trauma, and migraine. Drs. Chokroverty and Vertungo combined technical with clinical aspects of polysomnography and have made readily available to us numerous audio/video examples of sleep-related disorders. The chapters related to normal EEG through the ages and EEG recording in people with epilepsy have all been extensively updated and rewritten, reflecting the tremendous advances in both fields that have occurred since the prior edition. The chapters on normal EEG and the EEG findings in children with epilepsy were fused and many new collaborators joined the previous authors' team, namely Drs. Beal, Eisermann, Mizrahi, Pearl, and Plouin. Their combined efforts give these chapters a truly worldwide perspective. As noted earlier, examples of EEG findings seen in studies from people in different age groups and including playable recordings of seizures can be accessed directly from our online version of this book linked to the SCORE teaching system. Dr. Drislane and co-authors, working on chapters related to convulsive status epilepticus and nonconvulsive status, updated and extensively modified their work from the previous edition, as was the extensive rewrite of the chapter related to dementing disorders now authored by Dr. Babiloni and collaborators. Drs. LaFrance and Chen have authored a new chapter on "nonepileptic events." Almost all of our old favorites (e.g., HFOs, infraslow EEG, MEG, VEPs, BAERs, and SSEP) have been updated with many new examples. OUP is allowing all of the authors to have their color photos and examples appear in the related chapter instead of on "color plates" printed at a distance from their work, making the chapter just that much easier to read.

Finally, special thanks go out to Emily Samulski from OUP for her tireless support throughout the entire process getting this seventh edition ready to go to the production manager. Mary Ann Dobrata, a research scientist in my program, gave selflessly of her time and technical expertise to ensure all examples met or exceeded OUP expectations for delivery. Our sincere thanks goes out to her. Of course, both of us would still like to recognize Ernst Niedermeyer, not only for his foresight in identifying this book as a standard reference for the field of clinical neurophysiology, but also for his depth of understanding of all aspects of this field and the ability to write eloquently about it.

Donald L. Schomer, MD
Fernando H. Lopes da Silva, MD, PhD

CONTRIBUTORS

Florin Amzica, PhD
Department of Stomatology
Université de Montreal
Montreal, Canada

Jeffrey E. Arle, MD, PhD
Associate Professor of Neurosurgery,
    Harvard Medical School
Associate Chief, Neurosurgery
Beth Israel Medical Center
Chief Neurosurgery, Mt. Auburn Hospital
Boston, MA

Harald Aurlien, MD, PhD
Department of Neurology
Haukeland University Hospital
Department of Clinical Medicine
University of Bergen
Bergen, Norway

Claudio Babiloni, PhD
Department of Physiology and Pharmacology
    "Vittorio Erspamer"
University of Rome "La Sapienza"; and
Department of Neuroscience
IRCCS San Raffaele Pisana
Rome, Italy

Jules C. Beal, MD
Assistant Professor of Pediatrics and Neurology
Director of the Pediatric Neurohospitalist Service
Montefiore Medical Center
Albert Einstein College of Medicine
Bronx, NY

Sándor Beniczky, MD, PhD
Professor of Clinical Neurophysiology
Danish Epilepsy Centre, Dianalund
Aarhus University Hospital
Aarhus, Denmark

Adriana Bermeo-Ovalle, MD
Assistant Professor of Neurological Sciences
Director, EEG Laboratory
Department of Neurological Sciences
Rush University Medical College
Chicago, IL

Jan Brøgger, MD, PhD
Department of Neurology
Haukeland University Hospital
Department of Clinical Medicine
University of Bergen
Bergen, Norway

Clemens Brunner, PhD
Institute of Psychology
University of Graz
Graz, Austria

Ana Buján, PhD
Gerontology Research Group
Department of Biomedical Sciences, Medicine
    and Physiotherapy
Faculty of Health Sciences
University of A Coruña - INIBIC
A Coruña, Spain

Gastone G. Celesia, MD
Department of Neurology, Stritch School of Medicine
Loyola University of Chicago
Chicago Council for Science and Technology
Chicago, IL

Bernard S. Chang, MD, MMSc
Associate Professor, Harvard Medical School
Department of Neurology, Division of Epilepsy
    and Electroencephalography
Beth Israel Deaconess Medical Center,
    Harvard Medical School
Boston, MA

David K. Chen, MD
Assistant Professor of Neurology
Baylor College of Medicine
Director, Neurophysiology Services
Michael E. DeBakey VA Medical Center
Houston, TX

Sudhansu Chokroverty, MD
Professor, Neurology
New Jersey Neuroscience Institute at JFK
Edison, NJ

Marco Congedo, PhD
GIPSA-lab
CNRS (Centre National de la Recherche Scientifique)
Grenoble Institute of Technology
Grenoble-Alpes University
Grenoble, France

Nathan E. Crone, MD
Professor, Department of Neurology
Johns Hopkins University School of Medicine
Baltimore, MD

Frank W. Drislane, MD
Professor, Neurology, Harvard Medical School
Neurologist, Comprehensive Epilepsy Center
Beth Israel Deaconess Medical Center
Boston, MA

Barbara A. Dworetzky, MD
Associate Professor, Harvard Medical School
Chief, Division of Epilepsy
Department of Neurology
Brigham and Women's Hospital
Boston, MA

Jonathan C. Edwards, MD
Professor and Vice Chair for Clinical Affairs
Director MUSC Comprehensive Epilepsy Center
Medical Director, Clinical Neurophysiology Laboratories
The Medical University of South Carolina
Department of Neurology
Charleston, SC

Monika Eisermann, MD
Department of Clinical Neurophysiology
Necker Enfants Malades Hospital
Research Unit "Infantile Epilepsies and Brain Plasticity"
Inserm
Paris, France
University Paris Descartes
CEA
Gif sur Yvette, France

Ronald G. Emerson, MD
Department of Neurology
Professor of Neurology
Hospital for Special Surgery
Weill Cornell Medical College, Cornell University
New York, NY

Charles M. Epstein, MD
Professor of Neurology
Emory University School of Medicine
Emory Healthcare
Atlanta, GA

Joshua B. Ewen, MD
Department of Neurology and Developmental Medicine
Kennedy Krieger Institute
Department of Neurology
Johns Hopkins University School of Medicine
Department of Psychological and Brain Sciences
Johns Hopkins University
Baltimore, MD

Bruce J. Fisch, MD
Professor Emeritus of Neurology
Director, University of New Mexico Clinical MEG Center
Albuquerque, NM

John Gaitanis, MD
Chief, Pediatric Neurology Tufts Medical Center
Boston, MA

Marian Galovic, MD
Department of Clinical and Experimental Epilepsy
UCL Institute of Neurology
Queen Square
London, UK

Luis Garcia-Larrea, MD, PhD
NEUROPAIN—Intégration Centrale de la douleur
    chez l'Homme
INSERM, Centre de Recherche en Neurosciences
Groupement Hospitalier Est, Hôpital Neurologique
BRON Cedex, France

Howard Goodkin, MD
Shure Professor of Neurology and Pediatrics
University of Virginia
Charlottesville, VA

Jean Gotman, PhD
Professor, Montreal Neurological Institute
McGill University
Montreal, Quebec, Canada

Cecil D. Hahn, MD, MPH
Division of Neurology
The Hospital for Sick Children
Department of Paediatrics
University of Toronto
Toronto, Ontario, Canada

Eric Halgren, PhD
Departments of Radiology, Neurosciences, and Psychiatry
University of California at San Diego
La Jolla, CA

Mark Hallett, MD
Chief, Human Motor Control Section
National Institute of Neurological Disorders and Stroke
National Institute of Health
Bethesda, MD

Abeer J. Hani, MD
Assistant Professor, Pediatrics and Neurology
Gilbert and Rose-Marie Chagoury School of Medicine
Lebanese American University
Beirut, Lebanon

Riitta Hari, MD, PhD
Professor Emertia
Department of Art
School of Art, Design and Architecture, and
Department of Neuroscience and Biomedical Engineering
School of Science
Aalto University
Aalto, Finland

Adam L. Hartman, MD
Departments of Neurology and Pediatrics
Johns Hopkins School of Medicine
Baltimore, MD

Bin He, PhD
Department of Biomedical Engineering and Institute for
    Engineering in Medicine
University of Minnesota
Minneapolis, MN

Susan T. Herman, MD
Assistant Professor, Neurology, Harvard Medical School
Neurologist, Comprehensive Epilepsy Center
Beth Israel Deaconess Medical Center
Boston, MA

Lawrence J. Hirsch, MD
Professor of Neurology
Chief, Division of Epilepsy and EEG
Co-Director, Yale Comprehensive Epilepsy Center
Co-Director, Critical Care EEG Monitoring Program
Yale University
New Haven, CT

Aatif M. Husain, MD
Department of Neurology
Duke University Medical Center
Neurodiagnostic Center
Veterans Affairs Medical Center
Durham, NC

Stiliyan Kalitzin, PhD
Clinical Physicist
Principal Advisor in Medical Technology
Foundation Epilepsy Institute in The Netherlands (SEIN)
External Faculty
Image Sciences Institute
University Medical Center
Utrecht, The Netherlands

Andres M. Kanner, MD, FANA, FAES, FAAN
Professor of Clinical Neurology
Director, Comprehensive Epilepsy Center
Head, Epilepsy Division
Department of Neurology
University of Miami
Miller School of Medicine
Miami, FL

Peter W. Kaplan, MB, BS, FRCP
Department of Neurology, Johns Hopkins University
Johns Hopkins Bayview Medical Center
Baltimore, MD

Mena Kerolus, MD
Department of Neurosurgery
Rush University
Chicago, IL

Ryan Kochanski, MD
Department of Neurosurgery
Rush University
Chicago, IL

Vaishnav Krishnan, MD, PhD
Instructor, Harvard Medical School
Department of Neurology, Division of Epilepsy and
    Electroencephalography
Beth Israel Deaconess Medical Center
Harvard Medical School
Boston, MA

Ekrem Kutluay, MD
Professor of Neurology
Associate Director, MUSC Comprehensive Epilepsy Center
Medical Director, Neuro-Intraoperative Monitoring
The Medical University of South Carolina
Department of Neurology
Charleston, SC

W. Curt LaFrance, Jr., MD, MPH
Associate Professor of Psychiatry and Neurology
Brown University
Director, Neuropsychiatry and Behavioral Neurology
Rhode Island Hospital
Staff Physician
Providence VA Medical Center
Rhode Island Hospital, Brown University
Providence, RI

Alan D. Legatt, MD, PhD
Professor, Department of Neurology
Albert Einstein College of Medicine
Director of Intraoperative Monitoring
Department of Neurology
Montefiore Medical Center
Bronx, NY

Ronald P. Lesser, MD
Departments of Neurology and Neurosurgery
Johns Hopkins School of Medicine
Baltimore, MD

Fernando H. Lopes da Silva, MD, PhD
Emeritus Professor
Center of Neuroscience
Swammerdam Institute for Life Sciences
University of Amsterdam
Amsterdam, Netherlands
Department of Bioengineering
High Technical Institute
University of Lisbon
Lisbon, Portugal

François Mauguière, MD, PhD
Functional Neurology and Epilepsy Department
Hôpital Neurologique Pierre-Wertheimer
Hospices Civils de Lyon (HCL)
Lyon 1 University
Lyon, France

Douglas Maus, MD, PhD
Assistant Professor, Neurology, Harvard University
Department of Neurology
Massachusetts General Hospital
Boston, MA

Christoph M. Michel, PhD
Functional Brain Mapping Laboratory
Department of Basic Neuroscience
University of Geneva
Campus Biotech
Geneva, Switzerland

Sunita Misra, MD, PhD
Department of Pediatric Neurology
Baylor College of Medicine
Houston, TX

Eli M. Mizrahi, MD
Chief of the Neurophysiology Service
St. Luke's Episcopal Hospital
Chair, Department of Neurology
Professor, Neurology and Pediatrics
Baylor College of Medicine
Houston, TX

Solomon L. Moshe, MD
Professor of Neurology
The Saul R. Korey Department of Neurology
Professor of Pediatrics
Department of Pediatrics
Professor of Neuroscience
The Dominick P. Purpura Department of Neuroscience
Charles Frost Chair in Neurosurgery and Neurology
Albert Einstein College of Medicine
Director, Division of Pediatric Neurology
Director of Clinical Neurophysiology
The Saul R. Korey Department of Neurology
Director of the Division of Neurology
Department of Pediatrics
The Children's Hospital at Montefiore
Bronx, NY

Masatoshi Nakamura[†], MD
Emeritus Professor
Saga University Graduate School of Science
    and Engineering
Saga, Japan

Christa Neuper, PhD
Institute of Psychology
University of Graz
Graz, Austria

Douglas R. Nordli, Jr., MD
Chief, Division of Pediatric Neurology
Director of the Neurosciences Institute
Children's Hospital Los Angeles
Los Angeles, CA

Marc R. Nuwer, MD, PhD
Professor and Vice Chair, Department of Neurology
David Geffen School of Medicine at UCLA
Department Head, Department of Clinical
    Neurophysiology
Ronald Reagan UCLA Medical Center
Los Angeles, CA

Gamaleldin M. Osman, MD
ICU- EEG Research Fellow
Yale University
New Haven, CT
Assistant Lecturer of Neurology
Ain Shams University
Cairo, Egypt

J. Matias Palva, PhD
Neuroscience Center
Helsinki Institute of Life Science
University of Helsinki
Helsinki, Finland

Trudy Pang, MD
Assistant Professor, Neurology, Harvard University
Department of Neurology, Beth Israel Deaconess Medical Center
Beth Israel Deaconess Medical Center
Boston, MA

Alvaro Pascual-Leone, MD, PhD
Professor, Neurology, Harvard University
Director, Berenson-Allen Center for Noninvasive
    Brain Stimulation
Department of Neurology
Beth Israel Deaconess Medical Center
Boston, MA

Neal S. Peachey, PhD
Cole Eye Institute
Cleveland Clinic Foundation
Louis Stokes Cleveland VA Medical Center
Cleveland, OH

Phillip L. Pearl, MD
William G. Lennox Chair and Professor of Neurology
Director of Epilepsy and Clinical Neurophysiology
Department of Neurology, Boston Children's Hospital
Harvard Medical School
Boston, MA

Claudio Del Percio, PhD
Department of Integrated Imaging
IRCCS SDN
Napoli, Italy

Gert Pfurtscheller, PhD
Institute of Neural Engineering
Graz University of Technology
Graz, Austria

Perrine Plouin, MD
Department of Clinical Neurophysiology
Necker Enfants Malades Hospital
Paris, France

Ronit Pressler, MD, PhD, MRCPCH
Department of Clinical Neurophysiology
Great Ormond Street Hospital for Children NHS
    Foundation Trust
Clinical Neuroscience
UCL Institute of Child Health
London, UK

Claus Reinsberger, MD, PhD
Institute of Sports Medicine
Department of Sports and Health
Faculty of Science, Paderborn University
Paderborn, Germany

James J. Riviello, Jr., MD
Professor of Pediatrics
Associate Section Head for Epilepsy, Neurophysiology, and
    Neurocritical Care
Section of Pediatric and Developmental Neuroscience
Baylor College of Medicine
Blue Bird Clinic for Pediatric Neurology
Texas Children's Hospital
Houston, TX

Alexander Rotenberg, MD, PhD
Associate Professor, Neurology, Harvard University
Director, Neuromodulation Program
Department of Neurology
Fegan 9, Children's Hospital
Boston, MA

Sepehr Sani, MD
Assistant Professor, Department of Neurosurgery
Rush University
Chicago, IL

Bettina Schmitz, MD
Professor, Chair, Department of Neurology
Vivantes Humbolt-Klinikum
Berlin, Germany

Andrew Schomer, MD
Assistant Professor, University of Virginia
Department of Neurology
Divisions of Epilepsy and Neurocritical Care
University of Virginia
Charlottesville, VA

Donald L. Schomer, MD
Professor, Neurology, Harvard University
Director, Laboratory of Clinical Neurophysiology
Chief, Comprehensive Epilepsy Program
Department of Neurology
Beth Israel Deaconess Medical Center
Boston, MA

Stephan Schuele MD, MPH
Associate Professor, Department of Neurology
Feinberg School of Medicine, Northwestern University
Medical Director, Neurological Testing Center
Northwestern Memorial Hospital
Chicago, IL

Margitta Seeck, MD
EEG and Epilepsy Unit
Department of Clinical Neurosciences
University Hospital of Geneva
Geneva, Switzerland

Mouhsin M. Shafi, MD, PhD
Assistant Professor, Neurology, Harvard University
Department of Neurology
Division of Epilepsy and Clinical Neurophysiology
Beth Israel Deaconess Medical Center
Boston, MA

Hiroshi Shibasaki, MD
Kyoto University Graduate School of Medicine
Takeda General Hospital
Kyoto, Japan

Jay L. Shils, PhD, DABNM, FASNM, FACNS
Director of Intraoperative Neurophysiology
Associate Professor, Department of Anesthesia
Rush University
Chicago, IL

Laurent Spinelli, PhD
EEG & Epilepsy Unit
Department of Clinical Neurosciences
University Hospital of Geneva
Geneva, Switzerland

Travis Stoub, PhD
Associate Professor, Department of Neurological Science
Rush Epilepsy Center
Rush University Medical Center
Chicago, IL

Raoul Sutter, MD, PD
Department of Neurology and Intensive Care Medicine
University Hospital Basel
Basel, Switzerland

William O. Tatum, DO
Professor of Neurology
Mayo Clinic College of Medicine
Director, Comprehensive Epilepsy Center
Mayo Clinic
Jacksonville, FL

Barbara Tettenborn, MD
Professor, Chair, Department of Neurology
Kantonspital St. Gallen
St. Gallen, Switzerland

Philip D. Thompson, MD
Emeritus Professor of Neurology
University of Adelaide
Department of Neurology Royal Adelaide Hospital
Adelaide, Australia

Sampsa Vanhatalo, MD
Department of Clinical Neurophysiology
Children's Hospital
Department of Clinical Neurophysiology
HUS Medical Imaging Center
Helsinki University Central Hospital
University of Helsinki
Helsinki, Finland

Roberto Vetrugno, MD
Unit of Neurology and Neurophysiology
Casa di Cura Madre Fortunata Toniolo
Bologna, Italy

Wytse J. Wadman, PhD
Center of Neuroscience
Swammerdam Institute for Life Sciences
University of Amsterdam
Amsterdam, The Netherlands

Fabrice Wendling, Eng, PhD
LTSI—Inserm
Université de Rennes 1
Campus de Beaulieu
Rennes Cedex, France

M. Brandon Westover, MD, PhD
Assistant Professor, Neurology, Harvard University
Department of Neurology
Massachusetts General Hospital
Boston, MA

PART I | BASIC PRINCIPLES

1 | HISTORICAL ASPECTS OF ELECTROENCEPHALOGRAPHY

RAOUL SUTTER, MD, PD, PETER W. KAPLAN, MB, BS, FRCP,
AND DONALD L. SCHOMER, MD

ABSTRACT: Electroencephalography (EEG), a dynamic real-time recording of electrical neocortical brain activity, began in the 1600s with the discovery of electrical phenomena and the concept of an "action current." The galvanometer was introduced in the 1800s and the first bioelectrical observations of human brain signals were made in the 1900s. Certain EEG patterns were associated with brain disorders, increasing the clinical and scientific use of EEG. In the 1980s, technical advances allowed EEGs to be digitized and linked with videotape recording. In the 1990s, digital data storage increased and computer networking enabled remote real-time EEG reading, which made possible continuous EEG (cEEG) monitoring. Manual cEEG analysis became increasingly labor-intensive, calling for methods to assist this process. In the 2000s, complex algorithms enabling quantitative EEG analyses were introduced, with a new focus on shared activity between rhythms, including phase and magnitude synchrony. The automation of spectral analysis enabled studies of spectral content.

KEYWORDS: electroencephalography, EEG, action current, galvanometer, digital, continuous EEG, quantitative EEG, spectral analysis

PRINCIPAL REFERENCES

1. Caton R: The electric currents of the brain. B Med J 1875; 2:278
2. Berger H: Über das Elektrenkephalogramm des Menschen. Erster Bericht. Arch Psychiatr Nervenkr 1929; 87:527–580
3. Kornmüller AE: Der Mechanismus des epileptischen Anfalles auf Grund bioelektrischer Untersuchungen am Zentralnervensystem. Fortschr Neurol Psychiatry 1935; 7:391–400 and 414–432
4. Gibbs FA, Davis H, Lennox WG: The electroencephalogram in epilepsy and in conditions of impaired consciousness. Arch Neurol Psychiatry 1935; 34:1133–1148
5. Grass AM, Gibbs FA: A Fourier transform of the electroencephalogram. J Neurophysiol 1938; 1:521–526
6. Lindsley DB, Bowden JW, Magoun HW: The effect of subcortical lesions upon the electroencephalogram. Am Psychol 1949; 4:233–234
7. Knott JR, Hayne RA, Meyers HR: Physiology of sleepwave characteristics and temporal relations of human electroencephalograms recorded from the thalamus, the corpus striatum and the surface of the scalp. Arch Neurol Psychiatry 1950; 63:526–527
8. Gloor P: Hans Berger and the discovery of the electroencephalogram. Electroencephalogr Clin Neurophysiol 1969:Suppl 28:21–36
9. Niedermeyer E: The clinical relevance of EEG interpretation. Clin Electroencephalogr 2003; 34(3):93–98

1. THE DISCOVERY OF BIOELECTRICAL PHENOMENA

The history of electroencephalography (EEG) begins with the discovery of bioelectrical phenomena. The ancient Greeks (in about 1000 BC) started to open trade routes across the Black Sea, via the river Dnieper, to the Baltic region. Among many trade items that the Greeks obtained from the Baltic was a fossilized pine resin which they called "electron," but which we nowadays call amber. The ancient Greek philosopher Thales of Miletos, one of the pre-Socratic "natural philosophers" of Greece (around 620–550 BC), discovered that amber had the ability to attract light objects when it was rubbed with fur. For many centuries, this phenomenon was thought to be a unique property of amber. In Elizabethan times, the English physician William Gilbert (1544–1602), an English physician, physicist, and natural philosopher, began to study the electrical properties of various substances and coined the word "electric" to describe the above-mentioned effect. This was followed by the invention of a friction machine to create electrical fields by Otto von Guericke (1602–1686), a German scientist, inventor, and politician. This electrostatic generator eventually found its way into doctors' offices and even university hospitals, where the effects of the electrical field created a strong impression on patients by making their hair stand up. Throughout the 17th and 18th centuries, the friction machine demonstrated the attraction and repulsion of charged bodies and the electrical characteristics of conductors and nonconductors, and offered insights into the dualism of positive and negative electricity.

In 1746, a new and important piece of electrical equipment entered the scene when the Leyden jar was introduced by the Dutch scientist Pieter van Musschenbroek (1692–1761) (following the earlier work of Ewald von Kleist [1881–1954]), resulting in the pioneering storage of electricity. What the friction machine could generate, the Leyden jar could store. This condenser (or capacitor) turned into an indispensable part of modern electronics. The story of the bold experiment by Benjamin Franklin (1706–1790) involved trapping some of the electrical discharges from a thunderstorm in a Leyden jar.

In 1780, Luigi Galvani (1737–1798), an Italian physician, found that he could induce leg contractions in a dead frog within an electrical circuit connecting the preparation to an antenna during a thunderstorm. This experiment induced a serious scientific controversy in Italy between Galvani and Alessandro Volta (1745–1832) in which the views of Volta prevailed. Volta doubted the biological nature of the muscle contractions and placed the emphasis on physics—on his "pile," the first battery (around 1800). This bimetallic pile was a generator capable of producing a steady flow of electricity. The laws governing electrical flow were soon discovered in 1827 by Georg S. Ohm (1789–1854), a German physicist and mathematician.

After the discharges from condensers were used in a number of experiments (1), static electricity in medicine disappeared for about 150 years. In the 1950s and 1960s, William B. Kouwenhoven (1888–1975) and his coworkers reintroduced static electricity in clinical practice with the implementation of defibrillating cardioversion.

Nevertheless, Galvani's belief in "animal electricity" was not lost. There remained the ongoing question of the role of electricity in the function of nerves and muscles in animals.

2. FROM THE GALVANOMETER TO ELECTROPHYSIOLOGY

An important step in the field of neurophysiology was taken in 1825 by Leopoldo Nobili of Florence (1784–1835) with the introduction of the astatic galvanometer, an instrument for the detection of electric currents. This instrument was refined in 1858 by William Thompson (Lord Kelvin; 1824–1907), an English mathematical physicist and engineer (1). Although these galvanometers would faithfully demonstrate continuous electrical currents (Fig. 1.1) and their variations in intensity, they failed to detect brief electrical phenomena.

The earliest scientists to focus on neurophysiologically related phenomena were Carlo Matteucci (1811–1868), an Italian physicist and neurophysiologist, and Emil Du Bois-Reymond (1818–1896), a German physician and physiologist. Instigated by Galvani's work on bioelectricity, Matteucci in 1830 began experiments using the sensitive galvanometer of Nobili. With these studies, Matteucci proved that injured biological tissues were excitable and generated direct electrical currents, and that these currents could be multiplied so as to increase sensitivity. Du Bois-Reymond coined the term *negative variation* for a phenomenon of an unexpected decrease in current intensity measured by the galvanometer during active muscle contraction (1). This term was resurrected in earlier EEG research by Richard Caton (1842–1926; Fig. 1.2), an English scientist (2), and further supported by the discovery of the "contingent negative variation" by William Grey Walter (1910–1977), an American-born British neurophysiologist interested in robotics (3).

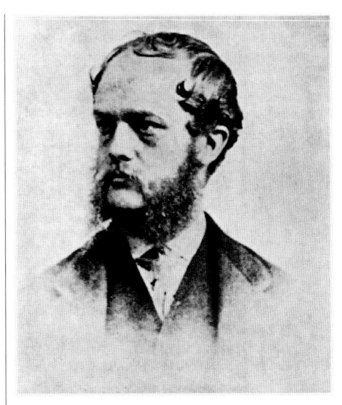

Figure 1.2. Richard Caton (1842–1926). (From Brazier MAB. A history of the electrical activity of the brain. The first half-century. London: Pitman; 1961, with permission from Macmillan.)

In 1849, Hermann von Helmholtz (1821–1894), a German physician and physicist, measured the speed at which electrical impulses were carried along nerve fibers. Du Bois-Reymond understood the importance of the use of electrodes for neurophysiological research and made them nonpolarizable. The concept of "action current" was introduced by Ludimar Hermann (1838–1914), a student of Du Bois-Reymond, who showed the existence of a wave of excitation, which he interpreted as a self-propagating state that is conveyed from one section of the nerve to the next. Julius Bernstein (1839–1917), a German physiologist, was the first to propose a membrane theory of nerve tissue, which ultimately was elucidated as late as 1939 and the following years by Alan Lloyd Hodgkin (1914–1998) and Andrew F. Huxley (1917–2012), two English physiologists and biophysicists who shared the 1963 Nobel Prize in physiology with John Eccles. With this foundation of electrophysiology of the nervous system, the first EEG observation of electrical brain activity took place.

3. UNCOVERING ELECTRICAL BRAIN ACTIVITY

Richard Caton (1842–1926) was an English physician who became deeply interested in electrophysiological phenomena and explored electrical phenomena of the exposed cerebral hemispheres of rabbits and monkeys. According to Brazier (4), Caton presented his findings to the British Medical Association on August 24, 1875, and published a short report of 20 lines in the *British Medical Journal* (2). This report was followed in

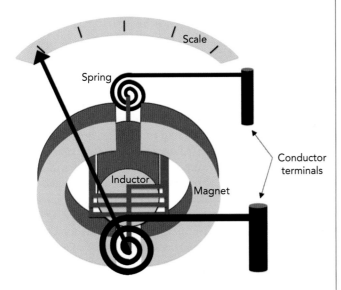

Figure 1.1. Scheme of a galvanometer.

1877 by a more detailed study of more than 45 rabbits, cats, and monkeys (5). These recordings of gray matter electrical activity would probably not have been possible without Du Bois-Reymond's high-quality electrodes, as earlier electrodes would have produced a significant amount of noise and artifacts, which in turn would likely have obscured the cortical electrical signals. Besides the nonpolarizable electrodes, Caton used a beam of light projected on the mirror of a galvanometer that reflected onto a large scale placed on the wall. In this way, he found "feeble currents of varying direction passing through the multiplier when the electrodes are placed on two points of the external surface, or one electrode on the grey matter, and one on the surface of the skull." Even though artifacts could have played a major role in these findings (as the galvanometer used by Caton had a very limited frequency response range from 0 to 6 Hz (6)), one can assume that it was the EEG phenomena that moved the needle in one direction or another. Caton further noted that the external surface of the cortical gray matter was positive compared to deep cerebral structures. In addition, he described electrical cerebral currents related to underlying neuronal function with variations associated with sleep and wakefulness, the presence of food, and anesthesia, and their absence in death (5). He further investigated several responses to the pinching of the skin of the lips and cheeks, thus gaining credit for being a pioneer in evoked potentials. Furthermore, the difference in polarity found between cortical surface and deeper areas could be interpreted as the discovery of the "steady potential" ("direct current [DC] potential"), although there is little other supporting evidence.

4. EARLY STUDIES OF ELECTRICAL BRAIN ACTIVITY ACROSS EUROPE

4.1. Eastern Europe

Concurrent with Caton's epochal work, physiologists across eastern Europe performed several studies of electrical brain activity. In 1870, Gustav T. Fritsch (1838–1927) and Julius Eduard Hitzig (1838–1907), two German physiologists, described the stimulation of the human cerebral cortex by electrical impulses in a joint study (7). This discovery was the consequence of an unusual observation by Fritsch, who observed contralateral muscle contractions during the dressing of an open brain wound acquired by his patient during the Prussian-Danish War in 1864 (1). This observation had a much greater impact on the early years of neuroscience in eastern Europe than Caton's demonstration of electrical brain activity had. In 1880, the work of Fritsch and Hitzig was followed by a study by David Ferrier (1843–1928) and Gerald F. Yeo (1845–1909), who performed electrical stimulations of the cerebrum in apes and also in a patient operated on for a brain tumor. The repercussions of these stimulation studies were considerable since many investigators of the time held the view that the entire cerebrum was a homogeneous organ that harbored the mental functions.

Studies especially in eastern Europe (i.e., Russian and Polish universities) demonstrated the response of the cerebral cortex to electrical stimuli and hence triggered further

investigations into spontaneous electrical phenomena. In 1877, Vasili Yakovlevich Danilevsky (1852–1939), a Ukrainian-born Russian physician and physiologist, finished his thesis on the electrical stimulation and spontaneous electrical brain activity in animals at the University of Kharkov (8). Danilevsky saw his high hopes unfulfilled as far as the spontaneous electrical activity of the brain was concerned (4). He had expected better correlation of electrical brain activity with psychic and emotional processes. Despite this initial disappointment, Danilevsky remained deeply involved in brain physiology.

Adolf Beck (1863–1939), a physician and physiologist at the University of Lwow (the Polish province of Galicia, at that time a part of the Austro-Hungarian Empire), investigated the spontaneous electrical activity of the brain in rabbits and dogs. He was the first neurophysiologist to describe the disappearance of rhythmic oscillations when the eyes were stimulated with light and thus became a forebear of Berger's discovery of the blocking of the basic alpha rhythm in the EEG. This observation became widely known through its publication in the *Centrallblatt*.

A profoundly important breakthrough came with the introduction by Willem Einthoven (1860–1927) in 1903 of the string galvanometer, a very sensitive instrument that required photographic recording and became the standard instrumentation for electrocardiography at the turn of the century. At that same time, Yurevich Kaufman (1877–1951), a Russian physiologist, hypothesized that an epileptic attack is associated with abnormal electrical discharges, and he pursued this idea by studying the effects of cortical electrical stimulation (4). In 1912, another Russian physiologist, Vladimir Vladimirovich Pravdich-Neminsky (1879–1952), began recording the electrical brain activity of animals with the string galvanometer (4) (Fig. 1.3). Pravdich-Neminsky recorded the EEG from the intact skull, the dura, and the brain of a dog. He described a 12- to 14-Hz rhythm under normal conditions and marked slowing during asphyxia. He coined the term *electrocerebrogram*. These studies were followed by an exciting report published in 1914 by Napoleon Cybulski (1854–1919), Beck's mentor in Krakow, providing photographic illustrations of EEG evidence of an epileptic seizure in the dog caused by electrical stimulation and recorded by a galvanometer with a photographic attachment (9).

4.2. Western and Central Europe

In contrast to the flourishing neurophysiological research activity in eastern Europe, EEG studies were scarce in western and central Europe in the 19th century. The ancestral lineage from Galvani to Du Bois-Reymond and Caton broke off and rivulets of a different orientation nourished the neurophysiological corpus. The work of Ernst von Fleischl-Marxow (1846–1891), an Austrian physiologist and physician, stands out in this emerging field. He described the cerebral electrical activity that he recorded over the visual cortex in a number of animal models but did not observe oscillatory activity. Von Fleischl-Marxow claimed priority when Beck in 1890 published his data but was not aware of the earlier work done by Caton and Danilevsky. The odd character of this episode is underscored

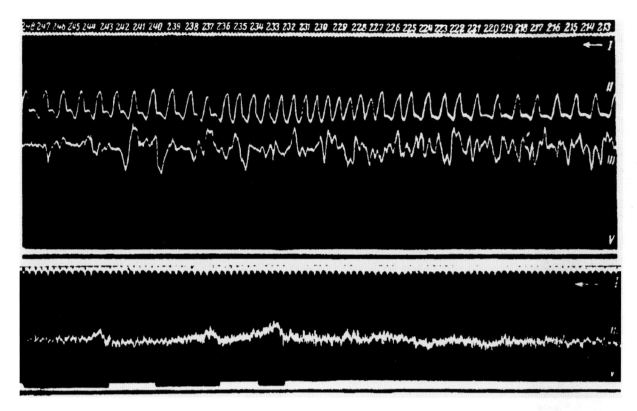

Figure 1.3. *The first photographs to be published of electroencephalograms. In the upper record Neminsky shows (in the third trace) the brain potentials of a curarized dog with the pulsations from an artery in the brain recorded above them. In the lower record the sciatic nerve is being stimulated from time to time, and the decrease in activity noted by Neminsky can be seen. The record reads from right to left, line I being a time marker in one fifth of a second, line III the galvanometer string, and line V the signal for stimulation. (From Pravdich-Neminsky VV. Ein Versuch der Registrierung der elektrischen Gehirnerscheinungen. Zbl Physiol 1913; 27:951–960, with permission from Dr. Mary Brazier and Macmillan.)*

by more recent historical accounts (1,4) that indicate that von Fleischl-Marxow's work was not of first-rate quality. Besides these observations of von Fleischl-Marxow, most Western neurophysiologists were caught in a dispute between "cerebral localizationists" and "antilocalizationists." In late 1888, Friedrich Leopold Goltz (1834–1902), a German physiologist, removed the cerebral hemispheres in a dog, leading to a state of extreme lethargy and mental inertia (10). Such studies aimed to investigate the working of the cerebral hemispheres as a whole and de-emphasized aspects of cortical localization, in contrast with the studies by Fritsch, Hitzig, Ferrier, and Yeo using cerebral stimulation techniques.

At the dawn of the 20th century, the studies by Charles Scott Sherrington (1857–1952), working in Liverpool and Oxford, were particularly influential in the development of a modern Western type of reflexology (11). This work, entitled *The Integrative Action of the Nervous System*, was based on a series of lectures held at Yale University in 1904 with the scope ranging from reflexology to decerebrate rigidity, and from motor cortex to sensory function. Aside from these areas of study, inhibition was one of the most important discoveries by Sherrington. Even Ramón y Cajal's net of independent synaptically connected neurons was a theory of neural excitation. (Incidentally, the term *synapse* was introduced by Sherrington.)

It is unfortunate that this neurophysiology pioneer lived a distance from electrophysiological thought; his work was centered chiefly on ablation techniques. His disciples—to name only Edward Liddell and Derek Ernest Denny-Brown—held similar views, while in Cambridge electrically oriented neurophysiology found its greatest proponent in Edgar Douglas Adrian (1889–1977), who is discussed in the following section in his relationship to Hans Berger's work.

5. HANS BERGER AND THE FIRST HUMAN EEG

Hans Berger (1873–1941; Fig. 1.4), the discoverer of the human EEG, was a German neuropsychiatrist. Although Berger was not thought of as a leader in either neurology or psychiatry, his work fundamentally pioneered EEG research. Berger was often described as a meticulous and conscientious person, somewhat aloof in his contact with his patients, a very strict and authoritarian department head, and a hard-working professor who hardly ever attended the annual meetings of the German neuropsychiatric society. In his first studies, Berger analyzed cerebral circulation using plethysmographic methods in patients with skull defects. From 1902 to 1910, he studied the electrical activity of the cerebrum in the dog with a capillary electrometer, with disappointing results. His cutting-edge EEG work was carried out in a small and very primitive laboratory. Berger was well aware of the scant pertinent literature from Caton to Cybulski and Pravdich-Neminsky when he started his studies on the human EEG. Filled with doubt, it took Berger almost

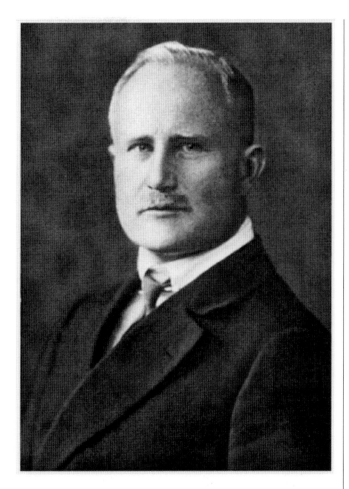

Figure 1.4. Hans Berger (1873–1941) (From Kolle K. Hans Berger. In: Kolle K, editor. Grosse Nervenärzte. Vol. 1. Stuttgart: Thieme; 1956, pp. 1–6, with permission.)

for strictly linguistic reasons: the mixture of Greek ("electro," "gram") and Latin ("cerebro") fragments. Berger proposed the German term *Elektrenkephalogram* since the root *enkephalo* from the Greek is linguistically more correct than *encephalo*.

For his studies of the human EEG, Berger used many different instruments following the latest technical advances. In 1910 he used a string galvanometer—first with the Einthoven type, later with the smaller Edelmann model, which was replaced in 1924 with the larger Edelmann model. In 1926, Berger started to use the more powerful Siemens double coil galvanometer (attaining a sensitivity of 130 μV/cm) (14). With this instrument and the use of nonpolarizable pad electrodes, Berger recorded the human EEG tracings shown in his first report of 1929 (12). The recordings from 1 to 3 minutes' duration were made on photographic paper. For his one-channel EEG tracings, Berger used a bipolar recording technique with fronto-occipital leads along with a time marking line generated with a sine wave of 10 Hz. In 1932, he received an oscillograph from Siemens but was unable to obtain further amplifiers with oscillographs that could be used to obtain multichannel recordings.

The first studies of the human EEG began in 1924 after World War I in Germany in several patients with large skull bone defects (Fig. 1.5). On July 6, 1924, the small Edelmann string galvanometer showed oscillations presumably coming from the underlying brain. This discovery was followed by the recognition that skull defects were not necessarily advantageous to obtaining a recording because of thickening of dura, postoperative adhesions, and so forth, and he found that recordings could be made just as well (or even better) through the intact skull and scalp. By using the double coil galvanometer between 1926 and 1929, Berger obtained several good records with oscillating waves in the alpha frequency range. The data were often unclear and, in 1928, according to his diary entries, Berger was beset with doubts concerning the authenticity of his observations (impressively outlined by Richard Jung (15)).

In his first report in 1929, Berger describes features of the alpha rhythm and the alpha blocking response (along with a description of the smaller and faster beta waves) (12). Chlorinated silver needle electrodes, platinum wires, and zinc-plated steel needles were used in those years. This report was largely ignored by the scientific community until Edgar Douglas Adrian (1889–1977), an English neurophysiologist, confirmed these findings in Cambridge in 1934 (16). Throughout the 1930s, Berger continued studying the human EEG and published several reports containing veritable gems: studies of fluctuation of consciousness, the first EEG

5 years to publish his report in 1929 that demonstrated the technique for recording the electrical activity of the human brain from the surface of the head (12). Interesting details in this context are compiled in the introduction to Pierre Gloor's authoritative translation of Berger's work (13).

Despite the importance of Berger's 14 reports, the acceptance of his work came very slowly, possibly explained by the cumbersome original German text and the rather simple title "On the Electroencephalogram of Man," which was the same for all 14 reports. Surely, a more attractive title would have helped. Berger's humanistic educational background becomes obvious in the rejection of the term *electrocerebrogram* of Pravdich-Neminsky

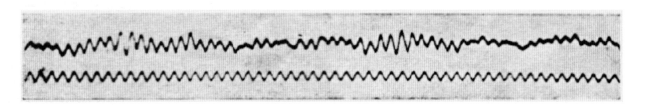

Figure 1.5. The first recorded electroencephalogram of a human. The lower line is a 10-Hz sine wave for use as a time marker. The upper line is the recording from Berger's young son made in 1925. (From Berger H. Über das Elektrenkephalogramm des Menschen. 1st report. Arch Psychiat Nervenkr 1929; 87:527–570, with permission from Dr. Mary Brazier and Macmillan.)

recordings during sleep to reveal sleep spindles, the effect of hypoxia on the human brain, a variety of diffuse and localized brain disorders, and even hints of epileptic discharges.

Computational techniques of wave analysis started early in the history of EEG with the first attempts also by Berger and his assistant Günther Dietsch, a German physicist, applying Fourier analysis to short EEG sections in 1932 (17).

In 1937, Berger was invited to an international congress of psychologists in Paris and to Bologna, where the bicentennial of Galvani's birthday was celebrated. Berger's relationship to the Nazi regime was not good and he was unceremoniously made a professor emeritus at earliest convenience in 1938 at the age of 65 (a few additional "years of honor" were granted to most retiring directors of university institutions). This was indeed a hard blow to his plans for further EEG studies and, in the wake of a flu-like disease, he evidently developed a severe endogenous depression, which remained undiagnosed. He ended his life by suicide on June 1, 1941, at the age of 68. Additional external factors may have contributed to Berger's depression: he felt deeply challenged by a group of independent EEG workers at the Institute of Brain Research at Berlin-Buch. This research group was led by Alois E. Kornmüller (1905–1968) and produced excellent experimental EEG work, which is discussed later. Kornmüller might have had better connections to the government institutions in Berlin, and the often insecure and highly sensitive Berger was afraid that his reputation and discovery were being taken away from him.

Berger was a very complex person and investigator. He did not excel clinically, either as psychiatrist or as neurologist (even though he was very interested in cerebral localization and particularly in the localization of brain tumors). Berger also developed very unscientific ideas about the nature of the EEG, even though he was a meticulous scientist in his EEG work. The driving force throughout his research was the quest for the nature of the all-powerful force of mental energy ("*psychische Energie*"). An early personal experience convinced Berger that such a mental energy—even capable of transmitting thoughts and emotions from person to person—existed. According to Berger's concept, which was significantly influenced by the Danish physiologist Alfred Georg Ludwig Lehmann (1858–1921) in 1901, mental energy is thought to be a partial product of metabolic energies, with warmth and electricity being the other two. This concept gives the EEG waves the eerie character of messengers within the mental process, even acting as messengers from person to person.

Behind the strict directorial facade of Berger was the gentle soul of a highly vulnerable man. It was the psychophysiologist Berger who searched for the correlate of mental energy and, on this voyage, he found the human EEG. It was one of those serendipitous discoveries that was made as a byproduct of a search in a different direction. According to Jung, Berger pursued his goal with the energy of a dilettante who has tumbled on an attractive concept (15). Specialists like the excellent physiologist (and electrophysiologist) Wilhelm Biedermann (1852–1929) in Jena were convinced that Berger's dilettantism would lead nowhere, but it was the dilettante and not the seasoned specialist who emerged victorious. Even though the EEG is not exactly what Berger assumed would be his important contribution, it was the greatest in the history of EEG.

6. MULTICHANNEL HUMAN EEG— GERMANY'S IMPULSES

The Institute of Brain Research (Hirnforschungs-Institut) in Berlin-Buch harbored a group of ambitious and energetic neuroscientists. Oskar Vogt (1870–1959), one of the great neuroanatomists and neuropathologists of his time and a remarkably independent thinker, was the director of the institute. In 1936 he lost his "directorship for lifetime" when the Nazi government became aware of his collaborations with a similar institute in Moscow and his reluctance to get rid of Jewish coworkers (18).

The Berliner Institute (a section of the Kaiser-Wilhelm Institutes) was composed of a variety of departments. The Departments of Physiology and Electrophysiology enjoyed the collaboration of an outstanding physicist and electronic engineer, Jan Friedrich Toennies (1902–1970), a friend of Oskar Vogt (both of whom came from the town of Husum in Holstein).

Toennies built the first ink-writing biological amplifier for the recording of brain potentials. While in New York as a fellow of the Rockefeller Foundation in 1932, he designed the differential amplifier—the still all-important principle of EEG amplification—but he shares this achievement with Brian Matthews, Lord Adrian's ingenious coworker, whose work is discussed in the next section.

The collaboration with Toennies gave the Berlin group a much better tool for EEG research in comparison with Berger's instrumentation. While single EEG scalp electrodes provided estimates of synaptic sources averaged over tissue masses containing up to 1 billion neurons, Kornmüller recognized the importance of recordings from a greater number of electrodes. His EEG studies in the human placed particular emphasis on the differences between given regions of the cerebrum ("*Hirnrindenfelder*") (19–22). His studies of the clinical significance of EEG in 1944 (23) paled somewhat beside the importance of his earliest experimental EEG work carried out with Max Heinrich Fischer and Hans Löwenbach. The latter then came to the United States, where he became one of the early EEG pioneers. In initial studies, focusing on epileptic manifestations and the demonstration of epileptiform spikes, the EEGs were obtained from the cerebral cortex of animals poisoned with convulsive substances (21,24–26).

In the 1930s, Oskar Vogt and his wife Cécile, a well-known neuropathologist, developed a concept of strict cerebral compartmentalization lying in sharply separated areas. He showed clear boundaries between healthy and diseased areas in the hippocampus (27) and conceived of the cortex as divided into some 200 regions with precise demarcation between fields, a concept that guided Vogt's coworkers and Kornmüller's EEG work.

Richard Jung (1911–1986), a German neurologist, joined this group in 1937 when Vogt lost his post. His replacement, Hugo Spatz, considerably changed the direction of the group's research. Toennies stayed with Herbert S. Gasser (1888–1963) at the Rockefeller Institute in New York, where he constructed the first cathode follower used to record from high-resistance electrodes. This in effect was the birth of microelectrode recording, which developed into an enormously powerful scientific tool in the 1950s and 1960s.

Kornmüller's work declined after World War II, when he appeared to be obsessed with a totally unproven theory of glia as the generator of slow brain potentials. In contrast, Jung developed into one of the greatest electroneurophysiologists of his time.

7. CLINICAL EEG—ITS INTRODUCTION INTO GREAT BRITAIN

Edgar Douglas Adrian (Baron of Cambridge and, as such, Lord Adrian) (1889–1977; Fig. 1.6) was one of the most influential electrophysiological neurophysiologists of the 20th century. He was already a neurophysiologist of great prestige when he confirmed Berger's data. He had been credited with the demonstration of single sensory nerve fiber potentials, and the analysis of unit activity, which resulted in the Adrian-Bronk law (28). (Incidentally, his collaborator, Detlef Bronk, became president of Johns Hopkins University in later years.) Prior to Matthews, Keith Lucas had been Adrian's brilliant electronic engineer and experimental coworker.

In 1933 Adrian became aware of Berger's work and immediately endeavored to confirm and promulgate his discoveries (16). He showed his colleagues his own EEG alpha rhythm and the blocking effect due to eye opening, but, alas, in contrast, his great electronic wizard, Brian Matthews, apparently had a low-voltage EEG with no alpha rhythm. Due to some strange quirk, Adrian's recording from the head ganglion of a water beetle happened to be indistinguishable from Adrian's alpha rhythm and was blocked in the same manner, namely by light falling

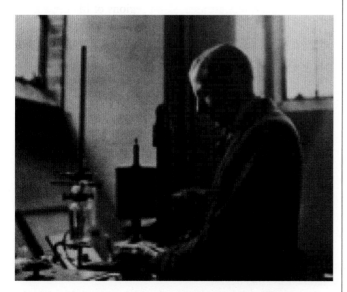

Figure 1.6. Edgar Douglas Adrian (1889–1977) in the laboratory (U.S. National Library of Medicine, Images from the History of Medicine Collection, photographer unknown, kindly provided by National Library of Medicine)

on the beetle's eyes. The Adrian/water beetle similarity and the Adrian/Matthews EEG dissimilarity must have been terribly confusing to the onlookers, a description given in the 1936 work entitled "The Berger rhythm in the monkey's brain" (29).

William Grey Walter (1910–1977) became the pioneer of clinical EEG in England, and his discovery of foci of slow activity (delta waves, named by Grey Walter) generated enormous clinical interest in the new method. Grey Walter, however, was a PhD, and this could have laid the foundation for the aversion of England's great neurologists to EEG, which in the years to follow was either ignored or left to PhD EEGers in the laboratory. We will find Grey Walter again in later decades. Let it be said that he was one of the most brilliant minds in all neurosciences—an independent thinker, a powerful writer, quite often a man who was almost consumed by the flame of his own brilliance. He founded a small but very effective school in Bristol at the Burden Institute.

8. BERGER'S EEG EXPLORES DIFFERENT STATES OF CONSCIOUSNESS—FROM FRANCE TO BELGIUM

France had its own proud neurophysiological schools in the 19th century, and the names of François Magendie (1783–1855) and, above all, Claude Bernard (1813–1878) belong in the pantheon of neuroscience.

In the 1930s, a fine school of early EEGers developed in Paris. Alfred Fessard (1900–1982) at the Collège de France must be mentioned as one of the most influential neurophysiologists. He also confirmed the results of Berger and even used EEG in the study of conditioned reflexes. Clinical EEG started in France under the aegis of Alphonse Baudouin (1876–1957) and Hermann Fischgold (1899–1982). Fischgold had come from Romania, developed into a leading clinical EEGer, and—in a curious quirk—also became a leader in neuroradiology. Baudouin was the key figure in the invitation of Berger to Paris in 1937.

Belgium was the home of the highly influential and emerging field of electrophysiological neurophysiology. Frederic Bremer (1892–1982), a Belgian neurophysiologist at the Université Libre of Brussels, early on recognized the usefulness of EEG methods in the experimental investigation of the brain. After his research in muscle tonus and the cerebellum, Bremer's curiosity pushed him toward studies recognizing the influence of afferent signals on the state of vigilance. He compared his feline preparation called "*cerveauisolé*" (with midbrain transection) with the "*encéphaleisolé*" resulting from transection at the boundary between the medulla oblongata and cervical cord. The former preparation would produce permanent coma; the latter would cause a variable state of vigilance, with waking and sleeping states demonstrated on the EEG. In other words, trigeminal-sensory, auditory, visual, and probably also olfactory influences would help to keep the (artificially ventilated) *encéphaleisolé* preparation in a waking/sleeping rhythm (30). The importance of his paper entitled "Cerebral and Cerebellar Potentials," published in 1958 (31), cannot be overemphasized.

9. DEVELOPMENTS IN OTHER PARTS OF EUROPE

Italy was one of the first countries where the EEG found fertile soil. Mario Gozzano (1898–1986), professor of clinical neurology in Bologna and later in Rome, published his first experiences with the EEG as early as 1935. Gozzano personifies the (none too common) example of a leading clinical neurologist assuming leadership in clinical EEG (32).

Agostino Gemelli (1878–1959) came from the opposite area of neurosciences. As a monk, psychologist, philosopher, historian, and president of the Catholic University in Milan, he reported his first studies of the human EEG in 1937. In this way, Gemelli represents the psychological wing of EEG research, which subsequently spawned a number of outstanding PhD EEGers.

Another EEGer from the same category as Gemelli was Hubert Rohracher (1903–1972), an Austrian chair of psychology at the University of Vienna. His early EEG studies can be dated back to 1938. He fell under the spell of the alpha rhythm and even made a "pilgrimage" to Hans Berger in Jena in the 1930s.

10. THE SPREAD OF AMERICAN EEG SCIENCE

Around 1935, the center of gravity in the emerging EEG science started to shift from Europe to North America, with European investigators starting to travel across the Atlantic. During the development of experimental EEG studies in Europe, America had not played a role. In 1918, Donald McPherson, a medical student at Harvard Medical School, worked under the eminent physiologist Alexander Forbes (1882–1965) (33). McPherson placed two electrodes on the exposed brain of a cat and ran the output through a string galvanometer and observed the rhythmic oscillating EEG activity of 10 Hz. This finding, however, was rejected as an artifact by Forbes. Was Forbes completely unaware of the work from Caton to Pravdich-Neminsky?

International fame was brought to American EEG science with the work of Hallowell Davis (1896–1992), Frederic A. Gibbs (1903–1992), and Erna L. Gibbs (1904–1987) at Harvard and also with the work of Herbert H. Jasper (1906–1999) at Brown University in Providence, Rhode Island. A. J. Derbyshire, a graduate student of Davis's, brought Berger's paper of 1929 to Davis's attention (1). Derbyshire, Pauline Davis, and H. N. Simpson then tried in vain to demonstrate their own alpha rhythms. In 1934, there were finally shouts of joy when Hallowell Davis himself was found to have a good alpha rhythm.

Starting with Howard Bartley (1901–1988) in the early 1930s in the United States, EEG was used in animal experiments for some years (34–36). Bartley did his work at Washington University in St. Louis, a place that had developed into a hotbed of neurophysiology due to the magnificent work of Herbert S. Gasser (1888–1963), Joseph Erlanger (1874–1965), and George Bishop (1889–1973)—a group that made excellent use of Braun's cathode ray oscilloscope (oscillograph)

in the study of peripheral nerve potentials. This excellent research group was joined later by James L. O'Leary (1904–1975), an outstanding neurophysiologist, EEGer, and neurologist. In the early 1930s several experimental EEG studies were done, mainly on the electrical changes in the brain to reflex activity (34,37–41). The work of Ralph W. Gerard (1900–1974) is linked with the introduction of a concentric needle electrode for the stereotaxic exploration of the brain in animal models.

American EEG studies in humans started at Harvard in Boston, at Brown in Providence (as noted above), and also at the University of Iowa in Iowa City, where Lee Edward Travis (1896–1987), an experimental psychologist who became the founder of the fourth American human EEG laboratory, played an important role. Travis was well aware of Berger's work from 1933, before it was confirmed by Adrian. Among the EEG pioneers trained by Travis were Herbert H. Jasper, Donald Lindsley, Charles Henry, and John Knott.

In 1934 the international breakthrough in clinical EEG came with studies of epileptic patients. Frederic A. Gibbs had come from Johns Hopkins University in Baltimore to join the Harvard group. He sought out William G. Lennox (1884–1960), who had already become a widely known epileptologist. Lennox had begun studies on the cerebral circulation by measuring the O_2 and CO_2 content in the blood of the jugular veins (42–44). Erna L. Gibbs, an immigrant from Germany, was the technical coworker of Lennox, married Frederic A. Gibbs, self-trained as one of the world's first EEG technicians, and became coauthor of numerous excellent papers, including the study of cerebral blood flow, a milestone in this field (44). In the following years, EEG began to preoccupy Lennox more than did cerebral blood flow.

Hardly any EEG finding has left such an indelible impression as the association of 3-Hz spike-wave complexes in petit mal absences, first described in the petit mal epilepsy study of 12 children performed by Lennox, Gibbs, Davis, and colleagues, now a perennial in the EEG cannon (45–47). In contrast to Berger, who was gripped by the oscillating rhythms, Frederic Gibbs's interest focused on paroxysmal EEG patterns such as spike-waves. This was followed by studies of EEG patterns in grand mal and psychomotor seizures reported by the same team (Gibbs, Lennox, and Gibbs), but the stretches of fast spikes in grand mal and the rhythmic 4- or 6-Hz activity in psychomotor seizures did not reach the same popularity as the 3-Hz spike-waves of petit mal. In contrast to their impact, the technical quality of the EEG tracings was limited. Hence, Dr. and Mrs. Gibbs visited Berger in Germany in the summer of 1935 and spent some time at the Berlin-Buch Institute to study the "polyneurograph" instrument of Toennies. Once in Europe, they also saw the instrumentation of Matthews in England. Frederic Gibbs then contracted Albert Grass (then at the Massachusetts Institute of Technology) to build a three-channel preamplifier, resulting in the Grass Model I, which went into use in 1935. This instrument, with three channels and an ink writer, recorded on rolls of paper. The era of commercial EEG had begun.

The Gibbs-Gibbs-Lennox era of the 1930s proved to be one of the most exciting and productive periods in the history of EEG. In those years, EEG found the domain of greatest effectiveness in the realm of the epileptic seizure disorders. EEG enormously accelerated epilepsy research; indeed, epileptology can be divided historically into two periods—before and after the advent of EEG. Insights into the nature of epileptic mechanisms greatly increased. What Fischer had started in 1931 with his experimental studies on picrotoxin and its effect on the cortical EEG in animals, the Gibbses and Lennox applied to human epilepsy, opening the door for investigations into epileptology for decades to come. It should be mentioned that Berger had cited in his seventh report examples of paroxysmal EEG discharges in a case of presumed petit mal attacks and also during a focal motor seizure in a patient with general paresis (48). However, these observations were noted only in passing and a great opportunity for a major breakthrough in neuroscience was missed.

In North America, Hallowell and Pauline Davis, two great EEG pioneers, produced fine work on the normal EEG and its variants, including the first observations during sleep. These first steps in electrophysiological research of sleep were followed by studies by Alfred Lee Loomis (1887–1975) and his coworkers, E. N. Harvey and G. A. Hobart, who methodically studied the human sleep EEG patterns and the stages of sleep. This research was done off the academic track in Tuxedo Park, New Jersey (49). The Davises eventually turned to audiology and moved to St. Louis. At Brown, Jasper studied the EEG in children with behavior disorders before he found his niche in basic and clinical epileptology at McGill University in Montreal in his epochal collaboration with Wilder G. Penfield (discussed later). Lee Travis gradually disappeared from the scene, but his foremost disciples, John R. Knott and Charles E. Henry (PhD EEGers with strong clinical interests), were to assume a very important role in America's EEG science. Their skill and supreme dedication turned them into the "conscience of EEG," steering developments in the right direction and correcting the course when there was danger of going astray. Donald B. Lindsey (1907–2003), a physiological psychologist at the University of California at Los Angeles best known as a pioneer in the field of brain function study, became one of the most influential investigators of maturational EEG aspects.

Following the first wave of American EEG pioneers and their immediate disciples and followers, it is difficult for the historian to do justice to the second wave, which began before the end of the 1930s. Robert Schwab at Harvard and at the Massachusetts General Hospital in Boston was prominent in his mastery of EEG, combined with great clinical neurological talents (especially in the field of myasthenia gravis, Parkinsonism, and epilepsy). Across the Charles River at the Massachusetts Institute of Technology, there was Warren McCulloch (1898–1969), a fiery genius like William Grey Walter in Bristol and a gifted thinker. His scope ranged well beyond the usual limits of EEG and neurophysiology (one must read his *Embodiments of Mind* to fathom his originality, although one may be inclined to disagree on many points). Earlier, at Northwestern University in Evanston, Illinois, outside Chicago, McCulloch had been involved with his mentor Dusser de Barenne in "neuronographic" work, an import from Utrecht in the Netherlands. This work was based on topical

strychnine poisoning of the cortex and exploration of transmitted spiking to other regions.

Clinical EEG research had already started to conquer certain scientific fields outside epileptology. Grey Walter's discovery of the delta focus located over hemispheric brain tumors had opened the search for further relationships between brain lesions and focal EEG correlates (50). This research was paralleled by studies of EEG patterns in patients with metabolic disturbances and especially hypoglycemia in the late 1930s (51).

After the first steps of EEG science in Europe, North America found itself in a leading position in the domain of EEG by the end of the 1930s. By contrast, EEG research in Europe slowed in the 1940s during World War II and was quite limited at the time.

11. THE IMPACT OF WORLD WAR II AND THE 1940S

During World War II (1939–1945), research and clinical EEG activities were constrained, particularly in Europe. There were some neurological laboratories where the EEG was used in the localization of traumatic brain lesions and epileptogenic foci. After World War II, the gap between North America and Europe was greater than ever before, and European EEG research found itself at a low point.

After the war, new activities started in England and France, while the situation in Germany looked desperate. Grey Walter with his collaborators V. J. Dovey and H. Shipton (a brilliant electronic engineer who later moved to Iowa City and then St. Louis) at the Burden Institute in Bristol discovered paroxysmal responses to flickering light in the critical frequency range between 10 and 20 Hz. Further work on epileptic photosensitivity immediately shifted from Bristol to Marseille, France, where the young and talented Henri Gastaut (1915–1995) used this method, in combination with intravenously administered pentylenetetrazol, to determine the individual threshold for paroxysmal responses ("*seuilépileptique*") (52,53). In 1947, the American EEG Society was founded and the first International EEG Congress was held in London, followed by a second congress in Paris in association with clinical neurology and other neurological disciplines (1949). At that time, Japan gained attention with the work of K. Motokawa, a researcher on EEG rhythms.

While activities in EEG research in Germany remained minimal, Switzerland started to develop its own profile with Marcel Monnier (1907–1996), a Swiss neurophysiologist and disciple of the Nobelist Walter R. Hess (1881–1973), who was instrumental in this regard. Hess had gained great prestige by the functional mapping of thalamus and hypothalamus with regard to autonomic responses to electrical stimulation.

The American EEG scene was bustling with activity. Frederic Gibbs and his coworkers produced another major study on the interictal anterior temporal spike or sharp-wave discharge in the interseizure interval in patients with psychomotor seizures (54). This was an important step in the elucidation of temporal lobe epilepsy, a work with far-reaching consequences for the entire development of EEG laboratories and the content of their routine work. Anterior temporal discharges were found to be prominent or indeed limited to the state of sleep, which has led to the current standard of obtaining a tracing that incorporates periods of sleep. This required electrodes attached by electrolyte paste (rather than by rubber bands or caps), the use of a much longer recording time, and a much smaller numerical output of recordings per EEG technician. However, transatlantic communication was very limited at the time and the expertise of American laboratories, enhanced by their inclusion of sleep in EEG studies, did not significantly influence their European counterparts.

Frederic Gibbs enjoyed enormous international prestige at the time as the world's leader in clinical EEG. Nevertheless, his position at Harvard was much less prestigious; he held the academic rank of an instructor (below the professorial ranks), even though a visit to his laboratory was the goal of many European colleagues. Robert Schwab did not fare much better at Harvard in spite of his fine clinical-neurological talents.

During the 1940s, many EEG instrument manufacturers appeared in the United States, Europe, and Japan. Commercial EEG systems provided new standard configurations including large consoles with paper feeders, and standardized reading tables. Toward the end of the 1940s, Jasper turned into a strong competitor of Gibbs. Jasper had moved to the Neurological Institute of McGill University in Montreal, starting his collaborations with Wilder G. Penfield (1891–1976), a neurosurgeon with a profound neuroscientific background. The rise of the Montreal group and the developments at that time (in the 1950s and 1960s) that led to more invasive EEG with the use of special depth electrodes and the exploration of deep intracerebral regions are discussed later.

Any discussion of the 1940s would be incomplete without mentioning the work of neurophysiologists, which was largely dominated by the use of EEGs. One of the most fascinating results in this regard was the demonstration of thalamocortical circuits, which had until then been explored solely on an anatomical basis (e.g., the study of the thalamus in 1938, which propelled A. Earl Walker [1907–1995] to great fame in the decades to come (55,56)). The work of Morison and Dempsey in 1942 on the recruiting response had a great impact on the neuroscientific world with the demonstration of cortical responses to relatively slow stimulation rates of the intralaminar structures of the thalamus in the cat (57). This work emphasized the role of the thalamus in cortical electrogenesis and broke the ground for the concept of a "centrencephalic epilepsy," a concept promoted by Penfield and Jasper in Montreal (somewhat naively understood as a concept of the thalamic origin of primary generalized epilepsy).

Even greater was the impact of the work of Horace W. Magoun (1907–1991), an American neuroanatomist and neurophysiologist. He had studied the effects of descending and mostly inhibitory influences of the brainstem reticular formation during his work at Northwestern University. Together with Giuseppe Moruzzi (1910–1986), a neurophysiologist from Pisa, Italy, and an investigator of basic epileptic mechanisms, Magoun started studying the ascending system of the brainstem reticular formation (chiefly at the midbrain level) and the effects of high-frequency electrical stimulation, consisting of EEG desynchronization and behavioral arousal, on cortical function. After Magoun had moved to the University of California at Los Angeles, he investigated the neurofunctional effects of acute lesions in the midbrain level reticular formation in cats in the late 1940s. These cats remained comatose and EEG uncovered the slowing of brain activity in spite of the electrical stimulation of the brainstem because of the destruction of the all-important ascending portion of the brainstem reticular formation (58). The effect of these studies on the world of neuroscience was critical: for the ensuing 10 to 15 years, the association of consciousness with reticular formation and Magoun's name was so strong that it even had considerable influence on the Pavlovian dogmatism of the Eastern Bloc countries.

The discussion of this experimental work clearly demonstrates the incredibly powerful role of EEG in the neurophysiology of the postwar period. Subsequently, experimental EEG work started to concentrate on single neurons while the study of "macro-EEG" gradually declined.

12. EEG—STANDARD EQUIPMENT IN THE 1950S

In the 1950s EEG became a "household word." During the early stretch of the decade, almost every academic tertiary medical care center had one or more EEG machines. At the end of the decade, EEG apparatuses had found their way into a large number of smaller hospitals and even into private practice. At university hospitals, central as well as departmental EEG laboratories emerged. The latter were usually restricted either to children or adults, and pediatric EEG units evolved (specialized neonatal EEG units followed about 10 years later). Some psychiatric departments took particular pride in their clinical and research-oriented EEG work. Psychiatry's domain was in need of organic or neurophysiological substrata of disorders and dysfunctions of a psychiatric or psychological nature. At that time, it had become clear that the majority of diseases affecting the central nervous system had more or less impressive EEG correlates, but the majority of neurologists remained either reserved or hostile to EEG. Neurosurgeons were interested as long as EEG could contribute to the determination of focal cerebral lesions and before EEG became overpowered by noninvasive neuroimaging techniques. Some epilepsy-oriented neurosurgeons like Wilder G. Penfield or A. Earl Walker remained interested in EEG and its use in the depth or cortex of the cerebrum.

The epilepsy-EEG work of Jasper and Penfield (Fig. 1.7) reached new heights, and Montreal reigned supreme as the place for the neurosurgical treatment of focal epilepsies. Penfield clearly proved to be far more than a neurosurgeon: his operations to remove epileptogenic foci and, in a later phase, large portions of affected cerebral lobes were associated with studies of the effects of electrical stimulation and a systematic study of behavioral consequences. At the time, local anesthesia was still widely used in neurosurgery. In contrast, Jasper was chiefly a neuroscientist and not merely an EEGer. Their book

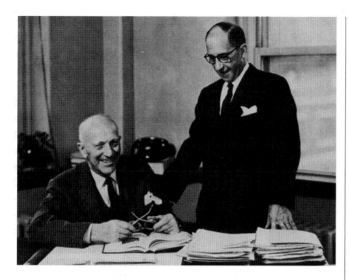

Figure 1.7. *Herbert H. Jasper (1906–1999) and Wilder G. Penfield (1891–1976) ("Wilder Penfield and Herbert Jasper at the time of publication of their monograph: Epilepsy and the Functional Anatomy of the Human Brain, (1954)" © Montreal Neurological Institute 2016. Thanks to Sandra McPherson, PhD, from the MNI for help in obtaining permission to reproduce here.)*

Epilepsy and the Functional Anatomy of the Human Brain was a result of this fruitful collaboration (59).

Very controversial, however, was their concept of a primary generalized form of epilepsy characterized by generalized synchronous paroxysmal EEG discharges and exemplified by the 3-Hz spike-waves of petit mal absences. Penfield and Jasper categorized these epilepsies as "centrencephalic," with the concept of "center of the encephalon" (i.e., "thalamic midline structures") serving as the starting point and promoter of the bilateral discharges. Henri Gastaut from Marseille and many others would follow the lead. Frederic Gibbs and a host of other EEGers and neuroscientists, however, became detractors of this centrencephalic concept.

It was not until the late 1960s that it became clear that the centrencephalic concept stood on very shaky ground and was ripe for being dismantled. Montreal's own Pierre Gloor (1923–2003; Fig. 1.8), one of the most influential scientists in the history of epilepsy, helped to do this in a cautious and diplomatic manner, while others buried the centrencephalic concept more bluntly.

Frederic Gibbs had moved to the University of Illinois School of Medicine in Chicago (where full professorship was given to him instantly after Harvard had denied him any promotion for more than a decade). The Chicago area—especially the University of Chicago but also Northwestern University and the University of Illinois—had started to play a world-leading role in neurological sciences. Percival Bailey (1892–1973), Paul Bucy (1904–1992), Roy Grinker (1900–1993), A. Earl Walker (1907–1995), Gerhardt Von Bonin (1890–1979), Charles J. Herrick (1868–1960), Frederic A. Gibbs (1903–1992), and many others give testimony to the glory of neurological science in Chicago at the middle of the century. In the field of EEG, the Chicago group, under the Gibbses, and the Montreal group, under Jasper and Gloor, were strong rivals throughout the 1950s, especially with respect to leadership in

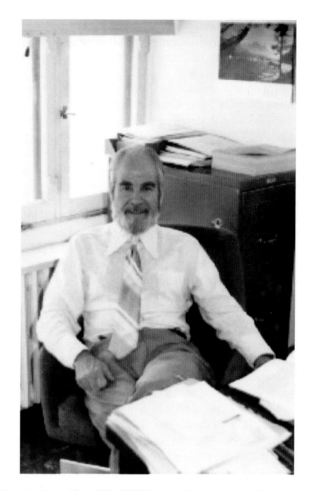

Figure 1.8. *Pierre Gloor (1923–2003) Thanks to Kenneth Laxer, MD, who took this picture at the end of our training at the MNI with Dr. Gloor, 1977.*

epilepsy-related EEG. One of the greatest scientists from the Chicago school, A. Earl Walker, came to the Johns Hopkins Hospital in Baltimore in 1947, introducing depth EEG, electrocorticography, epilepsy surgery, and a scientifically oriented approach to the study of epilepsy. Walker, who in 1972 moved to the University of New Mexico and who died in 1995, will always be remembered as one of the great scholars of neurosurgery and epileptology.

In the 1950s the Europeans made a strong comeback in the field of EEG research. Gastaut's intellectual brilliance was hard to match. In Marseille, disciples of great stature flocked to him, in particular Robert Naquet, Joseph Roger, and Annette Beaumanoir, to mention only the earliest nucleus of this group. At the great world centers of neurology, Salpêtrière Hospital and National Hospital, Queen Square, London, Antoine Rémond and William Cobb, respectively, represented EEG, but unfortunately remained too much in the shadow of the leading neurologists. Rémond later turned into a protagonist of the computerization of EEG data.

The eminent neurologists of both Queen Square and Salpêtrière thrived in a world of classic neurology. At Queen Square, the neurologists were more detached from EEG than their Parisian counterparts, perhaps due to the fact that Gastaut, from Marseille, arose to prominent neurological rank with his EEG achievements. Probably no other famous neurologist has expressed his opinion on EEG more scathingly than Francis M. R. Walshe. He was the brilliant Queen Square clinician who, it was said, knew everything about neurology except EEG. To Sir Francis, the electrical activity of the brain was "a bloodless dance of action potentials . . . hurrying to and fro of its molecules" (after Critchley (60)).

Fine EEG schools developed in the Netherlands with Otto Magnus (1913–2014) (son of a Nobel Prize–winning physiologist) in Wassenaar and Storm van Leeuwen in Utrecht. In Switzerland, Rudolf M. Hess (1913–2007) (also son of a Nobel-winning physiologist) created an important school of EEGers at the Zurich University Hospital. Giuseppe Pampiglione (1919–1993), from Italy, initiated pediatric EEG at the Hospital for Sick Children in London, concurrently with William Lennox's work at the Boston Children's Hospital. These European EEG centers had an international flavor with strong North American influence in contrast to the EEG laboratories in West Germany, which were dominated by the prestigious leader Richard Jung (1911–1986) in Freiburg. Jung's greatness pertained to experimental neurophysiology; he also had a great interest in the clinical fields and even in philosophy. This Renaissance man designed the outline for EEG training and the routine of the EEG laboratory—unfortunately not without shortcomings, which hamstrung the further development of clinical EEG in West Germany.

In the late 1950s, depth EEG with implanted intracerebral electrodes was used in the human for the first time by Meyers and Hayne (61) and Knott et al. (62) at the University of Iowa, Iowa City, and also by Hayne et al. (63) in Chicago. These short recordings were used to investigate EEG activity in the human basal ganglia and thalamus in patients with basal ganglia dyskinesias, and epilepsy. In the following years, deep brain structures were also explored in patients with psychiatric disorders until doubt was cast upon the ethical basis of this invasive approach. In the 1960s, depth EEG would find its best use in patients with refractory epilepsy who were considered candidates for epilepsy surgery.

The origin of intraoperative EEG dates back to 1935 with the work of Otfried Foerster (1873–1941) and H. Altenburger (64). Foerster, a German neurologist and neurosurgeon, was the mentor for Penfield, Bucy, and Bailey and for several other major leaders of neurosurgery. He was one of the first to use the EEG in the operating room and develop techniques for epilepsy surgery. Among several cutting-edge research activities, Foerster created his world-famous cytoarchitectonic map of the human cerebral cortex. He was nominated several times for the Nobel Prize in Physiology or Medicine without receiving it. However, Foerster was honored posthumously by German neurological and neurosurgical societies. In his last years during the Nazi regime, his activities were restricted because of his association with Russia as Lenin's physician and the Jewish ancestry of his wife. With the rise of the Nazis, these facts made him an outcast in Germany, and he died in Switzerland in exile in 1941. How was it possible that Foerster, perhaps one of the greatest clinical neurologists and an amazing self-taught master of neurosurgery, failed to recognize the future potential of EEG? Most of the work in electrocorticography remains associated with the Montreal Neurological Institute and the names of Penfield and Jasper.

The related fields of EEG started to bloom in the 1950s. In 1951, a study by George D. Dawson (1912–1983) from Queen Square, "A Summation Technique for Detecting Small Signals in a Large Irregular Background," reported the production of evoked potentials after electrical stimulation of the ulnar nerve (65), a study requiring advanced analog technology. Thus, Dawson became the father of evoked potential studies, which then developed into a major offshoot of EEG, eventually constituting a field of its own. Dawson's ingenious superimposition method was eventually superseded by the advent of computerized averaging methods in the 1960s.

After the computational techniques of wave analysis started with the first attempts by Berger in 1932 (as mentioned earlier), further work in this field was produced in the late 1930s. The first EEG frequency analyzer was a mechano-optical device constructed by Albert Grass and Frederick Gibbs. This instrument used a complex combination of mechanical and electrical technology. Using these new frequency analyzing systems, the Gibbs laboratory performed studies on the frequency spectrum of the EEG during an epileptic seizure (66), and during sleep in collaboration with Knott and Henry (67). At the Massachusetts Institute of Technology, Guillemin applied Fourier analysis to communication theory, and one of his students, Albert Grass, "could not wait to get the Gibbs interested" (14). The 1950s saw the early generation of automatic frequency analyzers, but interest in this sophisticated apparatus eventually waned.

With the introduction of the microelectrode technique in the early 1950s, EEG branched out into the world of single neurons. Microelectrodes can be made of metal such as tungsten with tips of 1 to 3 μm in diameter; glass electrodes filled with electrolytes such as KCl have tips of 0.5 μm or even less. Because of their characteristics, microelectrodes reach very high impedance values (1–60 megohm), which render conventional EEG recording techniques unsuitable. The introduction of the cathode follower by Toennies created the technical prerequisite for single-cell recordings.

Extracellular microelectrode recording was used on a larger scale in the early 1950s (68–70). About 10 years later, extracellular microelectrode studies were even done intraoperatively in humans. Far more revolutionary was the introduction of the extremely laborious intracellular microelectrode technology (Brock et al., in the spinal cord (71), and Phillips, in the cortex (72)). This technique opened the gates to a new world of neurobiochemical processes. These insights taught lessons in humility to the electrophysiological neurophysiologist: there was no doubt that the chemical changes were of primary significance, while the electrical phenomena were more or less byproducts.

Besides the increasingly invasive intracerebral EEG recordings, the new computational techniques, and the introduction of microelectrode recording, EEG-driven sleep studies advanced. At the University of Chicago, Nathaniel Kleitman (1895–1999) stood out as one of the world's leading investigators of the organization of sleep. Kleitman and his collaborators produced the first study of rapid eye movement (REM) sleep in 1953 (73). However, it must be pointed out that in 1937 Blake and Gerard described a "null stage" in the EEG of nocturnal sleep, thus indicating the desynchronization of EEG in REM sleep but without observing the accompanying ocular, muscular, and other autonomic changes (74). William C. Dement, a pioneering American sleep researcher and founder of the first sleep research center, continued the work of Kleitman and, following his move from Chicago to Stanford, became a world leader in the study of nocturnal sleep.

Sleep research gradually became based on polygraphic recording, and its share in the overall EEG research declined. This development led to a constantly widening gap between EEG and nocturnal sleep research in the 1960s and the following decades.

13. EEG SLEEP STUDIES IN THE 1960S

The rapid and incessant development of clinical and experimental EEG studies reached a high point around 1960 after 30 years, and research activities began to slow down. The interest of EEGers in academic institutions started to shift from the tracing, with all its waves and patterns, to automatic data analysis. Computerization was the new direction being sought—intimations of which reached back to Berger's coworker Dietsch (1932) but flourished in the 1960s and 1970s. In this context the names of Barlow, Brazier, Rémond, Lopes da Silva, Bickford, Saltzberg, Dumermuth, Matousek, D. O. Walter, Cooper, Künkel, Lehmann, Gasser, Burch, Hjorth, Schenk, Matejcek, and Low should be mentioned. In particular, Cooley and Tukey have been credited with the introduction of the fast Fourier transforms to extract the spectral or frequency content of a signal as the basis of power spectral analysis in 1965 (75). With their work EEG computerization reached new standards, and we were told that customary EEG reading would soon be replaced by fully automatic EEG interpretation systems. This new technique eventually enabled the field of quantitative EEG (qEEG) as we know it today. In the simplest form one speaks of qEEG when the EEG is submitted to spectral analysis. In this respect some EEGers prefer the term *normative EEG* to emphasize that the EEG not only should be submitted to spectral analysis but also needs to be compared to controls or normative databases.

The group led by Ross Adey at the UCLA Brain Research Institute throughout the 1960s and 1970s pioneered the use of qEEG. They were the first investigators to use digital computers in the analysis of EEG with the production of cerebral maps and developed the first normative library of brain maps. As part of the Space Biology Laboratory this group studied the effects of outer space and space travel on the human central nervous system. Thereby, Graham and Dietlein coined the term *normative EEG* (76). In the last decades, the availability of affordable computer equipment with increasing calculating power increased and the field of qEEG has expanded even further and has become available to many EEG laboratories.

The fears of many clinical EEGers were unfounded. So far, nobody became jobless, because such an automation of EEG reading was fictional. In the following years, it was found that EEG is far too complex for such automation and still depends on the interpretation that requires that wonderful computer that is located between the ears. One simply must consider that the methods of those years—frequency or time domain—were limited to an analysis of frequencies. Automatic spike detection had barely reached its earliest stage. The EEGers needed to be aware that all types of data computerization were nothing but the EEG in disguise—"an analog of an analog." Computerized frequency analysis was here to stay and would prove to be of enormous value not only in psychophysiological research but also in the assessment of neuropharmacological effects.

14. THE KNOCKOUT AND COMEBACK OF EEG IN THE 1970S AND 1980S

The events of the past four decades are too recent for the authors to see with the eyes of an historian. Nevertheless, modern trends are briefly discussed in this final section.

In the 1970s, the evoked potential technique progressed greatly, especially with the introduction of the pattern changer in the visual evoked potential technique significantly increasing the reliability of this method; the names of H. Speckrejse and R. Spehlmann ought to be mentioned in this context. In the field of auditory evoked potentials, the location of primary cortical discharge was elusive for many years, and the late vertex potential of limited clinical value. The introduction of the far field technique for the demonstration of the brainstem auditory evoked potentials by D. Jewell, however, proved to be extremely valuable. Analogous work in the field of somatosensory evoked potentials is associated with the names of Roger and Joan Cracco.

The 1960s and 1970s witnessed a regrettable alienation of EEG and epileptology, which had existed before in an almost perfect marriage. However, a sizable number of epileptologists lost interest in EEG studies. The reasons for this mysterious development can only be guessed at. Was the path to mastery of EEG becoming too laborious? Was it the emergence of modern neuroimaging techniques? This situation changed in the 1980s due to the rapidly increasing emphasis on EEG and related techniques in the presurgical workup of patients considered candidates for seizure surgery.

Ernst F. L. Niedermeyer (1920–2012; Fig. 1.9), an Austrian neurologist, psychiatrist, and neurophysiologist trained at Salpêtrière in Paris and a leading researcher, clinician, and pioneer in the field of EEG and its use in epilepsy, was instrumental in transforming EEG into an extremely useful diagnostic and research tool. After the end of World War II, he returned to Austria. At the Leopold-Franz University in Innsbruck, he was a docent in neurology and psychiatry and acting chief of the department. While he was in Innsbruck, Niedermeyer's hospital received an EEG under the postwar Marshall Plan, and when the technician who worked with it resigned, it became his task to learn how to operate the machine. Trained as a clinical EEGer, Niedermeyer moved to Baltimore, where he worked as an EEGer-in-chief at the Johns Hopkins Hospital and became an essential part of the epilepsy surgery program throughout the 1970s and 1980s. Among his numerous achievements, including several published papers and five books and four others he coauthored, he

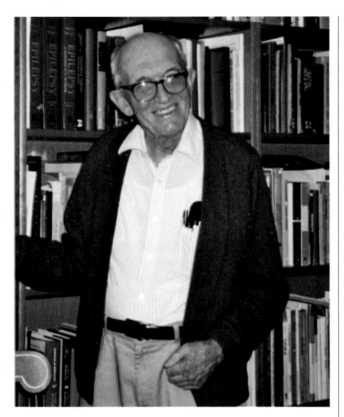

Figure 1.9. Ernst F. L. Niedermeyer (1920–2012) (From Krumholz A. Clin EEG Neurosci 2012; 43(4):255–256. Reprinted by Permission of SAGE Publications)

studied Lennox-Gastaut syndrome, a form of epilepsy that he named for the two doctors who had discovered it in 1968. His monumental contribution to the field of EEG, first published in 1982, was entitled *Electroencephalography*. It went through five editions under his direction together with his colleague, Fernando Lopes da Silva, followed by two editions now titled *Niedermeyer's Electroencephalography*.

The 1970s and 1980s saw brilliant structural neuroimaging techniques emerging, such as computed tomography and magnetic resonance imaging. This seemed to displace EEG as the principal player in the diagnosis of structural brain abnormalities. This displacement was arguably more apparent than real as the EEG, by its very nature, never was a structure-oriented test, but the only diagnostic tool providing very large-scale, robust real-time measures of neocortical dynamic function. The unfortunate result is that the neurologist of today seems to have lost interest in the realm of function and dysfunction. We believe that this tendency should be reversed.

Topical EEG diagnosis, however, has made a comeback of its own in the form of computerized brain mapping. This development has been much associated with the name of Frank Duffy. This "old EEG in new clothes" can only be understood by experts of the conventional EEG.

After compiling important historical events in the evolution of EEG over time (Fig. 1.10), our story is gradually approaching the present, and an historical outline must shy away from recent events that cannot yet be viewed from the advantage of time.

15. THE EEG TECHNICIANS

This historical overview is not complete without a few words about the EEG technicians who do the daily arduous work in the EEG laboratory. They are the ones who routinely have to place electrodes with the greatest accuracy so as to obtain a readable tracing, even under the most adverse conditions (especially in intensive care units).

John R. Knott and Charles E. Henry invested incredible energy into the founding of the American Society of Electroencephalographic (later Electroneurodiagnostic) Technologists, which came into being in 1962. Soon afterward, the first group of technicians underwent a stiff examination that made them registered EEG technologists. There have been similar developments in many other countries. This evolution has been helpful in giving EEG technologists the respect they

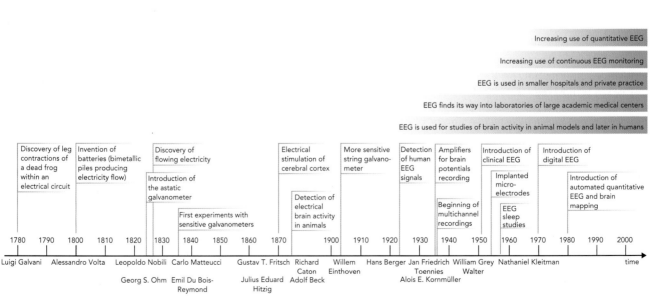

Figure 1.10. The evolution of electroencephalography over time.

deserve, but this process is far from being completed. With every record we read, we must be thankful for the work of our technical staff and invest some of our energies in their continued education and training for the sake of better and ongoing technical EEG quality and hence for the sake of our patients.

This historical overview remains a partial account because much remains untold in this story. However, it is hoped that the historical perspective this chapter brings to the reader will foster in our ranks insights that may help us avoid the mistakes of the past.

16. THOUGHTS ABOUT THE PRESENT AND FUTURE

16.1. Clinical EEG

The role of clinical EEG has been decreasing over the past 40 years except in the study of patients with epilepsy. In the latter, it has become a primary tool for video-EEG monitoring used to diagnose paroxysmal disorders of behavior and consciousness, and to establish the candidacy of patients for epilepsy surgery. Prolonged, computer-collected EEG monitoring produces an enormous accumulation of data that often warrant thorough analysis and interpretation—a highly time-consuming task that is often "farmed out" or subcontracted to outside readers with sometimes inadequate EEG expertise. Presence, number or absence of spikes, and spike-related discharges are not the only criteria; full justice must be done to all EEG abnormalities of nonparoxysmal character, and this task is a lot more difficult. Such expensive long-term recordings should be either artfully interpreted or arguably not done at all.

An urgently requested EEG nowadays deals mainly with the request to "rule out status epilepticus" (77). With the currently widespread uncertainties regarding the diagnosis and intensity of management of nonconvulsive status epilepticus, the answers need a sophisticated neurological–epileptological understanding and knowledge regarding the complexity of seizure patterns (78). Cases of acute cerebral anoxia (after cardiopulmonary arrest) may cause both convulsive and nonconvulsive pictures with massive paroxysmal EEG abnormalities that do not typically represent status epilepticus.

Outside the confines of epileptic conditions, the EEG contains much information on a great number of neurological diseases. It is most regrettable that this rich source of information has been greatly underused in most neurological teaching institutions and hospitals in general (79).

16.2. Continuous EEG Monitoring in Intensive Care

In the last three decades, the EEG has gained importance in intensive care. Critically ill patients often become confused or obtunded from a variety of critical illnesses. Excluding or uncovering nonconvulsive seizures or nonconvulsive status epilepticus, as well as the detection of focal slowing of EEG background activity as a correlate of acute brain lesions, and generalized slowing in more diffuse nonepileptic encephalopathies will depend on the EEG. Hence, in recent years, continuous EEG monitoring (cEEG) has been increasingly implemented in intensive care units.

The increasing use of cEEG may reveal clinically undetected epileptiform activity in up to 80% of critically ill patients with altered level of consciousness (80,81). Using cEEG, epileptic seizures have been detected in up to 15% of patients who are not neurocritically ill and in up to 50% of neurocritically ill patients (82). Status epilepticus can be found in 10% of patients with ischemic stroke, in about 15% with traumatic brain injury, in 20% with intracerebral hemorrhage, in 10% with subarachnoid hemorrhage, and in 30% after cardiac arrest (82).

Aside from seizure detection, some EEG characteristics, such as the degree of slowing brain activity and the presence of nonepileptic episodic transients, alert clinicians to direct further clinical investigation toward specific underlying etiologies and to provide important prognostic information in patients with acute nonepileptic encephalopathy. While most studies of patients with hypoxic-ischemic brain injury after cardiac arrest indicate that somatosensory evoked potentials are the most reliable outcome predictor (83), recent studies have revealed that the combination of clinical examination and EEG background reactivity offers the best prediction of outcome soon after postanoxic coma (84).

The recording over several hours to days, the challenges from patient- or intensive care equipment-related electrographic artifacts, and the interpretation by trained EEG readers are time-consuming and labor-intensive, calling for a targeted use in patients with defined risk profiles and effective methods to assist in rapid and accurate seizure detection. A recent investigation of an intensive care unit EEG analysis and seizure detection algorithm revealed promising results (85). Although most algorithms performed on cEEG recordings have a high sensitivity and a low false detection rate, there are several challenges to overcome before such new automated tools will be routinely integrated as reliable neurological monitoring systems in intensive care units.

16.3. EEG and Neurocognition

This area has become a fascinating area of EEG interest. Most of this research has been done with other tools such as functional magnetic resonance imaging, positron emission tomography scanning, and single photon emission computed tomography (methods demonstrating regional blood flow and metabolic needs). With the extension of EEG into the ultrafast frequency ranges, a powerful upswing in EEG-oriented neurocognitive research in animals and humans can be expected. Neurocognition has assumed the position of the "Holy Grail" of all neuroscience, and EEG stands a good chance to become a principal contributor. Newer work has addressed the interconnectivity of functional networks that are derived from brain imaging techniques. These study neuroelectromagnetic and hemodynamic signals derived from modalities such as functional magnetic resonance imaging, magnetoencephalography, and EEG. Analysis of these relationships provides a mathematical expression of a network of nodes and their interconnections, referred to as graph theory.

REFERENCES

1. O'Leary JL, Goldring S: Science and epilepsy. New York: Raven Press; 1976
2. Caton R: The electric currents of the brain. B Med J 1875; 2:278
3. Walter WG, Cooper R, Aldridge VJ, et al.: Contingent negative variation: an electric sign of sensorimotor association and expectancy in the human brain. Nature 1964; 203:380–384
4. Brazier MAB: A history of the electrical activity of the brain. The first half-century. London: Pitman Medical Publishing Company; 1961
5. Caton R: Interim report on investigation of the electric currents of the brain. Br Med J 1877; 1(Suppl):62
6. Geddes LA: What did Caton see? Electroencephalogr Clin Neurophysiol 1987; 67:2–6
7. Fritsch G, Hitzig E: Über die elektrische Erregbarkeit des Grosshirns. Arch Anat Physiol 1870; 37:300–332
8. Danilevsky VD: Investigations into the physiology of the brain: University Charkov 1877
9. Cybulski N, Jelenska-Macieszyna X: Action currents of the cerebral cortex. Bull Int Acad Cracov 1914:776–781
10. Goltz FL: Über die Verrichtungen des Grosshirns. Pflügers Arch Ges Physiol Rev 1888; 42:419–467
11. Sherrington CS: Integrative action of the nervous system. New Haven, CT: Yale University Press; 1906
12. Berger H: Über das Elektrenkephalogramm des Menschen. Erster Bericht. Arch Psychiatr Nervenkr 1929; 87:527–580
13. Gloor P: Hans Berger and the discovery of the electroencephalogram. Electroencephalogr Clin Neurophysiol 1969:Suppl 28:21–36
14. Grass AM: The electroencephalographic heritage until 1960. Am J EEG Technol 1984; 24(3):133–173
15. Jung R: Hans Berger und die Entdeckung des EEG nach seinen Tagebüchern und Protokollen. In: Werner R, editor. Jenenser EEG-Symposium: 30 Jahre Elektroenzephalographie. Berlin: Volk und Gesundheit; 1963
16. Adrian ED, Matthews BHC: The interpretation of potential waves in the cortex. J Physiol 1934; 88:440–471
17. Dietsch G: Fourier-Analyse von Elektrenkephalogrammen des Menschen. Pflugers Arch Ges Physiol 1932; 230:106–112
18. Hassler R: Cécile und Oskar Vogt. In: Kolle K, editor. Grosse Nervenärzte. Stuttgart: Thieme; 1959, pp. 45–64
19. Kornmüller AE: Architektonische Lokalisation bioelektriseher Erscheinungen auf der Grosshirnrinde. 1. Mitteilung: Untersuchungen am Kaninchen bei Augenbelichtung. J Psychol Neurol Clin 1932; 44:447–459
20. Kornmüller AE: Die Ableitung bioelektischer Effekte architektonischer Rindenfelder vom uneröffneten Schadel. J Psychol Neurol 1933; 45:172–184
21. Kornmüller AE: Der Mechanismus des epileptischen Anfalles auf Grund bioelektrischer Untersuchungen am Zentralnervensystem. Fortschr Neurol Psychiatry 1935; 7:391–400 and 414–432
22. Kornmüller AE: Die Bioelektrischer Erseheinungen der Hirnrindenfelder. Leipzig: Thieme; 1937
23. Kornmüller AE: Klinische Elektrenkephalographie. Munich: Lehmann; 1944
24. Fischer MH: Elektrobiologische Auswirkungen von Krampfgiften am Zentralnervensystem. Med Klin 1933; 29:15–19
25. Fischer MH, Löwenbach H: Aktionsströme des Zentralnervensystems unter der Einwirkung von Krampfgiften. 1. Mitteilung Strychnin und Pikrotoxin. Arch Exp Pathol Pharmakol 1934; 174:357–382
26. Fischer MH, Löwenbach H: Aktionsströme des Zentralnervensystems unter der Einwirkung von Krampfgiften. 2. Mitteilung: Cardiazol, Coffein und andere. Arch Exp Pathol Pharmakol 1934; 174:502–516
27. Vogt C, Vogt O: Sitz und Wesen der Krankheiten im Lichte der topistischen Hirnforschung und des Variierens der Tiere. Leipzig: Barth; 1937
28. Adrian ED, Bronk DW: The frequency of discharge in reflex and voluntary contractions. J Physiol 1929; 67:119–151
29. Adrian ED: The Berger rhythm in the monkey's brain. J Physiol 1936; 87:83–84
30. Bremer F: Cerveau isolé et physiologie du sommeil. C R Soc Biol (Paris) 1935; 118:1235–1241
31. Bremer F: Cerebral and cerebellar potentials. Physiol Rev 1958; 38:357–388
32. Mazza S, Pavone A, Niedermeyer E: Mario Gozzano: the work of an EEG pioneer. Clin Electroencephalogr 2002; 33:155–159
33. Schwab RS: Electroencephalography. Philadelphia: WB Saunders; 1951
34. Bartley SH: Analysis of cortical response to stimulation of the optic nerve. Am J Physiol 1932; 101:4P
35. Bartley SH, Newman EB: Recording cerebral action currents. Science 1930; 71:587
36. Bartley SH, Newman EB: Studies on the dog's cortex. Am J Physiol 1931; 99:1–8
37. Davis H, Saul LV: Action currents in the auditory tracts of the midbrain of the cat. Science 1931; 86:448–450
38. Travis LE, Dorsey JM: Action current studies of simultaneously active disparate fields of the central nervous system of the rat. Arch Neurol Psychiatr Pol 1932; 28:331–338
39. Travis LE, Herren RY: The relation of electrical changes in the brain to reflex activity. J Comp Psychol 1931; 12:23–29
40. Bishop GH, Bartley SH: Electrical study of the cerebral cortex as compared to the action potential of excised nerve. Proc Soc Exp Biol (New York) 1932; 29:698–699
41. Gerard RW, Marshall WH, Saul LJ: Cerebral action potentials. Proc Soc Exp Biol (New York) 1933; 30:1123–1125
42. Lennox WG: The oxygen and carbon dioxide content of blood from the internal jugular and other veins. Arch Intern Med 1930; 46:630–636
43. Lennox WG: The cerebral circulation. Arch Neurol Psychiatry 1931; 26:719–724
44. Lennox WG, Gibbs EL: The blood flow in the brain and the leg of man, and the changes induced by alteration of blood gases. J Clin Invest 1932; 1:1155–1177
45. Gibbs FA, Davis H, Lennox WG: The electroencephalogram in epilepsy and in conditions of impaired consciousness. Arch Neurol Psychiatry 1935; 34:1133–1148
46. Gibbs FA, Gibbs EL, Lennox WG: Epilepsy paroxysmal cerebral dysrhythmia. Brain 1937; 60:377–388
47. Gibbs FA, Davis H: Changes in the human electroencephalogram associated with loss of consciousness. Am J Physiol 1935; 113:49–50
48. Berger H: Über das Elektrenkephalogramm des Menschen. Siebter Bericht. Arch Psychiat Nervenkr 1933; 100:301–320
49. Loomis AL, Harvey EN, Hobart GA: Potential rhythms of the cerebral cortex during sleep. Science 1935; 82:198–200
50. Walter WG: The location of brain tumors by electroencephalogram. Proc R Soc Med 1936; 30:579–598
51. Hoagland H, Rubin MA, Cameron DF: The electroencephalogram of schizophrenics during insulin hypoglycemia and recovery. Am J Physiol Rev 1937; 120:559–570
52. Gastaut H: Effets des stimulations physiques sur l'E.E.G. de l'homme. Electroencephalogr Clin Neurophysiol Suppl 1949; 2:69–82
53. Gastaut H, Roger J, Gastaut Y: Les formes expérimentales d l'épilepsie humaine. L'épilepsie induite par la stimulation lumineuse intermittente ou épilepsie photogénique. Rev Neurol (Paris) 1948; 80:161–183
54. Gibbs EL, Fuster B, Gibbs FA: Peculiar low temporal localization of sleep-induced seizure discharges of psychomotor epilepsy. Arch Neurol Psychiatry 1948; 60:95–97
55. Blum M, Walker AE, Ruch TC: Localization of taste in the thalamus of Macaca mulatta. Yale J Biol Med 1943; 16(2):175–192 171
56. Walker AE: The primate thalamus. Chicago: University of Chicago Press; 1938
57. Morison RS, Dempsey EW: A study of thalamo-cortical relations. Am J Physiol Rev 1942; 135:281–292
58. Lindsley DB, Bowden JW, Magoun HW: The effect of subcortical lesions upon the electroencephalogram. Am Psychol 1949; 4:233–234
59. Penfield W, Jasper HH: Epilepsy and the functional anatomy of the human brain. Boston: Little, Brown; 1954
60. Critchley M: The ventricle of memory. New York: Raven Press; 1990
61. Meyers HR, Hayne R: Electrical potentials of the corpus striatum and cortex in Parkinsonism and hemiballism. Trans Am Neurol Assoc 1948; 73:10–14
62. Knott JR, Hayne RA, Meyers HR: Physiology of sleepwave characteristics and temporal relations of human electroencephalograms recorded from the thalamus, the corpus striatum and the surface of the scalp. Arch Neurol Psychiatry 1950; 63:526–527
63. Hayne R, Meyers R, Knott JR: Characteristics of electrical activity of human corpus striatum and neighboring structures. J Neurophysiol 1949; 12:185–195
64. Foerster O, Altenburger H: Elektrobiologische Vorgänge an der menschlichen Hirnrinde. Dtsch Z Nervenheilk 1935; 135:277–288
65. Dawson GD: A summation technique for the detection of small signals in a large irregular background. J Physiol 1951; 115:2P
66. Grass AM, Gibbs FA: A Fourier transform of the electroencephalogram. J Neurophysiol 1938; 1:521–526
67. Knott JR, Gibbs FA: A Fourier transform of the electroencephalogram from one to eighteen years. Psychol Bull 1939; 36:512–513
68. Jung R, Baumgarten RV, Baumgartner G: Mikroableitungen von einzelnen Nervzellen im optischen Cortex der Katze. Die lichtaktiviertcn B-Neurone. Arch Psychiat Z Ges Neurol 1952; 189:521–539

69. Li CL, Jasper HH, McLennan H: Décharge d'unités cellulaires en relation avec les oscillations électriques de l'écorce cérébrale. Rev Neurol Clin (Paris) 1952; 87:149–151

70. Moruzzi G: L'attività dei neuroni corticali durante il sonne e durante la reazione elettroencefalografica di risveglio. Ricerca Sci 1952; 22:1165–1173

71. Brock LG, Coombs JS, Eccles JC: The recordings of potentials from motor neurons with an intracellular electrode. J Physiol 1952; 117:413–460

72. Phillips CG. Some properties of pyramidal neurones of the motor cortex. In: Wolstenholme GEW, O'Conner M, editors. The nature of sleep. Boston: Little, Brown; 1961, pp. 4–24

73. Aserinsky W, Kleitman N: Regularly occurring episodes of eye motility and concomitant phenomena during sleep. Science 1953; 118:273–274

74. Blake K, Gerard RW: Brain potentials during sleep. Am J Physiol 1937; 119:692–703

75. Cooley JW, Tukey JW: An algorithm for the machine calculation of complex Fourier series. Math Comp 1965; 19:267–301

76. Graham MA, Dietlein LF: Technical details of data acquisition for normative EEG reference library. Analysis of central nervous system and cardiovascular data using computer methods. NASA SP-72 1965:433

77. Varelas PN, Spanaki MV, Hacein-Bey L, et al.: Emergent EEG: indications and diagnostic yield. Neurology 2003; 61(5):702–704

78. Sutter R, Kaplan PW: Electroencephalographic criteria for nonconvulsive status epilepticus: synopsis and comprehensive survey. Epilepsia 2012; 53 Suppl 3:1–51

79. Niedermeyer E: The clinical relevance of EEG interpretation. Clin Electroencephalogr 2003; 34(3):93–98

80. Oddo M, Carrera E, Claassen J, et al.: Continuous electroencephalography in the medical intensive care unit. Crit Care Med 2009; 37(6):2051–2056

81. Sutter R, Fuhr P, Grize L, et al.: Continuous video-EEG monitoring increases detection rate of nonconvulsive status epilepticus in the ICU. Epilepsia 2011; 52(3):453–457

82. Sutter R, Stevens RD, Kaplan PW: Continuous electroencephalographic monitoring in critically ill patients: indications, limitations, and strategies. Crit Care Med 2013; 41(4):1124–1132

83. Stevens RD, Sutter R: Prognosis in severe brain injury. Crit Care Med 2013; 41(4):1104–1123

84. Oddo M, Rossetti AO: Early multimodal outcome prediction after cardiac arrest in patients treated with hypothermia. Crit Care Med 2014; 42(6):1340–1347

85. Sackellares JC, Shiau DS, Halford JJ, et al.: Quantitative EEG analysis for automated detection of nonconvulsive seizures in intensive care units. Epilepsy Behav 2011; 22 Suppl 1:S69–73

2 | CELLULAR SUBSTRATES OF BRAIN RHYTHMS

FLORIN AMZICA, PHD AND FERNANDO H. LOPES DA SILVA, MD, PHD

ABSTRACT: The purpose of this chapter is to familiarize the reader with the basic electrical patterns of the electroencephalogram (EEG). Brain cells (mainly neurons and glia) are organized in multiple levels of intricate networks. The cellular membranes are semipermeable media between extracellular and intracellular solutions, populated by ions and other electrically charged molecules. This represents the basis of electrical currents flowing across cellular membranes, further generating electromagnetic fields that radiate to the scalp electrodes, which record changes in the activity of brain cells. This chapter presents these concepts together with the mechanisms of building up the EEG signal. The chapter discusses the various behavioral conditions and neurophysiological mechanisms that modulate the activity of cells leading to the most common EEG patterns, such as the cellular interactions for alpha, beta, gamma, slow, delta, and theta oscillations, DC shifts, and some particular waveforms such as sleep spindles and K-complexes and nu-complexes.

KEYWORDS: electroencephalogram, EEG, brain, alpha, beta, gamma, delta, theta

PRINCIPAL REFERENCES

ORIGINAL ARTICLES

1. Amzica F, Steriade M. Electrophysiological correlates of sleep delta waves. Electroencephalogr Clin Neurophysiol. 1998;107:69–83.
2. Buzsáki G. Theta oscillations in the hippocampus. Neuron. 2002;33:325–340.
3. Suffczynski P, Kalitzin, S, Pfurtscheller G, Lopes da Silva FH. Computational model of thalamo-cortical networks: dynamical control of alpha rhythms in relation to focal attention. Intl J Psychophysiol. 2001;43:25–40.
4. van Kerkoerle T, Self MW, Dagnino B, Gariel-Mathis MA, Poort J, van der Togt C, Roelfsema PR. Alpha and gamma oscillations characterize feedback and feedforward processing in monkey visual cortex. Proc Natl Acad Sci USA. 2014;111:14332–14341.
5. Somogyi P, Klausberger T. Defined types of cortical interneurone structure space and spike timing in the hippocampus. J Physiol. 2005;562:9–26.
6. Kroeger D, Florea B, Amzica F. Human brain activity patterns beyond the isoelectric line of extreme deep coma. PLoS One 2013;8(9):e75257.

REVIEW ARTICLES

1. Steriade M. Grouping of brain rhythms in corticothalamic systems. Neuroscience. 2006;137(4):1087–1106.
2. Lopes da Silva FH. EEG and MEG: relevance to neuroscience. Neuron. 2013;80:1112–1128.

RECOMMENDED BOOKS

1. Buzsáki G. Rhythms of the Brain. Oxford: Oxford University Press; 2006.
2. Steriade M. Neuronal Substrates of Sleep and Epilepsy. Cambridge: University Press; 2003.

Quasi-periodically recurring waves, henceforth termed oscillations, are, besides evoked potentials, one of the essential components of the electroencephalogram (EEG). The curiosity of understanding the cellular counterparts of EEG waves started almost simultaneously with the discovery and description of different EEG patterns during the early 1930s and 1940s as an effort to relate the global graphic aspect of the EEG with its more intimate cellular counterparts. In this chapter we will discuss how various patterns of oscillatory activity develop in cellular brain networks and are further reflected at the EEG level. The EEG is essentially an electric phenomenon; therefore, we will focus on the ionic currents active during various oscillating patterns but we will also identify the (minimal) anatomical structures necessary and sufficient for the genesis of the aforementioned activities. This approach has unavoidably oversimplifying virtues, while the EEG signal is a complex one. This reality will be recreated through the coalescence of various oscillations that coexist during a given behavioral context.[1]

From its very beginning, the EEG was characterized through its oscillatory nature; thus, the dominant frequency of an oscillation became its main descriptor. This trend was further enforced with the application of spectral analysis (e.g., Fourier transforms) and is still largely used nowadays. Although this might enclose certain advantages, it also contains numerous pitfalls that prevent the reaching of correct conclusions. This situation is generated by the fact that a given spectral component might ambiguously result either from the presence in the EEG of oscillations or from the contribution of particular waveforms, not necessarily rhythmic, to the EEG spectrum.

We will organize this chapter according to the frequency bands traditionally encountered in the EEG praxis, but emphasizing the possible sources of haziness related to the interpretation of EEG signals. Furthermore, as a section devoted to the understanding of the cellular mechanisms underlying the genesis of the oscillatory behavior of the EEG, the intracellular data constitute a very strong, although not absolute, source of knowledge. The reader should keep in mind that, when extrapolating from cellular data to EEG, one should not overlook essential details, such as the following:

1. Cellular recordings are almost exclusively performed in animals, whose philogenetical development and behavioral and structural peculiarities are often neglected.

---

[1] This chapter was initiated and written in the previous editions by the late Dr. Mircea Steriade (1924–2006). The present authors wish to pay tribute to his outstanding work, which has much advanced our understanding of the neuronal mechanisms underlying EEG rhythms. We hope to continue and preserve the spirit of his contributions.

2. The study of the intrinsic properties of cells is mostly carried out *in vitro* or in cultures, preparations that are as far as one can imagine from the complex reality of the whole brain, both in terms of network linkages and physiological state. At best, these preparations would correspond to a deeply comatose brain.

3. The study of the network interactions, however multisite they might be, are still based on recordings from spatially discrete and limited locations. The assumption of continuity should therefore bear reserve.

4. Anesthesia is often an unavoidable companion of animal studies, and the elimination of the pharmacological effect is time and again more complicated than a mere subtraction.

1. BASIC NEUROPHYSIOLOGICAL CONCEPTS

To have a comprehensive view of the nature of EEG signals it is important to incorporate concepts of cellular neurophysiology. These concepts are treated in detail in many basic neurophysiological textbooks. Instead of retaking such notions in a textbook form, we consider here a number of basic frequently asked questions that commonly arise in the realm of EEG. This gives the opportunity of bridging concepts of basic neurophysiology and the phenomenology of EEG. We will answer these questions:

1. Which sources of neuronal activity are reflected in electroencephalographic (EEG)/magnetoencephalographic (MEG) signals?

2. Besides postsynaptic potentials, do other types of membrane potentials, such as action potentials, also contribute to EEG signals?

3. What is the neurophysiological evidence underlying the equivalent dipole model, and is this model sufficient to account for EEG and MEG signals?

4. How does the transfer from the cortex to the scalp take place in order to be picked up by EEG electrodes?

5. Do glial cells also contribute to the EEG/MEG?

6. On the basis of the polarity of scalp EEG potentials, can one guess whether the sources are excitatory or inhibitory?

7. Which factors determine the size of a cortical area responsible for producing a measurable EEG/MEG signal on the scalp?

8. What is the range of frequencies of EEG signals?

1.1. Which Sources of Neuronal Activity Are Reflected in EEG/MEG Signals?

Local field potentials are the building blocks of neuronal activity that can be recorded extracellularly, and may be reflected in EEG/MEG signals.

The electrical activity underlying local field potentials is generated by ionic currents flowing through brain tissue. These ionic currents are generated by neurons (and possibly also by glial cells). Neurons are polarized cells, with an internal milieu that is negatively charged compared to the interstitial compartment. In this way, a neuron at rest has a membrane potential, in general, around −70 mV. This potential difference over the neuronal membrane is maintained by (1) the impermeability of the cellular membrane to proteins and other large molecules, generally negatively charged, and (2) the selective permeability of the neuronal membrane to some specific ions, most importantly Na^+, K^+, and Cl^-, such that they are unevenly distributed across the membrane (for the biophysical aspects see Chapter 4). Ion channels in the membrane regulate the flow of specific ion species through the membrane. The ion channels are proteins that can undergo conformational changes, which modulate their permeability. When the ion channels are in the open state, the corresponding ions can flow across the membrane according to the combined action of the corresponding concentration and electric gradients. This is what happens when an action potential is generated, because the membrane depolarizes above a certain threshold. The action potential is an all-or-none phenomenon where a very rapid (fraction of a millisecond) opening of Na^+ channels causes strong membrane depolarization that decays also rapidly, as Na^+ channels inactivate and K^+ channels open, leading to membrane repolarization and to the return to the resting membrane potential. Action potentials are generated mainly in the axon hillock and in axons, along which they propagate unidirectionally (from soma to the axonal terminal), but may also propagate in dendrites.

A neuron may be activated by appropriate presynaptic stimuli that generate postsynaptic potentials (PSPs) as a result of the opening or closing of specific ion channels depending on the neurotransmitter and on the receptors; these are usually present in the postsynaptic membrane but may also be situated presynaptically or extrasynaptically. The neurotransmitter binds to receptors, causing a series of biochemical processes that ultimately result in a modulation of the permeability of ion channels in the postsynaptic membrane. In this way, postsynaptic ionic currents and PSPs are generated. Typically, two major kinds of PSPs may be generated: excitatory (EPSPs), meaning that the postsynaptic membrane is depolarized, or inhibitory (IPSPs), meaning that the postsynaptic membrane is hyperpolarized (Fig. 2.1). In the case of an EPSP, a positive ionic current is directed toward the intracellular compartment (typically carried by Na^+ ions), while in the case of an IPSP a current is directed toward the extracellular milieu (typically caused by the entrance of negatively charged Cl^- ions, or the extrusion of K^+ ions). This means that at the level of an excitatory synapse, the local concentration of positively charged ions in the extracellular space decreases, therefore constituting what is called an active *sink*, whereas at the level of an inhibitory synapse there is a relative local increase of positively charged ions, thus called an active *source*. In this way net ionic currents flow across the membrane (transmembrane currents) and intracellularly; these

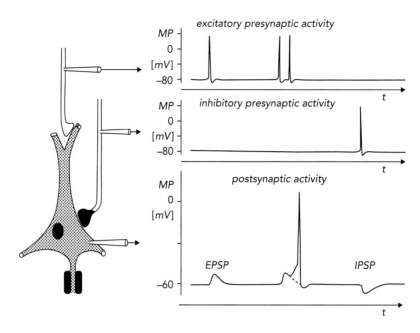

Figure 2.1. *Synaptic currents and potentials. Schematic pyramidal cell with two input fibers: one with an excitatory (terminal in white) and the other with an inhibitory synapse (terminal in black). The first trace shows the excitatory and the second trace the inhibitory presynaptic activity. Action potentials of the former cause EPSPs. The first pulse causes postsynaptic depolarization of the cell, which does not reach the threshold to elicit an action potential. Two pulses applied at a short interval from each other cause a summation of EPSPs such that the threshold is reached and an action potential is generated. Stimulation of the inhibitory fiber causes an IPSP (i.e., hyperpolarization of the postsynaptic membrane). (Modified with permission from Speckmann, Elger, and Gorgi, Chapter 2: Neurophysiologic basis of EEG and DC potentials. In: Schomer DL, Lopes da Silva FH, eds., Niedermeyer's Electroencephalography: Basic Principles, Clinical Applications and Related Fields, 6th ed. Philadelphia, PA: Lippincott Williams and Wilkins; 2011.)*

constitute the primary currents. It should be noted that there are cases (e.g., developing brains) in which, due to a different distribution of ions across the cellular membrane, the opening of GABA$_A$ receptors would be followed by Cl$^-$ ions leaving the neurons, generating EPSPs. A similar outcome occurs in normal glial cells, and in some pathological cases, namely in neurons belonging to an epileptogenic zone. The classic view is that local accumulation/depletion of ionic charges at the synapses does not occur since compensatory extracellular currents are generated in the extracellular space; these are called ohmic currents, assuming the extracellular medium to be purely resistive. In this way, and using a physical analogy, sink/source current dipoles are formed. In the case of an EPSP a negative pole is created in the region of the *active sink* and a positive one in the region of a *passive source*, with a zero potential somewhere in between. The adjective *active* is used to indicate that this current results from the active opening of ionic channels; the parts of the membrane where compensatory current flows in opposite direction are called *passive*, since their permeability does not change due to an active process. In the case of an IPSP there is a positive pole in the region of the *active source* at the level of the synapse and a negative pole at the level of the *passive sink* at a distance along the membrane. In both cases the extracellular potential generated by a sink/source configuration presents a polarity reversal along the cell (Fig. 2.2). This description summarizes the classic view, but recent more detailed studies by Riera et al. [1] found that extracellular potentials recorded in the rat barrel cortex do not sum to zero over the volume of a neocortical column. This suggests that besides ohmic or resistive currents,

it is necessary to also take into account currents due to ion diffusion, or diffusive currents; this implies that cortical current source monopoles may transiently coexist with dipolar sources at the microscopic scale. Monopoles, however, do not generate magnetic fields and are thus not seen in the MEG, contrary to the case of the EEG. These observations have been substantiated by modeling studies by Halnes et al. [2] that put in evidence that extracellular electric potentials, in addition to ohmic currents, may also receive contributions from diffusive currents, associated with ion concentration dynamics, mainly mediated by K$^+$ and Na$^+$ gradients (see more detailed discussion in the answer to question #3). The electric fields that result from these cellular processes may be detected at some distance in the brain or surrounding tissues, although attenuated with distance, and depend on the electric properties of these tissues (see also Chapter 4). The extracellular field potentials recorded near the cellular sources, typically by means of intracerebral electrodes, are commonly called local field potentials (LFPs). In summary, the latter constitute the building blocks of the electrocorticogram and consequently of the scalp EEG signals.

1.2. Besides PSPs, Do Other Types of Membrane Potentials, Such as Action Potentials, Also Contribute to EEG Signals?

In general, the contribution of action potentials to EEG signals, or more precisely of multiunit activity (MUA) consisting of spikes recorded from a population of cells, is considered limited, for two reasons.

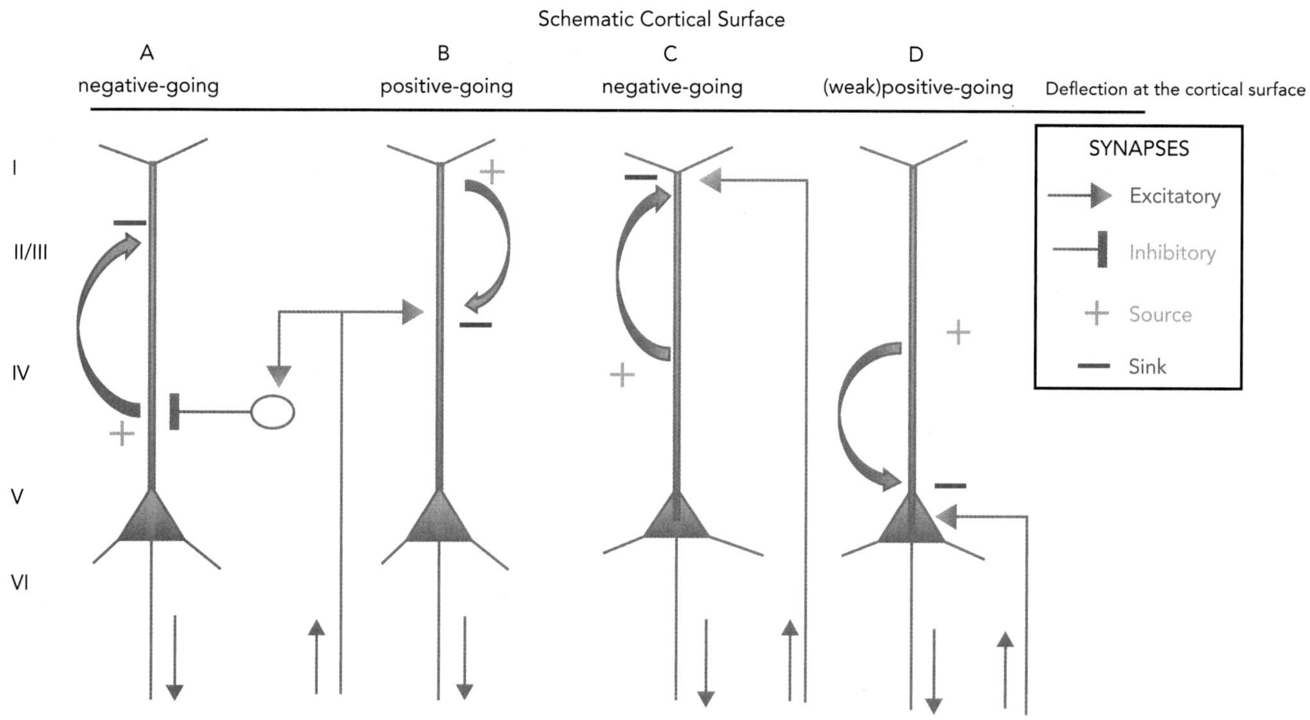

Figure 2.2. *Schematic representation of four typical cases of cortical generators of LFPs, elicited in one case by inhibitory (**A**) and in the other three (**B, C, D**) by excitatory synaptic activity, at different sites along the soma-dendritic membrane of a pyramidal cell with soma in layer V. The symbols representing excitatory and inhibitory synapses and sinks (-) and sources (+) are indicated in the inset on the right. The direction of extracellular currents is indicated by the curved arrows. **A:** Inhibitory synaptic activity (note the extracellular current pointing away from the synapse) causing an active source at the level of layers IV/V and a more superficial sink in layers II/III. At the cortical surface this would result in a negative-going deflection. Note that the interneuron (circle) represents a stellate cell that would generate an approximately closed field and would not generate a field potential far from its source. **B:** Excitatory synaptic activity on the apical dendrite of a pyramidal cell at the level of layers III/IV causing an extracellular active sink in the middle of the cortex and a passive source in superficial layers. This configuration would lead to a positive-going deflection at the cortical surface. **C:** Excitatory synaptic activity at the level of the distal apical dendrite causing an active sink in superficial layers and a deeper-lying passive source; this would result in a negative-going deflection at the cortical surface. **D:** Excitatory synaptic activation near the soma causes a local sink and a source in the middle cortical layers; this configuration would lead to a positive-going potential, but it would be relatively weak (smaller +) due to the distance from the source to the cortical surface. (Own scheme, inspired by [12].)*

First, the cellular sources of PSPs and of spikes differ appreciably in size. Indeed, the former (membrane depolarization or hyperpolarization) do not remain localized but spread (electrotonic propagation) over a relatively large portion of the neuronal membrane, typically in the order of the distance between the active synapses and the cell soma. In fact, the distance between the corresponding current sink and source is a main factor determining the size and shape of extracellular potentials [3]. In simplified terms, the equivalent current sources of PSPs can be described not in terms of a single dipole, but rather as a series of membrane current dipoles, forming a membrane dipole layer. On the contrary, in the case of an action potential the corresponding depolarization is localized to a much smaller piece of membrane and may be envisaged as constituting a single dipole, or even a quadrupole in some cases [4]; the latter has a steeper attenuation with distance.

What can an electrode pick up of these neuronal activities at a distance "r" from the cellular sources? A precise and detailed reply to this question has to take into consideration various factors, namely the geometry of the neuronal sources, the form of the cellular arborization, the localization of the synapses along the soma-dendritic tree, the extracellular resistivity, and the position of the recording electrode with respect to the cell. Here we consider only some elementary aspects;

according to general biophysical principles the potential of a single dipole decays as $1/r^2$, that of a quadrupole as $1/r^3$. Just to give a rough estimate, the amplitude of an action potential at a given distance from the cell, say at a couple of hundreds of μm, may have decayed about 10 times more than the amplitude of a PSP. Consequently, the latter has a much stronger contribution to a distant LFP than the former.

The interested reader may find a more extensive and biophysical handling of these issues in Chapter 4 and also, for example, in the study by Pettersen and Einevoll [3]. The latter showed, using model simulations, that the site of the sources along the soma-dendrite membrane can influence the attenuation of the extracellular potential as function of the distance: the amplitude of extracellularly recorded spikes decays with distance as $1/r^n$, with $1 \leq n \leq 2$ for dipolar sources close to the soma and $n \geq 2$ for sources far along the dendritic tree.

Second, the fact that PSPs and spikes differ considerably in duration and thus in frequency content is also important with respect to the question formulated above. While PSPs have durations that can vary from about 10 ms to multiples of this value, somatic action potentials correspond to much more rapid variations of the membrane potential in the order of 1 to 2 ms. While action potentials in their propagation suffer little attenuation due to their recurrent active regeneration (e.g., at Ranvier nodes), PSPs display a more complex reality both in time and space. Once they are generated in the dendrites, they activate a series of additional currents, some of which are Ca^{2+}-dependent, both low- and high-threshold, that can reach significant amplitudes and durations. Thereafter, through their electrotonic propagation they lose much of their amplitude and sharpness [5]. EPSPs and IPSPs generated by groups of neurons tend to overlap much more than action potentials. A population of neurons firing multiple action potentials generates MUA. The overlap and the degree of correlation within a neuronal population are of paramount importance with respect to the size of LFPs measured at a distance. Thus the contribution of elementary PSPS to LFPs recorded at a distance from the sources is, on average, more substantial than that of spikes, since the former tend to be much more strongly correlated. Nonetheless, experimental evidence indicates that synchronous spikes can also contribute to high-frequency components of EEG signals, for example when they tend to synchronize within a neuronal population by propagating through gap junctions (also termed electrical synapses). Thus a local field recording may gather contributions both of low-frequency activities comprising postsynaptic LFPs (<250 Hz), and higher-frequency activities (250–5,000 Hz) that include, among other high-frequency components, ripples and fast-ripples oscillations [6,9]. In cases in which the action potentials occur synchronously in clusters (e.g., when a group of fibers is excited by a short stimulus), the corresponding field may also be recorded at relatively large distances in the form of what is generally called a compound action potential.

It is often assumed that the extracellular medium could be described as homogenous and purely resistive. Is this assumption justified? In a first approximation the reply is positive, but the real situation appears to be more complicated, as pointed out by Freeman and Nicholson, who coined the term "tortuosity" to describe the fact that the extracellular medium is a medium where diffusion of ions is more restricted than in a free aqueous solution due to the complex microstructure of the medium (see also Nelson et al. [7]). Whether the extracellular medium may be considered strictly resistive or not is discussed in more detail in the reply to question #3.

Other relatively slow variations of the neuronal membrane potential caused by active membrane phenomena, such as those associated with depolarizing or hyperpolarizing after-potentials, owing, for example, to the activation of Ca^{2+}-dependent K^+ conductances, as well as dendritic events (e.g., Ca^{2+} spikes) that can be large and long-lasting, may also constitute sources of LFPs. In addition, the latter can reflect also other membrane active processes, as the ionic currents associated with voltage-dependent hyperpolarization-activated cyclic nucleotide-gated (HCN) I_h current, and low-threshold T-type Ca^{2+} currents, on condition that these would occur synchronously in a neuronal population [8,9]. In the answer to question #3 the contributions of active membrane phenomena, such as action potentials, to LFPs are further discussed.

1.3. What is the Neurophysiological Evidence Underlying the Equivalent Dipole Model, and Is This Model Sufficient to Account for EEG and MEG Signals?

In clinical neurophysiology the dipole model has been most often used to describe a source of neuronal activity recorded on EEG or MEG. Recent experimental findings and theoretical considerations have, however, added new dimensions to this model. To answer these questions we first examine the classic concept of the dipole model, or better the equivalent current dipole (ECD); subsequently we consider how this model is being revised to improve the representation of EEG and MEG signals.

At the macroscopic level, the cortical neuronal source of EEG or MEG signals, viewed from the far field, is commonly modeled as a set of current dipoles distributed within a given brain volume. The ECD model, however, should be seen as a rough simplification of reality (see Nunez and Srinivasan [10] and references and details in Chapter 45). This concept stems from the notion of a current dipole used in physics to represent a pair of electric charges of equal magnitude but opposite sign, separated by a small distance. To account for the neurophysiological basis of the ECD concept we have to move from the macroscopic EEG/MEG level to the mesoscopic level of the cortical tissue and down the microscopic level of the cortical neuron membrane.

At the mesoscopic level the common assumption is that postsynaptic activity in cortical neurons organized in palisades can be represented by dipole layers—that is, pairs of sinks and sources having an orthogonal dipolar configuration oriented with the axis perpendicular to the cortical surface. This configuration corresponds to an "open field" according to the classic denomination introduced by Lorente de Nó in 1947 [11]. The ECD would represent the weighted sum of these populations of dipoles. It should be noted that the degree of correlation between the activities of the neuronal elements plays an important role in the amplitude of the electric fields that can be measured at a distance. For the sake of simplicity, it may be assumed, in a first approximation, that configurations of electric fields other than dipolar ones may be neglected from the perspective of someone recording EEG/MEG fields at the level of the scalp. Further down we discuss, however, a number of observations that impose some constraints to this simple dipolar model. In answering question #2 we discussed the relations between the neuronal electric fields at the mesoscopic and at the microscopic levels. An insightful way of understanding these relations between potentials at the cortical surface and the underlying neuronal sources may be obtained by examining Figure 2.2, which shows a very simplified scheme with several patterns of cortical sinks and sources as a function of the configuration of synaptic contacts. This scheme shows that the polarity of a potential at the cortical surface depends not only on the nature of the synaptic potential (EPSP or IPSP) but also on the site where the active synapse contacts the soma-dendritic membrane. A precise analysis of the distribution of synaptic activities along the soma-dendritic membrane of a pyramidal cell can be obtained by means of the Current Source Density (CSD) analysis, as illustrated in Figure 2.3. CSD is the second-order spatial derivative of the local field potential (LFP) along the depth axis of a cortical column. The CSD corresponds

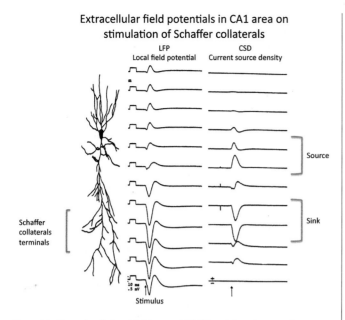

Extracellular field potentials in CA1 area on stimulation of Schaffer collaterals

LFP
Local field potential

CSD
Current source density

Source

Sink

Schaffer collaterals terminals

Stimulus

Figure 2.3. Example of a local field potential (LFP) and the corresponding current source density (CSD) analysis recorded in vivo in the anesthetized rat by means of a multichannel electrode probe consisting of 16 Ag/AgCl contacts of 25 x 25 μm, at an inter-electrode distance of 100 μm (upper and lower 2 sites are not displayed). Recordings are from the CA1 region of the dorsal hippocampus; single pulse electrical stimulation was applied to the Schaffer collaterals that project to the dendrite around electrodes 8-10, at the moment indicated by the arrow. Calibration pulse is included at the beginning of each trace. At the left-hand side the orientation of one cell of the population is schematically indicated. The middle column shows the LFP profile. The right column shows the corresponding calculated CSD. For this one-dimensional situation (only current flow parallel to the main dendrite is considered) the CSD is the second-order spatial derivative of the LFP (for further details see chapter 4). The CSD represents the net current between the local extracellular and intracellular compartments. At the site where synapses are activated, membrane conductance is enhanced and (in case of excitation) currents flow into the cell: we speak of an active sink. At other locations, where conductance is not changed, the change in transmembrane voltage results in current flow in the opposite direction; we call these sites passive sources. (Unpublished results from BPC Melchers, FH Lopes da Silva, WJ Wadman)

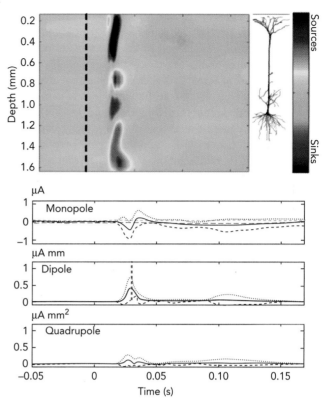

Figure 2.4. A CSD analysis from LFP (postsynaptic evoked activity) recorded from the rat barrel cortex elicited by whisker deflections. **Above:** Average CSD spatiotemporal map (mean values and standard deviations), based on a number of cortical barrels, showing sinks (blue) and sources (red). **Below:** The corresponding multipolar currents at the maximal postsynaptic activity are for the three components: −0.44 ± 0.20 μA for the monopolar, −0.43 ± 016 μA. mm for the dipolar, and 0.13 ± 0.06 μA.mm² for the quadrupolar components. To be comparable the dipolar and quadrupolar components must be divided by the cortical thickness, l and l2, respectively. The net charge at a large temporal scale (200 ms) was approximately zero. (Adapted from Riera JJ, Ogawa T, Goto T, et al. Pitfalls in the dipolar model for the neocortical EEG sources. J Neurophysiol. 2012;108:956–975, with permission.)

to the net current entering or leaving the extracellular space; in this way it gives an estimate of the location of *sinks* and *sources*. An active *sink* is where positive charges enter cells (e.g., activation of excitatory synapses), and it is coupled to passive *sources*, where compensatory positive charges exit cells. An active *source* is where positive charges arise (e.g., due to the activation of inhibitory synapses), and it is coupled to compensatory passive sinks, where positive charges diminish (for a classic account of the current source density CSD methodology see [12]).

As mentioned above, the interpretation that the sources of EEG/MEG signals would be simply dipolar has been put in question experimentally by the studies that Riera et al. [1] carried out in the barrel somatosensory cortex of the rat *in vivo*. These authors reported that the CSD estimated from the recorded extracellular potentials comprises not only dipolar but also monopolar and quadrupolar components (Fig. 2.4). The real existence of neuronal current-source monopoles, however, has been questioned by Gratiy et al. [13], who assumed that the neuronal system behaves as a homogenous conductor without capacitive effects. This proposal was in turn rebutted

by Bédard and Destexhe [14] who pointed out that the controversy concentrates on whether neurons and extracellular media are homogenous and resistive or not. In this context the following question should be considered: what are the biophysical processes behind the appearance of monopoles?

Bédard and Destexhe [14] in a theoretical study, proposed that this may be caused by the fact that ionic currents in the extracellular medium take a significant time to move such that the inward currents are not instantaneously balanced by the outward currents. This may cause a transient accumulation of ionic charges that are reflected in transient monopoles. It should be added that the contribution of the latter to signals recorded at a distance may be considerable since the attenuation of monopoles with distance r is proportional to $1/r$, compared with that of dipoles $1/r^2$ and quadrupoles $1/r^3$.

The controversy mentioned above was further cleared up by modeling studies. Two models are especially noteworthy in this respect: (1) Cabo and Riera [15] showed how neuronal activity can generate not only ohmic field currents but also ionic density imbalances (i.e., diffusional currents), leading to the appearance of monopolar contributions to CSD estimates performed at micrometer scales, as found experimentally for cortical cells [1] and (2) Halnes et al. [2] used multicompartmental neuron models and small networks to investigate the relative contributions to extracellular potentials of diffusive currents, associated with ion concentration dynamics, and ohmic currents, using realistic physiological parameters, although not including Na$^+$/K$^+$ pumps and glial buffering. These authors demonstrated that diffusion could contribute to extracellular potentials in accordance with experimental studies [16,17]. These simulations put also in evidence the difference in time course of ohmic currents, which can increase fast in milliseconds, and diffusive currents, which take much longer to build up. This implies that the latter can contribute mainly to the low-frequency components of the power spectra of extracellular potentials, with the strongest influence at frequencies around 1 Hz. At the time scale of EEG, it is possible that a current sink may temporarily appear as ions enter the cell to be compensated by a current source at a slightly later time as the charge leaves the cell. Thus the total electric charge is conserved, although it may first appear unbalanced. Furthermore, ion buffering due to ion pumps may contribute to imbalances in extracellular potentials, but the latter have probably a minor contribution for CSD unbalances because they operate at a much slower timescale. Also, shunting of electric currents by vessels and by axons may contribute to unbalances, but the relative contributions of the latter are not yet well established.

A directly related question is this: what are the contributions of different multipolar moments of intracortical current sources to evoked potentials recorded at the surface of the skull? Riera et al. [1] recorded evoked potentials over the rat barrel cortex and estimated inverse solutions, using least-squares dipolar fitting and the surface LORETA approach (for this methodology see Chapter 45). These solutions were analyzed with respect to the normalized multipolar moments using regression analysis. These authors found that current monopoles were the most significant source component of the evoked potential waveforms. Interestingly, it should be added that while monopoles can contribute to EEG signals, these do not contribute to MEG signals, since magnetic monopoles do not physically exist. This may explain differences that have been found between simultaneously recorded EEG and MEG signals, namely of interictal spikes in epileptic patients [18] that have been attributed to differences in the orientations of dipolar sources, although a possible contribution of monopolar fields to the EEG, and not to the MEG, may also be considered. The conclusion is that current monopoles, dipoles, and quadrupoles can constitute significant source components to EEG signals recorded at the scalp level.

This general statement has to be tapered taking into consideration that the cortex is a complex layered structure with different kinds and locations of pyramidal cells, stellate cells, and a diversity of types of interneurons situated at different intracortical levels and with different orientations, associated with fiber bundles organized in fascicles, some of which are oriented vertically and others horizontally. This heterogeneous structure makes the sources of electrical activities much more complex than simple neuronal models can account for. This is illustrated, for example, in the model study by Reimann et al. [9], who simulated local field potentials in a neocortical column including multicompartmental spiking pyramidal and basket cells of cortical layers IV and V with the corresponding ionic and synaptic currents. They found that spike-related currents can contribute more to local field potentials at relatively low frequencies than usually assumed.

In short, the answer to the initial question is that cellular neurophysiological measurements substantiate the general validity of multipolar models in accounting for EEG/MEG signals. Further experimental investigations are necessary to clarify the relative contribution of diverse combinations of modeling dimensions in relation to the specific microstructure of different cortical areas.

1.4. How Does the Transfer from the Cortex to the Scalp Take Place in Order to Be Picked Up by EEG Electrodes?

For LFPs to contribute to EEG signals recorded at some distance, a paramount condition must be fulfilled: the population of neurons generating the LFPs should consist of regularly arranged neurons that should be active in an approximately synchronous way, as described in question #3 (where we discussed the concept of equivalent cortical dipole and multipolar extensions). Here we concentrate on the question of how the transfer from the LFP at the level of the cortex to the scalp EEG takes place. This problem relies on the propagation of electric (and magnetic) fields in a volume of ill-conducting media. The physical properties, namely the resistivities of various tissues (brain, cerebrospinal fluid, skull, scalp) lying between cortex and scalp, play an essential role in this transfer. Estimates of these resistivities are presented in [19]. Knowledge of these properties is of great importance in constructing so-called *forward* models (i.e., calculating electric or magnetic fields at the scalp generated by sources within the brain). These forward models constitute the basis for solving the *inverse* problem (i.e., estimating from EEG or MEG signals the corresponding cerebral sources). These issues are dealt with in Chapters 4 and 45. Here we focus mainly on how the *orientation* of the dipole layers with respect to the cortical surface influences scalp potentials (Fig. 2.5). This cartoon shows a very simplified and schematic view of the distribution of dipole layers along gyri and sulci of the cortex. It emphasizes that the EEG recorded from the scalp is particularly sensitive to source layers situated along the convexity of gyri (see Fig. 2.5: *ab, de, gh*), where the equivalent sources are organized in a palisade perpendicular to the cortical surface, and less so to sources with opposing direction in a sulcus (*bcd, efg*), and to randomly oriented sources (*ijklm*). The situation is different in the case of the MEG, as further explained in Chapter 35.

1.5. Do Glial Cells Also Contribute to the EEG/MEG?

We may formulate two kind of answers to this question. First, in a general sense, glial cells do not only passively reflect neuronal activities but influence the excitability of the surrounding neuronal networks [20]. They have polarized membranes, which display significant variations (in the range of tens of

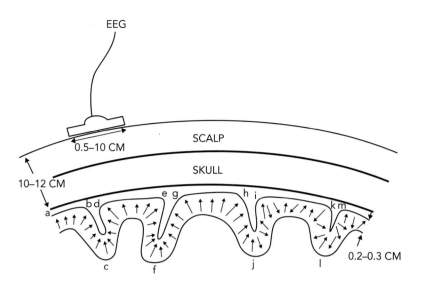

Figure 2.5. *Cartoon showing the distribution of cortical dipole layers with different orientations that result in different contributions to scalp EEG and MEG as explained in the text. (Modified from Nunez PL. Physical principles and neurophysiological mechanisms underlying event-related potentials. In: Rohrbaugh J, Johnson R, Parasuraman R, eds. Event-Related Potentials of the Brain. New York: Oxford University Press; 1990, with permission.)*

millivolts), and thus they may contribute to LFPs, and therefore to EEG signals. Second, glial cells have been shown to be involved in the generation of slow field potentials in the cortex [16,20], particularly evident during spreading depression, seizures [21], and sleep [22].

Glial cells are not only elements that support neurons, as first assumed (and as the name derived from the Greek word for "glue" suggests), but also contribute to the normal functioning of neurons. Glial cells also have polarized membranes and their membrane potential is typically more negative than that of most neurons, in the range of −80 to −90 mV due to the fact that these cells are preferentially permeable to K^+ ions. Glial cells play an important role in controlling the neuronal extracellular environment, the concentration of neurotransmitters, mainly in the synaptic cleft, and immunological responses in the central nervous system. Thus glial cells are not passive elements of the brain but are involved in signaling processes jointly with neurons. Furthermore, glial networks use a very efficient communication pathway by means of gap junctions, allowing ionic currents to flow over several millimeters. Whether such currents can generate noticeable dipoles is still unclear, but such a possibility would constitute a powerful contribution of glial cells to EEG/MEG.

1.6. On the Basis of the Polarity of Scalp EEG Potentials, Can One Guess Whether the Sources are Excitatory or Inhibitory?

An answer to this question is implicitly given by examining Figure 2.2, where the contribution of different configurations of cortical cellular generators to scalp potentials is schematically illustrated. In this figure one can see that an excitatory synaptic activation at the level of the dendrite of a pyramidal cell in layer III (see Fig. 2.2B) causes a positive deflection at the cortical surface, whereas if the excitatory synapse is situated at the distal apical dendrite (see Fig. 2.2C) of a similar cell, the result is a negative potential at the scalp level. Furthermore,

an inhibitory synapse at the level of the proximal dendrite of a similar cell results in a potential that is also negative at the cortical surface. These examples show that the polarity of scalp potentials in EEG, by itself, cannot provide reliable information with respect to the type of the intracortical sources— EPSPs or IPSPs. Thus, to unambiguously identify the nature of the source (excitatory or inhibitory) one has to have additional information about the site along the pyramidal cell where the synaptic current is initiated as can be obtained applying CSD analysis (Fig. 2.3). Furthermore, the orientation of the cellular source with respect to the recording site also influences the resulting electric field at the scalp (Fig. 2.5).

1.7. Which Factors Determine the Size of a Cortical Area Responsible for Producing a Measurable EEG/MEG Signal on the Scalp?

There have been several attempts to deal with this question, but giving a straight answer is not simple. A current assumption is that within the area occupied by the cortical cells that constitute the sources of the EEG/MEG signals, these cells would be synchronously active and arranged in the form of palisades according to the columnar organization of the cortex. Indeed, the columnar principle of the organization of the cortex proposed by Mountcastle in the 1970s [23] offers a useful concept to envisage how cortical cells are grouped. In the framework of the Blue Brain project [24], the template of a cortical column, or "Blue Column," is composed of about 10,000 neurons within a column about 500 μm in diameter and 1.5 mm in height, including different types of neurons. Using a similar cortical structure, consisting of more than 12,000 realistic interconnected neurons, Reimann et al. [9] developed a biophysical model, including synaptic and active ionic currents responsible for spiking, to get insight in how LFPs are generated. This model study showed that postsynaptic currents alone do not determine LFPs and that the presence of spike-related active currents influences the LFP characteristics. The degree of synchronization of the cellular activities on LFP amplitude plays a major role, such that increasing the correlation of inputs increases the radius (i.e., the spatial reach at which the LFP amplitude is close to the maximal amplitude).

In general, it may be stated, following Lindén et al. [25], that the amplitude generated by a population of neuronal sources picked up by an electrode at the cortical surface depends on three main factors: the *density* of neuronal sources in a given cortical column, the degree of *correlation* of these sources, and the *decay* of the potential from the neuronal sources with respect to the distance r. The latter depends on the kind of the spatial attenuation function $f(r)$: $1/r^2$ for a current dipole and $1/r$ for a monopolar source, as explained in the answer to question #3.

These three factors are thus important to determine the size of a cortical area responsible for a measurable EEG/MEG signal, but the question can be made more specific: is it possible to make *quantitative estimates* of the size of such cortical area?

This question may be simpler to tackle based on MEG rather than on EEG recordings, since the former are less distorted by inhomogeneities of the extracellular medium than the latter. In this respect relevant insights were revealed by Murakami and Okada [26], who combined a meta-analysis of physiological data and a theoretical analysis of the factors that determine the strength of current generators, based on MEG measurements. Since the magnetic vector generated by a neuron depends on the intracellular current, or primary current, MEG signals can be described in terms of the equivalent current dipole Q, the moment of which is expressed in nAm averaged over a population of neurons. Q depends on the size of active tissue, and thus on the degree of synchrony of the activated neurons. Specifically, they concluded that the value of Q per surface area of active cortex (i.e., the value of current dipole moment *density* $q_{primary}$) appears to have very similar values across brain areas and species, with a maximum value of $q_{primary}$ of about 1.0 nAm/mm². Several investigations of evoked MEG fields elicited by transcutaneous electric stimulation of peripheral nerves report values of Q varying between 10 and 50 nAm, corresponding to a cross-sectional area of the responsible cortical patch of about 10 to 50 mm². In the case of epileptic spikes, mean values Q of 137 ± 72 nAm in the frontal cortex and 275 ± 151 nAm in the temporal lobe, in two patients, were reported [26]. Assuming that the value of $q=1\ nAm/mm^2$ is valid for these brain areas also, the minimal size of the involved active area would be within the range of 137 to 275 mm².

Although these quantitative data give some hints about the size of the cortical sources of MEG signals, the situation appears to be more complex in the case of interpreting EEG signals. This complexity has been very clearly emphasized by the findings of Cosandier-Rimelé et al. [27], who compared the sensitivity of intracerebral and scalp EEG recordings with respect to the location and geometry of cortical sources. They showed that intracerebral electrodes are indeed much more sensitive to changes in the source position and orientation relative to the electrode than scalp EEG recordings. In contrast, intracerebral electrodes are capable of detecting small epileptic spikes arising from a cortical area of about 3 cm², which is of the same order of magnitude as the values based on MEG measurements mentioned above. In the case of scalp electrodes,

to record similar small EEG spike amplitudes, a cortical area of about 7 cm² would be required. It should be added that the detectability of an EEG signal at the scalp depends on the signal-to-noise ratio in the relevant frequency band (see also Chapter 33 for a discussion on how high-frequency oscillations can be recorded at the scalp).

Summing up, we may state that the factors that determine the size of a cortical area responsible for producing a measurable EEG/MEG signal at the cortical surface or at the scalp have been identified: the density of active neurons, the correlation among these, the decay function with distance. A quantitative correspondence between cortical source size and EEG signal amplitude is still precarious, although it appears to be somewhat simpler to estimate in the case of MEG signals.

1.8. What Is the Range of Frequencies of EEG Signals?

The frequency range of the EEG has no clear-cut limits both at the lower and the higher edges of the spectrum. The range of the clinically relevant EEG frequency components lies between 0.1 and 100 Hz and commonly in routine clinical settings it may be more restricted (i.e., between 0.1 and 70 Hz). Classically the following frequency bands are distinguished [28]:

Delta: below 3.5 Hz

Theta: 4 to 7.5 Hz

Alpha: 8 to 13 Hz

Beta: 14 to 30 Hz

Gamma: above 30 Hz

A question that should be asked is whether it is justifiable to make such a subdivision of frequency bands—that is, whether this subdivision is artificial or whether it has a physiological underpinning. Using factor analysis several groups arrived at the conclusion that EEG frequency bands can be grouped in a number of independent clusters, the frequency range of which shows an approximate overlap with the boundaries of the classic classification, although distinguishing within both the alpha and beta frequency bands two sub-bands [29]. Nonetheless, the definition of various frequency bands should preferentially rely on neurophysiological reality as revealed by distinct cellular mechanisms, and much less on arbitrary conventions. This chapter enlists the main cellular phenomena generating these various types of activities. It is equally noteworthy that pathological behavior might shift the limits of frequency bands, calling for additional consideration when performing "automated" spectral analysis of the EEG.

Following technical advances in EEG recording systems and new findings obtained in animal neurophysiology, the EEG frequency range of interest has considerably widened at both ends of the spectrum. This led to the coining of the term "full-bandwidth EEG" that has received much attention, as described in detail in Chapters 32 and 33. Indeed, the lower end of the frequency spectrum extends to ≤0.1 Hz (so-called ultra-slow activity); an upper limit is not precisely defined but it may extend beyond 300 Hz, the so-called high-frequency oscillations (HFOs), ripples and fast ripples. Practically, physical limitations (electrode impedances, electrode polarization, skin/electrolyte junction) do not allow recording EEG signals down to 0 Hz, which would correspond to real direct current (DC). Nonetheless, in practice, the effective frequency band can extend to very low frequencies in the order of 0.1 Hz, both for the EEG [30] and the MEG [31]. During slow-wave sleep EEG slow-frequency components, around 0.5 Hz, have been recorded in humans [32], as analyzed in detail by Steriade [33], where the importance of considering the coalescence between EEG frequency bands due to interactions in corticothalamic systems is put forward. Furthermore, it is well known that on the scalp very slow shifts of electric potential or of magnetic fields can be elicited under specific conditions such as the contingent negative variation (CNV), first described by Walter et al. [34] and the Bereitschaftspotential (readiness potential), first described by Kornhuber and Deecke [35].

The upper EEG frequency limit has expanded considerably with the discovery of HFOs extending from 80 to 500 Hz or even higher frequencies according to some authors [36]. An important limiting factor in recording such high frequencies on the scalp is the inherent experimental noise contamination from electrical muscle activity (electromyography, EMG). Therefore, HFOs are more reliably recorded intracranially by means of depth electrodes or grids placed over the cortex, although they have also been identified in scalp recordings [37,38]. Although the study of rhythmic activities of different frequency bands occupies a prominent position in the EEG field, recently some researchers have called attention to the arrhythmic EEG/MEG spectral components (also called *scale-free* behavior) of EEG signals, stimulated by the concept of scaling laws imported from physics. Indeed, EEG spectral power S(f) may obey scaling laws (i.e., it may follow a 1/f power law). This issue is further discussed in Chapter 44.

2. SLOW, DELTA RHYTHMS

Grey Walter in 1936 [39] was the first to assign the term "delta waves" to particular types of slow waves recorded in the EEG of humans. Although Walter introduced the term in correspondence to pathological potentials due to cerebral tumors, with time delta activities became more related to sleep and anesthesia. The International Federation of Societies for Electroencephalography and Clinical Neurophysiology (IFSECN) [40] defined delta waves as waves with a duration of more than 1/4 s (which implies a frequency band between 0 and 4 Hz). Thus the delta term is associated with frequency bands rather than with phenomena generating specific electrographic patterns. There have been various studies aiming at disclosing the relationship between cellular activities and EEG [41] and the sources of delta activities [42,43]. The following will emphasize that the frequency range of 0 to 4 Hz reflects more than one phenomenon and that definitions based exclusively on frequency bands may conceal the underlying mechanism. Studies in the last two decades have unveiled the electrophysiological substrates of several distinct activities in

the frequency range below 4 Hz during sleep and anesthesia. Their interaction within corticothalamic networks yields a complex pattern whose reflection at the EEG level takes the shape of polymorphic waves.

We stress from the beginning that delta activities cover two EEG phenomena, waves and oscillations, with no clear separations between the two as far as spectral analysis is concerned. The term "oscillation" designates a repeated variation of a parameter (e.g. current, voltage) between two extreme values, with an optional requirement of regularity of the variation. However, most of the biological phenomena resulting from large population interactions, such as the EEG, are rarely associated with clock-like rhythmicity. At the other limit of the definition is the wave, as a single variation of a parameter between two extreme values.

As of now, there are at least two cellular sources of delta activities: one originating in the thalamus and the other one in the cortex.

Thalamic delta oscillations have been found in a series of *in vitro* studies. These revealed that a clock-like oscillation within the delta frequency range is generated by the interplay of two intrinsic currents of thalamocortical cells. Whereas most brain oscillations are generated by interactions within networks of neurons, but also glial cells, the thalamic delta oscillation is an intrinsic oscillation depending on two inward currents of thalamocortical cells [44–47]. It was shown that thalamocortical neurons recorded *in vitro* display rhythmic bursts of high-frequency spikes with an interburst frequency of 1 to 2 Hz. This oscillation results from the interplay between two membrane currents: the transient calcium current (I_t) underlying the low-threshold spike (LTS) and a hyperpolarization-activated cation current (I_h). I_h is a non-inactivating inward (anomalous) rectifier carried by sodium and potassium. The model proposed for the genesis of this clock-like delta oscillation is depicted in Figure 2.6A: when the membrane potential hyperpolarizes (more negative than −70 mV), the I_h becomes activated and produces a depolarizing sag, which in turn will activate the I_t (de-inactivated by the hyperpolarized membrane). The ensuing LTS deactivates the I_h but also generates a hyperpolarizing overshoot that will reactivate the I_h, thus starting a new oscillatory cycle.

This oscillation was also found *in vivo*, in the thalamocortical neurons of the cat, after decortications [48–50]. Thalamocortical neurons from a variety of sensory, motor, associational, and intralaminar thalamic nuclei were able to display a clock-like delta rhythm either induced by imposed hyperpolarizing current pulses (see Fig. 2.6B) or spontaneously (see Fig. 2.6C). Interestingly, the deafferentation achieved through decortication, by removing the powerful depolarizing impingement from corticothalamic neurons and setting thalamic cells at a more hyperpolarized membrane potential (around −70 mV), was instrumental in permitting the delta oscillation to emerge. However, in intact preparations, with functional corticothalamic loops, the regular thalamic delta oscillation was absent or largely prevented by the ongoing cortical activity [51]. At the cellular level, the occurrence of the I_h was blocked during the depolarizing phases of the slow oscillation (<1 Hz; see below) due to the interference of synaptic

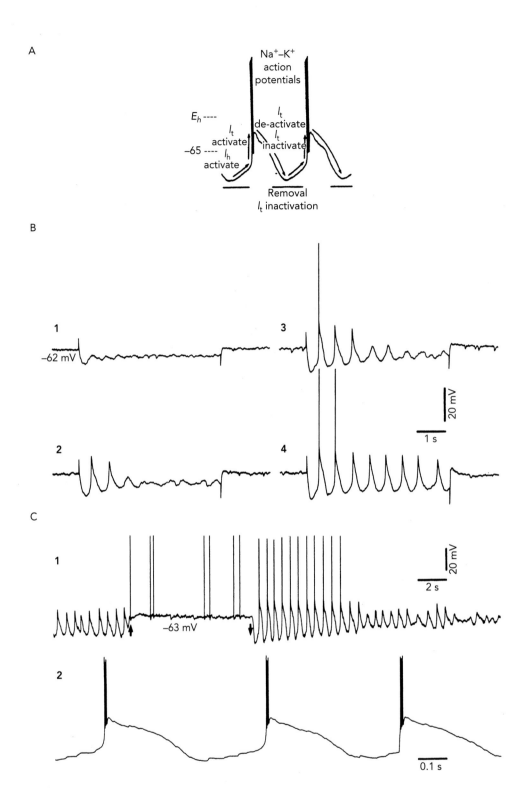

Figure 2.6. Delta oscillations in thalamocortical cells result from the interplay between two intrinsic currents, I_h and I_t. **A:** Proposed model for interaction between these intrinsic currents. Activation of the low-threshold calcium current, I_t, depolarizes the membrane toward threshold for a burst of sodium-dependent fast action potentials. The depolarization inactivates the portion of I_h that was active immediately before the calcium spike. Repolarization of the membrane due to I_t inactivation is followed by a hyperpolarizing overshoot due to the reduced depolarizing effect of I_h. The hyperpolarization in turn de-inactivates I_t and activates I_h, which depolarizes the membrane toward threshold for another calcium spike. **B:** Delta oscillation of cat ventrolateral thalamocortical cell triggered by hyperpolarizing current pulses (0.7 nA in 1, 1 nA in 2, 1.1 nA in 3, and 1.2 nA in 4). Note increasing number of cycles at a frequency of 1.6 Hz. **C:** Latero-posterior (LP) thalamocortical cell after decortication of areas projecting to LP nucleus. The cell oscillated spontaneously at 1.7 Hz. A 0.5-nA depolarizing current (between arrows) prevented the oscillation, and its removal set the cell back in the oscillatory mode. Three cycles after removal of depolarizing current in 1 are expanded in 2 to show high-frequency bursts crowning the low-threshold calcium spike. In this and following figures, polarity of EEG and field potentials is as for intracellular recordings (positivity up). (**A:** Modified from McCormick DA, Pape HC. Properties of a hyperpolarization-activated cation current and its role in rhythmic oscillation in thalamic relay neurones. J Physiol (Lond). 1990;431:291–318. **B** and **C:** Modified from Steriade M, Curró Dossi R, and Nuñez A. Network modulation of a slow intrinsic oscillation of cat thalamocortical neurons implicated in sleep delta waves: cortically induced synchronization and brainstem cholinergic suppression. J Neurosci. 1991;11:3200-3217, with permission.)

currents and the ensuing decreased membrane resistance with the intrinsically generated I_h. These more recent findings raised concerns as to the emergence of this intrinsically generated thalamic rhythm at the level of the EEG.

The existence of *cortical delta* oscillations was suggested on the basis that delta waves, at 1 to 2 Hz, survive in the EEG of athalamic cats [52]. Whether such procedures, which create a deafferentation of the cortex, generate a physiological or a pathological pattern remains an open question. Extracellular recordings of cortical activity during pathological delta waves (as obtained by lesions of the subcortical white matter, the thalamus, or the mesencephalic reticular formation) have shown a relationship between the firing probability and the surface-positive (depth-negative) delta waves, whereas the depth-positive waves were associated with a diminution in discharge rates [53]. These field-unit relationships led to the assumption that the depth-positive component of delta waves reflects the inhibition of pyramidal neurons by local circuit cells, implying maximal firing of inhibitory interneurons during the depth-positive delta waves. However, this has not been found. It was then suggested that, far from resulting exclusively from IPSPs, EEG delta waves are instead generated by summation of long-lasting after-hyperpolarizations produced by a variety of potassium currents in deep-lying pyramidal neurons [54,55].

The discovery of a novel slow-wave sleep- or anesthesia-related oscillation (around but generally less than 1 Hz) [56], together with its thorough investigation at the cellular level (see below), was the impetus for revisiting the cellular basis of delta rhythms. The frequency of the slow oscillation depends on the depth or type of anesthesia or the sleep stage: it is mainly between 0.3 and 0.6 Hz under urethane anesthesia, between 0.6 and 0.9 Hz under ketamine–xylazine anesthesia, and between 0.7 and ~1 Hz during natural sleep. This oscillation, termed *slow oscillation* by its authors, was first described in intracellular recordings from neocortical neurons in anesthetized animals and in EEG recordings from humans [56]. It was subsequently found during natural slow-wave sleep of animals [57] and humans [32,59–61].

The slow oscillation is generated within the cortex because it survives after thalamectomy [62], is absent from the thalamus of decorticated animals [63], and is present in cortical slices [64]. At the intracellular level, cortical neurons throughout layers II to VI (with physiologically identified thalamic and/or callosal inputs, and with projections to the thalamus and/or homotopic points of the contralateral hemisphere) displayed a spontaneous oscillation recurring with periods of between 1 to 1.5 and 5 seconds, depending on the anesthetic, and consisting of prolonged depolarizing and hyperpolarizing components (Fig. 2.7A). The long-lasting depolarizations of the slow oscillation consisted of EPSPs, fast prepotentials (FPPs), and fast IPSPs reflecting the action of synaptically coupled GABAergic local circuit cortical cells [56]. Data also demonstrated the contribution of both NMDA-mediated synaptic excitatory events and a voltage-dependent persistent sodium current, $I_{Na(p)}$, to the depolarizing component of the slow oscillation. The voltage dependence of these two currents explains the shortening of the depolarizing phase, and thus of the oscillating period, with deepening of sleep/anesthesia,

which is paralleled by membrane hyperpolarization. On the other hand, the long-lasting hyperpolarization, interrupting the depolarizing events, is associated with network disfacilitation in the cortex. This is supported by the fact that the membrane input resistance is highest during the long-lasting hyperpolarizing component of the slow oscillation [65]. The disfacilitation is probably achieved by a progressive depletion of the extracellular calcium ions during the depolarizing phase of the slow oscillation [66] (see Fig. 2.7B and C).

All major cellular classes in the cerebral cortex, as identified by electrophysiological characteristics and intracellular staining, display the slow oscillation: regular spiking and intrinsically bursting cells, as well as local circuit inhibitory basket cells [56,67,68]. All these neuronal types exhibit similar relationships with the EEG components of the slow oscillation: during the depth-positive EEG wave cortical neurons are hyperpolarized, whereas during the sharp depth-negative EEG deflection cortical neurons are depolarized (see Fig. 2.7A). The spectacular coherence between all types of cortical neurons and EEG waveforms raised the question of the underlying synchronizing mechanisms. Dual intracellular recordings *in vivo* revealed that intracellular potentials were highly synchronized among neurons [68,69]. This synchronization, displaying time lags as a function of the distance between cortical areas [70], mainly relies on the integrity of intracortical synaptic linkages. Although the coherence was impaired after local blockage of axonal transmission through local injections of lidocaine (Fig. 2.8), the slow oscillation survived at both locations and conserved a rudiment of synchronization, suggesting that, besides direct intracortical linkages, other projections, possibly cortico-thalamo-cortical, as well as networks of gap junctions (see below) might contribute to the synchronization of the slow oscillation.

Such cortical coherence is expected to equally involve the thalamus. Indeed, reticular (RE) thalamic cells exhibit similar and time-locked variations of their membrane potential, with prolonged depolarizations interrupted by prolonged hyperpolarizations [71] in reflection of the excitatory cortico-RE projections. The depolarizing component in RE neurons is transmitted to thalamocortical neurons, via GABAergic projections, where it triggers rhythmic IPSPs leading to rebound spike bursts (Fig. 2.9), which in turn will generate phasic excitations in the cortex, shaping the steady depolarization of cortical neurons.

The better comprehension of the mechanisms determining the pacing of the slow oscillations and the switch between depolarizing and hyperpolarizing phases came from experiments considering the possible dialogue between neurons and glial cells. Dual simultaneous intracellular recordings from neurons and adjacent glial cells were performed during sleep-like patterns produced by ketamine–xylazine anesthesia, exploring the possibility that glia may not only passively reflect, but also influence, the state of neuronal networks [72–74]. The behavior of simultaneously recorded neurons and glia is illustrated in Figure 2.10. During spontaneously occurring slow oscillations, the onset of the glial depolarization did, in the vast majority of the cases, follow the onset of the neuronal depolarization with an average time lag around 90 ms (see Fig. 2.10C).

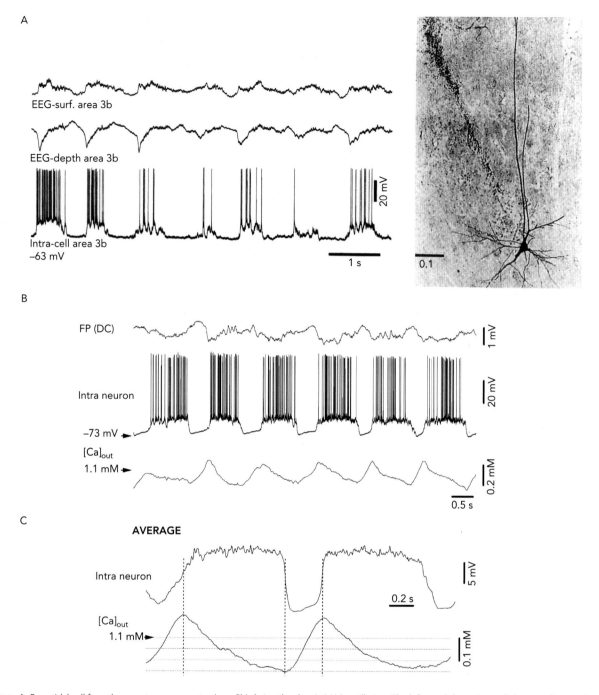

Figure 2.7. **A:** *Pyramidal cell from the somatosensory cortex (area 3b) during the slow (<1 Hz) oscillation. The left panel shows intracellular recordings and simultaneously recorded EEG in the vicinity (~1 mm) of the cell. The EEG was recorded by means of coaxial electrodes located on the surface and at a depth of ~0.6 mm. The cell oscillated at 0.9 Hz with depolarizing phases corresponding to depth-EEG negative (surface-positive) potentials. The right panel shows the corresponding cell stained with Neurobiotin (calibration bar in mm).* **B:** *Fluctuations during the slow oscillation. Relationships between intracellular membrane potential, extracellular calcium ([Ca]$_{out}$), and field potential. Periodic neuronal depolarizations triggering action potentials were interrupted by periods (300–500 ms) of hyperpolarization and silenced synaptic activity. [Ca]$_{out}$ dropped by about 0.25 mM during the depolarizing phase, reaching a minimum just before the onset of the hyperpolarization. Then, [Ca]$_{out}$ rose back until the beginning of the next cycle.* **C:** *Thirty cycles were averaged (spikes from the neuronal signal were clipped) after being extracted around the onset of the neuronal depolarization. The vertical dotted lines tentatively indicate the boundaries of the two phases of the slow oscillation. (*A: *Modified with permission from Contreras D, Steriade M. Cellular basis of EEG slow rhythms: a study of dynamic corticothalamic relationships. J Neurosci. 1995;15:604–622.* B *and* C: *Modified with permission from Massimini M, Amzica F. Extracellular calcium fluctuations and intracellular potentials in the cortex during the slow sleep oscillation. J Neurophysiol. 2001;85:1346–1350.)*

This time lag is, however, longer than the one obtained from pairs of neurons (around 10 ms in [70]). The glial depolarization reflects with virtually no delay the potassium uptake [75]. As potassium is also continuously recaptured by neurons through Na$^+$/K$^+$-ATP pumps, the actual onset of the glial depolarization may thus mark the moment where the increase of extracellular potassium concentration exceeds the capacity of the neuronal pumps. This behavior suggests that glial cells are essential for maintaining extracellular potassium levels within controlled values.

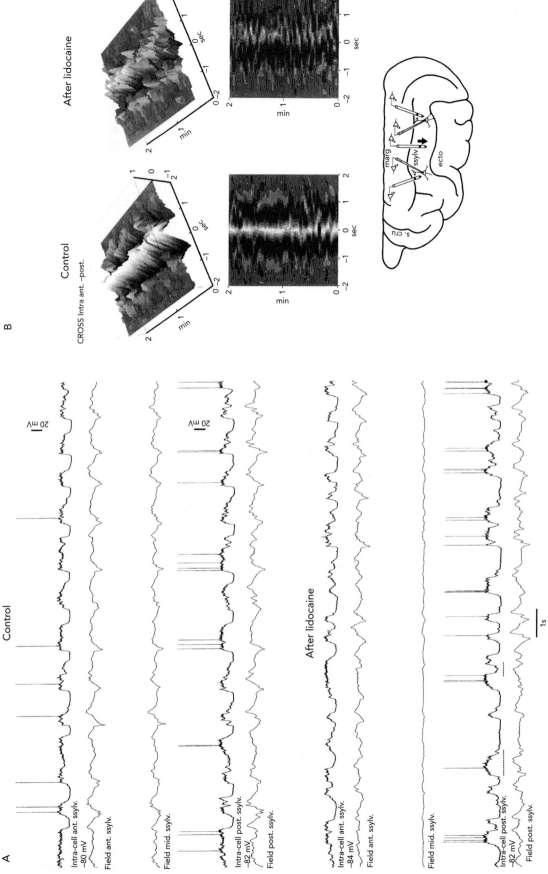

Figure 2.8. Effect of lidocaine inactivation on synchrony between intracellular activities and FPs. *A: Double intracellular recording in the anterior and posterior parts of the suprasylvian gyrus (see scheme). Synchrony was present between all three recording sites. Intracortical injection of lidocaine (40 μL, 20%; bottom) inactivated the electrical activity close to the cannula in the middle part of the gyrus and disrupted the synchrony between pools of neurons and between individual neurons. B: Sequential correlation analyses of intracellular and field potential data. Two periods lasting one minute each were analyzed with the sequential correlation method.* (Modified with permission from Amzica F, Steriade M. Disconnection of intracortical synaptic linkages disrupts synchronization of a slow oscillation. J Neurosci. 1995;15:4658–4677.)

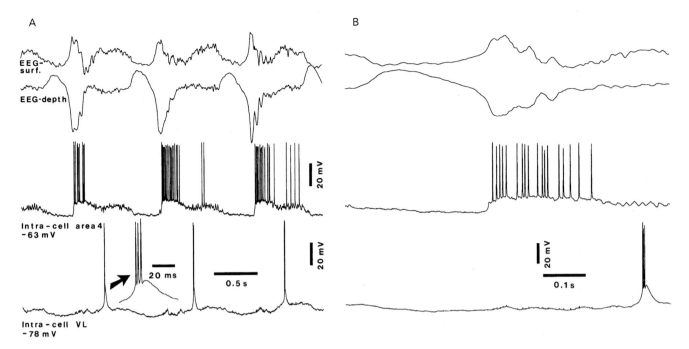

Figure 2.9. *The slow oscillation (about 0.9 Hz) in dual simultaneous intracellular recordings from a regular-spiking cell in cortical area 4 and a thalamocortical cell in the ventrolateral nucleus. Cat under ketamine-xylazine anesthesia. Arrow in **A** points to a low-threshold spike-burst. An expanded cycle is shown in **B**. Notes: (a) Depth-positive (upward) EEG waves are associated with hyperpolarization of cortical and thalamic cells, whereas the sharp depth-negatives are associated with depolarization and action potentials in cortical cell and the thalamic neuron displays a rebound spike-burst with a delay of 150–200 ms; (b) brief sequence of EEG spindles after depth-negative (surface-positive) sharp deflection; and fast depolarizing waves (40–50 Hz) in cortical neuron during the sustained depolarization. (Unpublished data by M. Steriade and D. Contreras.)*

Toward the end of the depolarizing phase, the glial membrane begins to repolarize before the neuronal membranes (see Fig. 2.10C) [74]. Interestingly, this observation may expose the mechanism ruling the onset of the hyperpolarizing phase of the slow oscillation. It was initially proposed that this hyperpolarization relies either on active GABA inhibition or on the activation of slow calcium-dependent potassium currents. In the first case, the release of GABA by neurons would depolarize glial cells either through direct action on $GABA_A$ receptors [76,77] or indirectly through the potassium output resulting from the neuronal activation of neuronal $GABA_B$ receptors. The alternative implication of calcium-dependent potassium currents should be discarded because the extracellular potassium level starts to drop before the onset of the hyperpolarizing phase. In addition, the glial membrane potential returns to control value at the end of each of the recurring oscillatory cycles, leading to the assumption that glial cells might control the pace of the oscillation through changes in the concentration of the extracellular potassium [75].

The overall synchronization of the slow oscillation in the cortex is also assisted by glial cells, which are imbedded in a gap junction-based network, through the phenomenon of spatial buffering [78–80]. Spatial buffering evens local increases of extracellular potassium by transferring it from the extracellular milieu to neighboring glial cells, then through gap junctions and along the potassium concentration gradient, at more distant sites with lower concentrations of potassium, where it is again expelled in the extracellular space. This pathway is preferred to the direct one through the extracellular space because of the tortuosity of the latter (reviewed in [81]). The

relationship between intracellular glial potentials and extracellular potassium concentrations [75] shows little accumulation of potassium in the extracellular space (<1.1 mM/cycle), and this causes a minimal imbalance between the extra- and intracellular potassium concentrations. Given that normally glial cells deal with low amounts of potassium but have a high propensity to uptake it [80,82,83], it is likely that spatial buffering would occur at a reduced spatial scale, thus contributing to a uniform distribution of the potassium around the membrane of neurons [75].

The local spatial buffering during slow oscillations might play two roles: (1) it contributes to the steady depolarization of neurons during the depolarizing phase of the slow oscillation in a Nernst-related manner, and (2) it modulates the neuronal excitability. The latter mechanism could favor the synaptic interaction within cortical networks at the onset of the depolarizing phase of the slow oscillation, but it could equally induce a gradual disfacilitation as the extracellular potassium reaches higher values toward the top of the glial depolarization. The amplitude of the potassium variations during the slow sleep oscillation ranges between 1 and 2 mM, which, when added to the physiological values of resting concentration (~3 mM), may assist cortical neurons in oscillating between hyper- and hypoexcitability [84–86]. This hypothesis was confirmed after testing the excitability of the neurons during the various phases of the slow oscillation cycle with cortical electric stimuli [74]. The results demonstrate that the neuronal excitability is maximal toward the beginning of the depolarizing cycle and almost zero toward the end of the depolarizing phase of the slow oscillation.

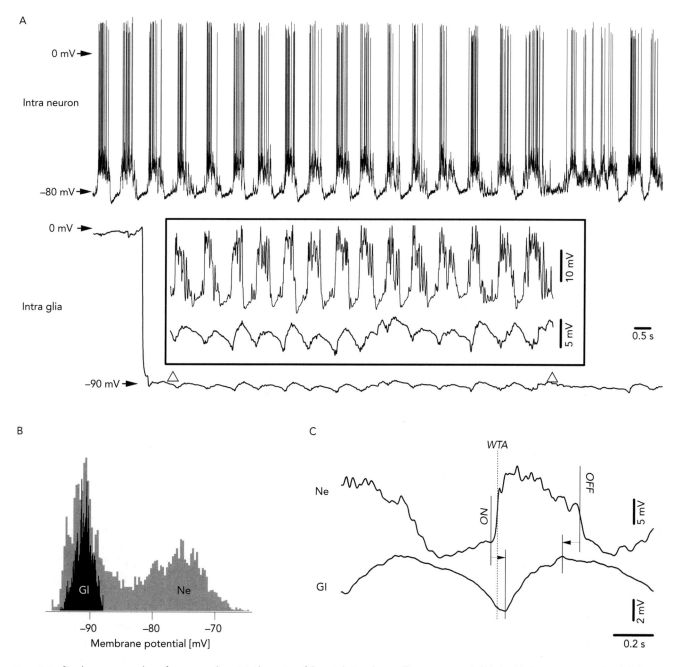

Figure 2.10. *Simultaneous recording of a neuron–glia pair in the cortex of the cat during slow oscillatory patterns. A: Relationship between neuronal and glial depolarizations on the one hand and between neuronal hyperpolarization and glial repolarizations on the other hand (note enlargement within the box). The glial impalement occurred during this period of the recording and is depicted as a brisk drop of the potential from the extracellular (0 mV) to the intracellular (−90 mV) level. B: Histogram of membrane potential variations in the neuron (in gray) and glial cell (in black). C: Typical time relationship between the onset and offset moments of the two phases of a slow oscillatory cycle. Note that the onset of the depolarizing phase starts in the neuron but that the end of this period is anticipated in the glia. (Modified with permission from Amzica F, Massimini M. Glial and neuronal interactions during slow-wave and paroxysmal activities in the neocortex. Cereb Cortex 2002;12(10):1101–1114.)*

3. THE SLOW OSCILLATION AND THE K-COMPLEX

One of the functional correlates of the slow cortical oscillation is the fact that, at the EEG level, each sequence of depolarizing–hyperpolarizing episodes within an oscillatory cycle corresponds to a waveform called K-complex. Although the phenomenon was first described in 1938 as a landmark of slow-wave sleep [87], its study remained at the EEG level for decades (see the excellent review [88]), during which researchers struggled with the inherent shape variability introduced by various bipolar electrode configurations, reference systems, and filter settings. These technical difficulties, together with the relative vagueness of the definition, often led to discordant conclusions and to difficult interpretations. The cellular mechanisms of the K-complex were only recently described [89] and disclosed that it is a recurrent event with the rhythmicity of the slow oscillation (less than but close to 1 Hz) and that, through its shape, it is one of the main contributors to the delta spectrum (Fig. 2.11) [58,72].

The rhythmicity of K-complexes during the onset of sleep is less obvious due to the lesser organization of the slow oscillation. This corroborates with the fact that bipolar recordings are often the only ones allowing the detection of K-complexes in the initial part of slow-wave sleep. However, with the deepening of sleep, the slow oscillation becomes more regular and faster (the frequency approaches 1 Hz). During late stages of sleep most of the K-complexes may be confounded with delta waves. The frequency shift (usually from 0.6 to 0.9 Hz) of the slow oscillation, as well as the shape modification of the K-complex (Fig. 2.12), accompanying the deepening of sleep can be explained by taking into account the intrinsic properties of the neuronal membrane. At sleep onset, neurons in the midbrain reticular formation and mesopontine cholinergic nuclei diminish their firing rate [90,91], thus removing a steady excitatory drive from thalamocortical neurons and allowing the membrane potential of cortical neurons to reach more hyperpolarized levels. The progressive hyperpolarization of thalamocortical neurons is a constant correlate of sleep deepening [92] and induces a gradual reduction of the duration of the depolarizing phase of the slow cortical oscillation together with the acceleration of the rhythm. The former action contributes mostly to the shape of the field potentials, while the second determines the oscillatory frequency.

Due to the controversial criteria for shape recognition, the study of K-complexes has relied mostly on evoked K-complexes because stimulation generally produces stereotyped responses. Although of certain experimental value, the evoked K-complexes have set a bias in the understanding of the underlying mechanisms because it was forgotten that the K-complex is mainly a spontaneous phenomenon [87]. The comparison at the cellular level between spontaneous and evoked K-complexes shows, in agreement with the original observation by Davis et al. [93], that the latter appears as a secondary discharge. Both spontaneous and evoked K-complexes display similar depth profiles and current source density distributions

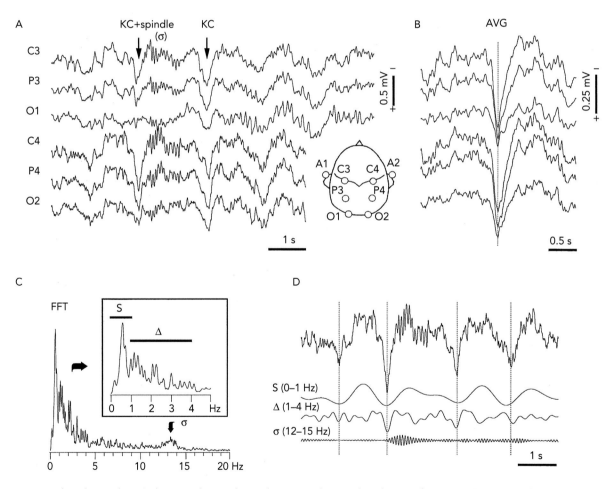

Figure 2.11. *K-complex in human sleep. Scalp monopolar recordings with respect to the contralateral ear (see figurine).* **A:** *Short episode from a stage 3 period of sleep. The two arrows point to a K-complex (KC) followed by a spindle sequence (σ) and to a KC in isolation. The two K-complexes are embedded into a slow oscillation at about 0.6 Hz. Note the synchrony of K-complexes in all recorded sites and the diminution of their amplitudes in the occipital area.* **B:** *Average of 50 K-complexes aligned on the positive peak (in this figure positivity is downwards) of the upper channel (vertical dotted line).* **C:** *Power spectrum of the C3 lead for a period of 80 seconds of stable stage 3 activity containing the period depicted in A. The three frequency bands (S, Δ, and σ; further illustrated in D) are represented in the power spectrum. Moreover, the slow (S) activity displays a high peak, distinct from the onset of delta (Δ) activity (see inset).* **D:** *Frequency decomposition of the C3 lead (upper trace) into three frequency bands: slow (S; 0–1 Hz), delta (Δ; 1–4 Hz), and sigma (σ; 12–15 Hz). It is shown that the K-complex results from a combination of slow and delta waves. (Modified with permission from Amzica F, Steriade M. The K-complex: its slow (<1 Hz) rhythmicity and relation to delta waves. Neurology 1997;49:952–959.)*

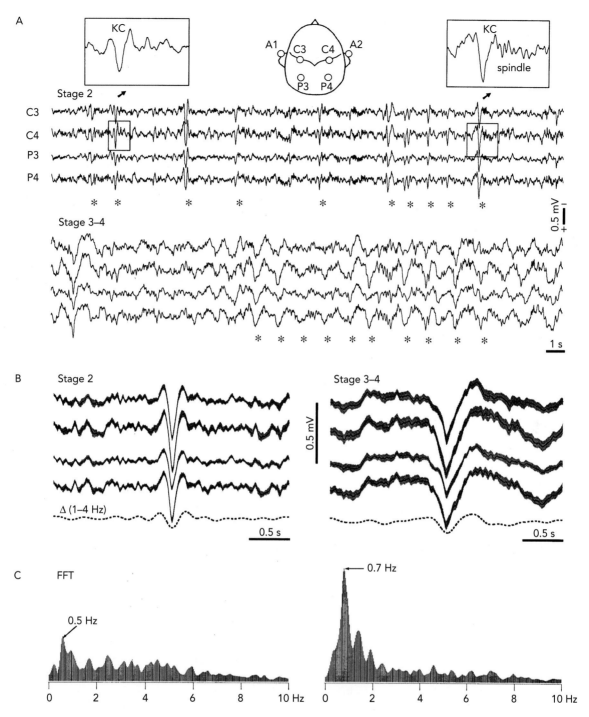

Figure 2.12. Rhythmic KCs in human EEG during natural slow-wave sleep. **A:** Four leads recorded from the two hemispheres during stage 2 sleep show quasi-rhythmic (around 0.5 Hz) KCs. The expanded insets display a simple KC (left) and a KC followed by a spindle (right). Stage 3-4 EEG (below) is characterized by a more regular oscillation of the KCs (0.7 Hz). Asterisks mark the most obvious KCs in order to suggest their rhythmicity. **B:** Averaged KCs (n = 200) from stages 2 (left) and 3-4 (right). The gray surface around the averaged KCs covers the standard deviation. The lowest trace (dotted line) results from the filtering of the average KC in the delta band (1–4 Hz). **C:** Power spectra of epochs lasting 2 minutes containing the ones displayed above. Note a principal peak at 0.5 Hz for the stage 2 episode (left), surrounded by other lower peaks as evidence for distributed rhythmicity. At variance, deep sleep shows a dominant peak at 0.7 Hz. The two FFT graphs are scaled with the same ordinate. (Modified with permission from Amzica F, Steriade M. The K-complex: its slow (<1 Hz) rhythmicity and relation to delta waves. Neurology 1997;49:952-959.)

[89], further supporting their common origin and generating mechanisms.

The complex electrographic pattern of slow-wave sleep results from the coalescence of the slow oscillation with sleep spindles (see below) and, possibly, thalamic delta oscillations

[94]. The weight of each of these major components is dynamically modulated during sleep by synaptic coupling, local circuit configurations, and the general behavioral state of the network. The discussion of the functional significance of the K-complex is determined by the role of the slow sleep oscillation of which

the K-complex is the electrographic reflection. Through its rhythmic occurrence at a frequency that is lower than the one of other sleep rhythms (spindles and delta), and due to its wide synchronization at the cortical level, the sharp onset of the K-complex provides a synchronous input to thalamic neurons, thus triggering and/or grouping sequences of spindles or delta oscillations.

4. THETA RHYTHMS

Theta waves are usually defined as occurring within the frequency range of 4 to 7.5 Hz. The normal theta activity should not be confused with pathological theta waves, described as a slowing down of alpha activity, expressed during cerebral blood flow reduction [95], or metabolic encephalopathies [96]. Rhythmic activities in the theta frequency range are conspicuous in limbic areas in various animal species, as extensively reviewed by Buzsáki [97].

4.1. Limbic Theta Rhythms in Humans

The presence of theta rhythms was first denied in humans [98,99], but they were later recorded in the hippocampus of epileptic patients with indwelling electrodes [100–102], or by way of mesio-temporal corticography with foramen ovale electrodes [103], and also using magnetoencephalography (MEG) in normal subjects [104,105]. In all these studies human hippocampal theta rhythm was studied under specific behavioral conditions. In the study by Arnolds et al. [100] the hippocampal activity was recorded while the subject was freely moving and performing a cognitive task; the frequency and rhythmicity of the hippocampal theta component while the subject was writing were consistently higher than while sitting or walking. In a word association task the amplitude, frequency, and rhythmicity showed a significant rise during the period of silent mental activity immediately following a verbal cue to which the subject was requested to give a verbal answer. Ekstrom et al. [102] found evidence for movement-related theta oscillations in human hippocampus and suggested that both cortical and hippocampal oscillations play a role in attention and sensorimotor integration. Kahana et al. [101] investigated hippocampal EEG activity using subdural recordings from epileptic patients during spatial navigation in computer-generated mazes and found that theta rhythm activity occurred more frequently when the subject was confronted with solving complex mazes. In addition, theta oscillations were more evident during recall trials than during learning trials. Bódizs et al. [103] recorded in the human hippocampus a rhythmic activity with frequency at the lowest end of the theta frequency range that presented a larger power spectrum during REM sleep than during other states; they suggested that this oscillation may be considered the counterpart of the hippocampal theta of mammalian REM sleep. Tesche and Karhu [104] recorded MEG signals in human subjects and reconstructed from these signals the corresponding hippocampal sources of theta rhythm activity. They reported that during the presentation of a memory task the duration of theta bursts increased with memory load, and they suggested a relation between "stimulus-locked hippocampal theta" and the processing of working memory. Using a whole-head 275-channel MEG system in normal subjects, Cornwell et al. [105] reported hippocampal and parahippocampal theta oscillations during a spatial navigation task (virtual reality Morris water maze). By carrying out source analyses they were able to show larger theta activity in the left anterior hippocampus and parahippocampal cortices during goal-directed navigation relative to aimless movements. Thus, similar to other species (see below), the human theta may represent a dynamic state emerging from hippocampal networks engaged in spatial navigation and in memory processes.

4.2. Limbic Theta Rhythms in Animals

Stewart and Fox [106], working on urethane-anesthetized primates, recorded hippocampal theta activity similar to that of rats but at a slightly higher frequency and appearing as relatively short bursts. Arnolds et al. [100] made a comparative study of hippocampal theta rhythms in cat, dog, and human and showed that all three displayed the same type of qualitative changes in spectral parameters (peak frequency, peak amplitude, and rhythmicity) in relation to behavioral tasks involving motor activities. Particularly in cat, remarkable relationships between theta spectral properties and vestibular stimulation (e.g., body acceleration) and/or eye movements were put in evidence. Theta rhythms appear conspicuously in rodents such as rabbits (first description of the rhythm by Green and Arduini [107]) and rats in relation with sensory processing and different types of movements [97] and have been recorded in several structures of the cortical limbic system [108,109]. Depending on species and conditions, these rhythmic may extend from between 3 to 4 Hz and 10 Hz, which is somewhat larger than the conventional range of the EEG theta rhythm (4–7.5 Hz). This is the reason why these limbic theta oscillations are also named "rhythmic slow activity (RSA)" in animal neurophysiology to avoid confusion with the classic human EEG theta frequency band. The two designations are commonly used in the literature.

In the rat, theta oscillations are most regular in frequency and present the largest amplitude in the stratum lacunosum-moleculare of the hippocampal CA1 region but are also found in the dentate gyrus and the CA3 region. In addition to the hippocampal formation, theta oscillations have been observed in the subiculum, entorhinal cortex, perirhinal cortex, amygdala, and cingulate cortex [110]. Although these areas are capable of displaying theta oscillations that can be recorded extracellularly, they are not able to generate theta activity on their own (i.e., isolated from the rest of the brain) unless manipulated by intracellular current injection or by the addition of pharmacological substances. In this respect it is interesting to mention that neurons of several limbic structures have intrinsic membrane properties that might facilitate their entrainment in theta oscillations as shown in vitro. This was demonstrated for some types of CA1 interneurons depolarized near spike threshold by current injection, which generated rhythmic firing at about 7 Hz [110], and also for neurons of the perirhinal cortex, which can display oscillations around 8 to 9 Hz when depolarized at threshold levels [111]. These intrinsic properties could facilitate the entrainment of these neurons in theta frequency oscillations.

4.3. Theta Rhythm Generation

Since the early years of this research line, several studies were carried out with the aim of finding a system that may act as theta "pacemaker." This search has led to controversial results. First it was claimed that the medial septo/diagonal band-hippocampal cholinergic system, driven by the brainstem reticular core, is the pacemaker of theta [112, 113]. The medial septum provides cholinergic and GABAergic input to the hippocampus. Whereas cholinergic neurons innervate both principal cells and interneurons, GABAergic projection neurons from the medial septum make synapses on hippocampal interneurons, including parvalbumin-positive basket cells [114].

More recent investigations revealed that hippocampal interneurons with long-range projections also innervate the cells of origin in the medial septum. Further, the supramammillary nucleus of the hypothalamus strongly connected to the medial septum, and to extended networks of the brainstem and diencephalon, has been proposed to play a role in pacemaking and modulating hippocampal theta [115].

The fact that theta rhythms survive after the blockade of cholinergic muscarinic inputs from the septal area using atropine brought to the fore the existence of an additional, non-cholinergic source of theta activity in the entorhinal cortex [116]. Indeed, a dipole of theta activity was found also in the entorhinal cortex, with two amplitude maxima, one superficial in layer I-II and the other in layer III [117-120]. We may conclude that the classic view of a septal/diagonal band pacemaker impinging rhythmic activity on the pyramidal cells of the hippocampus, within the theta frequency band, is too simplistic.

Many investigations analyzed the characteristics of the two types of hippocampal theta: one atropine sensitive, the other atropine resistant [121]. Removal of the entorhinal cortex makes hippocampal theta atropine-sensitive, so that it may be concluded that the atropine-resistant theta originates from the entorhinal inputs to the hippocampus [116,122]. These inputs are glutamatergic, and it was shown that NMDA synapses on the distal apical dendrites of CA1 pyramidal neurons are important sources of theta-generating inputs [109]. Which pathways are responsible for the atropine-sensitive theta component is still unclear in spite of many investigations using sophisticated methods such as high-density 96-site silicon probes enabling recordings simultaneously from the dentate gyrus and CA3 and CA1 areas [123].

Cholinergic inputs can cause excitation of interneurons, which may be responsible for theta rhythm discharges of hippocampal interneurons [114,124]. These interneurons, discharging at the theta frequency, can thus cause rhythmic IPSPs on their target pyramidal cells. Consequently, somatic outward currents at the level of the CA1 pyramidal layer can contribute to the theta extracellular field [116,125]. Further cholinergic agonists applied to hippocampal slices cause rhythmic depolarizations of lacunosum-moleculare interneurons at the theta frequency, which are blocked by atropine [126]. This indicates that muscarinic induction of theta-frequency membrane potential oscillations in lacunosum-moleculare interneurons may contribute to the generation of rhythmic inhibition that paces intrinsically generated theta activity in CA1 pyramidal cells. In addition, the CA3 can contribute to the generation of theta field potentials, since the recurrent network of CA3 pyramidal cells, and possibly hilar mossy cells, may form an intrahippocampal oscillator that may contribute to the atropine-sensitive component [109].

A classic view [127] is that hippocampal CA1 extracellular field during theta can be accounted for by a two-dipole model. According to this view the CA1 pyramidal cells receive rhythmic inputs in the theta frequency range from other sources that consist of atropine-sensitive and atropine-resistant inputs. The former would drive the somata and the latter the distal dendrites. The atropine-sensitive theta rhythm would be mainly caused by Cl^--mediated IPSPs on pyramidal cells [128,129]. Further intrinsic voltage-dependent membrane potential oscillations may modulate the response to a theta-frequency driving, although hippocampal pyramidal neurons do not oscillate in isolation [97]. However, they show, *in vitro*, resonant properties in the theta frequency range that are determined by the interplay between two main ionic currents with different kinetics, the I_h and I_m currents. The former is a hyperpolarization-activated cation current and the latter is a muscarinic K^+ current. In contrast, neurons of the entorhinal cortex layer II show subthreshold oscillations at the theta frequency that appear to result from the interplay of the I_h and the depolarization-activated persistent Na^+ current [97].

More recent studies [123], however, show that hippocampal theta is associated with multiple current sinks and sources with a wide range of phase relationships between the firing of pyramidal cells and of interneurons to the theta recorded extracellularly from different hippocampal layers.

4.4. Intrahippocampal Inhibitory System and Theta Generation

The phase relationship between spike firing and the polarity of the extracellular field depends on the relative strengths of the dendritic depolarization and somatic inhibition. The insightful review by Somogyi and Klausberger [130] summarizes the complex interrelationship between the firing of different populations of inhibitory interneurons and pyramidal cells during theta oscillations (Fig. 2.13). During theta oscillations several types of interneurons exhibited considerable variability in the relation between firing probability and the mean theta phase recorded extracellularly. Figure 2.13 shows the relationships of the firing of different kinds of interneurons not only with theta waves but also with high-frequency ripples and oscillations in the gamma frequency range. Here we limit ourselves to a description of the former. Axo-axonic cells displayed the highest firing rate around the positive peak of extracellular theta field recorded at the level of the pyramidal layer (i.e., when the average pyramidal cells are most hyperpolarized). Parvalbumin immunopositive basket cells fired during the descending phase of the theta oscillations recorded at the same level. Bistratified cells innervating strati radiatum and oriens fired during the

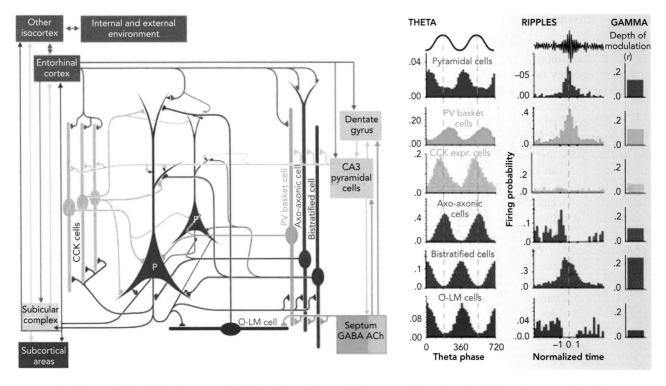

Figure 2.13. Spatiotemporal interaction between pyramidal cells and several classes of interneurons during network oscillations, shown as a schematic summary of the main synaptic connections of pyramidal cells (P), parvalbumin-positive (PV) expressing basket, axo-axonic, bistratified, oriens-lacunosum moleculare (O-LM), and three classes of cholecystokinin (CCK)-expressing interneurons. The firing probability histograms show that interneurons innervating different domains of pyramidal cells fire with distinct temporal patterns during theta and ripple oscillations, and their spike timing is coupled to field gamma oscillations to differing degrees. The same somatic and dendritic domains receive differentially timed input from several types of GABAergic interneuron. ACh, acetylcholine. (Modified with permission from Klausberger T, Somogyi P. Neuronal diversity and temporal dynamics: the unity of hippocampal circuit operations. Science 2008;321:53–57.)

trough of the extracellular theta in the pyramidal cell layer. The oriens-lacunosum moleculare cells terminating on the most distal dendrites in conjunction with the entorhinal input also fired during the trough of the theta field potential.

In addition, it should be noted that some inhibitory interneurons make synapses with other inhibitory interneurons such as described by Banks et al. [131], who demonstrated an interaction between two groups of CA1 interneurons defined according to the kinetics of the corresponding inhibitory postsynaptic currents (IPSCs): GABA$_A$ generating IPSPs with slow kinetics, and GABA$_A$ with fast kinetics, which may contribute to theta and gamma rhythms, respectively. Most interesting is the fact that incoming stimuli in stratum lacunosum moleculare do not only inhibit pyramidal cells, by activating "GABA-slow" IPSCs in these cells, but simultaneously inhibit "GABA-fast" interneurons. The authors hypothesize that this inhibitory–inhibitory interaction contributes to nested theta/gamma rhythms in the hippocampus. In Chapter 3 we describe that an alteration of this inhibitory interaction may constitute an important mechanism for the occurrence of epileptogenic activity in the hippocampus [132]. Fuentealba et al. [133] also described more recently a subpopulation of GABAergic interneurons expressing enkephalin that innervate parvalbumin-positive interneurons and thus may contribute to the organization of rhythmic activities in the CA1 area. The peak of the intracellular theta recorded in the dendrites of pyramidal cells slightly lags the peak of the extracellular theta in the pyramidal cell layer [134].

An important new finding [135] that further emphasizes the role of interneurons in the generation of hippocampal theta was obtained using transgenic mice where the fast synaptic GABAergic inhibition was removed from parvalbumin-positive interneurons. In CA1, these interneurons comprise bistratified and possibly oriens-lacunosum moleculare cells that target dendrites, basket cells that target somata, and axo-axonic cells [136]. Each of the perisomatic inhibitory parvalbumin-positive cells innervates more than 1,000 pyramidal cells [137] and causes IPSPs in the pyramidal cell layer. Via synaptic GABA$_A$ receptors, parvalbumin-positive basket cells reciprocally inhibit each other and receive inhibition from the medial septum and other local interneurons. Two groups, [135,138], found that this interneuron-specific ablation of the inhibitory septo-hippocampal projection can severely impair theta rhythm in the hippocampus. This study implies that the intrahippocampal systems of inhibition of parvalbumin-positive cells contribute to theta generation.

From all these data it emerges that to understand theta generation in the hippocampus and associated areas we must integrate single neuronal data with knowledge of local networks, their local synaptic wiring, and the corresponding dynamic properties. In other words, it is most useful to make explicit computational models [139] including networks of different types of interneurons as discussed in Chapter 3, as well as pyramidal neurons and granule cells; the latter should be simulated using compartmental models to account for the spatial distribution of specific inputs to dendrites and somata.

4.5. Alpha Rhythms

This section summarizes the few elements currently known about the mechanism(s) and origin(s) of alpha rhythm occurring in the frequency range of 8 to 13 Hz, mainly around 10 Hz. Its initial description [140] also marked the beginning of EEG. A more recent and exhaustive review of different EEG patterns of alpha rhythms in the waking adult can be found in Niedermeyer [141]. Besides the classic alpha rhythm of the visual cortex, there are rhythmic activities in the same frequency range that can be recorded from the somatosensory cortex (called the mu rhythm) and the temporal cortex (called the tau rhythm). Occipital alpha waves usually occur during reduced visual attention, while the mu rhythms of the sensorimotor cortex occur as the subject is in a state of muscular relaxation. In this way, the presence of dominant activity within the alpha frequency range has been interpreted, since Adrian and Matthews [142], as indicating an "idling state" of the brain, although paradoxical findings with alpha enhancement by attention tasks [143,144] were reported. These observations are now well understood since a number of findings, both of visual alpha and sensorimotor mu rhythms, have shown that enhancement and attenuation of these rhythmic activities can be recorded simultaneously at different sites and successively depending on a given task. This can be explained taking into consideration the interaction between different thalamocortical modules as explained in Chapter 40. In this respect, the experimental findings by Rihs et al. [145,146] showing enhancement of occipital alpha associated with active suppression of unattended positions during a visual spatial orienting task provide further evidence for the facilitating role of alpha-power decreases (event-related alpha desynchronization [ERD]) versus the inhibitory role of alpha-power enhancement (event-related alpha synchronization [ERS]) of attentional processes.

With few exceptions, the study of the cellular behavior underlying alpha oscillations was prevented mainly by the fact that alpha rhythms appear only during wakefulness and no valid anesthesia model was established. The fact that the alpha frequency band overlaps with another EEG phenomenon, the sleep spindles (or sigma rhythms, see next section) led to a legitimate although failed attempt to study it under barbiturate anesthesia [147]. Thus, most of our present knowledge is based on scalp recordings in humans and laminar profiles of cortical field potentials in animals.

4.6. Alpha Waves: Cortical Dipolar Sources and Thalamic Influences

In a series of experimental studies performed on dogs, Lopes da Silva et al. established that alpha rhythms are the undertaking of the cerebral cortex, mostly in the visual areas, although they can also be recorded in the visual thalamus (lateral geniculate and pulvinar nuclei) [148]. In the visual cortex, alpha waves are generated by an equivalent dipole layer centered at the level of the somata and basal dendrites of pyramidal neurons in layers IV and V (Fig. 2.14A) [149,150]. Furthermore, the coherence of alpha waves within the visual cortex was only partially dependent on thalamic sources measured in the same animal (see Fig. 2.14B) [150,151], leading to the conclusion that horizontal intracortical linkages are essential for the spread of alpha activities, with only moderate implication of the thalamus.

The cortical generator of alpha rhythms was confirmed and its functional properties were further analyzed in recent studies performed in awake monkeys, using fine microelectrode arrays implanted across the visual cortical areas V2 and V4 and the inferior temporal cortex by Bollimunta et al. [152] (Fig. 2.15). CSD analysis was combined with CSD-MUA coherence to identify intracortical alpha current generators. In V2 and V4, alpha current generators were found in all layers, with the infragranular neurons (layer V) acting as primary local generator. In contrast, in the inferior temporal cortex, alpha current generators were found in supragranular and infragranular layers, with the supragranular generator acting as the primary local generator. Granger causality analysis (see Chapter 44 for a definition) revealed that the influence of the infragranular on the supragranular cells had both a direct component as well as a component mediated by the granular layer cells. The analysis of the coherence between CSD sinks and local MUA in infragranular and granular layers showed that these cells are depolarized and tend to generate action potentials during the local current sinks; however, at the supragranular layer the coherence between CSD sinks and MUA was poor, suggesting that the cells of this layer are inhibited, possibly due to inhibitory inputs from layer V interneurons that innervate superficial pyramidal cells.

These properties were reanalyzed also in the awake monkey in more detail by van Kerkoerle et al. [153], who made CSD analyses and recorded MUA in primary visual area V1 during spontaneous activity. Applying measures of estimation of Granger causality, these authors reported that alpha waves are initiated in infragranular layer V, but also in supragranular layers I and II; alpha activity both from layer V and from layers I and II showed phase advance with respect to activity in layer IV, as illustrated in Figure 2.16. A study also using CSD and MUA in awake monkey described alpha current generators in the supragranular, granular, and infragranular layers [154]. These authors found that alpha LFP power was the strongest in the infragranular layers, while the CSD power was larger in the supragranular layers. These findings were not exclusive to the visual cortex but were also encountered in the somatomotor and auditory cortices. This is in line with the results of van Kerkoerle et al. [153], who also reported the strongest alpha LFP power in deep layers.

It is likely that previous findings [149] in visual cortex of dogs locating alpha generators predominantly in layer V may have been biased since these experiments were carried out with much less fine recording techniques, namely with a bundle of seven intracortical electrodes with inter-electrode distance of 200 μm, as compared to the array of 14 multielectrodes [154], or 23 or 24 multielectrodes [153], with 100-μm spacing. Nonetheless the dog's depth profile of alpha rhythms showed a 180-degree phase shift at about 1100 μm below the cortical surface, as determined with phase spectral analysis. It was then concluded that an alpha generator exists at the level

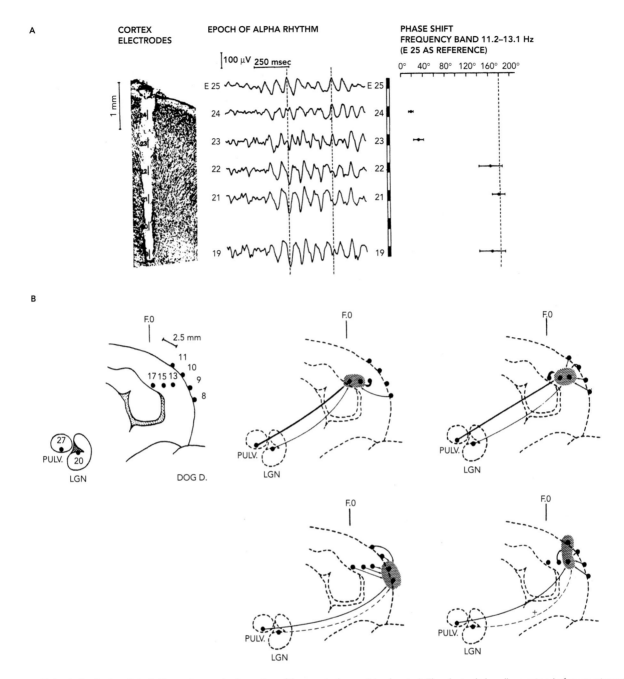

Figure 2.14. Alpha rhythm in dog. **A:** Left: Photomicrograph of a section of the marginal gyrus (visual cortex). The electrode bundle consisted of seven wires with a bare tip of 0.15 mm. Middle: An epoch of alpha activity recorded simultaneously from six sites corresponding to those at left, against a common frontal cranial reference (negativity upward). Note that there is a polarity change between the most superficial sites (E25, 24) and the deepest sites (E22, 21, 19). Right: Phase shift between the most superficial site (E25) and deeper-lying sites computed by using spectral analysis based on the average of a number of epochs within the frequency band 11.2–13.1 Hz. The mean values of the phase shift and the corresponding standard deviations are indicated. **B:** Schematic view of the relationship between thalamic and cortical alpha activity. The lines indicate the amount of influence that a thalamic signal has on the coherence between a pair of cortical signals (shaded area) recorded during alpha activity. This was measured by partializing the intercortical coherence on the thalamic signals from the lateral geniculate nucleus (LGN) and pulvinar (PULV) or other cortical signals. Even though PULV has an influence on cortico-cortical domains of alpha activity, the intercortical factors play a significant role in establishing cortical domains of alpha activity. (**A:** Modified from Lopes da Silva and Storm Van Leeuwen, 1977. **B:** Modified with permission from Lopes da Silva FH, Vos JE, Mooibroek J, van Rotterdam A. Relative contributions of intracortical and thalamo-cortical processes in the generation of alpha rhythms, revealed by partial coherence analysis. Electroencephalogr Clin Neurophysiol. 1980;50:449–456.)

of cortical layer V. In this early study it was noted, however, that this intracortical phase inversion may not yield sufficiently robust information concerning the exact location of the corresponding neuronal generators, due to the fact that different LFP sources with different spatiotemporal characteristics may coexist within the same cortical column. Interestingly, Haegens et al. noted that the intracortical distribution of alpha

generators may indicate that the sinks in the supragranular layers reflect synaptic inputs on the apical dendrites of layer V pyramidal cells, whereas the infragranular sinks would correspond to basal dendritic synaptic inputs [154]. For the interpretation of these rather complex findings a computational study, also discussed in Chapter 3, is particularly relevant because it integrates physiological data obtained using optogenetics

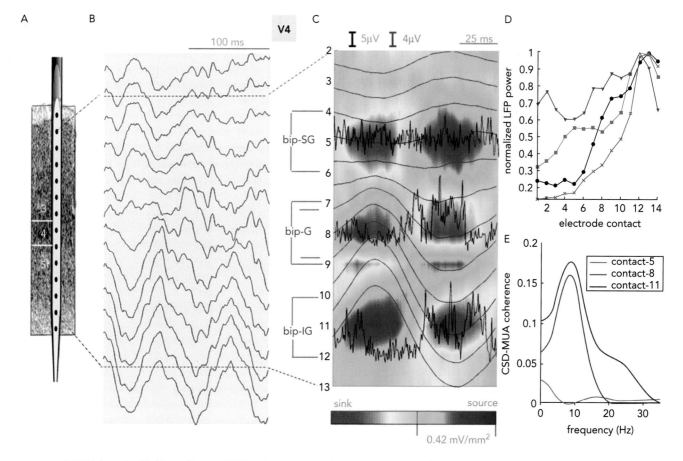

Figure 2.15. **A:** Multielectrode with 14 equally spaced (200 μm) contacts. **B:** A short segment (200 ms) of alpha rhythm. **C:** CSD displayed as a color-coded plot, with sinks in red and sources in blue. **D:** Spectra profiles shown for three sites. **E:** Coherence between CSD and MUA showing high coherence for the granular and infragranular layers, and in contrast with the superficial layer. (Modified with permission from Bollimunta A, Chen Y, Schroeder CE, Ding M. Neuronal mechanisms of cortical alpha oscillations in awake-behaving macaques. J Neurosci. 2008;28:9976–9988.)

and structural information about the main cortical neuronal populations [155]. A particularly interesting prediction of the model regarding the generation of alpha oscillations is that for alpha (peak at about 8 Hz) to be generated, neocortical Low

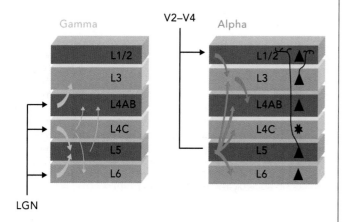

Figure 2.16. Schematic representation of Granger causality between layers for the γ- (left) and α-band (right). Thick arrows indicate Granger causality stronger than 0.015; thin arrows for the γ-band indicate Granger causality between 0.005 and 0.015 (not shown for the α-band to prevent crowding). (Modified with permission from van Kerkoerle T, Self MW, Dagnino B, et al. Alpha and gamma oscillations characterize feedback and feedforward processing in monkey visual cortex. Proc Natl Acad Sci USA 2014;111:14332–14341.)

Threshold Spiking (LTS) cells are necessary. In this model the thalamic input may drive LTS cells with cell bodies in non-granular layers, which would work as amplifiers of thalamic inputs at frequencies in the alpha band. Remarkably, during inattentive states, characterized by a low level of cholinergic activity, the thalamic alpha is dominant (synchronized state), which would lead to enhancement of LTS activity and of corti-cal alpha. On the contrary, during attentive states, with a high level of cholinergic activity, thalamic alpha drive input to the cortex decreases (desynchronized state, see also [156]) while LTS neurons are depolarized by nicotinic cholinergic recep-tors and tend to be asynchronously active. This may favor that the drive from fast-spiking (FS) cells on pyramidal cells may enhance gamma oscillations, depending on $GABA_A$ phasic inhibition.

Furthermore, Jones et al. [157] proposed a biophysi-cally based computational model to account for the specific properties of mu rhythm activities including alpha and beta frequency components as recorded from the primary somato-motor (S1) cortex using MEG. The model comprises a cortical network with distinct layers, excitatory and inhibitory neu-rons; feedforward connections represent the thalamic drive, and feedback ones represent cortical drive and inputs from non-lemniscal thalamic inputs. In this model mu rhythm is considered to arise from the combination of two stochastic signals, at the dominant frequency of about 10 Hz, that project to different cortical layers corresponding to thalamic feedforward and intracortical feedback inputs. In this model the main time constants characteristic of the mu rhythm were determined by the strength and timing of the exogenous rhythmic inputs and not by intrinsic cortical neuronal properties. This model approach would be more relevant if specific information about the activities of the thalamo-cortico-thalamic loops were taken into account.

The relationship between alpha and faster (mainly gamma) oscillations will be discussed later, after we introduce the cellular mechanisms of the latter rhythms.

4.7. Alpha Waves: Synaptic Processes Studied In Vitro

The nature of the synaptic processes underlying alpha frequency oscillations in the cortex was studied in *in vitro* preparations, although it is always a matter of discussion whether *in vitro* preparations that undergo pharmacological manipulations and display these kinds of oscillations provide reliable models of the situation in the intact brain, where the neurons are in different physiological conditions. Nonetheless, Flint and Connors [158] were able to obtain oscillations in the alpha frequency range when slices of rat somatosensory cortex were activated by low extracellular magnesium *in vitro*. These oscillations were N-methyl-D-aspartate (NMDA)-dependent since they were reversibly abolished by the NMDA receptor antagonist D-2-amino-5-phosphonovaleric acid (AP-5) but were relatively unaffected by the non-NMDA receptor antagonist 6,7-dinitroquinoxaline-2,3-dione (DNQX). This is in line with the results obtained *in vivo* by van Kerkoerle et al. [153] presented above. The duration of oscillatory events was increased by blocking $GABA_A$ receptors with bicuculline or by activating metabotropic glutamate receptors with trans-1-aminocyclopentane-1,3-dicarboxylic acid (trans-ACPD).

A similar kind of study, in slices of cat lateral geniculate nucleus maintained *in vitro* [159], showed that activation of the metabotropic glutamate receptors mGluR1a, which are postsynaptic to corticothalamic fibers, induces synchronized oscillations at alpha and theta frequencies in a subset of thalamocortical neurons that can be synchronized by gap junctions. The frequency of the oscillations, whether alpha (8–13 Hz) or theta (2–7 Hz), depended on the concentration of the agonist trans-ACPD. These oscillations are driven by a subset (~25%) of lateral geniculate thalamocortical neurons displaying high threshold burst activity occurring at membrane potentials more depolarized than −55 mV, which depends on Ni^{2+}-sensitive Ca^{2+} channels. In these *in vitro* conditions the alpha/theta oscillations do not appear to require chemical synapses because they can be sustained by coupling through gap junctions between thalamocortical neurons. These *in vitro* results suggest that activation of mGluRs of corticothalamic synapses may be an important mechanism for generating EEG alpha and theta activity but, as stated above, one should keep in mind that the mechanisms underlying oscillations in the alpha frequency range elicited in this kind of *in vitro* conditions may differ from those responsible for alpha rhythm generation in the intact brain. A comprehensive review of the basic findings with respect to the generation and organization of alpha rhythms, both *in vivo* and *in vitro*, can be found in Hughes and Crunelli [160].

Remarkably, in the last years interesting additional findings have enriched our understanding of how alpha rhythms are generated and posed some new challenges for further research. Lörincz et al. [161] confirmed in cat slices of the lateral geniculate nucleus and ventro-basal complex (somatosensory thalamus) that a sparse network of high threshold bursting thalamocortical cells coupled through gap junctions is capable of generating alpha rhythm activity. They also found that this activity can be induced in this preparation by administering a cholinergic agonist and can be abolished by muscarinic M3 receptor antagonists. However, this was evident in only about 26% of the thalamocortical cells. This raises the question of what happens in the remaining majority of thalamocortical cells. These authors suggest that the remaining cells are probably under phasic inhibition from local interneurons activated by the bursting thalamocortical cells. It remains unclear how these different neuronal populations behave in the intact brain where thalamocortical cells receive several important inputs from the cortex, reticular nucleus (RE) of the thalamus, and several brainstem sources that use various neurotransmitters in addition to acetylcholine, particularly serotonin, noradrenaline, and histamine that are mainly released during the waking state but not during REM sleep [162]. An important input to these thalamic nuclei is constituted by the cholinergic fibers that arise from brainstem and basal forebrain nuclear groups. It has been shown that cholinergic inputs are excitatory to thalamocortical cells, causing a direct depolarization associated with a decrease of a K^+ current; at the same time there is a decrease of the inhibitory input arising from the thalamic RE neurons, since the latter are hyperpolarized by cholinergic activation of a K^+ conductance, as was shown *in vitro* in guinea pig [163] and *in vivo* in cat [164,165]. In this way these cholinergic inputs favor the blockage of rhythmic spindles, a phenomenon that is generated in the thalamus and shares the same frequency range with alpha oscillations (see below). It is possible that the major effect of cholinergic inputs on thalamic oscillations *in vivo* may be to induce their blockage through muscarinic inhibition of thalamic RE neurons, although subtler effects appear to exist in some thalamic subpopulations, but the relevance of these effects for alpha oscillatory activity is not yet clear. These recent findings provide new insights, but it is evident that more research in *in vivo* conditions is necessary to achieve a deeper understanding of the mechanisms responsible for the generation of alpha oscillations of different kinds in the thalamocortical systems, including not only the lateral geniculate nucleus and ventrobasal complex [161] but also the pulvinar [151,166] and, of course, several cortical areas.

5. SPINDLE (SIGMA) RHYTHMS

Classically, spindles have been regarded as one of the first signs of EEG synchronization during the early stage of quiescent sleep. This type of oscillation is defined by the presence of two distinct rhythms: waxing and waning spindle waves at 7 to 14 Hz within sequences lasting for 1 to 2 seconds, and the periodic recurrence of spindle sequences with a slow rhythm, generally 0.2 to 0.5 Hz (Fig. 2.17A). Spindles are generated within the thalamus because they survive in the thalamus after decortications and high brainstem transection [167]. More radical procedures, including complete removal of the striatum and rhinencephalon, do not affect thalamic spindles either [52]. Sleep spindles have been mostly studied in cats (in vivo) and ferrets (in vitro). Humans and cats have similar sleep cycles, EEG patterns, and ultrastructural organization of their thalamus. Both intrinsic properties of various thalamic neurons

[168] and network linkages (for review, see [169]) contribute to the patterning of spindles.

As indicated above, the thalamic circuits comprise two main structures: (1) the dorsal thalamus, made up of several nuclei, each of them containing both relay (thalamocortical) and local circuit (inter-) neurons, and (2) the RE nucleus of the thalamus (see scheme in Fig. 2.17A). The latter is a thin sheet of GABAergic neurons that covers the rostral, lateral, and ventral surfaces of the thalamus [170]. It receives inputs mainly from the cerebral cortex and dorsal thalamus, but also from the rostral sector of the brainstem and basal forebrain. The RE-thalamic-cortical-RE loop constitutes a resonating circuit that reinforces the spindle

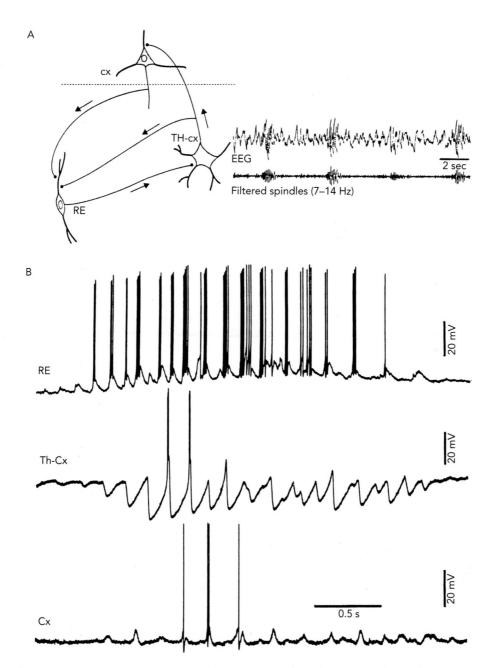

Figure 2.17. Spindle oscillations in reticular thalamic (RE), thalamocortical (Th-Cx, ventrolateral nucleus), and cortical (Cx, motor area) neurons. A: Circuit of three neuronal types and two rhythms (7–14 Hz and 0.1–0.2 Hz) of spindle oscillations in cortical EEG. B: Intracellular recordings in cats under barbiturate anesthesia. (Modified with permission from Steriade M, Deschênes M. Intrathalamic and brainstem-thalamic networks involved in resting and alert states. In: Bentivoglio M, Spreafico R, eds. Cellular thalamic mechanisms. Amsterdam: Elsevier; 1988:51–76.)

oscillation. Moreover, spindles generated within the RE nucleus travel along the dorsal thalamic relay pathway en route to the cortex, which probably is responsible for the genesis of the dipole that allows them to surface in the EEG. Interestingly, no spindles are recorded in the EEG of kittens during the first 6 to 7 days of life, although they are already present in thalamic recordings 3 to 4 hours after birth [171], suggesting that no viable dipole is generated in the thalamus. The brainstem and basal forebrain projections exert activating effects on the above-mentioned circuit, with the result of inhibiting spindles.

The RE nucleus has been pointed out as the pacemaker for spindle oscillations because spindles were abolished in the dorsal thalamus after disconnection from the RE [172] but were preserved in the rostral part of the RE nucleus severed from the dorsal thalamus [173]. Further support is provided by the fact that, in cat anterior nucleus, which does not receive inputs from the RE nucleus [174,175], spindles are absent [176]. Similarly, spindles are absent in the cingular cortex [177] and habenular nuclei, other structures that are devoid of RE inputs. Modeling studies of isolated RE neurons, with minimal or more realistic ionic models of RE cells [178–180], further strengthened the idea that the deafferented RE nucleus is a spindle "pacemaker."

Spindle oscillations, to produce a coherent pattern at the level of the target structures, need to be synchronized at the very site of their genesis. Besides the axonal projections allowing obvious connectivity between RE neurons, two other mechanisms have been proposed. The first relies on the dendro-dendritic GABAergic contacts between RE neurons [181–183], the second on the functional interconnection of RE neurons through gap junctions [184].

A fundamental question concerns how a spindle is triggered. Steriade et al. [173] have assumed that any excitatory drive stimulating RE cells would elicit the process. The decreased activity of brainstem cholinergic neurons at the onset of sleep [91] contributes to the overall hyperpolarization of thalamocortical cells, thus bringing the membrane potential in the range where bursting discharges can occur. Such clusters of high-frequency action potentials would excite the dendrites of RE neurons and would trigger the dendro-dendritic avalanche leading to the final synchronization of the whole RE nucleus. It should be emphasized that thalamic-RE loops may assist the onset of a spindle, but its synchronization cannot rely on the dorsal thalamic circuitry because there is scarce, if any, communication between thalamocortical neurons within dorsal thalamic nuclei [174,185].

Once a spindle has been started through one of the mechanisms mentioned above, the pacing of the actual oscillations within the spindle sequence depends on the RE–thalamic dialogue. This was investigated in ferret thalamic visual slices containing geniculate and perigeniculate (reticular) nuclei [186–188] and with multisite recordings within the thalamus [189,190]. It results that the bursting of RE neurons imposes powerful GABAergic IPSP on thalamocortical neurons. The end of this inhibition triggers a rebound LTS, crowned by a high-frequency burst of action potentials, which in turn will excite again the target RE cells. This is also the moment where intrinsic properties of thalamic, both thalamocortical and RE, neurons play an important role. The amount of

hyperpolarization of the thalamocortical cells determines the degree of de-inactivation of the LTS [191]. Another intrinsic property of thalamic cells is the voltage-dependent, non-inactivating or very slowly inactivating, persistent sodium current, $I_{Na(p)}$ [191], which modulates postinhibitory rebound depolarizations. The blockage of the $I_{Na(p)}$ by intracellular injection of quaternary derivatives of local anesthetics transformed spindles of thalamocortical cells into a single, long-lasting period of hyperpolarization (because unopposed by $I_{Na(p)}$) without any rhythmic rebounds within the frequency range of spindles [192]. Finally, the calcium-dependent potassium current, $I_{K(Ca)}$, or other voltage-dependent potassium currents [193,194] may prolong the long-lasting IPSPs generated in thalamocortical neurons by RE neurons and thus assist in the production of the LTS and in inducing rebound bursts in thalamocortical targets.

In an intact sleeping brain, the RE-thalamic network undergoes periodic, synchronized excitatory inputs from the cortex such as K-complexes (see above), which then shape and modulate the duration of spindles [195]. Cortico-thalamic stimuli produce shorter and waning spindles that lack the initial waxing component, probably because the volleys entrained from the very beginning large populations of thalamic cells. Moreover, the synchronization of spindles in the thalamus was widespread, with virtual zero time lag, in intact preparations, but dropped drastically after decortications [56,190] (Fig. 2.18). This result stands in some contrast to a propagating pattern of spindles in thalamic slices [196], likely due to the absence of corticothalamic inputs of this preparation and to the overall diminished synaptic activity of the slice.

The main functional correlate of sleep spindles is the blockage of incoming stimuli on their way to the cortex. This could result from the fact that thalamocortical neurons alternate between IPSPs and LTS bursts. Both events preclude the relaying of afferent synaptic signals, due to either the shunting nature of the former or the all-or-none feature of the latter. The functional blockage of sensory transmission at the thalamic level promotes the cortical deafferentation, further contributing to the process of falling asleep.

A final observation concerns the overlapping frequency range of spindles and alpha waves. It should be emphasized that the behavioral context of both phenomena and mechanisms are dissimilar. Alpha waves generally occur during relaxed wakefulness and are currently considered to regulate information flow and temporal coding in the visual system [197], as well as top-down attentional modulation [198]. Quite differently, spindle oscillations occur during unconsciousness, thus making the idea of an alpha-to-spindle continuum obsolete. Nonetheless, the same basic neural circuitries can be involved in both kinds of oscillatory activities—sleep spindles and alpha rhythms—but working according to different functional modes.

6. FASTER (BETA, GAMMA) RHYTHMS

At the opposite side of the EEG spectrum of slow sleep rhythms (<15 Hz) are fast oscillations (generally 20–40 Hz) that are

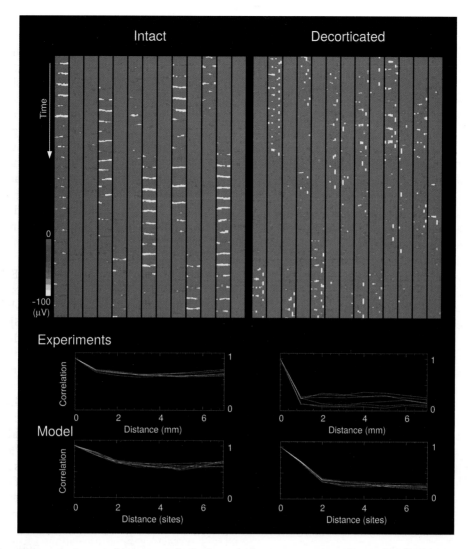

Figure 2.18. *Control of spatiotemporal coherence of thalamic spindles by the cerebral cortex in cat. Top panels: Disruption of the spatiotemporal coherence of thalamic oscillation after removal of the neocortex. Spatiotemporal maps of electrical activity across the thalamus were constructed by plotting time (time runs from top to bottom in each column; arrow indicates 1 second), space (from left to right, the width of each column represents 8 mm in the anteroposterior axis of the thalamus), and LFP voltage [from blue to yellow, color represents the amplitude of the negative deflection of thalamic LFPs; the color scale ranged in 10 steps from the baseline [blue] to 100 µV [yellow]). Time was divided into frames, each representing a snapshot of 4 ms of thalamic activity; a total of 40 s is represented (9,880 frames). Each frame consisted of eight color spots, each corresponding to the LFP of one electrode from anterior to posterior (left to right in each column). Middle panels (experiments): Decay of correlation with distance. Cross-correlations were computed for all possible pairs of thalamic sites, and the value at time zero from each correlation was represented as a function of the intersite distance for six different consecutive epochs of 20 s. Spatial correlation was calculated for thalamic recordings in the intact brain (left) and after removal of cortex (right). Bottom panel (model): Decay of correlation with distance (in units of sites). Similar computation of cross-correlations as in the above panel from experiments, in the presence of cortex (left) and after decortication (right). (Modified with permission from Contreras D, Destexhe A, Sejnowski TJ, Steriade M. Control of spatiotemporal coherence of a thalamic oscillation by corticothalamic feedback. Science 1996;274:771–774, and unpublished data by A. Destexhe, D. Contreras, T.J. Sejnowski and M. Steriade.)*

proper to vigilance states associated with wakefulness, but also paradoxical (REM) sleep. The brain substrate of EEG activation upon arousal has begun to be understood since the pioneering work of Moruzzi and Magoun [199]. They reported an "activation" response to the stimulation of brainstem structures consisting in the suppression of spindles and slower EEG rhythms. The cellular mechanisms of this suppressing mechanism have recently been analyzed: the blockage of spindles occurs at the very site of their genesis (the RE nucleus) through the action of acetylcholine, serotonin, and norepinephrine. Although acetylcholine hyperpolarizes GABAergic RE neurons [168,200], while serotonin and noradrenaline excite RE neurons [201], the combined action of these neurotransmitters is far from

being understood. The intrinsically generated thalamic delta oscillation is blocked through the depolarizing action of both acetylcholine [48] and monoamines [202] on thalamocortical cells. Finally, slow cortical delta activities are prevented by cholinergic actions of the nucleus basalis neurons [67,203].

6.1. Beta/Gamma Rhythms: Functional Implications

The disappearance of slow sleep waveforms during the activating response is also accompanied by the appearance of peculiar fast rhythms characterizing wakefulness [204]. Since this seminal paper several studies mentioned the presence of 20- to 40-Hz waves in various cortical areas, during different conditions of increased alertness. For instance, fast rhythms in the beta frequency range, with a spectral peak at about 18 or 26 to 27 Hz, depending on the cortical area with a relatively narrow spectral bandwidth, were observed in a canine subject in the occipital cortex while the dog paid intense attention to a visual stimulus [205], in the cortex of monkey during accurate performance of a conditioned response to a visual stimulus [206], and during tasks requiring fine finger movements and focused attention in monkey motor cortical cells [207]. Similar beta activity was observed as well during behavioral immobility associated with an enhanced level of vigilance while a cat was watching a visible but unseizable mouse [208]. Other studies have described stimulus-dependent oscillations in the frequency range of 25 to 45 Hz of the focal EEG and/or neuronal firing in the olfactory system [209] and visual cortex [210–214].

The underlying mechanism responsible for cortical gamma oscillations was furthered by demonstrating that synchronized gamma frequency oscillations are generated by the activation of acetylcholine muscarinic receptors, enhanced with arousal and attention [215], and also by electrical stimulation of the mesencephalic reticular formation [216].

The main functional implication of these rhythms in the cortex was proposed to rely on the degree of spatial and temporal synchronization, thus allowing, at a given moment, the aggregation of various cortical areas with the purpose of creating global and coherent properties of neuronal patterns, a prerequisite for scene segmentation and figure–ground distinction [217]. The issue of this "feature binding" has, however, been toned down by the fact that such fast rhythms are coherent also within thalamocortical and cortical networks during states such as sleep and deep anesthesia noted for the absence of any conscious behavior [57,218,219]. These studies established that thalamocortical cells do spontaneously oscillate within the beta-gamma frequency range and this occurs coherently with field potentials recorded from the related cortical areas (Fig. 2.19).

On the face of these findings we must conclude that there exist different kinds of beta/gamma rhythms with different properties and behavioral/cognitive associations. Since the report by Gray and Singer [211] that the firing probability of neurons of the visual cortex of the cat, in response to the presentation of appropriate visual stimuli, oscillates with a frequency in the gamma-frequency range, along with the observation that no evidence for similar oscillations was found in the thalamus, these gamma oscillations are considered to be generated intracortically. This observation led to the assumption that these gamma oscillations may reflect a general mechanism that is capable of binding together activities of spatially separate cortical areas [220]. In general, we may state that synchronization of neuronal networks by way of common oscillations in the gamma frequency range may enable fast routing and processing of information in the cortex [221]. In this context the current concept is that gamma-band synchronous oscillations can activate postsynaptic neuronal populations effectively, as would occur in systems recruited by selective attention, in order to promote a precise communication between the involved neuronal populations [222].

6.2. Genesis of Beta/Gamma Rhythms

The genesis of fast (beta-gamma) activities lies at the crossroads of intrinsic and network properties. Cortical neurons generate, upon depolarization, intrinsic oscillations in a range around 40 Hz [223,224]. This is equally valid for a subclass of rostral intralaminar thalamic neurons [225] (Fig. 2.20), a property that is in line with their implication in fast oscillations during activated states associated with neuronal depolarizations, waking, and REM sleep. Intralaminar nuclei are particularly fit for wide-range synchronization due to their widespread projections to the cerebral cortex [226], including the visual areas [227].

Despite these intrinsic properties that make neurons prone to generate fast oscillations, their imbedding in complex circuits, especially in the cortex, is required for the short- and long-range synchronization, in order to make the rhythm emerge at the EEG level. As examples of different kinds of circuits that may engage fast rhythmic activities we may mention the following two findings: (1) Freeman [209] postulated that the generation of 40- to 80-Hz activity in the olfactory bulb depends on feedback inhibitory circuits involving local circuit GABAergic neurons acting on output elements, the mitral cell, and (2) Chagnac-Amitai and Connors [228] showed that rat somatosensory slices with slightly reduced inhibition display activities around 37 Hz generated by networks of intrinsically pyramidal (excitatory) cells.

With respect to the cortical neuronal sources of gamma oscillations, initial studies pointed out the existence of several intracortical distributed microsinks and microsources as shown by CSD analyses [218]. Using laminar electrodes spanning the cortical depth with electrode contacts spaced 100 μm apart in the cortex of the awake monkey, van Kerkoerle et al. [153] revealed gamma oscillations (40–90 Hz) with largest power in layer III, while alpha oscillations were larger in layer V/VI. A CSD analysis showed that a cycle of gamma oscillation started with sinks in layer IV (i.e., the layer that receives thalamic feedforward inputs) and that the sinks propagated both to superficial (delay of 2 ms) and to deep (delay of 1 ms) cortical layers; layer IV sinks coincided with local spiking as measured by recording MUA. Estimation of Granger causality for gamma oscillations revealed the pattern shown in Figure 2.16: there was a strong directionality from layer IV to layer III and to layers V and VI.

Fast (beta-gamma) oscillations are mainly associated with increased levels of alertness, thus closely following the onset of activity in cholinergic aggregates of the brainstem and basal forebrain. The cholinergic activation induces a twofold increase of cortical EEG waves around 40 Hz, a potentiating effect that is mediated by muscarinic receptors as it is blocked by scopolamine [225]. Beyond the depolarizing effect exerted by acetylcholine on thalamocortical and cortical neurons, this neurotransmitter hyperpolarizes a subpopulation of cortical glial cells maintained in culture [229]. When tested *in vivo*, acetylcholine hyperpolarized most of the glial cells (Fig. 2.21), in parallel with an overall decrease in the extracellular potassium concentration [230] (see also next section). This effect was also accompanied by an increased cerebral blood flow,

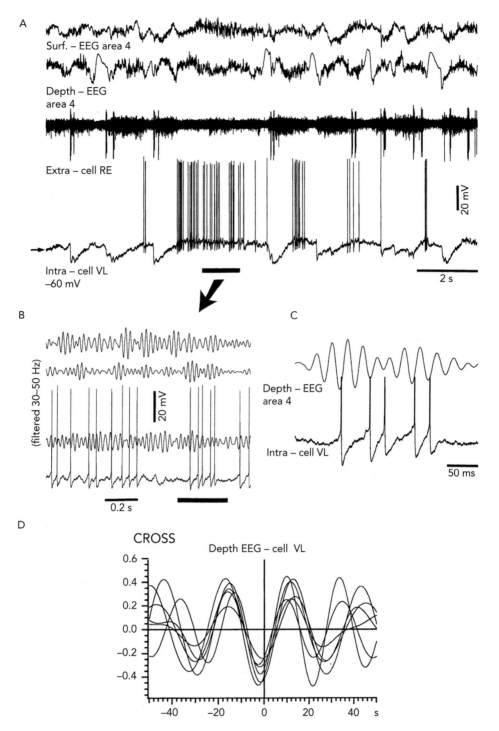

*Figure 2.19. Episodes of tonic activation are associated with coherent fast rhythms (40 Hz) in cortical EEG and intracellularly recorded thalamocortical neuron. Cat under ketamine-xylazine anesthesia. **A:** Four traces represent simultaneous recordings of surface and depth EEG from motor cortical area 4, extracellular discharges of neuron from the rostrolateral part of the thalamic reticular (RE) nucleus, and intracellular activity of thalamocortical neuron from ventrolateral (VL) nucleus. EEG, RE, and VL cells displayed a slow oscillation (0.7–0.8 Hz) during which the sharp depth-negative (excitatory) EEG waves led to IPSPs in VL cell, presumably generated by spike bursts in a cortically driven GABAergic RE neuron. Part marked by horizontal bar, taken from a short-lasting period of spontaneous EEG activation, is expanded in **B** (arrow), with EEG waves and field potentials from the RE nucleus filtered between 30 and 50 Hz; part marked by horizontal bar in this panel is further expanded in **C** to illustrate relations between action potentials of VL cell and depth-negative waves in cortical EEG at a frequency of 40 Hz. **D:** Cross-correlations (CROSS) between action potentials and depth-EEG shows clear-cut relation, with opposition of phase, between intracellularly recorded VL neuron and EEG waves. (Modified with permission from Steriade M, Amzica F, Contreras D. Synchronization of fast (30–40 Hz) spontaneous cortical rhythms during brain activation. J Neurosci. 1996;16:392–417.)*

leading to the interpretation that the glial hyperpolarization is due to a boosted transport of potassium across capillary membranes. This is further supported by the fact that EEG activation, when recorded with DC amplifiers, generally displays a persistent positive DC shift [230]. In addition, brain activation was accompanied in glial cells by a reduced membrane capacitance, suggesting that the interglial syncytium shuts down during wakefulness, preventing nonspecific synchronization

A   B (spontaneous)

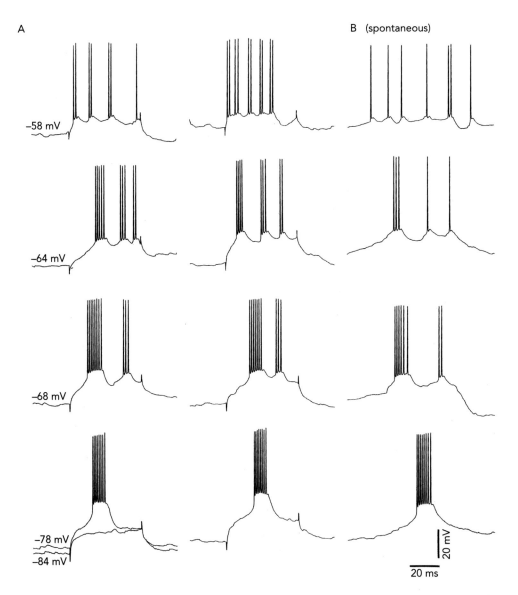

Figure 2.20. Fast oscillatory patterns of neuron recorded from the dorsolateral part of the centrolateral (CL) intralaminar thalamic nucleus, characterized by exceedingly high-frequency (800–1,000 Hz) spike bursts recurring rhythmically at 50 to 60 Hz. Intracellular recording in cat under barbiturate anesthesia. **A:** Activities triggered by depolarizing current pulses (+1.2 nA, 50 ms) at different levels of membrane potential (as indicated at left). Two examples are illustrated for each membrane potential level. At bottom, presence of LTS leading to high-frequency (800–1,000 Hz) spike burst at −78 mV and its absence at −84 mV. Note fast-recurring (50–60 Hz) spike doublets or spike triplets at relatively depolarized levels (−64 mV and −58 mV), a feature that is not seen in other types of thalamocortical neurons. **B:** Oscillatory patterns similar to those elicited by current injection occurred spontaneously at similar membrane potentials (from top to bottom, −58, −64, −68, and −78 mV). (Modified with permission from Steriade M, Curró Dossi R, Contreras D. Electrophysiological properties of intralaminar thalamocortical cells discharging rhythmic (approximately 40 Hz) spike-bursts at approximately 1000 Hz during waking and rapid eye movement sleep. Neuroscience 1993;56:1–9.)

through spatial buffering mechanisms (as mentioned previously). This feature may thus leave the synchronization of beta-gamma activities strictly confined to synaptic networks, achieving a more specific aggregation of the neuronal populations involved.

Recent studies in cortical slices revealed particularly interesting properties with respect to the cellular generators of gamma and beta rhythm activities. Roopun et al. [231] showed that gamma (30–70 Hz) rhythms could be generated in the superficial somatosensory cortical layers II/III, while beta rhythms (20–30 Hz) were generated in deep layer V mainly associated with the activity of FS interneurons, when kainate was applied to the slices. It is interesting to note that in

layer IV both activities may coexist (Fig. 2.22). A remarkable difference in the physiological mechanisms underlying these two types of cortical oscillations is that the beta rhythms of the deep layers are reduced by carbenoxolone, which blocks gap junction conductances, but are not affected by the blockade of synaptic transmission. In contrast, gamma rhythms in superficial layers are reduced by the blockade of chemical synaptic transmission. The fact that gamma and beta oscillations rely on different mechanisms is further emphasized in experiments with transverse cuts within the somatosensory cortical slices that completely separate layers I-II from layers V-VI. The gamma rhythm activity of the superficial layers and the beta rhythm activity of the deep layers survived the cut,

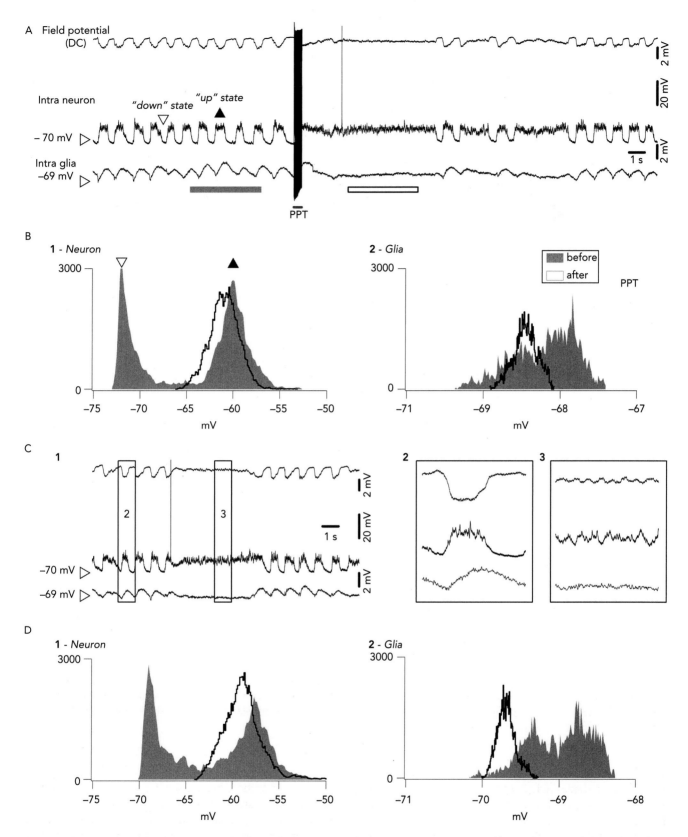

Figure 2.21. Comparison between electrically elicited and spontaneously occurring activation in a pair of simultaneously impaled neuron and glia in a cat under ketamine–xylazine anesthesia. **A**: Sequence of slow (<1 Hz) oscillation, brainstem cholinergic activation, and return to slow oscillation. Depolarizing phases of the slow oscillation are indicated with a black arrowhead (up state), while hyperpolarizing phases are marked with an empty arrowhead (down state). After activation, the sustained neuronal depolarization is accompanied by glial hyperpolarization and the DC field potential assumes rather positive values. **B**: Histograms of neuronal (panel 1) and glial (panel 2) V_m during the slow oscillation (in gray) and during activation (black trace). Histograms were calculated over the respective underlined epochs in **A**. They illustrate the incidence of different values of V_m, sampled at 20 kHz, over periods indicated by bar below traces. Note the bimodal histograms during sleep (up states correspond to the black arrowhead, down states to the empty arrowhead) and the unimodal histogram after activation, as well as the opposite evolution of glial and neuronal V_m (glia hyperpolarizes, neuron depolarizes). **C**: Similar pattern of activity in the same double intracellular recording during a period of spontaneous activation of the EEG (panel 1). Periods within rectangles are expanded at right (panels 2 and 3). **D**: Histograms from equivalent time periods before and after activation. (Modified with permission from Seigneur J, Kroeger D, Nita DA, Amzica F. Cholinergic action on cortical glial cells in vivo. Cereb Cortex 2006;16:655–668.)

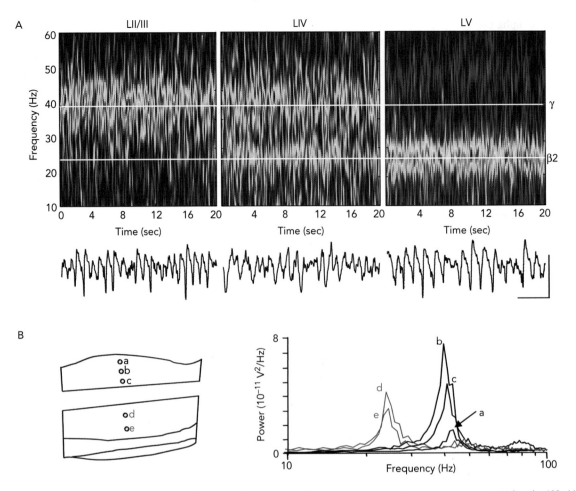

Figure 2.22. Beta2 rhythms are generated in deep layers of cortex. **A:** Spectrograms of field rhythms generated in somatosensory cortex slices by 400 nM kainate. Superficial layers generated gamma frequency (30–50 Hz) signals (layer II/III). Deep layers concurrently generated beta2 frequency signals (layer V, 20–30 Hz). Layer IV recordings show both frequency bands coexisting. Below each spectrogram are representative field potential traces (scale bars: 0.2 mV, 100 ms). **B:** Surgical separation of deep from superficial layers at the layer IV/V border abolished neither rhythm. Cartoon illustrates the electrode position for the power spectra taken from 60-s epochs of field potential data in the superficial layers (a–c, black lines) and deep layers (d and e, red lines). (Modified with permission from Roopun AK, Middleton SJ, Cunningham MO, et al. A beta2-frequency (20–30 Hz) oscillation in nonsynaptic networks of somatosensory cortex. Proc Natl Acad Sci USA 2006;103:15646–15650.)

showing that they can be maintained separately. The two kinds of rhythms also respond differently to pharmacological agents. While the blockage of GABA$_A$ receptors in these slices abolished gamma rhythms, it enhanced beta rhythms. This means that gamma oscillations depend on the discharge of pyramidal cells coupled to GABA-mediated local inhibitory circuits. We should emphasize, however, that demonstrations of these kinds of properties *in vitro* are not a guarantee that precisely the same mechanisms are also essential *in vivo*. Nonetheless, *in vitro* studies such as this one yield a proof-of-principle that such mechanisms can be operational in the cortex.

It was reported in the rat *in vivo* that benzodiazepines, which enhance GABA$_A$ receptor-mediated synaptic transmission, also increased beta oscillations in the EEG. In this sense, Mandema and Danhof [232] reviewed data showing that changes in the EEG spectral amplitude within the beta frequency band provide a remarkable quantitative indicator of the pharmacological effect of benzodiazepines. In addition to the classic beta and gamma oscillations, episodes of oscillations at high frequency (100–600 Hz) and short duration

(~50–100 ms) have been described in the brain of rodents and human, under both normal and epileptic conditions. These HFOs include the so-called *ripples* (see Fig. 2.15) or *fast ripples*, which are discussed in detail in Chapter 33; computational models of neuronal mechanisms responsible for these HFOs are presented in Chapter 3.

6.3. Relationship Between Alpha and Gamma Oscillations

In this section we will ask three central questions.

The first question is this: What is the distribution and interaction of alpha and gamma oscillations in the cortex? This was explicitly investigated in the cortex of the monkey using laminar LFP recordings to analyze simultaneously activities from the different cortical layers [233]. A conspicuous finding was the layer-specific entrainment of power of gamma oscillations (30–200 Hz), recorded mainly from superficial layers, by the phase of alpha waves (8–10 Hz) in infragranular deep layers. The amplitude of gamma oscillations was inversely related to the amplitude of alpha oscillations. A CSD analysis showed a consistent laminar pattern of sinks and sources of the alpha and gamma oscillations consisting of a low-frequency sink in the granular layer and a source immediately below during a burst of gamma oscillations. The burst was preceded, and followed, by the presence of sinks in infragranular layers, accompanied by sources in the granular layer. This can be interpreted as follows: alpha oscillations in deep layers modulate gamma oscillations in superficial layers by way of an intracortical pathway, since layer V pyramidal cells project to interneurons in the same layer that project to the superficial layers.

It is important to consider in some detail the main features of the intracortical networks that mediate the interactions described above. A major role is played by different kinds of interneurons [234]: in layer V the main classes of GABAergic interneurons are (1) the FS parvalbumin-positive cells, including basket cells, and (2) the LTS cells, which may express different neuropeptides alone or in combination (CCK, VIP, SST). These different classes of interneurons have distinct axonal arborizations: those of LTS are vertically oriented (intracolumnar) and make synaptic contact along the dendrites of pyramidal cells; FS are horizontally oriented (intercolumnar) and make synaptic contacts with the soma and axonal hillock of pyramidal cells. Particularly interesting is that these interneurons receive a diversity of subcortical inputs containing several kinds of neuromodulators. In this respect cholinergic inputs are especially important since these control the FS and LTS interneurons in opposite directions: while acetylcholine (Ach) depolarizes LTS cells through nicotinic receptors, it hyperpolarizes FS interneurons through muscarinic receptors. Thus the activation of cholinergic inputs by inhibiting FS-GABAergic and exciting LTS-GABAergic cells will result in the enhancement of intercolumnar excitation by freeing pyramidal cells from the inhibitory influence of FS cells, while suppressing intracolumnar excitation by activating LTS-mediated inhibition. In this way the information flow in cortical networks can be controlled by cholinergic modulation, constituting what Bacci et al. [234] appealingly called the "cholinergic switch." This functional feature is likely relevant for the powerful influence of Ach in controlling cortical oscillations. Indeed, cholinergic activation induces gamma oscillations in the cortex [67], while it reduces alpha oscillations in thalamus and cortex [156,162,235]. There are, in addition, several other kinds of interneurons and modulating neurotransmitters in the cortex that may also be relevant to these processes, but the mechanisms of action are still insufficiently known.

The second question is this: How do alpha and gamma oscillations propagate along cortical areas? A further study of cortical oscillations in both alpha and gamma frequency bands in the awake monkey focused on the interactions between cortical areas, namely visual cortex V1 and V4, and between different layers within V1 [153]. These authors revealed that alpha waves initiated in layer V and propagated to deep and to more superficial layers in opposite direction with respect to gamma waves. In addition, blocking NMDA receptors suppressed alpha oscillations while enhancing gamma, demonstrating that NMDA receptors are important for the generation of alpha oscillations. It appears that alpha oscillations originate in layer V, but there are also generators in layers I and II; in both deep (V and VI) and superficial (I–III) layers, alpha activity showed a phase advance in relation to layer IV. The opposite is the case for gamma oscillations: these originate in layer IV, where the feedforward inputs from the lateral geniculate nucleus terminate, propagating from there to superficial and deeper layers. Furthermore, the authors estimated the time relationships between primary visual area V1 and downstream V4 area and found a 9-ms lead of V4 with respect to V1 for alpha and a lead of 3 ms from V1 to V4 for gamma. These findings, associated with the study of responses to local microstimulation, allowed these authors to conclude that while alpha is a sign of feedback processing, gamma signals feedforward processing in the visual cortex.

From this study it emerges also that the alpha oscillations decrease when the animal focuses its eyes on a visual target but are enhanced when the animal views irrelevant information; the opposite occurs with the gamma oscillations. Moreover, as extensively explained in Chapter 48, alpha plays a role in the control of attention [152-154].

The third question concerns the general implications of the physiological findings on cortical alpha and gamma oscillations, described above, with respect to general brain functions. In an investigation with the aim of exploring neuronal activities of different visual cortical layers with respect to the effects of attention, Buffalo et al. [236] found a conspicuous difference between synchrony of gamma oscillations in the superficial cortical layers and alpha synchrony in deep layers: while the former increased with attention, the latter decreased (in line with the findings in [153]). The cortical functional and spatial organization of gamma and alpha oscillations can be very relevant in terms of brain operations since the superficial layers (II, III) and deep cortical layers (V, VI) reach different anatomical targets: from the former arise long-range connections providing feedforward signals to downstream areas; from the latter arise cortico-cortical feedback connections to upstream areas and subcortical connections to the superior colliculus, basal ganglia (from layer V), and thalamus (from layer VI).

6.4. Fast (Beta-Gamma) Rhythms in Human EEG

Whereas the mechanisms of generation of gamma and beta rhythms in cortical slices, *in vitro*, present clear different properties, the situation *in vivo* in humans is even more complex. On the one hand, beta EEG or MEG activities recorded over the Rolandic cortical area (about 15 and 30 Hz) display a close temporal relationship with peripheral EMG activity during isometric contractions, as shown using MEG recordings [237–239]. The MEG signals in the beta-frequency range lead the EMG signals in time, and the time lag increases with increasing brain–muscle distance. This implies that this beta rhythm activity is associated with rhythmic firing of neurons of the motor cortex that generate the commands to drive spinal motoneurons [240] (see also Chapter 35). On the other hand, there are other conditions where beta rhythms are not associated with a state of active neuronal firing in the sense described above. This is the case of an increase of beta activity after a finger movement (post-movement beta rebound at 16–21 Hz) or foot movement (19–26 Hz) [241] when the muscles relax. The combination of EEG recording with the application of transcranial magnetic stimulation showed that during this beta rebound the corticospinal excitability was diminished [242]. In general, stimulation of the motor cortex at beta frequencies slows the development of force during motor activity, and beta activity (13–30 Hz) is associated with static tonic or postural contractions, whereas normal voluntary movement is preceded by a suppression of beta activity [243]. This study proposes that for a normal state of motor activity there is an optimal level of beta neuronal synchrony, such that too low or too high levels correspond to impaired behavioral performance. The dynamics of changes of beta and gamma rhythms in relation to voluntary movements is further detailed in Chapter 40 on ERD/ERS [244].

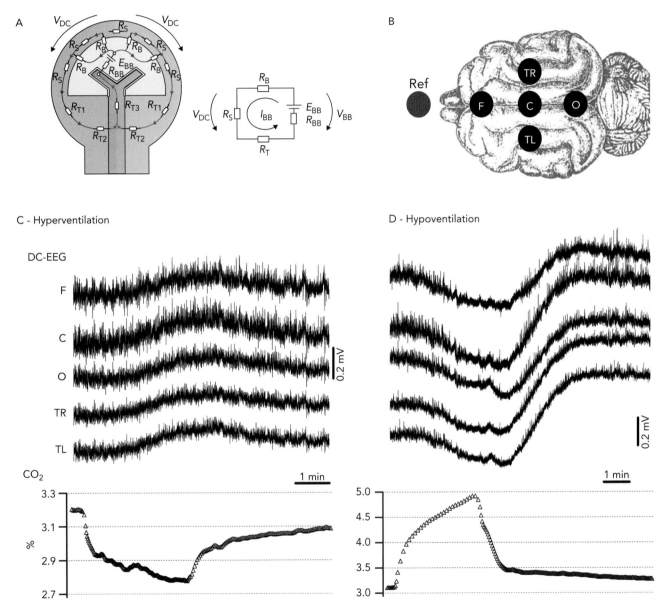

Figure 2.23. DC shift potentials generated in the EEG by variations of the systemic CO_2. **A,** left: Schematic drawing of the human head divided into four compartments: brain (yellow), blood (pink), the blood–brain or blood–cerebrospinal fluid barrier (black double line), and all other tissues (light green). E_{BB} = the electromotive force of the voltage source across the brain–blood interface; R_{BB}, its internal resistance. This voltage source generates a volume current (blue lines with arrowheads) that flows first through R_B (the distributed resistance that couples brain potential to the surrounding extracortical tissue layers) and R_S (the distributed resistance of the layers between brain surface and skin surface pooled together) and gives rise to the voltage drop V_{DC} that can be measured on scalp. Current returns back to the brain–blood interface through R_{T1} (resistance of wider tissue pathways below the level of cranial fossae), R_{T2} (access resistance to blood), and R_{T3} (resistance of blood). **A,** right: simplified equivalent circuit of the scheme depicted at left. I_{BB} represent the current that is driven in the circuit by the brain–blood potential difference (V_{BB}). **B:** Scheme with the position of the scalp electrodes with respect to the brain of the cat. DC shifts induced by hyperventilation (**C**) and hypoventilation (**D**) in a cat under ketamine–xylazine anesthesia. Below the EEG signals, variations of the CO_2 concentration in the expired air. Hyperventilation induced positive DC shifts, while hypoventilation was associated with negative DC shifts. (**A:** Modified with permission from [259]. **B–D:** Modified with permission from Nita DA, Vanhatalo S, Lafortune FD, Voipio J, Kaila K, Amzica F. Nonneuronal origin of CO_2-related DC EEG shifts: an in vivo study in the cat. J Neurophysiol. 2004;92:1011–1022.)

7. DC AND VERY LOW END EEG POTENTIALS

Although the chapter is devoted to oscillations in the brain, this section will briefly raise the issue of less conventional, very slow EEG signals, which are overwhelmingly left out of the clinical focus (see, however, [245,246] and a detailed discussion in Chapter 32, which focuses on the spectral range below 0.1 Hz, lately called infraslow potentials). Several studies have also demonstrated the involvement of glial cells in generating slow local field potentials during spreading depression [247,248], seizures [247,249–251]), and sleep [73]. Besides, pioneering studies in the early 1950s to the 1970s have proposed that some of the slow potential shifts are generated at the interface between cerebrospinal fluid and blood as a function of the partial pressure of CO_2 (PCO_2) [252–256]. Such potentials were suggested to originate across the blood–brain barrier [257–260]. The merit, but also the difficulty, of these studies consisted in introducing among the variables that condition brain phenomena extraneuronal parameters.

The basic aspects related to EEG potentials situated at the infraslow limit of the spectrum (DC to 0.01 Hz, although the upper limit is only informative) rely on the electrical scheme proposed by Voipio et al. [259] (Fig. 2.23A). It proved to be particularly useful to understand how large DC shifts that can be recorded on the scalp in response to hypo- or hypercapnia (see Fig. 2.23C, D) are not generated by networks of neurons and/or glia. This is in stark contrast with the prevailing view about the mechanisms generating ventilation-related DC shifts, which emphasized an almost exclusive role of cortical neurons and their dendritic tree [261]. Recent data [260]

demonstrate that such ventilation-induced DC shifts occurred in the absence of any parallel change in the neuronal or glial membrane potential. No extracellular, spatial polarity reversal of the DC shift responses was seen across or within the neocortex and the underlying white matter. This finding provides further support for the view that the DC shifts are not caused by cortical current dipoles generated in response to neuronal and/or glial activity. And finally, the breakdown of the blood–brain barrier produced itself a DC shift as a mark of the polarizing potential of the barrier. Once the blood–brain barrier was disrupted, ventilation-induced DC shifts were abolished (Fig. 2.24). These examples clearly state that, other than neurons and glia, a series of other parenchymal elements (blood flow, capillary epithelial cells) participate in the genesis of potentials that translate into EEG signals.

8. THE NU-COMPLEX, A GRAPHOELEMENT OF DEEP COMA

The plunging of a brain into coma, with notable etiological differences, follows certain characteristic patterns. At the beginning, during superficial comas, loss of consciousness is associated with EEG activities that are similar to sleep (from light to deep) and thus are dominated by continuous slow, ample waves (Fig. 2.25B). Deepening of the coma evolves into burst-suppression patterns (Fig. 2.25C). The EEG displays relatively short-lasting (few seconds), but ample, bursts of slow activities, alternating with periods of isoelectric potentials. This state marks a behavioral window of cortical hyperexcitability [262] due to at least partial suppression of cortical

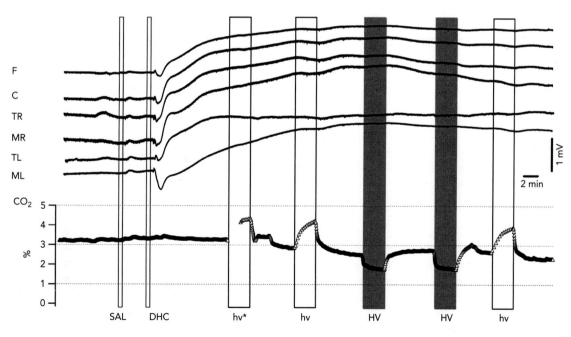

Figure 2.24. *DC shifts induced by the disruption of the blood–brain barrier. Scalp DC EEG recording in a cat under ketamine–xylazine anesthesia. After a control period, a volume of 3 ml saline (SAL) was slowly injected into the right carotid artery with no effect. Then an identical volume of sodium dehydrocholate (DHC; 17.5%) was injected in order to break the blood–brain barrier. This induced a clear positive DC shift, with right lateralization. During the period with open blood–brain barrier, the amplitude of the responses to hypo- and hyperventilation (hv/HV) maneuvers was drastically diminished. The asterisk during the first hypoventilation maneuver indicates that initially, for a period of about 1 minute, the respirator was stopped. (Modified with permission from Nita DA, Vanhatalo S, Lafortune FD, Voipio J, Kaila K, Amzica F. Nonneuronal origin of CO_2-related DC EEG shifts: an in vivo study in the cat. J Neurophysiol. 2004;92:1011–1022.)*

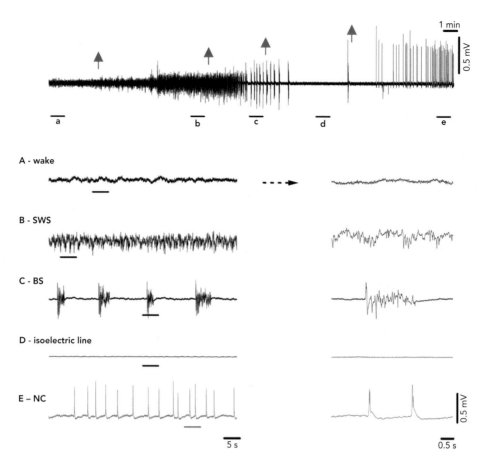

Figure 2.25. *EEG patterns during wakefulness and diverse degrees of loss of consciousness. Cat EEG recording during application of various concentrations of isoflurane. While the top-most panel depicts the complete sequence, with arrows indicating the applications of increasing anesthesia, the underlined epochs are expanded below. A: Undrugged preparation displaying low-amplitude, fast (mostly >15 Hz) EEG. B: Slow-wave sleep-like (SWS) pattern after 1% isoflurane, characterized by higher-amplitude slow waves dominated by delta oscillations (<4 Hz). C: Burst-suppression (BS) induced with 2% isoflurane showing alternating sequences of isoelectric line and bursting episodes. The latter are very similar to SWS patterns (see detail at right). D: A further increase in the isoflurane concentration (3%) establishes a stable isoelectric line portraying the absence of phasic events. Only very low-amplitude activities can be observed at high gain. E: Isoflurane at 4% elicits a revival of quasi-rhythmic spiky potentials of high amplitude, which we propose to call nu-complexes (νC). (Modified with permission from Kroeger D, Florea B, Amzica F. Human brain activity patterns beyond the isoelectric line of extreme deep coma. PLoS One 2013;8(9):e75257.)*

inhibition [263]. The bursts are evoked by "subthreshold" stimuli that do not trigger any overt responses in more superficial or deeper states of coma. During isoelectric episodes cortical neurons are silent, but spontaneous subcortical (e.g., thalamic) activities survive even during flat EEG patterns [264]. Beyond this depth of coma, cortical activities are continuously silenced, resulting in a flat (isoelectric) EEG (Fig. 2.25D). This was until recently the last frontier of a living brain. However, under particular conditions (see below), even deeper coma can be induced with anesthesia (e.g., isoflurane) resulting in a completely new, revived, EEG pattern characterized by a new waveform, called the nu-complex (Fig. 2.25E) [265].

This pattern was found both in animals (cats) and humans and proved to be perfectly reversible once the following condition was satisfied. The paramount condition for this comatose state relies on a relatively preserved cerebral tissue with adequate blood supply. If the previous, more superficial (isoelectric) coma is associated with compromised cerebral cells, then the nu-complex state cannot be induced.

Nu-complexes appear pseudo-rhythmically approximately every 10 s (average time interval of 9.3 ± 2.7 s). Simultaneous intracellular recordings in several subcortical regions and cortex have demonstrated that nu-complexes arise in the hippocampus as a result of an ongoing oscillatory activity within the delta frequency band (<4 Hz) also termed ripple activity (Fig. 2.26). Ripple oscillations occur during EEG isoelectric line and cannot disrupt the cortical unresponsiveness. However, from one ripple to the next, more hippocampal neurons are recruited and the oscillation becomes more robust, succeeding eventually to trigger a stronger excitatory potential in the hippocampus. While initial ripple oscillations cannot excite relay stations en route to the cortex, the nu-complex can overcome the high excitation threshold of the entorhinal cortex and trigger a full-blown nu-complex in the cortex [265].

The nu-complex state might have important clinical implications:

1. It represents the deepest form of coma obtained so far and demonstrates that the brain may remain operational beyond the EEG isoelectric line.

2. It demonstrates again that an isoelectric EEG does not necessarily reflect neuronal death, but merely cortical silence.

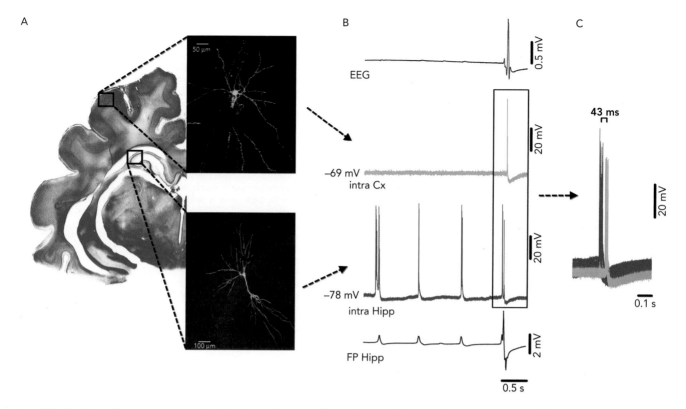

Figure 2.26. Cortical and hippocampal neuronal activity during νC state. **A:** *Neocortical pyramidal neuron from suprasylvian area 5 (above) and simultaneously recorded pyramidal CA3 hippocampal neuron filled with Lucifer Yellow and reconstructed with confocal microscopy. Their respective locations are schematically indicated on a Nissl-stained coronal section of the brain.* **B:** *From top to bottom: simultaneous recording of the EEG, intracellular cortical neuron (green), intracellular hippocampal neuron (blue), and adjacent hippocampal field potential (FP). Both hippocampal traces indicate the presence of two types of activities: delta ripples at about 1 Hz (small-amplitude positive potentials in the FP, accompanied by bursts of action potentials in the nearby neuron) and a νC (high-amplitude spiky multiphasic potential in the FP, which is paralleled by neuronal discharge). The EEG displays a continuous isoelectric line during hippocampal ripples but displays the νC during which the cortical neuron discharges bursts of action potentials. Delta ripples are not expressed in the neocortex.* **C:** *Time relationship between neuronal discharges for νC events indicating that the hippocampal discharges consistently precede the neocortical ones. (Modified with permission from Kroeger D, Florea B, Amzica F. Human brain activity patterns beyond the isoelectric line of extreme deep coma. PLoS One 2013;8(9):e75257.)*

3. While the debate about the use of EEG recordings in establishing brain death has been settled in many advanced countries, the discovery of the nu-complex state might open new ideas as to the assessment of the functional condition of a comatose brain. For example, an isoelectric EEG can ambiguously reflect a brain with massive neuronal loss or a silent cortex with active subcortical (thalamic, hippocampal) structures. Solving the dilemma might require deepening the coma to the point where nu-complexes are expected. If they were obtained, the balance would tilt toward the latter situation, while absence of nu-complexes would point toward brain death.

Finally, a conceptual breakthrough is called forth by the discovery of the nu-complex state. Wakefulness, as a state that hosts conscious processes and the domination of willful action, is characterized by a predominance of neocortical activity. As these functions fade at the onset of unconsciousness, the orchestrating powers are relinquished to more basic structures such as the thalamus (in the case of sleep) or the limbic system (coma). When these structures are released from neocortical influence, they begin to pursue activity patterns on their own and proceed to impose these patterns on other brain regions, including the neocortex [265].

REFERENCES

1. Riera JJ, Ogawa T, Goto, T, et al. Pitfalls in the dipolar model for the neocortical EEG sources. J Neurophysiol. 2012;108:956–975.
2. Halnes G, Mäki-Marttunen T, Keller D, Pettersen KH, Einevoll GT. The effect of ionic diffusion on extracellular potentials in neural tissue. 2015 arXiv: 1505.06033v2 [physics.bio-ph].
3. Pettersen KH, Einevoll GT. Amplitude variability and extracellular low-pass filtering of neuronal spikes. Biophys J. 2008;94(3):784–802.
4. Milstein JN, Koch C. Dynamic moment analysis of the extracellular electric field of a biologically realistic spiking neuron. Neural Computation. 2008;20(8):2070–2084.
5. Chitwood RA, Hubbard A, Jaffe DB. Passive electrotonic properties of rat hippocampal CA3 interneurones. J Physiol (Lond). 1999;515(3):743–756.
6. Simon A, Traub RD, Vladimirov N, et al. Gap junction networks can generate both ripple-like and fast ripple-like oscillations. Eur J Neurosci. 2014;30:46–60.
7. Nelson MJ, Bosch C, Venance L, Pouget P. Microscale inhomogeneity of brain tissue distorts electrical signal propagation. J Neurosci. 2013;33(7):2821–2827.
8. Buzsáki G, Anastassiou CA, Koch C. The origin of extracellular fields and currents-EEG, ECoG, LFP and spikes. Nat Neurosci Rev. 2012;13:407–420.
9. Reimann MW, Anastassiou CA, Perin R, Hill SL, Markram H, Koch C. A biophysically detailed model of neocortical local field potentials predicts the critical role of active membrane currents. Neuron. 2013;79:375–390.
10. Nunez PL, Srinivasan R. Electric Fields of the Brain: The Neurophysics of EEG. Oxford: Oxford University Press; 2006.
11. Lorente de Nó R. Action potential of the motoneurons of the hypoglossus nucleus. J Cell Comp Physiol. 1947;29:207–287.
12. Mitzdorf U. Current-source density method and applications in cat cerebral cortex: investigation of evoked potentials and EEG phenomena. Physiol Rev. 1985;65:37–100.

13. Gratiy SL, Pettersen KH, Einevoll GT, Dale AM. Pitfalls in the interpretation of multielectrode data: on the infeasibility of the current neuronal current-source monopoles. J Neurophysiol. 2013;109:1681–1682.
14. Bédard C, Destexhe A. Generalized theory for current-source-density analysis in brain tissue. Physical Rev. 2011;E 84, 041909.
15. Cabo A, Riera J. How the active and diffusional nature of brain tissues can generate monopole signals at micrometer sized measures. 2014;arXiv:1410.0274 [physics.bio-ph].
16. Dietzel I, Heinemann U, Lux H. Relations between slow extracellular potential changes, glial potassium buffering, and electrolyte and cellular volume changes during neuronal hyperactivity in cat. Glia. 1989;2:25–44.
17. Somjen GG, Kager H, Wadman WJ. Computer simulations of neuron-glia interactions mediated by ion flux. J Comput Neurosci. 2008;25:349–365.
18. Fernandes JM, Martins da Silva A, Huiskamp G, et al. What does an epileptiform spike look like in MEG? Comparison between coincident EEG and MEG spikes. J Clin Neurophysiol. 2005;22:68–73.
19. Gonçalves SI, de Munck JC, Verbunt PA, Bijma F, Heethaar RM, Lopes da Silva F. In vivo measurement of the brain and skull resistivities using an EIT based method and realistic models for the head. IEEE Trans BioMedical Eng. 2003;50(6):754–767.
20. Amzica F, Massimini M. Glial and neuronal interactions during slow-wave and paroxysmal activities in the neocortex. Cerebral Cortex. 2002;12(10):1101–1114.
21. Kager H, Wadman WJ, Somjen GG. Simulated seizures and spreading depression in a neuron model incorporating interstitial space and ion concentrations. J Neurophysiol. 2000;84(1):495–512.
22. Amzica F. Physiology of sleep and wakefulness as it relates to the physiology of epilepsy. J Clin Neurophysiol. 2002;19(6):488–503.
23. Mountcastle VB. The columnar organization of the neocortex. Brain. 1997;120(4):701–722.
24. Markram H. The Blue Brain project. Nat Neurosci Rev. 2006;7(2):153–160.
25. Lindén H, Tetzlaff T, Potjans TC, et al. Modeling the spatial reach of the LFP. Neuron. 2011;72(5):869–872.
26. Murakami S, Okada Y. Contributions of principal neocortical neurons to magnetoencephalography and electroencephalography signals. J Physiol (London). 2006;575(3):925–936.
27. Cosandier-Rimelé D, Merlet I, Badier JM, Chavel P, Wendling F. The neuronal sources of EEG: modeling of simultaneous scalp and intracerebral recordings in epilepsy. Neuroimage. 2008;42(1):135–146.
28. Chang BS, Schomer DL, Niedermeyer E. Normal EEG and sleep: adults and elderly. In: Schomer DL, Lopes da Silva FH, eds. Niedermeyer's Electroencephalography: Basic Principles, Clinical Applications and Related Fields. 6th ed. Philadelphia, PA: Lippincott Williams and Wilkins; 2011:183–214.
29. Lopes da Silva FH. Computer-assisted EEG pattern recognition and diagnostic systems. In: Schomer DL, Lopes da Silva FH, eds. Niedermeyer's Electroencephalography: Basic Principles, Clinical Applications and Related Fields. 6th ed. Philadelphia, PA: Lippincott Williams and Wilkins; 2011:1203–1225.
30. Vanhatalo S, Voipio J, Kaila K. Full-band (fbEEG): a new standard for clinical electroencephalography. Clin EEG Neurosci. 2005;36(4):311–317.
31. Leistner S, Sander T, Burhoff M, Curio G, Trahms L, Mackert BM. Combined MEG and EEG methodology for non-invasive recording of infraslow activity in the human cortex. Clin Neurophysiol. 2007;118(12):2774–2780.
32. Achermann P, Borbély AA Low-frequency (<1 Hz) oscillations in the human sleep electroencephalogram. Neuroscience. 1997;81(1):213–222.
33. Steriade M. Grouping of brain rhythms in corticothalamic systems. Neuroscience. 2006;137:1087–1106.
34. Walter WG, Cooper R, Aldridge VJ, et al. Contingent negative variation: an electric sign of sensorimotor association and expectancy in the human brain. Nature. 1964;203:380–384.
35. Kornhuber HH, Deecke L. Changes in the brain potential in voluntary movements and passive movements in man: readiness potential and reafferent potentials. Pflugers Archiv. 1965;284:1–17.
36. Waterstraat G, Telenczuk B, Burghoff M, Fedele T, Scheer HJ, Curio G. Are high-frequency (600 Hz) oscillations in human somatosensory evoked potentials due to phase-resetting phenomenon? Clin Neurophysiol. 2012;123(10):2064–2073.
37. Andrade-Valença LP, Dubeau F, Mari F, Zelmann R, Gotman J. Interictal scalp fast oscillations as a marker of the seizure onset zone. Neurology. 2011;77(6):524–531.
38. Zelmann R, Lina JM, Schulze-Bonhage A, Gotman J, Jacobs J. Scalp EEG is not a blur: it can see high frequency oscillations although their generators are small. Brain Topography. 2014;27(5):683–704.
39. Walter G. The location of cerebral tumors by electro-encephalography. Lancet. 1936;8:305–308.
40. IFSECN. A glossary of terms most commonly used by clinical electroencephalographers. Electroencephalogr Clin Neurophysiol. 1974;37:538–548.
41. Creutzfeldt OD, Watanabe S, Lux HD. Relations between EEG phenomena and potentials of single cortical cells. II. Spontaneous and convulsoid activity. Electroencephalogr Clin Neurophysiol. 1966;20:19–37.
42. Kellaway P, Gol A, Proler M. Electrical activity of the isolated cerebral hemisphere and isolated thalamus. Exp Neurol. 1966;14:281–304.
43. Rappelsberger P, Pockberger H, Petsche H. The contribution of the cortical layers to the generation of the EEG: field potential and current source density analyses in the rabbit's visual cortex. Electroencephalogr Clin Neurophysiol. 1982;53:254–269.
44. Leresche N, Jassik-Gerschenfeld D, Haby M, Soltesz I, Crunelli V. Pacemaker-like and other types of spontaneous membrane potential oscillations of thalamocortical cells. Neurosci Lett. 1990;113:72–77.
45. Leresche N, Lightowler S, Soltesz I, Jassik-Gerschenfeld D, Crunelli V. Low-frequency oscillatory activities intrinsic to rat and cat thalamocortical cells. J Physiol (Lond). 1991;441:155–174.
46. McCormick DA, Pape HC. Properties of a hyperpolarization-activated cation current and its role in rhythmic oscillation in thalamic relay neurones. J Physiol (Lond). 1990;431:291–318.
47. Soltesz I, Lightowler S, Leresche N, Jassik-Gerschenfeld D, Pollard CE, Crunelli V. Two inward currents and the transformation of low-frequency oscillations of rat and cat thalamocortical cells. J Physiol (Lond). 1991;441:175–197.
48. Steriade M, Curró Dossi R, Nuñez A. Network modulation of a slow intrinsic oscillation of cat thalamocortical neurons implicated in sleep delta waves: cortically induced synchronization and brainstem cholinergic suppression. J Neurosci. 1991;11:3200–3217.
49. Curró Dossi R, Nuñez A, Steriade M. Electrophysiology of a slow (0.5–4 Hz) intrinsic oscillation of cat thalamocortical neurones in vivo. J Physiol (Lond). 1992;447:215–234.
50. Nuñez A, Curró Dossi R, Contreras D, Steriade M. Intracellular evidence for incompatibility between spindle and delta oscillations in thalamocortical neurons of cat. Neuroscience. 1992;48:75–85.
51. Nita DA, Steriade M, Amzica F. Hyperpolarisation rectification in cat lateral geniculate neurons modulated by intact corticothalamic projections. J Physiol (Lond). 2003;552:325–332.
52. Villablanca J. Role of the thalamus in sleep control: sleep-wakefulness studies in chronic diencephalic and athalamic cats. In: Petre-Quadens O, Schlag J, eds. Basic Sleep Mechanisms. New York: Academic; 1974:51–81.
53. Ball GJ, Gloor P, Schaul N. The cortical electromicrophysiology of pathological delta waves in the electroencephalogram of cats. Electroencephalogr Clin Neurophysiol. 1977;43:346–361.
54. Steriade M, Gloor P, Llinás RR, Lopes de Silva FH, Mesulam MM. Report of IFCN Committee on Basic Mechanisms. Basic mechanisms of cerebral rhythmic activities. Electroencephalogr Clin Neurophysiol. 1990;76:481–508.
55. Steriade M, Buzsáki G. Parallel activation of thalamic and cortical neurons by brainstem and basal forebrain cholinergic systems. In: Steriade M, Biesold D, eds. Brain Cholinergic Systems. New York: Oxford University Press; 1990:3–62.
56. Steriade M, Nuñez A, Amzica F. A novel slow (< 1 Hz) oscillation of neocortical neurons in vivo: depolarizing and hyperpolarizing components. J Neurosci. 1993;13:3252–3265.
57. Steriade M, Amzica F, Contreras D. Synchronization of fast (30–40 Hz) spontaneous cortical rhythms during brain activation. J Neurosci. 1996;16:392–417.
58. Amzica F, Steriade M. The K-complex: its slow (<1 Hz) rhythmicity and relation to delta waves. Neurology. 1997;49:952–959.
59. Simon NR, Manshanden I, Lopes da Silva FH. A MEG study of sleep. Brain Res. 2000;860:64–76.
60. Mölle M, Marshall L, Gais S, Born J. Grouping of spindle activity during slow oscillations in human non-rapid eye movement sleep. J Neurosci. 2002;22:10941–10947.
61. Massimini M, Rosanova M, Mariotti M. EEG slow (approximately 1 Hz) waves are associated with nonstationarity of thalamo-cortical sensory processing in the sleeping human. J Neurophysiol. 2003;89:1205–1213.
62. Steriade M, Nuñez A, Amzica F. Intracellular analysis of relations between the slow (< 1 Hz) neocortical oscillation and other sleep rhythms of the electroencephalogram. J Neurosci. 1993;13:3266–3283.
63. Timofeev I, Steriade M. Low-frequency rhythms in the thalamus of intact-cortex and decorticated cats. J Neurophysiol. 1996;76:4152–4168.
64. Sanchez-Vives MV, McCormick DA. Cellular and network mechanisms of rhythmic recurrent activity in neocortex. Nat Neurosci. 2000;3: 1027–1034.

65. Contreras D, Timofeev I, Steriade M. Mechanisms of long-lasting hyperpolarizations underlying slow sleep oscillations in cat corticothalamic networks. J Physiol (Lond). 1996;494(Pt 1):251–264.

66. Massimini M, Amzica F. Extracellular calcium fluctuations and intracellular potentials in the cortex during the slow sleep oscillation. J Neurophysiol. 2001;85:1346–1350.

67. Steriade M, Amzica F, Nuñez A. Cholinergic and noradrenergic modulation of the slow (approximately 0.3 Hz) oscillation in neocortical cells. J Neurophysiol. 1993;70:1385–1400.

68. Contreras D, Steriade M. Cellular basis of EEG slow rhythms: a study of dynamic corticothalamic relationships. J Neurosci. 1995;15:604–622.

69. Amzica F, Steriade M. Disconnection of intracortical synaptic linkages disrupts synchronization of a slow oscillation. J Neurosci. 1995;15:4658–4677.

70. Amzica F, Steriade M. Short- and long-range neuronal synchronization of the slow (< 1 Hz) cortical oscillation. J Neurophysiol. 1995;73:20–38.

71. Steriade M, Contreras D, Curró Dossi R, Nuñez A. The slow (< 1 Hz) oscillation in reticular thalamic and thalamocortical neurons: scenario of sleep rhythm generation in interacting thalamic and neocortical networks. J Neurosci. 1993;13:3284–3299.

72. Amzica F, Steriade M. Electrophysiological correlates of sleep delta waves. Electroencephalogr Clin Neurophysiol. 1998;107:69–83.

73. Amzica F, Neckelmann D. Membrane capacitance of cortical neurons and glia during sleep oscillations and spike-wave seizures. J Neurophysiol. 1999;82:2731–2746.

74. Amzica F, Massimini M. Glial and neuronal interactions during slow wave and paroxysmal activities in the neocortex. Cereb Cortex. 2002;12:1101–1113.

75. Amzica F, Massimini M, Manfridi A. Spatial buffering during slow and paroxysmal sleep oscillations in cortical networks of glial cells in vivo. J Neurosci. 2002;22:1042–1053.

76. Bowman CL, Kimelberg HK. Excitatory amino acids directly depolarize rat brain astrocytes in primary culture. Nature. 1984;311:656–659.

77. Kettenmann H, Schachner M. Pharmacological properties of gamma-aminobutyric acid-, glutamate-, and aspartate-induced depolarizations in cultured astrocytes. J Neurosci. 1985;5:3295–3301.

78. Orkand RK, Nicholls JG, Kuffler SW. Effect of nerve impulses on the membrane potential of glial cells in the central nervous system of amphibia. J Neurophysiol. 1966;29:788–806.

79. Kettenmann H, Ransom BR. Electrical coupling between astrocytes and between oligodendrocytes studied in mammalian cell cultures. Glia. 1988;1:64–73.

80. Walz W. Role of glial cells in the regulation of the brain ion microenvironment. Prog Neurobiol. 1989;33:309–333.

81. Nicholson C. Extracellular space as the pathway for neuron-glial cell interaction. In: Kettenmann H, Ransom BR, eds. Neuroglia. New York: Oxford University Press; 1995:387–397.

82. Ballanyi K, Grafe P, ten Bruggencate G. Ion activities and potassium uptake mechanisms of glial cells in guinea-pig olfactory cortex slices. J Physiol (Lond). 1987;382:159–174.

83. Kettenmann H. K+ and Cl- uptake by cultured oligodendrocytes. Can J Physiol Pharmacol. 1987;65:1033–1037.

84. Kocsis JD, Malenka RC, Waxman SG. Effects of extracellular potassium concentration on the excitability of the parallel fibres of the rat cerebellum. J Physiol (Lond). 1983;334:225–244.

85. Rausche G, Igelmund P, Heinemann U. Effects of changes in extracellular potassium, magnesium and calcium concentration on synaptic transmission in area CA1 and the dentate gyrus of rat hippocampal slices. Pflugers Arch. 1990;415:588–593.

86. Hille B. Ion Channels of Excitable Membranes. Sunderland: Sinauer; 2001.

87. Loomis AL, Harvey EN, Hobart G. Distribution of disturbance patterns in the human electroencephalogram, with special reference to sleep. J Neurophysiol. 1938;1:413–440.

88. Colrain IM. The K-complex: a 7-decade history. Sleep. 2005;28:255–273.

89. Amzica F, Steriade M. Cellular substrates and laminar profile of sleep K-complex. Neuroscience. 1998;82:671–686.

90. Steriade M, Datta S, Paré D, Oakson G, Curró Dossi R. Neuronal activities in brain-stem cholinergic nuclei related to tonic activation processes in thalamocortical systems. J Neurosci. 1990;10:2541–2559.

91. Steriade M, Oakson G, Ropert N. Firing rates and patterns of midbrain reticular neurons during steady and transitional states of the sleep-waking cycle. Exp Brain Res. 1982;46:37–51.

92. Hirsch JC, Fourment A, Marc ME. Sleep-related variations of membrane potential in the lateral geniculate body relay neurons of the cat. Brain Res. 1983;259:308–312.

93. Davis H, Davis PA, Loomis AL, Harvey EN, Hobart G. Electrical reactions of the human brain to auditory stimulation during sleep. J Neurophysiol. 1939;6:500–514.

94. Steriade M, Amzica F. Coalescence of sleep rhythms and their chronology in corticothalamic networks. Sleep Res Online. 1998;1:1–10.

95. Ingvar DH, Sjölund B, Ardö A. Correlation between dominant EEG frequency, cerebral oxygen uptake and blood flow. Electroencephalogr Clin Neurophysiol. 1976;41:268–276.

96. Saunders MG, Westmoreland BF. The EEG in evaluation of disorders affecting the brain diffusely. In: Klass DW, Daly DD, eds. Current Practice of Clinical Electroencephalography. New York: Raven Press; 1979:343–379.

97. Buzsáki G. Rhythms of the Brain. Oxford: Oxford University Press; 2006.

98. Brazier MAB. Studies of the EEG activity of limbic structures in man. Electroencephalogr Clin Neurophysiol. 1968;25:309–318.

99. Halgren E, Babb TL, Crandall PH. Human hippocampal formation EEG desynchronizes during attentiveness and movement. Electroencephalogr Clin Neurophysiol. 1978;44:778–781.

100. Arnolds DE, Lopes da Silva FH, Aitink JW, Kamp A, Boeijinga P. The spectral properties of hippocampal EEG related to behaviour in man. Electroencephalogr Clin Neurophysiol. 1980;50:324–328.

101. Kahana MJ, Sekuler R, Caplan JB, Kirschen M, Madsen JR. Human theta oscillations exhibit task dependence during virtual maze navigation. Nature. 1999;399:781–784.

102. Ekstrom AD, Caplan JB, Ho E, Shattuck K, Fried I, Kahana MJ. Human hippocampal theta activity during virtual navigation. Hippocampus. 2005;15:881–889.

103. Bódizs R, Kántor S, Szabó G, Szucs A, Eross L, Hálasz P. Rhythmic hippocampal slow oscillation characterizes REM sleep in humans. Hippocampus. 2001;11:747–753.

104. Tesche CD, Karhu J. Theta oscillations index human hippocampal activation during a working memory task. Proc Natl Acad Sci USA. 2000;97:919–924.

105. Cornwell BR, Johnson LL, Holroyd T, Carver FW, Grillon C. Human hippocampal and parahippocampal theta during goal-directed spatial navigation predicts performance on a virtual Morris water maze. J Neurosci. 2008;28:5983–5990.

106. Stewart M, Fox SE. Hippocampal theta activity in monkeys. Brain Res. 1991;538:59–63.

107. Green JD, Arduini AA. Hippocampal electrical activity in arousal. J Neurophysiol. 1954;17:533–557.

108. Witter MP, Naber PA, van Haeften T, et al. Cortico-hippocampal communication by way of parallel parahippocampal-subicular pathways. Hippocampus. 2000;10:398–410.

109. Buzsáki G. Theta oscillations in the hippocampus. Neuron. 2002;33:325–340.

110. Chapman CA, Lacaille JC. Intrinsic theta-frequency membrane potential oscillations in hippocampal CA1 interneurons of stratum lacunosummoleculare. J Neurophysiol. 1999;81:1296–1307.

111. Bilkey DK, Heinemann U. Intrinsic theta-frequency membrane potential oscillations in layer III/V perirhinal cortex neurons of the rat. Hippocampus. 1999;9:510–518.

112. Petsche H, Stumpf C, Gogolak G. The significance of the rabbit's septum as a relay station between the midbrain and the hippocampus. The control of hippocampus arousal activity by septum cells. Electroencephalogr Clin Neurophysiol. 1962;14:202–211.

113. Petsche H, Gogolak G, van Zwieten PA. Rhythmicity of septal cell discharges at various levels of reticular excitation. Electroencephalogr Clin Neurophysiol. 1965;19:25–33.

114. Freund TF, Antal M. GABA-containing neurons in the septum control inhibitory interneurons in the hippocampus. Nature. 1988;336:170–173.

115. Vertes RP, Kocsis B. Brainstem-diencephalo-septohippocampal systems controlling the theta rhythm of the hippocampus. Neuroscience. 1997;81:893–926.

116. Buzsáki G, Leung LW, Vanderwolf CH. Cellular bases of hippocampal EEG in the behaving rat. Brain Res. 1983;287:139–171.

117. Mitchell SJ, Ranck JB Jr. Generation of theta rhythm in medial entorhinal cortex of freely moving rats. Brain Res. 1980;189:49–66.

118. Alonso A, Garcia-Austt E. Neuronal sources of theta rhythm in the entorhinal cortex of the rat. I. Laminar distribution of theta field potentials. Exp Brain Res. 1987;67:493–501.

119. Alonso A, Garcia-Austt E. Neuronal sources of theta rhythm in the entorhinal cortex of the rat. II. Phase relations between unit discharges and theta field potentials. Exp Brain Res. 1987;67:502–509.

120. Boeijinga PH, Lopes da Silva FH. Differential distribution of beta and theta EEG activity in the entorhinal cortex of the cat. Brain Res. 1988;448:272–286.

121. Vanderwolf CH, Buzsáki G, Cain DP, Cooley RK, Robertson B. Neocortical and hippocampal electrical activity following decapitation in the rat. Brain Res. 1988;451:340–344.

122. Vanderwolf CH, Leung LS. Hippocampal rhythmical slow activity: a brief history and effects entorhinal lesions and phencyclidine. In: Seifert W, ed. The Neurobiology of the Hippocampus. London: Academic Press; 1983:275–302.
123. Montgomery SM, Betancur MI, Buzsáki G. Behavior-dependent coordination of multiple theta dipoles in the hippocampus. J Neurosci. 2009;29:1381–1394.
124. Stewart M, Fox SE. Do septal neurons pace the hippocampal theta rhythm? Trends Neurosci. 1990;13:163–168.
125. Leung LW. Model of gradual phase shift of theta rhythm in the rat. J Neurophysiol. 1984;52:1051–1065.
126. Chapman CA, Lacaille JC. Cholinergic induction of theta-frequency oscillations in hippocampal inhibitory interneurons and pacing of pyramidal cell firing. J Neurosci. 1999;19:8637–8645.
127. Leung LS. Generation of theta and gamma rhythms in the hippocampus. Neurosci Biobehav Rev. 1998;22:275–290.
128. Buzsáki G, Czopf J, Kondákor I, Kellenyi L. Laminar distribution of hippocampal rhythmic slow activity (RSA) in the behaving rat: current-source density analysis, effects of urethane and atropine. Brain Res. 1986;365:125–137.
129. Soltesz I, Deschênes M. Low- and high-frequency membrane potential oscillations during theta activity in CA1 and CA3 pyramidal neurons of the rat hippocampus under ketamine-xylazine anesthesia. J Neurophysiol. 1993;70:97–116.
130. Somogyi P, Klausberger T. Defined types of cortical interneurone structure space and spike timing in the hippocampus. J Physiol (Lond). 2005;562:9–26.
131. Banks MI, White JA, Pearce RA. Interactions between distinct GABA(A) circuits in hippocampus. Neuron. 2000;25:449–457.
132. Wendling F, Bartolomei F, Bellanger JJ, Chauvel P. Epileptic fast activity can be explained by a model of impaired GABAergic dendritic inhibition. Eur J Neurosci. 2002;15:1499–1508.
133. Fuentealba P, Tomioka R, Dalezios Y, et al. Rhythmically active enkephalin-expressing GABAergic cells in the CA1 area of the hippocampus project to the subiculum and preferentially innervate interneurons. J Neurosci. 2008;28:10017–10022.
134. Kamondi A, Acsady L, Wang XJ, Buzsáki G. Theta oscillations in somata and dendrites of hippocampal pyramidal cells in vivo: activity-dependent phase-precession of action potentials. Hippocampus. 1998;8:244–261.
135. Wulff P, Ponomarenko AA, Bartos M, et al. Hippocampal theta rhythm and its coupling with gamma oscillations require fast inhibition onto parvalbumin-positive interneurons. Proc Natl Acad Sci USA. 2009;106:3561–3566.
136. Klausberger T, Somogyi P. Neuronal diversity and temporal dynamics: the unity of hippocampal circuit operations. Science. 2008;321:53–57.
137. Sik A, Penttonen M, Ylinen A, Buzsáki G. Hippocampal CA1 interneurons: an in vivo intracellular labeling study. J Neurosci. 1995;15:6651–6665.
138. Toth K, Freund TF, Miles R. Disinhibition of rat hippocampal pyramidal cells by GABAergic afferents from the septum. J Physiol (Lond). 1997;500 (Pt 2):463–474.
139. Rotstein HG, Pervouchine DD, Acker CD, et al. Slow and fast inhibition and an H-current interact to create a theta rhythm in a model of CA1 interneuron network. J Neurophysiol. 2005;94:1509–1518.
140. Berger H. Über das Elektroenkephalogramm des Menschen. 1st report. Arch Psychiat Nervenkr. 1929;87:527–570.
141. Niedermeyer E. The normal EEG of the waking adult. In: Niedermeyer E, Lopes da Silva FH, eds. Electroencephalography: Basic Principles, Clinical Applications, and Related Fields. Baltimore: Lippincott, Williams & Wilkins; 2005:167–192.
142. Adrian ED, Mathews BHC. The interpretation of potential waves in the cortex. J Physiol (Lond). 1934;81:440–471.
143. Creutzfeld O, Grünvald G, Simonova O, Schmitz H. Changes of the basic rhythms of the EEG during the performance of mental and visuomotor tasks. In: Evans CR, Mulholland TB, eds. Attention in Neurophysiology. London: Butterworth; 1969:148–168.
144. Ray WJ, Cole HW. EEG alpha activity reflects attentional demands, and beta activity reflects emotional and cognitive processes. Science. 1985;228:750–752.
145. Rihs TA, Michel CM, Thut G. Mechanisms of selective inhibition in visual spatial attention are indexed by alpha-band EEG synchronization. Eur J Neurosci. 2007;25:603–610.
146. Rihs TA, Michel CM, Thut G. A bias for posterior alpha-band power suppression versus enhancement during shifting versus maintenance of spatial attention. Neuroimage. 2009;44:190–199.
147. Andersen P, Andersson SA. Physiological Basis of the Alpha Rhythm. New York: Appleton-Century-Crofts; 1968.
148. Lopes da Silva FH, Van Lierop THMT, Schrijer CFM, Storm Van Leeuwen W. Organization of thalamic and cortical alpha rhythm: spectra and coherences. Electroencephalogr Clin Neurophysiol. 1973;35:627–639.
149. Lopes da Silva FH, Storm Van Leeuwen W. The cortical source of the alpha rhythm. Neurosci Lett. 1977;6:237–241.
150. Lopes da Silva FH, Storm Van Leeuwen W. The cortical alpha rhythm in dog: depth and surface profile of phase. In: Brazier MAB, Petsche H, eds. Architecture of the Cerebral Cortex, IBRO monograph series vol. 3. New York: Raven Press; 1978:319–333.
151. Lopes da Silva FH, Vos JE, Mooibroek J, van Rotterdam A. Relative contributions of intracortical and thalamo-cortical processes in the generation of alpha rhythms, revealed by partial coherence analysis. Electroencephalogr Clin Neurophysiol. 1980;50:449–456.
152. Bollimunta A, Chen Y, Schroeder CE, Ding M. Neuronal mechanisms of cortical alpha oscillations in awake-behaving macaques. J Neurosci. 2008;28:9976–9988.
153. van Kerkoerle T, Self MW, Dagnino B, et al. Alpha and gamma oscillations characterize feedback and feedforward processing in monkey visual cortex. Proc Natl Acad Sci USA. 2014;111:14332–14341.
154. Haegens S, Barczak A, Musacchia G, et al. Laminar profile and physiology of the alpha rhythm in primary visual, auditory, and somatosensory regions of neocortex. J Neurosci. 2015;35(42):14341–14352.
155. Vierling-Claassen D, Cardin JA, Moore CI, Jones SR. Computational modeling of distinct neocortical oscillations driven by cell-type selective optogenetic drive: separable resonant circuits controlled by low-threshold spiking and fast-spiking interneurons. Front Hum Neurosci. 2010;4:198.
156. Suffczynski P, Kalitzinb S, Pfurtscheller G, Lopes da Silva FH. Computational model of thalamo-cortical networks: dynamical control of alpha rhythms in relation to focal attention. Int J Psychophysiol. 2001;43:25–40.
157. Jones SR, Dominique I, Pritchett, L, et al. Quantitative analysis and biophysically realistic neural modeling of the MEG mu rhythm: rhythmogenesis and modulation of sensory-evoked responses. J Neurophysiol. 2009;102:3554–3572.
158. Flint AC, Connors BW. Two types of network oscillations in neocortex mediated by distinct glutamate receptor subtypes and neuronal populations. J Neurophysiol. 1996;75:951–957.
159. Hughes SW, Lörincz M, Cope DW, et al. Synchronized oscillations at alpha and theta frequencies in the lateral geniculate nucleus. Neuron. 2004;42:253–268.
160. Hughes SW, Crunelli V. Thalamic mechanisms of EEG alpha rhythms and their pathological implications. Neuroscientist. 2005;11:357–372.
161. Lörincz ML, Crunelli V, Hughes SW. Cellular dynamics of cholinergically induced alpha (8–13 Hz) rhythms in sensory thalamic nuclei in vitro. J Neurosci. 2008;28:660–671.
162. Steriade M. Neuronal Substrates of Sleep and Epilepsy. Cambridge: Cambridge University Press; 2003.
163. McCormick DA, Prince DA. Actions of acetylcholine in the guinea-pig and cat medial and lateral geniculate nuclei, in vitro. J Physiol (Lond). 1987;392:147–165.
164. Hu B, Steriade M, Deschênes M. The effects of brainstem peribrachial stimulation on neurons of the lateral geniculate nucleus. Neuroscience. 1989;31:13–24.
165. Hu B, Steriade M, Deschênes M. The effects of brainstem peribrachial stimulation on perigeniculate neurons: the blockage of spindle waves. Neuroscience. 1989;31:1–12.
166. Saalmann YB, Pinsk MA, Wang L, Li X, Kastner S. The pulvinar regulates information transmission between cortical areas based on attention demands. Science. 2012;337:753–756.
167. Morison RS, Bassett DL. Electrical activity of the thalamus and basal ganglia in decorticate cats. J Neurophysiol. 1945;8:09–314.
168. Steriade M, Llinás RR. The functional states of the thalamus and the associated neuronal interplay. Physiol Rev. 1988;68:649–742.
169. Steriade M. Cellular substrates of brain rhythms. In: Niedermeyer E, Lopes da Silva FH, eds. Electroencephalography: Basic Principles, Clinical Applications and Related Fields. Baltimore: Lippincott Williams & Wilkins; 2005:31–84.
170. Jones EG. The Thalamus. New York: Plenum; 1985.
171. Domich L, Oakson G, Deschênes M, Steriade M. Thalamic and cortical spindles during early ontogenesis in kittens. Brain Res. 1987;428:140–142.
172. Steriade M, Deschênes M, Domich L, Mulle C. Abolition of spindle oscillations in thalamic neurons disconnected from nucleus reticularis thalami. J Neurophysiol. 1985;54:1473–1497.
173. Steriade M, Domich L, Oakson G, Deschênes M. The deafferented reticular thalamic nucleus generates spindle rhythmicity. J Neurophysiol. 1987;57:260–273.
174. Steriade M, Deschênes M. The thalamus as a neuronal oscillator. Brain Res. 1984;320:1–63.

175. Velayos JL, Jimenez-Castellanos J Jr, Reinoso-Suarez F. Topographical organization of the projections from the reticular thalamic nucleus to the intralaminar and medial thalamic nuclei in the cat. J Comp Neurol. 1989;279:457–469.

176. Paré D, Steriade M, Deschênes M, Oakson G. Physiological characteristics of anterior thalamic nuclei, a group devoid of inputs from reticular thalamic nucleus. J Neurophysiol. 1987;57:1669–1685.

177. Leung LW, Borst JG. Electrical activity of the cingulate cortex. I. Generating mechanisms and relations to behavior. Brain Res. 1987;407:68–80.

178. Wang XJ, Rinzel J. Spindle rhythmicity in the reticularis thalami nucleus: synchronization among mutually inhibitory neurons. Neuroscience. 1993;53:899–904.

179. Destexhe A, Contreras D, Sejnowski TJ, Steriade M. A model of spindle rhythmicity in the isolated thalamic reticular nucleus. J Neurophysiol. 1994;72:803–818.

180. Golomb D, Wang XJ, Rinzel J. Synchronization properties of spindle oscillations in a thalamic reticular nucleus model. J Neurophysiol. 1994;72:1109–1126.

181. Deschênes M, Paradis M, Roy JP, Steriade M. Electrophysiology of neurons of lateral thalamic nuclei in cat: resting properties and burst discharges. J Neurophysiol. 1984;51:1196–1219.

182. Yen CT, Conley M, Hendry SH, Jones EG. The morphology of physiologically identified GABAergic neurons in the somatic sensory part of the thalamic reticular nucleus in the cat. J Neurosci. 1985;5:2254–2268.

183. Williamson AM, Ohara PT, Ralston DD, Milroy AM, Ralston HJ III. Analysis of gamma-aminobutyric acidergic synaptic contacts in the thalamic reticular nucleus of the monkey. J Comp Neurol. 1994;349:182–192.

184. Landisman CE, Long MA, Beierlein M, Deans MR, Paul DL, Connors BW. Electrical synapses in the thalamic reticular nucleus. J Neurosci. 2002;22:1002–1009.

185. Yen CT, Jones EG. Intracellular staining of physiologically identified neurons and axons in the somatosensory thalamus of the cat. Brain Res. 1983;280:148–154.

186. von Krosigk M, Bal T, McCormick DA. Cellular mechanisms of a synchronized oscillation in the thalamus. Science. 1993;261:361–364.

187. Bal T, von Krosigk M, McCormick DA. Role of the ferret perigeniculate nucleus in the generation of synchronized oscillations in vitro. J Physiol (Lond). 1995;483 (Pt 3):665–685.

188. Bal T, von Krosigk M, McCormick DA. Synaptic and membrane mechanisms underlying synchronized oscillations in the ferret lateral geniculate nucleus in vitro. J Physiol (Lond). 1995;483 (Pt 3):641–663.

189. Contreras D, Destexhe A, Sejnowski TJ, Steriade M. Control of spatiotemporal coherence of a thalamic oscillation by corticothalamic feedback. Science. 1996;274:771–774.

190. Contreras D, Destexhe A, Sejnowski TJ, Steriade M. Spatiotemporal patterns of spindle oscillations in cortex and thalamus. J Neurosci. 1997;17:1179–1196.

191. Jahnsen H, Llinás R. Electrophysiological properties of guinea-pig thalamic neurones: an in vitro study. J Physiol (Lond). 1984;349:205–226.

192. Mulle C, Steriade M, Deschênes M. The effects of QX314 on thalamic neurons. Brain Res. 1985;333:350–354.

193. McCormick DA. Functional properties of a slowly inactivating potassium current in guinea pig dorsal lateral geniculate relay neurons. J Neurophysiol. 1991;66:1176–1189.

194. Budde T, Mager R, Pape HC. Different types of potassium outward current in relay neurons acutely isolated from the rat lateral geniculate nucleus. Eur J Neurosci. 1992;4:708–722.

195. Contreras D, Steriade M. Spindle oscillation in cats: the role of corticothalamic feedback in a thalamically generated rhythm. J Physiol (Lond). 1996;490 (Pt 1):159–179.

196. Kim U, Bal T, McCormick DA. Spindle waves are propagating synchronized oscillations in the ferret LGNd in vitro. J Neurophysiol. 1995;74:1301–1323.

197. Jensen O, Gips B, Bergmann TO, Bonnefond M. Temporl coding organized by coupled alpha and gamma oscillations prioritize visual processing. Trends Neurosci. 2014;37(7):357–369.

198. Lopes da Silva FH. EEG and MEG: relevance to neuroscience. Neuron. 2013;80:1112–1128.

199. Moruzzi G, Magoun HW. Brain stem reticular formation and activation of the EEG. Electroencephalogr Clin Neurophysiol. 1949;1:445–473.

200. McCormick DA, Prince DA. Acetylcholine induces burst firing in thalamic reticular neurones by activating a potassium conductance. Nature. 1986;319:402–405.

201. McCormick DA, Wang Z. Serotonin and noradrenaline excite GABAergic neurones of the guinea-pig and cat nucleus reticularis thalami. J Physiol (Lond). 1991;442:235–255.

202. McCormick DA, Pape HC. Noradrenergic and serotonergic modulation of a hyperpolarization-activated cation current in thalamic relay neurones. J Physiol (Lond). 1990;431:319–342.

203. Buzsáki G, Bickford RG, Ponomareff G, Thal LJ, Mandel R, Gage FH. Nucleus basalis and thalamic control of neocortical activity in the freely moving rat. J Neurosci. 1988;8:4007–4026.

204. Bremer F, Stoupel N, Van Reeth PC. Nouvelles recherches sur la facilitation et l'inhibition des potentiels évoqués corticaux dans l'éveil réticulaire. Arch Ital Biol. 1960;98:229–247.

205. Lopes da Silva FH, van Rotterdam A, Storm van Leeuwen W, Tielen AM. Dynamic characteristics of visual evoked potentials in the dog. II. Beta frequency selectivity in evoked potentials and background activity. Electroencephalogr Clin Neurophysiol. 1970;29:260–268.

206. Freeman WJ, van Dijk BW. Spatial patterns of visual cortical fast EEG during conditioned reflex in a rhesus monkey. Brain Res. 1987;422:267–276.

207. Murthy VN, Fetz EE. Coherent 25- to 35-Hz oscillations in the sensorimotor cortex of awake behaving monkeys. Proc Natl Acad Sci USA. 1992;89:5670–5674.

208. Bouyer JJ, Montaron MF, Vahnee JM, Albert MP, Rougeul A. Anatomical localization of cortical beta rhythms in cat. Neuroscience. 1987;22:863–869.

209. Freeman WJ. Mass Action in the Nervous System. New York: Academic Press; 1975.

210. Eckhorn R, Bauer R, Jordan W, et al. Coherent oscillations: a mechanism of feature linking in the visual cortex? Multiple electrode and correlation analyses in the cat. Biol Cybern. 1988;60:121–130.

211. Gray CM, Singer W. Stimulus-specific neuronal oscillations in orientation columns of cat visual cortex. Proc Natl Acad Sci USA. 1989;86:1698–1702.

212. Gray CM, König P, Engel AK, Singer W. Oscillatory responses in cat visual cortex exhibit inter-columnar synchronization which reflects global stimulus properties. Nature. 1989;338:334–337.

213. Gray CM, Engel AK, König P, Singer W. Stimulus-dependent neuronal oscillations in cat visual cortex: receptive field properties and feature dependence. Eur J Neurosci. 1990;2:607–619.

214. Engel AK, König P, Gray CM, Singer W. Stimulus-dependent neuronal oscillations in cat visual cortex: inter-columnar interaction as determined by cross-correlation analysis. Eur J Neurosci. 1990;2:588–606.

215. Rodriguez R, Kallenbach U, Singer W, Munk MH. Short- and long-term effects of cholinergic modulation on gamma oscillations and response synchronization in the visual cortex. J Neurosci. 2004;24:10369–10378.

216. Munk MH, Roelfsema PR, König P, Engel AK, Singer W. Role of reticular activation in the modulation of intracortical synchronization. Science 1996;272:271–274.

217. von der Malsburg C, Schneider W. A neural cocktail-party processor. Biol Cybern. 1986;54:29–40.

218. Steriade M, Amzica F. Intracortical and corticothalamic coherency of fast spontaneous oscillations. Proc Natl Acad Sci USA. 1996;93:2533–2538.

219. Steriade M, Contreras D, Amzica F, Timofeev I. Synchronization of fast (30–40 Hz) spontaneous oscillations in intrathalamic and thalamocortical networks. J Neurosci. 1996;16:2788–2808.

220. Roelfsema PR, Engel AK, König P, Singer W. Visuomotor integration is associated with zero time-lag synchronization among cortical areas. Nature. 1997;385:157–161.

221. Fries P, Nikolic D, Singer W. The gamma cycle. Trends Neurosci. 2007;30:309–316.

222. Fries P. Rhythms for cognition: communication through coherence. Neuron. 2015;88: 220–235.

223. Llinás RR, Grace AA, Yarom Y. In vitro neurons in mammalian cortical layer 4 exhibit intrinsic oscillatory activity in the 10- to 50-Hz frequency range. Proc Natl Acad Sci USA. 1991;88:897–901.

224. Nuñez A, Amzica F, Steriade M. Voltage-dependent fast (20–40 Hz) oscillations in long-axoned neocortical neurons. Neuroscience. 1992;51:7–10.

225. Steriade M, Curró Dossi R, Paré D, Oakson G. Fast oscillations (20–40 Hz) in thalamocortical systems and their potentiation by mesopontine cholinergic nuclei in the cat. Proc Natl Acad Sci USA. 1991;88:4396–4400.

226. Jones EG. The Thalamus. New York: Plenum; 1985.

227. Cunningham ET, LeVay S. Laminar and synaptic organization of the projection from the thalamic nucleus centralis to primary visual cortex in the cat. J Comp Neurol. 1986;254:66–77.

228. Chagnac-Amitai Y, Connors BW. Synchronized excitation and inhibition driven by intrinsically bursting neurons in neocortex. J Neurophysiol. 1989;62:1149–1162.

229. Hösli L, Hösli E, Della BG, Quadri L, Heuss L. Action of acetylcholine, muscarine, nicotine and antagonists on the membrane potential of astrocytes in cultured rat brainstem and spinal cord. Neurosci Lett. 1988;92:165–170.

230. Seigneur J, Kroeger D, Nita DA, Amzica F. Cholinergic action on cortical glial cells in vivo. Cereb Cortex. 2006;16:655–668.
231. Roopun AK, Middleton SJ, Cunningham MO, et al. A beta2-frequency (20–30 Hz) oscillation in nonsynaptic networks of somatosensory cortex. Proc Natl Acad Sci USA. 2006;103:15646–15650.
232. Mandema JW, Danhof M. Electroencephalogram effect measures and relationships between pharmacokinetics and pharmacodynamics of centrally acting drugs. Clin Pharmacokinet. 1992;23:191–215.
233. Spaak E, Bonnefond M, Maier A, Leopold DA, Jensen O. Layer-specific entrainment of gamma-band neural activity by the alpha rhythm in monkey visual cortex. Curr Biol. 2012;22:2313–2318.
234. Bacci A, Huguenard JR, Prince DA. Modulation of neocortical interneurons: extrinsic influences and exercises in self-control. Trends Neurosci. 2005;28(11):602–610.
235. McCormick DA, Prince DA. Mechanisms of action of acetylcholine in the guinea-pig cerebral cortex in vitro. J Physiol (Lond). 1986;375:169–194.
236. Buffalo EA, Fries P, Landman R, Buschman TJ, Desimone R. Laminar differences in gamma and alpha coherence in the ventral stream. Proc Natl Acad Sci USA. 2011;108:11262–11267.
237. Salenius S, Salmelin R, Neuper C, Pfurtscheller G, Hari R. Human cortical 40 Hz rhythm is closely related to EMG rhythmicity. Neurosci Lett. 1996;213:75–78.
238. Salenius S, Portin K, Kajola M, Salmelin R, Hari R. Cortical control of human motoneuron firing during isometric contraction. J Neurophysiol. 1997;77:3401–3405.
239. Gross J, Tass PA, Salenius S, Hari R, Freund HJ, Schnitzler A. Corticomuscular synchronization during isometric muscle contraction in humans as revealed by magnetoencephalography. J Physiol (Lond). 2000;527 (Pt 3):623–631.
240. Hari R. Action-perception connection and the cortical mu rhythm. Prog Brain Res. 2006;159:253–260.
241. Pfurtscheller G, Neuper C, Andrew C, Edlinger G. Foot and hand area mu rhythms. Int J Psychophysiol. 1997;26:121–135.
242. Chen R, Yaseen Z, Cohen LG, Hallett M. Time course of corticospinal excitability in reaction time and self-paced movements. Ann Neurol. 1998;44:317–325.
243. Brittain JS, Sharott A, Brown P. The highs and lows of beta activity in cortico-basal ganglia loops. Eur J Neurosci. 2014;39:1951–1959.
244. Pfurtscheller G, Neuper C, Kalcher J. 40-Hz oscillations during motor behavior in man. Neurosci Lett. 1993;164:179–182.
245. Vanhatalo S, Tallgren P, Andersson S, Sainio K, Voipio J, Kaila K. DC-EEG discloses prominent, very slow activity patterns during sleep in preterm infants. Clin Neurophysiol. 2002;113:1822–1825.
246. Vanhatalo S, Holmes MD, Tallgren P, Voipio J, Kaila K, Miller JW. Very slow EEG responses lateralize temporal lobe seizures: an evaluation of non-invasive DC-EEG. Neurology. 2003;60:1098–1104.
247. Somjen GG. Electrogenesis of sustained potentials. Progr Neurobiol. 1973;1:201–237.
248. Somjen GG, Trachtenberg M. Neuroglial as generator of extracellular current. In: Speckmann EJ, Caspers H, eds. Origin of Cerebral Field Potentials. Stuttgart: Thieme; 1979:21–32.
249. Caspers H, Speckmann EJ, Lehmenkuler A. DC potentials of the cerebral cortex: seizure activity and changes in gas pressures. Rev Physiol Biochem Pharmacol. 1987;106:127–178.
250. Heinemann U, Walz W. Contributions of potassium currents and glia to slow potential shifts (SPSs). In: Laming PR, Sykova E, Reichenbach A, Haton GI, Bauer H, eds. Glial Cells: Their Role in Behaviour. Cambridge: Cambridge University Press; 1998:197–209.
251. Amzica F, Steriade M. Neuronal and glial membrane potentials during sleep and paroxysmal oscillations in the neocortex. J Neurosci. 2000;20:6648–6665.
252. Tschirgi RD, Taylor JL. Slowly changing bioelectric potentials associated with the blood-brain barrier. Am J Physiol. 1958;195:7–22.
253. Held D, Fencl V, Pappenheimer JR. Electric potential of cerebrospinal fluid. J Neurophysiol. 1964;27:942–959.
254. Kjällquist Å, Siesjö BK. Regulation of CSF pH-influence of the CSF/plasma potential. Scand J Clin Lab Invest. 1968;102:I:C.
255. Sorensen SC, Severinghaus JW. Effect of cerebral acidosis on the CSF-blood potential difference. Am J Physiol. 1970;219:68–71.
256. Hornbein TF, Sorensen SC. DC potential difference between different cerebrospinal fluid sites and blood in dogs. Am J Physiol. 1972;223:415–418.
257. Woody CD, Marshall WH, Besson JM, Thompson HK, Aleonard P, Albe-Fessard D. Brain potential shift with respiratory acidosis in the cat and monkey. Am J Physiol. 1970;218:275–283.
258. Revest PA, Jones HC, Abbott NJ. The transendothelial DC potential of rat blood-brain barrier vessels in situ. Adv Exp Med Biol. 1993;331:71–74.
259. Voipio J, Tallgren P, Heinonen E, Vanhatalo S, Kaila K. Millivolt-scale DC shifts in the human scalp EEG: evidence for a nonneuronal generator. J Neurophysiol. 2003;89:2208–2214.
260. Nita DA, Vanhatalo S, Lafortune FD, Voipio J, Kaila K, Amzica F. Nonneuronal origin of CO_2-related DC EEG shifts: an in vivo study in the cat. J Neurophysiol. 2004;92:1011–1022.
261. Speckmann EJ, Elger CE. Introduction to the neurophysiological basis of the EEG and DC potentials. In: Niedermeyer E, Lopes da Silva FH, eds. Electroencephalography: Basic Principles, Clinical Applications, and Related Fields. Baltimore: Lippincott, Williams & Wilkins; 2005:17–30.
262. Kroeger D, Amzica F. Hypersensitivity of the anesthesia-induced comatose brain. J Neurosci. 2007;27:10597–10607.
263. Ferron JF, Kroeger D, Chever O, Amzica F. Cortical inhibition during burst suppression induced with isoflurane anesthesia. J Neurosci. 2009;29:9850–9860.
264. Steriade M, Amzica F, Contreras D. Cortical and thalamic cellular correlates of electroencephalographic burst-suppression. Electroencephalogr Clin Neurophysiol. 1994;90:1–16.
265. Kroeger D, Florea B, Amzica F. Human brain activity patterns beyond the isoelectric line of extreme deep coma. PLoS One. 2013;8(9):e75257.

3 | DYNAMICS OF EEGS AS SIGNALS OF NEURONAL POPULATIONS: MODELS AND THEORETICAL CONSIDERATIONS

FABRICE WENDLING, ENG, PHD AND FERNANDO H. LOPES DA SILVA, MD, PHD

ABSTRACT: This chapter gives an overview of approaches used to understand the generation of electroencephalographic (EEG) signals using computational models. The basic concept is that appropriate modeling of neuronal networks, based on relevant anatomical and physiological data, allows researchers to test hypotheses about the nature of EEG signals. Here these models are considered at different levels of complexity. The first level is based on single cell biophysical properties anchored in classic Hodgkin-Huxley theory. The second level emphasizes on detailed neuronal networks and their role in generating different kinds of EEG oscillations. At the third level are models derived from the Wilson-Cowan approach, which constitutes the backbone of neural mass models. Another part of the chapter is dedicated to models of epileptiform activities. Finally, the themes of nonlinear dynamic systems and topological models in EEG generation are discussed.

KEYWORDS: electroencephalography, EEG, oscillations, models, neural mass model, epilepsy, nonlinear dynamics

PRINCIPAL REFERENCES

BOOKS

1. Malmivuo J, Plonsey R. Bioelectromagnetism—Principles and Applications of Bioelectric and Biomagnetic Fields. Oxford University Press, 1995.
2. Bower J, Beeman D. The Book of GENESIS: Exploring Realistic Neural Models with the General Neural Simulations System. Springer, 1995.
3. Gerstner W, Kistler WM. Spiking Neuron Models. Cambridge University Press, 2002.
4. Soltesz I, Staley KJ. Computational Neuroscience in Epilepsy. Academic Press, 2008.

REVIEW AND ORIGINAL ARTICLES

1. Wendling F, Benquet P, Bartolomei F, Jirsa V. Computational models of epileptiform activity. Journal of Neuroscience Methods. 2016;260:233–251.
2. Lytton WW. Computer modelling of epilepsy. Nature Reviews Neuroscience. 2008;9(8):626–637.
3. Deco G, Jirsa VK, Robinson PA, Breakspear M, Friston K. *The dynamic brain: from spiking neurons to neural masses and cortical fields.* PLoS Computational Biology. 2008;4(8):e1000092.
4. Suffczynski P, Wendling F, Bellanger J, Lopes da Silva FH. *Some insights into computational models of (patho)physiological brain activity.* Proceedings of the IEEE. 2006;784–804.
5. Wright JJ, Robinson PA, Rennie CJ, Gordon E, Bourke PD, Chapman CL, et al. *Toward an integrated continuum model of cerebral dynamics: the cerebral rhythms, synchronous oscillation and cortical stability.* BioSystems. 2001;63(1-3):71–88.

1. INTRODUCTION: MODELS OF EEG GENERATION

In Chapter 2 the neurophysiological basis of the electroencephalogram (EEG) was discussed, with special emphasis on phenomena at the cellular and membrane levels. In **Chapter 4**, the biophysical aspects of the generation of EEG signals are considered mainly in terms of electric and magnetic fields and volume conduction, but their dynamic properties of EEG patterns are only briefly mentioned. These dynamic properties, however, are essential for understanding EEG phenomena. In this chapter, EEG signals are considered as the result of the dynamic behavior of neuronal populations as revealed by modeling studies. According to this perspective, we must integrate experimental and theoretical results using models of neuronal networks and corresponding computer simulations. Paraphrasing the quote of the famous physicist Richard Feynman[1] "What I cannot create, I do not understand," we may state that the *creation* of computational models of EEG phenomena is a step forward in *understanding* how these phenomena are generated.

The mathematical treatment of such models has been avoided here; the interested reader is referred to a number of other publications that are cited for their thorough mathematical treatment of these issues. The fundamental assumption on which the following discussion is based is that EEG signals reflect the dynamics of electrical activity in populations of neurons, although attention must be paid to the detailed properties of neuronal membranes and synaptic processes. A property of such populations that is of essential importance for the generation of EEG signals is the capacity of the neurons to work in synchrony. This depends on the functional connectivity between the neurons that form a network.

2. MICROSCOPIC AND MACROSCOPIC MODELS OF GENERATION OF LOCAL FIELD POTENTIALS AND EEG SIGNALS

Local field potentials (LFPs) and EEG signals are signals collected at the level of electrodes positioned either on the head (scalp EEG) or on the cortical surface (ECoG), or directly

---

[1] Richard P. Feynman in Wikiquote.

embedded in the brain tissue (intracerebral EEG [iEEG]). These signals reflect summated currents generated by active cells within neuronal assemblies and flowing through the extracellular medium. As this medium is mainly characterized by its resistivity, a potential difference can be measured between two electrodes positioned either close (LFPs) or more distantly (EEG) from neuronal sources. These physiological and biophysical considerations show that measured potentials correspond to the superimposition of many current sources shaping the extracellular field.

Electrophysiological signals convey essential functional information about the activity of neurons (LFPs), neuronal assemblies (LFPs, iEEG, ECoG), brain areas (iEEG), and the whole brain (scalp EEG). Decoding this information is a difficult issue as many neurophysiological factors intervene in the generation of LFPs and EEG signals, and many biophysical factors are involved in their recording. Typically, synaptic transmembrane currents (either excitatory or inhibitory) are the main contributors to LFPs and EEG signals. However, depending on the recording technique, on the size of electrodes, and on the electrode position, configuration, and distance with respect to neurons, other sources like currents flowing through ion channels can also have an impact on the intracellular-LFP transfer function [1] and subsequently on collected signals. To better understand the complexity of this transfer between cellular phenomena and LFPs, computer modeling is strongly advised.

In these models, a crucial feature is the level of detail required to account for a particular activity or phenomenon occurring in neuronal assemblies. The choice of the level depends on the questions being addressed, on the mechanisms potentially involved in the considered phenomena, and on the nature of the available real observations. In essence a model is constructed to answer well-defined questions with respect to specific features of the phenomenon of interest. With respect to the working of neuronal networks the latter may be modeled at different levels of complexity. Accordingly, we may distinguish models of neuronal phenomena at the microscopic level built up from the properties of single neurons and assemblies of neurons, or at the macroscopic level of neural populations or neural masses based on averaged quantities related to neuronal properties and functions. In practical terms the computing cost may also be a factor to consider as simulations from detailed models may still need to be performed on high-performance computers, as compared with lumped-parameter models.

In the following sections, two complementary physiology-based modeling approaches are described. In the first one (Section 2.1), referred to as "microscopic," single neurons are accurately modeled regarding their structural components (dendrites, soma, axon) and functional properties (passive and active ion channels). Networks of neurons (Section 2.2) are then built from the interconnection (via synapses and/or gap junctions) of a relatively large number of cells (typically principal neurons and interneurons). From these networks, LFPs can be reconstructed from summated postsynaptic potentials (PSPs) generated at the level of principal neurons. Microscopic models offer the opportunity to analyze both cell-related and network-related factors that intervene in the generation of LFPs in particular oscillations; these factors include types of neurons, their firing patterns, the network size, the coupling and connectivity patterns between neurons, the synchronization processes, and others. Readers may refer to the book by Gerstner and Kistler [2], which addresses some of these issues through didactic material about detailed neuron and distributed network models.

The second approach (Section 2.3) is referred to as "macroscopic" or "lumped" as it directly considers the neuronal population level without explicit representation of specific properties of individual cells. This approach was initially proposed by Wilson and Cowan [3]. The key idea is to describe ensemble dynamics as reflected in LFPs through interactions (typically synaptic) among interconnected sub-populations of excitatory and inhibitory neurons, taking into account physiological data. Based on this idea, population models represent the temporal dynamics of neuronal aggregates while the spatial dimension is neglected. The assumption is that the relevant variables in these models are the average PSPs and average firing rate of each sub-population, contrasting with detailed models that explicitly represent individual spikes and PSPs.

2.1. Microscopic Models: Basic Principles, the Hodgkin and Huxley Approach

In this section, we present the basic principles of detailed models that consist of distributed networks of neurons. This section starts from the description of *models of single neurons* with special emphasis on the Hodgkin and Huxley formalism that is still largely used to develop neurophysiologically relevant neural network models. Then, some *network models* are presented, providing insights into the mechanisms of generation of oscillations, as reflected in LFP/EEG signals.

2.1.1. MODELS OF SINGLE CELL ACTIVITY: HODGKIN AND HUXLEY'S THEORY

To explain the initiation and propagation pattern of action potentials (APs) along the giant axon of the squid, Hodgkin and Huxley developed a seminal mathematical model (referred to as the HH model in the following) in the early 1950s [4]. Since then, the HH approach has been extended and extensively used to describe the ionic mechanisms involved in the generation of APs in excitable cells such as neurons and nervous fibers.

Hodgkin and Huxley's main discovery is that ionic channels are not purely passive. Indeed, to reproduce the features of actual APs, they assumed and modeled voltage-dependent ion channels governing the transmembrane potassium (I_K) and sodium (I_{Na}) currents, in addition to passive channels involved in leak currents (I_L).

Thus, according to the HH model, a small segment of neuron membrane is considered and treated as an equivalent electrical circuit. As illustrated in Figure 3.1A, this electrical circuit describes the biophysical mechanisms occurring across the cell lipid bilayer membrane—that is, the ion fluxes exchanged between the intracellular space (ICS) and the extracellular space (ECS).

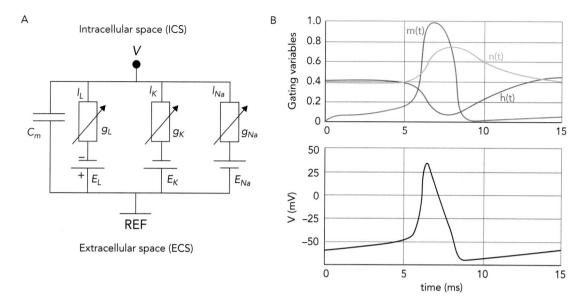

Figure 3.1. *The HH model describes the transmembrane currents flowing through ionic channels and the membrane capacitance C_m. **A:** It includes three types of currents: sodium (I_{Na}), potassium (I_K), and leakage (I_L), and the corresponding channel conductances (g_{Na}, g_K, and g_L) and equilibrium potentials (E_{Na}, E_K, and E_L). **B:** g_{Na} and g_K are "active" or "voltage-dependent" in contrast with the passive g_L. They depend on three gating variables (m, n, and h); upon stimulation the value of the gating variables dynamically changes with that of the membrane potential explaining, for instance, the firing and the time course of an AP (**B**, bottom) when the stimulus intensity is sufficiently large (simulation performed using equations 1, 2, and 3 with the following values: E_{Na} = 55 mV; E_K = −72 mV; E_L = −50 mV; C_m = 1 µF/cm²; I_{inj} = 9 µA/cm²; $\bar{g}_{Na}$ = 120 mS/cm²; $\bar{g}_K$ = 36 mS/cm²; $\bar{g}_L$ = 0.3 mS/cm²).*

As depicted in Figure 3.1A, any variation of the membrane potential V measured between the ICS and the ECS can be expressed as a function of the sum of ionic currents (I_L, I_K, I_{Na}) flowing through the cell membrane, itself characterized by (1) its capacitance (C_m), (2) the conductances associated with specific passive (g_L) and active (g_K and g_{Na}) ion channels, and (3) by ionic reversal (also called equilibrium) potentials (E_L, E_K, E_{Na}):

$$C_m \frac{dV}{dt} = \sum_{z=leak,K,N_a} g_z \left(V(t) - E_z\right) + I_{inj}(t), \quad \textbf{(Eq. 1)}$$

with

$$I_z(t) = g_z(V(t) - E_z) \quad \textbf{(Eq. 2)}$$

where I_{inj} denotes an injected current (synaptic current or experimentally injected current).

The "core" of the HH model is the nonlinear mathematical description of the time and the voltage dependence of Na and K conductances (g_K, g_{Na}). By performing voltage-clamp experiments, Hodgkin and Huxley were able to determine the time dependence, the maximum value, and the equilibrium value of sodium and potassium conductances at different voltages. Experimental measurements could then be accurately fitted by cubic and quadratic functions of so-called activation and inactivation variables, denoted by m, h, and n: $g_{Na} = \bar{g}_{Na} \cdot m^3 h$, $g_K = \bar{g}_K \cdot n^4$ (Eq. 3). These variables can be interpreted as a fraction of channel gates being in permissive state (hence, they can vary from 0 to 1), whereas $\bar{g}_{Na}$ and $\bar{g}_K$ represent maximal conductance values.

The value of activation and inactivation variables dynamically changes with that of the membrane potential

(conductance increases or decreases with depolarization). The kinetics of these changes, illustrated in Figure 3.1B, are given by the two following equations:

$$\frac{dn(V)}{dt} = \alpha_n(V)(1-n) - \beta_n(V)_n \quad \text{for K channels,}$$

and

$$\frac{dq(V)}{dt} = \alpha_q(V)(1-q) - \beta_q(V)_q \quad \left(q \text{ standing for } m, h\right) \text{ for NA channels.}$$

Functions α and β of V were empirically adjusted by Hodgkin and Huxley to fit the data of the giant axon of the squid (see Table 2.1 in [2] for α and β functions and for parameter values in the HH equations).

Several algorithms for the optimization of microscopic neuron models with respect to electrophysiological data have been developed. The interested reader can find more detailed analyses of such algorithms, such as the widely used "Neuron," a simulation environment for modeling individual neurons and networks, in [5], [6], and associated references. Here we only sketch some of the main features of the field.

2.1.2. FROM HH TO SINGLE CELL MODELS

Single cell models attempt to represent typical functional and/or structural features of real neurons. Most of these models use compartments to describe passive electrical (membrane capacitance, axial resistivity, leak conductance, membrane time constant, leak reversal potential) and active electrical (voltage-dependent ion channels, according to the HH model) properties that are usually specific to the considered cell type. By definition, these "multicompartment" models

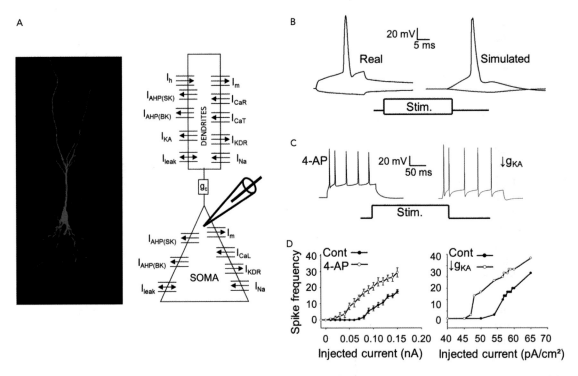

Figure 3.2. An example of a "reduced" neuron model for the hippocampal CA1 pyramidal cell. **A:** Two-compartment CA1 pyramidal neuron model. Both compartments include voltage-dependent sodium currents (I_{Na}), potassium delayed-rectifier currents (I_{KDR}), calcium-dependent potassium (I_{AHP}) currents, a muscarinic potassium current (I_m), and a nonspecific leak current (I_{Leak}). The soma adds an L-type calcium current (I_{CAL}). Dendrites have T- and R-type calcium currents (I_{CaT}, I_{CaR}), a fast inactivating potassium current (I_{KA}), and a hyperpolarization activated cationic current (I_h). Coupling between soma and dendrites is ensured by conductance g_c. **B:** Comparison between simulated and actual AP recorded from CA1 pyramidal cell upon supra-threshold stimulation. **C:** Comparison between experimental and simulated intracellular activity. Left: under 4AP (real case); right: by decreasing g_{KA} in the model. **D:** Firing rate as function of depolarizing current. Left: in real cells in control condition (Cont) or in the presence of 4AP; right: on simulated neurons. (Adapted from Demont-Guignard, S., et al., Analysis of intracerebral EEG recordings of epileptic spikes: insights from a neural network model. *IEEE Trans Biomed Eng*, 2009. 56(12): p. 2782–2795.)

treat the structural elements of neurons as multiple interconnected compartments with isopotential and spatially uniform properties. This spatial discretization has two major advantages. First, from the structural viewpoint, membrane non-uniformities such as variations in diameter can be accounted for. Second, and similarly, distinct functional properties (such as the different electrical features of dendrites, soma, and axon) can also be represented using different compartments. Coupling conductances between compartments ensure the propagation of changes of membrane potential from a given compartment to the neighbors. Based on this approach, very detailed neuron models (containing up to several thousands of compartments) were proposed, allowing the representation of complicated dendritic three-dimensional structures. These models vary according to ion currents represented at the level of dendrites, soma, or axon, and are used for many different purposes and applications, up to the "Blue Brain project," where this approach is extended to the level of the reconstruction and simulation of the anatomy and physiology of a complex neocortical circuit of the rat somatosensory cortex [7].

Besides "very detailed" multicompartment representations, "reduced" models were also proposed. Following Pinsky and Rinzel's approach [8], Demont-Guignard et al. [9] developed a two-compartment model of a CA1 pyramidal neuron (Fig. 3.2). In this section, this model will serve as an illustration

of some of the simulation results that can be obtained from single cell models. The proposed model is minimal but still biologically justified. Based on the HH formalism described above, the model includes distinct dendritic and somatic membrane properties (active and passive). As shown in Figure 3.2A, a number of ionic currents were implemented in both compartments, according to data from the literature and our own experimental data. As shown in Figure 3.2B, the shape of the simulated AP, mainly controlled by voltage-dependent sodium, potassium, and calcium currents (I_{Na}, I_{KDR}, I_{Ca}, low and high threshold), matches that of actual APs recorded in CA1 pyramidal cell. Parameters could also be adjusted to reproduce intracellular experimental data under conditions of hyperexcitability induced by 4-aminopyridine (4AP, a nonselective voltage-dependent K+-channel blocker). As depicted in Figure 3.2C, the decrease of g_{KA} causes the model to switch from normal to bursting activity, as also observed experimentally. Finally, the model reproduces quite well the average effect of different depolarizing pulses on CA1 pyramidal cell firing rate, both in the absence (control condition) or in the presence of 4AP as simulated by the decrease of g_{KA} value (see Fig. 3.2D).

2.1.3. NEURONAL INTRINSIC OSCILLATIONS

Some neurons may display *in vitro* "intrinsic oscillations" that appear without a specific stimulus and are independent of local network synaptic connections, aside from those oscillations that depend on the action of synaptic transmitters. Regarding "intrinsic oscillations" we should note that the HH model is a system of nonlinear equations constituted by time- and voltage-dependent conductances (g_K, g_{Na}). Nonlinear systems like this may have very different behaviors depending on even small changes of state variables such as of ionic conductances. In the case of the HH model, raising the value of g_{Na}, for example, can result in the neuron entering a limit cycle (i.e., displaying a self-sustained oscillation), or, according to terms used in physiology, generating an "intrinsic" or "pacemaker-like" oscillation. This is, for example, the case of the voltage-dependent oscillations reported by Leresche et al. [10] of thalamocortical cells *in vitro*. An advanced nonlinear analysis of neuronal subthreshold oscillations was presented by White et al. [11], who used nonlinear dynamic techniques to unravel the mechanisms underlying subthreshold oscillations in entorhinal cortical neurons. This modeling analysis revealed the conditions under which a persistent Na$^+$ current and a delayed K$^+$ current are able to generate subthreshold oscillations in those neurons; an I_h current (hyperpolarization-induced slow rectifying inward cation current) might be an alternative to the latter. In short, combinations of different membrane ionic currents can lead to intrinsic oscillations. The existence of interacting nonlinear conductances with opposite effects on membrane potential, given the appropriate time constants, may be sufficient to generate membrane potential oscillations. In addition, a neuron can also display resonance; in other words, it may respond preferentially to inputs within a specific frequency range due to the filtering properties of the corresponding neuronal membrane. Simple models of these dynamic properties are insightfully described by Hutcheon and Yarom [12].

2.2. Models of Detailed Neural Networks and Oscillations

For studies of network phenomena such as those involved in physiological and/or pathological oscillations, realistic network models have been proposed based on the interconnection of a number of single neuron models via synaptic or electrical (gap junction) couplings. Models of synapses incorporate transfer functions describing the variation of the membrane potential of the postsynaptic neuron Y upon occurrence of an AP in the presynaptic neuron X. This variation can be either positive (depolarization, typically mediated at glutamatergic synapses) or negative (hyperpolarization, typically mediated at GABAergic synapses). In general, synaptic currents are generated by ionic channels coupled to receptors at the postsynaptic level, generally written as $I_{syn} = g_{syn}(V - E_{syn})$ where V is the membrane potential, g_{syn} is the synaptic conductance, and E_{syn} is the equilibrium potential for the corresponding ion type.

In addition, electrical coupling models describe a physical connection between two neurons that allows for direct transfer of ions through gap junctions. Unlike models including chemical synapses, gap junction models are generally simple. They usually consist in an ohmic resistance $1/g_{XY}$ allowing for

current $I_{XY} = g_{XY}(V_Y - V_X)$ to flow between two membrane compartments with potential V_X and V_Y, respectively, the first one belonging to neuron X and the second one to neuron Y.

In the following, we briefly describe a number of studies based on detailed network models and aimed at explaining the genesis of *neuronal oscillations* at the network level observed under normal or pathological conditions.

In most of these models, the simulated extracellular field potential, or LFP, is calculated as the sum of membrane potentials generated at the level of principal cells, simply applying low-pass filtering to reduce the contribution of fast events (like APs). More sophisticated methods for reconstructing extracellularly recorded signals from network models were proposed, making use of the dipole theory and accounting for physical factors (cell orientation, cell–electrode distance) to solve the LFP forward problem [9].

2.2.1. MODELS OF SLOW OSCILLATIONS

Regarding physiological oscillations, detailed computational models were proposed to explain very slow activity (<1 Hz) as during slow-wave sleep, and in particular the characteristic oscillation made up of "up" and "down" states [13]. Here we describe two models that differ in that one simulates only cortical activity, while the other simulates a system including cortex and thalamus. The former [14] consists of a network of 1,024 pyramidal cells and 256 cortical interneurons interconnected by means of both excitatory and inhibitory (AMPA, NMDA, and GABA receptor-mediated) synaptic couplings. The latter, developed by Bazhenov et al. [15], consists of a network of 100 pyramidal cells and 25 interneurons in the cortex, and 50 thalamocortical cells and as many reticular neurons. In simple terms, both models can reproduce slow rhythmic activity (<1 Hz) as observed *in vitro* and *in vivo*. On the one hand, Compte et al.'s model [14] predicts that intrinsic bistability accounts for the switch between the up and down states. It predicts further that the up state is maintained by strong recurrent excitation among pyramidal cortical cells, and that the slow Na$^+$-dependent K$^+$ current (I_{KNa}) drives the transition to the down state. On the other hand, the thalamocortical model of Bazhenov et al.[15] shows that in the full thalamocortical model the active phases of slow wave sleep oscillations last longer, partly maintained by a depolarizing drive from the thalamocortical neurons.

2.2.2. MODELS OF THETA OSCILLATIONS

Theta oscillations (3–8 Hz) constitute a characteristic rhythm observed mainly in limbic structures like the hippocampus and entorhinal cortex in rodents, primates, and humans, although with some slight differences regarding the frequency band. According to the compartmental modeling approach reported by [16], the objective was to determine the necessary conditions for theta oscillations to emerge in the hippocampal CA1 circuitry. These authors built a detailed network model that included HH-based models of pyramidal cells, basket neurons, and OLM interneurons (OLM = stratum oriens–lacunosum moleculare of CA1 hippocampal area). Connectivity patterns were random and based on synaptic couplings only, either inhibitory (GABA$_A$ receptors) or excitatory (AMPA and NMDA receptors). Network simulations were performed with 15, 70, and 100 pyramidal, OLM, and basket cells, respectively. After detailed investigation of synchronization processes, the authors identified some key factors contributing to theta, including the precise AP timing in neuron populations, the role of the I_h current and NMDA receptors. Overall, results suggest that theta oscillations can be determined, to a large extent, by intrahippocampal circuitry. According to model predictions, theta frequency oscillations have been shown to be generated in the complete rat hippocampus *in vitro* without extrinsic inputs and that a feedback loop between CA1 pyramidal cells and local inhibitory interneurons can account for the generation of this *in vitro* theta rhythm [17]. It should be added that alternative mechanisms have been proposed to account for hippocampal theta rhythms [18].

2.2.3. MODELS OF ALPHA OSCILLATIONS

Brain oscillations in the alpha frequency band (8–12 Hz) have long been a topic of wide interest in neuroscience. Beside pioneering works based on lumped-parameter representations of cortical circuits (see Section 2.3 on alpha rhythm neural mass models), attempts were also made to explain the generation of such oscillations from networks of coupled multicompartmental model neurons. A representative illustration of this modeling approach can be found in [19]. In this study, up to 6,400 model neurons, incorporating as much neurophysiological realism as computationally tractable, were synaptically interconnected to build a network model subsequently used to investigate the conditions for emergence of cortical traveling waves. Among the identified dynamic regimes in this network model, two were shown to correspond to oscillatory states characterized by two different mean firing rates (low and high) indicating the presence of limit cycles, in the frequency range of alpha and beta rhythms (8–20 Hz). In the conclusion, these authors ask the crucial question of whether real alpha-like activity generated in the brain shares some mechanisms highlighted by the model. Although the model seems to accurately reproduce the features of the alpha rhythm, the authors emphasize a discrepancy related to the close coupling between firing of APs and alpha waves in the simulated LFP that occurs in the model but that would not be observed under physiological conditions. It should be noted, however, that recently a clear relationship between alpha oscillations in several cortical layers and the modulation of multiunit activity was demonstrated [20–22], in line with the model prediction.

2.2.4. MODELS OF GAMMA OSCILLATIONS

Gamma oscillations (30–90 Hz) and oscillations at higher frequencies (>90 Hz), usually known as high-frequency oscillations (HFOs), including ripples (≈100–200 Hz) and fast ripples (FRs; >200 Hz), although these frequency limits are arbitrary, have also been widely studied using computational models, in particular in models reproducing neuronal circuits of the hippocampus and cerebral cortex (see Section 3.2). Developed models range from mesoscopic and macroscopic representations (see Section 2.3.4) to highly detailed, biophysically plausible descriptions of hippocampal microcircuits. Traub, Kopell, and colleagues have extensively contributed to this topic with simple (single compartment) to very detailed (>60 compartments) biophysical models of pyramidal cells and interneurons, like fast-spiking (FS) basket cells and OLM cells, among others. With respect to gamma oscillations a complexity is that these can be produced under diverse *in vitro* and *in vivo* conditions. Three qualitatively different rhythms are reported in [18]: the gamma rhythm generated in interneuron networks (I-I), the gamma rhythm generated in pyramid-interneuron networks (E-I), and the pharmacologically induced persistent gamma rhythm [23]. These studies led to interesting theoretical speculations as, for instance, the possible role of electrical coupling via gap junctions in the generation of very fast oscillations both under normal and epileptic conditions [24,25].

Despite the great variety of possible mechanisms underlying gamma oscillations, detailed modeling studies of neuronal networks indicate that in the context of gamma oscillations, the increased firing of GABAergic synaptically coupled interneurons with fast kinetics is a common mechanism. In this context another remarkable EEG phenomenon is the strong association between "sharp waves" and ripples (SPW-Rs), first recorded in the hippocampus and thoroughly reviewed in [26]. They have been the object of several modeling studies, four of which are described by [27] as follows:

1. The first assumes that the input causing the sharp wave excites the interneuron network that enters into oscillation and thus entrains phasic spiking of pyramidal cells [28].

2. The second is based on an excitatory pyramidal-inhibitory interneuron network (PING) feedback loop [29].

3. The third assumes a pyramidal cell network connected by axo-axonal gap junctions where spikes are multiplied and propagate in the presence of a depolarizing input [30].

4. The fourth brings in a novel phenomenon that inputs impinging simultaneously, or at very short delays, on CA1 cells are capable of eliciting dendritic spikes on the basal dendrites of the latter, which sum nonlinearly such that the result is a rapid depolarization at the soma that is larger than the sum of the depolarizations caused by the distinct dendritic inputs. Memmesheimer's model [31] shows that in a network of coupled cells, this nonlinear amplification results in enhanced propagation of synchronous activity in the network such that both excitatory and inhibitory cells generate synchronous spikes; the latter generate spikes at rates around the ripple frequency of 200 Hz, due to their fast time constants.

We should note that all these different modeled mechanisms are not mutually exclusive [27], and combinations are likely to occur in reality.

Finally, regarding pathological activities, many studies have made use of computational models at cellular and network levels aimed to investigate pathological gamma HFOs observed in the context of epilepsy (see Section 3).

2.3. Macroscopic Models: Neural Mass Models of EEG Rhythms: The Wilson–Cowan Approach

In general, EEG signals are considered to result from the dynamic behavior of neuronal populations as revealed by model studies. A property of such populations that is essential for the generation of EEG signals is the capacity of neurons to work in synchrony.

This depends mainly on the connectivity among neurons that form networks. In the classic terminology of Freeman [32], groups of interacting populations of neurons constitute a *neural mass* that may occupy a few square millimeters of cortical surface or a few cubic millimeters of nuclear volume in the thalamus or brainstem. Typically, a neural mass consists of approximately 10^4 to 10^7 neurons. An essential feature of such a neural mass is the existence of multiple feedback and feedforward loops. Such a set of neurons can produce oscillatory phenomena. The main parameters that characterize the dynamic behavior of the set are (a) the synaptic time constants; (b) the length constants, which define the distance of the interactions between different neurons; (c) the gain factors—that is, the strength of interactions, either by way of chemical synapses or by direct electrical couplings (gap junctions); and (d) the properties of the intrinsic ionic and synaptic currents. Both inhibitory and excitatory feedback/feedforward loops play an important role.

In this section, macroscopic models of the generation of characteristic types of EEGs, including the spatial spread of rhythmic activity over the cortex, are presented. In these models, it is assumed that the dynamics of electroencephalographic/magnetoencephalographic (EEG/MEG) signals can be accounted by models of systems operating within spaces with relative low dimensions. This is the realm of neural mass models (NMMs) that use mean field concepts, where the properties of subpopulations of neurons are lumped together based on the fact that many neurons within a given neuronal system share the same basic properties.

The most general theoretical framework that can account for the fundamental properties of macroscopic models of EEG generation is the Wilson–Cowan approach, which describes NMMs based on the *mean-field approximation*. Wilson and Cowan in 1972 proposed a theoretical framework that emphasizes not the properties of individual cells but rather those of neuronal populations. The basic variable is the proportion of neurons of each population that are active at a given time, such that the relevant variable is not the single spike but the average spike frequency (or firing rate). The dynamics of the neural mass depends on the interaction of excitatory and inhibitory neuronal subpopulations. Accordingly, the model requires the use of two main variables, $E(t)$ and $I(t)$, describing the activity of the excitatory and inhibitory subpopulations, respectively, to characterize the state of the whole population. Based on these assumptions, the general Wilson and Cowan equations governing the dynamics of a localized population of neurons were derived:

$$E(t+r) = \left[1 - \int_{t-r}^{t} E(t')dt'\right] \cdot S_e \left\{\int_{-\infty}^{t} \alpha(t-t')\left[c_1 E(t') - c_2 I(t') + P(t')\right]dt'\right\}$$

and

$$I(t+r') = \left[1 - \int_{t-r'}^{t} I(t')dt'\right] \cdot S_i \left\{\int_{-\infty}^{t} \alpha(t-t')\left[c_3 E(t') - c_4 I(t') + Q(t')\right]dt'\right\}$$

This formalism describes the activities of the excitatory $E(t)$ and inhibitory $I(t)$ subpopulations; c_1–c_4 are the connectivity constants representing the average number of excitatory and inhibitory synapses for each subpopulation, $S_e(x)$ and $S_i(x)$ are the response functions that give the expected proportion of cells in a subpopulation that respond to a given level of excitation and are represented by sigmoid functions; $P(t)$ and $Q(t)$ are the external inputs to the excitatory and the inhibitory subpopulations, respectively; and r and r' are the refractory periods.

Based on this theoretical formalism introduced by Wilson and Cowan, Lopes da Silva et al. [34] constructed the first NMM that accounts for the generation of the alpha rhythm, described below.

2.3.1. NMM of Alpha Rhythm

With the general objectives mentioned above in mind, this section considers a few models of the generation of the alpha rhythm that have been elaborated in the past decades. We focus here on models at the mesoscopic and macroscopic levels. The past history is only very concisely presented (more detailed accounts of this part are given in previous editions of this book), while the emphasis lies on the most recent contributions.

The original study [34] had the main objective of testing whether a simplified model of two lumped subpopulations of interconnected excitatory and inhibitory neurons with properties of thalamocortical cells and interneurons of the reticular nucleus (Fig. 3.3A) was able to generate rhythmic activity with the characteristics of the alpha rhythm in the frequency band of 8 to 12 Hz as it can be recorded in the thalamus and also in the cortex.

The basic physiological parameters were presented and discussed in Chapter 2. The mathematical analysis was initially carried out for a linearized approximation of the neuronal network in order to express the transfer function of the network and the power spectrum of the average membrane potential, assuming that this is determined by the somadendritic membrane potential of the main cells. The latter was interpreted as the local EEG signal, which in this case consisted, indeed, of a predominant alpha rhythm (see Fig. 3.3).

The basic structure of the model is shown in the block diagram in Figure 3.3A (for the biophysical data and mathematical treatment, see [34]). It suffices to state here that to understand how oscillations may be generated in thalamic nuclei, we must consider the basic structure of these neuronal networks. Three main types of neurons can be distinguished in this system: the thalamocortical relay (TCR) neurons, whose axons project to the cortex; the RE nucleus neurons that cause the inhibitory feedback control of the former; and the local, intrinsic, neurons. In the original model the latter were not included for the sake of simplicity, since their behavior was considered less important regarding the main objective of the simulations.

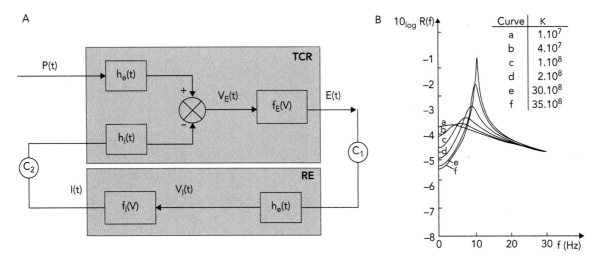

Figure 3.3. A: Block diagram of the lumped model for rhythmic activity of simplified alpha rhythm model. The TCR neurons are represented by two linear systems having impulse responses simulating an EPSP ($h_e(t)$) and an IPSP ($h_i(t)$), respectively, together with the static nonlinearity ($f_E(V)$) representing the spike-generating process. The interneurons (RE cells) are represented by one linear system ($h_e(t)$) and a nonlinearity ($f_i(V)$). C_1 represents the number of interneurons to which one TCR neuron projects; C_2 represents the number of TCRs to which one interneuron projects. B: Power spectra of the output of the lumped alpha rhythm model shown in A for different values of the feedback gain (K), which is mainly determined by the coupling constants representing the synaptic interactions within the neuronal set. As the synaptic interactions become stronger and K increases, the spectrum acquires a clear selectivity at the alpha frequency. (Adapted with permission from Lopes da Silva, F.H., et al., Model of brain rhythmic activity. The alpha-rhythm of the thalamus. Kybernetik, 1974. 15(1): p. 27–37)

Under white noise input the membrane potentials of thalamic cells oscillate within the alpha frequency range, as shown by the power spectrum of the simulated local EEG signal (see Fig. 3.3B) for different values of K, which represents a measure of the gain factor of the neuronal population. In the context of NMMs of alpha rhythms, Bhattacharya et al. [33] came forward with a refined NMM of the thalamo-cortico-thalamic system, based on the previous model [34], focusing on the visual pathways from the retina to the thalamic lateral geniculate nucleus and the visual cortex. In that study the authors used updated parameters to describe the thalamic populations according to the experimental data of [35]. Using this model Bhattacharya et al. made a parameter sensitivity analysis to study the effect of changing values of synaptic connectivities on alpha power and corresponding dominant frequency. Furthermore, Becker et al. [36] published an advanced NMM of a thalamocortical network of coupled nodes constituted by populations of spike-burst neurons with distributed parameters; these authors not only simulated realistic alpha rhythms but also were able to reproduce both the inverse relationship between alpha-rhythm power and functional magnetic resonance imaging (fMRI) BOLD signals, and the negative relationship between alpha rhythm and neuronal firing rates in different nodes. This model offers novel perspectives for more advanced studies on alpha rhythms both in terms of electrophysiology and the correlated hemodynamics. Though this is a very comprehensive model it does not include modulating inputs, such as cholinergic inputs from the brainstem.

2.3.2. Extension of the Original Alpha NMM in the Space Domain: Models of Van Rotterdam et al. and Suffczynski et al.

The original model described above, has served as the basis for a number of more elaborate models [37] that have been designed to test novel hypotheses and answer new questions. One of these models was proposed to answer the question (i) of how the *propagation of alpha rhythms along the cortex* can be accounted for. A second one (ii) was prompted by the interest in understanding the mechanism by which opposite changes of alpha power (increases and decreases) can be coupled while occurring in neighboring cortical areas in response to the same external event. This phenomenon was called *focal ERD-surround ERS* (ERD = event-related; D = desynchronization; S = synchronization); the assumption behind these expressions is that a desynchronization of the elements of the neuronal population results in a decrease of alpha power, while an increase of synchrony of those elements has the opposite effect.

Question (i) led to development of a *model of a chain of modules* [37], each one comprising pyramidal cells and interneurons interconnected; sequential modules were connected by means of recurrent excitatory collaterals and inhibitory fibers, with connectivity functions assumed to be homogenous while the strength of the connectivity was an exponentially decreasing function of distance. Subsequently these authors derived a mathematical expression in the form of a linear inhomogenous partial differential that accounts for voltage as a function of space and time. In this way they demonstrated that rhythmic components in the alpha band (~10–12 Hz) were less damped than frequency components outside the alpha band. Furthermore, the alpha rhythm activity propagates with a speed in the order of 0.3 m/s, which is in qualitative agreement with experimental data on alpha rhythm activity recorded from the visual cortex of dog [38].

Along a similar line Liley et al. [39] presented a mean field theory of electrocortical activity based on a set of nonlinear continuum field equations that accounts for the dynamics of neural activity in the cortex. This theoretical study emphasized that alpha rhythm traveling waves depend strongly on the integrity of inhibitory/inhibitory population interactions. Another example of continuous neural field models (NFMs) is that of Jirsa [40], which gives a very thorough theoretical account of how a set of state equations with parameter values based on physiology can account for the dynamics of cortical neuronal populations at different spatial scales: microscopic, mesoscopic, and macroscopic. At the microscopic level fast synaptic feedbacks appear to be crucial to the stability of the excited cortex. At mesoscopic scale the model shows how fields of synchrony can be established, and at macroscopic scale it shows how traveling waves may be generated in the cortex. The last two levels are particularly relevant with respect to the theory of the dynamics of EEG/MEG generation. The interested reader may find a thorough treatment of applications of this kind of formalism in the study of continuous field models in [41] and [42]. A similar problem has been mathematically elaborated by [43] and [44], who developed a model, also based on the existence of interconnections between different cortical modules, to account for the global wave pattern of the EEG recorded at the level of the scalp.

In reference to question (ii), another extension of the original model was constructed [45] to account for the phenomenon in which, in reaction to a given event (e.g., a finger movement), rhythmic activities in the alpha frequency range (also called mu rhythms, since these are recorded from the sensorimotor cortex) *decrease* in power within a given area of the cortex, while their power *increases* in a neighboring area, what is called the ERD-ERS phenomenon as described above [46] (for details see Chapter 40). The extended model of Suffczynski et al. [45] consists of a chain of coupled thalamocortical modules, themselves representing the systems responsible for hand and foot movements, respectively. These NMMs were able to show how this reciprocal ERD-ERS phenomenon takes place. The basic hypothesis was that "cross-talk" between the thalamocortical modules representing the hand and the foot would take place at the level of the reticular neurons (RE), since these form a sheet of interconnected inhibitory cells that surrounds most of those thalamic modules. Indeed, simulations revealed that the antagonistic ERD-ERS phenomenon [46] can result from the functional interaction between the populations of thalamocortical cells (TCR) and of the reticular nucleus cells (RE). Activation of one module (e.g., the hand module), for example by means of subcortical modulating inputs, results in deactivation of the neighboring module (e.g., the foot module).

2.3.3. NMMs of Spontaneous and Evoked Activities, and Beyond

An extension of the original NMM [34] was developed by Jansen and Rit [47], triggered by the question of how spontaneous cortical EEG rhythmic activities are related to visual evoked potentials. These authors introduced an NMM of cortical columns [48] consisting of a population of pyramidal cells interconnected with populations of excitatory and inhibitory interneurons, which displays different kinds of simulated EEG outputs when fed with random noise. Furthermore. this model accounted for the generation of visual evoked potentials, showing that in the first 100 to 200 ms these potentials are due primarily to a combination of phase reorganization and processing of primary afferent inputs.

Based on the results obtained with NMMs generating rhythmic activities within the alpha frequency range, several researchers extended these models to account for different EEG frequency bands besides the alpha rhythm. In this respect, David and Friston [49] described a lumped model that generates various rhythmic activities ranging from delta to gamma, according to the kinetics of the populations included in the model.

With the aim of investigating how different cortical regions can display complex EEG frequency spectra and several patterns of functional connectivity, Zavaglia et al. [50] also developed interconnected lumped models. They showed that three populations, each consisting of four subpopulations (pyramidal neurons, excitatory, slow, and fast inhibitory interneurons), arranged in parallel, are sufficient to account for complex EEG spectra with dominant frequency ranging from theta to alpha and gamma. This model is akin to the comprehensive NMM introduced by Wendling et al. [51] to account for the generation of different kinds of neural activities and the corresponding EEG signals, including epileptic activity, as described in more detail in Section 3. In addition to the lumped NMMs developed with the objective of understanding the mechanisms of generation of EEG rhythmic activities, described above, similar models were developed with the aim of reproducing EEG combined with fMRI BOLD signals. Valdés-Sosa et al. [52] proposed an approach where the summed PSPs generated by an NMM of a cortical area are used in the forward mode to estimate the primary current density distribution of a cortical area, as applied also by Bojak et al. [53].

An essential feature of these models is that the summed PSPs generated by the NMM are transformed into a local vasomotor feedforward signal that is then further transformed by way of a temporal convolution with the hemodynamic response function into a simulated BOLD signal. In this way the information obtained from the EEG signal and from the corresponding fMRI BOLD signal recorded from the same region of interest can be merged. Although this approach opens interesting novel perspectives it needs further elaboration, since it is based on concepts that are still insufficiently established.

2.3.4. NMMs of Specific EEG Rhythms Other than Alpha

In addition to the detailed neural networks models described in Section 2.2, the approach inspired by Wilson and Cowan has also been used to model the main properties of different kinds of rhythmic activities besides alpha rhythms, namely cortical slow, theta, beta, and gamma oscillations. These EEG models are less detailed with respect to cellular properties. However, they have the advantage, in comparison to the detailed neuronal network models described in Section 2.2, that they permit investigating *population dynamic properties*, namely the influence of modulating systems, and their reflection on EEG spectral properties, as these may be recorded *in vivo* in different behavioral contexts. Thus we will emphasize here the dynamic properties of a few neuronal systems responsible for specific EEG oscillations based on specific NMMs.

2.3.4.1. NMMs of Slow Oscillations

There are several kinds of slow, and very slow, oscillations that not only are associated with sleep but that occur also in the awake state. Those EEG phenomena are the main topic of Chapter 32. Here we pay attention only to models of neuronal populations that elucidate the dynamics of such phenomena (NFMs). In this respect a comprehensive study is that by Zhao et al. [54], which includes modeling of EEG activities in the corticothalamic system, namely the dynamics of cortical up (depolarized) and down (hyperpolarized) states [13] coupled to the dynamics of bursting neurons in the reticular thalamic nucleus. In this model two slow variables occupy an important place: one represents the conductance of slow Ca^{2+} that mediates bursting of the reticular neurons, the other a slow feedback inhibition. According to this model these variables modulate the switching between "on and off" firing of the bursting neurons of the reticular nucleus. An interpretation of these results is that the occurrence of up/down oscillations depends on the interaction between thalamocortical network properties and the bursting dynamics of the thalamic reticular nucleus. The effects of circadian, homeostatic, and brainstem modulating factors, however, are not explicitly considered in this model. A comprehensive overview of phenomenological models of sleep dynamics is that by Booth and Behn [55].

2.3.4.2. NMMs of the Dynamics of Beta and Gamma Oscillations Associated with Movement

A general experimental observation is that the power in the beta frequency band (13–25 Hz) decreases (ERD) below baseline level during the preparation of a finger brisk movement but increases (ERS) after movement execution, the so-called rebound beta. In addition, a surge of gamma power may appear just before the movement, as described in detail in Chapter 40. How can these dynamic properties be accounted for? Grabska-Barwinska and Zygierewicz [56] developed an NMM with the objective of answering this question. Similarly to other NMMs this one consists of two interacting populations of cortical neurons: pyramids and interneurons. The cellular properties are mainly based on the physiological data reported in [57], which describes the activity-dependent facilitation of synaptic transmission between pyramidal and FS interneurons. In the NMM these authors introduce this dynamic property in terms of the probability of synaptic facilitation growing as the level of excitation delivered to the presynaptic pyramidal neuron increases. This NMM can display beta (≈ 24 Hz) or gamma (≈ 37 Hz) oscillations. When the external inputs are weak the NMM displays bursts of beta, whereas when the input and the functional coupling between pyramidal and interneurons are strong, gamma oscillations occur.

2.3.4.3. NMMs of the Dynamics of Gamma Oscillations

An early NMM of spontaneous gamma oscillations, as recorded in the hippocampus of the rat, is the model of Leung [58]. One question that this model was able to investigate was this: What is the mechanism underlying the dependency of the oscillation at gamma frequency (≈ 40 Hz) on input intensity (assuming that the latter is white noise of wide bandwidth)? The NMM comprises two neuronal populations, pyramids and

interneurons, with a recurrent path from the former to the latter that includes a time delay and a nonlinear element, as well as a modulating influence representing inputs arising from the brainstem. An interesting property of this NMM is that it reproduces the dynamics of the dependency of the oscillations on input intensity, as reflected in local EEG signals.

A more recent model of neocortical networks consisting of a number of columns, constructed based on anatomical data of different cortical layers, was shown to generate oscillations at different frequencies, including gamma oscillations [59]. In this model the emergence of the latter appeared to depend particularly on the existence of "hubs" (i.e., cells with many more connections than average) in cortical layers 2/3. Indeed, different neuronal mechanisms can give rise to different kinds of gamma oscillations.

At a more general level, we should mention the mean field model of Bojak and Liley [60], which describes the dynamics of a large population of cortical neurons based on two-dimensional nonlinear partial differential equations. According to this approach the cortex would be in a state of marginal stability, as reflected by the presence of alpha activity, but a shift from alpha to higher frequencies may occur, particularly due to an increase in the mean inhibitory/inhibitory connectivity enhancing the presynaptic release of GABA, such that a 40-Hz state may emerge. This mechanism could operate through the influence of thalamic afferents on cortical inhibitory interneurons in layer IV. These predictions may be tested experimentally.

2.3.4.4. NMMs of Cross-Frequency Coupling (Theta and Gamma and Others)

Noteworthy examples of the coupling between EEG oscillations at different frequencies are the demonstrations of such coupling in memory tasks [61,62], namely between theta and gamma oscillations, that have been found in the CA3 area of the rat hippocampus and associated cortical areas [63,64], and also between gamma and alpha [65]. In these cases the phase of a low-frequency activity (e.g., theta or alpha rhythm) modulates the amplitude of a higher-frequency oscillation (e.g., gamma rhythm). This kind of phase-amplitude coupling (PAC) is not restricted to a specific combination of frequencies. Mainly theta–gamma and alpha–gamma PAC have been the object of more elaborated NMM studies. Onslow et al. [66] adopted an NMM approach to investigate how an input signal at the theta frequency received either by the excitatory or the inhibitory population can lead a network, consisting of pyramidal and interneuron populations, to generate "intrinsic" gamma-frequency (≈ 55 Hz) oscillations, modulated periodically at the theta frequency. In this way the gamma oscillations appear nested within the theta rhythm displaying PAC.

Instead of theta rhythm, also alpha–beta rhythms can be modulators, as has been proposed by, among others, Jensen et al. [65]. Ursino et al. [67] modified the NMM introduced by Wendling et al. [51] and constructed a model of a cortical region consisting of four interconnected neuronal populations (pyramidal cells, excitatory, and two types of GABAergic inhibitory interneurons, with slow and fast kinetics). In this way it was shown that the model can produce several combinations of oscillations at different frequencies (beta and gamma, alpha and gamma). Sotero [68] reviewed several model studies focused on the analysis of PAC combinations, paying special attention to those based on an NMM approach. One of the models consists in the simulation of a cortical column comprising four different neuronal populations: two excitatory (intrinsically bursting and regulatory spiking cells) and two inhibitory (FS and low-threshold-spiking [LTS] cells) grouped in four layers, two of which with all four populations and the other two with only regulatory spiking, FS, and LTS cells; these populations are interconnected by a complex matrix of excitatory and inhibitory connections. With a given input, which can be any arbitrary function including white noise, the model can generate different PAC combinations, such as theta and gamma or alpha and gamma. Notwithstanding the interest of these models for generating EEG coupled oscillations similar to some experimental findings, we need to develop more specific networks with more elaborate elementary properties in order to test well-defined hypotheses.

3. MODELS OF EPILEPTIFORM ACTIVITY

By definition, epileptiform activity is the activity recorded from the brain during epileptic events. These events refer mainly to seizure episodes, but not exclusively, as a variety of abnormal transient signals also occur during interictal periods (i.e., outside seizures)—for instance, interictal epileptic spikes (IESs) or HFOs in partial epilepsies. Due to unmatched time resolution, electrophysiological techniques remain the gold standard for recording epileptiform activity at either a global level (EEG signals, scalp electrodes) or a local level (intracellular, multiunit activity [MUA], LFPs, and iEEG signals using microelectrodes and/or macroelectrodes). Depending on the level of recording (from intracellular to whole brain), electrophysiological signals convey different, although complementary, types of information. In general, the difficulty of interpreting these signals in terms of underlying mechanisms increases with the size of the neuronal system whose activity is "captured" by the electrodes. Typically, in the context of epilepsy, scalp EEG signals are more difficult to decode than iEEG signals directly recorded with depth electrodes. Nevertheless and whatever the recording techniques, epileptiform signals remain difficult to analyze, and their interpretation, in terms of underlying pathophysiological mechanisms, is a challenging issue that has received much attention during the past decades. Many questions arise when one is carefully reviewing the often very complicated electrophysiological signals recorded from epileptic brain:

How and why do neuronal networks *switch* to seizure activity?

How do these seizures *start, propagate,* and *terminate*?

What are the cellular and network mechanisms governing the generation of IESs and/or HFOs?

In this context, the field of computational modeling in epilepsy has grown rapidly over the past decades. Soltesz and Staley (2008, listed in the principal references) edited a comprehensive book dedicated to the achievements of the field of computational epilepsy research up to 2007. Computational modeling is now recognized as an efficient way to reveal relevant mechanisms potentially involved in the generation of epileptiform activity as reflected in signals collected at the level of sensors, and to formulate hypotheses that may be tested experimentally. Numerous computational models have been proposed to investigate (1) the pathophysiological factors leading to the occurrence of seizures (ictogenesis) and (2) the progression of the disease from an initial brain insult (epileptogenesis). Since the early developments in the 1970s, these models have progressively gained acceptance by the community of epileptologists and are now viewed as "integrative" tools, allowing us to bridge the gap between the micro- and mesoscopic level of neuronal networks and the macroscopic level of EEG signals. For instance, detailed models of HFOs, possibly biomarkers of epileptogenic zones, can lead to hypotheses regarding how epileptogenicity may be linked to abnormal firing patterns of pyramidal cells and interneurons and to alterations of synaptic transmission in small clusters of neurons. In this section, we review some of the many computer models that have been developed at various levels of description, from small-scale networks (detailed models) to larger-scale systems (NMMs and NFMs), to reproduce and explain epileptiform activity. Readers will also find complementary information in reviews on the same topic [69–71] or available online (http://www.scholarpedia.org/article/Models_of_epilepsy).

3.1. Models of Interictal Activity: Epileptic Spikes

During interictal periods, sporadic transient epileptiform events (spikes, polyspikes, sharp waves, spike-waves, spike-bursts) occur very frequently. Among these events, IESs have been a topic of broad interest as they are observed in most human partial epilepsies [72] as well as in most experimental models of focal epilepsy [73]. A number of experimental studies also reported the appearance of IESs during the latent period in experimental models of epileptogenesis [74,75]. Although IESs are, to some extent, polymorphic events, they always present with a sharp initial component (the spike), sometimes followed by a slower, more or less pronounced, component of opposite polarity (the wave) (see Fig. 3.4D). For instance, in an *in vivo* model of epileptogenesis, Chauvière et al. [76] distinguished two types of interictal spikes—type 1 (spike followed by a long-lasting wave) and type 2 (spike without wave)—and could relate these morphological features to the impending occurrence of spontaneous seizures characterizing the chronic epileptic state. Next we describe a number of computational models that have been developed to improve our understanding of the mechanisms underlying IESs, as reflected in LFPs or EEG recordings.

3.1.1. DETAILED NETWORK MODELS OF EPILEPTIC SPIKES
At the single neuron level, *sustained depolarizations* and *paroxysmal depolarizing shifts* (PDSs) are recorded during epileptiform activity. At the network level, these abnormal depolarizations are associated with IESs simultaneously

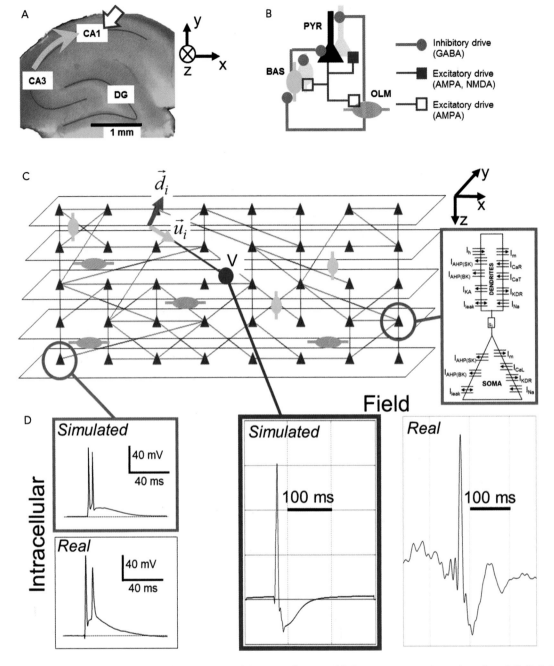

Figure 3.4. Detailed modeling of IESs. **A:** The activity of the hippocampal CA1 network was modeled in response to excitatory input from CA3. **B, C:** Pyramidal (PYR), basket (BAS), and OLM multicompartment neuron models were interconnected using excitatory and inhibitory synapses to reproduce the CA1 three-dimensional network. **D:** From this network, the cellular activity (D, left) of principal neurons (PYR) and interneurons (BAS, OLM) in response to input from CA3 could be simulated, simultaneously with the LFP (V) recorded by an extracellular point electrode and simulated using the dipole theory. For increased excitability (altered glutamatergic and GABAergic synaptic transmission), simulated signals (D, middle) resemble actual IESs (D, right) recorded from hippocampus (with depth electrodes) in patients with epilepsy.

observed in LFPs. A six-compartment single neuron model of increasing physiological and morphological detail level was elaborated to investigate sustained depolarizations and PDSs [77]. Findings suggested the dominance of neuronal membrane physiological processes (calcium-related transmembrane currents, in particular) over specific morphological features, namely the structure of dendritic trees, in the generation and shaping of those types of epileptiform activity.

Based on the two-compartment model presented in Figure 3.2, a model of a realistic neural network (principal cells, interneurons, and corresponding synaptic connectivity) reproducing the main physiological features of the CA1 subfield of the hippocampus was reported [9]. This model is illustrated in Figure 3.4. The objective was to identify the key parameters that account for the morphological features of IES components (the spike and the wave) in response to a stimulation that mimics an afferent volley of APs from the CA3 area via the Schaffer collaterals to the CA1 subfield of the hippocampus (see Fig. 3.4A). Both glutamatergic (AMPA and NMDA) and GABA$_A$ergic synapses were included in the network (see Fig. 3.4B). The percentage of simulated cells and the connectivity patterns were defined in accordance with basic knowledge about structural and functional features of the CA1 circuitry [78], although some cellular and synaptic features, such as $GABA_B$ synaptic actions, are not included in this simplified model.

An interesting aspect in the modeling approach reported in [9] relates to the computation of the simulated LFP (i.e., the signal generated by the three-dimensional network activity and recorded by an extracellular electrode positioned at a point in its center). Unlike the classic approach, which makes use of the total transmembrane current [79–82], this computation was based on the dipole concept and on three main assumptions:

1. Pyramidal cells were considered to be the main contributors to the LFP due to their spatial arrangement in palisades.

2. The synaptic activation of each pyramidal cell was represented as a current dipole formed by a sink and a source.

3. The volume conductor was considered as homogeneous.

Under these assumptions, Figure 3.4D provides an example of IES as reflected in the simulated LFP (center) along with a real IES (right) recorded from CA1 in an *in vivo* kainate model of epilepsy in mouse. As depicted, the general shape of the simulated event approximates the two components of the real IES. In both cases, the sharp spike is followed by a slower wave component of opposite polarity.

A unique feature of these detailed models is that they offer the opportunity to relate the extracellular field activity to the simultaneously generated intracellular activity of pyramidal cells and interneurons. Interestingly, the model shows that during the interictal spike, pyramidal cells generate a PDS-like activity, as also observed experimentally (see Fig. 3.4D, left). The model also predicts that the dramatic increase of the firing rate of interneurons (especially basket cells) corresponds to the slow wave by the sustained activity of interneurons generating feedback inhibition; the real situation may be, however, more complex, as discussed below regarding changes occurring during epileptogenesis [92].

Thus, a number of predictions could be made regarding the cellular and network mechanisms favoring the generation of IESs. First, the model highlights the major contribution of APs generated at the soma of CA1 pyramidal cells, in response to stimulation from CA3, to the sharp component of IESs. Second, the model predicts that the AMPA conductance plays a key role both in the generation of the spike component and in its amplitude, in line with experimental data showing that spontaneous interictal bursts in CA1 can be completely abolished following addition of AMPA/kainate receptor antagonists [83].

Another detailed network model of IESs in CA1 was recently reported [84]. Here, data concerning glutamatergic pyramidal cells, basket cells. and oriens-alveus were taken from the literature [85–87]. As in the model described above, the detailed network comprised 80% excitatory neurons and 20% inhibitory neurons. AMPA and $GABA_A$ conductances were included for synaptic transmission. An increase of the average number of pyramidal-to-pyramidal synapses was used to represent axonal sprouting. The conditions under which neuronal synchronization is able to evoke PDS events in CA1 pyramidal cells were determined. Experimental measurements of PDS burst width and PDS after-hyperpolarization duration were used to adjust model parameters. Results show that this model can nicely reproduce spontaneous interictal spikes when the sprouting-induced recurrent connectivity of the CA1 is sufficiently increased, regardless of the synchronization level of the Schaffer collateral input.

3.1.2. NMMs AND NFMs OF EPILEPTIC SPIKES

The first attempt to reproduce paroxysmal spikes in an NMM dates back to the 1980s [88]. At that time, an electronic hardware circuit was built to model and accurately analyze the waveforms of output signals under both stable and unstable conditions. The model was intended to represent a local neuronal assembly comprising three subsets of neurons (two excitatory and one inhibitory). As in today's computer implementations of NMMs, this model was a nonlinear dynamic system with positive (excitatory) and negative (inhibitory) feedback loops, each containing a linear dynamic transfer function and a nonlinear static element. The analysis of this nonlinear dynamic system revealed that the input noise level can change the network stability and lead to the appearance of limit cycles. As a very interesting prediction, this bifurcation analysis brought up the hypothesis that *epileptic spikes are generated in a population of neurons that operate close to instability* and that *spikes may be viewed as borderline cases between normal background activity and seizure activity*, corroborating some real observations typical of hippocampal activity in mesial temporal lobe epilepsy, in which large-amplitude spikes (so-called preictal discharges) often precede the seizure onset [89].

NMMs have also been used to gain insight into epileptogenesis itself, defined as the ensemble of structural and functional alterations occurring in the brain and leading to recurrent spontaneous seizures. Indeed, in most experimental animal models of epileptogenesis, epileptic spikes constitute an early electrophysiological marker appearing during the latent period (defined as the time period spanning from the brain initial insult to the appearance of the first spontaneous seizures). In the pilocarpine animal model of temporal lobe epilepsy [90], recordings performed early (3 days after injection), late (10 days after injection), and at chronic stage (characterized by recurrent spontaneous seizures) were modeled in an NMM of the CA1 hippocampal region to explain how the changes in both the glutamatergic and GABAergic processes have an impact on the observed interictal-like activity (with respect to spike morphology and frequency of occurrence) during epileptogenesis [91]. Extensive simulations were performed for a series of model parameters (excitatory and inhibitory postsynaptic potentials [EPSPs and IPSPs] amplitude, rise and decay time constants) localized along the soma and dendrites of the pyramidal cell subpopulation. Simulations showed that a sufficient condition for the appearance of sporadic epileptic spikes is an increase of glutamatergic/GABAergic drive ratio, which also affects their shape and frequency of occurrence.

In the kainate model, some studies also reported the presence of epileptic spikes with an increase of frequency of occurrence during epileptogenesis [92]. Huneau et al. [93] reported the development of an NMM to investigate which factors condition spike frequency, as well as spike morphological features. These authors first designed signal processing techniques to automatically detect epileptic spikes and extract shape features (spike amplitude, wave area) over long durations (30 days). The observed changes, quantified as functions of time, were then reproduced in an NMM comprising two subsets of neurons (pyramidal cells and interneurons). Parameters with major influence on the morphological features of epileptic spikes were identified on the basis of extensive stimulations. Results indicated that the increase of the wave area following the spike component is directly related to the progressive diminution of $GABA_A$ergic inhibition. The question, however, is this: How can this increase of the wave area be explained while $GABA_A$ergic inhibition decreases? This finding implies that with the progression of epileptogenesis some changes occur in dendritic inhibition; we may hypothesize that several factors, not yet included in the model, may contribute to these changes, as, for example, shifts in $GABA_A$ reversal potential [92] and contributions of plastic changes [74]. This case provides an example of how modeling simulations that do not entirely account for some experimental findings can lead to new hypotheses that can be further tested. Notwithstanding these limitations, based on these results, a novel electrophysiological marker of progressive epileptogenicity was devised from the LFPs. This marker was shown to provide useful practical information about the progress of the process of epileptogenicity after the initial insult induced by intra-hippocampal kainic acid microinjection.

A single NMM can only account for the temporal dynamics of a local population of neurons. This limitation is removed in NFMs, which can account for the spatiotemporal evolution of coarse-grained variables such as synaptic or firing rate activity in coupled populations of neurons. An NFM [94] was developed to help interpret IESs recorded using depth-EEG electrodes in patients who were possible candidates for surgery. In this model (Fig. 3.5), an extended source (corresponding to a neocortical patch) is considered. To simulate the LFPs collected at the level of intracranial electrode contacts, the depth-EEG forward problem was solved based on dipole theory. First, the temporal dynamics of neuronal sources within the patch were represented by coupled NMMs. Second, distributed current dipoles with different spatial locations and orientations (assumed to be orthogonal to the cortical surface) were simulated and their contributions to the electric fields recorded at the level of electrode contacts were calculated. This model offered the opportunity to include, in the simulation of

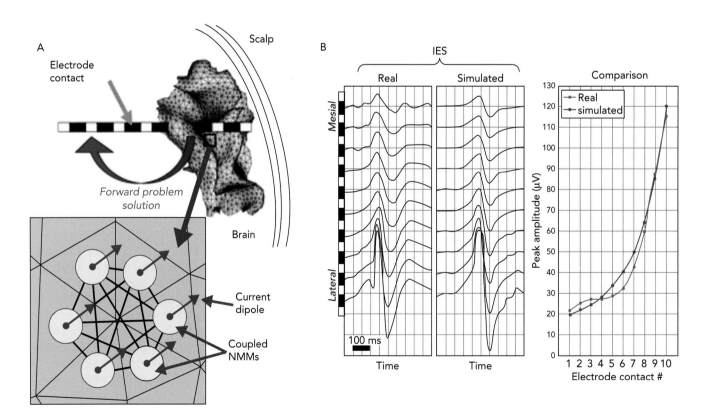

Figure 3.5. Simulation of IESs from an NFM. **A:** A neocortical patch composed of coupled NMMs (i.e., an NFM) is modeled. To simulate depth-EEG signals recorded at the level of a multi-contact intracerebral electrode, the contribution of each neuronal assembly is modeled by an equivalent current dipole with orientation normal to the cortical surface. **B:** Comparison between a real (left) and simulated (middle) IES obtained for increased excitation and connectivity in the NFM. For a sufficiently extended source, the model accurately reproduces the IES as well as its amplitude gradient along the electrode (right). (Adapted from Cosandier-Rimele, D., et al., A physiologically plausible spatio-temporal model for EEG signals recorded with intracerebral electrodes in human partial epilepsy. IEEE Trans Biomed Eng, 2007. **54**(3): p. 380–388)

depth-EEG signals, physical factors like the distance from the current dipole sources to the electrode contacts, their orientation and moment, as well as the volume conductor properties (resistivity of the different brain tissue layers). This NFM was used to investigate various factors associated with the sources of the signals collected by the electrodes (the neocortical patch). Some key parameters like the excitability level within the local neuronal populations, the connectivity and synchronization degree of the latter, and the geometry and spatial extent of the source could be separately analyzed.

As depicted in Figure 3.5B, some parameter configurations led to the simulation of realistic IESs as compared with those actually recorded by depth electrodes. In the displayed example, after parameter fitting, the model accurately approximates the temporal dynamics, the amplitude (in μV), and the amplitude gradient (along the electrode track) of a real IES recorded from the temporal region (electrode located in the middle temporal gyrus) in a patient with temporal lobe epilepsy. In this case, typical of large-amplitude spikes, a high coupling degree between neuronal populations with increased excitability was realized in the model. In addtion,with a volume conductor which accounted for the three main tissues of the head (brain, skull, and scalp) and with a brain conductivity value chosen to be equal to 32×10^{-5} S/mm, the cortical surface of the patch involved in the generation of the IES was estimated to be about 25 cm².

3.2. Models of Interictal Activity: Fast Ripples

The past decade has witnessed an increasing interest in HFOs (>90 Hz) in the general context of electrophysiology and FRs (>200 Hz) in the particular context of epilepsy. A comprehensive description of the general properties of HFOs and related phenomena is given in Chapters 23 and 33. Here we focus on the modeling approaches that have been developed to account for these phenomena in epilepsy. To date, at least five different computational models have been developed to understand the pathophysiological mechanisms underlying the generation of HFOs and FR in particular in the context of epilepsy.

The first model consists of a cortical column model comprising 4,750 multicompartment cortical neurons [95]. These model neurons included three main membrane compartments (soma, axon initial segment, and dendrites) with Na⁺, K⁺, Ca²⁺, and rectifier conductances. Main excitatory neurons were interconnected with interneurons (basket, axo-axonic, low threshold spiking, and neuroglial cells) through glutamatergic excitatory synapses (AMPA receptors) and inhibitory synapses (GABA$_A$ receptors). In addition, two types of gap junctions (at interneuron dendrites and between axons of homologous types of glutamatergic neurons) were introduced in the network. The computational model was used to explain experimental recordings performed in human temporal neocortical slices indicating that the occurrence of interictal very fast oscillations (up to 400 Hz) is not affected by the reduction of the GABA$_A$ receptor function but is significantly reduced by the nonspecific blocker carbanoxolone (CBX); see also the remarks below about the fact that there are no specific gap-junction blockers [96]. The model simulations confirmed this

result, indicating a major contribution of nonsynaptic couplings (key role of gap junctions between excitatory cells) to the origin of HFOs in epileptic human neocortex.

The second computational model of FRs as recorded experimentally in the epileptic rat hippocampus [97] is that proposed by Ibarz et al. [98]. This model consisted of a network of 120 model pyramidal neurons (based on [99]), each composed of 19 compartments representing the soma and the basal and the apical dendrites. The main objective was to study the effect of a pattern of "out-of-phase" firing on the occurrence of FRs. Thus, the authors simulated two clusters of 60 neurons bursting at different delays. Interestingly, this model was able to produce FRs with faster Na⁺ dynamics but without gap junctions or depolarizing GABA (reversal potential for GABA$_A$-like synaptic currents was −75 mV). Two different firing regimens were identified. In the first one, referred to as "in-phase" neuronal firing, the model produces oscillations in the FR frequency band (>250 Hz) when single cells in the two clusters fire synchronously. However, if clustered bursting neurons are slightly desynchronized, then the LFP oscillations occur at much higher frequency. In this second regimen, the "out-of-phase" firing mode of two small clusters of neurons generate FRs at higher frequency (>400 Hz).

The third model was initially designed to explore the mechanisms underlying both epileptic spikes and FRs in the hippocampus [100]. The whole network included 1,182 pyramidal neurons, 52 OLM interneurons, 52 basket cells, and 52 bistratified cells, connected via inhibitory GABAergic and excitatory glutamatergic (AMPA/NMDA) synapses. Interestingly, this model allowed the researchers to determine which conditions were sufficient for the generation of FRs. First, groups of "hyperexcitable" pyramidal cells, from small to large (Fig. 3.6A), could be simulated by increasing the reversal potential of GABAergic-mediated IPSPs at synapses of clustered neurons. This depolarizing GABA effect modified the firing pattern of model neurons that depolarize and trigger a few APs before hyperpolarization (see Fig. 3.6B), as observed during PDSs. Second, synaptic transmission was modified by increasing the conductance of AMPA/NMDA-receptor-mediated currents and by lowering those associated with GABAergic currents. Under these conditions, the model was shown to produce realistic FRs (see Fig. 3.6C) only for small clusters of neurons and for moderate alteration of synaptic transmission. In this case, simulated firing patterns were found to be weakly synchronized and out of phase (see Fig. 3.6B, right), in line with the previously described model [98]. Interestingly, epileptic spikes could also be simulated, but in larger groups of hyperexcitable cells and for higher levels of network excitability. In this case, simulated firing patterns were highly synchronized. Importantly, the model predictions were experimentally verified on organotypic slices. Experiments confirmed that a normal LFP (i.e., a field response evoked by a single electrical pulse) under control condition changes into an FR oscillation (350 Hz) under moderately increased AMPA/NMDA-ergic currents and decreased GABAergic currents. This field impulse response evolved into large amplitude spikes with further increase of the network excitability.

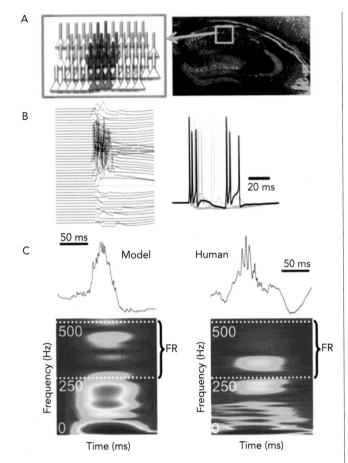

Figure 3.6. Simulation of FRs from a detailed model of the CA1 hippocampal circuit. **A:** Small clusters of hyperexcitable neurons are modeled by adding a depolarizing GABA effect and by altering synaptic transmission. **B:** Under these conditions, neurons depolarize and trigger a few APs before hyperpolarization. **C:** For weakly synchronized firing patterns, the simulated field activity (left) exhibits HFOs, typically in the FR frequency band (>250 Hz). Such oscillations (right) can be observed in actual depth-EEG signals recorded with intracerebral electrodes in patients. (Adapted from Wendling, F., et al., Computational models of epileptiform activity. J Neurosci Methods, 2016. 260: p. 233–251)

The fourth detailed model described in this section [101] was used to study the transition from ripples (<100–200 Hz) to FRs. These authors started from a pyramidal neuron model [102] comprising soma, branching dendrites, and a 24-compartment axon with gap junctions localized in the distal axonal branch. The network activity was generated by spreading waves and/or cycles of axonal firing. In this model, results showed that ripples are amplified when APs are conducted from an axon to another through electrical coupling, while FRs are elicited by ectopic spikes that randomly occur. It is noteworthy, however, that this model of transition between ripples and FRs did not include interneurons, unlike other studies that showed that interneuron firing and consecutive depolarizing GABA appear to play a key role in the generation of FRs [100,103–105].

The fifth model addressed specifically the question of how FRs may be related to seizure generation, using a cascade of two computational models, one at the detailed compartmental neuronal scale and the other at the NMM scale. In this model the probability of generating epileptic-type activity increases gradually with the increase of the density of axonal–axonal gap junctions. The latter can generate FRs and simultaneously shift the operational point of the NMM from a steady-state network into bistable behavior that can autonomously generate epileptic seizure activity. In this model the pathological FRs consist of transient bursts of APs arising from a relatively quiet baseline [106].

In conclusion, these five models demonstrate that FR oscillations may emerge according to different mechanisms: through a major contribution of nonsynaptic gap junctions between excitatory cells (first and fifth models; when clustered bursting neurons are slightly desynchronized or, even more, exhibit out-of-phase firing (second model); as a consequence of an increase in AMPA/NMDA-mediated synaptic transmission associated with lowering of GABAergic currents leading also to out-of-phase firing (third model); and ripples can occur as amplified APs that are conducted from an axon to another through electrical coupling, while FRs are elicited by ectopic spikes that randomly occur (fourth model). Further experimental validation of these alternative hypotheses is necessary. Although these models focused on FRs as they emerge in epileptic tissues, we should note that it is not yet possible to make a clear distinction between the specific characteristics of normal and pathological ripples— possible markers of epileptogenic tissue—as discussed in more detail in Chapter 33.

3.3. Models of Ictal Activity in Partial Epilepsies

In partial epilepsies, the onset of seizures is often characterized by the emergence of fast oscillations that can be directly observed in EEG signals. Typically, in human neocortical epilepsies, rapid discharges observed at seizure onset (sometimes referred to as "chirps" [107]) range from 70 to 120 Hz. In mesial temporal lobe epilepsies, fast oscillations at seizure onset were also observed in the hippocampus, amygdala, and entorhinal cortex [108] but are usually associated with lower frequencies (in the beta and low gamma range, 20–40 Hz). These fast oscillations constitute a hallmark of focal seizures characterized by a noticeable increase of intracerebral EEG signal frequency as compared with the preictal ongoing background activity [109,110].

3.3.1. Models of HFOs (Gamma, High Gamma) at Seizure Onset

For the specific case of gamma and other HFOs ranging from 40 to 120 Hz (gamma and high-gamma frequency bands) typically observed at the onset of neocortical seizures, NMMs [111], detailed models [112–114], and formal mathematical models [115] were elaborated. Interestingly, these modeling approaches (described below) are based on two fundamentally different assumptions that are still controversial. According to the former, HFOs are produced by synchronous firing of FS interneurons. The LFP basically reflects IPSPs generated onto pyramidal neurons, as also reported experimentally. According to the latter, HFOs are caused by nonsynaptic electrical couplings among pyramidal axons; this is compatible with the experimental observation that they may persist under conditions where chemical synaptic transmission is blocked but would disappear under the influence of gap junction blockers. Nonetheless, it should be noted, as mentioned above, that the lack of selective gap junction blockers makes rigorous experimental testing of this model assumption difficult [96].

According to the first assumption mentioned above (that HFOs are produced by synchronous firing of FS interneurons), an NMM was developed [110] to specifically assess the mechanisms underlying the generation of HFOs (>80 Hz) typically observed on depth-EEG electrodes at the onset of neocortical seizures. These authors followed the classic NMM approach and included two subsets of cells in the model: one subset of pyramidal neurons and one subset of FS interneurons targeting the perisomatic region of pyramidal cells, where fast GABAergic currents are activated. The simulation of a fast-onset activity that reproduces the actual seizure-onset pattern (in term of frequency, energy, and bandwidth) could be obtained only under the following scenario: dramatic increase of both the average amplitudes of EPSPs and IPSPs generated at the pyramidal cell level, followed by a slow and gradual decrease of these same PSPs to approximate the chirp aspect. In addition, simulations indicated that mutual inhibition is a key parameter in the tuning of the frequency of seizure-onset oscillations. These results are in line with previous experimental studies suggesting that a possible substrate for fast activity (gamma range) reflected in LFPs is the presence of mutual $GABA_A$-mediated synaptic inhibition within the interneuron network ([86], reviewed in [116]).

According to the second assumption, very fast EEG oscillations (HFOs) occurring at the onset of focal seizures were the object of a number of related network models by Traub et al. in which gap junctions play a prominent role. In [114], the model included 3,072 pyramidal cells and 384 interneurons interconnected through both synaptic and gap junctional couplings. Simulations from this model could replicate actual data when chemical synapses were blocked while axonal gap junctions between principal neurons were present. It is noteworthy that HFOs could also be simulated in interneuron networks when axonal gap junctions were included between interneurons. Based on extensive computer simulations, these authors concluded that gap junctions may play a crucial role in the emergence of very fast EEG oscillations similar to those observed in patients with drug-resistant epilepsy. Later, in another detailed network model by the same group [112], simulated field and intracellular patterns close to those observed experimentally could be obtained only when gap junctions were preserved. Interestingly, as in actual recordings, simulated signals exhibited more spikelets on somatic membrane potentials than full APs. The contribution of electrical couplings among neurons to the emergence of HFOs was also investigated on theoretical grounds [117,118].

More abstract network models inspired by the "cellular automata" used in physics were also developed by Traub et al. [110], particularly to further test the hypothesis of the role of electrical coupling between pyramidal cell axons. The specific purpose was to reproduce the sudden appearance of "blobs" of HFO activity, as seen in human seizures of frontal onset. These models consisted of 120,000 to 5,760,000 elements called "cells" to keep the biological signature; "cells" change states (e.g., firing, refractory, excitable) according to certain deterministic or stochastic rules. A basic feature is that inputs to the "cells" consist of non-rectifying symmetrical gap junctions that represent the electrical coupling between cortical layer 5 pyramidal cell axons. These models were able to reproduce the sudden appearance of "blobs" of HFO activity. These blobs evolve as spreading wavefronts that may coalesce but never pass through each other, as described by Lewis and Rinzel [117] in cellular automaton models. These models allowed the formulation of a number of predictions regarding the importance of gap junctions between axons of layer 5 pyramidal neurons localized in the vicinity of each other in the generation of HFOs prior to seizures. These predictions are being tested. Finally, following a similar modeling approach, some theoretical results were published regarding the influence of several factors on these blobs, such as the network topology and the connection length [115].

3.3.2. MODELS OF FOCAL SEIZURES: TRANSITION FROM INTERICTAL TO ICTAL ACTIVITY AND SEIZURE PROPAGATION

In contrast with generalized seizures in which both hemispheres are involved (see Section 3.7), focal (or "partial") seizures are limited to a relatively well-circumscribed area of the brain, referred to as the epileptogenic zone. Many studies based on the stereotaxic exploration of epilepsies [119] reported that this zone very often involves several distinct and distant brain areas, not only at seizure onset but also during seizure propagation [108]. Therefore, the notion of "epileptic focus" has evolved toward the now well-accepted concept of an epileptogenic network [120]. From the signal processing viewpoint (see also Chapter 44), many methods have been developed to identify epileptogenic networks and to characterize their dynamics from depth-EEG recordings. Some of these methods are based on functional connectivity, typically quantified by association/synchronization measures among signals [121–124]), while some other methods are based on the computation of "epileptogenicity" indices [125]. From the modeling viewpoint, the description of focal seizure dynamics (initiation, propagation, and termination) has long been—and is still—a topic of wide interest. Over the past years, models were proposed at any level of description, as exemplified in the following.

3.3.2.1. NMMs OF FOCAL SEIZURES

More than 25 years ago, Freeman et al. showed that the NMM that they initially proposed for the olfactory system could also produce realistic epileptiform EEG signals that simulated actual EEGs recorded from rats during seizures initiated by electrical stimulation [126]. The relevance of NMMs, which may also be called "nonlinear lumped-parameter models," in the analysis of depth-EEG epileptic signals was then emphasized by Wendling et al. [127], who published a series of papers showing that NMMs can produce epileptiform signals strikingly similar to those recorded in mesial temporal lobe epilepsy. A paramount example would be the model studies reported in [51,128] that focused on limbic seizures characterized by the appearance of HFOs (beta and gamma frequency bands) that constitute one of the most characteristic EEG patterns in focal seizures of human epilepsy, especially those in which the epileptogenic zone includes the hippocampus and associated limbic cortical areas [129,130]. This model starts from the hypothesis that networks of inhibitory interneurons with different properties are essential for the generation of gamma frequency oscillations [131]. Unlike the "generic" NMM that classically includes one interneuron type, this lumped model includes different kinds of neuronal populations, in particular two kinds of GABAergic neurons with different kinetics, GABA$_A$ fast and GABA$_A$ slow populations; the former cause IPSPs with fast time constants on the soma of pyramidal neurons, while the latter cause IPSPs with slow time constants on the dendrites of these neurons. Furthermore, as demonstrated experimentally by Banks et al. [132], both classes interact: GABA$_A$ slow cells inhibit not only pyramidal cells but also GABA$_A$ fast interneurons. The model is based on the important experimental observation that a nonuniform alteration of GABAergic inhibition underlies the generation of epileptiform activity in hippocampus and associated areas of the limbic brain, namely a reduced dendritic inhibition and increased somatic inhibition [133]. The simulations show that strikingly realistic activities are produced by the model (Fig. 3.7) when compared to real EEG signals recorded with intracerebral electrodes in patients with temporal lobe epilepsy [134]. Importantly, this model, reviewed in [69,104], explains the transition from interictal to ictal activity by a progressive decrease of slow dendritic inhibition leading to disinhibition of the GABA$_A$ fast interneurons. This model prediction was confirmed by some experimental results obtained later in an ex vivo model of limbic seizures (isolated brain) based on transient perfusion of bicuculline [135] as well as in the in vitro 4-aminopyridine model [136].

Following the same approach, NMMs were then elaborated to describe the transition from interictal to ictal activity in the entorhinal cortex from recordings performed in the isolated brain preparation [137,138].

Formally, NMMs are nonlinear dynamic systems. In this respect, NMMs reproducing the various patterns encountered during the transition to seizure activity have also been used as topics of theoretical studies aimed at analyzing the system's behavior with respect to endogenous or exogenous parameter changes. Typically, stability and bifurcation studies were conducted both in the generic NMM and in Wendling's model [139,140]. Similar models were used to investigate various scenarios involved in the generation of seizures. In [141], a novelty consisted in the simulation of several interconnected neuronal populations, with one representing a set of excitatory pyramidal cells and the other representing inhibitory interneurons. The main objective was to determine whether model parameters are correlated with the observable features of the simulated EEG signals (covariance functions), assuming that the connectivity between neuronal populations controls the dynamic spectrum of the system. These authors introduced a signal measure called "ictality" that quantifies the length and amplitude of the ictal phase. A number of scenarios were identified to explain how a neuronal system exhibiting multi-stability can switch from a "normal ongoing activity" state to a "paroxysmal EEG activity" state and then to an "epileptic seizure" state.

3.3.2.2. NFMs of Focal Seizures

NMMs have been able to simulate realistic epileptiform signal dynamics and transitions efficiently. In the classic format, however, NMMs cannot account for the spatial features of epileptogenic networks that often involve several distant and extended brain areas. This limitation motivated the development of NFMs, which take into account the multiplicity of interconnected brain sources, their complex geometry (folded cortical surface), and their synchronization level. In addition to the temporal dynamics of each source, these factors contribute to the solution of the EEG forward problem and thus have an impact on signals collected at the level of intracerebral or scalp electrodes. In [142], an NFM was proposed to study the relationships between the spatiotemporal features of neuronal generators (convoluted cortical dipole layers) and the corresponding EEG signals recorded at the scalp. This model was based on coupled neurophysiologically relevant NMMs and allowed researchers to investigate several factors regarding the location, area, geometry, and synchronization of neocortical sources as represented by neuronal populations. This permitted the joint analysis and interpretation of simultaneously recorded depth and scalp EEG signals, which remains a difficult task.

3.3.2.3. Detailed Network Models of Focal Seizures

Early modeling studies by Traub et al. [143] at the neuronal level in the CA2 and CA3 subfields of the hippocampus, combined with in vitro data, provided evidence for the impact of three important parameters on the generation of synchronized epileptiform after-discharges: the synaptic strength, the synaptic density, and the refractoriness of neurons following a period of excitation In brief, the authors constructed a network of CA3 neurons interconnected by excitatory synaptic connections where a chain reaction of excitation can be shown to spread over the whole network, depending on whether the excitatory interconnectivity is sufficiently dense and the synaptic interactions are sufficiently strong. A good fit between simulated and experimentally recorded epileptiform transients was obtained. For sustained repetitive after-discharges to occur in the model, some form of pacing inhibitory process was needed. This was accomplished by incorporating in the model (1) a slow voltage-dependent K$^+$ conductance (M current) and (2) an axonal refractoriness located at the axonal initial segment, at branch points, or at presynaptic terminals, which causes intermittent conduction from one to the next depolarized cell. Furthermore, a number of loops allowing reentrant paths within the neuronal population are important for maintaining a series of after-discharges. Using this kind of model, in a number of studies Traub et al. [144] investigated the role of several factors in inducing epileptiform oscillations similar to those observed in brain slices in vitro, namely synaptic-mediated activation of NMDA dendritic synapses and intrinsic voltage-dependent conductances.

Following this pioneering work on hippocampal area CA3, which has been one of the most extensively studied brain regions with respect to computational models of epileptiform activity (review in [145]), a number of detailed models were developed to investigate the network mechanisms underlying

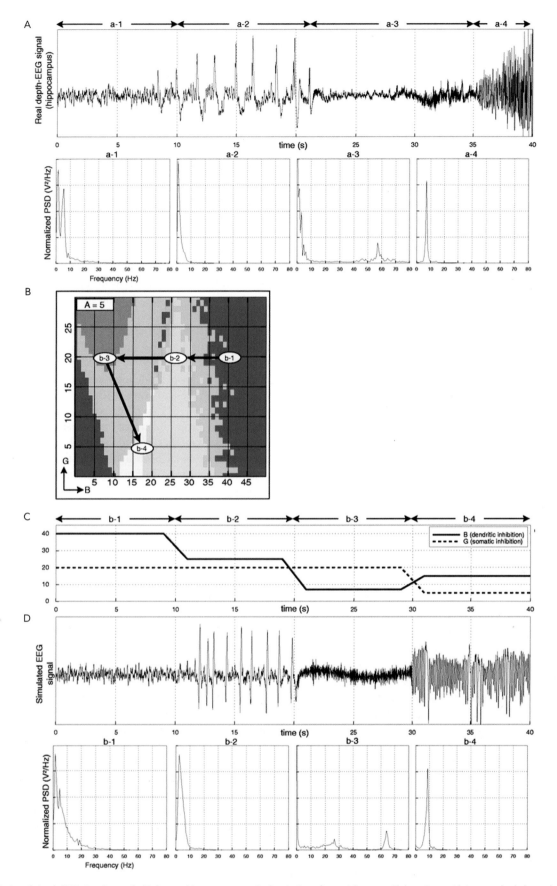

Figure 3.7. **A:** *A real depth-EEG signal recorded in human hippocampus at the beginning of a partial temporal lobe seizure with intracerebral electrodes (SEEG). Four phases (a-1 to a-4) are distinguished according to the pseudo-stationary nature of the activities reflected by the signal: normal background activity (a-1), discharge of rhythmic spikes (a-2), low-voltage rapid discharge (a-3), and high-amplitude quasi-sinusoidal slowing down activity (a-4). The normalized power spectral density (PSD) shows that part of the activity corresponding to phase a-3 belongs to the gamma band (55–60 Hz). **B:** A candidate path on the activity map, for a value of excitation (A = 5) and different values of slow (B) and fast (G) inhibition, showing the transitions between different types of activity observed in the real signal (a-1 → a-2 → a-3 → a-4). **C:** Slow and fast inhibitory synaptic gain profiles defined by the candidate path and used in the model to simulate a time-series signal with transitions in dynamics. **D:** Simulated EEG signal obtained with the model when the synaptic gains vary as a function of time and PSDs computed on the four periods of 10 seconds (b-1 to b-4). (With permission from Wendling, F., et al., Epileptic fast activity can be explained by a model of impaired GABAergic dendritic inhibition. Eur J Neurosci, 2002. 15(9): p. 1499–1508)*

focal seizure initiation and propagation in other brain structures. Van Drongelen et al. [146] developed a model to evaluate the relationship between network connectivity and seizure-like activity patterns generated by neocortical networks. This network included 656 excitatory and inhibitory neuron models (HH formalism) of four types: bursting pyramidal, regular-firing pyramidal, basket cell, and chandelier cell. In this model the essential parameter changes necessary to generate seizure activity were investigated. The network model was found to exhibit a large variety of behaviors that critically depended on the strength of synaptic connections. Interestingly, and in contrast to the common belief that strong excitatory coupling is needed to synchronize bursting, results obtained from computational modeling studies indicated that neural networks can generate and sustain seizure-like activity even if the excitatory coupling strength falls below a critical value.

3.4. Models of Ictal Activity in Generalized Epilepsies

3.4.1. Models of Spike-and-Waves and Absence Seizures

Thalamic neurons can display different modes of activity, including rhythmic bursting, that are akin to the spike-and-wave discharges characteristic of generalized epilepsies. In this respect the *single neuron model* of a thalamic relay neuron of Wang [147], which shows both 10- and 3-Hz bursting dynamic modes, is particularly instructive. This model demonstrates clearly how distinct oscillatory modes depend on different balances of sets of ion currents. In this model the emergence of 3-Hz bursts, which resemble the 3-Hz oscillations seen in human generalized epilepsies, depends on the value of the hyperpolarization-activated cationic current, I_h (the so-called sag current), although the T-type Ca^{2+} current also plays an important role. According to this model the 10-Hz oscillatory mode is maintained, at the level of a single neuron, by the dynamics of the low-voltage activated Ca^{2+} current, I_T. Under normal conditions the neuronal membrane does not hyperpolarize sufficiently to activate the I_h current. Indeed, if the neuronal membrane were deeply hyperpolarized, it would stay in such a condition in case only I_T were active, because the latter current is not sufficient to overcome a strong hyperpolarization. However, the presence of I_h allows the neuron to escape this strong hyperpolarized state. Thus, the transition between the 10- and the 3-Hz modes depends on the level of hyperpolarization. This single neuron model is completely deterministic and it may display "strange attractors" typical of a chaotic dynamic state.

A model of a *thalamic neuronal network* that is closer to the reality of epileptic discharges than the single neuron model described above was developed to account for spike and-wave seizures at the level of a neuronal population. A basic physiological phenomenon simulated was that during spike-and-wave discharges the reticular nucleus neurons (RE) discharge with long spike bursts riding on a depolarization, whereas the TCR neurons are either entrained into the seizure oscillation or are quiescent; cortical stimulation can trigger a transition between these two modes [148]. The spatial model of these neuronal populations predicts that in the focus of seizure activity there will be intense RE activity and TCR quiescence; further, this focus will be surrounded by an area where the TCR neurons are less hyperpolarized such that low-threshold oscillatory spikes may occur. This surrounding area will be the forefront of a wave of propagating seizure activity. The model shows that the complex nonlinear dynamics of the neuronal network depends critically on the low-voltage-activated (LVA or LTS) Ca^{2+} current I_T that can produce intrinsic repetitive bursting in TCR neurons. In this context it is also interesting to note that in the genetic model of absence epilepsy GAERS (genetic absence epilepsy rats of Strasbourg), the presence of a significantly enhanced LVA (or LTS) current in thalamic neurons was reported [149]. It is also noteworthy that drugs such as ethosuximide that depress I_T can suppress seizure initiation. However, further studies showed that ethosuximide acts also on the non-inactivating Na^+ current and on a Ca^{2+}-activated K^+ current [150]. The level of hyperpolarization of TCR cells, which appears to be a crucial determinant of the dynamic behavior of the neuronal population, depends on the level of synaptic inputs.

Along the line of modeling studies of thalamocortical oscillations and spike-and-wave discharges at the neuronal level, Destexhe et al. [151] investigated the role of corticothalamic feedback in promoting these oscillations, in contrast with most previous studies, where the emphasis was on the role of intrathalamic mechanisms. The model indicated that corticothalamic feedback is of crucial importance and that it acts through excitation of GABAergic RE neurons leading to the inhibition of TCR cells that can show rebound firing. Among other predictions (for a comprehensive overview of these models see [152]), the model also reveals that the upregulation of I_h current, induced by an increase of $[Ca^{2+}]_i$, mediates the termination of absence seizures. Interestingly, the role of I_h current in terminating a burst of spike-and-wave discharges was also analyzed in the modeling study by Koppert et al. [153] using a quite different approach, as presented below. Although the models of spike-and-wave discharges described above focus on neuronal activities at the level of the thalamus, it has now been shown that the driver of these discharges in absence seizures is constituted by a neocortical network, situated in the area of the face representation in rat (WAG/Rij in [154], GAERS in [155], see also discussion in [156]). However, the properties of this cortical driving system have not yet been incorporated in a computational model.

3.4.2. Models of Dynamics of Neural Systems in Absence Seizures

The models discussed above have given us insight into some basic neuronal mechanisms underlying spike-and-wave discharges but do not address specifically an essential issue of the dynamics of this type of epileptic activity: namely what causes absence seizures *to start and to stop*? A thalamocortical system can display both kinds of activity—normal EEG and spike-and-wave discharges; that is, possesses *bistability*. This means that the dynamics of this system may undergo a transition or a bifurcation between those two states, depending on some specific conditions. In this context two essential questions can be formulated:

1. What is the nature of the set of parameters that make this system more prone to undergo such transitions in epileptic patients than in normal subjects?

2. What are the mechanisms responsible for *transitions* from the normal state of activity to the paroxysmal state characterized by the presence of spike-and-wave discharges?

To answer those questions, a computational model of absence epilepsy focusing on the *dynamic behavior of the networks* was constructed [157,158]. This model consisted of four interacting neural populations: TCR, RE, cortical pyramidal cells, and interneurons integrating synaptic and network properties at the mesoscopic and macroscopic levels. The model's output signal can display a waxing and waning "spindle-like" oscillation of relatively low amplitude having a spectrum with a peak at approximately 11 Hz, simulating the normal-state EEG, or a high-amplitude "seizure-like" oscillation at a frequency around 9 Hz, which is characteristic of absence seizures in the rat (WAG/Rij or GAERS) (Fig. 3.8).

Thus, for a given set of neuronal parameters, the model is in a "bistable regimen" where it may generate both normal and paroxysmal oscillations and spontaneous transitions between these two types of behavior, depending on exogenous and/or endogenous fluctuations. A parameter sensitivity analysis in this computational model revealed the critical parameters responsible for lowering the threshold for the transition between normal and spike-and-wave discharge states, as occurs in absence epilepsy [157]:

1. The level of cortical GABA$_A$ inhibition

2. The slope of the sigmoid transfer function of cortical interneurons

3. Changes of Ca^{2+} currents in RE and TCR neurons

4. A decrease of cholinergic activation, which corresponds to the observation that spike-and-wave discharges tend to occur at the transition between waking state and sleep and when attention and the level of activity are reduced.

These model results underscore the concept that there are several routes to epilepsy [159].

This model facilitated making the prediction that the probability distributions of interictal intervals and of ictal durations should follow a gamma distribution:

$$y = C\,x^{\alpha-1}e^{-x/\beta}$$

where *C* is a normalization constant and the distribution's parameters are α, the shape parameter, and β, the scale parameter of the distribution. The value of the shape parameter α = 1 indicates that transitions occur according to a random exponential, Poisson process. Values of α < 1 may arise due to a continuous random walk process. The prediction that the distribution of *interictal* intervals may follow a gamma distribution with α = 1 was verified experimentally, both in WAG/Rij rat and GAERS, in human absence seizures, and also in an *in vitro* model [158].

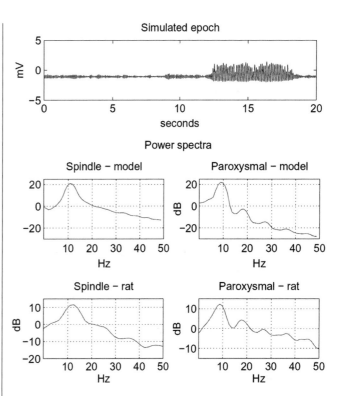

Figure 3.8. Example of the output of the model of absence seizures. Upper panel: Simulated EEG signals showing an epoch of normal ongoing EEG followed by a spontaneously occurring paroxysmal episode. Lower panels: EEG power spectra of normal spindle EEG (left) and paroxysmal EEG (right) simulated with the model and recorded from a WAG/Rij epileptic rat. (With permission from Suffczynski, P., et al., Epileptic transitions: model predictions and experimental validation. J Clin Neurophysiol, 2005. **22**(5): p. 288–299)

Regarding *ictal durations*, however, it emerged that values of α > 1 gave a better fit, indicating the presence of deterministic, time-dependent or use-dependent, homeostatic mechanisms that act to abort the current spike-and-wave discharge state. Koppert et al. [153] explored this issue further in a similar model and demonstrated that the most likely homeostatic mechanism controlling seizure duration is the hyperpolarization-dependent cationic (I_h) current, as also mentioned above [152]. An additional prediction of the model is that paroxysmal oscillations can be annihilated by a well-timed pulse; this was experimentally demonstrated later in animal models using different stimulation paradigms [160,161].

3.5. Models of Status Epilepticus

In adults, status epilepticus is defined as a continuous seizure lasting more than 30 minutes, or two or more seizures without full recovery of consciousness in between. Readers may refer to [162] for a description of the electroclinical features of status epilepticus. In contrast with focal seizures, spike-and-wave discharges, or absence seizures, computational modeling approaches of status epilepticus have been developed only recently.

In the low-dose lithium–pilocarpine model (rat), the entire course of status epilepticus was investigated using an NMM [163]. The authors started from status epilepticus induced in rats where a sequence of abnormal behaviors, such as chewing, forelimb clonus, and continuous clonic activity of four limbs and tail, could be observed. EEG spectral features were analyzed and EEG segments were classified according to observed animal behaviors. The authors reported that most EEG patterns recorded during status epilepticus (except narrow-band waves in the theta range) could be simulated using Wendling's model [51], by tuning only a few parameters. Some experimental results in the literature could support the reported model-based findings.

4. RELEVANCE OF NONLINEAR DYNAMIC SYSTEMS AND NETWORK TOPOLOGY IN EEG GENERATION

4.1. Nonlinear Dynamic Systems

Computational models of complex neuronal networks, where parameters and variables are easily identifiable with physiological phenomena, in general are particularly attractive for the neuroscientific community. These models, however, are often too constrained and confined to the set of specific parameters chosen, such that the general dynamic properties of these networks may be difficult to put in evidence. This restriction does not apply to formal mathematical models like nonlinear dynamic systems. The latter have the advantage of enabling the extensive exploration of the network's dynamic behavior: all possible states (stable, multistable) as well as transitions (bifurcations) can be determined and theoretically investigated, albeit at the expense of detail. However, the links between computational and experimental variables are less straightforward and require deeper extrapolation.

Two representative examples of this kind of analytical computational model in the study of neural dynamics and resulting oscillations at the EEG level were published recently. Kalitzin et al. [164] introduced a formal mathematical model (the Z6 model) that corresponds indirectly to realistic neuronal processes (excitatory and inhibitory synaptic interactions, AP generation). It provides an insightful contribution to understanding oscillatory states in "epileptic" neuronal networks; it also proposes specific methods for optimal reactive control able to force transitions from one state (attractor) into another.

The second example of the potential interest of formal nonlinear dynamic systems in the analysis of neural dynamics in the context of epilepsy is the phenomenological model called the Epileptor [165]. Acknowledging the different time scales present in seizure evolution, Jirsa et al. used the theory of fast–slow systems in nonlinear dynamics to account for this evolution, namely the generation of fast oscillations, of interictal spikes and of the spike-and-wave complexes close to seizure offset. A slow permittivity variable accounts for the extracellular effects on network dynamics, related to energy and oxygen consumption, and captures details of the autonomous slow evolution of interictal and ictal phases, as well as various features of seizure evolution during each phase.

4.2. Topological Models and Impact of Network Structural/Functional Models

One particular kind of models has been proposed as having potential relevance for epilepsy studies, namely large-scale structural and functional models that focus on a specific brain area, in particular the dentate gyrus of the hippocampus, where morphological changes, as found in epileptogenic tissue, are integrated with functional properties (namely sclerosis and mossy fiber sprouting). A noteworthy example of such models was published by Dyhrfjeld-Johnsen et al. [166]. The approach is computationally heavy and consists of a structural model containing eight kinds of neurons (considered "nodes" in the nomenclature of graph theory) linked by cell type–specific connection probabilities. The "epileptogenic" condition, corresponding to the sclerosis of the dentate gyrus ("end-folium"), was simulated by removing hilar cells and adding mossy fiber sprouted contacts. Based on this structural model a functional model was derived. It was then scaled down for simplicity, and a number of measures by means of which a state of hyperexcitability could be estimated were explored. Although neither the appearance of interictal epileptiform spikes nor of seizure activity was analyzed, this model revealed that the removal of a small fraction of hilar cells is sufficient to reach a state of hyperexcitability in the network, which is in line with experimental observations.

Another model where the effects of structural changes on epileptogenesis were investigated is that of Volman et al. [167]. In this case the change in network excitability represents the effects of trauma. This model consists of a two-dimensional network of 6,400 interconnected neurons, 80% of them pyramidal cells and 20% inhibitory interneurons, with the adequate biophysical properties. The effect of trauma was simulated by deafferentation and the consequent reduction of afferent inputs: only a small number of neurons (1–5%) preserved their external afferents, the so-called intact neurons. The simulations showed that the appearance and the rate of epileptiform paroxysmal discharges depend mainly on the distribution of these intact neurons in the network (i.e., their spatial density) but not on the network topology as such. However, the link between the results from this model and the occurrence of epileptic seizures needs to be made more explicit and requires further investigation.

5. CONCLUSION: MODELS FOCUSING ON NORMAL AND EPILEPTIFORM NEURAL ACTIVITIES

The number of studies making use of modeling approaches to investigate neuronal systems, both under normal and epileptic conditions, has considerably expanded, particularly over the past two decades. For the large panel of issues addressed in this review, we were able to find modeling attempts, either at neural mass, neural field, or detailed network, or more abstract, mathematical levels. All described models were developed to investigate a specific issue, in a specific context, at a specific level of description. To a large extent, these models have *face validity*, as they appear to reasonably replicate actual neuronal activity, either normal or epileptiform. However, this is only a first step toward the validation of model assumptions. Indeed, with a bit of effort, any dynamic system, even purely abstract and disconnected from neurophysiology, can approach some morphological features or signatures reflected in electrophysiological signals. Therefore, the reproduction of actual data should not be the sole purpose of computational models of neuronal activities. An equally important, or even more important, ability is when models explicitly include properties (wide sense) that are likely to play a role in the real system and may be shown to underlie specific features. This ability is sometimes referred to as the model's *constructive value*.

The ability of computational models to replicate and explain neurophysiological observations is, however, not sufficient to guarantee that the embedded ingredients and mechanisms are key to the behavior of real neuronal systems. Further model validation is always required, and this is certainly the most difficult issue. In some of the reported studies, this issue is addressed using a *prediction-validation loop*. The general idea is to generate predictions that can further be tested experimentally in order to increase confidence in the model. If predictions are verified, the model gains power and acceptance; conversely, inconsistencies highlight the need for model improvements. In this perspective, combined theoretical and experimental approaches provide an ideal framework to test the model's *predictive value* and to elaborate progressively more "valid" models [168].

Winding up, we note that models with detailed biological realism can only be investigated through extensive and usually computationally expensive simulations, up to the extreme dimension of the Blue Brain Project [7]. This still does not guarantee, from a formal standpoint, that all possible behaviors will be uncovered. This stands in contrast to abstract formal mathematical models that may permit exploring all possible states (stable, multistable) as well as transitions (bifurcations) of the dynamics of neuronal networks, at the cost, however, of a less explicit match between model and physiological variables. Therefore, we favor combining models based on biological realism with formal analytical models to enhance the potential of each one in yielding insightful interpretations of neuronal phenomena.

ACKNOWLEDGMENTS

The authors wish to thank Dr. Julien Modolo for the critical reading of the final version of this chapter.

REFERENCES

1. Bedard, C., H. Kroger, and A. Destexhe, *Model of low-pass filtering of local field potentials in brain tissue.* Phys Rev E Stat Nonlin Soft Matter Phys, 2006. **73**(5 Pt 1): p. 051911.
2. Gerstner, W. and W. Kistler, *Spiking Neuron Models.* Cambridge University Press, 2002.
3. Wilson, H.R. and J.D. Cowan, *Excitatory and inhibitory interactions in localized populations of model neurons.* Biophys J, 1972. **12**(1): p. 1–24.
4. Hodgkin, A.L. and A.F. Huxley, *A quantitative description of membrane current and its application to conduction and excitation in nerve.* J Physiol, 1952. **117**(4): p. 500–544.
5. Hines, M.L. and N.T. Carnevale, *NEURON: a tool for neuroscientists.* Neuroscientist, 2001. **7**(2): p. 123–135.
6. Brette, R., M. Rudolph, N. T. Carnevale, et al., *Simulation of networks of spiking neurons: a review of tools and strategies.* J Comput Neurosci, 2007. **23**(3): p. 349–398.
7. Markram, H., et al., *Reconstruction and simulation of neocortical microcircuitry.* Cell, 2015. **163**(2): p. 456–492.
8. Pinsky, P.F. and J. Rinzel, *Intrinsic and network rhythmogenesis in a reduced Traub model for CA3 neurons.* J Comput Neurosci, 1994. **1**(1-2): p. 39–60.
9. Demont-Guignard, S., P. Benquet, U. Gerber, and F. Wendling, *Analysis of intracerebral EEG recordings of epileptic spikes: insights from a neural network model.* IEEE Trans Biomed Eng, 2009. **56**(12): p. 2782–2795.
10. Leresche, N., D. Jassik-Gerschenfeld, M. Haby, I. Soltesz, and V. Crunelli, *Pacemaker-like and other types of spontaneous membrane potential oscillations of thalamocortical cells.* Neurosci Lett, 1990. **113**(1): p. 72–77.
11. White, J.A., T. Budde, and A.R. Kay, *A bifurcation analysis of neuronal subthreshold oscillations.* Biophys J, 1995. **69**(4): p. 1203–1217.
12. Hutcheon, B. and Y. Yarom, *Resonance, oscillation and the intrinsic frequency preferences of neurons.* Trends Neurosci, 2000. **23**(5): p. 216–222.
13. Steriade, M., D. Contreras, R. Curro Dossi, and A. Nunez, *The slow (< 1 Hz) oscillation in reticular thalamic and thalamocortical neurons: scenario of sleep rhythm generation in interacting thalamic and neocortical networks.* J Neurosci, 1993. **13**(8): p. 3284–3299.
14. Compte, A., M.V. Sanchez-Vives, D.A. McCormick, and X.J. Wang, *Cellular and network mechanisms of slow oscillatory activity (<1 Hz) and wave propagations in a cortical network model.* J Neurophysiol, 2003. **89**(5): p. 2707–2725.
15. Bazhenov, M., I. Timofeev, M. Steriade, and T.J. Sejnowski, *Model of thalamocortical slow-wave sleep oscillations and transitions to activated States.* J Neurosci, 2002. **22**(19): p. 8691–8704.
16. Orban, G., T. Kiss, and P. Erdi, *Intrinsic and synaptic mechanisms determining the timing of neuron population activity during hippocampal theta oscillation.* J Neurophysiol, 2006. **96**(6): p. 2889–2904.
17. Goutagny, R., J. Jackson, and S. Williams, *Self-generated theta oscillations in the hippocampus.* Nat Neurosci, 2009. **12**(12): p. 1491–1493.
18. Kopell, N., C. Borgers, P. Pervouchine, P. Malerba, and A. Tort, *Gamma and theta rhythms in biophysical models of hippocampal circuits.* V. Cutsuridis et al. (eds.), Hippocampal Microcircuits, Springer Series in Computational Neuroscience 5, 2010: p. 423–457.
19. Liley, D.T., D.M. Alexander, J.J. Wright, and M.D. Aldous, *Alpha rhythm emerges from large-scale networks of realistically coupled multicompartmental model cortical neurons.* Network, 1999. **10**(1): p. 79–92.
20. Bollimunta, A., J. Mo, C.E. Schroeder, and M. Ding, *Neuronal mechanisms and attentional modulation of corticothalamic alpha oscillations.* J Neurosci, 2011. **31**(13): p. 4935–4943.
21. van Kerkoerle, T., M.W. Self, B. Dagnino, et al., *Alpha and gamma oscillations characterize feedback and feedforward processing in monkey visual cortex.* Proc Natl Acad Sci U S A, 2014. **111**(40): p. 14332–14341.
22. Haegens, S., A. Barczak, G. Musacchia, et al., *Laminar profile and physiology of the alpha rhythm in primary visual, auditory, and somatosensory regions of neocortex.* J Neurosci, 2015. **35**(42): p. 14341–14352.
23. Buzsaki, G., C.A. Anastassiou, and C. Koch, *The origin of extracellular fields and currents—EEG, ECoG, LFP and spikes.* Nat Rev Neurosci, 2012. **13**(6): p. 407–420.
24. Perez Velazquez, J.L. and P.L. Carlen, *Gap junctions, synchrony and seizures.* Trends Neurosci, 2000. **23**(2): p. 68–74.
25. Galarreta, M. and S. Hestrin, *A network of fast-spiking cells in the neocortex connected by electrical synapses.* Nature, 1999. **402**(6757): p. 72–75.
26. Buzsaki, G., *Hippocampal sharp wave-ripple: a cognitive biomarker for episodic memory and planning.* Hippocampus, 2015. **25**(10): p. 1073–1188.
27. Jahnke, S., M. Timme, and R.M. Memmesheimer, *A unified dynamic model for learning, replay, and sharp-wave/ripples.* J Neurosci, 2015. **35**(49): p. 16236–16258.
28. Buzsaki, G. and J.J. Chrobak, *Synaptic plasticity and self-organization in the hippocampus.* Nat Neurosci, 2005. **8**(11): p. 1418–1420.
29. Borgers, C. and N. Kopell, *Synchronization in networks of excitatory and inhibitory neurons with sparse, random connectivity.* Neural Comput, 2003. **15**(3): p. 509–538.
30. Traub, R.D., D. Schmitz, J.G. Jefferys, and A. Draguhn., *High-frequency population oscillations are predicted to occur in hippocampal pyramidal neuronal networks interconnected by axoaxonal gap junctions.* Neuroscience, 1999. **92**(2): p. 407–426.
31. Memmesheimer, R.M., *Quantitative prediction of intermittent high-frequency oscillations in neural networks with supralinear dendritic interactions.* Proc Natl Acad Sci U S A, 2010. **107**(24): p. 11092–11097.
32. Freeman, W., *Mass Action in the Nervous System.* New York: Academic Press, 1975.
33. Bhattacharya, B.S., D. Coyle, and L.P. Maguire, *A thalamo-cortico-thalamic neural mass model to study alpha rhythms in Alzheimer's disease.* Neural Netw, 2011. **24**(6): p. 631–645.

34. Lopes da Silva, F.H., A. Hoeks, H. Smits, and L.H. Zetterberg, *Model of brain rhythmic activity. The alpha-rhythm of the thalamus.* Kybernetik, 1974. **15**(1): p. 27–37.

35. Sotero, R.C., N.J. Trujillo-Barreto, Y. Iturria-Medina, F. Carbonell, and J.C. Jimenez, *Realistically coupled neural mass models can generate EEG rhythms.* Neural Comput, 2007. **19**(2): p. 478–512.

36. Becker, R., S. Knock, P. Ritter, and V. Jirsa, *Relating alpha power and phase to population firing and hemodynamic activity using a thalamo-cortical neural mass model.* PLoS Comput Biol, 2015. **11**(9): p. e1004352.

37. van Rotterdam, A., F. Lopes da Silva, J. van den Ende, M. Viergever, and A. Hermans, *A model of the spatio-temporal characteristics of the alpha rhythm.* Bull. Math. Biology, 1982. **44**(2): p. 283–305.

38. Lopes da Silva, F.H., J.E. Vos, J. Mooibroek, and A. Van Rotterdam, *Partial coherence analysis of thalamic and cortical alpha rhythms in dog: a contribution towards a general model of the cortical organization of rhythmic activity.* In: Pfurtscheller G, Buser P, Lopes da Silva FH, eds. Rhythmic EEG Activities and Cortical Functioning. Amsterdam: Elsevier, 1980: p. 33–59.

39. Liley, D.T., P.J. Cadusch, and M.P. Dafilis, *A spatially continuous mean field theory of electrocortical activity.* Network, 2002. **13**(1): p. 67–113.

40. Jirsa, V.K., *Neural field dynamics with local and global connectivity and time delay.* Philos Trans A Math Phys Eng Sci, 2009. **367**(1891): p. 1131–1143.

41. Deco, G., V.K. Jirsa, P.A. Robinson, M. Breakspear, and K. Friston, *The dynamic brain: from spiking neurons to neural masses and cortical fields.* PLoS Comput Biol, 2008. **4**(8): p. e1000092.

42. Harrison, L.M., O. David, and K.J. Friston, *Stochastic models of neuronal dynamics.* Philos Trans R Soc Lond B Biol Sci, 2005. **360**(1457): p. 1075–1091.

43. Nunez, P.L., *Generation of human EEG by a combination of long and short range neocortical interactions.* Brain Topogr, 1989. **1**(3): p. 199–215.

44. Nunez, P.L., *Neocortical Dynamics and Human EEG Rhythms.* New York: Oxford University Press, 1995.

45. Suffczynski, P., S. Kalitzin, G. Pfurtscheller, and F.H. Lopes da Silva, *Computational model of thalamo-cortical networks: dynamical control of alpha rhythms in relation to focal attention.* Int J Psychophysiol, 2001. **43**(1): p. 25–40.

46. Pfurtscheller, G. and F.H. Lopes da Silva, *Event-related EEG/MEG synchronization and desynchronization: basic principles.* Clin Neurophysiol, 1999. **110**(11): p. 1842–1857.

47. Jansen, B.H. and V.G. Rit, *Electroencephalogram and visual evoked potential generation in a mathematical model of coupled cortical columns.* Biol Cybern, 1995. **73**(4): p. 357–366.

48. Jansen, B.H., G. Zouridakis, and M.E. Brandt, *A neurophysiologically-based mathematical model of flash visual evoked potentials.* Biol Cybern, 1993. **68**(3): p. 275–283.

49. David, O. and K.J. Friston, *A neural mass model for MEG/EEG: coupling and neuronal dynamics.* Neuroimage, 2003. **20**(3): p. 1743–1755.

50. Zavaglia, M., L. Astolfi, F. Babiloni, and M. Ursino, *A neural mass model for the simulation of cortical activity estimated from high-resolution EEG during cognitive or motor tasks.* J Neurosci Methods, 2006. **157**(2): p. 317–329.

51. Wendling, F., F. Bartolomei, J.J. Bellanger, and P. Chauvel, *Epileptic fast activity can be explained by a model of impaired GABAergic dendritic inhibition.* Eur J Neurosci, 2002. **15**(9): p. 1499–1508.

52. Valdes-Sosa, P.A., J.M. Sanchez-Bornot, R.C. Sotero et al., *Model-driven EEG/fMRI fusion of brain oscillations.* Hum Brain Mapp, 2009. **30**(9): p. 2701–2721.

53. Bojak, I., T.F. Oostendorp, A.T. Reid, and R. Kotter., *Connecting mean field models of neural activity to EEG and fMRI data.* Brain Topogr, 2010. **23**(2): p. 139–149.

54. Zhao, X., J.W. Kim, and P.A. Robinson, *Slow-wave oscillations in a cortico-thalamic model of sleep and wake.* J Theor Biol, 2015. **370**: p. 93–102.

55. Booth, V. and C.G. Diniz Behn, *Physiologically-based modeling of sleep-wake regulatory networks.* Math Biosci, 2014. **250**: p. 54–68.

56. Grabska-Barwinska, A. and J. Zygierewicz, *A model of event-related EEG synchronization changes in beta and gamma frequency bands.* J Theor Biol, 2006. **238**(4): p. 901–913.

57. Thomson, A.M. and J. Deuchars, *Synaptic interactions in neocortical local circuits: dual intracellular recordings in vitro.* Cereb Cortex, 1997. **7**(6): p. 510–522.

58. Leung, L.S., *Generation of theta and gamma rhythms in the hippocampus.* Neurosci Biobehav Rev, 1998. **22**(2): p. 275–290.

59. Neymotin, S.A., H. Lee, E. Park, A.A. Fenton, and W.W. Lytton., *Emergence of physiological oscillation frequencies in a computer model of neocortex.* Front Comput Neurosci, 2011. **5**: p. 19.

60. Bojak, I. and D.T. Liley, *Axonal velocity distributions in neural field equations.* PLoS Comput Biol, 2010. **6**(1): p. e1000653.

61. Osipova, D., A. Takashima, R. Oostenveld, G. Fernandez, E. Maris, and O. Jensen, *Theta and gamma oscillations predict encoding and retrieval of declarative memory.* J Neurosci, 2006. **26**(28): p. 7523–7531.

62. Sauseng, P., W. Klimesch, K.F. Heise, et al., *Brain oscillatory substrates of visual short-term memory capacity.* Curr Biol, 2009. **19**(21): p. 1846–1852.

63. Colgin, L.L., *Theta-gamma coupling in the entorhinal-hippocampal system.* Curr Opin Neurobiol, 2015. **31**: p. 45–50.

64. Tort, A.B., R. Komorowski, H. Eichenbaum, and N. Kopell, *Measuring phase-amplitude coupling between neuronal oscillations of different frequencies.* J Neurophysiol, 2010. **104**(2): p. 1195–1210.

65. Jensen, O., M. Bonnefond, T.R. Marshall, and P. Tiesinga, *Oscillatory mechanisms of feedforward and feedback visual processing.* Trends Neurosci, 2015. **38**(4): p. 192–194.

66. Onslow, A.C., M.W. Jones, and R. Bogacz, *A canonical circuit for generating phase-amplitude coupling.* PLoS One, 2014. **9**(8): p. e102591.

67. Ursino, M., F. Cona, and M. Zavaglia, *The generation of rhythms within a cortical region: analysis of a neural mass model.* Neuroimage, 2010. **52**(3): p. 1080–1094.

68. Sotero, R.C., *Modeling the generation of phase-amplitude coupling in cortical circuits: from detailed networks to neural mass models.* Biomed Res Int, 2015. **2015**: p. 915606.

69. Lytton, W.W., *Computer modelling of epilepsy.* Nat Rev Neurosci, 2008. **9**(8): p. 626–637.

70. Wendling, F., *Computational models of epileptic activity: a bridge between observation and pathophysiological interpretation.* Expert Rev Neurother, 2008. **8**(6): p. 889–896.

71. Wendling, F., P. Benquet, F. Bartolomei, and V. Jirsa, *Computational models of epileptiform activity.* J Neurosci Methods, 2016. **260**: p. 233–251.

72. de Curtis, M. and G. Avanzini, *Interictal spikes in focal epileptogenesis.* Prog Neurobiol, 2001. **63**(5): p. 541–567.

73. Schwartzkroin, P.A. and H.V. Wheal, *Electrophysiology of Epilepsy.* Academic Press, 1984.

74. Staley, K.J. and F.E. Dudek, *Interictal spikes and epileptogenesis.* Epilepsy Currents/American Epilepsy Society, 2006. **6**: p. 199–202.

75. Avoli, M., G. Biagini, and M. De Curtis, *Do interictal spikes sustain seizures and epileptogenesis?* Epilepsy Currents/American Epilepsy Society, 2006. **6**: p. 203.

76. Chauviere, L., T. Doublet, A. Ghestem, et al., *Changes in interictal spike features precede the onset of temporal lobe epilepsy.* Ann Neurol, 2012. **71**(6): p. 805–814.

77. Heilman, A.D. and J. Quattrochi, *Computational models of epileptiform activity in single neurons.* Biosystems, 2004. **78**(1-3): p. 1–21.

78. Andersen, P., R. Morris, D. Amaral, T. Bliss, and J. O'Keefe, *The Hippocampus Book.* New York, 2007.

79. Almeida, A.C., V.M. Fernandes de Lima, and A.F. Infantosi, *Mathematical model of the CA1 region of the rat hippocampus.* Phys Med Biol, 1998. **43**(9): p. 2631–2646.

80. Varona, P., J.M. Ibarz, L. Lopez-Aguado, and O. Herreras., *Macroscopic and subcellular factors shaping population spikes.* J Neurophysiol, 2000. **83**(4): p. 2192–2208.

81. Erdi, P., Z. Huhn, and T. Kiss, *Hippocampal theta rhythms from a computational perspective: code generation, mood regulation and navigation.* Neural Netw, 2005. **18**(9): p. 1202–1211.

82. Traub, R.D., D. Contreras, and M.A. Whittington, *Combined experimental/simulation studies of cellular and network mechanisms of epileptogenesis in vitro and in vivo.* J Clin Neurophysiol, 2005. **22**(5): p. 330–342.

83. Bausch, S.B. and J.O. McNamara, *Synaptic connections from multiple subfields contribute to granule cell hyperexcitability in hippocampal slice cultures.* J Neurophysiol, 2000. **84**(6): p. 2918–2932.

84. Ratnadurai-Giridharan, S., R.A. Stefanescu, P.P. Khargonekar, P.R. Carney, and S.S. Talathi., *Genesis of interictal spikes in the CA1: a computational investigation.* Front Neural Circuits, 2014. **8**: p. 2.

85. Golomb, D., C. Yue, and Y. Yaari, *Contribution of persistent Na⁺ current and M-type K⁺ current to somatic bursting in CA1 pyramidal cells: combined experimental and modeling study.* J Neurophysiol, 2006. **96**(4): p. 1912–1926.

86. Wang, X.J. and G. Buzsaki, *Gamma oscillation by synaptic inhibition in a hippocampal interneuronal network model.* J Neurosci, 1996. **16**(20): p. 6402–6413.

87. Wang, X.J., *Pacemaker neurons for the theta rhythm and their synchronization in the septohippocampal reciprocal loop.* J Neurophysiol, 2002. **87**(2): p. 889–900.

88. Zetterberg, L.H., L. Kristiansson, and K. Mossberg, *Performance of a model for a local neuron population.* Biol Cybern, 1978. **31**(1): p. 15–26.

89. Huberfeld, G., L. Menendez de la Prida, J. Pallud, et al., *Glutamatergic pre-ictal discharges emerge at the transition to seizure in human epilepsy.* Nat Neurosci, 2011. **14**(5): p. 627–634.

90. Curia, G., D. Longo, G. Biagini, R.S. Jones, and M. Avoli., *The pilocarpine model of temporal lobe epilepsy.* J Neurosci Methods, 2008. **172**(2): p. 143–157.

91. El-Hassar, L., L., M. Milh, F. Wendling, N. Ferrand, M. Esclapez, and C. Bernard, *Cell domain-dependent changes in the glutamatergic and GABAergic drives during epileptogenesis in the rat CA1 region.* J Physiol, 2007. **578**(Pt 1): p. 193–211.

92. White, A., P.A. Williams, J.L. Hellier, S. Clark, F.E. Dudek, and K.J. Staley., *EEG spike activity precedes epilepsy after kainate-induced status epilepticus.* Epilepsia, 2010. **51**(3): p. 371–383.

93. Huneau, C., P. Benquet, G. Dieuset, A. Biraben, B. Martin, and F. Wendling., *Shape features of epileptic spikes are a marker of epileptogenesis in mice.* Epilepsia, 2013. **54**(12): p. 2219–2227.

94. Cosandier-Rimele, D., J.M. Badier, P. Chauvel, and F. Wendling, *A physiologically plausible spatio-temporal model for EEG signals recorded with intracerebral electrodes in human partial epilepsy.* IEEE Trans Biomed Eng, 2007. **54**(3): p. 380–388.

95. Roopun, A.K., J.D. Simonotto, M.L. Pierce, et al., *A nonsynaptic mechanism underlying interictal discharges in human epileptic neocortex.* Proc Natl Acad Sci U S A, 2010. **107**(1): p. 338–343.

96. Jefferys, J.G., L. Menendez de la Prida, F. Wendling, et al., *Mechanisms of physiological and epileptic HFO generation.* Prog Neurobiol, 2012. **98**(3): p. 250–264.

97. Foffani, G., Y.G. Uzcategui, B. Gal, and L. Menendez de la Prida., *Reduced spike-timing reliability correlates with the emergence of fast ripples in the rat epileptic hippocampus.* Neuron, 2007. **55**(6): p. 930–941.

98. Ibarz, J.M., G. Foffani, E. Cid, M. Inostroza, and L. Menendez de la Prida., *Emergent dynamics of fast ripples in the epileptic hippocampus.* J Neurosci, 2010. **30**(48): p. 16249–16261.

99. Traub, R.D., R.K. Wong, R. Miles, and H. Michelson, *A model of a CA3 hippocampal pyramidal neuron incorporating voltage-clamp data on intrinsic conductances.* J Neurophysiol, 1991. **66**(2): p. 635–650.

100. Demont-Guignard, S., P. Benquet, U. Gerber, A. Biraben, B. Martin, and F. Wendling, *Distinct hyperexcitability mechanisms underlie fast ripples and epileptic spikes.* Ann Neurol, 2012. **71**(3): p. 342–352.

101. Simon, A., R.D. Traub, N. Vladimirov, et al., *Gap junction networks can generate both ripple-like and fast ripple-like oscillations.* Eur J Neurosci, 2014. **39**(1): p. 46–60.

102. Traub, R.D., D. Schmitz, N. Maier, M.A. Whittington, and A. Draguhn., *Axonal properties determine somatic firing in a model of in vitro CA1 hippocampal sharp wave/ripples and persistent gamma oscillations.* Eur J Neurosci, 2012. **36**(5): p. 2650–2660.

103. Pallud, J., M. Le Van Quyen, F. Bielle, et al., *Cortical GABAergic excitation contributes to epileptic activities around human glioma.* Sci Transl Med, 2014. **6**(244): p. 244ra89.

104. Wendling, F., F. Bartolomei, F. Mina, C. Huneau, and P. Benquet, *Interictal spikes, fast ripples and seizures in partial epilepsies—combining multi-level computational models with experimental data.* Eur J Neurosci, 2012. **36**(2): p. 2164–2177.

105. Alvarado-Rojas, C., G. Huberfeld, M. Baulac, et al., *Different mechanisms of ripple-like oscillations in the human epileptic subiculum.* Ann Neurol, 2015. **77**(2): p. 281–290.

106. Helling, R.M., M.M. Koppert, G.H. Visser, and S.N. Kalitzin, *Gap junctions as common cause of high-frequency oscillations and epileptic seizures in a computational cascade of neuronal mass and compartmental modeling.* Int J Neural Syst, 2015. **25**(6): p. 1550021.

107. Schiff, S.J., D. Colella, G.M. Jacyna, et al., *Brain chirps: spectrographic signatures of epileptic seizures.* Clin Neurophysiol, 2000. **111**(6): p. 953–958.

108. Bartolomei, F., F. Wendling, J.J. Bellanger, J. Regis, and P. Chauvel, *Neural networks involving the medial temporal structures in temporal lobe epilepsy.* Clin Neurophysiol, 2001. **112**(9): p. 1746–1760.

109. Lee, S.A., D.D. Spencer, and S.S. Spencer, *Intracranial EEG seizure-onset patterns in neocortical epilepsy.* Epilepsia, 2000. **41**(3): p. 297–307.

110. Wendling, F., F. Bartolomei, J.J. Bellanger, J. Bourien, and P. Chauvel, *Epileptic fast intracerebral EEG activity: evidence for spatial decorrelation at seizure onset.* Brain, 2003. **126**(Pt 6): p. 1449–1459.

111. Molaee-Ardekani, B., P. Benquet, F. Bartolomei, and F. Wendling, *Computational modeling of high-frequency oscillations at the onset of neocortical partial seizures: from 'altered structure' to 'dysfunction'.* Neuroimage, 2010. **52**(3): p. 1109–1122.

112. Traub, R.D., R. Duncan, A.J. Russell, et al., *Spatiotemporal patterns of electrocorticographic very fast oscillations (> 80 Hz) consistent with a network model based on electrical coupling between principal neurons.* Epilepsia, 2010. **51**(8): p. 1587–1597.

113. Traub, R.D., S.J. Middleton, T. Knopfel, and M.A. Whittington, *Model of very fast (> 75 Hz) network oscillations generated by electrical coupling between the proximal axons of cerebellar Purkinje cells.* Eur J Neurosci, 2008. **28**(8): p. 1603–1616.

114. Traub, R.D., M.A. Whittington, E.H. Buhl, et al., *A possible role for gap junctions in generation of very fast EEG oscillations preceding the onset of, and perhaps initiating, seizures.* Epilepsia, 2001. **42**(2): p. 153–170.

115. Vladimirov, N., R.D. Traub, and Y. Tu, *Wave speed in excitable random networks with spatially constrained connections.* PLoS One, 2011. **6**(6): p. e20536.

116. Bartos, M., I. Vida, and P. Jonas, *Synaptic mechanisms of synchronized gamma oscillations in inhibitory interneuron networks.* Nat Rev Neurosci, 2007. **8**(1): p. 45–56.

117. Lewis, T.J. and J. Rinzel, *Self-organized synchronous oscillations in a network of excitable cells coupled by gap junctions.* Network, 2000. **11**(4): p. 299–320.

118. Munro, E. and C. Borgers, *Mechanisms of very fast oscillations in networks of axons coupled by gap junctions.* J Comput Neurosci, 2010. **28**(3): p. 539–555.

119. Talairach, J., J. Bancaud, A. Bonis, G. Szikla, and P. Tournoux, *Functional stereotaxic exploration of epilepsy.* Confin Neurol, 1962. **22**: p. 328–331.

120. Nair, D.R., A. Mohamed, R. Burgess, and H. Luders, *A critical review of the different conceptual hypotheses framing human focal epilepsy.* Epileptic Disord, 2004. **6**(2): p. 77–83.

121. Pijn, J.P., P.C. Vijn, F.H. Lopes da Silva, W. Van Ende Boas, and W. Blanes, *Localization of epileptogenic foci using a new signal analytical approach.* Neurophysiol Clin, 1990. **20**(1): p. 1–11.

122. Schindler, K., H. Leung, C.E. Elger, and K. Lehnertz., *Assessing seizure dynamics by analysing the correlation structure of multichannel intracranial EEG.* Brain, 2007. **130**(Pt 1): p. 65–77.

123. Lehnertz, K., S. Bialonski, M.T. Horstmann, et al., *Synchronization phenomena in human epileptic brain networks.* J Neurosci Methods, 2009. **183**(1): p. 42–48.

124. Wendling, F., P. Chauvel, A. Biraben, and F. Bartolomei, *From intracerebral EEG signals to brain connectivity: identification of epileptogenic networks in partial epilepsy.* Front Syst Neurosci, 2010. **4**: p. 154.

125. Andrzejak, R.G., O. David, V. Gnatkovsky, et al., *Localization of epileptogenic zone on pre-surgical intracranial EEG recordings: toward a validation of quantitative signal analysis approaches.* Brain Topogr, 2015. **28**(6): p. 832–837.

126. Freeman, W.J., *Simulation of chaotic EEG patterns with a dynamic model of the olfactory system.* Biol Cybern, 1987. **56**(2-3): p. 139–150.

127. Wendling, F., J.J. Bellanger, F. Bartolomei, and P. Chauvel, *Relevance of nonlinear lumped-parameter models in the analysis of depth-EEG epileptic signals.* Biol Cybern, 2000. **83**(4): p. 367–378.

128. Wendling, F., A. Hernandez, J.J. Bellanger, P. Chauvel, and F. Bartolomei, *Interictal to ictal transition in human temporal lobe epilepsy: insights from a computational model of intracerebral EEG.* J Clin Neurophysiol, 2005. **22**(5): p. 343–356.

129. Allen, P.J., D.R. Fish, and S.J. Smith, *Very high-frequency rhythmic activity during SEEG suppression in frontal lobe epilepsy.* Electroencephalogr Clin Neurophysiol, 1992. **82**(2): p. 155–159.

130. Bragin, A., J. Engel, Jr., C.L. Wilson, I. Fried, and G.W. Mathern, *Hippocampal and entorhinal cortex high-frequency oscillations (100–500 Hz) in human epileptic brain and in kainic acid–treated rats with chronic seizures.* Epilepsia, 1999. **40**(2): p. 127–137.

131. White, J.A., M.I. Banks, R.A. Pearce, and N.J. Kopell, *Networks of interneurons with fast and slow gamma-aminobutyric acid type A (GABAA) kinetics provide substrate for mixed gamma-theta rhythm.* Proc Natl Acad Sci U S A, 2000. **97**(14): p. 8128–8133.

132. Banks, M.I., J.A. White, and R.A. Pearce, *Interactions between distinct GABA(A) circuits in hippocampus.* Neuron, 2000. **25**(2): p. 449–457.

133. Cossart, R., C. Dinocourt, J.C. Hirsch, et al., *Dendritic but not somatic GABAergic inhibition is decreased in experimental epilepsy.* Nat Neurosci, 2001. **4**(1): p. 52–62.

134. Bartolomei, F., P. Chauvel, and F. Wendling, *Epileptogenicity of brain structures in human temporal lobe epilepsy: a quantified study from intracerebral EEG.* Brain, 2008. **131**(7): p. 1818–1830.

135. Gnatkovsky, V., L. Librizzi, F. Trombin, and M. de Curtis, *Fast activity at seizure onset is mediated by inhibitory circuits in the entorhinal cortex in vitro.* Ann Neurol, 2008. **64**(6): p. 674–686.

136. Shiri, Z., F. Manseau, M. Levesque, S. Williams, and M. Avoli, *Interneuron activity leads to initiation of low-voltage fast-onset seizures.* Ann Neurol, 2015. **77**(3): p. 541–546.

137. Labyt, E., et al., *Modeling of entorhinal cortex and simulation of epileptic activity: insights into the role of inhibition-related parameters.* IEEE Trans Inf Technol Biomed, 2007. **11**(4): p. 450–461.

138. Labyt, E., P. Forgerais, L. Uva, J.J. Bellanger, and F. Wendling., *Realistic modeling of entorhinal cortex field potentials and interpretation of epileptic activity in the guinea pig isolated brain preparation.* J Neurophysiol, 2006. **96**(1): p. 363–377.

139. Touboul, J., F. Wendling, P. Chauvel, and O. Faugeras., *Neural mass activity, bifurcations, and epilepsy.* Neural Comput, 2011. **23**(12): p. 3232–3286.

140. Blenkinsop, A., A. Valentin, M.P. Richardson, and J.R. Terry, *The dynamic evolution of focal-onset epilepsies—combining theoretical and clinical observations.* Eur J Neurosci, 2012. **36**(2): p. 2188–2200.

141. Kalitzin, S., M. Koppert, G. Petkov, D. Velis, and F.Lopes da Silva., *Computational model prospective on the observation of proictal states in epileptic neuronal systems.* Epilepsy Behav, 2011. **22 Suppl 1**: p. S102–109.

142. Cosandier-Rimele, D., I. Merlet, F. Bartolomei, J.M. Badier, and F. Wendling, *Computational modeling of epileptic activity: from cortical sources to EEG signals.* J Clin Neurophysiol, 2010. **27**(6): p. 465–470.

143. Traub, R.D., W.D. Knowles, R. Miles, and R.K. Wong, *Synchronized afterdischarges in the hippocampus: simulation studies of the cellular mechanism.* Neuroscience, 1984. **12**(4): p. 1191–1200.

144. Traub, R.D., W.D. Knowles, R. Miles, and R.K. Wong, *Models of the cellular mechanism underlying propagation of epileptiform activity in the CA2-CA3 region of the hippocampal slice.* Neuroscience, 1987. **21**(2): p. 457–470.

145. Lytton, W.W., R. Orman, and M. Stewart, *Computer simulation of epilepsy: implications for seizure spread and behavioral dysfunction.* Epilepsy Behav, 2005. **7**(3): p. 336–344.

146. van Drongelen, W., H.C. Lee, M. Hereld, Z. Chen, F.P. Elsen, and R.L. Stevens, *Emergent epileptiform activity in neural networks with weak excitatory synapses.* IEEE Trans Neural Syst Rehabil Eng, 2005. **13**(2): p. 236–241.

147. Wang, X.J., *Multiple dynamical modes of thalamic relay neurons: rhythmic bursting and intermittent phase-locking.* Neuroscience, 1994. **59**(1): p. 21–31.

148. Lytton, W.W., D. Contreras, A. Destexhe, and M. Steriade, *Dynamic interactions determine partial thalamic quiescence in a computer network model of spike-and-wave seizures.* J Neurophysiol, 1997. **77**(4): p. 1679–1696.

149. Tsakiridou, E., L. Bertollini, M. de Curtis, G. Avanzini, and H.C. Pape, *Selective increase in T-type calcium conductance of reticular thalamic neurons in a rat model of absence epilepsy.* J Neurosci, 1995. **15**(4): p. 3110–3117.

150. Leresche, N., H.R. Parri, G. Erdemli, et al., *On the action of the antiabsence drug ethosuximide in the rat and cat thalamus.* J Neurosci, 1998. **18**(13): p. 4842–4853.

151. Destexhe, A., D. Contreras, and M. Steriade, *Mechanisms underlying the synchronizing action of corticothalamic feedback through inhibition of thalamic relay cells.* J Neurophysiol, 1998. **79**(2): p. 999–1016.

152. Destexhe, A. and T.J. Sejnowski, *Interactions between membrane conductances underlying thalamocortical slow-wave oscillations.* Physiol Rev, 2003. **83**(4): p. 1401–1453.

153. Koppert, M.M., S. Kalitzin, F.H. Lopes da Silva, and M.A. Viergever., *Plasticity-modulated seizure dynamics for seizure termination in realistic neuronal models.* J Neural Eng, 2011. **8**(4): p. 046027.

154. Meeren, H.K., J.P. Pijn, E.L. Van Luijtelaar, A.M. Coenen, and F.H. Lopes da Silva, *Cortical focus drives widespread corticothalamic networks during spontaneous absence seizures in rats.* J Neurosci, 2002. **22**(4): p. 1480–1495.

155. Polack, P.O., I. Guillemain, E. Hu, C. Deransart, A. Depaulis, and S. Charpier., *Deep layer somatosensory cortical neurons initiate spike-and-wave discharges in a genetic model of absence seizures.* J Neurosci, 2007. **27**(24): p. 6590–6599.

156. Gurbanova, A.A., R. Aker, K. Berkman, F.Y. Onat, C.M. van Rijn, and G. van Luijtelaar, *Effect of systemic and intracortical administration of phenytoin in two genetic models of absence epilepsy.* Br J Pharmacol, 2006. **148**(8): p. 1076–1082.

157. Suffczynski, P., S. Kalitzin, and F.H. Lopes Da Silva, *Dynamics of nonconvulsive epileptic phenomena modeled by a bistable neuronal network.* Neuroscience, 2004. **126**(2): p. 467–484.

158. Suffczynski, P., F.H. Lopes da Silva, J. Parra, et al., *Dynamics of epileptic phenomena determined from statistics of ictal transitions.* IEEE Trans Biomed Eng, 2006. **53**(3): p. 524–532.

159. Lopes da Silva, F.H., W. Blanes, S.N. Kalitzin, J. Parra, P. Suffczynski, and D.N. Velis., *Dynamical diseases of brain systems: different routes to epileptic seizures.* IEEE Trans Biomed Eng, 2003. **50**(5): p. 540–548.

160. Berenyi, A., M. Belluscio, D. Mao, and G. Buzsaki., *Closed-loop control of epilepsy by transcranial electrical stimulation.* Science, 2012. **337**(6095): p. 735–737.

161. Luttjohann, A. and G. van Luijtelaar, *Thalamic stimulation in absence epilepsy.* Epilepsy Res, 2013. **106**(1-2): p. 136–145.

162. Treiman, D.M., *Electroclinical features of status epilepticus.* J Clin Neurophysiol, 1995. **12**(4): p. 343–362.

163. Chiang, C.C., M.S. Ju, and C.C. Lin, *Description and computational modeling of the whole course of status epilepticus induced by low dose lithiumpilocarpine in rats.* Brain Res, 2011. **1417**: p. 151–162.

164. Kalitzin, S., M. Koppert, G. Petkov, and F.Lopes da Silva, *Multiple oscillatory states in models of collective neuronal dynamics.* Int J Neural Syst, 2014. **24**(6): p. 1450020.

165. Jirsa, V.K., W.C. Stacey, P.P. Quilichini, A.I. Ivanov, and C. Bernard, *On the nature of seizure dynamics.* Brain, 2014. **137**(Pt 8): p. 2210–2230.

166. Dyhrfjeld-Johnsen, J., V. Santhakumar, R.J. Morgan, R. Huerta, L. Tsimring, and I. Soltesz, *Topological determinants of epileptogenesis in large-scale structural and functional models of the dentate gyrus derived from experimental data.* J Neurophysiol, 2007. **97**(2): p. 1566–1587.

167. Volman, V., T.J. Sejnowski, and M. Bazhenov, *Topological basis of epileptogenesis in a model of severe cortical trauma.* J Neurophysiol, 2011. **106**(4): p. 1933–1942.

168. Suffczynski, P., F. Lopes Da Silva, J. Parra, and S. Kalitzin, *Epileptic transitions: model predictions and experimental validation.* J Clin Neurophysiol, 2005. **22**(5): p. 288–299.

4 | BIOPHYSICAL ASPECTS OF EEG AND MEG GENERATION

WYTSE J. WADMAN, PHD AND FERNANDO H. LOPES DA SILVA, MD, PHD

ABSTRACT: This chapter reviews the essential physical principles involved in the generation of electroencephalographic (EEG) and magnetoencephalographic (MEG) signals. The general laws governing the electrophysiology of neuronal activity are analyzed within the formalism of the Maxwell equations that constitute the basis for understanding electromagnetic fields in general. Three main topics are discussed. The first is the forward problem: How can one calculate the electrical field that results from a known configuration of neuronal sources? The second is the inverse problem: Given an electrical field as a function of space and time mostly recorded at the scalp (EEG/MEG), how can one reconstruct the underlying generators at the brain level? The third is the reverse problem: How can brain activity be modulated by external electromagnetic fields with diagnostic and/or therapeutic objectives? The chapter emphasizes the importance of understanding the common biophysical framework concerning these three main topics of brain electrical and magnetic activities.

KEYWORDS: electroencephalogram, EEG, magnetoencephalogram, MEG, electrophysiology, electromagnetic, forward problem, inverse problem, reverse problem, brain activity

PRINCIPAL REFERENCES

1. Somjen GG, Kager H, Wadman WJ. Computer simulations of neuron–glia interactions mediated by ion flux. *J Comput Neurosci.* 2008;25:349–365.
2. Einevoll GT, Kayser C, Logothetis NK, et al. Modelling and analysis of local field potentials for studying the function of cortical circuits. *Nature Rev Neurosci.* 2013;14(11):770–785.
3. Gonçalves SI, de Munck JC, Verbunt JPA, Bijma F, Heethaar RM, Lopes da Silva FH. In vivo measurement of the brain and skull resistivities using an EIT-based method and realistic models of the head. *IEEE Trans Biomed Eng.* 2003;50:754–767.
4. Murakami S, Okada Y. Invariance in current dipole moment density across brain structures and species: physiological constraint for neuroimaging. *NeuroImage.* 2015;111:49–58.
5. Rahman A, Reato D, Arlotti M, Gasca F, Datta A, Parra LC, Bikson M. Cellular effects of acute direct current stimulation: somatic and synaptic terminal effects. *J Physiol.* 2013;591:2563–2578.
6. Reimann MW, Anastassiou CA, Perin R, Hill SL, Markram H, Koch C. A biophysically detailed model of neocortical local field potentials predicts the critical role of active membrane currents. *Neuron.* 2013;79:375–390.
7. Di Lazzaro V, Ziemann U, Lemon RN. State of the art: physiology of transcranial motor cortex stimulation. *Brain Stim.* 2008;1:345–362.
8. Nicholson C. Diffusion and related transport mechanisms in brain tissue. *Reports on Progress in Physics.* 2001;64(70):815–884.
9. Jefferys JGR. Nonsynaptic modulation of neuronal activity in the brain: electric currents and extracellular ions. *Physiol Rev.* 1995;75(4):689–723.
10. Plonsey R. The nature of sources of bioelectric and biomagnetic fields. *Biophys J.* 1969;39:309–315.
11. Hille B. *Ion Channels of Excitable Membranes.* 3rd ed. Sunderland, MA: Sinauer Assoc. Publishers, 2001.

1. BIOPHYSICAL ASPECTS OF EEG AND MEG GENERATION

The electroencephalographic (EEG) / magnetoencephalographic (MEG) signal reflects the activity of millions of neurons located in a multitude of brain structures. The neurons can be subdivided into many classes and are organized in highly complex networks that maintain multiple interactions. Although this complexity may appear tantalizing, the essential properties that account for the generation of EEG/MEG signals are based on well-understood and straightforward physical principles. In this chapter we review the biophysical principles that govern EEG/MEG generation. The chapter builds upon the two previous chapters, in which basic notions of the physiology of neuronal electromagnetic activity were presented.

In Chapter 2 the properties of neurons as polarized cells with selective permeability for specific ions were discussed, along with some general questions that neurophysiologists frequently ask about the relationship between neuronal sources in the brain and EEG/MEG signals recorded at the scalp. In Chapter 3 general laws governing the electrophysiology of neuronal activity were analyzed within the framework of the Hodgkin–Huxley description of voltage-dependent ionic membrane currents. The electric currents generated through the ionic channels in the membrane are directly responsible for the electrical fields that are manifest at some distance from the cellular sources. The precise form of the fields also depends on the electric properties of the different tissues lying between the sources and the recording sites.

Extracellular field potentials recorded in the neighborhood of their cellular sources are commonly called local field potentials (LFPs). In turn they constitute the building blocks of the electrocorticogram and of the scalp EEG and MEG signals. The general question central in this chapter is: How does one go from neuronal sources to LFPs, and ultimately to the EEG/ MEG?

We consider three distinct classes of problems, each with specific physical underpinnings:

1. The *forward problem*: Can we calculate the electrical field that results from a known configuration of neuronal sources? This sounds like an academic question, but solving it helps us to understand the fundamental properties of EEG/MEG generation and allows the validation of the solutions proposed for questions 2 and 3.

2. The *inverse problem* is clinically the most relevant one: Given an electrical field as a function of space and time, mostly (but not always) on the scalp, such as the EEG, can the underlying generators be reconstructed? In 1855 the German physicist Herrmann Helmholtz [1] proved that there is no unique solution to this question.

Intuitively this is easy to comprehend, as any "perfect" solution can always be replaced by a more complicated equivalent one. In practice, the search is for the "simplest" solution that is adequate within the appropriate boundary conditions. The suitability of such a solution will strongly depend on the clinical question to answer and is extensively dealt with in Chapter 45.

3. The last problem, the *reverse problem*, deals with the question of how external electromagnetic fields modulate and/or interfere with brain function. The biophysical foundations of this problem are not commonly considered jointly with the previous two but merit being discussed here. They include diagnostic electrical stimulation, stimulation with therapeutic aims, such as deep brain stimulation, transcranial direct current stimulation, and transcranial magnetic stimulation, but also potential hazardous interferences by electromagnetic fields today originating from communication antennas, mobile phones, and/or digital enhanced cordless transmitted phones.

2. THE FORWARD PROBLEM

When a distributed set of electrical charges is placed in a spatial configuration, it creates an electromagnetic field, which can be observed at any point in space. If the charges move (moving charges are generally called currents), the field will continuously change and reflect these movements; the currents will also generate a magnetic field. In one of the most famous (negative) experiments in physics, Michelson and Morley showed that an electromagnetic field travels with the speed of light, which is constant in all directions, and also that there is no "ether" medium necessary for this propagation. That is the reason why we can talk to a man on the moon over the radio. The electromagnetic waves (light is one form of them) propagate, even in vacuum, with the absolute speed of light as opposed to, for example, sound, which needs air (or water) to propagate (with a much lower, medium-dependent velocity). The complete classical description of the electromagnetic fields was unified and formulated by Maxwell in his set of famous equations (Box 4.1). Later-developed formalisms that also take into account relativistic aspects are not relevant in the context of our EEG/MEG discussion, where all speeds involved are well below the speed of light. For a more in-depth fundamental discussion on electromagnetic theory, the reader is referred to one of the many classical textbooks, such as that of Plonsey [2].

As opposed to, say, copper wires, where electrons are the charge carriers, all currents in the brain use ions as charge carriers. Na^+ and Cl^- are the prominent ones in the extracellular space, and K^+ and Cl^- are the most prominent ones intracellularly. Luckily the transport numbers of those pairs of ions (in simple terms, the ease with which they diffuse through the extracellular/intracellular solution) are quite similar, so that local accumulation of charge/ions hardly occurs. For currents that pass the neuronal membrane the situation is more complex, as many different and ion-selective channels are involved

BOX 4.1. BASIC LAWS OF ELECTRODYNAMICS: THE MAXWELL EQUATIONS

The Maxwell equations describe the electrical field $\vec{E}(\vec{r},t)$ and the magnetic field $\vec{H}(\vec{r},t)$ as a function of place and time and relate them to the charges and currents present in space. Within the context of EEG/MEG recordings electromagnetic waves propagate with speeds close to infinity, which implies that all fields are instantaneously observed at all locations in space. In other words, the time and space components of the electrical field can be reliably separated and solved. The electrical vector field $\vec{E}$, which has a *direction and a value* at each location, is defined as the gradient of the scalar potential field (V), which has only a *value* at each location:

$$\vec{E} = -grad(V) \tag{Eq. B1}$$

If we assume (for now) uniform homogeneous conductance σ, the relation between the current density $\vec{J}$ anywhere in the medium and the injected current $\vec{J}_i$ and the field $\vec{E}$ by (a generalized form of Ohm's law):

$$\vec{J} = \vec{J}_i + \sigma\vec{E}$$

If we take the divergence of both sides and realize that current cannot accumulate or disappear in the brain (i.e., $div\,\vec{J} = 0$) we end up with:

$$div\,E = \frac{-div\,\vec{J}_i}{\sigma}$$

which after substitution of Eq. B1 gives:

$$div\,grad\,V = \frac{div\,\vec{J}_i}{\sigma} \tag{Eq. B2}$$

which describes how the extracellular potential field V is generated by the currents, injected, for example, by neurons in the extracellular space. The operators *grad* and *div* can also be specified in Cartesian coordinates:

$$grad\,V = \left(\frac{\delta V}{\delta x}, \frac{\delta V}{\delta y}, \frac{\delta V}{\delta z}\right)$$

and

$$div\,\vec{J}\,dxdydz = \left(\frac{\delta J_x}{\delta x}dydz\right)dx + \left(\frac{\delta J_y}{\delta y}dxdz\right)dy + \left(\frac{\delta J_z}{\delta z}dxdy\right)dz$$

Every electrical current generates a magnetic field $\vec{H}(\vec{r},t)$ proportional to the induction field $\vec{B}(\vec{r},t)$ according to $\vec{B}(\vec{r},t) = \mu\vec{H}(\vec{r},t)$ where μ is the magnetic permeability of the brain. The relation between current density $\vec{J}$ and magnetic field is given by

$$curl\,\vec{H} = \vec{J}$$

As in the case of the electrical field $div\,\vec{B} = 0$, in words: magnetic monopoles do not exist in the brain. The curl operator represents the well-known corkscrew rule in physics: a linear current generates a circular magnetic field around it, clockwise in the direction of the current, which is easier visualized in Cartesian coordinates:

$$curl\,\vec{H} = \left(\frac{\delta H_y}{\delta z} - \frac{\delta H_z}{\delta y}, \frac{\delta H_z}{\delta x} - \frac{\delta H_x}{\delta z}, \frac{\delta H_x}{\delta y} - \frac{\delta H_y}{\delta x}\right)$$

BOX 4.1. CONTINUED

Mathematically it can be shown that ($div\,\vec{B} = 0$) is equivalent to the assumption that $\vec{B}$ originates from a vector potential $\vec{A}$ according to:

$$\vec{B} = curl\,\vec{A} \qquad \text{(Eq. B3)}$$

After some straightforward algebra we find for the relation between the vector field $\vec{A}$ and the imposed current $\vec{J}_i$:

$$div\,grad\,\vec{A} = -\mu\,\vec{J}_i \qquad \text{(Eq. B4)}$$

Equations B2 and B4 (with Eq. B3) are the desired solutions of the forward problem. They provide us the electrical and the magnetic fields that are generated by any set of currents that neurons inject into the extracellular space under the assumption of linear superposition.

---

in that process. Despite this complexity the major carriers of electric charges through neuronal membranes are also Na^+ and K^+ and to a lesser extent Cl^-. In a first approximation, the extracellular space can be considered as a conductive medium with uniform scalar conductivity. Injecting current into a uniform conductive medium with conductance σ creates potential gradients, as described by the Maxwell equation (see Box 4.1). For the simplest one-dimensional case the expression reduces to the well-known Ohm's law:

$$I = \sigma\,dV \qquad \text{(Eq. 1)}$$

which states that in a uniform conductor with conductance (σ), the current (I) and the voltage gradient (dV) that generates it, are proportional. In physics, current is defined as the movement of positive charge, even though in the brain it may consist of negative ions moving in the opposite direction. To avoid confusion we ignore this detail in the following explanations.

2.1. What Are the Generators of the Electric Fields in the Brain and Where Are They Located?

All cell membranes effectively separate the internal medium of the cell from the external world, allowing the active buildup of differences in ionic composition. Neurons are specialized as sources of electrical activity and use energy-driven pumps to maintain ionic concentration gradients over their membrane for the cations Na^+ and K^+. There are also gradients for Cl^- and Ca^{2+}, which are essential for neuronal function but less important for the electrical balance that we discuss here first.

When two compartments are separated by a semipermeable membrane (one that only conducts ion X and contains different concentrations for ion X, say $[X]_o$ on one side and $[X]_i$ on the other), diffusion through the membrane sets up a voltage gradient that forms an electrical driving force that perfectly matches the diffusion driving force. The resulting thermodynamic equilibrium is described by the Nernst equation:

$$E_X = \frac{RT}{zF}\ln\frac{[X]_o}{[X]_i} \qquad \text{(Eq. 2)}$$

which relates the equilibrium voltage (E_X) over the membrane to the ion concentrations in both compartments. The ion X has a valence z; R is the gas constant, T is the absolute temperature in Kelvin, and F is the constant of Faraday (the charge of a Mole of ions). For a monovalent ion this results in a voltage gradient of about 58 mV for each decade of concentration difference. The situation described above for a single ion is a real equilibrium where no current flows once it is reached. Most neurons, however, contain specific membrane conductances for Na^+ as well as K^+; the resulting equilibrium potentials, about +60 for sodium and −90 mV for potassium, are quite different. For this situation the resulting membrane voltage is given by the Goldman equation:

$$V_m = \frac{RT}{F}\ln\left(\frac{P_K\left[K^+\right]_0 + P_{Na}\left[Na^+\right]_o + P_{Cl}\left[Cl^-\right]_i}{P_K\left[K^+\right]_i + P_{Na}\left[Na^+\right]_i + P_{Cl}\left[Cl^-\right]_o}\right) \qquad \textbf{(Eq. 3)}$$

which relates the membrane potential V_m to the concentrations of the participating monovalent ions Na^+, K^+, and Cl^- and their permeabilities (P_{Na}, P_K, and P_{Cl}). Permeability is related to conductance and can best be described as the possibility to conduct; it results in measurable conductance only if there are ions that can pass. Thus, conductance depends on the actual ion concentrations, while permeability does not.

The Goldman equation describes an equilibrium where there is no *net* electrical current flow through the membrane, but because V_m is a compromise between all E_X's of the individual ions, they are each left with a driving force ($E_X - V_m$) and the equilibrium only implies zero net electrical current. For each ion there will be a membrane current (I_X) given by Ohm's law:

$$I_X = g_X\left(E_X - V_m\right) \qquad \textbf{(Eq. 4)}$$

where g_X represents the specific membrane conductance for ion X. This simple equation is sufficient to qualitatively understand most aspects of current flow through the neuronal membrane; for more quantitative calculations, however, the reader is advised to use the Goldman-Hodgkin-Katz current equation, which defines the membrane currents for non-equilibrium situations [3].

The ("leak") ionic currents that flow in the Goldman equilibrium with multiple ionic gradients need to be compensated by active energy-driven pumps in order to keep a sustainable stable situation and the neurons alive. The most important pump is the ATP-driven Na/K exchanger, which exchanges two K^+ ions against three Na^+ ions and therefore transports one electric charge at each cycle. It thus creates a measurable electrical current. Thus, at rest the currents through the K^+ and Na^+ channels are counterbalanced by the pump and instead of being equal, they should have a ratio of two against three.

Most channel- and receptor-mediated ionic currents are active only a small fraction of the time. Action potentials typically last about 1 ms and are then silent for a longer period; synaptic currents last longer but are substantially smaller. As the ion pumps work continuously, they can under most practical conditions keep up with the counteracting flows. In most electrophysiological discussions we may therefore ignore pump activity and replace their presence by the assumption that intracellular ion concentrations do not substantially change over time. However, this is not always the case, as discussed by Somjen et al. [4] and Wei et al. [5], who modeled and analyzed ionic changes during epileptic seizures and anoxic spreading depression.

In short, membrane potential in neuronal (and all other) cells is determined by the relative conductances for the most important ions, and changing these conductances will change membrane potential: e.g. increasing Na$^+$ conductance will depolarize the membrane. Neurotransmitters and neurohormones modulate neuronal activity by manipulating specific conductances, either directly or via one of the many indirect (intracellular) routes.

More remarkable is that many Na$^+$ and K$^+$ conductances in excitable (neuronal) membranes depend on the membrane voltage that they establish themselves. Most Na$^+$ and K$^+$ channels open (conductances increase) upon depolarization of the membrane. In the case of K$^+$ this creates a situation of stabilizing feedback (the opening of K$^+$ channels drives the membrane potential back into negative direction as $E_K \sim -90$ mV), while in the case of Na$^+$ depolarization evokes more depolarization ($E_{Na} \sim +60$ mV), leading to regenerative activity. These properties explain the generation of all-or-none action potentials (for details see Hille [3]). Thus, during the action potential the fast regenerative opening of voltage-dependent Na$^+$ channels strongly depolarizes the membrane, driving it into the direction of the reversal potential for Na$^+$. This opens the slowly activating K$^+$ channels and inactivates the Na$^+$ channels; both of these actions will bring V_m back to its resting value. Because K$^+$ channels close slowly, V_m often goes through a period of hyperpolarization after the action potential, the so-called after-hyperpolarization, a period where the neuron is less excitable.

2.2. From Neuronal Activity to Electrical Fields

From the previous discussion it is clear that neuronal activity is associated with (fast changes in) current flow through the cellular membrane; these currents are the generators of the electrical fields. In first approximation we assume that the superposition principle holds: for example, the field generated by a population of neurons is the linear summation of the contributions of all neurons in the population. How much each individual neuron contributes depends on the amplitude of its currents and on its morphology. Physics imposes an important limitation here in that it requires that the net current flow into a neuron is zero; for the relevant time scales (longer then milliseconds) we can ignore the currents that charge the membrane capacitance because they are small and extremely transient.

Spherical symmetrical neurons with uniform conductance contribute very little to the field, since all injected currents cancel. This condition also applies to stellate neurons with large dendritic trees that ramify symmetrically in all directions. They generate noticeable fields only within the realm of these dendrites; farther away, their contribution is negligible. In contrast, polarized neurons with distal synaptic activation counteracted by somatic current flow generate a much larger net electrical field, even if their actual membrane currents are

not much different. Cellular morphology dictates that the far field, where LFPs and ultimately EEG signals become manifest, is strongly dominated by currents generated in polarized neurons, although many more neurons with less favorable morphologies may also be active, but their net membrane currents go unnoticed at a distance. At the cellular level polarized neurons are clearly in the lead over spherical symmetrical neurons, and the classical pyramidal neurons with their strict dendritic polarized orientation likely have the strongest contribution to the far field.

What holds for single cell morphology also holds for the organization of large neuronal populations. Intuitively one can understand that in a structure constituted by randomly oriented neurons, a large fraction of the contributions of individual neurons will cancel out. In contrast, in a very regular network of polarized neurons, as found in cortical layers where neurons are organized in palissades, the contributions of different neurons will summate, even more so if their activity is to some extent synchronized.

2.3. The Concept of Open and Closed Fields

In layered organized cortex an important proportion of neurons is constituted by pyramidal cells, which present a rather long, vertically oriented apical dendrite that ramifies in the most superficial layers of the cortex, and by basal dendrites distributed around the soma; the axon runs vertically downward to the white matter. The macroscopic field generated in such palissades of neurons can be mimicked by that of a dipole layer (see below). Lorente de Nó, in a classic study [6], named this type of potential field the "open field" (Fig. 4.1C). In contrast, he called fields generated by neurons with dendritic arborizations radially distributed about the soma "closed fields" (see Fig. 4.1A,B). The configuration of the radially oriented neurons represents a central source (current outflow) surrounded by spherically distributed sinks (current inflow into the cells) or, depending on the type of synapses (see below), a central sink surrounded by peripheral sources. It can be intuitively understood that, under these circumstances, not only the tangential but also the radial components of the currents cancel in the far field. In short, cellular morphology as well as the spatial organization of the neurons in a structure determines how much they contribute to the EEG fields measured at a distance.

In the discussion on basic neurophysiological concepts in Chapter 2 we pointed out (in Figs. 2.1 and 2.2) that synaptic activity either directly, in the case of ionotropic receptors, or indirectly, in the case of metabotropic receptors, results in a localized change in conductance in the postsynaptic membrane. The direction of the resulting transmembrane current depends on the type of conductance that is activated. Excitatory synapses, which open up either sodium (reversal potential +60 mV) or nonselective (reversal potential 0 mV) conductances, generate an inward current (a *sink*, Fig. 4.2), typically carried by Na$^+$ ions (which are the extracellular majority ions). Inhibitory synapses either open up potassium channels, resulting in an outward current, carried by K$^+$ ions (reversal potential −90 mV and the intracellular majority ion),

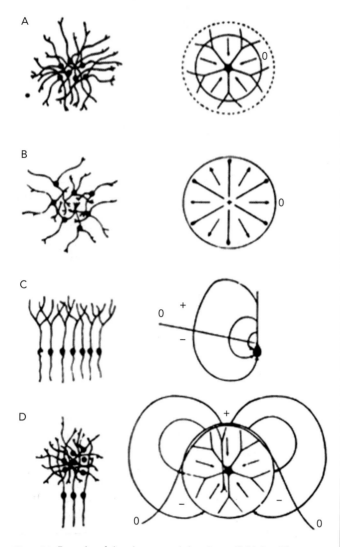

Figure 4.1. Examples of closed, open, and closed-open fields for different types of neuron pools in the central nervous system. Left: The populations are drawn. Right: Neurons representing the simultaneously activated pools are shown together with the arrows representing the lines of flow of current at the instant when the impulses have evaded the cell bodies. The zero isopotential lines are also indicated. A: Oculomotor nucleus represented schematically by only one neuron with dendrites oriented radially outward. The isopotential lines are circles; the currents flow entirely within the nucleus, resulting in a closed field (all points outside the nucleus remain at zero potential). B: Superior olive represented by neurons each having a single dendrite oriented radially inward. The currents result in a closed field. C: Accessory olive consisting of a palissade of neurons with a single long aligned dendrite. The arrangement of sources and sinks in this structure permits the spread of current in the volume of the brain and thus results in an open field. D: Two structures mixed together, generating an open-closed field. A similar arrangement exists in the neocortex and hippocampus. (Modified from Lorente de Nó R. Action potential of the motoneurons of the hypoglossus nucleus. J Cell Comp Physiol. 1947;29:207–287; Hubbard JI, Llinas R, Quastel DMJ. Electrophysiological Analysis of Synaptic Transmission. London: Edward Arnold Ltd., 1969.)

or they open chloride channels and produce an inward current of negative Cl⁻ ions. In physics we also call the latter current an outward electrical current. For the extracellular space both variants function as a current *source*. The excitatory postsynaptic current results in a depolarization of the membrane and brings membrane voltage closer to firing threshold (i.e., the excitatory postsynaptic potential). The inhibitory postsynaptic current mostly (see below) results in a hyperpolarization of

the membrane (i.e., the inhibitory postsynaptic potential). In both situations the sink/source is the result of an *active* change in membrane conductance; therefore, the sinks/sources at the site of the conductance change are called *active*. The locally induced change in membrane potential, however, is not restricted to the active site; the depolarization propagates over the cell membrane, decaying with distance, and often reaching the soma. At all membrane locations where the voltage is changed but the conductance is not, there remains a driving force resulting in a current in the opposite direction than the one in the active region (see Fig. 4.2). According to the basic rule of physics that the net current into each cell must be zero, active sinks are always accompanied by *passive* sources, while active sources are accompanied by *passive* sinks. In polarized neurons this is also the ideal configuration to make a dipole.

The current distribution over the cell depends on the relative conductances over the remaining surface of the cell. Active sinks/sources are restricted to the small region in the neuron where the active conductance (ion channel) is localized, while balancing passive current will flow everywhere else in the cell as long as the local transmembrane potential is affected. Currents in active sink/source configurations are generated by a change in conductance, while the currents in passive regions are generated by a change in driving force.

The transmembrane currents that are generated by sinks and sources are injected into the conductive extracellular (and intracellular) space. They constitute a current flow from source to sink, which in accordance with Ohm's law sets up a voltage gradient in the extracellular space that is proportional to the local resistance. Important to note is that the amplitude and polarity of the field change with location but (for a simple sink/source configuration) the time course of the voltage change is everywhere the same and reflects the transmembrane current flow (but see the discussion below). That is why extracellular potentials give us quite a good impression of what actually happens at the membrane level. The amplitude depends on the resistance of the medium but also on how well the centers of gravity of the sink and the source are separated. In a polarized (pyramidal) neuron with a strong synaptic sink in the dendrite and the major source in the soma, the configuration resembles that of a *dipole*.

An electrical dipole is a configuration of two charges of equal but opposite valence ($+q$) and ($-q$) separated by an "infinitely small" distance (d). The dipole moment (p) is given by $p = q \times d$. In practice d is never infinitely small, but as long as it is much smaller than the distance from the point of observation to the dipole, this approximation is valid. As long as the superposition principle holds (no interference between the charges), it is relatively easy to calculate the electrical fields generated by any artificial charge configuration (Box 4.2). In a first approximation we may ignore the existence of electrical monopoles in the brain (see, however, next section), and the dipole is the first realistic configuration in the brain to be used to describe an extracellular field. But the dipole is also the first-order term of the multipole expansion in which higher-order terms (quadrupole, etc.) can be used to approximate much more complex charge configurations. One can compare this approach to the Taylor expansion, in which sufficient

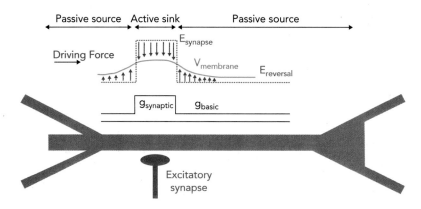

Passive source   Active sink   Passive source

Figure 4.2. *Currents generated in a synaptically activated neuron. An excitatory synapse located in the dendritic region of the neuron is activated by afferent fibers and induces a local region of high conductance. At rest the conductance level is defined as g_{basic}, uniform everywhere in the neuron and resulting in a uniform membrane voltage $E_{reversal}$. At the peak of the synaptic activity, the conductance at the activated region is $g_{synaptic}$ and for an excitatory synapse the reversal potential in the activated region rises to $E_{synapse}$. Because the membrane is a strongly connected cable, the membrane voltage (here indicated by the green line) does not reach $E_{synapse}$ and everywhere else the membrane voltage is higher than $E_{reversal}$. The end result is an inward current due to a large driving force and located in the synaptic region; this is called the active sink, because that is the region where the membrane conductance is actively changed. The rest of the cell where the driving force is outward behaves as a passive source.*

derivatives allow the evaluation of even the most complicated function at a specific point. In practice, the higher-order terms of the physically correct multipole expansion are little used in describing EEG signals.

2.4. Which Membrane Conductances Contribute to LFPs and EEG Signals?

The physical law that states that the net current in a cell should be zero has as a direct consequence that at scales larger than ~100 μm electrical monopoles cannot exist in the brain. As described above, all transmembrane currents present in neurons will contribute at least dipolar components to the electrical field, as they always consist of a sink and an associated source. How much each component contributes to the field at a certain distance depends on at least four aspects:

1. The distance to the observation site

2. The amplitude of the current

3. The dipole moment of the resulting configuration (more precisely, the separation of the [balanced] positive and negative currents)

4. The spatial configuration and temporal synchronization of all similar components in the generating population, as the source rarely consists of a single neuron.

In addition to synaptic currents and currents that generate the action potential, relatively slow membrane currents (e.g., those involved in depolarizing or hyperpolarizing after-potentials or dendritic events such as calcium action potentials) are also possible sources of extracellularly measurable potentials.

In Chapter 2 we noted that mainly due to the membrane filtering characteristics, the cellular dipoles of postsynaptic potentials and of action potentials differ appreciably in size. A membrane depolarization or hyperpolarization that results

from a local change in conductance does not remain localized but spreads over the rest of the cell membrane according to its electrotonic properties (for electrotonic propagation, see [7,8]). For membrane changes that are slower than the typical membrane time constant (5–10 ms), the spread is mainly determined by the electrotonic size, and these changes will spread over a large fraction of the neuronal membrane, typically in the order of the distance between the active synapses and the cell soma. For faster signals, like action potentials (<1 ms), the spread is limited by the filter characteristics of the membrane, resulting in dipoles with a relative small dipole moment. Thus, the distance between the corresponding current sinks and sources is an important factor determining the size and shape of the extracellular field.

Computer simulations have helped to estimate the relative contribution of the involved membrane currents [9–11]. The computational model of Reimann [10] was developed in the framework of the "Blue Brain Project" simulating the fields generated by thousands of cortical neurons and millions of synapses. Among many other things the model illustrates how the power spectral density (PSD) of the extracellular electric field depends on the spatial distribution of the neuronal sources. It describes how the PSD of the electric field decays as a function of distance r from the membrane sources, according to a power law of the form $PSD(r) \approx 1/r^{\Upsilon}$. For very small distances ($r \ll 100$ μm), postsynaptic sources appear as monopoles and scale with $\Upsilon \approx 1$; at more relevant distances, most sources scale as dipoles with $\Upsilon \approx 2$ (see also Box 4.2). At larger distances, the widespread passive currents also contribute, resulting in an additional pole; for those situations the value for the exponential decay Υ increases to about 3. The latter observation implies that local populations have a finite reach beyond which their influence on the field is not very relevant [10].

As most fields are composed of the linear superposition of currents from a large number of neurons, their "synchrony" (overlap in time) constitutes an important issue. Intuitively it is clear that, in a neuronal system with timing accuracies in the order of 1 ms, synaptic potentials with a duration 10 to

A spatial distribution of dipoles $p(r_0)$ observed at distance r can be summarized by:

$$p(r) = \int_{Vol} p(r_0)(r_0 - r)d^3r_0$$

where integration is over the volume (Vol) using d^3r_0 as a three-dimensional elementary volume.

The simplest form of such a configuration is the electric monopole (charge q), whose electrostatic potential and electrical field are only of academic interest and at a distance r are given by:

$$V(r) = \frac{1}{4\pi\varepsilon_0}\left(\frac{q}{r}\right) \quad \text{and} \quad \vec{E}(r) = \frac{1}{4\pi\varepsilon_0}\left(\frac{q}{r^2}\right)$$

For the dipole the approximation (the dipole is not ideal) of both terms is:

$$V(r) \approx \frac{1}{4\pi\varepsilon_0}\left(\frac{qd}{r^2}\right) \quad \text{and} \quad \vec{E}(r) \approx \frac{1}{4\pi\varepsilon_0}\left(\frac{qd}{r^3}\right)$$

while quadrupole configurations obey:

$$V(r) \approx \frac{1}{4\pi\varepsilon_0}\left(\frac{qd^2}{r^3}\right) \quad \text{and} \quad \vec{E}(r) \approx \frac{1}{4\pi\varepsilon_0}\left(\frac{qd^2}{r^4}\right)$$

And we can continue with the octupole

$$V(r) \approx \frac{1}{4\pi\varepsilon_0}\left(\frac{qd^3}{r^4}\right) \quad \text{and} \quad \vec{E}(r) \approx \frac{1}{4\pi\varepsilon_0}\left(\frac{qd^3}{r^5}\right)$$

From this series it is clear that higher-multipole components fall off faster with distance.

An important consequence of this behavior is that different components weight in a different manner, depending on the distance to the configuration, or in other words the contribution of more complex charge configurations vanishes with distance r.

---

100 ms are much easier to synchronize than action potentials that last less than 1 ms. Nevertheless, experimental evidence indicates that synchronous action potentials can still contribute substantially to high-frequency components of the EEG signal, for example when neurons are synchronized through gap junctions (electrical synapses that couple them galvanically). Thus a local field may represent low-frequency activities originating from postsynaptic currents (<250 Hz) and also high-frequency components (250–5,000 Hz) often indicated as high-frequency oscillations, such as ripples and fast ripples associated with spiking activity (see Chapter 33 for a discussion of these phenomena).

Using microelectrodes, Ray et al. (12) recorded single units (spikes) and LFPs in the somatosensory cortex of monkeys. They found that high-gamma power (60–200 Hz) of LFPs was strongly correlated with the mean firing rate of the spikes, whereas the correlation between firing rate and low-gamma power (40–80 Hz) was much smaller. They also carried out computer simulations of the electrocorticogram, which indicated that the increases in firing rate and in neuronal synchrony were related to an increase in high-gamma power; synchrony had a stronger contribution than firing rate.

In principle, all current components present in the brain contribute to the EEG and MEG, irrespective of their origin, and although neurons are electrically the most active and versatile current generators, other current sources could also contribute. At least two are worth mentioning here. Astrocytes were for a long time considered just as the support cells in the brain; their total number is an order of magnitude larger than the neuron count, and although they are not excitable in the sense that they cannot generate action potentials, they have a large conductance for potassium and can carry considerable ionic current. In recent years it has also become clear that astrocytes might be more involved in modulating neuronal communication than originally thought [13]. An important functional aspect is their role in redistributing potassium ions extruded by neurons, in particular during strong activity, the so-called potassium buffering [14–16]. Two factors explain why, despite their large conductance and huge numbers, astrocytes contribute relatively little to the fields: their basic morphology is not strongly polarized and the cells are small, so they cannot form a substantial dipole moment. Astrocytes are also mostly randomly organized as a syncytium, which cancels the majority of their contributions. Finally, astrocytes are electrically predominantly responsive cells in that they are most active when neurons demand them to be. Thus, when they contribute, they mostly do so in the presence of strong and dominant neuronal fields. However, there is one aspect of glia organization that might be taken into consideration in this respect: astrocytes are strongly electrically coupled by gap junctions and the syncytium thus formed could act as an aggregated dipole with a relatively large dipole moment. This concept is worth being studied experimentally or modeled computationally.

In the brain all currents are carried by ions, which leads in two ways to charge separation. First, the voltage gradients cause electrodiffusion in the extracellular space and push/pull positive as well as negative ions. Difference in transport number (diffusion coefficient) for the oppositely charged ions could lead to the buildup of charge. Second, the majority charge carrier extracellularly is sodium, while intracellularly it is potassium. This could also lead to separation of charges. Actually, both effects are quite small compared to all other sources that influence the field, but they can be calculated [14,16].

A last relevant question within the current framework is: Can there be strong neuronal activity that does not show up in the electrical field? We have seen above that, for example in randomly organized neurons, a lot of activity will cancel in the far field. To evaluate such activity we must, in general, record as close to the population as possible or revert to a different recording modality such as MEG (see below) or to single unit activity. An even more compelling example of strong activity without much representation in the electrical field is the so-called shunting inhibition [17]. In this case the released neurotransmitter GABA activates a very strong inhibitory conductance in the postsynaptic membrane, but the membrane voltage is very close to the reversal potential for Cl^-, which is the relevant ion for the activated $GABA_A$ receptor. Due to the absence of a substantial driving force, even a strong increase in membrane conductance will not result in a large current. Functionally such an inhibition can be extremely effective as it "clamps" the membrane, at very little metabolic cost, at a voltage where spikes can no longer be generated.

2.5. How Do Neuronal Populations Contribute to MEG?

Physics dictates that electrical currents generate radial magnetic fields (see Box 4.1). The calculation of the magnetic field generated by an action potential in an isolated frog axon performed by Swinney and Wikswo [18], compared well with experimental data [19,20]. The authors concluded that the magnetic field resulting from the axial intracellular current flow was two orders of magnitude larger than the one generated by the more distributed return currents in the extracellular space surrounding the axon, while the contribution of the transmembrane currents was negligible.

As the magnetic field and the electrical field can both be independently and exactly calculated from the current distribution in the tissue, an important practical issue is whether the MEG contains any additional information that is not already contained in the EEG. To settle this point, Swinney [21] described a theoretical dipole configuration where the MEG resolves an ambiguous EEG configuration and where MEG and EEG thus contain supplementary information. The key here is the morphological organization; it is straightforward to design dipole configurations where components in the EEG cancel while those in the MEG do not [21].

More recently Murakami and Okada [22] designed a computer model aimed at simulating the MEG and EEG of a cortical network of excitatory and inhibitory neurons. Such a model helps to interpret scalp EEG and MEG recordings. Each pyramidal neuron was implemented as a three-dimensional compartmental model with characteristic geometry, passive electrical properties, and voltage-dependent ionic conductances. Stimulation of these neurons was accomplished by current injection in the soma. Next the intracellular current, relevant for the magnetic field, was quantified by the current dipole moment (q), and the orthogonal component at the cortical surface of the population Q was aggregated by vectorial summation of all q's. The same was done for currents in the inhibitory neurons. The magnetic field B and the electrical potential V at the scalp can be expressed as functions of, respectively, the intracellular currents and the extracellular return currents. The magnetic field is assumed to be generated by the tangential component of Q, with respect to the inner skull surface, whereas the electric field is due to both the tangential and radial components. This implies that B is mainly caused by neuronal activity in sulci, since Q is directed perpendicularly to the pial surface, whereas both radial and tangential components contribute to the electric field.

In their study Murakami and Okada [22] came to the remarkable conclusion that although the values of the net equivalent dipole moment Q are quite variable and depend on the size of the active tissue, the value of the current dipole moment density reaches about 1 to 2 nAm/mm² and seems to be rather similar over regions and species. This number also matches with theoretical predictions.

For a dipole moment Q of 0.2 pA.m *per cortical pyramidal neuron*, a population of 50,000 synchronously active cells generates a field with a magnitude of 10 nA.m, which, according to Hämäläinen et al. [23], corresponds closely to the smallest measurable value in the human cortex. If we assume that a cortical mini-column with a diameter of 40 μm contains 100 cells, the cortical surface of 50,000 cells is a patch with an area of about 0.63 mm² and a diameter of 0.9 mm.

Several investigations of evoked MEG fields elicited by transcutaneous electric stimulation of peripheral nerves report values of Q in the range of 10 to 50 nA.m, corresponding to a cross-sectional area of the responsible cortical patch of about 10 to 50 mm². In the case of epileptic spikes, the mean value of Q was reported to be 137 ± 72 nA.m in the frontal cortex and 275 ± 151 nA.m in the temporal lobe [22]. Assuming the dipole moment density of 1 nA.m/mm², the minimal size of the involved active region would amount to 137 to 275 mm².

2.6. Influence of Inhomogeneity in the Extracellular Space

The discussion so far has assumed a scalar uniform conductance for the whole brain, which is only an approximation. To analyze the consequences of inhomogeneities with respect to the resulting fields we need to distinguish at least three different spatial scales.

The first scale involves very local differences at a fast time scale. In Chapter 2 (Section 3) we pointed out that controversy exists over whether the extracellular media may be considered resistive and homogenous. Destexhe and Bédard [24], in a theoretical study, proposed that the extracellular medium in close proximity to the neuronal membrane is not homogenous and purely resistive due to the fact that ionic currents are not instantaneously balanced as diffusion is involved. This causes a transient accumulation of charge, which is reflected in transient potential changes. Indeed, electrical neutrality is not instantaneous and holds only on a time scale in the order of milliseconds. In the direct surroundings of the membrane the situation is even more complex due to the presence of charged layers (biophysical details can be found in Hille [3]).

At a larger spatial scale, inhomogeneity and anisotropy are induced by variations in cell density, the extracellular matrix, fiber orientation, and the like. In the discussion so far we have considered the generation of electrical fields in a homogenous isotropic medium with uniform scalar conductance σ using the simplified Poisson equation B2, which relates the electrical potential field V to the current density $\vec{J}$ and originates from the general form:

$$div\, \overset{\leftrightarrow}{\sigma}\, grad\, V = div\, \vec{J} \qquad \text{(Eq. 5)}$$

The difference to note is that we now use the symbol $\overset{\leftrightarrow}{\sigma}$ to indicate that conductance in reality is not a scalar but a tensor, its value is location-dependent (non-homogeneity), and it may also have a different value in each direction (anisotropy) at each location; thus, it has to be defined as a three-dimensional matrix. The consequence of this complication can be easily illustrated for the one-dimensional case: assuming σ, V, and $\vec{J}$ to be functions of z and zero currents in the x and y direction, Eq. 5 reduces to:

$$\frac{d}{dz}\left(\sigma(z)\frac{d}{dz}V(z)\right)=\frac{d}{dz}\vec{J}(z)$$

which can be worked out as (applying the chain rule for differentiation and leaving out the dependence on z for clarity):

$$\sigma\frac{dV}{dz}+V\frac{d\sigma}{dz}=\frac{d}{dz}\vec{J} \qquad \textbf{(Eq. 6)}$$

This equation for the one-dimensional case illustrates not only that the location dependence of $\vec{\vec{\sigma}}$ position-dependently scales the voltage gradients $\left(\frac{dV}{dz}\right)$, but that ignoring it will introduce artificial sinks and sources at locations where a large voltage (V) coincides with substantial gradients in conductance $\left(\frac{d\sigma}{dz}\right)$. Luckily, Eq. 6 shows that the errors in the field either are proportional to the conductance, and thus are relatively easy to understand, or they occur where large gradients in conductance coincide with large fields, which rarely happens.

In addition (equation not given here), an often-ignored consequence in the one-dimensional simplification is that extracellular currents in the x and y direction, which are assumed to be zero, will show up as sinks and sources in the z direction. To the best of our knowledge there are very few to no measurements that succeed in quantifying the complete tensor $\vec{\vec{\sigma}}$ for a brain structure.

The extracellular medium is most often considered a fluid with constant extracellular ionic composition. Because conductance is proportional to ionic strength, this implies that changes in ionic concentrations (e.g., potassium extrusion from neurons during activity) lead to variation in conductance. Except for extreme pathological conditions, such as spreading depression [25], these variations are small and can be ignored.

When measuring conductance values in real tissue, two additional corrections need to be made. Currents can pass through only the *extracellular* fraction of the volume, not through the high-resistance membranes of the cells. Therefore, resistivity scales with the extracellular volume fraction [26], which can be quite distinct and varies between 0.1 in very dense cell layers and 0.8 in regions that contain only sparse dendrites. As currents in the extracellular space are carried by diffusing ions, hindering diffusion is equivalent to increasing the extracellular resistance. The extracellular matrix induces a kind of tortuosity in the extracellular space [27], which elongates the diffusion distance that ions need to move by up to a factor 2 in comparison to plain fluid diffusion. This tortuosity is location-dependent and a second source of inhomogeneities.

The third time scale we need to consider involves the fact that, specifically in the case of scalp EEG, the skull and skin form a strong barrier. They are located completely outside the region where the field is generated, so their consequence is mainly one of filtering. For an interpretation of field potentials measured at the scalp, it is important to take into consideration the three layers that lie around the brain: the cerebrospinal fluid (CSF), the skull, and the scalp. These layers account, at least in part, for the attenuation of EEG signals measured at the scalp as compared to those recorded at the underlying cortical surface. To solve the forward problem (i.e., to calculate the potential distribution at the surface of the scalp caused by a dipole placed within the brain), we must compute the potential distribution at the surface of each shell (i.e., solve the boundary value problem). In classic circle symmetrical models, typically three concentric spheres were used that had radii of 78, 83, and 90 mm. The values of the conductivities of the three layers were proposed by Geddes and Baker [28]: for the brain 0.33, for the skull 0.0042, and for the scalp 0.33 Sm⁻¹; in case the CSF was included, it had a conductivity of 1.0 Sm⁻¹. Recently more precise estimates of these conductivities were obtained by way of measurements in vivo, using the method of electric impedance tomography (EIT) combined with a realistic model of the head. The results of the study by Gonçalves et al. [29] showed that the ratio between the conductivities of the skull and the brain lies between 20 and 50 (for six subjects) rather than the traditionally assumed value of 78. The authors reported a mean value of 0.33 Sm⁻¹ for the brain and 0.0081 Sm⁻¹ for the skull. There was considerable intersubject variation for these values: a factor of 2.4 was found between subjects with respect to the extreme values of the ratio of conductivities. This implies that the values of conductivity should be estimated for each individual to obtain reliable measurements.

In addition, it is known that the conductivity of the various tissues is not homogeneous: the conductivity of the skull varies with its thickness and bone structure. Law et al. [30] showed that there is an inverse relation between skull resistivity and thickness. Cuffin [31] and Eshel et al. [32] investigated the effects of varying the conductivity of the skull. The former study determined that the effect of local variations in skull and scalp thickness was slightly larger on the EEG than on the MEG, while the latter showed a correlation between interhemispheric asymmetry in skull thickness and the amplitude of the scalp EEG. The very thorough studies by Haueisen [33] on the influence of various combinations of conductivities on both the EEG and MEG showed that the scalp EEG was most influenced by the conductivities of the skull and the scalp, while the MEG was most influenced by the conductivities of the brain tissue and the CSF. We should note that the conductivity of the tissues of the head can also present anisotropy. Indeed, it is known that in brain tissue, the conductivity measured in a direction parallel to a fiber tract can be 10 times larger than in the perpendicular direction. However, it is difficult to integrate this finding in global models of the whole head, since fiber tracts are organized in a most complex way within the anatomical constraints of the folds of the brain. Nevertheless, De Munck [34], using a model consisting of five concentric shells, solved the forward problem in an analytic form for the case in which the skull and the cortex had anisotropic properties. The effects of the anisotropic conductivity of the skull were determined by Yvert et al. [35] and by Van den Broek et al. [36]. The latter showed that the anisotropy of the skull causes the smearing out of the distribution of the EEG over the scalp, whereas the normal component of the MEG is not affected (for the specific properties of the MEG see Chapter 35). In addition, it is relevant to emphasize that the skull does not have a homogeneous surface, due to the existence of regions with different thickness, the occipital opening, and the eye sockets. The existence of holes in the skull (e.g., due to surgical interventions) also influences the distribution of the EEG over the scalp [35]. Since the late 1980s, realistically shaped models were gradually introduced and applied. This was made possible by using magnetic resonance imaging (MRI), which allows us to make realistic estimates of the three-dimensional geometry of the brain and surrounding tissues. To solve the forward problem in a realistically shaped volume of the head, we must apply numerical methods. Examples of the latter are the finite-volume, the finite-difference, and the finite-element methods (for details see [37]). These methods are powerful, but they need reliable information about the structure of the brain and surrounding tissues obtained from MRI scans, and of the corresponding conductivities, to be applied in a sensible way. They are particularly suited for calculating the influence of specific inhomogeneities such as the influence of the cerebral ventricles filled with CSF and anisotropic conductivities. These and more advanced approaches for solving the volume conductor problem are presented and discussed in Chapter 45.

3. THE INVERSE PROBLEM

The forward problem, discussed above, has a large academic context and boils down to basic physics. The more relevant clinical question is often defined as the inverse problem: Given a recorded potential distribution, what can we deduct about the sources that generated it? If we can again separate space and time and know the location of all the sources (the "exact" inverse problem!), it is straightforward to calculate the time patterns. However, in practice, the most important question is often to estimate also the location of an unknown number of sources. Notwithstanding the fundamental proof presented by Helmholtz [1] that there is no unique solution to this problem, a lot of effort has been invested in developing models to obtain estimates of a solution, where everything depends on choosing the appropriate boundary conditions (Box 4.3).

The classical physics solution to the general problem is the multipole expansion described in Box 4.2, which locates as many higher-order poles at a particular site as is necessary to describe the voltage at another site within the experimental accuracy. For the brain that approach is hardly useful, as the main problem is to find a reasonable solution within the boundaries of an unknown multitude of current sources. The problem becomes the unsolvable Helmholtz problem if we do not have a completely sampled three-dimensional voltage profile but only a set of recordings of electrical fields at the scalp (as a function of space and time).

For LFPs the question of source localization is often tackled using CSD analysis, originally formulated by Nicholson and Freeman [38,39]. Here we have measured the spatial voltage profile in one, two, or three dimensions and need to estimate the generating current sources. Realizing that the extracellular current is equal to the voltage gradient and that the desired CSD is the current gradient that links the transmembrane current I_m (the sources and sinks for the LFP) to the recorded spatial field V through conductivity tensor σ as described in Box 4.1:

$$I_m(x,y,z) = div\, \vec{\bar{\sigma}}\, grad\, V(x,y,z)$$

For the simplified one-dimensional case (i.e., currents flow only in the z direction and are identical in the infinitely large x-y plane), this equation simplifies for uniform conductivity σ to:

$$I_m = \sigma \frac{d^2}{dz^2} V$$

and for non-homogeneous tissue to:

$$I_m = \sigma \frac{d^2}{dz^2} V + \frac{d\sigma}{dz} \frac{dV}{dz}$$

The complications arise when we realize that the volume of the activity is limited, that the activity is not in one direction, and that sampling is most often quite limited. The reader is referred to sources that deal extensively with these problems [40,41].

The general approach is to decompose the volume conductor in a mesh consisting of a relatively large number of discrete elements. The accuracy of the method increases with the spatial resolution of the sampling, but the necessary computational effort increases much faster. If the neuronal activity of interest is restricted to a well-defined brain region, it is called the "source localization problem." These methods need reliable information about the structure of the brain and surrounding tissues, obtained from MRI scans, as described further in Chapter 45, where different approaches such as "dipole source localization," "distributed source imaging," and "multimodal integration of EEG with fMRI" are presented. The latter issue is also dealt with in Chapter 46.

The final outcome of all these analyses is a description of the local current sources that are responsible for the observed field. The last step is to interpret these aggregated variables in terms of synaptic components, action potentials, and all the other elements that were extensively described concerning the forward problem, while realizing that currents that canceled out can never be reconstructed without the help of other modalities (e.g., MEG!). This most difficult step is essential for understanding the functional meaning of the measurements made. For example, if the current represents excitatory synaptic activity, it is very likely to reflect the (synaptic) *input* to the structure under investigation, but if it reflects action potential activity, it is more likely linked to the *output* of the structure. This makes a huge difference for the functional meaning of an observation.

4. THE REVERSE PROBLEM

The third important question in the field of brain biophysics is the reverse of the forward problem: Can electromagnetic fields imposed from outside the brain modulate neuron and brain function? The biophysical foundations of this problem are not commonly considered jointly with the forward and inverse problems but merit being discussed here since both approaches share fundamental biophysical aspects. Mostly according to scale, we distinguish several levels at which electrical modulation can be exerted.

First, the classical way of manipulating neuronal function is by direct current injection using an electrode placed inside the cell. Current forced into the cell and through the resistive membrane will change membrane voltage according to Ohm's law and thus will depolarize or hyperpolarize (depending on the sign of the current) the membrane (Fig. 4.3A). This allows us to measure the (voltage-dependent) conductance of the membrane and to induce cell firing. There are various forms of forcing current through the membrane, even if there is no intracellular electrode present (for examples and in-depth treatment of the topic, see [3]).

Although the observed effect may often look the same, artificially injecting current through the membrane is not identical to activating afferent fibers. In the latter case the neurotransmitter alters membrane conductance (by opening channels) and the driving force leads to the current flow. The change in membrane conductance also affects the dynamics of the response. In addition, there is quite a distinction in the ions that are involved in both cases of activation.

Molecular tools have recently been invented that force genetically specified neurons to express light-sensitive ion channels in their membranes ("optogenetics"). When activated by light these channels respond in a very similar way as receptor-operated channels do; because these tools are very cell-specific, they open a huge realm for network stimulation and analysis [42].

Second, most invasive electrostimulation in the brain uses extracellular electrodes that set up a voltage gradient in the extracellular compartment by directly injecting current (see Fig. 4.3B). Long axons keep their transmembrane voltage at resting level (say, −65 mV in respect to zero voltage outside). The current injected in the extracellular space creates a relative positive potential around the anode and a negative one around the cathode, proportional to the stimulation current, if we assume uniform extracellular conductivity. This implies a (virtual) depolarization of the axonal membrane around the cathode (therefore, the transmembrane potential is reduced, which we call depolarization) and, vice versa, a hyperpolarization around the anode. At the cathode we have brought the transmembrane potential closer to firing threshold and thus increased excitability that might induce an action potential, while around the anode we could encounter "anodal block". It is much more difficult to generate an action potential at the anode. The efficacy of the stimulation depends on how strong the axonal membrane near the cathode can be depolarized. Correct alignment of the field with the axons improves stimulation efficacy; in other words, the orientation of the stimulus electrode will in part determine the efficacy with which fibers with different orientation are stimulated. This principle of activation holds for vagal nerve stimulation, for deep brain stimulation and also for transcranial magnetic stimulation, where a changing magnetic flux induces a response current in the brain (for practical details see Chapter 28). Refining the stimulus electrode into an array of electrodes that can be properly controlled gives the clinician the possibility to optimize stimulation for a preferred set of axons [43], for example in deep brain stimulation for Parkinson's disease.

Third, in brain regions that contain large palissades of polarized neurons (e.g., the hippocampus or the cortex), the principle explained in the previous paragraph has a consequence. These neuronal layers can set up LFPs that reach voltage gradients of several millivolts, sometimes larger, and under

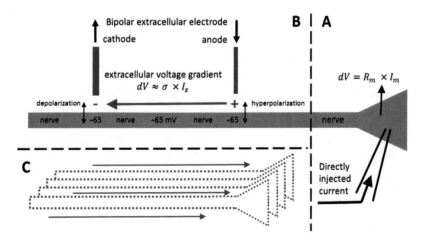

Figure 4.3. *Three basic forms of stimulation in neuronal tissue. A: Direct current injection into the cell through an intracellular electrode (or other advanced method) forces current through the membrane and so manipulates membrane voltage. B: Extracellular stimulation forces a current through the extracellular space from anode to cathode and thereby sets up a voltage gradient between these two electrodes. Biophysics dictates that the intracellular voltage in the axon is almost equipotential (−65 mV in this example), which implies that due to the extracellular gradient, the transmembrane voltage difference near the cathode decreases (depolarization and enhanced excitability), while it increases near the anode (hyperpolarization and reduced excitability). C: If a palissade of neurons generates a laminar field of sufficient strength, this field acts like an external field for the neurons and can modulate/synchronize them.*

pathological conditions much larger (e.g., seizures, spreading depression). Such fields fulfill the same role as the extracellular field set up by the stimulation, explained above. The result is that they have a strong synchronizing effect on the neuronal population (see Fig. 4.3C). Such interactions between similarly oriented neurons are called ephaptic interactions [44,45].

Fourth, based on the principles explained above, a large class of diagnostic and therapeutic techniques has been developed. Two methods will be discussed here: transcranial direct current stimulation and transcranial magnetic stimulation. Chapter 28 deals with cortical stimulation techniques and the corresponding clinical applications in detail; here we just point out how these techniques are linked to the two biophysical principles explained above. Two questions are related to the biophysical principles that underlie these forms of stimulation:

1. How can the stimulation (current) affect the axonal membranes, enhance excitability, and most often induce action potentials?

2. How is the efficacy (in space and time) of the stimulation affected by the electrical properties of the volume conductor of the head?

4.1. Biophysics of Transcranial Direct Current Stimulation

In transcranial electric stimulation, which encompasses transcranial direct current stimulation, transcranial alternating current stimulation, and transcranial random noise stimulation, the electric current is applied to the head using two surface electrodes on the scalp. Only a fraction of the applied current will actually reach the brain and create a voltage gradient at the desired location. Detailed voltage profiles can only be predicted with computational models that take into account the physical properties of all the volume conductor elements that are relevant. Since the seminal modeling studies by Miranda et al. [46], models with increasing degrees of complexity have been put forward. Bikson et al. [47] list 17 models, from the early simple concentric four-sphere models to high-resolution models based on personalized MRIs. The latter involve accurate reproduction of detailed segmented MRIs, including scalp, skull, CSF, gray and white matter, down to the gyrus level. In this way a surface mesh is constructed that represents the boundaries between the different tissues (e.g., the white–gray matter boundary). The outer boundaries are assumed to be insulating; transcranial direct current stimulation electrodes are placed at standard or at desired locations. Next, this volume mesh is imported into a finite element program that computes the electrical field that results from current injected via the electrodes into the brain, or alternatively from an applied controlled voltage [48,49]. The electrical field in the brain is calculated using the rules explained in Box 4.1, taking into account the spatially well-defined non-homogeneous σ mesh. In the last step, the model determines the effect of the local field potentials on the (axonal) membrane potential: Is it depolarizing (exciting) or hyperpolarizing (inhibiting)? Electrical fields as weak as ±1 mV/mm can already influence

neuronal membrane cortical activity [44,50], and the position and the orientation of the electrical field with respect to the soma-dendritic membrane of the neuron must be considered.

The experimental and modeling studies reported by Merlet et al. [48] and by Rahman et al. [50] demonstrate the relevance of radial and tangential electrical fields with respect to the cortical surface. *Radial fields* target mainly somatic compartments; in contrast, *tangential fields* target mainly processes that are oriented along the tangential direction, such as horizontally directed axon terminals (Fig. 4.4).

The comprehensive study by Rahman et al. [50] demonstrated that radial cortical current flow induces somatic polarization and modulates synaptic efficacy, while tangential cortical current flow induces polarization of axon synaptic terminals (including cortico-cortical afferents). The latter polarize more than the soma of pyramidal cells. In the human case both components must be taken jointly into account, although the tangential fields tend to dominate. The modeling results appear to be consistent with those obtained in cortical slices in vitro; thus, tangential electric fields that produce synaptic terminal hyperpolarization/depolarization lead to facilitation/inhibition of synaptic efficacy. The hyperpolarization of presynaptic terminals may lead to the enhancement of transmitter release [50]. In real life, the complexity of the folded cortical surface makes unlikely the presence of pure radial and tangential fields in the sense of the definition above. Therefore, we must be cautious in simplifying the interpretation of transcranial direct current stimulation.

4.2. Biophysics of Transcranial Magnetic Stimulation

In transcranial magnetic stimulation a very strong current pulse delivered to a coil placed above the subject's head generates a time-varying magnetic field $\vec{B}(t)$, which in turn induces a circular electric field $\vec{E}(t)$ in the brain. The latter field sets up voltage gradients that influence membrane potentials of local neurons, similar to that described for transcranial direct current stimulation in the previous paragraph. The relation between $\vec{E}$ and $\vec{B}$ is given by the Maxwell–Faraday law of induction:

$$curl\,\vec{E} = -\frac{\partial \vec{B}}{\partial t} \qquad \textbf{(Eq. 7)}$$

which has a general solution of the form (see also Box 4.1):

$$\vec{E} = -\frac{\partial \vec{A}}{\partial t} - grad\,V \qquad \textbf{(Eq. 8)}$$

The first right-hand term is the primary vector field $\vec{A}$ induced by the current in the magnetic coil, while the second term represents the secondary field with scalar potential V, determined by the boundary conditions. (For a comprehensive treatment of this topic see Nummenmaa et al. [51].) The total field $\vec{E}$ is responsible for inducing electrical currents in the brain tissue.

Once the magnetically induced electrical field is known, the next steps, preferably using fine-mesh spatial models,

MACROSCOPIC

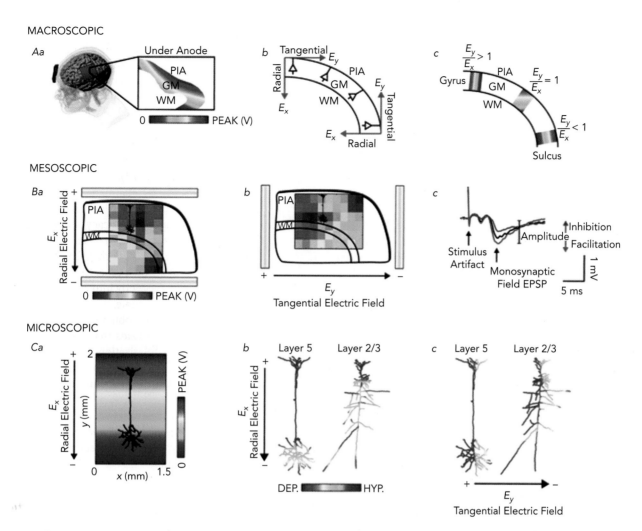

Figure 4.4. *Effects of uniform electric field (EF) directionality at the macroscopic (Aa), mesoscopic (Ba), and microscopic (Ca) levels, according to two components of the electric field: E_x = radial and E_y = tangential components. **Aa:** Gyri-precise finite element models (FEM) of current flow during transcranial direct current stimulation (tDCS) indicate a uniform voltage gradient in cortical gray matter (GM) directly under the anode. **Ab:** The induced electric field in the cortex can be decomposed into a component parallel to the somatodendritic axis (Ex) and a component orthogonal to the somatodendritic axis (Ey). **Ac:** The relative occurrence of radial and tangential fields in cortical gray matter is expressed as the ratio of Ey to Ex. **Ba and Bb:** The voltage gradient is superimposed on a schematic of a sagittal slice of the rat primary motor cortex. Compare voltage gradients in **Aa** (macroscopic) and **Ba** (mesoscopic). **Bc:** The field excitatory postsynaptic potential provides a measure of synaptic efficacy through facilitation or inhibition of the response amplitude. **Ca:** Compartment model simulations of morphologically reconstructed neocortical pyramidal neurons used to provide a description of axon terminal polarization in a uniform electric field. **Cb:** The polarization profile of a layer V pyramidal neuron in a radially directed uniform electric field indicating soma depolarization (red) corresponds to apical dendrite hyperpolarization (blue). Layer 2/3 neurons have a more complex polarization profile, with long processes reaching maximal depolarization independent of the neuronal body. **Cc:** Neurons in a uniform electric field directed tangential to the somatodendritic axis preferentially affect processes that are oriented along the tangential field. WM, white matter; PIA, pia mater. (Adapted, with permission, from Rahman A, Reato D, Arlotti M, Gasca F, Datta A, Parra LC, Bikson M. Cellular effects of acute direct current stimulation: somatic and synaptic terminal effects. J Physiol. 2013;591(10):2563–2578, Fig. 1, p. 2566.)*

should be similar to the ones described in the previous paragraph for transcranial direct current stimulation using a realistic volume conductor model based on anatomical MRI. This implies considerable computational costs, which is why it is not generally done in real-time transcranial magnetic stimulation. A comparison of different volume conductor models for transcranial magnetic stimulation navigation is given by Nummenmaa et al. [51], who propose a realistically shaped boundary element head model.

Empirical observations in human and experimental work in animals gave some clues about the kind of transcranial magnetic stimulation setups that may be more efficient in stimulating neuronal populations in the human brain. Nonetheless, the physiological basis of how these stimuli can interact with

neuronal populations and activate the latter is still a matter of debate. Major advances have been made with respect to the stimulation of cortical motor populations. It is well known that the application of an electrical stimulus to the motor cortex in animals can evoke neuronal activity that can be recorded at the level of the spinal cord. This activity has been characterized as consisting of a series of events, the characteristics of which depend on the way transcranial magnetic stimulation is applied. Current in the brain that is induced in the posterior-to-anterior direction activates preferentially cortico-cortical circuits projecting onto the corticospinal neurons, thus evoking high-frequency (~600 Hz) repetitive discharges of corticospinal fibers. These discharge bursts are called indirect waves, or I-waves, because they result from *indirect* activation of corticospinal cells through the activation of neuronal elements that are presynaptic to corticospinal cells. In contrast, D-waves are produced by *direct* stimulation of corticospinal axons at a short latency. We cannot go into the details of cortical physiology underlying these phenomena; a comprehensive review of the physiology of these processes can be found in Terao and Ugawa [52] and Di Lazzaro et al. [53].

The final level at which electrical modulation can be exerted involves the use of wireless equipment such as mobile phones, digital enhanced cordless transmitted phones, and Wi-Fi installations. The recent exponential increase in the use of such technology has raised concerns about its potential interference with human health, mostly whether these fields can induce cancer. Although this seems very unlikely based on the large gap between the energy in the electromagnetic waves and the energy needed for DNA damage, some epidemiological studies report very weak associations. The complete lack of any mechanistic explanation, except for very weak temperature effects, makes interpretations of these findings highly speculative.

Direct interference of antenna fields with neurons can be studied using computational models. The frequencies of the radio signals are in the range of 300 MHz to 300 GHz, and so quite outside everything we have discussed so far. If we also include signals from digital enhanced cordless transmitted phones, the frequency content becomes even more difficult to establish. Exposing cells to fields of strength in the order of 100 V/m creates measurable signals around their membrane [54], although they are in general orders of magnitude smaller than the ephaptic interactions mentioned above. The fields at these frequencies have wavelengths in the order of centimeters; thus, size matters, and one must be very careful in extrapolating, for example, data obtained in small rodents to humans.

5. FINAL REMARKS

The laws of basic physics that describe the relation between current generators and the resulting electrical fields are quite straightforward, which implies that the *forward problem* can be solved, assuming one has sufficient computing power at one's disposal. It is the bewildering morphological complexity of the head that makes the *inverse problem*, namely how to estimate the brain generators of an electrical field distribution measured at the scalp level, a real challenge in terms of deciding on the boundary conditions. Advances have been made using realistic models that take into account the effects of inhomogeneity and anisotropy (further worked out in other chapters of this volume). Understanding the consequences of such complexity is essential while dealing with the *reverse problem*, namely how to apply current or magnetic stimuli in order to enhance or suppress activity in well-defined regions of the brain for therapeutic reasons. In short, we must recognize the importance of understanding the common basic framework concerning these three main topics of brain physics: the forward, inverse, and reverse problems.

REFERENCES

1. Helmholtz H. Ueber einige Gesetze der Verteilung elektrischer Ströme in Körperlichen Leitern mit Anwendung auf die thierischelektrischen Versuche. *Prog Ann Physik Chemie.* 1855;89:211–233, 353–377.
2. Plonsey R. The nature of sources of bioelectric and biomagnetic fields. *Biophys J.* 1969;39:309–315.
3. Hille B. Ion Channels of Excitable Membranes. 3rd ed. Sunderland, MA: Sinauer Assoc. Publishers, 2001.
4. Somjen GG, Kager H, Wadman WJ. Computer simulations of neuron-glia interactions mediated by ion flux. *J Comput Neurosci.* 2008;25:349–365.
5. Wei Y, Ullah G, Schiff SJ. Unification of neuronal spikes, seizures, and spreading depression. *J Neurosci.* 2014;34(35):11733–11743.
6. Lorente de Nó R. Action potential of the motoneurons of the hypoglossus nucleus. *J Cell Comp Physiol.* 1947;29:207–287.
7. Rall W. Core conductor theory and cable properties of neurons. *Compr Physiol.* 2011, Supplement 1: Handbook of Physiology, The Nervous System, Cellular Biology of Neurons: 39–97.
8. Johnston D, Wu SM-S. *Foundations of Cellular Neurophysiology.* Cambridge, MA: MIT Press, 1994.
9. Einevoll GT, Kayser C, Logothetis NK. Modelling and analysis of local field potentials for studying the function of cortical circuits. *Nature Rev Neurosci.* 2013;14(11):770–785.
10. Reimann MW, Anastassiou CA, Perin R, Hill SL, Markram H, Koch C. A biophysically detailed model of neocortical local field potentials predicts the critical role of active membrane currents. *Neuron.* 2013;79:375–390.
11. Lindén H, Tetzlaff T, Potjans TC, Pettersen KH, Grün S, Diesmann M, Einevoll GT. Modeling the spatial reach of the LFP. *Neuron.* 2011;72:859–872.
12. Ray S, Crone NE, Niebur E, Franaszczuk PJJ, Hsiao SS. Neural correlates of high-gamma oscillations (60–200 Hz) in macaque local field potentials and their potential implications in electrocorticography. *J Neurosci.* 2008;28(45):11526–11536.
13. Araque A, Parpura V, Sanzgiri RP, Haydon PG. Tripartite synapses: glia, the unacknowledged partner. *Trends Neurosci.* 1999;22(5):208–215.
14. Dietzel I, Heinemann U, Lux H. Relations between slow extracellular potential changes, glial potassium buffering, and electrolyte and cellular volume changes during neuronal hyperactivity in cat brain. *Glia.* 1989;2(1):25–44.
15. Gardner-Medwin A. Analysis of potassium dynamics in mammalian brain tissue. *J Physiol.* 1983;335:393–426.
16. Halnes G, Ostby I, Pettersen KH, Omholt SW, Einevoll GT. Electrodiffusive model for astrocytic and neuronal ion concentration dynamics. *PLoS Comput Biol.* 2013;9(12):e1003386.
17. Mann EO, Paulsen O. Role of GABAergic inhibition in hippocampal network oscillations. *Trends Neurosci.* 2007;30(7):343–349.
18. Swinney KR, Wikswo JP Jr. A calculation of the magnetic field of a nerve action potential. *Biophys J.* 1980;32(2):719–731.
19. Barach JP, Freeman JA, Wikswo JP. Experiments on the magnetic-field of nerve action-potentials. *J Appl Physics.* 1980;51(8):4532–4538.
20. Irimia A, Swinney KR, Wikswo JP. Partial independence of bioelectric and biomagnetic fields and its implications for encephalography and cardiography. *Phys Rev E.* 2009;79(5):051908.
21. Swinney KR, Irimia A, Wikswo JP. The partial independence of bioelectric and biomagnetic fields and its implications for encephalography and cardiography. *Phys Rev E Stat Nonlin Soft Matter Phys.* 2009;79(5):051908.
22. Murakami S, Okada Y. Invariance in current dipole moment density across brain structures and species: Physiological constraint for neuroimaging. *NeuroImage.* 2015;111:49–58.
23. Hämäläinen MS, Hari R, Ilmoniemi R, Magneto-encephalography: theory, instrumentation and applications to the noninvasive study of human brain function. *Rev Med Physics.* 1993;65:413–497.
24. Destexhe A, Bédard C. Do neurons generate monopolar current sources? *J Neurophysiol.* 2012;108:953–955.
25. Somjen GG. Mechanisms of spreading depression and hypoxic spreading depression-like depolarization. *Physiol Rev.* 2001;81(3):1065–1096.
26. Nicholson C, Phillips IM, Gardner Medwin AR. Diffusion from an iontophoretic point source in the brain—role of tortuosity and volume fraction *Brain Res.* 1979;169 (3):580–584.
27. Nicholson C. Diffusion and related transport mechanisms in brain tissue. *Rep Progr Physics.* 2001;64(70):815–884.
28. Geddes LA, Baker LE. The specific resistance of biological; materials—a compendium of data for the biomedical engineer and physiologist. *Med Biol Eng.* 1967;5:271–293.
29. Gonçalves SI, de Munck JC, Verbunt JPA, Bijma F, Heethaar RM, Lopes da Silva FH. In vivo measurement of the brain and skull resistivities using

an EIT-based method and realistic models of the head. *IEEE Trans Biomed Eng.* 2003;50:754–767.

30. Law SK, Nunez PL, Wijesinghe RS. High-resolution EEG using spline generated surface Laplacians on spherical and ellipsoidal surfaces. *IEEE Trans Biomed Eng.* 1993;40:145–153.

31. Cuffin BN. Effects of local variations in skull and scalp EEG's and MEG's. *IEEE Trans. Biomed Eng.* 1993;40:42–48.

32. Eshel Y, Witman S, Rosenfeld M, Abboud, S. Correlation between skull reflects the direction of the current densities. *IEEE Trans Biomed Eng.* 1995;42:232–249.

33. Haueisen J, Ramon C, Czapski P, Eiselt M. On the influence of volume currents and extended sources on neuromagnetic fields: a simulation study. *Ann Biomed Eng.* 1995;23:728–739.

34. De Munck JC. The potential distribution in a layered anisotropic spheroidal volume conductor. *J Appl Physics.* 1988;64:464.

35. Yvert B, Bertrand O, Echallier JF, Pernier J. Improved dipole localization using local mesh refinement of realistic head geometries: an EEG simulation study. *Electroenceph Clin Neurphysiol.* 1996;99:79–89.

36. Van den Broek SP, Reinders F, Donderwinkel M, Peters MJ. Volume conduction effects in EEG and MEG. *Electroenceph Clin Neurophysiol.* 1988;106(6):522–534.

37. Van Uitert R, Weinstein D, Johnson C. Volume currents in forward and inverse magnetoencephalographic simulations using realistic head models. *Ann Biomed Eng.* 2003;31(1):21–31.

38. Nicholson C, Freeman JA. Theory of current source-density analysis and determination of conductivity tensor for anuran cerebellum. *J Neurophysiol.* 1975;38(2):356–368.

39. Freeman JA, Nicholson C. Experimental optimization of current source-density technique for anuran cerebellum. *J Neurophysiol.* 1975;38(2):369–382.

40. Herreras O, Makarova J, Makarov VA. New uses of LFPs: pathway-specific threads obtained through spatial discrimination. *Neuroscience.* 2015;310:486–503.

41. Einevoll GT, Kayser C, Logothetis NK, Panzeri S. Modelling and analysis of local field potentials for studying the function of cortical circuits. *Nat Rev Neurosci.* 2013;14(11):770–785.

42. Ritter LM, Golshani P, Takahashi K, Dufour S, Valiante T, Kokaia M. Optogenetic tools to suppress seizures and explore the mechanisms of epileptogenesis. *Epilepsia.* 2014;55(11):1693–1702.

43. Teplitzky BA, Zitella LM, Xiao Y, Johnson MD. Model-based comparison of deep brain stimulation array functionality with varying number of radial electrodes and machine learning feature sets. *Front Comput Neurosci.* 2016;10:58–63.

44. Jefferys JGR. Nonsynaptic modulation of neuronal activity in the brain: electric currents and extracellular ions. *Physiol Rev.* 1995;75(4):689–723.

45. Frohlich F, McCormick DA. Endogenous electric fields may guide neocortical network activity. *Neuron.* 2010;67(1):129–143.

46. Miranda PC, Lomarev M, Hallett M. Modeling the current distribution during transcranial direct current stimulation. *Clin Neurophysiol.* 2006;117:1623–1629.

47. Bikson M, Rahman A, Datta A. Computational models of transcranial direct current stimulation. *Clin EEG Neurosci.* 2012;43(3):176–183.

48. Merlet I, Birot G, Salvador R, Molaee-Ardekani B, Mekonnen A, Soria-Frish A, Ruffini G, Miranda PC, Wendling F. From oscillatory transcranial current stimulation to scalp EEG changes: a biophysical and physiological modeling study. *PLoS One.* 2013;8(2):e57330.

49. Ruffini G, Wendling F, Merlet I, Molaee-Ardenaki B, Mekonne A, Salvador R, Soria-Frisch A, Grau C, Dunne S, Miranda PC. Transcranial current brain stimulation (tCS): models and technologies. *IEEE Trans Neural Systems Rehab Eng.* 2013;21(3):333–345.

50. Rahman A, Reato D, Arlotti M, Gasca F, Datta A, Parra LC, Bikson M. Cellular effects of acute direct current stimulation: somatic and synaptic terminal effects. *J Physiol.* 2013;591:2563–2578.

51. Nummenmaa A, Stenros M, Ilmoniemi RJ, Okada YC, Hämäläinen M, Raij T. Comparison of spherical and realistically shaped boundary element head models for transcranial magnetic stimulation. *Clin Neurophysiol.* 2013;124:1995–2007.

52. Terao Y, Ugawa Y. Basic mechanisms of TMS. *J Clin Neurophysiol.* 2002;19(4):322–343.

53. Di Lazzaro V, Ziemann U, Lemon RN. State of the art: physiology of transcranial motor cortex stimulation. *Brain Stim.* 2008;1:345–362.

54. Vanegas-Acosta JC, Lancellotti V, Zwamborn APM. Numerical investigation of proximity effects on field gradients in biological cells, *Proceedings of the 8th European Conference on Antennas and Propagation, EUCAP 2014*, 1664–1668.

5 | RECORDING PRINCIPLES: ANALOG AND DIGITAL PRINCIPLES; POLARITY AND FIELD DETERMINATIONS; MULTIMODAL MONITORING; POLYGRAPHY (EOG, EMG, ECG, SAO₂)

DONALD L. SCHOMER, MD, CHARLES M. EPSTEIN, MD, SUSAN T. HERMAN, MD, DOUGLAS MAUS, MD, PHD, AND BRUCE J. FISCH, MD

ABSTRACT: This chapter reviews the technical aspects of recording and reviewing clinical electroencephalograms (EEGs) and related biopotentials. While advances in engineering technology have revolutionized EEG machines, the basic principles underlying accurate representation of brain activity are largely unchanged. The first section reviews the analog EEG components, and the second section discusses analog-to-digital conversion, digital filters, and display and storage parameters. Digital EEG machines are now less expensive and their capabilities far surpass those of analog machines. The third section reviews how electrode positions and systems of signal display (montages) can be used to determine the polarity and field of EEG signals. The final section describes how other biopotentials are acquired and displayed. Polygraphy can provide crucial information on other physiological processes that can impact EEG activity and can help identify potential artifactual signals. We highlight recent advances that allow the recording of a broader range of EEG frequencies and spatial distribution.

KEYWORDS: electroencephalogram, EEG, analog, digital, biopotential, polygraphy, artifact

PRINCIPAL REFERENCES

1. Kuratani J, Pearl PL, Sullivan L, et al. American Clinical Neurophysiology Society Guideline 5: Minimum Technical Standards for Pediatric Electroencephalography. *J Clin Neurophysiol*. 2016;33(4):320–323.
2. Sinha SR, Sullivan L, Sabau D, et al. American Clinical Neurophysiology Society Guideline 1: Minimum Technical Requirements for Performing Clinical Electroencephalography. *J Clin Neurophysiol*. 2016;33(4):303–307.
3. Ebner A, Sciarretta G, Epstein CM, Nuwer M. EEG instrumentation. The International Federation of Clinical Neurophysiology. *Electroencephalogr Clin Neurophysiol Suppl*. 1999;52:7–10.
4. Nuwer MR, Comi G, Emerson R, et al. IFCN standards for digital recording of clinical EEG. The International Federation of Clinical Neurophysiology. *Electroencephalogr Clin Neurophysiol Suppl*. 1999;52:11–14.
5. Acharya JN, Hani A, Cheek J, Thirumala P, Tsuchida TN. American Clinical Neurophysiology Society Guideline 2: Guidelines for Standard Electrode Position Nomenclature. *J Clin Neurophysiol*. 2016;33(4):308–311.
6. Halford JJ, Sabau D, Drislane FW, Tsuchida TN, Sinha SR. American Clinical Neurophysiology Society Guideline 4: Recording Clinical EEG on Digital Media. *J Clin Neurophysiol*. 2016;33(4):317–319.
7. International Electrotechnical Commission. IEC 60601-1-11:2015: Medical electrical equipment—Part 1-11: General requirements for basic safety and essential performance, 2015.
8. Stecker MM, Sabau D, Sullivan L, et al. American Clinical Neurophysiology Society Guideline 6: Minimum Technical Standards for EEG Recording in Suspected Cerebral Death. *J Clin Neurophysiol*. 2016;33(4):324–327.
9. Acharya JN, Hani AJ, Thirumala PD, Tsuchida TN. American Clinical Neurophysiology Society Guideline 3: A Proposal for Standard Montages to Be Used in Clinical EEG. *J Clin Neurophysiol*. 2016;33(4):312–316.
10. Fisch BJ. *Fisch and Spehlmann's EEG Primer: Basic Principles of Digital and Analog EEG*. 3rd ed. Amsterdam: Elsevier B.V.; 1999.
11. Fisch BJ. EEG localization and interpretation. In: Fisch BJ, ed. *Epilepsy and Intensive Care Monitoring*. New York: Demos Medical Publishing; 2010:57–76.
12. Venables PH, Martin I. *A Manual of Psychophysiological Methods*. Amsterdam: North Holland; 1967.

1. ANALOG PRINCIPLES

1.1. Analog Recording

Digital analysis and storage have transformed modern neurophysiology in ways that could only be imagined and envied by the founders of electroencephalography (EEG). But the "front end" of all recording systems, the portion that interfaces with the patient, remains analog. Understanding the operation of analog components can also give insight into aspects of signal processing that are now performed mostly by digital techniques. *Analog* refers to methods of handling data that are physically similar to the original signal. For example, the moving pens and ink traces of the original EEGs produced waveforms that mirrored the electrical potential differences on the scalp. Simple amplification of the microvolt potentials in EEG is an analog process. Analog data "look like" the original signal, whereas digital representations do not. Ideally, each type of data processing would produce a perfect reflection of the original waveforms. In practice, however, each is subject to its own limitations and potential for inaccuracy, which will be discussed. More detailed discussion of this material can be found online in the Guidelines of the American Clinical Neurophysiology Society (ACNS)[1,2] and in those of the International Federation of Clinical Neurophysiology.[3,4]

1.2. The Hostile World of Clinical Neurophysiology

Figure 5.1 shows the approximate amplitudes of electromlographic (EMG) activity, EEG, and evoked potential (EP) signals in relation to the many sources of noise that constantly threaten to overwhelm them. This vast range of voltages requires the use of a logarithmic scale. So, for example, an electrocardiogram (ECG) recorded *from the head* can be a thousand times larger than a brainstem EP. Within electrified

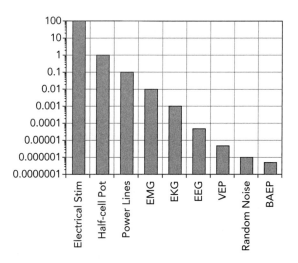

Figure 5.1. Potential sources of noise in neurophysiologic recording. Sources may represent noise in some contexts and signals in others. Note the logarithmic scale.

buildings, the 50- or 60-Hz electric field on human bodies can be 10,000 times larger than the EEG. Some physiological signals, such as EMG, can also represent noise in relation to smaller signals that we need to see behind them.

At first glance, it may seem impossible that any interpretable recording could be performed through noise that is orders of magnitude larger than the signal of interest. This chapter discusses some of the ubiquitous artifacts in Figure 5.1, the features of the analog front end that are designed to defeat them while allowing faithful recording of the desired signal, and the ways in which they may make an unwanted appearance in EEG and other neurophysiological recordings. The major entry points and barriers to noise consist of the electrode interface, the amplifier inputs, and analog filters. The following sections describe in a logical sequential order the different components of the recording system and the features that contribute to an accurate reproduction of the neurophysiologic signals.

1.3. Electrodes

EEG and other recording electrodes provide an interface between lead wires and human tissue. Because cutaneous oils and keratin are good insulators, placing dry metal electrodes directly on dry skin is usually ineffective. Keratin is often removed by rubbing the skin gently with mild abrasives. Sometimes oils are removed separately with alcohol wipes. Despite such preparations, the epidermis remains the single greatest barrier to current flow between the body and the recording system. In addition, an ionic solution, or electrolyte, is placed between the skin surface and the electrode. As with human extracellular fluids, the most abundant ions in the electrolyte are sodium and chloride. The consistency of the electrolyte ranges from free-flowing solutions to thick sticky pastes. The latter are used to help hold cup electrodes mechanically against the scalp. The former are chosen when the cup is attached by other means and must be filled with electrolyte through a small hole in the middle. Contact between the electrolyte and the electrode causes opposite charges to

line up at the metal–ionic boundary. The simplest model for this arrangement is the "electrical double layer," first proposed in the 1850s by Helmholtz. The double layer contributes to the stability of the interface and represents a capacitance that augments the apparent current flow. At times, especially with new electrodes, the electrical double layer undergoes sudden, poorly understood transitions that produce electrode "pops" and a variety of bizarre oscillations.

The junction between the metal electrode and the ionic electrolyte also develops a half-cell potential, which reflects the electrical force of incipient chemical reactions between them. It represents half of an electrical battery. The half-cell potential can be much smaller than that in a flashlight battery and still be enormously larger than the EEG itself. Ideally this would not be problem, because the half-cell potentials on any pair of matching electrodes would be identical and thus would simply cancel out when those electrodes are connected to an amplifier. However, half-cell potentials can be altered in a number of ways, including drying out of the electrolyte, its dilution by sweat or other fluids, relative differences in temperature, or exposure of different metallic surfaces by wear and tear. These potentials are also affected by movement of the electrode against the electrolyte and the skin, which disrupts the electrical double layer. The effect of movement is reduced by using cup-shaped electrodes, which hold a larger reservoir of moist electrolyte. Chemical interactions at the electrode surface consist of redox reactions, in which an electron is donated or removed from an ion. Since the product of such interactions is commonly a toxic species, such as hydroxyl ions or chlorine gas, care must be taken to avoid injury of the underlying tissues. The safest operating zone for recording and stimulating electrodes is one where they carry only a limited alternating or balanced pulse current, small enough to be transmitted entirely through the double-layer capacitance rather than through redox reactions. Passage of direct current through the double layer will more readily produce chemical changes at the metal surface, including electrical *polarization*, which impedes the free flow of current in one direction more than another, increases impedance at low frequencies, and may be associated with a substantial change in the half-cell potential.

Scalp electrodes typically consist of a conductive contact such as a cup, disc, wire, pad, or sponge. The electrodes are attached to a long, insulated, flexible, and conductive lead wire, which ends in a safety connector pin that plugs into the jackbox of the EEG machine. Commercially available electrodes are made of gold, silver coated with a layer of silver chloride, platinum, tin, or plastic with silver chloride inserts, wires, or epoxy coatings. Silver–silver chloride electrodes are the most stable electrode available for neurophysiological applications; when combined with a chloride electrolyte, they are resistant to polarization and have the best characteristics for low-frequency and direct-current recording.[5] Occasionally the exposure of metallic silver to the light pulse from photic stimulators produces synchronous photoelectric discharges, which may be puzzling to novice interpreters. Cup electrodes are available in 4- to 10-mm diameters and may have a hole on top for periodic refilling with electrolyte conductive gel. Cups may be shallow or deep; shallow cups cause less pressure on the scalp, while deep cups hold more electrolyte. Other conformations such as flat discs or webs are sometimes used when skin breakdown is a concern. Disposable stick-on electrodes almost always use a silver–silver chloride interface.

Several semi-invasive electrode types are available for rapid application. These do not require scalp abrasion, but the scalp should be cleaned with alcohol prior to insertion. Single-use disposable stainless-steel needle electrodes may cause patient discomfort, have inferior recording characteristics (attenuate low-frequency signals), and pose a risk for needle-stick injury if dislodged. They are generally not recommended[2] but may be appropriate for rapid application and brief recording in some comatose patients.[6] Subdermal wire electrodes are single-use disposable Teflon-coated silver wire with a 3- to 5-mm silver chloride tip. They are placed subcutaneously with a small-gauge hypodermic needle introducer, which is then removed. They may reduce skin breakdown in long-term recordings and are imaging compatible.[7] Similar but longer wire electrodes can be used for sphenoidal electrode placement using aseptic technique.

When a patient undergoing long-term EEG monitoring is likely to require repeated neuroimaging studies, electrodes compatible with computed tomography (CT) and/or magnetic resonance imaging (MRI) should be considered. These electrodes can remain in place during imaging, reducing time spent removing and reapplying electrodes, and may also reduce skin breakdown caused by frequent electrode removal and reapplication.[8] For CT compatibility, electrodes must be low density and non-metal to avoid "starburst" artifacts from scattering of x-rays. These are typically carbon or plastic electrodes coated or impregnated with small amounts of silver–silver chloride. For MRI compatibility, specialized electrodes and techniques are needed to avoid thermal or radiofrequency burns as well as artifact. These include nonmagnetic electrodes (plastic with conductive silver epoxy), short electrode wires, specialized connectors, and careful avoidance of electrode wire coils.[9]

Once applied, several methods can be used to hold electrodes in place. For short recordings in cooperative patients, electrode paste alone may be sufficient. For longer recordings, tape, adhesive gauze, or adhesive pastes on a gauze square placed over the electrodes is usually necessary. EC2 paste dries to a hard shell over the electrode and can be removed by rubbing with warm water. Collodion is a pyroxylin glue in ether or alcohol that dries in several minutes with compressed air. Collodion is flammable, should be used only in well-ventilated areas, and must be removed with acetone or specialized non-acetone solutions. Finally, a variety of electrode caps, elastic templates, and electrode nets are available for more rapid electrode application and prolonged recordings.

Intracranial electrodes, including subdural and depth electrodes, are typically made from platinum or stainless steel. The more favorable electrical properties of platinum tend to be offset by its greater cost. With modern amplifiers the high impedance and polarization of stainless steel represent less of a problem than they did in the past. Subdural strip and grid electrodes are arrays of small (2.3–5 mm in diameter) discs embedded in thin flexible Silastic (plastic) strips or grids. Depth electrodes consist of a plastic tube with four to 10 2.3-mm cylindrical electrodes spaced 5 to 10 mm apart. Additional details of intracranial electrodes can be found in Chapter 29.

Most scalp EEG electrodes are reusable and must be adequately disinfected after each use with intermediate- to high-level disinfection or sterilization.[10] Disposable scalp electrodes should be strongly considered for patients with open scalp wounds or infections.[2] Needle electrodes and intracranial electrodes are typically for single use and are disposable.[10]

1.4. Lead Wires, Jackbox, and Cables

The lead wires, jackbox, and cables are basically passive components whose function is transparent. The lead wires from each scalp location are plugged into the corresponding jackbox input according to the International 10-20 System[11] or other labeling system. Excessive separation of the lead wires should be avoided. The capacitance of extremely long cables can attenuate very high frequencies. These effects can be ameliorated by placing the amplifiers inside the jackbox or even directly on the electrodes and by using fiber-optic connections to replace electrical cables. In exceptional circumstances, such as inside the bore of a high-field MRI system, resistors should be placed in series with every electrode lead to prevent induction of excessive current. When troubleshooting, it is worth remembering that if things mysteriously go wrong, the most common culprit is a bad lead wire, cable, or connector.

1.5. Elementary Electronics

Classically the building blocks of the EEG front end are amplifiers, filters, switches, and potentiometers. The top portions of Figures 5.2 through 5.6 sketch the simplified "transfer functions" of an amplifier, a voltage divider, a high filter (which, confusingly, an engineer would call a low *pass* filter), and a low filter (LF) (which an engineer would call a high *pass* filter). The amplifier (Fig. 5.2) makes the desired signal larger. The purpose of the LF is to block frequencies so low that they carry more noise than signal, and thus are better removed. The high filter blocks frequencies so high that they carry more noise than signal. These simple functions remain the basic components of analog recording. For this discussion the amplifier will remain mostly a "black box," which is the way electrical engineers prefer to use modern integrated circuits anyway. The voltage divider and filters are represented in the form of their simplest analog components: resistors and capacitors.

Amplifiers (see Fig. 5.2) have the primary purpose of magnifying the signal from a range measured in microvolts up to several volts, which, in turn, can do something useful such as moving mechanical pens or undergoing analog-to-digital conversion to a stream of numbers. The ratio of the signal coming out of the amplifier to its size going in is called *gain*. For both analog and digital systems, gain should be in the range of 100,000 or more. In neither case is gain easily apparent from the system output. This is because the EEG signal is universally shown in terms of *sensitivity*, the ratio of microvolts to millimeters on a paper or electronic display.

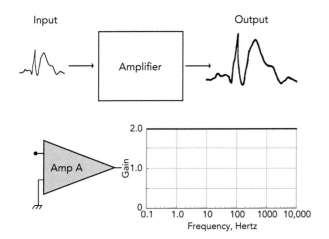

Figure 5.2. Amplifier. The top sketch shows the amplifier as just a "black box" that magnifies the size of the signal. At bottom left is the standard circuit symbol for an amplifier, with two inputs on the left and an output on the right. At bottom right is a graph of the output. It shows a straight line representing a gain of 2.0 at the top of the y-axis, because the gain is the same at all frequencies. This simple "single-ended" amplifier has asymmetric inputs: one terminal is "hot" and the other is usually connected to system ground (bent trident symbol). The inherent asymmetry prevents accurate rejection of noise signals, even when they are equal at both inputs.

Figure 5.3 shows a simple voltage divider or potentiometer in the form of a two-resistor network. A *resistor* is a circuit element with two characteristics: (1) it partially blocks the flow of current according to Ohm's law (voltage = current × resistance), and (2) this relationship is independent of signal frequency. Potentiometers are useful when, for any reason, voltage must be reduced rather than increased (i.e., the gain should be less than 1). The signal enters the two-resistor network as the AC voltage source at the top and passes through the resistors to system ground. According to Ohm's law, if the resistors share the same current and have equal values, the voltage output at the middle of the network must be half the voltage at the top. Since the function of the resistors is the same at all frequencies, the graph shows a steady gain of 0.5 all the way across.

The middle and bottom of Figure 5.4 show an LF composed of one resistor and one capacitor. A *capacitor* consists basically

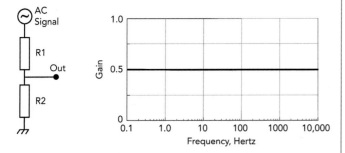

Figure 5.3. Resistance bridge. The circuit symbol for a resistor [R] is a cylinder. The two resistors here are labeled R1 and R2, and both have the same value. Current from the AC input signal at the top flows through the resistors to system ground (bent trident symbol) at the bottom. The output voltage graph is a straight line with a gain of 0.5, because a pure resistive circuit has the same gain at all frequencies.

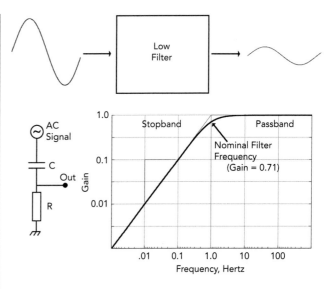

Figure 5.4. Low filter (LF). The low-frequency waveform coming out is smaller than the one going in. The circuit symbol for the capacitor (C) is a pair of parallel lines. Current from the AC input signal at the top flows through the capacitor and the resistor [R] to system ground at the bottom. The log–log output voltage graph shows a horizontal line indicating a gain of one on the right side, where frequencies are above the cutoff. Below the cutoff frequency, gain drops steadily as frequency increases.

of two metal plates that are close together but separated by an insulator. Current cannot cross the insulator directly, but positive and negative charges attract and repel electrostatically on the plates, producing AC current flow in and out of the capacitor. The behavior of the capacitor changes predictably with frequency according to the equation $Z = 1/(2\pi FC)$. Here Z represents the impedance of the capacitor to current flow. *Impedance*, which is a generic term for all obstacles to electric current, goes down as either frequency F or capacitance C goes up.

LF gain changes strikingly with frequency. The right side of the graph in Figure 5.4 shows a value of 1, meaning that the signal passing through is unchanged. On the left side of the graph, the signal comes through at lower and lower amplitude as the frequency drops—essentially, low frequencies are filtered out. In the middle of the graph is a break point where the impedance of the capacitor matches the resistance of the resistor. This break point is the nominal filter frequency, cutoff frequency, or 3-decibel (dB) point. Readers familiar with decibel notation may notice that the output of the resistor–capacitor (RC) filter is reduced by only the square root of 2 when the resistive impedance equals the capacitive impedance, whereas it is attenuated by a factor of 2 in the two-resistor network. Explaining the difference requires the use of imaginary numbers, which will not be attempted here.

The behavior of analog filters far from the cutoff frequency is sketched for an LF in Figure 5.5. It may be understood most easily by remembering the equivalence of the capacitor impedance and the resistor resistance at the cutoff point in Figure 5.4. At lower frequencies the impedance of the capacitor is so high that the AC signal has less and less influence on the output terminal, and the output approaches a short circuit to system ground. At higher frequencies, however, the impedance of the capacitor

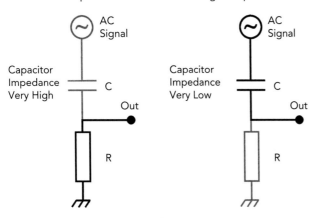

A At Low Frequencies

AC Signal

Capacitor Impedance Very High

C

Out

R

B At High Frequencies

AC Signal

Capacitor Impedance Very Low

C

Out

R

Figure 5.5. Sketch of how changing frequencies produce the LF behavior graphed in Figure 5.4. At low frequencies (A) the capacitor impedance becomes very high, so the capacitor and signal source practically drop out of the circuit. At high frequencies (B) the capacitor impedance becomes very low, and the resistor practically drops out of the circuit.

becomes much lower than the resistance, so that the system ground has less and less influence on the output terminal—which is now practically short-circuited to the signal source. The flat passband with a gain of 1.0 reflects this short circuit.

The high-filter (HF) circuit (Fig. 5.6) and its transfer function are simply the reverse of the LF. The elegant symmetry of the filter curves is seen only in log–log displays, which is one reason for preferring this type of graph over linear representations. Merging the HF and LF curves would form a complete passband of 1.0 to 100 Hz.

1.6. Amplifiers for Neurophysiology

Modern amplifiers are small, low-power, single-chip multi-channel devices with solid-state integrated circuits. In addition

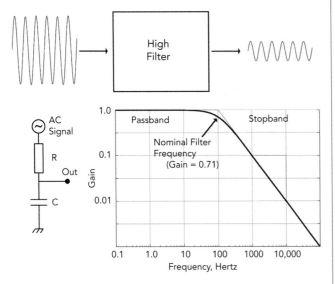

Figure 5.6. High filter (HF). The circuit is simply an inverted LF. The high-frequency waveform coming out is smaller than the one going in. The log–log output voltage graph is a horizontal line for a gain of one on the left side, where frequencies are below the cutoff. Above the cutoff frequency, gain drops steadily as frequency decreases.

to gain, neurophysiologic amplifiers require three other essential properties: (1) linearity and flatness across the entire frequency range of possible signals, (2) high common-mode signal rejection, and (3) high input impedance. Any reasonable commercial device should have excellent linearity. The other requirements are explained below.

Prior to digitization, the microvolt EEG signals must be amplified. This may be done via one or more cascaded amplifiers, with the output of one amplifier becoming the input to the next. Preamplifiers raise the signal into a range where stray device noise (powerline, television, radio) is negligible and so cannot disturb the signal. Commercial analog-to-digital converters (ADCs) have an expected input range, such as ±5 V. To take full advantage of the amplitude resolution of the ADC, input signals must be brought up to this voltage range by amplification (though not over it, since this would "clip" the signal).

Removing the enormous fields caused by AC wiring and by other electrical noise (see Fig. 5.1) is the purpose of the Faraday cages used with the earliest EEGs and of shielded rooms still required for many modern magnetoencephalograms. As an alternative, patients have occasionally been connected directly to earth ground. Faraday cages are unacceptably clumsy and grounding patients is prohibitively dangerous in medical environments, so more practical alternatives have been found. The key to effective recording of small neurophysiological signals is the fact that, large as the noise may be, *most sources of electrical noise are of similar amplitude in nearby regions of the body.* Thus the ECG potentials at adjacent EEG electrodes are almost identical, at least, in most normal individuals. The large alternating current (AC) field produced by capacitive coupling between protoplasm and AC power systems is similar all over the body. Potentials that are similar at different electrode sites are called *common-mode signals.* Common-mode signals are removed by very precisely subtracting the whole combination of potentials at one electrode site from the combination of potentials at another, leaving behind only those potentials that are different at the two electrodes. This is the so-called *differential-mode signal.* This process is illustrated in Figure 5.7. The simpler amplifiers used in radios, stereos, and other familiar electronics, sometimes referred to as single-ended amplifiers, are incapable of the very precise subtraction needed. Thus, all neurophysiologic amplifiers have some version of the symmetrical inputs in Figure 5.7. The latter are called differential, balanced, or instrumentation amplifiers to distinguish them from the single-ended variety. The two "hot" inputs in Figure 5.7 are symmetrical and equally active, despite the universal practice of labeling one of them as "active" and the other as "reference" in many EEG recording montages and in EMG/nerve conduction velocity (NCV) studies. Their electrical behavior is indistinguishable; the only difference is in terminology. The "ground" or neutral connection in Figure 5.7 is normally present during all neurophysiological recording, although modern amplifiers may appear to function passably without it.

In EEG, a single "ground" or system reference is shared by all recording channels and is almost universally placed on the forehead. The ground must be distinguished from the *recording*

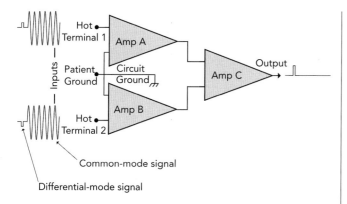

Figure 5.7. Differential amplifier with balanced "hot" inputs and system ground. The vertical symmetry of this more complicated circuit allows precise rejection of large common-mode signals that are equal at both "hot" inputs. The relatively small differential-mode signal—the small square at the far left—is the only signal that passes through the amplifier.

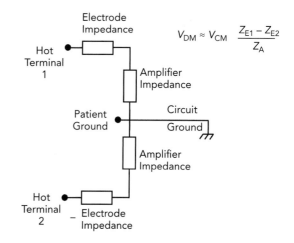

$$V_{DM} \approx V_{CM} \frac{Z_{E1} - Z_{E2}}{Z_A}$$

Figure 5.8. Model of the differential amplifier showing the impedances of the electrodes and the two amplifier inputs. Making some reasonable approximations, the equation at the upper right represents the way in which unequal electrode impedances Z_{E1} and Z_{E2} convert a portion of the common-mode noise voltage V_{CM} into a differential-mode voltage V_{DM}, which passes through the amplifier.

reference, used in constructing referential EEG montages. The "reference" in referential montages is the second hot terminal of the three-terminal differential amplifier, *not* ordinarily the "ground." With modern electronics, it is possible to use a single digital recording reference or one of the regular scalp electrodes, rather than a separate recording reference and ground. Noise rejection will be better using both, provided there is provision for them in the jackbox.

The classic differential amplifier takes the common-mode noise signal as it comes, whatever its size, and attempts to subtract it out. But smaller common-mode voltages would make the task easier. A more recent technique takes the common-mode signals seen by all of the amplifiers on the head, averages and inverts them, and injects the result back into the body through the former "ground" electrode. Since the necessary currents are measured in microamperes, no risk is involved. This method, still referred to anachronistically from its original ECG usage as "driven right leg," can cancel and reduce excess noise in some applications. It also removes the "ground" label and with it the possibility for a misunderstanding that could lead to harm to the patient; see Section 1.9.

The ability of an amplifier to pass differential-mode signals and block common-mode signals is described by its *common-mode rejection ratio* (CMRR) and is usually expressed in decibels (dB). Thus an amplifier that reduces the common-mode signal by a factor of 100,000 (10^5) relative to the differential-mode signal has a CMRR of 100 dB. Modern integrated circuit amplifiers can come off the assembly line with CMRR specifications of 120 dB (1,000,000:1) or higher. However, many extraneous factors can defeat them and allow noise to get through despite the nominal superb performance of the differential amplifier. One mundane consideration is simply that common-mode noise is not absolutely identical at different electrode sites, and the difference grows larger as the electrodes are moved farther apart. Another example is the induction of AC potentials in the electrode lead wires if they become widely separated and form an open loop. A third example is the stimulus artifact from the electrical stimulators used in NCV studies and EPs. At hundreds of volts, the latter can produce an enormous difference at the two hot amplifier inputs. Very

commonly, as discussed below, poor electrode application can defeat the differential amplifier.

An ideal amplifier senses electrical potentials without any current actually passing through the inputs. This perfect device would have infinite input impedance.[12] Although perfect amplifiers do not exist, the highest practical impedance is preferred for neurophysiological recording. Figure 5.8 shows why. Imagine an amplifier in which the two inputs have an impedance of 10,000,000 Ω, connected to two "hot" electrodes with impedances Z_{E1} of 1,000 and Z_{E2} of 10,000 Ω, respectively. Both electrodes are picking up an equal 60-Hz common-mode noise signal of 10 mV. Assuming that the input impedances of the amplifier are still much larger than the electrode impedances, the simplified equation in Figure 5.8 allows calculation of the result. The unequal electrode impedances will produce a differential-mode noise signal at the amplifier inputs of 0.01 × (10,000 − 1,000)/10,000,000 = 0.000009 V or 9 μV. This noise will be faithfully magnified by the differential amplifier to produce visible widening of the EEG tracings—just as seen in Figure 5.9B.

Since it would be impossibly cumbersome to make all the electrode impedances exactly equal, we make sure all electrode impedances are low, in which case the difference between them cannot get too large, and make the amplifier input impedances as high as practical. Recent guidelines specify that the differential input impedance of the amplifier must be at least 100 MΩ[2]. The high input impedance of modern amplifiers allows electrode impedances up to 10,000 ohms[2]. If electrode impedance is higher, such as in dry electrode systems or electrodes not requiring scalp abrasion, then the input impedance of the EEG amplifier must be even higher.

The CMRR should be at least 90 dB (30,000:1) at the highest sensitivity of the amplifier when the common-mode signal is applied between both inputs and neutral.[2] Amplifier input impedances higher than this can be obtained without much difficulty, but their performance is liable to be degraded by the capacitance between conductors in the lead wires and cables.

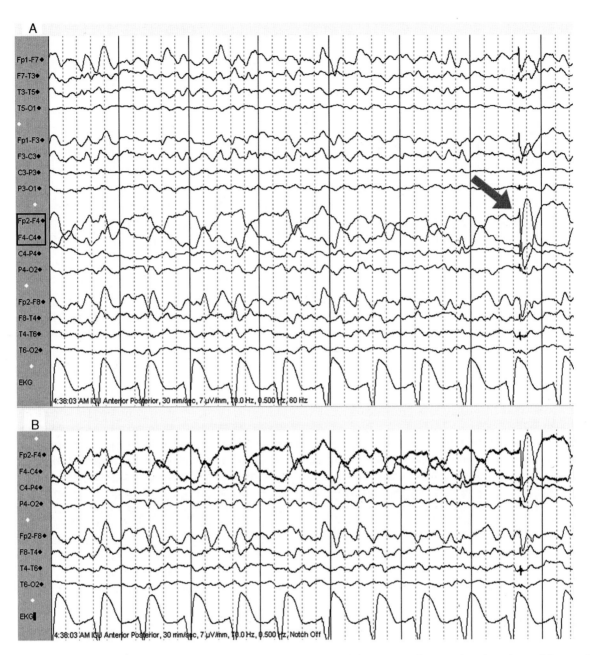

Figure 5.9. Intensive care unit EEG study with ground recording artifacts in the F4 channels, including apparent slowing and a spike at the tip of the arrow (A). 60-Hz noise with the notch filter off (B) is an important clue to the existence of a serious problem. See text for further discussion.

If the only problem caused by unbalanced (i.e., excessively large) electrode impedance were 50- or 60-Hz noise, it would be easy to deal with using notch filters. But Figure 5.9 illustrates a far more insidious consequence. Panel A of this intensive care unit recording appears to show focal delta slowing involving electrode F4, culminating in an apparent spike-wave discharge. Panel B, with the 60-Hz notch filter turned off, indicates that in fact there is a poor, high-impedance connection at F4 and that 60-Hz common-mode AC noise has entered the involved channels. The crucial message of Figure 5.9 is that *the apparent focal abnormalities also represent common-mode noise.* The F4 slowing is actually time-locked to the ECG and reflects an obscure component of the t-wave. The apparent spike is due to the small phasic EMG artifact seen in other leads, picked up by the ground lead on the forehead and magnified across

the now-unbalanced amplifier inputs. Recognizing the presence of ground recording artifacts, and the importance of AC power line artifacts in assisting that recognition, is vital exactly because these artifacts may not be obvious. One corollary of the preceding discussion is noteworthy for being even more counterintuitive. Poor, high-impedance electrode connections do *not* generally reduce the size of the EEG signal. Indeed, as in Figure 5.9, channels 9 to 10, they commonly make it look bigger.

1.7. Analog Filters

After amplification, the EEG signal is filtered to exclude frequencies outside the range of interest. This allows the EEG signal to be reproduced without contamination by extraneous signals. The amplifiers of analog EEG machines contain an HF, an LF, and a notch filter. The 60-Hz or notch filter attenuates electrical artifact produced by AC line frequencies (60 Hz in the United States, 50 Hz in Europe). This filter is sharply tuned to attenuate the amplitude of sine waves at 60 Hz, but it does have some effect on frequencies above and below 60Hz. It should not be used routinely, as it may mask high-impedance electrodes and affect the sharpness of epileptiform discharges. Control over each of the three filter actions is provided by individual channel controls. A master switch allows selection of the same filter settings for all amplifiers. Typical filter settings for analog EEG are LF 1 Hz, HF 70 Hz, and notch filter off. In analog EEG, the filter settings permanently affect how the EEG signal is displayed; once filtered, the original signal cannot be recovered.

Digital EEG instruments also incorporate analog filters prior to ADC. Filters may be controlled by software and can be applied to individual channels or for all channels simultaneously using a master command. In contrast to analog machines, digital EEGs are acquired and stored using broad bandpass analog filter settings, typically low filter (LF) 0.1 to high filter (HF) 100 Hz or higher, so that the original EEG signal is affected as little as possible by the analog filters. For specialized applications, however, the bandpass may include very low frequencies (0.001 Hz) or even direct current (DC), as well as high frequencies up to 3000 to 10,000 Hz.[13] After conversion of the analog signal into a digital signal, software filters are applied during review (see the section on digital filters below). DC recording is not commonly used in clinical EEG but may be used for research purposes. In most commercial systems, therefore, analog filters are inserted to remove the DC (constant) and very-low-frequency components (<0.1 Hz), which make the record harder to read and require a larger magnitude resolution for the ADC. These have the additional benefit of maximally exploiting the ADC resolution, since the average signal is then zero, and the greatest positive and negative excursions can be designed to fit within the digitizer input range to take full advantage of the magnitude resolution of the ADC. Another filter that may appear before digitization is a power line "notch" filter, which is specifically tuned to eliminate the frequencies matching that of the power line: 60 Hz in the United States, 50 Hz in Europe and other countries. More commonly, however, the notch filter is achieved using digital filters. Digital EEG instruments typically use a steep analog HF (6–24 dB), producing more abrupt attenuation of signals above the cutoff frequency. Such analog anti-aliasing filters may be designed according to Butterworth or Chebyshev topologies,[14] and eliminate frequency components above the Nyquist frequency (see the section on ADC below). ACNS guidelines recommend a sampling rate three times the HF setting, or anti-aliasing filter cutoff at 66% of the Nyquist frequency.[15]

1.8. Random Background Noise

In addition to the physiologic and manmade artifacts described above, several sources of random noise can interfere with recording of very small electrical signals. Of these the most irreducible is thermal or "Johnson" noise, which represents

TABLE 5.1. Minimum System Noise Under Representative Recording Conditions

MODALITY	BANDWIDTH (HZ)	ELECTRODE RESISTANCE (Ω)	THERMAL NOISE (MV)
EEG	35	1,000	0.024
EEG	70	10,000	0.13
Brainstem auditory evoked potential	1,000	1,000	0.13
Brainstem auditory evoked potential	3,000	10,000	0.72
EMG[a]	10,000	100,000	4.1

[a] Concentric needle electrode.

Brownian movement of electrons in resistive conductors. The magnitude of thermal noise increases with temperature, circuit resistance, and recording bandwidth. At body temperature, with a high filter of 70 Hz and total electrode resistances of 1,000 Ω, thermal noise is about 0.035 μV and unlikely to make any difference in recording. But in a brainstem auditory EP or concentric needle EMG study, high electrode resistance can raise the minimum noise to the approximate magnitude of the desired signal. Some examples of possible recording conditions are given in Table 5.1. Note that other noise sources in the amplifier may increase actual noise figures several times above those listed. Recent guidelines specify that the noise level of an EEG amplifier should be less than 1 μV peak to peak at any frequency between 0.5 and 100 Hz.[15]

1.9. Electrical Safety and Ground

Patients and operators must not be harmed when using a medical device. The degree of electrical risk depends on the type, amount, and entry point of current and whether the patient is connected to other electrical devices. Requirements for safety are specified in International Electrotechnical Commission (IEC) IEC 60601-1-11:2015: Medical electrical equipment—Part 1-11: General requirements for basic safety and essential performance[16] and IEC 60601-2-26: Particular safety of electroencephalographic equipment. An isolation transformer prevents a direct connection between the ground electrode and power line ground. For electrically sensitive patients, use of an electrically or optically isolated jackbox provides further safety.

In electronic circuits "ground" is a reference point that remains at a virtual zero voltage. Without such a reference point, circuit operation easily becomes unstable. Many years ago the circuit ground, and with it the ground electrode on the head, was actually connected to real earth ground through metal plumbing or other low-resistance conduits. Earth ground is a wonderful zero-reference point representing a near-infinite reservoir of electrons that will never be changed by local circuit operation. It is also an unacceptable connection for human bodies, especially in medical environments.

This is because one of the two wires in AC power lines is almost always connected to earth ground at the power station. Grounding of the power line is necessary because of the astonishingly large voltage gradients that can develop at different elevations in the atmosphere and over long distances across the earth's surface. In modern neurophysiology, this feature of the power system is the most important concept for electrical safety. To operate electrical devices plugged into the AC wall jack, current flows from the "hot" wire of the power line to the "neutral" wire at earth ground. *If patients are connected to earth ground, any stray currents, especially those from the hot power line, will happily flow through the patient on the way there.* A third wire, which represents a second and more direct earth ground connection, is required in hospital equipment as well. This additional ground, commonly referred to as "the" ground, increases safety in some situations but also constitutes a risk if the patient is connected to it. *Modern safety standards require that the recording ground on the patient cannot form a direct connection to the power line ground(s) or to other sources of earth ground, including "the" ground wire.*

Traditionally discussions of electrical safety have focused on "ground loops," which may be formed when the patient is connected to more than one ground electrode through different pieces of medical equipment. Decades ago, currents flowing through the power line ground system could place the different components of that system at somewhat different voltages—in which case the voltages would attempt to equalize through the body of the patient. But the modern requirement that recording ground on the patient must never be connected to earth ground means that ground loops can seldom present a safety risk using commercial systems. However, ground loops may contribute substantially to electrical noise.

1.10. Full Analog Recording

Prior to the digital era, the vast amount of information contained in even a routine EEG could be stored only on paper. The original signal was amplified up to 1,000,000 times, enough to power an electromagnetic coil that moved a long mechanical pen that carried ink onto fanfold paper. Mechanical pens could move only so fast, setting the upper frequency limit around 70 Hz. They could move only so far, causing the waveforms to "square off" at the limits of the pen range (Fig. 5.10). Special circuitry was used to prevent pens from colliding and tangling together. The fanfold paper advanced from one tray to another via a mechanical chart drive with rollers, which could move at speeds of 15, 30, and 60 mm/sec. The paper was prone to ripping or jamming. Ordinarily, EEGs were recorded at 30 mm/sec on pages 300 mm wide. The resulting scale of 10 sec/page has been carried over to digital systems. The obsolete designation of paper speed in mm/sec is so engrained in older technologists and electroencephalographers that even now computer displays are labeled anachronistically in the same manner.

In fully analog EEG systems, constructing different montages requires the use of elaborate mechanical switches. Rows of individual switches are also needed for every channel to set gain, HF and LF, and AC notch filters. The available range of settings is consequently limited, most notably to the legendary

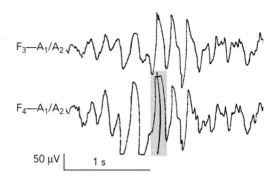

Figure 5.10. *Detail of two channels from an analog paper write-out. During a burst of high-voltage frontal theta, the pen in the second channel reaches the limits of its mechanical range, causing the waveform to "square off" in the vicinity of the shaded area. Within the shaded area is a very narrow spike-like artifact, apparently caused by the collision-avoidance system meant to protect the EEG pens. Note the curvature of the high-voltage waveforms and of the artifact, due to the radial nature of the pen movement.*

HF choices of 15, 35, and 70 Hz. A few generations of "hybrid" systems are likely to still be in use. In hybrid systems switching and the associated notations are done electronically, but the final write-out remains pen and ink.

To produce a comprehensive overview of cerebral activity, several montages must be used during each analog recording. Because the physical settings are not noted automatically on the paper record, analog interpreters rely on the technologist to write by hand every setting and every change in parameters at the time of recording. Traditionally, every combination of parameters is then replicated during a terminal calibration. Producing a true calibration, which faithfully displays the performance of the entire pathway from inputs to write-out, is a virtue of analog recording that not every digital system properly duplicates. On the other hand, the mechanical write-out, the weakest link in the analog recording chain, has been abolished from digital systems. Perhaps the greatest limitation of analog recording is the dependence on the technologist to make notations accurately, to recognize abnormalities "online," and to optimize their display for the reader by making appropriate changes in montages and recording parameters. This feature does, however, have a silver lining: the technologist by necessity is far more engaged in the recording and its eventual interpretation. Other virtues of paper should not be entirely dismissed. The spatial resolution of paper EEG is in the range of 100 dots/cm, as compared to about 30 pixels/cm for conventional computer monitors. To give equivalent resolution, while leaving room for data labeling, digital monitors would have to be about a meter wide and incorporate pixel counts that only now are being approached by high-definition systems. Furthermore, paper can easily be unfolded to provide an overview of several minutes' data while maintaining the same exquisite detail. The inability of computer displays to show more than 10 seconds worth of data without severe compromise in frequency resolution is an underappreciated handicap. It can be overcome only by knowledgeable adjustment of the display on the part of interpreters who understand its limitations for slowly evolving activity. Finally, there is no recorded instance of an entire paper EEG tracing vanishing forever on its way to the server, when somebody accidentally pushed the "delete" button or when the operator forgot to hit "record." The recent history of digital recording media suggests that ancient paper records will still be quite readable when many digital studies can only be viewed in a museum.

1.11. Artifacts Unique to Analog Recording

Artifacts related to the electrode interface, poor common-mode rejection, and ground recording have been discussed previously. Mechanical pen writers are subject to radial displacement due to the pens moving in an arc rather than in a straight line (see Fig. 5.10), at times causing inaccurate alignment of high-voltage, sharp-contoured waveforms. The ink may skip or puddle on the page. The moving paper can transiently slip or jam on the roller, stretching or compressing the EEG waveforms. Figure 5.10 also shows an unusual artifact apparently caused by the collision-avoidance system in a hybrid EEG. What appeared at first glance to be spike wave consists only of high-voltage theta slowing plus a spike-like artifact. When the pen reaches the limit of movement, it paradoxically moves across its full range in the opposite direction and quickly back. We have observed this behavior in several different brands of paper EEG, where it was misinterpreted as evidence of epilepsy.

2. DIGITAL PRINCIPLES

2.1. Introduction and History of Digital EEG

Digital EEG refers to the recording, storage, and review of the EEG on digital equipment (i.e., computers). The process requires conversion of the continuous analog EEG signal, as described above, into discrete numerical values. Over the past 20 years, digital EEG has gradually replaced analog systems and is now the standard for clinical EEG. Digital acquisition and processing of EEG allows many advantages but at the same time imposes limitations that should be understood by the clinician to avoid inaccurate interpretation. The practical advantages of digital EEG over analog EEG are summarized in Table 5.2. In this section, we will outline the principles of digital signal acquisition and processing that are important in the design and proper use of clinical EEG.

Clinical digital EEG represents the convergence of two scientific fields that evolved in parallel for the last 70 years. In 1929, Hans Berger first reported his studies on the EEG.[17] Its utility for clinical diagnosis was quickly established, and EEG has flourished as a tool of neurologists. Practical digital computation began with the development of ENIAC around 1943 to 1944.[18] As early as the 1950s, the potential advantages of computer analysis of EEG were foreseen.[19] However, the routine use of computers for EEG acquisition and analysis required several decades for commercial digital electronics to achieve benchmarks that equal or surpass the capabilities of analog EEG recording apparatus. Reliable, power-efficient computation began with the semiconductor transistor, invented at Bell Labs by William Shockley in 1947. The development of integrated circuits in the 1950s permitted mass production and

TABLE 5.2. Advantages of Digital EEG

Efficiency	Computer-based display generally permits quick review of many studies.
Nondestructive processing	Raw data are stored digitally, allowing reconstructed display with different montages, different filters, and different sensitivity.
Precision	Can precisely measure frequencies and amplitudes for longitudinal or intergroup comparisons
Archiving	Easily make *exact* copies, retain for easy access on disk drive, or save on optical media (CD, DVD)
Transmission/ comparison	Digital copies can be easily and quickly transmitted for second opinion or conferences.
Increased frequency range	Current and near-future digital sampling rates easily exceed the frequency range accessible by traditional analog EEG.
Reliability	Use of stable and reliable electronics, controlled by microprocessors, decreases likelihood of technical artifacts compared to analog equipment requiring manual calibration for each channel.
Portability	Amplifiers can be small enough for patients to carry during ambulatory and long-term studies.
Digital signal processing	Allows extensive online or post-acquisition analysis, such as automated detection of spikes and seizures, topographic maps, and graphical displays of quantitative EEG
Associated software	May include patient information databases, report-writing programs, and integration with hospital electronic medical records

commercialization. A notable computer algorithm for spectral analysis, the Tukey–Cooley version of the discrete fast Fourier transform (FFT), was published in 1965.[20] First-generation digital EEG systems, with limited digitization technology and screen resolution, could not match the display properties of paper-based EEG,[21] but digital electronics gradually achieved fast sampling rates and larger data throughput. Finally, in the late 1990s, digitization rates and computer storage available for reasonably priced digital commercial products were sufficient to match routine analog EEG machines.

Rapid advances in digital technology have greatly improved the efficiency and reliability of clinical EEG recordings and offer new possibilities for research applications. New electrode systems that use dry electrodes or require limited skin preparation may allow recordings to be initiated easily in nontraditional locations, such as the emergency room, ambulances, or even patients' homes.[22-24] EEG data could then be transmitted wirelessly to central locations for access and review by electroencephalographers. Small, light, wireless amplifiers may allow recording of ambulatory patients over weeks to months, analogous to cardiac monitoring with implantable loop recorders. Such data could help to elucidate patterns of seizure occurrence or the development of epileptiform activity or seizures after potentially epileptogenic brain injuries. Current network and remote access solutions allow rapid EEG review from any location, making "real-time" monitoring of brain activity (e.g., for critically ill neurology patients) an achievable goal.[25] The decreased cost and the increased capacity of storage media allow collection and archiving of vast amounts of EEG data. Modern ADCs can sample at thousands of times per second from hundreds of channels, facilitating collection of multi-channel EEG from microelectrodes to reveal pathophysiological mechanisms of epilepsy and other neuronal activity at the single neuron or localized network level. Finally, EEG data can be analyzed by an ever-increasing array of signal analysis techniques, co-registered with imaging procedures for source localization, or used to create statistical databases of normal and abnormal findings. These techniques are described below and in detail in later chapters.

2.2. Overview of Digital EEG Components

Figure 5.11 shows the basic components of the digital EEG signal path from the electrodes to the display. Several components (i.e., jackbox, differential amplifier, display) parallel those encountered in analog EEG machines. The features of these components that differ from analog EEG will be highlighted in the sections below. Components unique to digital EEG systems include (i) the ADC, which samples the analog EEG signal and converts it into discrete digital data; (ii) the computer or microprocessor, which stores and manipulates the digital data for optimal review; (iii) monitors for display of EEG data; and (iv) digital storage devices and networking equipment, which allow archiving of EEG data and transmission to remote sites. Most systems contain video processors and sound cards for simultaneous acquisition and synchronization of video and audio data. The hardware and software capabilities of current digital EEG systems vary significantly between vendors. This review cannot describe all possible digital system specifications but aims to provide a summary of the most important features.

2.3. Electrodes and Electrode Impedance Testing

Along the signal acquisition path, we turn to the first component, the electrodes. These are discussed in detail above. As with analog EEG, a good recording depends on low-impedance electrical contact with the scalp. As discussed above, the resistance, or impedance, between electrode and tissue should be small compared with the input impedance of the amplifier. Most current commercial EEG acquisition machines have functionality for checking electrode impedances. In general,

these are software automated. For each electrode, the impedance is estimated by forming a complete circuit, starting with that electrode, then creating a return path with all the other electrodes joined, so that section of the circuit has an impedance equivalent to all other electrodes in parallel, and thus small. A small (microvolt) voltage (typically oscillatory, on the order of 30 Hz) is applied, and the current is measured. The impedance of that single electrode contact is thereby estimated by the voltage (known) divided by the current (measured). For standard scalp electrodes applied with electrolytic paste, impedances should be less than 10 kΩ[2]. This technique relies, of course, on the assumption that at least some of the electrodes are well connected. If all electrodes have poor contact, spurious results can be obtained. Since impedance varies with frequency, 10- to 30-Hz signals are used to accurately test frequencies typically seen with surface EEG. Impedance results are displayed as numbers on the EEG monitor. The values should be stored with the digital EEG. The ACNS guidelines suggest the individual electrodes should have impedances between 100 and 10,000 ohms[2]. Mismatched impedance between electrodes compromises the ability of EEG amplifiers to reject common-mode signals (potentials that are the same at both amplifier inputs).[26,27] Channels with mismatched electrode impedances are therefore more susceptible to environmental artifacts, particularly 60-Hz artifact.[28]

Routine digital EEG has no requirements for specialized electrodes. Current protocols for *experimental* digital EEG acquisition at high sampling rate with intracranial implantation may derive benefit from specialized microelectrodes. These have a smaller contact area and may be able to detect spatially localized multiunit or even single-unit firing trains. High-density microelectrode arrays allow recording of high-frequency oscillations and high-resolution cortical mapping for research purposes but are uncommonly used in clinical intracranial recordings. Microelectrodes are available either as standalone arrays[29,30] or hybrid electrodes that combine standard macroelectrodes with microelectrode arrays.[31] These microelectrodes have high impedances, which can result in high levels of noise and other artifacts when used with standard clinical EEG amplifiers.[32]

2.4. Electrode Jackbox

The standard number of inputs for clinical digital EEG is 32, plus ground electrode. This allows full 10-20 recording plus recording of some additional electrodes, such as inferior temporal chain electrodes of the 10-10 system and polygraphy

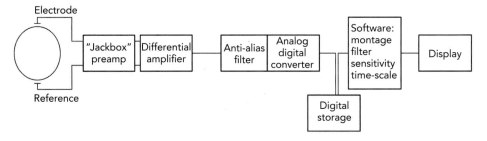

Figure 5.11. The schematic of a digital EEG machine shows components of the signal path from the electrode to the display.

channels.[11] Jackboxes for digital EEG typically have a greater number of electrode inputs; jackboxes accepting 64, 128, or even 256 inputs are common for epilepsy monitoring and intracranial EEG recordings. Additional inputs can accommodate additional EEG electrodes, such as 10-10 modified International System placements,[11] as well as electro-oculogram (EOG), EMG, or other polygraphic inputs.[2] Jackbox inputs are labeled with the location of the electrode on the head according to the International 10-20 System[11] or numbered. In addition, there are inputs for ground and for a *machine reference*, sometimes called *recording reference*, electrode, which is usually placed in a location not susceptible to large artifacts, such as the midline central-parietal region.

In contrast to analog systems using electrode selectors, most digital amplifiers are "hard-wired," with the signal from each jackbox position going to Input 1 of a specific amplifier. Input 2 for all amplifiers is the machine reference electrode. Some digital systems have electronically switched jackboxes to allow amplifier input channels to be switched among different electrodes. Because all EEG activity is acquired in relation to the machine reference electrode, the data in all channels may be distorted if this reference electrode is of high impedance. With a high-impedance reference, external noise may overwhelm the EEG signal, producing a very low-amplitude recording with little signal. This is different from effects of high impedance in any other electrode, which can *increase* the apparent EEG amplitude through ground reference recording, in addition to showing the noise. To prevent this problem, the EEG should be reviewed during the recording in a machine reference montage to check for excessive noise in the reference electrode.

Digital EEG jackboxes may be housed in the same enclosure as other digital components, such as preamplifiers (see Section 2.5 on amplifiers). The short distance between the scalp electrode and this first amplification step reduces electrical interference and artifact in the EEG signal. ADCs may also be present in the jackbox itself, as in systems for ambulatory recording.[33] The jackbox also contains or is connected to an impedance meter to allow measurement of electrode impedance (see Section 2.3 on electrodes) without unplugging the electrode wires from the electrode input panel.

2.5. Amplifiers

For EEG, one of the most important aspects of the amplification stage is the use of *differential* amplifiers. Both analog and digital EEG employ differential amplifiers. Differential amplifiers have three input connections: (i) inverting input; (ii) noninverting input; and (iii) ground, typically placed on the forehead, and a single output. The output is the difference between the two inputs multiplied by some constant, the amplification factor, or *gain*. Gain for clinical EEG machines is usually in the range of 2000 to 20,000 but can be up to 1,000,000. The gain equals output voltage divided by input voltage. Gain is typically expressed as a logarithmic ratio in dB, with gain (dB) = $20(\log(V_{out}/V_{in}))$. For instance, with inputs of 106 μV (noninverting) and 104 μV (inverting), and amplification factor (gain) of 20, the output will be 40 μV. In our figures, we show the electrical symbol for an *op-amp*, short for operational amplifier. Op-amps do amplify the difference between their inputs, but this is a simplification. Actual hardware differential amplifiers are more complex circuits, using a combination of op-amps with other circuit elements, specifically designed and tuned to amplify the difference in voltage even when both voltages may be quite large in absolute value. See more about *common-mode rejection* below.

In analog EEG, the montage is fixed at acquisition time by the fact that the electrodes are mechanically connected to a set of differential amplifiers for that montage. Figure 5.12 shows a simple diagram of the arrangement of differential amplifiers for analog EEG for a longitudinal bipolar montage. Digital EEG also employs differential amplifiers, but with a significant distinction. Instead of determining the difference between electrode inputs at acquisition time, each electrode is acquired relative to one fixed common electrode, the *machine reference*. These individual electrode channels are then digitized and stored. Later review with tracings displayed in different montages can be performed by digitally reconstructing the montages. Figure 5.13 shows a simple diagram highlighting this difference from analog EEG. Note that the vertical dashed line separates the fixed, unalterable acquired data on the left from computations on the right showing the data in one of many

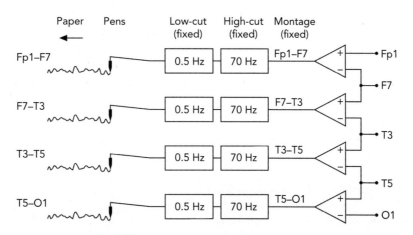

Figure 5.12. Schematic of amplifier inputs for analog EEG for a longitudinal bipolar montage. One additional electrode input—the ground—is omitted for simplicity.

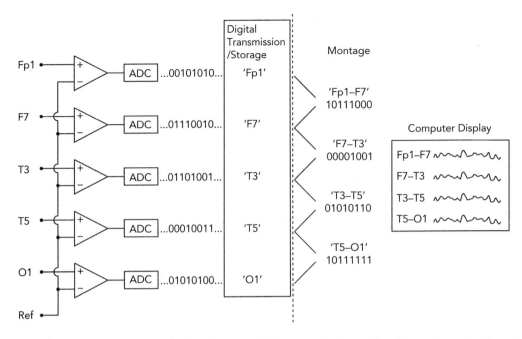

Figure 5.13. Differential amplifiers for digital EEG, with each electrode input amplified compared to the machine reference. Computer software then converts this referential montage to a longitudinal bipolar montage. See text for details. The ground electrode is omitted for simplicity.

possible different montages, which can be easily reconstructed. Also note that the input to the inverting contact for each differential amplifier is the machine reference for *all* the electrode channels recorded.

There are several other aspects of amplifiers that could impact the data acquisition. The CMRR is a measure of how well the differential amplifier reflects the difference between the inputs, especially when both inputs are large in magnitude. Real differential amplifiers can be best modeled as generating an output voltage V_0 as

$$V_0 = A_D\left(V_+ - V_-\right) + \frac{1}{2}A_s\left(V_+ - V_-\right)$$

The coefficient A_d is the differential gain and A_s is called the common-mode gain. The common-mode rejection ratio is

$$CMRR = 20\log_{10}\left(\frac{A_d}{|A_s|}\right)$$

So, a CMRR of 90 dB, as recommended by the ACNS,[2] indicates that the amplifier will begin to lose accuracy when the absolute magnitude is 30,000 times the difference in magnitudes. Most of the common-mode signal is 60-Hz noise, and the magnitude of that noise is determined more by the electrode impedances than circuit specifications.

2.6. Analog Filters

Prior to digitization, analog electrical filtering is applied. The fundamentals of analog filter design are discussed above. In contrast to analog machines, digital EEGs are acquired using broad bandpass filter settings, typically 0.1 to 70 or 100 Hz. However, for specialized applications, the bandpass may include very low frequencies (0.001 Hz) or even DC, as well as high frequencies up to 3,000 to 10,000 Hz.[13]

The most important filter in this stage is the anti-aliasing filter as described below. This requires a low-pass filter (i.e., passes low-frequency signals but attenuates high-frequency ones). The simplest low-pass analog filter is a resistor (R) and capacitor (C) in series, with the voltage across the capacitor transmitted to the next stage, as diagrammed in Figure 5.14. This first-order low-pass filter will attenuate high frequencies and has a cutoff frequency (in Hz) of $1/(2\pi RC)$. Commercial anti-alias filters may be this simple but are often engineered with more components to achieve a faster roll-off in the transition band, thus a "sharp" cutoff. Such analog filters may be designed according to Butterworth or Chebyshev topologies.[14]

Other filters can be inserted prior to digitization. DC is not commonly used in clinical EEG but may be used for research purposes. In most commercial systems, filters are inserted to remove the DC (constant) and very low-frequency components (<0.5 Hz), which make the record harder to read and require a larger-magnitude resolution for the ADC. These have the additional benefit of maximally exploiting the ADC resolution, since the average signal is then zero, and the greatest positive and negative excursions can be designed to fit within the digitizer

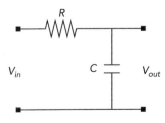

Figure 5.14. A low-pass analog filter is a resistor (R) and capacitor (C) in series, with the voltage across the capacitor transmitted to the next stage.

input range to take full advantage of the magnitude resolution of the ADC. Another filter that may appear before digitization is a power line "notch" filter, which is specifically tuned to eliminate the frequencies matching that of the power line: 60 Hz in the United States, 50 Hz in Europe and other countries.

2.7. Analog-to-Digital Conversion

Once amplified and analog bandpass-filtered, the analog EEG signal is converted to a digital representation by the ADC or digitizer. The act of digitization assigns discrete values to an EEG signal in two independent axes: time and magnitude. The stage of conversion of the analog signal to digital representation is the most crucial step in the digital acquisition process. Design of an acquisition system requires that the components be matched and appropriate as a whole, so that the final data are not hindered by poor design of any one element in the path. Because parameters of the digitization impact acquisition components both earlier and later in the signal path, thorough understanding of digitizer capabilities and limitations is crucial. The act of digitization collapses an EEG signal in two independent axes: time and magnitude.

2.7.1. TIME

Typically, a time-varying signal is digitized at fixed (constant) discrete intervals. The time intervals are described by sampling rates. Typical sampling rates are on the order of several hundred to several thousand samples per second (Hz). For 200 Hz, this implies that samples are taken every 5 msec. The time interval between two successive samples, or *dwell time*, is the inverse of the sampling rate. Current commercially available systems can sample 256 to 512 channels at rates between 2,000 and 16,000 Hz. Specialized research equipment may be able to sample 256 channels or more at up to 30 kHz. Very high sampling rates are necessary to record high-frequency oscillations and unit potentials.

The choice of sampling rate impacts how well the obtained data reflect the analog source, with faster sampling roughly giving more fine detail. A reasonable question is: How fast is fast enough? A well-known theorem from signal processing literature provides a quantitative answer to this question. The Nyquist theorem states that the highest frequency distinguishable is one-half the sampling frequency. The downside of more rapid sampling is the creation of larger EEG files. Armed with the Nyquist theorem, one knows the limitations of what signal components in the source can be captured, but the question is naturally raised as to the consequence of signals that are above this Nyquist limit. If these were simply eliminated, the issue would be moot, but sadly high-frequency components above the Nyquist can actually create nefarious artifacts in the digitized output. Figure 5.15A shows an example of a pure sinusoid at 11 Hz (the dashed curve) being sampled at 16 samples per second (Nyquist frequency of 8 Hz). The sampled data points can be seen to equivalently match a sinusoid at 5 Hz (solid curve). Indeed, in practice, when displayed on a screen (connected by straight lines), these points would more closely match the 5-Hz sinusoid than the original 11-Hz sinusoid. This phenomenon is known as "aliasing." Figure 5.15B shows the pattern by which frequencies above the Nyquist are "folded back" into the range

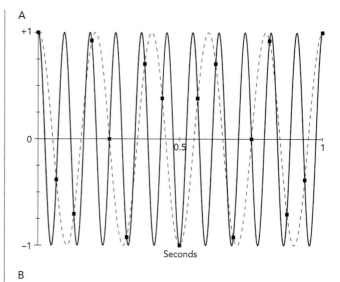

A

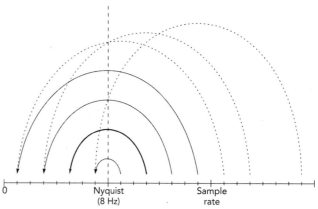

B

Figure 5.15. Aliasing. A: A pure sinusoid at 11 Hz (solid curve) sampled at 16 samples per second (Nyquist frequency is then 8 Hz). The sampled data points can be seen to equivalently match a sinusoid at 5 Hz (dashed curve). When displayed on a screen (connected by straight lines), these points would more closely match the 5-Hz sinusoid than the original 11-Hz sinusoid. B: Frequencies above the Nyquist are "folded back" across the Nyquist, as if the paper were folded with the crease at the Nyquist frequency—best exemplified by the solid curves of the frequencies between the Nyquist and the sampling rate. The heavily darkened curve represents the aliasing of 11 to 5 Hz from A.

between 0 and the Nyquist frequency, with the example of 11 Hz being folded back to 5 Hz at sampling rate of 16 samples per second emphasized with the bold arc.

Figure 5.16 shows the deleterious effect of noise above the Nyquist frequency. Fortunately, methods to eliminate this artifact are quite simple. Electrical filters—specially designed circuits composed of elements such as resistors and capacitors—can be used to eliminate undesired frequencies in the analog signal prior to digitization. In particular, ADC systems incorporate an analog low-pass filter prior to digitization, with this filter designed to pass frequencies below the Nyquist frequency and eliminate those above it. Such a low-pass filter in this context is termed an "anti-aliasing" filter.

The anti-alias filter and ADC in Figure 5.11 are deliberately joined. The analog hardware anti-alias filter must obviously precede the ADC. The anti-alias filter cutoff must be appropriate for the sampling rate of the joined ADC. The filter must adequately attenuate frequencies above the Nyquist, or else

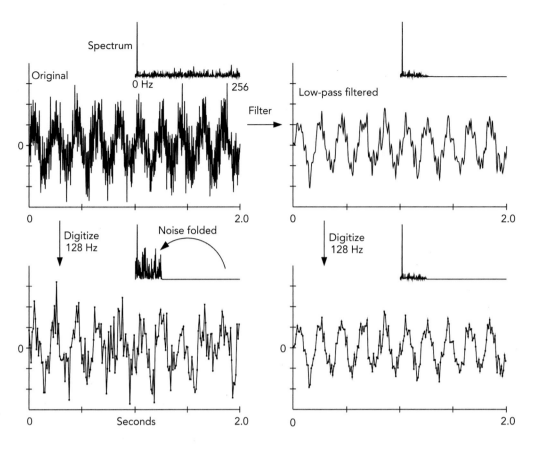

Figure 5.16. *Deleterious effect of noise above the Nyquist frequency. Top-left panel shows 2 seconds of "original" (simulated) data composed of a signal at 5 Hz, plus noise with significant components up to 256 Hz. The inset (just above and to right) shows the power spectrum of this data, showing the white noise and the large signal at 5 Hz. Bottom left panel shows what would be the result of naïve direct digitization at 128 samples per second, rendering the signal at 5 Hz nearly unrecognizable within the abundant noise. The signal-to-noise ratio (SNR) has actually been worsened because the noise above the Nyquist limit (64 Hz = half of 128 samples per second) has been folded back, adding to the noise in the frequencies below the Nyquist, as illustrated in its power spectrum. The right-side panels show how anti-aliasing filtering prior to digitization can prevent this problem. Top-right panel shows the tracing after a low-pass filter (modeled as Butterworth third order) with cutoff at 50 Hz has been applied. Bottom-right panel shows the result of digitization (again at 128 samples per second) of this filtered tracing. Frequencies above the Nyquist (64 Hz) have been attenuated by the low-pass filter and are therefore not folded back, so digitization in this case yields a faithful reproduction of the signal.*

high-frequency noise will be aliased into the digitized signal. If the cutoff is too low, then signals with frequencies above this cutoff and below the Nyquist will be unnecessarily attenuated and lost, and expense will have been wasted in using an ADC with higher sampling rate than necessary.

Another point regarding the time axis regards the "frequency resolution," a factor important for quantitative analysis of EEG. The sampling rate does not impact whether one can distinguish a signal as being one of two closely spaced frequencies, for example 8.3 Hz versus 8.4 Hz. Frequency resolution is determined by the *duration* of the acquired signal. In general, the duration required is approximately the inverse of the difference in frequency. This reflects the fact that two sinusoids with some difference in frequency will become out of phase with each other over that time frame. For instance, to reliably distinguish a 0.1-Hz difference in frequency requires a total acquired signal on the order of 1/(0.1 Hz) = 10 seconds. This applies irrespective of the absolute frequency—that is, distinguishing 8.3 from 8.4 Hz and distinguishing 124.7 from 124.8 Hz both require approximately 10 seconds of acquisition.

2.7.2. Magnitude or Amplitude

Digitization occurs along the magnitude axis as well. In this respect, the effect of digitization is typically discussed in terms of digitization "depth." Digitizers presume that each successive point is at a known time interval, so this time interval does not need to be stored. Instead, only the value or magnitude at each successive point is stored. Digital equipment is optimized when storing each successive magnitude in a predefined length. To be concrete, the output is a stream of 0's and 1's. The number of binary digits (bits) set aside for each measurement is the same. This storage length can differ between equipment manufacturers. Early digitizers used 8, 10, or 12 bits to store each measurement; digitizers now routinely use 16 to 24 bits. The number of bits determines explicitly the number of distinguishable magnitudes of the measurements. For example, 8 bits per measurement can store up to $2^8 = 256$ different values (0 to 255 unsigned, or -127 to $+127$ signed two's complement system). Figure 5.17 illustrates the practical effect of 4-, 6-, and 8-bit digitization depth.

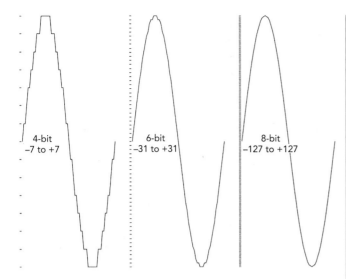

Figure 5.17. *The practical effect of 4-, 6-, and 8-bit digitization depth. Note that for the 6-bit depth, the digital step is most apparent at the peak and trough, where for each time step the voltage change is small, but these changes are smaller than the smallest discrete step and so cannot be represented.*

The three parameters, maximum value (or dynamic range), minimum distinguishable difference, and digitization depth, are interconnected and not independent; choosing any two specifies the third. With a 12-bit linear digitizer (2^{12} = 4,096 different levels), in order to be able to represent magnitudes up to ±1 mV, then the "resolution"—the smallest detectable difference in magnitude—will be (2,000 μV/4,096) ~0.5 μV. Values between this difference are rounded to the nearest allowable magnitude value. With a 16-bit ADC and a dynamic range of ±10 mV, resolutions would be 20,000 μV/(2^{16} − 1) = ~0.31 μV. The more bits available, the more accurate each sample. For very low-amplitude signals (e.g., electrocerebral inactivity recordings), ADC resolution less than 0.5 μV is necessary.[4,34]

2.7.3. ADC Effects on File Size
Sampling rate, digitization depth, and number of channels all have an impact on acquired file sizes. For example, for 32 channels with digitization of 16 bits (2 bytes) per sample and a sampling rate of 512 samples per second, 1 hour of EEG (3,600 seconds) will generate (32 × 2 × 512 × 3,600) = 117,964,800 bytes = 115,200 kB = 112.5 MB. A full day of EEG with these settings would generate ~2.7 GB. The downside of improved amplifiers and ADCs is the creation of larger EEG files. Increasing the sampling rate to 1,000 Hz would increase the file sizes by 2, generating ~5.14 GB per day, while acquiring 256 channels at 1,000 Hz would yield more than 41 GB per day. Large files sizes are less problematic today, given the low cost and large size of local and network storage resources, but can still test the limits of file storage and transfer. Lossless and near-lossless compression techniques can also reduce file sizes without distortion of the original signal.

2.7.4. ADC Guidelines
A recent ACNS guideline updates the minimum requirements of digital EEG acquisition, specifically touching on digitization.[15] The guideline suggests that 16-bit depth (including sign bit) is the minimum. The minimum amplitude resolution is recommended to be 0.5 μV. These minimum standards yield a dynamic range of ±1.638 mV, sufficient for display of EEG, electrocorticography, and artifacts. The minimum recommended sampling rate is 256 samples per second,[15] but higher sampling rates are preferred to avoid aliasing on high-resolution computer monitors. The minimum rate "is selected to be more than three times the high-frequency filter setting, assuming a typical 70 Hz HFF setting," which is equivalent to saying that for a given sampling rate, the anti-aliasing filter cutoff should be at two-thirds the Nyquist frequency. Since the ADC rate and anti-aliasing filter are hardware determined, these are under the control of the manufacturer but should be investigated and documented clearly when purchasing decisions are considered. Some systems allow the sampling rate, and consequently the anti-aliasing filter cutoff, to be selected via software controls.

2.7.5. ADC Hardware
Some of the basic principles of ADC hardware are worth mentioning. First, no ADC operates instantaneously. The input voltage is typically measured over some finite time (obviously less than the time between samples). The time over which the signal is actually measured is called the *conversion time*. Sampling skew, or loss of time axis integrity, can occur if the ADC samples each channel sequentially, since it takes some time to sample one channel and convert the amplitude to a numerical value before it moves on to the next channel's sample. Sampling skew is most problematic with high-frequency activity and may cause misalignment of high-frequency events such as spikes between the first and the last channels sampled. Most ADCs use an input circuit called a sample-and-hold, employing a capacitor to "hold" the voltage during this conversion time. Then, comparator circuits are applied to bracket the "held" voltage to the desired precision. A second method is to have a series of ADCs, one for each channel, all triggered by a single computer command. Some digital instruments have combinations of these two methods, with ADCs for blocks of four to eight channels using the "sample-and-hold" method. Since large ADCs with high throughput are expensive, multiple ADCs may be more cost-efficient.

Various ADC hardware structures are available. These structures include direct conversion or flash, successive approximation, ramp-compare, delta-encoded, pipeline, and sigma–delta. Some of these structures actually involve complex combinations of simpler ADC designs. For example, the sigma–delta converter first oversamples at a very high rate, digitally filters and may use a Flash ADC, then finally downsamples to the desired sampling rate.

The most obvious tradeoff of ADCs is between sampling rate and number of channels. The product (rate × channels) is basically a fixed constant, with this constant being proportional to the expense of the digitizer. With current hardware digitizers, it is often possible to sample very fast (2 kHz) on a handful (~16) of channels, or at slow rates (256 Hz) on several dozen channels (64–256). Most commercial EEG machines aim for a compromise with the ability to monitor

32 to 64 channels at sampling rates of 256 to 1,024 Hz, and these rates can be programmed by the user according to the task at hand.

2.8. Calibration

Digital calibration differs significantly from analog calibration. The ADC must be calibrated so that it "knows" how large to represent each voltage point. A 50- or 100-μV signal (usually a 30-Hz sine wave) is passed through each amplifier. The ADC takes the amplifier outputs and assigns the appropriate value in microvolts to the peak of each channel. All other amplitude values are determined based on this initial calibration. Calibration information is saved with each EEG record. The digital EEG software should contain a voltage cursor that allows the user to determine the voltage of individual waveforms. This cursor is then applied to the known signal from the signal generator to determine whether the system is properly calibrated.

Square-wave calibration pulses can sometimes be generated using a digital EEG machine to verify the amplifier and analog filter functioning. The calibration signal should be time-locked to the ADC clock.[35] The square-wave calibration should be examined in the machine reference montage with all digital filters off. Since the jackbox of digital EEG machines is hardwired for each electrode position, biological calibration may not be possible with digital EEG machines.

2.9. Ambulatory and Long-Term EEG Portable Recorders

Systems for acquisition of long-term EEG (hours to days) can have a variety of configurations. Early systems recorded four channels of EEG on a portable cassette recorder for 24 hours,[36] but systems are now fully digital. Portable ambulatory recorders are designed for home EEG recording. They are small lightweight enclosures, approximately 6 × 4 × 2 inches and less than 2 lbs., containing an electrode input panel (EEG and polygraphic channels), amplifiers, ADC, batteries, and data storage.[37,38] The enclosure is placed in a pouch with a shoulder harness or belt so patients are truly ambulatory and can maintain their regular activities of daily living. An event button allows patients to mark segments of the EEG when clinical events of interest occur. The number of hours of EEG that can be stored depends on the number of channels recorded, memory storage type and capacity, and recorder battery life. Some systems record continuous EEG, while others utilize computer-assisted spike and seizure detection and sampling algorithms to record epochs of EEG data of greatest interest. Modern systems can store up to 96 hours of continuous 16- to 32-channel EEG data, so limited recording is typically no longer performed. Removable storage (compact flash memory cards) allow longer recordings to be performed. Battery life is the main limitation to duration of recording, but many systems now feature easily removable batteries that can be changed by the patient. When recording is complete, data are downloaded to a computer via a universal serial bus (USB) or proprietary connection for review. Most amplifiers can also be used with a laptop or desktop computer and acquisition software in "tethered" or host connection mode. Many systems now include synchronous digital video recording via a camera with a wide-angle lens, further increasing the utility of home EEG recording by capturing behavioral manifestations as well as EEG.[39,40]

In systems for long-term monitoring of epilepsy, amplifiers/ADCs can be connected directly to a computer via USB, Ethernet, or other cable, or have TCP/IP connectivity that allows the amplifier to be plugged into a network jack near the patient and to stream data to an acquisition machine anywhere on the network. Advanced long-term monitoring recorders may have Bluetooth connectivity and can wirelessly stream data to nearby storage[41] and often have battery backup and local storage to allow patients increased mobility while ensuring uninterrupted data acquisition.

2.10. Video and Audio Acquisition

Simultaneous video and audio recording is most commonly done in long-term monitoring for epilepsy and in the intensive care unit, to allow correlation of EEG features with behavioral events.[25,42,43] Most digital EEG systems today utilize digital cameras and store EEG and video data to computer hard drives, although some older systems with analog video and audio recorded to videotape are still in operation.[44] Early proprietary video capture systems have been replaced by standard digital video recording equipment, markedly decreasing the cost and increasing the efficiency of video acquisition and review. Digital video recorded directly to hard drives can be accessed randomly, allowing the reviewer to quickly jump to any portion of the record rather than having to fast-forward or rewind a series of videotapes. Video equipment can be customized to optimize recording for specific types of monitoring. Camera options include analog versus digital, color versus black-and-white, low light versus infrared, fixed versus pan-tilt, and wide-angle versus remote zoom. Many systems have controls for remote pan-tilt and zoom functions. While early systems required custom cabling for video, modern systems can transmit and control digital video over standard TCP/IP cables.

Video and audio are usually encoded into AVI, MPEG, MPEG2, or MPEG4 formats. These are standard formats for digital video, differing in resolution and compression algorithms. All data should include time markers so that EEG, video, and audio can be synchronized precisely.[45,46] Video should be synchronized to EEG in the millisecond range, or frame by frame. Video files contain large amounts of data; 24 hours of video recording can be 8 to 30 GB, depending on resolution (usually 320 × 240 pixels or 640 × 480 pixels), color depth, frame rate, and data compression algorithm. EEG machines for video-EEG recording should be able to store at least 24 hours of continuous video and EEG data. Currently available systems, with hard drive capacities of 200 GB or more, may allow continuous recording for more than a week. Because of the size of video files, the entire video is not usually archived; rather, video segments of interest (seizures and behavioral events) are clipped and archived.

2.11. Computer and Software

The EEG acquisition and digitization devices described above are connected to a central computer, which can be either a standard desktop personal computer or a laptop computer. The computer contains a central processing unit (CPU) that performs calculations, random access memory (RAM) that holds data temporarily while they are being manipulated, and a hard disk drive for permanent data storage, as well as a monitor, keyboard, mouse, network connectivity devices, and various connections for removable media such as CDs, DVDs, and external hard drives. Most EEG vendors currently use standard commercially available computers, running on commonly used software platforms such as Microsoft Windows, Macintosh, or Linux operating systems.

Most of the variability in modern digital EEG systems comes from proprietary software applications that allow customization of EEG acquisition as well as manipulation and display of the EEG and video data through a graphical user interface (GUI). Features of review software are discussed in more detail below. In addition, vendor-provided software applications may include databases for patient and study information, interfaces to hospital patient information systems, report-generation software, security packages, and a variety of post-acquisition signal processing software. Because the central machine is a standard computer, review stations can also run other software that may enhance laboratory productivity such as word processors, voice recognition software, and hospital electronic medical record systems.

2.12. Display

Digital EEG can be displayed in a variety of methods. The recorded signal can be output to an oscilloscope, printed out on paper, reconverted to analog signal via digital-to-analog conversion and written by traditional pen-writing systems, or viewed on a computer monitor. The most practical and versatile method is display on a computer monitor. Monitors must have adequate temporal and spatial resolution for the EEG data being displayed.

Visual display on screen is also a digital process. Whether displayed on older CRT or modern digital LCD screens, images are drawn as discrete pixels. In fact, current display pixel resolution may be the limiting factor impeding precise representation of the signal characteristics to the electroencephalographer.[47] The EEG signal consists of points discretized in time and voltage but obviously not necessarily in adjacent pixels, so intermediate pixels are filled to construct lines connecting the points. The top diagram in Figure 5.18 is an idealized example of a set of such points and where they might lie on a pixel display. Modern software draws lines between these points using line-drawing routines based on Bresenham's algorithm.[48]

Screen resolution is described in terms of the number of horizontal and vertical points or pixels. In 2016, typical mid-range display monitors for EEG have 1,600 pixels across with 1,200 pixels vertically. We examine horizontal resolution first. Display of 10 seconds of EEG on a screen implies each second being allotted 160 pixels, if no space is taken for channel labels

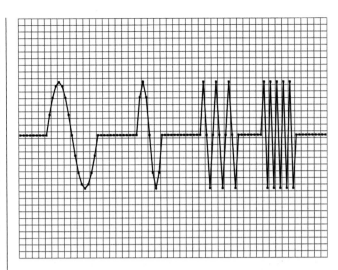

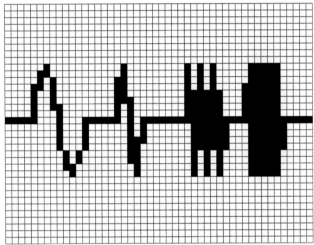

Figure 5.18. Effects of horizontal pixel resolution on EEG display. Supposing two time steps per pixel-width (e.g., 200-Hz digital sampling rate and 1000 pixel-widths for 10 seconds = 100 pixel-widths per second). Top panel shows idealized signals at 12.5, 25, 50, and 100 Hz (the digitization Nyquist frequency). Bottom panel shows how these frequencies would be actually drawn with pixels. As can be seen, 50 Hz is the highest frequency that can be visualized with these pixel settings (and not terribly well), with frequencies above 50 Hz appearing "smudged." In analogy with the digitization Nyquist frequency, the highest frequency represented by pixels can be said to be half the number of pixels per second (100 pixel-widths per second can represent signals up to 50 Hz).

or other screen elements. At a sampling rate of 256 samples per second, then horizontally there would be 1.6 EEG points per pixel. Suppose there were (for simplicity) 100 pixels per second, and an EEG channel sampled at 200 Hz, with signals up to 100 Hz (which is at the Nyquist frequency, and representable in the digitized data stream). Figure 5.18 shows a set of points with sine waves up to 100 Hz. Unfortunately, by the Bresenham line-drawing algorithm, these signals will not be able to be traced out, instead resulting in blurred uninterpretable lines, as shown at the bottom of Figure 5.18. In general, the maximum frequency that can be faithfully represented on a pixel display is one-half the number of pixels per second. In this case, that would be (100/2) = 50 Hz.

Display of EEG on monitors with inadequate resolution (i.e., lower than the sampling rate) can result in aliasing, the introduction of spurious waveforms caused by "undersampling" the EEG signal.[49] This is analogous to violating the Nyquist theorem when choosing a sampling rate. Aliasing artifacts typically occur when viewing fast-frequency activity, such as 60-Hz artifact or EMG activity, and can occur even when following recommended guidelines for video resolution. When such video aliasing artifacts are suspected, decreasing the number of seconds displayed per page (e.g., from 10 to 5 seconds) or increasing screen resolution will allow display of all samples in each second and resolve the artifact, as demonstrated in Figure 5.19.

We now turn to the vertical display resolution. The required vertical resolution depends on the number of channels displayed. The dimension of pixels on current LCD screens is on the order of 0.25 mm. If we try to replicate the vertical scale of analog EEG, then 7 µV/mm translates into 7 µV over 4 pixels. Thus, each pixel spans about 2 µV in vertical height. With current digitizers (12- or 16-bit), the amplitude resolution is typically better than 0.5 µV, perhaps as low as 0.03 µV. Figure 5.20 shows an idealized example with a low-amplitude signal that ranges from +1 µV to −1 µV. This variation is lost with pixels of 0.25 mm at a sensitivity of 7 µV/mm, resulting in a flat line. Conversely, to achieve 0.5 µV per pixel requires setting the sensitivity to 2 µV/mm. With our 1.024 pixels in the vertical dimension, and viewing 20 channels, we see that we have approximately 50 pixels per channel. Using our standard 7 µV/mm, EEG signals of ±50 µV can be displayed. Signals larger than ±50 µV will begin to spill over into adjacent channel display, causing overlap of tracings in adjacent channels and making the EEG more difficult to interpret.

Several methods can be used to improve signal display. Screen size for review stations should measure 20 inches diagonally or more. Dot pitch (the diagonal distance between display pixels) should be as small as possible. Display is best when the monitor's "native" screen resolution is used. Large (20 or 24 inches) monitors with high resolution (1,600 × 1,200 pixels, or widescreen 1,920 × 1,200 pixels) are currently reasonably priced, and higher-resolution larger monitors are available for those with larger budgets (Table 5.3). ACNS guidelines recommend standard horizontal scaling of 25 to 35 mm per second of EEG, with a minimum resolution of 128 data points per second.[15] The minimum horizontal resolution would therefore be 1,280 pixels. For vertical scaling, at least 10 mm should be available per channel, for up to 21 channels. For lower-resolution monitors, decreasing the number of seconds per screen can allow display of every data sample point. Similarly, for vertical resolution, one can reduce the number of channels displayed or use a "zoom" feature to hone in on waveforms of interest. Dual monitor displays may be a particularly attractive option, offering the ability to view raw EEG and quantitative EEG simultaneously, view longer segments of EEG during electrographic seizures, or compare two segments of EEG simultaneously. Two side-by-side 24-inch widescreen WUXGA monitors, rotated 90 degrees, give an effective resolution of 2,400 × 1,920 pixels. This allows viewing of nearly every data point in 10 seconds of EEG sampled at 250 samples per second.

Digital EEG signals can also be printed on paper. Printers using fanfold paper allow printing of a continuous EEG record similar to that acquired with analog systems. Laser jet printers should be able to print at resolutions of 600 dots per inch (DPI), or approximately 350 samples per second. Optimally, the system should be able to print a subset of channels on each page to maximize vertical resolution.

2.13. Computer Acquisition and Review

Digital EEG has several advantages over analog recordings.[50] In routine clinical practice, the ability to reformat montages, change sensitivities and "paper speed," and manipulate filter settings during EEG review are some of the major advantages. For analog EEG, what the technologist records is what the electroencephalographer reviews, with no ability to change or reformat data to better localize abnormalities or exclude artifacts. Digital EEG allows review of the data "as acquired" (i.e., as the technologist viewed the data as they were being recorded) or with a nearly limitless array of post hoc montage, sensitivity, and filter settings.

Digital reformatting improves EEG interpretation. Levy et al.[51] demonstrated that interrater agreement for "as-acquired" digital EEG was the same as for paper EEG, with weighted kappa scores of approximately 0.65 (good agreement). When electroencephalographers were given the ability to reformat the digital EEG, however, interpreter agreement improved to kappa scores of 0.8 (very good agreement). Montage reformatting was most useful for distinguishing normal variants from abnormal patterns, identifying artifacts, and classifying abnormalities as focal or generalized. Correlation of digital EEG with simultaneously recorded video also enhances the ability to detect and correctly identify environmental and biological artifacts. Digital EEG can be reviewed page by page, usually 10 seconds per page, or in continuous "scroll" mode. Scroll mode is typically used during acquisition or when reviewing simultaneous video and EEG, and page mode is used during review. Page mode is much faster; up to 5 to 10 pages can be presented each second. Only superficial features of the EEG can be determined with this rapid paging speed, but it may be useful for screening for seizures or determination of sleep states. In page mode, EEG abnormalities or comments at the edge of the page may be missed. This can be avoided by overlapping the pages by several seconds.

2.13.1. PATIENT INFORMATION
At a minimum, the patient's name, date of birth, medical record number, laboratory EEG number, and the date the study was performed should be recorded and stored with the EEG.[15] This information can be stored in the same file as the EEG data itself, as a separate text file, or in a database linked to the EEG data file. Most systems allow recording of more detailed information including patient history, medications, and recording conditions. More advanced systems may include report-generation software, allowing reports to be stored with the digital EEG record.

2.13.2. DATA LABELING
During recording, the EEG data should be automatically labeled with time of day; all montage, sensitivity, and filter

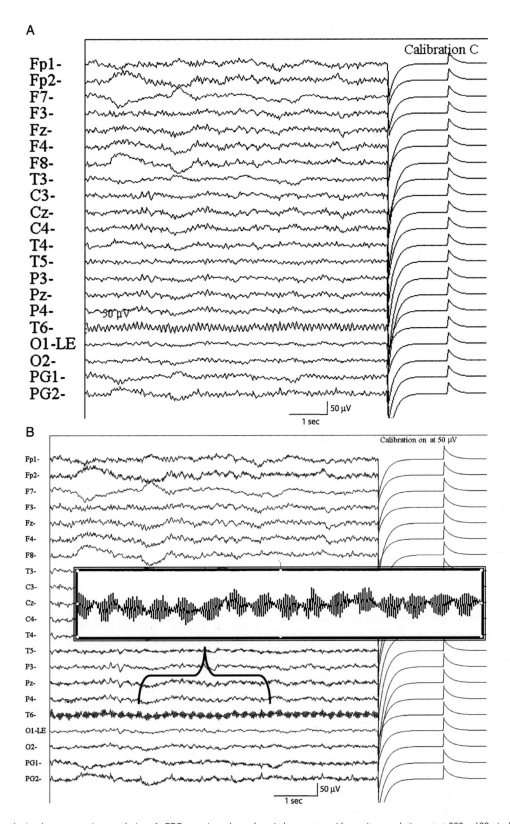

Figure 5.19. *Aliasing by inadequate monitor resolution.* **A:** *EEG was viewed on a hospital computer with monitor resolution set at 800 × 600 pixels. An unusual 9.5-Hz artifact is seen in channel T6—reference.* **B:** *When the EEG was viewed on a monitor with screen resolution 1,600 × 1,200 pixels, this signal is seen to be a sinusoidal 60-Hz artifact.*

settings used by the technologist during recording; and start and end of procedures such as photic stimulation and hyperventilation. The system should support entry of comments by the technologist, both as stored "codes" for common events (e.g., "eyes open," "awake," or "seizure") and as free text. Comments can also be generated by digital analysis programs, such as spike and seizure detection algorithms.

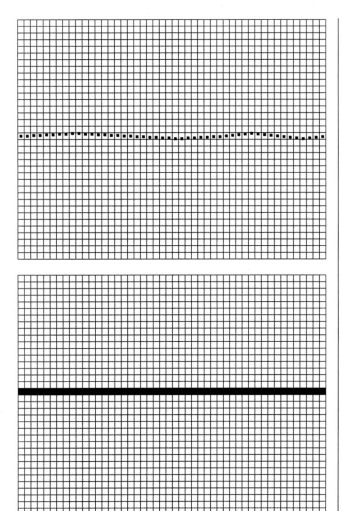

Figure 5.20. Effects of vertical display resolution on EEG. Idealized example with a low-amplitude signal that ranges from +1 to −1 μV. This variation is lost with pixels of 0.25 mm at a sensitivity of 7 μV/mm, resulting in a flat line.

TABLE 5.3. Commonly Used Computer Monitor Resolutions

CODE	NAME	ASPECT RATIO	RESOLUTION
VGA	Video Graphics Array	4:03	640 × 480
SVGA	Super Video Graphics Array	4:03	800 × 600
XGA	eXtended Graphics Array	4:03	1,024 × 768
SXGA	Super eXtended Graphics Array	5:04	1,280 × 1,024
WXGA	Widescreen eXtended Graphics Array	16:09	1,366 × 768
UXGA	Ultra eXtended Graphics Array	4:03	1,600 × 1,200
WSXGA+	Widescreen Super eXtended Graphics Array Plus	16:10	1,680 × 1,050
WUXGA	Wide Ultra eXtended Graphics Array	16:10	1,920 × 1,200
WQXGA	Wide Quad eXtended Graphics Array	16:10	2,560 × 1,600
WQUXGA	Wide Quad Ultra eXtended Graphics Array	16:10	3,840 × 2,400

During review, the electroencephalographer should be able to view all notations made during acquisition, as well as add comments. A scrollable list of comments can allow the reviewer to immediately find an EEG segment of interest. A particularly useful feature is the ability to create a "context-sensitive" comment, which stores both a text annotation and the montage, sensitivity, and filter settings at which the EEG was originally viewed.

2.13.3. MONTAGE REFORMATTING

Since digital EEG data are acquired using a hard-wired referential montage (Input 2 for all channels is the machine reference, or REF), the computer can perform calculations on the stored data to create any desired montage nearly instantaneously. For example, transforming the recorded montage to a bipolar montage requires the calculations in Table 5.4.

Montage reformatting allows the electroencephalographer to mentally reconstruct the three-dimensional EEG by combining views of three or more montages, such as longitudinal bipolar, transverse bipolar, and referential montages. Additional reference montages can be easily constructed by taking the average of data from two or more electrodes.[52]

Laplacian montages (source current density montages) are also easy to implement using "nearest neighbor" methods to approximate the Laplacian.[53] Montages can include electrodes of the modified 10-10 International System, as well as other physiological monitors such as EOG, ECG, oxygen saturation, and EMG.

In addition to changing montages, digital EEG software usually allows the reviewer to optimize vertical resolution by selecting only certain channels or groups of channels for display or "hiding" channels contaminated by artifact. Individual or groups of channels can be moved or reordered to improve comparisons between homologous brain regions. Extra space or "gaps" between channel groups can facilitate review, albeit at the expense of vertical resolution. Using different colors (red vs. blue) for left versus right hemisphere channels can help the

TABLE 5.4. Montage Reformatting

CHANNEL	RECORDING MONTAGE	CALCULATIONS	DISPLAY MONTAGE
1	Fp1-REF	Fp1-REF – Fp1-F7	(F7-REF)
2	F7-REF	F7-REF – F7-T3	(T3-REF)
3	T3-REF	T3-REF – T3-T5	(T5-REF)
4	T5-REF	T5-REF – T5-O1	(O1-REF)
5	O1-REF		

electroencephalographer quickly localize waveforms but may introduce subtle visual illusions that can mislead the interpreter.

2.13.4. SENSITIVITY CHANGES

In analog EEG, sensitivity is the input voltage (μV) divided by the output pen deflection (mm). For example, a 50-μV signal at a sensitivity of 7 μV/mm would be 7.1 mm high. In digital EEG, the same waveform on the display may not actually measure 7.1 mm; rather, the amplitude scale is displayed as a vertical icon (calibration line) on the monitor, and the amplitude of EEG signals is determined relative to this reference amplitude. The scale can be changed to provide a variety of sensitivity settings.

Sensitivity changes can be performed in two ways with a digital EEG machine. Rarely, the technician can use a software sensitivity switch during EEG acquisition to change the actual amplifier sensitivity (e.g., for intracranial vs. surface EEG recordings). More commonly, the display sensitivity is changed during acquisition or review. To decrease the amplitude of the waveforms on the page, the software program plots each data point on the monitor as if it were half as large. Sensitivity changes can be made for a single channel, groups of channels, or the entire page.

2.13.5. TIME SCALE CHANGES

Most EEG software programs display EEG at 10 seconds per screen or, for larger or widescreen monitors, 25 to 35 mm per second. The number of seconds displayed per page can be adjusted, however, to optimize interpretation. For example, displaying 20 seconds or more per page will enhance slow activity and allow analysis of slow periodic complexes or prolonged events such as seizures. Spreading out the EEG to show only 2 to 5 seconds per page will spread out faster frequencies, similar to increasing the paper speed on an analog machine. This allows more precise analysis of time relationships of signals in adjacent channels, for example to analyze the propagation of epileptiform spikes. In addition, time cursors can usually be placed on the screen to measure time relationships exactly. Many software programs allow the number of seconds per page to be varied from 1 to 100 seconds. Unfortunately, even the largest monitors cannot adequately display more than 20 to 30 seconds of EEG, limiting simultaneous analysis of long segments of EEG (e.g., evolution of seizures over several minutes). Printing the EEG to fanfold paper may enhance the interpretation of long EEG epochs. Alternatively, most EEG software programs allow split-screen views to allow side-by-side comparison of noncontiguous segments of EEG.

2.13.6. WAVEFORM MEASUREMENTS

Waveforms can be measured in several ways. Some software displays the maximal "peak-to-peak" amplitudes available for each channel. Others contain a calibration icon that shows the size of a 50- or 100-μV signal. The calibration icon can be moved around the screen and compared to various waveforms. Most programs also contain a feature that allows a user to draw a line from peak to trough of any given waveform to get a numerical value for the amplitude in microvolts, or the

TABLE 5.5. Time Domain Digital Filters

FILTER TYPE	PROS	CONS
FIR	Absolutely stable	Computationally more expensive
	Linear phase, constant group delay (peaks and other features of wave shapes will have the same delay in two channels processed by the same filter)	Require higher order for equivalent performance
		Difficult to reproduce effect of analog filters
IIR	Computationally cheaper	Potentially unstable (stable in typical practice)
	Can obtain good performance with low order	Nonlinear phase, group delay is frequency dependent
	Can simply and exactly reproduce analog filters	

duration in milliseconds. Finally, more advanced waveform measurements may include average amplitude or frequency for a selected segment of a channel of EEG, or even a spectrogram of the component frequencies.

2.13.7. DIGITAL FILTERING

One of the major advantages of digital EEG is the ability to apply, remove, and reapply a variety of digital filters to enhance or minimize activity in certain frequency bands without altering the original EEG data.[54] This is analogous to inserting electrical filters in the acquisition path. The field of digital time domain filters is vast and complex, but some basic principles are important to illustrate (Table 5.5).

The three common methods of digital filtering include two time domain methods (finite impulse response [FIR] and infinite impulse response [IIR]) and one frequency domain method using the FFT. While most commercial systems do not incorporate all the filter choices discussed below, it is important to understand how different digital filter types can be designed to mimic (or improve upon) the analog filters. Signal processing programs and toolboxes used for quantitative EEG analysis (e.g., MatLab) will incorporate a larger number of filters and the ability to design custom digital filters.

2.13.7.1. TIME DOMAIN FILTERS

Processing discrete time sequences to accentuate or diminish frequency bands is made possible by a technique called digital filtering. We begin with an extremely simple example, the two-point moving average. If one takes a sequence and replaces each value by the average of it and the previous value, one generates a new sequence. If x_k is the input at time t_k and y_k is the output at t_k, then

$$y_k = 1/2\left(x_k + x_{k-1}\right)$$

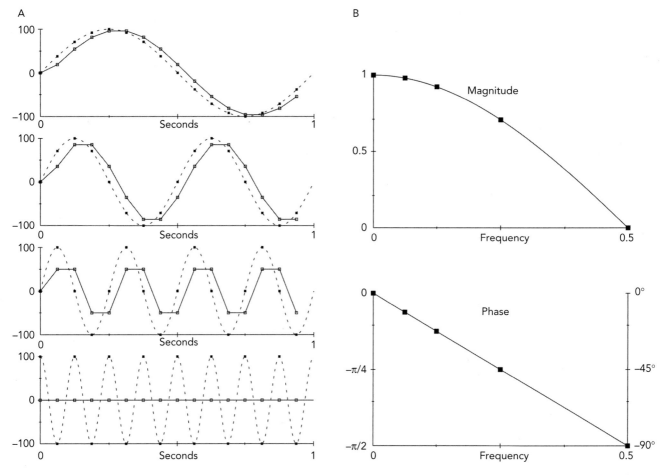

Figure 5.21. *Filtering by finite impulse response (FIR) filter, two-point moving average. See text for explanation.*

Figure 5.21A shows this concept applied to pure sinusoids of several different frequencies, up to the Nyquist limit. The squares (connected by solid curve) are the original data points. The circles, connected by dashed curve. are the points that result from the two-point moving average. We note several features:

1. For an input of a pure sinusoid, the amplitude of the output may be altered, but the frequency of the output is the *same* as the input. This is a general feature.

2. The amplitude of the output diminishes with higher frequency. This is specific to our example. Other filters might attenuate low frequencies and preserve high frequencies.

3. The output is shifted to the right. In particular, the peaks in the output are all shifted a half-point to the right relative to the input sinusoid. However, the apparent shift in *phase* increases with higher frequency.

4. At the Nyquist frequency, the output is identically zero, for this example.

Figure 5.21B shows graphs of these effects. The top shows the ratio of the output amplitude over the input amplitude, as a function of frequency (in this case, the absolute frequency

divided by the sampling frequency, as this effect does not depend on absolute sampling rate, so 0.5 is the Nyquist frequency). The bottom shows the phase delay (in radians and degrees) as a function of (reduced) frequency. Note also that the phase shift is a straight line (linear). This simple algorithm (average of 2 points) acts as a filter that attenuates higher-frequency inputs and preserves low frequencies and is thus termed a low-pass filter. A four-point moving average would act similarly but would more dramatically attenuate high frequencies. A simple filter that would attenuate low frequencies and preserve high frequencies would be a two-point difference filter, computing the difference between the current input point and the previous input point.

The graph of the magnitude of the output as a function of the input frequency is known as the *transfer function*. Several different regions or bands in this transfer function have specific names. The frequency band in which the output is preserved (ratio of output to input near 1) is called the *passband*. The frequency band in which the output is severely attenuated (ratio near 0) is termed the *stopband*. The frequency band in between is known as the *transition band*. The slope of the transfer function in the transition band is called the *roll-off*. The graph of the phase shift versus frequency is known as the *phase plot*. There is a delay in the output, the *group delay*, generally expressed in number of sample points. The group delay may vary as a function of frequency. In general, the group delay at a given frequency is the (negative) slope of the phase plot at that frequency. The *order* of a digital filter is the number of prior input values used in computing the output. Thus, a two-point average is first order and a four-point moving average is third order. These are the principal features that are compared and contrasted between different digital filters.

2.13.7.1.1. Finite Impulse Response

The examples described so far are part of a class known as FIR filters. When the input consists of an "impulse"—a single nonzero input value in a sequence of zero inputs—the output sequence (response) will be nonzero for only a finite number of elements before it necessarily returns to zero. This is a direct consequence of the fact that the output y_k depends only on current and prior inputs x_k, x_{k-1}. This feature defines the FIR class of filters. FIR filters can be designed to be low-pass, high-pass, bandpass, and many other forms. A particular feature of the FIR class of filters is that the phase shift is a linear function of frequency, and thus the slope is constant, so the group delay is the same at all frequencies.

2.13.7.1.2. Infinite Impulse Response

The other class of digital filters is known as IIR filters. They are also known by other names, such as autoregressive or recursive. A simple example is

$$y_k = \frac{1}{5} x_k + \frac{4}{5} y_{k-1}$$

That is, the output (y_k) is computed as one-fifth the current input (x_k) plus four-fifths the prior *output*.

Using prior output values is what gives this filter class its important characteristics. For an input sequence that contains an impulse (a single nonzero value), this filter will yield an output that continues to have nonzero outputs. Figure 5.22A shows such an IIR (though the values trend toward and approach zero).

This filter applied to another input sequence known as a step function is shown in Figure 5.22B. This plot will probably remind many readers of the graph of voltage charging a capacitor, and in fact this filter is the digital analogy of a simple single resistor and capacitor circuit arranged as a low-pass filter. Digital filters are specified by the coefficients that multiply prior inputs and output to compute the current output. Given a set of coefficients, it is straightforward (though possibly complicated) to determine the transfer function and phase plot. In general, the equation for a filter of order n follows:

$$y_k = \{b_0 x_{k-0} + b_1 x_{k-1} + b_2 x_{k-2} + \ldots b_n x_{k-n}\} + \{a_1 y_{k-1} + a_2 y_{k-2} + \ldots + a_n y_{k-n}\}$$

The transfer function (H) and phase are generated by calculating (or having a graphing program display)

$$|H| = \left| \frac{\{b_0 + b_1 e^{-i2\pi x} + b_2 e^{-2i2\pi x} \ldots\}}{\{1 - a_1 e^{-i2\pi x} - a_2 e^{-2i2\pi x} - \ldots\}} \right|$$

and

$$phase = \tan^{-1} \left\{ \frac{\text{Im}ag(H)}{\text{Re}al(H)} \right\}$$

For our simple example, $b_0 = 0.2$ and $a_1 = 0.8$. With these coefficients, the transfer function (solid) and phase (dashed, in radians) are graphed in Figure 5.22C. It demonstrates that these choices yield a low-pass filter. Note that these coefficients yield a small passband and a cutoff near 0.05; in other words, low frequencies below 0.05 × sampling rate are passed, but frequencies above 0.1 × sampling rate are mostly attenuated. In this manner, given a set of filter coefficients, one can compute the transfer function and phase plot. There are algorithms for generating the coefficients corresponding to traditional analog circuits (e.g., Butterworth, Chebyshev type 1 and 2, Bessel) with a given cutoff frequency. The inverse problem, having a desired transfer function, and computing the required order and coefficients, is beyond the scope of this chapter. For details, see reference[55].

In general, for IIR filters, phase shift is nonlinear, so group delay varies with frequency. In fact, particular coefficients for IIR filters can create a situation in which two finite sinusoidal signals of different frequencies can appear reversed in order after being filtered, compared to the input sequence. Techniques to mitigate group delay for both FIR and IIR filters are discussed below.

2.13.7.2. Undesired Effects

Group delay can produce unexpected distortions in digital signals, particularly for multichannel comparisons, as with EEG. Figure 5.23 shows the distorting effect of different filter settings when visually comparing channels. Group delay can be problematic, and it affects both FIR and IIR filters. As mentioned previously, the group delay generally increases with increasing order of the filter. Since FIR filters typically require significantly higher orders to obtain the same transfer function attenuation as IIR filters, group delay can quickly become very problematic for FIR filters. Techniques to eliminate it have been developed. Filters that are *acausal* can eliminate group delay. Acausal filters are ones in which *future* time points as well as past time points are included in the computation, as opposed to the filters discussed previously that include *only* past time points, which are called *causal*. While causal filers can be used to filter live on a point-by-point basis (but introducing the group-delay artifact), acausal filters cannot be implemented live. They can, however, be implemented with a short delay.

If the entire time series of points is known and immutable, having been acquired and stored, then acausal filters are simple to implement and can completely eliminate the group delay. In fact, a simple scheme is to filter the entire time series in the forward direction, then reverse and use the same filter coefficients in the backward direction. This eliminates the group delay and can even eliminate the phase distortion, achieving zero-phase distortion. This forward–backward zero-phase filtering works for both FIR and IIR filters. A further trick can be employed

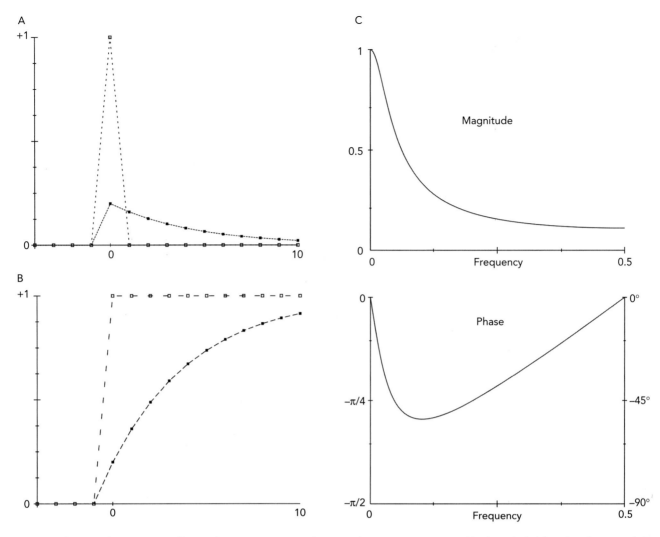

Figure 5.22. Infinite impulse response (IIR) filter. **A:** *Filter response to an impulse input. The* open squares connected by the wide-dash line *show the input, which is zero everywhere except time point 0, where it is 1, and the* filled squares connected by narrow-dash line *plot the output, which approaches but never reaches zero, having a persisting, infinite response to an impulse input, thus the term "infinite impulse response."* **B:** *IIR filter applied to another input sequence known as a step function. Again, the* open squares connected by wide-dash line *show the input, and the* filled squares connected by narrow-dash line *plot the output.* **C:** *Transfer function and phase plot of IIR low-pass filter. See text for details.*

to minimize transients at the end of the time series, producing the same result whether filtering forward first or backward first.[56]

2.13.7.3. FREQUENCY DOMAIN FILTERS

Frequency domain filters use FFT to remove unwanted frequencies from the signal.[57] According to Fourier's theorem, any time series waveform can be modeled as the sum of a set of sinusoidal waveforms, each with different frequency, amplitude, and phase. In frequency filtering, the input signal is broken into short segments and then transformed into its component sine wave signals using FFT. To filter the signal, the coefficients of the unwanted frequencies above or below a specified cutoff frequency are set to zero, and the inverse Fourier transform is then computed to obtain the original EEG signal minus the unwanted frequencies, as seen in Figure 5.24.

Frequency domain filters have several limitations. Frequency filtering cannot be performed until the full epoch to be filtered has been acquired, precluding true real-time filtering. To improve computational speed, certain limitations may be placed on the time series, such as a requirement to contain exactly 2^n members, where n is a positive integer. Finally, if the EEG signal is not stationary (i.e., has variable frequency components) over the epoch, the FFT may introduce artifactual high-frequency noise.[58] For this reason, frequency domain filtering is typically performed over short epochs (e.g., 1 second) to improve the likelihood that the signal will remain stationary during the entire epoch. Breaking the EEG into short epochs, however, may introduce discontinuities between subsequent epochs. "Windowing" procedures can minimize such discontinuities. Windowing is the application of a weighting function (e.g., Hamming window) to taper the ends of each epoch toward zero. Because windowing necessarily loses some information at the ends of the epochs, analysis is commonly performed on multiple epochs overlapping each other by 25% to 75%. The length of the analyzed epoch, the windowing function utilized, and the degree of overlap all influence the computational speed of frequency domain filtering.

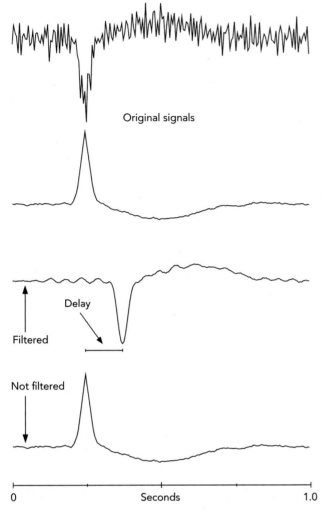

Figure 5.23. *Distorting effect of different filter settings when visually comparing channels. The top panel shows (synthesized) traces for two sequential channels from a bipolar derivation with an idealized sharp-and-slow wave complex, but with significant noise on the top channel. It is tempting to try to eliminate the noise in that one channel by selectively applying a low-pass filter. The bottom panel shows the result of an FIR low-pass (cutoff 25 Hz) filter, with order of 50 (a not unreasonable order for an FIR filter). The high-frequency noise is indeed reduced, but a delay is induced by the filter. The (downgoing) peak of the top tracing is delayed by 1/8th of a second. All traces are 1-second duration at 200 samples per second.*

2.14. Digital Analysis and Data Reduction

Digital EEGs can be very rapidly reviewed by displaying pages at rates of 1 to 10 pages (10 seconds of EEG) per second. The maximal speed of review is determined by the speed of the network, computer processor, and graphics card. Even at very rapid review speeds, however, review of an entire 24-hour EEG (8,640 10-second pages) will take 15 to 60 minutes or more. A variety of data-reduction methods can be used to identify EEG segments of interest for more rapid interpretation.

Digital EEG can be analyzed quantitatively to assist interpretation, automatically detect events, and produce graphical displays.[59,60] A full discussion of these techniques is beyond the scope of this chapter, but they are included in later chapters. Signal processing can be performed either online, as EEG is acquired, or offline. Online analyses are limited to those that can be performed in real time by the computer processor, while offline analyses can be more complex. Digital processing can highlight specific features of the EEG using graphical displays, remove or correct artifacts, or detect common patterns such as seizures or sleep states.

2.14.1. AUTOMATED ARTIFACT IDENTIFICATION

Several online and offline techniques have been developed to remove artifactual segments of EEG, either to improve visual review and analysis or as a preprocessing step for further digital analysis.[61] Some techniques automatically reject short segments of EEG if the segment exceeds predefined thresholds in simple measures such as amplitude, numbers of zero crossings, or 60-Hz artifact.[62] These automatic rejection techniques will not identify all possible artifacts, especially for ambulatory patients or in electrically hostile environments. Since the entire EEG segment is rejected if the threshold is exceeded, some useful EEG may be eliminated. Other methods aim to identify artifact and to remove only the artifact from the recording, leaving a "clean" EEG for digital analysis. These techniques may result in distortion of the EEG signal, as some normal brain signals may be subtracted. Source decomposition techniques aim to break EEG signals down into individual components that represent EEG and others that represent artifact. Once the artifactual component is identified, it is removed and the remaining signal is recomposed. Examples of these methods include spatial filtering,[63] principal component analysis, and independent component analysis.[64] Wavelet-based and neural network algorithms[65] allow adaptation of this method to a wider variety or artifact types.

2.14.2. SPIKE AND SEIZURE DETECTION

Algorithms to detect spikes and seizures are commonly used in long-term video-EEG monitoring, intensive care unit monitoring, and ambulatory EEG. The algorithms are designed to detect specific features in the digital data, such as the sharpness and field of an epileptiform discharge or the change in frequencies or amplitude at the beginning of a seizure.[66,67] Other methods use neural networks that can be trained and updated with a database of seizures to improve detection accuracy.[68,69] The detection algorithms mark the sections of data that contain events of interest. The electroencephalographer can then review this prescreened data rather than the entire EEG recording. The detection algorithms are not perfect and may either miss seizures or spikes or have high numbers of false detections.

2.14.3. TOPOGRAPHIC DISPLAY (MAPPING)

Topographic maps display the EEG voltage at various locations on the head.[70] To construct smoothed maps, interpolation techniques such as spline interpretation or nearest neighbor rules are used.[71,72] The maps are most accurate when large numbers of electrodes are used. Topographic maps can be used to display the voltage topography of epileptiform activity.[73]

2.14.4. ELECTRICAL SOURCE MODELING

This technique aids in localizing the generators of EEG events, such as epileptiform discharges.[74,75] Multichannel digital EEG is modeled as being generated by a single dipole source (or

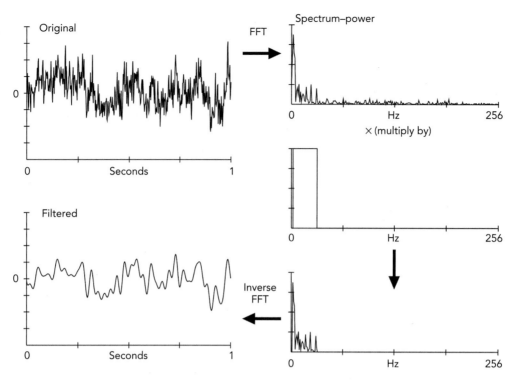

Figure 5.24. *Filtering in the frequency domain. The top left shows the original signal (this example has 512 samples per second). The fast (discrete) Fourier transformation converts this signal into a frequency domain representation (top right). The spectrum is multiplied by a desired filter function (middle right), in this case preserving all frequencies between 2 and 32 Hz—a bandpass—and zeroing all other frequency components. The resulting spectrum (bottom right) is then inverse Fourier transformed back into the time domain, yielding the filtered signal (bottom left). The Fourier domain representation also has phase information but this has been omitted for clarity of illustration.*

a small number of them). Each dipole source produces particular scalp voltage waveforms when placed in a mathematical model of the head. The locations and orientations of the dipoles are adjusted to produce the best fit between the mathematical model and the actual EEG. Source localizations can be co-registered with data from MRI, which is especially useful in planning epilepsy surgery.[76–78]

2.14.5. Spectral Analysis/Graphical Displays of Quantitative EEG (QEEG)

Spectral analysis involves analyzing the various frequencies that make up the digital EEG signal.[79] Typically, the FFT is used to calculate the frequencies present in the EEG, or mean or median amplitude is determined over short segments of EEG. The spectral analysis of a segment of EEG can then be plotted on a topographic map or displayed as a graph of power in a particular frequency versus time. Commonly used QEEG trends include color density spectral array, amplitude integrated EEG, alpha-delta ratios, and asymmetry indices. This application can help to speed review of long EEG recordings in the epilepsy monitoring and intensive care units, but raw EEG tracings must always be available for review and confirmation of the quantitative findings.[80–82]

2.15. Data Sharing, Storage, and Networking

2.15.1. EEG File Formats and Data Sharing

EEG files acquired with current commercial EEG systems are typically stored in proprietary formats that require vendor-specific software to open and view the files. Files consist of patient identifying information (e.g., name, gender, birthdate) and recording information (e.g., start date and time, equipment name, duration), then the type of signal, channel labels, units of measurement, and sampling rate, and well as annotations and event codes. Use of proprietary formats can cause significant problems in transferring data between different EEG laboratories for review, and even for maintaining readable archives as file formats are changed over time. Unfortunately, no universally accepted standard format exists, and there may be variations even in commonly used open formats. There are several approaches to overcome this Tower of Babel problem.[83] Most commercial systems can export EEGs to a compact disk (CD) or digital video disk (DVD) with a limited-function version of the EEG reader software, so the disk becomes a self-contained reader station usable on any computer. Others provide a "light" version of review software that can be installed on multiple computers at low cost. Some allow EEGs to be converted to open-source formats (e.g., European Data Format [EDF], European Data Format plus [EDF+],[84] Extensible Biosignal [EBS],[85] ASCII,[86] or the ACNS's Technical Standard 1[87]) that can be read by a variety of freely available reader programs and some commercial systems. These open formats may not replicate all of the features available in the original EEG software, and most have been adopted by only a few vendors. Finally, there are several commercial programs that can read EEG files collected by different commercial EEG systems, but these may not read all EEG file types and can be quite expensive. Labs should have policies and procedures for archive types, and for conversion of archives when old formats become obsolete. These should be in compliance with local and state requirements for medical record retention.

For research, EEG software should provide the ability to export de-identified (with patient identifiers removed to meet Health Insurance Portability and Accountability Act of 1996 [HIPAA] standards) data. Freely available, expertly scored EEG data in a common data format would help to advance research efforts in epilepsy and other neurological conditions.[88]

2.15.2. DATA STORAGE

Once the EEG is reviewed, video and EEG data are typically clipped for events of interest and archived to long-term storage. Archiving schemes vary; most labs save all routine EEGs but only clips of significant events for long-term video-EEG monitoring. Some save all continuous 24-hour EEG data, but continuous video files are too large to store in a cost-effective manner. A laboratory performing 2,000 routine EEGs, 1,000 video-EEG studies, and 500 ambulatory EEGs will produce more than a terabyte of digital data each year.

EEGs can be archived on a variety of media, including CD, DVD, Blu-ray BD-R or BD-RE, tape, hard drives (internal or external), servers, or network-attached storage devices. These media vary greatly in size (i.e., the amount of data that can be stored), cost, convenience (i.e., the time required to archive and ease of use), and durability. Use of digital media has significantly decreased the space requirements and cost of EEG storage. CDs (storing up to 700 MB) and DVDs (4.7 GB, dual layer 9 GB) are most commonly used when EEGs need to be transferred to another electroencephalographer for interpretation. Archiving to removable optical media is low in cost but inefficient, as each disk holds only a small amount of data, must be "burned" individually, must be placed back in the computer for the data to be reviewed, and may become unreadable over years. More importantly, these media may become obsolete over the next few years; optical disk data will need to be re-recorded to other media or may become unreadable. External tape drive storage devices have a large capacity and rapid backup, but data retrieval can be slow because the tape must be transferred back to the review station hard drive before review. Tapes may also deteriorate over time. USB flash drives are larger and faster than optical disks, but still more expensive per MB. External hard drives are inexpensive and provide more rapid access to data than tape drives. Hard drive costs have decreased significantly over recent years, making storage of large amounts of data on servers or network-attached storage devices economically feasible. EEG data stored on a server can be rapidly retrieved from any computer on the network. Maintaining digital EEG archives (e.g., updating to new media or to new file formats) can be costly and time-consuming. Locating EEG archives on hospital servers managed by information technology staff has several advantages, including improved lab efficiency, regular data backups, and optimal security and audit trails.

The size of an EEG file depends on the number of channels recorded, the sampling rate of the ADC, and the duration of the recording. One hour of 32-channel EEG sampled at 200 samples per second produces an approximately 50-MB file, while 1 hour of video data can be nearly 1 GB, depending on resolution and compression. Compression techniques can be used to reduce the number of bits necessary to represent information by removing repeated bits. For example, instead of encoding 10 binary 1 and 5 binary 0 values, the compression method encodes that a binary 1 value is repeated 10 times and binary 0 value 5 times (1111111111100000 vs. 10-1 5-0). The destination computer then decodes the information and expands it back to the original number of bits. While it is possible to compress digital EEG signals slightly, in general the savings are small and may not justify computing overhead (decompressing data) in these systems. Digital video compression is essential, and this technology continues to evolve.

2.15.3. NETWORKING

One of the most useful features of digital EEG is the ability to connect acquisition machines to computer networks for data transmission and communication. A network is a group of computers and other devices that are connected to facilitate the transfer of information and sharing of resources. The type of network and its bandwidth, or speed, will determine how quickly EEG studies can be accessed and reviewed (Table 5.6). Wired networks are typically faster (100–1,000 Mbits/sec) and more reliable than wireless networks (bandwidth 11 to >100 Mbits/sec), although the latter does not incur the high costs of running cable to all EEG locations and may be adequate for low-volume laboratories.

An efficient and organized network requires careful planning, usually in conjunction with trained and certified hospital network managers. The design of a network for EEG is determined by a few basic principles: (i) function, (ii) geography (number of users, distance of the farthest users from the server), (iii) speed or bandwidth, (iv) budget, (v) expandability/flexibility, and (vi) requirements for network administration. The first step is to identify the purpose(s) of the network, such as (i) data acquisition, (ii) transmission of data to central review area, (iii) provision of access to data from multiple locations, sometimes simultaneously, (iv) interpretation of studies, (v) generation of reports, and (vi) data archiving.

A server, a computer specialized for the storage, transmission, and security of data, can provide a central repository of files, most importantly EEG and video files, EEG databases, and EEG reports, which can then be accessed from multiple network locations. The EEG can be streamed continuously to the server as it is acquired or transferred after the study is completed. Having the data in a central location facilitates security measures and improves the efficiency of data backups and archiving. The server is typically located locally in the EEG laboratory or in the hospital's server farm.

Networks used in hospitals usually consist of a long length of very high-bandwidth cable media that connects the servers, called the *backbone*, with branches off the backbone called *segments* (Fig. 5.25). Segments (such as to EEG labs) usually consist of lower-bandwidth cable media, which again branch to individual users. EEG machines connected to the network can be accessed remotely to review ongoing studies, update patient databases, and adjust recording parameters (e.g., montage,

TABLE 5.6. Transmission Speed of Digital EEG and Video

TYPE	DATA RATE	EEG TRANSFER TIME	EEG REAL TIME	VIDEO TRANSFER TIME	VIDEO REAL TIME
Wired					
Gigabit Ethernet	1 Gbps	0.5 sec	Yes	5.3 sec	Yes
T4 (fiber-optic trunk line)	274.76 Mbps	1.7 sec	Yes	19.2 sec	Yes
Fast Ethernet	100 Mbps	4.8 sec	Yes	52.8 sec	Yes
Ethernet	10 Mbps	48 sec	Yes	8 min 48 sec	Yes
Cable modem	2.5–6 Mbps	1 min 20 sec–3 min 12 sec	Yes	14 min 40 sec–35 min 20 sec	Yes
T1 (trunk line)	1.54 Mbps	5 min 20 sec	Yes	57 min 8 sec	Yes
DSL	1–3 Mbps	2 min 40 sec–8 min	Yes	29 min 20 sec–88 min	Maybe
Modem	56 kbps	2 hr 38 min	No	26 hr 20 min	No
Wireless					
802.11n	100 Mbps	4.8 sec	Yes	52.8 sec	Yes
802.11a/g	54 Mbps	8.9 sec	Yes	1 min 38 sec	Yes
801.11b	11 Mbps	43.6 sec	Yes	8 min	Yes
4G cellular	6–100 Mbps	4.8 sec–1 min 20 sec	Yes	52.8 sec–14 min 40 sec	Yes
3G cellular	144 kbps–2.4 Mbps	3 min 20 sec–55 min 33 sec	Yes	36 min 20 sec–10 hrs 10 min	Maybe

Digital EEG, 32 channels, 16-bit resolution, sampled at 256 Hz, 1 hour = 60 MB = 480 Mbit.
MPEG4 color video, 640 pixels × 480 pixels resolution, 30 frames per second, compressed,
1 hour = 660 MB = 5280 Mbit.

camera position). The bandwidth (or speed) of the network will determine the speed of remote review.

Finally, the need to review data from several different sites (e.g., remote EEG labs, physicians' offices, home) may require additional resources, such as remote access servers, as well as Internet service providers outside the hospital or healthcare facility.[89] Users can access the network using nearly any device with Internet access, such as a home computer, laptop, wireless personal digital assistant, or digital cellular telephone. Cellular wireless systems are slower than cable or DSL connections but may be adequate to quickly review emergency studies.

Remote access allows users to connect to the network and perform tasks as if they were directly connected to the network,

even when they are far away. Remote access can be accomplished via a dial-up connection to a remote access server or via a virtual private network (VPN) tunneled through the Internet. The VPN tunnel maintains the confidentiality of the data through encryption. Transmission of EEG data to remote locations may be very slow (see Table 5.6). A terminal server system such as Windows Terminal Server or Citrix Metaframe allows multiple remote users to run applications from anywhere with an Internet connection, nearly identical to when sitting in front of a computer on the network. The remote user logs in and is authenticated, then can open the EEG software application. The terminal server sends remote keystroke and mouse movements to the application and sends screenshots of the application to the remote user. Because only screenshots, not the actual EEG data, are transmitted, review is typically much faster.

An information technology specialist or network administrator is often helpful for troubleshooting computer and software problems and providing network security and disaster protection/recovery. Network security is especially important if patient information is stored in the network, as law protects patient confidentiality. The security architecture must be compliant with HIPAA guidelines. Adequate security measures must protect against unauthorized users, computer viruses, accidental destruction of files, and other forms of attack. Sensitive files may need to be encrypted both on the computer disk and during network transmission. Networks connected to the Internet or other outside connections are especially vulnerable to outside attack and need a firewall or proxy to create a barrier around the internal network. Protecting data from catastrophic data loss includes several considerations: (i) power backup with surge protectors or universal power supplies, (ii) data backup on a regular and reliable schedule, (iii) maintenance of backup files in a secure location separate from the original files, (iv) disk fault tolerance by providing multiple copies of the same information on an array of hard drives, and (v) server fault tolerance by providing multiple servers in case of server malfunction.

2.15.4. SECURITY

HIPAA[90] instituted a set of rules (the "Security Standard") that impact digital EEG storage, review, transmission, and archiving. The U.S. Department of Health and Human Services (HHS) has published a guideline document that provides a concise description of many of the issues that relate to HIPAA rules on network transmission and storage of protected health information (PHI) and that can be applied directly to digital EEG.[91] We review some general issues and recommendations and describe some of the specifics of the HHS guideline.

One goal of HIPAA was protection of patient privacy and prevention of abuse of patient information. While the vast majority of data in digital EEG files are the digitized voltage time series and are fairly useless to identity thieves, some portions of the files (depending on the vendor) can contain electronic PHI, such as name, date of birth, address, doctor, and diagnoses. These pieces of information could be used to harm patients if obtained by individuals with ill intent. Strategies for protecting this information must be addressed by the modern

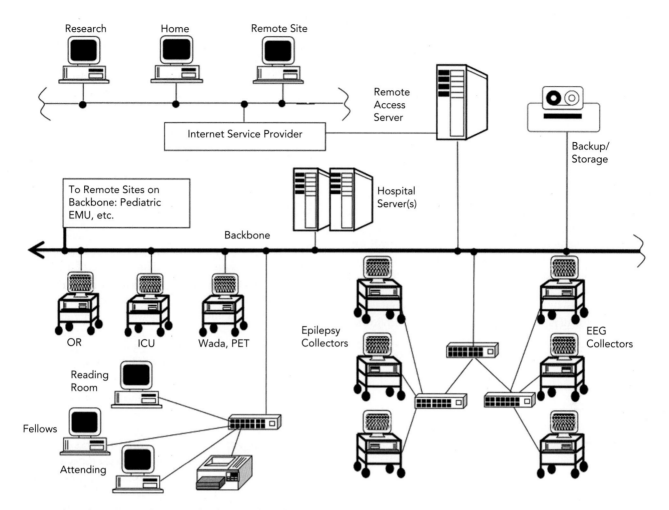

Figure 5.25. A complex EEG network connected to the hospital backbone. EEG data are collected from patients in various locations and sent to a central server. The backbone provides for high-speed transmission of files, so the review location can be quite distant from the collection locations. The network also provides remote access for users outside the hospital. The hospital server can provide a backup for the EEG server.

digital EEG laboratory. The HHS guideline groups electronic processing into three areas: *accessing, storing,* and *transmitting.*

2.15.4.1. Accessing

With regard to digital EEG, an example relating to accessing might be the login accounts of acquisition and reviewing workstations. Unauthorized persons might access patient information by directly viewing unsecured workstations, or obtaining passwords written on the stations themselves, keystroke capture malware, or social engineering (requesting passwords from authorized personnel by using the pretense of being an information technology employee). Some strategies applicable to digital EEG to mitigate these risks include the following:

Computers on which EEG data are stored must be password protected.

Automatic logins, in which a login password is bypassed on computer startup, should be disabled.

Each user should have an individual password.

Vendors of EEG acquisition and reading stations should work toward the goal of avoiding the practice of a common username and password for all technicians and

physicians using the stations. Ideally, each user should have an individual account, with shared configuration settings placed in shared folders and personalized preferences stored in individual accounts.

Antivirus and anti-malware software should be installed and kept current on each workstation to mitigate the possibility of keystroke capture of passwords.

2.15.4.2. Storing

Digital EEG involves storing/archiving vast amounts of data, and while PHI is again a small minority, risks remain. Laptops containing digital EEG could be stolen. Portable hard drives could likewise be stolen. Digital EEG records could be recovered from local cached files when accessed from computers outside the hospital. Strategies to minimize these risks include the following:

Laptops and desktops could be stored in locked rooms when not in use.

Laptops could be secured by "locking mechanisms" to fixed walls.

Laptops (and even desktops) could have full hard disk drive encryption. Without the disk encryption password, the plaintext information would not be recoverable. Of course, this leads to additional passwords, so a clear password policy and password management system becomes even more necessary.

Prevention of cached records on outside computers is more difficult and would likely involve software implementation by vendors.

2.15.4.3. TRANSMITTING

This is probably the aspect of security with digital EEG that requires the most attention. There is no doubt that remote access (e.g., physicians who are offsite, home, conferences) and distant second opinions could add much value to patient care. However, remote access then requires careful consideration of protection from data security breaches. Electronic PHI could be intercepted when in network transit, either outside the hospital network (external) or even within it (internal). Strategies to minimize the risk of network interception include the following:

Digital EEG data transmitted over networks should be encrypted. For external network access, most sites use VPN protocols.

Ideally, automated network analysis by the hospital information technology staff should prompt alerts for unusual traffic, such as frequent logins, simultaneous logins from disparate locations, logins from other continents, and so on.

Web-based (HTTP) protocols are also used. For these, at a minimum HTTPS (HTTP-secure) should be used. For HTTPS, modern browsers use TLS (transport layer security, which superseded the older SSL/secure sockets layer protocol) for bidirectional encryption.

3. POLARITY AND FIELD DETERMINATIONS

3.1. Introduction

Accurate EEG interpretation is not possible without a thorough understanding of EEG scalp localization. In contrast to most other aspects of EEG interpretation, the process of scalp localization is deductive and does not present the problem of reasonable disagreement between readers. The development of digital EEG recording has made it possible to view the same segment of recording retrospectively using different frequency filters and spatial filters (montages). This retrospective analysis greatly increases the ability of the electroencephalographer to localize the electrical fields of the scalp EEG and thereby provide more accurate interpretation. There are several reasons why localizing EEG activity is an essential skill:

1. The identification and classification of EEG activity is always based to some degree on localization. For example, a high-amplitude, sharply contoured, anterior temporal waveform that clearly stands out from the background and is activated by sleep has a high likelihood of being an abnormal epileptiform spike. However, the same waveform appearing over the central head region during sleep is far more likely to be a benign vertex wave of normal sleep.

2. Localization is often the only feature that allows the electroencephalographer to determine if an activity is cerebral in origin or an artifact. A sharp rhythmic pattern that evolves in frequency and morphology over a left frontal head region may be likely an electrographic seizure, whereas the same pattern that appears simultaneously over both the left frontal head region and the right occipital head region without involvement of electrodes between these regions is far more likely to be an artifact.

3. The clinical correlation portion of EEG interpretation always depends on the cortical localization of the EEG findings. Localization is the one skill that greatly increases the likelihood of correctly interpreting an EEG pattern the reader has never encountered before.

3.2. The EEG Signal: Cortically Generated Scalp Currents

The skill of localization in routine clinical EEG interpretation consists of two steps: localizing EEG activity to specific electrode positions on the scalp and then relating the scalp localization to the likely source in the underlying cerebral cortex. To perform the latter requires an understanding of how the EEG signal arises and is conducted to the scalp. The relationship between the scalp signal and its origin within the brain is a complex topic that has been approached by a variety of mathematical models and was covered in greater detail in Chapters 2, 3, and 4. In routine practice localization is approximated according to a basic understanding of cortical anatomy and volume conduction theory.

The spontaneous EEG signal in the routine scalp recorded EEG arises from cortical pyramidal cell postsynaptic potentials. Although other sources (e.g., other neurons and glial cells) and other forms of electrical potentials (e.g., action potentials within the cortex) exist, their contributions to extracranial electrical fields appear to be very limited. Pyramidal cells that generate postsynaptic potentials have the biophysical advantage of firing in synchrony (i.e., they summate in time) and with similar radial orientation (i.e., they are aimed in the same direction toward the cortical surface) and similar long duration, making them ideal for producing a large enough signal to be conducted through the skull and recordable at the scalp. As illustrated in Figure 5.26, this usually means that the recording electrode that detects the highest-amplitude signal is overlying the cortical source.[92] However, there are contributions from the walls of cortical sulci that are not oriented perpendicular to the scalp and may affect adjacent electrode positions. More notable exceptions to this simple spatial relationship can occur, particularly if:

1. The source is in a fissure

2. The source is primarily in sulci

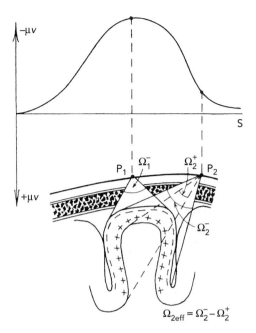

Figure 5.26. Volume conductor theory for a cortical source that occupies a gyrus. The distribution of the amplitude of the voltage that reaches the scalp surface is shown in line S. The current that reaches the electrode from the cortical source is equivalent to the area contained by the lines that begin at the cortex and converge on the electrodes P1 or P2. For P1, the gyral convexity source projects only negativity. For P2, the source projects both negativity from the outer cortex and positivity from the inner cortex of the sulcus (shown by the area between the dashed lines that converge on P2). The cancellation effect of the inner cortex and the outer cortex (negativity added to positivity; the area within the dashed lines subtracted from that within the solid lines converging on P2) reduces the voltage of the signal detected by P2 as shown in line S. Although the figure is drawn in two dimensions, it is intended to represent three-dimensional space with the lines leading from the cortex to electrodes representing the sides of an approximately conical space. The amount of current reaching P1 and P2 then depends on the solid angle (signified by the omega characters in the figure) subtending the volume. (From Gloor P. Neuronal generators and the problem of localization in electroencephalography: application of volume conductor theory to electroencephalography. J Clin Neurophysiol. 1985;2:327–354.)

3. Cortical anatomy and orientation have been altered (e.g., in cerebral palsy)

4. Skull thickness has been altered. There is relative thinning as in early infancy, thickening as in certain bone diseases, or a gap in the skull from prior trauma or surgery.

The way in which electrical current is transmitted throughout the body is referred to as *volume conductor theory*. Figure 5.26 illustrates an example of volume conductor theory applied to EEG in which the outer layers of the cortex are producing a momentary signal that is negatively charged. In the example, the EEG source involves an entire gyrus. Because the pyramidal cell postsynaptic potentials generate a circuit of current flow throughout the length of each cell, one end of the pyramidal cell always has the opposite electrical polarity from the other (in Fig. 5.26 the outer cortex is negative and the inner cortex is positive). In Figure 5.26, the addition of all polarities oriented toward the recording electrode determines the final voltage at the scalp. Typically, there is negativity in the outer cortex pointing toward the recording electrodes, and positive in the deeper cortex.

The scalp EEG can be imagined as a constantly changing relief map in which the map is composed of hills and valleys whose height or depth represents a particular voltage that is determined by the changing currents arising from underlying pyramidal cell postsynaptic potentials. Electrode placement is used to accurately map the contours of the changing voltages over the scalp surface. Each electrode, therefore, represents a spatial voltage sample point. The more electrodes used, the more faithfully they will map the actual contours of the scalp potentials. If too few electrodes are used, then the presence or absence of EEG changes in some areas of the scalp may be missed. This is somewhat analogous to digital sampling of EEG or audio signals: if too few samples are taken, then high-frequency waveforms cannot be recorded, but if too few electrodes are used, then voltage changes over areas in between will be completely missed. A certain number of electrodes is necessary to avoid spatial undersampling.

3.3. Electrode Positions

Routine EEG recording uses 21 scalp electrode positions. These are placed according to the International 10-20 System of electrode placement described in Figure 5.27.[11,93,94] Although this is sufficient for routine clinical recording, to accurately sample the scalp surface for the detection of small signals generated by EP recordings, or for research in quantitative EEG analysis and intracranial localization, it is estimated that at least 100 electrodes would be needed.[95]

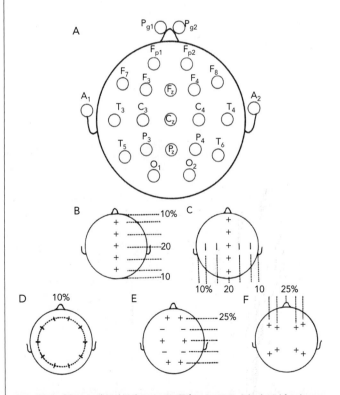

Figure 5.27. Steps outlined in the text (A–F) for measuring the head for the placement of the 10-20 system. (From Fisch BJ. Fisch and Spehlmann's Digital and Analog EEG Primer. Amsterdam: Elsevier; 1999.)

Spatial sampling in neonates also follows the 10-20 system, but because of the reduced head size fewer electrodes are used. F7, F3, F8, F4, P7, P3, P8, and P4 are excluded. Fp1 and Fp2 may be replaced by more posterior electrodes, Fp3 located midway between Fp1 and F3 and Fp4 located midway between Fp2 and F4, consistent with the relatively more posterior location of the frontal lobes in relation to skull measurements at that age.[1,11] If A1 and A2 cannot be applied to the earlobe, then the mastoid position (M1, M2) is used.[96,97] As illustrated in Figures 5.27 and 5.28, each recording electrode is named with a letter indicating the head region and a subscript number indicating the side of the head, with odd numbers on the left and even numbers on the right and "z" for the midline. The further the electrodes are placed laterally from the midline, the higher the subscript number (e.g., P7 is lateral to P3). Measurements of the head are made with a measuring tape. Calipers or other methods should never be used. Measurements are all based on four landmarks: the nasion (lower forehead between the eyes), the inion (bone protuberance in the midline back of the head), and the left and right preauricular point (immediately anterior to the auditory canal). Measurements are made sequentially as shown in Figure 5.27 and summarized as follows:

1. The midline distance between the inion and nasion is measured. Beginning at 10% of the total distance above the inion (or nasion), a scalp mark is placed with a wax pencil. Then three more marks are placed at intervals of 20% of the total nasion-to-inion distance to establish the positions for Fz, Cz, and Pz.

2. The coronal distance between the left and right preauricular points intersecting with Cz is measured. Points at 20% and 40% of the total distance are then placed from Cz on the left and right to mark the positions for C3, C4, T7, and T8.

3. The distance around the head that passes through T7, T8, and the points 10% above the inion and nasion is measured by placing the measuring tape around the patient's head. Once that measurement is obtained, Fp1 is placed at 5% of the total distance on the circumferential line to the left of the midline. Then marks are placed at intervals of 10% of the total distance around the head, with the last mark at the Fp2 position. These marks establish the positions for F7, T7, P7, O1, O2, P8, T8, F8, and Fp2.

4. The front-to-back distance from Fp1 and Fp2 running through C3 and C4 to O1 and O2, respectively, is measured on each side. At half the distance between Fp1 and C3 on the left, and Fp2 and C4 on the right, F3 and F4 positions are marked, respectively. Similarly, the midpoints

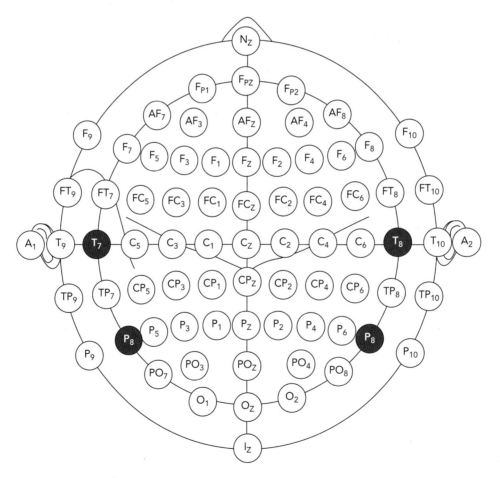

Figure 5.28. *The 10% system of electrode placement is shown, with T7, T8, P7, and P8 replacing the formerly named T3, T4, T5, and T6 electrodes to maintain naming consistency. The added electrodes at 10% distances are named according to the surrounding 10-20 electrodes. Note that in recording an anterior temporal source that FT9 and FT10 placement is usually superior to F7 and F8, which are located over the posterior lateral frontal lobes.*

between C3 and O1 on the left and C4 and O2 on the right give the positions for P3 and P4.

5. Next, the measurements are taken from F7 to F8 through Fz to define the transverse coordinates for F3 at the midpoint between F3 and Fz, and for F4 halfway between Fz and F8. Similarly, measurements from T5 to T6 through Pz locate the transverse coordinates for P3 midway between T5 and Pz and for P4 midway between Pz and T6.

If an electrode cannot be placed (due to scalp defects, bandages, or monitors), then the nearest available electrode site of the "10-10" combinatorial system should be used, and the corresponding electrode on the other side of the head should be moved to the same mirror image position. The electroencephalographer should keep in mind that there is no substitute for the careful approach to measure the head outlined above. Unfortunately, it is also the procedure in which some technologists take shortcuts. With the advent of digital EEG and video, it is reasonable to request that the technologist include the electrode measurement and application process in the video recording of each EEG as a quality control measure. In some clinical situations (e.g., presurgical epilepsy monitoring), better localization may require using more than 21 electrodes. In such cases, selected additional electrodes are placed according to the 10-10 system described in Figure 5.28.

Several common electrode positions are not defined by the 10-20 or combinatorial 10-10 system. Ground electrodes are generally placed at Fpz and recording reference electrodes in regions not susceptible to artifact, generally near the parietal vertex (e.g., CPz or linked P1 and P2). Additional electrodes can be placed to better define activity arising from the anterior temporal regions. T1 and T2 are placed by measuring the distance between the external auditory meatus and the outer canthus of the eye, then placing each electrode one-third of this distance anterior to the tragus and up 1 cm.[98] Sphenoidal electrodes (Chapter #6) are thin flexible wire electrodes placed using a small-gauge hypodermic introducer needle, which is then removed. These electrodes can also improve recording from the anterior temporal regions, but their added value compared to basal temporal scalp electrodes such as T1 and T2 is small.[99] Sphenoidal electrodes are inserted below the zygomatic arch between the coronoid and condylar processes of the mandible, about 2.5 cm anterior to the tragus, to a depth of approximately 4 cm.[100]

With 10-20 system placement, interelectrode distances are between 4 and 6 cm. The advent of digital EEG allows recording from a higher number of electrodes simultaneously. Higher electrode density (typically 64, 128, or 256 electrodes) can improve spatial resolution of EEG signals and source localization techniques.[11] The most commonly used expanded electrode position system, the 10-10 system (see Fig. 5.28), defines locations and a modified combinatorial nomenclature for additional electrodes (77 electrodes total) placed between and below positions of the 10-20 system.[11] This improves spatial sampling, especially for inferolateral and basal temporal, orbitofrontal, and occipital regions (Fig. 5.28). The 10-10 system replaces the names of T3/T4 and T5/T6 with more consistent T7/T8 and P7/P8 (see Fig. 5.28, black electrode positions). As

a result of this change, all electrode positions along the same sagittal line have the same postscripted number. In addition, all electrodes designated by the same letter lie in the same coronal line. Electrodes between 10-20 positions are named by combining the letters for the electrodes anterior and posterior to the intervening position and/or the numbers on either side of the intervening position; for instance, an electrode between C3 and P3 becomes CP3, an electrode between Cz and C3 becomes C1, and an electrode in the center between Cz, Pz, C3, and P3 becomes CP1. The first intermediate transverse positions are designated AF rather than FpF. Subtemporal chain electrodes (F9/F10, T9/T10, and P9/P10) are located 10% inferior to standard frontotemporal electrodes. An extension of the 10-10 system describes additional posterior positions 10% below posterior temporal and occipital electrodes (PO9/PO10, O9/O10) as well as another row of electrodes 10% inferior to the subtemporal chain (F11/F12, FT11/FT12, T11/T12, TP11/TP12, P11/P12, PO11/PO12, and O11/O12).[11]

There is no accepted standard electrode placement for high-density EEG with more than 10-10 electrodes.[11] A 10-5 system has been proposed, extending up to 345 electrode locations,[101] but has not been accepted as a standard. Because of the time required to measure and place so many electrodes, most high-density EEG systems utilize caps or nets with embedded electrodes. The locations of electrodes are determined by digitization in three-dimensional space using electromagnetic digitizers or multiple-camera photogrammetry systems.[102]

The exact role of expanded electrode systems in clinical EEG remains unclear.[11] Currently, the most common use is in presurgical evaluation for patients with drug-resistant epilepsy. Additional electrodes are useful for localization of epileptiform activity and particularly for source localization techniques.[76,103] The precision of source localization, however, appears to plateau at around 100 electrodes for distributed inverse models,[104] although advanced conductivity models and surface Laplacian estimates may increase the utility of higher-density arrays.[95] It is not known whether high-density EEG increases the yield of epileptiform activity in patients with epilepsy compared to standard EEG. High-density EEG may have disadvantages. Placement of additional electrodes can be time-consuming for technologists and uncomfortable for patients. Higher electrode numbers may not provide clinically useful information in patients undergoing EEG for indications other than epilepsy. Because vendors of commercial EEG systems rarely include 10-10 nomenclature in jackboxes, creation of electrode input protocols and montages may be difficult and prone to error. In some systems, electrodes may be labeled only with numbers, making it difficult to visualize the relationships between neighboring electrodes and to underlying brain regions. Visual review of more than 32 channels of EEG is cumbersome and often slow, and readers may default to a limited channel view, defeating the purpose of increased spatial sampling.

3.4. Differential Amplification, Electrode Derivations, and Polarity

Physiological electrical currents are detected using differential amplifiers. Each amplifier has two electrode inputs, named

Input Terminal 1 and Input Terminal 2. The amplifiers subtract the voltage of the Input 2 electrode from the Input 1 electrode (Input 1 − Input 2 = recorded EEG signal), hence *differential* amplification. Differential amplification is used for the recording of all bioelectrical signals, including ECG, EMG, and EEG. The advantage of differential amplifiers is that they cancel external noise. The most common sources of noise arise from other electrical devices. In environments where current is provided at 60 or 50 cycles/sec, the electrical interference nearly equally contaminates both Input 1 and 2 electrode wires with 60- or 50-cycle signals. Because the differential amplifier subtracts the Input 2 signal from the Input 1 signal, the electrical interference that is equal in both inputs cancels out and is removed from the signal. However, because differential amplification is used, the absolute voltage value at electrodes attached to either Input 1 or 2 is never known; only the difference between them is known. Fortunately, by comparing a number of electrode positions, the EEG can give a good approximation of the activity at a particular scalp location relative to other locations.

As noted above and illustrated in Figure 5.26, the currents flowing through the scalp have a polarity that is either positive or negative. The comparison of electrodes by differential amplification yields a difference in voltage and assigns the output a polarity (negative or positive). As described above, the signal output and its polarity are achieved by subtracting the voltages between Input 1 and 2. The voltage is displayed on the EEG monitor or recording paper by the distance the signal deviates from the zero baseline. The polarity is displayed according to the direction the waveform deflects (above or below the baseline). If the voltage in the electrode in Input 1 is −50 μV and the voltage in the electrode in input 2 is +50 μV, then the EEG signal will be Input 1 minus Input 2, or in this case (−50) − (+50) = −100 μV. In addition to knowing that Input 1 is subtracted from Input 2, the electroencephalographer has to understand how the amplifier orients the direction of the waveforms upward or downward to indicate the relative polarity of the signal.

As shown in Figure 5.29, the convention for biological recording is that if Input 1 is more negative than Input 2, the output signal will deflect upward, whereas if Input 1 is more positive than Input 2, then the output signal will deflect downward. This is the same as stating that if Input 2 is more positive than Input 1, then the signal will deflect upward, and if Input 2 is more negative than Input 1, then the signal will deflect downward. Also, if the polarity and voltage in the Input 1 electrode are the same as in the Input 2 electrode, then the output signal will be a flat line (zero).

At this point readers should test their understanding of the information presented in Figure 5.29 by answering the following question:

A potential of −70 μV in Input 1 and −80 μV in Input 2 of an EEG amplifier yields what voltage and what direction of signal deflection?

(A) +10 and downward
(B) −10 and upward
(C) −150 and downward
(D) −150 and upward

Differential Amplification
    (Input 1) − (Input 2) = EEG signal

Polarity Convention
    Input 1 < Input 2 ⟶ Upward signal deflection
    Input 1 > Input 2 ⟶ Downward signal deflection
    Input 1 = Input 2 ⟶ No signal change (flat line)

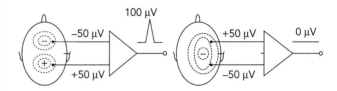

Figure 5.29. Biological amplifiers use differential amplification in which the voltage in the electrode plugged into Input 2 is subtracted from the voltage in the electrode(s) plugged into Input 1. In EEG, EMG, and EP recording, by convention if the relative voltage difference is negative, the signal will deflect upward, and if positive, downward. However, as shown in the figure, the voltage source in the brain can produce opposite deflections depending on whether the Input 1 or Input 2 electrode is closer to the scalp source.

The answer is located at the very end of the section; do not look until you have tried to answer the question on your own.

3.5. Scalp Current Field Localization: Spatial Filtering

Scalp potential fields overlap and vary in size and location. Widely distributed fields are often higher in amplitude than fields that occupy a small area of the scalp. When viewed simultaneously, smaller fields are frequently obscured by or lost in the higher-amplitude widespread fields. However, there is a way to spatially filter out the more widespread fields so that the more localized ones can be easily seen. The use of spatial filters is extremely important because many EEG signals, such as epileptiform spikes, often occupy small scalp areas.

The electrodes in Inputs 1 and 2 of each line of amplified EEG signal channel displayed are referred to as the *electrode derivation*. Derivations are written with the name of the electrode in Input 1 followed by the name of the electrode in Input 2, separated by a hyphen (e.g., Fp1-F3). All derivations are also mathematical expressions. In Fp1-F3, the output of the differential amplifier displayed on the monitor screen will be the voltage detected at Fp1 minus the voltage detected at F3 or Fp1-F3.

A derivation is referred to as *bipolar* if it consists of adjacent electrodes on the scalp. Fp1-F3 is therefore a bipolar derivation because Fp1 and F3 are located next to each other. In contrast to bipolar derivations, those with longer interelectrode distances are referred to as *referential*. An example of a typical referential derivation is Fp1-A1.

A display that consists of a combination of derivations is referred to as a *montage*. Montages that use long interelectrode distances are referential montages, whereas those that use bipolar derivations are referred to as bipolar montages. The use of bipolar versus reference montages allows the electroencephalographer to visualize localized versus widespread scalp fields.

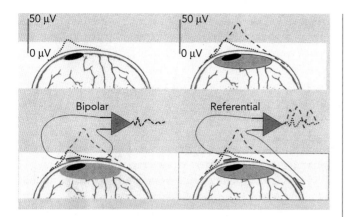

Figure 5.30. Filtering effects of interelectrode distance on the recording of underlying EEG scalp potential fields. The more closely spaced bipolar electrodes (left) filter out the more widespread field (gray cortical area) because both inputs see the same voltage. The more localized field (black cortical area) is clearly displayed. The more widely spaced referential electrodes display a combination of both fields in which the more localized field (black cortical area) is obscured by the larger field (gray cortical area) but the larger field is now seen (see also the discussion in the text).

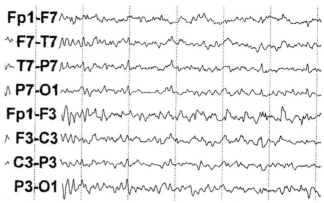

Figure 5.31. A longitudinal bipolar montage records a left hemisphere seizure that is not visible. (From Fisch BJ, Padin-Rosado J. EEG localization and interpretation. In: Fisch BJ, ed. Epilepsy and Intensive Care Monitoring. New York: Demos Medical Publishing; 2010:57–76.)

The concept of spatial filtering is illustrated in Figure 5.30. The bipolar derivation (closely spaced electrodes) on the left side of Figure 5.30 shows the electrode in Input 1 immediately overlying a cortical generator represented by the black oval area, and the Input 2 electrode is outside the area of the black cortical generator. Both electrodes are within the field of the larger underlying cortical generator represented by the gray oval area. As Input 2 is subtracted from Input 1, the activity in the black area is accurately represented as the difference between the two electrodes (black dashed line waveform at the amplifier output). In contrast, the larger gray field produces a similar voltage at both Input 1 and 2 electrodes in the bipolar derivation and is therefore filtered out by cancellation.

The referential derivation on the right side of Figure 5.30 has a much larger interelectrode distance. The Input 1 electrode is within the field of both the small black cortical area and the larger gray cortical area, whereas the Input 2 electrode is outside of both fields. This means that it will amplify a summation of both fields. The advantage is that it "sees" the signal from the larger gray cortical generator that is eliminated from the bipolar recording. The disadvantage is that by combining the two generators, the localized black field is obscured in the larger signal produced by the gray field. The spatial filtering effect shown in Figure 5.30 explains how widespread fields can be removed from the recording. It also illustrates that overall EEG amplitude increases with increasing interelectrode distances. This tends to occur with distances up to about 10 cm. This is also the reason why EEGs performed for the determination of electrocerebral inactivity (brain death) are recorded with long interelectrode distances. Early in the history of EEG, clinical schools developed that strongly stressed the exclusive use of either bipolar or referential recording. Neither is superior to the other; they are simply viewed as different spatial filters that emphasize different aspects of the scalp topography of EEG voltage fields. Montages are constructed in either a linear anterior-to-posterior or transverse pattern across the scalp

to simplify interpretation. Bipolar montages are constructed in overlapping chains (e.g., Fp1-F3 followed by F3-C3) in either an anterior-to-posterior direction (*longitudinal bipolar montages*) or in a transverse left-to-right direction (*transverse bipolar montages*). Referential montages are usually displayed with electrodes in successive channels in an anterior-to-posterior direction, with the same reference electrode (or electrodes) in Input 2 of every channel.

Longitudinal and transverse bipolar montages are both used because scalp voltage fields can be asymmetrical along either anterior-to-posterior or transverse axis. Such asymmetries can only be reliably assessed by either using both a longitudinal and a transverse bipolar montage, or by using one bipolar montage and reference montage. This is dramatically illustrated in Figures 5.31 through 5.33.[105] Each figure shows the same epoch of EEG recording. A widespread left frontal seizure is not visible in the longitudinal bipolar montage (Fig. 5.31) but becomes easily visible in the transverse bipolar montage (Fig. 5.32) and in the referential montage (Fig. 5.33). The Input 2 reference of the referential montage consists of an electrode placed at the top of the sternum and an electrode placed over the C6 vertebral protuberance and is referred to as a noncephalic neck–chest reference. It has the advantage of eliminating reference contamination by the scalp but is sometimes overwhelmed by the ECG signal. This illustration also makes the important point that for some patients it is not sufficient to review the record using only one montage because important electrographic events can be missed.

3.6. Selecting Spatial Filters: Montage Design

There are five commonly used montage designs, and each has a unique spatial filtering characteristic. The montages that can produce the severest filtering of widespread fields and the greatest enhancement of highly localized fields are the longitudinal bipolar and transverse bipolar montages (described earlier). These montages are followed, in order of greatest to least in filtering of widespread fields, as follows: the Laplacian montage, the average reference montage, and the common reference montage.

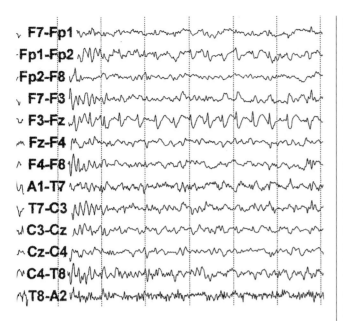

Figure 5.32. *The same recorded epoch as in Figure 5.31 using a transverse bipolar montage now clearly reveals the presence of an electrographic seizure most easily seen in the fifth channel (F3-Fz). (From Fisch BJ. EEG localization and interpretation. In: Fisch BJ, ed. Epilepsy and Intensive Care Monitoring. New York: Demos Medical Publishing; 2010:57–76.)*

The *Laplacian montage* is implemented as a local average reference montage in which the electrode in Input 1 is referred to a combination of the immediately surrounding electrodes in Input 2—for example, Cz − ¼ (Fz + C3 + Pz + C4). Each channel of the montage has a different reference combination in Input 2 that depends on the location of the electrode in Input 1. The Laplacian montage complements the bipolar one when identifying highly localized fields with low amplitude, such as a focal electrographic seizure onset. A reduced filtering effect that produces less suppression of regional fields can be achieved by a Laplacian montage that incorporates all electrodes on the scalp except the Input 1 electrode into the

reference. This is done by weighting the contributions of the reference electrodes according to their distances from the Input 1 electrode—in other words, the farther away the Input 2 electrode is from the Input 1 electrode, the less it contributes to the combined voltage of the Input 2 electrodes. This montage is not commercially available but can be implemented on many systems using a spreadsheet.[106]

The *average reference montage* consists of a single electrode in Input 1 referred to a combination of all or most of the remaining scalp electrodes. The average reference montage is good for viewing highly localized medium- to high-amplitude fields and somewhat more widespread regional fields. When a high-amplitude or very widespread activity occurs, the average reference itself will contain that activity, sometimes producing a confusing picture. For example, eye movement waveforms that typically have a voltage field maximum at Fp1 and Fp2 will often appear upside-down simultaneously in the occipital electrodes O1 and O2, not because there are eye movement potentials in O1 and O2 but because the activity is actually coming from the reference electrodes that include the activity detected by Fp1 and Fp2. Therefore, it is important to be aware that waveforms that appear upside-down in distant head regions in an average reference montage are likely to be due to reference contamination. However, *the electrodes with the highest amplitude are almost always closest to the true source of the activity.*

The *common reference montage* consists of the same one or two electrodes in Input 2 in all channels of the montage. The common reference montage produces the least attenuation of widespread fields, particularly when the reference electrodes are not placed on the head (e.g., noncephalic neck–chest reference). A widely used reference montage uses the A1 and A2 ear reference electrodes. All left-sided electrodes are often referenced to A1, with all right-sided electrodes referenced to A2. A1 and A2 reference electrodes are particularly useful during sleep when high-amplitude activity is occurring over the central head regions that would otherwise contaminate the

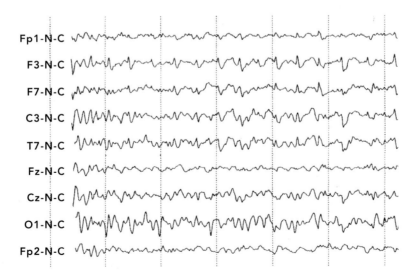

Figure 5.33. *The same recorded epoch as in Figures 5.31 and 5.32 using a noncephalic neck–chest electrode pair reference reveals the widespread seizure with maximal amplitude epileptiform spikes at F3 and very little activity at Fz. (From Fisch BJ. EEG localization and interpretation. In: Fisch BJ, ed. Epilepsy and Intensive Care Monitoring. New York: Demos Medical Publishing; 2010:57–76.)*

reference electrodes with excessive activity. In contrast, during wakefulness, a common reference montage using Cz is often used because central activity is generally low in amplitude and the relative absence of muscle at the vertex makes it less likely that Cz will be contaminated with muscle artifact. The advantage of the common reference montage, particularly the noncephalic neck–chest reference, is that it produces a simple view of the scalp field, where the Input 1 electrode whose channel has the highest amplitude identifies the scalp location with the field maxima. As will be seen in the following section, this works well unless the reference electrode is within the field of interest (reference contamination).

ACNS guidelines propose a minimum set of simple, linear montages that are sufficient for localization and at the same time facilitate standardization across EEG laboratories.[52] Guideline recommendations include the following:

Use of both bipolar and referential montages, with at least 16 channels of simultaneous recording, incorporating all 21 electrodes of the 10-20 system

Clear labeling of each channel of the montage by electrode derivations

Organization in straight unbroken lines with equal interelectrode distances

Placement of anterior derivations above posterior and left derivations above right

Inclusion of an ECG channel.

Additional montages are suggested for 10-10 system and/or sphenoidal electrodes.[52]

3.7. Localizing Current Fields: Phase Changes and Differential Amplification

Localization using bipolar montages is accomplished by analyzing phase orientation (the upward or downward deflection of the waveform) and amplitude. Localization using reference montages is accomplished mainly by analyzing amplitude. Bipolar localization depends on changes in phase between channels. Phase refers to the upward or downward direction of a waveform. A phase reversal has occurred if the phase has changed direction from up to down or from down to up. Figure 5.34 shows an example of a phase reversal between Channels 1 (derivation Fp1-F3) and 2 (derivation F3-C3).

The rules for localization in bipolar montages are summarized in Box 5.1. Examples of these rules are illustrated in Figures 5.34 through 5.37. The electrodes in these figures are shown as black circles and the lines leading from them plug into Input 1 (the higher line going into the derivation) or Input 2 (the lower line going into the derivation). They are arranged as a longitudinal bipolar montage.

Figure 5.34 shows an instrumental phase reversal between channels with the derivations Fp1-F3 and F3-C3. The field over the scalp is displayed by the dashed lines with the highest voltage not covered by an electrode. The field potential is negative. Therefore, the Channel 1 deflection is downward (Input 1 is

more positive than Input 2) but the deflection in Channel 2 is upward (Input 1 is more negative than Input 2) (see Fig. 5.29). The third channel deflection is also upward because Input 1 is more negative than Input 2. The last channel shows no deflection because both electrodes, P3 and O1, are the same. *The electrode common to both channels that reverse phase localizes the maximum field potential to that common electrode.* In this case that is F3.

Figure 5.34 illustrates the concept of *instrumental phase reversal* because it is the instrument (i.e., the way the electrodes are arranged with the Input 2 electrode becoming the Input 1 electrode in the next channel) that causes the phase reversal. In contrast, a true phase reversal would mean that two different polarities are simultaneously present in adjacent cortical areas. The occurrence of a true phase reversal of cortical polarity would produce two instrumental phase reversals in a linear chain of bipolar electrodes. In the event that there is no phase reversal in a bipolar chain (i.e., all the waveforms point in the same direction), then the field maximum is closest to the electrode at the end of the chain that shows the most rapid change in voltage (highest amplitude) in successive channels. This is referred to as the end-of-chain phenomenon. It is localizing to the electrode at the end of the electrode chain and does not suggest the source is deep in the brain.

Figure 5.35 illustrates an instrumental phase reversal with cancellation in an intervening channel. The field on the scalp has a negative polarity with maximal voltage in the center of the dashed lines. The first channel deflection is downward because Input 1 is more positive than Input 2. The second

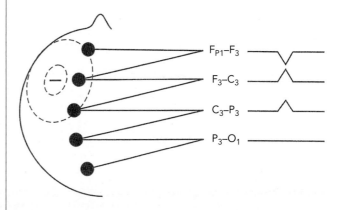

Figure 5.34. Instrumental phase reversal.

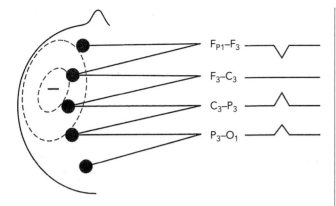

Figure 5.35. Instrumental phase reversal with cancellation in an intervening channel.

channel is flat because the Input 1 and 2 electrodes, F3 and C3, see the same voltage. The third channel deflects upward and is reversed from the first channel because Input 1 is more negative than Input 2. *The intervening channel with cancellation (F3-C3) localizes the field maximum on the scalp to be between the electrodes F3-C3. This phenomena is referred to as a zone of isopotentiality.*

Figure 5.36 illustrates the end-of-chain phenomena with cancellation. Channel 1 electrodes detect the highest voltage, but because it is the same in both electrodes the output is zero, a flat line. As in Figure 5.29 this localizes the field maximum between those two electrodes (Fp1 and F3) at the end of the bipolar chain. The next channel shows an upward deflection because Input 1 is more negative than Input 2. The same applies to the third channel. The fourth channel is flat because there is no voltage difference between those electrodes.

Without the accompanying head figure it is reasonable to ask why the changes in this montage are not interpreted as a positive field in the back of the head instead of a negative field in the front of the head. While that is possible, it is unlikely. The rate of change in voltage (i.e., the amplitude of the waveform) between two electrodes is usually greatest near the field maximum and least at a distance from it. In this case, the presence of a higher amplitude in Channel 2 than in Channel 3 localizes the signal source (field maximum) to the front of the head.

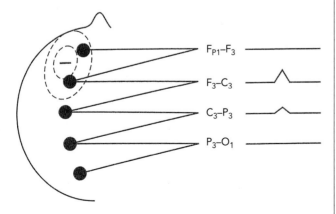

Figure 5.36. End-of-chain phenomena with cancellation.

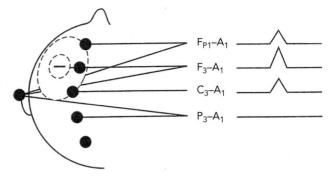

Figure 5.37. Ipsilateral ear reference with the negative field maximum closest to F3.

A true phase reversal is shown in Figure 5.38. True phase reversals are rarely encountered except in situations where the cortical anatomy has been disturbed (e.g., cerebral palsy) or more often as an identifying feature of benign childhood epilepsy with centro-midtemporal spikes (BCECTS). In these patients the epileptiform spike arises at an angle that is parallel to the cortical surface, allowing both the negativity from the outer cortex and the positivity from the deeper cortex to be seen simultaneously. In BCECTS the positivity projects anteriorly, for example appearing as an upward deflection in Fp1-F3 and downward in F3-C3 (positivity at F3). The negativity appears more posteriorly and in this example would appear as a downward deflection in C3-P3 and upward in P3-O1 (negativity at P3). The anterior positivity is typically lower in voltage than the posterior negativity and may require increasing the gain or the use of a neck–chest reference to be visualized.

As noted above, common reference montages are most useful for identifying widespread scalp fields and least useful for identifying highly localized low-amplitude fields. Although localization is usually simple with a reference montage, a confusing picture arises when the reference electrode(s) are within

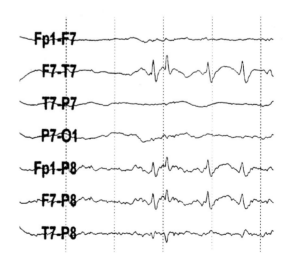

Figure 5.38. Tangential dipole with cancellation in bipolar derivations and true phase reversal in common reference derivations; anterior maximal negativity with posterior positivity. (From Fisch BJ, Padin-Rosado J. EEG localization and interpretation. In: Fisch BJ, ed. Epilepsy and Intensive Care Monitoring. New York: Demos Medical Publishing; 2010:57–76.)

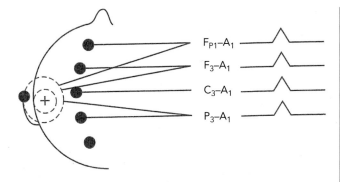

Figure 5.39. *Ipsilateral ear reference with reference contamination. The signal is from the reference electrode as the other electrodes are outside of the scalp field.*

the field of the activity of interest. In that case, the activity in a channel may be coming from the reference instead of the Input 1 electrode. If the reference is not in the scalp field of interest, then the channel with the highest amplitude identifies the Input 1 electrode closest to the field maximum. If all channels containing a reference show the same signal output then the activity is coming from the reference, not the Input 1 electrode.

Figure 5.37 illustrates a reference recording of a negative field in which the reference electrode, A1, is outside of the scalp field. In this case, the derivation with the highest-amplitude signal shows the Input 1 electrode that is closest to the field maximum (F3). The deflections are all upward because Input 1 is more negative than Input 2.

Figure 5.39 illustrates reference contamination. In this example, the reference electrode A1 is within the positive scalp field; the other electrodes are outside of the field. Therefore, the deflection seen in all channels is the same and is upward because for each channel, Input 1 is more negative than Input 2.

Figure 5.40 illustrates how confusing the picture can become when the reference is contaminated with activity also detected by the Input 1 electrodes. Channel 1 deflects downward because the reference is relatively negative (Input 1 is more positive than Input 2). Channel 2 is flat because Input 1 and Input 2 see the same negative voltage. Channel 3 deflects upward because Input 1 is more negative than Input 2, and Channel 4 deflects downward because Input 1 is more positive than Input 2.

A field with a single polarity will not produce waveforms of opposite phase in a referential recording between adjacent

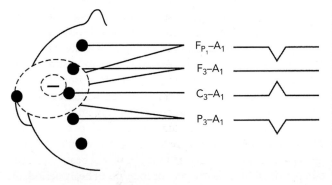

Figure 5.40. *Reference contamination.*

channels unless the reference is contaminated. Two phase reversals as shown in Figure 5.40 (Channel 1 vs. Channel 3 and Channel 3 vs. Channel 4) virtually always assure the reader that reference electrode contamination is occurring. A single-phase reversal in a common reference recording without reference contamination, as shown in the lower three channels in Figure 5.38, represents a true (not instrumental) phase reversal, in that it indicates the presence of a horizontal (tangential) cortical dipole.

An example of how to approach localization is shown in Figure 5.38. In the initial longitudinal bipolar recording epileptiform spikes are present in only one channel, creating a complex problem in localization. The problem is quickly solved by using a reference montage. At the time of EEG interpretation new derivations were selected using a distant reference electrode unlikely to be contaminated by the field of the epileptiform activity. In this case the EEG reader selected the most distant electrode, P8 (opposite side of the head, lateral and posterior) for the reference to explore the activity in Fp1, F7, and T7. The added derivations are in the last three channels in Figure 5.38. They show that there are similar-amplitude spikes in Fp1 and F7. This explains why the first channel is relatively flat (very low-amplitude upward deflections are present): there is cancellation between Fp1 and F7 (if Input 1 and Input 2 are nearly equal, the output is nearly zero). T7-P8 demonstrates a phase reversal with positivity arising from T7. If opposite polarities are subtracted, as shown in the left lower part of Figure 5.29, then the resulting signal will summate to create a higher-amplitude signal than that in either input alone. This effect creates the high-amplitude spikes in Channel 2 (F7-T7). T7 and P7 share a similar-amplitude positivity and therefore cancel out in the third channel. The positivity of P7 in relation to O1 can barely be seen in the fourth channel P7-O1.

3.8. EEG Instruction in Localization

Those who teach EEG should be aware that many, if not most, physicians who read EEGs do not understand how to localize EEG findings. It is a disservice to patients with neurological disorders when teachers fail to emphasize the importance of localization and practicing physicians continue to believe that EEG interpretation is only a matter of pattern recognition. Although it is not possible to reach physicians who have completed their training and are already out in practice, it is possible to improve the skills of those currently being trained.

When training residents and fellows in EEG localization it is helpful to ask certain questions that assess their progress.

1. What is the polarity of an upward deflection in a single channel of recording? Most students initially believe that an upward deflection in a channel is negative. Of course, the correct answer is that there is no way of knowing. In a single channel one never knows if an upward deflection is caused by a negative potential in Input 1 or a positive potential in Input 2. Any misconceptions can usually be further resolved by a discussion of positive occipital sharp transients of sleep (POSTS), because they always deflect upward in the longitudinal bipolar montages.

2. Is a phase reversal an abnormal finding? It is a surprising how often students believe phase reversals are abnormal. This occurs because the student never understood the importance of studying localization and the teacher invoked the concept of phase reversal only in the setting of EEG abnormalities. This situation can be quickly resolved by discussing phase reversals of vertex waves (or other normal waveforms) in bipolar montages.

3. What is the difference between an instrumental phase reversal and a true phase reversal?

Students who can correctly answer these basic questions are well on their way to understanding EEG localization.

Lastly, never allow students to speak in terms of head regions when localizing EEG findings. Instead, insist that they speak in terms of actual scalp spatial sampling points by only using electrode names.

(The answer to the question in the section on differential amplification and polarity is A.)

4. POLYGRAPHY

4.1. Introduction

Polygraphy denotes the simultaneous recording of several physiological and/or behavioral variables. The main reasons for simultaneously recording several variables are to obtain information on behavioral aspects and to differentiate artifacts in the EEG data. These objectives usually do not require precise representation; in many instances, the relevant information concerns only the occurrence of a certain phenomenon or is easily obtained from clearly discernible characteristics of a variable. Therefore, most polygraphic data of interest in EEG studies can be obtained using simple recording methods that allow appreciable distortion of the original data. If, however, the polygraphic variables are of primary concern, then sophisticated and precise recording methods are necessary. In view of the techniques used and the interpretation of the recorded data, these methods go far beyond the simple polygraphic methodology commonly applied to EEG studies. This section of the chapter discusses these simple methods and presents a number of examples of variables that are of interest in certain EEG studies. A classic survey of variables of interest in polygraphic studies and of corresponding recording methods can be found in *Manual of Psychophysiologic Methods*, edited by Venables and Martin.[107]

In practice, polygraphic recordings are made with an EEG apparatus; this may be of primary interest for determining the temporal relations between the EEG and the other signals, which reflect different physiological functions and/or behavioral states. Unfortunately, the frequency characteristics and the magnitude ranges of many signals of interest for polygraphic studies fall outside those provided by a conventional EEG recording system; moreover, they might not be recordable due to the electrical characteristics of the input circuit of the EEG recorder. Such signals, therefore, require special provisions, such as the use of specialized preamplifiers or input couplers to obtain an adaptation or a conversion; in this way, the recording of such signals can be carried out with the EEG apparatus. Many variables of interest in polygraphic studies, such as blood pressure, respiratory parameters, temperature, and electrodermal signals, vary slowly as a function of time; therefore, their recording requires highly sensitive universal DC amplifiers that are equipped with means of sensitivity control and adjustable high- and low-pass filters for selection of the appropriate frequency response. Modern EEG recorders have low-sensitivity auxiliary input terminals that also permit DC recording; these inputs can be used to record other signals of sufficiently large amplitude (e.g., in Fig. 5.48, the traces indicated by EDG, STIM, BUTTON PRESS, and TIME CODE). When the EEG is used to record different physiological and/or behavioral variables simultaneously, employing separate recording systems, the time relations between the various types of signals must be preserved by using a form of time indexing or time marking on both recording media.

4.2. Cardiovascular Variables: ECG and Heart Rate

There are several reasons for recording the ECG simultaneously with the EEG. It may be desirable in specific cardiovascular or cerebrovascular studies. In most cases, however, the ECG recording is not intended to carry out a vascular study but only serves as an indicator of ECG artifacts in EEG records or as a general parameter of vegetative functions; in these latter circumstances, one is mainly interested in the heart rate. An ECG can be recorded perfectly using an EEG system because the electrical characteristics of its input circuit and the provisions commonly available for adjustment of frequency response and gain are adequate. The bandwidth required for appropriate ECG recording goes from 0.8 to 60 Hz; the recording sensitivity required is approximately 1 mV/cm using conventional ECG electrode placements. When the ECG electrodes are placed on the chest wall, a higher sensitivity may be necessary. The subject's behavioral activities might lead to artifacts in the ECG record owing to muscular activity or electrode motion. The latter can be reduced significantly by using an appropriate type of electrode, such as cup electrodes with a jelly bridge between skin and electrode surface. Interference caused by EMG potentials can be minimized by choosing electrode positions carefully and lowering the high-frequency response of the recording system (20 Hz; 3 dB) in order to attenuate the high-frequency EMG potentials. High-frequency filtering can be obtained by means of the EEG apparatus's adjustable HFFs.

Heart rate recording is best carried out by using a series of pulses generated at the top of clearly distinguishable R waves of the ECG. If, however, owing to less favorable electrode positions, the R wave cannot be easily distinguished, extra signal processing must be applied. This processing may consist of high-pass filtering and/or the introduction of a refractory period, during which the instrument is insensitive. Commercially available heart frequency meters or heart rate counters usually have such provisions. Heart rate measurements may be given in terms of the number of beats over a certain period of time (heart rate) or in terms of heart period, the average interval between a number of successive heartbeats.

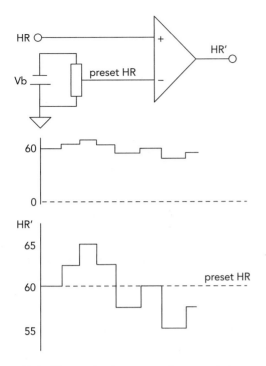

Figure 5.41. *Method for recording instantaneous heart rate; the momentary heart period value, transformed into heart rate, is plotted in relation to an adjustable preset mean heart rate value.*

Because heart rate and heart period are reciprocal, the instrument, although calibrated in terms of heart rate, may have a meter deflection or another output signal proportional to T_{int}, the interval between successive heartbeats. In the available instruments, heart rate is more commonly presented than heart period. In some applications of polygraphy, the main interest is not in the nominal heart rate but rather in heart rate changes and the relation to other physiological, psychological, or behavioral variables. So that relatively small heart rate changes can be distinguished, the recording is best carried out with a preadjusted preset heart rate value. The model given in Figure 5.41 demonstrates a simple method for subtracting a preset value from the heart rate meter's electrical output.

4.3. Plethysmography

Plethysmography is the measurement of the variations in organ or limb volume due to changes in the quantity of blood it contains. Because such volume changes are related to increased or decreased blood flow, plethysmographic methods can be used to obtain estimates of the mean blood flow rate and of pulsatile and transient flow changes. Plethysmography may be of interest in psychophysiological studies because mental processes and behavioral responses are often accompanied by changes in cardiovascular parameters such as blood flow, accompanied by measurable changes in limb volume. Continuous measurement of the latter is known as pulse volume plethysmography; under certain restricted conditions, an index of the blood flow rate can also be obtained in this way.[108] In most psychophysiological studies, however, the variable of interest relates to changes in blood volume and in blood volume pulses. The most common methods for measuring limb volume changes are pneumatic

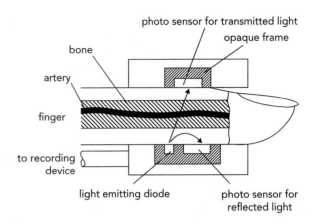

Figure 5.42. *Principle of finger photophethysmography for transmission and reflection of light.*

and photoelectric. Pneumatic methods are more complicated and are not suited to psychophysiological studies. Therefore, although providing more precise information, they are much less frequently used in polygraphy. Figure 5.42 shows the principle of finger photoplethysmography. Two photosensors measure the transmission and reflection of the light emitted from a light-emitting diode. The fraction of transmitted light through the tissue and the fraction of reflected light from the tissue depend on the amount of blood in the tissue. Extensive discussions of the measuring principles, amplifier recorder requirements, and recorded waveforms have been provided by Lader[109] (pneumatic plethysmography) and Weiman[110] (photoplethysmography).

Impedance plethysmography of the thorax for impedance cardiography is the basis for noninvasive beat-to-beat monitoring of the stroke volume.[111] An electric current is introduced into the thorax and the corresponding voltage is measured. The ratio of voltage to current yields the impedance (Z) that varies (in a very simplified model) with the amount and distribution of blood in the thorax. Based on the ECG, the phonocardiogram, and the impedance cardiogram, the stroke volume can be determined noninvasively (Fig. 5.43).

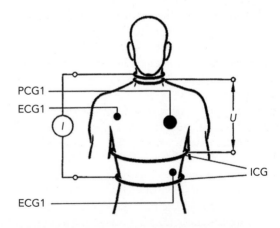

Figure 5.43. *Principle of impedance cardiography. (Adapted from Gratze G, Fortin J, Holler A, et al. A software package for noninvasive, real-time beat-to-beat monitoring of stroke volume, blood pressure, total peripheral resistance and for assessment of autonomic function. Comp Biol Med. 1998;28:121–142.)*

4.4. Blood Pressure

The catheter-manometer system is, at present, the fundamental method for continuous accurate measurement of the full arterial pressure waveform. It is, however, an invasive procedure and should be avoided unless the introduction of a catheter into an artery is necessary. The Riva–Rocci–Korotkoff method (using an upper-arm cuff and a stethoscope) is noninvasive and commonly used, but it does not provide continuous blood pressure information. However, most automatic methods developed for determining blood pressure have been based primarily on the Riva–Rocci–Korotkoff method. For instance, Roy and Weiss[112] described a technique for providing intermittent determinations of the systolic and diastolic blood pressure obtained over several heartbeats. Such systems have also become commercially available. The method indicated above, however, is sensitive to motion artifacts and not continuous.

Penaz[113] developed an important improvement in the noninvasive determination of blood pressure, using continuous measurement of the blood pressure in the finger. This method uses a finger cuff. By means of a servosystem the cuff pressure is maintained equal to the arterial pressure. This is achieved by minimizing arterial diameter changes using a photoelectric plethysmographic feedback method. The working principle is shown in the block diagram of Figure 5.44. The further development and evaluation of methods based on this approach[114,115] are of great interest to those interested in the continuous

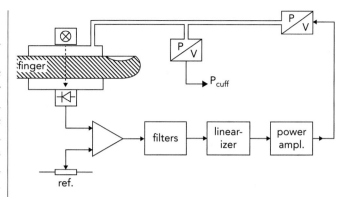

Figure 5.44. Block diagram of a system for noninvasive continuous recording of blood pressure based on the Penas principle. *(From Wesseling KH, van Bemmel RA, van Dieren A, et al. Two methods for the assessment of hemodynamic parameters for epidemiology. Acta Cardiol. 1978;33:84–87.)*

measurement and recording of beat-to-beat diastolic, systolic, and mean arterial pressure. This is indicated in Figure 5.45 by the similarity between continuous blood pressure and curves recorded simultaneously by way of noninvasive and invasive methods.

The noninvasive blood pressure measurement was first applied during anesthesia[116] and was also used for long-term sleep monitoring in patients with systemic hypertension and sleep-related breathing disorders.[117] The new system gives

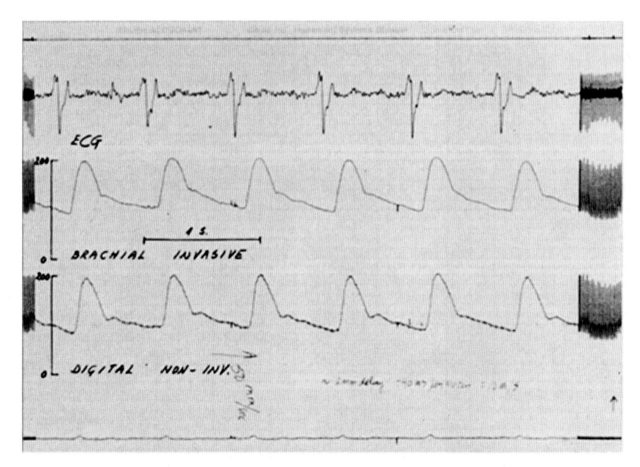

Figure 5.45. Example of a comparison of continuous recordings of blood pressure, simultaneously obtained by an invasive (intra-arterial) and a noninvasive method. The latter was performed according to the method introduced by Penaz.

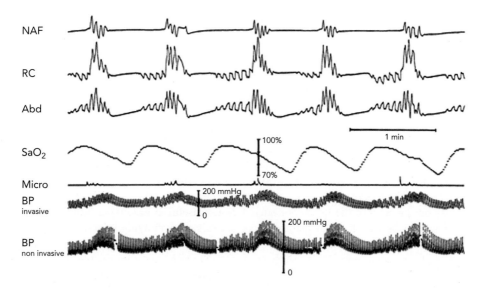

Figure 5.46. *Recording of a patient with obstructive apneas and systemic hypertension. The trace of nasal airflow (NAF) shows complete cessation of respiratory flow, whereas rib cage (RC) and abdominal (Abd) movement show obstructive efforts. Noninvasive (FINA-PRES) and invasive BP were recorded in parallel. SaO₂, oxygen saturation; micro, snoring noise. (From Penzel T, Ducke E, Peter JJ, et al. Noninvasive monitoring of blood pressure in a sleep laboratory. In: Ruddel H, Curio I, eds. Non-invasive Continuous Blood Pressure Measurement. Frankfurt am Main: Peter Lang; 1991.)*

valuable results if the position of the finger cuff is carefully controlled. An example of blood pressure recordings combined with respiratory measurements is displayed in Figure 5.46. A review of noninvasive continuous blood pressure measurements is found in Ruddel and Curio[118] and more recently in Parati et al.[119]

The capacity for measuring acute and immediate changes in autonomic, EEG, and hemodynamic physiological variables during different sleep stages on a continuous basis has played an important role in enabling us to understand the interplay between changes in EEG and changes in circulatory variables and in autonomic neural functions. In this way the possibility of recording, simultaneously with the EEG, heart rate variability and blood pressure, among other cardiovascular physiological variables, has advanced our understanding of mechanisms linking sleep and cardiovascular physiology.[120]

4.5. Respiration

The polygraphic recording of respiration patterns is usually carried out to obtain information on frequency or changes in inhalation depth. Changes in thoracic volume due to respiratory movements are usually estimated in terms of changes in the perimeter of the chest; this can be measured easily using transducers working on the principle of a strain gauge. This type of respiration transducer, which is commercially available, consists of a tube with an inner diameter of a few millimeters; the tube is elastic and is filled with an electrically conductive liquid substance with measurable electrical resistance. The tube forms part of a belt strapped around the chest; changes in resistance resulting from changes in chest perimeter are measured by means of the Wheatstone bridge circuit. The rather smooth slow respiration rhythm can be recorded with most EEGs without further measures; in case of insufficient frequency response of the apparatus, an AC voltage can

be applied to the measuring bridge instead of a DC voltage. If respiration must be recorded from moving subjects, chest size changes not related to respiration can easily occur; in these cases other methods should be chosen.

A simple and easily implemented solution is to use a thermistor or equivalent temperature-sensitive device placed in the mouth and/or nostrils. Such a device works as a respiration transducer by signaling the characteristic differences in temperature of the inspired and expired air. With such methods, information is obtained on frequency and depth of chest movements. Other methods should be used to obtain exact information concerning respiratory volume.

For information concerning respiratory volume and thoracic and abdominal diameter, variations can be measured by using elastic strips provided with strain gauges that encircle the thorax and abdomen at the level of the nipple and umbilicus, respectively. Using both measurements, the respiratory volume can be calculated. This method of spirometry determines the contributions of the chest and abdomen separately, then adds them together to mimic the total spirometric volume. As the chest and abdominal volumes change during breathing, changes in electrical impedance of the bands are related to changes in the spirometric volume contributions using a calibration and gain adjustment procedure. A combination of techniques is commonly used, namely the measurement of oral and nasal airflow and, in parallel, of abdominal and thoracic movements (see Fig. 5.44). The best method to analyze the respiratory effort is the use of an esophageal pressure probe.[121]

Pulse oximetry is a noninvasive method to measure the arterial hemoglobin oxygen saturation (SaO₂). Continuous pulse and oxygen saturation measurements are obtained by ear, finger, or soft probes (Fig. 5.44 contains an example). The widely used pulse oximeter quantifies the SaO₂ as a percentage based on spectrophometric and photoelectric plethysmography.[122]

The SaO_2 measurement yields information about the effectiveness of respiration and is recommended for all types of sleep monitoring.[123]

4.6. Electrodermal Activities

The variations of skin electrical properties in relation to psychological variables, commonly known as the galvanic skin response or psychogalvanic response, consist of changes of the electrical conductivity of the skin or of the electrical skin potential, which can be measured by means of electrodes placed on the palms or the soles in reference to an electrode placed elsewhere, such as on the back of the hand. For such measurements, the skin should be intact; when placing the electrodes, the skin must not be abraded. The skin potential can be recorded easily, but it is unstable and of little use; therefore, skin electrical conductance is much more useful in this respect. It can be estimated by applying a constant voltage across two electrodes and by measuring the resulting electrical current. This is, of course, equivalent to estimating the skin's electrical resistance by applying a constant current through the electrodes and measuring the voltage across the electrodes. Skin resistance can vary considerably among subjects, assuming values from kilo- to mega-ohms. Transient skin resistance responses related to sudden changes in psychological state are in the order of 100 ohms. In practice, it is preferable to measure the skin's electrical conductance by applying a constant voltage instead of measuring resistance by applying a constant electrical current. The circuit of Figure 5.47A illustrates a constant voltage measuring procedure. An example of electrodermal responses recorded during the performance of a contingent negative variation (CNV) paradigm from a normal subject is shown in Figure 5.48. Classic extensive basic and practical information about electrodermal response recording can be found in the publications by Venables and Martin[124] and Montagu[125] on skin resistance potential. Interesting applications of the galvanic skin response in psychophysiological studies have been published by Deschaumes-Molinaro et al.[126] and Vernet-Maury et al.[127]

4.7. Eye Movements

In various behavioral studies, particularly in sleep research for the recognition of sleep stages, eye movement recording (i.e., by means of the EOG) is necessary. Eye movement recording is also useful in EEG recording for identifying eye movement artifacts and studying lambda waves. An example of the former is the recording of eye movement in relation to that of the CNV; in this case, it is possible either to reject the EEG epochs in which the amount of eye movement exceeds a certain predetermined threshold in order to carry out selective averaging,[128] or to average the EOG along with the CNV to obtain an indication of the reliability of the latter. Preferably, the method chosen for identifying eye movement artifacts will make use of the electrical field generated by the eyes.

The EOG is, in general, easy to measure. The usual principle of EOG measurement is demonstrated by the model in Figure 5.49. As a result of the corneoretinal standing potential (the cornea is positive relative to the fundus), a DC potential difference can be measured either between the pair of electrodes (EH) placed in a horizontal plane near the canthi of the eyes or between the two electrodes (EV) placed in a vertical plane, depending on the position of the eyeballs. Any change in eyeball position results in a corresponding change of these two potential differences. DC recording is necessary to measure exact eye positions, whereas AC recording suffices for determining changes in eye position.

To carry out a DC recording of the EOG, nonpolarizable electrodes must be used, and the drift of the electrodes' offset potential should be taken into account. To obtain sufficiently high recording sensitivity, the electrodes must be placed as close to the eye as possible. To record horizontal movements, the electrodes should be placed near the external canthus of each eye; for vertical movements, the electrodes should be placed closely above and below one or both eyes. The EOG measured in this way has an amplitude of about 20 μV per degree of eyeball rotation. A frequency response up to about 30 Hz is adequate to record the most rapid eye movements, and thus an EEG recording channel can be used without further provision (see, e.g., trace EOG (HOR) in Fig. 5.48).

Other principles for monitoring eye movement in clinical EEG are the measurement of changes in impedance related to eye movements[129] and use of a pressure transducer system.[130] In the latter system, a thin membrane covering one end of a tube held in a spectacle frame is adjusted to touch the closed eyelid lightly. A pressure transducer connected at the other end of the tube detects pressure changes from eye movements. Robinson[131] describes eye movement recording systems that also provide information on exact eye position; eye position is determined from the voltage generated by an alternating magnetic field in a coil embedded in a scleral contact lens worn by

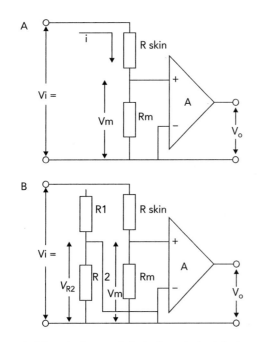

*Figure 5.47. **A:** Schematic diagram of a basic electronic circuit for the recording of electrodermal conductance using a constant voltage source. **B:** Bridge circuit for the recording of relatively small changes in electrodermal conductance.*

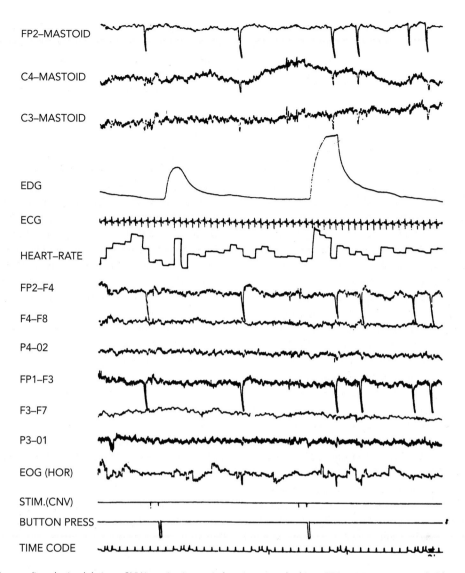

Figure 5.48. Polygraphic recording obtained during a CNV investigation carried out in a normal subject. EEG activities were recorded from three direct-coupled CNV derivations (FP$_2$, C$_4$, and C$_3$ against linked mastoids) and six anteroposterior symmetrical derivations. Other variables recorded were electrodermogram (EDG), ECG, instantaneous heart rate, EOG horizontal eye movements [EOG (HOR)], CNV stimulus presentation [STIM (CNV)], the button press, and a time code (1-second intervals).

the subject. A similar photoelectric device[132] consists of four small infrared-detecting cells mounted on a light spectacle frame together with a miniature infrared (9,000 Å)-emitting diode. This system, which preserves maximum vision field size,

has a resolution less than 1 minute of arc, a bandwidth of 1,000 Hz, and 5% linearity of the maximum range. Currently, systems are available for recording and analysis of a wide range of eye movements, both saccadic and smooth pursuit movements,

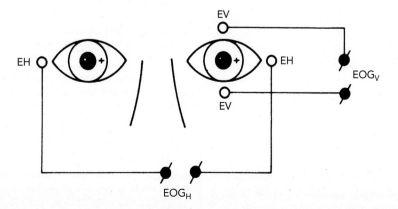

Figure 5.49. Positions of EOG electrodes for recording horizontal and vertical movements.

where these are measured using a scleral reflection technique (IRIS instrument).[133] Saccades are rapid eye movements that move the line of sight between successive points of fixation; they are among the best understood of movements, possessing dynamic properties that are easily measured.[134] Saccades have become a popular means to study motor control and cognitive functions, particularly in conjunction with other techniques such as EEG, EPs, functional imaging, and transcranial magnetic stimulation.

4.8. Muscle Activity (EMG) and Body Movements

4.8.1. EMG Activity

Part of the electrical activity of muscles (EMG) can be recorded easily by means of either surface electrodes placed on the surrounding skin or needle electrodes inserted into muscle. The frequency range of EMG potentials, particularly those recorded by means of intramuscular needles, goes far beyond the frequency response of most EEG recording systems. Even an EEG apparatus having an ink-jet writing system with a frequency response of up to 1,000 Hz does not provide a faithful representation of EMG potentials. However, by using a filter giving the highest possible EEG frequency response (usually 70–100 Hz), the recording of EMG activity in most instances adequately indicates the presence of muscular activity and may even provide a rough quantitative measure of the amount of such activity. In certain applications, the latter can be better obtained by passing the EMG potentials through a two-way rectifier, the output of which is integrated with a specified time window. In this way, a rectified smoothed EMG record is obtained. It is important to recognize that the recording of EMG along with EEG signals may be necessary for the interpretation of some specific features of the latter, particularly in those applications such as EEG-based brain–computer interfaces that rely on automated measurements of EEG features.[135]

In behavioral studies, EMG activity is often used to monitor the onset of certain motor activities such as limb movements. Another way of determining limb movements and tremor[136] makes use of displacement transducers or accelerometers. A special form of tremor is the microtremor (microvibration), which is a phenomenon of the sensorimotor system that is modulated by central mechanisms.[137] This microtremor is in the frequency range of 8 to 12 Hz (amplitudes of 1–10 μm) and can be recorded by an accelerometer fixed, for example, at the wrist. The measurement range of such an accelerometer should be between −5 and +5 g, such that the microtremor in the range of 10 mV/g can be recorded. Using accelerometry and EMG recordings of the forearm, the characteristics of physiological tremor have been studied.[138] In addition to the microtremor, ballistic movements also be measured with this technique.

4.8.2. Body Movements

The detection of limb or whole-body movements can be of interest in sleep studies. With a simple wrist actigraph, a discrimination between sleep and wakefulness is possible.[139] Actigraphy has been found to be reliable for evaluating sleep patterns in patients with insomnia, for studying the effect of treatments designed to improve sleep, and in the diagnosis of circadian rhythm disorders, including shift work.[140] Such a wrist actigraph can be used not only in the sleep laboratory but also with outpatients to obtain a picture of the degree of sleep disturbances within, for example, a 24-hour period.[123] The recording of movements along with the EEG can also be important in differentiating authentic EEG activity from movement artifacts,[141] which, on the basis of their waveforms and amplitude, cannot easily be identified as noncerebral. When monitoring movements of epileptic patients to determine the occurrence of seizures during the night, transducers indicating global body movements may be used. With this objective, conventional pressure or displacement transducers or other special methods developed for the detection of whole-body[142] or limb movements[143] have been used. Another method used for recording body movements is the static charge-sensitive bed, which consists of a mattress with two electrically active layers[144] with the use of filters; the ballistocardiogram, respiratory signals, and movement signals can be differentiated. For movement quantification in epileptic seizures, advanced video analysis methods can be applied.[145] Markers at landmark points are attached to the patient. Then EEG is acquired and the movement of the body parts is monitored using special cameras. Quantified motion trajectories of body parts can be extracted based on the fiducial markers. The trajectories reflect the motion pattern of patients during seizures, yielding additional movement information that cannot be obtained from standard video-EEG analysis.

4.9. Temperature

Temperature can be measured with sensors placed on the skin or with a rectal probe. Temperature measurements are especially important in sleep studies. Detailed studies of rectal temperature recordings over 24 hours are reported by Stephan and Dorow.[146] Experiments with long-term isolation of subjects have revealed a relationship between the body temperature and the duration and stage of sleep.[147] To assess core temperature, for instance during monitoring under anesthesia, tympanic temperature may be recorded.

REFERENCES

1. Kuratani J, Pearl PL, Sullivan L, et al. American Clinical Neurophysiology Society Guideline 5: Minimum Technical Standards for Pediatric Electroencephalography. *J Clin Neurophysiol*. 2016;33(4):320–323.
2. Sinha SR, Sullivan L, Sabau D, et al. American Clinical Neurophysiology Society Guideline 1: Minimum Technical Requirements for Performing Clinical Electroencephalography. *J Clin Neurophysiol*. 2016;33(4):303–307.
3. Ebner A, Sciarretta G, Epstein CM, Nuwer M. EEG instrumentation. The International Federation of Clinical Neurophysiology. *Electroencephalogr Clin Neurophysiol Suppl*. 1999;52:7–10.
4. Nuwer MR, Comi G, Emerson R, et al. IFCN standards for digital recording of clinical EEG. The International Federation of Clinical Neurophysiology. *Electroencephalogr Clin Neurophysiol Suppl*. 1999;52:11–14.
5. Cooper R. Electrodes. *Am J EEG Technol*. 1963;3:91–101.
6. Kolls BJ, Olson DM, Gallentine WB, Skeen MB, Skidmore CT, Sinha SR. Electroencephalography leads placed by nontechnologists using a template system produce signals equal in quality to technologist-applied, collodion disk leads. *J Clin Neurophysiol*. 2012;29(1):42–49.

7. Young GB, Ives JR, Chapman MG, Mirsattari SM. A comparison of subdermal wire electrodes with collodion-applied disk electrodes in long-term EEG recordings in ICU. *Clin Neurophysiol.* 2006;117(6):1376–1379.

8. Vulliemoz S, Perrig S, Pellise D, et al. Imaging compatible electrodes for continuous electroencephalogram monitoring in the intensive care unit. *J Clin Neurophysiol.* 2009;26(4):236–243.

9. Mirsattari SM, Davies-Schinkel C, Young GB, Sharpe MD, Ives JR, Lee DH. Usefulness of a 1.5 T MRI-compatible EEG electrode system for routine use in the intensive care unit of a tertiary care hospital. *Epilepsy Res.* 2009;84(1):28–32.

10. Scott NK. Infection prevention: 2013 review and update for neurodiagnostic technologists. *Neurodiagnostic J.* 2013;53(4):271–288.

11. Acharya JN, Hani A, Cheek J, Thirumala P, Tsuchida TN. American Clinical Neurophysiology Society Guideline 2: Guidelines for Standard Electrode Position Nomenclature. *J Clin Neurophysiol.* 2016;33(4):308–311.

12. Van Drongelen W. *Signal Processing for Neuroscientists.* Burlington, MA: Academic Press; 2007.

13. Vanhatalo S, Voipio J, Kaila K. Full-band EEG (FbEEG): an emerging standard in electroencephalography. *Clin Neurophysiol.* 2005;116(1):1–8.

14. Horowitz P, Hill W. *The Art of Electronics.* 2nd ed. Cambridge, England: Cambridge University Press; 1989.

15. Halford JJ, Sabau D, Drislane FW, Tsuchida TN, Sinha SR. American Clinical Neurophysiology Society Guideline 4: Recording Clinical EEG on Digital Media. *J Clin Neurophysiol.* 2016;33(4):317–319.

16. International Electrotechnical Commission. IEC 60601-1-11:2015: Medical electrical equipment—Part 1-11: General requirements for basic safety and essential performance 2015.

17. Berger H. Uber das Elektrenkephalogramm des Menschen IV. (English translation by P. Gloor: On the Electroencephalogram of Man, *Electroenceph Clin Neurophysiol.* 1969, Suppl 28). *Arch Psychiat Nervenheil.* 1929;97:6–26.

18. Burks AW, Burks AR. The ENIAC: first general-purpose electronic computer. 1981. *MD Comput.* 1995;12(3):206–212.

19. Farley B, Clark W, Gilmore J, Frishkopf L. *Computer Techniques for the Study of Patterns in the Electroencephalogram.* Lincoln Laboratories, MIT; 1957.

20. Cooley JW, Tukey JW. An algorithm for the machine calculation of complex Fourier series. *Math Comput.* 1965;19:297–301.

21. Technology and equipment review: digital electroencephalographs. *J Clin Neurophysiol.* 1993;10(3):378–392.

22. Halford JJ, Schalkoff RJ, Satterfield KE, et al. Comparison of a novel dry electrode headset to standard routine EEG in veterans. *J Clin Neurophysiol.* 2016;33(6):530–537.

23. Wyckoff SN, Sherlin LH, Ford NL, Dalke D. Validation of a wireless dry electrode system for electroencephalography. *J Neuroengineering Rehab.* 2015;12:95.

24. Ladino LD, Voll A, Dash D, et al. StatNet electroencephalogram: a fast and reliable option to diagnose nonconvulsive status epilepticus in emergency setting. *Can J Neurol Sci.* 2016;43(2):254–260.

25. Herman ST, Abend NS, Bleck TP, et al. Consensus statement on continuous EEG in critically ill adults and children, part II: personnel, technical specifications, and clinical practice. *J Clin Neurophysiol.* 2015;32(2):96–108.

26. Usakli AB. Improvement of EEG signal acquisition: an electrical aspect for state of the art of front end. *Comput Intell Neurosci.* 2010:630649.

27. Gordon M. Artifacts created by imbalanced electrode impedance. *Am J EEG Technol.* 1980;20:149–160.

28. Ferree TC, Luu P, Russell GS, Tucker DM. Scalp electrode impedance, infection risk, and EEG data quality. *Clin Neurophysiol.* 2001;112(3):536–544.

29. Park YS, Hochberg LR, Eskandar EN, Cash SS, Truccolo W. Early detection of human focal seizures based on cortical multiunit activity. *Conf Proc IEEE Eng Med Biol Soc.* 2014;2014:5796–5799.

30. Escabi MA, Read HL, Viventi J, et al. A high-density, high-channel count, multiplexed muECoG array for auditory-cortex recordings. *J Neurophysiol.* 2014;112(6):1566–1583.

31. Van Gompel JJ, Stead SM, Giannini C, et al. Phase I trial: safety and feasibility of intracranial electroencephalography using hybrid subdural electrodes containing macro- and microelectrode arrays. *Neurosurg Focus.* 2008;25(3):E23.

32. Stacey WC, Kellis S, Greger B, et al. Potential for unreliable interpretation of EEG recorded with microelectrodes. *Epilepsia.* 2013;54(8):1391–1401.

33. Schomer DL. Ambulatory EEG telemetry: how good is it? *J Clin Neurophysiol.* 2006;23(4):294–305.

34. Stecker MM, Sabau D, Sullivan L, et al. American Clinical Neurophysiology Society Guideline 6: Minimum Technical Standards for EEG Recording in Suspected Cerebral Death. *J Clin Neurophysiol.* 2016;33(4):324–327.

35. Blum DE. Computer-based electroencephalography: technical basics, basis for new applications, and potential pitfalls. *Electroencephalogr Clin Neurophysiol.* 1998;106(2):118–126.

36. Bridgers SL, Ebersole JS. Ambulatory cassette EEG in clinical practice. *Neurology.* 1985;35(12):1767–1768.

37. Gilliam F, Kuzniecky R, Faught E. Ambulatory EEG monitoring. *J Clin Neurophysiol.* 1999;16(2):111–115.

38. Schomer DL. Advances in EEG telemetry. *Suppl Clin Neurophysiol.* 2004;57:477–484.

39. Seneviratne U, Mohamed A, Cook M, D'Souza W. The utility of ambulatory electroencephalography in routine clinical practice: a critical review. *Epilepsy Res.* 2013;105(1-2):1–12.

40. Patel AC, Thornton RC, Mitchell TN, Michell AW. Advances in EEG: home video telemetry, high frequency oscillations and electrical source imaging. *Journal of neurology.* 2016;263(10):2139–2144.

41. Budinger TF. Biomonitoring with wireless communications. *Ann Rev Biomed Engineering.* 2003;5:383–412.

42. Guideline 12: guidelines for long-term monitoring for epilepsy. *Am J Electroneurodiagnostic Technol.* 2008;48(4):265–286.

43. Michel V, Mazzola L, Lemesle M, Vercueil L. Long-term EEG in adults: Sleep-deprived EEG (SDE), ambulatory EEG (Amb-EEG) and long-term video-EEG recording (LTVER). *Neurophysiol Clin.* 2015;45(1):47–64.

44. Ives JR. Video recording during long-term EEG monitoring of epileptic patients. *Adv Neurol.* 1987;46:1–11.

45. Burgess RC. Design and evolution of a system for long-term electroencephalographic and video monitoring of epilepsy patients. *Methods.* 2001;25(2):231–248.

46. Ives J. 'Time-scribe': a universal time writer for any EEG/polygraph chart recorder. *Electroencephalogr Clin Neurophysiol.* 1984;57(4):388–391.

47. Risk WS. Viewing speed and frequency resolution in digital EEG. *Electroencephalogr Clin Neurophysiol.* 1993;87(6):347–353.

48. Bresenham J. Algorithm for computer control of a digital plotter. *IBM Systems J.* 1965;4(1):25–30.

49. Epstein CM. Aliasing in the visual EEG: a potential pitfall of video display technology. *Clin Neurophysiol.* 2003;114(10):1974–1976.

50. Swartz BE. The advantages of digital over analog recording techniques. *Electroencephalogr Clin Neurophysiol.* 1998;106(2):113–117.

51. Levy SR, Berg AT, Testa FM, Novotny EJ, Jr., Chiappa KH. Comparison of digital and conventional EEG interpretation. *J Clin Neurophysiol.* 1998;15(6):476–480.

52. Acharya JN, Hani AJ, Thirumala PD, Tsuchida TN. American Clinical Neurophysiology Society Guideline 3: A Proposal for Standard Montages to Be Used in Clinical EEG. *J Clin Neurophysiol.* 2016;33(4):312–316.

53. Klein SA. Inverting a Laplacian topography map. *Brain Topogr.* 1993;6(1):79–82.

54. Widmann A, Schroger E, Maess B. Digital filter design for electrophysiological data: a practical approach. *J Neurosci Methods.* 2015;250:34-46.

55. Oppenheim AV, Shafer P, Buck JR. *Discrete-Time Signal Processing.* 2nd ed. Englewood Cliffs, NJ: Prentice-Hall, Inc.; 1998.

56. Gustafsson F. Determining the initial states in forward-backward filtering. *IEEE Trans Signal Processing.* 1996;44(4):988–992.

57. Brigham EO. The fast Fourier transform and its applications. In: Prentice Hall Signal Processing Series; Oppenheim AV, ed. Englewood Cliffs: Prentice Hall; 1988.

58. Cook EW, 3rd, Miller GA. Digital filtering: background and tutorial for psychophysiologists. *Psychophysiology.* 1992;29(3):350–367.

59. Duffy FH, Hughes JR, Miranda F, Bernad P, Cook P. Status of quantitative EEG (QEEG) in clinical practice, 1994. *Clin Electroencephalogr.* 1994;25(4):VI–XXII.

60. Nuwer MR, Lehmann D, da Silva FL, Matsuoka S, Sutherling W, Vibert JF. IFCN guidelines for topographic and frequency analysis of EEGs and EPs. The International Federation of Clinical Neurophysiology. *Electroencephalogr Clin Neurophysiol Suppl.* 1999;52:15–20.

61. Uriguen JA, Garcia-Zapirain B. EEG artifact removal: state-of-the-art and guidelines. *J Neural Eng.* 2015;12(3):031001.

62. Barlow JS. Automatic elimination of electrode-pop artifacts in EEG's. *IEEE Trans Biomed Eng.* 1986;33(5):517–521.

63. Ille N, Berg P, Scherg M. Artifact correction of the ongoing EEG using spatial filters based on artifact and brain signal topographies. *J Clin Neurophysiol.* 2002;19(2):113–124.

64. Astolfi L, Cincotti F, Mattia D, et al. Removal of ocular artifacts for high-resolution EEG studies: a simulation study. *Conf Proc IEEE Eng Med Biol Soc.* 2006;1:976–979.

65. Robert C, Gaudy JF, Limoge A. Electroencephalogram processing using neural networks. *Clin Neurophysiol.* 2002;113(5):694–701.

66. Gotman J. Automatic detection of seizures and spikes. *J Clin Neurophysiol.* 1999;16(2):130–140.

67. Qu H, Gotman J. A seizure warning system for long-term epilepsy monitoring. *Neurology.* 1995;45(12):2250–2254.

68. Wilson SB. A neural network method for automatic and incremental learning applied to patient-dependent seizure detection. *Clin Neurophysiol.* 2005;116(8):1785–1795.

69. Wilson SB, Turner CA, Emerson RG, Scheuer ML. Spike detection II: automatic, perception-based detection and clustering. *Clin Neurophysiol.* 1999;110(3):404–411.

70. Nuwer MR. The development of EEG brain mapping. *J Clin Neurophysiol.* 1990;7(4):459–471.

71. Perrin F, Pernier J, Bertrand O, Echallier JF. Spherical splines for scalp potential and current density mapping. *Electroencephalogr Clin Neurophysiol.* 1989;72(2):184–187.

72. Soong AC, Lind JC, Shaw GR, Koles ZJ. Systematic comparisons of interpolation techniques in topographic brain mapping. *Electroencephalogr Clin Neurophysiol.* 1993;87(4):185–195.

73. Ebersole JS, Wade PB. Spike voltage topography identifies two types of frontotemporal epileptic foci. *Neurology.* 1991;41(9):1425–1433.

74. Gotman J. Noninvasive methods for evaluating the localization and propagation of epileptic activity. *Epilepsia.* 2003;44(Suppl 12):21–29.

75. Scherg M, Ebersole JS. Brain source imaging of focal and multifocal epileptiform EEG activity. *Neurophysiol Clin.* 1994;24(1):51–60.

76. Mouthaan BE, Rados M, Barsi P, et al. Current use of imaging and electromagnetic source localization procedures in epilepsy surgery centers across Europe. *Epilepsia.* 2016;57(5):770–776.

77. He B, Sohrabpour A. Imaging epileptogenic brain using high-density EEG source imaging and MRI. *Clin Neurophysiol.* 2016;127(1):5–7.

78. Feng R, Hu J, Pan L, et al. Application of 256-channel dense array electroencephalographic source imaging in presurgical workup of temporal lobe epilepsy. *Clin Neurophysiol.* 2016;127(1):108–116.

79. Alarcon G, Binnie CD, Elwes RD, Polkey CE. Power spectrum and intracranial EEG patterns at seizure onset in partial epilepsy. *Electroencephalogr Clin Neurophysiol.* 1995;94(5):326–337.

80. Scheuer ML, Wilson SB. Data analysis for continuous EEG monitoring in the ICU: seeing the forest and the trees. *J Clin Neurophysiol.* 2004;21(5):353–378.

81. Haider HA, Esteller R, Hahn CD, et al. Sensitivity of quantitative EEG for seizure identification in the intensive care unit. *Neurology.* 2016;87(9):935–944.

82. Topjian AA, Fry M, Jawad AF, et al. Detection of electrographic seizures by critical care providers using color density spectral array after cardiac arrest is feasible. *Pediatr Crit Care Med.* 2015;16(5):461–467.

83. Rapoport DM, Ayappa I, Norman RG, Herman ST. NPSG data interchange: dealing with the Tower of Babel. *Sleep.* 2006;29(5):599–600.

84. Kemp B, Olivan J. European data format 'plus' (EDF+), an EDF alike standard format for the exchange of physiological data. *Clin Neurophysiol.* 2003;114(9):1755–1761.

85. Hellmann G, Kuhn M, Prosch M, Spreng M. Extensible biosignal (EBS) file format: simple method for EEG data exchange. *Electroencephalogr Clin Neurophysiol.* 1996;99(5):426–431.

86. ASTM. ASTM E1467-94 Standard specification for transferring digital neurophysiological data between independent computer systems. Available from: ASTM, 1916 Race Street, Philadelphia, PA 19103.

87. Guideline TS1: Standard for transferring digital neurophysiological data between independent computer systems. Acns.org/pdf/guidelines/technical-standard-1.pdf. 2008.

88. Wagenaar JB, Worrell GA, Ives Z, Matthias D, Litt B, Schulze-Bonhage A. Collaborating and sharing data in epilepsy research. *J Clin Neurophysiol.* 2015;32(3):235–239.

89. Sauleau P, Despatin J, Cheng X, et al. National French survey on teletransmission of EEG recordings: more than a simple technological challenge. *Neurophysiol Clin.* 2016;46(2):109–118.

90. Health Insurance Portability and Accountability Act of 1996, Public Law 104-191.

91. U.S. Department of Health and Human Services. HIPAA administrative simplification: regulation text. 45 CFR parts 160,162 and 164. 2013; http://www.hhs.gov/sites/default/files/hipaa-simplification-201303.pdf, 2016.

92. Gloor P. Neuronal generators and the problem of localization in electroencephalography: application of volume conductor theory to electroencephalography. *J Clin Neurophysiol.* 1985;2(4):327–354.

93. Klem GH, Luders HO, Jasper HH, Elger C. The 10-20 electrode system of the International Federation of Clinical Neurophysiology. *Electroencephalogr Clin Neurophysiol Suppl.* 1999;52:3–6.

94. Fisch BJ. *Fisch and Spehlmann's EEG Primer: Basic Principles of Digital and Analog EEG.* 3rd ed. Amsterdam: Elsevier B.V.; 1999.

95. Srinivasan R, Nunez PL, Tucker DM, Silberstein RB, Cadusch PJ. Spatial sampling and filtering of EEG with spline Laplacians to estimate cortical potentials. *Brain Topogr.* 1996;8(4):355–366.

96. Park KL, Nordli DR. Special considerations in neonatal monitoring. In: Fisch BJ, ed. *Epilepsy and Intensive Care Monitoring.* New York: Demos Medical Publishing; 2010:91–103.

97. Tsuchida TN, Wusthoff CJ, Shellhaas RA, et al. American Clinical Neurophysiology Society standardized EEG terminology and categorization for the description of continuous EEG monitoring in neonates: report of the American Clinical Neurophysiology Society Critical Care Monitoring Committee. *J Clin Neurophysiol.* 2013;30(2):161–173.

98. Silverman D. The anterior temporal electrode and the 10-20 system. *Electroencephalogr Clin Neurophysiol.* 1960;12:735–737.

99. Schomer DL. The sphenoidal electrode: myth and reality. *Epilepsy Behav.* 2003;4(2):192–197.

100. Cherian A, Radhakrishnan A, Parameswaran S, Varma R, Radhakrishnan K. Do sphenoidal electrodes aid in surgical decision making in drug-resistant temporal lobe epilepsy? *Clin Neurophysiol.* 2012;123(3):463–470.

101. Oostenveld R, Praamstra P. The five percent electrode system for high-resolution EEG and ERP measurements. *Clin Neurophysiol.* 2001;112(4):713–719.

102. Kaiboriboon K, Luders HO, Hamaneh M, Turnbull J, Lhatoo SD. EEG source imaging in epilepsy: practicalities and pitfalls. *Nature Rev Neurol.* 2012;8(9):498–507.

103. Wang G, Worrell G, Yang L, Wilke C, He B. Interictal spike analysis of high-density EEG in patients with partial epilepsy. *Clin Neurophysiol.* 2011;122(6):1098–1105.

104. Michel CM, Lantz G, Spinelli L, De Peralta RG, Landis T, Seeck M. 128-channel EEG source imaging in epilepsy: clinical yield and localization precision. *J Clin Neurophysiol.* 2004;21(2):71–83.

105. Fisch BJ. EEG localization and interpretation. In: Fisch BJ, ed. *Epilepsy and Intensive Care Monitoring.* New York: Demos Medical Publishing; 2010:57–76.

106. Lemos MS, Fisch BJ. The weighted average reference montage. *Electroencephalogr Clin Neurophysiol.* 1991;79(5):361–370.

107. Venables PH, Martin I. *A Manual of Psychophysiological Methods.* Amsterdam: North Holland; 1967.

108. Melrose DG, Lynn RB, Rainbow RLG, Wherrell AG. A sensitive digital plethysmograph. *Lancet.* 1964;263(6816):810–812.

109. Lader MH. Pneumatic plethysmography. In: Venables PH, Martin I, eds. *A Manual of Psychophysiological Methods.* Amsterdam: North Holland; 1967:159–183.

110. Weiman J. Photoplethysmography. In: Venables PH, Martin I, eds. *A Manual of Psychophysiological Methods.* Amsterdam: North Holland; 1967:185–217.

111. Gratze G, Fortin J, Holler A, et al. A software package for non-invasive, real-time beat-to-beat monitoring of stroke volume, blood pressure, total peripheral resistance and for assessment of autonomic function. *Comput Biol Med.* 1998;28(2):121–142.

112. Roy R, Weiss M. Automatic blood pressure indicator. *IRE Trans Biomed Electron.* 1962;9:244–246.

113. Penaz J. Photoelectric measurement of blood pressure volume and flow in the finger. In: Alben R, Vogt W, Helbig W, eds. *Digest of the 10th International Conference on Medicine and Biological Engineering.* Vol. 104. Dresden, 1973.

114. Reeben V, Epler M. Detection and many-side use of signals from controlled counter pressure finger cuffs. *Proc Biocapt Paris.* 1975;1:265–270.

115. Wesseling KH, van Bemmel RA, van Dieren A, et al. Two methods for the assessment of hemodynamic parameters for epidemiology. *Acta Cardiol.* 1978;33:84–87.

116. Wesseling KH, Settels JJ, de Wit B. The measurement of continuous finger arterial pressure noninvasively in stationary subjects. In: Schmidt TH, Dembroski TM, Blumchen G, eds. *Biological and Psychological Factors in Cardiovascular Disease.* Berlin: Springer-Verlag; 1986:355–375.

117. Penzel T, Ducke E, Peter JJ. Non-invasive monitoring of blood pressure in a sleep laboratory. In: Ruddel H, Curio I, eds. *Non-invasive Continuous Blood Pressure Measurement: Methods, Evaluations and Applications of the Vascular Unloading Technique.* Frankfurt am Main: Peter Lang; 1991.

118. Ruddel H, Curio I. *Non-invasive monitoring of blood pressure in a sleep laboratory.* Frankfurt am Main: Peter Lang; 1991.

119. Parati G, Ongaro G, Bilo G, et al. Non-invasive beat-to-beat blood pressure monitoring: new developments. *Blood Press Monit.* 2003;8(1):31–36.

120. Murali NS, Svatikova A, Somers VK. Cardiovascular physiology and sleep. *Front Biosci.* 2003;8:s636–652.

121. Roberts S, Davies WL. Comparison of simple (slope based) and more complex (simple syntactic) algorithms for central apnoea detection. In: Chase MH, Lydic R, O'Connor C, eds. *Sleep Research.* Vol. 398. Los Angeles: Brain Information Service/Brain Research Inst.; 1989.

122. West P, George CF, Kryger MH. Dynamic in vivo response characteristics of three oximeters: Hewlett-Packard 47201A, Biox III, and Nellcor N-100. *Sleep.* 1987;10(3):263–271.

123. Penzel T, Stephan K, Kubicki S, Herrmann WM. Integrated sleep analysis, with emphasis on automatic methods. *Epilepsy Res Suppl.* 1991;2:177–204.

124. Venables PH, Martin I. Skin resistance and skin potential. In: Venables PH, Martin I, eds. *A Manual of Psychophysiological Methods.* Amsterdam: North Holland; 1967:53–102.

125. Montagu JD. The psycho-galvanic reflex: a comparison of DC and AC methods of measurement. *J Psychosom Res.* 1964;8:49–65.

126. Deschaumes-Molinaro C, Dittmar A, Vernet-Maury E. Autonomic nervous system response patterns correlate with mental imagery. *Physiol Behav.* 1992;51(5):1021–1027.

127. Vernet-Maury E, Alaoui-Ismaili O, Dittmar A, Delhomme G, Chanel J. Basic emotions induced by odorants: a new approach based on autonomic pattern results. *J Auton Nerv Syst.* 1999;75(2-3):176–183.

128. Papakostopoulos D, Winter A, Newton P. New techniques for the control of eye potential artefacts in multichannel CNV recordings. *Electroencephalogr Clin Neurophysiol.* 1973;34(6):651–653.

129. Sullivan GH, Weltman G. Impedance oculograph: a new technique. *J Appl Physiol.* 1963;18:215–216.

130. Winter AL. A simple eye movement monitoring system for clinical electroencephalography. *Electroencephalogr Clin Neurophysiol.* 1974;37(2):182–184.

131. Robinson DA. A method of measuring eye movement using a scleral search coil in a magnetic field. *IEEE Trans Biomed Eng.* 1963;10:137–145.

132. Gauthier GM, Volle M. Two-dimensional eye movement monitor for clinical and laboratory recordings. *Electroencephalogr Clin Neurophysiol.* 1975;39(3):285–291.

133. Muir SR, MacAskill MR, Herron D, Goelz H, Anderson TJ, Jones RD. EMMA: an eye movement measurement and analysis system. *Australas Phys Eng Sci Med.* 2003;26(1):18–24.

134. Leigh RJ, Kennard C. Using saccades as a research tool in the clinical neurosciences. *Brain.* 2004;127(Pt 3):460–477.

135. Goncharova, II, McFarland DJ, Vaughan TM, Wolpaw JR. EMG contamination of EEG: spectral and topographical characteristics. *Clin Neurophysiol.* 2003;114(9):1580–1593.

136. Oppel F, Umbach WU. A quantitative measurement of tremor. *Electroencephalogr Clin Neurophysiol.* 1977;43(6):885–888.

137. Burne JA, Lippold OC, Pryor M. Proprioceptors and normal tremor. *J Physiol.* 1984;348:559–572.

138. Elble RJ. Characteristics of physiologic tremor in young and elderly adults. *Clin Neurophysiol.* 2003;114(4):624–635.

139. Sadeh A, Alster J, Urbach D, Lavie P. Actigraphically based automatic bedtime sleep-wake scoring: validity and clinical applications. *J Ambul Monit.* 1989;2(3):209–216.

140. Ancoli-Israel S, Cole R, Alessi C, Chambers M, Moorcroft W, Pollak CP. The role of actigraphy in the study of sleep and circadian rhythms. *Sleep.* 2003;26(3):342–392.

141. Buchthal F, Dahl K, Trojaborg W. Simultaneous recording of acceleration and brain waves. *Electroencephalogr Clin Neurophysiol.* 1973;34(5):550–552.

142. van Nimwegen C, Boter J, van Eijnsbergen B. A method for detecting epileptic seizures. *Epilepsia.* 1975;16(5):689–692.

143. Kripke DF, Mullaney DJ, Messin S, Wyborney VG. Wrist actigraphic measures of sleep and rhythms. *Electroencephalogr Clin Neurophysiol.* 1978;44(5):674–676.

144. Alihanka J, Vaahtoranta K, Saarikivi I. A new method for long-term monitoring of the ballistocardiogram, heart rate, and respiration. *Am J Physiol.* 1981;240(5):R384–392.

145. Li Z, Martins da Silva A, Cunha JP. Movement quantification in epileptic seizures: a new approach to video-EEG analysis. *IEEE Trans Biomed Eng.* 2002;49(6):565–573.

146. Stephan K, Dorow R. Circadian variations of core body temperature, performance, and subjective ratings of fatigue in "morning" and "evening" types. In: Redfern PA, Campall IC, Davies JA, eds. *Circadian Rhythms in the Central Nervous System.* Weinheim: Verlagssgesellschaft; 1985:233–236.

147. Zulley J, Wever R, Aschoff J. The dependence of onset and duration of sleep on the circadian rhythm of rectal temperature. *Pflugers Arch.* 1981;391(4):314–318.

6 | ANTEROTEMPORAL, BASAL TEMPORAL, NASOPHARYNGEAL, AND SPHENOIDAL ELECTRODES AND HIGH-DENSITY ARRAYS

ANDREW SCHOMER, MD, PD, MARGITTA SEECK, MD, ANDRES M. KANNER, MD, FANA, FAES, FAAN, TRAVIS STOUB, PHD, AND DONALD L. SCHOMER, MD

ABSTRACT: Temporal lobe epilepsy is the most frequent type of epilepsy of focal origin in adults. Electroencephalographic evaluation for surgical treatment requires accurate localization of epileptic foci. The yield of detection with scalp electrodes depends on three variables: source and extent of the epileptogenic area relative to the scalp electrodes' position; electric field generated by the epileptiform activity and the electric vectors' orientation; and extent of propagation of the epileptiform activity from mesial to temporal lateral regions. Recordings of epileptiform activity of presumed mesial-temporal origin should include additional electrodes such as anterior temporal or basal temporal electrodes or a subtemporal chain. Nasopharyngeal electrodes appear to yield no advantage over anterior temporal or basal temporal electrodes or a subtemporal chain and are associated with discomfort. Sphenoidal electrodes should be considered in special circumstances; reliability is improved if placed under fluoroscopy. High-density scalp recordings allow for even greater resolution and improved spatial sampling.

KEYWORDS: electroencephalography, epilepsy, electrode, temporal lobe, fluoroscopy, scalp

PRINCIPAL REFERENCES

1. Homan RW, Jones MC, Rawat S. Anterior temporal electrodes in complex partial seizures. *Electroencephalogr Clin Neurophysiol.* 1988;70(2):105–109.
2. Goodin DS, Aminoff MJ, Laxer KD. Detection of epileptiform activity by different noninvasive EEG methods in complex partial epilepsy. *Ann Neurol.* 1990;27(3):330–334.
3. Jones D. Recording of the basal electroencephalogram with sphenoidal electrodes. *Electroencephalogr Clin Neurophysiol.* 1951;3(1):100.
4. Rovit RL, Gloor P, Rasmussen T. Sphenoidal electrodes in the electrographic study of patients with temporal lobe epilepsy. An evaluation. *J Neurosurg.* 1961;18:151–158.
5. Ives JR, Gloor P. Update: chronic sphenoidal electrodes. *Electroencephalogr Clin Neurophysiol.* 1978;44(6):789–790.
6. Kanner AM, Ramirez L, Jones JC. The utility of placing sphenoidal electrodes under the foramen ovale with fluoroscopic guidance. *J Clin Neurophysiol.* 1995;12(1):72–81.
7. Sperling MR, Mendius JR, Engel J. Mesial temporal spikes: a simultaneous comparison of sphenoidal, nasopharyngeal, and ear electrodes. *Epilepsia.* 27(1):81–86.
8. Leijten FSS, Huiskamp G-JM, Hilgersom I, Van Huffelen AC. High-resolution source imaging in mesiotemporal lobe epilepsy: a comparison between MEG and simultaneous EEG. *J Clin Neurophysiol.* 20(4):227–238.
9. Plummer C, Harvey AS, Cook M. EEG source localization in focal epilepsy: where are we now? *Epilepsia.* 2008;49(2):201–218.
10. Grieve PG, Emerson RG, Isler JR, Stark RI. Quantitative analysis of spatial sampling error in the infant and adult electroencephalogram. *NeuroImage.* 2004;21(4):1260–1274.

1. INTRODUCTION

Temporal lobe epilepsy (TLE) is the most frequent type of epilepsy of focal origin in adults. It is a heterogeneous type of epilepsy as the epileptogenic zone can be restricted to mesial temporal structures and/or involve temporal lateral neocortex. Accordingly, the yield of detection of epileptiform activity with scalp electrodes depends on the following variables: (i) the source and extent of the epileptogenic area relative to the position of the scalp electrodes, (ii) the electric field generated by the epileptiform activity and the orientation of the electric vectors, and (iii) the extent of propagation of the epileptiform activity from mesial to temporal lateral regions. For example, epileptiform discharges originating in temporal lateral neocortex would be readily recorded with the standard 10-20 mid-temporal scalp electrodes. Unfortunately, such electrodes often fail to detect epileptiform activity of mesial-temporal origin. For one, the amygdala nucleus is not a laminar structure and, therefore, it generates very restricted electrical field potentials. Likewise, the hippocampus, with its "double C shape," appears as a closed loop electrically and generates epileptiform discharges with a vertical dipole that might only be detected by frontotemporal and temporal lateral electrodes if the epileptiform activity were to propagate to those regions.

Several studies have shown that the standard International 10-20 System of scalp electrode placement often fails to identify epileptiform activity of mesial-temporal lobe origin.[1-4] The overall findings of these studies suggest that the lateral and anterior portion of the temporal lobe is not adequately covered using the standard 10-20 system. In the 10-20 system, electrodes F7, F8, T7, T8 (also known as T3-T4), and A1-A2 have been used to record anterior temporal electrical activity. More specifically, electrodes F7 and F8 are positioned over the inferior frontal gyrus and the rostral pars triangularis,[1] while electrodes T7 and T8 are positioned over the middle and superior temporal gyri posterior to the rolandic fissure.[1] Therefore, the angle subtended by these electrodes relative to the mesial temporal source of the epileptiform discharges may often be inadequate (unless it propagates to temporal lateral regions).

This problem was recognized in the first half of the 20th century and led to the development of sphenoidal electrodes

(SEs) and nasopharyngeal electrodes (NPEs). Later on, antero-temporal electrodes (ATEs), mini-sphenoidal electrodes (MSEs), and basal-temporal (scalp) electrodes (BTEs) started to be used in an attempt to avoid the inconvenience and discomfort associated with the insertion of SEs. A subtemporal chain of electrodes, placed inferior to the standard temporal chain, often yields similar resolution without the need for needle placement. More recently, complex, high-density arrays of electrodes have been developed that allow for even greater spatial sampling.

Studies carried out in the 1980s and 1990s reported that SEs and ATEs identified a significantly greater number of epileptiform discharges that were not recorded with the standard temporal electrodes included in the 10-20 system. The noninvasive and user-friendly placement of ATEs led to their use in most epilepsy centers. This chapter reviews the conditions in which SEs, NPEs, ATEs, subtemporal chains, and high-density arrays should be used in patients suspected of suffering from TLE of mesial-temporal origin.

2. TECHNICAL ASPECTS

2.1. Sphenoidal Electrodes

Jones, in 1950, was the first to report the use of SEs.[5] At that time, the electrodes consisted of a fine insulated needle electrode inserted under local anesthesia. The point of entry was under the zygomatic arch through the mandibular notch; the target was a position under the base of the skull lateral to the foramen ovale (FO). In 1957, Marshall introduced SEs made of flexible wire, initially made of stainless steel to allow for longer periods of recording, particularly during presurgical evaluations.[6] More recently, SEs consisted of multistranded silver and platinum wires, the latter to avert its lateral displacement.[7]

Typically, SEs are inserted at the bedside under local anesthesia with lidocaine. The SE wire is mounted on a 22-gauge lumbar puncture needle and the recording end is inserted into the lumen of the needle. The needle is inserted through the skin at a point 3 cm anterior to the external auditory canal, beneath the zygomatic arch, and through the mandibular notch oriented in a 10-degree posterior direction targeting the lateral border of the FO (Fig. 6.1). The tip of the needle is advanced to a depth of 4 to 5 cm beneath the skin's surface, or until the patient reports mandibular pain.[8]

Blind insertion of SEs has several problems that may negate any advantage of their use. First, when SEs are inserted blindly, the recording tips may end up in a position at a distance from the FO, either anterior or posterior to it. Recordings from SEs positioned posterior to the FO are hampered by recording through the thick (2 cm) petrous pyramid, while a position anterior or lateral to the foramen has the additional disadvantage of recording through bone and at an increased distance from target mesial-temporal structures. To overcome this potential problem it has been suggested to insert the SE under fluoroscopic guidance (Fig. 6.2, left and right panels).[9,10] This technique ensures that the recording tip is positioned inferior to the FO (Fig. 6.3). Furthermore, the variable shape of the sphenoid wing among patients can result in an obstacle to the insertion of the needle when done blindly, which in turn results in additional discomfort to patients. Insertion under fluoroscopic guidance averts this problem but must be weighed against the higher costs associated with fluoroscopic guidance.

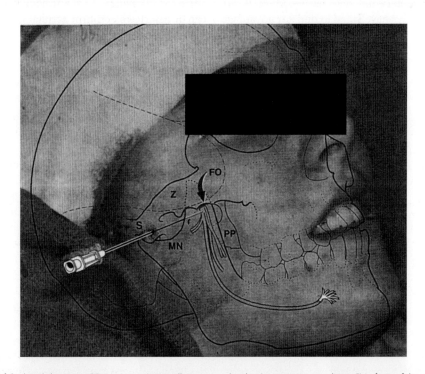

Figure 6.1. Phantom image of the head showing a 22-gauge carrier needle entering the skin (concentric target lines, S) in front of the condylar process of the mandible passing under the zygomatic arch (Z) and through the mandibular notch (MN), en route to V3 emerging from the FO (seen on the edge). PP, pterygoid plate. The SE that is mounted on the superior surface of the needle is not shown. (Reprinted with permission from Kanner AM, Ramirez L, Jones JC. The utility of placing electrodes under the foramen ovale with fluoroscope guidance. J Clin Neurophysiol. 1995;12:72–81.)

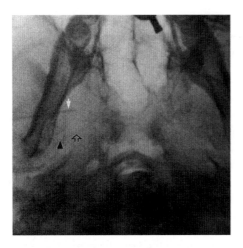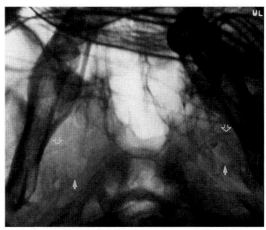

Figure 6.2. Left panel: Submental-vertex radiograph shows the normal relationship of the FO (open arrow) to the foramen spinosum (arrowhead). The electrode/ needle system (solid arrow) is positioned anterior and slightly lateral to the FO. Right panel: Submental-vertex radiograph shows the position of both SE wires (open arrows) anterior and lateral to their respective FO (solid arrows). (Left panel reprinted with permission from Kissani N, Alarcon G, Dad M, et al. Sensitivity of recordings at sphenoidal electrode site for detecting seizure onset: evidence from scalp, superficial and deep foramen ovale recordings. Clin Neurophysiol. 2001;112:232–240. Right panel reprinted with permission from Fenton DS, Geremia GK, Dowd AM, et al. Precise placement of sphenoidal electrodes via fluoroscopic guidance. Am J Neuroradiol. 1997;18:776–778.)

2.2. Mini-sphenoidal Electrodes

MSEs were introduced by Laxer in 1984 as an alternative to SEs. In a study of 100 patients, 34 of whom had epileptiform activity of temporal lobe origin, the epileptiform activity was detected only by MSEs in 21 of these patients.[11] MSEs consist of stainless-steel 0.5-cm needles inserted under the zygomatic arch. Insertion is associated with less discomfort than that of SEs.[12] A study of 100 patients found that MSEs and SEs yielded comparative data in nine patients; however, SEs identified interictal epileptiform activity not detected by MSEs in six patients.[12] Additional studies have failed to find any advantage of MSEs over ATEs.[3,13]

2.3. Nasopharyngeal Electrodes

In 1948, Roubicek and Hill introduced NPEs, and the increased yield of localization of epileptiform activity of mesial-temporal origin was confirmed by several authors.[3,14] These electrodes consist of a solid silver rod with a small silver ball at the tip of 0.67 and 0.055 inches in diameter for use in adults and children, respectively.[15,16] The shaft is flexible and malleable and is insulated up to the ball tip with six or seven coats of insulex varnish. The distal 1 inch is angled about 20 degrees, but the angle can be changed to fit any nasal passage. Unlike SEs, NPEs can be inserted by electroencephalograph (EEG) technologists through the nasal cavity to target the posterior pharyngeal

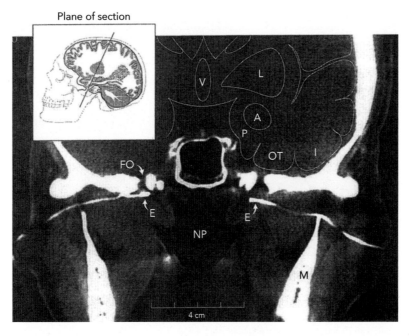

Figure 6.3. Coronal computed tomography scan through FO, showing the relation between the SE (E) and the inferomesial temporal lobe. M, mandible; A, amygdala; P, parahippocampal gyrus; OT, occipitotemporal gyrus; I, inferior temporal gyrus; V, third ventricle; NP, nasopharynx; L, lentiform nucleus.

wall. When positioned optimally, the ball tip is expected to lie in an area beneath the foramen lacerum.

2.4. Scalp Anterotemporal, Basal-Temporal Electrodes, and the Subtemporal Chain

In 1960, Silverman suggested a position for scalp electrodes outside of the International 10-20 System aimed at recording electrical activity of anterotemporal origin.[17] These ATEs, labeled T1 and T2, are positioned "one centimeter above a point one third of the distance along a line from the external auditory meatus to the outer canthus of the ipsilateral eye." A disadvantage of T1 and T2 is that their locations are not proportional to 10-20 or 10-10 system positions and thus display disproportionate voltages when used in bipolar derivations (Fig. 6.4). Accordingly, referential derivations may be preferable when using these electrodes (Figs. 6.5 and 6.6). Use of ATEs significantly improved detection of the epileptiform activity of mesial-temporal origin compared to the standard temporal electrodes.[2,3]

In addition to T1 and T2 electrodes, scalp BTEs that are part of the 10-10 system have been used with increasing frequency to record epileptiform activity of mesial-temporal origin. BTEs are located in the coronal plane defined by their superior counterparts (i.e., F9 and F10 are in the plane defined by F7, F3, Fz, F4, and F8 [see Fig. 6.4]). Interelectrode distances within the coronal plane are determined by the superior electrodes as well (i.e., F9–F7 is 2.5 cm when F7–F3 is 5 cm). Distances between basal electrodes should be as equidistant as possible (T9 and T10 usually have to be placed either anterior or posterior to their ideal position to avoid the ear auricles).

Many labs now include an entire subtemporal chain of electrodes placed 10% inferior to the standard temporal chain with scalp electrodes designated as F9/F10, T9/T10, and P9/P10. Recording from adjacent electrodes (Fp1-F9, F9-T9, T9-P9, P9-O1 and Fp2-F10, F10-T10, T10-P10, P10-O2) adds additional resolution from anterior and mesial temporal structures beyond the standard 10-20 recording and is believed to have similar resolution to sphenoidal recordings without the need for any needle placement.[18]

2.5. Choice of Electrodes

Several studies have compared the localizing yield of ATEs, NPEs, SEs, and MSEs over the 10-20 scalp temporal electrodes in the recording of interictal and ictal epileptiform activity of mesial-temporal origin. These studies have confirmed that any of these electrodes are superior to the standard 10-20 temporal electrodes in recording epileptiform activity of mesial-temporal origin.

Studies that have compared the effectiveness of spike detection between NPEs and ATEs showed that ATEs are as good as or better than NPEs at detecting epileptiform activity.[4,17,19] One study showed that NPEs detected significantly fewer spikes.[4] Additionally, most of these studies report patient discomfort with NPEs and more muscle and movement artifact associated with NPEs than ATEs. Given these data, ATEs have essentially replaced NPEs in most epilepsy centers.

When only two ATEs are being placed, T1 and T2 may be preferable to 10-10 system electrodes because of their ease of placement. The closest counterparts to T1 and T2 in the 10-10 system are electrodes FT9 and FT10. Locating FT9 and FT10

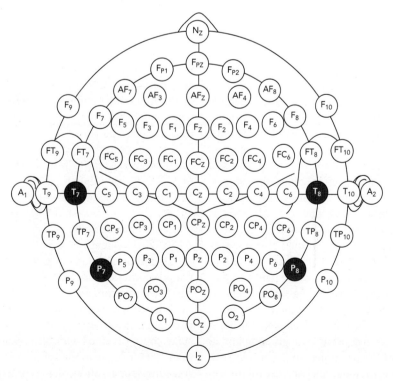

Figure 6.4. Position of ATE and BTE within the 10-10 electrode placement system.

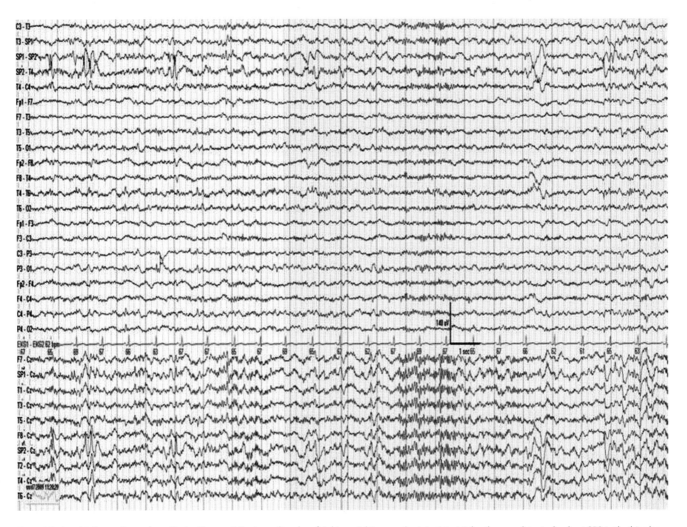

Figure 6.5. *Interictal recordings of a patient with a partial seizure disorder of right mesial-temporal origin. Interictal spikes are detected only at SP2 in the bipolar montage, while in the referential montages sharp transients can be identified at T2 and T4 electrodes in the first two discharges.*

requires the calculation of at least four other coordinates in the 10-10 system.

ATEs and scalp BTEs are included today in EEG and video-EEG studies in patients with presumed epilepsy of mesial-temporal origin in all major epilepsy centers worldwide. A debate remains on whether the use of SEs adds any localizing yield to the interictal and ictal data obtained with ATEs and BTEs. Table 6.1 summarizes the data from studies that compared the localizing yield of interictal and ictal foci with SEs and ATEs.[9,10,20–29] As seen from the table, some studies show some advantage of SEs over ATEs, while others do not.

Such discrepant findings are likely due to practice variations at the majority of epilepsy centers. Because SEs are often inserted under blind conditions, the recording tips commonly end up in a position that is at a distance from the FO (either anterior or posterior to it). As stated above, the petrous pyramid is interposed between the SE recording tip and mesial-temporal structures when it ends up in a posterior position to the FO, while a position anterior or lateral to the foramen has the disadvantage of recording through bone and at an increased distance from the presumed epileptogenic area. A large electric field of interictal and ictal activity minimizes the impact of longer electrode–generator distances and the

effect of bone attenuation. In such circumstances, recordings obtained with SEs positioned at a distance from the FO would look the same as ATE/BTE recordings. In addition, SEs placed anterior to the FO and ATE/BTE yield comparable subtended angles to mesial-basal generators; hence, epileptiform activity would not differ at either electrode, no matter the extent of its electric field.

The question that needs to be asked is not whether SEs are superior to ATEs or BTEs in recording epileptiform activity of mesial-temporal origin but rather the circumstances in which SEs should be used. Data from three studies may provide answers.[9,10,29] The first study included 17 patients with TLE of mesial-temporal origin in which SEs inserted blindly (SEB) and ATEs failed to identify a focal ictal onset.[9] Recordings with SEs inserted under fluoroscopy (SEF) detected a unilateral anterotemporal interictal focus in four patients in whom SEB/ATEs had failed to record any interictal spikes and detected bitemporal independent interictal foci in one patient where SEB/ATEs had only identified unilateral spikes. In nine other patients, the spike count obtained with SEF recordings increased by more than 100% relative to the spike count obtained with SEB/ATE recordings. In addition, SEF recorded seizures with an anterotemporal focal onset pattern in 10 patients where SEB/ATEs

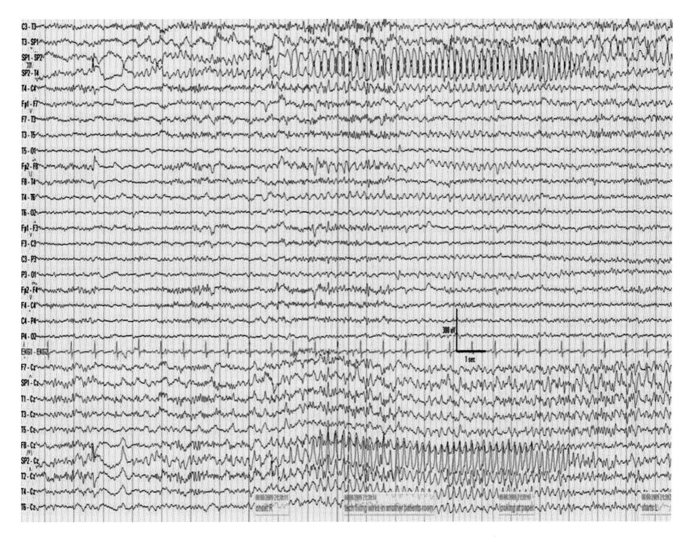

Figure 6.6. Ictal recordings of a patient with a partial seizure disorder of right mesial-temporal origin. The ictal onset was identified 6 seconds at SP2 before it was recorded at the ATE.

had failed to do so. These data raised the hypothesis that the detection of interictal and ictal activity with only SEF was related to a restricted electric field of the activity recorded with SEF (see Figs. 6.5 and 6.6). A second study, carried out using the interictal data of the previous study, consisted of a comparison of spike voltages at SEF, SEB, and ATEs in sets of five randomly selected spikes per interictal focus, recorded in the course of the two monitoring studies.[10] The voltage differences were expressed as ratios, $V_{ATE/SEF}$ and $V_{ATE/SEB}$, and for each spike set a mean ratio was calculated. The spike voltages were almost identical at SEB and ATE (mean $V_{ATE/SEB} = 0.94$) but were significantly higher at SEF than at ATE (mean $V_{ATE/SEF} = 0.66$; $p < .001$). In the SEF recordings, the narrowest electric field contours were found among interictal foci that had only been recorded with SEF, which, in turn, were significantly smaller than those of interictal foci in which SEF yielded an increment of more than 100% in spike counts (relative to those obtained with SEB/ATEs). These, in turn, had a significantly smaller contour than those of the interictal foci where SEF failed to yield any advantage over SEB/ATEs ($p < .001$). In addition, $V_{ATE/SEF}$ of interictal foci in which SEF recorded seizures with a focal onset pattern were significantly lower than those of foci

where SEF failed to do so ($p = .016$). Finally, $V_{ATE/SEF}$ did not differ from $V_{ATE/SEB}$ among interictal foci where SEF failed to yield any advantage over SEB/ATEs in either interictal ($p = .240$) or ictal ($p = .311$) recordings. The data of the second study confirmed our hypothesis and proved that SEs inserted under fluoroscopic guidance yield additional localizing data when recording epileptiform activity with a restricted field, provided that the recording tip is positioned below the FO. When distant from the FO, SEs can be expected to yield comparable data to those obtained with ATEs.

The question of when SEs should be inserted was addressed in a third study by determining the frequency with which SEs inserted under fluoroscopic guidance detected localizing data not obtained with ATE/BTE recordings in a group of 40 unselected patients whose presurgical evaluation had demonstrated a unilateral ($n = 32$) seizure focus or bilateral independent ($n = 8$) seizure foci in anterotemporal regions.[29] The study consisted of a comparison of the ictal onset pattern of 156 seizures obtained with SEF and ATE/BTEs by four electroencephalographers who reviewed the 312 ictal recordings independently, and who were blind to the patients' identity, to any presurgical data, and to whether the recordings' montage

TABLE 6.1. Comparison of Interictal and Ictal Recordings Among ATEs, SEs, and NPEs

AUTHORS	ELECTRODES COMPARED	RESULTS
Sperling and Engel[20]	Interictal discharges at SEs, earlobe electrodes, and NPEs	99% of discharges were detected with SEs, 57% with NPEs, and 54% with earlobe electrodes.
Binnie et al.[21]	Interictal discharges at multipolar SEs and surface electrodes (near current T1 and T2 sites)	SEs offer no improvement in sensitivity compared with surface electrodes.
Sperling et al.[22]	Interictal discharges at SEs and invasive electrodes	SEs were synchronous with invasive electrodes in the neocortical areas but not in the amygdala or hippocampus.
Binnie et al.[23]	Interictal discharges at SEs stereotactically placed into the FO and surface electrodes	4% of discharges were seen at SEs only, while 3% were seen at surface electrodes only.
Sperling and Engel[24]	Ictal onset at SEs and scalp electrodes	19% of the seizure onset was seen only at SEs. The SEs led the scalp electrodes by more than 5 seconds in 70% of the seizure onsets.
Fernández Torre et al.[25]	Ictal onset at SEs, infrazygomatic electrodes, ATEs, and surface temporal electrodes	Ictal onset was seen earliest at the SEs and then at infrazygomatic and ATE leads.
Ives et al.[26]	Ictal onset at SEs and T1/T2 electrodes	40% of the seizures were seen first at SEs and 60% of the seizures were seen at both recording sites.
Wilkus et al.[27]	Ictal onset at SEs, T1/T2 electrodes, and ATEs	No difference was seen between electrodes.
Pacia et al.[28]	Ictal onset at FO-placed SEs and ATEs	Improved identification and timing at the SEs 7% of the time
Kanner et al.[9]	Interictal and ictal activity with SEs placed with fluoroscopic guidance just below the FO and standard blind-placed SEs	Fluoroscopically placed SEs added additional information, such as increased spike count and better seizure onset localization.
Kanner and Jones[10]	Interictal and ictal activity at SEs placed with fluoroscopic guidance just below the FO, standard blind-placed SEs, and ATEs	Significantly higher voltage spikes and significantly narrower electric field contour were seen during ictal and interictal activity recorded from fluoroscopic-guided SEs, adding additional data.
Mintzer et al.[29]	Ictal onset at SEs placed with fluoroscopic guidance just below the FO and ATEs	Fluoroscopically placed SEs increased rater reliability, increased the number of seizures correctly localized, and detected seizures ≥5 seconds before they were seen at the ATEs in 43% of the seizures.

included ATEs or SEF. Inter-rater agreement among the four raters was significantly greater with SEF than ATE recordings ($p < .0001$). The number of seizures correctly localized by at least three raters was significantly greater with SEF ($n = 144$) than ATEs ($n = 99$; $p < .0001$). All the seizures ($n = 36$, or 23%) originating from 14 ictal foci (29%) in 11 patients (27.5%) were localized only with SEF. This was a significantly more common occurrence in patients with bilateral independent ictal foci ($p = .04$). The ictal onset was detected at SEF 5 or more seconds earlier than at ATEs in 67 seizures (43%) originating from 33 (69%) foci in 30 patients (75%). In addition, SEF had a significant advantage over ATEs in the recording of seizures of patients with bilateral independent foci and with normal magnetic resonance imaging (MRI), but not in seizures of patients with a structural lesion. These data suggested that SEs placed with fluoroscopic guidance facilitate the localization of anterotemporal ictal onset, and *in about one fourth of patients* SEs placed under fluoroscopy identify ictal data not localized, or mislocalized, with ATE recordings.

The following conclusions can be derived from these data:

1. If SEs are to be inserted, they should be placed under fluoroscopic guidance.

2. SEs need not be inserted in all patients with suspected TLE of mesial-temporal origin.

3. The indications to insert SEs under fluoroscopy are as follows:

   In case of hippocampal atrophy, the decision to insert SEs under fluoroscopy can be delayed until the first seizure is recorded and the interictal recordings of the first 24 hours have been reviewed. SE insertion under fluoroscopy will not be necessary in patients with unilateral atrophy if ATE recordings demonstrate that (i) the majority of spikes are ipsilateral to the atrophic hippocampus and (ii) the first seizure has a focal or regional onset pattern (provided that all of the patient's seizures are identical by history). However, SEF should be inserted if (i) ATE interictal recordings reveal bilateral independent spike foci with a relative frequency of 50/50 to 60/40; (ii) ATE recordings reveal an ictal onset pattern that is lateralized or not localized; (iii) the patient's seizures are not identical by history (excluding complex partial seizures that also evolve to secondarily generalized tonic–clonic seizures); and (iv) there is bilateral hippocampal atrophy.

In case of a unilateral anterotemporal structural lesion, the same criteria as outlined above can be used.

In case of a normal brain MRI, SEs should be inserted under fluoroscopy.

2.6. The Advantage of Joint Use of SEs and ATE/BTEs

As stated above, epileptic seizures of TLE may originate in mesial-temporal structures or temporal lateral neocortex. With the widespread availability of digital EEG systems, a spatial-temporal analysis of epileptiform discharges with SEs and ATEs may help establish the source in mesial structures by demonstrating the initial negativity at the SE. On the other hand, a synchronous discharge at SEs and ATE/BTEs does not exclude a mesial source.

2.7. High-Density Scalp Electrodes

Standard routine EEG is recorded with 19 electrodes (eight electrodes on each hemisphere and three midline electrodes). This allows determining the presence or absence of encephalopathy, coma monitoring, and a first view of an epileptogenic focus,

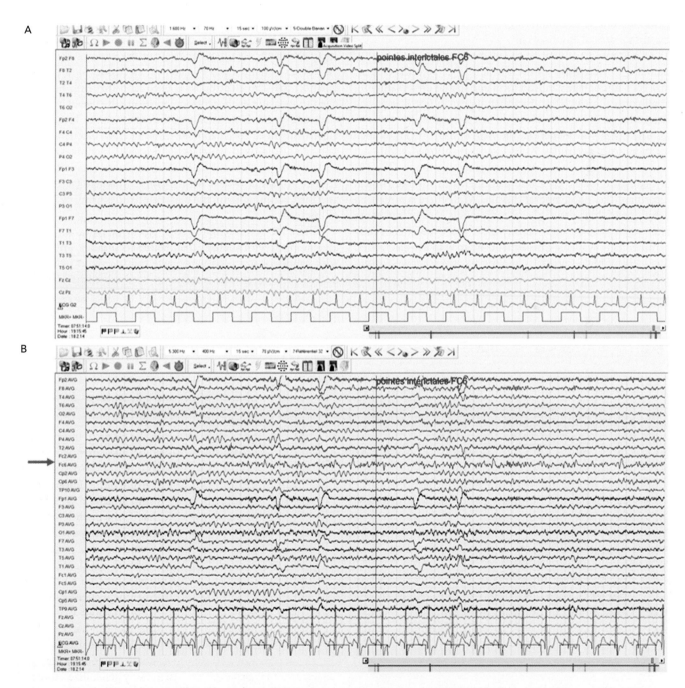

Figure 6.7. A 13-year-old patient with nonlesional extratemporal lobe epilepsy and nocturnal seizures. A: Standard "double banana" EEG is unrevealing. B: By adding more scalp electrodes, very focal spikes become apparent in FC6, only occasionally propagating to F8.

provided that the 19 electrodes cover the area of the focus and the focus is not too limited. By using simultaneous recording of 26 scalp electrodes and 46 to 98 intracranial subdural electrodes, it has been demonstrated that a cortical area of at least 10 cm^2 is necessary to produce a visible scalp spike. Increasing this resolution is possible through the use of additional scalp electrodes. According to a study with simultaneous scalp and intracranial EEG, when using 64 scalp electrodes, the median area necessary to generate a visible scalp spike was 6 cm^2.[30] This would imply that that in half of the 14 patients with focal cortical dysplasia, the area is even smaller than 6 cm^2. An example of the crucial role of additional electrodes can be seen in Figures 6.7 through 6.9. In this case, the interictal focus is quite focal—that is, essentially seen in only one electrode of the 31 electrode setup (for long-term monitoring)—and corresponds to a cortical surface area of around 4 cm^2.

In a transparent view of the electrode position using the standard 19 electrodes (or even with a 26 or 30), it is evident that such a montage can lead to major spatial undersampling of all cortical areas. Thus, foci that appear in just one or few electrodes, as in Figure 6.10, could be easily missed.

The easiest way to increase the yield of scalp EEG is by adding more scalp electrodes. As previously mentioned, additional electrodes can be placed over the sphenoidal bone (T1, T2) or below the lowest electrode placements in routine clinical recordings (i.e., subtemporal chains). While there is no official definition of "high density," electrode counts of 64 or higher are often referred to as "high-density EEG" (HD-EEG). Currently commercially available EEG systems offer 64 to 256 electrodes. The yield of higher spatial sampling has been shown in several studies and reviews.[31–33] Adequate spatial sampling of EEG

in small children requires more electrodes than in adults, as shown in a simulation study.[34] The reason is that the skull is thinner and therefore there is less blurring of the EEG activity.

As seen in Figure 6.8, significantly more regions are covered by 256 contacts, allowing a comprehensive view of additional brain activity. Interhemispheric or other deeply buried cortex like operculum are still obscured; this is a limitation of HD-EEG due to anatomy, and similar to low-montage scalp EEG. Scalp EEG, including HD-EEG, "sees" foci of both radial and tangential orientation, compared to magnetoencephalography, which sees only tangential foci.[35] There is still discussion of how deep the scalp EEG can localize sources. Based on recent studies, it appears that foci as deep as 5 to 7 cm can be picked up by scalp EEG and this is more likely if sampled with more electrodes.[30,36,37]

The practical problem remains the workload needed to apply the electrodes, but for most of the systems this could be solved. Usually a cap or net with electrodes in a prefixed position (64–256 electrodes) is used, and this eliminates the need to measure each electrode position. The use of averaged electrode position is usually sufficient if source localization algorithms need to be applied. Alternatively, electrode position can be digitized, which is not practical in clinical routine. Visual analysis of the EEG is of course possible, which may require an initial review with a simple montage (screening), and then zooming in on the dense electrodes array of the area of interest.

There are several high-density electrode types. Electrodes are equipped with sponges that, before recordings, are soaked with saline, or are used with paste that needs to be applied under each electrode, similar to well-established routine

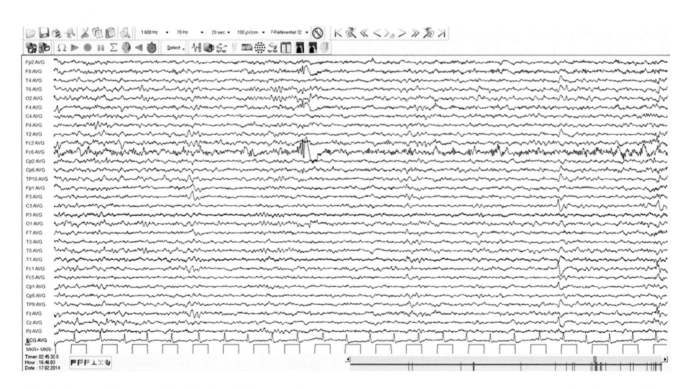

Figure 6.8. Increase of discharges during light sleep. AVG, average reference.

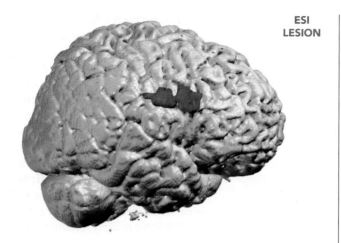

Figure 6.9. Co-registration of the source of the interictal discharges and the lesion, which became "visible" after review of the MRI (right frontal transmantle dysplasia).

clinical setups. With the saline solution, recordings of large electrode counts are obtained quite rapidly (i.e., within 15–20 minutes); however, recording times are limited to 1 to 1.5 hours, as the saline solution quickly dries. Applying paste or gel under each contact takes more time, but excellent recording quality can be obtained for 24 hours or more. Setup time depends on the experience of the technician. We calculated the total duration for a 256-electrode set on five patients (Geodesic

inc®). On average, putting on the cap took 5 minutes and applying the gel under each contact another 45 minutes. Together with verifying key electrode positions (e.g., Cz, Nasion), applying a bandage to keep the cap in place (in particular in small children), and entering patient data in the machine, the entire setup can take 60 minutes. While this is too long to be done on a routine basis, it compares favorably with the typical procedure for patients admitted for a presurgical evaluation, which requires individual measurement and positioning of 30 to 40 electrodes. MRI-compatible HD-EEG systems allow simultaneous recording of the EEG and functional MRI and can be valuable to shorten the presurgical evaluation.[38]

3. CONCLUDING REMARKS

Recordings of epileptiform activity of presumed mesial-temporal origin should always include ATE/BTEs or a sub-temporal chain. Available data do not appear to support the use of NPEs, which yield no advantage over ATE/BTEs or sub-temporal chain and are associated with discomfort. SEs should be considered in special circumstances, and their reliability is significantly improved if they are placed under fluoroscopic guidance. High-density scalp recordings allow for even greater resolution and improved spatial sampling. The use of HD-EEG should also be considered in the presurgical evaluation.

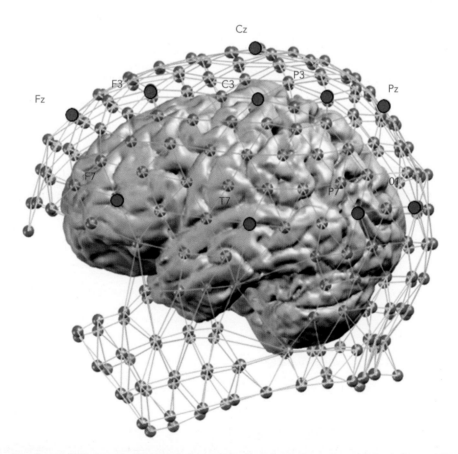

Figure 6.10. A transparent view of a net of 256 electrodes (blue) on the brain of a healthy volunteer (reconstructed from a high spatial 3T MRI). Electrodes (red) are highlighted and are the typical electrodes used in the routine EEGs. As can be seen, most cortical areas are not covered by the red electrodes, so the additional electrodes can improve the yield of scalp EEG.

REFERENCES

1. Homan RW, Herman J, Purdy P. Cerebral location of International 10-20 System electrode placement. *Electroencephalogr Clin Neurophysiol.* 1987;66(4):376–382.
2. Homan RW, Jones MC, Rawat S. Anterior temporal electrodes in complex partial seizures. *Electroencephalogr Clin Neurophysiol.* 1988;70(2):105–109.
3. Goodin DS, Aminoff MJ, Laxer KD. Detection of epileptiform activity by different noninvasive EEG methods in complex partial epilepsy. *Ann Neurol.* 1990;27(3):330–334.
4. Sadler RM, Goodwin J. Multiple electrodes for detecting spikes in partial complex seizures. *Can J Neurol Sci.* 1989;16(3):326–329.
5. Jones D. Recording of the basal electroencephalogram with sphenoidal electrodes. *Electroencephalogr Clin Neurophysiol.* 1951;3(1):100.
6. Marshall C. Sphenoidal electrodes: an effort toward their popularization. *Electroencephalogr Clin Neurophysiol.* 1957;9(2):379–382.
7. Rovit RL, Gloor P, Rasmussen T. Sphenoidal electrodes in the electrographic study of patients with temporal lobe epilepsy. An evaluation. *J Neurosurg.* 1961;18:151–158.
8. Ives JR, Gloor P. Update: chronic sphenoidal electrodes. *Electroencephalogr Clin Neurophysiol.* 1978;44(6):789–790.
9. Kanner AM, Ramirez L, Jones JC. The utility of placing sphenoidal electrodes under the foramen ovale with fluoroscopic guidance. *J Clin Neurophysiol.* 1995;12(1):72–81.
10. Kanner AM, Jones JC. When do sphenoidal electrodes yield additional data to that obtained with antero-temporal electrodes? *Electroencephalogr Clin Neurophysiol.* 1997;102(1):12–19.
11. Laxer KD. Mini-sphenoidal electrodes in the investigation of seizures. *Electroencephalogr Clin Neurophysiol.* 1984;58(2):127–129.
12. Buchhalter JR, Schomer DL, Schachter SC. Standard sphenoidal and mini-sphenoidal electrodes: A direct comparison. *J Epilepsy.* 1991;4(1):29–31.
13. Chu NS. Surface sphenoidal electrode for recording anterior temporal spikes. *Clin Electroencephalogr.* 1992;23(4):190–195.
14. Roubicek J, Hill D. Electroencephalography with pharyngeal electrodes. *Brain.* 1948;71(1):77–87.
15. DeJesus PV, Masland WS. The role of nasopharyngeal electrodes in clinical electroencephalography. *Neurology.* 1970;20(9):869–878.
16. Kashnig DM, Celesia GG. Letter: Nasopharyngeal electrodes in the diagnosis of partial seizures with complex symptoms. *Arch Neurol.* 1976;33(7):519–520.
17. Silverman D. The anterior temporal electrode and the ten-twenty system. *Electroencephalogr Clin Neurophysiol.* 1960;12:735–737.
18. Acharya JN, Hani A, Cheek J, Thirumala P, Tsuchidak TN. American Clinical Neurophysiology Society Guideline 2: Guidelines for Standard Electrode Position Nomenclature. doi:10.1097/WNP.0000000000000316.
19. Nowack WJ, Janati A, Metzer WS, Nickols J. The anterior temporal electrode in the EEG of the adult. *Clin Electroencephalogr.* 1988;19(4):199–204.
20. Sperling MR, Engel J. Electroencephalographic recording from the temporal lobes: a comparison of ear, anterior temporal, and nasopharyngeal electrodes. *Ann Neurol.* 1985;17(5):510–513.
21. Binnie CD, Dekker E, Smit A, Van der Linden G. Practical considerations in the positioning of EEG electrodes. *Electroencephalogr Clin Neurophysiol.* 1982;53(4):453–458.
22. Sperling MR, Mendius JR, Engel J. Mesial temporal spikes: a simultaneous comparison of sphenoidal, nasopharyngeal, and ear electrodes. *Epilepsia.* 1986;27(1):81–86.
23. Binnie CD, Marston D, Polkey CE, Amin D. Distribution of temporal spikes in relation to the sphenoidal electrode. *Electroencephalogr Clin Neurophysiol.* 1989;73(5):403–409.
24. Sperling MR, Engel J. Sphenoidal electrodes. *J Clin Neurophysiol.* 1986;3(1):67–73.
25. Fernández Torre J, Alarcón G, Binnie C, Polkey C. Comparison of sphenoidal, foramen ovale and anterior temporal placements for detecting interictal epileptiform discharges in presurgical assessment for temporal lobe epilepsy. *Clin Neurophysiol.* 1999;110(5):895–904.
26. Ives JR, Drislane FW, Schachter SC, et al. Comparison of coronal sphenoidal versus standard anteroposterior temporal montage in the EEG recording of temporal lobe seizures. *Electroencephalogr Clin Neurophysiol.* 1996;98(5):417–421.
27. Wilkus RJ, Vossler DG, Thompson PM. Comparison of EEG derived from sphenoidal, infrazygomatic, anterior temporal, and midtemporal electrodes during complex partial seizures. *J Epilepsy.* 1993;6(3):152–161.
28. Pacia S V, Jung W J, Devinsky O. Localization of mesial temporal lobe seizures with sphenoidal electrodes. *J Clin Neurophysiol.* 1998;15(3):256–261.
29. Mintzer S, Nicholl JS, Stern JM, Engel J. Relative utility of sphenoidal and temporal surface electrodes for localization of ictal onset in temporal lobe epilepsy. *Clin Neurophysiol.* 2002;113(6):911–916.
30. Koessler L, Cecchin T, Colnat-Coulbois S, et al. Erratum to: Catching the invisible: mesial temporal source contribution to simultaneous EEG and SEEG recordings. *Brain Topogr.* 2015;28(4):646.
31. Brodbeck V, Spinelli L, Lascano AM, et al. Electroencephalographic source imaging: a prospective study of 152 operated epileptic patients. *Brain.* 2011;134(Pt 10):2887–2897.
32. Leijten FSS, Huiskamp G-JM, Hilgersom I, Van Huffelen AC. High-resolution source imaging in mesiotemporal lobe epilepsy: a comparison between MEG and simultaneous EEG. *J Clin Neurophysiol.* 20(4):227–238.
33. Plummer C, Harvey AS, Cook M. EEG source localization in focal epilepsy: where are we now? *Epilepsia.* 2008;49(2):201–218.
34. Grieve PG, Emerson RG, Isler JR, Stark RI. Quantitative analysis of spatial sampling error in the infant and adult electroencephalogram. *NeuroImage.* 2004;21(4):1260–1274.
35. Ebersole JS, Ebersole SM. Combining MEG and EEG source modeling in epilepsy evaluations. *J Clin Neurophysiol.* 2010;27(6):360–371.
36. Yamazaki M, Tucker DM, Fujimoto A, et al. Comparison of dense array EEG with simultaneous intracranial EEG for interictal spike detection and localization. *Epilepsy Res.* 2012;98(2):166–173.
37. Ramantani G, Dümpelmann M, Koessler L, et al. Simultaneous subdural and scalp EEG correlates of frontal lobe epileptic sources. *Epilepsia.* 2014;55(2):278–288.
38. Grouiller F, Delattre BMA, Pittau F, et al. All-in-one interictal presurgical imaging in patients with epilepsy: single-session EEG/PET/(f)MRI. *Eur J Nucl Med Mol Imaging.* 2015;42(7):1133–1143.

PART II | NORMAL EEG

7 | NORMAL EEG IN WAKEFULNESS AND SLEEP: PRETERM; TERM; INFANT; ADOLESCENT

PHILLIP L. PEARL, MD, JULES C. BEAL, MD, MONIKA EISERMANN, MD,

SUNITA MISRA, MD, PHD, PERRINE PLOUIN, MD, SOLOMON L. MOSHE, MD,

JAMES J. RIVIELLO, JR., MD, DOUGLAS R. NORDLI, JR., MD, AND

ELI M. MIZRAHI, MD

ABSTRACT: Electroencephalogram (EEG) interpretation depends on accurate pattern recognition. One of the first lessons the novice electroencephalographer learns is that EEG pattern interpretation must take into account the patient's age and the level of vigilance, or state. EEG patterns vary according to central nervous system development and maturation. This process evolves over time, starting with the early development and maturation of the nervous system (an evolution) to a peak of maturity, followed by an involution. Basic differences exist between the ascending (developmental) and descending (involutional) portions of this curve. This chapter discusses pediatric EEG, from the dramatic ontogenic transitioning of the neonate, premature and term, to infants, children, and adolescents.

KEYWORDS: electroencephalography, EEG, pediatric, neonate, infant, child, adolescent

PRINCIPAL REFERENCES

1. Petersén I, Selldén U, Eeg-Olofsson O. The evolution of the EEG in normal children and adolescents from 1 to 21 years. In: Remond A, Lairy GC, eds. *Handbook of Electroencephalography and Clinical Neurophysiology.* Vol. 6B. Amsterdam: Elsevier; 1975:31–68.
2. Dreyfus-Brisac C. The electroencephalogram of the premature infant and full-term newborn: Normal and abnormal development of waking and sleeping patterns. In: Kellaway P, Petersén I, eds. *Neurological and Electroencephalographic Correlative Studies in Infancy.* New York: Grune & Stratton; 1964:186–206.
3. Koszer SE, Moshe SL, Holmes GL. Visual analysis of the neonatal electroencephalogram. In: Holmes GL, Moshe SL, Jones HR, Jr., eds. *Clinical Neurophysiology of Infancy, Childhood, and Adolescence.* Philadelphia, PA: Butterworth-Heinemann; 2006:70–86.
4. Koszer SE, Zacharowicz L, Moshe SL. Visual analysis of the pediatric electroencephalogram. In: Holmes GL, Moshe SL, Jones HR, Jr., eds. *Clinical Neurophysiology of Infancy, Childhood, and Adolescence.* Philadelphia, PA: Butterworth-Heinemann; 2006:99–129.
5. Shellhaas RA, Chang T, Tsuchida T, et al. The American Clinical Neurophysiology Society's Guideline on Continuous Electroencephalography Monitoring in Neonates. *J Clin Neurophysiol.* 2011;28(6):611–617.
6. Tsuchida TN, Wusthoff CJ, Shellhaas RA, et al. American Clinical Neurophysiology Society standardized EEG terminology and categorization for the description of continuous EEG monitoring in neonates: report of the American Clinical Neurophysiology Society critical care monitoring committee. *J Clin Neurophysiol.* 2013;30(2):161–173.
7. Ohtahara S. Development of electroencephalogram during infancy and childhood. *Proc Jpn EEG Soc.* 1964:18–23.
8. Samson-Dollfus D, Nogues B, Delagree E. [EEG recording during drowsiness in normal babies aged 2 to 12 months (author's transl)]. *Rev Electroencephalogr Neurophysiol Clin.* 1981;11(1):23–27.

1. GENERAL PRINCIPLES

Electroencephalogram (EEG) interpretation depends on accurate pattern recognition. One of the first lessons the novice electroencephalographer learns is that EEG pattern interpretation must take into account the patient's age and the level of vigilance, or state. EEG patterns vary according to central nervous system (CNS) development and maturation. This process evolves over time, starting with the early development and maturation of the nervous system (an evolution) to a peak of maturity, followed by an involution. Basic differences exist between the ascending (developmental) and descending (involutional) portions of this curve. This chapter discusses pediatric EEG, from the dramatic ontogenic transitioning of the neonate, premature and term, to infants, children, and adolescents.

2. HISTORICAL ASPECTS

Berger[1] performed the first EEG studies in children (starting with his own son!) and discovered age-dependent changes. The EEG evolution from infancy to adolescence in a large number of healthy adolescents has been extensively studied by Swedish authors,[2–6] whose work set the standards for developmental EEG. In a remarkable study of 1,416 healthy subjects with an age range from 6 to 39 years using quantitative EEG, Matsuura et al.[7] investigated the development of various frequency ranges over the occipital, central, and frontopolar regions. Gasser et al.[8,9] investigated the development of the EEG in children and adolescents by frequency analysis and topography.

A number of investigators have, over the years, contributed to our understanding of the normal neonatal EEG, beginning with the pioneering work of the French school.[10–14] More recent discussions of normal neonatal EEG include those by Hrachovy et al.,[15] Watanabe et al.,[16] Clancy et al.,[17] Mizrahi et al.,[18] Plouin et al.,[19] Vecchierini et al.,[20] André et al.,[21] and Mizrahi et al.[22] Table 7.1 provides a condensed presentation of a number of EEG variables and their developmental aspects from the neonatal period, beginning with extreme prematurity and extending to term, through infancy, childhood, and

TABLE 7.1 A Condensed View of EEG Maturation

	PREMATURE (24–27 WK)	PREMATURE (28–31 WK)	PREMATURE (32–35 WK)	FULL-TERM NEWBORN (36–41 WK)
Continuity	Discontinuous, long flat stretches	Discontinuous	Continuous in waking state and REM sleep, discontinuous in non-REM sleep	Continuous except for trace alternant in non-REM (quiet) sleep
Interhemispheric synchrony	Short bursts in synchrony	Mostly asynchronous activity leads	Partly synchronous, especially in occipital	Minor asynchronies still present
Differentiation of waking and sleeping	Undifferentiated	Undifferentiated	Waking distinguished from sleep early in the period, them differentiation of non-REM and REM sleep	Good
Posterior basic (alpha) rhythm	None	None	None	None
Slow activity (awake)	Very slow bursts, high voltage (state of vigilance undifferentiated)	Very slow activity predominant	Slow (delta) with occipital maximum	Slow (delta), mostly of moderate voltage
Temporal theta	Present and increasing	Prominent	Decreasing and disappearing	Disappearing or absent
Occipital theta	Prominent	Decreasing	Decreasing	Absent
Fast activity (awake)	Very little beta activity	Frequent ripples or brushes around 16 per second	Frequent ripples or brushes (16–20 per second)	Decreasing ripples, sparse fast activity
Low voltage	Long flat stretches	Flat stretches, mainly asynchronous	Low-voltage record suspect of serious cerebral pathology	Very low voltage records are due to severe cerebral pathology, prognosis ominous
Hyperventilation	Not feasible	Not feasible	Not feasible	Not feasible
Intermittent photic stimulation	Unknown	Unknown	Unknown	Driving reponse below 4 flashes/second may occur, not easily elicited
Drowsiness	Undifferentiated	Undifferentiated	Undifferentiated	Undifferentiated
Trace alternant	None	None	Present in non-REM (quiet) sleep	Present in non-REM (quiet) sleep
Spindles	None	None (but ripples present)	None (but ripples present)	None (but scanty ripples)
Vertex waves and K complexes	None	None	None	None
Positive occipital sharp transients of sleep	None	None	None	None
Slow and fast activity in sleep	Slow activity of high voltage, little slow activity (stage of vigilance undifferentiated)	Much slow activity, more irregular, little fast activity	Irregular slow activity of occipital predominance	Much delta and theta activity, continuous in REM sleep

INFANCY (2–12 MO)	EARLY CHILDHOOD (12–36 MO)	PRESCHOOL AGE (3–5 YR)	OLDER CHILDREN (6–12 YR)	ADOLESCENTS (13–20 YR)
Continuous	Continuous	Continuous	Continuous	Continuous
No significant asynchrony	No significant asynchrony	No significant asynchrony	No significant asynchrony	No significant asynchrony
Good	Good	Good	Good	Good
Starting at age 3–4 mo at 4 per second, reaching about 6 per second at 12 mo	Rising from 5–6 per second to 8 per second (seldom 9 per second)	Rising from 6–8 per second to 7–9 per second	Rising 10 per second at age 10 yr	Averaging 10 per second
Considerable	Considerable	Marked admixture of posterior slow activity (to alpha rhythm)	Varying degree of posterior slow activity mixed with alpha	Posterior slow activity diminishing
None	None	None	None	None
None	None	None	None	None
Very moderate	Mostly moderate	Mostly moderate	Mostly moderate	Mostly, except for low voltage fast records
Uncommon, usually abnormal	Uncommon, usually abnormal	Uncommon, usually abnormal	Seldom as variant of normalcy	Occasionally and (at end of teenage period more often) as variant of normalcy
Not feasible	Mostly not feasible	Often marked delta response	Often marked delta response	Delta responses become less impressive
Improving driving to low flash rates after age 6 mo	Often good driving response to low flash rates	Often good driving response to low flash rates	Often good driving response, chiefly at medium flash rates (8–16 per second)	Often good driving response, chiefly at medium flash rates
Around age 6 mo, appearance of rhythmical theta	Marked "hypnagogic" rhythmical theta (4–6 per second)	Rhythmical theta gradually vanishing, other types of slow activity predominant	Gradual alpha dropout with increasing slow activity	Gradual alpha dropout with low-voltage stretches (mainly slow)
Disappears in first (seldom second) month	None	None	None	None
Appear after second month; 12–15 per second, sharp, shifting	In second year, sharp and shifting, then symmetrical with vertex maximum	Typical vertex maximum	Typical vertex maximum	Typical vertex maximum
Appear mainly at 5 mo fairly large, blunt	Large, becoming more pointed	Large with an increasingly impressive sharp component	Large with a prominent sharp component	Not quite as large, sharp component not quite as prominent
None	Poorly defined	Poorly defined	Still poorly defined but gradually evolving	Often very well developed
Much diffuse 0.75–3 per second activity with poster or maximum; moderate fast activity	Marked posterior maximum of slow activity; often a good deal of fast activity	Predominant slowing but less prominent posterior maximum	Much diffuse slowing, slightly decreasing voltage	Much diffuse slowing with further attenuation of voltage

(continued)

TABLE 7.1. CONTINUED

	PREMATURE (24–27 WK)	PREMATURE (28–31 WK)	PREMATURE (32–35 WK)	FULL-TERM NEWBORN (36–41 WK)
REM sleep	Undifferentiated	Undifferentiated	Continuous slow activity; oculographically, REM present	Continuous slow activity, REM in EOG (more REM or "active" than non-REM sleep)
Rhythmical frontal theta activity (6–7 per second)	None	None	None	None
14 and 6 per second positive spikes	None	None	None	None
Psychomotor variant (marginal abnormality)	None	None	None	None
Sharp waves, spikes	Some intermixed sharp activity in bursts (normal)	Some intermixed sharp activity (normal)	Often prominent sharp waves or spikes (normal)	Some minor sharp transients (normal) (abnormal spikes more consistent and prominent)

adolescence. An orderly approach to analysis of the neonatal and pediatric EEG can also be found in other sources.[23,24]

3. NEONATAL EEG

The interpretation of the neonatal EEG consists of related phases of analysis that are mostly conducted in parallel. Initially, the EEG is assessed to determine the conceptional age (CA) of the infant. In concert with this, the background activity is assessed to determine whether it is normal and, if not, to characterize the abnormal features. In addition, the determination of CA provides the basis for understanding the range of both diffuse and focal abnormalities that may be anticipated within each age-dependent epoch. Thus, visual analysis of the neonatal EEG begins with recognition of the CA-dependent features characteristic of specific epochs of development. This is followed by inspection for EEG abnormalities based upon an understanding of possible CA-dependent findings. Taken together, these aspects of visual analysis of the neonatal EEG provide the basis for determining the infant's CA and assessing the degree to which the EEG is normal.

Two additional principles of interpretation of the neonatal EEG relate to CA-dependent changes over time and to findings of indeterminate significance. Typically, the EEG-determined age of the infant is given in terms of CA, which represents the gestational age (GA) plus the legal age. The GA is synonymous with the menstrual age, or the time elapsed from the first day of the last normal menstrual period to the time of birth.[25] The legal age is the time from birth to the time of the EEG. The CA is the GA plus the legal age. The American Academy of Pediatrics has recommended the term *post-menstrual age* for the period that electroencephalographers have traditionally called CA or GA, and strictly speaking, postmenstrual age is correct. This terminology required clarification based on the cognizance that while historically most women knew the date of their prior menstrual period as opposed to ovulation, the availability of assistive reproductive technology allows for precise knowledge of the date of conception. Thus, electroencephalographers should recognize that terminology referring to newborns based on number of weeks is based on postmenstrual age (i.e., GA) and not *postconceptional* age in the strict sense of number of weeks following conception (i.e., fertilization).

The second basic principle of neonatal interpretation is that the EEG graphoelements develop at the same rate whether in utero or following delivery. Thus, the EEG recorded several weeks after an infant was born prematurely would have similar features to an EEG recorded on the first day of life of infant whose CA equaled the GA plus the legal age of the premature infant. Another important consideration is that the clinical significance has not been determined for all features of the neonatal EEG. Thus, the challenge is to differentiate the known from the unknown, and focus interpretation on those aspects of the EEG for which accurate data are available.

INFANCY (2–12 MO)	EARLY CHILDHOOD (12–36 MO)	PRESCHOOL AGE (3–5 YR)	OLDER CHILDREN (6–12 YR)	ADOLESCENTS (13–20 YR)
REM portion decreasing; mostly slow activity	Mostly slow, starting to become more desynchronized	Slow activity with some desynchronization	Less slowing and increasing desynchronization	Mature desynchronization
None	Seldom in third year of life	May occur, not very common	A bit more common	A bit more common, declining at end of period
None	Rare	May occur, not very common	Fairly common	Fairly common
None	None	Probably none	Uncommon	More common (although relatively rare)
Essential as abnormal phenomena	Spikes in seizure-free children, mainly occipital (mild abnormalities)	Spikes in seizure-free children, mainly occipital, also Rolandic (slight abnormalities)	Spikes in seizure-free children, mainly Rolandic (central-mid-temporal), slight to moderate abnormalities; physiological occipital spikes in congenitally blind children	Benign Rolandic spikes usually disappear before beginning of this period

3.1. Technical Considerations

The general principles of recording the EEG in neonates are similar to those of older children and adults, with some important additions and exceptions. Guidelines for the recording of the neonatal EEG have been established by the American Clinical Neurophysiology Society (ACNS)[26] and the International Federation of Clinical Neurophysiology,[27] with a more recent guideline on continuous EEG monitoring in neonates.[28]

Critical to the recording of neonatal EEG is a well-trained staff of electroneurodiagnostic technologists with expertise in the recording of newborns and young infants. To ensure maximal clinical relevance, the technologist should obtain basic information about each neonate to be recorded, including standard demographic data, description of the recording environment, documentation of reason for referral, details of the medical history, a list and timing of medications, and the specifics of the infant's general medical condition. In addition, the technologist must consider the state of each infant and determine the best method to make the infant as comfortable as possible in order to obtain a complete recording. This may require having the infant fed, having diapers changed, adjusting room temperature, and, often, just prolonging the recording until the infant becomes comforted.

The International 10-20 System of Electrode Placement has been modified for recording neonates. Some laboratories prefer a full 10-20 array, while others use a reduced array, especially for premature infants or neonates with small head sizes. The ACNS guidelines suggest a minimum reduced array as comprising Fp1, Fp2, C3, C4, CZ, T7 (T3), T8 (T4), O1, O2, A1, and A2. If the earlobes are too small, mastoid leads may be substituted, designated M1 and M2. Alternative frontal placements are also recommended, such as Fp3 (AF3) and Fp4 (AF4), halfway between electrodes Fp1 and F3, and Fp2 and F4 positions, respectively. Use of the alternative Fp3 and Fp4 creates unequal interelectrode distances in montages. A ground electrode is placed either at mid-forehead or on a mastoid region. Since digital recordings are fundamentally referential, an additional reference electrode position may be needed (typically noncephalic), although some instruments provide an "internal" reference. Placement of all of the standard electrodes of the International System could result in such close spacing on the neonate's scalp that electrode recording may overlap, with redundant electrical fields. Paste, not collodion, is used for electrode placement. While electrode impedances of <5 kOhms are standard in pediatric recordings, more liberal impedance measurements of 5 to 10 kOhms are acceptable in neonates to avoid excessive manipulation or abrasion of tender skin.[26] Marked differences among impedances between electrodes should be avoided.

At least 16 channels are recommended for routine neonatal EEG recordings. Polygraphic measures are integral to the recording of the EEG in order to assist in characterizing sleep states, eye movements, muscle contractions, cardiac rhythms,

TABLE 7.2. Initial Instrument Settings for Recording Neonatal EEG

EEG Channels

Sensitivity	7 µV/mm
Time-constant	0.3 sec
High-frequency filter	70 Hz
Notch filter (60 Hz, 50 Hz)	Off

Display time

Paper speed	30 mm/sec*
Screen display	10 sec/"page"*

Polygraphic Channels

	EOG**	EMG***	Respir.***	ECG***
Sensitivity	7 µV/mm	7 µV/mm	7 µV/mm	300 µV/mm
Time-constant	0.3 sec	0.01 sec	0.3 sec	0.3 sec
High-frequency filter	70 Hz	70 Hz	70 Hz	70 Hz
Notch filter (60 Hz, 50 Hz)	Off	Off	Off	Off

*Some laboratories may choose to record at "half paper speed" with a paper speed setting of 15 mm/sec or a screen display of 20 sec/"page/"
**EOG settings remain the same as EEG settings for comparison of simultaneously recorded waveforms.
*** EMG, respiratory (pneumograph), and ECG settings may be adjusted to optimize display.

and respiratory patterns and to help identify noncephalic artifact. The polygraphic measures include the electro-oculogram (EOG), submental electromyogram (EMG), electrocardiogram (ECG), and respiratory monitors such as a strain gauge, bipolar electrodes, or pneumograph.

The recording of the neonatal EEG includes the documentation of wake/sleep cycles, the characterization of reactivity of the record to stimulation, and identification of age-dependent waveforms and other features. These are best achieved using a single, bipolar montage with broad coverage over the scalp. Digital recording provides the opportunity to examine various waveforms with different montages after recordings are complete.

Instrument settings used at the onset of recording are listed in Table 7.2. The filter settings and sensitivity of the EEG channels should be the same as that for EOG in order to allow accurate comparison of waveforms to differentiate cerebral activity from that of ocular origin. The time base may be set at 30 mm/sec (10 sec/screen or "page"), although some electroencephalographers will prefer the slower speeds (e.g., 15 mm/sec [20 sec/screen]) to better appreciate the graphoelements representing the various patterns of wake and sleep states.

The most successful and clinically relevant neonatal EEG recordings are those in which objectives and strategies are identified prior to the beginning of each study. The basic tasks are to obtain historical data, determine reason for referral, initiate technical recordings, examine the EEG with accompanying video, observe the infant for clinical behaviors,

record the infant in sleep and wakefulness, and attempt to provoke abnormal paroxysmal clinical events when clinically indicated. Close observation of the infant at all times is particularly important when recording a neonatal EEG. The record should be annotated when behavioral or autonomic changes occur or when other events happen that may affect the record.

A final technical consideration relates to the duration of the neonatal EEG recording. There are two considerations: the time it may take for the infant to experience the full cycles of sleep and wakefulness and a sufficient period of time for the infant to experience clinical or electrical events. The typical minimum duration of recording for a standard neonatal EEG is 1 hour, although in many circumstances the recording will be in the context of more prolonged duration, depending upon clinical indications.

3.2. Age-Dependent Developmental Features

Initial analysis includes the assessment of the degree of continuity and interhemispheric synchrony of background activity. Further analysis consists of inspection for specific age-dependent waveforms and patterns, or graphoelements (Table 7.3), and the presence and character of sleep/wake cycles. In addition, there is recognition of some special waveforms and patterns that occur in the near-term or term infant that are considered developmental milestones and variations of the normal EEG.

TABLE 7.3. Age-Dependent Features of the Neonatal EEG

C.A, (WEEKS)	CONTINUITY	SYNCHRONY	LANDMARKS	WAKE/SLEEP CYCLES	REACTIVITY	IBI DURATION (SECS)*
24–26	Discontinuous (tracé discontinu)	Asynchronous	Beta-delta complexes may be present, although absence is not abnormal	Limited behavioral or polygraphic changes No cyclical EEG changes	No reaction to stimulation	46–60 sec
27–28	Discontinuous Interburst intervals are CA-dependent and less than preceding epoch	Asynchronous Traditionally characterized as an epoch of hypersynchrony	Beta-delta complexes first appearing in the central regions Temporal theta bursts (rudimentary)	Limited behavioral or polygraphic changes No cyclical EEG changes	No reaction to stimulation	38–46 sec
29–30	Discontinuous Interburst intervals are CA-dependent and less than preceding epoch Some brief periods of relative continuity	Asynchronous >50% activity asynchronous on the two sides	Beta-delta complexes in the central regions Temporal theta bursts (most consistent during this epoch)	Tendency for greater continuity of background activity during behavioral REM sleep	No reaction to stimulation	35 sec
31–33	Discontinuity during wakefulness Continuity during behavioral sleep	Asynchronous Degree of synchrony greater than previous epoch	Beta-delta complexes more prominent in temporal and occipital regions Temporal theta bursts until 32 weeks CA Temporal alpha bursts replace theta bursts at 33 weeks CA	Continuity during REM sleep Discontinuous during wakefulness and NREM sleep	No reaction to stimulation	20 sec
34–35	Discontinuity during NREM, less than the previous epoch Continuity during wakefulness and REM sleep	Asynchronous Degree of synchrony greater than previous epoch	Frontal sharp transients (enchoches frontales) Beta-delta complexes in occipital-temporal region, most often in NREM sleep	EEG and physiological features of wakefulness, REM and NREM sleep clearly defined	Background activity is reactive to stimulation—state-dependent	10 sec
36–37	Continuity during wakefulness and REM sleep Episodes of discontinuity during NREM sleep	Residual asynchrony Degree of synchrony ~80% on the two sides	Frontal sharp transients persist Beta-delta complexes become less frequent Bifrontal delta may be present	EEG and physiological features of wakefulness, REM and NREM sleep clearly defined	Background activity is reactive to stimulation—state-dependent	6–10 sec
38–40	Continuity in all states	Synchronous on the two sides by 40 weeks CA	Frontal sharp transients persist Beta-delta complexes disappear from NREM sleep	EEG and physiological features of wakefulness, REM and NREM sleep clearly defined Appearance of tracé alternant	Background activity is reactive to stimulation—state-dependent	6 sec
41–44	Continuity in all states	Synchronous on the two sides	Frontal sharp transients persist No other immature waveforms are present	EEG and physiologic features of wakefulness, REM and NREM sleep clearly defined Tracé alternant begins to resolve by 44 weeks CA	Background activity is reactive to stimulation—state-dependent	2–4 sec

*Based upon data from Vecchierini et al.[36] (24–26 weeks CA); Selton et al.[31] (26–28 weeks CA); Hahn et al.[30]; and Clancy et al.[17] (30–40 weeks CA).

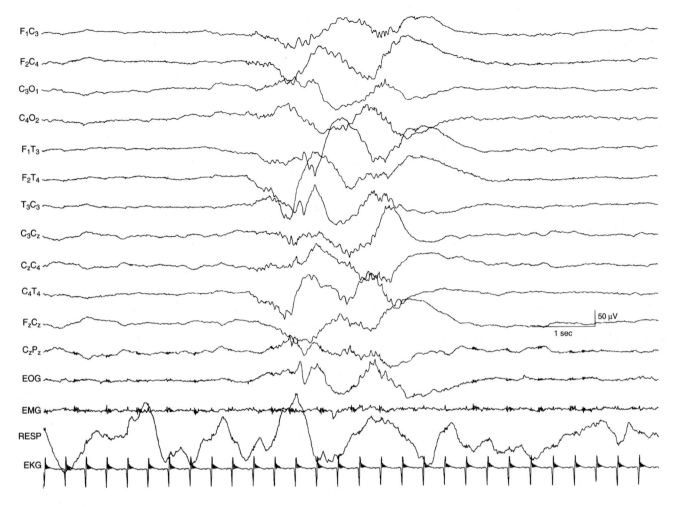

Channel labels (top to bottom): F_1C_3, F_2C_4, C_3O_1, C_4O_2, F_1T_3, F_2T_4, T_3C_3, C_3C_z, C_zC_4, C_4T_4, F_zC_z, C_zP_z, EOG, EMG, RESP, EKG

50 µV

1 sec

Figure 7.1. 26 to 27 weeks CA. This EEG demonstrates a tracé discontinu pattern with a burst of bilateral polyfrequency activity. The burst is somewhat asynchronous and has features of beta-delta complexes. (Reprinted with permission from Mizrahi EM, Hrachovy RA, Kellaway P. Atlas of Neonatal Electroencephalography. 3rd ed. Philadelphia, PA: Lippincott Williams & Wilkins; 2004.)

3.2.1. CONTINUITY

The earliest appearance of electrical activity on the EEG is characterized by a pattern of discontinuity, with long periods of quiescence (Fig. 7.1). This pattern may be present in all states of waking and sleep depending upon CA and has been referred to as *tracé discontinu*. As the CA increases, periods of inactivity shorten. The identification of interburst intervals (IBIs) is primarily based upon the degree of attenuation between bursts, although there is no real consensus among investigators regarding a definition of the maximum amplitude of the IBI; definitions range from 30 µV[29] to 15 µV[30], with 30 µV recommended as the upper limit.[31]

Several groups of investigators have measured IBIs to establish normative data at the various CAs. Although all have noted the trend of shortened IBIs with increasing CA, there is much variation in mean and maximum IBI values at the earliest CAs.[10,11,29–34] The variation in findings may relate to methodology differences, which include the amplitude of activity during the IBI (the lower the allowable amplitude, the shorter the attenuated interval), localization of attenuated activity of IBI (all channels simultaneously vs. allowable activity in some channels), the method of measurement of burst onset, and the

presence and degree of underlying CNS dysfunction such as hypoxia-ischemia (which may prolong IBIs, even at subclinical levels).

In most studies of IBI duration the earliest CA characterized has been ~27 to 28 weeks. There are limited data concerning the IBIs of younger neonates. Hayakawa et al.[35] studied infants beginning as young as 21 to 22 weeks CA and observed that the mean and maximum IBI duration also deceased with increasing CA. Vecchierni et al.[36] concluded that in neurologically normal infants with a CA of 24 to 26 weeks, IBIs do not exceed 60 sec. In addition, Clancy et al.[17] suggested that a starting point for mean IBI in the very premature infant (24 weeks CA) is 10 sec. The maximum duration of the IBI is based upon a composite of various studies,[37] beginning with a CA of ~26 weeks. Within an individual recording the duration of IBIs may vary, but in clinical practice, the IBIs with the longest duration are the most clinically relevant.

At ~30 weeks CA, continuous activity first appears, but it is state-dependent: it is present only during active sleep, the forerunner of rapid eye movement (REM) sleep. At ~34 weeks CA, the EEG also becomes continuous in the apparent awake state. By 37 to 38 weeks CA, continuity appears in the behavioral sleep state characterized as quiet sleep, the forerunner of non-REM (NREM). However, from that time until ~5 to 6 weeks postterm, during periods of quiet sleep the EEG demonstrates semiperiodic episodes of generalized voltage attenuation, not quiescence, lasting from 3 to 15 sec; this pattern has been called *tracé alternant*. These periods of attenuation differ from those of *tracé discontinu*: *tracé alternant* is characterized by persistence of waveforms at lower voltage, while *tracé discontinu* features periods of electrical quiescence with virtual absence of electrical activity.

3.2.2. BILATERAL HEMISPHERIC SYNCHRONY
It has often been reported that at or prior to 27 to 28 weeks CA, bursts of activity in the two hemispheres between periods of quiescence occur as generalized bisynchronous bursts with a discontinuous background.[11,33] However, others have reported that at 27 to 28 weeks CA the activity is generally asynchronous in homologous regions of the hemispheres.[18] The greater the recording distance from the midline, the greater the degree of asynchrony. With increasing maturity, the degree of asynchrony diminishes. The degree of asynchrony reflects not only maturation but also the wake/sleep state of the infant. Asynchrony is most prominent in quiet sleep and is least prominent in active sleep. The only exception to these general rules is that from the time frontal sharp waves first appear, at about 35 weeks CA, they are bilaterally synchronous.

3.2.3. AGE-DEPENDENT WAVEFORMS
There is an orderly appearance and disappearance of specific waveforms and patterns with increasing CA. These age-dependent waveforms are referred to as graphoelements and are essential landmarks in assessing CA and determining the degree to which the background EEG is normal.

3.2.3.1. BETA-DELTA COMPLEXES
These constitute the principal landmarks of prematurity. Various names have been given to these complexes: spindle-delta bursts, brushes, spindle-like fast waves, and ripples of prematurity. Dreyfus-Brisac et al.,[12] who first described the complexes, referred to them as rapid bursts, emphasizing the fast component of the complexes.

They are present from ~26 to 38 weeks CA and consist of randomly occurring 0.3- to 1.5-Hz waves of 50 to 250 μV, with superimposed bursts of low- to moderate-voltage fast activity (Fig. 7.2). The frequency of the fast activity may vary, even in the same infant. Two frequencies predominate: 8 to 12 Hz and, more commonly, 18 to 22 Hz. The voltage of the fast activity varies throughout each burst but rarely exceeds 75 μV. Until 32 weeks CA, the fast component has a predominant frequency of 18 to 22 Hz; thereafter, the slower frequency is most often present.

The complexes first appear as a dominant feature in the EEG at ~26 weeks CA. When first present they occur infrequently, predominantly in the central regions. During the next 5 to 6 weeks they become progressively more persistent, and the voltage of the fast component usually increases. From 29 to 33 weeks CA, the pattern is a prominent feature during active sleep. The spatial distribution of the beta-delta complexes is also age-dependent, becoming more prominent in the occipital and temporal areas with increasing age. Beta-delta complexes typically occur asynchronously in derivations from homologous areas and show a variable voltage asymmetry on the two sides.

At 33 weeks CA, beta-delta complexes are maximally expressed in quiet sleep and appear more prominently in the temporal-occipital areas. From 33 to 38 weeks CA, beta-delta complexes continue to occur primarily in quiet sleep. The disappearance of the beta-delta complexes when the infant appears behaviorally awake constitutes one marker of 36 to 37 weeks CA.

3.2.3.2. TEMPORAL THETA AND ALPHA BURSTS
Temporal theta bursts appear at ~26 weeks CA and are maximally expressed between 30 and 32 weeks (see Fig. 7.2). They then rapidly disappear and are replaced by temporal alpha bursts, a very specific marker for 33 weeks CA. Temporal theta bursts are characterized by rhythmic 4.5- to 6.0-Hz waves occurring independently in short bursts of rarely more than 2 sec from the left and right midtemporal areas. Voltage varies from roughly 20 to 200 μV. Some individual waves often have a sharp configuration. Temporal alpha bursts have similar features, except the frequency of their waveforms is greater than 6.0 Hz (Fig. 7.3).

In practical terms, strongly expressed temporal theta bursts can serve as a useful developmental landmark in determining CA between 30 and 32 weeks, particularly when considered in relation to other developmental features. The occurrence of temporal alpha bursts defines a more narrow CA range at 33 weeks.

3.2.3.3. FRONTAL SHARP WAVES
These are characterized as isolated sharp but bluntly configured waves. They usually have an initial surface-negative phase followed by a surface-positive phase. They have been referred to as *enchoches frontales*. Frontal sharp waves may first appear at 34 weeks CA but attain maximum expression at ~35 weeks CA (Fig. 7.4). When they initially appear they are low voltage and infrequent in occurrence, with a less well-defined waveform than when they are maximally expressed later. After 44 weeks CA they diminish in number and voltage and are only rarely seen in infants older than 6 weeks postterm.

Frontal sharp transients are bilaterally synchronous and symmetrical from the time of their first appearance. The initial surface-negative component lasts ~200 msec. The succeeding surface-positive component lasts somewhat longer and is variable. Although typically blunt in configuration, when they are maximally expressed, the waveforms may be quite sharp in morphology. Frontal sharp transients typically occur randomly as single events, predominantly in transitional rather than in active or quiet sleep. However, they may also recur in brief runs and may also be mixed with bifrontal delta activity, which is another normal feature of near-term infants (see below).

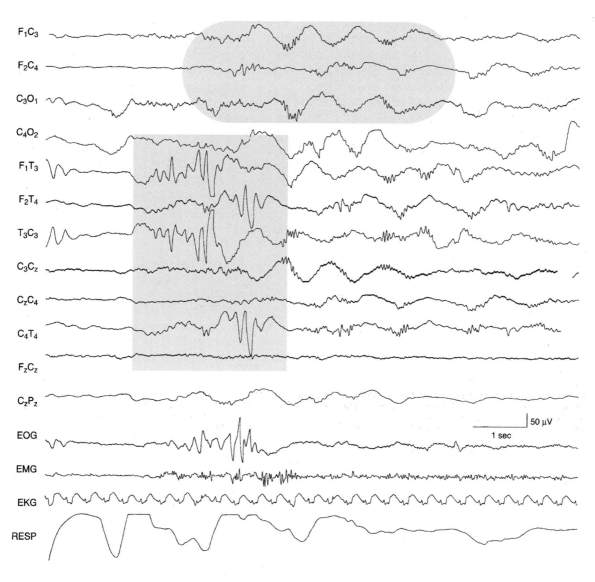

Figure 7.2. 29 to 30 weeks CA. Beta-delta complexes are present predominantly in the left central region (shaded oval). Temporal theta bursts are present independently on the left and right (shaded square). The EEG is discontinuous and asynchronous. (Reprinted with permission from Mizrahi EM, Hrachovy RA, Kellaway P. Atlas of Neonatal Electroencephalography. 3rd ed. Philadelphia, PA: Lippincott Williams & Wilkins; 2004.)

3.3. State Changes

3.3.1. THE EEG IN WAKEFULNESS AND SLEEP

Until 36 to 37 weeks CA, distinguishing the various states of the wake/sleep cycle is based upon infant behavior and findings of polygraphic recordings rather than EEG features, although there may be EEG changes associated with behavioral state changes before that epoch. Eye opening is associated with the awake state and eye closure is associated with sleep. Regular respiration, random eye movements, and variable muscle tone are associated with quiet sleep. Irregular respiration, rapid eye movements, and decreased muscle tone are associated with active sleep.

3.3.2. WAKEFULNESS

At ~30 weeks CA, the background activity is continuous in behavioral and polygraphic determined active sleep, and discontinuous during wakefulness and behavioral and polygraphic quiet sleep. In all states, beta-delta complexes are present with their age-dependent characteristics of abundance, spatial distribution, and degree of synchrony. By 36 to 37 weeks CA, there is a clear distinction between the waking EEG and the sleep EEG, without reliance on clinical or polygraphic recordings (Fig. 7.5). In the awake EEG age-dependent features persist and the background activity consists chiefly of continuous polyfrequency activity. This polyfrequency activity is characterized by random, very slow, low-voltage activity best described as baseline shifting, with superimposed semirhythmic 4- to 8-Hz activity in all regions. In addition there may be very-low-voltage 18- to 22-Hz activity and very-low-voltage 2- to 3-Hz activity in frontal regions. At 36 to 37 weeks, during wakefulness, the beta-delta complexes are no longer present.

3.3.3. QUIET SLEEP

Prior to ~36 weeks CA, the background activity in behavioral and polygraphic determined quiet sleep is discontinuous. Between 36 and 38 weeks CA, two patterns of quiet

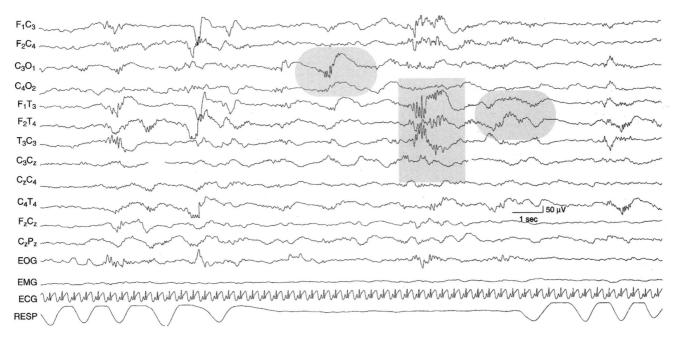

Figure 7.3. 33 weeks CA. Temporal alpha bursts are present on the left (shaded square) and beta-delta complexes are present in the occipital (shaded oval) and temporal regions (shaded oval). The EEG is discontinuous and asynchronous. (Reprinted with permission from Mizrahi EM, Hrachovy RA, Kellaway P. Atlas of Neonatal Electroencephalography. 3rd ed. Philadelphia, PA: Lippincott Williams & Wilkins; 2004.)

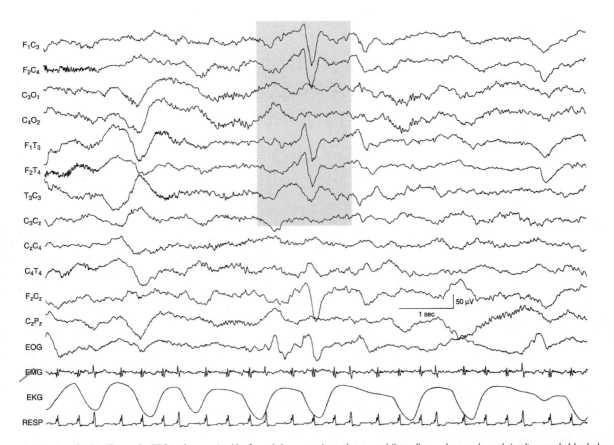

Figure 7.4. 36 to 37 weeks CA. The awake EEG is characterized by frontal sharp transients that occur bilaterally, synchronously, and simultaneously (shaded square). The background activity is continuous and synchronous, with some persistent beta-delta complexes in occipital regions. (Reprinted with permission from Mizrahi EM, Hrachovy RA, Kellaway P. Atlas of Neonatal Electroencephalography. 3rd ed. Philadelphia, PA: Lippincott Williams & Wilkins; 2004.)

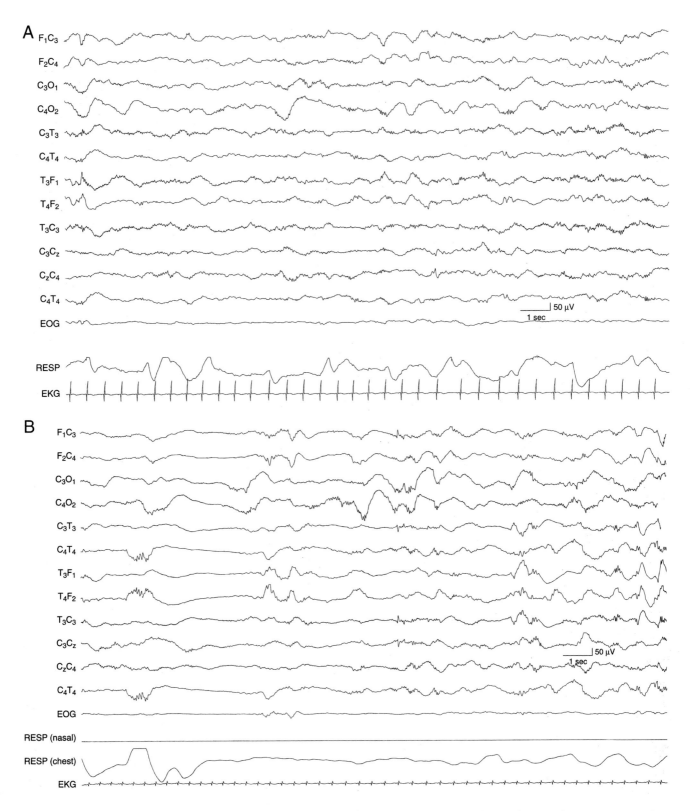

Figure 7.5. 34 to 35 weeks CA. **A:** Awake: The background activity is continuous with intermittent beta-delta complexes in the occipital regions (same recording as **B**). **B:** NREM sleep: Discontinuity during NREM sleep with otherwise similar developmental features as during wakefulness (same recording as **A**). (Reprinted with permission from Mizrahi EM, Hrachovy RA, Kellaway P. Atlas of Neonatal Electroencephalography. 3rd ed. Philadelphia, PA: Lippincott Williams & Wilkins; 2004.)

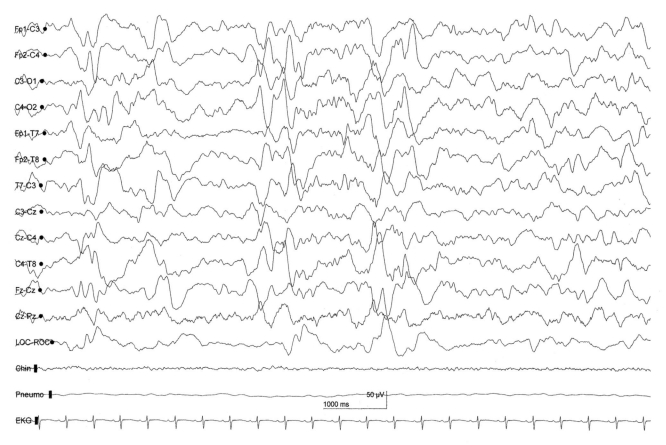

Figure 7.6. 40 to 44 weeks CA. The EEG is characterized by NREM sleep. The fluctuating amplitude of the background activity is typical of the tracé alternant pattern of quiet sleep. (Reprinted with permission from Mizrahi EM, Hrachovy RA, Kellaway P. Atlas of Neonatal Electroencephalography. 3rd ed. Philadelphia, PA: Lippincott Williams & Wilkins; 2004.)

sleep emerge: continuous high-voltage slow-wave activity in all regions and *tracé alternant* (Fig. 7.6). The latter is characterized by modulation of activity with alternating periods of high- and low-voltage activity. This pattern may be present up to 44 weeks CA. Thereafter, quiet sleep is characterized by continuous slow-wave activity with the eventual emergence of sleep spindles after ~46 weeks CA (although rudimentary spindles may occur earlier).

3.3.4. ACTIVE SLEEP

The character of the EEG during active sleep is similar to that of the awake recording beginning from ~30 weeks CA. Infant behaviors and polygraphic recordings of respiration, eye movements, and submental EMG are used to distinguish the awake state from active sleep.

3.3.5. TRANSITIONAL OR INDETERMINATE SLEEP

These terms are used to characterize the EEG when the state of the infant cannot be precisely determined. This may occur in the transition from wakefulness to sleep and can be a relatively brief period or more prolonged between states.

3.3.6. REACTIVITY TO STIMULATION

Between 33 and 34 weeks CA, changes in EEG activity in response to stimuli appear. By 37 weeks CA, these responses may be easily and more reliably elicited. Typically, the response to a stimulus is related to the character of the ongoing activity at the time of the stimulus. If high-voltage, very slow activity is present, an effective stimulus produces abrupt and pronounced generalized attenuation of voltage lasting up to several seconds (Fig. 7.7). In addition, there may be spontaneous episodes of attenuation associated with self-arousal. These may occur in infants until ~2 weeks postterm and should not be interpreted as evidence of immaturity or be confused with the repetitive episodes of generalized or regional attenuation that occur in neonatal encephalopathies.

3.4. Special Waveforms and Patterns

Some special waveforms and patterns are present, particularly in the near-term and term infant, which are considered to be within the range of normal variation.

3.4.1. BIFRONTAL DELTA ACTIVITY

Bifrontal delta activity appears in the near-term or term infant as intermittent semirhythmic 1.5- to 2-Hz moderately high to high voltage activity in the frontal regions bilaterally (Fig. 7.8). These waveforms may occur in close association with frontal sharp transients and are most prominent during transitional sleep. Although the pattern has been referred to as anterior dysrhythmia, it does not suggest, nor has it been associated with, any abnormality.

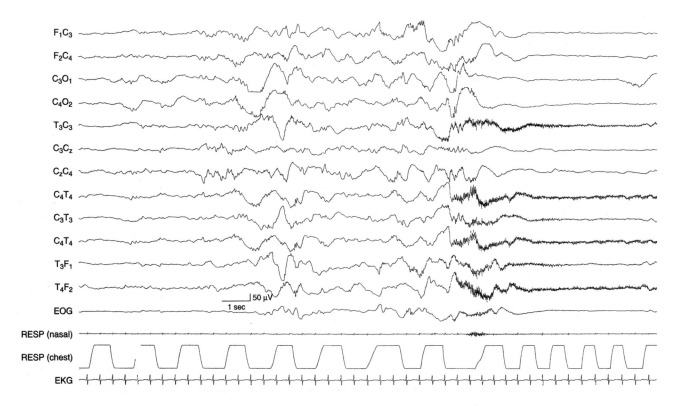

Figure 7.7. 38 to 40 weeks. A transient arousal is characterized by a brief episode of generalized voltage attenuation. The background activity is consistent with NREM sleep before and after the arousal. (Reprinted with permission from Mizrahi EM, Hrachovy RA, Kellaway P. Atlas of Neonatal Electroencephalography. 3rd ed. Philadelphia, PA: Lippincott Williams & Wilkins; 2004.)

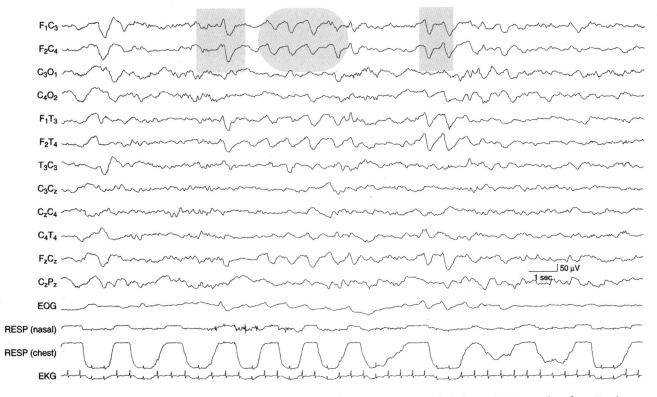

Figure 7.8. 38 to 40 weeks. Bifrontal delta activity is present (shaded oval) mixed with frontal sharp transients (shaded square) in this recording of transitional or indeterminant sleep. The EEG is continuous and synchronous on the two sides. There are no immature features. (Reprinted with permission from Mizrahi EM, Hrachovy RA, Kellaway P. Atlas of Neonatal Electroencephalography. 3rd ed. Philadelphia, PA: Lippincott Williams & Wilkins; 2004.)

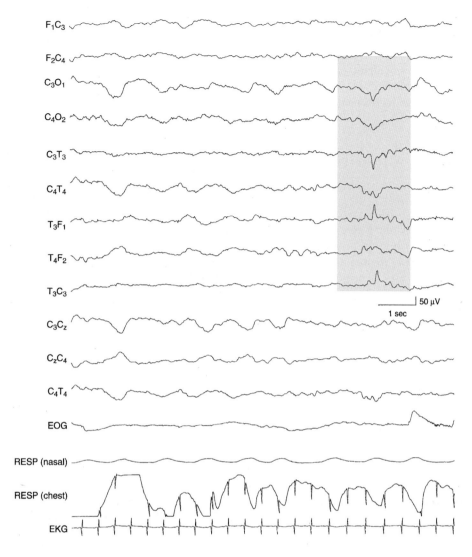

Figure 7.9. *38 to 40 weeks. A temporal sharp wave is present on the left (shaded square). It is randomly occurring, moderate in voltage, and simple in morphology, occurring during transitional or indeterminant sleep. The background activity is within the range of normal for CA. (Reprinted with permission from Mizrahi EM, Hrachovy RA, Kellaway P. Atlas of Neonatal Electroencephalography. 3rd ed. Philadelphia, PA: Lippincott Williams & Wilkins; 2004.)*

3.4.2. SHARP WAVE TRANSIENTS

Physiological sharp wave transients are seen in neonatal EEG and are considered normal when they meet certain criteria: negative polarity to the initial and predominant deflection; 100- to 200-ms discharges against a normal background for corrected age; most abundant in the midtemporal, central, and centrotemporal regions; and mostly single and only occasionally seen in brief trains or runs (Fig. 7.9). They should be distributed symmetrically, typically involving homologous regions, and randomly instead of being predominant in one region. Quantification during the more continuous portions of the tracing (i.e., wakefulness and active sleep) has led to the recommendation in consensus criteria that having 11 or less per hour in a preterm infant, and 13 or less per hour in a term infant, is considered nonpathological, assuming the other criteria are met.[38] Brief rhythmic discharges (BRDs), of less than ten seconds duration and sometimes referred to as BIRDS (brief interictal/ictal rhythmic/repetitive discharges) or BERDS (brief epileptiform rhythmic discharges), are rarely seen in isolation in normal neonatal EEG and are more consistent with pathology.

3.5. Transition from Neonatal to Infantile Patterns

Neonatal EEG patterns generally end between 46 and 48 weeks CA and transition to predominantly infantile EEG patterns by 3 months of age. The *tracé alternant* pattern, the EEG correlate of quiet sleep (non-REM sleep), is common during the first 1 to 3 weeks of life in a full-term newborn. The majority of sleep time in the term newborn is spent in active sleep. Quiet sleep onset is well established 1 month after full-term delivery and gradually emerges as the predominant type of sleep with the development of the non-REM sleep stages. *Tracé alternant* patterns disappear about 3 to 4 weeks after full-term birth,[39] although they have been observed up to day 47.[40] Intervening CNS insults, either primary or secondary (systemic), may interfere with CNS function and temporarily cause developmental regression, which may be expressed with a return to a less mature EEG pattern.

With the disappearance of neonatal EEG patterns and the emergence of patterns such as the posterior basic (posterior dominant) rhythm, the forerunner of alpha rhythm, and sleep spindles, the EEG begins to demonstrate the more mature patterns seen in older children and adults. During the waking state, a generally rhythmic 3- to 4-Hz posterior activity occurs, a precursor of the posterior alpha rhythm. This posterior rhythm demonstrates reactivity to eye opening and closing, characterized by blocking with eye opening and activation with eye closing.

4. EEG IN INFANCY (2–12 MONTHS)

It is challenging to obtain a waking EEG recording in the infant. As infants tend to keep their eyes open, in order to obtain a posterior dominant rhythm, gentle passive occlusion of the eyes (passive eye closure) for short periods may be helpful to activate the posterior basic rhythm. Temporary use of a short time constant (0.1 sec) may be helpful to separate the posterior rhythm from movement artifacts. This rhythm may be present in a crying infant (associated with forceful closure of eyes and concomitant frontal muscle artifact) as well as in a quiet infant with open eyes. The infant usually closes the eyes as a sign of impending drowsiness.

There are two basic philosophies to EEG recording in infancy. In the first, the recording is started in a sleeping baby. Spontaneous sleep is desirable, and this may be achieved when the recording is scheduled shortly after feeding. The second approach is to start the recording with the patient awake. It is difficult to place electrodes in an awake infant although some technologists become experienced in the art of handling an awake infant and obtain both waking and spontaneous sleep recordings. Conscious sedation for all practical purposes is no longer used, and sleep deprivation and placement in a bed or in the mother's arms is frequently done.[41–43]

The International 10-20 System should be used for electrode placement, using a full set of 21 EEG electrodes (19 scalp electrodes and two ear reference electrodes).[26] It is helpful to use ocular leads, respiratory monitoring, and ECG in detecting artifacts, as well as in assessing sleep stages. Although some laboratories use rubber caps in small infant sizes, this technique is not conducive to sleep, and collodion or commercial pastes are preferable.

4.1. EEG Characteristics in the Waking State

In early infancy (age ~2 months), irregular delta activity of 2 to 3.5 Hz and medium to high voltage (50–100 µV) is widely preponderant. As noted above, rhythmic occipital 3- to 4-Hz activity is often noted at age 3 to 4 months; this activity can be blocked by eye opening.

This posterior basic (dominant) rhythm becomes more stable at age 5 months and increases over time, first to 5 Hz[39] and subsequently to an average frequency of 6 to 7 Hz (occasionally 8 Hz) by age 12 months. The amplitudes range from 50 to 100 µV.

Some rhythmic rolandic (central) activity of 5 to 8 Hz may be present as early as age 3 months, with an amplitude around 25 to 50 µV. This activity is the precursor of the mu rhythm and is stable during the first year of life,[39] but it may be dependent on somatosensory stimulation.[44] These visual analysis findings have been confirmed with quantitative EEG.[45–47]

4.2. EEG Characteristics in Drowsiness

Prior to the age of 5 to 8 months, the transition from the waking state to sleep is a gradual process characterized by progressive slowing into the delta frequency range. No specific drowsy state is identified in this smooth progression of slow activity to the sleep stage. Drowsiness is recognized by a distinct pattern between ages 6 and 8 months: a hypersynchronous rhythm in the lower theta range, around 4 Hz, with gradual acceleration to 5 and 6 Hz over the ensuing months. This impressive theta rhythmicity is known as hypnagogic hypersynchrony.[48]

This drowsy pattern seems to develop from the posterior basic (dominant) rhythm. The transition from wakefulness to drowsiness is associated with a change in the amplitude distribution. The maximum rhythmic theta activity moves into the centroparietal region, where amplitudes commonly reach 100 to 250 µV. EEG amplitude values depend on the interelectrode distance and may vary from montage to montage; they are best measured with a referential montage.

According to Dreyfus and Curzi-Dascalova,[39] the occipital rhythm may be somewhat slower than the diffusely predominant theta rhythm (possibly indicating a basic difference between two coexisting rhythmic theta patterns). In rare cases, hypnogogic hypersynchrony may not occur.

4.3. Sleep EEG and Non-REM Sleep

EEG and polygraphic data indicate sleep onset with active (REM) sleep in neonates and gradual evolution of sleep onset with quiet (NREM) sleep during the ensuing weeks. The "slow" sleep of the infant is dominated by diffuse 0.75- to 3-Hz activity with a maximum amplitude (100–150 or 200 µV) over the occipital area, "occipital delta." This occipital delta activity may be quite prominent during the first year of life. The amplitudes increase with deepening slow sleep. There are some intermixed theta, alpha, and beta frequencies of smaller amplitudes.

Sleep spindles usually appear during the second month of life; occasionally spindle fragments may be seen somewhat earlier.[49,50] The spindle frequency ranges from 12 to 15 Hz, with 14 Hz the most commonly encountered frequency. Throughout infancy, spindles are maximal over central and parietal areas with shifting asymmetries. A clear-cut midline (vertex) maximum does not exist at this age. Spindles of infancy usually show a negative sharp component, whereas the positive component is rounded. The sharp spindle configuration[51] is a typical hallmark of sleep in infancy. The comblike shape of these runs may be erroneously interpreted as 14-Hz positive spikes, but a careful analysis of polarity clearly shows the negativity of the spiky components. The spatial distribution also is different: spindles are rolandic, whereas 14-Hz positive spikes are predominantly in a posterotemporal location. Finally, the 14- Hz or 14- and 6-Hz positive spike pattern is extremely rare before the age of 2 years and virtually nonexistent during the first year of life (Fig. 7.10).

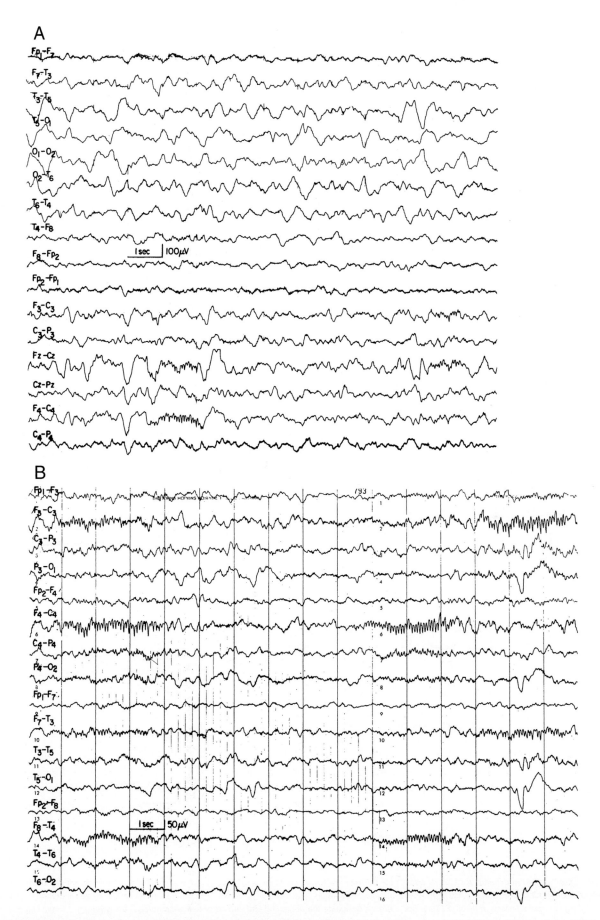

Figure 7.10. A: Patient age 10 months. Light NREM sleep. Typical spindles of infancy, sharp and shifting. Normal posterior voltage maximum of slow activity (channels 3–7 from the top). **B:** Patient age 9 months. More prolonged trains of infantile spindles.

Spindles may show sharp negative and positive phases after age 6 months.[52] This sharp positive spindle polarity is less common than spindles with a strictly negative sharp component. The spindle train duration varies with age. Spindle trains are of short duration and low voltage during the second month. With the third month, the amplitude increases and the duration of the runs becomes much longer.[53] The intervals between spindle trains become shorter, and at times they may appear almost continuous.[46] Spindle bursts may reach a duration of 10 sec in the second half of the first year, but there is a decreased duration of each spindle run, while the overall number of runs increases.

Dreyfus and Curzi-Dascalova[39] report that the complete absence of spindles at age 3 to 8 months represents a severe abnormality. However, this finding should be interpreted with great caution, as enough sleep must have been obtained during the recording in order "to give the baby a chance to produce spindles." At this age, there is still a fair chance that the sleep recording is limited to stage REM; this demonstrates the importance of oculographic and pneumographic recording. An excellent demonstration of the development of sleep spindles from age 10 weeks to 1 year was presented by Hughes[54] (Fig. 7.11).

Vertex waves and *K-complexes* are usually seen around the age of 5 months, although rudiments may occur much earlier. Vertex waves may be quite large at age 5 to 6 months. At this age, K-complexes are of considerable voltage, but the initiating sharp component is poorly developed and somewhat "blunted."[55] In contrast, Metcalf et al.[56] have stressed the comparatively low voltage of K-complexes in infancy. These authors also noticed the appearance of K-complexes in infants age 5 to 6 months, but the complexes may be obscured by background activity (Figs. 7.12 and 7.13). A vertex wave may be frontally dominant or extend into the lateral frontal regions; this is sometimes called an F-wave[57] (Fig. 7.14). In normal infants in the first year of life, Ellingson et al.[58] recorded brief apneic episodes ("respiratory pauses" lasting 3–10 sec) during sleep. These pauses are more common in REM sleep.

4.4. Sleep EEG and REM Sleep

REM sleep abundance decreases during the first year of life:[59,60] it is ~50% at birth and falls to 40% at 3 to 5 months and 30% between 12 and 24 months.

Dittrichova et al.[61] and Dreyfus and Curzi-Dascalova[39] reported the occurrence of sharply contoured occipital activity in the REM sleep of infants. This activity shows a frequency around 2 Hz at 6 weeks and 2 to 4 Hz at 12 to 16 weeks of age. Some intermixed delta and theta activity is associated with the occipital sharp transients.

The REM sleep latency (time span from sleep onset to the first REM period) gradually lengthens during the first year of life. Schulz et al.[62] have shown that the REM sleep latency underlies diurnal rhythmic changes, with the longest latencies between noon and 4 p.m. and the shortest between 4 a.m. and 8 a.m.

4.5. Reactivity

The blocking response of the posterior basic (dominant) rhythm (obtained by passive eye closure) is usually present at age 3 to 4 months. The central mu rhythm does not react to eye opening, which permits differentiation when there is anterior spreading of the posterior dominant rhythm. A true rolandic mu rhythm cannot be identified during the first year of life, although forerunners of this activity are likely to be present. Mu rhythm has been seen as young as 20 months of age.[63] A photic driving response to flickering light may be obtained as early as 3 to 4 months of age; the responses are most prominent in the theta band.[64,65] Occipital lambda wave activity occurs rarely during the first year of life.

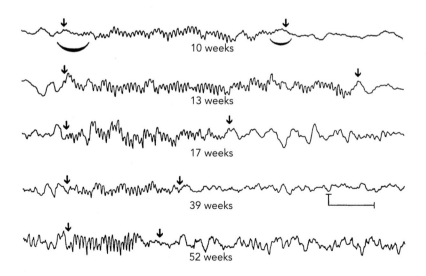

Figure 7.11. *Sleep spindles at different ages. At 10 weeks note the very low amplitude at the beginning and end of the burst (underlined) with a duration of 5 sec; at 13 weeks a long-lasting spindle of 6.5 sec; at 17 weeks, 3.5 sec; at 39 weeks, 2 sec; and at 52 weeks, 1.5 sec. Time (1 sec) and voltage calibration (50 µV) are shown. Montage is bipolar linkage of the C₃-P₃ electrodes. Arrows designate the beginning and ending of typical spindles at the given age. (From Hughes JR. Development of sleep spindles in the first year of life. Clin Electroencephalogr. 1996;27:107–115.)*

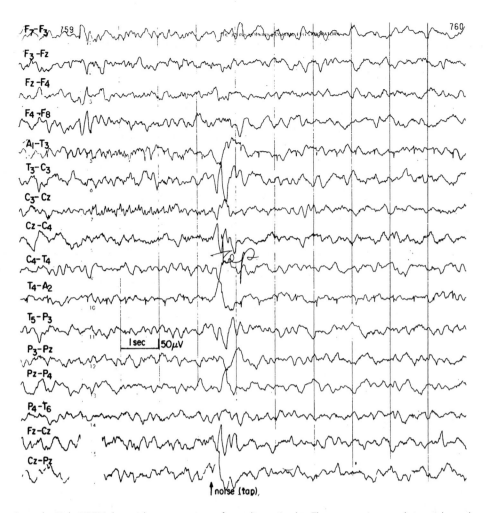

Figure 7.12. Patient age 9 months. Light NREM sleep. A large vertex wave after auditory stimulus. The response is somewhat complex and resembles a K-complex.

5. EEG IN EARLY CHILDHOOD (12–36 MONTHS)

5.1. Waking Record

Readable waking records are challenging to obtain in the second and third years of life. At this age, many children resent being placed in a supine position for electrode placement and recording and may be too heavy to be comfortably held. These children may successfully fight sleepiness and sleep, and if sedated, the waking portion is a postarousal tracing, in which it must be determined that the child is truly awake. Some children may pull off their electrodes almost immediately after awakening.

The *posterior basic (dominant) rhythm* increases from the upper theta to the lowest alpha range and is most commonly found between 6 to 7 Hz during the second year and 7 to 8 Hz during the third year of life. The blocking response to eye opening intensifies, although the degree of this reactivity, a more impressive response, is considerably determined by the darkness or brightness of the recording room. The posterior basic (dominant) rhythm frequency is subject to considerable variation in the second and third year of life. According to Lindsley,[66] a frequency range from 5 to almost 10 Hz can be observed in the second year, whereas Eeg-Olofsson[2] reported a surprisingly high mean frequency of 8 Hz at this age.

Eye blinks are associated with a biphasic (negative-positive) potential of medium to high voltage in bilateral synchrony over occipital areas.[67]

Fast activity (18–25 Hz) may be very prominent, especially in sleep, and not necessarily related to sedative medication. *Frequencies slower than the posterior basic (dominant) rhythm* are practically always noted in the waking state at this age, mostly in the 2- to 5-Hz range and widely scattered. The amount of this activity is also quite variable and may be accentuated by crying, due to a hyperventilation effect.

The reactivity of the waking EEG becomes more prominent; the blocking response of the posterior basic rhythm is more clearly demonstrable than in the first year. Mu rhythm over the rolandic regions may be identifiable in the second year of life.[63] The photic driving response to the strobe light remains accentuated in the low-frequency range.

5.2. Drowsiness

Generalized high-voltage (mostly 4–6 Hz) theta activity is the hallmark of the drowsy state in early childhood. This drowsy

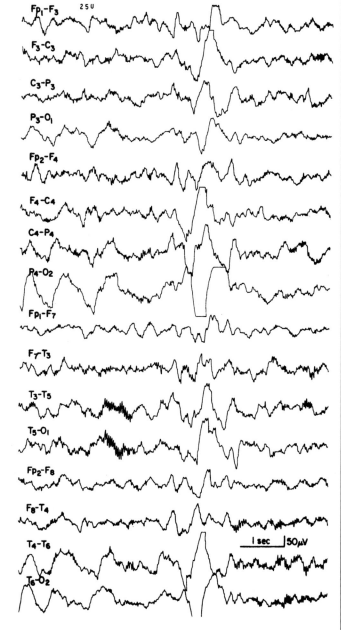

Figure 7.13. A K-complex in a patient age 13 months; quite large with a blunted sharp component.

must refrain from calling these discharges epileptiform or spike-wave complexes. Brandt and Brandt[69] determined that these admixed sharp or spiky components occur in a small percentage (~5–10%) of normal children at all ages. This was confirmed by Eeg-Olofsson et al.[2] Unless unquestionable spikes are detectable, the presence of such small spiky potentials is harmless, does not represent a definite abnormality, and should be interpreted as a normal finding. The mature form of drowsy EEG activity with dropout of the posterior dominant rhythm and general decline of the voltage output is quite common at this age.

5.3. Sleep Record

Sleep begins with NREM sleep. Because of the usual relatively short duration of a sleep recording in the EEG laboratory in daytime, REM stages are usually not observed. The hypnagogic hypersynchrony of drowsiness is replaced by diffusely preponderant, irregular, high-voltage (1–3 Hz) and medium- to high-voltage (4–6 Hz) activity. The maximum amplitude is almost invariably found over the occipital area, where 0.75- to 2-Hz waves may reach very high voltage (see Fig. 7.10). A different type of voltage distribution or even an anterior voltage maximum should warn the electroencephalographer; residual damage to the posterior regions is a possibility, although none of the typical EEG abnormalities may be present (Fig. 7.16). This anterior-to-posterior amplitude difference is referred to as the frequency amplitude gradient.[70]

The varying degree of intermixed fast activity without premedication was mentioned earlier. *Spindle activity* in the 12- to 14-Hz range is now found in a transitional stage; the shifting spindle runs occurring over centroparietal areas with a negative spiky component are gradually replaced by symmetrical spindle activity with a maximum over the vertex. A 14-Hz spindle type appears first over the vertex and with deepening sleep (transition stage 2 to 3); spindles in the 12-Hz range appear over frontal midline and upper frontal regions. Both types of spindles may occur concomitantly, but they have a different spatial distribution.

Vertex waves, formerly known as biparietal humps,[68] are quite prominent at this age; their amplitude is impressive, but their rise is not as abrupt and the configuration is not as sharp as in later years (ages 4–12). This same is true for *K-complexes,* which are abundantly noted in the stages of NREM sleep. *Positive occipital sharp transients of sleep* (occipital positive sharp activity, lambdoid activity) are absent or very poorly developed at this age. *REM sleep* at this age rarely occurs during a standard EEG but is seen during a standard sleep study; it starts to show signs of EEG desynchronization, but slow activity (mostly 2–5 Hz, according to Cadilhac[71]) is still preponderant (Fig. 7.17).

5.4. Unusual and Variant Patterns in Sleep

Extreme spindles[72,73] represent an unusual variant of sleep spindle activity with high voltage, a wide frequency range (6–18 Hz), and occasional paroxysmal traits. In a diminutive form,

pattern is called hypnogogic hypersynchrony. It is most pronounced in the central and parietal leads, is less impressive over the temporal areas, and is sometimes least developed over the occipital region. The rhythmicity may assume a quite monotonous character; the in-phase character of the ubiquitous pattern makes it tempting to theorize about an enormously extended generator area (Fig. 7.15).

Gibbs and Gibbs[68] paid special attention to a variant of the rhythmic theta activity of drowsiness. In a large number of small children, bursts of 4- to 5-Hz activity may be present instead of the steady rhythmic theta activity. This pattern extends into the fourth year of life and shows mild paroxysmal activity without representing a true abnormality. Occasionally, small sharp or spiky discharges may be interspersed between the theta waves; the electroencephalographer

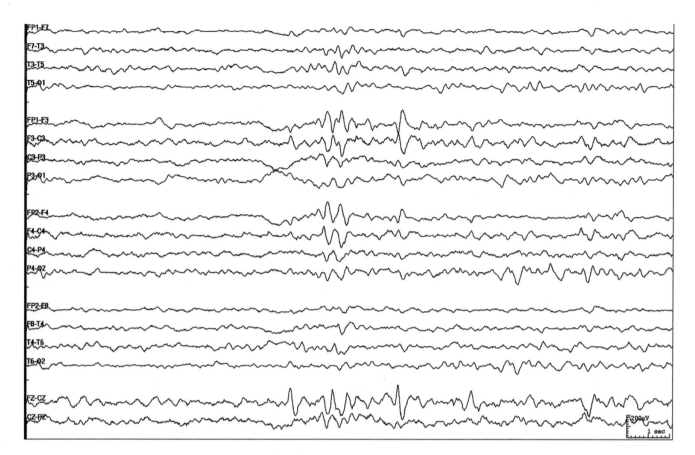

Figure 7.14. *The F-wave: a more frontal (anterior) vertex wave.*

these spindles may even occur while the child is awake (coexisting with a posterior alpha rhythm) (Fig. 7.18).

According to Gibbs and Gibbs,[73] this pattern occurs in 0.05% of normal children, but the prevalence reaches 5% to 18% in children with intellectual deficiency or cerebral palsy. This pattern is seen from age 1 to 12 years, with a peak at age 3; after age 12, the incidence falls to almost zero.

Following the original studies by Gibbs and Gibbs, there have been very few reports dealing with this pattern. When clearly separable from typical spindle activity, extreme spindles might represent a mild abnormality.

The *fast spiky spindle variant*[74] is a very rare pattern (about one case in 2,000–3,000 EEGs of children). It consists of spindle-like activity in the range of 16 to 20 Hz and may occur

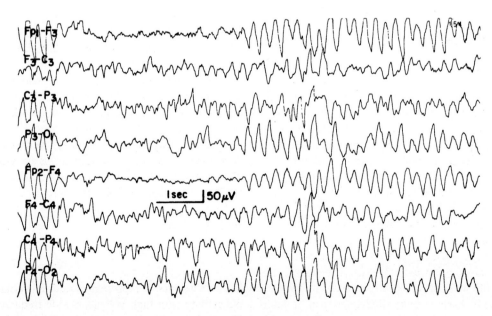

Figure 7.15. *Patient age 3 years. Drowsiness. Rhythmic hypnagogic theta activity, 4 to 5 per second.*

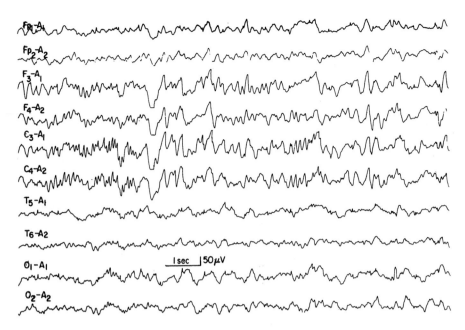

Figure 7.16. Patient age 9 months. Cerebral palsy, diplegic. Lack of posterior voltage maximum. Otherwise a normal record with sharp spindles of infancy.

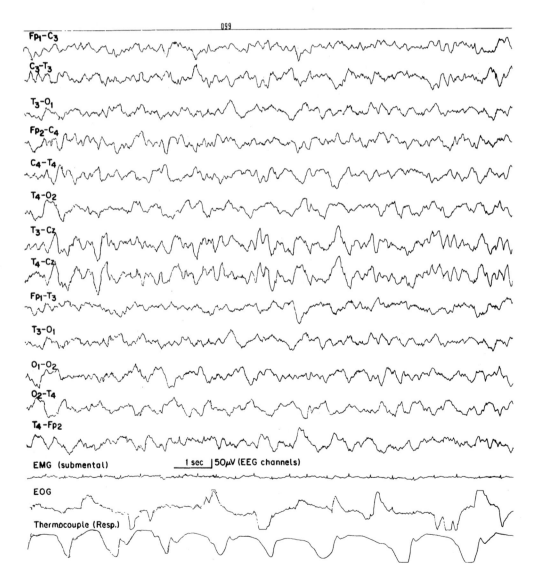

Figure 7.17. Patient age 22 months. REM sleep.

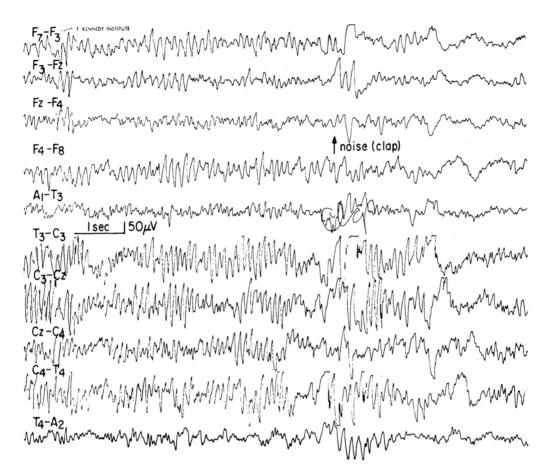

F Kennedy Institute

F7–F3

F3–Fz

Fz–F4

F4–F8

↑ noise (clap)

A1–T3

T3–C3 |1 sec |50 μV

C3–Cz

Cz–C4

C4–T4

T4–A2

Figure 7.18. Patient age 22 months. Extreme spindles over central region; a somewhat slower type of spindles over the frontal area.

over a variety of areas (central, parietal, vertex, or midtemporal) in stage 2 or 3 of sleep. It is seen mainly in early childhood (around age 3) but also occurs in older children and adolescents. This fast spiky spindle variant is usually seen in children with static or progressive brain dysfunction and probably indicates a mild abnormality.

The *14- and 6-Hz positive spike discharge, or 16- and 6-Hz positive burst,* is very uncommon before age 3.

5.5. Arousal from Sleep

Arousal from sleep is characterized by a similar marked and prolonged high-voltage 4- to 6-Hz activity in all leads with some intermixed slower frequencies.[75,76] This is called hypnopompic hypersynchrony and is considered a normal variant (Fig. 7.19). White and Tharp[77] reported the observation of prolonged rhythmic sharp or spiky activity over the frontal areas in children between ages 2 and 12 years during arousal. This "frontal arousal rhythm" is maximal over the frontal midline and generally considered a normal variant, although an ictal example was reported in which this frontal arousal rhythm was associated with a clinical seizure consisting of eyelid flutter and chewing.[78]

5.6. Occurrence of Minor and Major Abnormalities in Early Childhood (Scarcity of Minor Abnormalities During the First 2 Years of Life)

When abnormalities are carefully and consistently graded as minimal, slight, moderate, marked, and severe, there is a statistically significant ($p < .001$) small number of minor (i.e., minimal, slight, and moderate) abnormalities prior to the age of 21 months. In other words, there is no real continuum of various forms of minor abnormalities between normal records on one side and markedly abnormal records on the other side.[79] After the age of 21 months (~2 years), minor abnormalities become much less frequent, and the aforementioned continuum of graded abnormalities is present. Thus, there is a relatively silent period, following the neonatal period, during which EEG detects relatively few abnormalities until the end of the second year of life, when EEG abnormalities tend to reappear.

A hypothesis is that there is a limited number of EEG responses to cerebral impairment prior to the age of 21 months, associated with a lack of fine intermediate nuances of abnormality. It is possible that minor abnormalities are not so rare after all, and that new valid criteria will

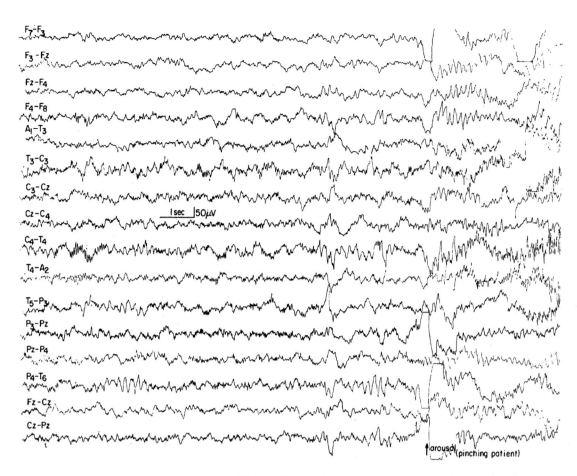

Figure 7.19. *Patient age 16 months. Arousal from sleep. Pronounced rhythmic 6/sec activity with a sharp component, maximal over frontal midline.*

evolve for the interpretation of the EEG in infancy and early childhood. Progress in neonatal EEG has shown that classical signs of abnormality such as spikes, focal or diffuse slowing, or local voltage depression cannot serve as the only guideline; the sequences of sleep stages and their adequacy for the GA are important criteria for the newborn. In the older child and adult, an additional criterion for normality vis-à-vis the background organization would be the integrity of the frequency amplitude gradient.

6. PRESCHOOL-AGE EEG (3–5 YEARS)

6.1. Waking Record

A waking record is much easier to obtain at this age, and with good handling by the technologist, many children are quite cooperative. At age 3, the *posterior basic (dominant) rhythm* has reached 8 Hz and thus the alpha range. The alpha amplitude is almost always higher than in adolescence and adulthood. Leissner et al.[80] correlated the alpha amplitude with skull thickness by ultrasound. The alpha amplitude may reach 100 µV and tends to increase from age 3 to a peak at 8 or 9 years. As with adults, amplitudes are usually higher over the right hemisphere.

The train of posterior alpha waves is frequently interrupted by admixed slow waves, mostly in the range of 1.5 to 4 Hz,

extending from occipital into the posterior temporal and, less impressively, into the parietal regions. These admixed slow waves, fused with overriding alpha, are called posterior slow waves of youth. Alpha voltage, distribution, and admixture of slow activity create a picture that makes the tracing almost immediately identifiable as a record of childhood.

Posterior slowing may show a variety of forms. Most common is the irregularly interspersed type of slow activity. These slow waves are often preceded by a sharply contoured potential that blends together with the ensuing "slow fused transients."[81] Posterior slow activity can reach abnormal degrees, especially with towering amplitudes or abnormal rhythmicity such as prolonged trains of rhythmic slow waves. The differentiation of such abnormal forms from physiological posterior slow activity is usually not difficult. Posterior slow waves of youth react to eye opening and closing, as does the posterior dominant, or alpha, rhythm.

In the *absence of posterior slow activity*, the posterior alpha rhythm assumes a more "mature" character with unbroken prolonged stretches. Eeg-Olofsson[3] and Petersén and Eeg-Olofsson[6] list such tracings as "supernormal," which is a term comprehensible to electroencephalographers but of no particular clinical significance. Such records perhaps suggest a hastened process of maturation, and a 5-year-old child may show the adult features of posterior alpha.

Anterior rhythmic 6- to 7-Hz theta activity is not uncommonly found at preschool age but reaches its peak somewhat later. The clinical significance of this pattern is discussed in the next section. *Rolandic mu rhythm* becomes increasingly manifest at this age before peaking early in the second decade of life. At this age, *low-voltage records* with activity consistently below 25 to 30 μV are not seen as a variant of normalcy; such tracings have been associated with underlying static encephalopathy.[73] *Excessively fast records* usually represent drug effect; otherwise, such records fall into the mildly to moderately abnormal range.

6.2. Activation Patterns

At age 4 years, children usually become very cooperative for *hyperventilation*, although one seldom finds a cooperative 3-year-old. Four-year-olds seem to enjoy the test and are sometimes hard to stop. The use of a pinwheel is very helpful.

High-amplitude slowing to hyperventilation can be very pronounced at this age and must be considered normal unless unequivocal epileptic discharges or marked asymmetries are found. Protracted slowing (either as rhythmic delta bursts or as continuous irregular delta-theta activity) after termination of hyperventilation usually indicates that the child continues overbreathing. In such cases, the effect of hypoglycemia must also be taken into consideration; it may be important to document the time of the last meal. Special studies in this field were done by Gibbs et al.[82] and by Petersén and Eeg-Olofsson.[6] A prolonged response to hyperventilation may indicate vascular disease, as has been specifically reported in Moya-Moya syndrome.[83]

The occipital driving response to *intermittent photic stimulation* is quite often best obtained with a flash frequency in the lower flicker frequency range; responses are most prominent below 8 Hz.[6] Paroxysmal responses to flicker (even in the normal child) are more likely to occur in school-age children.

6.3. EEG Findings in Drowsiness

Past 3 years of age, the previously mentioned hypnagogic hypersynchrony disappears; it is seldom seen in healthy children at age 6. Paroxysmal theta bursts are also on the decline. The admixture of posterior slow activity tends to increase in early drowsiness, and increased delta and theta activity soon occurs in all leads.

Anterior rhythmic 6- to 7-Hz theta activity increases in early drowsiness but disappears in deep drowsiness. This pattern occurs more often in school-age children and is discussed below. The *14- and 6-Hz positive burst* manifests itself in deep drowsiness and vanishes in light sleep. This pattern is not very common at this age and will be discussed below.

6.4. Sleep EEG Records

The posterior maximum of diffusely predominant delta (1–3 Hz) activity is not as pronounced as in infancy and early childhood. *Sleep spindles* have lost their sharp and bilaterally shifting feature of infancy and now show a well-defined maximum over the vertex. Frequencies around 14 Hz are seen before more anterior spindles in the 10- to 12-Hz range occur with deepening sleep. *Vertex waves* and *K-complexes* show a more prominent sharp component than in earlier years. *Positive occipital sharp transients of sleep* (lambdoid activity) are absent or very poorly delineated at this age. *REM sleep* is rarely recorded under regular laboratory conditions. The EEG shows little desynchronization at this age.

7. EEG IN OLDER CHILDREN (6–12 YEARS)

7.1. General Considerations

Normal children are fairly cooperative. Complete records with a resting awake portion, hyperventilation, intermittent photic stimulation, and sleep are easily obtained.

This is a well-explored age range. The most authoritative studies in this field were carried out in Göteborg, Sweden, by Eeg-Olofsson[2] and Petersén and Eeg-Olofsson[6] (also see Petersén et al.[4]). To secure a population of truly healthy children, a remarkable set of strict criteria was used, excluding those with even minute signs of neurological, autonomic, and psychological dysfunction.

7.2. Waking Record

The *posterior alpha rhythm* gradually reaches a mean frequency of ~10 Hz, which equals the mean frequency of the mature adult EEG. This frequency is reached around the age of 10 years. In the work by Petersén and Eeg-Olofsson,[6] the mean value of 9 Hz was reached at age 7 and 10 Hz at 15 years. These authors reported an increase of the alpha amplitude during early childhood until a peak was reached at age 6 to 9 years, with subsequent gradual decline. There was no gender difference. The alpha amplitude was determined by a bipolar occipitotemporal array, and a mean of 56 μV was found; such precise values are completely dependent on electrode selection and interelectrode distance.

The posterior alpha rhythm is usually of higher amplitude over the right side. According to Petersén and Eeg-Olofsson,[6] these asymmetries seldom exceed 20 μV. These authors were also unable to correlate alpha asymmetries with handedness.

Although the mature alpha frequency of 10 Hz may be reached at age 10 or at least at age 15, there is still a considerable admixture of posterior slow activity interspersed between trains of alpha waves. The maturational process of the second decade of life is thus characterized by the gradual disappearance of the admixed posterior slow activity, excluding a few other minor changes in EEG evolution (Fig. 7.20).

Posterior slow activity is still quite prominent between ages 6 and 12 years; "slow fused transients"[84] with sharp transients preceding single large slow waves are quite common. In addition to the common type of posterior slowing as randomly intermixed slow potentials, there are also other and more rhythmic forms of posterior slow activity.

Waveforms of *posterior slow activity* are broken down into arrhythmic and rhythmic slowing. This division also applies in adolescence and adulthood, although certain forms of posterior slowing are more common in children and others in adults.[4,85,86]

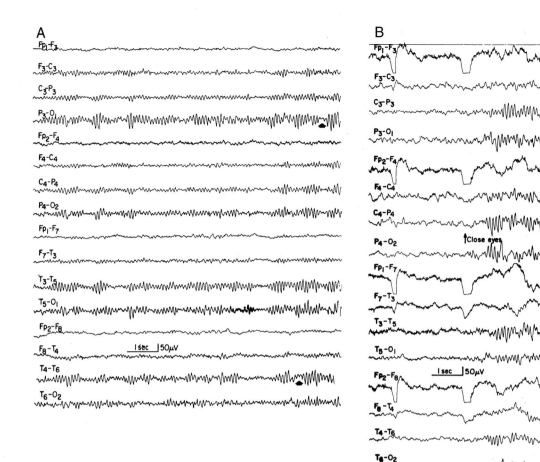

Figure 7.20. **A:** *"Supernormal" posterior alpha rhythm in a patient age 9 years. The only intermingled slow waves are indicated by an arrow.* **B:** *Patient age 8 years. Considerable intermixed posterior slowing, mostly 2.5 to 3.5/sec.*

In the age range from 6 to 12 years, posterior slow waves of youth, or the arrhythmic type of "slow, posterior waves found predominantly in youth,"[85] are most commonly encountered. This pattern consists of waves in the delta and theta range, of variable form, lasting 0.35 to 0.5 sec or longer without any consistent periodicity. Alpha waves are almost always intermingled or superimposed. Posterior slow waves of youth react to eye opening with blocking, similar to the posterior dominant rhythm.

Among the rhythmic forms, the slow alpha variant represents a subharmonic of the alpha frequency (mostly 4–5 Hz), often with intermixed alpha waves. Unilateral alpha subharmonics (left side, 4.5 Hz) were noted[87] in a neurologically normal 10-year-old girl. Forms of pronounced rhythmic high-voltage 3- to 4-Hz activity over occipital areas and adjacent regions are not uncommon at this age; these waves are often sharply contoured, and the moderately paroxysmal character of these slow runs places this activity into the mildly abnormal range. According to the extensive work by Kuhlo et al.,[88] the 4- to 5-Hz rhythm, which is a special entity of posterior slowing, is not demonstrable during the first decade. Very rhythmic high-voltage 3- to 4-Hz waves may occur in prolonged runs in children with absence epilepsy; this is referred to as occipital intermittent rhythmic delta activity (OIRDA).[89] This pattern is abnormal and is discussed in Chapter 18 on epileptiform EEG patterns.

Figure 7.20B shows slow waves often preceded by a sharply contoured large alpha wave (fused forms). The record is within normal limits of variability for age. *Fast activity* usually does not play a major role at this age. *Rolandic mu rhythm* steadily increases until a peak is reached between ages 11 and 15 years.[63] Occipital *lambda waves* are demonstrated more easily in older than in younger children but still lack the crisp and unmistakable contour of adulthood.

The prevalence of *anterior rhythmic 6- to 7-Hz theta activity* increases between ages 6 and 12 years before reaching a peak at age 13 to 15 (Fig. 7.21).[90] While earlier authors considered a potential pattern with "epileptological implications," the presence of anterior theta rhythms has been documented in healthy young individuals and would be considered a normal pattern.[4]

Low-voltage records as a variant of normal are rare at this age; Petersén and Eeg-Olofsson[6] did not find a single case in their series.

7.3. Activation Patterns

Hyperventilation shows particularly pronounced high-amplitude slowing at this age. The slowing may start over posterior areas and gradually becomes diffusely distributed with a frontal maximum; rhythmic slow activity usually ranges from

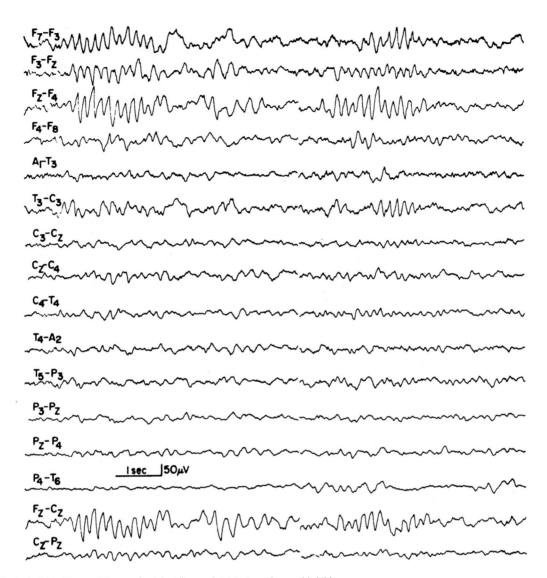

Figure 7.21. Rhythmical 6 to 7/sec activity over frontal midline and vicinity in a 12-year-old child.

1.5 to 4 Hz. A variety of responses have been reported by Daute et al.[91] (with concomitant evaluation of pH and pCO_2 changes) and by Petersén and Eeg-Olofsson.[6] The normal character of the rhythmic and arrhythmic slow responses cannot be overemphasized [see the section on Activations (Adolescents) below for more details].

Intermittent photic stimulation shows a more mature type of occipital driving response, less prominent at low flash rates and more impressive in the medium range (6–16 Hz). The work by Herrlin,[92] Doose et al.,[93] and Petersén and Eeg-Olofsson[6] has been essential in the investigation of these responses.

7.4. Drowsiness

Drowsiness is characterized, at this age, by increasing theta and delta frequencies along with gradually fading posterior rhythmic alpha activity. The mature type of onset of drowsiness with gradual alpha dropout and mixed low-voltage slow and fast activity usually does not occur in the first decade and slowly makes its appearance in early adolescence. Alternatively, the hypnagogic hypersynchrony seen in early childhood usually disappears around the age of 6 years.

7.5. Sleep

Under regular EEG laboratory conditions (leaving aside nocturnal or all-day sleep studies), NREM sleep in its various stages is almost exclusively found unless the recording is prolonged to 1 hour or more. Prior to the appearance of the first spindle trains, *vertex waves* are noted (transition from stage 1 to 2). These vertex waves are of remarkably high voltage and may have a very sharply contoured morphology; at times, their sharp character may be poignant, bordering on spikes. These potentials were also known as biparietal humps because, in the montages of Gibbs and Gibbs,[68] the maximum was over the parietal region, because neither vertex nor strictly central-rolandic electrodes were used (Fig. 7.22).

In school-age children, vertex waves may show asymmetries of moderate (seldom considerable) amplitude with

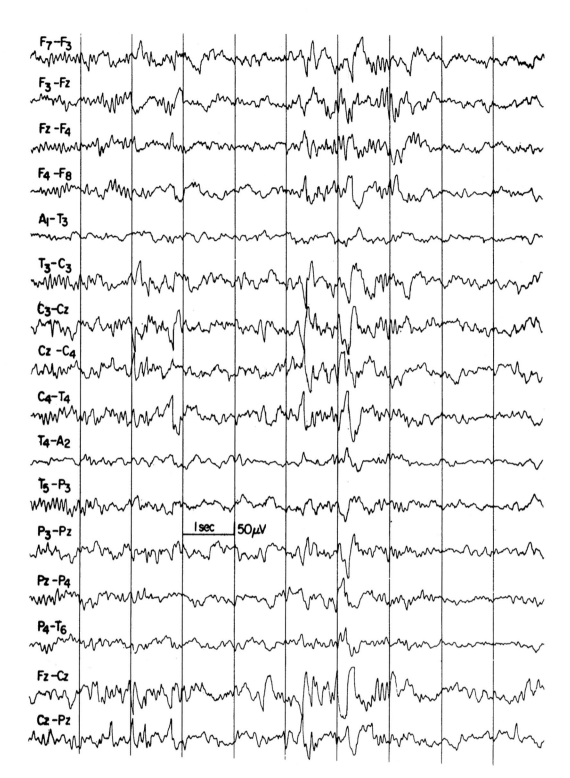

Figure 7.22. Patient age 10 years, NREM sleep stage 2. Well-developed spindles, vertex waves, and K-complexes.

asymmetrical spread into the vicinity. Under these circumstances, the physiological vertex activity may be confused with cerebral (rolandic) spikes; with greater experience, however, such errors can be avoided. The distinction between vertex waves and rolandic spikes, usually picked up by electrodes C_3 or C_4 over central areas, may occasionally arise from the vertex itself. When such a coexistence of vertex potentials exists, the physiological vertex waves are usually of longer duration and of somewhat higher voltage than the abnormal spikes.

Prior to onset of stage 2 (light sleep), *positive occipital sharp transients of sleep* may already be noticeable. This pattern, however, is less common and less prominent in children than in adolescents and adults. A more detailed discussion is presented in the section below dealing with the sleep EEG in general.

Sleep spindles show the features of maturity, with a well-defined vertex maximum. Their initial frequency of 14 Hz or 12 to 14 Hz may decrease to 10 to 12 Hz with deepening sleep; the superior frontal electrodes (F3, F4) may show the spindles somewhat better than the central electrodes (C3, C4). The spindle activity maximum remains over the midline; a vertex maximum may or may not be replaced by a maximum over frontal midline (F_z) with deepening sleep (transition from stage 2 to 3). The spindle trains are usually shorter than 1 sec. The waves are rounded; the physiological negative spiky spindle character has disappeared much earlier (age 2) (see Fig. 7.22).

K-complexes are often seen in association with spindles. K-complexes and vertex waves represent fascinating responses to intrinsic or extrinsic stimuli discussion (Fig. 7.23).

REM sleep (rarely seen in a routine outpatient study but readily apparent with prolonged monitoring) shows less slow activity and increasing desynchronization with mixed activities in the theta, alpha, and beta frequency range.

Arousal from sleep is characterized by an increasingly shorter transition from sleep to the waking state and decreasing length of high-voltage theta activity.

7.6. Variant Patterns of Uncertain Clinical Significance in Drowsiness and Sleep

There are EEG waveforms that are now considered normal variants. These waveforms typically occur in a rhythmic manner, with an admixed "epileptiform" morphology.

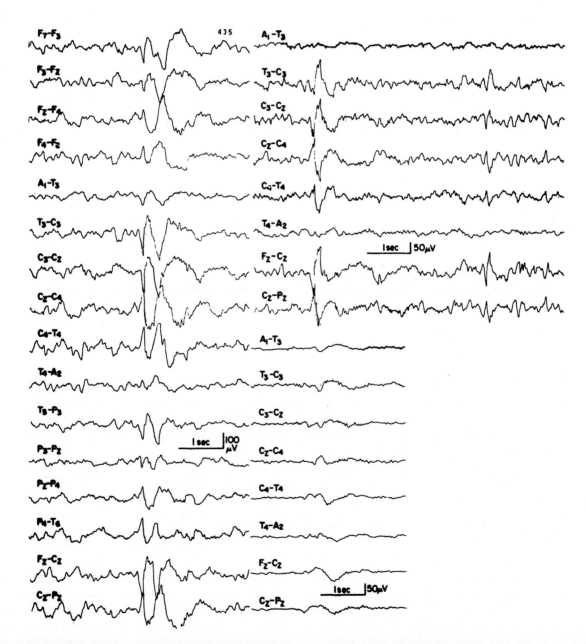

Figure 7.23. *Evolutional and involutional phases of the K-complex. Left tracing, patient age 5 years. Prominent initiating sharp component. Upper right tracing, patient age 8 years. Note very pronounced sharp component of K-complex. Far right, a single vertex wave is shown. Lower right, patient age 47 years. K-complex of moderate voltage; the initiating sharp component is markedly blunted. The slow component is inconspicuous; superimposed spindles are barely visible. This decline in the K-complex suggests some cerebral pathology.*

These may represent a superimposition of background frequencies.[94] These patterns are now referred to as normal variants, benign variants, or patterns of uncertain clinical significance.[95,96]

The 14- and 6-Hz positive burst, also termed ctenoids due to their resemblance to a comb, is a common finding at this age. These are morphologically surface-positive comblike spikes maximally distributed over the posterior temporal (T5/ P7, T6/P8) regions. They are typically less than 1 sec in duration and occur at bimodal frequency patterns of 6 Hz (actually 5–7 Hz) and 14 Hz (range of 3–17 Hz). The faster range is common, although the slower-range discharges can occur in longer bursts. Ctenoids had been considered an abnormality after the first report by Gibbs and Gibbs[97] but are currently recognized as a normal variant. They can be unilateral or bilaterally asynchronous and often have shifting hemispheric predominance, although it is not unusual for one hemisphere to be more affected. Their detection is maximized using a contralateral ear referential montage given the longer interelectrode distances.

Rhythmic temporal theta bursts of drowsiness, also known as the *psychomotor variant* pattern,[73,98,99] are predominantly seen in adolescents and young adults but are not uncommon in older children. The pattern is marked by runs of 5- to 7-Hz activity that is maximal in the midtemporal regions but sometimes detected in parietal or occipital regions. They are seen bilaterally or independently over either hemisphere and may be asymmetrical in distribution. The waves may have a flat, notched, or very sharp pattern but do not evolve into an ictal signature.[95]

8. EEG IN ADOLESCENTS (13–20 YEARS)

8.1. General Considerations

Although the transition from childhood to puberty is a major step in biological development, EEG maturation shows no dramatic changes in these years. In other words, there are no striking differences between the record of a healthy teenager and a healthy older child. Nevertheless, there are a number of subtle changes.

Eeg-Olofsson[3] carried out a special study of the EEG development of normal adolescents and selected 185 persons from ages 16 to 21 years, using the same strict criteria that were applied to the younger children. Earlier studies mostly included mixed ages, both adolescents and children.

8.2. Waking Record

The *posterior alpha rhythm* shows a mean frequency around 10 Hz; according to Petersén and Eeg-Olofsson.[6] The entire alpha range, as reported by Petersén and Eeg-Olofsson, stretches from 8 to 12 Hz; these authors observed a case of 8-Hz alpha rhythm in a healthy 17-year-old boy (this would raise the suspicion of a minimal abnormality, in the opinion of

some electroencephalographers). With the use of frequency analysis, Samson-Dollfus and Goldberg[100] found mean alpha frequencies from 9.64 to 9.94 Hz in subjects at age 15.

The posterior alpha rhythm is of moderately higher amplitude than in adulthood, but a slight decline from the height of alpha waves in childhood is noticeable. Alpha waves may show a negative sharp component (classically present in mu rhythm) that is due to a hidden or overt admixture of fast activity. Such sharp alpha waves are common in older children, adolescents, and young adults; this pattern is perfectly normal, a fact already stressed by Gibbs and Gibbs.[68] Amplitude asymmetries are the rule, with amplitudes usually somewhat higher on the right side, but, according to Petersén and Eeg-Olofsson,[6] the difference seldom exceeds 20% of the greater amplitude.

The admixture of *posterior slow activity* constantly diminishes during adolescence. In general, the amount of intermixed delta-theta activity (between alpha waves) lies around 10% to 15%, but slightly or moderately higher figures are still considered normal. Healthy adolescents' slow frequencies may show a wider distribution and their peak over the posterior regions is not quite as impressive as in older children.

Another form of rhythmic posterior slow activity consists of *rhythmic 3- to 4-Hz waves of high voltage over the occipital region* and its immediate vicinity. This is referred to as OIRDA and has also been called the phi rhythm.[101] The pattern is activated by hyperventilation as well as drowsiness, photic stimulation, and eye closure following a latency period of 300 to 500 msec. The rhythmic 3- to 4-Hz waves exhibit a more or less obvious sharp component, sometimes a "notch" in the slow wave. The pattern has been documented in children and adolescents from age 6 to 16 years and reported in patients with and without a history of epilepsy,[102] although it is widely recognized as an interictal pattern in patients with epilepsy, especially in patients with a history of generalized absence epilepsy that may be in remission.[89,103,104]

Fast activity is more widely seen in adolescents than in older children. The maximum fast activity is most commonly found over the frontal areas. Well-defined and circumscribed beta waves over the rolandic regions are seen, usually in conjunction with central mu rhythm. The *rolandic mu rhythm* is fairly common in adolescents and gradually declines from a peak reached between ages 11 and 15 years.[63] *Occipital lambda waves* show their typical mature configuration. *Anterior rhythmic 6- to 7-Hz theta activity* gradually decreases from its peak prevalence (age 13–15).

Given the prevalence of texting on smartphones in the current era, electroencephalographers need to be aware of the recently described "texting rhythm," which is time-locked to text messages and appears to represent an electrocerebral response to texting on smartphones and rarely on computer tablets.[105,106] Although originally described as a generalized monomorphic 5- to 6-Hz theta burst induced by active text

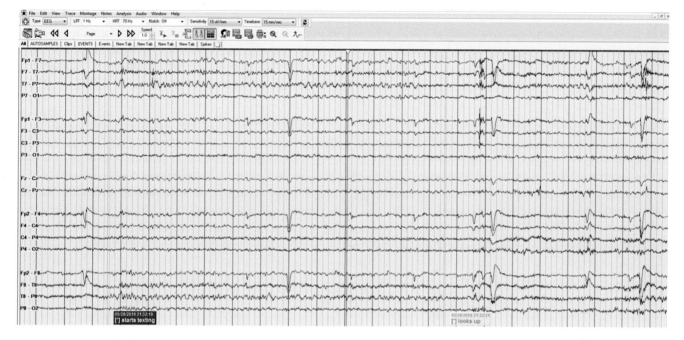

Figure 7.24. Texting rhythm in 18-year-old adolescent with time-locked monomorphic theta pattern restricted to active texting on a smartphone.

messaging, we have seen a similar pattern most prominent over the temporal regions (Fig. 7.24).[107] Such rhythms are likely to be seen during prolonged studies, especially ambulatory ones that may not have accompanying video, and should not be misconstrued as ictal patterns despite the rhythmicity and persistence.

Low-voltage records, very rare in childhood, are more common in adolescents and may occur in about 5% of patients; these records are usually dominated by beta frequencies. This type of low-voltage fast record has been found more often in females.[6,108–110] Vogel[110] investigated the role of predisposing genetic factors. Despite hereditary predisposition, the fact remains that such low-voltage tracings do not manifest themselves until a certain age around puberty. In healthy adults, the prevalence of low-voltage records increases to 11.6%.[68]

8.3. Activation

Hyperventilation does not yield the dramatic high-amplitude slowing seen in children. Marked bilateral synchronous delta activity was found in 22% of the healthy adolescents studied by Petersén and Eeg-Olofsson.[6] Hyperventilation is a poorly standardized procedure in which motivation and effort play a paramount role.

Intermittent photic stimulation shows essentially the mature type with a peak driving response in the medium and fast rate of flicker (mostly 6–20/sec). In addition to occipital driving responses, photomyoclonic responses, characterized by myogenic contractions of the eyelids and orbicularis oculi,

are normal phenomena, to be distinguished from an epileptiform photoparoxysmal response.

8.4. Drowsiness

The transition from wakefulness to sleep (stage 1) shows, in general, the mature adult type with gradual alpha dropout and long stretches of a diffuse low-voltage pattern with mixed slow and fast activity. With deepening drowsiness, vertex waves appear, and positive occipital sharp transients of sleep may be present.

8.5. Sleep

In the commonly observed NREM sleep onset recording in the EEG laboratories, there is little difference from the activity found in adults. The sleep spindle amplitude is somewhat greater than in adulthood, and this is also generally true for the amplitude of vertex waves and K-complexes. Their sharp component is not quite as sharp as in older children. Positive occipital transients of sleep may be abundant in stage 2. REM sleep and arousal from sleep show the mature type with very rapid transition from sleep patterns to waking activity.

8.6. Variant Patterns of Uncertain Clinical Significance

The *14- and 6-Hz positive burst pattern*, described above, is common in adolescents. The age-related incidence changes

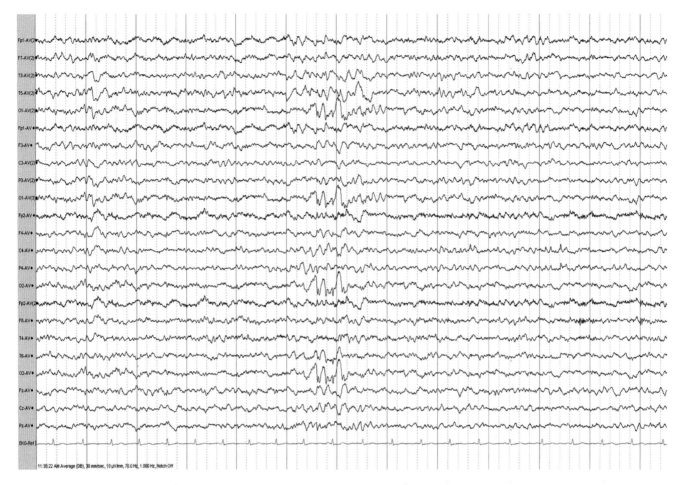

Figure 7.25. *Phantom spike-wave complex. The high-amplitude wave is the prominent component of the spike-wave complex.*

from approximately 16% at age 5 to 9 to 20% at 10 to 14; this declines to 8% to 10% between ages 20 and 24 and 1% to 2% between 25 and 29.[2,73] Another study found ctenoids in nearly 60% of 13- to 15-year-old normal high school boys.[111]

The adult EEG variant of the *6-Hz spike-wave complex*, also known as *phantom spike and wave*, is occasionally seen in adolescents. These are associated with brief (typically 1–2 sec) bursts of spike-wave of 5 to 7 Hz with low-voltage spikes (<25 microvolts) of brief duration (<30 msec). Two variants have been described: FOLD (female, occipital, low amplitude, drowsiness) and WHAM (waking, high amplitude, anterior, male). The higher amplitude of the wave compared to the spike leads to the designation of "phantom spike and wave" (Fig. 7.25).

The rhythmic temporal theta bursts of drowsiness (*psychomotor variant*), described above, occur in adolescence and were reported as occurring in 0.4% at the age range of 15 to 19 years.[73]

9. CONCLUSION

This chapter provides a condensed description of EEG maturation from birth through young adulthood. The basic rules of this EEG maturation are not carved in stone and must be viewed with a certain degree of flexibility. It is strongly recommended that terms such as *within broad (or very broad) normal limits of variability for age* be used in mildly deviant but not definitely abnormal tracings rather than making rigid distinctions between the "normal" and "abnormal" character of a given record.

The "clinician within ourselves" will demand statements concerning the clinical significance of mild deviations or definite abnormalities in the maturational process. The aforementioned normal variant patterns, such as the 14- and 6-Hz positive spike discharge, rhythmic temporal theta bursts of drowsiness, and 6-Hz spike-wave discharges, must be interpreted in a prudent and circumspect manner.

Interpretation of the neonatal and pediatric EEG is based upon the recognition of age-dependent features. For the neonate with an ultimately normal EEG, the recording provides a basis for determination of CA (postmenstrual age) and the assessment of expected background features and graphoelements. In addition, the understanding of chronological age–dependent features will suggest the range of both diffuse and focal abnormal features that may be present at specific epochs. Overall, it may be very difficult to make a firm and solidly founded statement as to whether deviations from the rules of

EEG maturation (e.g., excessive posterior slowing at a given age) are simply a sign of immaturity or a sign of possible sustained structural insult to the brain.

ACKNOWLEDGMENTS

The authors acknowledge the contributions of Richard A. Hrachovy and the late Ernst Niedermeyer to the prior versions of this chapter.

SCORE EEG SOFTWARE

Further examples related to the topics addressed in this chapter can be found in the interactive online Niedermeyer Educational Platform. EEG recordings with illustrative examples can be opened and browsed. Features are marked and described using the SCORE EEG software. The users can see the features marked by experts, they can score these features themselves, and then compare them with the scorings of the experts.

The Niedermeyer Educational Platform can be accessed at: www.scoreEEG.com/academy.

REFERENCES

1. Berger H. Über das Elektroenzephalogramm des Menschen. V. Mitteilung. *Arch Psychiatr Nervenkr.* 1932 98:231–254. [English translation: Gloor, P. 1969. Hans Berger. *On the Electroencephalogram of Man.* Amsterdam: Elsevier (see pp. 1157–1160)].
2. Eeg-Olofsson O. The development of the electroencephalogram in normal children from the age of 1 through 15 years. 14 and 6 Hz positive spike phenomenon. *Neuropadiatrie.* 1971;2(4):405–427.
3. Eeg-Olofsson O. The development of the electroencephalogram in normal adolescents from the age of 16 through 21 years. *Neuropadiatrie.* 1971;3(1):11–45.
4. Petersén I, Selldén U, Eeg-Olofsson O. The evolution of the EEG in normal children and adolescents from 1 to 21 years. In: Remond A, Lairy GC, eds. *Handbook of Electroencephalography and Clinical Neurophysiology.* Vol. 6B. Amsterdam: Elsevier; 1975:31–68.
5. Eeg-Olofsson O, Petersen I, Sellden U. The development of the electroencephalogram in normal children from the age of 1 through 15 years. Paroxysmal activity. *Neuropadiatrie.* 1971;2(4):375–404.
6. Petersén I, Eeg-Olofsson O. The development of the electroencephalogram in normal children from the age of 1 through 15 years. Non-paroxysmal activity. *Neuropadiatrie.* 1971;2(3):247–304.
7. Matsuura M, Yamamoto K, Fukuzawa H, et al. Age development and sex differences of various EEG elements in healthy children and adults—quantification by a computerized wave form recognition method. *Electroencephalogr Clin Neurophysiol.* 1985;60(5):394–406.
8. Gasser T, Jennen-Steinmetz C, Sroka L, Verleger R, Mocks J. Development of the EEG of school-age children and adolescents. II. Topography. *Electroencephalogr Clin Neurophysiol.* 1988;69(2):100–109.
9. Gasser T, Verleger R, Bacher P, Sroka L. Development of the EEG of school-age children and adolescents. I. Analysis of band power. *Electroencephalogr Clin Neurophysiol.* 1988;69(2):91–99.
10. Dreyfus-Brisac C. The electroencephalogram of the premature infant. *World Neurol.* 1962;3:5–15.
11. Dreyfus-Brisac C. The electroencephalogram of the premature infant and full-term newborn: Normal and abnormal development of waking and sleeping patterns. In: Kellaway P, Petersén I, eds. *Neurological and Electroencephalographic Correlative Studies in Infancy.* New York: Grune & Stratton; 1964:186–206.
12. Dreyfus-Brisac C, Fischgold H, Samson-Dollfus D, Sainte-Anne-Dargassies S, Monod N, Blanc C. Veille, sommeil, réactivité sensorielle chez le prématuré, le nouveau-né et le nourrisson. *Electroencephalogr Clin Neurophysiol.* 1957;6(Suppl.):417–440.
13. Dreyfus-Brisac C, Monod MD. Sleeping behaviour in abnormal newborn infants. *Neuropadiatrie.* 1970;1(3):354–366.
14. Dreyfus-Brisac C, Larroche JC. [Discontinuous electroencephalograms in the premature newborn and at term. Electro-anatomo-clinical correlations]. *Rev Electroencephalogr Neurophysiol Clin.* 1971;1(1):95–99.
15. Hrachovy RA, Mizrahi EM, Kellaway P. Electroencephalography of the newborn. In: Day DD, Pedley TA, eds. *Current Practice of Clinical Electroencephalography.* 2nd ed. New York: Raven Press; 1990:201–242.
16. Watanabe K, Hayakawa F, Okumura A. Neonatal EEG: a powerful tool in the assessment of brain damage in preterm infants. *Brain Dev.* 1999;21(6):361–372.
17. Clancy RR, Bergqvist C, Dlugos DJ. Neonatal electroencephalography. In: Ebersole JS, Pedley TA, eds. *Current Practice of Clinical Electroencephalography.* 3rd ed. Philadelphia, PA: Lippincott Williams & Wilkins; 2003:160–234.
18. Mizrahi EM, Hrachovy RA, Kellaway P. *Atlas of Neonatal Electroencephalography.* 3rd ed. Philadelphia, PA: Lippincott Williams & Wilkins; 2004.
19. Plouin P, Kaminska A, M. M, Soufflet C. *L'EEG en pediatrie.* United Kingdom: John Libbey; 2005.
20. Vecchierini MF, Andre M, d'Allest AM. Normal EEG of premature infants born between 24 and 30 weeks gestational age: terminology, definitions and maturation aspects. *Neurophysiol Clin.* 2007;37(5):311–323.
21. Andre M, Lamblin MD, d'Allest AM, et al. Electroencephalography in premature and full-term infants. Developmental features and glossary. *Neurophysiol Clin.* 2010;40(2):59–124.
22. Mizrahi EM, Hrachovy RA. *Atlas of Neonatal Electroencephalography.* 3rd ed. Philadelphia, PA: Demos Medical; 2016.
23. Koszer SE, Moshe SL, Holmes GL. Visual analysis of the neonatal electroencephalogram. In: Homes GL, Moshe SL, Jones HR, Jr., eds. *Clinical Neurophysiology of Infancy, Childhood, and Adolescence.* Philadelphia, PA: Butterworth-Heinemann; 2006:70–86.
24. Koszer SE, Zacharowicz L, Moshe SL. Visual analysis of the pediatric electroencephalogram. In: Homes GL, Moshe SL, Jones HR, Jr., eds. *Clinical Neurophysiology of Infancy, Childhood, and Adolescence.* Philadelphia, PA: Butterworth-Heinemann; 2006:99–129.
25. Engle WA, American Academy of Pediatrics Committee on Fetus and Newborn. Age terminology during the perinatal period. *Pediatrics.* 2004;114(5):1362–1364.
26. American Clinical Neurophysiology Society. Guideline 2: Minimum technical standards for pediatric electroencephalography. *J Clin Neurophysiol.* 2006;23(2):92–96.
27. De Weerd AW, Despland PA, Plouin P. Neonatal EEG. The International Federation of Clinical Neurophysiology. *Electroencephalogr Clin Neurophysiol Suppl.* 1999;52:149–157.
28. Shellhaas RA, Chang T, Tsuchida T, et al. The American Clinical Neurophysiology Society's Guideline on Continuous Electroencephalography Monitoring in Neonates. *J Clin Neurophysiol.* 2011;28(6):611–617.
29. Biagioni E, Bartalena L, Boldrini A, Cioni G, Giancola S, Ipata AE. Background EEG activity in preterm infants: correlation of outcome with selected maturational features. *Electroencephalogr Clin Neurophysiol.* 1994;91(3):154–162.
30. Hahn JS, Monyer H, Tharp BR. Interburst interval measurements in the EEGs of premature infants with normal neurological outcome. *Electroencephalogr Clin Neurophysiol.* 1989;73(5):410–418.
31. Selton D, Andre M, Hascoet JM. Normal EEG in very premature infants: reference criteria. *Clin Neurophysiol.* 2000;111(12):2116–2124.
32. Monod N, Tharp B. [The normal E.E.G. of the neonate (author's transl)]. *Rev Electroencephalogr Neurophysiol Clin.* 1977;7(3):302–315.
33. Anderson CM, Torres F, Faoro A. The EEG of the early premature. *Electroencephalogr Clin Neurophysiol.* 1985;60(2):95–105.
34. Connell JA, Oozeer R, Dubowitz V. Continuous 4-channel EEG monitoring: a guide to interpretation, with normal values, in preterm infants. *Neuropediatrics.* 1987;18(3):138–145.
35. Hayakawa M, Okumura A, Hayakawa F, et al. Background electroencephalographic (EEG) activities of very preterm infants born at less than 27 weeks gestation: a study on the degree of continuity. *Arch Dis Child Fetal Neonatal Ed.* 2001;84(3):F163–167.
36. Vecchierini MF, d'Allest AM, Verpillat P. EEG patterns in 10 extreme premature neonates with normal neurological outcome: qualitative and quantitative data. *Brain Dev.* 2003;25(5):330–337.

37. Hrachovy RA. Development of the normal electroencephalogram. In: Levin KH, Luders HO, eds. *Comprehensive Clinical Neurophysiology*. Philadelphia, PA: WB Saunders; 2000:387–413.

38. Tsuchida TN, Wusthoff CJ, Shellhaas RA, et al. American Clinical Neurophysiology Society standardized EEG terminology and categorization for the description of continuous EEG monitoring in neonates: report of the American Clinical Neurophysiology Society critical care monitoring committee. *J Clin Neurophysiol*. 2013;30(2):161–173.

39. Dreyfus C, Curzi-Dascalova L. The EEG during the first year of life. In: Remond A, ed. *Handbook of Electroencephalography and Clinical Neurophysiology*. Vol. 6B. Amsterdam: Elsevier; 1975:24–30.

40. Ellingson RJ. EEGs of premature and full-term newborns. In: Klass DW, Daly DD, eds. *Current Practice of Electroencephalography*. New York: Raven Press; 1979:149–177.

41. Sweeney D, Beckman D, Calmese F, Kreis A. The use of modified sleep deprivation to facilitate pediatric electroencephalographic recordings. *Am J END Technol*. 1997;37:218–230.

42. Brown V, Haak N, Egel RT. Technical tips: Age-specific sleep deprivation guidelines. *Am J END Technol*. 1997;37(3):231–235.

43. Ong HT, Lim KJ, Low PC, Low PS. Simple instructions for partial sleep deprivation prior to pediatric EEG reduces the need for sedation. *Clin Neurophysiol*. 2004;115(4):951–955.

44. Stroganova TA, Orekhova EV, Posikera IN. EEG alpha rhythm in infants. *Clin Neurophysiol*. 1999;110(6):997–1012.

45. Hagne I. Development of waking EEG in normal infants during the first year of life. In: Kellaway P, Petersén I, eds. *Clinical Electroencephalography of Children*. New York: Grune & Stratton (Stockholm: Almqvist & Wiksell); 1968:97–118.

46. Hagne I, Persson J, Magnusson R. Spectral analysis via fast Fourier transform of waking EEG in normal infants. In: Kellaway P, Petersén I, eds. *Automation of Clinical EEG*. New York: Raven Press; 1972:3–48.

47. Ohtahara S. Development of electroencephalogram during infancy and childhood. *Proc Jpn EEG Soc*. 1964:18–23.

48. Samson-Dollfus D, Nogues B, Delagree E. [EEG recording during drowsiness in normal babies aged 2 to 12 months (author's transl)]. *Rev Electroencephalogr Neurophysiol Clin*. 1981;11(1):23–27.

49. Metcalf DR. The effect of extrauterine experience on the ontogenesis of EEG sleep spindles. *Psychosom Med*. 1969;31(5):393–399.

50. Ellingson RJ. Electroencephalograms of normal, full-term newborns immediately after birth with observations on arousal and visual evoked responses. *Electroencephalogr Clin Neurophysiol*. 1958;10(1):31–50.

51. Fois A. *The Electroencephalogram of the Normal Child*. Springfield, IL: Charles C Thomas; 1961.

52. Katsurada ML. [Electroencephalographic study of sleep in infants and young children. I. Development of spindle waves]. *Ann Paediatr Jpn*. 1965;2:391–394.

53. Lenard HG. The development of sleep spindles in the EEG during the first two years of life. *Neuropadiatrie*. 1970;1(3):264–276.

54. Hughes JR. Development of sleep spindles in the first year of life. *Clin Electroencephalogr*. 1996;27(3):107–115.

55. Niedermeyer E. *The Generalized Epilepsies*. Springfield, IL: Charles C Thomas; 1972.

56. Metcalf DR, Mondale J, Butler FK. Ontogenesis of spontaneous K-complexes. *Psychophysiology*. 1971;8(3):340–347.

57. Westmoreland BF. Electroencephalography: adult, normal, and benign variants. In: Rubin DI, Daube JR, eds. *Clinical Neurophysiology*. 3rd ed. Oxford: Oxford University Press; 2009:119–136.

58. Ellingson RJ, Peters JF, Nelson B. Respiratory pauses and apnea during daytime sleep in normal infants during the first year of life: longitudinal observations. *Electroencephalogr Clin Neurophysiol*. 1982;53(1):48–59.

59. Roffwarg HP, Muzio JN, Dement WC. Ontogenetic development of the human sleep-dream cycle. *Science*. 1966;152(3722):604–619.

60. Stern E, Parmelee AH, Akiyama Y, Schultz MA, Wenner WH. Sleep cycle characteristics in infants. *Pediatrics*. 1969;43(1):65–70.

61. Dittrichova J, Paul K, Pavlikova E. Rapid eye movements in paradoxical sleep in infants. *Neuropadiatrie*. 1972;3(3):248–257.

62. Schulz H, Salzarulo P, Fagioli I, Massetani R. REM latency: development in the first year of life. *Electroencephalogr Clin Neurophysiol*. 1983;56(4):316–322.

63. Niedermeyer E, Koshino Y. My-Rhythmus: Vorkommen und klinische Bedeutung. *Z EEG-EMG*. 1975;6:69–78.

64. Hrbek A, Vitova Z, Mares P. Optic evoked potentials in children, using different stimulation frequencies. *Physiol Bohemoslov*. 1966;15(3):201–204.

65. Vitova Z, Hrbek A. Developmental study on the responsiveness of the human brain to flicker stimulation. *Dev Med Child Neurol*. 1972;14(4):476–486.

66. Lindsley DB. A longitudinal study of the alpha rhythm in normal children: frequency and amplitude standards. *J Genet Psychol*. 1939;55:197–213.

67. Westmoreland BF, Stockard JE. The EEG in infants and children: normal patterns. *Am J EEG Technol*. 1977;17:187–206.

68. Gibbs FA, Gibbs EL. *Atlas of Electroencephalography*. Vol. 1. Cambridge, MA: Addison-Wesley; 1950.

69. Brandt S, Brandt H. The electroencephalographic patterns in young healthy children from 0 to five years of age; their practical use in daily clinical electroencephalography. *Acta Psychiatr Neurol Scand*. 1955;30(1-2):77–89.

70. Slater GE, Torres F. Frequency-amplitude gradient: a new parameter for interpreting pediatric sleep EEGs. *Arch Neurol*. 1979;36(8):465–470.

71. Cadilhac J. Ontogenesis and phylogenesis of sleep. In: Remond A, Passouant P, eds. *Handbook of Electroencephalography and Clinical Neurophysiology*. Vol. 7A. Amsterdam: Elsevier; 1975:18–25.

72. Gibbs EL, Gibbs FA. Extreme spindles: correlation of electroencephalographic sleep pattern with mental retardation. *Science*. 1962;138(3545):1106–1107.

73. Gibbs FA, Gibbs EL. *Atlas of Electroencephalography*. Vol. 3. Reading, MA: Addison-Wesley; 1964.

74. Niedermeyer E, Capute AJ. A fast and spikey spindle variant in children with organic brain disease. *Electroencephalogr Clin Neurophysiol*. 1967;23(1):67–73.

75. Hess R. The Electroencephalogram in Sleep. *Electroencephalogr Clin Neurophysiol*. 1964;16:44–55.

76. Kellaway P, Fox BJ. Electroencephalographic diagnosis of cerebral pathology in infants during sleep. I. Rationale, technique, and the characteristics of normal sleep in infants. *J Pediatr*. 1952;41(3):262–287.

77. White JC, Tharp BR. An arousal pattern in children with organic cerebral dysfunction. *Electroencephalogr Clin Neurophysiol*. 1974;37(3):265–268.

78. Hughes JR. The frontal arousal rhythm (FAR) is an ictal pattern: a case report. *Clin Electroencephalogr*. 2003;34(1):13–14.

79. Niedermeyer E, Yarworth S. Scarcity of minor EEG abnormalities during the first two years of life. *Clin Electroencephalogr*. 1978;9(1):20–28.

80. Leissner P, Lindholm LE, Petersen I. Alpha amplitude dependence on skull thickness as measured by ultrasound technique. *Electroencephalogr Clin Neurophysiol*. 1970;29(4):392–399.

81. Kellaway P. Ontogenetic evolution of the electrical activity of the brain in man and animals. *Trans IVth Int Congr Electroencephalogr Clin Neurophysiol Acta Med Belg*. 1957:141–154.

82. Gibbs FA, Gibbs EL, Lennox WG. Electroencephalographic response to overventilation and its relation to age. *J Pediatr*. 1943;23:497–505.

83. Sunder TR, Erwin CW, Dubois PJ. Hyperventilation- induced abnormalities in the electroencephalogram of children with Moyamoya disease. *Electroencephalogr Clin Neurophysiol*. 1980;49(3-4):414–420.

84. Kellaway P, Crawley JW, Kagawa N. A specific electroencephalographic correlate of convulsive equivalent disorders in children. *J Pediatr*. 1959;55:582–592.

85. Aird RB, Gastaut Y. Occipital and posterior electroencephalographic rhythms. *Electroencephalogr Clin Neurophysiol*. 1959;11:637–656.

86. Kuhlo W. Slow posterior rhythms. In: Remond A, ed. *Handbook of Electroencephalography and Clinical Neurophysiology*. Vol. 6A. Amsterdam: Elsevier; 1976:89–104.

87. Attarian HP, Pacquiao PA, Erickson SM. Unilateral alpha subharmonics: a case report. *Clin Electroencephalogr*. 2001;32(1):32–35.

88. Kuhlo W, Heintel H, Vogel F. The 4-5 c-sec rhythm. *Electroencephalogr Clin Neurophysiol*. 1969;26(6):613–618.

89. Riviello JJ, Jr., Foley CM. The epileptiform significance of intermittent rhythmic delta activity in childhood. *J Child Neurol*. 1992;7(2):156–160.

90. Palmer FB, Yarworth S, Niedermeyer E. Frontal midline theta rhythm. *Electroencephalogr Clin Neurophysiol*. 1976;7:131–138.

91. Daute KH, Frenzel J, Klust E. Über den unspezifischen Hyperventilationseffekt im EEG des gesunden Kindes. I. Stärkegrad. *Zeitschrift für Kinderheilkunde*. 1968;104(3):197–207.

92. Herrlin KM. EEG with photic stimulation: a study of children with manifest or suspected epilepsy. *Electroencephalogr Clin Neurophysiol*. 1954;6(4):573–589.

93. Doose H, Gerken H, Hien-Volpel KF, Volzke E. Genetics of photosensitive epilepsy. *Neuropadiatrie*. 1969;1(1):56–73.

94. Klass DW, Westmoreland BF. Nonepileptogenic epileptiform electroencephalographic activity. *Ann Neurol*. 1985;18(6):627–635.

95. Westmoreland BF. Benign EEG variants and patterns of uncertain clinical significance. In: Ebersole JS, Pedley TA, eds. *Current Practice of Clinical Electroencephalography*. 3rd ed. Philadelphia, PA: Lippincott Williams and Wilkins; 2003:235–245.

96. Tatum WO, Husain AM, Benbadis SR, Kaplan PW. Normal adult EEG and patterns of uncertain significance. *J Clin Neurophysiol*. 2006;23(3):194–207.

97. Gibbs EL, Gibbs FA. Electroencephalographic evidence of thalamic and hypothalamic epilepsy. *Neurology*. 1951;1(2):136–144.

98. Gibbs FA, Rich CL, Gibbs EL. Psychomotor variant type of seizure discharge. *Neurology*. 1963;13:991–998.

99. Lipman IJ, Hughes JR. Rhythmic mid-temporal discharges. An electroclinical study. *Electroencephalogr Clin Neurophysiol*. 1969;27(1):43–47.

100. Samson-Dollfus D, Goldberg P. Electroencephalographic quantification by time domain analysis in normal 7–15-year-old children. *Electroencephalogr Clin Neurophysiol*. 1979;46(2):147–154.

101. Silbert PL, Radhakrishnan K, Johnson J, Klass DW. The significance of the phi rhythm. *Electroencephalogr Clin Neurophysiol*. 1995;95(2):71–76.

102. Belsh JM, Chokroverty S, Barabas G. Posterior rhythmic slow activity in EEG after eye closure. *Electroencephalogr Clin Neurophysiol*. 1983;56(6):562–568.

103. Brigo F. Intermittent rhythmic delta activity patterns. *Epilepsy Behav*. 2011;20(2):254–256.

104. Watemberg N, Linder I, Dabby R, Blumkin L, Lerman-Sagie T. Clinical correlates of occipital intermittent rhythmic delta activity (OIRDA) in children. *Epilepsia*. 2007;48(2):330–334.

105. Tatum WO, DiCiaccio B, Kipta JA, Yelvington KH, Stein MA. The texting rhythm: a novel EEG waveform using smartphones. *J Clin Neurophysiol*. 2016;33(4):359–366.

106. Tatum WO, DiCiaccio B, Yelvington KH. Cortical processing during smartphone text messaging. *Epilepsy Behav*. 2016;59:117–121.

107. Tomko S, Loddenkemper T, Pearl PL. Texting rhythm with temporal predominance. *J Clin Neurophys*. 2016;33:570.

108. Mundy-Castle AC. Theta and beta rhythm in the electroencephalograms of normal adults. *Electroencephalogr Clin Neurophysiol*. 1951;3(4):477–486.

109. Vogel F, Fujiya Y. The incidence of some inherited EEG variants in normal Japanese and German males. *Humangenetik*. 1969;7(1):38–42.

110. Vogel F, Goetze W. [Statistical observations on the beta-waves in human electroencephalography]. *Dtsch Z Nervenheilkd*. 1962;184:112–136.

111. Lombroso CT, Schwartz IH, Clark DM, Muench H, Barry PH, Barry J. Ctenoids in healthy youths. Controlled study of 14- and 6-per-second positive spiking. *Neurology*. 1966;16(12):1152–1158.

8 | NORMAL EEG IN WAKEFULNESS AND SLEEP: ADULTS AND ELDERLY

VAISHNAV KRISHNAN, MD, PHD, BERNARD S. CHANG, MD, MMSC, AND DONALD L. SCHOMER, MD

ABSTRACT: The normal adult electroencephalogram (EEG) is not a singular entity, and recognizing and appreciating the various expressions of a normal EEG is vital for any electroencephalographer. During wakefulness, the posterior dominant rhythm (PDR) must display a frequency within the alpha band, although an absent PDR is not abnormal. A symmetrically slowed PDR, excessive theta activity, or any delta activity during wakefulness is abnormal and a biomarker of encephalopathy. Low-voltage EEGs have been associated with a variety of neuropathological states but are themselves not abnormal. During non-rapid eye movement sleep, a normal EEG will display progressively greater degrees of background slowing and amplitude enhancement, which may or may not be associated with specific sleep-related transients. In contrast, the EEG during rapid eye movement sleep more closely resembles a waking EEG ("desynchronized") in amplitude and background frequencies. Across both wakefulness and sleep, significant asymmetries in background frequencies and amplitude are abnormal.

KEYWORDS: electroencephalogram, EEG, adult, posterior dominant rhythm, sleep, theta, delta, rapid eye movement

PRINCIPAL REFERENCES

1. Noachtar, S., C. Binnie, J. Ebersole, F. Mauguiere, A. Sakamoto, and B. Westmoreland, *A glossary of terms most commonly used by clinical electroencephalographers and proposal for the report form for the EEG findings. The International Federation of Clinical Neurophysiology.* EEG Clin Neurophysiol Supplement, 1999. 52: p. 21–41.
2. Davis, P.A., *Effects of acoustic stimuli on the waking human brain.* J Neurophysiol, 1939. 2: p. 494–499.
3. Saper, C.B., *The neurobiology of sleep.* Continuum, 2013. 19: p. 19–31.
4. Rodin, E.A., E.D. Luby, and J.S. Gottlieb, *The electroencephalogram during prolonged experimental sleep deprivation.* EEG Clin Neurophysiol, 1961. 14: p. 544–551.
5. Davis, H., P.A. Davis, A.L. Loomis, E.N. Harvey, and G. Hobart, *Changes in human brain potentials during the onset of sleep.* Science, 1937. 86: p. 448–450.
6. Cobb, W.A., The normal adult EEG, in *Electroencephalography*, D. Hill and G. Parr, eds. 1963. Macmillan: New York, p. 232–249
7. Walter, W.G. and V.J. Dovey, *Electro-encephalography in cases of subcortical tumour.* J Neurol Neurosurg Psychiatry, 1944. 7, p. 57–65.
8. Adams, A., *Studies on the flat electroencephalogram in man.* EEG Clin Neurophysiol, 1959. 11, p. 35–41.
9. Davis, H. and P.A. Davis, *Action potentials of the brain in normal persons and in normal states of cerebral activity.* Arch Neurol Psychiatry (Chicago), 1936. 36: p. 1214–1224.
10. Duffy, F.H., M.S. Albert, G. McAnulty, and A.J. Garvey, *Age-related differences in brain electrical activity of healthy subjects.* Ann Neurol, 1984. 16: p. 430–438.

1. INTRODUCTION

There is perhaps nothing as compellingly beautiful to a clinical neurophysiologist as the appearance of a normal

adult electroencephalogram (EEG) recording, in wakefulness and sleep. But the relative order, symmetry, and transitions that populate such a recording and are so welcome to the clinically trained eye can lead us to forget the fundamentally remarkable phenomena that electrical activity from the human brain can indeed be measured routinely by electrodes placed only on the scalp; that defined, well-catalogued abnormalities in the resulting measurements can be identified and interpreted with clinical meaning; and that our entire understanding of this field has essentially arisen within only the past century.

Ernst Niedermeyer, 1920–2012

The goal of this chapter is to define and describe certain expected elements in a human adult electroencephalogram (EEG) that would conventionally be recognized as *normal*, a weighted term that deserves some clarification:

- First and foremost, a *normal* EEG does not necessarily imply *normal* neuropsychiatric health. Instead, it should be interpreted as the electroencephalographer's general impression of observed EEG waveforms during a specific recording epoch, which itself may capture only a single state.

- Second, a *normal* EEG is by no means a unique entity: there are indeed several quantitative and qualitative variations in *normal* background activity. Thus, some electroencephalographers would define *normality* on an EEG as being simply the *absence* of identifiable *abnormalities*.

- Third, there are a series of EEG patterns that are neither *normal* nor *abnormal*. These include the benign variants of uncertain clinical significance, for instance subclinical rhythmic electrographic discharges in adults, and are discussed extensively in Chapter 12.

2. EEG FREQUENCIES

A typical scalp recording in an adult captures a wide spectrum of EEG frequency activity. However, for clinical diagnostic purposes, the electroencephalographer must pay particular attention to activity that lies within a clinically relevant frequency range that lies between 0.1 to 0.3/sec (or cycles per second [cps] or Hz) to 70 to 100 Hz. These frequencies have been further divided into the following bands or ranges [1]:

Delta: <4 Hz

Theta: 4–7.5 Hz

Alpha: 8–13 Hz

Beta: 14–40 Hz

Gamma: >40 Hz

The sequence of Greek letters that have been used to label these primary frequency bands is not logical and can be understood only in a historical view. The terms *alpha* and *beta* rhythm or waves were introduced by Berger [2,3]. *Gamma rhythm* was a term coined by Jasper and Andrews [4] to designate frequencies above 30 or 35/sec; these were essentially 35- to 45-Hz waves that were superimposed on the occipital alpha rhythm [5]. This term was temporarily abandoned, and *gamma* frequencies became a part of the beta range. The term *delta rhythm* was introduced by Walter [6] to designate all frequencies below the alpha range. Walter also found a need to introduce a special designation for the 4 to 7.5/sec range and used the letter *theta*. He thus bypassed the letters *epsilon, zeta,* and *eta* and chose *theta* because he presumed a thalamic origin of these waves [7].

Other Greek letters have been used in EEG terminology to depict specific cerebral rhythms or waveforms rather than raw frequency ranges. The *mu* rhythm and *lambda* waves are discussed later in this chapter. *Zeta* waves simply denote a sharply contoured larger amplitude delta wave with a "Z"-like configuration [8,9]. Dutertre devised the term *pi rhythm* to designate posterior slow rhythms (3–4/sec) that are nonharmonic to the posterior dominant rhythm [5]. Separately, the term *phi rhythm* was suggested to designate posterior rhythmic delta waves occurring within 2 seconds of eye closure [10,11]. The term *kappa rhythm* has been used to depict bursts of alpha and theta frequencies in the anterior temporal regions [12,13] during mental activity, though the cerebral origin of this activity is considered unproven [1]. Kugler championed the term *sigma activity*, which described what is now conventionally referred to as *sleep spindles*. He also applied the term *sigma rhythm* for activity in the 11 to 15/sec range [14]. Similarly, positive occipital sharp transients of sleep (POSTS) used to be called *rho waves* [15]. The use of several of these terms has either been discouraged (e.g., kappa rhythm) or not acknowledged (e.g., rho or zeta waves) by the International Federation of Societies for Electroencephalography and Clinical Neurophysiology (IFSECN) [1].

Scalp EEG can also be used to record *ultraslow* and *ultrafast* frequencies. On a typical scalp EEG, rhythmic activity below 1 Hz (typically 0.3–0.5 Hz) is most often related to two main noncerebral sources: (i) slow roving eye movements of drowsiness or (ii) high electrode impedance caused by the formation of a salt bridge, typically due to local sweat ("sweat sway")

(see Chapter 11 on EEG artifacts). True *ultraslow*-frequency activity, which ranges from ~0.3 Hz down to very slow EEG oscillations (just slightly greater than 0 Hz, termed *direct current potential shifts* or DC shifts), requires a different amplifier and nonpolarizable electrodes. These slow shifts in local field potential have been shown to aid in lateralizing temporal lobe seizures [16] and have also been in identified in the EEGs of preterm infants [17]. Cyclic but slow changes in gross excitability during sleep have been shown to be synchronous with faster-frequency EEG activity, including interictal spikes [18]. Interest in EEG activity within the *ultrafast* range (80–1,000 Hz) has been surging over the past two decades. Physiological high-frequency oscillations may serve as an important biomarker of memory and reconsolidation processes, while pathological high-frequency oscillations, particularly those identified by intracranial EEG recordings, are potential biomarkers of highly epileptogenic tissue and may guide a resective surgical procedure [19,20]. A complete discussion of the physiology of ultraslow and high-frequency oscillations is included in Chapters 32 and 33.

3. EEG AMPLITUDE

Ultimately, an EEG is a depiction of local field potentials (voltage) plotted against time. Intracranial EEG recordings with subdural "strip" or "grid" electrodes placed directly on the cortical surface (*electrocorticography*) reveal amplitudes of 500 to 1,500 μV (0.5–1.5 mV). The passage of this cortical EEG signal through cerebrospinal fluid, layers of the meninges, bone, galea, and scalp results in an attenuating effect on the original signal [21], such that the amplitude (voltage) of scalp EEG in adults is comparatively reduced, measuring between 20 and 100 μV.

To a large extent, interindividual differences in the overall absolute amplitude of an adult EEG are clinically irrelevant, as they are affected by a series of variables, most notably interelectrode distance (varying proportionally to amplitude) and skull thickness (varying inversely to amplitude). We discuss the issue of "low-voltage records" in greater detail later in this chapter: in these individuals, typical waking scalp EEG amplitudes are less than 20 μV, a feature considered to be a variant of normalcy. In contrast to benign variations in overall "average" amplitude, interhemispheric differences in EEG amplitude, particularly if greater than 50%, are indeed abnormal, signifying the presence of either an obstructive lesion over the attenuated hemisphere (e.g., subdural hemorrhage) or an attenuation defect over the hemisphere that displays relatively higher amplitudes (e.g., following prior craniotomy or craniectomy), which may or may not be associated with the presence of a "breach rhythm" [22]. Additionally, reductions in EEG voltage during a recording, either asymmetrical or global, may be related to life-threatening reductions in cerebral perfusion and/or elevations in intracranial pressure. Finally, focal or global changes in EEG amplitude, associated with prominent increases in rhythmicity, are a critical component of the electrographic signature of the excessive hypersynchrony of seizures (discussed in Chapter 19).

4. BASIC EEG PATTERNS SEEN IN WAKEFULNESS

On scalp EEG, wakefulness can be inferred from the presence of eye blinks. In addition, myogenic artifact/electromyelographic (EMG) artifact (transmitted primarily from frontalis and temporalis muscles) is normally enhanced during wakefulness. Two requisite features of a normal waking EEG are *organization* and *continuity*. EEG activity during wakefulness typically displays an anteroposterior gradient such that faster-frequency activity (beta/gamma) is seen frontally and more posterior regions display higher-amplitude alpha activity ("organized"). The anteroposterior gradient is often less pronounced in low-voltage EEGs (see below). An EEG is reported as *discontinuous* when the normal *continuous* arrangement of EEG frequencies is interrupted by periods of voltage attenuation or suppression (see Chapters 20, 21, and 22 for discussions of burst suppression, an extreme example of discontinuity).

4.1. Alpha Rhythm/Posterior Dominant Rhythm (Berger Rhythm)

4.1.1. Definition

IFSECN defines the alpha rhythm as an 8- to 13-Hz rhythm occurring during wakefulness over the posterior regions of the head, typically occipital areas, that is best appreciated with the eyes closed and without fixed gaze, during physical relaxation and mental inactivity. Importantly, the alpha rhythm demonstrates *reactivity*, in that it is attenuated (or *desynchronized*) with eye opening or mental effort [1] (Fig. 8.1). This committee also has pointed out that the term *alpha rhythm* must be restricted to rhythms fulfilling all of the above criteria. The mu rhythm, for instance, may have the same frequency range (see below), but it has a distinct topography and reactivity. Importantly, in certain conditions (which can be broadly generalized as *encephalopathy*), the alpha rhythm frequency may lie below the alpha frequency band. Thus, many electroencephalographers prefer the term *posterior dominant rhythm* (PDR) and/or may use these terms interchangeably.

4.1.2. Frequency

The PDR is either absent or imperceptible at birth. Around the age of 4 months, an approximately 4/sec posterior rhythm can be detected. This rhythm shows a progressive frequency increase, with average values of around 6/sec at age 12 months and 8/sec at age 3 years. At this age, as noted above, the PDR now lies within the alpha frequency band and thus there is justification for the use of the term *alpha rhythm*. The frequency reaches a mean of about 10/sec at age 10 years. At this age (and lower), the PDR is often obscured by intermixed posterior slow activity that does

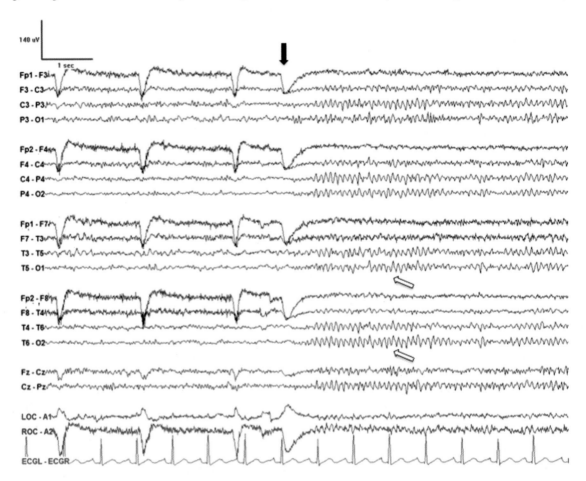

Figure 8.1. The posterior dominant rhythm (PDR) or alpha rhythm (white arrows) is reactive in that it is attenuated and obscured during states of eye opening and mental activity. A brief period of sustained eye closure (black arrow) is typically sufficient to enhance PDR amplitude when the true PDR frequency can be ascertained.

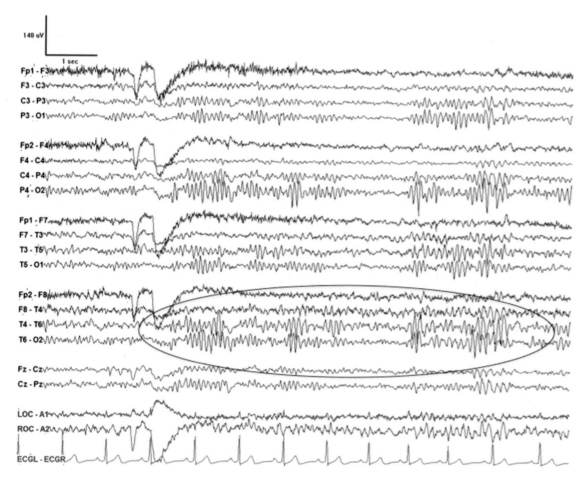

Figure 8.2. The amplitude of the PDR may itself be sinusoidally modulated over time.

decline over the next decade, such that by the third decade of life, the PDR is often described as "well-formed" or "well-regulated," to connote the presence of relatively long stretches of intact uninterrupted alpha rhythm, the amplitude of which is itself sinusoidally modulated (Fig. 8.2). A detailed discussion of the normal EEG maturation from preterm to adult is found in Chapter 7.

Petersen and Eeg-olofsson measured an average alpha rhythm frequency of 10.2 ± 0.9 Hz in healthy adults [23], a figure that probably stabilizes in the mid-adolescent years [24]. Some controversy exists about whether the "normal" PDR frequency range is truly narrower than the alpha frequency band, as a variety of cross-sectional studies of PDR frequency in healthy adolescents and young adults have shown that 80% to 90% of individuals lie between a range of between 8.5 and ~11 Hz (nicely summarized in [24]). Accordingly, some have argued for a more stringent lower "normal" limit of ~8.5 Hz [25]. In contrast, PDRs measuring above 11.5 Hz may be related to a medication-induced enhancement in beta activity, discussed further below [24].

Elderly individuals as a group tend to have a slightly slower measured PDR, although there is little evidence to suggest that this is a feature of normal aging. A true age-related decline in PDR frequency, the unambiguous demonstration of which would require serial measurements over several decades, likely reflects some degree of cerebral pathology, typically related to vascular insufficiency or mild neurodegeneration, neither of which may necessarily correlate with overall intellectual or executive function. Many healthy elderly individuals may show little or no alpha frequency decline [26,27].

PDR frequencies measured in an EEG laboratory may be susceptible to various acute modulating effects. As an example, sinusoidally modulated light (distinct from photic stimulation, which are *square* waves) can frequency-stabilize the PDR [28]. Early reports suggested that extreme upward gaze [29] and extreme lateral gaze may increase PDR frequencies [30], but this may be related ultimately to the effect of alterations in visual input [31]. PDR frequency may temporarily be increased immediately following eye closure by ~1 Hz [32, 33], a phenomenon known as the "alpha squeak" effect. Finally, and perhaps most importantly, transitions from wakefulness to drowsiness are classically said to display an "alpha dropout," when the alpha rhythm is *replaced* by a slower posterior rhythm that is typically in the high theta range (7–8 Hz), discussed further below. By definition, the PDR, when observed, is a feature of the waking EEG, and therefore ascertaining the true PDR frequency must be carried when the EEG demonstrates clear signs of wakefulness, including eye blinks and general reactivity.

While the amplitudes of several EEG frequency bands, including alpha activity, may vary with the circadian rhythm

[34,35], PDR frequencies have not been shown to reliably demonstrate diurnal fluctuations [36]. Similarly, there have been several attempts to understand how various frequency bands are modulated by the menstrual cycle, though reported changes in alpha rhythm frequency have been subtle, inconsistent, and not universal by any means [36–38].

4.1.3. AMPLITUDE

Berger found alpha rhythm voltages of 15 to 20 uV [3]. These are small values when one considers the large interelectrode distances of a fronto-occipital recording technique, and likely reflected the limitations of his Edelmann string galvanometer (see Chapter 1). Across individuals, PDR amplitude may vary between 10 and 100 uV [39,40]. Additionally, this value may vary from moment to moment within an individual. The electroencephalographer should look for stretches of optimal PDR output. A referential montage to the ipsilateral ear is usually most suitable for the determination of the PDR amplitude, but interelectrode distances must always be considered. The maximum alpha rhythm voltage is usually over the occipital region, but a bipolar montage with a parasagittal array may obscure rather than reveal the true alpha maximum. At times, PDR amplitude may be quite small in the channels displaying P_3–O_1 and P_4–O_2 because of massive homophasic activity resulting in phase cancellation. In some patients, alpha rhythm amplitudes during stretches of relaxed wakefulness show a sinusoidal waxing and waning of amplitude.

A mild-to-moderate asymmetry in PDR amplitude, with a higher voltage on the right hemisphere, has been repeatedly demonstrated in healthy patients and can also be considered normal [23,39–43]. This asymmetry may be related to differences in skull thickness rather than true relationships between hemispheric *dominance* or handedness [42].

4.1.4. MORPHOLOGY, SPATIAL DISTRIBUTION, AND REACTIVITY

The alpha rhythm is usually characterized by rounded or sinusoidal waves, but a sizeable minority of individuals have a more "sharp" alpha configuration. In such cases, the negative component appears to be sharp and the positive component appears to be rounded, similar to the wave morphology of rolandic mu rhythm. This is by no means abnormal and likely is related to an admixture of beta activity (discussed further below).

Berger had originally wrongly concluded that the alpha rhythm was a global cerebral rhythm [3], perhaps related to his fronto-occipital bipolar recording technique. The alpha rhythm is typically appreciated to be maximal over the occipital regions, and to a lesser extent in the parietal and posterior temporal regions. It may extend into central areas, the vertex, and also the midtemporal region. When the central region is strongly involved, the alpha rhythm must be distinguished from possibly coexisting rolandic mu rhythm. This is usually easily demonstrable with eye opening, which should lead to attenuation of the alpha rhythm but not the mu rhythm. The alpha rhythm occasionally extends slightly into the superior frontal leads (F_3, F_4). Apparent alpha rhythm in the frontopolar leads may be very prominent in referential (unipolar) montages if the referential ear electrode picks up the posterior alpha rhythm. This is particularly common when the mastoid region is used instead of the earlobe. Alpha-frequency eyelid flutter may also give rise to the apparent presence of the alpha rhythm in frontopolar leads (previously referred to as the *kappa* rhythm).

The PDR is *reactive* to various sensory stimuli that may be as simple as an influx of light (eye opening), as well as other afferent stimuli that may promote mental activity. Thus, the PDR has been often termed the *idling* rhythm of the posterior head regions. The degree of reactivity can vary; the alpha rhythm may be completely blocked, suppressed, or attenuated in voltage. This phenomenon, first described by Berger [3], came as somewhat of a surprise for investigators who were searching for cerebral "action potentials" and hence would have expected enhancement of EEG voltage with influx of light. To explain this phenomenon, Berger described a theoretical zone of inhibition surrounding the area of excitation by the afferent stimulus [44].

4.1.5. BENIGN AND PATHOLOGICAL INTERINDIVIDUAL DIFFERENCES

When Adrian and Matthews displayed their own EEGs on May 12, 1934, at a meeting of the members of the Physiological Society in Cambridge, England, it was found that Adrian's 10/sec alpha rhythm was quite "impressive" whereas Matthews produced "no regular waves" [45]. Indeed, in a minority of patients, the PDR may be poorly visualized or only intermittently visualized. It may also be discerned only during voluntary hyperventilation, which may ultimately be related to a calming/relaxation effect. Thus, for any specific EEG epoch containing wakefulness, the absence of a PDR is not abnormal by any means. Based on the percentage of intact alpha rhythm observed during wakefulness, Davis and Davis [46] distinguished four types of records: (a) dominant alpha (>75% of the record, found in 20% of healthy adults); (b) subdominant alpha (50–75% of the record, 35% of adults); (c) mixed alpha (25–50% of the record, 20% of adults); and (d) rare alpha (<25% of the record, in 25% of adults). Similarly, Golla et al. [47] distinguished three alpha types: M for minus or "minimal" (where the alpha rhythm appears to be completely absent), P for "persistent" (implying only a brief attenuation to eye opening), and R for "responsive" (indicating a more sustained attenuation to eye opening (see [40]). Since marked similarities in alpha rhythm morphology have been seen in identical twins, these morphological traits of the alpha rhythm may be, to some degree, genetically transmitted [46,48–50].

Historically, in an attempt to objectively describe certain psychological traits or states, there have been several reports suggesting relationships between the alpha rhythm and personality traits [51–57], but with little evidence of reproducibility of findings. Voluntary control of the alpha rhythm and the use of alpha feedback methods have been widely discussed topics since the late 1960s. This work was prompted by the observation of well-modulated alpha during meditation practiced by yogis [58] and Zen Buddhists [59]. These findings have been summarized nicely by Fingelkurts [60] and demonstrate that EEG alterations may ultimately depend upon the style of meditation implemented, and that the most consistent effects were an increase in alpha power (amplitude) and an increase in alpha coherence. There may be no consistent EEG pattern associated with successful or unsuccessful meditation [61]. Stigsby showed that the EEG spectrum displayed by healthy individuals during Transcendental Meditation was situated between wakefulness and drowsiness, with an overall ~1/s reduction in mean EEG frequency [62]. More recent EEG power spectral analyses performed on experienced meditators have shown that in contrast to a wakeful closed-eyes state, a state of "thoughtless emptiness" displayed less delta and theta activity, suggesting that meditative states may be electroencephalographically distinct from wakefulness *or* drowsiness [63].

In clear distinction to variations in PDR morphology, symmetrical reductions in PDR frequency to the theta range represent a clear abnormality and are consistent with the presence of an *encephalopathy*, a term that has been broadly used to depict diffuse cerebral dysfunction. This may be either an *acute* encephalopathy (aka delirium or acute confusional state [64]) or a more *chronic* encephalopathy, as seen in a range of conditions associated with dementia and intellectual disability [65]. In both conditions, PDR slowing is often accompanied by more diffuse delta or theta frequency activity. The unilateral absence of the alpha rhythm or a comparatively slowed alpha rhythm over one hemisphere conveys the presence of an ipsilateral structural lesion, which may be broadly situated.

4.1.6. Cerebral Generators of the Alpha Rhythm

The alpha rhythm reflects a cortical phenomenon that requires interactions between thalamocortical pathways and corticocortical connections [66]. The theory of a thalamic pacemaker function was spurred by the work of Berger [3], who presumed a cortical genesis but thalamic governance of the alpha rhythm. At around the same time, Bishop [67] proposed a concept of corticothalamic reverberating circuits. Various experimental models have been implemented to study the cerebral generators of the alpha rhythm [66]. Andersen and Andersson [68] began this work in the cat model by studying the formation of spindles that occur under barbiturate anesthesia. These spindles bore some semblance to alpha waves, though overall this model was appropriately felt to display poor face and construct validity. According to this theory, the alpha rhythm is driven by presynaptic input to cortical neurons from the thalamic level. This concept has been challenged by Lopes da Silva et al. [69,70], who showed in awake dogs that alpha rhythms of the same frequency, bandwidth, and reactivity can be recorded from the visual cortex as well as visual thalamic regions, namely the pulvinar and lateral geniculate nucleus [66].

Important new vistas were opened with the demonstration of some degree of interhemispheric asynchrony between alpha waves [71], leading to the suspicion that there may be more than one alpha generator [72]; this was further substantiated by depth-EEG studies in the human [73]. More recent studies from patients with severe thalamic pain syndromes implanted with thalamic depth electrodes [74,75] have shown that the alpha rhythm can be recorded from various thalamic subnuclei, including the pulvinar nucleus. Overall, however, our comprehension of alpha rhythm genesis has not strikingly

increased in the past several decades; it seems likely that there are corticocortical and thalamocortical systems that interact in the generation of cortical alpha rhythms. See Chapter 2 for a full discussion of cerebral rhythm generators.

4.2. Mu Rhythm

The *mu* rhythm is defined as 7- to 11-Hz activity, composed of arch-shaped waves occurring over the central and centroparietal regions of the scalp during wakefulness. It is blocked or attenuated most clearly by contralateral movement, the thought of movement, readiness to move, or tactile stimulation [1]. The mu rhythm is often similar to the alpha rhythm in frequency and amplitude, but its topography and physiological significance are quite different (Fig. 8.3). Historically, the existence of a special central alpha frequency rhythm was first reported as a "precentral alpha rhythm" by Jasper and Andrews [4], and later as "high voltage rolandic alpha" by Schütz and Müller [76]. Gastaut first identified the mu rhythm as *rhythme rolandique en arceau* [77], with the epithet *en arceau* alluding to the arc- or arch-shaped wave morphology, which has also prompted the term *wicket rhythm* [78], to be distinguished from temporal *wickets* or *wicket spikes*. Other terms that have been used include *arcade rhythm, comb rhythm*, and *somatosensory alpha rhythm*.

4.2.1. Age and Prevalence

Central mu rhythm used to be considered scarce. The introduction of the 10-20 montage has contributed to a much greater awareness of this pattern as the C_3 and C_4 electrodes are located over the precentral gyrus in an optimal location for picking up central mu rhythm. Gastaut et al. [78] found mu rhythm in 10% of their adult patients, and similar findings have been reported by other groups. In the patients of Niedermeyer and Koshino [79], the prevalence of mu rhythm was 8.1% (182 of 2,248); broken down into age ranges, there were 9.0% between ages 0 and 10 years, 13.8% between 11 and 20 years, 8.4% between 21 and 40 years, and 4.5% above 41 years. These authors demonstrated the presence of a rolandic mu rhythm in a 20-month-old child; this was thought to be an exceptionally early manifestation of mu rhythm, although the data of Stroganova et al. [80] demonstrated central mu rhythm (during a state of attention) in the tracing of an 8-month-old baby with a frequency of ~6 to 8.8/sec. The authors speculated that mu rhythm tends to appear before the occipital alpha equivalent because, unlike visual stimulation, somatosensory stimulation is present within the uterus. With the use of frequency analysis, the prevalence of mu rhythm probably reaches closer to 100% [81]. Familial occurrence of mu rhythm has been reported by Koshino and Isaki [82].

4.2.2. Morphology, Frequency, and Spatial Distribution

Older synonyms such as *rhythme en arceau* or *wicket rhythm* pertain to the wave morphology; the mu rhythm in most instances displays a sharp (or spiky) negative phase and a rounded positive phase. The posterior alpha rhythm may have

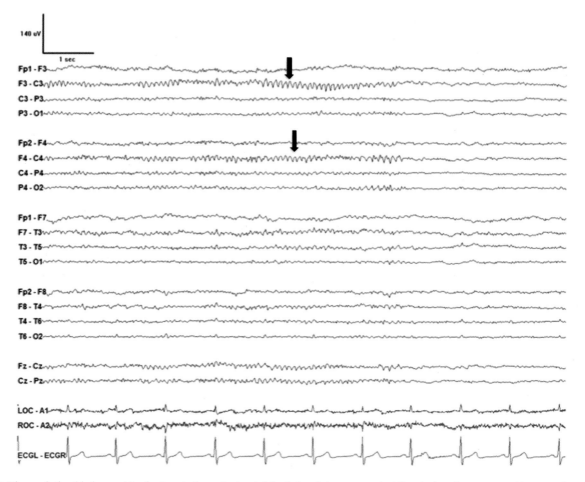

Figure 8.3. *The mu rhythm (black arrows) is a frontocentrally predominant alpha rhythm that represents the idling rhythm of somatosensory/motor regions. Unlike the alpha rhythm, which is reactive to eye opening, the mu rhythm is reactive to movement, the thought of movement, or certain tactile stimuli. With training, some individuals are able to voluntarily modulate the amplitude of the mu rhythm, providing for a means of biofeedback that can be implemented into brain–computer interface techniques.*

a similar configuration. The amplitudes of the mu rhythm are comparable to those of the posterior alpha rhythm.

Mu rhythm usually occurs in short stretches lasting several seconds each. Mu frequencies are typically slightly higher than alpha frequencies and always bilaterally incoherent [83], indicating distinct generators for the alpha rhythm and mu rhythms. The spatial distribution is essentially confined to the precentral–postcentral regions; some spread into parietal leads is not uncommon. The C_3 and C_4 electrodes are mostly involved. Occasionally, a vertex (C_z) maximum is noted: a distinct *vertex mu rhythm* with a distinct reactivity pattern has been described by Farnarier et al. [84]. In most persons, the mu rhythm can be appreciated bilaterally but may shift from side to side. The occurrence of a strictly unilateral mu rhythm (or that which demonstrates only unilateral reactivity) must be scrutinized for the possibility of an ipsilateral rolandic disturbance such as a parasagittal meningioma, an arteriovenous malformation, or other neoplasms. In such cases, the possibility of a contralateral rolandic lesion must be taken into consideration [77]. More importantly, the possibility of a local cranial bone defect, surgical or traumatic, must be ruled out. A single burr hole in the rolandic region can enable an otherwise hidden mu rhythm to become manifest on the scalp.

4.2.3. REACTIVITY

The mu rhythm is attenuated by movements of the contralateral limb and can also be similarly reactive to the thought of movement, the mental state of readiness to move, or tactile stimulation [1,77,78]. The mu rhythm has thus been considered to be an *idling* or resting rhythm of sensorimotor regions. Movements may be active (voluntary), passive, or reflexive. The attenuating effect is bilateral but more pronounced on the rolandic region contralateral to the site of movement; the effect appears prior to the onset of muscular contraction [85]. In Chatrian's studies [86], after the initiation of the spontaneous flexion of the contralateral thumb, delays of 50 msec to 7.5 sec (average of ~1.5 sec) could occur prior to the onset of the mu blocking effect, with the ipsilateral lagging behind the contralateral response. Mu blocking responses have also been demonstrated in persons with amputations of extremities [85].

4.2.4. CEREBRAL GENERATORS OF THE MU RHYTHM

Jasper and Penfield [87] found strictly localized 20-Hz activity over the human motor cortex with electrocorticographic recording techniques in locally anesthetized patients. This rhythm could be blocked like mu rhythm with movement, especially contralateral movement, and also with thinking about the execution of movement. This cortical activity is felt to be a harmonic variant of the scalp-recorded rolandic mu rhythm, and similar patterns were recorded by Gastaut [77]. While the scalp mu rhythm (typically 10/sec) and electro-corticographically measured fast activity (~20 Hz) appear to be harmonically related, a similar relationship does not exist between scalp-recorded mu rhythm and rolandic beta activity, when present [88].

4.2.5. FEEDBACK TRAINING AND CLINICAL SIGNIFICANCE

With training, individuals can learn to voluntarily modulate the power of the mu rhythm. With the help of a closed-loop system, power in the mu range can be measured in real time using power spectral analysis and feedback can be provided to the participant. Such mu rhythm feedback training has been used for various purposes, including the treatment of epileptic seizure disorders [89–92] and mild autistic traits in children [93]. Since this type of EEG-based brain–computer communication does not require motor output, mu feedback training has become an essential element of early features of brain–computer interfaces designed for quadriplegic/quadra-paretic individuals. Results so far indicate that with learning/training, individuals can modulate their mu power to answer simple yes/no questions [94] or turn left or right in complex three-dimensional simulated environments [95].

Pure rolandic mu rhythm as such is categorically within normal limits. In some cases spiky discharges may be present and even single spikes may stand out. Children with benign rolandic epilepsy may gradually develop mu rhythm when rolandic spike activity subsides and the seizures appear to be under control. In some cases, rolandic spikes can be blocked by contralateral movements in the same manner as mu rhythm is blocked [96]. Finally, since the mu rhythm may also attenuate with the observation of a movement [97], the presence and modulation of the mu rhythm has been interpreted as a read-out of the mirror neuron system, which itself is thought to be disrupted in various neuropsychiatric disorders that involve abnormalities of social perception, such as autism, bipolar disorder, or schizophrenia [98–101].

4.3. The "Third Rhythm"

In intracranial EEG, rhythmical background activity in the 6- to 11-Hz range can be picked up from epidural electrodes over the midtemporal regions. Niedermeyer recognized this temporal 6- to 11-Hz activity, typically in the alpha range, as the *third* alpha frequency rhythm (distinct from the posterior dominant rhythm and the mu rhythm) [102–104]. On scalp EEG, the third rhythm is visualized rarely: in a study of ~4,900 healthy adults, it was identified in 15 individuals (0.3%), only half of whom had a skull/bone defect [105]. Perhaps due to its rarity and questionable significance, this rhythm has not been recognized by the IFSECN [1]. Admixed theta/alpha activity in the temporal region constitutes an important element of the breach rhythm [22] but may not be clearly evident without power spectral analyses due to the typical background disorganization and chaotic mixed frequency activity that is also seen in classical breach patterns. If present, the third rhythm may be seen in wakefulness, drowsiness, and early slow-wave sleep. No clear pattern of reactivity has been identified, and as such, the presence or absence of this rhythm confers no pathological significance [102].

4.4. Beta Rhythm

Historically, the discovery of beta activity is closely linked to the first description of the alpha rhythm by Berger. In his first report on the human EEG [2], Berger wrote that "the electro-encephalogram represents a continuous curve with continuous oscillations in which . . . one can distinguish larger first-order waves with an average duration of 90 sigma [msec] and smaller second-order waves of an average duration of 35 sigma" [44]. In his second report [106], Berger pointed out: "For the sake of brevity I shall subsequently designate the waves of first order as alpha waves, the waves of second order as beta waves." By his 14th report [107], Berger pointed out "that the beta waves and not the alpha waves of the EEG are the concomitant phenomena of mental activity."

Rhythmic activity that lies within 14 to 40 Hz is broadly termed the *beta* rhythm (or beta activity) and is typically of relatively low amplitude, mostly below 30 uV [1]. In modern digital EEG recordings, which often automatically apply a 70-Hz digital high-frequency filter (or low-pass filter), beta activity typically undergoes a further 10% to 20% reduction in amplitude. Beta activity is encountered chiefly over the frontal and central regions. Such beta activity may be seen prominently only during wakefulness or only during transitions to drowsiness. In certain patients, a prominent central beta rhythm can be a manifestation of the rolandic mu rhythm and can be blocked by motor activity or tactile stimulation, as described above.

Scalp-recorded beta activity may be enhanced diffusely by a variety of psychoactive medications (chiefly benzodiazepines and barbiturates [108]), various anticonvulsant agents [109], and other sedative-hypnotics (e.g., propofol [110]). Symmetrical increases in beta activity may be seen in some subtypes of major depression [111] and may be correlated with high anxiety states [112]. Focal or asymmetrical increases in faster activity, typically in the beta range, may be seen over bone defects as one part of the breach rhythm [22]. With the exception of beta activity that clearly evolves into an electroclinical seizure ([113], discussed in Chapter 19), neither the prominent absence nor a prominent "excess" of beta activity is sufficient to interpret an EEG as abnormal. Beta activity is found in every healthy adult EEG. The relative amplitude of beta activity may be conspicuously enhanced or attenuated depending upon other morphological features of the EEG background as well as filter settings. There is no clear consensus about the physiological role of beta activity. According to a theory by Engel and Fries, beta band activity may be expressed more strongly when there is a need to maintain the "current" sensorimotor or behavioral state, and it appears to be pathologically enhanced in certain states of motor or cognitive inflexibility, such as Parkinson's disease [114].

4.5. The Low-Voltage Record

A *low-voltage EEG* is formally defined as a waking record in which the amplitude of EEG activity over *all* head regions is not greater than 20μV [1]. While asymmetrical or global reductions in voltage occurring during an EEG are clearly abnormal (as described earlier), a true persistent low-voltage EEG pattern identified during wakefulness is entirely compatible with perfect CNS functioning (Fig. 8.4). The small amplitudes are ultimately the result of a lesser degree of synchronization of cortical electrical activity at the neuronal level. This pattern was previously referred to as a *desynchronized EEG*, but the use of this term has been discouraged. This cortical desynchronization is in fact an active process, coordinated by a series of brainstem nuclei that have together been labeled the *ascending reticular activating system* or the *ascending mesodiencephalic reticular formation*, among other terms. Our understanding of this phenomenon dates back to the original work of Bremer [115], who identified a synchronized slow-wave-sleep–like EEG pattern in cats following a transection between the inferior and superior colliculi (*cerveau isolé*). In contrast, cats with a transection between the spinal cord and the caudal medulla displayed normal sleep–wake cycles and a normal EEG. We now know that the ascending reticular activating system is made up of two main components: (i) a cholinergic system, made up of the pedunculopontine and laterodorsal tegmental regions that innervate relay and reticular thalamic nuclei, and (ii) a broad and diverse monoaminergic system, consisting of serotonergic (raphe complex), noradrenergeic (locus coeruleus), dopaminergic (ventral tegmental area), histaminergic (tuberomammillary nucleus), and additional combined GABAergic and cholinergic inputs (basal forebrain) to cortical regions [116]. During rapid eye movement (REM) sleep, activation of the cholinergic afferents to the thalamus occurs in the absence of monoaminergic input to the cortex, resulting in a desynchronized EEG pattern that enters the cortex into a "dreaming-like" state [116]. On the other hand, during sleep, the activity of both systems is inhibited by GABAergic input from the ventrolateral preoptic and median preoptic regions of the hypothalamus, both of which display high rates of activity only during sleep [117]. See Chapter 36 for a more detailed discussion.

Early studies of low-voltage tracings were carried out by Davis and Davis [46], Jasper et al. [118], and Finley [119]. Jasper and others have often used the term *flat EEG*, a term that should now be reserved for truly isoelectric records that reflect electrocerebral inactivity [1]. Overall, this low-voltage EEG pattern has been reported at rates of 3% to 13% in generally healthy adults (reviewed in [120]). Gibbs, Gibbs, and Lennox [121] found a low-voltage EEG in 11.6% of 1,000 normal adult subjects. Adams studied 427 normal individuals and

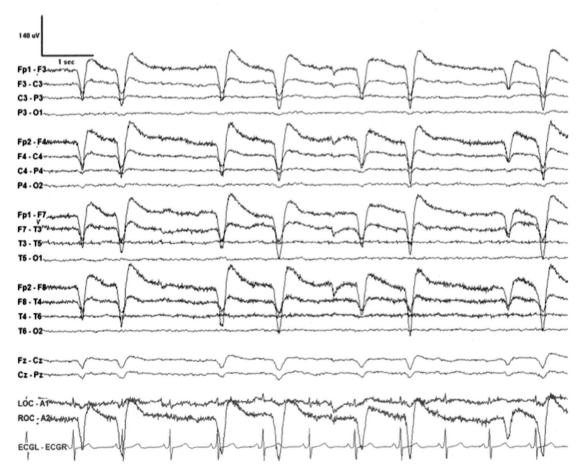

Figure 8.4. *Approximately 10% of normal healthy adults display a low-voltage EEG, characterized by diffusely low-amplitude EEG signal that is typically less than 20 μV. Predominant background frequencies lie in the beta range (14–40 Hz), and the PDR is usually absent or visualized only during voluntary hyperventilation.*

found the incidence of a low-voltage EEG (he also used the term "flat EEG") to be approximately 8% overall, but the prevalence of this pattern rose with age: 1% between ages 0 and 20, 7% between 20 and 39, and 11% between 40 and 69 years of age [122]. An age-related increased incidence of low-voltage EEGs has also been demonstrated by others [123–125].

In Adams' original study, he simultaneously examined 2,000 "neurological and psychiatric" patients who were not age-matched to his healthy control cohort. In this population, the low-voltage EEG pattern was not found in any patients with epilepsy (either "symptomatic" or "idiopathic"), but an increased incidence of a "flat EEG" was observed in patients with endocrine disorders (18%) or "psychopathy and neurosis" (19%) [122]. Congruently, Pine and Pine [126] studied 74 consecutive patients with low-voltage EEGs and showed that 64% of these patients had a "primary psychiatric disorder," most commonly "psychoneurosis with tension headache." Among more recent studies, an increased incidence of low-voltage EEG records has been observed in patients with Huntington's chorea [127] and alcohol dependence (extensively reviewed in [128]). Finally, in some patients, a low-voltage EEG pattern may be inherited as an autosomal dominant trait, and a number of genetic loci have been determined (i.e., genetic heterogeneity), each with a degree of incomplete penetrance [120].

4.6. Theta Rhythm

Activity in the 4- to 8-Hz frequency band is termed *theta* activity [1]. The term was introduced by Walter and Dovey [129,130], who observed that superficial tumors (presumably with cortical involvement) that spread inward were associated with local 1- to 3-Hz EEG activity, whereas subcortical tumors (or "deep" tumors with or without superficial involvement) displayed a characteristic ipsilateral parietotemporal 6/sec activity, which they termed *theta*.

The normal adult waking record may contain a small amount of theta frequency activity that is typically predominantly in anterior derivations (Fig. 8.5) and should not display any form of an organized theta rhythm. Theta frequencies and theta rhythms feature prominently in the EEG of infancy and childhood (see Chapter 7), as well as in adults during states of drowsiness and sleep. Larger or more continuous stretches of theta activity in the waking adult EEG, either symmetrical or asymmetrical, are abnormal and can be seen in various pathological conditions, not necessarily limited to subcortical tumors. Certainly, the presence of a theta frequency PDR is abnormal and conveys the presence of an encephalopathy, albeit mild and etiologically nonspecific. Finally, intermittent bursts of asymmetrical theta frequency slowing may be the only sign of "subcortical dysfunction," a

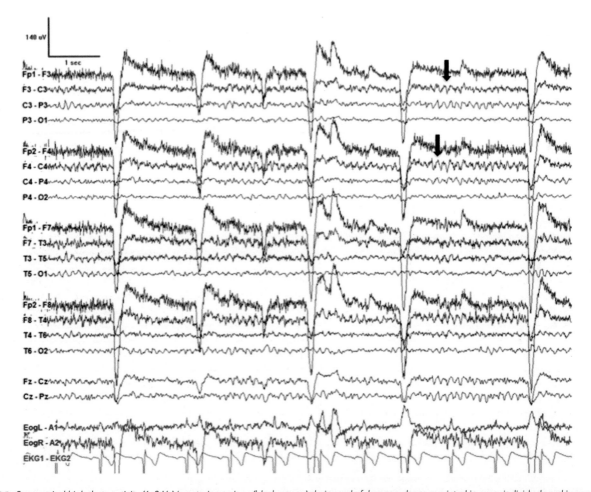

Figure 8.5. Symmetrical high theta activity (6–8 Hz) in anterior regions (black arrows) during wakefulness can be appreciated in some individuals and is normal. In stark contrast, a slowed PDR to the theta range is categorically abnormal, whether symmetrical or asymmetrical.

rather broad term that may correlate with the presence of leu-koaraiosis, demyelinating lesions, or other structural lesions and may be a biomarker of paroxysmal seizure-like symptoms in patients following a closed head injury [131–133]. Finally, polymorphic sharply contoured theta-alpha activity (6–11 Hz) often constitutes the predominant background frequency of a breach rhythm [22].

4.7. Lambda Waves

4.7.1. Definition and Historical Aspects
Lambda waves are diphasic sharp transients, with the main component being positive, occurring over the occipital regions of the head during visual exploration [1]. These visually induced occipital discharges were first described by Gastaut in 1949 [134], with subsequent studies presented by Cobb and Pampiglione [135], Evans [136], and Roth and Green [137].

4.7.2. Prevalence and Mechanism
Lambda waves are unmistakably present in some records and are not readily demonstrable in others (Fig. 8.6). They are most prominent in waking patients intently viewing an illuminated visual field. The true prevalence of lambda waves may depend upon the length of EEG studies and whether any emphasis has

been placed on demonstrating this phenomenon. In Chatrian's original review, lambda waves were reported to be most common between ages 3 and 12 years (82.3%); their prevalence declined to 72% between 18 and 30 years and to 36.4% between 31 and 50 years [138]. In more recent work by Tatum et al., lambda waves were found in 50% of patients who displayed visual scanning, and the presence of lambda waves was strongly correlated with a PDR >8.5 Hz, suggesting that their presence may be used to exclude an encephalopathy [139]. Lambda waves often resemble POSTS, and the two are often correlated [140,141].

4.7.3. Morphology, Spatial Distribution, and Reactivity
Lambda waves are biphasic waves, with the more prominent phase being positive. Their form has been described as triangular or sawtooth-shaped, with amplitudes that are slightly larger than that of the PDR. These waves are often repetitive, usually at intervals from 200 to 2,000 msec. Lambda waves are most prominent in, or confined to, the occipital leads. Spread into parietal and posterotemporal areas is common and, in certain cases, the maximum may be found in areas adjacent to the occipital lobe [136,137]. Lambda activity is strictly bilaterally synchronous. With the use of depth electrodes, Perez-Borja et al. [73] demonstrated multiple foci of lambda waves,

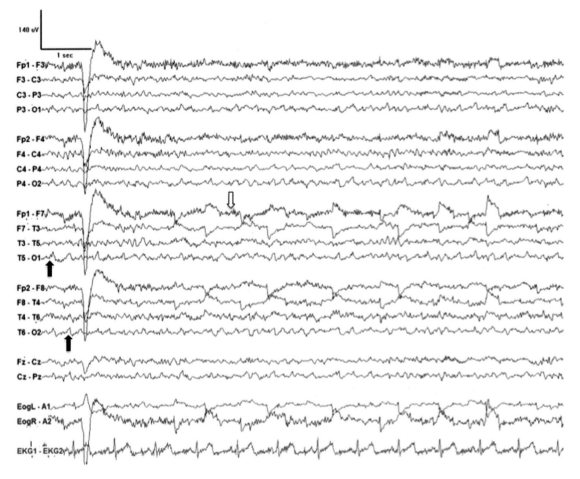

Figure 8.6. *Symmetrical positive biphasic sharp transients can be seen during wakefulness in posterior regions and are termed lambda waves (black arrows). They are generally brought on by visual scanning. This EEG also identifies the presence of lateral eye movement artifact in bilateral frontopolar/frontotemporal regions (white arrow).*

either in or near the calcarine region or more laterally in the occipital lobes.

Voluntary scanning eye movements, exploratory saccades, play a very important role in the generation of lambda waves [142]; indeed, it is no surprise that they are often triggered by watching television [140]. Most lambda waves follow an exploratory eye movement with a latency of 67 to 85 msec (mean, 78 msec) [143]. Lambda waves are best found in brightly lit laboratories and cannot be elicited in darkness. The size of a given pattern and its distance and color are further variables. Binocular viewing of a picture may or may not produce larger lambda waves than monocular viewing [144,145], and the presentation of a previously unfamiliar visual object enhances lambda production [138,146], though lambda activity does not seem to be related to recognition of objects [143]. Finally, no correlation between lambda waves and any neurological or psychiatric disorder has been demonstrated.

5. BASIC EEG PATTERNS SEEN DURING SLEEP

EEG recordings of sleep have been performed for several decades. EEG during nocturnal sleep is automatically captured during 24-hour-long recordings (e.g., inpatient EEG telemetry studies or outpatient ambulatory studies). In addition, a significant majority of "routine" EEGs, defined here as short-duration studies that are 20 to 60 minutes long, also capture brief epochs of sleep, which are basically naps. For many epilepsies, the incidence of interictal epileptiform discharges (IEDs) increases during sleep (discussed further below), and in many patients, IEDs occur only during sleep [147–151]. Thus, allowing sleep to occur during a short EEG is a provocative technique, akin to hyperventilation and photic stimulation. Certain paroxysmal events typically occur only during nocturnal sleep—for example, nocturnal frontal lobe seizures or parasomnias, such as night terrors or somnambulism. While patients with suspected primary sleep disorders are typically referred for polysomnography in formal sleep laboratories, an ambulatory EEG may be the first test of choice in a patient with abnormal spells during sleep and in whom the distinction between a parasomnia and nocturnal seizures may not be clear. Ambulatory EEG monitoring may offer a more convenient and better-tolerated modality to obtain several sequential days of sleep-containing recordings, which may in turn provide a higher yield for more rarely occurring sleep-related paroxysms [152,153].

In the mid-1930s, Hobart's group [154,155] was the first to provide an EEG-based staging system to classify individual sleep stages. In these studies, subjects were instructed to lie down and fall sleep with a rubber bulb in one hand. They were asked to squeeze the bulb *once* whenever they felt that they had "just drifted or floated off for a moment" and *twice* when they felt that they had awakened from a "real sleep." With these subjective markers of state transition, they characterized six distinct sleep stages as follows:

A—"*Alpha*": at rest but awake, typically with an alpha rhythm

B_1—"*Low voltage, alpha rhythm lost*": corresponding to the drowsy or "floating" state

B_2—"*Low voltage, delta waves appearing*": merging into sleep

C—"*Spindles and moderate delta waves*": real sleep

D—"*Spindles plus random*": with increased sleep spindles and longer delta waves

E—"*Random*": rare spindles, delta waves continue to increase in voltage [154]

It was only in the mid-1950s that REM sleep was discovered by Kleitman's group, who noticed "jerky eye movements" occurring during sleep in both adults and infants, typically associated with mild increases in heart and respiration rate [156,157]. In 1968, the first consensus-based sleep EEG staging guidelines were developed under the leadership of Rechtschaffen and Kales [158] (often abbreviated as "R&K rules"), with the following definitions:

Waking: 50% of the page (epoch) consists of alpha (8–13 Hz) activity or low-voltage, mixed-frequency (2–7 Hz) activity

Stage 1: 50% of the epoch consists of relatively low-voltage mixed (2–7 Hz) activity, and <50% of the epoch contains alpha activity. Slow rolling eye movements lasting several seconds often seen in early stage 1.

Stage 2: Appearance of sleep spindles and/or K-complexes and <20% of the epoch may contain high-voltage (>75µV, <2 Hz) activity. Sleep spindles and K-complexes each must last >0.5 sec.

Stage 3: 20–50% of the epoch consists of high-voltage (>75 µV), low-frequency (<2 Hz) activity

Stage 4: >50% of the epoch consists of high-voltage (>75 µV) <2 Hz delta activity

REM sleep: Relatively low-voltage, mixed-activity (2–7 Hz) EEG with episodic REMs and absent or reduced chin EMG activity

The committee recommended a minimum of a single central EEG channel, usually C3 or C4 referenced to the opposite mastoid, in addition to other modalities, including chin EMG. A 30-second-long epoch-based scoring system was implemented, such that for every 30 sec of the sleep record, a single sleep stage was assigned. Over the ensuing several decades, a number of limitations of the R&K system were noted (reviewed in [159]). Chiefly, as it pertains to the staging of sleep, interrater accuracy was high for REM sleep but poor for stage 1 sleep and slow-wave sleep (specifically, discriminating between stage 3 and 4). Accordingly, the American Academy of Sleep

Medicine (AASM) proposed a revised set of rules for sleep staging in 2007 that provided greater detail and also proposed clear guidelines for transitions between sleep stages (Box 8.1) [160]. Importantly, stages 3 and 4 of the R&K system are now together labeled as simply stage N3 (slow-wave sleep). These rules also provide an approach to accurately stage wakefulness and transitions to drowsiness in patients who do not display a clear alpha rhythm. Of note, the AASM rules now also recommend greater EEG spatial coverage, calling for the inclusion of frontal and occipital leads in addition to central leads.

With the AASM rules, which we follow for the remainder of the chapter, the improvement in interrater reliability has been minimal to negligible [161]. Disagreements persist about stage N1 (drowsiness, often scored either as W or N2) and stage N3 (often alternatively scored as N2). Such consistent diagnostic disagreements across scoring systems perhaps demonstrate that the division of non-REM sleep into such discrete stages may not accurately reflect what is truly a continuum of electrographic changes associated with sleep. As we shall see below, many graphoelements of sleep persist across several different stages. In some EEGs, a distinction between drowsiness and mild encephalopathy can be quite challenging when mild background slowing and/or bursts of mild generalized slowing are seen.

In an appropriately darkened and quiet room, most children and adults fall asleep readily. To enhance the chances of obtaining sleep in a routine EEG, patients can be asked to remain sleep-deprived prior to the study. However, there are no internationally recognized consensus guidelines that provide a clear recommendation on the precise duration of sleep deprivation that would provide the highest yield, or even whether the initial routine EEG should be universally performed with sleep deprivation [162]. Previously, relatively prolonged periods of sleep deprivation were employed. Mattson and colleagues showed retrospectively that 26- to 28-hour-long forced sleep deprivation resulted in an enhanced rate of IED detection in individuals who previously had a normal EEG (with a history consistent with a single seizure) as well as in patients known to have epilepsy with IEDs present on baseline routine EEGs [163]. This finding was confirmed prospectively [164] and was shown to remain true even in the presence of anticonvulsant therapy [165]. More recently, *partial* sleep deprivation has gained more popularity, whereby adult patients are instructed to sleep for no more than 4 hours, or approximately half of their typical nocturnal sleep duration [166,167]. Kubicki showed, using an age-corrected partial sleep deprivation protocol, that sleep, of various stages, was achieved in 79% of patients referred for a routine EEG [166]. Sleep-deprived routine EEGs appear to display a better sensitivity for the detection of generalized epileptiform discharges as opposed to focal IEDs [168]. However, following a single suspected or witnessed seizure, appreciating such an electroclinical distinction may not be obvious, particularly since a proportion of patients with idiopathic generalized epilepsy syndromes report "focal" seizure symptoms [169]. In contrast to adults, sleep deprivation has been reported to have more modest diagnostic gains in pediatric populations [170,171].

Might sleep deprivation itself lead to epileptiform discharges in patients who otherwise may not have an enduring

BOX 8.1. TRANSITIONS BETWEEN SLEEP STAGES

I. Stage W
   A. Score epochs as stage W when >50% of the epoch has alpha rhythm over the occipital region.
   B. Score epochs without visually discernible alpha rhythm as stage W if any of the following are present:
      (1) Eye blinks at a frequency of 0.5–2 Hz
      (2) Reading eye movements
      (3) Irregular conjugate rapid eye movements associated with normal or high chin muscle tone

II. Stage N1
   A. In subjects who generate alpha rhythm, score stage N1 if alpha rhythm is attenuated and replaced by low-amplitude, mixed-frequency activity for >50% of the epoch.
   B. In subjects who do not generate alpha rhythm, score stage N1 commencing with the earliest of any of the following phenomena:
      (1) Activity in the range 4–7 Hz with slowing of background frequencies by ≥1 Hz from those of stage W
      (2) Vertex sharp waves
      (3) Slow eye movements

III. Stage N2
   A. The following rule defines the start of a period of stage N2 sleep:
      (1) Begin scoring stage N2 (in absence of criteria for N3) if 1 or both of the following occur during the first half of that epoch or the last half of the previous epoch:
         a. One or more K-complexes unassociated with arousals
         b. One or more trains of sleep spindles
   B. The following rule defines continuation of a period of stage N2 sleep:
      (1) Continue to score epochs with low-amplitude, mixed-frequency EEG activity without K-complexes or sleep spindles as stage N2 if they are preceded by:
         a. K-complexes unassociated with arousals or
         b. Sleep spindles
      (2) End stage N2 sleep when 1 of the following events occurs:
         a. Transition to stage W
         b. An arousal (change to stage N1 until a K-complex unassociated with an arousal or a sleep spindle occurs)
         c. A major body movement followed by slow eye movements and low-amplitude, mixed-frequency EEG without non-arousal-associated K-complexes or sleep spindles
         d. Transition to stage N3
         e. Transition to stage R

IV. Stage N3
   Score N3 when 20% or more of an epoch consists of slow-wave activity (waves of frequency 0.5–2 Hz and

BOX 8.1. CONTINUED

peak-to-peak amplitude >75 μV, measured over the frontal regions), irrespective of age

V. Stage R

A. Score stage R sleep in epochs with all the following phenomena:

a. Low-amplitude, mixed-frequency EEG

b. Low chin EMG tone

c. Rapid eye movements

B. Continue to score stage R sleep, even in the absence of rapid eye movements, for epochs following 1 or more epochs of stage R as defined in A above, if the EEG continues to show low-amplitude, mixed-frequency activity without K-complexes or sleep spindles and the chin EMG tone remains low

C. Stop scoring stage R sleep when 1 or more of the following occur:

a. There is a transition to stage W or N3

b. An increase in chin EMG tone above the level of stage R is seen and criteria for stage N1 are met

c. An arousal occurs followed by low-amplitude, mixed-frequency EEG and slow eye movements

d. A major body movement followed by slow eye movements and low-amplitude, mixed-frequency EEG without non-arousal-associated K-complexes or sleep spindles

e. One or more non-arousal-associated K-complexes or sleep spindles are present in the first half of the epoch in the absence of rapid eye movements, even if chin EMG tone remains low

D. Score epochs at the transition between stage N2 and stage R as follows:

(1) In between epochs of definite stage N2 and definite stage R, score an epoch with a distinct drop in chin EMG in the first half of the epoch to the level seen in stage R as stage R if all of the following criteria are met, even in the absence of rapid eye movements:

a. Absence of non-arousal-associated K-complexes

b. Absence of sleep spindles

(2) In between epochs of definite stage N2 and definite stage R, score an epoch with a distinct drop in chin EMG in the first half of the epoch to the level seen in stage R as stage N2 if all of the following criteria are met:

a. Presence of non-arousal-associated K-complexes or sleep spindles

b. Absence of rapid eye movements

(3) In between epochs of definite stage N2 with minimal chin EMG tone and definite stage R without further drop in chin EMG tone, score epochs as stage R if all of the following are met, even in the absence of rapid eye movements:

a. Absence of non-arousal-associated K-complexes

b. Absence of sleep spindles

predisposition to epilepsy? Rodin et al. [172] provided a highly illustrative study of the EEG of 16 healthy male adults who were asked to remain sleep-deprived for up to 120 hours. After 48 hours of voluntary wakefulness, the alpha rhythm became progressively less sustained, only seen for about 1 to 3 sec at a time immediately following eye closure after ~120 hours of sleep deprivation. A slight decrease in amplitude was observed, and in six patients, a 1-cps *increase* in frequency was seen. In five patients, 1-sec-long bursts of high-voltage diffuse paroxysmal activity occurred "[as] seen in some patients with convulsive disorders of *deep level* origin." This was observed at the 24- to 48-hour stage but decreased subsequently as sleepiness progressed. With progressively greater sleep deprivation, two patients developed epileptiform changes following photic stimulation, but hyperventilation did not appear to provoke the recording in these patients. Finally, consistent with the known effects of sleep deprivation on seizure threshold, a majority of subjects displayed a lower threshold for epileptiform changes following the administration of the proconvulsant agent megimide (a barbiturate GABA antagonist), with one patient demonstrating a convulsive seizure of the "centrencephalic type." Nevertheless, aside from these studies of extreme sleep deprivation, the incidence of electroclinical seizures occurring during routine EEGs is quite low (45 out of 1,000) [147]. A partially sleep-deprived EEG may thus be a safe and useful strategy to enhance the yield of IED detection in an individual who has previously had a normal routine non-sleep-deprived study.

Whenever a sleep recording is desirable and cannot be obtained naturally, the use of sedated sleep may be necessary. This is particularly relevant for pediatric populations, where mild sedation may also assist in the safe placement of electrodes in patients who may be quite agitated or fearful. Classically, chloral hydrate has been employed as a sedative [173]. A number of alternatives to chloral hydrate have also been proposed, including dexmedetomidine (an alpha-2 adrenergic agonist) [174], hydroxyzine (a first-generation antihistamine) [175], melatonin [176], and music therapy [177]. Chloral hydrate is typically safe but may alter the presence of epileptic activity [178]. In adults, the use of sedation may rarely be associated with a change in clinical care, and given the confounds associated with changes in EEG activity associated with sedative-hypnotics, simple sleep deprivation is probably a better first approach [179]. Sedation may still ultimately be necessary to obtain artifact-free recordings of sleep *and* wakefulness in patients who display disruptive behaviors.

6. ELECTROGRAPHIC FEATURES OF SLEEP STAGES

6.1. Drowsiness (Stage N1)

Phenomenologically, drowsiness is a state of diminished and/or fluctuating vigilance, intermediate between wakefulness and sleep. This is a state that is distinct from encephalopathy and associated reductions in consciousness. Drowsiness or stage N1 can have a remarkably varied EEG appearance, particularly across the age spectrum. Fleeting and brief episodes of very light drowsiness are common in waking records. Boredom, fatigue, and monotony may quickly induce such periods in a patient instructed to relax during the test. In addition to being both variable and brief, electrographic correlates of drowsiness can also be quite subtle. Often, the first signs of drowsiness are reflected in three main EEG changes that are unrelated to cerebral EEG activity: (i) decreased or absent eye blinks, (ii) diminished muscle or myogenic artifact, and (iii) the presence of slow roving eye movements (Fig. 8.7). In the early stages of drowsiness, the presence of one or more of these elements may be the only clue that the patient has entered a drowsy state.

Drowsiness-related changes in "cerebral" background activity can take several forms, each of which may or may not be present. Classically, drowsiness is characterized by an "alpha dropout" whereby the alpha rhythm is often *replaced* by a slower rhythm in the high theta band (5–8 Hz). While the term "dropout" (not recognized by the IFSECN [1]) may indicate a stepwise "drop" in posterior frequencies, in practice this is rarely observed and a more gradual reduction in posterior frequencies is seen. In addition to background slowing, there may or may not be a voltage decline associated with enhanced beta activity, which in some individuals may resemble a desynchronized or "low-voltage" EEG. This should be strictly separated from periods of enhanced alertness after

eye opening or those caused by mental or emotional stress, associated with alpha attenuation. Particularly in patients with low-voltage EEG patterns, the onset of early drowsiness may be quite poorly defined or may reveal a gradual subtle increase in overall amplitude.

Progressively "deeper" stages of drowsiness are associated with a mild enhancement in the amplitude of slower frequencies. Long trains of frontocentrally predominant theta activity may be seen. In addition, brief 1- to 2-sec-long bursts of mixed-frequency slowing may be seen, and these are normal if they are symmetrical and primarily in the theta range (Fig. 8.8). In addition to these changes in background activity, the EEG of stage N1 sleep may display two additional graphoelements that often persist into stage 2 sleep, vertex waves and POSTs.

6.2. Vertex Waves or Vertex Sharp Transients

Vertex sharp transients are defined as sharp potentials, maximal at the vertex, negative relative to other areas, apparently occurring spontaneously during sleep or in response to a sensory stimulus during sleep or wakefulness [1] (Fig. 8.9). Vertex waves were first described by Liberson [180] and represent a compounded potential: a small spike discharge of positive polarity precedes the large following negative wave, which is almost always the most prominent feature of the discharge. Another small positive spiky discharge usually follows.

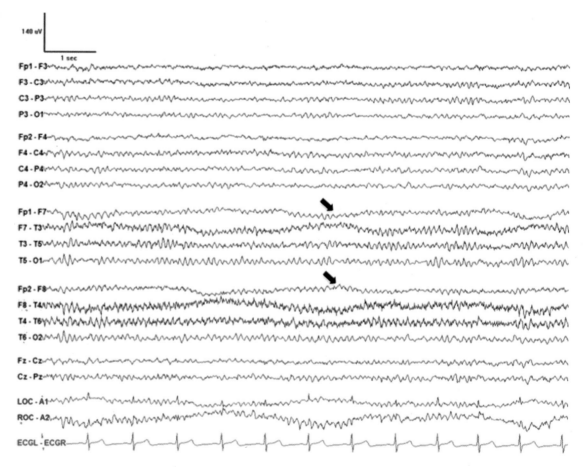

Figure 8.7. In addition to changes in background EEG activity, the state of drowsiness is associated with slow lateral roving eye movements that are reflected as slow deviations in voltage (<1 Hz) that are out of phase across left and right frontal regions (black arrows).

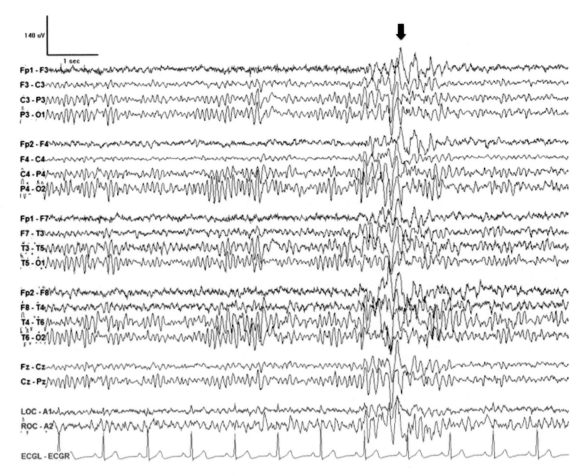

Figure 8.8. Theta band activity is an important element of the sleep EEG. In addition to background theta slowing, isolated bursts of diffuse symmetrical theta slowing can be a normal feature of drowsiness.

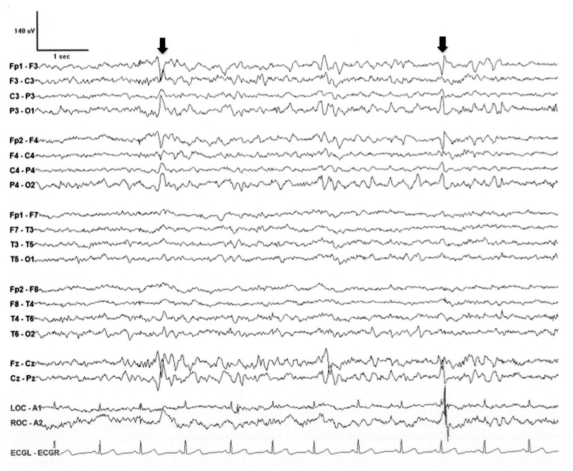

Figure 8.9. During N1 and N2 stages of sleep, centrally maximal surface negative sharp transients (typically maximal at Cz) are termed vertex waves (black arrows).

Vertex sharp transients are typically isolated events, but trains of repetitive vertex waves may occur in some individuals (Fig. 8.10). Their amplitudes are usually significantly larger than the remainder of EEG activity and are typically maximal at the vertex (Cz). Slightly anterior or laterally oriented vertex waves are not categorically abnormal; however, in concert with other electrographic signs of asymmetrical cerebral dysfunction, such anatomically deviated vertex waves may reflect structural pathology in the dysfunctional hemisphere. Truly epileptogenic spikes may occur over the vertex [181,182] and may be a result of a midline epileptogenic lesion [183]. Vertex waves may become small and inconspicuous in aged individuals.

POSTS are sharp transients that are maximal over the occipital regions, are positive relative to other areas, may occur spontaneously during sleep, and may be single or repetitive [1] (Fig. 8.11). They are typically bilaterally synchronous. This discharge was described first by Gibbs and Gibbs as "positive spike-like waves in occipital areas" [123]. They are found most commonly in adolescents and young and middle-aged adults. Its prevalence declines after the age of 70 years [184]. Similarities to occipital lambda waves were pointed out in several studies [73,137,185], where the term *lambdoid* activity was used (now discouraged [1]). Vignaendra et al. studied the distribution of these potentials in relation to the nocturnal sleep cycle, stressing their abundance in N2 and N3 stages

and scarcity or absence in REM sleep, introducing the term *positive occipital sharp transients of sleep* [186]. Vignaendra and others proposed that POSTs are unrelated to dreaming (which occurs primarily during REM sleep): instead, they may signify the offline "playback" of visual information with the intent of sorting and rejecting redundant visual information collected during wakefulness. In line with these assumptions, POSTS are often absent in blind or severely amblyopic individuals [187].

6.3. Stage N2

N2 sleep is defined by the presence of two main graphoelements: K-complexes and spindles, described in detail below. Aside from these two findings, stage N2 sleep can have a very variable background pattern, which, when compared with a normal waking background, displays background disorganization and a marked increase in theta and delta activity (Fig. 8.12). Overall EEG amplitudes tend to rise, and this may be quite prominent for individuals with low-voltage EEG patterns. POSTS and vertex waves are also often seen. However, just as background patterns alone may not clearly distinguish N1 from N2 sleep stages, there are no characteristic clinical or physiological findings to ascertain entry into stage N2 sleep. Snoring, for instance, may occur in various stages of non-REM sleep, including drowsiness.

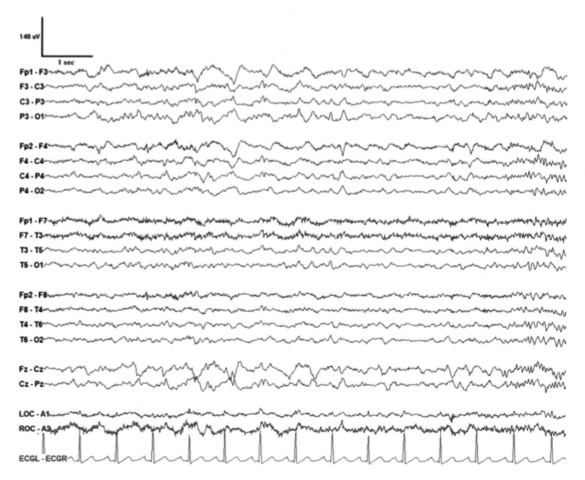

Figure 8.10. Vertex waves may also be repetitive or at times rhythmic, and this can be a normal feature of N1 and N2 stages of sleep.

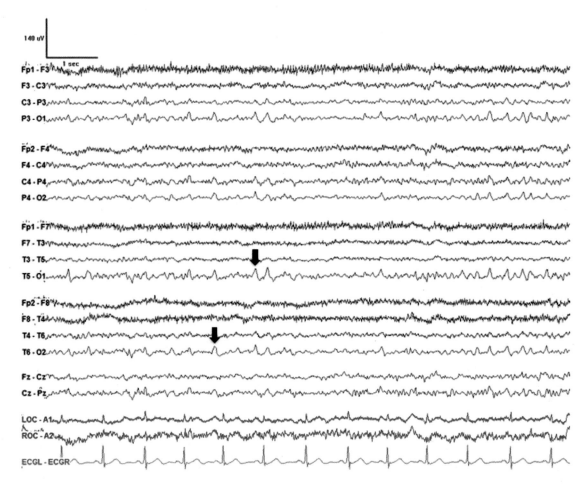

Figure 8.11. POSTS resemble lambda waves morphologically but are distinguished by the state in which they occur (drowsiness and N2 sleep). POSTS can also be repetitive.

6.3.1. Sleep Spindles

Sleep spindles, often referred to as simply "spindles," are bursts of 11- to 15-Hz activity that are generally diffuse but centrally predominant and occur during the N2 and N3 stages of sleep (Fig. 8.13) [1]. These were previously referred to as *sigma waves* or *sigma activity*. The IFSECN also separately recognizes the term *spindle*, perhaps best used as a modifier, to connote the presence of a "spindle-like" gradual increase and then decrease in the amplitude of a rhythmic burst. Sleep spindles may or may not display a clear spindle morphology. The observation of sleep spindles dates back to the work of Loomis [155,188], who identified sleep spindles as a distinct EEG phenomenon from the "random" activity that dominated his early two-channel sleep EEG recordings. Gibbs and Gibbs [123] made remarkable contributions to the early descriptions of sleep spindles and demonstrated their central predominance. Spindles are most impressive in childhood and adolescence; their voltage tends to become smaller throughout adulthood, similar to vertex sharp transients and K-complexes. Sleep spindles have been reported to be more frequent in women than in men [189,190] and appear to vary with the menstrual cycle in parallel with changes in core body temperature [191].

Sleep spindles are thought to relate to synchronous cortical and thalamic activity that is generated in the absence of cholinergic activation during non-REM sleep [192]. In combined intracranial/scalp EEG recordings, sleep spindles were observed in deep frontal cortical regions as well as in thalamic regions. In some cases, sleep spindles in these depth recordings were seen even during wakefulness and drowsiness, and they typically preceded the onset of scalp-visualized sleep spindles, suggesting that a greater degree of synchronization is required to visualize spindles on scalp EEG [193]. There are at least two distinct recognized sleep spindle types. *Slow spindles* (12–14 Hz) are more anteriorly predominant and *fast spindles* have a posterior distribution [194]. These topographical and frequency differences have been confirmed with intracranial EEG [195].

Since the topography and density of sleep spindles can be quite consistent for any given individual across multiple nights of sleep, some have proposed that spindle characteristics may serve as an electrophysiological "fingerprint" [196]. The relationships between sleep spindles and memory and consolidation are complex (reviewed extensively in [194]). Gibbs and Gibbs showed that intellectually disabled children less than 12 years of age displayed exaggerated or high-voltage spindles that were more continuous; the presence of these extreme spindles did not appear to correlate with epilepsy [197]. In contrast, among individuals with normal intelligence, sleep spindle densities have been shown to correlate with various

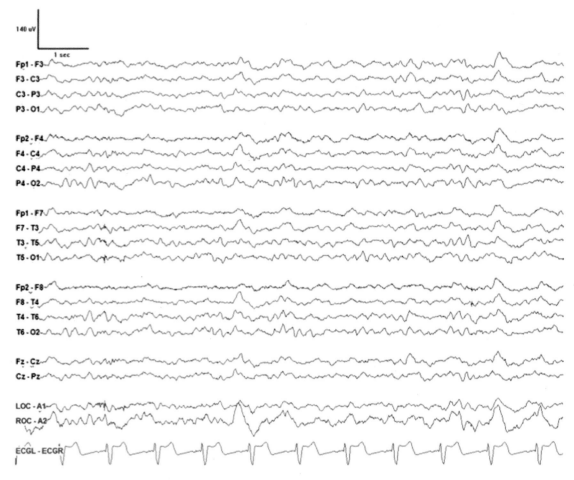

Figure 8.12. Theta activity and delta activity predominate in background activity in N2 sleep, without a clear anteroposterior gradient.

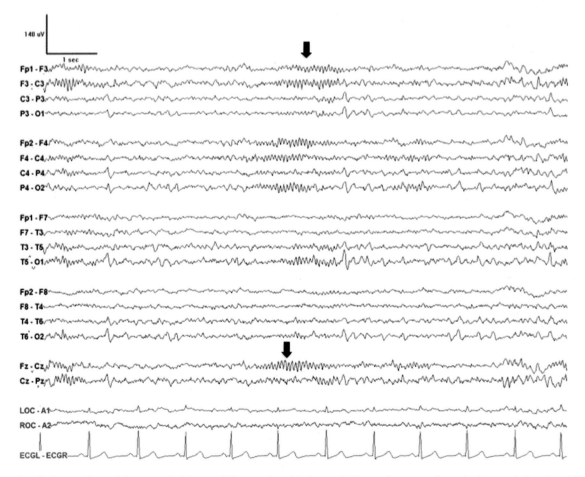

Figure 8.13. Spindles (or spindle activity) are a cardinal feature of N2 stage sleep (black arrows). They are frontocentrally predominant and often sinusoidal in amplitude and occur at a frequency of 12 to 16 Hz.

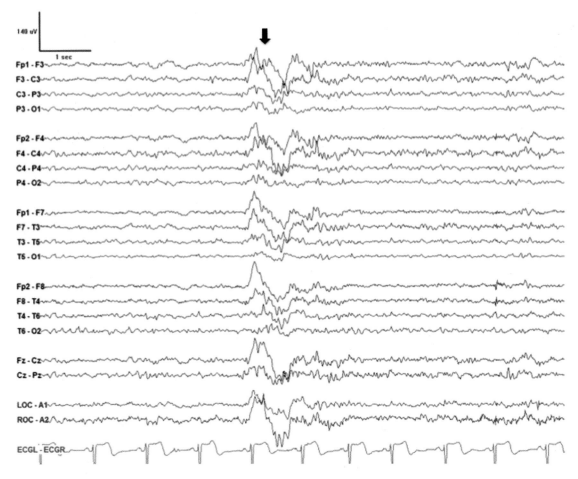

Figure 8.14. *During N2 sleep, one may observe large-amplitude biphasic or triphasic frontally predominant transients with superimposed fast activity, termed K-complexes (black arrow). Like POSTS and vertex waves, K-complexes can also present in a repetitive/rhythmic fashion on a continuum of delta-predominant activity as the main feature of slow-wave sleep.*

measures of attention and memory [194]. More recently, in a study of nocturnal polysomnography employing a larger population of individuals more broadly distributed in intelligence quotient (IQ) scores, correlations with intelligence were found in women but not men [192].

6.3.2. K-COMPLEXES

K-complexes are frontally predominant transients that consist of a high-voltage negative deflection followed by a smaller positive slow wave, often superimposed with a sleep spindle [1] (Fig. 8.14). K-complexes were first described by Loomis [198] and Davis [199,200], who demonstrated that during sleep, mostly during stage C sleep, the presentation of a mild tone resulted in a centrally maximal diphasic potential. This auditory "on-effect," a term now recognized as *evoked potential*, was typically much larger and more consistent during sleep. The reason for calling them "K-complexes" remains obscure: there have been reports that the naming was made on the spur of the moment without attaching any significance to the letter K. Others assume that "K" stands for "knock complex," since K complexes can be precipitated by sound and are often but not always followed by a brief arousal [201] (Fig. 8.15).

The physiological function of K-complexes has been debated over the years. Some have argued that evoked K-complexes, particularly during slow-wave sleep, may serve to prevent an arousal [202], thereby assigning a nonthreatening value to an external (or internal) stimulus during sleep. In depth-EEG recordings, spontaneous K-complexes have been recorded from lateral thalamus [203]. EEGs of patients with fatal familial thalamic degeneration do not display spindles or K-complexes [204], consistent with a prominent role of the thalamus in generating a variety of sleep-related potentials. With micro- or macroelectrode cortical arrays in patients undergoing epilepsy surgery evaluation, spontaneous K-complexes were detected in widespread cortical regions and were temporally associated with decreased neuronal firing [205], thereby briefly suppressing synaptic activity during sleep. Intracranial electrical stimulation studies have shown that K-complex–like responses were elicited with electrical stimulation of the cingulate cortex (dorsocaudal anterior cingulate), during both sleep and wakefulness, suggesting that activity within the cingulate may initiate a more widespread potential shift [206].

As with other sleep elements, K-complexes are largest in older children and in early adolescence; with advancing age, K-complexes shows a decline of voltage and often degenerate into an insignificant slow potential with tiny superimposed spindle-like waves.

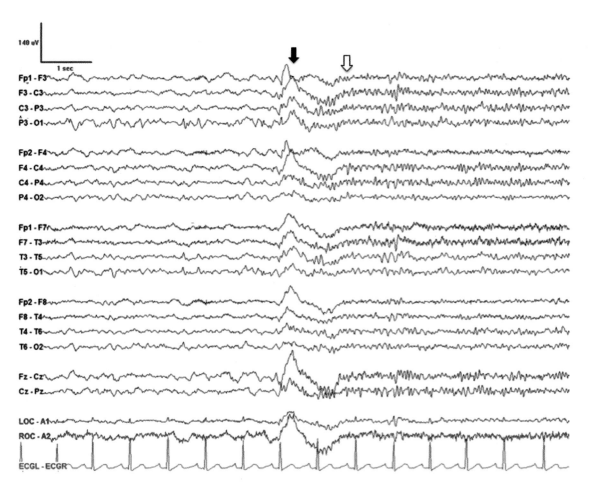

Figure 8.15. Often, but not always, a K-complex (black arrow) is followed by a brief electrographic and/or clinical arousal (white arrow), illustrated here by an increase in faster background frequencies (alpha/beta activity) and myogenic artifact.

6.4. Deep Sleep (Stage N3)

R&K stages 3 and 4 now together make up a single stage of sleep labeled stage N3. This stage is defined primarily by the presence of high-amplitude delta waves that occupy at least 20% of a particular epoch (Fig. 8.16). In routine EEGs, stage N3 sleep is rarely seen and may require a more prolonged period of sleep deprivation to be observed in short EEG studies. In our experience, the occurrence of slow-wave sleep in inpatient telemetry studies (in the epilepsy monitoring unit) is seen more frequently though not universally, perhaps due to medication effects and/or frequent interruptions to sleep that may be encountered in an inpatient setting. In stage N3, delta frequencies in the range of 0.75 to 3 Hz are particularly prominent over the anterior regions, often with superimposed 5- to 9-Hz activity. Sleep spindles can also be found but may dwindle in frequency when more pronounced delta activity is present. The AASM guidelines also impose a voltage requirement for these delta waves (i.e., >75 μV). As we have discussed before, absolute overall EEG amplitudes can vary across individuals for a variety of reasons. Such interindividual variations should be taken into consideration when applying a broad voltage criterion to stage N3 sleep.

In addition to rhythmic delta slowing, the EEG during N3 sleep may show "mitten waves," described first by Leemhuis and Stamps in patients with parkinsonism [207–209]. Later, Gibbs and Gibbs reported that mitten waves occurred in only 3% of 1,000 healthy control EEGs and in up to 42% of patients with epilepsy and psychosis [210]. This anteriorly predominant synchronous complex transient is formed by (i) a thumb, made up of the last wave of a sleep spindle, and (ii) a subsequent "hand," made up of a broad bluntly contoured frontal slow wave, together providing a "mitten"-like appearance. Based on the frequency of the initial "thumb" wave, A- and B-mittens were distinguished and attributed to various neuropsychiatric processes, including schizophrenia and the propensity to develop tardive dyskinesia [211–213]. Because this pattern was detectable only in deep sleep stages and was not consistently or specifically associated with any single neuropsychiatric condition, interest in mitten waves diminished over the years [214].

Slow-wave sleep plays an important role in memory consolidation [215,216]. However, this is perhaps an oversimplification: different stages of sleep may be involved in the strengthening of various types of memories (e.g., procedural, semantic, fear-related [217,218]). It is in stage N3 sleep when the bulk of *non-REM-related parasomnias* occur, which are a spectrum of clinical conditions characterized by the inappropriate transition out of non-REM sleep [219]. These primarily

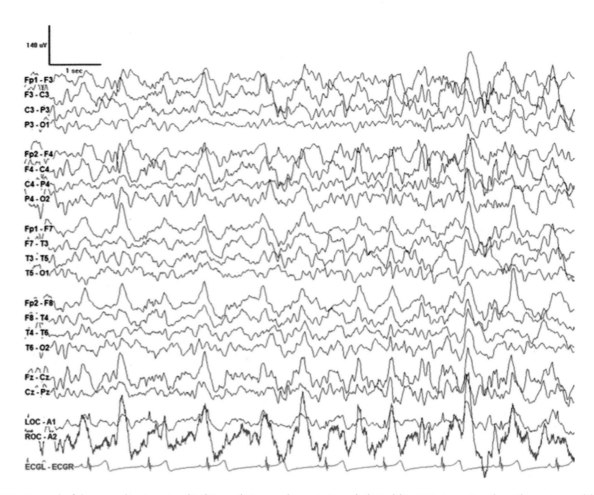

Figure 8.16. An epoch of slow-wave sleep is captured in this sample image, where prominent rhythmic delta activity is seen together with superimposed theta activity and spindles.

include confusional arousals, somnambulism, sleep terrors, and their variants. These disorders constitute an important contribution to sleep-related injury and may be difficult to distinguish from nocturnal seizures due to their stereotyped nature.

6.5. REM Sleep (Stage R)

During transitions from N3 to lighter stages of sleep, the EEG may abruptly display a desynchronized pattern associated with intermittent REMs and atonia, termed REM sleep [117] (Fig. 8.17). In normal individuals, REM sleep is rarely observed during routine EEGs and requires a long waiting period, as the first entry into REM sleep occurs only 60 to 90 minutes after sleep onset, often more prolonged with sedation). Further, entry into REM sleep is more prominent during the latter half of nocturnal sleep. REM stages may be seen commonly in afternoon naps, provided they are long enough. Finally, dreaming occurs predominantly during REM sleep [220].

Overnight EEGs, including ambulatory or inpatient telemetry studies, may capture REM sleep. Without simultaneous separate chin EMG recordings, entry into stage R may be ascertained by (i) the presence of characteristic eye movement artifacts (in frontopolar and anterior temporal leads), (ii) a relative loss of EMG tone (which may be subtle), and (iii) background activity demonstrating a relatively low-voltage EEG pattern with some alpha and beta activity but without the alpha rhythm. "Sawtooth waves" may be seen, which are bursts of 2- to 5-Hz activity over the vertex with a sawtooth appearance, often occurring in conjunction with eye movements [221].

The occurrence of REM sleep at sleep onset may suggest the presence of narcolepsy [222] but may also be a nonspecific marker of sleep disruption, and may be seen with drug withdrawal and sleep deprivation [223]. In contrast to somnambulism or night terrors, which occur during stage N3, the main REM-related parasomnia is termed *REM sleep behavior disorder*. It is characterized by a paradoxical absence of atonia during REM sleep; thus, patients may "act out" their dreams and display vocalizations or complex motor movements [224]. Spontaneous REM sleep behavior disorder is most often caused by alpha-synuclein–mediated degeneration of pontine nuclei involved in the control of REM sleep and can presage a later more pervasive neurodegenerative condition such as Parkinson's disease.

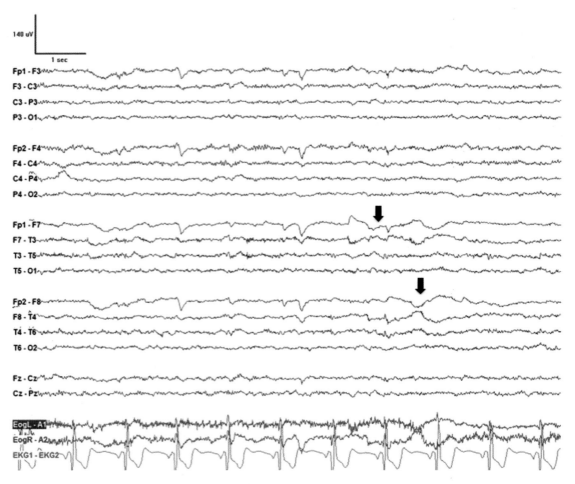

Figure 8.17. *Identified most easily by the characteristic electrographic signature of rapid lateral or vertical eye movement artifacts (black arrows), the background activity of REM sleep is typically made up of lower-voltage alpha and beta activity.*

SCORE EEG SOFTWARE

Further examples related to the topics addressed in this chapter can be found in the interactive online Niedermeyer Educational Platform. EEG recordings with illustrative examples can be opened and browsed. Features are marked and described using the SCORE EEG software. The users can see the features marked by experts, they can score these features themselves, and then compare them with the scorings of the experts.

The Niedermeyer Educational Platform can be accessed at: www.scoreEEG.com/academy

REFERENCES

1. Noachtar, S., et al., *A glossary of terms most commonly used by clinical electroencephalographers and proposal for the report form for the EEG findings. The International Federation of Clinical Neurophysiology.* Electroencephalogr Clin Neurophysiol Suppl, 1999. 52: p. 21–41.
2. Berger, H., *Über das Elektrenkephalogramm des Menschen.* Arch Psychiatr Nervenkr, 1929. 87: p. 527–570.
3. Berger, H., *Über das Elektrenkephalogramm des Menschen. Sechste Mitteilung (6th report).* Arch Psychiatr Nervenkr, 1933. 99: p. 555–574.
4. Jasper, H.H. and H.L. Andrews, *Electroencephalography III. Normal differentiation of occipital and central regions in man.* Arch Neurol Psychiatry, 1938. 39: p. 96–115.
5. Dutertre, F., *Catalogue of the main EEG patterns,* in *Handbook of Electroencephalography and Clinical Neurophysiology.* 1977, Elsevier: Amsterdam. p. 40–79.
6. Walter, W.G., *The location of cerebral tumors by electroencephalography.* Lancet, 1936. 2: p. 305–308.
7. Knott, J.R., *The theta rhythm,* in *Handbook of Electroencephalography and Clinical Neurophysiology.* 1976, Elsevier: Amsterdam.
8. Magnus, O. and M. Van der Holst, *Zeta waves: a special type of slow delta waves.* Electroencephalogr Clin Neurophysiol, 1987. 67(2): p. 140–146.
9. Siepman, T.A., P.J. Cherian, and G.H. Visser, *Zeta waves, an unusual EEG finding in structural brain lesions: report of two patients.* Am J Electroneurodiagnostic Technol, 2004. 44(1): p. 24–29.
10. Silbert, P.L., et al., *The significance of the phi rhythm.* Electroencephalogr Clin Neurophysiol, 1995. 95(2): p. 71–76.
11. Belsh, J.M., S. Chokroverty, and G. Barabas, *Posterior rhythmic slow activity in EEG after eye closure.* Electroencephalogr Clin Neurophysiol, 1983. 56(6): p. 562–568.
12. Laugier, H. and W.T. Liberson, *Contribution á l'étude de l'EEG humain.* CR Soc Biol (Paris), 1937. 125: p. 13–17.
13. Suenaga, K., T. Endo, and N. Ohki, *Influence of kappa-rhythm when assessing drowsiness.* Psychiatry Clin Neurosci, 2002. 56(3): p. 263–264.
14. Kugler, J., *Elektroenzephalographie in Klinik und Praxis.* 3rd ed. 1981: Thieme.
15. Kugler, J. and M. Laub, *"Puppet show" theta rhythm.* Electroencephalogr Clin Neurophysiol, 1971. 31: p. 532–533.
16. Vanhatalo, S., et al., *Very slow EEG responses lateralize temporal lobe seizures: an evaluation of non-invasive DC-EEG.* Neurology, 2003. 60(7): p. 1098–1104.
17. Vanhatalo, S., et al., *DC-EEG discloses prominent, very slow activity patterns during sleep in preterm infants.* Clin Neurophysiol, 2002. 113(11): p. 1822–1825.

18. Vanhatalo, S., et al., *Infraslow oscillations modulate excitability and interictal epileptic activity in the human cortex during sleep.* Proc Natl Acad Sci U S A, 2004. 101(14): p. 5053–5057.

19. Engel, J., Jr. and F.L. da Silva, *High-frequency oscillations—where we are and where we need to go.* Prog Neurobiol, 2012. 98(3): p. 316–318.

20. Cimbalnik, J., M.T. Kucewicz, and G. Worrell, *Interictal high-frequency oscillations in focal human epilepsy.* Curr Opin Neurol, 2016. 29(2): p. 175–181.

21. Cooper, R., et al., *Comparison of subcortical, cortical and scalp activity using chronically indwelling electrodes in man.* Electroencephalogr Clin Neurophysiol, 1965. 18: p. 217–228.

22. Cobb, W.A., R.J. Guiloff, and J. Cast, *Breach rhythm: the EEG related to skull defects.* Electroencephalogr Clin Neurophysiol, 1979. 47(3): p. 251–271.

23. Petersen, I. and O. Eeg-Olofsson, *The development of the electroencephalogram in normal children from the age of 1 through 15 years. Non-paroxysmal activity.* Neuropadiatrie, 1971. 2(3): p. 247–304.

24. Marcuse, L.V., et al., *Quantitative analysis of the EEG posterior-dominant rhythm in healthy adolescents.* Clin Neurophysiol, 2008. 119(8): p. 1778–181.

25. Zifkin, B. and R. Cracco, *An orderly approach to the abnormal electroencephalogram*, in *Current practice of clinical electroencephalography*, J. Ebersole and T. Pedley, Editors. 2003, Lippincott Williams and Williams: Philadelphia. p. 288–302.

26. Duffy, F.H., et al., *Age-related differences in brain electrical activity of healthy subjects.* Ann Neurol, 1984. 16(4): p. 430–438.

27. Hubbard, O., D. Sunde, and E.S. Goldensohn, *The EEG in centenarians.* Electroencephalogr Clin Neurophysiol, 1976. 40(4): p. 407–417.

28. Townsend, R.E., A. Lubin, and P. Naitoh, *Stabilization of alpha frequency by sinusoidally modulated light.* Electroencephalogr Clin Neurophysiol, 1975. 39(5): p. 515–518.

29. Mulholland, T. and C.R. Evans, *An unexpected artefact in the human electroencephalogram concerning the alpha rhythm and the orientation of the eyes.* Nature, 1965. 207(992): p. 36–37.

30. Fenwick, B.B.C. and S. Walker, in *Attention in Neurophysiology: An International Conference.* 1969, Butterworths: London. p. 100–127.

31. Chapman, R.M., S.A. Shelburne, Jr., and H.R. Bragdon, *EEG alpha activity influenced by visual input and not by eye position.* Electroencephalogr Clin Neurophysiol, 1970. 28(2): p. 183–189.

32. Westmoreland, B.F. and D.W. Klass, *Unusual EEG patterns.* J Clin Neurophysiol, 1990. 7(2): p. 209–228.

33. Storm Van Leeuwen, W. and D.H. Bekkering, *Some results obtained with the EEG-spectrograph.* Electroencephalogr Clin Neurophysiol, 1958. 10(3): p. 563–570.

34. Lafrance, C. and M. Dumont, *Diurnal variations in the waking EEG: comparisons with sleep latencies and subjective alertness.* J Sleep Res, 2000. 9(3): p. 243–248.

35. Cacot, P., B. Tesolin, and C. Sebban, *Diurnal variations of EEG power in healthy adults.* Electroencephalogr Clin Neurophysiol, 1995. 94(5): p. 305–312.

36. Harding, G.F.A. and C.R.S. Thompson, *EEG rhythms and the internal milieu*, in *Handbook of Electroencephalography and Clinical Neurophysiology.* 1976, Elsevier. p. 176–194.

37. Creutzfeldt, O.D., et al., *EEG changes during spontaneous and controlled menstrual cycles and their correlation with psychological performance.* Electroencephalogr Clin Neurophysiol, 1976. 40(2): p. 113–131.

38. Leary, P.M. and K. Batho, *Changes in the electro-encephalogram related to the menstrual cycle.* S Afr Med J, 1979. 55(17): p. 666.

39. Cobb, W.A., *The normal adult EEG*, in *Electroencephalography*, D. Hill and G. Parr, Editors. 1963, Macmillan: New York. p. 232–249.

40. Simon, O., *Das Elektroenzephalogramm.* 1977, Urban und Schwarzenberg: Munich.

41. Brazier, M.A. and J.E. Finesinger, *Characteristics of the normal electroencephalogram. I. A study of the occipital cortical potentials in 500 normal adults.* J Clin Invest, 1944. 23(3): p. 303–311.

42. Cabral, R. and D.F. Scott, *The degree of alpha asymmetry and its relation to handedness in neuropsychiatric referrals.* Acta Neurol Scand, 1975. 51(5): p. 380–384.

43. Kiloh, L.G., A.J. McComas, and J.W. Osselton, in *Clinical Electroencephalography.* 1972, Butterworths: London.

44. Gloor, P., *The work of Hans Berger*, in *Handbook of Electroencephalography and Clinical Neurophysiology*, A. Remond, Editor. 1971, Elsevier: Amsterdam. p. 11–24.

45. Adrian, E.D., *The discovery of Berger*, in *Handbook of Electroencephalography and Clinical Neurophysiology*, A. Remond, Editor. 1971, Elsevier: Amsterdam. p. 5–10.

46. Davis, H. and P.A. Davis, *Action potentials of the brain in normal persons and in normal states of cerebral activity.* Arch Neurol Psychiatry (Chicago), 1936. 36: p. 1214–1224.

47. Golla, F., E.L. Hutton, and W.G. Walter, *The objective study of mental imagery I. Physiological concomitance. Appendix on new method of electroencephalographic analysis.* J Ment Sci, 1943. 89: p. 216–223.

48. Travis, L.E. and A. Gottlober, *Do brain waves have individuality?* Science, 1936. 84(2189): p. 532–533.

49. Lennox, W.G., F.A. Gibbs, and E.L. Gibbs, *The brain wave pattern, an hereditary trait. Evidence from 74 "normal" pairs of twins.* J Hered., 1945. 36: p. 233–243.

50. Smit, C.M., et al., *Genetic variation of individual alpha frequency (IAF) and alpha power in a large adolescent twin sample.* Int J Psychophysiol, 2006. 61(2): p. 235–243.

51. Lemere, F., *The significance of individual differences in the Berger rhythm.* Brain, 1936. 59: p. 366–375.

52. Saul, L.J., H. Davis, and P.A. Davis, *Correlations between electroencephalograms and the psychological organization of the individual.* Trans Am Neurol Assoc, 1937. 63: p. 167–169.

53. Lindsley, D.B., *Electrical potentials of the brain in children and adults.* J Gen Psychol, 1938. 19: p. 285–306.

54. Wall, T.L., et al., *EEG alpha activity and personality traits.* Alcohol, 1990. 7(5): p. 461–464.

55. Antognini, J.F., et al., *Preserved reticular neuronal activity during selective delivery of supra-clinical isoflurane concentrations to brain in goats and its association with spontaneous movement.* Neurosci Lett, 2004. 361(1-3): p. 94–97.

56. Nowak, S.M. and T.J. Marczynski, *Trait anxiety is reflected in EEG alpha response to stress.* Electroencephalogr Clin Neurophysiol, 1981. 52(2): p. 175–191.

57. Vogel, F. and E. Schalt, *The electroencephalogram (EEG) as a research tool in human behavior genetics: psychological examinations in healthy males with various inherited EEG variants. III. Interpretation of the results.* Hum Genet, 1979. 47(1): p. 81–111.

58. Anand, B.K., G.S. China, and B. Singh, *Some aspects of electroencephalographic studies in yogis.* Electroencephalogr Clin Neurophysiol, 1961. 13: p. 452–456.

59. Gastaut, H., *Vom Berger-Rhythmus zum Alpha-Kultund zur Alpha-Kultur.* Z EEG-EMG, 1974. 5: p. 189–199.

60. Fingelkurts, A.A., A.A. Fingelkurts, and T. Kallio-Tamminen, *EEG-guided meditation: A personalized approach.* J Physiol Paris, 2015.

61. Pagano, R.R., et al., *Sleep during Transcendental Meditation.* Science, 1976. 191(4224): p. 308–310.

62. Stigsby, B., J.C. Rodenberg, and H.B. Moth, *Electroencephalographic findings during mantra meditation (Transcendental Meditation). A controlled, quantitative study of experienced meditators.* Electroencephalogr Clin Neurophysiol, 1981. 51(4): p. 434–442.

63. Hinterberger, T., et al., *Decreased electrophysiological activity represents the conscious state of emptiness in meditation.* Front Psychol, 2014. 5: p. 99.

64. Jacobson, S. and H. Jerrier, *EEG in delirium.* Semin Clin Neuropsychiatry, 2000. 5(2): p. 86–92.

65. Malek, N., et al., *Electroencephalographic markers in dementia.* Acta Neurol Scand, 2016.

66. Steriade, M., et al., *Report of IFCN Committee on Basic Mechanisms. Basic mechanisms of cerebral rhythmic activities.* Electroencephalogr Clin Neurophysiol, 1990. 76(6): p. 481–508.

67. Bishop, G.H., *The interpretation of cortical potentials.* Cold Spring Harb Symp Quant Biol, 1936. 4: p. 305–319.

68. Andersen, P. and S.A. Andersson, *Physiological mechanisms of alpha waves*, in *Clinical Electroencephalography in Children*, P. Kellaway and I. Petersen, Editors. 1968, Grune and Stratton: New York. p. 31–48.

69. da Silva, F.H., et al., *Organization of thalamic and cortical alpha rhythms: spectra and coherences.* Electroencephalogr Clin Neurophysiol, 1973. 35(6): p. 627–639.

70. da Silva, F.H., et al., *Essential differences between alpha rhythms and barbiturate spindles: spectra and thalamo-cortical coherences.* Electroencephalogr Clin Neurophysiol, 1973. 35(6): p. 641–645.

71. Aird, R.B. and B. Garoutte, *Studies on the cerebral pacemaker.* Neurology, 1958. 8(8): p. 581–589.

72. Walter, D.O., et al., *Comprehensive spectral analysis of human EEG generators in posterior cerebral regions.* Electroencephalogr Clin Neurophysiol, 1966. 20(3): p. 224–237.

73. Perez-Borja, C., et al., *Electrographic patterns of the occipital lobe in man: a topographic study based on use of implanted electrodes.* Electroencephalogr Clin Neurophysiol, 1962. 14: p. 171–182.

74. Ohmoto, T., et al., *Thalamic control of spontaneous alpha-rhythm and evoked responses.* Appl Neurophysiol, 1978. 41(1-4): p. 188–192.

75. Gucer, G., E. Niedermeyer, and D.M. Long, *Thalamic EEG recordings in patients with chronic pain.* J Neurol, 1978. 219(1): p. 47–61.

76. Schutz, E. and H.W. Muller, *Uber ein neues Ziechen zentralnervoser Erregbarkeitssteigerung im Elektroencephalogramm.* Klin Wochenschr, 1951. 29: p. 22–23.

77. Gastaut, H., *Etude electrocorticographique de la reativity des rhythmes rolandiques.* Rev Neurol (Paris), 1952. 87: p. 176–182.

78. Gastaut, H., M. Dongier, and G. Courtois, *On the significance of "wicket rhythms" ("rhythmes en arceau") in psychosomatic medicine.* Electroencephalogr Clin Neurophysiol, 1954. 6: p. 687.

79. Niedermeyer, E. and Y. Koshino, *My-Rhythmus: vorkommen und klinische Bedeutung.* Z EEG-EMG, 1975. 6: p. 69–78.

80. Stroganova, T.A., E.V. Orekhova, and I.N. Posikera, *EEG alpha rhythm in infants.* Clin Neurophysiol, 1999. 110(6): p. 997–1012.

81. Schoppenhorst, M., et al., *The significance of coherence estimates in determining central alpha and mu activities.* Electroencephalogr Clin Neurophysiol, 1980. 48(1): p. 25–33.

82. Koshino, Y. and K. Isaki, *Familial occurrence of the mu rhythm.* Clin Electroencephalogr, 1986. 17(1): p. 44–50.

83. van Leeuwen, W.S., et al., *Lack of bilateral coherence of mu rhythm.* Westmoreland Clin Neurophysiol, 1978. 44(2): p. 140–146.

84. Farnarier, G., J.P. Mattei, and R. Naquet, *[The mu rhythm of the vertex and its reactivity: an infrequent observation (author's transl)].* Rev Electroencephalogr Neurophysiol Clin, 1980. 10(4): p. 357–365.

85. Klass, D.W. and R.G. Bickford, *Observations on the rolandic arceau rhythm.* Electroencephalogr Clin Neurophysiol, 1957. 9: p. 570.

86. Chatrian, G.E., M.C. Petersen, and J.A. Lazarte, *The blocking of the rolandic wicket rhythm and some central changes related to movement.* Electroencephalogr Clin Neurophysiol, 1959. 11(3): p. 497–510.

87. Jasper, H.H. and W. Penfield, *Electrocorticograms in man: effects of voluntary movement upon the electrical activity of the precentral gyrus.* Arch Psychiatr Nervenkr, 1949. 183.

88. Pfurtscheller, G., *Central beta rhythm during sensorimotor activities in man.* Electroencephalogr Clin Neurophysiol, 1981. 51(3): p. 253–264.

89. Finley, W.W., H.A. Smith, and M.D. Etherton, *Reduction of seizures and normalization of the EEG in a severe epileptic following sensorimotor biofeedback training: preliminary study.* Biol Psychol, 1975. 2(3): p. 189–203.

90. Kuhlman, W.N., *EEG feedback training: enhancement of somatosensory cortical activity.* Electroencephalogr Clin Neurophysiol, 1978. 45(2): p. 290–294.

91. Kuhlman, W.N., *EEG feedback training of epileptic patients: clinical and electroencephalographic analysis.* Electroencephalogr Clin Neurophysiol, 1978. 45(6): p. 699–710.

92. Sterman, M.B., L.R. Macdonald, and R.K. Stone, *Biofeedback training of the sensorimotor electroencephalogram rhythm in man: effects on epilepsy.* Epilepsia, 1974. 15(3): p. 395–416.

93. Pineda, J.A., et al., *Neurofeedback training produces normalization in behavioural and electrophysiological measures of high-functioning autism.* Philos Trans R Soc Lond B Biol Sci, 2014. 369(1644): p. 20130183.

94. Miner, L.A., D.J. McFarland, and J.R. Wolpaw, *Answering questions with an electroencephalogram-based brain-computer interface.* Arch Phys Med Rehabil, 1998. 79(9): p. 1029–1033.

95. Pineda, J.A., et al., *Learning to control brain rhythms: making a brain-computer interface possible.* IEEE Trans Neural Syst Rehabil Eng, 2003. 11(2): p. 181–184.

96. Niedermeyer, E., *The Generalized Epilepsies*, 1972, Charles C Thomas: Springfield, IL.

97. Hari, R., *Action-perception connection and the cortical mu rhythm.* Prog Brain Res, 2006. 159: p. 253–260.

98. Brown, E.C., et al., *Reward modulates the mirror neuron system in schizophrenia: a study into the mu rhythm suppression, empathy, and mental state attribution.* Soc Neurosci, 2016. 11(2): p. 175–186.

99. Andrews, S.C., et al., *Reduced mu suppression and altered motor resonance in euthymic bipolar disorder: evidence for a dysfunctional mirror system?* Soc Neurosci, 2016. 11(1): p. 60–71.

100. Mitra, S., et al., *Mu-wave activity in schizophrenia: evidence of a dysfunctional mirror neuron system from an Indian study.* Indian J Psychol Med, 2014. 36(3): p. 276–281.

101. Oberman, L.M., V.S. Ramachandran, and J.A. Pineda, *Modulation of mu suppression in children with autism spectrum disorders in response to familiar or unfamiliar stimuli: the mirror neuron hypothesis.* Neuropsychologia, 2008. 46(5): p. 1558–1565.

102. Niedermeyer, E., *Alpha-like rhythmical activity of the temporal lobe.* Clin Electroencephalogr, 1990. 21(4): p. 210–224.

103. Niedermeyer, E., *The "third rhythm": further observations.* Clin Electroencephalogr, 1991. 22(2): p. 83–96.

104. Niedermeyer, E., *Alpha rhythms as physiological and abnormal phenomena.* Int J Psychophysiol, 1997. 26(1-3): p. 31–49.

105. Shinomiya, S., T. Fukunaga, and K. Nagata, *Clinical aspects of the "third rhythm" of the temporal lobe.* Clin Electroencephalogr, 1999. 30(4): p. 136–142.

106. Berger, H., *Uber das Elektrenkephalogramm des Meschen. Zweite Mitteilung (2nd report).* J Psychol Neurol (Leipzig), 1930. 40: p. 160–179.

107. Berger, H., *Uber das Elektrenkephalogramm des Meschen. Vierzehnte Mitteilung (14th report).* Arch Psychiatr Nervenkr, 1938. 108: p. 407–431.

108. Fink, M., et al., *Blood levels and electroencephalographic effects of diazepam and bromazepam.* Clin Pharmacol Ther, 1976. 20(2): p. 184–191.

109. Cho, J.R., et al., *Effect of levetiracetam monotherapy on background EEG activity and cognition in drug-naive epilepsy patients.* Clin Neurophysiol, 2012. 123(5): p. 883–891.

110. Borgeat, A., et al., *Propofol and spontaneous movements: an EEG study.* Anesthesiology, 1991. 74(1): p. 24–27.

111. Matousek, M., *EEG patterns in various subgroups of endogenous depression.* Int J Psychophysiol, 1991. 10(3): p. 239–243.

112. de Carvalho, M.R., et al., *Frontal cortex absolute beta power measurement in panic disorder with agoraphobia patients.* J Affect Disord, 2015. 184: p. 176–181.

113. Westmoreland, B.F., *The EEG findings in extratemporal seizures.* Epilepsia, 1998. 39 Suppl 4: p. S1–8.

114. Engel, A.K. and P. Fries, *Beta-band oscillations—signalling the status quo?* Curr Opin Neurobiol, 2010. 20(2): p. 156–165.

115. Bremer, F., *[Physiologic bases of electroencephalography].* Rev Neurol (Paris), 1950. 83(1): p. 6–8.

116. Posner, J.B., et al., Pathophysiology of signs and symptoms of coma, in *Plum and Posner's Diagnosis of Stupor and Coma.* 2007, Oxford University Press.

117. Saper, C.B., *The neurobiology of sleep.* Continuum (Minneap Minn), 2013. 19(1 Sleep Disorders): p. 19–31.

118. Jasper, H.H., C.P. Fitzpatrick, and P. Solomon, *Analogies and opposites in schizophrenia and epilepsy.* Am J Psychiatry, 1939. 95(4): p. 835–851.

119. Finley, K., *On the occurrence of rapid frequency potential changes in the human electroencephalogram.* Am J Psychiatry, 1944(101): p. 194–200.

120. Anokhin, A., et al., *A genetic study of the human low-voltage electroencephalogram.* Hum Genet, 1992. 90(1-2): p. 99–112.

121. Gibbs, F.A., E.L. Gibbs, and W.G. Lennox, *Electroencephalographhic classification of epileptic patients and control subjects.* Arch Neurol Psychiatry (Chicago), 1943. 50: p. 111–128.

122. Adams, A., *Studies on the flat electroencephalogram in man.* Electroencephalogr Clin Neurophysiol, 1959. 11(1): p. 35–41.

123. Gibbs, E.L. and F.A. Gibbs, *Atlas of Electroencephalography.* Vol. 1. 1950, Addison-Wesley: Cambridge, MA.

124. Lucioni, R. and G. Penati, *[On the frequency in psychiatry of so-called flat tracings].* Riv Neurol, 1966. 36(2): p. 200–208.

125. Panzani, R. and M. Turner, *[Electroencephalographic study of asthma; correlation of EEG and clinical manifestations; hypothesis on the pathogenesis].* Presse Med, 1952. 60(83): p. 1826–1828.

126. Pine, I. and H.M. Pine, *Clinical analysis of patients with low voltage EEG.* J Nerv Ment Dis, 1953. 117(3): p. 191–198.

127. Scott, D.F., et al., *The EEG in Huntington's chorea: a clinical and neuropathological study.* J Neurol Neurosurg Psychiatry, 1972. 35(1): p. 97–102.

128. Ehlers, C.L., et al., *Low-voltage alpha EEG phenotype is associated with reduced amplitudes of alpha event-related oscillations, increased cortical phase synchrony, and a low level of response to alcohol.* Int J Psychophysiol, 2015. 98(1): p. 65–75.

129. Walter, W.G. and V.J. Dovey, *Electro-encephalography in cases of subcortical tumour.* J Neurol Neurosurg Psychiatry, 1944. 7(3-4): p. 57–65.

130. Walter, W.G. and V.J. Dovey, *Delimitation of subcortical tumours by direct electrography.* Lancet, 1946. 1(6384): p. 5–9.

131. Roberts, R.J., K. Franzen, and N.R. Varney, *Theta bursts, closed head injury, and partial seizure-like symptoms: a retrospective study.* Appl Neuropsychol, 2001. 8(3): p. 140–147.

132. Varney, N.R., et al., *Neuropsychiatric correlates of theta bursts in patients with closed head injury.* Brain Inj, 1992. 6(6): p. 499–508.

133. Maynard, S.D. and J.R. Hughes, *A distinctive electrographic entity: bursts of rhythmical temporal theta.* Clin Electroencephalogr, 1984. 15(3): p. 145–150.

134. Gastaut, Y., *[A little-known electroencephalographic sign: occipital points occurring during opening of the eyes].* Rev Neurol (Paris), 1951. 84(6): p. 635–640.

135. Cobb, W. and G. Pampiglione, *Occipital sharp waves responsive to visual stimuli.* Electroencephalogr Clin Neurophysiol, 1952. 4: p. 110–111.

136. Evans, C.C., *Spontaneous excitation of the visual cortex and association areas; lambda waves.* Electroencephalogr Clin Neurophysiol, 1953. 5(1): p. 69–74.

137. Roth, M., *The lambda wave as a normal physiological phenomenon in the normal electroencephalogram.* Nature, 1953. 172(4384): p. 864–866.

138. Chatrian, G.E., *The lambda wave as a normal physiological phenomenon in the human electroencephalogram,* in *Handbook of Electroencephalography and Clinical Neurophysiology,* A. Remond, Editor. 1976, Elsevier: Amsterdam. p. 123–149.

139. Tatum, W.O., et al., *Lambda waves and occipital generators.* Clin EEG Neurosci, 2013. 44(4): p. 307–312.

140. Alvarez, V., M. Maeder-Ingvar, and A.O. Rossetti, *Watching television: a previously unrecognized powerful trigger of lambda waves.* J Clin Neurophysiol, 2011. 28(4): p. 400–403.

141. Egawa, I., K. Yoshino, and Y. Hishikawa, *Positive occipital sharp transients in the human sleep EEG.* Folia Psychiatr Neurol Jpn, 1983. 37(1): p. 57–65.

142. Brigo, F., *Lambda waves.* Am J Electroneurodiagnostic Technol, 2011. 51(2): p. 105–113.

143. Green, J., *Some observations on lambda waves and peripheral stimulation.* Electroencephalogr Clin Neurophysiol, 1957. 9(4): p. 691–704.

144. Bickford, R.G. and D.W. Klass, *Eye movements and the electroencephalogram,* in *The Oculomotor Systems,* M.B. Bender, Editor. 1964, Hoeber: New York. p. 293–302.

145. Scott, D.F., U.C. Groethuysen, and R.G. Bickford, *Lambda responses in the human electroencephalogram.* Neurology (Minneapolis), 1967. 17: p. 770–778.

146. Green, J., *Lambda waves in the EEG and their relation to some visual tasks.* Proc EPTA, 1954. 5: p. 3.

147. Angus-Leppan, H., *Seizures and adverse events during routine scalp electroencephalography: a clinical and EEG analysis of 1000 records.* Clin Neurophysiol, 2007. 118(1): p. 22–30.

148. Marsan, C.A. and L.S. Zivin, *Factors related to the occurrence of typical paroxysmal abnormalities in the EEG records of epileptic patients.* Epilepsia, 1970. 11(4): p. 361–381.

149. Martins da Silva, A., et al., *The circadian distribution of interictal epileptiform EEG activity.* Electroencephalogr Clin Neurophysiol, 1984. 58(1): p. 1–13.

150. Burkholder, D.B., et al., *Routine vs extended outpatient EEG for the detection of interictal epileptiform discharges.* Neurology, 2016. 86(16): p. 1524–1530.

151. Delil, S., et al., *The role of sleep electroencephalography in patients with new-onset epilepsy.* Seizure, 2015. 31: p. 80–83.

152. Lawley, A., et al., *The role of outpatient ambulatory electroencephalography in the diagnosis and management of adults with epilepsy or nonepileptic attack disorder: a systematic literature review.* Epilepsy Behav, 2015. 53: p. 26–30.

153. Seneviratne, U., et al., *The utility of ambulatory electroencephalography in routine clinical practice: a critical review.* Epilepsy Res, 2013. 105(1-2): p. 1–12.

154. Davis, H., et al., *Changes in human brain potentials during the onset of sleep.* Science, 1937. 86(2237): p. 448–450.

155. Loomis, A.L., E.N. Harvey, and G. Hobart, *Further observations on the potential rhythms of the cerebral cortex during sleep.* Science, 1935. 82(2122): p. 198–200.

156. Aserinsky, E. and N. Kleitman, *Regularly occurring periods of eye motility, and concomitant phenomena, during sleep.* Science, 1953. 118(3062): p. 273–274.

157. Dement, W. and N. Kleitman, *Cyclic variations in EEG during sleep and their relation to eye movements, body motility, and dreaming.* Electroencephalogr Clin Neurophysiol, 1957. 9(4): p. 673–690.

158. Rechtschaffen, A. and A. Kales, *A Manual of Standardized Terminology, Techniques and Scoring System for Sleep Stages of Human Subjects.* 1968, U.S. Government Printing Office: Washington DC.

159. Silber, M.H., et al., *The visual scoring of sleep in adults.* J Clin Sleep Med, 2007. 3(2): p. 121–131.

160. Iber, C., et al., *The AASM Manual for the Scoring of Sleep and Associated Events: Rules, Terminology and Technical Specifications,* 2007: American Association of Sleep Medicine, Westchester, IL.

161. Rosenberg, R.S. and S. Van Hout, *The American Academy of Sleep Medicine inter-scorer reliability program: sleep stage scoring.* J Clin Sleep Med, 2013. 9(1): p. 81–87.

162. Glick, T.H., *The sleep-deprived electroencephalogram: evidence and practice.* Arch Neurol, 2002. 59(8): p. 1235–1239.

163. Mattson, R.H., K.L. Pratt, and J.R. Calverley, *Electroencephalograms of epileptics following sleep deprivation.* Arch Neurol, 1965. 13(3): p. 310–315.

164. Pratt, K.L., et al., *EEG activation of epileptics following sleep deprivation: a prospective study of 114 cases.* Electroencephalogr Clin Neurophysiol, 1968. 24(1): p. 11–15.

165. Degen, R., *A study of the diagnostic value of waking and sleep EEGs after sleep deprivation in epileptic patients on anticonvulsive therapy.* Electroencephalogr Clin Neurophysiol, 1980. 49(5-6): p. 577–584.

166. Kubicki, S., W. Scheuler, and H. Wittenbecher, *Short-term sleep EEG recordings after partial sleep deprivation as a routine procedure in order to uncover epileptic phenomena: an evaluation of 719 EEG recordings.* Epilepsy Res Suppl, 1991. 2: p. 217–230.

167. Bagic, A.I., et al., *American Clinical Magnetoencephalography Society Clinical Practice Guideline 1: recording and analysis of spontaneous cerebral activity.* J Clin Neurophysiol, 2011. 28(4): p. 348–354.

168. Renzel, R., C.R. Baumann, and R. Poryazova, *EEG after sleep deprivation is a sensitive tool in the first diagnosis of idiopathic generalized but not focal epilepsy.* Clin Neurophysiol, 2016. 127(1): p. 209–213.

169. Seneviratne, U., et al., *Focal seizure symptoms in idiopathic generalized epilepsies.* Neurology, 2015. 85(7): p. 589–595.

170. DeRoos, S.T., et al., *Effects of sleep deprivation on the pediatric electroencephalogram.* Pediatrics, 2009. 123(2): p. 703–708.

171. Gilbert, D.L., S. DeRoos, and M.A. Bare, *Does sleep or sleep deprivation increase epileptiform discharges in pediatric electroencephalograms?* Pediatrics, 2004. 114(3): p. 658–662.

172. Rodin, E.A., E.D. Luby, and J.S. Gottlieb, *The electroencephalogram during prolonged experimental sleep deprivation* Electroencephalogr Clin Neurophysiol, 1961. 14: p. 544–551.

173. Rumm, P.D., et al., *Efficacy of sedation of children with chloral hydrate.* South Med J, 1990. 83(9): p. 1040–1043.

174. Gumus, H., et al., *Comparison of effects of different dexmedetomidine and chloral hydrate doses used in sedation on electroencephalography in pediatric patients.* J Child Neurol, 2015. 30(8): p. 983–988.

175. Bektas, O., et al., *Chloral hydrate and/or hydroxyzine for sedation in pediatric EEG recording.* Brain Dev, 2014. 36(2): p. 130–136.

176. Ashrafi, M.R., et al., *Melatonin versus chloral hydrate for recording sleep EEG.* Eur J Paediatr Neurol, 2010. 14(3): p. 235–238.

177. Loewy, J., et al., *Sleep/sedation in children undergoing EEG testing: a comparison of chloral hydrate and music therapy.* Am J Electroneurodiagnostic Technol, 2006. 46(4): p. 343–355.

178. Thoresen, M., et al., *Does a sedative dose of chloral hydrate modify the EEG of children with epilepsy?* Electroencephalogr Clin Neurophysiol, 1997. 102(2): p. 152–157.

179. Britton, J.W. and S.C. Kosa, *The clinical value of chloral hydrate in the routine electroencephalogram.* Epilepsy Res, 2010. 88(2-3): p. 215–220.

180. Liberson, W.T. and C.W. Liberson, *Protracted vertex and frontal waves during drowsy states.* Electroencephalogr Clin Neurophysiol, 1967. 23(1): p. 94–95.

181. Wittenbecher, H. and S. Kubicki, *["Epileptic" spiked vertex potentials in brief sleep after sleep reduction].* EEG EMG Z Elektroenzephalogr Elektromyogr Verwandte Geb, 1982. 13(3): p. 133–137.

182. Bourgeois, M., et al., *[Vertex spikes in newborn infants in acute cerebral anoxia. Prognostic value].* Arch Fr Pediatr, 1991. 48(10): p. 697–701.

183. McLachlan, R.S. and J.P. Girvin, *Electroencephalographic features of midline spikes in the cat penicillin focus and in human epilepsy.* Electroencephalogr Clin Neurophysiol, 1989. 72(2): p. 140–146.

184. Wright, E.A. and R.L. Gilmore, *Features of the geriatric EEG: age-dependent incidence of POSTS.* Clin Electroencephalogr, 1985. 16(1): p. 11–15.

185. Prior, P.F. and P.A. Deacon, *Spontaneous sleep in healthy subjects in long-term serial electroencephalographic recordings.* Electroencephalogr Clin Neurophysiol, 1969. 27(4): p. 422–424.

186. Vignaendra, V., R.L. Matthews, and G.E. Chatrian, *Positive occipital sharp transients of sleep: relationships to nocturnal sleep cycle in man.* Electroencephalogr Clin Neurophysiol, 1974. 37(3): p. 239–246.

187. Brenner, R.P., D.W. Zauel, and T.J. Carlow, *Positive occipital sharp transients of sleep in the blind.* Neurology, 1978. 28(6): p. 609–612.

188. Loomis, A.L., E.N. Harvey, and G. Hobart, *Potential rhythms of the cerebral cortex during sleep.* Science, 1935. 81(2111): p. 597–598.

189. Gaillard, J.M. and R. Blois, *Spindle density in sleep of normal subjects.* Sleep, 1981. 4(4): p. 385–391.

190. Huupponen, E., et al., *A study on gender and age differences in sleep spindles.* Neuropsychobiology, 2002. 45(2): p. 99–105.

191. Driver, H.S., et al., *Sleep and the sleep electroencephalogram across the menstrual cycle in young healthy women.* J Clin Endocrinol Metab, 1996. 81(2): p. 728–735.

192. Ujma, P.P., et al., *Sleep spindles and intelligence: evidence for a sexual dimorphism.* J Neurosci, 2014. 34(49): p. 16358–16368.

193. Jankel, W.R. and E. Niedermeyer, *Sleep spindles.* J Clin Neurophysiol, 1985. 2(1): p. 1–35.
194. Fogel, S.M. and C.T. Smith, *The function of the sleep spindle: a physiological index of intelligence and a mechanism for sleep-dependent memory consolidation.* Neurosci Biobehav Rev, 2011. 35(5): p. 1154–1165.
195. Andrillon, T., et al., *Sleep spindles in humans: insights from intracranial EEG and unit recordings.* J Neurosci, 2011. 31(49): p. 17821–17834.
196. De Gennaro, L., et al., *An electroencephalographic fingerprint of human sleep.* Neuroimage, 2005. 26(1): p. 114–122.
197. Gibbs, E.L. and F.A. Gibbs, *Extreme spindles: correlation of electroencephalographic sleep pattern with mental retardation.* Science, 1962. 138(3545): p. 1106–1107.
198. Loomis, A.L., E.N. Harvey, and G. Hobart, *Distribution of disturbance-patterns in the human electroencephalogram with special reference to sleep.* J Neurophysiol, 1938. 1: p. 413–430.
199. Davis, H., et al., *Electrical reactions of the human brain to auditory stimulation during sleep.* J Neurophysiol, 1939. 2: p. 500–514.
200. Davis, P.A., *Effects of acoustic stimuli on the waking human brain.* J Neurophysiol, 1939. 2: p. 494–499.
201. Roth, M., J. Shaw, and J. Green, *The form voltage distribution and physiological significance of the K-complex.* Electroencephalogr Clin Neurophysiol, 1956. 8(3): p. 385–402.
202. Bastien, C.H., C. Ladouceur, and K.B. Campbell, *EEG characteristics prior to and following the evoked K-complex.* Can J Exp Psychol, 2000. 54(4): p. 255–265.
203. Jurko, M.F. and O.J. Andy, *The K-complex in thalamic depth recordings.* Clin Electroencephalogr, 1978. 9(2): p. 80–89.
204. Tinuper, P., et al., *The thalamus participates in the regulation of the sleep-waking cycle. A clinico-pathological study in fatal familial thalamic degeneration.* Electroencephalogr Clin Neurophysiol, 1989. 73(2): p. 117–123.
205. Cash, S.S., et al., *The human K-complex represents an isolated cortical down-state.* Science, 2009. 324(5930): p. 1084–1087.
206. Voysey, Z., et al., *Electrical stimulation of the anterior cingulate gyrus induces responses similar to K-complexes in awake humans.* Brain Stimul, 2015. 8(5): p. 881–890.
207. Winfield, D.L. and P.J. Sparer, *The electroencephalogram in paralysis agitans.* Dis Nerv Syst, 1954. 15(4): p. 114–117.
208. Lyketsos, G., L. Belinson, and F.A. Gibbs, *Electroencephalograms of nonepileptic psychotic patients awake and asleep.* AMA Arch Neurol Psychiatry, 1953. 69(6): p. 707–712.
209. Leemhuis, A.J. and F. Stamps, *Mitten patterns in electroencephalogram of patients with Parkinsonism,* in *Proceedings of the American EEG Society.* 1949: Atlantic City, NJ.
210. Gibbs, F.A. and E.L. Gibbs, *The mitten pattern: an electroencephalographic abnormality correlating with psychosis.* J Neuropsychiatr, 1963. 4: p. 6–13.
211. Struve, F.A. and D.R. Becka, *The relative incidence of the B-mitten EEG pattern in process and reactive schizophrenia.* Electroencephalogr Clin Neurophysiol, 1968. 24(1): p. 80–82.
212. Kane, J., J. Wegner, and F. Struve, *The mitten pattern as a potential EEG predictor of tardive dyskinesia [proceedings].* Psychopharmacol Bull, 1978. 14(2): p. 35–36.
213. Struve, F.A., D.R. Becka, and D.F. Klein, *B-mitten EEG pattern and process and reactive schizophrenia. A replication.* Arch Gen Psychiatry, 1972. 26(2): p. 189–192.
214. Boutros, N.N., *Psychiatric correlates of the B-mitten EEG pattern,* in *Standard EEG: A Research Roadmap for Neuropsychiatry.* 2014, Springer: Switzerland.
215. Sarkis, R.A., et al., *Sleep-dependent memory consolidation in the epilepsy monitoring unit: A pilot study.* Clin Neurophysiol, 2016. 127(8): p. 2785–2790.
216. Pace-Schott, E.F. and R.M. Spencer, *Age-related changes in the cognitive function of sleep.* Prog Brain Res, 2011. 191: p. 75–89.
217. Stickgold, R., *Sleep-dependent memory consolidation.* Nature, 2005. 437(7063): p. 1272–1278.
218. Menz, M.M., J.S. Rihm, and C. Buchel, *REM sleep is causal to successful consolidation of dangerous and safety stimuli and reduces return of fear after extinction.* J Neurosci, 2016. 36(7): p. 2148–2160.
219. American Academy of Sleep Medidine, *International Classification of Sleep Disorders* 2014, American Academy of Sleep Medicine: Illinois.
220. Brown, R.E., et al., *Control of sleep and wakefulness.* Physiol Rev, 2012. 92(3): p. 1087–1187.
221. Schwartz, B.A., *[EEG and ocular movements in night sleep].* Electroencephalogr Clin Neurophysiol, 1962. 14: p. 126–128.
222. Burgess, C.R. and T.E. Scammell, *Narcolepsy: neural mechanisms of sleepiness and cataplexy.* J Neurosci, 2012. 32(36): p. 12305–12311.
223. Gangadhara, S., et al., *The significance of REM sleep on routine EEG.* Neurodiagn J, 2016. 56(1): p. 37–40.
224. Howell, M.J. and C.H. Schenck, *Rapid eye movement sleep behavior disorder and neurodegenerative disease.* JAMA Neurol, 2015. 72(6): p. 707–712.

9 | VALIDATING BIOMARKERS AND DIAGNOSTIC TESTS IN CLINICAL NEUROPHYSIOLOGY: DEVELOPING STRONG EXPERIMENTAL DESIGNS AND RECOGNIZING CONFOUNDS

JOSHUA B. EWEN, MD AND SÁNDOR BENICZKY, MD, PHD

ABSTRACT: There has been an explosion in the development of electroencephalogram (EEG)-based biomarkers and clinical tests. This upsurge is likely due to an increase in therapies rooted in biological mechanisms rather than behavioral descriptions, as well as to the democratization of computational power and the lower cost of EEG compared with competing methodologies. This increase in motivation and opportunity demands an increased responsibility for proper validation studies. Fields including laboratory medicine and psychometrics have paved the way for rigorous validation methodology. This chapter reviews a systematic methodology for biomarker/clinical test validation, translating approaches from other fields to the specific characteristics of EEG-based metrics. A checklist is provided to help readers design high-quality diagnostic validation studies of EEG-based biomarkers.

KEYWORDS: electroencephalogram, EEG, biomarkers, clinical test, diagnostic, validation

PRINCIPAL REFERENCES

1. Biomarkers Definitions Working Group. Biomarkers and surrogate endpoints: preferred definitions and conceptual framework. *Clin Pharmacol Ther*. 2001;69(3):89–95.
2. Bossuyt PM, Reitsma JB, Bruns DE, et al. STARD 2015: an updated list of essential items for reporting diagnostic accuracy studies. *BMJ*. 2015;351:h5527.
3. Morris SE, Cuthbert BN. Research Domain Criteria: cognitive systems, neural circuits, and dimensions of behavior. *Dialogues Clin Neurosci*. 2012;14(1):29–37.
4. Nuwer M. Assessment of digital EEG, quantitative EEG, and EEG brain mapping: report of the American Academy of Neurology and the American Clinical Neurophysiology Society. *Neurology*. 1997;49(1):277–292.

1. INTRODUCTION

The electroencephalograph (EEG) has been used for the better part of a century as a clinical test, and for many decades as an important research technique for uncovering mechanisms of brain function in both health and disease. In recent years, some mechanistic findings have begun to re-enter the realm of clinical utility as biomarkers. The requirements for validating biomarkers to make judgments about a single patient, however, are in many ways more rigorous than the original group studies that investigated mechanisms. The purpose of this chapter is to review the key elements of diagnostic test/biomarker validation studies that provide rigorous proof of the accuracy and utility of these important clinical tools.

A *clinical (diagnostic) test* provides information, within a specified clinical scenario, that is not already known—about whether a patient has a particular disease/disorder, or to predict natural history of clinical signs/symptoms, or to predict responsiveness to a treatment. Additionally, a clinical test may serve as surrogate endpoint in clinical studies (1). The quantity measured by the diagnostic test may or may not have a known mechanistic relationship to the disease process. A *biomarker*, on the other hand, is "a characteristic that is objectively measured and evaluated as an indicator of normal biologic processes, pathogenic processes, or pharmacological responses to a therapeutic intervention" (1–3). Inherent in the definition of a biomarker is that it reflects a known mechanism of the disease. Although the sets of laboratory studies covered by the terms "diagnostic tests" and "biomarkers" are not identical, there is considerable overlap. Many biomarkers may be used as diagnostic tests, and the mechanistic underpinnings of many diagnostic tests are sufficiently well characterized to qualify them as biomarkers. Because the experimental design considerations for diagnostic tests and biomarkers are similar, the terms are used interchangeably in the text, unless specifically noted.

As a first pass, validation studies attempt to demonstrate that the test under study is *accurate*—that the test result is positive when the disease or mechanism of interest is present and negative when the disease or mechanism is absent. If a test accurately reflects the presence of the disease (or mechanism) and has low rates of false negatives, then it is called *sensitive*. If it accurately reflects the absence of disease/mechanism and has low rates of false positives, then it is called *specific*. But sensitivity and specificity do not represent the full story. It is important to consider that these tests are used in a context. First, diagnostic tests are typically used to decide between two entities that are clinically similar, such as epilepsy and certain movement disorders. *Specificity* therefore encompasses the ability to differentiate the diagnosis of interest from the mimics that the physician is trying to decide between, and not just the presence of the disorder from its absence in asymptomatic patients.

We also note that a diagnostic test or biomarker must be able to give information that is not already known or not knowable from easier (more widely available, less invasive, or less expensive) methods (4). It is not sufficient for a clinical test to be sensitive and specific; the information it provides must also get the attending clinician closer to correct diagnosis than he or she was prior to learning the results of the test. The information provided by the test therefore must not be redundant to what is already known by history, physical exam, or earlier testing.

An example of a good biomarker is blood sugar for diabetes mellitus (DM). Not only has hyperglycemia been shown to be an accurate (sensitive and specific) indicator of the presence or absence of DM—the characteristics of a good diagnostic test—but blood glucose is directly related to the physiology of DM and its consequences. Hyperglycemia is not a perfectly specific indicator of DM, however, as other conditions can cause hyperglycemia (e.g., medication effects, cortisol-related effects, and endocrine tumors). By comparison, the Westergren erythrocyte sedimentation rate (ESR) is perhaps a less specific test *in general* and can be affected by a number of disorders, such as systematic lupus erythematosus, vasculitides, and infections. In certain situations, it may be a practically useful diagnostic test, but it cannot be considered a biomarker because of the lack of specific information about the pathogenic mechanism reflected by the ESR. The test characteristics (sensitivity, specificity) for any one of these disorders can be studied in the context of patients who have other signs and symptoms of these disorders.

Unlike *group* studies (e.g., clinical group *vs.* control), biomarker and diagnostic test validation studies need to pass the higher statistical hurdle of saying something valid about *an individual*. In the case of group studies, interindividual variance is averaged out in group statistics. In test validation studies, the signal must be able to overcome this interindividual noise. It is this higher hurdle that necessitates many of the requirements of a validation study, which are the focus of this chapter.

Several other fields have recognized the need for enhanced experimental design for the validation of clinical tests and biomarkers. Psychometrics and laboratory medicine have a long tradition of this type of research. The Standard for Reporting of Diagnostic Accuracy (STARD) initiative (5,6) was started in the 1990s in laboratory medicine in response to the recognition of methodological errors and inconsistencies, as well as lack of reproducibility in validation studies. Concerns about reproducibility have plagued research generally (7,8), and these concerns have come to the fore in diagnostic testing. Negative experiences (e.g., with the use of biomarkers in clinical trials) have spurred increased scrutiny of methodology in validation studies (1,2). The recommendations of the STARD Consortium serve only as a necessary-but-insufficient starting place for validation studies. Indeed, a number of groups have extended the STARD requirements to meet the specific needs of their subfields (9).

Now is a critical time to adapt these rigorous methods to EEG. With advances in personal computing and signal processing technology, we live in an era in which EEG-based biomarker technologies are rapidly expanding. A simple PubMed search for "EEG AND biomarker" reveals that the first reference was published in 1976, but the median date was 2011.

New techniques hold the promise of delivering useful and reliable clinical tests that fill clinical needs that have existed for decades. Further, there has been much progress in revealing pathophysiological mechanisms using explorative studies, which, in turn, could provide the substrates for clinical tests. This expansion of EEG-based biomarkers and clinical tests motivates a close look at the experimental design of test validation as applied to neurophysiology.

EEG-based biomarkers are based on some aspect of the signal. It is not correct to say that "the EEG" or "the EEG signal" is a biomarker for any process or a diagnostic test for any disorder. Rather, some specific element of the EEG signal—or an explicit combination of elements, or pattern—may be relevant to the diagnosis in question. For example, epileptiform discharges are relevant to the diagnosis of epilepsy, while focal slowing is relevant to the localization of tumors. The EEG signal is complex, and extracting just the right bit of information to answer any single clinical question is a nontrivial enterprise. Identifying a clinical need and using computational brawn to better understand its physiological substrates, and actually identifying biomarkers that truly make a positive impact on clinical care, can be successfully traversed only via solid experimental design.

The concepts derived from a century of experience in clinical test development must be applied to novel EEG techniques in order to ensure that novel metrics intended for clinical use provide clinicians with information that means what we believe it to mean. Stories from the long history of the development of EEG provide warning tales. The rise and fall of the particular EEG features that are now considered normal variants or patterns of uncertain significance demonstrate the traps of careless biomarker validation.

The 14-and-6-per-second positive spike discharges were initially described by Gibbs and Gibbs, who considered that these reflected "evidence of thalamic and hypothalamic epilepsy" (10). These patterns were later associated with a variety of pathologies (e.g., behavioral disorders, autonomic nervous system dysfunction) (11). In the end, it turned out that these patterns were even more common in normal individuals than initially appreciated (12), illustrating the trouble that can come with insufficient prospective random sampling practices and/or control groups.

A similar example is the case of the small sharp spikes or benign epileptiform transients of sleep. Two thirds of the patients showing this pattern had a history of epileptic seizures. However, when a neurologically typical control population was investigated, they were found in almost 8% of the normal adult control subjects (13).

1.1. Why Do We Need EEG Biomarkers?

Over the last decade, there has been an increasing interest in biomarkers in general, and EEG-based biomarkers more specifically. There are a number of compelling needs that have spurred this interest in biomarkers. A biomarker may give information about diagnosis, response to therapy, or outcome—earlier, less invasively, in a more widely available fashion, or less expensively than alternative methods.

Biomarkers in clinical trials are used as surrogate endpoints, to assess outcomes before they can be recorded clinically (1). Another driver of biomarkers is the promise of reduction of human subjectivity, both on the part of the clinician and in the information provided by patients. In mathematical terms, this subjectivity is *noise* or *error*—variation in the measurement that is unrelated to whatever we hope to measure.

Take the example of behavioral/affective disorders. Typical clinical tests (or biomarkers) include diagnostic interviews and rating scales. In each case, the personality and mindset of the reporter (patient or family member) can bias the results significantly, incorporating statistical error that is not relevant to the question that the clinical test is attempting to answer. Indeed, two raters of the same patient can give results that lead to significantly different conclusions. We see this all the time in parent versus teacher rating scales in attention-deficit/hyperactivity disorder (ADHD). It is not only patients and their caregivers who can inject subjective noise into the clinical test or judgment, but the clinician's interpretation inevitably adds an element of subjectivity, as a matter of normal human cognitive biases. Further, any particular clinician will have more or less expertise (training, certification, experience) with a particular chief complaint or with a diagnostic entity on the differential. In situations in which the required clinical expertise is not widespread, such as with rare disorders or in cases where there are insufficient specialists to meet clinical need, biomarkers may be designed to recapitulate (and thus will be validated against) specialized human expertise. The hope is that physiological biomarkers can remove much or all of this subjectivity, both on the part of the patient and on the part of the clinician, or to replace human expertise that is otherwise widely unavailable.

"Unmonitored" biomarkers—those that require no human input—should be most effective at addressing these concerns. Not all quantitative EEG biomarkers are unmonitored, however, and many rely on human operators for rejection of artifact or for selection of clean epochs of signal. Unless masked appropriately, human operators involved in the EEG-based biomarker can introduce biases into the results. Even under conditions that remove humans to the greatest degree possible, any EEG-based biomarker will ultimately still be dependent on humans: the ability of the technologist who applies the electrodes and the state of the patient at the time of recording can have profound effects on the signal produced by the brain.

Another clear benefit of physiology-based biomarkers over behavioral measures is in cases in which patients cannot give a behavioral response, either because they are locked-in or are in a minimally conscious/persistent vegetative state (14,15). In some examples, neuropsychological or simpler behavioral tasks tests may be presented during recording of the EEG. Consider one approach, in which task-related responses in the EEG signal are used to provide evidence of cognitive processing of the stimuli (event-related potentials [ERPs]), in lieu of pencil-and-paper or other behavioral responses. Such tasks can demonstrate fairly complex cognitive processing, for example by monitoring ERPs that differentiate "match" and "mismatch" EEG responses for vocabulary words matched (correctly or incorrectly) to corresponding pictures. Future developments of similar techniques may be relevant for individuals with developmental disabilities who have severe motor limitations, whose level of cognitive processing is hard to determine, and in whom it is difficult to perform neuropsychological testing. These approaches are fundamentally equivalent to the implementation of brain–computer interfaces in patients with severe motor disabilities.

A final legitimate reason for the current interest in biomarkers is a bit more abstract. It is motivated by the lack of 1:1 correspondence (degeneracy) between biological factors that may be relevant to treatment selection and clinically observable phenomena. Psychiatry in particular is in the midst of a paradigm shift from behaviorally categorized diagnoses to neurobiologically categorized diagnoses, necessitating valid measures that report on neurobiology directly (16). Take the example of genetic and clinical diagnoses of developmental disabilities. The clinician can describe developmental disabilities in terms of behavioral syndromes, such as intellectual disability, autism spectrum disorders, specific learning disabilities, language disorders, and ADHD. Each of these behavioral syndromes could be caused by a host of genetic disorders, among other causes. Conversely, genetic disorders such as tuberous sclerosis and Fragile X may manifest in a variety of different ways, resulting in different behavioral syndromes in different individuals (i.e., there is degeneracy between genetic and behavioral diagnoses). While educational therapies may be tailored to the behavioral syndrome, biological therapies are likely to depend on the underlying genetic etiology. As more biological therapies come online for developmental disabilities, there is a need for biological tests that can point clinicians to the appropriate therapy for an individual. (This example is admittedly poor, in that clinicians would certainly use genetic testing to diagnose a genetic disorder, not EEG-based testing. But the example does illustrate the point, discussed later, that there is little point to using a biomarker whose read-out can be assessed more easily or readily by other means. Psychiatric researchers have for decades recognized inconsistent responses of behaviorally defined and diagnosed psychiatric conditions to medical therapies.) As psychiatric genetics has evolved, the concept of *endophenotypes* or intermediate phenotypes has attempted to bridge the non-1:1 relationship between behavioral syndromes and genetics (17), with the thought that treatment may be best focused at a level between genetics and behavior. It is hoped that physiological markers, such as those derived from EEG, may help stratify patients at the level of the intermediate phenotype in a way that is optimal for identifying and tracking the most effective biological therapies (16).

We also need to be conscious of less legitimate motivations for physiological biomarkers. When demonstrably adequate clinical tools exist, an unreasoned deference to technology may cause physiological biomarkers to be misinterpreted as being more reliable or valid than more "low-tech" diagnostic approaches, like taking a thoughtful history, performing a thorough physical exam, or reasoning through the differential diagnosis. Unfounded biases toward technological approaches may be seen in juries, medical payers, and scientific reviewers.

1.2. Potential Advantages and Challenges of EEG

Given legitimate motivating factors toward physiological biomarkers in appropriate contexts, there are a number of features that make EEG a promising tool in a range of applications. In particular, technological developments have opened the door to a renaissance of interest in EEG as a physiological biomarker. New sensor technologies hold the promise of quicker electrode application times with less dependence on technologist skill. Marked advances in computational power and signal processing techniques have enabled software packages that expand what the EEG can "see" and simultaneously decrease dependence on analyst skill. Nevertheless, these developments must not, at this stage, be oversold. Those of us who perform translational science using EEG signals understand the difficulties involved in characterizing novel effects in the EEG signal, even in group data, obsessively examining the same dataset with a range of methods and analysis parameters to ensure that the particular effect is not a spurious artifact of a particular analysis method. While software is progressively better able to achieve results formerly attempted only by experienced EEG signal processing researchers, any turnkey software solution at the current time that purports to do an excellent job of circumventing extensive training and experience should be evaluated critically.

EEG competes with other physiology-measuring technologies, such as functional magnetic resonance imaging (fMRI), positron emission tomography (PET), and single photo emission computed tomography (SPECT). fMRI is, in many instances, the most directly competing technology, but EEG has a number of benefits over fMRI. First, EEG systems are far less expensive: tens of thousands of dollars versus millions. This leads to increased availability of EEG systems. (Note, however, that in contexts in which behavioral responses are adequate, reflex hammers, pencils and paper, and computer-based behavioral testing systems are still less expensive than an EEG machine.) Because the EEG is silent, the study of the auditory system is far more feasible than with MRI. Because EEG has excellent (millisecond) time resolution, as compared with second-level resolution in fMRI (and even then with a number of technical assumptions), dynamic patterns of brain activation that unfold over a period of seconds or even milliseconds can be differentiated with EEG but not with fMRI. EEG measures the direct electrical activity of ensembles of neurons, whereas fMRI BOLD signals represent metabolic/vascular coupling to neuronal activity. EEG activity reflects inhibitory and excitatory activity differentially, whereas the metabolic activity captured indirectly by fMRI may be the same for both inhibitory and excitatory activity. The oscillations that are reliably measured with EEG (sub-Hertz frequencies, to the gamma range of $\geq$40 Hz in some investigators' hands) are believed to be more directly related to computational processing in the brain (18,19) than the ultraslow oscillations (0.1–0.01 Hz) measured by fMRI. Whereas there are known compatibility issues among results from fMRI scanners of different vendors, such issues have not been noted to the same degree in EEG. The implication of head movement is somewhat different between the two techniques.

On the other hand, fMRI is capable of examining the entire brain, including deep and closed-field structures, with far greater spatial resolution, and the setup time for fMRI is far shorter than in EEG.

In cognitive research, EEG/magnetoencephalography (MEG) and fMRI often provide complementary information. In clinical epilepsy, anatomical MRI, PET, and SPECT provide information complementary to that of the EEG. The topics covered in this chapter represent, in a sense, a very basic case of integration of medical information. That is, the current discussion covers only the integration of pretest clinical information with the results of a single test to find a probability of a single clinical outcome. The integration of multiple sources of information, from multiple aspects of the clinical exam and from multiple testing modalities, is more complex by an order of magnitude. To an extent, when we diagnose seizure syndromes, we are integrating multiple sources of information: clinical, imaging, diagnostic testing, and genetic. Integration of information from multiple modalities is a topic of current interest and is covered in Chapter 46.

2. CRITICAL CONCEPTS IN BIOMARKER VALIDATION

Validation studies differ fundamentally from the vast majority of clinical studies. Most studies aim to say something about the shared characteristics of a particular *group*. To that end, patients within the clinical group are assumed to be the same in terms of the dependent variable; individual variation within that group is assumed to be measurement error and cancels itself out across subjects. The same assumption holds for the control group. In such cases, we use inferential statistics to demonstrate whether the averages of some measure differ between groups. These results give us important insights into the nature of the disorder.

Validation studies, however, need to pass a higher statistical bar. In validation studies, it is an *individual patient*—with his or her individual variability—who needs to be classified correctly. The clinical test does not have the luxury of relying on large groups to smooth out interindividual differences that are unrelated to the patient's clinical status. While the criterion of demonstrating a group difference ($p < .05$) may be sufficient in the first type of study, it is necessary but insufficient for a clinical test validation study. Clinical biomarkers therefore typically require a much higher signal-to-noise ratio than measures in group studies. The presence of a novel and perhaps incredibly important mechanistic EEG finding in a certain disorder does not necessarily mean that this same EEG measure will have an adequate signal-to-noise ratio to be effective as a biomarker or clinical test.

The course for developing a biomarker should proceed approximately as follows:

1. Assess the well-posed clinical question to be answered by the test.

2. Find a reference standard ("gold standard") that best represents the outcome of interest.

3. Construct a clinical group and a control group whose inclusion and exclusion criteria match the clinical

scenarios that the test will face "in the real world" (training set) (retrospective), or randomly sample the population of all possible patients who would receive the test (prospective).

4. If the EEG metric relies on human operators (and almost all do), specify the "inclusion and exclusion" characteristics of potential operators who will use the technique "in the real world" (e.g., training, experience, and certification requirements). The study should in principle sample randomly from all operators meeting these requirements.

5. Specify test collection parameters, such as time of day and length of recording.

6. Determine what aspect of the EEG signal to measure.

7. Apply the metric to the training set and determine the optimal threshold for the EEG metric that will differentiate between a positive and negative result.

8. On a separate population (validation or test set), using similar inclusion and exclusion criteria to #3, and using the threshold developed in #7, assess the classification accuracy of the metric, along with its sensitivity, specificity, positive predictive value, and negative predictive value.

9. Assess utility, in two senses:

   a. The ability of the test to answer a question more easily than the "current standard of care" test, and

   b. The ability of the test to provide information that is not redundant to other clinical information.

10. When possible, assess whether the use of the test improved patient outcomes.

As an example, consider if we were validating the presence of 3-Hz spike-wave complexes for the diagnosis of absence epilepsy. We may initially (1) define the question as: *How well does the presence of 3-Hz spike-waves on EEG define the presence of childhood absence epilepsy (CAE)?* This question, however, may not adequately define a realistic clinical scenario; we do not run around town performing EEGs on randomly selected children to see if they have absence epilepsy. A better-posed question might be: *Can the presence of 3-Hz spike-wave complexes on the EEG specify which children with staring spells have CAE versus nonepileptic spells?* Or, *Can the presence of 3-Hz spike-wave complexes on EEG specify which children with staring spells have CAE versus focal seizures?*

When (2) defining the reference standard, we may choose a certain clinical definition, such as parent-reported, uninterruptable staring spells, of which the patient has no recollection, which occur at least daily and last 5 to 30 sec, and which are responsive to treatment with ethosuximide, valproate, or lamotrigine. If we were to use only a clinical definition, without including responsiveness to therapy, then there would be essentially no point in conducting the study, since we could never demonstrate that performing the EEG would add value beyond asking those simple clinical questions that a physician

would do before ordering an EEG anyway. Further, we might consider adding the clinical requirement of resolution in adolescence, but this would make the study difficult to do: EEG data would have to be collected at the time at which the EEG is most likely to be performed clinically (say, 5–7 years of age), and the patients would have to be followed prospectively into adolescence to see if they meet our reference standard.

When we construct our (3) inclusion and exclusion criteria, we must consider the clinical question. Our inclusion and exclusion criteria would then include children with staring spells in such a way as to capture those with CAE as well as those with either nonepileptic staring spells or focal seizures. Of course, if clinical history were able to adequately differentiate the two groups, then there would be little reason to perform an EEG. The goal of the study is to demonstrate that the clinical test helps clinicians determine which of the patients who meet the inclusion and exclusion criteria also meet the reference standard. Exclusion criteria may include focal findings on the MRI. In this case, once the test is validated using these criteria, we could not properly use the test on patients who have a focal MRI. Finally, to reiterate, when defining the control group, it makes little sense to include those who have no clinical symptoms, as the test will not be performed clinically on children who have no clinical symptoms.

We may then specify (4) that EEGs will be recorded by registered technologists (R.EEG.T credential, in the United States) and read by electroencephalographers who are board-certified in clinical neurophysiology. We may next specify (5) that the EEG must run for at least 30 minutes and must contain at least 3 minutes of hyperventilation with good effort (6 and 7). If we had prior observations (preliminary data) that motivated the selection of 3-Hz spike-wave complexes, we would be aware of important variables, incomplete forms (*formes frustes*), and potential confounds, such as frequency range, burst duration, morphology, voltage criteria, presence of evolution, symmetry requirements, topographical distribution, and presence of alternate findings that may contradict the particular diagnosis (e.g., consistent focality). In the initial (training) set, we could determine which ranges of parameters best differentiate subjects who meet the reference standard for CAE from those without. We would then (8) collect a new sample of subjects with identical inclusion and exclusion criteria (validation/test set), and rerun the study using those parameters as defined from the training set. From this, sensitivity, specificity, positive and negative predictive values, and overall accuracy may be determined. (9) If we have data on pretest probability (clinical judgment of a clinician prior to the EEG being performed), we can then define utility both in cases in which the test is positive and in cases in which the test is negative. Over time, it may be possible to assess (10) the degree to which including EEG in the assessment of possible CAE would help patient outcomes.

2.1. The EEG in Clinical Use

Since most readers are likely experienced in the standard clinical interpretation of EEG, it may be effective to raise critical points in clinical test development through a case-study examination both of the history of the practice of EEG interpretation and underexplored assumptions in the current practice of EEG interpretation. Before starting, we should point out that the clinical EEG, as it is currently interpreted, is in fact many clinical tests occurring in parallel or independently in different contexts. EEG is used to assess the probability that the patient has epilepsy, given the presence of certain spells. It is used to determine the type of epilepsy. It is used to document organic encephalopathies. It has been used to localize tumors. Each of these independent functions should be validated independently, in each relevant clinical context. What is the evidence for the validity of these EEG functions, or do they mainly rely on "expert opinion"? We will discuss a few examples here, highlighting aspects that are usually ignored in most clinical teaching materials. These examples illustrate many of the issues of current relevance to novel biomarker development.

Interictal epileptiform discharges (IEDs) are the most commonly used EEG markers for epilepsy (see Chapters 18 and 19). The general belief is that IEDs have high specificity for epilepsy (98–99%) but low sensitivity (~50%) and that repeated EEG recordings, including sleep EEGs, can increase the sensitivity to 80% to 90% (20,21). Although this may be generally true, several critical considerations should also be taken into account when IEDs are set into their clinical context. Specificity depends both on the clinical question at hand (differentiating epilepsy *vs.* mimics), but also on the patient exclusion/exclusion criteria. The data on high specificity are derived from studies on healthy subjects, without any complaints, who were screened as candidates for aircrew training. However, this population is very different from the patients referred for clinical EEG recordings who are later determined not to have epilepsy. The specificity of IEDs is somewhat lower among patients with neurological or psychiatric symptoms, and there are certain subgroups where the specificity is very low, with up to 30% false positives (patients with intellectual disability, perinatal brain injury, and brain tumors) (22). Moreover, specificity was not investigated properly when examining the contribution of repeated EEGs, including sleep recordings. There are some data suggesting that the specificity of sleep recordings is lower compared to the standard, wake recordings (23).

Hypsarrhythmia (see Chapter 18) is considered by most experts to be a sensitive and specific biomarker for West syndrome. However, the classical hypsarrhythmia pattern is observed in only 7% to 75% of patients with West syndrome (24). Sensitivity can be increased by including hypsarrhythmia variant patterns (modified hypsarrhythmia) (25). However, the effect on specificity of the extension of the hypsarrhythmia definition has not been systematically investigated yet. Another problematic aspect is the surprisingly low interrater reliability (26). As discussed below, the validity of a test/biomarker (i.e., its ability to accurately determine whether or not a diagnosis is present) is limited by imperfect reliability (i.e., consistency between readers or test/retest consistency; discussed below).

Slow spike-wave complexes, with frequency ranging between 1 and 2.5 Hz, are generally considered to be the hallmark of Lennox-Gastaut syndrome (see Chapter 18). Gibbs et al. described the poor prognosis in children with "petit mal variant" showing this interictal EEG pattern (27). However, this pattern is seen in many other conditions (i.e., nonspecificity).

It is less widely discussed that the International League Against Epilepsy classification requires the presence of 10- to 12-Hz bursts during sleep to diagnose Lennox-Gastaut, to increase specificity against other conditions that can also show slow spike-wave (28). Sleep recordings, including polygraphic channels (surface electromyelographic [EMG] electrodes), are necessary to demonstrate the presence of these EEG patterns.

High-frequency oscillations (HFOs) (see Chapter 33) seem to be a promising corticography-based biomarker for identifying the seizure-onset zone in patients with focal epilepsy evaluated for surgery (29). However, HFOs occur also at contacts outside the seizure-onset zone, and in a clinical setting, it is extremely difficult to distinguish epileptic from physiological HFOs. A recent Cochrane review concluded that no reliable conclusions on the role of HFOs in presurgical evaluation can be drawn from the limited evidence that exists at present, and that the quality of evidence for all outcomes was very low (30). Most of the studies addressing this issue were retrospective, and the prospective studies were nonrandomized, with no control group and no blinding. The combined results from the included prospective studies showed that only 55% of the patients whose resection was based on HFOs had an Engel class I outcome. Further, well-designed studies are needed to elucidate the clinical value of the HFOs. Automated detection of HFOs seemed to be a promising tool in a small-scale study (31). If intracranially ascertained HFOs are shown to be a reliable indicator of the seizure-onset zone, it is possible that surface EEG or MEG could be studied subsequently as a less invasive method for detection and localization of HFOs, using intracranial HFOs or even postresection seizure freedom as a reference standard.

In *Alzheimer's disease* (AD), Poil et al. (32) developed an EEG-based test that predicts the conversion to AD of individuals with mild cognitive impairment (MCI). In the experimental design, the investigators performed EEGs on individuals with MCI and then observed them prospectively over nearly 2 years. They then looked for analyses and combinations of analyses that best distinguished those patients who converted to AD versus those who did not. The resulting test has nontrivial potential, as foreknowledge of which patients with MCI are at greatest risk of developing AD may be both clinically useful and relevant to the design of clinical trials for therapies that may halt the advance of MCI. On the other hand, the study as reported is missing a validation group, so actual sensitivity and specificity are unknown.

A study of the *error-related negativity* (ERN) (33) provides an example of a study that is useful in the progress of the development of a biomarker but is nevertheless not itself a validation study. The ERN is an ERP that is produced when the subject makes an error in a time-locked psychological test. The ERN has been used for decades to study several aspects of cognitive function, and more recently to study forms of anxiety, in which there may be greater sensitivity to making errors. The paper in question, however, does not look at diagnostic *validity*—the ability of the test to determine which subject has anxiety, or to correlate with a dimensional measure of anxiety. Rather, this study assesses even more basic characteristics of the test: reliability (i.e., test/retest stability) and the relative internal consistency of two different cognitive paradigms for eliciting the ERN. Not all studies important to biomarker validation are themselves validation studies.

2.2. The Well-Posed Clinical Question: What Do Clinical Tests Do?

Clinical tests and biomarkers answer a well-formed question. Relevant questions include the following:

What is the probability that this individual has this disorder? (This is also equivalent to risk stratification.)

What is the probability that this individual will develop this disorder (1)?

What is the prognosis for this individual (i.e., what is the probability that this individual will have a certain outcome)?

What is the probability that this individual will respond to this therapy?

What is the severity of the patient's disorder? Has the patient's condition worsened or improved over time?

Just because a biomarker may be able to answer one of these questions adequately does not mean that it can answer any other adequately. As noted in an earlier section, it is not relevant to say that the standard clinical, visually interpreted EEG is a validated tool *in general*. Rather, it has been studied, more or less, with regard to each of the individual questions that it can help answer:

How well does the EEG determine whether or not a patient is having epileptic seizures?

How well does the EEG differentiate patients with generalized epilepsy from those with focal epilepsy?

How well does the EEG determine the focal onset zone of a patient's epilepsy?

Does treating to the EEG results or to clinical seizure persistence lead to better outcomes in infantile spasms?

How well does the EEG predict whether an individual is likely to have a recurrence of seizure once antiseizure medications are stopped?

How well does the EEG now demonstrate that the patient's epilepsy is better controlled than it was at the time of the last EEG?

How well does the EEG predict neurological outcome in an anoxic patient?

Such questions are moreover answered in the context of particular patient characteristics (validation study inclusion and exclusion criteria), as described below. The EEG needs to be validated separately for its ability to answer each of these questions. Similarly, future biomarkers and clinical tests each need to be validated separately for each of its functions.

2.3. The Gold Standard

In biomarker validation, the "gold standard" means only one thing: the absolute, operational arbiter of whether or not the patient has the disorder in question. Formally called the *reference standard* and often referred to as "ground truth," it is the independent variable against which the accuracy of the *index test* (the new test, which is being validated) is assessed. An index test is, in essence, always replacing a different source of the same information. The degree to which the index test accurately reflects the reference standard defines the properties of the test. If the index test faithfully reports the conclusions of the reference test, it is said to be *valid*. The motivation for developing the index test is that it should be less invasive, less expensive, or more widely available than the reference test, or that it can report the same information before the reference test can. In some cases, a biomarker or clinical test will be used to predict events that have not happened yet, such as prognosis or response to a medication. In other cases, an automated biomarker will be used to substitute for the capabilities of a trained expert whose skills are not widely available. In yet other cases, a novel biomarker will be studied as a replacement for a more invasive or expensive biomarker. In each of these cases, the validation study would use the strongest currently available outcome—however difficult to assess—as the independent variable: the eventual outcome, the actual response to medication, the expert opinion, or the more invasive test.

If the reference test is easy to perform and widely available, then there is little reason to develop the new test. Consider a hypothetical EEG test for an affective disorder that is validated against the reference standard of a structured psychiatric interview. The EEG-based test can never be shown using this methodology to be more accurate than the interview (as described in the following paragraphs), and since the interview can be conducted as easily as or more easily than the EEG-based test, there is little motivation to develop the EEG-based test.

A common yet irredeemable fallacy is a belief that a new test or biomarker can better discern a diagnosis or create subtypes than any currently existing method. While one can sympathize with the hope that new methods can tease heterogeneous clinical groups apart better than previous methods, unless there is some standard against which to judge the "ground truth" relevance of these new subgroups or assess the accuracy of the new test, on what basis would we be able to say that the new test is accurate or not?

By similar reasoning, improved accuracy over the reference standard can never be a motivation for the development of an index test. *The index test can never be proven to be more accurate than the reference test, since the reference test is taken as infallible for the purposes of the validation study.* For this reason, the selection of the best possible reference standard is critical. Consider a made-up example of using fMRI to assess the laterality of language networks prior to resective epilepsy surgery. fMRI is being developed as a less-invasive replacement for some of the aspects of the Wada test (34). The most appropriate reference standard would be language outcomes after surgery, as that is the information (prediction) that an epileptologist would want to know when using the fMRI test.

Because outcome studies take a long time, a research group instead elects to use Wada results as the surrogate reference standard in the study. Imagine that Wada results predict actual postsurgical outcome with 90% validity. Imagine further that the fMRI results are shown to correlate with Wada results 90% of the time. It is possible that fMRI is actually a better test than Wada and is actually correct (as compared with postsurgical outcome) 100% of the time. On the other hand, the fMRI may be a worse test, correct only 85% of the time as compared with postsurgical outcomes. In both cases, the only data we have is that fMRI and Wada achieve the same results in 90% of subjects. Only a validation study that actually uses postoperative outcomes would be able to discern the difference.

This is not to say that the selection of a reference standard is always clear-cut. At times, there may be controversies regarding current diagnostic regimens. A reference test may be a more or less good representation of a more abstract concept. For example, in a validation study of a novel test for the diagnosis of a psychiatric disorder, study designers may use expert opinion or *Diagnostic and Statistical Manual of Mental Disorders* (DSM) criteria or a particular rating scale as the reference test. Reviewers and readers may agree or disagree about whether the selected reference standard actually reflects the concept being studied. *For the purposes of the validation study, however, the selected reference standard is taken as infallible.*

Responsiveness to treatment is often a natural reference standard. Because nosology is ultimately directed toward providing therapy and, to a lesser degree, prognosis, responsiveness to treatment or outcome may serve as the reference standard in cases where no other obvious reference standard exists.

Sometimes issues with the gold standard cannot be easily solved. An example that illustrates the difficulties of finding a proper reference standard is the source localization of epileptiform EEG discharges for presurgical evaluation. There is no single test or even criterion that reliably can localize the epileptogenic zone, and thus there is no absolute gold standard that would satisfy all critics. In studies used to validate new technologies to localize epileptiform discharges, investigators often use, as a reference test, the consensus decision of the multidisciplinary epilepsy surgery team (MDT) who combine several modalities/tests (35–37). Nevertheless, since only half to two thirds of the patients become seizure-free, this MDT reference standard is suboptimal. A better option might be to use the outcome after surgery as the reference standard: if the index test localized discharges to the resected area in seizure-free patients, then the test is considered validated. However, there are several drawbacks with this approach too. Surgical outcome can be affected by factors unrelated to the accuracy of localization. Due to complications or incomplete resection of the epileptogenic zone, the surgical outcome can be unfavorable despite correct source localization. Inversely, when large areas are resected (as in cases of temporal lobe epilepsy), the patient might become seizure-free although the source localization result was only in the vicinity of the real focus. An incomplete or too short follow-up time would also lead to erroneously good results of the study. After removing the seizure-onset zone correctly localized by the index test, the patient might develop new seizure types from a previously dormant second focus. In this case the patient is not seizure-free, although the index test correctly localized the previously active focus. In such cases, the relevance and the accuracy of the index test are limited by the theoretical concerns involved in selecting a reference standard.

Several studies of the utility of MEG illustrate creative approaches to defining a reference standard when none is immediately apparent. For example, one might wonder how adequate information from the MEG is to suggest a resection target in epilepsy surgery. It would, however, be unethical to subject patients to a resection based solely on an inadequately tested methodology. What the authors of these MEG studies did was to assess the incremental information supplied by MEG within a specific phase of operative planning: the determination of grid placement (38,39). They were then able to follow how the addition of these intracranial electrodes changed the resection plan, as compared with what the plan would have been had those additional electrodes not been included. In both studies, MEG influenced the resection plan in about 10% of patients.

The reference standard should be contrasted with a different concept: the current "standard of practice" clinical test. Unlike the reference standard, the "standard of practice" is not necessarily the most rigorous diagnostic method for the disorder currently available. Instead, it is the "compromise" that is most widely available, perhaps because the reference standard is expensive, invasive, relatively unavailable, or immediately unknowable (in the case of prognosis). The goal of the index test, then, is to be as convenient as (or more so than) the "standard of practice" and as accurate as the reference standard. Consider the example of the theta/beta ratio in the diagnosis of ADHD (40) (see also (41)). The authors used as their reference standard a multidisciplinary expert evaluation—an evaluation they considered to be the most rigorous possible behavioral diagnosis of ADHD, though one that is expensive and not sufficiently widely available to meet the demand of the number of children who are evaluated for ADHD. The current "standard of practice" is a clinical evaluation by a primary care provider. Their experimental design was set up to demonstrate that the theta/beta ratio, in combination with the "standard of practice" primary care evaluation, would better approximate the results of the reference standard multidisciplinary expert evaluation than did the primary care evaluation alone. The anticipated benefit of the index test, then, is to be as informative as the reference standard while being as noninvasive, inexpensive, and widely available as the "standard of practice" test.

2.4. Study Populations

In summary, the subject sample for a validation study should optimally be a prospective random sampling of individuals in the same clinical situation as those for whom the test will be applied. Contrapositively, the test is not formally valid for patients who do not meet the validation study's inclusion and exclusion criteria.

As with many types of studies, one approach is to prospectively recruit large and relatively heterogeneous groups for the validation study, one that is randomly sampled and has approximately the same distribution of relevant factors as in the population on whom the test will be used. Another approach is to recruit smaller but more homogenous groups, often defined retrospectively by the presence of the target condition and clinically relevant mimics. In the first case, the test may then be applied clinically to a wider range of patients. In the second case, while the test may be more restricted in its use, it is reasonable to believe that the accuracy could be higher (i.e., lower variance). In either case, information should be provided documenting how many potential subjects were excluded and why, so that reviewers and readers can understand potential biases in the data. Other information, such as disease severity, patient demographics, comorbidities, and treatments, are critical for subsequent clinicians to understand whether the sample recruited matches the clinical population on whom they are running the test.

The STARD criteria require that the setting of recruitment be stated explicitly, as the proportion of patients with or without the disorder may vary from community settings to academic medical centers. The prospective versus retrospective nature of the recruitment and study must also be stated.

Take a hypothetical example of a test intended to differentiate patients with major depressive disorder (MDD) from those with adjustment disorder in a primary care setting. The sample used should be a random sampling of all patients to whom the test would ultimately be applied—say, all patients with unipolar depressive symptoms who enter a community psychiatric clinic. The index test (our EEG biomarker) is applied to these patients, as is our reference test (for example, an expert assessment by specialist psychiatrists). We then examine the ability of our novel test to sort patients into the groups as defined by our reference standard.

If the patient and control groups do not recapitulate those to whom the test will actually be applied, validation studies can lead to incorrect conclusions. One common issue is when studies use highly refined control groups—ones comprising patients who would never undergo testing in a real-world setting. In our example, this would occur if we used one clinical group (MDD) along with control subjects who have no depressive symptoms. Because it is entirely plausible that EEG features could be shared between individuals with MDD and those who have adjustment disorder, a study that demonstrates that the index test can differentiate between subjects with MDD and asymptomatic control subjects does not recapitulate the actual use in a clinic and does not therefore prove that the test can differentiate between MDD and adjustment disorder. And no clinician is likely to need a test that differentiates only between patients with MDD and those without depressive symptoms, as that information can be ascertained in easier ways. In other instances, researchers use proxy clinical or control groups who also do not recapitulate the subjects who will undergo testing. Recent studies that have attempted to use EEG to predict the development of autism spectrum disorder (ASD) have used subjects at high clinical risk versus those at low risk, rather than subjects who went on to develop ASD versus those who did not. Risk in this case was based on the presence of siblings who have ASD. (We should note that this study

does not claim to be a validation study but rather a "proof of principle" that the EEG analysis employed may be useful in assessing brain pathophysiology associated with ASD.) In this case, the test can only be shown to separate high-risk from low-risk infants. A validation study formulated this way can say little about the test's ability to differentiate infants who will develop ASD from those who will not. And since risk status is known through easier means (taking a family history), the information provided by the EEG-based test is entirely redundant in a clinical setting.

It may be beneficial for a test to specify exclusion criteria for subjects who may not validly use the test. For example, an EEG-based test that looks at hemispheric asymmetries related to ischemia may specifically exclude any subject who has had skull surgery, which would lead to artifacts from a breach rhythm. These same exclusion criteria should then be applied when the test is actually used in a clinical setting.

2.5. Test Operators: The Second Study Population

EEG-based tests have some aspect of operator dependence. In the minimal case, the ability of a technologist to apply electrodes properly and engage the subject is at issue in all studies. In more complex cases, the results of a study may depend on the complex judgments of an expert. (Those of us who perform mechanistic research using EEG know we can spend two years looking at the same dataset in many different ways before we are convinced that the results are valid.) It is not realistic to expect that all interpreting clinicians who perform the test "in the real world" will be able to reach the same level of validity (or reliability) as an expert who has, for example, spent decades describing and refining the technique.

Reliability is defined as the extent to which a test yields the same result when administered multiple times, assuming no change in the patient condition. Imagine running an analysis on 5 minutes of EEG and obtaining one result. Rerunning the same analysis on the next 5 minutes of EEG from the same subject would yield a slightly different result. The amount of variation in the absence of a clinically important change is the reliability.

When applied to the discussion of different operators, *interrater reliability* refers to the extent to which different operators will give the same results. Reliability can be assessed with statistical tests such as Cohen's kappa for tests with binary results and interclass correlation for tests with continuous results. *The upper bound of the validity of a test is set by the reliability.* That is, if there is inherent noise in the measurement that is independent of the patient's state (presence/absence/severity of a disease), then we can never know the patient's state with a precision that is greater than the bounds set by this noise. In the case of different operators (interrater reliability), if we know that different operators routinely give results that are 20% different from each other, we could not expect to draw the conclusions that a 5% change in test scores from different raters represents an improvement or worsening, since the noise factor is too large. This uncertainty sets bounds on how fine a discrimination we can make in the test results. Other forms of reliability are relevant in other test/retest scenarios.

It is therefore necessary to describe inclusion and exclusion criteria for the professionals who will be running the test and collecting the data as well as the interrater reliability. Such criteria might include training, certification, and experience requirements. Optimally, a validation study would sample study personnel randomly from all practitioners who could perform this test. More commonly, studies will report interrater reliability alongside validity data.

Further, studies should describe how all personnel are masked (blinded) to diagnosis or to other data that may be correlated with diagnosis (e.g., risk factors, history, other test results). Although disclosure of the actual diagnosis is less of a concern in prospective studies, additional clinical and paraclinical information (e.g., history, seizure semiology, MRI, PET) can bias the results of EEG analysis, provided the operator is not blinded to these data.

2.6. What to Measure?

The EEG signal is complex, and there is a broad range of tools available to quantify aspects of the signal. These issues are discussed in detail in Chapter 44 (43,44). Of thousands of possible metrics, choosing which element is most likely to correlate with the reference standard is a daunting task. No single approach will provide optimal guidance in all circumstances, but some concepts may be helpful. Prior mechanistic research into the condition in question can serve as a guide. Analyses span the full range of mathematics, including time-domain and frequency-domain methods; linear and nonlinear analyses; and univariate, bivariate, and multivariate analyses.

The EEG signal is highly dimensional in terms of topography, frequency space, and evolution over multiple time scales and subject state. Indeed, the EEG is not just one signal but several, partially co-varying signals from across the scalp. The EEG time series also depend on choice of montage and reference, or of method of source localization (see Chapter 46), when used. Filter selection and parameters can also affect the results.

Many EEG studies are performed on spontaneous (or "resting state") data (i.e., without the subject/patient performing defined tasks). Standard clinical EEG is recorded spontaneously, with the exception of activation procedures such as hyperventilation and photic stimulation, and noting the fact that data may be collected in a variety of states (alert waking, drowsiness, eyes open vs. closed, rapid eye movement, N1, N2, N3, seizure). Other data are task-related, particularly as they relate to cognitive applications.

For the clinical neurophysiologist, the most familiar and basic type of task-related EEG data is the evoked potential (visual and somatosensory evoked potentials, brainstem auditory evoked responses). As with fMRI, however, a wide range of cognitive tasks can be applied to the EEG. Indeed, many clinical electroencephalographers are unaware that EEG-based techniques have been, for the better part of a century, a key tool in the toolbox of the cognitive psychologist, and more recently of the systems neuroscientist. Many key discoveries regarding human cognitive processing have been achieved through basic scientists using EEG in combination with well-designed and well-controlled experimental tasks. For many cognitive psychologists, event-related potentials (ERPs), such as the well-known P3 (aka P300), have been the tool of choice (45,46). More recently, work on the genesis and behavioral significance of cortical oscillations and their modulation (event-related spectral perturbations) has begun to tie together cellular and behavioral levels of analysis (see Chapters 44 and 46) (18,19). Although it is beyond the scope of this chapter to summarize the rich body of insights into human cognitive function provided to date from the EEG, we can draw a few lessons from this literature in terms of guiding the development of diagnostic tests and biomarkers.

The first is that fine-grained dissection of human cognition takes place only with well-designed cognitive experiments that tap disorder-related abilities, taking into account the literature related to that particular cognitive domain. Such tasks may also be accompanied by a series of control tasks designed to address potential confounds. The second is a related point: that individual ERP components or particular oscillations rarely have a simplistic relationship to a particular cognitive domain. As a result, merely evoking a certain ERP or inducing the event-related spectral perturbation (ERSP) cannot be interpreted to reflect a particular psychological domain. Rather, the ERP or ERSP needs to be assessed within the task-relevant context in which it is produced. As an example, the P3 is perhaps the most widely known ERP component. Experiments leveraging the P3 effect have been used to draw important conclusions regarding sensory discrimination, attention, working memory, language processing, and conscious awareness, among other domains, each through a series of "custom built" experimental paradigms designed to carefully elicit an unambiguous effect of interest. It is therefore disheartening to see prospective attempts at EEG-based biomarkers that use a fairly nonspecific P3-evoking paradigm that the developers purport will say something about some neuropsychological domain or other. Further, most cognitive psychological experiments use groups of healthy subjects and are based on the assumption that one person (or brain) performs the task similarly to all others; individual differences are assumed to be measurement error and are averaged out. Biomarker validation studies, on the other hand, are focused on the interindividual difference. This is not to say that it is impossible to derive valid and reliable biomarkers from task-related EEG data, but a review of the ERP literature in ADHD (47) gives some sense of the magnitude of the challenges posed.

The advantage of spontaneous data is that they do not require equipment that can synchronize the EEG recording with stimulus presentation and patient responses. The advantage of task-related data is that far more specific conclusions can be made relative to a single cognitive process. Additionally, in the experience of one of the authors (JBE), comparing two task conditions within the same individual may increase signal-to-noise by eliminating an error term that is consistent between conditions.

In some cases, a biomarker may incorporate multiple metrics or patterns of metrics. In this case, regression-based approaches can help determine which variables are most important to predicting a particular outcome. Dimensional reduction methods, such as principal component analysis, independent component analysis, and factor analysis, can create a statistical structure in which several variables are reduced to a single variable. In most cases, it is necessary to have the biomarker output a single variable. Other approaches that make binary (positive/negative) judgments using multiple inputs but without reporting a single, intermediate variable include machine learning techniques, such as neural networks and support vector machines.

Because the EEG signal is so rich in aspects that can be measured, an initial form of output is likely to include many variables, such as amplitude in each of four frequency bands (delta, theta, alpha, beta) × 19 electrodes. Some quantitative EEG measures reach thousands of output variables (48). It is likely that only some of these variables will be relevant. It is further likely that many of these variables co-vary with each other and that some of the *patterns* of variables will be important. Without some method to find these patterns, statistics requires correction for all of the variables—the many that are potentially irrelevant (type I error) as well as those that may be relevant. This requirement increases the risk of a type II error—that actually useful patterns will be falsely dismissed. Dimensional reduction approaches locate those patterns that are most relevant to the independent variable. Think of it this way: if we want to represent a three-dimensional object as a two-dimensional pattern (i.e., photograph), certain perspectives will be most helpful. Say we want to find a representation of a toy horse that most people can identify properly. If we cast a shadow on the toy from the side, the profile shadow would be identifiable to most people. If we cast a shadow from a light source at a different angle—say, from above—the pattern would be much more difficult to identify. In this way, we project a multidimensional pattern into one of fewer dimensions in a way that allows us to highlight features important to identifying the pattern and obscures the features that are unimportant.

As an example, the work of one of the authors with collaborators (JBE) is seeking to find patterns in sleep EEG that are relevant to the diagnosis of insomnia. Input variables include amplitude data from six EEG channels × 60 frequency bands × 5 wake/sleep states = 1,800 variables. One approach would be to look at each of the 1,800 variables independently. This would require correction for 1,800 variables; effect sizes would have to be far greater than what is typically seen in EEG. But we can specifically find the most relevant patterns within the variables. As you can imagine, there is correlation within a patient between the amplitudes from the theta band as compared with the delta band on one hand and with the alpha band on the other, and from one channel to the adjacent channels on each side. Principal component analysis and independent component analysis can find the least number of variables that can explain the greatest amount of the variance in the data by identifying patterns of covariance. Classification techniques can then identify which of the components (principal components or independent components) best separate out patients with insomnia versus those without (49).

Given this complexity of things we *could* measure, how do we make progress in finding what we *should* measure? One approach relies on data-driven or data-mining approaches.

We use preliminary data from subjects whose clinical characteristics echo those of the patients who will ultimately benefit from the test, as described in the next section. This is called the *training set*. The gold-standard diagnosis (independent variable), as described above, must be known. Data-mining techniques are then used to search for EEG-related variables that accurately classify the patients of the training set into the correct reference standard-derived groups. There is a danger in focusing on too many possible metrics, even at this stage. *Overspecification* refers to having too many variables, statistically, for the number of subjects. Given the tradeoffs inherent in statistical techniques, mining too many variables inevitably means that spurious correlations between some EEG variables and clinical group will be found (type I error). To assess for spurious correlations in the training set, whatever the number of variables, it is necessary to run the same analysis on a fresh set of similar subjects—the *validation (or test) set*.

A second, less agnostic approach is to base the selection of which EEG variables to use from prior knowledge. EEG benefits from a rich "basic science" literature that associates oscillatory and transient aspects of MEG/EEG signals with phenomena on many levels of analysis, from molecular and cellular events on one hand to neutrally instantiated computation and behavior on the other. In combination with genetic methods, optogenetics, cellular neurophysiology, electrocorticography, fMRI, and behavioral techniques, the EEG has played a major role in modern systems neuroscience. We can use the knowledge derived from this literature to increase the chances that a variable we pick will demonstrate useful clinical test characteristics.

2.7. Defining a Threshold

The clinical question is set, as is the reference standard. The EEG metric is chosen. The inclusion and exclusion criteria are defined, and the training set population is recruited. Data from the training sent are collected. The next challenge is to define where to set the threshold between a normal (negative) and abnormal (negative) test result. While the data fed into a clinical test or biomarker are often continuous, such as the measurement of the amplitude of an EEG signal, most clinical tests output a binary judgment (positive or negative). Some tests output ordinal risk strata (e.g., low, medium, high risk), but a binary judgment is the simplest case.

The performance of the test is defined in terms of *sensitivity* and *specificity*. The actual sensitivity and specificity of any test are ultimately defined by running the test on the validation set using the threshold developed on the training set. Before this, we must define the optimal threshold, and we do so using the data of the training set. Although specific procedures vary based on the type of data being analyzed, a typical approach begins with proposing the most clinically useful tradeoff between sensitivity and specificity. The optimal tradeoff will differ based on, for example, whether the index test is being developed as a screening test or a confirmatory test, and the practical implications of erring on the side of over-identifying or under-identifying a disorder. Next, preliminary sensitivities and specificities (let's call these *training sensitivity* and *training specificity*) are computed iteratively as the threshold is varied systematically. The optimal threshold is chosen based on the training sensitivity and training specificity that best meet the optimal clinical tradeoff.

Sensitivity and training sensitivity are computed as follows. If we took all patients who have the disorder (positive reference test), sensitivity is the percentage of those who have a positive result on the index test. Specificity is the proportion of subjects without the disease who have a negative result on the index test to all subjects without the disease. Specificity is used in the context of the sample being studied, which is, as discussed earlier, a random sample of *all subjects on whom the test could be run in the clinical setting.* Imagine an accelerometer-based test used to give information about whether a patient has nocturnal convulsive epilepsy. Imagine further the clinical scenario in which a physician may order the test, such as to determine between nocturnal seizures and a nocturnal movement disorder. It would be ecologically unlikely for a physician to order this test in a scenario in which the patient was having no nocturnal movements. When we say that this test is *specific,* we mean that it registers negative in the case of patients who have a nocturnal movement disorder, not just in the case of patients who are completely well.

The threshold below which the test is reported as negative and above which the test is reported positive is, in the end, determined intentionally by the researcher, and on the data from the training set. While good tests may simultaneously have excellent sensitivity and excellent specificity, and while poor tests may have both fair sensitivity and fair specificity, there is a natural tradeoff between sensitivity and specificity in all tests.

One choice of threshold may be advantageous over another for a variety of reasons. Screening tests, for example, intentionally have high sensitivities (at the expense of specificity) in order to catch the greatest reasonable number of individuals with the disorder. Receiver operating characteristic (ROC) curves are used both to demonstrate the classification ability of the metric and to allow the developer to select a threshold either for an optimal training sensitivity/training specificity tradeoff (i.e., that has the highest overall accuracy) or a biased tradeoff (e.g., in the example of a screening test).

2.8. Validation

Validation is the heart of the matter. Whereas we broadly refer to the entire enterprise as validation, in this instance we refer to the more specific procedure of assessing the test performance against the reference standard, in the validation (test) set, using the threshold defined in the training set. This is what allows the actual test characteristics to be determined. From these results, we compute the test's actual sensitivity and specificity, which characterize true versus false positives and true versus false negatives. As described in the STARD criteria, sensitivity and specificity should be reported with magnitude of uncertainty (e.g., 95% confidence intervals).

When thinking about validation and the ultimate clinical use of a test, it is important to go beyond sensitivity and specificity. Sensitivity and specificity are based on already

knowing whether or not the patients have the disease. If a clinician already knew whether or not the patient has the disease (as defined by the reference standard), there would be no reason to perform the test in the first place. Instead, the clinician knows the test results; what he or she wants to know is whether the patient has the disease. If the result is negative, the clinician will want to know the *negative predictive value*—the likelihood that the patient has the disorder if the test is negative. If the result is positive, the clinician will want to know the *positive predictive value.* These factors take into account both the sensitivity and specificity as well as the prevalence of the disorder. Prevalence can greatly change the interpretation of a test. A positive result in a rare disorder has a good chance of being a false positive, even with a highly specific test. For the sake of argument, the specificity of EEG for interictal epileptiform discharges is 99%. Assuming a prevalence of epilepsy of 1% and a sensitivity of 50%, the positive predictive value of epileptiform discharges (i.e., the probability that someone who has epileptiform discharges on an EEG has epilepsy) is only 33% (though see additional considerations regarding the specificity of IEDs in Section 2.1).

This assumes that the clinician knows nothing else about the patient, but in reality, a clinician interprets a test result in the context of a lot of other information about the patient: history and physical findings, perhaps a video of the spells he or she is having, the results of other tests. A clinical test is useful only if it provides *unique* information that is not already known. If the information from a biomarker is accurate but highly correlated with other information, it may add little value. We can think about a test in the context of Bayesian statistics. A clinician will use a broad range of information, including overall disease prevalence, presence of risk factors, history, and physical exam findings, as well as prior testing, to create a *pretest probability* that the patient has the disease. In Bayesian statistics, this is called the "prior." The test characteristics, combined with the test results (positive/negative), will then allow us to determine the *posttest probability* (the "posterior"). The test results may adjust the pretest probability a lot or a little; the amount depends on how unexpected the test results were and how compelling the test information is known to be relative to the other clinical information.

As an example, after listening to the patient's history, seeing his MRI with mesial temporal sclerosis, and watching a video of what very much appears to be the patient having a temporal lobe seizure, a neurologist may have assign the pretest probability of the patient having epilepsy as over 95%. The patient then has an EEG, which is normal. Knowing that interictal EEG is often falsely negative (insensitive) in patients who have focal epilepsy, the physician assigns a posttest probability of the patient having epilepsy at still over 95%. In this case, because the test is weak relative to the preponderance of other evidence, the test has not contributed much to the care of the patient, as it has not modified the pretest probability very much at all.

The same doctor's second patient of the day has a story that is very compelling for absence epilepsy. The doctor thinks that the child has an 85% pretest probability of having absence.

Despite capturing good hyperventilation and sleep, an EEG in this patient is negative. Knowing that the sensitivity of the EEG for absence is very high, the doctor concludes that the posttest probability is very low. In this case, the EEG results were unexpected and compelling, and the EEG contributed greatly to the care of the patient.

The back-and-forth letters to the editor regarding a study by Gilbert and Buncher (50) illustrate this issue. The point of the study was to simulate the *unique* contribution of EEG after a first seizure. Through data simulation, they demonstrated statistically (under certain assumptions) that the EEG added little to clinical knowledge following a first seizure. Letter writers rebutted that the EEG was predictive of further seizures. The authors countered that, while this was true, most of the predictive data contained in the EEG co-vary with (and are therefore redundant to) clinical information obtained through other means (baseline recurrence risk, other factors from history and physical). A test that is correct may still be unhelpful if it merely tells you what you already knew.

A final aspect of test validation is the extent to which using a test (versus not using the test, or versus using alternative tests) improves patient outcomes. Such a metric depends on not only the test's validity but also its utility (i.e., its ability to provide information that is not obtained through other means) and the treating clinician's ability to integrate the test results meaningfully into the patient's care.

2.9. Communication of Test Results

The extent to which a test improves patient outcomes is based not only on the test characteristics but also on how the test results are communicated to the referring clinician and how appropriately the referring clinician integrates those results into the management plan. There is always the concern in clinical EEG, for example, that a non-neurologist referring doctor may misunderstand the negative predictive value of EEG for focal epilepsy and may believe that the negative results are more reassuring than they actually are. See Chapter 26 on the SCORE initiative to help communicate EEG results in the clearest form.

3. COMMUNICATION OF TEST VALIDATION DATA

The way clinical validation studies are reported is essential for conveying a clear picture about the value, feasibility, and utility of the diagnostic test/biomarker. This applies not only to EEG or clinical neurophysiology but to any diagnostic test. That is why, in 2003, the STARD criteria for reporting diagnostic studies were published in several scientific journals, including *BMJ, Radiology, Annals of Internal Medicine*, and *Clinical Chemistry* (6). The STARD rubric was updated in 2015 (5).

The goal of the STARD initiative is to improve the accuracy and completeness of reporting of studies of diagnostic accuracy and to help readers assess the potential for bias in the study (internal validity) and evaluate its generalizability (external validity). STARD comprises a checklist of 30 items and a prototypical flow diagram, describing the design of the study and the patient flow.

The STARD checklist is structured according to the usual items of original research papers (title, abstract, methods, results, and discussion) (Table 9.1). For each of these, a set of items that must be included in the paper is listed. A Word file with the STARD checklist is available; in the last column one can specify the page number in the manuscript where the item can be found (http://www.equator-network.org/reporting-guidelines/stard/).

These criteria are directly applicable to reporting EEG studies as well. All 30 items and the flowchart can be adapted to EEG studies on validating diagnostic tests or biomarkers. Unfortunately, up to this point, only a handful of clinical neurophysiology papers have used these criteria.

4. PROPOSAL OF CHECKLIST FOR DIAGNOSTIC TRIALS AND VALIDATION OF BIOMARKERS IN CLINICAL EEG

Although the STARD checklist provides an excellent template for reporting diagnostic studies, there is a need for guidelines early in the planning phase, when designing the study. We propose here a list of essential items that should be systematically considered while planning a validation study of a diagnostic test or biomarker. The general theme is that the experimental conditions must mimic the actual clinical context in which the test will be used.

These criteria could be implemented in an interactive way into an online database. Similar to therapeutic trials, studies on clinical validation of EEG biomarkers could be registered in this database at the beginning of the study. Furthermore, the possibility of depositing data/results into this database throughout the studies would further increase their value, minimizing the risk of bias. Well-designed studies using this template and the online database would provide compelling evidence for changing/improving clinical practice by implementing the validated biomarkers.

4.1. Define the Clinical Question

A well-posed clinical question is essential for a good quality diagnostic study. First, define the aim of the study: *What do you want to know?*

i. A certain diagnosis (outcome: yes/no)

ii. Severity (define the scale in advance)

iii. Endophenotype (define the categories/subtypes in advance)

iv. Localization (specify at what level of spatial resolution; add a list with the possible location categories, when applicable)

v. Prognosis/change over time (define the scale in advance)

TABLE 9.1. The STARD Checklist

SECTION AND TOPIC	ITEM #		ON PAGE #
TITLE OR ABSTRACT	1	Identification as a study of diagnostic accuracy using at least one measure of accuracy (such as sensitivity, specificity, predictive values, or AUC)	
ABSTRACT	2	Structured summary of study design, methods, results, and conclusions (for specific guidance, see STARD for Abstracts)	
INTRODUCTION	3	Scientific and clinical background, including the intended use and clinical role of the index test	
	4	Study objectives and hypotheses	
METHODS			
Study design	5	Whether data collection was planned before the index test and reference standard were performed (prospective study) or after (retrospective study)	
	6	Eligibility criteria	
	7	On what basis potentially eligible participants were identified (such as symptoms, results from previous tests, inclusion in registry)	
	8	Where and when potentially eligible participants were identified (setting, location and dates)	
	9	Whether participants formed a consecutive, random or convenience series	
Test methods	10a	Index test, in sufficient detail to allow replication	
	10b	Reference standard, in sufficient detail to allow replication	
	11	Rationale for choosing the reference standard (if alternatives exist)	
	12a	Definition of and rationale for test positivity cut-offs or result categories of the index test, distinguishing pre-specified from exploratory	
	12b	Definition of and rationale for test positivity cut-offs or result categories of the reference standard, distinguishing pre-specified from exploratory	
	13a	Whether clinical information and reference standard results were available to the performers/readers of the index test	
	13b	Whether clinical information and index test results were available to the assessors of the reference standard	
Analysis	14	Methods for estimating or comparing measures of diagnostic accuracy	
	15	How indeterminate index test or reference standard results were handled	
	16	How missing data on the index test and reference standard were handled	
	17	Any analyses of variability in diagnostic accuracy, distinguishing pre-specified from exploratory	
	18	Intended sample size and how it was determined	
RESULTS			
Participants	19	Flow of participants, using a diagram	
	20	Baseline demographic and clinical characteristics of participants	
	21a	Distribution of severity of disease in those with the target condition	
	21b	Distribution of alternative diagnoses in those without the target condition	
	22	Time interval and any clinical interventions between index test and reference standard	
Test Results	23	Cross tabulation of the index test results (or their distribution) by the results of the reference standard	
	24	Estimates of diagnostic accuracy and their precision (such as 95% confidence intervals)	

TABLE 9.1. Continued

SECTION AND TOPIC	ITEM #		ON PAGE #
	25	Any adverse events from performing the index test or the reference standard	
DISCUSSION			
	26	Study limitations, including sources of potential bias, statistical uncertainty, and generalizability	
	27	Implications for practice, including the intended use and clinical role of the index test	
OTHER INFORMATION			
	28	Registration number and name of registry	
	29	Where the full study protocol can be accessed	
	30	Sources of funding and other support; role of funders	

vi. Response to therapy (define the scale in advance)

vii. Probability of potential complication

Each is a separate question and needs to be addressed independently,

Then, define the added value of the study: *What do you want to know that you don't already know?* Baseline clinical and basic laboratory data already provide some information about the probability of a diagnosis (or other outcome). The investigators must show that the test provides additional information beyond what is already known (i.e., the pretest probability). This aspect can be addressed using one of the following approaches:

i. Report sampling methods. Do these methods randomly sample (prospectively) from the population of individuals on whom the test is likely to be run in the future?

ii. Calculate the baseline incidence/prevalence of the diagnosis/condition you are working with. Does the sampling result in a distribution of the independent variable that is similar to that in the general population (prospectively or retrospectively)?

iii. Log the pretest probability before applying the index test. Then include the information from the index test and monitor whether the conclusion changes.

4.2. Define the Patient Populations

In the best case, the novel test would be studied prospectively—meaning that any future patient likely to undergo the test clinically would meet the inclusion and exclusion criteria for the study population. The test would then be studied against patients who were ultimately diagnosed with one condition versus another. Most studies are retrospective, however. In these cases, there is a tendency to test a clinical population against a pure control. While this approach may be good for mechanistic studies, it is an impediment to test validation studies. Specify the inclusion criteria, exclusion criteria, and any other factors influencing the patient selection.

Report whether an initial training-set evaluation was performed. Report the validation methodology. An unvalidated study means relatively little, as the training sensitivity and specificity of the original sample (training set) are defined by the researchers; the actual sensitivity and specificity are determined in the validation set. Ask whether the study was validated using a patient population different from the one used for training, and the degree to which the validation patient population corresponded to the clinical scenario in which the test will be used.

4.3. Describe the Methodology

The methodology for carrying out the test needs to be explicitly laid out, providing all details so that it can be reproduced in another laboratory. Specify the measured parameter, quantification/metric, threshold/decision-making algorithm (e.g., ROC, supporting vector machine) (1). Provided there is any technician/clinician whose performance will affect the outcome of the test, specify the following:

i. What is the certification/experience of the clinician/technologist and/or interpreter? Interrater reliability is necessary for any test that depends on human performance.

ii. Blinding of the interpreter to clinical data and the gold standard; potentials for bias.

iii. Was test/retest reliability addressed? Test/retest characteristics are necessary for determining sensitivity to differences for longitudinal testing or for stratified testing.

4.4. Define the Reference Standard for the Study and Explain the Rationale for Choosing It

A solid, well-chosen reference standard is critical. Many studies fail because the reference standard is either easily obtainable (i.e., no less expensive, available, or invasive than the test being proposed) or because the reference standard is not well defined.

4.5. Report the Test Characteristics

State the diagnostic accuracy (sensitivity, specificity, positive and negative predictive value, risk/odds ratio). Note the clinical utility (whether the test results will change the clinician's diagnostic or therapeutic decisions). For a very threatening condition, a test result may incrementally reduce the estimated probability of a diagnosis by a small amount, but that amount may not change the approach at all.

Explain how the use of the test will affect the clinical outcome. Enhanced patient outcomes are the ultimate test, as these results incorporate not only the validity/accuracy of the test but also the technologist/physician's skill, the communication to the clinician of the test results, and the clinician's ability to integrate the results into clinical care.

4.6. Produce a Flowchart for the Validation Study

This flowchart accounts for dropouts and patients for whom reference standard ("gold standard") is not obtained, just like in drug trials. The flowchart also shows how and when clinical decisions are influenced by the index test

5. EXAMPLES

5.1. Example 1

We will illustrate implementation of these criteria using a diagnostic study on electromagnetic source imaging (EMSI) in the presurgical evaluation of patients with focal epilepsy.

5.1.1. Define the Clinical Question

The aim of the study is to assess the accuracy of localization of epileptiform discharges (EDs) and to assess the changes in the conclusion of the MDT on the localization of the focus. A set of 29 brain regions is defined at a sub-lobar level and localization results are logged using these regions. The MDT's conclusions on localization are logged before knowing the EMSI results; then the possible changes are logged after presenting the results of the EMSI.

5.1.2. Define the Patient Populations

All patients enrolled in presurgical evaluation for possible surgical treatment of focal epilepsy who are refractory to treatment with antiepileptic drugs will be included. Patients who did not have EDs during the presurgical evaluation will be excluded. The number of excluded patients is included in the validation flowchart. Since the methods of source imaging will be typically available from previous studies, in this case the validation of the EMSI method is done on a separate patient population than the one used for developing the method.

5.1.3. Describe the Methodology

The methods are described in detail, including selection and preprocessing, filtering of EEG data, visual identification of EDs versus spike/seizure detection algorithms, averaging of EDs, selection of the time point for the analysis, head model,

and inverse solution. The method for classifying the source solutions into the 29 brain regions is described.

5.1.4. Define the Reference Standard/Report the Test Characteristics

The reference standard for calculating diagnostic accuracy is the final conclusion of the MDT. The following categories are defined: "concordant," "non-localizable," and "discordant." For calculating positive and negative predictive value, the clinical outcome (Engel classification) one year after surgery will be used. From these outcome measures, 2×2 tables are constructed: concordant/discordant versus seizure-free/not seizure-free. Odds ratios are calculated from this table.

5.2. Example 2

The other example, automated seizure detection, needs a different approach, yet the validation checklist can be applied to this case too.

5.2.1. Define the Clinical Question

The clinical question is when the seizure occurs. Thus the question is not whether a certain diagnosis is true or not, but when (precise timing) a certain pathophysiological condition associated with the diagnosis occurs. The starting point for all patients is a known diagnosis (epilepsy); the question (what we do not know in advance) is when the seizure occurs.

5.2.2. Define the Patient Population

Although in principle this question is relevant for all patients with epilepsy, for the study we must limit the patient populations to those who are admitted to long-term video-EEG monitoring, given the need for a reference standard. The inclusion criteria will also depend on the methodology of seizure detection and the type of seizures that are to be detected. For example, an accelerometer or a surface-EMG-based seizure detection can aim at detecting only convulsive seizures. An EEG-based or electrocardiogram (ECG)-based algorithm can target complex partial seizures. It is important that the whole recorded period is scanned/monitored using the algorithm, not only selected epochs. Cases in which the long-term video-EEG monitoring cannot provide a definite conclusion about an event should be excluded.

Some seizure-detection algorithms are "generic"—that is, they are meant to work on all patients or all patients in a certain group. Other algorithms are patient-tailored, and they need some baseline physiological (normal background) and/or pathophysiological data (recorded during a seizure). All these aspects have to be clarified and fixed before starting the clinical validation.

5.2.3. Describe the Methodology

When describing the methodology, besides the details about recording the signals and the detection algorithm, in a study it is important to specify whether the detection is going to run in real time or offline. It is important that operators of the seizure-detection system are blinded to the clinical data, and clinicians making decision about the presence/absence of seizures during the long-term monitoring are blinded to the results of the algorithm.

5.2.4. DEFINE THE REFERENCE STANDARD

The best available reference standard for this clinical question is the long-term video-EEG monitoring. Since this is extremely resource-demanding, it will limit the inclusion of patients. To extrapolate data from the monitoring unit to the "real-life"/home environment of the patient, we might try to reproduce some conditions that could elicit false positives (e.g., physical exercise in the case of EMG-based algorithms). An optimal study would collect data at home as the index test and compare the results against the gold standard of inpatient long-term monitoring.

5.2.5. REPORT THE TEST CHARACTERISTICS

The outcome measures are sensitivity and the rate of false positives. Sensitivity is calculated as the ratio between the true-positive automated seizure detections and the total number of seizures in the reference standard. Rate of false positives is calculated as the average number of false seizure detections in a 24-hour period.

6. INTEGRATING MULTIPLE DIAGNOSTIC TESTS

A central theme of this chapter has been that the design of diagnostic test validation studies and the interpretation of test accuracy (sensitivity/specificity) and utility depend on situating the test in the precise context in which it will be used clinically. The job of the clinician is to synthesize all of this information—that from general prevalence rates, from the history (including presence of risk factors), physical exam, our test of interest and all other test results . . . and perhaps a dose of intuition. If we were programmers developing an expert system to integrate all of this information, we would need many, many data points to assess not only the probabilities associated with each question in the history, maneuver in the exam, and test result, but the extent to which certain exam findings correlate with certain test results. For example, if we are assessing the probability that a patient with brief staring spells and an EEG with unilateral temporal sharp waves has temporal lobe epilepsy (TLE), we could look at the probability of the patient having TLE given the presence of staring spells, and perhaps a higher probability given the patient having staring spells that cannot be interrupted. Separately, a patient with an EEG with unilateral temporal sharp waves (and unknown history) has only a certain probability of having TLE. Also separately—and critically to this discussion—there is a certain probability of a patient with staring spells having an EEG with temporal sharp waves. The probability that a patient with uninterruptable staring spells and an EEG with temporal sharp waves has TLE is not just a combination of the probability that a patient with a positive EEG has TLE and the probability that a patient with staring spells has TLE, given that having a positive EEG and having staring spells are not independent events.

The upshot is that it takes a lot of data to combine multiple diagnostic tests (given the correlation structure) and that such assessments are beyond the range of all but the largest datasets. Expert systems are beginning to meet these needs.

7. CONCLUSIONS

A systematic approach for validating diagnostic studies/EEG biomarkers is essential for providing compelling evidence for the new methods. Each stage of the process—posing a clinical question, selecting a reference standard, defining inclusion and exclusion criteria, defining operator characteristics, selecting an aspect of the EEG signal to be analyzed, setting a threshold, and assessing test performance—is fraught with potential (and common) fallacies and pitfalls. In this chapter, we propose a set of steps and criteria that should help in designing and implementing these studies. These criteria attempt to minimize the sources of bias and error.

The checklist we propose here could be a starting point for the web-based tool that could help users in designing their diagnostic studies. The tool would be used before starting the study and would provide a prospective database of ongoing studies, similar to what is broadly accepted for therapeutic trials. Such an approach should increase the quality and reliability of diagnostic studies. However, this initiative would be feasible only if supported by editors of scientific journals publishing diagnostic studies, and by the relevant international medical associations.

REFERENCES

1. Wagner JA, Atkinson AJ, Jr. Measuring biomarker progress. *Clin Pharmacol Ther*. 2015;98(1):2–5.
2. Biomarkers Definitions Working Group. Biomarkers and surrogate endpoints: preferred definitions and conceptual framework. *Clin Pharmacol Ther*. 2001;69(3):89–95.
3. Port RG, Anwar AR, Ku M, Carlson GC, Siegel SJ, Roberts TP. Prospective MEG biomarkers in ASD: pre-clinical evidence and clinical promise of electrophysiological signatures. *Yale J Biol Med*. 2015;88(1):25–36.
4. Moons KG, de Groot JA, Linnet K, Reitsma JB, Bossuyt PM. Quantifying the added value of a diagnostic test or marker. *Clin Chem*. 2012;58(10):1408–1417.
5. Bossuyt PM, Reitsma JB, Bruns DE, et al. STARD 2015: an updated list of essential items for reporting diagnostic accuracy studies. *BMJ*. 2015;351:h5527.
6. Bossuyt PM, Reitsma JB, Bruns DE, et al. Towards complete and accurate reporting of studies of diagnostic accuracy: the STARD initiative. *BMJ*. 2003;326(7379):41–44.
7. Open Science Collaboration. Estimating the reproducibility of psychological science. *Science*. 2015;349(6251):aac4716.
8. Ioannidis JP. Why most published research findings are false. *PLoS Med*. 2005;2(8):e124.
9. Noel-Storr AH, McCleery JM, Richard E, et al. Reporting standards for studies of diagnostic test accuracy in dementia: The STARDdem Initiative. *Neurology*. 2014;83(4):364–373.
10. Gibbs EL, Gibbs FA. Electroencephalographic evidence of thalamic and hypothalamic epilepsy. *Neurology*. 1951;1(2):136–144.
11. Boutros N, Fristad M, Abdollohian A. The fourteen and six positive spikes and attention-deficit hyperactivity disorder. *Biol Psychiatry*. 1998;44(4):298–301.
12. Little S. A general analysis of the fourteen and six per second dysrhythmia. Paper presented at: 6th International Congress Electroencephalography and Clinical Neurophysiology, 1965, Vienna.

13. Gibbs FA, Gibbs EL. *Atlas of electroencephalography*. Vol. 3. Reading, MA: Addison-Wesley; 1964.
14. Connolly JF, Marchand Y, Major A, D'Arcy RC. Event-related brain potentials as a measure of performance on WISC-III and WAIS-R NI similarities sub-tests. *J Clin Exp Neuropsychol*. 2006;28(8):1327–1345.
15. Landsness E, Bruno MA, Noirhomme Q, et al. Electrophysiological correlates of behavioural changes in vigilance in vegetative state and minimally conscious state. *Brain*. 2011;134(Pt 8):2222–2232.
16. Morris SE, Cuthbert BN. Research Domain Criteria: cognitive systems, neural circuits, and dimensions of behavior. *Dialogues Clin Neurosci*. 2012;14(1):29–37.
17. Jeste SS, Frohlich J, Loo SK. Electrophysiological biomarkers of diagnosis and outcome in neurodevelopmental disorders. *Curr Opin Neurol*. 2015;28(2):110–116.
18. Cannon J, McCarthy MM, Lee S, et al. Neurosystems: brain rhythms and cognitive processing. *Eur J Neurosci*. 2014;39(5):705–719.
19. Kopell NJ, Gritton HJ, Whittington MA, Kramer MA. Beyond the connectome: the dynome. *Neuron*. 2014;83(6):1319–1328.
20. Binie C. Epilepsy in adults: diagnostic EEG investigation. In: Kimura J, Shibasaki H, eds. *Recent advances in clinical neurophysiology*. Amsterdam: Elsevier; 1996:217–222.
21. Salinsky M, Kanter R, Dasheiff RM. Effectiveness of multiple EEGs in supporting the diagnosis of epilepsy: an operational curve. *Epilepsia*. 1987;28(4):331–334.
22. Zivin L, Marsan CA. Incidence and prognostic significance of "epileptiform" activity in the EEG of non-epileptic subjects. *Brain*. 1968;91(4):751–778.
23. Beun AM, van Emde Boas W, Dekker E. Sharp transients in the sleep EEG of healthy adults: a possible pitfall in the diagnostic assessment of seizure disorders. *Electroencephalogr Clin Neurophysiol*. 1998;106(1):44–51.
24. Hrachovy RA, Frost JD, Jr. Infantile epileptic encephalopathy with hypsarrhythmia (infantile spasms/West syndrome). *J Clin Neurophysiol*. 2003;20(6):408–425.
25. Hrachovy RA, Frost JD, Jr., Kellaway P. Hypsarrhythmia: variations on the theme. *Epilepsia*. 1984;25(3):317–325.
26. Hussain SA, Kwong G, Millichap JJ, et al. Hypsarrhythmia assessment exhibits poor interrater reliability: a threat to clinical trial validity. *Epilepsia*. 2015;56(1):77–81.
27. Gibbs F, Davis H, Lennox W. The influence of the blood sugar level on the wave and spike formation in petit mal epilepsy. *Arch Neurol Psychiatry*. 1939;47:1111–1116.
28. Berg AT, Berkovic SF, Brodie MJ, et al. Revised terminology and concepts for organization of seizures and epilepsies: report of the ILAE Commission on Classification and Terminology, 2005-2009. *Epilepsia*. 2010;51(4):676–685.
29. Zijlmans M, Jiruska P, Zelmann R, Leijten FS, Jefferys JG, Gotman J. High-frequency oscillations as a new biomarker in epilepsy. *Ann Neurol*. 2012;71(2):169–178.
30. Gloss D, Nolan SJ, Staba R. The role of high-frequency oscillations in epilepsy surgery planning. *Cochrane Database Syst Rev*. 2014;1:CD010235.
31. Dumpelmann M, Jacobs J, Schulze-Bonhage A. Temporal and spatial characteristics of high frequency oscillations as a new biomarker in epilepsy. *Epilepsia*. 2015;56(2):197–206.
32. Poil SS, de Haan W, van der Flier WM, Mansvelder HD, Scheltens P, Linkenkaer-Hansen K. Integrative EEG biomarkers predict progression to Alzheimer's disease at the MCI stage. *Front Aging Neurosci*. 2013;5:58.
33. Meyer A, Bress JN, Proudfit GH. Psychometric properties of the error-related negativity in children and adolescents. *Psychophysiology*. 2014;51(7):602–610.
34. Balsamo LM, Gaillard WD. The utility of functional magnetic resonance imaging in epilepsy and language. *Curr Neurol Neurosci Rep*. 2002;2(2):142–149.
35. Weller SC, Mann NC. Assessing rater performance without a "gold standard" using consensus theory. *Med Decis Making*. 1997;17(1):71–79.
36. Beniczky S, Lantz G, Rosenzweig I, et al. Source localization of rhythmic ictal EEG activity: a study of diagnostic accuracy following STARD criteria. *Epilepsia*. 2013;54(10):1743–1752.
37. Rosenzweig I, Fogarasi A, Johnsen B, et al. Beyond the double banana: improved recognition of temporal lobe seizures in long-term EEG. *J Clin Neurophysiol*. 2014;31(1):1–9.
38. Knowlton RC, Razdan SN, Limdi N, et al. Effect of epilepsy magnetic source imaging on intracranial electrode placement. *Ann Neurol*. 2009;65(6):716–723.
39. Sutherling WW, Mamelak AN, Thyerlei D, et al. Influence of magnetic source imaging for planning intracranial EEG in epilepsy. *Neurology*. 2008;71(13):990–996.
40. Snyder SM, Rugino TA, Hornig M, Stein MA. Integration of an EEG biomarker with a clinician's ADHD evaluation. *Brain Behav*. 2015;5(4):e00330.
41. Arns M, Conners CK, Kraemer HC. A decade of EEG theta/beta ratio research in ADHD: a meta-analysis. *J Atten Disord*. 2013;17(5):374–383.
42. Bosl W, Tierney A, Tager-Flusberg H, Nelson C. EEG complexity as a biomarker for autism spectrum disorder risk. *BMC Med*. 2011;9:18.
43. Cohen M. *Analyzing neural time series data: theory and practice*. Cambridge, MA: MIT Press; 2014.
44. Thakor NV, Tong S. Advances in quantitative electroencephalogram analysis methods. *Annu Rev Biomed Eng*. 2004;6:453–495.
45. Luck S. *An introduction to the event-related potential technique*. 2nd ed. Cambridge, MA: MIT Press; 2014.
46. Luck S, Kappenman E. *The Oxford handbook of event-related potential components*. Oxford: Oxford University Press; 2013.
47. Barry RJ, Johnstone SJ, Clarke AR. A review of electrophysiology in attention-deficit/hyperactivity disorder: II. Event-related potentials. *Clin Neurophysiol*. 2003;114(2):184–198.
48. Nuwer M. Assessment of digital EEG, quantitative EEG, and EEG brain mapping: report of the American Academy of Neurology and the American Clinical Neurophysiology Society. *Neurology*. 1997;49(1):277–292.
49. Gunnarsdottir K, Kang Y, Kerr M, et al. A look at the strength of micro and macro EEG analysis for distinguishing insomnia within an HIV cohort. Paper presented at: Engineering in Medicine and Biology Society, 37th Annual International Conference of the IEEE, 2015; Milan, Italy.
50. Gilbert DL, Buncher CR. An EEG should not be obtained routinely after first unprovoked seizure in childhood. *Neurology*. 2000;54(3):635–641.

10 | EEG ACTIVATION METHODS

MOUHSIN M. SHAFI, MD, PHD AND M. BRANDON WESTOVER, MD, PHD

ABSTRACT: Activation procedures are commonly employed to increase the diagnostic yield of electroencephalography (EEG) in patients with suspected epilepsy. This chapter reviews the effects and utility of hyperventilation, intermittent photic stimulation, and color/pattern stimulation on the EEG in patients with epilepsy and other neurological disorders. In theory, the greater the number of different activation methods used in EEG evaluation of an epilepsy patient, the greater the chance of obtaining abnormal findings. However, the specificity of these findings for epilepsy is uncertain. Furthermore, from a practical point of view, desirable activations are those methods that can be carried out easily and systematically, in a short time frame, with affordable equipment, without undesirable side effects for patients, and with reliable and predictive results. At this time, hyperventilation and intermittent photic stimulation are the most widely used activation methods and have an extensive body of literature supporting them.

KEYWORDS: electroencephalography, EEG, hyperventilation, photic stimulation, epilepsy, pattern stimulation

PRINCIPAL REFERENCES

1. Achenbach-Ng J, Siao TC, Mavroudakis N, Chiappa KH, Kiers L. Effects of routine hyperventilation on PCO2 and PO2 in normal subjects: implications for EEG interpretations. *J Clin Neurophysiol.* 1994;11(2):220–225.
2. Jonas J, Vignal J-P, Baumann C, et al. Effect of hyperventilation on seizure activation: potentiation by antiepileptic drug tapering. *J Neurol Neurosurg Psychiatry.* 2011;82(8):928–930.
3. Benbadis SR, Johnson K, Anthony K, et al. Induction of psychogenic non-epileptic seizures without placebo. *Neurology.* 2000;55(12):1904–1905.
4. Kasteleijn-Nolst Trenité D, Rubboli G, Hirsch E, et al. Methodology of photic stimulation revisited: updated European algorithm for visual stimulation in the EEG laboratory. *Epilepsia.* 2012;53(1):16–24.
5. Waltz S, Christen H-J, Doose H. The different patterns of the photoparoxysmal response—a genetic study. *Electroencephalogr Clin Neurophysiol.* 1992;83(2):138–145.
6. Wolf P, Goosses R. Relation of photosensitivity to epileptic syndromes. *J Neurol Neurosurg Psychiatry.* 1986;49(12):1386–1391.
7. De Bittencourt PR. Photosensitivity: the magnitude of the problem. *Epilepsia.* 2004;45(s1):30–34.
8. Quirk JA, Fish DR, Smith SJ, Sander JW, Shorvon SD, Allen PJ. Incidence of photosensitive epilepsy: a prospective national study. *Electroencephalogr Clin Neurophysiol.* 1995;95(4):260–267.
9. Wilkins AJ, Bonanni P, Porciatti V, Guerrini R. Physiology of human photosensitivity. *Epilepsia.* 2004;45(Suppl 1):7–3.
10. Fisher RS, Harding G, Erba G, Barkley GL, Wilkins A, Epilepsy Foundation of America Working Group. Photic- and pattern-induced seizures: a review for the Epilepsy Foundation of America Working Group. *Epilepsia.* 2005;46(9):1426–1441.

1. INTRODUCTION

Activation procedures are commonly employed to increase the diagnostic yield of electroencephalography (EEG) in patients with suspected epilepsy. In this chapter, we review the effects and utility of hyperventilation (HV), intermittent photic stimulation (IPS), and color/pattern stimulation on the EEG in patients with epilepsy and other neurological disorders.

2. HYPERVENTILATION

Precipitation of seizures by HV was known prior to discovery of human EEG.[1] Therefore, EEG activation by HV has been widely used in almost all clinical EEG laboratories since its introduction, and early studies showed the provocative efficacy of generalized-synchronous paroxysmal discharges and of absence seizures produced by this test.[2] This method consists of deep and regular respiration at a rate of about 20/min for a period of 2 to 5 minutes.[3]

An understanding of the time course and magnitude of the systematic changes in blood gases produced by routine HV in adults is important for clinical interpretations of EEGs. Achenbach-Ng et al.[4] studied these changes in adults and children and found that during 3 minutes of HV, the pCO_2 fell a mean of 18 mm Hg and the pO_2 rose 7 mm Hg, the former with a near-linear response curve (Fig. 10.1). Note that pCO_2 reached its nadir 30 seconds after the end of the 3 minutes of HV. From this point, after the command to "breathe normally," pCO_2 rose linearly to return to resting levels in about 5.5 minutes, more slowly for children. As pCO_2 rose during this post-HV period, pO_2 fell to 25 mm Hg below resting values at 5.2 minutes after cessation of HV, and then rose to resting levels over the following 11.6 minutes (see Fig. 10.1). Any perturbation of ventilation in the post-HV period (e.g., talking) prolonged these steps. These findings minimize the clinical importance of slowing in the EEG that outlasts the HV period and correlate with the "re-buildup" of post-HV slowing seen in Moyamoya disease.

The characteristic EEG response to HV, most prominent in children, consists of a fluctuating increase of bilaterally synchronous slow activity and slowing of alpha and beta rhythms (Fig. 10.2). In normal adults, although the slowing is generally not marked, there are wide differences among individuals. Aside from diffuse slowing, HV may induce diffuse sharp waves or spike-wave discharges of epileptogenic significance; it is particularly effective in eliciting bilaterally synchronous spike-wave discharges in patients with generalized epilepsies. Dalby[5] found that patients with absence seizures were more sensitive to HV than patients with non-absence seizures, with the incidence of spike-wave paroxysms (Fig. 10.3) being 50% in the former and 25% in the latter. In general, latent abnormalities are likely to be activated by HV. Slow-wave foci associated with localized lesions may also be aggravated; abnormalities in temporal regions are more prone to accentuation than those elsewhere.[6]

The utility of HV in patients with suspected focal epilepsy has been debated. Miley and Forster[7] reported that vigorous

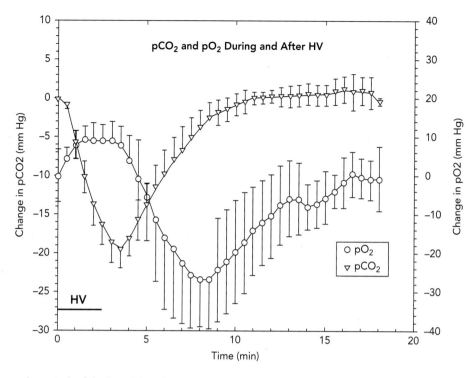

Figure 10.1. *Time course and magnitude of absolute pCO$_2$ and pO$_2$ changes with 3 minutes of HV in nine normal adult subjects. The error bars represent 1 standard deviation. A transcutaneous heated membrane technique was used for the blood gas measurements. (Achenbach-Ng J, Siao TC, Mavroudakis N, Chiappa KH, Kiers L. Effects of routine hyperventilation on pCO$_2$ and pO$_2$ in normal subjects: implications for EEG interpretations. J Clin Neurophysiol. 1994;11[2]:220–225.)*

HV of longer duration induced abnormal discharges with or without clinical seizures in 11% of epilepsy patients with complex partial seizures. However, Klein et al.[8] reported that 5 minutes of HV had no effect on interictal epileptiform discharge frequency in 20 patients with focal (predominantly temporal lobe) epilepsy. In 384 patients with proven localization-related epilepsy, a single 5-minute session of HV produced an increase in interictal discharges and/or seizures in 3.6%[9]; the authors interpreted this finding as evidence that "localization-related epilepsies . . . are relatively resistant to routine HV activation in adults and adolescents." A similar finding was reported for 3 minutes of HV in patients admitted for long-term video EEG monitoring. In contrast, Guaranha et al.[10] reported that HV (performed repeatedly for 5 minutes every 3 hours from 6 a.m. to midnight) was associated with seizure activation in 24 of 97 patients with medically refractory focal epilepsy admitted to an epilepsy monitoring unit for continuous video-EEG monitoring, with a higher probability of HV-elicited seizures in patients with a temporal focus. Some clarification was provided in another study of predominantly (>90%) focal epilepsy patients admitted for video-EEG monitoring, in which the rate of activated seizures was approximately nine times higher during HV periods versus the non-HV period[11]; a significant effect was seen primarily during antiepileptic drug tapering (as opposed to before tapering). Taken together, these studies suggest that HV does indeed increase the incidence of epileptiform abnormalities and seizures in focal epilepsies, but that the impact is not as substantial or reliable as in the generalized epilepsies, and is likely modulated by the presence of antiseizure medications. However, given that HV is generally a very

safe procedure,[12] repeated sessions to maximize the likelihood of capturing seizures is a reasonable procedure in patients admitted to epilepsy monitoring units.[13]

With regard to the underlying mechanism of HV's provocation of slowing and seizure discharges, Gibbs et al.[14] suggested that diffuse slowing is caused by inadequate compensatory vasoconstriction of the cerebrum in response to systemic hypocapnia. According to Gotoh et al.,[15] diffuse slowing is considered to be the direct result of cerebral ischemic anoxia resulting from hypocapnic cerebral vasoconstriction. Yamatani et al.,[16] measuring cerebral blood flow in the right carotid artery during HV, reported that decreased pCO$_2$ and cerebral blood flow were the fundamental factors causing EEG slowing. This finding was confirmed by Duarte et al.,[17] who found that end-tidal CO$_2$ concentration and cerebral blood flow velocity in the middle cerebral artery were tightly coupled, and EEG slowing was correlated with but lagged behind decreases in flow velocity. Fisch and So[18] summarized the physiological basis of the EEG response to HV as the following: alteration of pCO$_2$, rather than pH or partial pressure of oxygen (PO$_2$), is the most important factor in producing EEG response to HV, whereas the most obvious and dramatic physiological effect of HV is decreased cerebral blood flow. Sherwin[19] attributed the diffuse slowing to synchronous activity in the nonspecific thalamocortical projecting systems, which become more active in hypocapnia. Patel and Maulsby[20] raised the possibility that hypocapnia induced by HV decreased activity in mesencephalic reticular formation, which then caused EEG slowing, just as drowsiness and sleep produce EEG slowing. Similar mechanisms to those described above are considered

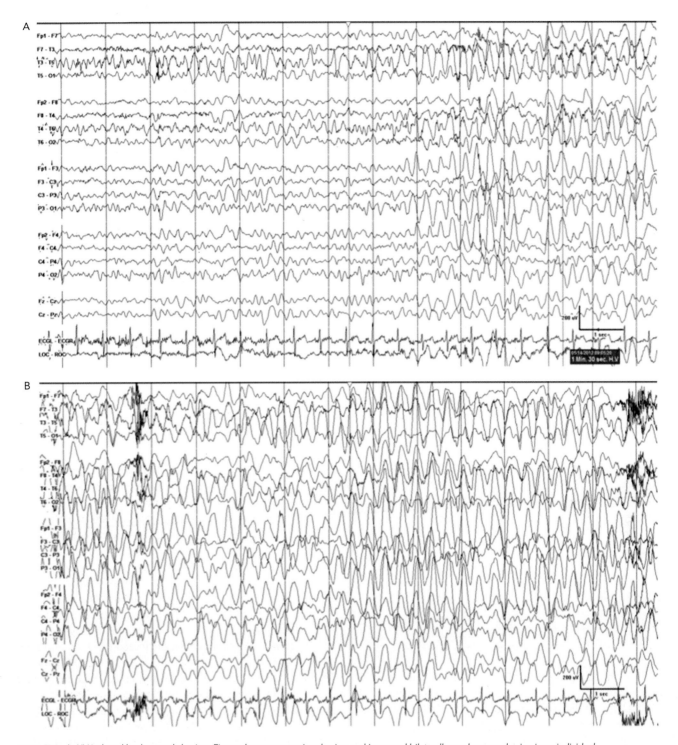

Figure 10.2. A: *HV-induced background slowing. Figure shows progressive slowing and increased bilaterally synchronous slowing in an individual undergoing HV.* **B:** *Continuation of EEG recording showing progression of HV-induced slowing and hypersynchrony.*

to be important for provoking paroxysmal discharges[21]; hyperexcitability of neurons may be induced by respiratory alkalosis.[22] However, the change from the pure delta response to the appearance of intermixed spikes and clear-cut spike-wave discharges remains obscure. Interestingly, it has been reported that intravenous administration of diazepam prevented HV-induced spike patterns, though it failed to attenuate the delta response.[23] More recently, it has also been reported that valproate reduces HV-induced spike-wave discharges, but not

the photoparoxysmal response.[24] Furthermore, HV with supplemental 5% CO_2 can also suppress HV-induced absence seizures and spikes,[25] highlighting the role of hypocapnia in producing epileptiform abnormalities.

The magnitude of HV response depends upon a number of factors.[26] First, vigorous exchange of air can enhance activation effects. For the purpose of routine examination with HV, however, it is suggested that the rate of breathing be as close as possible to that of the resting rhythm (15–20 breaths/min).[26]

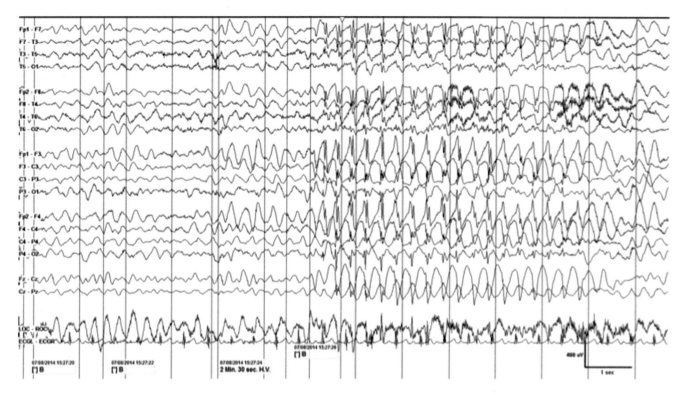

Figure 10.3. 3-Hz generalized spike-and-wave discharges induced by HV in a patient with absence seizures. "B" indicates a breath by the patient.

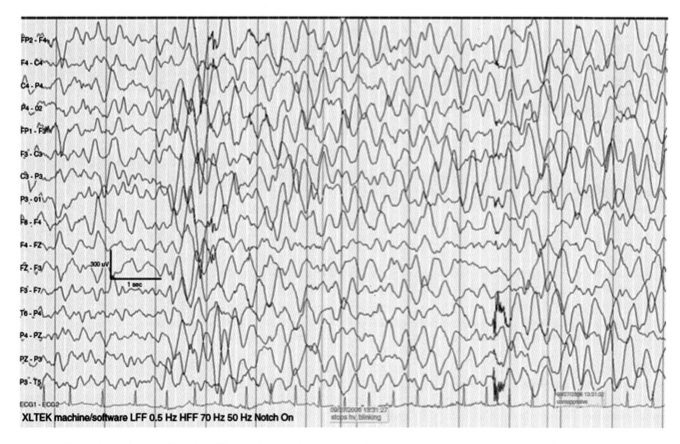

Figure 10.4. EEG during an episode of HV-induced high-amplitude rhythmic slowing activity associated with alteration of awareness. (Figure 1 in Barker A, Ng J, Rittey CD, Kandler RH, Mordekar SR. Outcome of children with hyperventilation-induced high-amplitude rhythmic slow activity with altered awareness. *Dev Med Child Neurol.* 2012;54[11]:1001–1005.)

Second, age is an important factor. Slow waves appear much more abruptly, are more pronounced, and persist longer in children than in adults. The degree and abruptness of the response are related directly to age.[27] The most dramatic EEG responses to HV usually occur between the ages of 8 and 12 years.[28] According to Gibbs et al.[14], in children between 3 and 5 years of age, 97% of epilepsy patients and 70% of normal subjects showed diffuse slowing with HV; after 20 years of age, more than 40% of epilepsy patients but less than 10% of normal subjects showed diffuse slowing. The areas most affected by HV in children are occipitotemporal regions.[29] Delta waves tend to appear initially in the posterior regions and spread forward in the younger age group, whereas they tend to appear in the frontal regions and spread backward in the older age group.[30]

Third, blood glucose level is important in determining the degree of HV response. In adults, a low blood glucose level (<80 mg/dL) tends to enhance the appearance of slow waves; a high level (>120 mg/dL) tends to inhibit or prevent such an effect.[31] Delta waves induced by HV can occasionally be the first indication of pathological hypoglycemia secondary to an islet cell tumor in a patient referred for an EEG.[30]

Fourth, an erect position as compared to a reclining position enhances the effect of HV; EEG slowing occurs earlier and with greater intensity. This is thought to be a result of relative cerebral anoxia.[32] Diffuse slowing induced by HV usually disappears rapidly after ceasing HV; it may persist up to 30 seconds in normal adults.

HV may also be useful in identifying and characterizing other conditions. Unusually prolonged post-HV high-voltage slowing may be seen in patients with syncopal attacks of various etiologies.[33] Buildup of slow waves after the end of HV ("re-buildup") may be a diagnostic finding in children with Moyamoya disease.[34] In a study that addressed three cases of Moyamoya disease,[35] it was reported that this EEG re-buildup was noted about 5 minutes after HV cessation; moreover, corresponding decreases in cerebral blood flow and PO_2 were documented with it. Such a post-HV hypoxia 5 minutes after cessation of HV was also found in a study of nine normal adult subjects.[4] Note that it is suggested that HV should be avoided in patients with Moyamoya disease,[36] although a recent study in 127 pediatric Moyamoya patients reported no adverse clinical ischemic events.[37]

HV may be particularly beneficial in assessing patients with suspected psychogenic nonepileptic spells. In combination with suggestion and photic stimulation, HV can produce a typical psychogenic nonepileptiform spell in up to 84% of patients,[38] without the need for deception used in other suggestive maneuvers such as an intravenous saline infusion. The potential utility of hyperventilation in activating psychogenic nonepileptic events has since been replicated in numerous other studies.[13,39–41]

The American Clinical Neurophysiology Society Guidelines Committee in 2016 proposed[42] the following minimum technical requirements:

Hyperventilation should be used routinely unless medical or other justifiable reasons (e.g., a recent intracranial hemorrhage, significant cardiopulmonary disease, sickle cell disease or trait, or patient inability or unwillingness to cooperate) contraindicate it. It should be performed for a minimum of 3 min, with continued recording for at least 1 min after cessation of overbreathing. At times, hyperventilation must be performed for a longer period in order to obtain adequate activation of the EEG. To evaluate the effects of this activation technique, at least 1 min of recording with the same montage should be obtained before overbreathing begins.

Some studies[43] suggest that 5 minutes of HV may reveal epileptiform abnormalities in more patients than 3 minutes of HV. While the American Clinical Neurophysiology Society Guidelines suggest continued recording for at least 1 minute after cessation of overbreathing, the slow time course of the recovery of pCO_2 levels discussed previously[4] and the findings in the Moyamoya patients[35] indicate that at least 6 minutes of post-HV recording would be prudent.

Regarding the clinical interpretation of EEG changes seen during HV, a few simple principles should be kept in mind as guidelines, and any clinical interpretation that exceeds these guidelines should have a firm, rational basis for the variance. These guidelines are as follows:

1. HV-induced slowing may be of any amplitude, location, rhythmicity, and time course and should still be considered to be within normal limits unless it is significantly asymmetrical or contains definite spikes.

2. As with most amplitude asymmetry considerations in clinical EEG interpretations, there are no precise values available for normal limits in HV-induced slowing, but a 2:1 ratio is definitely abnormal and any asymmetry greater than 1.5:1 is probably abnormal.

3. HV-induced slowing can persist for several minutes after the command to breathe normally, as discussed above, and this persistence or reappearance is only very rarely abnormal.

Regarding a clinical interpretative declaration stating that there are HV-induced spikes in the EEG, a very conservative approach needs to be employed. As in most other sections of the EEG, the admixture and interaction of different, nonepileptiform frequencies can sum to produce a waveform with an epileptiform appearance that is not a true spike with the pathophysiological significance of that cortical event. This is especially true with HV-induced slowing and its superimposed faster frequencies, and even more so in childhood, since that age has the most complex mixture of frequencies and the highest amplitudes of all of those components, including the HV-induced slowing. In the pediatric age group both paroxysmal drowsy hypersynchrony and HV-induced bursts of slowing may contain admixed components with a spike-like appearance that are, despite their superficial appearance, normal variants. This differentiation constitutes the major challenge in the interpretation of pediatric EEGs.

In addition, the presence of altered responsiveness in association with high-amplitude rhythmic slowing (HIHARS;

see Fig. 10.4) with HV is not abnormal.[44] In the latter study, eight of 12 healthy nonepileptic children (mean age 9.6 years) exhibited impaired verbal recall and failed to respond to repeated auditory clicks. Furthermore, Lum et al.[45] studied 77 episodes of HIHARS with loss of awareness from 22 children and 107 absence seizures during HV from another 22 children; eye opening and eyelid flutter were seen more frequently in absence seizures whereas fidgeting, smiling, and yawning occurred more frequently during HIHARS episodes, and arrest of activity, staring, and oral and manual automatisms were observed in both groups, so that the EEG is the only reliable means of differentiating the two conditions (i.e., epileptic vs. nonepileptic). A long-term follow-up study of 15 children with HIHARS[46] found that all nine children presenting with only "blank spells" on history and with only HIHARS on EEG did not subsequently receive a diagnosis of epilepsy, whereas the six children eventually diagnosed with epilepsy all presented with a history of either convulsive or motor seizures, and five of the six had epileptiform abnormalities on interictal EEG.

3. INTERMITTENT PHOTIC STIMULATION

The effect of IPS on the human EEG was first studied by Adrian and Matthews,[47] who used sinusoidal IPS derived from a constant light source in front of which a disk with cutout sectors was rotated. After this earliest report, similar instruments were used for more than a decade.[48] Walter et al.[49] were the first to report activation of paroxysmal discharges by IPS with an electronic strobe light. After this pioneering work, the method of IPS using a strobe light became popular.

While the details of IPS use in routine examination vary greatly between EEG laboratories, recent methodological papers have attempted to standardize IPS delivery across EEG laboratories.[50] The three main EEG changes induced by IPS are the photic driving response (PDR), the photomyogenic response (PMR), and the photoparoxysmal response (PPR), the latter of which is considered to be indicative of epilepsy-related photosensitivity.

3.1. Methodology of Photic Stimulation

In a recent methodology algorithm for assessing patients for IPS,[50] the authors recommended using a lamp with a circular reflector that delivers flashes with an intensity of at least 0.70 (and preferably 1.0) Joules, applied at a viewing distance of 30 cm in a dimly lit room with simultaneous video recording to assist in characterization of events. It was suggested that IPS sensitivity be assessed with separate trains of flashes of 5-sec duration during eye closure, eyes closed and eyes open conditions; alternatively, if not enough time is available, 7 sec of stimulation at each flash frequency could be applied with closure of the eyes (the most provocative eye condition) on command at the start of the flash train. The technologist must be alert to stop stimulation immediately upon identifying a PPR, since prolonged stimulation can trigger a generalized tonic-clonic seizure in a sensitive patient. It was recommended that IPS be carried out with the following frequencies in this order: 1, 2,

8, 10, 15, 18, 20, 25, 40, 50, and 60 Hz. If a generalized PPR is provoked, the authors recommended skipping the remainder of the series, starting again at 60 Hz, and going down in frequencies (e.g., 60, 50, 40 Hz, . . .) until again a generalized PPR response occurs, to establish the upper threshold for the PPR. Once the upper and lower thresholds for eliciting a PPR have been definitely identified, further stimulation should not be attempted as these patients may become more sensitive as stimulation continues or is repeated, and may launch into a seizure with little warning. The additional information gained from repeated stimulation is not worth the risk to the patient.

3.2. Photic Driving Response

The PDR is a physiological response consisting of rhythmic activity elicited over the posterior regions of the head by IPS frequencies of about 5 to 30 Hz (Fig. 10.5). The term PDR should be limited to activity that is time-locked to the stimulus and is of a frequency identical or harmonically related to the stimulus frequency.[51] Entrainment is typically maximal around individual alpha frequency, and at subharmonics, and may be more prominent with magnetoencephalographic (MEG) recordings.[52]

As a rule, PDR is found over posterior regions. In infants, PDR can be elicited a few hours after birth,[53] but it remains relatively small up to about 6 years of age.[54] In older children, PDR becomes much larger, particularly at low frequencies.[6] The amplitude of PDR is usually higher in children than in adults and again tends to increase in elderly people. Regardless of age, however, an exaggerated PDR to low flash frequencies (0.5–3 Hz) usually signifies acute or subacute neuronal dysfunction[55]; examples include MELAS (mitochondrial myopathy, encephalopathy, lactic acidosis, and stroke-like episodes)[18] and the late infantile form of ceroid lipofuscinosis.[56,57]

Large positive occipital sharp transients of sleep (POSTS) and lambda waves in response to scanning a complex pattern are predictive of a prominent PDR.[18,58,59] Destructive cortical lesions may cause unilateral PDR depression, whereas irritative lesions, such as those associated with epileptic scars, may produce increased PDR on the side of the lesion.[30] Interpretation suggesting abnormal PDR should be made carefully because a minor and inconsistent asymmetry of PDR is seen even in normal subjects. Some authors[60] claim that an asymmetry in amplitude only, in the absence of other EEG changes, should not be viewed as abnormal. Very-low-voltage or absent PDRs are of little diagnostic significance because some normal persons are not responsive to IPS.[55] At a group level, decreases in photic driving, particularly in the alpha band, have been reported in patients with Alzheimer's disease[61,62] and schizophrenia,[63,64] whereas increases in photic driving have been reported in patients with migraine[65–67] and major depression.[64] However, these differences are likely not consistent or large enough to be clinically useful.[68,69]

3.3. Photomyoclonic Response (Photomyogenic Response)

The PMR is a response to IPS characterized by appearance of brief repetitive muscle spikes over anterior regions of the head. These often increase gradually in amplitude as stimulation

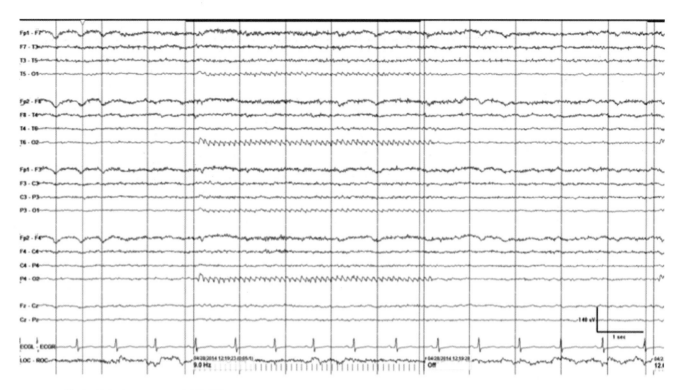

Figure 10.5. Photic driving in response to 9.0-Hz IPS.

continues and cease promptly when the stimulus is withdrawn (Fig. 10.6). The response is associated frequently with eyelid flutter, a vertical oscillation of the eyelids and eyeballs; sometimes it is associated with discrete jerking, mostly involving musculature of the face and head.[51] Principal features of this response were first described by Gastaut and Rémond[70] and Bickford et al.,[71] who introduced the term PMR, which differs from PPR. Occasionally, a PMR can be seen with a PPR. The most effective triggering IPS frequency lies between 12 and 18 Hz.[72] The PMR tends to appear in conjunction with muscular tension. It occurs less often in children than in adults. Gastaut et al.[73] reported that PMR was found in 0.3% of normal subjects, 3% of patients with epilepsy, 13% of patients with brainstem lesions, and 17% of patients with psychiatric disorders. However, the incidence of PMR was lower, ranging from 0.1% to 0.8%, in other studies.[74–77] The PMR is considered to be a nonspecific finding that is not significant for ruling out a seizure disorder.[78] The PMR can be enhanced in early stages of alcohol withdrawal in chronic alcoholics,[79] although the incidence is likely still low (<5%),[80] or after sudden withdrawal from barbiturates and related sedatives.[81] A symptomatic transient PMR secondary to a metabolic disorder (severe hypocalcemia) can occur.[82,83]

3.4. Photoparoxysmal Response (Photoconvulsive Response)

The PPR (Fig. 10.7) is a response to IPS that is characterized by spike-and-wave and multiple spike-and-wave complexes that are traditionally bilaterally synchronous, symmetrical, and generalized; they may outlast the stimulus by a few seconds. There may be associated with impairment of consciousness and brisk jerks involving musculature of the whole body, most predominantly that of the upper extremities and head.[51] Newmark and Penry[78] state that generalized slow activity and posterior spikes are not accepted universally as a PPR, but the significance of these discharges increases if they continue after stimulation is discontinued; however, this has been debated.[84–86] Generalized PPR may be most pronounced in the frontal, central, or occipital regions. Hishikawa et al.[87] classified generalized PPR in photosensitive epilepsy patients into two groups: (1) patients in whom the PPR appears first in the occipital area and (2) those in whom the PPR occurs simultaneously over all areas or appears earlier over anterior regions. In the former group, an augmented visual evoked response could be obtained. Generalized PPRs in children are usually rhythmic and higher in amplitude than those seen in adults. Occipital spikes as a sole response to IPS may not be indicative of epilepsy.[88] Unilateral occipital spikes are rarely induced by IPS. These patients, as opposed to patients with generalized PPR, often have a history of a local posterior lesion, mostly traumatic. In a genetic study of patients with photosensitivity and their relatives, Waltz et al.[89] classified the PPR into four types (Fig. 10.8): type 1, spikes with occipital rhythm; type 2, parieto-occipital spikes with a biphasic slow wave; type 3, parieto-occipital spikes with a biphasic slow wave and spread to the frontal region; type 4, generalized spikes and waves or polyspikes and waves. They found that patients with a history of generalized idiopathic epilepsy had type 4 (generalized) discharges more often than the control patients with a PPR but without a history of epilepsy, who were more likely to have discharges of types 1 to 3.

Although PPRs in photosensitive epilepsy patients are elicited by a broad range of IPS frequencies from 1 to 65 Hz,[90] the

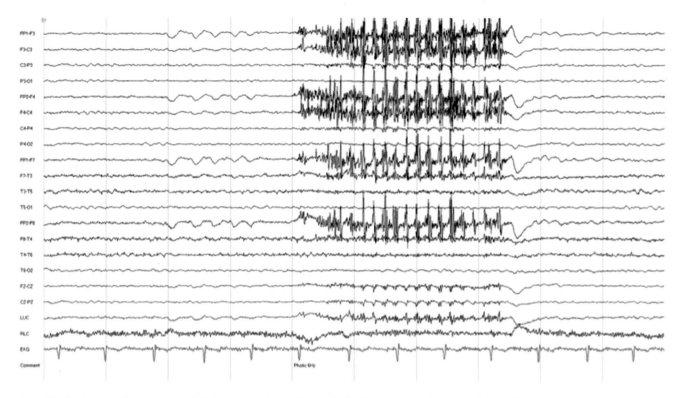

Figure 10.6. *Photomyoclonic response to IPS. Note the increasing frontally predominant response over the course of stimulation.*

most epileptogenic frequencies are typically within the range of 15 to 20 Hz,[90,91] with 18 Hz as the single most epileptogenic frequency,[91] although this may vary as a function of whether IPS is done with the eyes open, eyes closed, or with eye closure upon initiation of IPS. Some studies have suggested PPRs may be more likely to be induced by eye closure.[92,93] Patients with PPRs are less sensitive to IPS when asleep.[87,94] When IPS is used with eyes open, careful attention to eye movement and position is needed because a directional change from central to lateral gaze diminishes the effect of IPS in evoking PPRs. This effect is greater than the diminution effect with monocular IPS stimulation as compared with binocular IPS stimulation in

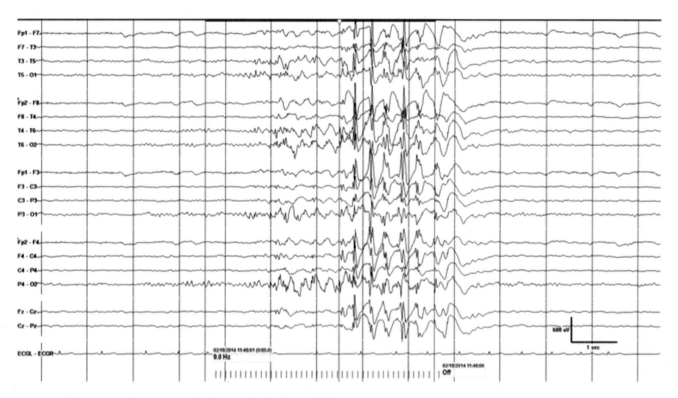

Figure 10.7. *Photoparoxysmal response to IPS, with generalized spike-wave discharges.*

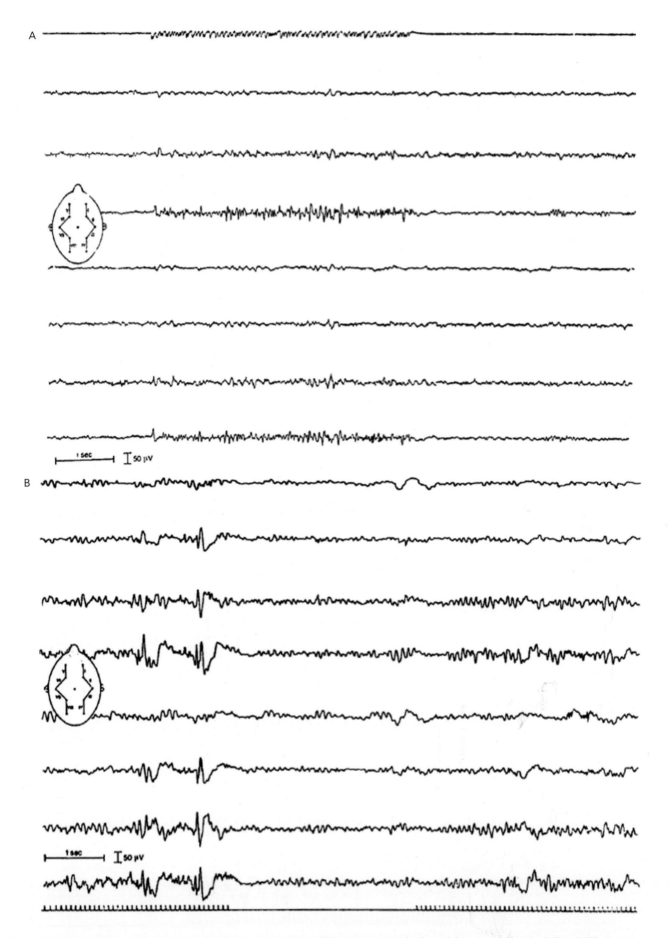

Figure 10.8. A: Type 1 PPR[89]: spikes within the occipital rhythm only. **B:** Type 2 PPR: parieto-occipital spike-and-slow-wave discharges. **C:** Type 3 PPR: parieto-occipital spike-and-slow-wave discharges with frontal spread. **D:** Type 4 PPR: generalized spike-wave discharges.

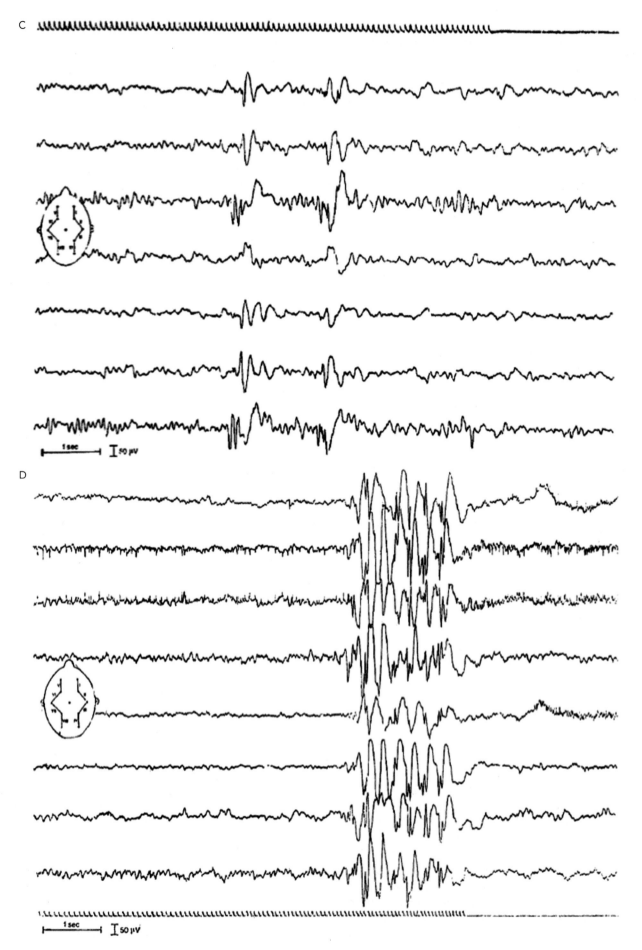

C

D

Figure 10.8. Continued

eliciting PPRs.[95] Regarding levels of ambient light, with high-intensity IPS, the effects of normal ambient lighting may be negligible,[96] although performance of the IPS procedure in dim lighting is still recommended in most guidelines.[50] Stimulators with energy output close to 1 Joule may be more effective in eliciting PPRs than lower-intensity stimulators.[97]

The prevalence of PPR varies widely as a function of the age, gender, epilepsy diagnosis, and inclusion criteria of the study population. PPRs are most often detected in adolescents ages 7 to 20, and with a higher (approximately 2:1) prevalence in females.[93,98-100] In healthy children, a PPR has been reported in 1.3% to 8% of subjects,[99,101-103] although the higher numbers are typically from older studies that included focal spikes in the category of PPR. In healthy adults, screening of aircrew candidates has typically identified PPR in 0.4% to 0.7% of applicants,[104-107] although rates as high as 2.2% have been reported.[107,108] For patients referred for EEG examination, somewhat similar to higher numbers have been reported. Jeavons[109] found a PPR in 2.8% of the patients referred for EEG examination, a figure similar to that of Gastaut et al.,[73] whereas Wadlington and Riley[98] reported a PPR in 1.25%. Subsequent studies have generally reported PPRs in 0.8% to 2% of patients referred for EEG.[110-114] Of note, ethnic differences in PPR have been reported, with lower rates noted specifically for black patients than for white, Asian, or mixed-race patients in studies conducted in sub-Saharan Africa.[110,115]

A few studies have attempted to assess the incidence of PPRs in consecutive patients referred for EEG evaluation after the development of seizures. Danesi[116] evaluated 408 consecutive patients (almost all adult) investigated after a single seizure and reported PPRs in 6.4%; this number was similar to the prevalence of PPRs (5.9%) seen in 3,161 patients with confirmed epilepsy in that same center. The most comprehensive and rigorous study of the incidence of photosensitivity was by Quirk et al.,[117] who conducted a prospective nationwide study to determine the incidence of photosensitive epilepsy over a 3-month period in Great Britain, and included results from ~90% of all EEGs conducted during this time period. A total of 191 cases with a PPR were identified, including 143 with a type 4 PPR (Waltz[89] criteria). Based on these results, the annual incidence of cases of epilepsy in which patients had type 4 PPRs on their first EEG was conservatively estimated to be 1.1 per 100,000, representing ~2% of all new cases of epilepsy. In patients ages 7 to 19 years (an age range prespecified by the authors based on the known high prevalence of photosensitivity in this population), the annual incidence was 5.7 per 100,000, representing approximately 10% of all new cases of epilepsy.

The prevalence of PPRs in patients with epilepsy clearly varies as a function of the specific epilepsy diagnosis. A number of early studies have established that PPRs are seen primarily in patients with generalized epilepsy. Specifically, Gastaut et al.[73] reported that the PPR is almost entirely confined to patients with primary generalized epilepsy and that it occurs in 40% of cases with absence seizures and in 20% of cases with generalized tonic-clonic seizures. A PPR occurred in 53% of patients with nonfocal seizures in the study by Stevens[118] but in only 3% of patients with focal seizures. Similarly, Wolf and

Goosses evaluated 4,007 EEGs in 1,062 patients with epilepsy over an 8-year period and reported a PPR in 9.9% of them[100]; 88% of the patients with a PPR had a generalized epilepsy. A PPR was seen in 30% of patients with juvenile myoclonic epilepsy, 18% of patients with childhood absence epilepsy, 17% of patients with West and Lennox syndromes, and 13% of patients with grand mal on awakening. In patients with focal epilepsy, PPRs occurred primarily in patients with versive seizures with visual hallucinations. A subsequent study in Japan[111] also found a higher rate of PPRs in patients with idiopathic generalized epilepsy (5.6%) than in patients with focal epilepsy (0.7%), with a particularly higher prevalence in patients with juvenile myoclonic epilepsy (17.4%) and grand mal on awakening (7.6%). This study also found that in patients with focal epilepsy, PPRs were primarily seen in patients with occipital lobe epilepsy (6.1%). Other studies have also reported a high rate of PPRs in patients with idiopathic generalized epilepsy,[119] with rates as high as 90% reported in with juvenile myoclonic epilepsy.[120] A high incidence of photosensitivity has also been reported in patients with the progressive myoclonic epilepsies Unverricht-Lundborg disease, Lafora body disease, and the neuronal ceroid lipofuscinoses.[121-123]

With regard to focal epilepsies, Guerrini et al.[124] proposed a concept called *idiopathic photosensitive occipital lobe epilepsy* based on detailed analysis of 10 patients with recurrent episodes of visually induced occipital seizures; all seizures were stimulus-related (mostly television and computer screen) and began with elementary visual symptoms, followed in most patients by a slow clustering of cephalic pain, epigastric discomfort, and vomiting, with either normal or only mildly impaired responsiveness: all of them showed PPRs of types 1 to 4. PPRs are also seen in eyelid myoclonia with absences,[125] which has generally been considered to be an idiopathic generalized epilepsy syndrome, but recent studies have suggested it may be occipitally generated.[126-128]

Patients whose seizures are induced by visual stimuli such as viewing a visual pattern or television[129] or eye closure are particularly sensitive to IPS and tend to demonstrate PPR. For epileptic seizures triggered by television, photosensitivity remains the most common single mechanism.[90] Patients with seizures triggered by electronic screen games (ESGs) such as video, console, and computer games have also been reported.[130-134] Quirk et al.[135] conducted a nationwide study to identify patients who had a first seizure during or shortly after playing an ESG during two three-month periods. A total of 118 such patients were identified, 103 of whom were 7 to 19 years old. Within that age group, the annual incidence of first seizure triggered by playing ESGs (71 patients altogether) was estimated to be 1.5/100,000, representing approximately 3% of all new patients with epilepsy in this age range. Of 71 patients, 46 showed type 4 PPR, whereas 18 showed types 1 to 3 PPR (the other seven had no PPR but had recurrent seizures triggered by ESGs). Although photosensitivity is thought to play the most important role in engendering ESG-induced seizures, other circumstances, acting either singly or in combination, should be taken into consideration.[136] Examples include (1) seizure precipitation by specific cognitive activities, decision making, hand movements, and so forth; (2) seizure precipitation by nonspecific emotional factors relating to the subjects' engagement in games, such as anxiety or excitement; (3) lowering of the seizure threshold by fatigue or sleep deprivation; and (4) chance occurrence of a spontaneous seizure in a person with epilepsy while playing ESGs.

Spontaneous epileptiform abnormalities (SEAs) are reported to occur in up to 65% of patients with a PPR. Gilliam and Chiappa[137] examined seizure classifications and SEAs in 115 consecutive patients who had a PPR. A PPR was the only epileptiform abnormality in 47 patients (41%), 27 (24%) had focal SEAs, and 41 (36%) had only generalized SEAs. Seventeen patients (15%) had partial seizures and 40 (35%) had only generalized seizures, and seizure classification was strongly associated with the type of SEA. Although the PPR is often presumed to signify primary generalized epilepsy, most patients with a PPR and focal SEAs have partial seizures.

The ictal events that may accompany PPR are predominantly absence seizures, generalized tonic-clonic seizures, and myoclonic jerks, especially of the eyelids or arms.[138] Gambardella et al.[139] reported a 17-year-old girl with pure photosensitive epilepsy who showed photic-induced epileptic negative myoclonus (PPR was accompanied by loss of postural tone in both arms). They claim that negative myoclonus should be included among the ictal phenomena accompanying PPR.

Several stimulation features are known to alter the likelihood of eliciting a PPR. As described above, PPR is often associated with eye closure and is most likely to occur immediately after eye closure.[92] This effect may also result from movement of the eyelids or of the eyes themselves. In addition, eye closure may produce activation by suddenly eliminating the visual pattern and by causing the field of vision to become red-hued.[140,141]

With regard to color, saturated long-wavelength red light facilitates induction of PPR,[142,143] with the 660- to 720-nm wavelength spectrum being the only visible spectrum essential for provoking PPRs in patients with wavelength dependence.[144,145] With regard to pattern, when stimuli are presented with the eyes open, a patterned field of vision (or flickering geometric pattern) has sometimes been found to be more effective than a homogeneous field (or white-light flicker) in eliciting PPR[146–149] (see Section 4.2 below for further details).

Especially in adults without previous seizures and without a family history of seizures, PPR usually suggests a toxic, metabolic, or drug withdrawal state.[55,81,150,151] Symmetrical posterior high-amplitude spikes can be evoked at slow IPS rates in patients with diffuse encephalopathies, such as progressive myoclonic epilepsy or Creutzfeldt-Jakob disease.[60,152,153]

Several studies have demonstrated that there is a strong genetic component for photosensitivity, with recent work demonstrating that PPR may actually be an inheritable endophenotype. Doose and Gerken[99] first reported that a photoconvulsive reaction is significantly more common in the siblings of probands with a photoconvulsive reaction than in the siblings of those without (19.3% vs. 3.4%). Similarly, in the study by Waltz et al.[89] that originally categorized PPR into four types, type 4 PPRs were more prevalent in patients with epilepsy than in patients without epilepsy in whom a PPR was incidentally noted on EEG. Notably, a type 4 PPR was also noted in a high proportion (46%) of the asymptomatic siblings of patients with

epilepsy. A follow-up study showed that if one of the parents of a patient with epilepsy and PPR also had a PPR, then the asymptomatic sibling of the patient was significantly more likely to have a PPR (50%) than if neither of the parents had a PPR (15%). Recent work has begun to identify specific genes that convey risk for PPR.[154,155]

The pathophysiological mechanisms underlying PPR are unclear, but recent studies have provided some clues. A number of studies employing spatial patterns in patients with photosensitivity have suggested that PPRs are triggered from visual cortex.[156] Based on the observation that gratings that drift continuously toward the center of gaze do not provoke epileptiform discharges but those that repeatedly change their direction or phase do,[157] it has been argued that epileptiform discharges result from hypersynchrony of visual cortex.[158] Studies in patients with idiopathic photosensitive occipital epilepsy have shown significantly increased visual evoked potential amplitude, again consistent with hypersynchrony,[159,160] and these patients also have abnormally large visual evoked potential amplitudes and abnormal latencies for high-contrast visual stimuli, suggesting a failure of cortical gain control[161] (Fig. 10.9). This finding was replicated in a subsequent study in patients with idiopathic generalized epilepsy, which also found that patients show less saturation of the visual evoked potential response amplitudes at high stimulus contrasts in comparison to controls, and suggested that this may be consistent with diminished inhibition from surrounding neurons in patients, possibly due to reduced GABAergic inhibition.[162] An increase in gamma band synchronization during IPS may also occur in patients with PPR.[163–165]

Two prior studies[166,167] used EEG in combination with functional magnetic resonance imaging (fMRI) and magnetic resonance spectroscopy to study the metabolic and hemodynamic consequences of photic-stimulation-triggered and spontaneous generalized epileptiform discharges in normal subjects and patients with PPR. While there were no fMRI abnormalities specifically associated with the brief PPR seen in the patients, these patients did show four unique findings compared with normal subjects: (1) lactate levels were slightly but significantly increased in the occipital cortex in the resting state; (2) there was an increased area of visual cortex activation with photic stimulation; (3) simultaneous with the occipital cortex stimulus-induced increased fMRI signal, there were noncontiguous areas of signal attenuation, most prominent in perirolandic regions; and 4) a marked decrement (undershoot) of fMRI signal intensity occurred immediately after the photic stimulation in the occipital cortex and in the region of the posterior cingulate gyrus. These findings suggest abnormal interictal metabolism and increased vascular reactivity in the photosensitive patients. A subsequent EEG-fMRI study[168] that captured PPR in six patients with an IGE showed PPR-related increases in BOLD signal 3 seconds before the onset of the PPR, in five of the six patients involving the parietal cortex in the vicinity of the intraparietal sulcus and the premotor cortex (Fig. 10.10), followed by a deactivation of the BOLD signal at the onset of the PPR. Studies using transcranial magnetic stimulation (TMS) have demonstrated that patients with PPR have lower phosphene thresholds and steeper stimulus–response

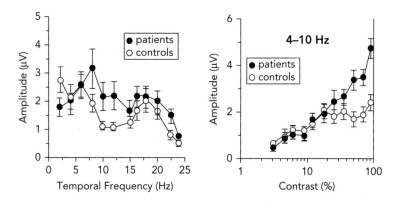

Figure 10.9. Lack of cortical contrast gain control in patients with photosensitive epilepsy. Steady-state visual evoked potentials (VEPs) were recorded as patients and control subjects were presented with flickering luminance-contrast horizontal sinusoidal black and white gratings at 2 cycles per degree. Left: Average VEP amplitude as a function of temporal flicker frequency. Control subjects have amplitude peaks at low and high frequencies, with a local minimum at 10 to 12 Hz. In contrast, photosensitive patients had substantially more activity at intermediate frequencies (10–12 Hz). Right: In the 4- to 10-Hz range, there is a marked difference in VEP amplitudes at medium-higher contrasts, with a lack of saturation of the VEP response in photosensitive patients. Error bars depict standard errors. (Porciatti V, Bonanni P, Fiorentini A, Guerrini R. Lack of cortical contrast gain control in human photosensitive epilepsy. Nat Neurosci. 2000;3[3]:259–263.)

curves than individuals without PPR or with occipital spikes only, whereas no differences were found with stimulation of motor cortex, consistent with increased excitability of the occipital but not motor cortex in these individuals.[169] Studies combining TMS of motor cortex with TMS or visual stimulation of occipital cortex have demonstrated abnormal visuomotor interactions.[170,171] Taken together, these studies suggest that the PPR is due to abnormal occipital cortex excitability that affects other regions via network interactions.

4. OTHER VISUAL STIMULATION

4.1. Eye Movements and Fixation

Various visual stimuli other than IPS may provoke paroxysmal discharges akin to PPR in susceptible individuals. For example, eye closure can provoke paroxysmal discharges in patients with photosensitivity[92,172]; indeed, eye-closure–induced paroxysmal discharges are a defining feature of some epilepsy syndromes, such as eyelid myoclonia with absences.[125,173] Spike-wave

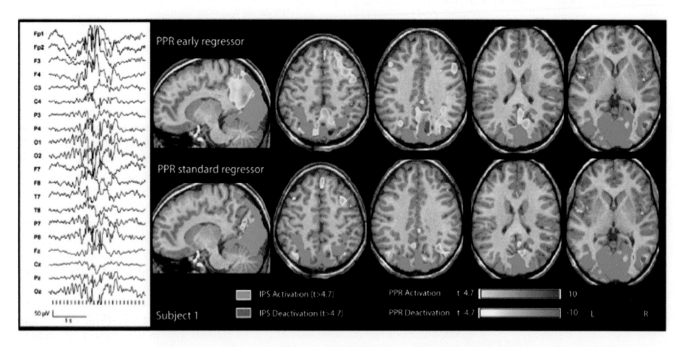

Figure 10.10. EEG-triggered fMRI showing IPS- and PPR-related changes in BOLD signal in a patient with photosensitive epilepsy. Left: EEG recording of a characteristic example of PPR during fMRI, displayed in a referential montage. Right: color-coded statistical parametric t-score maps showing IPS-related increases (green) or decreases (brown) in BOLD signal as well as PPR-related increases (yellow/red) or decreases (blue/white). The upper row shows the BOLD signal changes in association with a regressor set 3 sec before the onset of the PPR. The bottom row shows BOLD signal changes with a regressor set at the time of the PPR. IPS leads to activation of the primary visual cortex. An early PPR-related BOLD signal increase is present in the parietal cortex, more prominent on the right (consistent with the EEG in this patient), and in the right premotor cortex. With the PPR, there is deactivation in the right premotor and R>L parietal regions that were activated prior. (Moeller F, Siebner HR, Ahlgrimm N, et al. fMRI activation during spike and wave discharges evoked by photic stimulation. NeuroImage. 2009;48[4]:682–695.)

discharges associated with seizures can rarely be induced by a single-flash light stimulus.[140] Darkness may also induce paroxysmal discharges.[174,175] In particular, in fixation-off sensitivity,[176,177] paroxysmal discharges occur when the eyes are closed, in complete darkness, or when subjects are wearing Ganzfeld lenses or other devices that prevent fixation, and resolve when fixation is possible. Fixation-off sensitivity is suspected if EEG abnormalities appear and persist as long as the eyes remain closed and disappear when the eyes are opened. Fixation-off sensitivity may be as common as PPR in children younger than 12 years of age[177] and is typically seen in conditions such as idiopathic childhood epilepsy of Gastaut and Panayiotopoulos syndrome, although it has also been reported in a wide variety of other epileptic syndromes.[176–178]

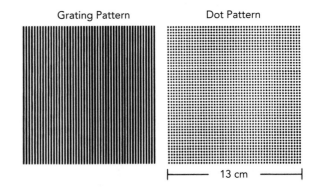

Figure 10.11. Geometric patterns used for square-type strobe-filter method. Each pattern was presented 30 cm before the eyes, resulting in its spatial frequency at 2 cycles/degree; pattern contrast is 0.98.

4.2. Pattern, Pattern Flicker, and Red Flicker Stimulation

Geometric patterns often provoke paroxysmal discharges in photosensitive epilepsy patients.[129,179–182] The incidence of paroxysmal discharges in photosensitivity patients varies widely across studies, from 5% to 72%, depending on the precise stimulation protocol[140,183]; a more recent large study of 387 patients[133] with suspected photosensitivity reported epileptiform discharges provoked by patterns in 28%, versus by IPS in 85%. However, patients who respond to patterns (particularly oscillating ones) but not IPS have also been reported.[184] The patterns that are most effective for activation consist of closely spaced lines or dots with sharply contrasting interfaces that are arranged geometrically.[185] Parallel lines or stripes with sharp edges are more epileptogenic than dot patterns[186] (Fig. 10.11), checkerboard patterns,[187] or wavy lines.[188] Studies have suggested that line patterns must have a spatial frequency between 1 and 4 cycles per degree of the visual field to induce paroxysmal discharges, and the epileptogenicity of a line pattern is also related to its contrast (between black and white lines) and overall size.[186,187] There is no clear orientation sensitivity across subjects, although individual patients may show a particular orientation selectivity.[187] Oscillation of a grating pattern greatly enhanced provocation of paroxysmal discharges; gratings oscillating in a direction orthogonal to the lines were the most effective, and the optimal oscillation frequency was in the range of 15 to 20 Hz.[157] In contrast, gratings drifting in one direction with a constant velocity were noted to be less effective in provoking epileptiform discharges.[157] Flickering gratings are also effective in provoking a photoconvulsive response, with one study demonstrating that 15-Hz flickering gratings were much more effective than 15-Hz IPS.[148] For dot patterns, a spatial frequency of 1.5 to 2.1 cycles/degree (Fig. 10.12) and a flicker frequency of 15 to 20 Hz is optimal for evoking discharges.[189] Paroxysmal discharges induced by viewing usually arise from the occipital area, suggesting that they may arise primarily in an epileptogenic visual cortex.[141,180,186] A study exploring cortical oscillatory patterns in response to static gratings in normal subjects demonstrated that gratings of 2 to 4 cycles/degree that are most likely to produce epileptiform discharges in photosensitive epilepsy patients also produce maximal gamma synchronization (in comparison to other spatial frequencies) and visual discomfort in healthy subjects with no prior neurological history.[190]

Paroxysmal discharges may be evoked by red light alone.[184,191] It has also been demonstrated that full-field red-flicker stimuli are particularly effective in provoking a paroxysmal response in photosensitive epilepsy patients,[142,147,148,192,193] even when stimulation is applied at a decreased luminance of 10 to 20 cd/m²; as discussed previously, the 660- to 720-nm

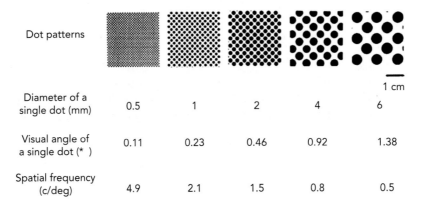

Dot patterns					
Diameter of a single dot (mm)	0.5	1	2	4	6
Visual angle of a single dot (°)	0.11	0.23	0.46	0.92	1.38
Spatial frequency (c/deg)	4.9	2.1	1.5	0.8	0.5

Figure 10.12. Dot patterns used to assess photosensitivity. The optimal spatial frequency for elicitation of PPR is 1.5 to 2.1 cycles/degree. (Takahashi T, Tsukahara Y. Photoparoxysmal response elicited by flickering dot pattern stimulation and its optimal spatial frequency of provocation. Electroencephalogr Clin Neurophysiol. 1998;106[1]:40–43.)

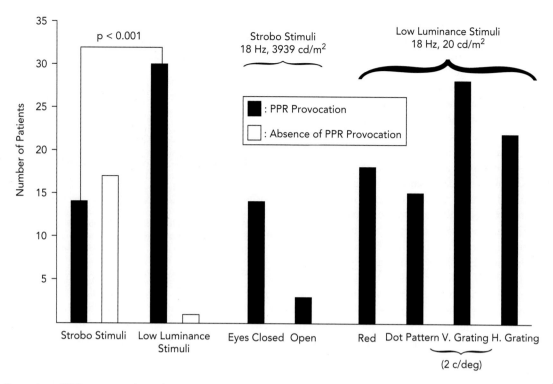

Figure 10.13. Comparison of PPR provocation by stroboscopic IPS and low-luminance visual stimuli (flickering full-field red light, dot pattern, vertical and horizontal gratings) in 31 photosensitive patients. Stroboscopic IPS failed to elicit PPR in 17 of the 31 patients, whereas low-luminance visual stimuli elicited PPR in all but one. (Takahashi T, Nakasato N, Yokoyama H, Tsukahara Y. Low-luminance visual stimuli compared with stroboscopic IPS in eliciting PPR in photosensitive patients. Epilepsia. 1999;40[Suppl 4]:44–49.)

wavelength spectrum is the only visible spectrum essential for provoking PPRs in patients with wavelength dependence.[144,145] Red-flicker stimuli of 15 Hz are significantly more effective in provoking a photoconvulsive response than 15-Hz IPS, at least with the eyes open,[147] or light of any other color.[142] Of note, red light with a wavelength of more than 600 nm is required, as red light at shorter wavelengths (580 nm) does not have increased provocative effects.[188]

The utility of an approach combining IPS with flickering low-luminance color and pattern stimuli was demonstrated by Takahashi et al.,[194] who reported that low-luminance flickering (18 Hz) red light, flickering dot, or flickering vertical or horizontal gratings produced a type 4 PPR in 30 of 31 photosensitive patients, whereas conventional 18-Hz IPS (with eyes both open and closed) produced a type 4 PPR in only 14 of 31 patients (Fig. 10.13). The importance of flickering color/pattern stimuli was also demonstrated in the Pokémon (Pocket Monsters) incident in Japan in December 1997, when a TV cartoon containing a 4-sec red/blue sequence flashing at 12 Hz caused simultaneous seizures in 685 Japanese children,[195] only 24% of whom had ever suffered a prior seizure. Subsequent studies in photosensitive patients demonstrated that alternating red/cyan flicker is more likely to produce a PPR than simple red flicker[196,197] or other colors or color combinations, particularly when the stimulation occurs at lower frequencies (<20 Hz[197]). The latter study thus supported the hypothesis that there are two pathophysiological mechanisms for human photosensitivity that may contribute to a PPR: one dependent purely on quantity of light or luminance changes, and the other dependent on the wavelength.[145]

5. OTHER STIMULATION

Epileptic seizures are referred to as *reflex* if they are objectively and consistently evoked by a specific sensory or cognitive stimulus.[198] Visually evoked seizures are by far the most common; in one large case series of 1,000 consecutive outpatients, 6.5% were found to have reflex seizures, and 5% were photosensitive.[199] A prevalence of 8.9% has been reported in a study from Asian countries, with the most common provoking factors being eating, mental calculations, and bathing.[200] Overall, a wide variety of epileptogenic stimuli have been reported, ranging from simple stimuli such as auditory tones or somatosensory tactile stimulation, more complex stimuli such as hot water or eating, or stimuli with a cognitive component such as startle, music, reading, or praxis, all presumably leading to seizures due to changes in cerebral structural and functional connectivity.[198,200,201] Although the effects of these different stimuli on the EEG of epilepsy patients have been explored across a variety of studies, systematic protocols for testing these other domains have not been defined (although see Matsuoka et al.[202]), the reliability of EEG activation with repeated exposures for single subjects at a population level is unclear, and an organized, quantitative understanding of the rate of provocation of epileptiform abnormalities and the sensitivity and specificity of these tests across different epilepsy conditions is not available. Consequently, these other activation procedures are not widely, routinely, or systematically used, although certainly tailored stimulation can be attempted in individual patients who report specific reliable seizure-inducing stimuli.

An additional stimulation procedure that could be used to directly test cortical excitability is TMS,[203] particularly when combined with EEG. Preliminary TMS-EEG studies have suggested that patients with epilepsy may have abnormalities in TMS-evoked EEG potentials in comparison to healthy controls.[204–207] However appealing in theory,[208] the utility of TMS-EEG in the diagnosis and management of epilepsy needs significant further study.

6. CONCLUDING REMARKS

In theory, the greater the number of different activation methods used in EEG evaluation of an epilepsy patient, the greater the chance of obtaining abnormal findings. However, the specificity of these findings for epilepsy is uncertain. Furthermore, from a practical point of view, desirable activations are those methods that can be carried out easily and systematically, in a short time frame, with affordable equipment, without undesirable side effects for patients, and with reliable and predictive results. At this time, HV and IPS are the most widely used activation methods and have an extensive body of literature supporting them. Visual types of stimulation with flickering patterns and red lights also are useful, particularly when evaluating patients with presumed photosensitive epilepsy. While a wide variety of further activation methods are possible, the clinical utility of these procedures needs further study before widespread implementation can be recommended. However, specific activation procedures may be useful in patients who report consistent provoking stimuli, as in various reflex epilepsies.

REFERENCES

1. Foerster O. Hyperventilationsepilepsie. *Zbl Ges Neurol Psychiatr.* 1924;38:289–293.
2. Nims LF, Gibbs EL, Lennox WG, Gibbs FA, Williams D. Adjustment of acid-base balance of patients with petit mal epilepsy to overventilation. *Arch Neurol Psychiatry.* 1940;43(2):262–269.
3. Morrice JKW. Slow wave production in the EEG, with reference to hyperpnoea, carbon dioxide and autonomic balance. *Electroencephalogr Clin Neurophysiol.* 1956;8(1):49–72.
4. Achenbach-Ng J, Siao TC, Mavroudakis N, Chiappa KH, Kiers L. Effects of routine hyperventilation on PCO2 and PO2 in normal subjects: implications for EEG interpretations. *J Clin Neurophysiol.* 1994;11(2):220–225.
5. Dalby MA. Epilepsy and 3 per second spike and wave rhythms. A clinical, electroencephalographic and prognostic analysis of 346 patients. *Acta Neurol Scand.* 1969:Suppl 40:3+.
6. Kiloh LG, McComas AJ, Osselton JW. *Clinical Electroencephalography.* Oxford: Butterworth-Heinemann; 1972.
7. Miley CE, Forster FM. Activation of partial complex seizures by hyperventilation. *Arch Neurol.* 1977;34(6):371–373.
8. Klein KM, Knake S, Hamer HM, Ziegler A, Oertel WH, Rosenow F. Sleep but not hyperventilation increases the sensitivity of the EEG in patients with temporal lobe epilepsy. *Epilepsy Res.* 2003;56(1):43–49.
9. Holmes MD, Dewaraja AS, Vanhatalo S. Does hyperventilation elicit epileptic seizures? *Epilepsia.* 2004;45(6):618–620.
10. Guaranha MSB, Garzon E, Buchpiguel CA, Tazima S, Yacubian EMT, Sakamoto AC. Hyperventilation revisited: physiological effects and efficacy on focal seizure activation in the era of video-EEG monitoring. *Epilepsia.* 2005;46(1):69–75.
11. Jonas J, Vignal J-P, Baumann C, et al. Effect of hyperventilation on seizure activation: potentiation by antiepileptic drug tapering. *J Neurol Neurosurg Psychiatry.* 2011;82(8):928–930.
12. Kane N, Grocott L, Kandler R, Lawrence S, Pang C. Hyperventilation during electroencephalography: safety and efficacy. *Seizure.* 2014;23(2):129–134.
13. Arain AM, Arbogast PG, Abou-Khalil BW. Utility of daily supervised hyperventilation during long-term video-EEG monitoring. *J Clin Neurophysiol.* 2009;26(1):17–20.
14. Gibbs FA, Gibbs EL, Lennox WG. Electroencephalographic response to overventilation and its relation to age. *J Pediatr.* 1943;23(5):497–505.
15. Gotoh F, Meyer JS, Takagi Y. Cerebral effects of hyperventilation in man. *Arch Neurol.* 1965;12(4):410–423.
16. Yamatani M, Konishi T, Murakami M, Okuda T. Hyperventilation activation on EEG recording in childhood. *Epilepsia.* 1994;35(6):1199–1203.
17. Duarte J, Markus H, Harrison MJG. Changes in cerebral blood flow as monitored by transcranial Doppler during voluntary hyperventilation and their effect on the electroencephalogram. *J Neuroimag.* 1995;5(4):209–211.
18. Fisch BC, So EL. Activation procedures. In: Ebersole JS, Pedley TA, eds. *Current Practice of Clinical Electroencephalography.* 3rd ed. Philadelphia, PA: Lippincott Williams & Wilkins; 2003:246–270.
19. Sherwin I. Hyperventilation: mode of action and application in electroencephalography. *Am J EEG Technol.* 1984;24(4):201–211.
20. Patel VM, Maulsby RL. How hyperventilation alters the electroencephalogram: a review of controversial viewpoints emphasizing neurophysiological mechanisms. *J Clin Neurophysiol.* 1987;4(2):101–120.
21. Niedermeyer E. *The Generalized Epilepsies; a Clinical Electroencephalographic Study.* Springfield, IL: Charles C Thomas; 1972.
22. Esquivel E, Chaussain M, Plouin P, Ponsot G, Arthuis M. Physical exercise and voluntary hyperventilation in childhood absence epilepsy. *Electroencephalogr Clin Neurophysiol.* 1991;79(2):127–132.
23. Niedermeyer E. Focal and generalized seizure discharges in the electroencephalogram and their response to intravenous diazepam. *Int Med Dig.* 1972;7:49–61.
24. Muhle H, Ettle E, Boor R, Stephani U, Siniatchkin M. Valproate reduces spontaneous generalized spikes and waves but not photoparoxysmal reactions in patients with idiopathic generalized epilepsies. *Epilepsia.* 2011;52(7):1297–1302.
25. Yang X-F, Shi X-Y, Ju J, et al. 5% CO_2 inhalation suppresses hyperventilation-induced absence seizures in children. *Epilepsy Res.* 2014;108(2):345–348.
26. Bostem F. Hyperventilation. In: Rémond A, ed. *Handbook of Electroencephalography and Clinical Neurophysiology: Vol. 6: The Normal EEG Throughout Life: Part A: The EEG of the Waking Adult.* Amsterdam: Elsevier; 1976:74–88.
27. Ziegler DK, Hassanein RS, Dick AR. Effect of age and depth of hyperventilation on a quantitative electroencephalographic response. *Clin EEG Neurosci.* 1975;6(4):184–190.
28. Petersén I, Eeg-Olofsson O. The development of the electroencephalogram in normal children from the age of 1 through 15 years—Non-paroxysmal activity. *Neuropediatrics.* 1971;2(03):247–304.
29. Kellaway P. An orderly approach to visual analysis: parameters of the normal EEG in adults and chilren. In: Klass DW, Daly DD, eds. *Current Practice of Clinical Electroencephalography.* New York: Raven Press; 1979:69–147.
30. Bickford RG. Activation procedures and special electrodes. In: Klass DW, Daly DD, eds. *Current Practice of Clinical Electroencephalography.* New York: Raven Press; 1979:269–305.
31. Davis HH, Wallace WL. Factors affecting changes produced in electroencephalogram by standardized hyperventilation. *Arch Neurol Psychiatry.* 1942;47(4):606–625.
32. Billinger TW, Frank GS. Effects of posture on EEG slowing during hyperventilation. *Am J EEG Technol.* 1969;9(1):22–27.
33. Engel J. A practical guide for routine EEG studies in epilepsy. *J Clin Neurophysiol.* 1984;1(2):109–142.
34. Kodama N, Aoki Y, Hiraga H, Wada T, Suzuki J. Electroencephalographic findings in children with moyamoya disease. *Arch Neurol.* 1979;36(1):16–19.
35. Kameyama M, Shirane R, Tsurumi Y, et al. Evaluation of cerebral blood flow and metabolism in childhood Moyamoya disease: an investigation into "re-build-up" on EEG by positron CT. *Childs Nerv Syst.* 1986;2(3):130–133.
36. Dlamini N, Goyal S, Jarosz J, Hampton T, Siddiqui A, Hughes E. Paroxysmal episodes, "re-build up" phenomenon and Moyamoya disease. *Epileptic Disord.* 2009;11(4):324–328.
37. Cho A, Chae J-H, Kim HM, et al. Electroencephalography in pediatric moyamoya disease: reappraisal of clinical value. *Childs Nerv Syst.* 2013;30(3):449–459.
38. Benbadis SR, Johnson K, Anthony K, et al. Induction of psychogenic non-epileptic seizures without placebo. *Neurology.* 2000;55(12):1904–1905.

39. McGonigal A, Oto M, Russell AJC, Greene J, Duncan R. Outpatient video EEG recording in the diagnosis of non-epileptic seizures: a randomised controlled trial of simple suggestion techniques. *J Neurol Neurosurg Psychiatry*. 2002;72(4):549–551.

40. Hoepner R, Labudda K, Schoendienst M, May TW, Bien CG, Brandt C. Informing patients about the impact of provocation methods increases the rate of psychogenic nonepileptic seizures during EEG recording. *Epilepsy Behav EB*. 2013;28(3):457–459.

41. Popkirov S, Grönheit W, Wellmer J. Hyperventilation and photic stimulation are useful additions to a placebo-based suggestive seizure induction protocol in patients with psychogenic nonepileptic seizures. *Epilepsy Behav EB*. 2015;46:88–90.

42. Sinha SR, Sullivan L, Sabau D, et al. American Clinical Neurophysiology Society. http://www.acns.org/UserFiles/file/EEGGuideline1Tech_final-rev20160411clean_v1.pdf. Accessed September 18, 2016.

43. Craciun L, Varga ET, Mindruta I, et al. Diagnostic yield of five minutes compared to three minutes hyperventilation during electroencephalography. *Seizure*. 2015;30:90–92.

44. Epstein MA, Duchowny M, Jayakar P, Resnick TJ, Alvarez LA. Altered responsiveness during hyperventilation-induced EEG slowing: a non-epileptic phenomenon in normal children. *Epilepsia*. 1994;35(6):1204–1207.

45. Lum LM, Connolly MB, Farrell K, Wong PK. Hyperventilation-induced high-amplitude rhythmic slowing with altered awareness: a video-EEG comparison with absence seizures. *Epilepsia*. 2002;43(11):1372–1378.

46. Barker A, Ng J, Rittey CD, Kandler RH, Mordekar SR. Outcome of children with hyperventilation-induced high-amplitude rhythmic slow activity with altered awareness. *Dev Med Child Neurol*. 2012;54(11):1001–1005.

47. Adrian ED, Matthews B. The Berger rhythm: potential changes from the occipital lobes in man. *Brain*. 1934;57:355–385.

48. Bickford RG, Daly D, Keith HM. Convulsive effects of light stimulation in children. *AMA Am J Dis Child*. 1953;86(2):170–183.

49. Walter WG, Dovey VJ, Shipton H, others. Analysis of the electrical response of the human cortex to photic stimulation. *Nature*. 1946;158(4016):540–541.

50. Kasteleijn-Nolst Trenité D, Rubboli G, Hirsch E, et al. Methodology of photic stimulation revisited: updated European algorithm for visual stimulation in the EEG laboratory. *Epilepsia*. 2012;53(1):16–24.

51. Chatrian GE, Bergamini L, Dondey M, Klass DW, Lennox-Buchthal M, Petersen I. A glossary of terms most commonly used by clinical electroencephalographers. *Electroencephalogr Clin Neurophysiol*. 1974;37(5):538–548.

52. Schwab K, Ligges C, Jungmann T, Hilgenfeld B, Haueisen J, Witte H. Alpha entrainment in human electroencephalogram and magnetoencephalogram recordings. *Neuroreport*. 2006;17(17):1829–1833.

53. Ellingson RJ. Cortical electrical responses to visual stimulation in the human infant. *Electroencephalogr Clin Neurophysiol*. 1960;12(3):663–677.

54. Walter VJ, Walter WG. The effect of physical stimuli on the EEG. *EEG Clin Neurophysiol*. 1949;(Suppl. no. 2):60.

55. Kooi KA, Tucker RP, Marshall RE. *Fundamentals of Electroencephalography*. New York: HarperCollins Publishers; 1978.

56. Pampiglione G, Harden A. So-called neuronal ceroid lipofuscinosis neurophysiological studies in 60 children. *J Neurol Neurosurg Psychiatry*. 1977;40(4):323–330.

57. Pinsard N, Livet MO, Saint-Jean M. [A case of cerebral lipidosis with an atypical presentation (author's transl)]. *Rev Électroencéphalographie Neurophysiol Clin*. 1978;8(1):175–179.

58. Shih JJ, Thompson SW. Lambda waves: incidence and relationship to photic driving. *Brain Topogr*. 1998;10(4):265–272.

59. Tatum WO, Ly RC, Sluzewska-Niedzwiedz M, Shih JJ. Lambda waves and occipital generators. *Clin EEG Neurosci*. 2013;44(4):307–312.

60. Coull BM, Pedley TA. Intermittent photic stimulation. Clinical usefulness of non-convulsive responses. *Electroencephalogr Clin Neurophysiol*. 1978;44(3):353–363.

61. Drake ME, Shy KE, Liss L. Quantitation of photic driving in dementia with normal EEG. *Clin EEG Electroencephalogr*. 1989;20(3):153–155.

62. Politoff AL, Monson N, Hass P, Stadter R. Decreased alpha bandwidth responsiveness to photic driving in Alzheimer disease. *Electroencephalogr Clin Neurophysiol*. 1992;82(1):45–52.

63. Rice DM, Potkin SG, Jin Y, et al. EEG alpha photic driving abnormalities in chronic schizophrenia. *Psychiatry Res*. 1989;30(3):313–324.

64. Jin Y, Potkin SG, Sandman CA, Bunney WE. Electroencephalographic photic driving in patients with schizophrenia and depression. *Biol Psychiatry*. 1997;41(4):496–499.

65. Golla FL, Winter AL. Analysis of cerebral responses to flicker in patients complaining of episodic headache. *Electroencephalogr Clin Neurophysiol*. 1959;11(3):539–549.

66. Smyth VO, Winter AL. The EEG in migraine. *Electroencephalogr Clin Neurophysiol*. 1964;16:194–202.

67. Simon RH, Zimmerman AW, Tasman A, Hale MS. Spectral analysis of photic stimulation in migraine. *Electroencephalogr Clin Neurophysiol*. 1982;53(3):270–276.

68. Gronseth GS, Greenberg MK. The utility of the electroencephalogram in the evaluation of patients presenting with headache: a review of the literature. *Neurology*. 1995;45(7):1263–1267.

69. Fogang Y, Gérard P, De Pasqua V, et al. Analysis and clinical correlates of 20 Hz photic driving on routine EEG in migraine. *Acta Neurol Belg*. 2015;115(1):39–45.

70. Gastaut H, Rémond A. L'activation de l'electroencephalogramme dans les affections cerebrales non epileptogenes (vers une neurophysiologie clinique). *Rev Neurol*. 1949;81:594–598.

71. Bickford RG, Sem-Jacobsen CW, White PT, Daly D. Some observations on the mechanism of photic and photometrazol activation. *Electroencephalogr Clin Neurophysiol*. 1952;4(3):275–282.

72. Niedermeyer E, Fineyre F, Riley T, Bird B. Myoclonus and the electroencephalogram, a review. *Clin EEG Electroencephalogr*. 1979;10(2):75–95.

73. Gastaut H, Trevisan C, Naquet R. Diagnostic value of electroencephalographic abnormalities provoked by intermittent photic stimulation. *Electroencephalogr Clin Neurophysiol*. 1958;10:94–195.

74. Melsen S. The value of photic stimulation in the diagnosis of epilepsy. *J Nerv Ment Dis*. 1959;128(6):508–519.

75. Kooi KA, Thomas MH, Mortenson FN. Photoconvulsive and photomyoclonic responses in adults An appraisal of their clinical significance. *Neurology*. 1960;10(12):1051–1051.

76. Small JG. Photoconvulsive and photomyoclonic responses in psychiatric patients. *Clin Electroencephalogr*. 1971;2:78–88.

77. Reilly EL, Peters JF. Relationship of some varieties of electroencephalographic photosensitivity to clinical convulsive disorders. *Neurology*. 1973;23(10):1050–1057.

78. Newmark ME, Penry JK. *Photosensitivity and Epilepsy: A Review*. Philadelphia, PA: Lippincott Williams & Wilkins; 1979.

79. Victor M. The role of alcohol in the production of seizures. In: Niedermeyer E, ed. *Modern Trends in Pharmacopsychiatry*. Vol. 4. Basel: S. Karger AG; 1970:185–199.

80. Fisch BJ, Hauser WA, Brust JCM, et al. The EEG response to diffuse and patterned photic stimulation during acute untreated alcohol withdrawal. *Neurology*. 1989;39(3):434–434.

81. Wikler A, Essig CF. Withdrawal seizures following chronic intoxication with barbiturates and other sedative drugs. In: Niedermeyer E, ed. *Modern Trends in Pharmacopsychiatry*. Vol. 4. Basel: S. Karger AG; 1970:170–184.

82. De Stegge BM, van Putten MJ. A patient with a transient photomyogenic response. *Clin Neurophysiol*. 2010;121(1):118–120.

83. Moccia M, Erro R, Nicolella E, Striano P, Striano S. Extreme startle and photomyoclonic response in severe hypocalcaemia. *Epileptic Disord*. 2014;16(1):84–87.

84. Jayakar P, Chiappa KH. Clinical correlations of photoparoxysmal responses. *Electroencephalogr Clin Neurophysiol*. 1990;75(3):251–254.

85. Puglia JF, Brenner RP, Soso MJ. Relationship between prolonged and self-limited photoparoxysmal responses and seizure incidence: study and review. *J Clin Neurophysiol*. 1992;9(1):137–144.

86. Nagarajan L, Kulkarni A, Palumbo-Clark L, et al. Photoparoxysmal responses in children: their characteristics and clinical correlates. *Pediatr Neurol*. 2003;29(3):222–226.

87. Hishikawa Y, Yamamoto J, Furuya E, Yamada Y, Miyazaki K, Kaneko Z. Photosensitive epilepsy: relationships between the visual evoked responses and the epileptiform discharges induced by intermittent photic stimulation. *Electroencephalogr Clin Neurophysiol*. 1967;23(4):320–334.

88. Maheshwari MC, Jeavons PM. The clinical significance of occipital spikes as a sole response to intermittent photic stimulation. *Electroencephalogr Clin Neurophysiol*. 1975;39(1):93–95.

89. Waltz S, Christen H-J, Doose H. The different patterns of the photoparoxysmal response—a genetic study. *Electroencephalogr Clin Neurophysiol*. 1992;83(2):138–145.

90. Harding GFA, Harding PF. Televised material and photosensitive epilepsy. *Epilepsia*. 1999;40(s4):65–69.

91. Topalkara K, Alarcón G, Binnie CD. Effects of flash frequency and repetition of intermittent photic stimulation on photoparoxysmal responses. *Seizure*. 1998;7(3):249–255.

92. Panayiotopoulos CP. Effectiveness of photic stimulation on various eye-states in photosensitive epilepsy. *J Neurol Sci*. 1974;23(2):165–173.

93. Kasteleijn-Nolst Trenité DG. Photosensitivity in epilepsy. Electrophysiological and clinical correlates. *Acta Neurol Scand Suppl*. 1989;125:3–49.

94. Sato S, Dreifuss FE, Penry JK. Photic sensitivity of children with absence seizures in slow wave sleep. *Electroencephalogr Clin Neurophysiol.* 1975;39(5):479–489.

95. Jeavons PM, Harding GF. *Photosensitive Epilepsy: A Review of the Literature and a Study of 460 Patients.* London: Heinemann Educational Books; 1975.

96. Van Egmond P, Binnie CD, Veldhuizen R. The effect of background illumination on sensitivity to intermittent photic stimulation. *Electroencephalogr Clin Neurophysiol.* 1980;48(5):599–601.

97. Specchio N, Kasteleijn-Nolst Trenité DGA, Piccioli M, et al. Diagnosing photosensitive epilepsy: fancy new versus old-fashioned techniques in patients with different epileptic syndromes. *Brain Dev.* 2011;33(4):294–300.

98. Wadlington WB, Riley HD. Light-induced seizures. *J Pediatr.* 1965;66(2):300–312.

99. Doose H, Gerken H. On the genetics of EEG anomalies in childhood(1)—IV. Photoconvulsive reaction. *Neuropediatrics.* 1973;4(02):162–171.

100. Wolf P, Goosses R. Relation of photosensitivity to epileptic syndromes. *J Neurol Neurosurg Psychiatry.* 1986;49(12):1386–1391.

101. Eeg-Olofsson O, Petersén I, Selldén U. The development of the electroencephalogram in normal children from the age of 1 through 15 years—Paroxysmal activity. *Neuropediatrics.* 1971;2(04):375–404.

102. Papatheophilou R, Turland DN. The electroencephalogram of normal adolescent males: visual assessment and relationship with other variables. *Dev Med Child Neurol.* 1976;18(5):603–619.

103. De Bittencourt PR. Photosensitivity: the magnitude of the problem. *Epilepsia.* 2004;45(s1):30–34.

104. Gregory RP, Oates T, Merry RT. Electroencephalogram epileptiform abnormalities in candidates for aircrew training. *Electroencephalogr Clin Neurophysiol.* 1993;86(1):75–77.

105. Hendriksen IJ, Elderson A. The use of EEG in aircrew selection. *Aviat Space Environ Med.* 2001;72(11):1025–1033.

106. Roy AK, Pinheiro L, Rajesh SV. Prevalence of photosensitivity—an Indian experience. *Neurol India.* 2003;51(2):241–243.

107. Kasteleijn-Nolst Trenité DG. Intermittent photic stimulation as an activation method for electroencephalographic screening of aircrew applicants. *Epilepsy Behav EB.* 2005;6(1):21–26.

108. Trojaborg W. EEG abnormalities in 5,893 jet pilot applicants registered in a 20-year period. *Clin EEG Electroencephalogr.* 1992;23(2):72–78.

109. Jeavons PM. The use of photic stimulation in clinical electroencephalography. *Proc Electrophysiol Technol Assoc.* 1969;16:225.

110. Adamolekun B, Familusi JB, Olayinka B, Levy LF. The influence of racial and environmental factors on EEG photoparoxysmal responses in Zimbabwe. *Acta Neurol Scand.* 1998;97(1):8–12.

111. Shiraishi H, Fujiwara T, Inoue Y, Yagi K. Photosensitivity in relation to epileptic syndromes: a survey from an epilepsy center in Japan. *Epilepsia.* 2001;42(3):393–397.

112. Hughes JR. The photoparoxysmal response: the probable cause of attacks during video games. *Clin EEG Neurosci.* 2008;39(1):1–7.

113. Binelli S, Ragona F, Canafoglia L, et al. Electroencephalographic (EEG) photoparoxysmal responses under 5 years of age: diagnostic implications and peculiarities. *J Child Neurol.* 2015;30(13):1824–1830.

114. Whitehead K, Sherratt M, Kandler R, Lawrence S, Pang C. Photic stimulation during electroencephalography: efficacy and safety in an unselected cohort of patients referred to UK neurophysiology departments. *Seizure.* 2016;34:29–34.

115. De Graaf AS, Lombard CJ, Claassen DA. Influence of ethnic and geographic factors on the classic photoparoxysmal response in the electroencephalogram of epilepsy patients. *Epilepsia.* 1995;36(3):219–223.

116. Danesi MA. Photoparoxysmal discharges among patients investigated after a single seizure. *Electroencephalogr Clin Neurophysiol.* 1987;67(6):588–590.

117. Quirk JA, Fish DR, Smith SJ, Sander JW, Shorvon SD, Allen PJ. Incidence of photosensitive epilepsy: a prospective national study. *Electroencephalogr Clin Neurophysiol.* 1995;95(4):260–267.

118. Stevens JR. Central and peripheral factors in epileptic discharge: clinical studies. *Arch Neurol.* 1962;7(4):330–338.

119. Stephani U, Tauer U, Koeleman B, Pinto D, Neubauer BA, Lindhout D. Genetics of photosensitivity (photoparoxysmal response): a review. *Epilepsia.* 2004;45(s1):19–23.

120. Appleton R, Beirne M, Acomb B. Photosensitivity in juvenile myoclonic epilepsy. *Seizure.* 2000;9(2):108–111.

121. Rubboli G, Meletti S, Gardella E, et al. Photic reflex myoclonus: a neurophysiological study in progressive myoclonus epilepsies. *Epilepsia.* 1999;40:50–58.

122. De Haan G-J, Halley DJJ, Doelman JC, et al. Univerricht-Lundborg disease: underdiagnosed in the Netherlands. *Epilepsia.* 2004;45(9):1061–1063.

123. Guerrini R, Genton P. Epileptic syndromes and visually induced seizures. *Epilepsia.* 2004;45(s1):14–18.

124. Guerrini R, Dravet C, Genton P, et al. Idiopathic photosensitive occipital lobe epilepsy. *Epilepsia.* 1995;36(9):883–891.

125. Appleton RE, Panayiotopoulos CP, Acomb BA, Beirne M. Eyelid myoclonia with typical absences: an epilepsy syndrome. *J Neurol Neurosurg Psychiatry.* 1993;56(12):1312–1316.

126. Viravan S, Go C, Ochi A, Akiyama T, Carter Snead O, Otsubo H. Jeavons syndrome existing as occipital cortex initiating generalized epilepsy. *Epilepsia.* 2011;52(7):1273–1279.

127. Vaudano AE, Ruggieri A, Tondelli M, et al. The visual system in eyelid myoclonia with absences. *Ann Neurol.* 2014;76(3):412–427.

128. Giráldez BG, Serratosa JM. Jeavons syndrome as an occipital cortex initiated generalized epilepsy: further evidence from a patient with a photic-induced occipital seizure. *Seizure.* 2015;32:72–74.

129. Wilkins AJ, Darby CE, Binnie CD, Stefansson SB, Jeavons PM, Harding GF. Television epilepsy—the role of pattern. *Electroencephalogr Clin Neurophysiol.* 1979;47(2):163–171.

130. Rushton DN. "Space invader" epilepsy. *Lancet Lond Engl.* 1981;1(8218):501.

131. Ferrie CD, De Marco P, Grünewald RA, Giannakodimos S, Panayiotopoulos CP. Video game-induced seizures. *J Neurol Neurosurg Psychiatry.* 1994;57(8):925–931.

132. Fylan F, Harding GF, Edson AS, Webb RM. Mechanisms of video-game epilepsy. *Epilepsia.* 1999;40 Suppl 4:28–30.

133. Kasteleijn-Nolst Trenité DG, da Silva AM, Ricci S, et al. Video-game epilepsy: a European study. *Epilepsia.* 1999;40 Suppl 4:70–74.

134. Kasteleijn-Nolst Trenité DGA, Martins da Silva A, Ricci S, et al. Video games are exciting: a European study of video game-induced seizures and epilepsy. *Epileptic Disord.* 2002;4(2):121–128.

135. Quirk JA, Fish DR, Smith SJ, Sander JW, Shorvon SD, Allen PJ. First seizures associated with playing electronic screen games: a community-based study in Great Britain. *Ann Neurol.* 1995;37(6):733–737.

136. Binnie CD, Harding GF, Richens A, Wilkins A. Video games and epileptic seizures—a consensus statement. Video-Game Epilepsy Consensus Group. *Seizure.* 1994;3(4):245–246.

137. Gilliam FG, Chiappa KH. Significance of spontaneous epileptiform abnormalities associated with a photoparoxysmal response. *Neurology.* 1995;45(3 Pt 1):453–456.

138. Kasteleijn-Nolst Trenité DG, Binnie CD, Meinardi H. Photosensitive patients: symptoms and signs during intermittent photic stimulation and their relation to seizures in daily life. *J Neurol Neurosurg Psychiatry.* 1987;50(11):1546–1549.

139. Gambardella A, Aguglia U, Oliveri RL, Pucci F, Zappia M, Quattrone A. Photic-induced epileptic negative myoclonus: a case report. *Epilepsia.* 1996;37(5):492–494.

140. Bickford RG, Klass DW. Sensory precipitation and reflex mechanisms. In: Jasper HH, Ward, AA Pope A, eds. *Basic Mechanisms of the Epilepsies.* Boston, MA: Little, Brown and Company; 1969:543–564.

141. Takahashi T, Tsukahara Y. Generalized paroxysmal discharges induced by visual stimuli and eye movements. *Tohoku J Exp Med.* 1975;115(1):1–10.

142. Takahashi T, Tsukahara Y. Influence of color on the photoconvulsive response. *Electroencephalogr Clin Neurophysiol.* 1976;41(2):124–136.

143. Takahashi T, Tsukahara Y. Usefulness of blue sunglasses in photosensitive epilepsy. *Epilepsia.* 1992;33(3):517–521.

144. Takahashi Y, Fujiwara T, Yagi K, Seino M. Wavelength specificity of photoparoxysmal responses in idiopathic generalized epilepsy. *Epilepsia.* 1995;36(11):1084–1088.

145. Takahashi Y, Fujiwara T, Yagi K, Seino M. Wavelength dependence of photoparoxysmal responses in photosensitive patients with epilepsy. *Epilepsia.* 1999;40:23–27.

146. Jeavons PM, Harding GFA, Panayiotopoulos CP, Drasdo N. The effect of geometric patterns combined with intermittent photic stimulation in photosensitive epilepsy. *Electroencephalogr Clin Neurophysiol.* 1972;33(2):221–224.

147. Takahashi T, Tsukahara Y. Photoconvulsive responses induced by use of "visual stimulator." *Tohoku J Exp Med.* 1980;130(3):273–281.

148. Takahashi T, Tsukahara Y, Kaneda S. EEG activation by use of stroboscope and visual stimulator SLS-5100. *Tohoku J Exp Med.* 1980;130(4):403–409.

149. Takahashi T, Tsukahara Y, Kaneda S. Influence of pattern and red color on the photoconvulsive response and the photic driving. *Tohoku J Exp Med.* 1981;133(2):129–137.

150. Solomon S, Fine D. The precipitation of seizures by photic stimulation in a patient with hypoparathyroidism. *J Nerv Ment Dis.* 1960;130(3):253–260.

151. Victor M, Brausch C. The role of abstinence in the genesis of alcoholic epilepsy. *Epilepsia.* 1967;8(1):1–20.

152. Gastaut H. Introduction to the study of organic generalized epilepsies. In: Gastaut H, Jasper H, Bancaud J, Waltregny A, eds. *The Physiopathogenesis of the Epilepsies.* Springfield, IL: Charles C Thomas; 1969:147–157.
153. Lee RG, Blair RDG. Evolution of EEG and visual evoked response changes in Jakob-Creutzfeldt disease. *Electroencephalogr Clin Neurophysiol.* 1973;35(2):133–142.
154. Lorenz S, Taylor KP, Gehrmann A, et al. Association of BRD2 polymorphisms with photoparoxysmal response. *Neurosci Lett.* 2006;400(1-2):135–139.
155. Galizia EC, Myers CT, Leu C, et al. CHD2 variants are a risk factor for photosensitivity in epilepsy. *Brain J Neurol.* 2015;138(Pt 5):1198–1207.
156. Wilkins AJ, Bonanni P, Porciatti V, Guerrini R. Physiology of human photosensitivity. *Epilepsia.* 2004;45(Suppl 1):7–13.
157. Binnie CD, Findlay J, Wilkins AJ. Mechanisms of epileptogenesis in photosensitive epilepsy implied by the effects of moving patterns. *Electroencephalogr Clin Neurophysiol.* 1985;61(1):1–6.
158. Wilkins AJ, Binnie CD, Darby CE, Trenité DK-N. Inferences regarding the visual precipitation of seizures, eye strain, and headaches. In: Avoli M, Gloor P, Kostopoulos G, Naquet R, eds. *Generalized Epilepsy: Neurobiological Approaches.* Basel: Birkhauser; 1990:314–326.
159. Guerrini R, Bonanni P, Parmeggiani L, et al. Induction of partial seizures by visual stimulation. Clinical and electroencephalographic features and evoked potential studies. *Adv Neurol.* 1998;75:159–178.
160. Siniatchkin M, Moeller F, Shepherd A, Siebner H, Stephani U. Altered cortical visual processing in individuals with a spreading photoparoxysmal EEG response. *Eur J Neurosci.* 2007;26(2):529–536.
161. Porciatti V, Bonanni P, Fiorentini A, Guerrini R. Lack of cortical contrast gain control in human photosensitive epilepsy. *Nat Neurosci.* 2000;3(3):259–263.
162. Tsai JJ, Norcia AM, Ales JM, Wade AR. Contrast gain control abnormalities in idiopathic generalized epilepsy. *Ann Neurol.* 2011;70(4):574–582.
163. Parra J, Kalitzin SN, Iriarte J, Blanes W, Velis DN, Lopes da Silva FH. Gamma-band phase clustering and photosensitivity: is there an underlying mechanism common to photosensitive epilepsy and visual perception? *Brain J Neurol.* 2003;126(Pt 5):1164–1172.
164. Visani E, Varotto G, Binelli S, et al. Photosensitive epilepsy: spectral and coherence analyses of EEG using 14Hz intermittent photic stimulation. *Clin Neurophysiol.* 2010;121(3):318–324.
165. Varotto G, Visani E, Canafoglia L, Franceschetti S, Avanzini G, Panzica F. Enhanced frontocentral EEG connectivity in photosensitive generalized epilepsies: a partial directed coherence study. *Epilepsia.* 2012;53(2):359–367.
166. Chiappa KH, Hill RA, Huang-Hellinger F, Jenkins BG. Photosensitive epilepsy studied by functional magnetic resonance imaging and magnetic resonance spectroscopy. *Epilepsia.* 1999;40(Suppl 4):3–7.
167. Hill RA, Chiappa KH, Huang-Hellinger F, Jenkins BG. Hemodynamic and metabolic aspects of photosensitive epilepsy revealed by functional magnetic resonance imaging and magnetic resonance spectroscopy. *Epilepsia.* 1999;40(7):912–920.
168. Moeller F, Siebner HR, Ahlgrimm N, et al. fMRI activation during spike and wave discharges evoked by photic stimulation. *NeuroImage.* 2009;48(4):682–695.
169. Siniatchkin M, Groppa S, Jerosch B, et al. Spreading photoparoxysmal EEG response is associated with an abnormal cortical excitability pattern. *Brain J Neurol.* 2007;130(Pt 1):78–87.
170. Suppa A, Rocchi L, Li Voti P, et al. The photoparoxysmal response reflects abnormal early visuomotor integration in the human motor cortex. *Brain Stimulat.* 2015;8(6):1151–1161.
171. Strigaro G, Falletta L, Varrasi C, Rothwell JC, Cantello R. Overactive visuomotor connections underlie the photoparoxysmal response. A TMS study. *Epilepsia.* 2015;56(11):1828–1835.
172. Darby CE, Korte RA, Binnie CD, Wilkins AJ. The self-induction of epileptic seizures by eye closure. *Epilepsia.* 1980;21(1):31–42.
173. Giannakodimos S, Panayiotopoulos CP. Eyelid myoclonia with absences in adults: a clinical and video-EEG study. *Epilepsia.* 1996;37(1):36–44.
174. Panayiotopoulos CP. Conversion of photosensitive to scotosensitive epilepsy: report of a case. *Neurology.* 1979;29(11):1550–1554.
175. Lugaresi E, Cirignotta F, Montagna P. Occipital lobe epilepsy with scotosensitive seizures: the role of central vision. *Epilepsia.* 1984;25(1):115–120.
176. Panayiotopoulos CP. Inhibitory effect of central vision on occipital lobe seizures. *Neurology.* 1981;31(10):1330–1333.
177. Panayiotopoulos CP. Fixation-off, scotosensitive, and other visual-related epilepsies. *Adv Neurol.* 1998;75:139–157.
178. Brigo F, Rossini F, Stefani A, et al. Fixation-off sensitivity. *Clin Neurophysiol.* 2013;124(2):221–227.
179. Bickford RG, Klass DW. Stimulus factors in the mechanism of television-induced seizures. *Trans Am Neurol Assoc.* 1961;87:176–178.
180. Chatrian GE, Lettich E, Miller LH, Green JR. Pattern-sensitive epilepsy. *Epilepsia.* 1970;11(2):125–149.
181. Binnie CD, Wilkins AJ. Visually induced seizures not caused by flicker (intermittent light stimulation). *Adv Neurol.* 1998;75:123.
182. Fisher RS, Harding G, Erba G, Barkley GL, Wilkins A, Epilepsy Foundation of America Working Group. Photo- and pattern-induced seizures: a review for the Epilepsy Foundation of America Working Group. *Epilepsia.* 2005;46(9):1426–1441.
183. Stefánsson SB, Darby CE, Wilkins AJ, et al. Television epilepsy and pattern sensitivity. *Br Med J.* 1977;2(6079):88–90.
184. Forster FM. *Reflex Epilepsy, Behavioral Therapy, and Conditional Reflexes.* Springfield, IL: Charles C Thomas Pub Limited; 1977.
185. Klass DW, Fischer-Williams M. Sensory stimulation, sleep and sleep deprivation. In: Remond A., ed. *Handbook of Electroencephalography and Clinical Neurophysiology.* Vol. 3D. Amsterdam: Elsevier; 1976:5–73.
186. Wilkins AJ, Binnie CD, Darby CE. Visually-induced seizures. *Prog Neurobiol.* 1980;15(2):85–117.
187. Wilkins AJ, Darby CE, Binnie CD. Neurophysiological aspects of pattern-sensitive epilepsy. *Brain J Neurol.* 1979;102(1):1–25.
188. Harding GFA, Jeavons PM. *Photosensitive Epilepsy.* Cambridge, UK: Cambridge University Press; 1994.
189. Takahashi T, Tsukahara Y. Photoparoxysmal response elicited by flickering dot pattern stimulation and its optimal spatial frequency of provocation. *Electroencephalogr Clin Neurophysiol.* 1998;106(1):40–43.
190. Adjamian P, Holliday IE, Barnes GR, Hillebrand A, Hadjipapas A, Singh KD. Induced visual illusions and gamma oscillations in human primary visual cortex. *Eur J Neurosci.* 2004;20(2):587–592.
191. Takahashi T, Tsukahara Y. EEG activation by red color. *Igaku No Ayumi.* 1972;83:25–26.
192. Carterette EC, Symmes D. Color as an experimental variable in photic stimulation. *Electroencephalogr Clin Neurophysiol.* 1952;4(3):289–296.
193. Takahashi T. Techniques of intermittent photic stimulation and paroxysmal responses. *Am J EEG Technol.* 1989;29(3):205–218.
194. Takahashi T, Nakasato N, Yokoyama H, Tsukahara Y. Low-luminance visual stimuli compared with stroboscopic IPS in eliciting PPR in photosensitive patients. *Epilepsia.* 1999;40 Suppl 4:44–49.
195. Harding GRA. TV can be bad for your health. *Nat Med.* 1998;4(3):265–267.
196. Shirakawa S, Funatsuka M, Osawa M, Fujita M, Oguni H. A study of the effect of color photostimulation from a cathode-ray tube (CRT) display on photosensitive patients: the effect of alternating red–cyan flicker stimulation. *Epilepsia.* 2001;42(7):922–929.
197. Parra J, Lopes da Silva FH, Stroink H, Kalitzin S. Is colour modulation an independent factor in human visual photosensitivity? *Brain J Neurol.* 2007;130(Pt 6):1679–1689.
198. Wolf P, Koepp M. Reflex epilepsies. *Handb Clin Neurol.* 2012;107:257–276.
199. Symonds C. Excitation and inhibition in epilepsy. *Brain.* 1959;82(2):133–146.
200. Kasteleijn-Nolst Trenité DGA. Provoked and reflex seizures: surprising or common? *Epilepsia.* 2012;53 Suppl 4:105–113.
201. Koepp MJ, Caciagli L, Pressler RM, Lehnertz K, Beniczky S. Reflex seizures, traits, and epilepsies: from physiology to pathology. *Lancet Neurol.* 2016;15(1):92–105.
202. Matsuoka H, Takahashi T, Sasaki M, et al. Neuropsychological EEG activation in patients with epilepsy. *Brain J Neurol.* 2000;123 (Pt 2):318–330.
203. Barker AT, Jalinous R, Freeston IL. Non-invasive magnetic stimulation of human motor cortex. *Lancet.* 1985;1(8437):1106–1107.
204. Valentin A, Arunachalam R, Mesquita-Rodrigues A, et al. Late EEG responses triggered by transcranial magnetic stimulation (TMS) in the evaluation of focal epilepsy. *Epilepsia.* 2008;49(3):470–480.
205. Del Felice A, Fiaschi A, Bongiovanni GL, Savazzi S, Manganotti P. The sleep-deprived brain in normals and patients with juvenile myoclonic epilepsy: a perturbational approach to measuring cortical reactivity. *Epilepsy Res.* 2011;96(1-2):123–131.
206. Shafi MM, Vernet M, Klooster D, et al. Physiological consequences of abnormal connectivity in a developmental epilepsy: cortical connectivity. *Ann Neurol.* 2015;77(3):487–503.
207. Ter Braack EM, Koopman A-WE, van Putten MJAM. Early TMS evoked potentials in epilepsy: a pilot study. *Clin Neurophysiol.* 2016;127(9):3025–3032.
208. Kimiskidis VK. Transcranial magnetic stimulation (TMS) coupled with electroencephalography (EEG): biomarker of the future. *Rev Neurol (Paris).* 2016;172(2):123–126.

11 | ARTIFACTS OF RECORDING AND COMMON ERRORS IN INTERPRETATION

WILLIAM O. TATUM, DO, CLAUS REINSBERGER, MD, PHD, AND BARBARA A. DWORETZKY, MD

ABSTRACT: This chapter examines the fundamental neurophysiological principles involved in determining electroencephalographic (EEG) artifact and provides general instructions for minimizing the risk of error during clinical interpretation. Examples from EEG recordings are given to illustrate common artifacts that may be challenging to the reader because they mimic epileptiform pattern associated to people with epilepsy. Emerging techniques used to detect and reduce artifact without altering the electrocerebral signal are being developed to limit the contamination. While many artifacts are easy to recognize, more complex waveforms may confuse even the most experienced reader. Constant vigilance and a team effort to minimize artifact will help to ensure a proper interpretation of the EEG for optimal patient care.

KEYWORDS: artifact, electroencephalogram, EEG, errors, contamination, waveform

PRINCIPAL REFERENCES

1. Nuwer MR, Comi G, Emerson R, et al. IFCN standards for digital recording of clinical EEG. International Federation of Clinical Neurophysiology. Electroencephalogr Clin Neurophysiol. 1998;106(3):259–261.
2. Lesser RP, Luders H, Dinner DS, Morris H. An introduction to the basic concepts of polarity and localization. J Clin Neurophysiol. 1985;2(1):45–61.
3. Beniczky S, Conradsen I, Moldovan M, et al. Automated differentiation between epileptic and nonepileptic convulsive seizures. Ann Neurol. 2015;77(2):348–351.
4. Tatum WO, Dworetzky BA, Freeman WD, Schomer DL. Artifact: recording EEG in special care units. J Clin Neurophysiol. 2011;28(3):264–277.
5. Gaspard N, Hirsch LJ. Pitfalls in ictal EEG interpretation: critical care and intracranial recordings. Neurology. 2013;80(1, Suppl 1):S26–42.
6. Tatum WO, Dworetzky BA, Schomer DL. Artifact and recording concepts in EEG. J Clin Neurophysiol. 2011;28(3):252–263.
7. Tatum WO. Normal "suspicious" EEG. Neurology. 2013;80(1, Suppl 1):S4–11.
8. Hamaneh MB, Chitravas N, Kaiboriboon K, Lhatoo SD, Loparo KA. Automated removal of EKG artifact from EEG data using independent component analysis and continuous wavelet transformation. IEEE Trans Biomed Eng. 2014;61(6):1634–1641.
9. Gao J, Yang Y, Sun J, Yu G. Automatic removal of various artifacts from EEG signals using combined methods. J Clin Neurophysiol. 2010;27(5):312–320.
10. Beniczky S, Aurlien H, Brogger JC, et al. Standardized computer-based organized reporting of EEG: SCORE. Epilepsia. 2013;54(6):1112–1124.

1. INTRODUCTION

Electroencephalographic (EEG) artifact may appear as a single waveform, burst, or series of waveforms that originate from a source outside the brain obscuring the electrocerebral activity beneath it. Recording the electrical activity from the brain requires recording, amplifying, and displaying the waveforms. In this process the "brainwaves" are subject to extracerebral interference or "artifact" and the EEG may become "contaminated" when the amount is excessive enough to interfere with interpretation.[1] The patterns of artifact may range from being obvious and so commonly observed that every reader will recognize them almost instantaneously, to those uncommon or unique artifacts that defy even the most discerning expert. Artifact is found ubiquitously on every EEG and may be derived from a variety of sources. Artifact may obscure the signals generated by the cortex to create an electrical interference due to the sensitivities used during recording in order to adequately visualize the extremely low-voltage neuronal activity. Artifact may also lead to the problem of misinterpreting a normal EEG[2] as abnormal by mimicking epileptiform abnormalities associated to people with epilepsy. This may then lead to mistreatment with antiseizure drugs before the error is recognized at an epilepsy center.[3,4]

The ideal EEG is devoid of artifact to solely represent cerebral activity. When an EEG is performed by a qualified EEG technologist, artifact may be reduced to minimize the risk of "contamination" by "noise" that might be misleading. Guidelines are available to perform minimal technical standards in performing EEG to assist with optimal recording and minimize confusion.[5,6] However, while artifact is critical for interpreting normal activity and state changes, it can lead to disaster when associated with misinterpretation. It is therefore very important to have a systematic approach to artifact, recognizing, identifying, and eliminating it so that the interpretations are as accurate as possible. Properly trained EEG technologists skilled in careful placement and monitoring of the electrodes and the patient for artifacts[7] is the first line of defense against misinterpreting extraneous artifact as an abnormality. An experienced EEG technologist, therefore, is critical and can be enormously helpful. The EEG reader must be continuously on the lookout for waveforms that do not occupy a cerebral physiological field. The use of video to supplement EEG recording enhances interpretation and can be applied both on an inpatient and outpatient basis. EEG with synchronized video adds significantly to the process of identifying a behavioral semiology as well as rhythmic patterns that can mimic seizures. In this chapter, we provide some basic as well as some complex examples of unusual artifacts in the EEG to challenge readers in various settings and degrees of complexity.

2. GENERAL PRINCIPLES

The brain sources that form the basis of the EEG are generated by neurons producing electrical dipoles directed within a three-dimensional sphere. EEG, however, is represented by a two-dimensional graph. Although the EEG is designed to record three-dimensional electrical sources from the brain, it also records signals generated outside the brain. Artifact is generated through a variety of sources, divided into physiological (those originating from the body) and nonphysiological (those originating from the equipment or environment) generators (Table 11.1). A source must follow the physical principles that apply to a physiological field by obeying the rules of polarity and convention for source distribution to be credible. Many common physiological artifacts can and should be recognized by the reader based upon the characteristic EEG waveform morphology, polarity, and spatial characteristics underlying a credible electrocerebral field. Eye movements are one of the most common and simple forms of artifact; in fact, it is present in nearly every recording (Fig. 11.1). The change in the direction and amplitudes of eye movement artifact may suggest an important change in the level of arousal (e.g., drowsiness and rapid eye movement [REM] sleep). They are easily recognizable and may be aided with the use of eye movement monitors (Fig. 11.2).

Other common artifacts, such as artifact in the EEG "contaminated" by the electrocardiogram (ECG; Fig. 11.3) or pulse artifact (Fig. 11.4), may appear. These are suspected by the characteristic periodic appearance. It is only by recording the ECG during EEG that the time-locked relationship between the periodic QRS waveforms of the ECG is apparent. In contrast, the time-locked relationship of the waveforms present from ECG artifact separates it from pathological generalized periodic discharges (Fig. 11.5) or lateralized periodic discharges.

Myogenic artifact is another common artifact observed in the EEG. On occasion this artifact may appear quite "spiky" and mimic an epileptiform discharge associated to people with epilepsy (Fig. 11.6). Therefore the appearance of ocular, ECG,

TABLE 11.1. Artifact Generated through Physiological and Nonphysiological Generators

SOURCE	POTENTIAL GENERATOR & TYPE	EXAMPLES
Physiological	Patient	
	Eye (ocular)	- Vertical eye blink - Lateral rectus spikes - Electroretinogram
	Oropharynx (glossokinetic)	- Swallow
	Heart (cardiogenic)	Electrocardiogram
	Muscle (myogenic)	- Simple: frontalis/temporalis single motor unit potentials - Complex: focal seizures; chewing, talking, bruxism, or deglutition
	Lungs (respiratory)	- Respiration - Cough
	Skin (thermoregulatory)	- Sweat
	Body movement (environmental)	- Simple: tremor, myoclonus - Complex: body rolling, head movement
Nonphysiological	EEG	
Electrodes	Electrodes and their jackbox connections	- Electrode "pop" or lead wire sway - High or mismatched impedance - Salt bridge
Instrumental	Machines/electromechanical sources and computer	- Electrical: cable movement (capacitance) - Digital: aliasing, "sticky bit"
External Environment	60 Hz	- alternating current (50 or 60 Hz)
	Nearby activity/People and devices	- Patient contact (e.g., patting, suction, percussion) - Electrostatic forces from bedsheets
	Electrical devices	- Intravenous drip (inductance) - Dialysis, ventilator, bed motors, monitors and mechanical devices
Internal Devices	Bioelectric devices	- Cerebral: responsive neurostimulator, deep brain stimulator - Extracerebral: vagus nerve stimulator, bladder stimulator, cardiac pacemakers, implantable defibrillators, ventricular assist devices, pain pumps

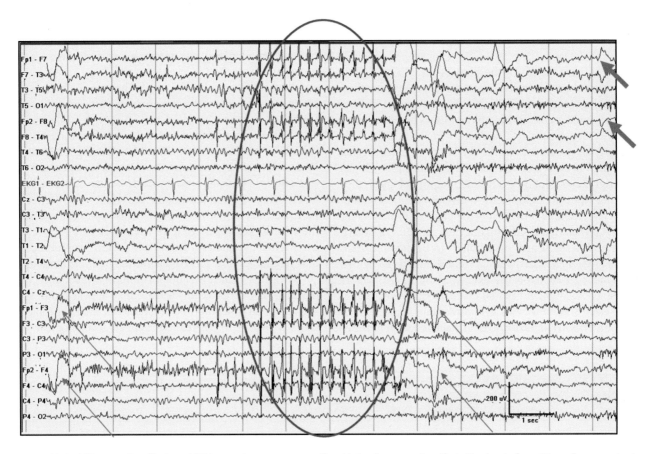

Figure 11.1. Vertical (thin arrows) and horizontal (thick arrows) eye movement artifact. Notice the myogenic artifact with a burst of repetitive spikes appearing in seconds 6–9 (oval). Sensitivity 7 uV/mm; filter settings 1–70 Hz; display speed 30 mm/sec.

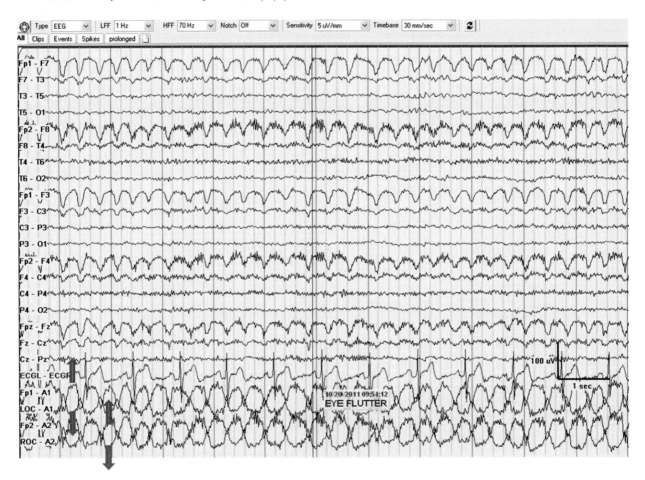

Figure 11.2. Continuous vertical eye flutter artifact. Note the "out of phase" polarity signified by the red arrows (downward deflection) and blue arrows (upward deflection) in the lower four channels, reflecting eye movement monitors. This identifies the eye as the generator versus brain (e.g., FIRDA), which would appear "in phase." Borrowed with permission from Tatum WO. Handbook of EEG Interpretation. 2014:14. Courtesy of Demos Publishers Inc.

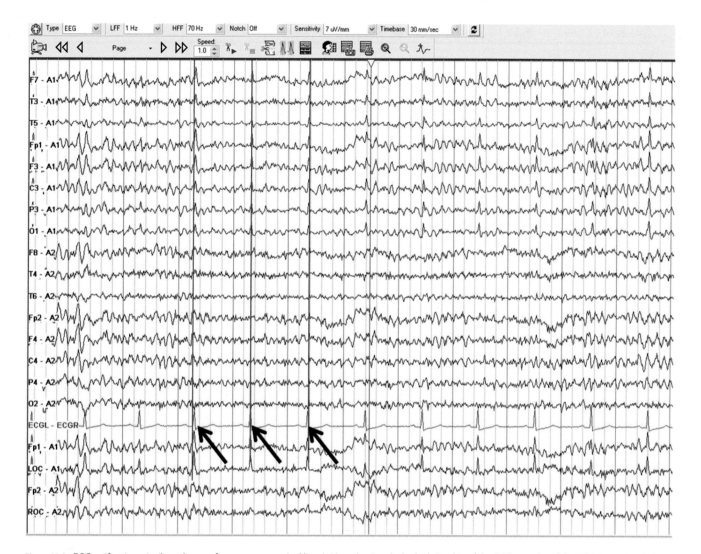

Figure 11.3. ECG artifact in an ipsilateral ears reference montage (red lines). Note the time-locked relationship of the QRS complex of the ECG (arrows) with the periodic discharges in the EEG.

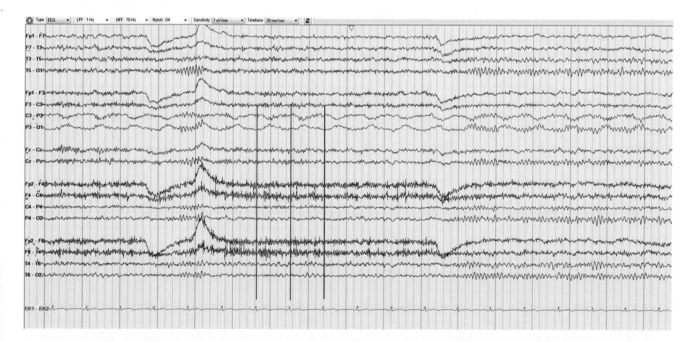

Figure 11.4. Pulse artifact in channel P3-O1. Note the 1:1 relationship of the red lines that coincide with the QRS complex on the ECG.

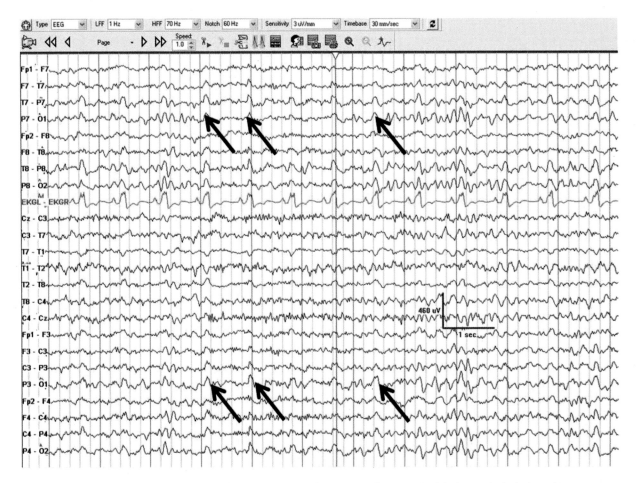

Figure 11.5. Bilateral posterior dominant periodic potentials in the EEG appear due to ECG artifact (arrows). While the time-locked relationship is apparent, lateralized and generalized periodic discharges may be confused with ECG artifact due to the periodicity.

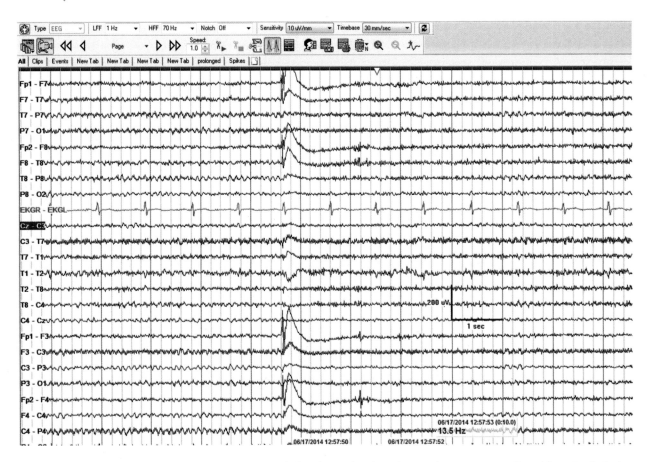

Figure 11.6. Pseudo-poly-spike-and-wave created by superimposition of a frontalis muscle spike and a vertical eye movement artifact as the patient looks down.

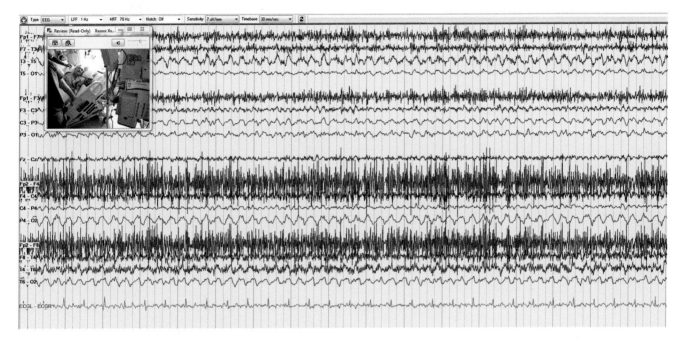

Figure 11.7. Head tremor in the ICU mimicking rhythmic activity occurring at 3 to 3.5 Hz.

and myogenic artifact merits special consideration. These common sources of artifact may be monitored by electro-oculogram (EOG), ECG, and electromyelographic (EMG) electrodes in addition to other movement monitors to define the source of a waveform as artifact. Some artifacts may be more uncommon and specific for certain situations (Fig. 11.7) or settings.[8] Nonphysiological artifacts induced by electrical equipment or complex patient movements (Fig. 11.8) may be rarely encountered during a routine scalp EEG that is recorded in the outpatient setting. However, these artifacts may be commonly observed during continuous EEG (cEEG) recordings observed in the epilepsy monitoring unit (EMU) or the intensive care unit (ICU) and during ambulatory long-term EEG recordings. The etiology of complex waveforms can often be identified only with the use of simultaneous video recordings and documentation of an activity at the same time by the technologist, nursing personnel, or an outpatient diary. EEG interpreters, however, need to be familiar with EEG patterns that raise concern for artifact in certain cases, even when the exact source cannot be identified by the EEG waveform alone.

Some artifacts are very common and appear in nearly every EEG. While their recognition is essential for both the

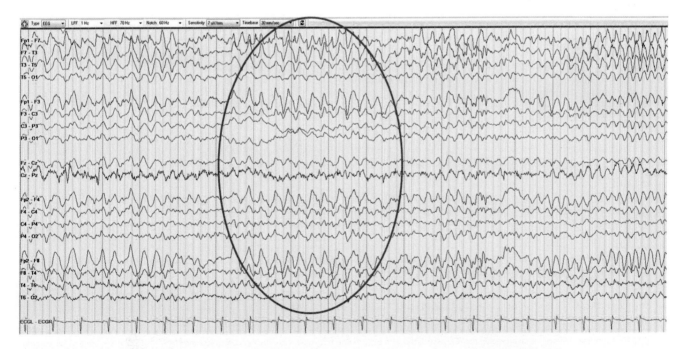

Figure 11.8. Mouth-washing artifact present during EEG recording in the EMU. Note the similarity to intermittent bursting of theta/delta.

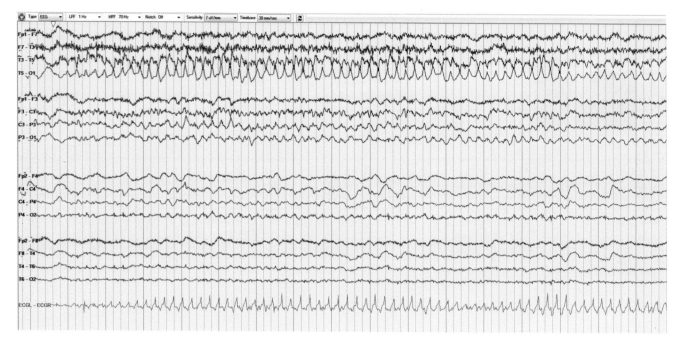

Figure 11.9. Complex environmental artifact present in left posterior temporal channel associated with "patting" the patient by nursing personnel. Note the involvement of the extracerebral channel (ECG) mimicking ventricular tachycardia.

technologist and the EEG reader, more complex artifacts may be encountered that challenge the interpreter when reviewing the EEG independently (Fig. 11.9). With advances in digital EEG systems that permit the acquisition, analysis, management, transfer, and storage of EEG information, longer durations of EEG monitoring are being performed, predisposing records to an increase in the amount of artifact present. The greater use of cEEG monitoring in criticallly ill patients (either in the ICU or emergency department), in addition to patients with complex EEG patterns during video-EEG monitoring, have revealed new and unusual artifacts with increasing regularity (Fig. 11.10). These environments are significantly different than the EEG lab or EMU, with unique types of artifact that may be seen. Common equipment that produces artifact in the hospital or ICU can be generated by either an extrinsic or intrinsic source. One extrinsic source of artifact may be an automatic programmable intravenous infusion pump. This type of artifact typically is characterized by very brief

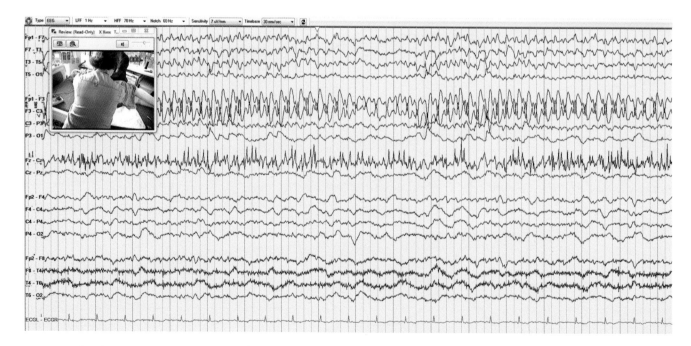

Figure 11.10. Complex environmental artifact in the ICU associated with positioning of the patient. The head contacts the mattress to create a continuous pseudo-spike-and-wave pattern in F3.

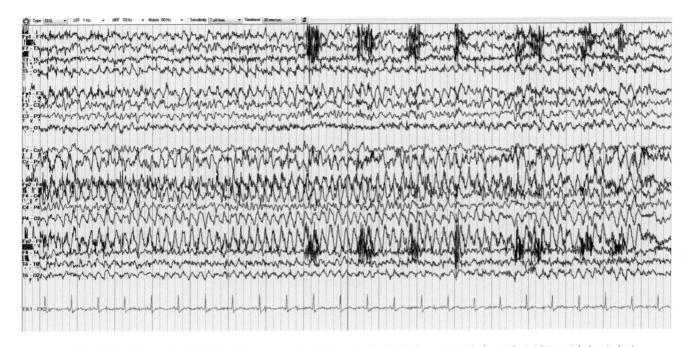

Figure 11.11. Right-sided artifact associated with rhythmic tremor and audible banging from behind a curtain in the hospital mimicking a right hemispheric electrographic seizure.

spiky transients, which are stereotyped and repeat at regular intervals; this activity can be constant or intermittent and can mimic epileptic patterns (Fig. 11.11). Slow components may also be present, creating a pseudo-spike-and-wave appearance (see Fig. 11.6). Pneumatic boots are unique to hospital settings and may produce periodic waveforms that might be difficult to interpret. In essence, any piece of equipment with a motor can produce an artifact due to the switching of magnetic fields within the motor. Intrinsic sources include pacemakers, ventricular assist devices, implantable stimulators and medication pumps, and other devices. In critically ill patients who are mechanically ventilated, a favorable chance of survival is more likely with the use of cEEG recording instead of a routine EEG.[9] This has led to an increasing number of cEEG recordings being performed in the ICU. Therefore, more frequent and unique artifacts are being identified that are exclusive to this setting (Fig. 11.12). These artifacts are important to recognize. Clinical situations involving only alteration of consciousness

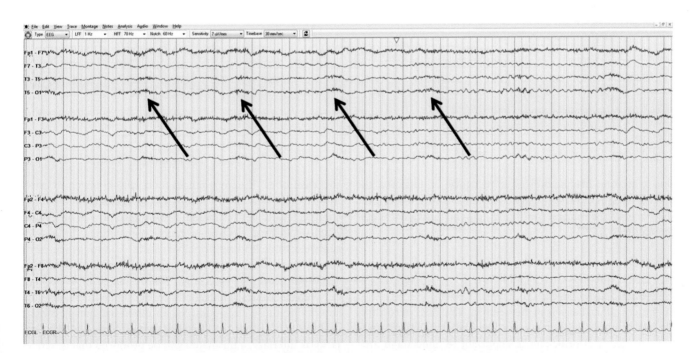

Figure 11.12. Ventilator artifact (arrows) producing slow waveforms at the same rate as the ventilator (24 breaths/minute). The endotracheal tubing is closest to the forehead and therefore mechanical respiration creates an anterior dominant field.

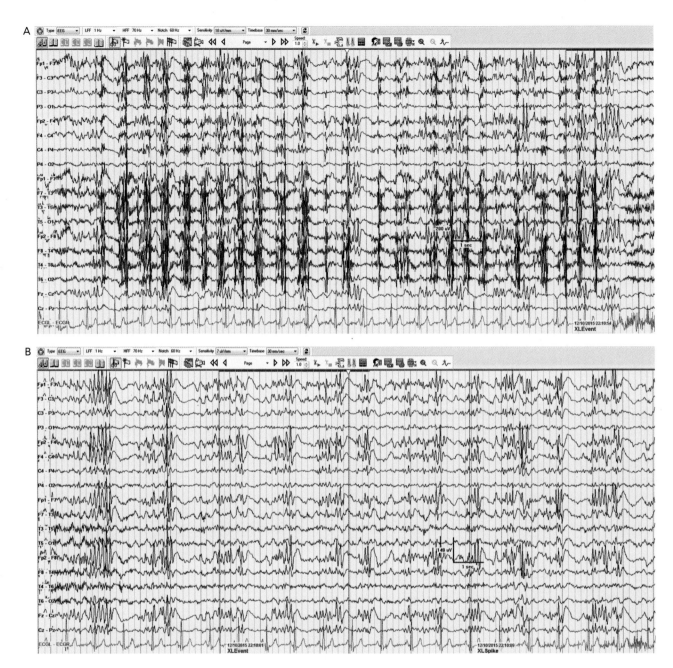

Figure 11.13. **A:** *Nonconvulsive status epilepticus partially obscured by myogenic (chewing) artifact in a 62-year-old with an acute right frontal lobe intracerebral hemorrhage.* **B:** *Nonconvulsive status epilepticus with artifact eliminated after neuromuscular blockade disclosing the nearly continuous generalized polyspike discharges.*

due to seizures may be difficult to recognize. In this case, the EEG is essential to reveal diagnostic patterns such as periodic discharges, subclinical seizures, and non-convulsive status epilepticus (Fig. 11.13).

3. ELECTRICAL POTENTIALS

A variety of artifacts can be seen in any EEG recording, though recognizing artifact is an acquired skill. Basic knowledge of electrical principles is important to understand artifact. The instruments used to record EEG utilize differential amplifiers. Each channel provides input to the amplifier from two electrodes. The impedances must closely match to minimize artifact. Any electrical activity that is confined to a single channel should be considered artifact until proven otherwise. High-impedance electrodes, faulty connections, or a fractured electrode lead are principal causes. Minimum standards require individual electrodes to have impedances less than 5,000 ohms during recording.[5] The mismatch of impedance between electrodes will distort the EEG signal in the channels subserving those electrodes. When dissimilar metals contact each other, at either the electrode–wire interface or the pin–jackbox interface, a mismatch will be produced that generates an artifactual potential. Silver amalgamated dental fillings with dissimilar metals can create a spiky-appearing artifact when the

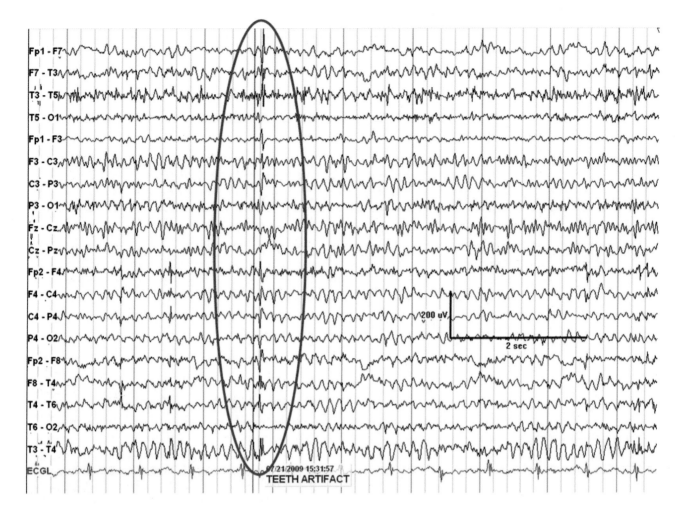

Figure 11.14. *Dental artifact (oval) created by dental fillings (mercury amalgam) and a crown (gold) that touched. Sensitivity 7 uV/mm; filter settings 1–70 Hz; display speed 30 mm/sec.*

metals touch during chewing or speaking (Fig. 11.14). High-impedance electrodes can cause falsely high (or falsely low) amplitudes and alter the normal frequency components on the EEG. Furthermore, EEG channels with mismatched electrode impedances are more susceptible to the secondary effects of environmental electrical signals, particularly 60-Hz artifact (50-Hz artifact in European countries). High-impedance electrodes may cause a photoelectric (photovoltaic) artifact during photic stimulation (Fig. 11.15). Each flash produces a photochemical reaction at the electrode site. This may appear as a spike-like transient in the high-impedance electrodes simultaneously with the flash. Photoelectric artifact can be identified and confirmed by its ability to be eliminated (or "blocked") by covering the involved electrodes.

The process of visual analysis, remontaging, and the use of digital filters allows for the identification of most of the artifact on EEG. Using a different montage for a particular waveform may enlighten the reader as to the nonanatomical/nonphysiological nature of the waveform. Digital EEG machines utilize a single reference electrode and all montages are created and reformatted based on this recording. The impedance of the machine reference electrode(s) is therefore of critical importance to ensure proper recording (Fig. 11.16). Newer digital EEG machines with amplifiers that are hardwired to each channel reduce the likelihood of previous analog problems seen with switches. EEG may be acquired with filters beyond 1 to 70 Hz to include infra-slow activity in the lower- and high-frequency oscillations in the bandwidth that is sampled.

Digital EEG is not without artifacts, however, and in fact has created new types. Digital filters can be applied without significantly altering the original signal. Our reliance upon software has not eliminated errors in sensitivity, filters, or montages, which can still result in spurious displays.[10] Digital artifacts include aliasing that results from an inadequate sampling rate, errors in analog-to-digital conversion, skew errors, multiplexing artifacts, and blocking.[11] Aliasing, which occurs when signals are sampled at a rate less than twice the highest frequency present in the signal, can introduce spurious slower frequencies into the EEG. Multiplexing artifacts occur when the samples from multiple amplifiers are combined. Blocking can occur when the amplifier is saturated (Fig. 11.17). This produces a characteristic squared-off waveform at the limits of amplifier resolution. Displaying a digital signal may also produce pitfalls that lead to artifact. Using video display monitors with inadequate display resolution can produce aliasing and introduce spurious slow frequencies into the display; they can be resolved by using a higher screen resolution.[12]

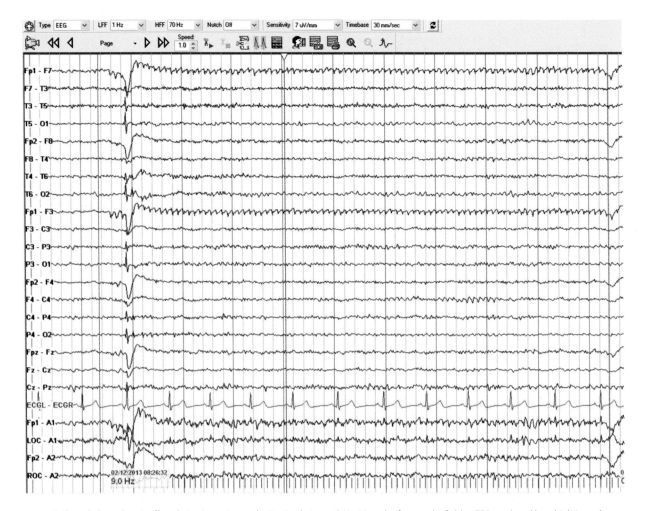

Figure 11.15. *Unilateral photoelectric effect during intermittent photic stimulation at 9 Hz. Note the frontopolar field at FP1 produced by a high-impedance electrode.*

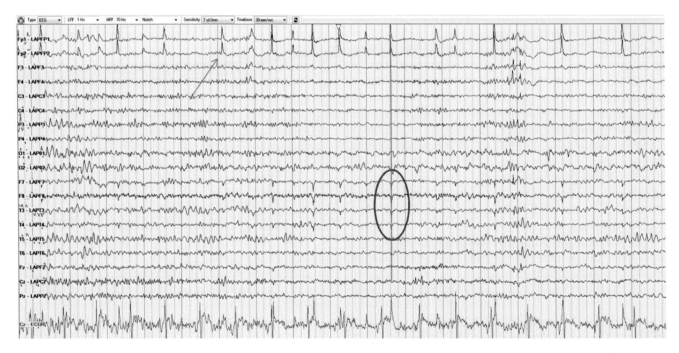

Figure 11.16. *Frontopolar electrode artifact (arrow) from frontalis motor unit potentials in a Laplacian montage during body movements (oval). Note involvement of ECG (line).*

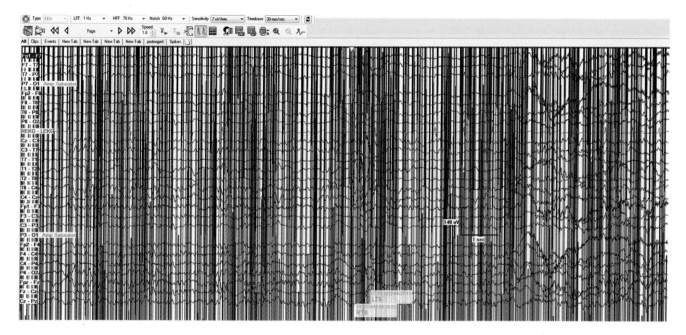

Figure 11.17. Amplifier saturation from the O1 electrode being disconnected from the patient. This led to complete obliteration of EEG.

4. RECOGNITION

Recognizing artifact is the first step to identifying the source and is an acquired skill. Artifact does not respect the principles that govern a realistic electrophysiological head model. Physiological activity should be localizable and have the proper polarity and spatial distribution to implicate a cerebral origin. Some basic concepts of polarity and localization are also necessary to distinguish a source of artifact.[13] During the routine interpretation of the EEG, the reader must appreciate essential concepts of EEG recording in order to suspect artifact (Table 11.2). These concepts serve as a guide to optimize the interpretation of physiological waveforms and recognize electrical potentials that are extracerebral. To recognize the nonphysiological nature of artifact in the EEG, the reader must be acquainted with some basic concepts, such as excluding waveforms that (i) are confined to a single channel, (ii) appear at the end of an electrode chain, (iii) have a complex morphology, (iv) appear as noncontiguous activity, (v) have alternating double and triple phase reversals in adjacent electrodes, (vi) manifest atypical generalized waveforms, (vii) have very slow or very fast frequencies, and (viii) appear periodic, with a precise interdischarge interval.[14] All of these features should make the reader suspicious for artifact. This is crucial so that these waveforms may be eliminated from the visual analysis. Both physiological and nonphysiological electrical generators can create artifact that obscures the underlying electrocerebral activity of interest.

Some artifacts actually provide important information required for interpretation and do not interfere with correct interpretation of the EEG. For example, physiological vertical eye blink artifact orients the reader to wakefulness, slow rolling eye movements signify drowsiness, and rapid eye movements indicate REM sleep. This "good" type of artifact has a notable influence on signifying the level of arousal and stages of sleep in the background activity. However, many "bad" nonphysiological artifacts exist and can contaminate the record, thus limiting the reader's ability to correctly interpret the recording.

Perhaps the most common source of artifact is generated by a nonadherent electrode. This can produce an alternating

TABLE 11.2. Interpretation of EEG Features

FEATURE IN THE EEG	INTERVENTION
Activity or waveform confined to a single channel	Check impedances, re-gel, or replace electrode.
Complex waveforms with alternating double and triple phase reversals present in the recording	When a credible cerebral field inherent to all physiological electrical generators is absent, troubleshoot the precise type of artifact for correction.
Activity at the end of a chain of electrodes within the montage	Apply extracerebral electrodes to demonstrate the absence of a field disclosing the source as artifact.
Noncontiguous activity in an electrode array or head region	Non-homologous electrode contacts in isolation may indicate artifact, and impedance testing and changes in montage may elucidate a nonphysiological field.
Atypical generalized waveforms or potentials	Check the reference electrode, ground, and preamplifier connections.
Very high or very slow frequencies (<1 Hz or >70 Hz)	Apply filter settings of 1 Hz to reduce the low frequencies or use the 60-Hz notched filter in the ICU to help reduce artifact.
Metronomic periodic patterns	Assess the internal and external environment for synchrony with an electrical generator.

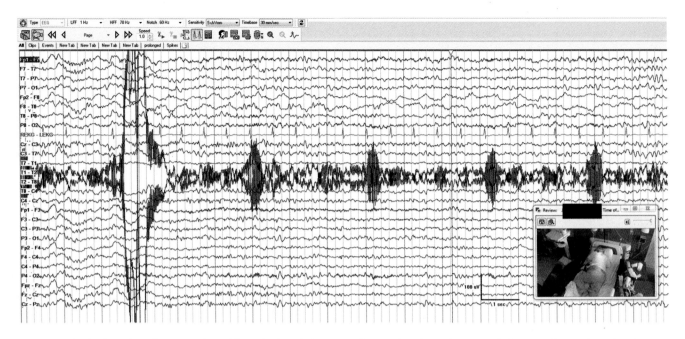

Figure 11.18. Single-electrode artifact at T2 with variable amplitude and phase reversals. Note the pulse artifact in F8 with the patient lying on his right side (picture insert).

polarity and a nonphysiological morphology that are readily visible (Fig. 11.18). However, morphologically, these artifacts can occasionally mimic an epileptiform "discharge" (Fig. 11.19). The clue is the restricted electrophysiological field that is limited to a single electrode derivation.

Noting a spatial distribution of a waveform in the EEG is important. When it is present, periodic artifact may have a temporal relationship between waveforms in the EEG and those originating from an ECG, intravenous fluid drips, or mechanical pumps and would suggest a non-brain source for their presence or obscure the underlying cerebral activity. Monitoring these artifacts can provide essential information to identify the source, which can then help lead to elimination.

The temporal-spatial evolution of artifact may have diagnostic value (Fig. 11.20). Evolution is a characteristic of epileptic seizures and may provide useful information in individuals with recurrent paroxysmal episodic events.[15]

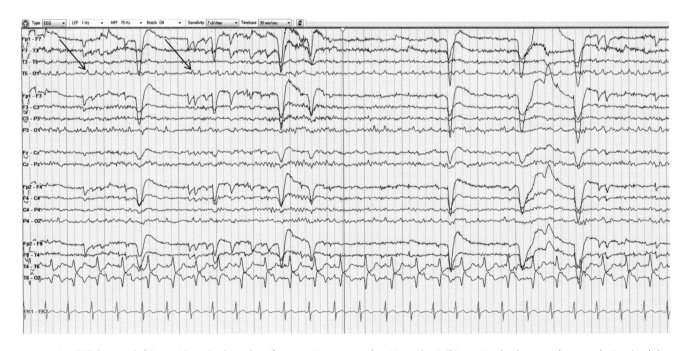

Figure 11.19. EEG during wakefulness with single-electrode artifact appearing as a run of positive spikes in T6 associated with temporal artery pulsation. Lambda waves are also present during scanning eye movements (arrows).

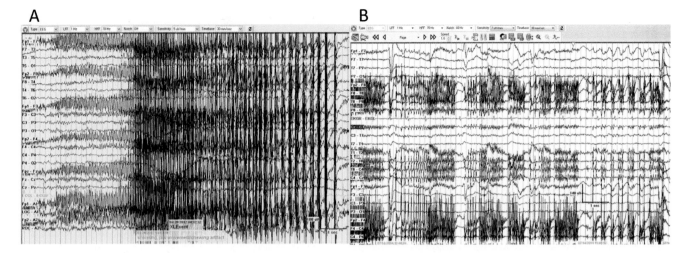

Figure 11.20. **A**: The EEG during a right frontal seizure out of sleep accompanied by left face hemiclonic jerking. **B**: The EEG of a patient with hemifacial spasm. Note the evolution in the pattern of myogenic artifact generated by the focal seizure in **A** and the intermittent pattern in **B**.

5. SOURCE IDENTIFICATION

Identifying artifact requires the reader to distinguish a physiological cerebral potential from one that is nonphysiological. The reader needs to identify the source of an extracerebral generator and detect unusual fields of distribution in order to locate the source of artifact. These patterns typically lack an "anatomical" electrical field generated by the brain. Therefore, the reader must seek factors that govern believable cerebral fields and polarities of these sources to distinguish a physiologic source from artifact.[16] Neurosurgical procedures may produce breach rhythms that demonstrate changes in amplitude, making the EEG appear "spikier" to mimic epileptiform discharges associated to people with epilepsy, especially when myogenic artifact is superimposed. When identified, single-channel abnormalities, periodic patterns, nonadjacent electrode involvement, and involvement of the extracerebral channels (e.g., EOG, ECG) all suggest the presence of artifact. When periodic artifact is encountered, compressing the display speed may help identify the precise regularity and distribution of the waveform in question, making artifact easier to identify.

6. GENERATORS OF ARTIFACT

6.1. Physiological

The physiological sources of artifacts apparent on every EEG are generated by the biological properties of the patient. Many sources within the body can serve as electrical dipoles. The most common and important sources are the eyes, the muscles of the head and face, and the heart. Other important physiologic generators of artifact include the tongue and pharyngeal muscles, respiration, and potentials generated in the skin by the sweat glands (see Table 11.1). In addition, patient movement, especially when it is rhythmic, may be a source of artifact. Placing an extra electrode on or near a moving body part may demonstrate the extracerebral physiological origin by recording the same waveforms as the one in question in the EEG. Using synchronized video analysis may allow the reader to confirm the extracerebral origin of an artifact by revealing body movement with the same frequency as the waveform in question. These artifacts may appear isolated or in combination, creating complex patterns. Recognizing these patterns as artifact is of considerable importance, especially during long-term inpatient video-EEG or ambulatory EEG recordings. In addition, EEG can be contaminated by various physiological activities that can obscure waveforms of interest.

However, as we noted above, not all artifact is unhelpful. When myogenic artifact is seen during seizures, separation between the tonic and the clonic phases of a seizure can provide a group difference between psychogenic nonepileptic seizures and epileptic seizures using surface EMG.[17] Convulsive epileptic seizures have a characteristic pattern (see Fig. 11.20A). An evolving frequency during time-frequency mapping helps separate epileptic seizures from the stable, non-evolving pattern of myogenic artifact seen with convulsive psychogenic nonepileptic seizures.[15] Analyzing patterns of artifact may result in a device that can detect seizures, during both wakefulness and sleep. In combination with other types of biosensors, myogenic artifact that normally "contaminates" the EEG may ultimately function as a seizure detector that can help reduce injury and sudden unexpected death in epilepsy.[18,19]

6.2. ECG

Some extracerebral electrophysiological signals such as the ECG occur as useful artifact. The ECG needs to be interpreted to address the impact of brain–cardiac physiological function during the EEG recording. ECG artifact may be a dominant waveform in low-voltage recordings (e.g., electrocerebral inactivity [ECI] recordings). Due to the trajectory of the cardiac vector generated by the ventricles, the QRS complex may become prominent in the temporal electrode derivations of the EEG. In addition, referential montages often accentuate ECG artifact. This is especially true when using ipsilateral ear reference with long interelectrode distances (see Fig. 11.3). A linked ears montage will reduce this artifact but may not eliminate it. Patients with short or stocky necks (e.g., those who are overweight or infants) are predisposed to ECG artifact. This is because the

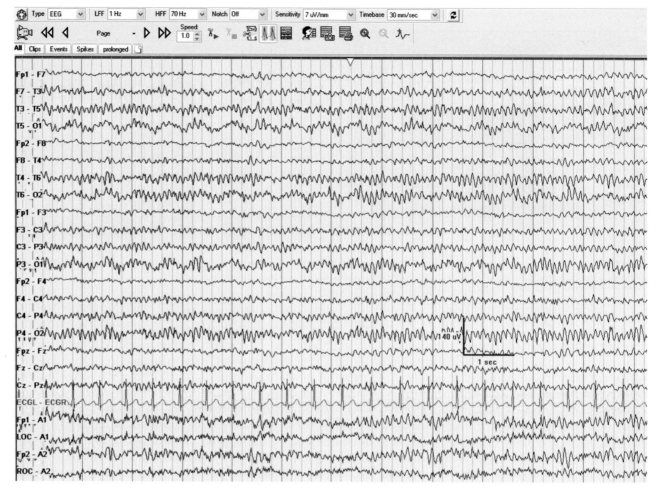

Figure 11.21. Ballistocardiographic effect with slow head movement associated with a more rapid heartbeat.

electrical dipole is situated closer to the recording electrodes and is therefore better able to transmit the higher-voltage electrical current to the recording electrodes on the head. This can be reduced in some patients by altering the head position. The channels used to record the ECG are governed by electrodes that link the left and right chest (approximating V2 axis in the ECG) using bipolar recording to identify the QRS complex. ECG interference may be noted as a single potential recurring at a rate of one per second. In isolation ECG artifact can mimic an interictal epileptiform discharge. In succession it can mimic generalized or lateralized periodic discharges (see Fig. 11.5). Bipolar montages may reveal apparent interictal epileptiform discharges that are "focal" diphasic waveforms predominately in the temporal derivations of the left hemisphere due to the vector created by the electrical conduction of the heart. Opposite polarities of the R-wave in the QRS complex may demonstrate ECG artifact on the left as a negative potential and on the right as a positive potential in the ear electrodes. ECG can be readily identifiable as the source because of the periodic regularity and time-locked ECG and EEG waveform synchrony.

As a corollary to ECG artifact, when an electrode is positioned over an artery, the pulsation of blood moving through the cranial blood vessels produces regular, rhythmic, slower periodic waveforms that are time-locked to the QRS complex of the cardiac rhythm. These waveforms appear approximately 200 msec following the QRS complex (see Fig. 11.4). Pulse artifact can be eliminated easily by moving the electrode off the artery. Occasionally, repositioning the head or placing a towel under the neck can eliminate the artifact by modifying the pulse pressure. A ballistocardiographic effect may occur from hyperdynamic cardiac conditions that produce head or body movement associated with cardiac contractions. Artifact stems from regular movement of the head or body from the mechanical effect of blood pulsating through large vessels to the head. This artifact has a slight time delay for the traveling pulse that is still linked to the ECG.[20] These are usually the dependent electrodes (e.g., occipital electrodes) when ballistocardiographic artifacts are seen (Fig. 11.21).

6.3. Myogenic Artifact

The muscles are another commonly observed source of artifact in the EEG. Myogenic artifact is characterized by high-frequency activity that may be very "spiky" and mimic epileptiform discharges in patients without epilepsy (see Fig. 11.1). However, myogenic potentials are <20 msec and thus are too brief to suspect interictal epileptiform discharges. Prominent myogenic artifact is observed more often while the patient is awake and may obscure critical portions of the EEG during seizure monitoring (e.g., during hypermotor seizures). The frontalis and

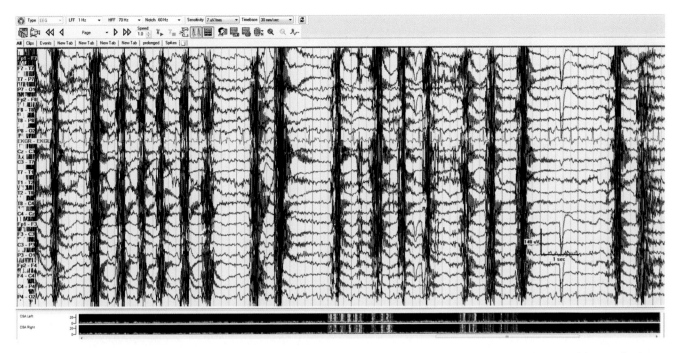

Figure 11.22. Chewing artifact. Note the episodic pattern in the compressed spectral array for high frequencies elicited by a muscle source while eating lunch.

temporalis muscles are principal sites on the head that generate myogenic artifact. Frontalis muscle becomes most involved with forced eye closure and photic stimulation.[10] The temporalis muscles become active with chewing, jaw clenching, or bruxism appearing as repetitive bursts of bitemporally predominant "polyspikes" or fast activity (Fig. 11.22). Technologists can ask the patient to stop chewing, open the mouth, or relax the jaw to diminish this artifact. Frontalis muscle contraction during periocular movement may elicit sustained or individual motor unit potentials that can appear like railroad tracks. Repetitive contraction of the jaw muscles may produce a visible tremor, creating a rhythmic artifact (Fig. 11.23). Lateral rectus muscle spikes representing single motor unit potentials recorded from the lateral orbit may simulate an interictal epileptiform discharge in the lateral eye leads at F7/F8 (Fig. 11.24). During intermittent photic stimulation, eye flutter artifact at frequencies of <6 Hz may mimic generalized spike-and-wave when coupled with myogenic potentials. Superimposition of background frequencies can create a "pseudo-photoparoxysmal response" (Fig. 11.25) when myogenic spikes generated by the frontalis muscles are time-locked to the flash frequency.

Myogenic artifacts may also obscure cerebral activity in a clinically decisive way. For example, during ictal recordings in the EMU, seizure onset may be obscured, limiting localization through scalp EEG recording (Fig. 11.26). Studies using surface EMG demonstrate muscle activation during convulsive seizures that increases in amplitude, reaching a significant peak in high frequencies of 64 to 256 Hz during the tonic phase to distinguish a convulsion.[21]

6.4. Eye Movement

Eye movement artifact is seen in virtually every routine EEG. Eye movement produces a bilateral, synchronous deflection that appears on the EEG due to its anterior location linking both eyes. The eye generates a constant polarized bioelectric signal unrelated to light that that is detected even when the eyes are closed or the patient is asleep. It reflects a fixed dipole, with the positive pole present at the cornea and a negative source at the retina. When the eyeballs move, the inherent bioelectrical dipole between the positively charged cornea and the negatively charged retina also moves as long as there is an intact cornea and retina (Fig. 11.27). This yields a large surface positive (or negative) extracerebral potential that is governed by the direction and rate of the movement. In general, it is symmetric as long as lead placement is correct, the patient has both eyeballs, both retinas are functional, and the frontal bones are intact to secure the electrodes.[22] Eye movement monitors placed above and below the eye using one or two channels help identify the relative polarity of the potentials generated by the eye (see Fig. 11.2). When the signals are *in phase* with one another, the signal arises from the brain; when they are *out of phase*, it indicates the eye as the source.[23] Eye movement artifact is important for determining a normal waking background with vertical eye blink artifact that is characteristic of wakefulness (Fig. 11.28). Additionally, eye movements are crucial to correctly identify the level of alertness and the stages of sleep. Slow rolling eye movement artifact in the delta bandwidth appears in the lateral eye leads during N1 sleep, though alternating eye movements may appear during wakefulness in the same distribution (Fig. 11.29 🎥 Video 11.1). Not only is the eye a dipole, but activation of the lateral rectus muscles produces motor unit potential artifact during rapid eye movements in the F7 and F8 electrode derivations (see Fig. 11.24). Normal eye blinking produces the Bell's phenomenon, where the eyelids close and the eyeballs roll upward. The positive dipole created by the cornea produces a relative electropositivity in the scalp EEG electrodes on the forehead (FP1/FP2). This

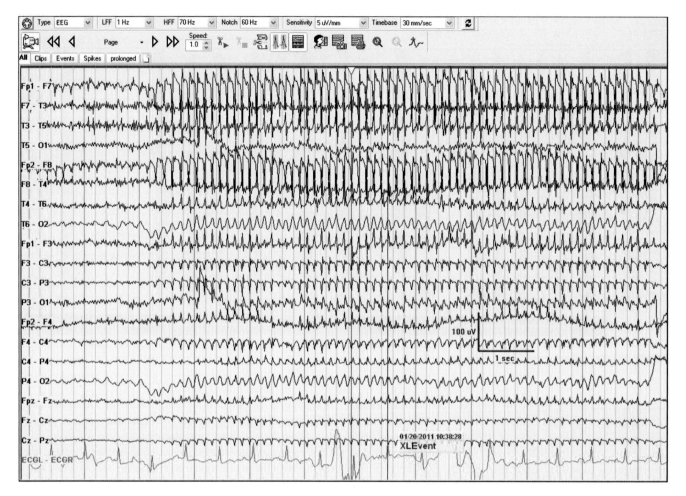

Figure 11.23. Chin and jaw rhythmic tremor artifact in a patient in the ICU.

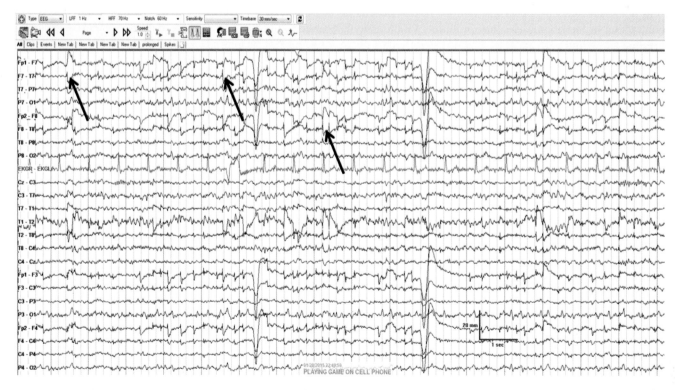

Figure 11.24. Lateral rectus spikes (arrows) during rapid eye movement while playing a game on a cellular telephone.

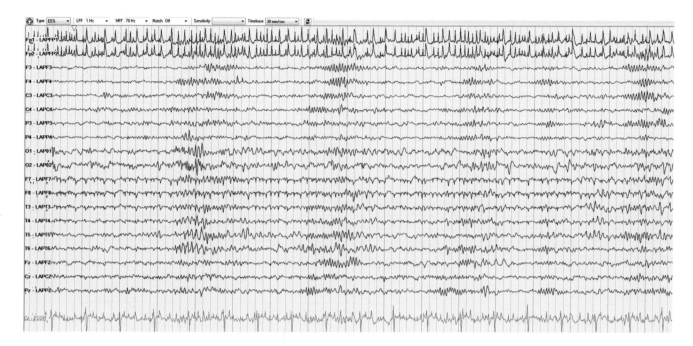

Figure 11.25. Spikes and polyspikes due to frontalis muscle motor unit potentials.

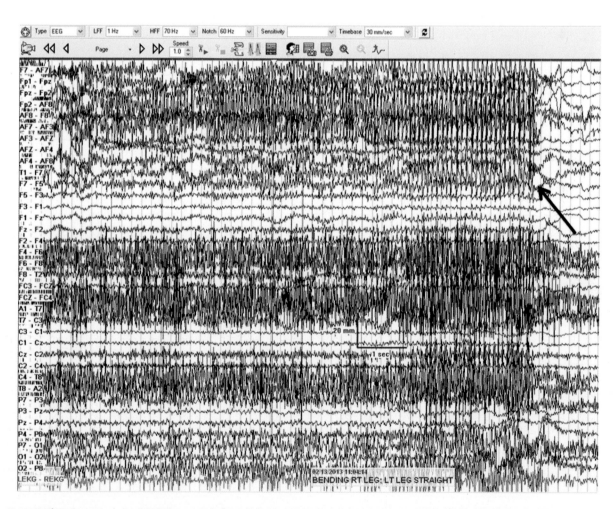

Figure 11.26. Artifact obscuring the ictal EEG during a right frontal lobe seizure. Note the phasic myogenic artifact during clonic jerking and the paroxysmal offset of the seizure (arrow).

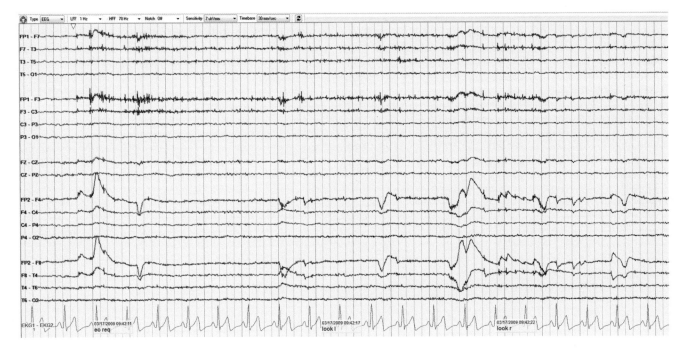

Figure 11.27. The eye as a dipole: the cornea is relatively electropositive compared with the electronegative retina. Note the lack of eye movement artifact in a patient with a left glass eye.

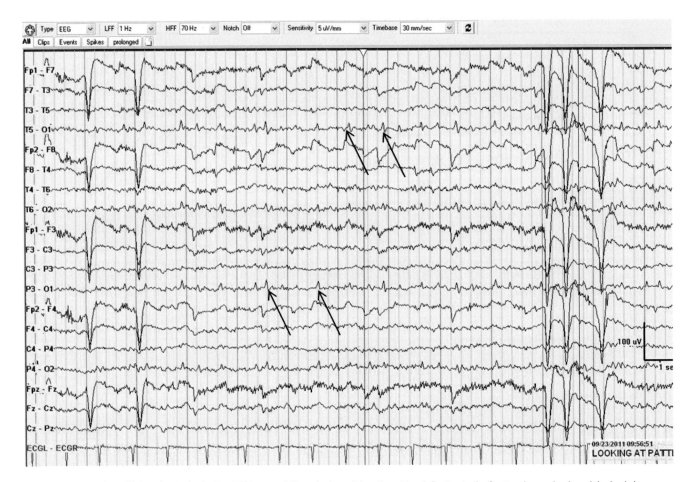

Figure 11.28. Vertical eye blink artifact in the 2nd and 11th second. Note the large "sharp" positive deflection in the frontopolar eye leads and the lambda waves from scanning eye movements (arrows).

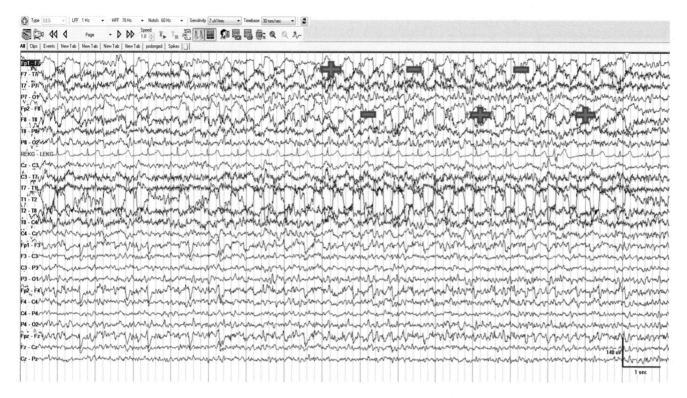

Figure 11.29. A burst of alternating lateral eye movements seen during concentration. The positive phase reversals in the anterior temporal derivations on the EEG have a corresponding negative phase reversal in the homologous channel in the opposite hemisphere.

then produces the downward deflection that is recognized as vertical eye blink artifact on the EEG (see Fig. 11.1). Eye movements can be rapid with fluttering eyelids, up to 13 Hz. They can also be in the delta range, mimicking abnormal patterns such as frontal intermittent rhythmic delta activity (FIRDA); these can be easily clarified by eye movement monitors placed above and below the eye (see Fig. 11.2). With horizontal eye movements the artifact is generated over the lateral eye leads, F7 and F8. The side of the positive phase reversal indicates the direction of the fast component of the nystagmus. With leftward eye movement, the F7 electrode "sees" the positive phase reversal produced by the cornea. Because conjugate eye movements occur in the same direction, the F8 electrode reveals the complementary negative phase reversal at the same time. It can be quite striking, as in the case of lateral gaze nystagmus, generally noted more prominently on the side generating the fast phase.[10] The characteristic deflection that includes a rapid rise and more gradual fall with the corrective phase of the eye movement is quite easy to recognize (Fig. 11.30).

6.5. Glossokinetic Artifact

The tongue is composed of a large muscle (genioglossus) in the midline within the head. Similar to the eye, the tongue generates a bioelectric dipole, with the tip of the tongue electronegative (Fig. 11.31) relative to the root.[10] During oropharyngeal motion, a direct current (DC) potential is produced that is often seen in all the EEG channels, with frontal and temporal predominance.[10] This produces delta frequency waveforms that may mimic FIRDA, which is distinguished by the

superimposed myogenic artifact. Similar artifact may be reproduced when patients are asked to say "lilt" or "ta ta ta," to accentuate lingual and labial movement, when attempting to identify the source of an undetermined pattern as artifact more conclusively (Fig. 11.32). Cephalocaudad motions may be produced by tongue movements involuntarily while speaking or when swallowing and create a pseudo-spike-and-wave pattern when combined with intermittent myogenic artifact (Fig. 11.33). Horizontal tongue movements (i.e., tongue in cheek) can create unilateral artifact on the EEG that may be confusing due to the anticipated symmetry from tongue movement (Fig. 11.34 Video 11.2). It may also appear as a quasi-periodic waveform mimicking generalized periodic discharges if the pharyngeal muscles are involved, such as during singultus (hiccups; Fig. 11.35). Furthermore, when eye movement monitors are used, the waveforms will appear in phase because the location of the tongue generating the movement is below the monitoring electrodes. Validation is possible through application of tongue movement monitors with electrodes placed above and below the mouth over the cheek in a fashion similar to eye movement monitors (see Fig. 11.31). This may be necessary to distinguish artifact from waveforms that can mimic an abnormality if the video is unrevealing. Using a bipolar montage, positive phase reversals are evident with tongue movement in a similar fashion to those recorded during eye movements.[24]

6.6. Thermoregulatory

Scalp perspiration (sweat) will also produce artifact by creating unwanted electrical connection between two electrodes.

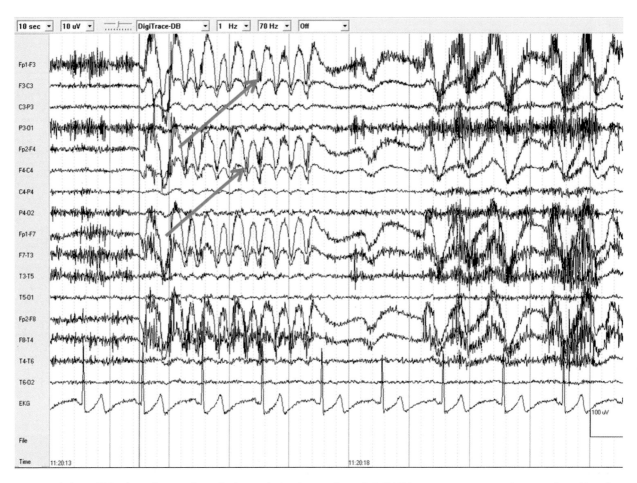

Figure 11.30. Ambulatory EEG with eye flutter artifact in the frontopolar head regions (seconds 3–5). Without eye movement monitors, superimposition of myogenic artifact produces a pseudo-spike-and-wave pattern (arrows).

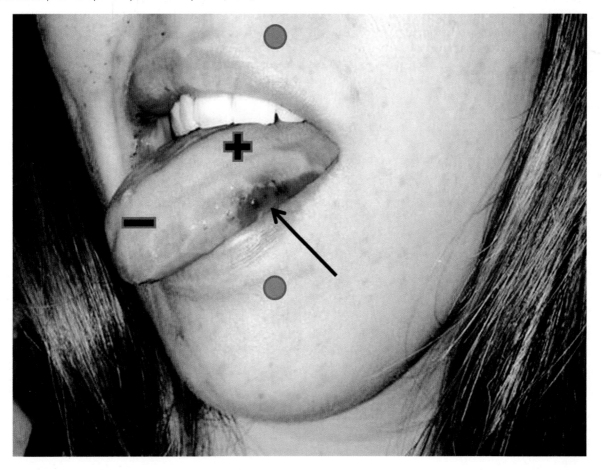

Figure 11.31. The tongue is a dipole, with the tip electronegative and root positive. Note the left posterolateral contusion from a convulsion (arrow). Blue dots signify the position of tongue movement electrodes in the EEG.

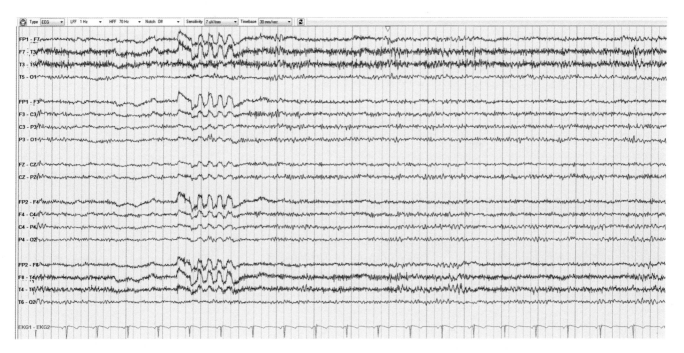

Figure 11.32. Glossokinetic artifact in second 5–6 that is reproduced when speaking the phrase "lalala." Sensitivity 7 uV/mm; filter settings 1–70 Hz; display speed 30 mm/sec.

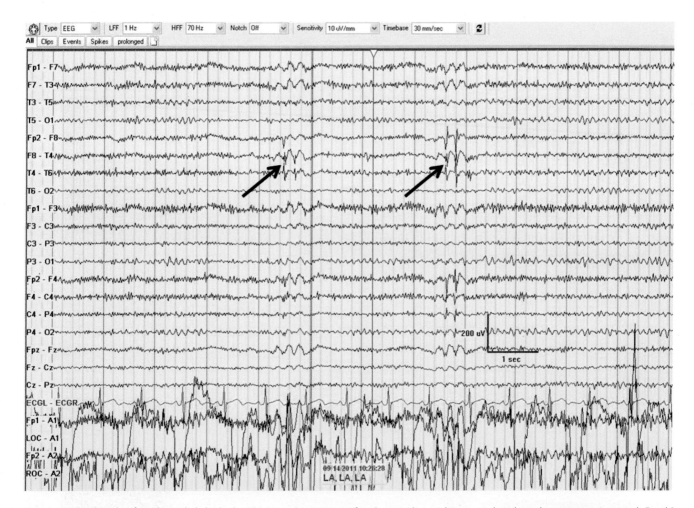

Figure 11.33. Combined artifacts that include both glossokinetic and myogenic artifact that together produce a pseudo-spike-and-wave pattern in seconds 5 and 8 (arrows). Sensitivity 7 uV/mm; filter settings 1–70 Hz; display speed 30 mm/sec.

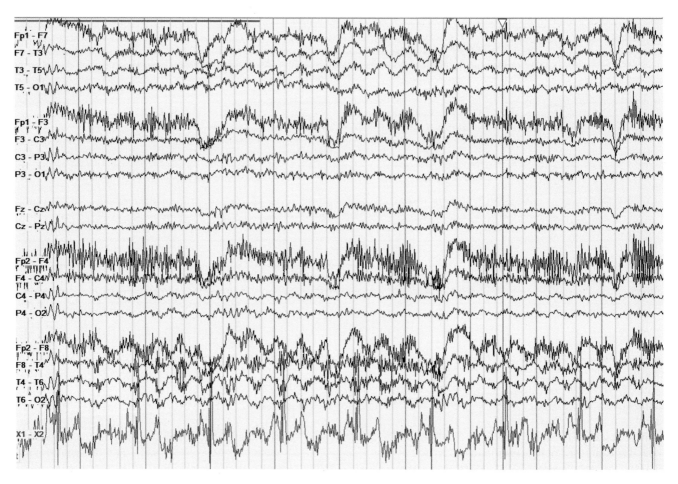

Figure 11.34. *Milk-swishing artifact manifest as a rhythmic burst. Note the alternating polarity in the temporal derivations from alternating cheek movement. Sensitivity 7 uV/mm; filter settings 1–70 Hz; display speed 30 mm/sec.*

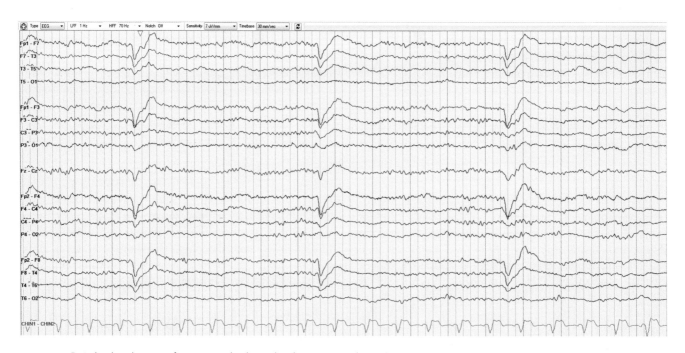

Figure 11.35. *Periodic glossokinetic artifact associated with singultus (hiccups). Note the similarity to generalized periodic discharges. Sensitivity 7 uV/mm; filter settings 1–70 Hz; display speed 30 mm/sec.*

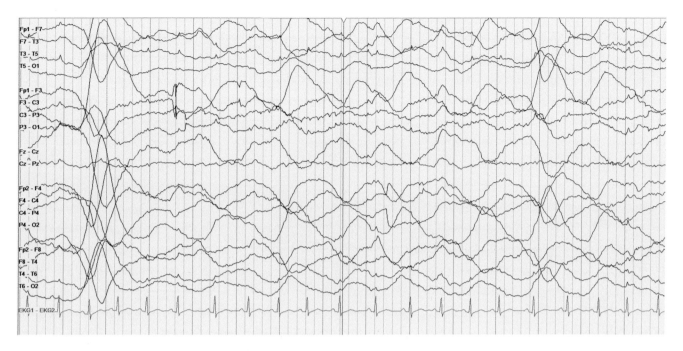

Figure 11.36. Sweat artifacts due to perspiration collecting on the scalp. Note the multiple electrodes and ultraslow potentials in different areas of the EEG. Sensitivity 7 uV/mm; filter settings 1–70 Hz; display speed 30 mm/sec.

Artifact from the skin may vary in magnitude of the amplitude but is always a slow-frequency potential. Sweat artifact from perspiration typically appears as an ultraslow frequency (<0.5 Hz) composed of low-amplitude undulating waveforms. Changes in the DC electrode potential from perspiration may result in an unstable baseline ("sweat sway") that crosses over into adjacent channels (Fig. 11.36). Sweat artifacts are usually seen in multiple adjacent channels or over the entire scalp and may limit interpretation by functionally connecting adjacent electrodes and creating a nonphysiological salt bridge (Fig. 11.37). Sweat artifact can be reduced by making sure the patient is comfortable and by using a fan or wiping the patient with an alcohol pad to cool him or her during the EEG. If sweat artifact becomes resistant to cooling techniques, the technologist can change the low-frequency setting on the EEG to eliminate the artifact for a brief period of the tracing. It can also be potentially eliminated by drying the scalp and reapplying electrodes after cooling the patient with a fan.

6.7. Patient Movements

Patient movement may be complex. During patient movement, a physiological source may produce a complex nonphysiological artifact by moving the electrodes and the lead wires (Fig. 11.38). This is especially true for awake and ambulatory patients undergoing long-term EEG recordings.[25] However, movement-associated artifact is also notable in patients who are agitated, confused, or critically ill. Synchronous video has been inordinately helpful in discerning the variety of patient movements.[26] Regular and rhythmic patient movements such as tremor may manifest at different frequencies and amplitudes. For example, the regular 6-Hz tremor of Parkinson's disease (Fig. 11.39) or scratching or patting near an electrode may appear as an episodic or fluctuating artifact ipsilateral to the

side of involvement (Fig. 11.40). Movements that produce artifact may be identified when extra electrodes are placed on the involved limb to confirm an identical frequency of a movement or tremor when in doubt. High-amplitude tremor or complex movements will produce the same rhythmic frequency that may be readily apparent in the ECG lead (see Fig. 11.7). Sudden or rapid patient movements may include shaking from a psychogenic nonepileptic seizure or movement of the body via peripheral motion (Fig. 11.41). Physiological shivering or spasm (Fig. 11.42) can also mimic the paroxysmal quality of an electrographic seizure. However, neither usually evolves over time to show progression of the artifact like a seizure does. When high sensitivities are required, such as during electrocerebral inactivity recordings, ballistocardiographic, pulse, and ECG artifact can become more prominent. Stabilizing the head with towels under the neck often eliminates ballistocardiographic artifact by stabilizing the neck. Artifact due to respiration, mechanical ventilation, or other complex movements in the ICU may also generate movement of the body or the head (Fig. 11.43 ⏺ Video 11.3). This may occur in the posterior head region during hyperventilation in a conscious person and in the anterior head regions in a comatose patient who requires mechanical ventilation. A technologist can observe the breathing rhythm and rate, annotating the recording to indicate where inhalation and exhalation occur. In the EMU, the technologist is away from the patient, but continuous video and the ability to transmit and display the time-locked behavior with EEG usually leads to accurate interpretation. Technical guidelines for recording in the EMU have been developed by the American Clinical Neurophysiology Society.[27] Long-term EEG monitoring increases the likelihood that there will be deterioration of the patient–electrode interface. Drying out of the electrolytic gel or nonadherence of the electrodes will predispose to artifact that may obscure interpretation during

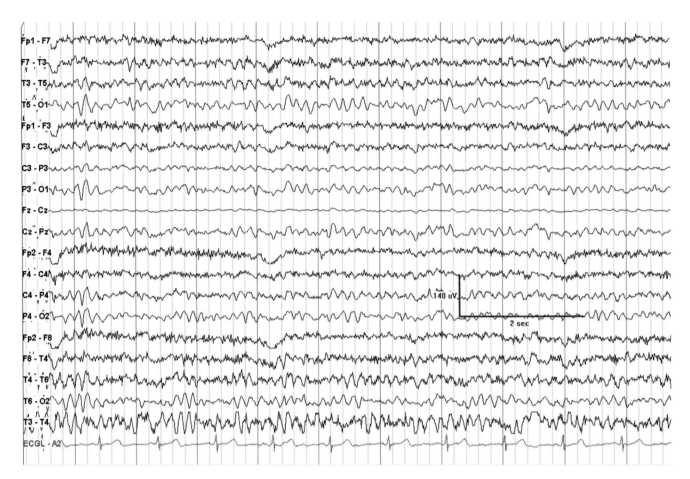

Figure 11.37. Salt bridge produced at Fz-Cz due to similar voltages from "bridging" of the electrodes by EEG paste.

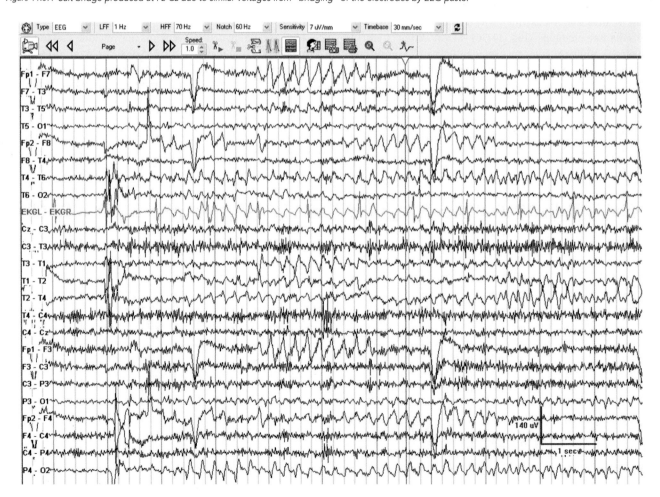

Figure 11.38. Complex artifact seen during alternating leg bouncing from restlessness that occurred during long-term video-EEG epilepsy monitoring. Note the lack of homologous frontotemporal deflections expected with nystagmus and the presence of a similar artifact in the ECG.

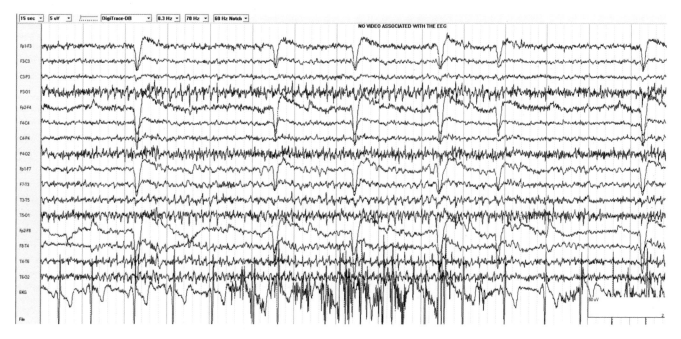

Figure 11.39. Tremor artifact that was misinterpreted as occipital spikes.

behavioral events. Artifact in the EMU is not uncommon. Approximately 20% to 25% of patients with episodes will be manifest as psychogenic nonepileptic attacks.[28] This diagnosis is predicated upon the absence of an ictal EEG change during unresponsiveness. However, artifact may impair the ability to identify subtle EEG changes (Fig. 11.44), failing to demonstrate an ictal pattern specific for epilepsy.[15] It is essential to recognize and identify the source for artifact to prevent misdiagnosis of patients with psychogenic nonepileptic attacks. This is especially true when there is "pseudo-evolution" of an artifactual pattern that simulates a true ictal recording. In the ICU,

periodic patterns of artifact may occur to distinguish a seizure from an interictal finding (Fig. 11.45). Most complex artifacts produced by patient movements can be easily identified when the video recordings demonstrate a similar frequency of the periodic or rhythmic activity in question.

6.8. Nonphysiological Sources

A variety of generators produced by nonphysiological sources may arise during an EEG. This may deceive the interpreter into thinking the apparent source is pathological and generated by

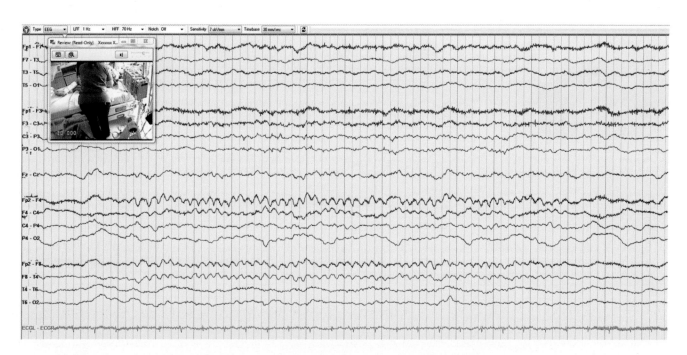

Figure 11.40. Right-sided artifact on EEG. The patient was on his right side during chest percussion therapy in the ICU.

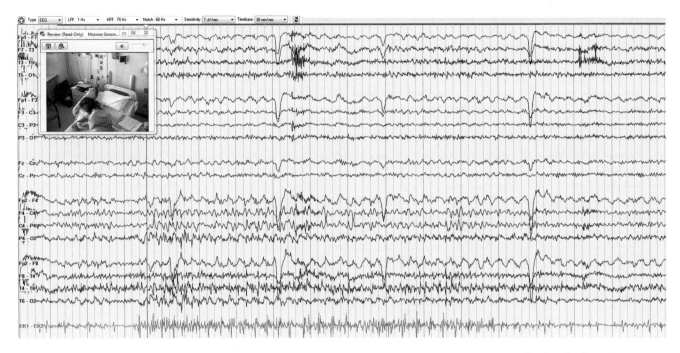

Figure 11.41. *Right hemispheric artifact associated with scrubbing the right foot with a pumice stone. Note the rhythmic burst of artifact of different frequencies mimicking a right temporal seizure.*

the brain. When in doubt, the EEG interpreter should assume that a questionable source is an artifact until proven otherwise. In our experience, if the waveform remains in question for longer than 5 minutes, it is best to interpret it as normal or nonspecific (personal communication, WOT).

6.9. Electrode and Connections

Electrode artifact is probably the most commonly encountered nonphysiological artifact. The characteristic electrode "pop" occurs with a subtle electrode movement that disturbs the electrical double layer, creating a DC potential similar to discharging a capacitor.[29] Electrode artifact may occur due to drying of the electrode gel or paste, a poor connection of the electrode to the wire, a broken lead wire, or a faulty connection between the electrode pin and the jackbox. This type of artifact usually shows an initially steep high-voltage deflection followed by an exponential decay due to the amplifier's low-frequency filter (Fig. 11.46). The morphological characteristics of an electrode "pop" often resemble those of the calibration waveform, with "mirror images" of a positive phase reversal seen in other channels where the electrode is common to them.

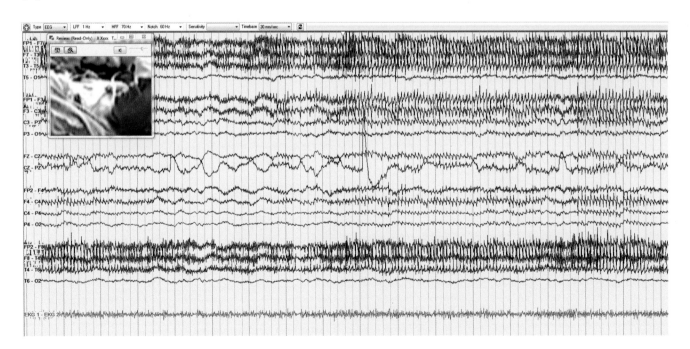

Figure 11.42. *Shiver artifact created by myogenic sources associated with medication in the ICU.*

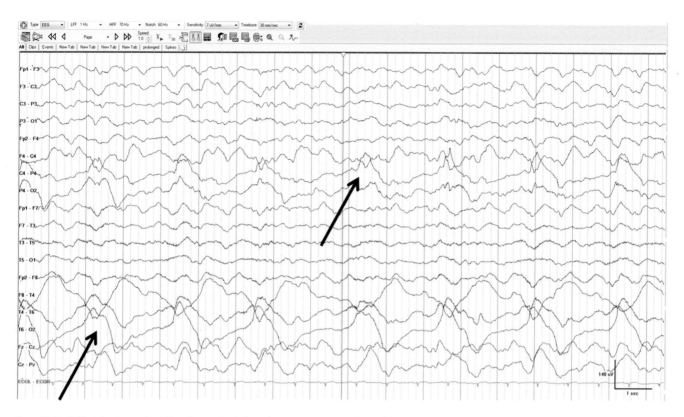

Figure 11.43. Artifact due to overbreathing the mechanical respirator at a preset rate (arrows).

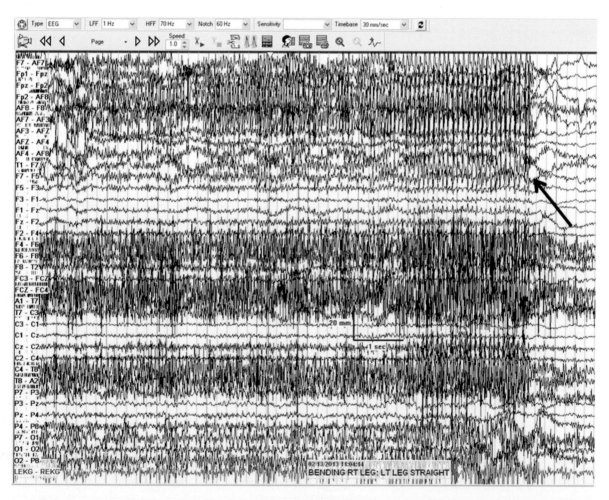

Figure 11.44. Artifact obscuring the ictal EEG during a right frontal lobe seizure. Note the phasic myogenic artifact during clonic jerking and the paroxysmal offset of the seizure (arrow).

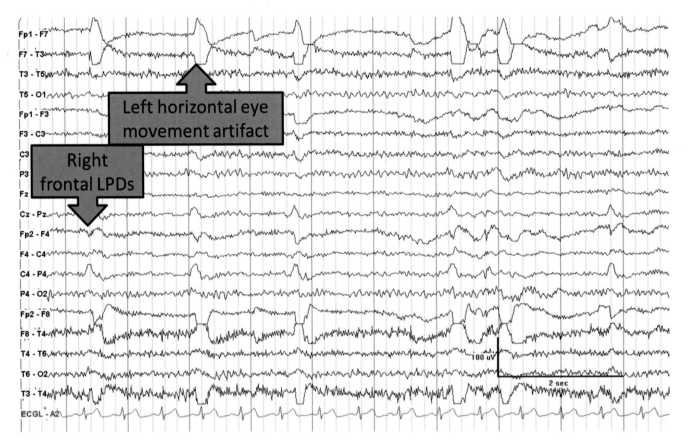

Figure 11.45. *Right frontal lateralized periodic discharges coupled with left horizontal eye movements in a patient with seizures from a right frontal lobe brain tumor (glioblastoma multiforme). Sensitivity 7 uV/mm; filter settings 1–70 Hz; display speed 30 mm/sec.*

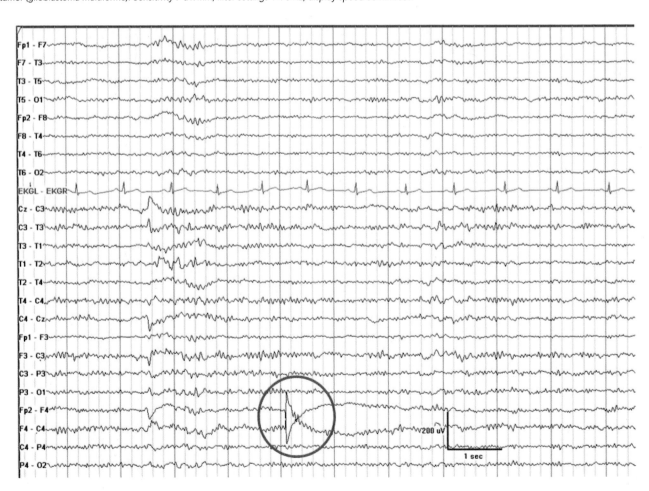

Figure 11.46. *Single electrode "pop" artifact identified at F4 in second 5 (circle). Sensitivity 7 uV/mm; filter settings 1–70 Hz; display speed 30 mm/sec.*

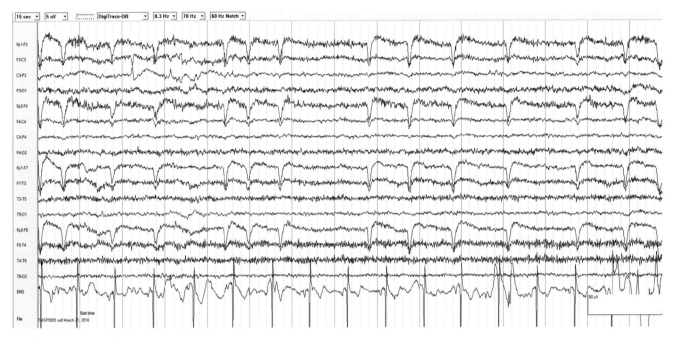

Figure 11.47. Single-electrode artifact at C3 mimicking an interictal epileptiform discharge. Note the lack of involvement in adjacent channels and therefore the absence of a credible spatial field.

Pops may appear as a single deflection and mimic an interictal epileptiform discharge in a bipolar montage (Fig. 11.47); this can be clarified as a single-electrode artifact by converting to a reference montage (Fig. 11.48). Single-electrode artifact may also appear as a repetitive discharge (Fig. 11.49) and can be caused by a faulty electrode or wire, disrupted scalp–electrode interface, or inadequate conductive gel to secure an electrode connection. Some high-impedance electrode pairs (>10 kohms) may produce exaggerated bizarre waveform morphologies that can mimic abnormal epileptiform discharges.[30]

Electrode artifact can produce a sudden burst of electropositive or alternating positive and negative waveforms but occurs without a credible or discernible electrophysiological field. In some cases, the poor or fluctuating contact between the electrode and scalp results in rhythmic activity that simulates focal slowing or mimics a focal seizure (Fig. 11.50).

Proper electrode application and maintenance is the best way to reduce electrode artifact. Good electrode contact should be ensured by adequate skin preparation to remove surface oils. Electrode impedance should be measured and

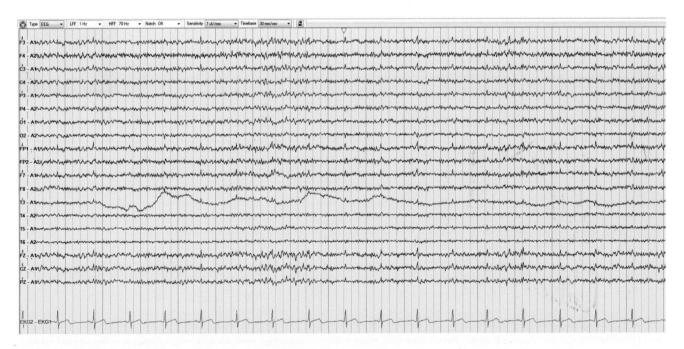

Figure 11.48. Single-electrode artifact at T3 clarified by use of an ipsilateral reference montage.

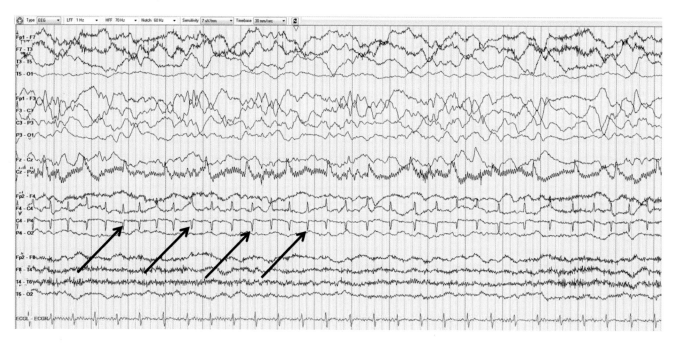

Figure 11.49. C4 single-electrode artifact in the EEG (arrows). Note the lack of a credible field but the ability to mimic a lateralized periodic discharge.

verified to be <5,000 ohms.[5] Any extra electrode paste between electrodes should be removed. Securing the electrodes with collodion or EC2 paste minimizes small movements of the electrode and slows the drying process of the electrode paste. Electrode wires should be kept close together to prevent movement and excessive tension on electrodes. Electrodes should be cleaned well and inspected regularly for signs of corrosion between the electrode and conducting wire, damaged insulation, or broken lead wires, and faulty electrodes should be discarded. If silver–silver chloride electrodes are

used, maintenance should be done on a regular schedule to optimize their ionic charge.

Waveforms that occur at the end of an electrode chain or those restricted to a single electrode should be considered single-electrode artifact until proven otherwise.[14] When a repeated abnormality is encountered, an impedance test should be performed and corrected when it is >10 kohms. The problem may be eliminated by reapplying conductive gel or paste at the electrode site or replacing the electrode, subsequently eliminating the electrode artifact. However, some

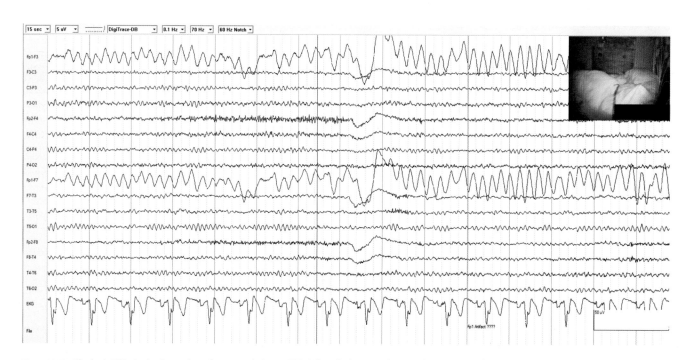

Figure 11.50. Rhythmic FP1 single-electrode artifact on ambulatory EEG. When rhythmic or changing frequencies occur, single-electrode artifact may mimic a focal seizure. In this case the EEG electrode was nonadherent to the patient.

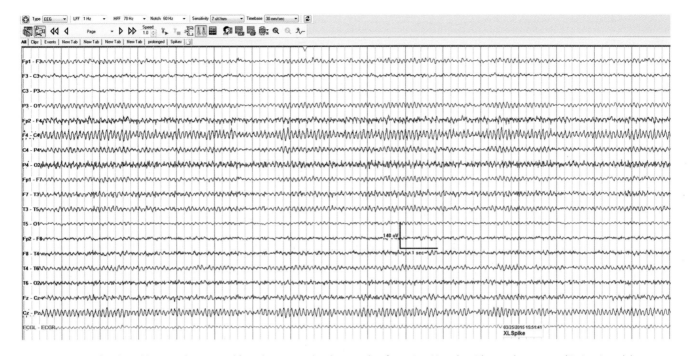

Figure 11.51. EEG after the jackbox was disconnected from the patient when he was taken for testing. Note the widespread, monomorphic, invariant alpha frequency.

neuronal migrational disorders can produce electropositive epileptiform transients and runs of bizarre electrocerebral activity, even manifesting atypical spatial fields.[31]

Artifacts caused by electrodes or their connections (Fig. 11.51) require troubleshooting by the technologist to discover the source of the problem and eliminate it from the recording to avoid compromising interpretation.

When single-electrode artifact is encountered, if reapplication of the electrode does not eliminate the artifact, the technologist can try recording from another electrode placed close to the electrode with suspected artifact. This can determine if the activity is artifactual by eliminating the presence of a credible field due to cerebral activity. If artifact remains after changing electrodes, the technologist should assess the jackbox by switching electrode pins to help isolate the artifact to a single channel in the jackbox. This is verified when, despite switching electrode pins, the artifact does not "move" and remains in the same malfunctioning channel of the jackbox. Prompt replacement of the faulty jackbox will eliminate the problem of channel-specific artifact. Occasionally, electrode leads placed into the incorrect jack inside the head box can yield spurious electrophysiological fields.

Ground lead recordings are another system artifact that occurs when a very high-impedance (or disconnected) electrode exceeds the input impedance of the recording system.[11] In this case, the ground electrode is substituted for the malfunctioning electrode, leading to aberrant or bizarre waveforms (Fig. 11.52).

Salt bridges occur when electrode paste or gel is smeared between two electrode locations (see Fig. 11.37). EEG activity recorded from each electrode therefore becomes the sum of the activity from the two electrodes, leading to spuriously low-amplitude recordings that may appear "flat." This type of artifact is more likely to occur when closely spaced electrodes are used, as in the International 10-10 modified system or when using the full 10-20 placement in neonates.

6.10. Photoelectric Effect

During photic stimulation, light from the flash stimulus may produce artifact in the frontopolar head regions (Fig. 11.53). This artifact is generated in FP1/FP2 by a nonphysiological source, usually associated with electrodes that have high impedance. A photocell is created that generates an artifact that is time-locked to intermittent photic stimulation. This effect should not be mistaken for photic driving because the photoelectric effect is located in the frontal electrodes, not in the occipital region. The source should also not be confused with the normal physiologic electroretinogram (ERG) produced by the retina in response to photic stimulation. The ERG is associated with a brief delay following the photic stimulus and may be difficult to separate from the nonphysiological artifact due to the photoelectric effect. The amplitude of the ERG is usually low voltage; it appears in the anterior head regions and will fatigue with time at high rates of intermittent photic stimulation. Covering the eyes with a towel will block the input to the retina (and therefore the ERG from being elicited). Covering the frontopolar electrodes will eliminate the photoelectric effect but not the ERG if the eyes are left uncovered.

6.11. Instrumental Artifacts

Malfunction of the instruments for recoding may involve almost any part of the EEG machine to produce artifact. Improved design of the machines, the nearly universal use of digital technology, and the portability of equipment has

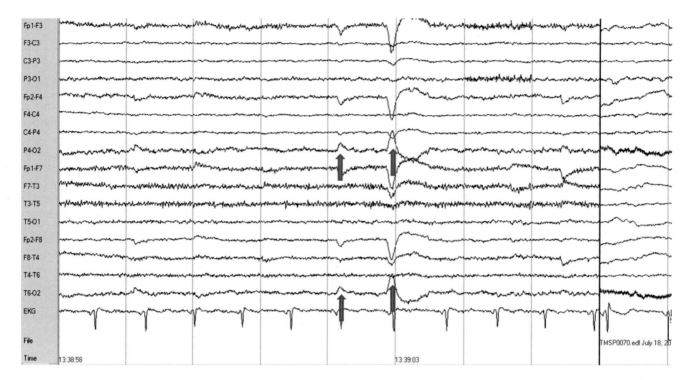

Figure 11.52. Ground lead recording at O2. In this case a very high-impedance electrode at O2 causes the ground electrode placed at FPz to serve as input terminal 2. This produces the inverted eye blink morphology at the P4-O2 and T6-O2 channels. Sensitivity 7 uV/mm; filter settings 1–70 Hz; display speed 30 mm/sec.

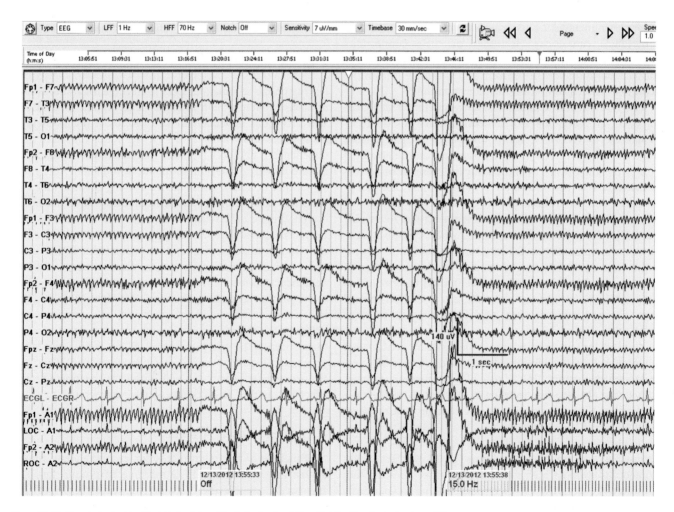

Figure 11.53. The photoelectric effect during intermittent photic stimulation. Not the time-locked nature of the appearance.

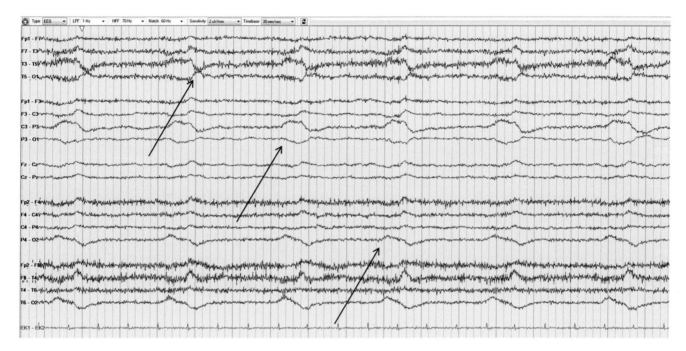

Figure 11.54. Low-voltage EEG (2 uV/mm) following trauma performed for electrocerebral inactivity with a subsequent double-distance electrode recording confirmed brain death. Note the background "noise" and respirator artifact (arrows).

reduced the likelihood of equipment malfunction. Nonetheless, this still occurs frequently enough that both the EEG technologists and the interpreter must have a thorough understanding of the most common technical artifacts. Portable equipment is more susceptible to mechanical wear and tear, when motion from vibration or jolting of the machine induces a loss of system integrity that predisposes to artifact. Loose wiring and loosening of circuit board connections are probably the most common sources of artifact and may cause loss of the signal or intermittent failure to record computer-assisted ambulatory EEG.

Modern amplifiers are small, low-power, single-chip multichannel devices with solid-state integrated circuits. Amplifier "noise" is caused by thermal reverberation of the amplifier circuits. This noise contains components at all frequencies and therefore increases with the bandwidth of the amplifier. Noise levels should be <2 microvolts in amplitude measured peak to peak.[5] The effect from intrinsic noise is typically problematic only when the EEG is recorded at higher sensitivities (Fig. 11.54). An example is during brain death recordings, when a level of 2 microvolts per millimeter is used to demonstrate electrocerebral inactivity producing artifact.[32] A malfunctioning amplifier component (e.g., capacitor, resistor, or transistor) can produce noise that is of higher amplitude than the background activity to disrupt or distort cerebral activity. Artifact may arise from inadequate sampling rates of the computer within the EEG machine. When analog-to-digital conversion occurs, faster frequencies may be misrepresented with low sampling rates. This creates a false representation of the waveform as a slower frequency (aliasing) and may be subject to misinterpretation.

Failure of components common to all channels often causes lack of power or 50/60-Hz artifact. Excessive 50/60-Hz artifact is usually caused by a faulty or absent ground connection to the patient but may also be caused by defects in the power supply or other parts of the instrument (Fig. 11.55). Digital recording may produce artifacts during analog-to-digital conversion. When data points are inaccurately sampled, information from a channel may be lost; this is referred to as a "sticky" bit. The display is clearly artifact and should not be confused with an interictal epileptiform discharge. Similarly, when two digital instruments are close to one another, instrumental artifact may occur. Additionally, when the instrument is turned off and then on, artifacts may occur that mimic high-frequency oscillations (Fig. 11.56). When digital equipment records multiple channels, multiplexing artifacts and other artifacts from digital recording may be present (Fig. 11.57), regardless of the type of amplifier. This usually occurs when only some of the channels are sampled that are governed by the amplifier. An error in the timing of display occurs, and this may result in errors in channel display. Display resolution may also be subject to aliasing if the screen resolution is too low (Fig. 11.58). This produces an undersampling of the waveforms and may eliminate higher frequencies to make them appear as an alias falsely represented by lower frequencies.[33]

6.12. Environmental Artifacts

A wide variety of artifacts may arise from electrical sources generated by devices located in the environment surrounding the patient. The vast and complex array of artifacts involving various frequencies and morphologies can make recognition a challenge and identification of the source even more difficult. Environmental artifacts are especially common in the ICU. In a hostile environment,[34] an experienced technologist and video associated with the EEG recording are indispensable.

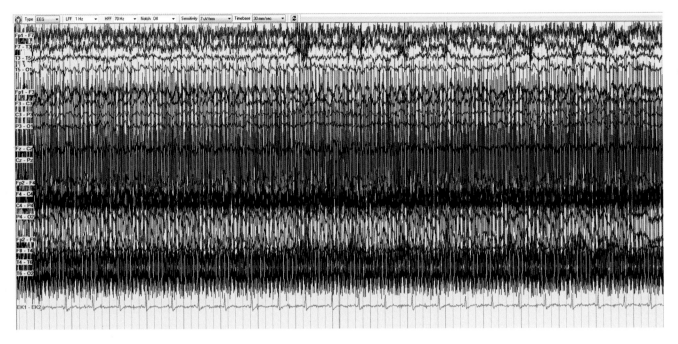

Figure 11.55. 60-Hz artifact obscuring the EEG. Resolution was seen when the notched filter was turned on.

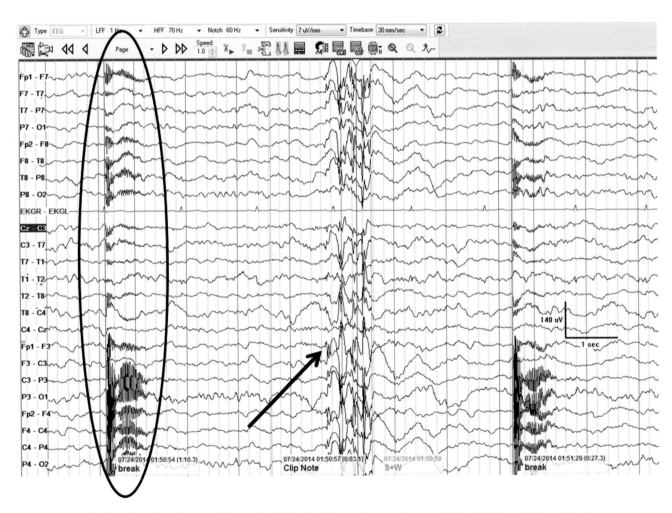

Figure 11.56. Digital artifact during intermittent machine use (oval). Note the difference between the generalized epileptiform discharges (arrow).

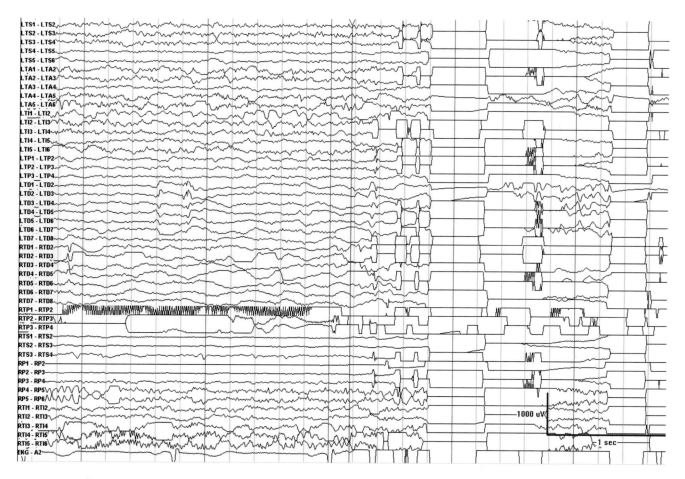

Figure 11.57. Digital artifact may occur with multiplexing during intracranial EEG recording. Note the amplifier saturation that occurs in multiple channels.

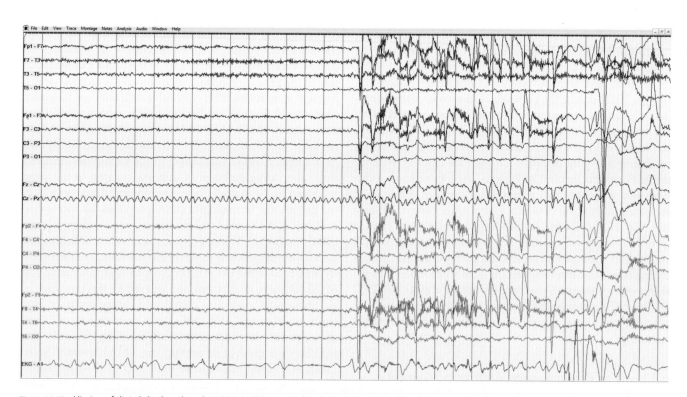

Figure 11.58. Aliasing of digital display when the 1920 × 1080 monitor falsely identifies a high-frequency signal from Pz as a lower ("alias") frequency. Screen resolution 1920 × 1080; high-frequency filter 70; low-frequency filter 1; notch OFF; sensitivity 7 uV/mm; time base 15 mm/sec. EEG courtesy of Dr. Jonathan Edwards.

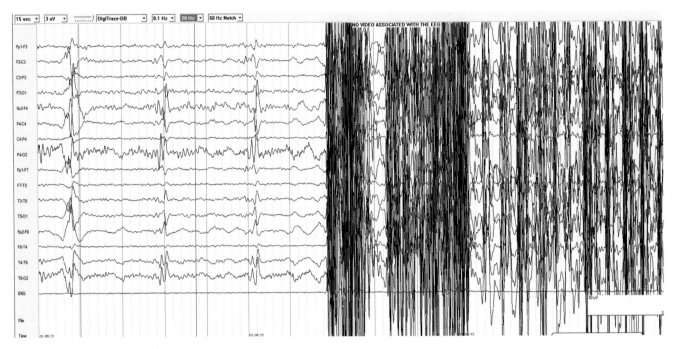

Figure 11.59. Artifact mimicking generalized periodic discharges due to a dialysis machine. In the latter half of the recording artifact obscured the tracing when the bed motor was activated to lower the patient. The computer detection software identified the artifact as a seizure.

Typically, artifactual waveforms from external devices show significantly different morphologies that readily distinguish them from cerebral activity. Waveforms that appear monomorphic, lack a believable electrophysiological field, or appear in the extracerebral channels (e.g., ECG) are highly suspect for artifact. They may often be identified as artifact even if the exact source cannot be isolated to attempt elimination (Fig. 11.59). Nevertheless, some may be difficult to identify due to the unique electrophysiological characteristics of the waveform.

The ICU environment is different from the EEG laboratory and the EMU due to the presence of numerous signals from multiple electrical generators that may be present, producing unique and peculiar artifacts. During cEEG in the ICU there are many extrinsic sources, including mechanical ventilators, cooling or warming blankets, feeding tube delivery systems, the ECG monitor, central and arterial lines, intravenous infusion pumps, continuous pressure devices, and intracranial pressure monitors, all of which may produce bizarre artifacts (see Fig. 11.59). Simultaneous video recording can help to identify some environmental artifacts. Movement of people and objects around the patient, including chest percussion during physiotherapy, may become clear when video is available to define simultaneous motion during a rhythmic EEG finding.[35] The prolonged EEG recordings often used in the ICU are subject to greater technical issues than short routine EEG recordings.

6.13. Mains Power Supply (Alternating Current Artifact)

The most common instrumental source of artifact is generated by the alternating electrical interference from mains power supply. The frequency of the artifact occurs at 60 Hz in the United States (see Fig. 11.55) and 50 Hz in Europe. Electrical interference from mains power supplies can be either electrostatic or electromagnetic. In most neurophysiology labs, the power lines are adequately grounded and significant electrical interference is rarely problematic. If necessary, interference can be reduced by shielding the power cables; this is done by connecting the outer metal braided wire to a ground. It may also be done by using a shielded room or by removing the patient from the source of artifact in the room.[10] In areas outside of the EEG lab ("hostile environments") such as the ICU and operating room, other medical instruments are frequently encountered that can interfere with EEG recordings and produce artifact. The 60-Hz (50-Hz in Europe) alternating current can cause artifact in the EEG via its electrostatic effects. Power lines couple to other conductors in the vicinity and induce a small alternating potential of opposite polarity to the signal produced by the main.[10] These environmental sources may be the patient, the technologist, other people in the room, electrode wires, mechanical objects or devices, and even stationary metal bed frames. While these potentials are small, they may be relatively large when compared to the voltage of EEG activity measured in microvolts. Ensuring an adequate connection of the patient to an earth ground will reduce this potential.

Sixty-cycle artifact is commonly caused by poor electrode application.[36] This artifact can be reduced keeping all the electrode wires and cables short, bundling electrode wires together in a group, and unplugging all unnecessary equipment. A notched filter can be used to preferentially remove excessive 60-Hz/50-Hz artifact. However, the notched filter will also remove signals of interest around 50 or 60 Hz and so should not be used routinely. Other pieces of electrical equipment near the patient can cause electromagnetic interference from current flowing through cables, nearby transformers, or motorized devices. The intensity of the magnetic flux produced is proportional to current that may interfere with the EEG recording. Common hospital equipment that can create artifact can stem from the use of photic stimulators, portable air pumps, monitoring devices, lights and lamps, fans, air conditioning, pneumatic boots, electric beds, intravenous infusion pumps, feeding delivery systems, or nearby elevators, computers, telephones, diathermy, and x-ray equipment.[10] The electrical field generated by the equipment is inductively coupled to the electrode wires, usually producing an out-of-phase harmonic of 60 Hz (in the United States). However, other frequencies outside the narrow range of the notched filter, such as 60-Hz harmonics, will not be completely eliminated.

The technologist may reduce electromagnetic artifact by (i) ensuring that all equipment has a shielded metal case and is connected to ground, (ii) plugging all equipment into the same connection point, and (iii) ensuring that power cables do not run in parallel and are remote from electrode wires and cables used to record the EEG.

Some 60-Hz (50-Hz outside the United States) artifact is present in small amounts in nearly all EEG recordings. However, this is usually of low amplitude because differential amplifiers used to amplify the EEG signal use common mode rejection algorithms to remove most of the artifact. When there are high or mismatched impedances in electrodes, the amplifier's ability to cancel out noise is reduced, and 60- Hz/50-Hz artifact will appear in the channels that include the high-impedance electrodes. These electrodes should be reapplied as soon as possible. If 50-Hz/60-Hz artifact is seen in all channels, this usually indicates a problem with the ground electrode or the ground of the EEG machine. This should be investigated before performing clinical EEG to ensure no electrical safety hazard is passed on to the patient.[22] Analysis of spectral power using the fast Fourier transformation available with most standard EEG reading software and compressed spectral analysis during continuous EEG monitoring can readily identify this artifact by demonstrating a steady peak of power at frequencies of 60 Hz/ 50 Hz on a power spectrogram. The appearance of an increase in the power in this bandwidth is often readily observable and serves as a means of detecting high-impedance electrodes during continuous EEG recordings.

6.14. Electrostatic Artifacts

Electrostatic forces may induce currents in electrode wires or cables. Movement of the electrode wires may cause regional or widespread slow waves that occur at the same frequency as the movement of the wires. Using short electrode wires and bundling the wires together, either in plastic wrap or with gauze, will reduce this type of artifact. Movement of the input cable between the electrode jackbox and the amplifier can also cause capacitance coupling and can transfer energy between adjacent cables, producing artifact in a widespread distribution involving cerebral and extracerebral channels and creating unusual electrical fields (Fig. 11.60). Artifact may also be induced by rhythmic movement of the electrode wires. Scratching the

head or neck, rubbing the eyes, chest percussion, cardiopulmonary resuscitation, patting or tapping (Fig. 11.61), and burping infants may cause rhythmic movement-induced artifact. Semirhythmic and repetitive artifact may be produced by similar movement of the electrode wires or from patient movement. These patient movements may occur from ventilators, anti-bedsore beds, intra-arterial balloon pumps, ventricular assist devices, and especially oscillatory ventilators and tubing. The morphology of the artifact may vary, and the appearance depends on the frequency of activity produced by the electromechanical device. It is commonly a mixture of frequencies superimposed on a slow wave that is typically stereotyped or monomorphic. Percussive beds or oscillatory ventilators may cause periodic and rhythmic artifact in the theta or alpha bandwidth, usually best seen in the electrodes at the back of the head or the ones in contact with the bed. An extra lead can be applied to the ventilator tubing or mechanical device; this will reveal the source that produces a similar discharge to show that the waveform is an artifact.

Movement of nearby people or objects in the environment may induce electrostatic artifacts, and this may occur even if the wires themselves do not move. Environmental sources of artifact can include movements of nurses and EEG technologists around the patient's bed, external contact of clothing or bedding by staff (especially synthetic fabrics), swaying of tubing near the patient, or movement of fluid in intravenous lines or respirator tubing near the scalp electrode wires or input cable.[10] These waveforms may appear high voltage with complex morphologies that conform to nonphysiological fields. Water movement in the respirator tubing connected to the patient results in periodic high-voltage slow waves with superimposed fast components on the EEG (Fig. 11.62) after a "breath" has been delivered by the ventilator. This typically occurs with a widespread field over the frontal regions on the side of the head nearest the respiratory tubing. Similarly, electrostatic charges on drops of fluid in intravenous macro-drips may cause spike-like potentials coinciding with the drip rate of the infusion (Fig. 11.63). This is less common now with the greater use of micro-drips.

Piezoelectricity is an electrical charge generated by the mechanical deformation of polymeric materials. Artifact may also result from electric infusers that create static electricity between the polyvinyl chloride tubing of the intravenous line and the pump roller head.[10] Unusual artifacts may also be produced by continuous venous hemofiltration and dialysis machines. These artifacts arise from a combination of static and piezoelectric currents in pumps rotating between 50 and 600 rpm, causing currents to flow into the patient (and then to electrodes) via fluid in the tubing.[37]

The technologist should make every effort to minimize movements around the patient and note any changes in the EEG associated with movement. In addition, the technologist should attempt to correlate unusual or periodic EEG transients with equipment function when present (e.g., respirator function or intravenous drips). Briefly turning off a machine or disconnecting the respirator tubing during the EEG can confirm the origin of the rhythmic artifact if the suspicious waveform disappears.

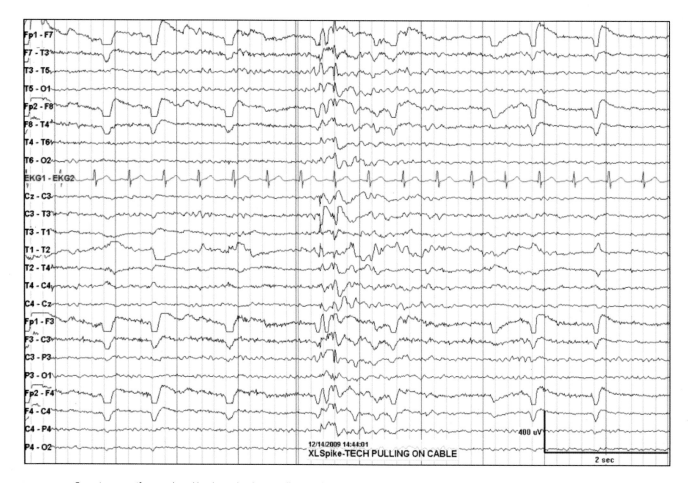

Figure 11.60. Capacitance artifact produced by the technologist pulling on the cable. In this case the cable acts like a discharging capacitor. When multiple insulated wires are compressed, the cable discharges like a capacitor, resulting in a high-voltage transient mimicking a spike-wave artifact on the EEG. Sensitivity 7 uV/mm; filter settings 1–70 Hz; display speed 30 mm/sec.

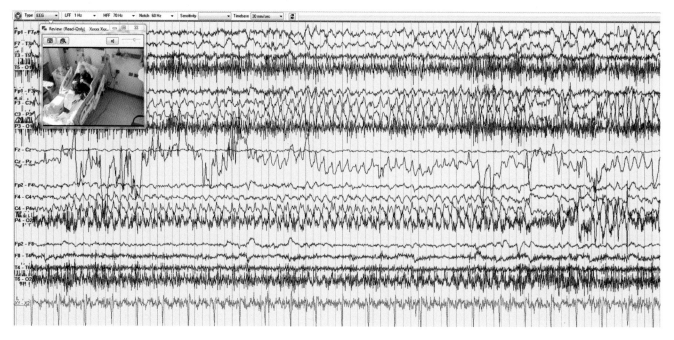

Figure 11.61. Physiological artifact from tapping movement (with "muscle") and nonphysiological artifacts arising from the electrodes.

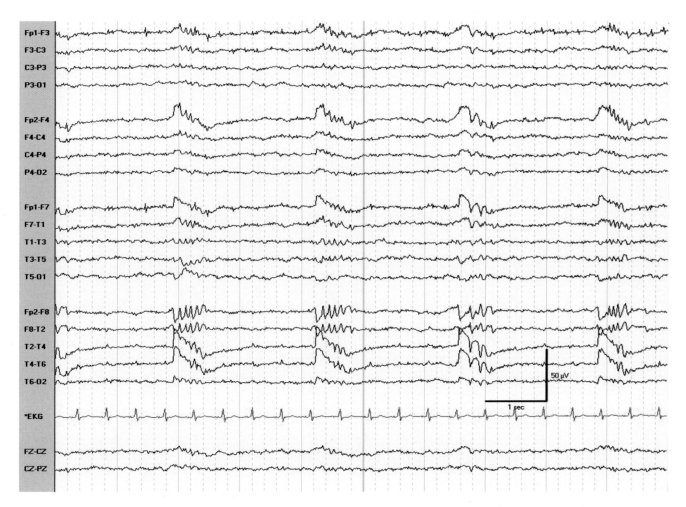

Figure 11.62. Water movement in the respirator tubing producing periodic high-voltage slow waves with superimposed fast components on the EEG. Sensitivity 7 uV/mm; filter settings 1–70 Hz; display speed 30 mm/sec.

6.15. Electromagnetic Artifacts

With electromagnetic artifacts, interference is seen in all channels. High-frequency interference from television and radio towers or stations in close proximity is an infrequent cause of artifact but can be difficult to eliminate when it is encountered. Hospital paging systems and walkie-talkies using radiofrequency carriers may introduce artifact into the EEG. Noncellular telephones may cause artifacts during the ring tone; this is related to the voltage change that develops in the telephone lines during the ringing.[10] Portable and cellular telephones can generate artifact in the EEG even when not being used.[38] The impact of cell phones in terms of producing artifact on the EEG depends on the proximity to the electrodes and the operating frequency and form of technology used. Cell phones may create repetitive sharp and slow-wave complexes mimicking an interictal epileptiform discharge. The nonphysiological distribution will mark these waveforms as artifact. They can be widespread but appear higher voltage in electrodes nearest the telephone (Fig. 11.64). Many of these high- or mixed-frequency artifacts are eliminated by the EEG machine's common mode rejection features and its anti-aliasing high-frequency filter. Nevertheless, some may cause bizarre intermittent artifacts.

Microwave ovens near the EEG lab may also produce radiofrequency interference. Televisions and computer screens can cause high-frequency interference at the screen refresh rate when they are near the patient. In the operating room, electrocautery devices generate high-voltage, high-frequency signals that travel through the body to the recording electrodes, including the EEG and ECG.[39] An artifact due to a train-of-four stimulus to verify the depth of anesthesia will be obvious on the EEG and demonstrates the integrity of the stimulation (Fig. 11.65). If the EEG machine is operating while electrocautery is being applied, bizarre artifacts may be present in the EEG. Even high-frequency electrocautery used in adjacent unshielded rooms may produce interference.[10]

Line isolation monitors, common safety devices present in the ICU and operating room, scan electrical outlets for leakage currents. They generate low-voltage artifact that may be noticeable in EEGs recorded at increased sensitivities, such as in comatose or anesthetized patients.[39]

6.16. Electrical Stimulators

Electrical devices may produce high-frequency artifact that interferes with recording an EEG. Pacemakers can produce very short-duration spiky, high-voltage artifact. Pacer spikes are best

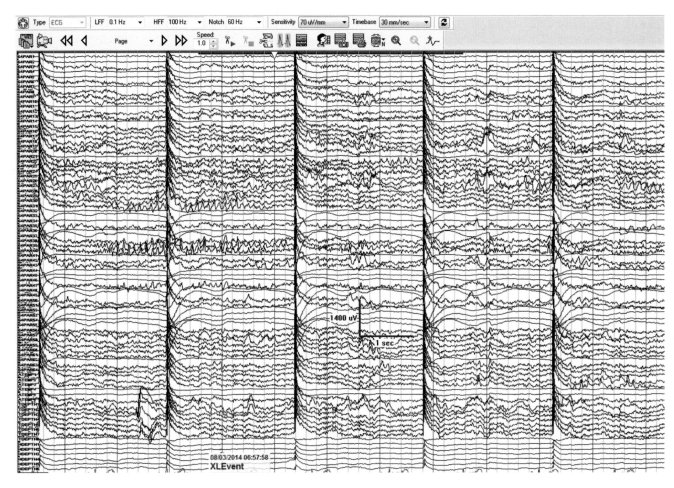

Figure 11.63. *Intravenous drip artifact on intracranial EEG. Note the regularity and periodicity.*

seen in the ECG channel but occasionally show a field extending to EEG electrodes, especially in patients with short necks. Artifacts can occur with deep brain stimulators, vagal nerve stimulators, responsive neurostimulators, spinal cord stimulators, and other nonneurological stimulators. The vagal nerve stimulator produces an artifact characterized by a high-amplitude, surface-negative evoked potential on scalp EEG (Fig. 11.66). This electrical potential is produced in the mid-cervical region of the neck and therefore can be recorded in the scalp EEG as well as the ECG.[40] With the greater availability of brain stimulation techniques and devices, these artifacts may be encountered more often and may be confused with an abnormality.

7. PITFALLS IN PHYSICIAN INTERPRETATION

There are many pitfalls in the interpretation of EEG. Misinterpretation usually occurs due to lack of experience and training, leading to overinterpretation of nonepileptiform potentials as epileptiform and potentially leading to unwarranted treatment. From a practical standpoint, this may be more likely to occur when a limited or confusing history is coupled with a lack of clinical expertise. This can lead to an overreliance on an EEG interpretation that is made without taking into account the patient's clinical situation.[41] It is well known that a normal interictal EEG does not exclude a clinical diagnosis of epilepsy.[42] However, even if the EEG records a brief focal seizure, there may be no scalp electrographic pattern that is identifiable. This is especially true in patients with extra-temporal seizures or when a deeper or smaller seizure focus exists to defy diagnosis. EEG has been a major contributor to the misdiagnosis of epilepsy when an EEG is misread as abnormal.[3,4,42] In a survey of 47 clinical neurophysiologists attending a symposium at the American Clinical Neurophysiology Society's annual meeting, all but one had encountered artifact that was misinterpreted as an epileptiform discharge.[43] Repeated EEGs increase the yield of recovery of an abnormality up to 80% to 90% but also increase the cumulative amount of artifact.[42] An "abnormality" that is misidentified in the EEG could ultimately lead to mistreatment, with a profound adverse impact upon patient care.[4,44] Artifact of any source that produces spiky waveforms may be misinterpreted. The EEG may become obscured by myogenic or movement artifact to mask an epileptic origin (see Fig. 11.44). In addition to artifact, there are variations in the expression of normal waveforms, and a number of normal variants may be misidentified as abnormal (Box 11.1). In addition, myogenic sources may be superimposed upon normal background and suggest that a waveform is "potentially epileptogenic." Because the presence of an interictal epileptiform discharge on EEG following a first unprovoked seizure has class A evidence for a high risk

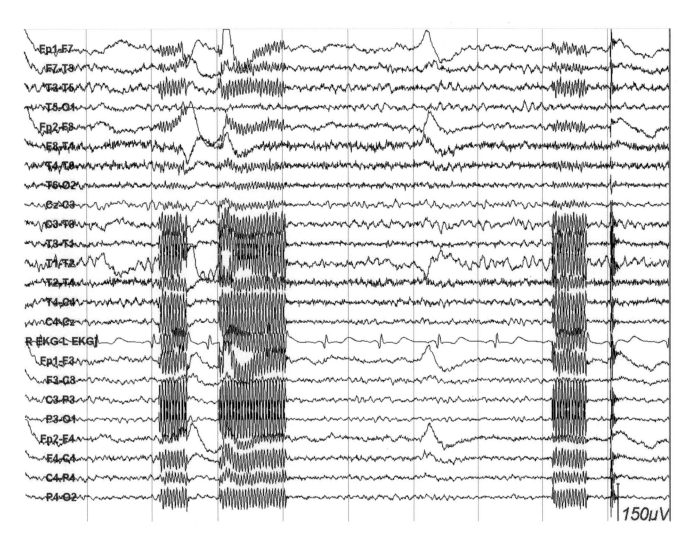

Figure 11.64. Intermittent artifact created by ringing of a nearby telephone. Sensitivity 7 uV/mm; filter settings 1–70 Hz; display speed 30 mm/sec.

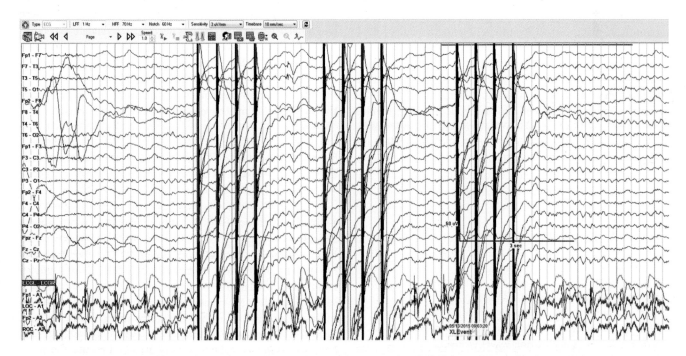

Figure 11.65. Characteristic train-of-four artifact produced in the operating room during carotid endarterectomy to ensure adequate anesthesia.

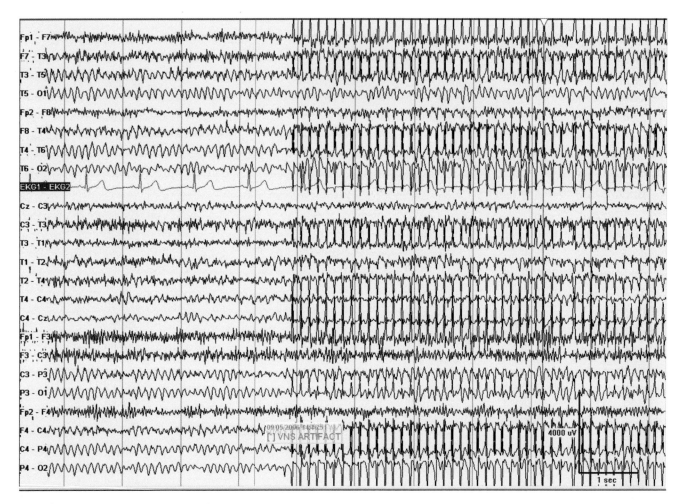

Figure 11.66. *Vagal nerve stimulator artifact during the "on time" of stimulation.* Borrowed with permission from Demos Publishers. In: Tatum WO, ed. *Handbook of EEG Interpretation.* 2nd Edition. New York: Demos Publishers; 2014:1–361.

of recurrence,[45] the emphasis on correct interpretation is paramount to ensuring correct treatment of a single seizure as epilepsy.[46] By falsely interpreting an EEG in the context of a first seizure or in a patient with nonepileptic events, inappropriate treatment can ensue for years before a correct diagnosis is realized through video-EEG monitoring. Patients identified with a definitive diagnosis of psychogenic nonepileptic seizures often have at least one EEG that was misinterpreted as abnormal.[47]

The reasons for misinterpretation of an EEG are unclear and complex. Applying basic recording concepts to the EEG lies at the foundation for arriving at the correct interpretation.[48] It is important to obtain and review the "abnormal" EEG, not just the report, when the finding does not agree with the clinical diagnosis (e.g., syncope). This is necessary to validate the epileptiform finding that has been reported. Verifying the true nature of an interictal epileptiform discharge or attributing the finding to an artifact or normal variant is essential, since multiple normal EEGs that may subsequently be performed do not eliminate the one EEG that may have demonstrated an abnormality.

8. COMMON ARTIFACTS THAT MIMIC EPILEPTIFORM ABNORMALITIES ASSOCIATED TO PEOPLE WITH EPILEPSY

Artifact can mimic nearly any abnormal pattern. Both physiological and nonphysiological sources of artifact may serve as pitfalls to physician interpretation (see Table 11.1). The process of recognizing an EEG finding that is "suspicious" for abnormality requires knowledge of the wide range of normal waveforms and variants as well as the types of artifact that may occur.[49] During routine scalp EEG recordings, patterns mistaken for epileptiform discharges associated to people with epilepsy commonly include nonspecific fluctuations of background activity.[47] Eye movements change the electric fields around the eyes and affect the scalp EEG and may mimic "frontal sharp waves," especially

---

BOX 11.1. BENIGN EPILEPITFORM PATTERNS

Wicket spikes
Breach rhythm
Benign epileptiform transients of sleep
Rhythmic midtemporal theta of drowsiness (sharp form)
6-Hz generalized spike-and-waves ("phantom spikes")
Vertex sharp (or "spiky" vertex) waves (adolescents)
Positive occipital sharp transients of sleep (POSTS)
Artifacts (such as overfiltered muscle potentials)

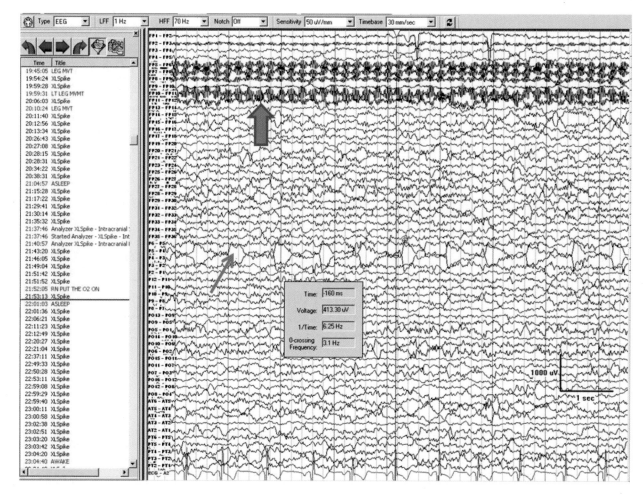

Figure 11.67. Artifact on intracranial EEG with physiological pulse artifact (thin blue arrow) and nonphysiological electrode artifact (thick blue arrow).

in patients who are encephalopathic. In addition, as a result of the topographic distribution, EEG recordings may be significantly distorted, leading to problems of interpretation. There is a common misconception that "phase reversals" indicate abnormality. Even intracranial EEG may be subject to artifact (Fig. 11.67). Despite the higher fidelity of the signal-to-noise ratio that is present to reduce intracranial electrode noise, extracranial sources may generate patterns on intracranial EEG that could be confused with seizures.[50] Artifacts are particularly relevant in prolonged and ambulatory recordings (Fig. 11.68) and cEEG monitoring in the ICU, where they are more abundant and diverse. These may be very misleading and in this scenario an "over-read" EEG can be dangerous. In the critically ill population, EEG is the sole test for nonconvulsive status epilepticus.[35] When this leads to a wrong diagnosis, it is usually accompanied by significant treatment intensity that may be not only unnecessary but associated with significant morbidity. Certain common artifacts during cEEG are common to all EEG recordings (ECG, eye movements, muscle activity, sweating, electrode instability, etc.), with certain patterns providing challenges to correct recognition. The main one of these includes periodic patterns that mimic generalized (see Fig. 11.35) and lateralized periodic discharges (see Fig. 11.43), challenging the interpreter. Other artifacts that should be directly eliminated by the technologist include pulse, sweat, electrode pops, ground

lead recordings, 60 Hz, and other technical nonphysiological artifacts, including those that occur during shivering, intravenous infusions that drip, dialysis, mechanical beds, and other machines that can occur in this "hostile" environment. From a technical standpoint, the improper use of high-frequency filters that restrict the bandpass may result in an inappropriate display of waveforms that modifies the morphology, making artifact appear "sharp."[3] This in turn may lead to misinterpretation and misdiagnosis.

The growing number of artifacts seen increases with the use of cEEG monitoring. Similarly, quantitative EEG and trending, networking, and invasive EEG monitoring may also contain artifact that may result in misidentification of seizures.[35] In addition, before judging whether periodic activity on quantitative EEG is epileptiform, it is essential to analyze the raw EEG to assess the original waveforms and exclude artifact. While trends to identify artifact are emerging, many algorithms have a greater sensitivity for seizures than for detecting artifact.

9. TRAINING AND STANDARDS

Not all neurologists are skilled at interpreting EEGs. Recognizing artifact has a significant learning curve. Identifying artifact can be challenging when pattern recognition alone is used to

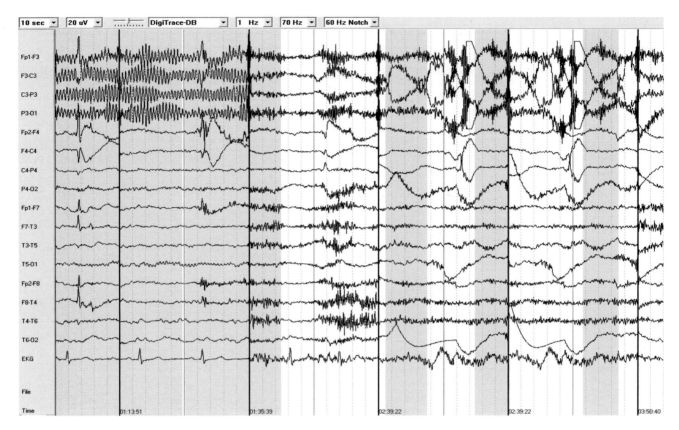

Figure 11.68. A variety of artifact identified on computer-assisted ambulatory EEG. Automated spike detections taken every 2 seconds that identify nonphysiological artifact as abnormality.

interpret an EEG. Strict criteria to define epileptiform discharges associated to people with epilepsy are limited, and therefore room for qualitative error exists in determining whether a discharge is of epileptic significance. Some misreadings may be due to the desire to find an abnormality when patients have an episode of unexplained loss of consciousness,[51] fear of missing a diagnosis and being responsible for event-related consequences, and limited training or experience in interpretation. Many introductory primers, atlases, and comprehensive textbooks are available for would-be readers who are interested in learning how to interpret EEGs.

Even though neurologists are the designated experts who interpret EEGs, at present there is no requirement by the Accreditation Council for Graduate Medical Education for a neurologist to receive education in EEG interpretation. Dedicated training in EEG reading during neurology residency typically includes very limited exposure, with most programs offering 0 to 3 months during a 4-year postgraduate training period. It is widely believed that neurologists are trained to read EEGs competently and that the result represents an absolute parameter to be used in treatment. Even though training may be absent, any neurologist is able to submit bills for interpreting an EEG and need not prove competence to be able to receive remuneration. There is little incentive for a general clinical neurologist to receive further training in neurophysiology or EEG, which has been mainly focused on academic neurologists.[52]

While the incidence of misdiagnosis in a general neurology practice is unknown, it is likely to be a common occurrence. Misinterpretations are often due to the lack of experience or

training. Interpreters who have not seen a large number of normal tracings may not appreciate the wide range of normal EEG variability and may not apply strict criteria for sharply contoured nonepileptiform variants or artifacts. The less experience achieved, the lower the threshold for misidentifying a waveform as an abnormality. Therefore, validating a potentially misread EEG requires that the tracing be recovered to confirm the nonpathological nature of the finding that was identified. Medical records may not be easy to obtain, or may in fact have been destroyed. When misinterpretation of the EEG occurs, it can go unchallenged for many years until the typical event is recorded during video-EEG monitoring. A general neurologist might prefer to start treating a possible seizure rather than taking the more conservative approach of always under-reading the EEG and waiting to be absolutely sure of the diagnosis before starting the patient on medication.

Solutions include defining and ensuring the EEG competency of neurologists who read EEGs, and perhaps providing a confirmatory reading by an electroencephalographer, as is done for ECGs.[53] Requiring a structured educational course of study for neurology residents is a goal for good training programs. Competence and ultimately board certification in clinical neurophysiology would be the anticipated outcome for trainees who intend to use their skills in EEG during clinical practice. Maintenance of certification is now available for electroencephalographers who are board-certified to ensure ongoing learning.[54] However, for neurologists who have limited or no formal training in EEG, a gap exists to ensure appropriate competence when seeking hospital privileges to read EEGs.

10. CASE PRESENTATION

The patient was a 73-year-old female being evaluated for "blackouts." A past medical history included cardiomyopathy with congestive heart failure, generalized anxiety disorder, fibromyalgia, degenerative joint disease, and chronic low back pain. She presented to the emergency department after an episode of lightheadedness upon standing that progressed to nausea, diaphoresis, and "tunnel vision." She was diagnosed in the emergency department with syncope and was then evaluated by cardiology, where she was diagnosed with vasovagal syncope following evaluation. She also seen by neurology and a brain MRI and EEG were obtained. The brain MRI demonstrated periventricular white matter microvascular ischemic changes but was without focal or acute changes. An EEG was performed and captured "seizure activity" during photic stimulation. She was treated with rapidly escalating doses of oxcarbazepine to 600 mg orally twice daily. Within 2 weeks she presented to the hospital with malaise, nausea and vomiting, and dizziness. Her serum sodium level was 123 mEq/dL. She underwent overnight video-EEG while oxcarbazepine was abruptly discontinued with cardiac telemetry. Her symptoms resolved, though on cardiac telemetry, prolonged sinus pauses were evident, and a permanent pacemaker was implanted. The abnormal EEG describing epileptic activity was requested and revealed only myogenic artifact in a generalized distribution that mimicked a generalized epileptic discharge (Fig. 11.69).

Commentary: This case highlights the negative consequences of a misinterpreted EEG and illustrates the potential pitfall of misinterpreting a normal photomyogenic response as abnormal epileptic activity. It also emphasizes the importance of selecting an appropriate antiseizure medication and highlights the potential for any treatment to produce a serious consequence. In this case, the mistreatment led to an adverse event—severe hyponatremia—that required hospitalization. Even if the artifact contained in the EEG was considered to be an abnormal photoparoxysmal response, oxcarbazepine was a poor choice for an antiseizure medication: generalized seizures may be aggravated because a photoparoxysmal response is characteristically associated with genetic generalized epilepsy. Even worse, the mistreatment could have camouflaged or worsened a potentially fatal cardiac arrhythmia that was heralded by syncope. While fortunately this was discovered during hospitalization, the morbidity (and potential mortality), in addition to the discomfort, time, and expense borne by the patient, could have been avoided had the EEG been correctly interpreted in the context of the clinical presentation.

Fortunately in this case the EEG could be obtained and the artifactual nature of the finding could be resolved. In addition. a photomyogenic response was reproduced to confirm the "typical" event that was previously recorded. Overall, the outcome was favorable after oxcarbazepine was withdrawn and the issue of an abnormal EEG was put to rest.

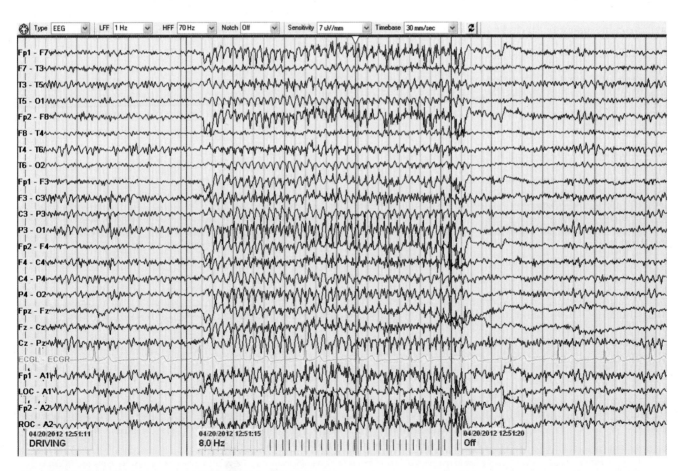

Figure 11.69. Photomyoclonic response in an elderly woman with hyponatremia.

11. ARTIFACT ELIMINATION

Eliminating the many patient- and technology-generated artifacts requires a team approach during EEG recording and interpretation. This team involves the technologist, nursing and medical personnel, and the interpreter to ensure the integrity of the patient's recording prior to interpretation of the EEG.[48] Current digital EEG systems typically include video with EEG capable of acquiring large quantities of information. These systems allow remontaging and use software applications such as spike and seizure detection, quantitative EEG, and trends and artifact reduction programs to optimize interpretation of the EEG. Digital recording allows easy post-hoc manipulation of the montage, filter settings, display, and review speed to eliminate or modify artifact. It is often possible after acquiring an EEG to clean up the recording when excessive artifact is present. However, this may lead to overuse of the digital filters and alteration of the waveforms; this is especially true when employing high-frequency low-pass filters. For example, when muscle activity is filtered with excessive use of high-frequency filters, the morphology may be altered and may falsely appear as epileptiform discharges associated to people with epilepsy (Fig. 11.70). Despite the advantages of digital EEG, artifacts unique to a computer-based recording may arise (see Fig. 11.57).

To eliminate artifact from the EEG before interpretation, it first must be recognized and the cause accurately identified. An experienced technologist who is always mindful of artifact during the performance and record review used to be the sole means of minimizing artifact. Ensuring adequate electrode and machine integrity (including ground) and identifying or monitoring patient and environmental sources of artifact is essential. The American Society of Electroneurodiagnostic Technologists Inc. has set standards for technologists who record EEG. The presence of a competent technologist during an EEG recording is essential for reducing artifact and the misinterpretation that might ensue. The technologist can actively search for artifacts and try to troubleshoot and eliminate them by re-gelling the electrodes, encouraging the patient to relax, and ensuring the integrity of the recording system. Artifact reduction may occur after the recording is complete, but it is the responsibility of the technologist during the study to try to minimize or eliminate, camouflage, or annotate artifact that may interfere with interpretation. Even expert readers have difficulty interpreting a poor-quality EEG recording. The American Clinical Neurophysiology Society has established guidelines for recording EEG on digital media, standards of practice in clinical EEG, and reporting.[55]

Special care units that use continuous EEG, such as an EMU, or critical care EEG monitoring in the ICU can generate large amounts of artifact over long periods of time. cEEG is less amenable to proactive artifact elimination because the technologist is not present during the majority of the recording. In addition, special care units are "hostile" environments due to the multiple sources that can interfere with recording cerebral activity. Video recording is very helpful to elucidate artifact during cEEG monitoring by demonstrating movements synchronous with the frequency of the artifact. Even intracranial EEG recordings performed for epilepsy are subject to artifact despite less electrode artifact than scalp EEG recording (see Fig. 11.67).[35] Computer-assisted ambulatory EEG and ICU EEG recordings are associated with a high exposure to environmental sources in addition to instrumental sources.[56]

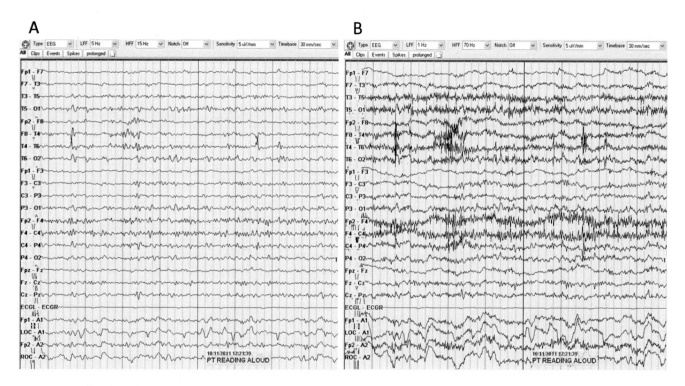

Figure 11.70. **A:** *Filtered muscle activity using a low-frequency high-pass filter of 15 Hz and (**B**) standard parameters with filters of 1–70 Hz. Note the T8 "spike" created by the digital filtering.*

12. ARTIFACT REDUCTION TECHNIQUES

Manual rejection techniques require identification and elimination of artifacts during the EEG recording. Using this technique, the EEG technologist or EEG interpreter visually reviews the entire EEG recording and marks segments that contain artifact. This is a reliable method and may detect some complex artifact that would otherwise be missed by automated techniques. However, this method is time-consuming and impractical in most settings, and reader fatigue may become problematic for multichannel EEG recordings over long periods of time. In addition, subtle or brief artifacts can be missed because different interpreters have different thresholds for rejection. This method cannot be used for real-time digital EEG recording and is used only in offline analysis. These labor-intensive methods of artifact removal require a human element. When segments containing artifact are identified, they are then eliminated from the analysis before the final interpretation is rendered. Unfortunately, eliminating segments of artifact also removes physiological signals, and therefore important underlying EEG signals may also be lost.

Automated *subtraction* is a technique that rejects short segments of EEG when they exceed the preset parameter thresholds. This technique may be applied using online or offline subtraction of artifact. Thresholds can be set by simply analyzing the EEG channels themselves to determine parameter cutoffs based upon amplitude, numbers of zero crossings, or frequency (e.g., 60 Hz). Segments may be identified by an individual waveform or series of waveforms exceeding the predefined threshold and are subsequently eliminated from the recording. Artifact regression is a software-based method performed by selectively subtracting specific patterns that represent artifact. This may be performed relative to either the time or frequency domain. This method can be used in EEG to focus on eye movements, "regressing" the EOG activity from the recording based upon the frequency domain. This inevitably involves subtracting a relevant portion of the EEG signal from the recording. While common artifacts such as eye movements and ECG artifact may be amenable to this technique, non-stereotyped artifacts produced by myogenic or mechanical sources (e.g., electrode artifact) do not have a singular reference channel, so the regression methods cannot be used to remove them. In these cases, it may be necessary to camouflage the artifacts rather than expecting elimination of the source. Eye movements, cardiac signals, myogenic sources, and line noise present serious problems for EEG interpretation and analysis.[57] Some techniques use additional channels employing special electrodes to identify artifact signals, including EOG, EMG, ECG, or use of accelerometers. If the signal in these channels exceeds a predetermined threshold, the segment of EEG will be rejected. These automatic subtraction techniques cannot identify all possible artifacts because of the multiplicity and complexity of the different waveforms.

Artifact *rejection* is a technique that uses post hoc manipulation of the recorded EEG. Digital filtering, montage selection, adjustment in sensitivity, and alteration of the display speeds enhance the ability to recognize artifact and identify the source for elimination.[3] Low-pass and high-pass digital filtration can be individualized based upon the frequency and used intermittently. In the case of 60-Hz artifact, application of the notched filter may be used throughout a recording. Digital filters can be used and removed, leading to improved visibility of the waveform in question. However, filter use can distort waveforms by removing the sharpness or by producing a falsified rhythmicity. It is therefore always important to return to the raw EEG waveform for corroboration. Amplitude may be changed by adjusting the sensitivity, and this can permit clearer interpretation of a field that may be obscured. Altering other parameters of the recording, such as slowing the display speed, may enhance the ability to identify extracerebral potentials by clarifying nonphysiological features. Caution is advisable when using automated rejection software because there is a considerable loss of acquired information from the EEG signal at the time of artifact rejection. Rejecting contaminated EEG segments and filtering artifactual waveforms can result in an unacceptable loss of useful information. Several methods have been used to remove common artifacts such as blink and other eye movement artifact from EEG recordings.

Although there are several techniques used in artifact reduction from the EEG, most of them have relied upon targeting a specific source of artifacts or use simulated artifacts that may markedly differ in morphology from patient data. Software is continuously being improved to implement new algorithms that permit the filtering of common types of artifacts generated by the eye, skeletal muscles, and ECG.[58] Newer methods of artifact reduction separate the electrical sources identified by the scalp sensors using *independent component analysis* or analysis of the principal component analysis.[59] ICA is a technique that uses statistical principles to represent independent components of a predetermined signal. Applying independent component analysis to multiple channels of the EEG recording can identify, select, and remove a wider variety of artifacts by selectively eliminating the contributions of artifact sources to the electrocerebral signals that are recorded on the scalp.[57] Newer artifact reduction algorithms using the technique of *blind source separation*–based algorithms[60] also separate original signals into the underlying components. By applying a set of advanced neural networks to the signal, the individual components of the signal that arise from various sources may be identified.[61] These components of a signal, such as eye movement, ECG, electrode, and myogenic artifact, can thus be identified and removed. Substantial artifact reduction is therefore possible.

While automated artifact reduction systems continue to evolve, it is clear that eliminating more than a single type of artifact is most advantageous.[62] Wider application of quantitative EEG using the fast Fourier transform in spectral analysis and other panel trends incorporating signal power in ICU-EEG monitoring will require new methods of artifact reduction. It is crucial to improve mathematical calculations that provide frequency components and indexes so that pure cerebral activity can be more appropriately represented. As a result, a greater degree of confidence will be possible when using the absolute numerical values in EEG and artifact intensity trends when artifact reduction software is applied.

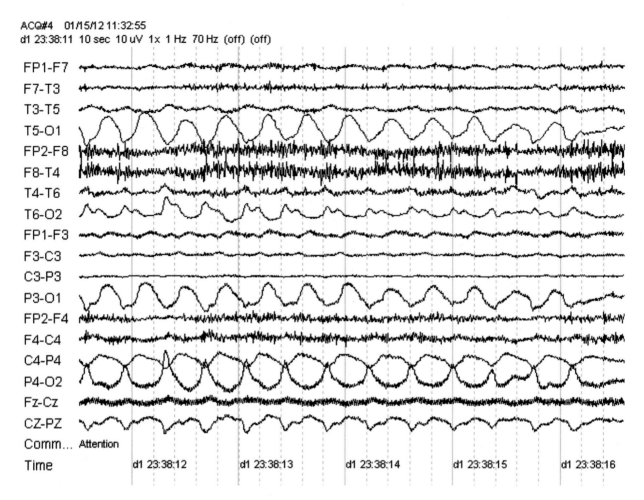

ACQ#4 01/15/12 11:32:55
d1 23:38:11 10 sec 10 uV 1x 1 Hz 70 Hz (off) (off)

FP1-F7
F7-T3
T3-T5
T5-O1
FP2-F8
F8-T4
T4-T6
T6-O2
FP1-F3
F3-C3
C3-P3
P3-O1
FP2-F4
F4-C4
C4-P4
P4-O2
Fz-Cz
CZ-PZ
Comm... Attention
Time   d1 23:38:12   d1 23:38:13   d1 23:38:14   d1 23:38:15   d1 23:38:16

Figure 11.71. EEG artifact on a smartphone "seizure alert" caused by cardiopulmonary resuscitation after cardiac arrest in the ICU. The artifact was produced by head movement from chest compressions. Courtesy William D. Freeman, M.D.

13. CONCLUSIONS

The EEG is designed to record cerebral activity, but it also frequently records electrical activity arising from extracerebral sites. Some physiological artifacts reflect functions that are crucial for appropriate interpretation of an EEG,[1] but many sources may obscure the record. Recognition of artifact should be followed by identification of the source, if at all possible, with subsequent attempts at elimination when it interferes with interpretation. Other artifacts may mimic an abnormality and can serve as pitfalls for the interpreter by leading to misinterpretation of the EEG and then to inappropriate treatment. While it is impossible to eliminate all diagnostic errors from the treatment decision-making process,[63] minimizing misinterpretation of the EEG by improved artifact recognition and reduction techniques is a critical step in the process. Newer systems of remote interpretation (Fig. 11.71), guidelines for reporting,[64] and digital scoring of the EEG may help bridge the gap between the classical method of visual analysis and the computerized means of identifying and quantifying recorded artifact.[65]

ACKNOWLEDGMENT

We wish to thank our chief technologists, Kirsten Yelvington, R.EEG T., CLTM, and Paul Dionne, R.EEG T., for their help in acquiring samples of EEG artifact.

Chapter #11: Artifacts of Recording and Common Errors in Interpretation

SCORE EEG SOFTWARE

Further examples related to the topics addressed in this chapter can be found in the interactive online Niedermeyer Educational Platform. EEG recordings with illustrative examples can be opened and browsed. Features are marked and described using the SCORE EEG software. The users can see the features marked by experts, they can score these features themselves, and then compare them with the scorings of the experts.

The Niedermeyer Educational Platform can be accessed at: www.scoreEEG.com/academy

REFERENCES

1. Aurlien H, Gjerde IO, Aarseth JH, et al. EEG background activity described by a large computerized database. Clin Neurophysiol. 2004;115(3):665–673.
2. Tatum WO, Husain AM, Benbadis SR, Kaplan PW. Normal adult EEG and patterns of uncertain significance. J Clin Neurophysiol. 2006;23(3):194–207.
3. Tatum WO. EEG interpretation: common problems. Clin Practice. 2012;9(5):527–538.
4. Benbadis SR, Tatum WO. Overinterpretation of EEGs and misdiagnosis of epilepsy. J Clin Neurophysiol. 2003;20(1):42–44.
5. Sinha SR, Sullivan L, Sabau D, et al. American Clinical Neurophysiology Society Guideline 1: Minimum Technical Requirements for Performing Clinical Electroencephalography. J Clin Neurophysiol. 2016;33: 303–307.
6. Nuwer MR, Comi G, Emerson R, et al. IFCN standards for digital recording of clinical EEG. Electroencephalogr Clin Neurophysiol. 1998;106(3):259–261.
7. American Society of Electroneurodiagnostic Technologists Inc. Minimum Educational Requirements for Performing Electroneurodiagnostic Procedures. https://www.aset.org/files/public/Min_Education_Requirements_for_Performing_EEG.pdf. Accessed March 12, 2016.
8. Young B, Osvath L, Jones D, Socha E. A novel EEG artifact in the intensive care unit. J Clin Neurophysiol. 2002;19(5):484–486.
9. Ney JP, van der Goes DN, Nuwer MR, Nelson L, Eccher MA. Continuous and routine EEG in intensive care: utilization and outcomes, United States 2005–2009. Neurology. 2013;81(23):2002–2008.
10. Dworetzky B, Herman S, Tatum WO. Artifacts of recording. In: Schomer DL, Lopes da Silva FH, eds. Niedermeyer's Electroencephalography: Basic Principles, Clinical Applications, and Related Fields. 6th ed. Philadelphia: Wolters Kluwer Health/Lippincott Williams & Wilkins; 2011:239–266.
11. Blum DE. Computer-based electroencephalography: technical basics, basis for new applications, and potential pitfalls. Electroencephalogr Clin Neurophysiol. 1998;106(2):118–126.
12. Epstein CM. Aliasing in the visual EEG: a potential pitfall of video display technology. Clin Neurophysiol. 2003;114(10):1974–1976.
13. Lesser RP, Luders H, Dinner DS, Morris H. An introduction to the basic concepts of polarity and localization. J Clin Neurophysiol. 1985;2(1):45–61.
14. Maulsby RL. Guidelines for assessment of spikes and sharp waves in EEG tracings. Am J EEG Technol. 1971;11(1):3–16.
15. Vinton A, Carino J, Vogrin S, et al. "Convulsive" nonepileptic seizures have a characteristic pattern of rhythmic artifact distinguishing them from convulsive epileptic seizures. Epilepsia. 2004;45(11):1344–1350.
16. Ebersole JS, Hawes-Ebersole S. Clinical application of dipole models in the localization of epileptiform activity. J Clin Neurophysiol. 2007;24(2):120–129.
17. Beniczky S, Conradsen I, Moldovan M, et al. Automated differentiation between epileptic and nonepileptic convulsive seizures. Ann Neurol. 2015;77(2):348–351.
18. Poh MZ, Loddenkemper T, Reinsberger C, et al. Convulsive seizure detection using a wrist-worn electrodermal activity and accelerometry biosensor. Epilepsia. 2012;53(5):e93–97.
19. Patterson AL, Mudigoudar B, Fulton S, et al. SmartWatch by SmartMonitor: assessment of seizure detection efficacy for various seizure types in children, a large prospective single-center study. Pediatr Neurol. 2015;53(4):309–311.
20. Stern JM, Engel JJ. Artifacts. In: Stern JM, Engel JJ, eds. Atlas of EEG Patterns. Philadelphia: Lippincott, Williams & Wilkins; 2005:55–86.
21. Conradsen I, Moldovan M, Jennum P, Wolf P, Farina D, Beniczky S. Dynamics of muscle activation during tonic-clonic seizures. Epilepsy Res. 2013;104(1-2):84–93.
22. Fisch BJ. Fisch and Spehlmann's EEG Primer: Basic Principles of Digital and Analog EEG. 3rd ed. Amsterdam: Elsevier; 1999.
23. Croft RJ, Barry RJ. Removal of ocular artifact from the EEG: a review. Neurophysiol Clin. 2000;30(1):5–19.
24. Sirven JI. EEG in focal encephalopathies: cerebrovascular disease, neoplasms, and infections. In: Ebersole JS, Husain AM, Nordli D, eds. Current Practice of Clinical Electroencephalography. 4th ed. Philadelphia: Wolters Kluwer; 2014:242.
25. Seneviratne U, Mohamed A, Cook M, D'Souza W. The utility of ambulatory electroencephalography in routine clinical practice: a critical review. Epilepsy Res. 2013;105(1-2):1–12.
26. Chen DK, Graber KD, Anderson CT, Fisher RS. Sensitivity and specificity of video alone versus electroencephalography alone for the diagnosis of partial seizures. Epilepsy Behav. 2008;13(1):115–118.
27. Guideline twelve: guidelines for long-term monitoring for epilepsy. J Clin Neurophysiol. 2008;25(3):170–180.
28. Benbadis SR, Agrawal V, Tatum WO. How many patients with psychogenic nonepileptic seizures also have epilepsy? Neurology. 2001;57(5):915–917.
29. Ferree TC, Luu P, Russell GS, Tucker DM. Scalp electrode impedance, infection risk, and EEG data quality. Clin Neurophysiol. 2001;112(3):536–544.
30. Gordon M. Artifacts created by imbalanced electrode impedance. Am J EEG Technol. 1980;20(4):149–160.
31. Alarcon G, Binnie CD, Garcia Seoane JJ, et al. Mechanisms involved in the propagation of interictal epileptiform discharges in partial epilepsy. Electroencephalogr Clin Neurophysiol Suppl. 1999;50:259–278.
32. Stecker MM, Sabau D, Sullivan L, et al. American Clinical Neurophysiology Society Guideline 6: Minimum Technical Standards for EEG Recording in Suspected Cerebral Death. J Clin Neurophysiol. 2016;33:324–327.
33. Schevon CA, Thompson T, Hirsch LJ, Emerson RG. Inadequacy of standard screen resolution for localization of seizures recorded from intracranial electrodes. Epilepsia. 2004;45(11):1453–1458.
34. Tatum WO, Dworetzky BA, Freeman WD, Schomer DL. Artifact: recording EEG in special care units. J Clin Neurophysiol. 2011;28(3):264–277.
35. Gaspard N, Hirsch LJ. Pitfalls in ictal EEG interpretation: critical care and intracranial recordings. Neurology. 2013;80(1, Suppl 1):S26–42.
36. Klem GH. Artifacts. In: Ebersole JS, Pedley TA, eds. Current Practice of Clinical Electroencephalography. 3rd ed. Philadelphia: Lippincott, William & Wilkins; 2003:271–287.
37. McGrath B, Columb M. Renal replacement therapy causing ECG artifact mimicking atrial flutter. Br J Intens Care. 2004;14:49–52.
38. Sethi PK, Sethi NK, Torgovnick J. Mobile phone artifact. Clin Neurophysiol. 2006;117(8):1876–1878.
39. Patel SI, Souter MJ. Equipment-related electrocardiographic artifacts: causes, characteristics, consequences, and correction. Anesthesiology. 2008;108(1):138–148.
40. Tatum WO. Normal EEG. In: Tatum WO, ed. Handbook of EEG Interpretation. 2nd Edition. New York: Demos Publishers; 2014:1–361.
41. Chadwick D. Diagnosis of epilepsy. Lancet. 1990;336(8710):291–295.
42. Fowle AJ, Binnie CD. Uses and abuses of the EEG in epilepsy. Epilepsia. 2000;41(Suppl 3):S10–18.
43. Tatum WO. How not to read an EEG: concluding statements. Neurology. 2013;80(1, Suppl 1):S52–53.
44. Krauss GL, Abdallah A, Lesser R, Thompson RE, Niedermeyer E. Clinical and EEG features of patients with EEG wicket rhythms misdiagnosed with epilepsy. Neurology. 2005;64(11):1879–1883.
45. Krumholz A, Wiebe S, Gronseth GS, et al. Evidence-based guideline: management of an unprovoked first seizure in adults: Report of the Guideline Development Subcommittee of the American Academy of Neurology and the American Epilepsy Society. Neurology. 2015;84(16):1705–1713.
46. Fisher RS, Acevedo C, Arzimanoglou A, et al. ILAE official report: a practical clinical definition of epilepsy. Epilepsia. 2014;55(4):475–482.
47. Benbadis SR. Errors in EEGs and the misdiagnosis of epilepsy: importance, causes, consequences, and proposed remedies. Epilepsy Behav. 2007;11(3):257–262.
48. Tatum WO, Dworetzky BA, Schomer DL. Artifact and recording concepts in EEG. J Clin Neurophysiol. 2011;28(3):252–263.
49. Tatum WO. Normal "suspicious" EEG. Neurology. 2013;80(1, Suppl 1):S4–11.
50. Goodkin HP, Quigg M. Toothbrushing EEG artifact recorded from chronically implanted subdural electrodes. Neurology. 2010;75(20):1850.
51. Zaidi A, Clough P, Cooper P, Scheepers B, Fitzpatrick AP. Misdiagnosis of epilepsy: many seizure-like attacks have a cardiovascular cause. J Am Coll Cardiol. 2000;36(1):181–184.
52. Natus Neurology. Neurology Diagnostics EEG—2014 Reimbursement Information. 2014; http://www.natus.com/documents/Neurology%20 Diagnostics%20EEG%202014.pdf. Accessed March 12, 2016.
53. Benbadis SR. "Just like EKGs!" Should EEGs undergo a confirmatory interpretation by a clinical neurophysiologist? Neurology. 2013;80(1, Suppl 1):S47–51.
54. American Board of Psychiatry and Neurology Inc. Clinical Neurophysiology. 2015; http://www.abpn.com/maintain-certification/moc-exams/taking-a-moc-exam/subspecialty-moc-exams/clinical-neurophysiology/. Accessed March 12, 2016.

55. American Clinical Neurophysiology Society. Guidelines and Consensus Statements. 2006; http://www.acns.org/practice/guidelines. Accessed April 10, 2016.
56. Shih JJ, Tatum WO. Computer-assisted ambulatory EEG. In: Rubin DI, Daube JR, eds. Clinical Neurophysiology. 4th ed. New York: Oxford University Press; 2016.
57. Jung TP, Makeig S, Humphries C, et al. Removing electroencephalographic artifacts by blind source separation. Psychophysiology. 2000;37(2):163–178.
58. Hamaneh MB, Chitravas N, Kaiboriboon K, Lhatoo SD, Loparo KA. Automated removal of EKG artifact from EEG data using independent component analysis and continuous wavelet transformation. IEEE Trans Biomed Eng. 2014;61(6):1634–1641.
59. Akhtar MT, Mitsuhashi W, James CJ. Employing spatially constrained ICA and wavelet denoising, for automatic removal of artifacts from multichannel EEG data. Signal Processing. 2012;92(2):401–416.
60. Romero S, Mananas MA, Barbanoj MJ. A comparative study of automatic techniques for ocular artifact reduction in spontaneous EEG signals based on clinical target variables: a simulation case. Comput Biol Med. 2008;38(3):348–360.
61. Persyst. Persyst Artifact Reduction—detect and reduce artifact with the touch of a button. http://www.persyst.com/technology/artifact-reduction/. Accessed March 12, 2016.
62. Gao J, Yang Y, Sun J, Yu G. Automatic removal of various artifacts from EEG signals using combined methods. J Clin Neurophysiol. 2010;27(5):312–320.
63. Newman-Toker DE, Pronovost PJ. Diagnostic errors—the next frontier for patient safety. JAMA. 2009;301(10):1060–1062.
64. Tatum WO, Selioutski O, Ochoa JG, et al. American Clinical Neurophysiology Society Guideline 7: Guidelines for EEG Reporting. J Clin Neurophysiol. 2016;33:328–332.
65. Beniczky S, Aurlien H, Brogger JC, et al. Standardized computer-based organized reporting of EEG: SCORE. Epilepsia. 2013;54(6):1112–1124.

PART III | CLINICAL EEG: GENERAL TOPICS

12 | PATTERNS OF UNCLEAR SIGNIFICANCE

JONATHAN C. EDWARDS, MD AND EKREM KUTLUAY, MD

ABSTRACT: Accurate interpretation of electroencephalograms requires knowledge and experience with a wide range of findings. Misinterpretation is common and may result from insufficient inexperience, incomplete training, or simply human error. However, misinterpretation may also arise from the relative rarity of some findings, and also from the evolution and necessary change in our understanding of the significance of these findings. One of the most common sources of reader error is in dealing with patterns that have some hallmarks of abnormalities but are actually normal findings. We refer to these findings as variants, or "patterns of unclear significance." This chapter reviews several of the common and uncommon patterns (fast or slow alpha variant, alpha squeak, rhythmic midtemporal theta bursts of drowsiness, midline theta rhythm, subclinical rhythmic electrographic discharge in adults, 14- and 6-Hz positive bursts, 6-Hz spike-and-wave bursts, benign sporadic sleep spikes, wickets, frontal arousal rhythm), emphasizing characteristics that can optimize interpretation.

KEYWORDS: variant, electroencephalogram, patterns, unclear significance, misinterpretation

PRINCIPAL REFERENCES

1. Westmoreland BF, Klass DW. Unusual EEG patterns. J Clin Neurophysiol. 1990;7:209–228.
2. Gibbs FA, Rich CL, Gibbs EL. Psychomotor-variant type of seizure discharge. Neurology. 1963;13: 991–998.
3. Santoshkumar B, Chong JJ, Blume WT, et al. Prevalence of benign epileptiform variants. Clin Neurophysiol. 2009;120:856–861.
4. Cigánek L. Theta-discharges in the middle line: EEG symptom of temporal lobe epilepsy. Electroencephalogr Clin Neurophysiol. 1961; 13:669–673.
5. Westmoreland BF, Klass DW. A distinctive rhythmic EEG discharge of adults. Electroencephalogr Clin Neurophysiol. 1981;51:186–191.
6. Gibbs FA, Gibbs EL. Fourteen and six per second positive spikes. Electroencephalogr Clin Neurophysiol. 1963;15:553–558.
7. Klass DW, Westmoreland BF. Nonepileptogenic epileptiform electroencephalographic activity. Ann Neurol. 1985;18:627–635.
8. Tatum WO, Husain AM, Benbadis SR et al. Normal adult EEG and patterns of uncertain significance. J Clin Neurophysiol. 2006;23:194–207.
9. Benbadis SR, Tatum WO. Overinterpretation of EEGs and misdiagnosis of epilepsy. J Clin Neurophysiol. 2003;20:42–44.
10. Krauss GL, Abdallah A, Lesser R, et al. Clinical and EEG features of patients with EEG wicket rhythms misdiagnosed with epilepsy. Neurology. 2005;64:1879–1883.

1. INTRODUCTION

The subject of patterns of unclear significance encompasses a selection of electroencephalographic (EEG) findings that may look abnormal but usually are not. These variants, which can be challenging and commonly lead to misinterpretation, can be mainly grouped into two types: variant *rhythms* and variant *transients*. Table 12.1 provides a summary of the patterns that will be discussed here. Some of these findings will also be discussed in the chapters on the normal EEG (Chapters 7 and 8).

The difficulties of interpretation posed by these variants arise for several reasons. These patterns possess features that are similar in some ways to abnormal patterns. Beginning with variant rhythms, as a general rule, a few common features help distinguish these rhythms from definitely abnormal findings:

1. The variant rhythms are, for the most part, **monomorphic**. The term "monomorphic" simply means that each of the waves in the rhythm looks distinctly like the other waves in the rhythm. The waves have a characteristic shape, or "morphology," that repeats.

2. Most of the variants have an **arch-shaped** appearance, although some of the normal rhythms may have **notches** in some or all of the waves.

3. Most importantly, the variant rhythms for the most part **do not evolve**.

One important source of misinterpretation of these patterns may simply be that many of these patterns are uncommon. A significant number of clinicians who read EEGs in clinical practice may have only 2 or 3 months of closely supervised EEG training, and the chances of seeing a rare pattern are quite low during this short training. Without extensive preparation in the fundamentals of EEG and extensive supervised experience, misinterpretation of a rare pattern would not be surprising.

Finally, some confusion may arise from the fact that many of these patterns have changed names since first being described. In some cases, the nomenclature has changed numerous times. For some of the patterns, numerous names are still concurrently in use today (Table 12.2).

A particular challenge in assessing the true prevalence and clinical significance of these patterns is the tendency toward subject bias. Most patients who undergo EEG are doing so because of neurological symptoms, and many of these patients have a clinical history suggestive of epilepsy. While a few studies have looked at these findings in a general population, most have reviewed their presence in a clinical population. Since EEG is used to help diagnose epilepsy or other neurological conditions, the true predictive value of these findings may be biased.

2. FAST ALPHA VARIANT/SLOW ALPHA VARIANT

At times, harmonics or subharmonics of the background rhythm are seen. When this occurs, the resultant appearance

TABLE 12.1. Summary: Patterns of Unclear Significance

FINDING	AGE	STATE	LOCATION	FREQUENCY	DURATION	CHARACTERISTICS
Slow or fast alpha variant	Children and adults	Awake, eyes closed	Occipital	Half or double the posterior dominant rhythm	Brief or lasting many seconds	Sinusoidal, archiform, notched, flat-topped
Alpha squeak	Children and adults	Awake, immediately upon eye closure	Occipital	Initially fast (beta) slowing rapidly to the posterior dominant rhythm	Typically 0.5–2 sec	Sinusoidal, spindle-shaped
Rhythmic midtemporal theta bursts of drowsiness (RMTD)	Younger to middle-aged adults	Drowsiness, light sleep	Midtemporal, at times with spread to parasagittal or occipital-temporal region. Bilateral or independent over the right or left side.	5–7 Hz	Several seconds, or up to a minute or more	Arched, notched, flat-topped. Notches may give the waves a sharply contoured appearance.
Midline theta rhythm (Cigánek rhythm)	Children and adults	Common in drowsiness and during mental activation; less common in resting wakefulness	Midline (CZ, FZ), parasagittal	4–7 Hz	Brief or lasting many seconds	Arched, notched, flat-topped
Subclinical rhythmic electrographic discharge in adults (SREDA)	Adults, mostly age 40s to 80s (mean 60s)	Drowsiness and resting wakefulness (rare cases reported in sleep)	Maximal in temporal and parietal regions. Usually bilateral, but may be asymmetric.	May begin with delta frequency, but then increases to 4–7 Hz	Brief or lasting minutes	Sharply contoured, archiform, notched, flat-topped
14- and 6-Hz positive bursts	Childhood and adolescence	Drowsiness, light sleep	Posterior temporal	14 or 6 Hz	0.5–1 sec	Archiform, comb-like, low amplitude
6-Hz spike-and-wave bursts	Children and adults	Drowsiness, light sleep	Highest amplitude over fronto-central regions	5–6 Hz	1–2 sec	Usually low amplitude (<25 μV) and short duration (<30 msec) spike component
Benign sporadic sleep spikes (BSSS)	Mainly in adults; also reported in children and adolescents	Drowsiness, light sleep	Anterior- and mid-temporal	Sporadic	Usually <50 msed	Mono- or diphasic spike with steep descending arm
Wickets	Adults	Awake, sleep	Temporal regions	6–11 Hz if they occur in runs	Average of 2- to 4-sec bursts in sleep	Archiform, monophasic
Frontal arousal rhythm (FAR)	Children	Awakening, arousal from sleep	Frontal	6.5–8.5 Hz	Up to 13 sec	Monomorphic

is of a rhythm that is twice as fast or half as fast as the awake background. When the appearance is of a rhythm that is twice the frequency of the awake background, it is referred to as a "fast alpha variant" (1,2). A "slow alpha variant" has an apparent frequency that is about half that of the awake background (1–3). These harmonics often have a notched appearance, as if many of the waves are simply being cut in half, but only partly so. Slow and fast alpha variants are reactive to eye opening and closure.

Fast alpha variant is easy to detect, since awake posterior background rhythms in the middle to upper beta range would be quite unusual. True beta rhythms are most often seen in the frontal, central, and parietal regions. When a posterior background rhythm of 16, 18, or 20 is seen, it is easy to think of fast alpha variant. However, slow alpha variant is more challenging and may easily be misinterpreted as occipital slowing. This tendency to misread slow alpha variant as abnormal stems mostly from the fact that slowing is such an easily recognized abnormality, and all electroencephalographers look for signs of slowing. As a general rule, any time you see occipital slowing, think of slow alpha variant first before calling the record abnormal. Look for a sample of normal awake background within the record. If the slowing is approximately half the frequency of the patient's awake

TABLE 12.2. Nomenclature over Several Decades

EEG PATTERN	OTHER TERMS USED PREVIOUSLY
Rhythmic midtemporal theta bursts of drowsiness (RMTD)	Psychomotor variant (7) Rhythmic midtemporal discharge (8) Rhythmic theta bursts of drowsiness (1) Rhythmic temporal theta bursts of drowsiness
Midline theta rhythm	Theta discharges in the middle line (16) Electrographic theta discharges in the midline (19) Cigánek rhythm Rhythmical midline theta (24)
Subclinical rhythmic EEG discharge of adults (SREDA)	Paroxysmal discharge of the temporo-parieto-occipital junction (25)
14- and 6-Hz positive bursts	14- and 6-Hz positive spikes (34), Ctenoids (35)
6-Hz spike-and-wave bursts	Spike and wave phantom (47)
Benign sporadic sleep spikes (BSSS)	Small sharp spikes (33), Benign epileptiform transients of sleep (55)
Wickets	Wicket spikes (63)
Frontal arousal rhythm (FAR)	Frontal arousal rhythm (71)

background, then the slowing is probably just a slow alpha variant. An additional clue can be small notches in some of the "slow waves," but bear in mind that the notches can be quite subtle (Figs. 12.1 and 12.2).

3. ALPHA SQUEAK

Immediately upon eye closure, the awake background is sometimes initially faster and of lower voltage. Over ~0.5 to 2 seconds, the background slows and increases in amplitude to become the normal awake background. This initial "speeding up" of the background immediately upon eye closure, referred to as an "alpha squeak," is a normal finding (2,4–6) (Fig. 12.3).

4. RHYTHMIC MIDTEMPORAL THETA BURSTS OF DROWSINESS

First described by Gibbs and Gibbs (1941), this pattern has been given several names over nearly six decades (7). Its earlier name, "psychomotor variant," is still commonly used. "Psychomotor" is an older term for a complex partial seizure, typically of temporal lobe origin. RMTD has commonly been referred to as "psychomotor variant" because it was thought to have a strong resemblance to a temporal lobe seizure. Subsequent names have included rhythmic midtemporal discharge (8), rhythmic theta bursts of drowsiness, and rhythmic temporal theta bursts of drowsiness (1).

The name "rhythmic midtemporal theta bursts of drowsiness" (RMTD) is widely accepted and quite clear in listing the most distinctive characteristics. RMTD is seen mostly during drowsiness and light sleep, although it may rarely be seen during wakefulness. It occurs in bursts or trains of rhythmic 5- to 7-Hz activity. RMTD is maximal in the midtemporal leads and may at times spread to the parasagittal regions, or more posteriorly to the occipital-temporal region. Like mu rhythm, RMTD may be seen bilaterally or may be independent over the

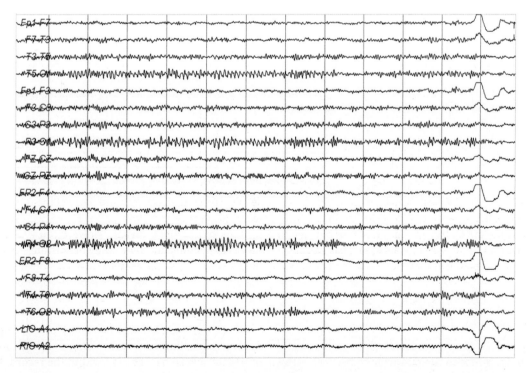

Figure 12.1. Fast alpha variant.

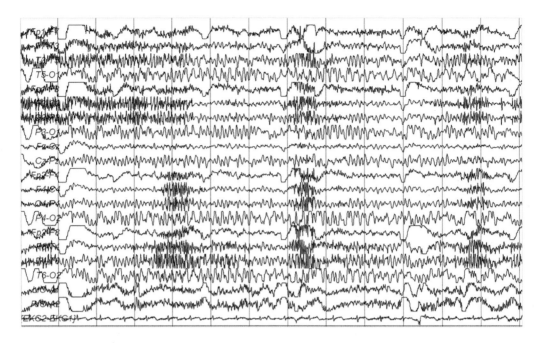

Figure 12.2. Slow alpha variant.

right or left side. Like most rhythmic variants, it is typically arch-shaped and is often notched. These notches may give the waves a somewhat sharply contoured appearance, which may be mistaken for a sharp wave. At times, the notched arches may have a flat-topped appearance (1,7,8). RMTD may occur in runs that last several seconds, or even up to a minute or more. The rhythmic nature and temporal location can lead to misinterpretation as seizure activity (9). However, like other normal rhythms, RMTD can be clearly distinguished from seizure activity because it is monomorphic and monorhythmic and does not evolve.

The reported overall prevalence of RMTD is quite low, ranging from 0.1% to 2% of records (10–14). The prevalence appears to be lower in age-matched normal controls than it is in EEGs performed in neurological patients (10). While some studies (8) have reported that a significant number of patients who are found to have RMTD may have epilepsy, the majority of patients with this finding will not. RMTD has been reported in the presence of a structural abnormality (15). The overall clinical significance of this finding is unclear. It is most commonly considered a normal variant (Fig. 12.4).

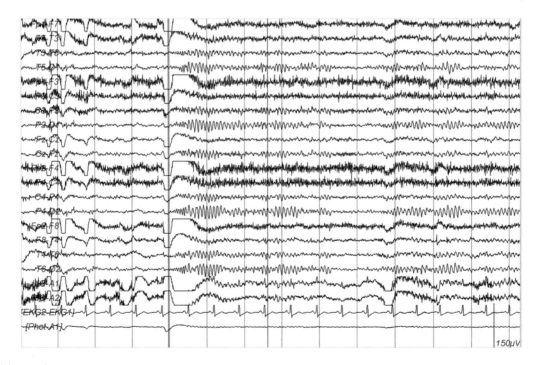

Figure 12.3. Alpha squeak.

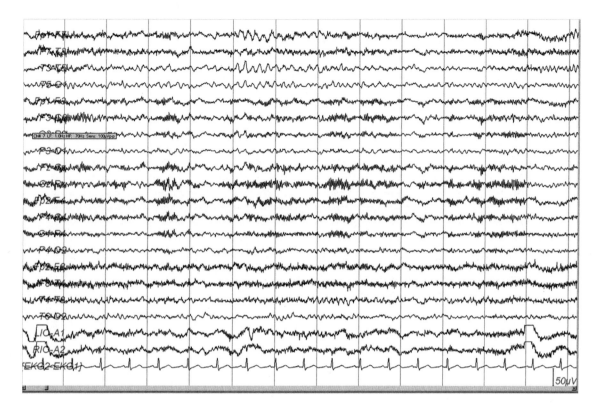

Figure 12.4. Rhythmic midtemporal theta bursts of drowsiness.

5. MIDLINE THETA RHYTHM (CIGÁNEK RHYTHM)

Midline theta rhythm was first described by Cigánek (1961) and is still commonly referred to as "Cigánek rhythm" (16). As is the case with many variant rhythms, the midline theta rhythm was originally thought to be indicative of epilepsy but was later found to be present in normal subjects also. Cigánek's 1961 report is actually titled "Theta-discharges in the middle line: EEG symptom of temporal lobe epilepsy." Midline theta is seen during wakefulness and drowsiness. Similar to RMTD, the midline theta rhythm is typically a 4- to 7-Hz arch-shaped or sinusoidal rhythm that may be notched or flat-topped (17). The main difference in appearance from RMTD is the location (typically maximum over CZ) and presence in wakefulness

The reported prevalence of midline theta rhythm has been highly variable, ranging from 2% to 35% of subjects (18,19). This wide disparity is in part accounted for by subject selection. Maulsby included the presence of midline theta during drowsiness and determined that it was present in 35% of normal adults. Many others have reported midline theta during mental tasks in a high number of patients (20–23). With the exclusion of midline theta rhythm that is seen only during drowsiness of mental activation, the prevalence has been reported to be low in normal controls and higher in patients with epilepsy. A more recent study (24) suggested that when drowsiness and mental activation are excluded, midline theta rhythm was common (26% overall) in patients with epilepsy and uncommon (0/54) in controls. Interestingly, in the same series, and using the same

exclusion criteria, midline theta rhythm was seen much more frequently in frontal lobe epilepsy (48.1%) than in temporal lobe epilepsy (3.7%).

The clinical significance of midline theta rhythm is not universally agreed upon (17,24). It is typically regarded as a nonspecific finding and is generally read as normal. Midline theta rhythm during the awake recording and without mental tasks may warrant further study. A potential practical challenge and confounding variable would be in actually knowing what a subject is doing mentally in an awake, at-rest recording, and ruling out that particular mental tasks are taking place. Most evidence suggests that the presence of midline theta rhythm during drowsiness or during mental task is not an abnormality (Fig. 12.5).

6. SUBCLINICAL RHYTHMIC ELECTROGRAPHIC DISCHARGE IN ADULTS

Subclinical rhythmic electrographic discharge in adults (SREDA) is a fairly rare pattern that can be easily misinterpreted. It is perhaps the most challenging pattern among those that are considered normal variants. First described in 1961 by Naquet et al., this pattern was originally thought to be associated with hypoxia (25). Westmoreland and Klass described 65 patients who had 142 EEG recordings and provided the name "subclinical rhythmic EEG discharge in adults." In this series, SREDA was seen in patients aged 42 to 80, with an average age of 61 (26).

The pattern is seen mostly during relaxed awake or drowsy states, although it can be seen during sleep (26,27). The typical

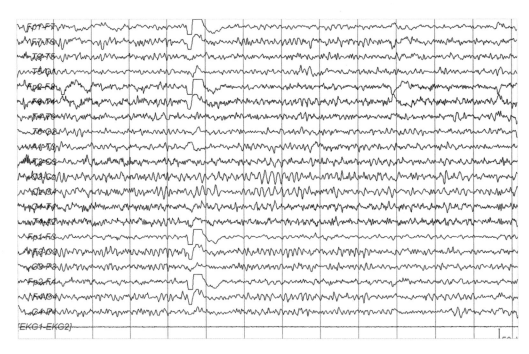

Figure 12.5. Midline theta rhythm.

appearance is a diffuse, sharply contoured, theta rhythm that is usually maximal in the temporal and parietal regions. While SREDA is usually bilateral, it may be asymmetric. An interesting feature of SREDA is that it often occurs in long runs, such as 15 seconds to a minute or more (26). The appearance on visual inspection is of a monomorphic rhythm. However, a more recent detailed digital study using frequency spectral analysis and Laplacian montages suggests that SREDA is "composed of a complex mixture of multiple rapidly shifting frequencies predominantly in the theta range, which show poor spatial and temporal resolution" (28).

This pattern has a distinctive feature that is different from other nonepileptic variants and that makes it especially difficult to recognize and easy to misdiagnose: it may initially evolve. SREDA may begin with a single sharp transient or a series of sharp transients, initially at delta frequencies, then increasing to theta, before becoming a well-defined 4- to 7-Hz rhythm. A smaller number of cases remain in the 2- to 4-Hz frequency range. After the initial period in which the rhythm is established, however, SREDA does not continue to evolve, despite the fact that it may be seen in prolonged runs of 20 seconds to several minutes. The rhythm ends abruptly in about half of patients; in the other cases, it gradually dissipates and merges with ongoing normal background rhythms. Unlike seizures, SREDA is not followed by "postictal" slowing, and no clinical changes accompany it.

While this pattern may easily be mistaken for an ictal pattern, evidence suggests that it has no clear association with seizures (14,26,29,30). In a large series, there was not only a low incidence of clinical history of seizures or subsequent development of seizures but also a "uniform lack of any clinical accompaniment during the bursts, even with the involvement of both hemispheres and persistence of several minutes" (26). A report of SREDA during video-EEG monitoring demonstrated that SREDA can be suppressed by the administration of lorazepam. Hence, a response to benzodiazepine administration cannot be used to distinguish electrographic seizure from SREDA (31). One study of ictal single-photon emission computed tomography demonstrated no significant changes in uptake during the bursts, further suggesting that the pattern is not ictal (32) (Fig. 12.6).

7. 14- AND 6-HZ POSITIVE BURSTS

Like many other variants, this unique EEG phenomenon was also described by Gibbs and Gibbs (33,34). Although it was previously called 14- and 6-Hz positive spikes, the current preferred term is 14- and 6-Hz positive bursts. Lombroso et al. also proposed the name "ctenoids" due to their appearance and complex morphology resembling a comb (*ktenos* in Greek translates to "comb") (35).

The typical bursts last between 0.5 and 1 sec and usually occur during light sleep or drowsiness (36–38). However, a few cases with occurrence in REM sleep have also been reported (39). The bursts can be unilateral or bilateral but usually show a shifting predominance if enough bursts are recorded in the same patient (36–38). Although the laterality of these bursts can appear to shift, the maximum amplitude is expressed over the posterior temporal head regions (36–38). The bursts are usually small in amplitude; therefore, referential or long-distance electrode montages reveal better waveforms (36–38). A referential montage to the contralateral ear or the use of additional temporal derivations (such as T1-T5 and T2-T6) is recommended to improve visualization of 14- and 6-Hz bursts (40,41).

There seems to be strong age predilection. This activity initially starts to appear during early childhood and peaks during

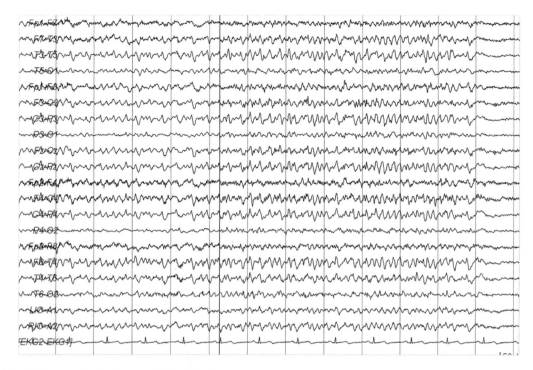

Figure 12.6. Subclinical electrographic discharges of adults (SREDA).

adolescence (36–39). The coexistence of 14- and 6- Hz positive bursts and 6-Hz spike-and-wave bursts was also reported. Silverman hypothesized that a maturational sequence might be responsible for this co-occurrence, and that most of the 6-Hz spike-and-wave bursts are part of the 14- and 6-Hz positive bursts (42). Fourteen- and 6-Hz positive bursts are still seen during adulthood, but the incidence decreases with advanced age (36). Lombroso reported the highest incidence of 58% in the literature in boys ages 13 to 16 years (35). In adults, the incidence is much lower; an incidence as low as 4% was seen in a group of psychiatric patients (43), whereas a study of EEG in asymptomatic normal adults revealed a rate of around 12% (44). In fact, the authors of the latter study claimed that 14- and 6-Hz positive bursts was the most common pattern of uncertain significance in their series of 100 asymptomatic adults (44).

Several reports have been published correlating the coexistence of this pattern with certain symptoms and illnesses. A wide variety of psychiatric conditions and neurovegetative symptoms were subjected to research (35,36,45). Epilepsy was also thought to be more common in patients with 14- and 6-Hz positive bursts (46). However, most of the patients with behavioral symptoms and organic central nervous system impairment were children or adolescents, which is the age of peak incidence for this phenomenon (43). One study suggests that a majority of patients with seizures and 14- and 6-Hz positive spikes also showed other epileptiform abnormalities in their EEGs (46).

This controversial pattern seems to be an age-related phenomenon. Although there are arguments that it has pathological significance, the reported incidence of up to 58% in normal teenagers and 12% in healthy adults makes this relatively hard to prove (Fig. 12.7).

8. 6-HZ SPIKE-AND-WAVE BURSTS

Six-Hz spike-and-wave bursts were first described in 1950 as "wave and spike phantom" (34,47). The first collected cases revealed a unique EEG pattern of 1-sec bursts of 5- to 6-Hz spike-and-waves (47). The average amplitude of the discharge was low (~25 μV or less), with the spike component <30 msec in duration (47–49). This pattern can be seen in both children and adults, with amplitude usually higher over the fronto-central regions (47,48). These bursts were mostly seen during drowsiness and light sleep but were also seen during full wakefulness (47). Bursts are usually diffuse but may show anterior or posterior predominance. Marshall suggested the comparison linkage, which measures the potential difference between analogous scalp areas for better viewing rather than traditional bipolar or referential montages (47).

The average incidence of 6-Hz spike-and-wave bursts is 1% to 2.5% of all EEG recordings (14,47,48,50,51). Several authors tried to link this controversial pattern to specific complaints, ranging from simple fainting to vegetative or dysautonomic pathologies, and from psychiatric disturbances to seizures (43,47,48,52). However, occurrence in normal people and absence of clinical symptoms during the bursts make it difficult to label these discharges as a specific indicator of any certain disease (36,52). As mentioned earlier, Silverman suggested that there is relationship as a maturational sequence and waveform spectrum between 6-Hz spike-and-wave bursts and 14- and 6-Hz positive bursts (42). He claimed that most of the 6-Hz spike-and-wave bursts are part of the 14- and 6- Hz positive bursts and that transition between these two types may lead to the occurrence of both patterns in the same person (42).

Upon investigating more than 60,000 EEGs over 30 years, Hughes proposed two distinct subtypes of this pattern (51).

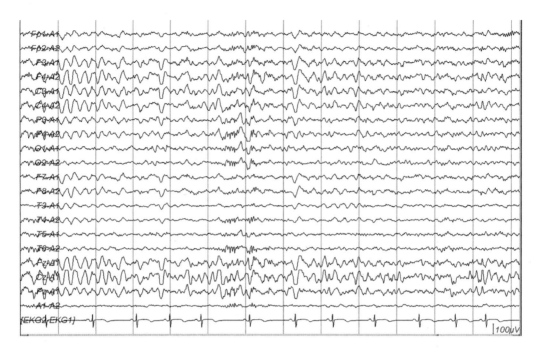

Figure 12.7. 14- and 6-Hz positive bursts.

The features of these two variants were summarized by acronyms WHAM (**W**ake, **H**igh amplitude, **A**nterior location, **M**ale gender) and FOLD (**F**emale gender, **O**ccipital location, **L**ow amplitude, **D**rowsiness) (51). Hughes indicated that these two variants are more extreme forms, and also suggested that the more components of the WHAM form that exist in a single person, the more likely is the association with seizures (51). Current consensus is that this EEG pattern is of unclear clinical significance; however, high amplitude of the spikes, a rate slower than 6 Hz, and persistence of the discharges in deeper stages of sleep is more likely associated with seizures (37,53).

Overinterpretation of benign EEG variants as epileptiform activity is a common problem during daily practice. In particular, 6-Hz spike-and-wave bursts are notorious for mimicking generalized spike-and-wave discharges (54). However, the special characteristics described above should help the interpreter to distinguish these benign discharges from epileptiform activity (Fig. 12.8).

9. BENIGN SPORADIC SLEEP SPIKES

Small sharp spikes, the term originally used by Gibbs and Gibbs, are also known as benign epileptiform transients of sleep or benign sporadic sleep spikes (BSSS) (34,36,55). The latter has recently become the preferred term. These spikes are short in duration and low in amplitude. Although they are usually <50 msec and <50 µV, the duration can be slightly longer and the amplitude can be slightly higher depending on the recording circumstances and montage used (36–38). The shape is rather simple and consists of mono- or diphasic spike with a steep descending arm (36,37). An aftergoing slow wave is not prominent and usually is lower in amplitude than the spike component (36,37,55). Background activity at the region of BSSS is not disrupted (36,37). These discharges are best seen during drowsiness and light sleep (stage

I and II) and are best displayed over anterior and midtemporal or ear electrodes (36,37). Although they have been reported in children and adolescents, BSSS are mainly seen in adults (37,56).

The origin and cortical location of the BSSS have been the subject of a few investigations. Recording with depth electrodes in two patients revealed a similarity to surface findings (57). Invasively recorded spikes had widespread distribution and similar simple morphological appearance (58). They occurred as single sporadic transients without disrupting the ongoing background activity; however, the amplitude was higher than surface recordings (57). Another study with subdural electrodes showed that BSSS were more widespread than on surface recordings and were mainly seen over the posterior mesial temporal area (58).

BSSS are generally not thought to be related to any certain disease and are accepted as a variant of normal EEG activity (37,55,59). However, over the years, several reports tried to find a connection between BSSS and seizures or certain psychiatric conditions. BSSS were thought to be a sign of epileptogenicity. Different authors reported higher incidence of BSSS in patients with seizures, particularly in younger patients (56,60). One study indicated that the highest incidence is seen in patients younger than 20 years, with a gradual decrease with advanced age leading to complete disappearance after age 80 (60). Still other studies claimed a relationship between BSSS and certain psychiatric conditions. Positive correlations were reported with manic depressive psychosis and psychotic depressive episodes as well as during acute mania (61,62).

BSSS were first described about half a century ago. They are very common EEG findings, seen in up to 25% of the normal population (38,55). Although several studies reported an increased frequency of BSSS in certain psychiatric conditions and seizures, because of their high incidence in the normal population we believe that this peculiar EEG activity is of unknown clinical significance and has no statistical relationship to a certain disease (Fig. 12.9).

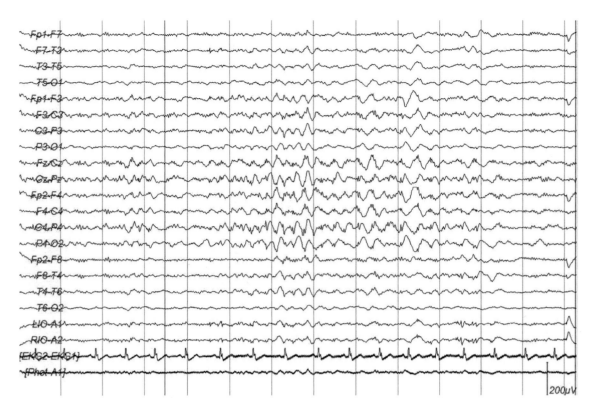

Figure 12.8. 6-Hz spike-and-wave discharges.

10. WICKETS

Wickets are archiform waveforms first described as wicket spikes by Reiher and Ebel in 1977 (63). They are simple mono-phasic waveforms with surface negativity (63). Initial descriptions revealed that wicket spikes are found both in awake and sleep EEGs (63). Because of the intermixed background activities during the awake state, they are better recognized during sleep (63,64). They are best seen during initial stages of sleep but also reported during rapid-eye-movement sleep (63,65,66). Their location remains unchanged during differ-ent stages of sleep (65). Wickets can occur as isolated "spikes"

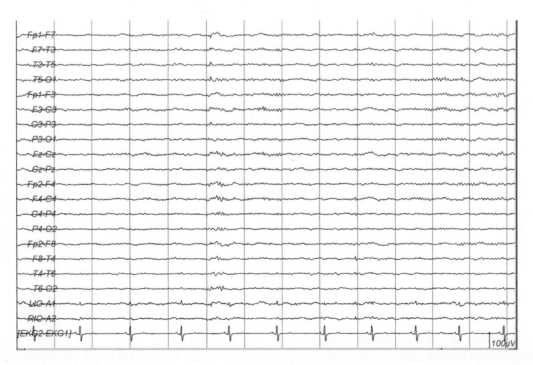

Figure 12.9. Benign sporadic sleep spikes (BSSS).

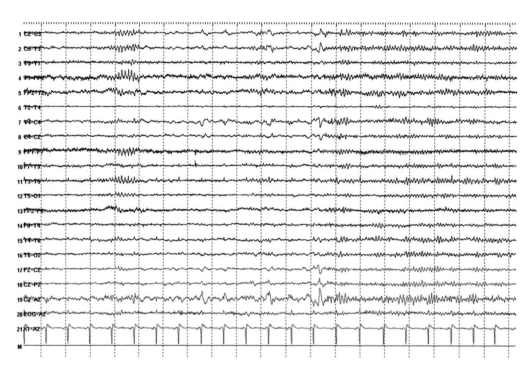

Figure 12.10. Wickets.

or they may come in runs (36,38,63). If they occur in runs, the usual frequency is between 6 and 11 Hz. The amplitude of a wicket spike may range between 60 and 210 µV and is maximally expressed over the temporal regions (36,38,63). Although they shift sides, often one side is more dominant than the other (63). However, prolonged recordings with continuous EEG suggest that they are more often lateralized to the left than the right (67,68).

Wickets are usually seen in adults (63). They are almost exclusively reported in adults 30 years or older; however, cases as young as 20 years have also been reported (13,38,63). Wickets are reported to be an uncommon EEG pattern. Their incidence in large EEG series has been reported to be <1%, ranging between 0.03% and 0.96% (13,14,63). In adults 30 years and older the incidence may rise to 2.9% (63).

Wickets are considered to be a normal variant. In Reiher and Lebel's original description, wickets occurred four times more in patients with no history of seizures than in those with a history of seizures (63). An experienced electroencephalographer can differentiate wickets from temporal sharp waves easily by the lack of aftergoing slow waves and the absence of distortion of the background activities (38,53,63). However, one can also overread or misinterpret wickets as epileptiform sharp waves, especially if they occur in isolation (69,70). The clues mentioned above, as well as observation of runs of wicket spikes elsewhere in the same EEG, should alert the reader that this is a nonepileptiform variant (69) (Fig. 12.10).

11. FRONTAL AROUSAL RHYTHM

Frontal arousal rhythm (FAR) is a unique EEG pattern that was first described by White and Tharp in 1974, although the pattern was first recognized in 1969 (71). In their original report, the authors described eight cases out of 4,780 EEGs reviewed over a 4-year period. The four boys and four girls had a mean age of 6.6 years, ranging from 2 to 14 years. Their initial diagnoses were mild cerebral dysfunction and/or seizure disorder. Representative EEG samples showed normal awake and sleep patterns. However, during arousal from stage 2 sleep, a 6.5- to 8.5-Hz rhythm was seen over the frontal regions involving mainly the F3 and F4 electrodes, with little or no spread to adjacent regions. The overall amplitude of this activity was between 30 and 150 µV, with duration of up to 13 sec. This pattern was originally described in children with evidence of minimal cerebral dysfunction and seizures, but the authors noted that the incidence in a normal population was unknown at the time of the publication (71).

Twenty-five years after the initial description of this rare and unusual EEG pattern, Hughes and Daaboul discussed their findings in 50 cases (72). The incidence of FAR was 0.22% in their series of 22,500 patients seen over an 8-year period. The characteristics of the pattern were similar to those described before. While FAR was the only atypical pattern in 58% of these patients, nearly half (42%) also showed other abnormalities, including focal and generalized epileptiform activity. Clinically, 70% of the children had a seizure disorder, and 56% had both seizures and cognitive/behavior disorders. Only 6% of the reported patients had neither seizure nor cognitive/behavior disorders. However, the incidence of cognitive/behavior disorders was not statistically different from their control group whose EEG did not show a FAR pattern. Their conclusion was that FAR is related to seizures. To support this view, a recent case report described a 6-year-old boy with mental retardation and possible seizure disorder (73). A typical FAR pattern was seen during a few episodes associated with eye fluttering followed by chewing, increased inspiration, and upper lip quivering. These episodes were all recorded during

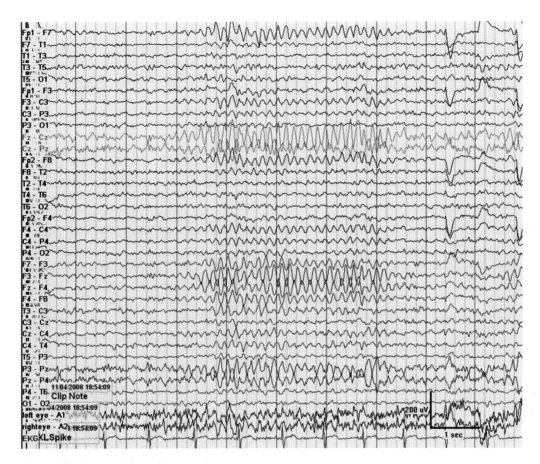

Figure 12.11. Frontal arousal rhythm (FAR). Courtesy of Dr. William Tatum.

arousal from sleep and no clinical changes were seen when the patient was awakened without the FAR pattern present.

Few illustrative reports are available in the literature. The incidence of FAR in the general population is unknown. The consensus is that FAR is more of a nonspecific EEG pattern with unknown clinical significance (2,35). However, the reported case series as well as demonstration of FAR as an ictal pattern in a reported case warrants careful review for other interictal activity and detailed questioning for possible seizure-like activity (Fig. 12.11).

SCORE EEG SOFTWARE

Further examples related to the topics addressed in this chapter can be found in the interactive online Niedermeyer Educational Platform. EEG recordings with illustrative examples can be opened and browsed. Features are marked and described using the SCORE EEG software. The users can see the features marked by experts, they can score these features themselves, and then compare them with the scorings of the experts.

The Niedermeyer Educational Platform can be accessed at: www.scoreEEG.com/academy

REFERENCES

1. Chatrian GE, Bergamini L, Dondey M, et al. A glossary of terms most commonly used by clinical electroencephalographers. Electroencephalogr Clin Neurophysiol. 1974; 37:538–548.

2. Westmoreland BF, Klass DW. Unusual EEG patterns. J Clin Neurophysiol. 1990;7:209–228.
3. Goodwin JE. The significance of alpha variants in the EEG, and their relationship to an epileptiform syndrome. Am J Psychiatry. 1947;104:369–379.
4. Bekkering D, Kamp A, Storm van Leeuwen W, Werre PF. Example of the use of the spectrograph and the magnetograph: the squeak phenomenon. Electroencephalogr Clin Neurophysiol. 1956; 8:721.
5. Storm van Leeuwen W, Bekkering D. Some results obtained with the EEG spectrograph. Electroencephalogr Clin Neurophysiol. 1958;10:563–570.
6. Storm van Leeuwen W, Kamp A, Kniper J Concerning the "squeak" phenomenon of the alpha rhythm. Electroencephalogr Clin Neurophysiol. 1960;12:244.
7. Gibbs FA, Gibbs EL. Atlas of Electroencephalography. 1st ed. Cambridge, MA: Lew A. Cummings, 1941:55, 109.
8. Lipman IJ, Hughes JR. Rhythmic midtemporal discharges: an electroclinical study. Electroencephalogr Clin Neurophysiol. 1969;27:43–47.
9. Beiske KK, Kostov KH, Kostov H. Rhythmic midtemporal discharge in a youth during light sleep. Neurodiagn J. 2016;56:32–36.
10. Gibbs FA, Rich CL, Gibbs EL. Psychomotor-variant type of seizure discharge. Neurology. 1963;13: 991–998.
11. Gibbs EL, Gibbs FA. Psychomotor-variant type of paroxysmal cerebral dysrhythmia. Clin Eectroencephalogr. 1989;20: 147–152.
12. Maulsby RL. EEG patterns of uncertain diagnostic significance. In: Klass DW, Daly DD. Current Practice of Electroencephalography. New York: Raven Press; 1979:411–419
13. Radhakrishnan K, Santoshkumar B, Venugopal A Prevalence of benign epileptiform variants observed in an EEG laboratory from South India. Clin Neurophysiol. 1999;110:280–285.
14. Santoshkumar B, Chong JJ, Blume WT, et al. Prevalence of benign epileptiform variants. Clin Neurophysiol. 2009;120:856–861.
15. Hennessy MJ, Koutroumanidis M, Hughes E, Binnie CD. Psychomotor EEG variant of Gibbs: an association with underlying structural pathology. Clin Neurophysiol. 2001;112:686–687.
16. Cigánek L. Theta-discharges in the middle line: EEG symptom of temporal lobe epilepsy. Electroencephalogr Clin Neurophysiol. 1961; 13:669–673.
17. Westmoreland BF, Klass DW. Midline theta rhythm. Arch Neurol. 1986;43:139–141.

18. Maulsby R. The normative electroencephalographic data reference library. Final report, contract NAS 9-1200. National Aeronautics and Space Administration, Washington DC, 1968.
19. Mokráň V, Cigánek L, Kabátnik Z. Electrographic theta discharges in the midline. Eur Neurol. 1971;5:288–293.
20. Gevins A, Smith ME, McEvoy L, Yu D. High-resolution EEG mapping of cortical activation related to working memory: effects of task difficulty, type of processing, and practice. Cereb Cortex. 1997;7:374–385.
21. Okada S, Urakami Y. Midline theta rhythm revisited. Clin Electroencephalogr. 1993;24:6–12.
22. Takahashi N, Shinomiya S, Mori D, Tachibana S. Frontal midline theta rhythm in young healthy adults. Clin Electroencephalogr. 1997;28:49–54.
23. Inanaga K. Frontal midline theta rhythm and mental activity. Psychiatry Clin Neurosci. 1998;52:555–566.
24. Beleza P, Bilgin Ö, Noachtar S. Interictal rhythmical midline theta differentiates frontal from temporal lobe epilepsies. Epilepsia. 2009;50:550–555.
25. Naquet R, Louard C, Rhodes J, Vigouroux M. A propos de certaines décharges paroxystiques du carrefour temporo-pariéto-occipital. Leur activation par l'hypoxie. Rev Neurol. 1961;105:203–207.
26. Westmoreland BF, Klass DW. A distinctive rhythmic EEG discharge of adults. Electroencephalogr Clin Neurophysiol. 1981;51:186–191.
27. Fleming WE, Avidan A, Malow BA. Subclinical rhythmic electrographic discharge of adults (SREDA) in REM sleep. Sleep Med. 2004;5:77–81.
28. O'Brien TJ, Sharbrough FW, Westmoreland BF, Busacker NE. Subclinical rhythmic electrographic discharges of adult (SREDA) revisited: a study using digital EEG analysis. J Clin Neurophysiol. 1998;15:493–501.
29. Begum T, Ikeda A, Takahashi J, et al. Clinical outcome in patients with SREDA (subclinical rhythmic EEG discharge of adults). Intern Med. 2006;45:141–144.
30. Westmoreland BF, Klass DW. Unusual variants of subclinical rhythmic electroencephalographic discharge of adults. Electroencephalogr Clin Neurophysiol. 1997;102:1–4.
31. Carson RP, Abou-Khalil BW. Density spectral array analysis of SREDA during EEG-video monitoring. Clin Neurophysiol. 2012;123:1096–1099.
32. Thomas P, Migneco O, Darcourt J, Chatel M. Single-photon emission computed tomography study of subclinical rhythmic electrographic discharge in adults. Electroencephalogr Clin Neurophysiol. 1992;83:223–227.
33. Gibbs FA, Gibbs EL. Fourteen and six per second positive spikes. Electroencephalogr Clin Neurophysiol. 1963;15:553–558.
34. Gibbs FA, Gibbs EL. Atlas of Electroencephalography. Vol. 3. Addison Wesley, 1964.
35. Lombroso CT, Schwartz IH, Clark DM, et al. Ctenoids in healthy adults. Controlled study of 14- and 6-per-second positive spiking. Neurology. 1966;16:1152–1158.
36. Klass DW, Westmoreland BF. Nonepileptogenic epileptiform electroencephalographic activity. Ann Neurol. 1985;18:627–635.
37. Ebersole JS, Pedley TA. Current Practice of Clinical Electroencephalography. 3rd ed. Philadelphia, PA: Lippincott Williams & Wilkins, 2003.
38. Tatum WO, Husain AM, Benbadis SR et al. Normal adult EEG and patterns of uncertain significance. J Clin Neurophysiol. 2006;23:194–207.
39. Beun AM, van Emde Boas W, Dekker E. Sharp transients in the sleep EEG of healthy adults: a possible pitfall in the diagnostic assessment of seizure disorders. Electroencephalogr Clin Neurophysiol. 1998;106:44–51.
40. Sullivan L. Waveform window #16. 14 and 6 Hertz positive spikes. Am J Electrodiagnostic Technol. 2010;50:67–72.
41. Velizarova R, Crespel A, Serafini A, Gelisse P. A new approach for the detection of the fourteen- and six-Hertz positive bursts (6-14 Hz): the lower temporal line. Clin Neurophysiol. 2011;122:1272.
42. Silverman D. Phantom spike-waves and the fourteen and six per second positive spike pattern: a consideration of their relationship. Electroencephalogr Clin Neurophysiol. 1967;23:207–213.
43. Small JG, Sharpley P, Small IF. Positive spikes, spike-wave phantoms, and psychomotor variants. A survey of these EEG patterns in psychiatric patients. Arch Gen Psychiatr. 1968;18:232–238.
44. Jabbari B, Russo MB, Russo ML. Electroencephalogram of asymptomatic adults. Clin Neurophysiol. 2000;111:102–105.
45. Boutros N, Fristad M, Abdollohian A. The fourteen and six positive spikes and attention-deficit hyperactivity disorder. Biol Psychiatry. 1998;44:298–301.
46. Hughes JR, Cayaffa JJ. Positive spikes revisited in the adult. Clin Elecroencephalogr. 1978;9:52–59.
47. Marshall C. Some clinical correlates of the wave and spike phantom. Electroencaphalogr Clin Neurophysiol. 1955;7:633–636.
48. Tharp BR, Arsenal E. The 6-per-second spike and wave complex. The wave and spike phantom. Arch Neurol. 1966;15:533–537.
49. Tharp BR. The six per second spike and wave complex (the wave and spike phantom). Electroencephalogr Clin Neurophysiol. 1967;23:291.
50. Olson SF, Hughes JR. The clinical symptomatology associated with the 6 c/sec spike and wave complex. Epilepsia. 1970;11:383–393.
51. Hughes JR. Two forms of the 6/sec spike and wave complex. Electroencephalogr Clin Neurophysiol. 1980;48:535–550.
52. Thomas JE, Klass DW. Six-per-second spike-and-wave pattern in the electroencephalogram. Neurology. 1968;18:587–593.
53. Westmoreland BF. Epileptiform electroencephalographic patterns. Mayo Clin Proc. 1996;71:501–511.
54. Azzam R, Bhatt AB. Mimickers of generalized spike and wave discharges. Neurodiag J. 2014;54:156–162.
55. White JC, Langston JW, Pedley TA. Benign epileptiform transients of sleep. Clarification of the small sharp spike controversy. Neurology. 1977;27:1061–1068.
56. Saito F, Fukushima Y, Kubota S. Small sharp spikes: possible relationship to epilepsy. Clin Electroencephalogr. 1987;18:18:114–119.
57. Westmoreland BF, Reiher J, Klass DW. Recording of small sharp spikes with depth electroencephalography. Epilepsia. 1979;20:599–606.
58. McLachlan RS, Lubus N. Cortical location of benign paroxysmal rhythms in the electrocorticogram. Can J Neurol Sci. 2002;29:154–158.
59. Reiher J, Klass DW. "Small sharp spikes" (SSS): electroencephalographic characteristics and clinical significance. Electroencephalogr Clin Neurophysiol. 1970;28:94.
60. Hughes JR, Gruener G. Small sharp spikes revisited: further data on this controversial pattern. Clin Electroencephalogr. 1984;15:208–213.
61. Small JG. Small sharp spikes: EEG signals of psychiatric significance. Electroencephalogr Clin Neurophysiol. 1970;28:417–422.
62. Inui K, Motomura E, Okushima R, et al. Electroencephalographic findings in patients with DSM-IV mood disorder, schizophrenia, and other psychotic disorders. Biol Psychiatry. 1998;43:69–75.
63. Reiher J, Lebel M. Wicket spikes: clinical correlates of a previously undescribed EEG pattern. Can J Neurol Sci. 1977;4:39–47.
64. Waveform Window #11. Wicket spikes. Am J Electroneurodiagnostic Technol. 2008;48:52–55.
65. Gelisse P, Kuate C, Coubes P, et al. Wicket spikes during rapid eye movement sleep. J Clin Neurophysiol. 2003;20:345–350.
66. Serafini A, Crespel A, Velizarova R, Gelisse P. Activation of wicket spikes by REM sleep. Neurophysiol Clin. 2014;44:245–249.
67. Vallabhaneni M, Baldassari LE, Scribner JT, et al. A case-control study of wicket spikes using video-EEG monitoring. Seizure. 2013;22:14–19.
68. Azzam RH, Arain AM, Azar NJ. Revisiting the laterality of wicket spikes with continuous EEG. J Clin Neurophysiol. 2015;32:e8–11.
69. Benbadis SR, Tatum WO. Overinterpretation of EEGs and misdiagnosis of epilepsy. J Clin Neurophysiol. 2003;20:42–44.
70. Krauss GL, Abdallah A, Lesser R, et al. Clinical and EEG features of patients with EEG wicket rhythms misdiagnosed with epilepsy. Neurology. 2005;64:1879–1883.
71. White JC, Tharp BR. An arousal pattern in children with organic cerebral dysfunction. Electroencephalogr Clin Neurophysiol. 1974;37:265–268.
72. Hughes JR, Daaboul Y. The frontal arousal rhythm. Clin Electroencephalogr. 1999;30:16–20.
73. Hughes JR. The frontal arousal rhythm (FAR) is an ictal pattern: a case report. Clin Electroencephalogr. 2003;34:13–14.

13 | THE EEG IN DEGENERATIVE DISORDERS OF THE CENTRAL NERVOUS SYSTEM: CONGENITAL MALFORMATIONS, NEUROCUTANEOUS DISORDERS, INHERITED DISORDERS OF METABOLISM, CEREBRAL PALSY, AND AUTISM SPECTRUM DISORDERS

JOHN GAITANIS, MD, PHILLIP L. PEARL, MD, AND HOWARD GOODKIN, MD

ABSTRACT: Nervous system alterations can occur at any stage of prenatal or postnatal development. Any of these derangements, whether environmental or genetic, will affect electrical transmission, causing electroencephalogram (EEG) alteration and possibly epilepsy. Genetic insults may be multisystemic (for example, neurocutaneous syndromes) or affect only the brain. Gene mutations account for inborn errors of metabolism, channelopathies, brain malformations, and impaired synaptogenesis. Inborn errors of metabolism cause seizures and EEG abnormalities through a variety of mechanisms, including disrupted energy metabolism (mitochondrial disorders, glucose transporter defect), neuronal toxicity (amino and organic acidopathies), impaired neuronal function (lysosomal and peroxisomal disorders), alteration of neurotransmitter systems (nonketotic hyperglycinemia), and vitamin and co-factor dependency (pyridoxine-dependent seizures). Environmental causes of perinatal brain injury often result in motor or intellectual impairment (cerebral palsy). Multiple proposed etiologies exist for autism, many focusing on synaptic development. This chapter reviews the EEG findings associated with this myriad of pathologies occurring in childhood.

KEYWORDS: electroencephalogram, EEG, inborn errors of metabolism, autism, cerebral palsy, neurocutaneous, epilepsy

PRINCIPAL REFERENCES

1. Scriver CR, Beaudet AL, Sly WS, et al., eds. The Metabolic and Molecular Bases of Inherited Disease. Vol. II. New York: McGraw-Hill; 2001.
2. Chu-Shore CJ, Major P, Camposano S, et al. The natural history of epilepsy in tuberous sclerosis complex. Epilepsia. 2010;51(7):1236–1241.
3. Korf BR1, Carrazana E, Holmes GL. Patterns of seizures observed in association with neurofibromatosis 1. Epilepsia. 1993;34(4):616–620.
4. Ostendorf AP, Gutmann DH, Weisenberg JLZ. Epilepsy in individuals with neurofibromatosis type 1. Epilepsia. 2013;54:1810–1814.
5. Matsuo M, Maeda T, Sasaki K, et al. Frequent association of autism spectrum disorder in patients with childhood onset epilepsy. Brain Dev. 2010;32:759–763.
6. Woolfenden S, Sarkozy V, Ridley G, et al. A systematic review of two outcomes in autism spectrum disorder—Epilepsy and mortality. Dev Med Child Neurol. 2012;54:306–312.
7. Silva ML, Cieuta C, Guerrini R, et al. Early clinical and EEG features of infantile spasms in Down syndrome. Epilepsia. 1996;37:977–982.
8. Laan LAEM, Renier WO, Arts WFM, et al. Evolution of epilepsy and EEG findings in Angelman syndrome. Epilepsia. 1997;38:195–199.
9. Glaze DG, Frost JD Jr, Zoghbi HY, et al. Rett's syndrome: correlation of electroencephalographic characteristic with clinical staging. Arch Neurol. 1987;44:1053–1056.
10. Wallace SJ. Epilepsy in cerebral palsy. Dev Med Child Neurol. 2001;43:713–717.

1. INTRODUCTION

Inborn errors of metabolism frequently involve the central nervous system (CNS) and may manifest predominantly or solely as encephalopathy, including epilepsy and epileptic encephalopathies. Thus, electroencephalography (EEG) is an integral tool in the diagnosis, assessment, and management of affected patients. These disorders predominantly present in early life, especially during the neonatal and infantile periods, although later ages of onset occur and manifestations vary by age. In terms of epilepsy, the presence of early life seizures poorly responsive to traditional antiseizure medicines, myoclonic seizures or infantile spasms, associated encephalopathy, progressive or intermittent course, and family history of consanguinity rank among the typical clues toward an inborn metabolic error. The clinical presentation may be nonspecific—that is, a neonate with decreasing feeding, hypotonia, lethargy, respiratory distress, or lactic acidosis. Seizures may be subtle and may be characterized only as apnea, erratic eye movements, facial movements, or grunting.

The typical EEG in a metabolic disorder will have background disturbance, often with slowing and disorganization, as well as epileptiform features including multifocal spike discharges, generalized sharp waves or spike-wave patterns, hypsarrhythmia, and also burst-suppression. There are some EEG patterns with more specific association with certain metabolic disorders, including the comb-like rhythm of maple syrup urine disease, fast central spikes of Tay–Sachs disease, vanishing background of neuronal ceroid lipofuscinosis type 1, and repetitive high-amplitude delta activity with polyspike discharges of polymerase gamma-1 disorders (including Alpers–Huttenlocher syndrome) (Table 13.1). Certain seizure types are associated to at least some degree with particular metabolic disorders, although these are not specific (Table 13.2).

Inborn errors of metabolism can be classified in several instructive ways. One clinically useful approach is based on their major neuroanatomical distribution at presentation or maximum severity—for example, cerebral cortical disorders (e.g., lysosomal storage disorders), leukodystrophies (e.g.,

TABLE 13.1. EEG Patterns Associated with Inborn Errors of Metabolism

Comb-like rhythm	Maple syrup urine disease, priopionic acidemia
Fast central spikes	Tay–Sachs disease, biotinidase deficiency
Rhythmic vertex-positive spikes	Sialidosis (type 1)
Vanishing EEG	Ceroid lipofuscinosis 1 (PPT deficiency)
High-amplitude (16–24 Hz) activity	Infantile neuroaxonal dystrophy
Giant SSEPs	Progressive myoclonus epilepsy
Marked photosensitivity	Lafora body, ceroid lipofuscinosis 2
Burst-suppression	Neonatal adrenoleukodystrophy, citrullinemia, D-glyceric acidemia, glycine encephalopathy, holocarboxylase synthetase deficiency, Leigh disease, molybdenum co-factor deficiency, Menkes, methylene tetrahydrofolate reductase (MTHFR) deficiency, pyruvate dehydrogenase complex/pyruvate carboxylase (PDH/PC) deficiency, priopionic acidemia, pyridoxine dependency, sulfite oxidase deficiency
Hypsarrhythmia	Neonatal adrenoleukodystrophy, congenital disorders of glycosylation, glycine encephalopathy, hyperornithinemia, hyperammonemia, and hypercitrullinemia (HHH), Menkes disease, neuroaxonal dystrophy, pyruvate dehydrogenase complex (PDH) deficiency, progressive encephalopathy with edema, hypsarrhythmia, and optic atrophy (PEHO), phenylketonuria, Zellweger syndrome
Low-amplitude slowing	Urea cycle defects (carbamoyl phosphate synthetase, ornithine transcarbamylase, arginosuccinate synthetase)
Repetitive high-amplitude delta activity with poly-spikes (RHADS)	POLG mutations

TABLE 13.2. Metabolic Disorders: Major Seizure Types

Neonatal seizures	Hypoglycemia, pyridoxine dependency, PNPO deficiency, glycine encephalopathy, organic acidurias, urea cycle defects, neonatal adrenoleukodystrophy, Zellweger syndrome, folinic acid dependency, holocarboxylase synthase/biotinidase deficiency, molybdenum co-factor deficiency, sulfite oxidase deficiency
Infantile spasms	Biotinidase deficiency, Menkes disease, mitochondrial disorders, organic acidurias, amino acidopathies
Myoclonic seizures	Glycine encephalopathy, mitochondrial disorders, GLUT1 deficiency, storage disorders
Progressive myoclonus epilepsy	Lafora disease, MERRF, MELAS, Unverricht–Lundborg Baltic myoclonus, sialidosis
Generalized tonic–clonic seizures	GLUT1 deficiency, neuronal ceroid lipofuscinoses 2 and 3, storage diseases, mitochondrial disorders
Astatic-myoclonic seizures	GLUT1 deficiency, neuronal ceroid lipofuscinosis 2
Absence seizures	GLUT1 deficiency
Multifocal seizures	GLUT1 deficiency, neuronal ceroid lipofuscinosis 3 and others
Epilepsia partialis continua	Mitochondrial disorders, especially POLG and MELAS

or externally. Lysosomal storage disorders occur when there is deficiency of one or more of these enzymes. Undegraded material accumulates, leading to cellular and organ dysfunction. Most of these conditions exhibit autosomal recessive inheritance.

3. GM2 GANGLIOSIDOSES/TAY–SACHS DISEASE

The infantile form of Tay–Sachs disease is named for the British ophthalmologist Warren Tay, who, in 1881, described the cherry-red spot, and the American neurologist Bernard Sachs, who reported on the clinical features and the enlarged pyramidal neurons of the condition. The biochemical understanding came about when Ernst Klenk found a novel group of glycolipids in the brains of these patients, which was later discovered to be GM2 ganglioside. Its accumulation in neurons results from a deficiency of the lysosomal enzyme hexosaminidase A. The hexosaminidase enzyme comprises alpha and beta subunits. Hexosaminidase A consists of one alpha and one beta subunit and hexosaminidase B is composed of two beta subunits. In Tay–Sachs disease, there is loss of the alpha subunit, resulting in absence of hexosaminidase A. The result is a neurologically devastating disease that begins in the first months of life. The initial symptom is excessive startle myoclonus to noise, sound, or touches. The startle does not attenuate

Krabbe disease, metachromatic leukodystrophy, adrenoleukodystrophy), and extrapyramidal system (Leigh syndrome, neuroferritinopathy, Wilson disease). Another approach is in the traditional biochemical classification of small-molecule disorders (e.g., amino acids, organic acids, vitamins, neurotransmitters, glucose) versus large-molecule disorders (e.g., congenital disorders of glycosylation, peroxisomal disorders, lysosomal storage). This chapter proceeds with an organelle-based approach, a common lens through which metabolic disorders are classified and studied.

2. LYSOSOMAL DISORDERS

Lysosomes are membrane-bound organelles that function as the digestive system of the cell. They contain enzymes that break down macromolecules originating either internally

with subsequent exposures, distinguishing it from a normal Moro response. The myoclonic movements consist of arm and leg extension. As the disease progresses, motor, visual, and intellectual impairments develop. The affected infant develops axial hypotonia with appendicular spasticity and increased reflexes. Motor skills, such as head control, rolling, and purposeful hand movements, are lost. Visual loss ensues as lipid accumulates in the retinal ganglion cells, resulting in a whitish discoloration around the fovea—the characteristic cherry-red spot. With intraneuronal accumulations of GM2 ganglioside, macrocephaly develops. The children experience progressive cognitive impairment and seizures. Feeding and autonomic disturbances develop. Between 3 and 5 years of age, the patient succumbs to cachexia or aspiration pneumonia.

The disease affects multiple regions of the brain. The basal ganglia and cerebral white matter show low-density signal on CT in early stages and enlargement of the caudate nucleus later in the disease course (1). Early into the disease, the interictal EEG may be normal. By age 1, there is a rapid and progressive deterioration of the EEG (2). Fast central spikes may become prominent and widespread spike and sharp waves are seen during myoclonic seizures (3). A progressive decline in voltage occurs in later stages of the disease, likely resulting from continued neuronal loss. The electroretinogram remains normal even in advanced stages (2,4), since only the ganglion cell layer of the retina is affected. Progressive loss of the visual evoked potential (VEP) occurs between 9 and 15 months (2).

Sandhoff disease, resulting from mutations of the beta subunit of hexosaminidase A, is phenotypically similar to Tay–Sachs disease, the only differences being the presence of hepatosplenomegaly, cardiomyopathy, or N-acetylglucosamine–containing oligosaccharides in the urine of patients with Sandhoff disease. The AB variant occurs when there is a deficiency of the GM2 activator, which is necessary for hydrolysis of GM2 gangliosides by hexosaminidase A. Its phenotype is indistinguishable from the infantile form of Tay–Sachs (5). Late-onset variants of Tay–Sachs also exist and can manifest in childhood, adolescence, or adulthood. They may result in a wide constellation of symptoms, including spastic paraparesis, ataxia with cerebellar atrophy, seizures, or psychiatric symptoms. Psychosis and depression can even be the initial manifestation in adult patients (6). EEG changes in late-onset GM2 gangliosidosis are variable and unrelated to age or enzyme defect (2).

4. GM1 GANGLIOSIDOSIS

GM1 gangliosidosis results from a deficiency of β-galactosidase, which is responsible for cleavage of the terminal galactose of GM1. The result is neuronal storage of monosialoganglioside GM1. Histopathology reveals a marked decrease in the number of oligodendrocytes and myelin sheaths. As a result, spasticity, tonic spasms, and pyramidal signs predominate. As in Tay–Sachs disease, a cherry-red spot is seen and the electroretinogram (ERG) remains normal (2). The EEG also shows a progressive deterioration as it does in GM2 patients. EEGs universally reveal abnormal slowing, which worsens as the disease

advances. By 2 to 3 years of age, 4- to 5-cycle/sec rhythmic activity is seen in the temporal regions. Paroxysmal discharges, however, are not commonly observed in GM1 patients (7).

5. NEURONAL CEROID LIPOFUSCINOSES

The neuronal ceroid lipofuscinoses are a group of neurodegenerative conditions caused by intralysosomal accumulation of ceroid and lipofuscin (8). Originally described as a form of "amaurotic familial idiocy," the group of disorders was renamed "neuronal ceroid lipofuscinoses" by Zeman to better distinguish them from gangliosidoses (9). Clinically, the disease group is characterized by cognitive decline, progressive myoclonic epilepsy, and motor regression. Some forms also cause visual failure (8). The four originally described phenotypes are organized according to age of onset: infantile (INCL), late infantile (LINCL), juvenile (JNCL), and adult (ANCL). Patients with INCL are normal at birth and exhibit developmental delays or myoclonic seizures between 6 and 24 months of age. In LINCL, patients experience developmental regression and epilepsy between 2 and 4 years. JNCL develops between age 4 and 10 years, with visual loss being the initial symptom and epilepsy following shortly afterwards. ANCL appears sometime around age 30 years and presents with progressive myoclonic epilepsy, dementia, behavioral abnormalities, ataxia, and pyramidal or extrapyramidal signs (10). These disorders are inherited in an autosomal recessive pattern and there are at least seven genes responsible for the clinical phenotypes. The infantile form is now recognized as secondary to palmitoyl-protein thioesterase-1 (PPT-1) deficiency and the late infantile form to tripeptidyl peptidase 1 (TPP1) deficiency.

Magnetic resonance imaging (MRI) findings in INCL include cerebral atrophy, callosal thinning, T2-weighted hyperintensities in the thalami, and cerebellar atrophy. After 4 years of age, the atrophy is severe and the entire white matter shows abnormally high signal intensity. Single-photon emission computed tomography (SPECT) studies show progressive cerebral and cerebellar hypoperfusion with relative sparing of the basal ganglia. LINCL and JNCL reveal lesser degrees of atrophy (11).

The EEG findings reflect the predominance of cortical abnormalities on MRI and SPECT. In INCL, the EEG initially shows a lack of attenuation to eye opening and a disappearance of sleep spindles. The background activity gradually attenuates and becomes flat by 3 years of age, producing the so-called vanishing EEG. ERGs are unrecordable by age 3 and VEPs are unrecordable by age 4. There is progressive attenuation of cortical somatosensory potentials (12). In LINCL, seizures are the presenting symptom, and the EEG reveals occipital spike-waves in response to photic stimulation at 1 to 2 Hz. The ERG is abnormal at presentation and extinguishes in time. VEPs are enhanced but diminish in the final stages of the disease (13). In JNCL, the EEG shows disorganization and spike- and slow-wave complexes. ERG and VEPs are abnormal early into the course of the disease. The EEG abnormalities of ANCL are nonspecific (14). In one case series, the frequency of background slowing in all types of NCL was 94.6% and epileptiform discharges were seen in 81.1% (15). Slow-frequency photic stimulation elicited a response in 5 out of 22 patients, a giant somatosensory evoked potential (SSEP) was seen in 7 of 25 patients, and slow or absent waveforms were seen in 9 of 25 patients on VEP (15).

6. MUCOPOLYSACCHARIDOSES

The mucopolysaccharidoses are a heterogeneous group of disorders caused by deficiency of a lysosomal enzyme involved in the degradation of glycosaminoglycans (16). As glycosaminoglycans accumulate in lysosomes, cell and organ dysfunctions result. Seven types exist. The age of onset and severity vary, but most exhibit a chronic, progressive course characterized by multisystemic involvement, coarse facies, organomegaly, and bony defects (dysostosis multiplex) (16). The more severe forms (MPS I, MPS II, and MPS VIII) result in progressive mental retardation, whereas patients with MPS IV and MPS VI have normal cognition, even when somatic manifestations are severe (16). The only variant without somatic symptoms is MPS III, of which there are four subtypes. MPS III presents between 1 and 6 years of age with delayed psychomotor development and behavioral problems. Progressive dementia, sleeplessness, and epilepsy follow (17). In MPS III, the EEG is normal in half of patients but shows diffuse slowing in the rest (18). Low-amplitude 12- to 15-Hz activity is seen intermixed with generalized delta frequencies (19). These findings correspond to the severe cortical involvement seen pathologically (19). VEPs and brainstem auditory evoked potentials (BAEPs) are almost always normal (18). Enzyme replacement therapy and hematopoietic stem cell transplantation offer potential benefit in these conditions (20,21).

7. SIALIDOSIS TYPES I AND II (NEURAMINIDASE DEFICIENCY)

In sialidosis, a deficiency of the enzyme neuraminidase leads to progressive storage of sialidated glycopeptides and oligosaccharides. Sialidosis bears clinical and histopathological resemblance to the mucopolysaccharidoses in that patients exhibit mild Hurler-like facies, skeletal dysplasia, and psychomotor retardation. Sialidosis is divided into types I and II (22). Type I has a later age of onset and patients exhibit little if any dysmorphology. Visual failure, cherry-red spots, ataxia, and myoclonus are common features (23,24). Type II patients have an earlier age of onset and demonstrate coarse facies, hepatosplenomegaly, and skeletal anomalies (dysostosis multiplex and spinal deformities) (25). MRI findings include atrophy of the cerebral hemispheres, cerebellum, and pontine region (26).

EEG findings in sialidosis types I and II are indistinguishable (27). In type I, the background is low voltage and rhythmic spikes are observed over the vertex, which increase in frequency during sleep (27). Spike-wave discharges precede myoclonic jerking in both types I and II (28,29). VEPs demonstrate low amplitudes and prolonged latencies in type I (28),

while sensory evoked potentials (SEPs) exhibit giant potentials in both conditions (28,29).

8. NIEMANN–PICK DISEASE

Niemann–Pick disease occurs when a deficiency of the enzyme acid sphingomyelinase causes sphingomyelin to accumulate within cells of the monocyte–macrophage system (30). Four phenotypic subtypes exist. In type A (NPD-A), infants present in the first few weeks or months of life with failure to thrive and hepatomegaly. Psychomotor regression follows, with head lag, inability to sit, and loss of interest in surroundings. In time, rigidity and opisthotonos predominate. Death occurs in the second or third year. Startle myoclonus, like that seen in Tay–Sachs, is not observed and there are no coarse features, like those present in mucopolysaccharidosis. In type B (NPD-B), visceral involvement predominates without significant neurological impairment (31). An intermediate form between NPD-A and NPD-B may also exist with retinal degeneration and slowed nerve conduction presenting in adolescence or adulthood (30). In type C (NPD-C), patients present between ages 3 and 8 years with ataxia, vertical supranuclear gaze palsy, and hepatosplenomegaly. In time, they experience dementia, dystonia, and seizures (32). Cataplexy occurs late in the disease course (33). Type D (NPD-D) occurs in French Canadian patients who share a common founder mutation (34).

In late-childhood or adult-onset NPD-C, the EEG may reveal generalized slowing (35). Late into the course of NPD-C, abnormally high-voltage and diffuse alpha activity is seen and is enhanced by intermittent photic stimulation. In a patient with myoclonus, EEG–electromyelographic (EMG) frequency analysis demonstrated a cortical origin for the myoclonus (36) (Fig. 13.1).

9. GAUCHER DISEASE

Gaucher disease is the most common lysosomal storage disorder. It results from a deficiency of the lysosomal enzyme beta-glucocerebrosidase, resulting in accumulation of glucocerebroside in the mononuclear phagocyte system (37). The characteristic features include hepatosplenomegaly, bony disease, and neurological decline. Three phenotypic subtypes exist. Type I has minimal if any neurological impairment. Bulbar symptoms predominate in type II patients (38). In type III patients, ocular motor apraxia is often the initial finding. The pathological hallmark of the disorder is the Gaucher cell, an enlarged macrophage with cytoplasmic linear inclusions resulting from excessive lysosomal accumulation of glucocerebroside (38). Enzyme replacement therapy with recombinant glucocerebrosidase (Cerazyme) is the mainstay of treatment in Gaucher disease (39) but is not effective for the neurological symptoms since it does not cross the blood–brain barrier.

MRI in type II disease is often normal, but cerebral atrophy is commonly observed in type III patients (40). Brainstem auditory evoked responses (BAERs) and SSEPs can demonstrate

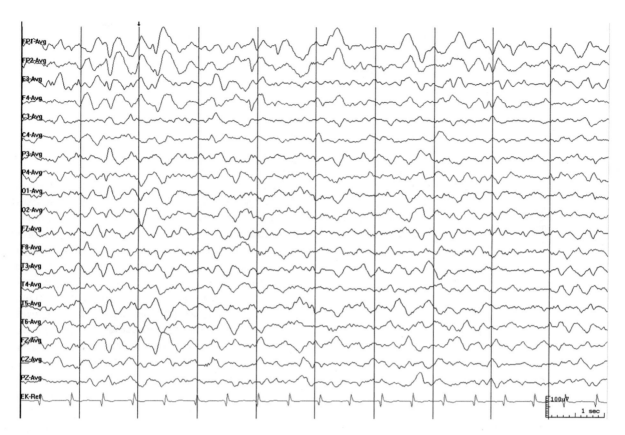

Figure 13.1. EEG in a 10-year-old boy with Niemann–Pick type C. Note the frontal slowing with intermixed sharp waves bilaterally.

abnormalities, even when no lesions are detectable by MRI (41). EEGs show rhythmic sharp waves (6–10/sec), polyspikes, and spike-wave discharges in type III patients (42). These features are diffuse but have a posterior predominance. EEGs are commonly normal in type II patients. Reduced amplitude can also be an EEG feature of some patients (41).

10. FABRY DISEASE

Fabry disease is the only X-linked lysosomal disorder; the others are inherited in an autosomal recessive fashion. Hence, the disease affects men more severely than it does women (43). It results from a deficiency of alpha-galactosidase A. This leads to storage of glycosphingolipids in a variety of tissues, producing cellular dysfunction, inflammation, and fibrosis. Symptoms begin in early childhood with peripheral neuropathy and burning pain of the hands and feet, which can remain disabling throughout life (43). Hypohydrosis, nausea, and postprandial diarrhea are also seen in childhood. By adulthood, proteinuria and renal failure develop. Left ventricular hypertrophy and coronary artery disease are also common. Angiokeratomas develop on the skin. Neurologically, cryptogenic strokes occur. Enzyme replacement therapy can clear microvascular endothelial deposits from the kidneys, heart, and skin, reversing the pathogenesis (44). MRI scans reveal gray and white matter lesions. The anterior circulation generally appears normal, but tortuous basilar arteries are common (45). EEGs can reveal either focal or diffuse slowing (46).

11. METACHROMATIC LEUKODYSTROPHY

Metachromatic leukodystrophy is characterized by an inability to degrade sulfated glycolipids due to a deficiency of the lysosomal enzyme arylsulfatase A. The disorder affects central and peripheral myelin. There is widespread loss of myelinated oligodendroglia in the CNS and segmental demyelination of peripheral nerves (47). Clinically, it presents with motor regression and ataxia at around 2 years of age (47) and leads to a decerebrate state some years after the initial onset of symptoms. Epileptic seizures can occur late into the course of the illness. A late-onset form exists and presents in the third decade with psychiatric symptoms.

Earlier into the course of metachromatic leukodystrophy, EEGs are often normal. If abnormalities are seen at presentation, they consist of mild slowing of the background activity (48). As the clinical severity of the disease progresses, so does the degree of slowing. Later into the course of the illness, as the patients develop epileptic seizures, focal spike-waves appear. In the final stages of the disease course, hypersynchronous activity is seen (49). Both the clinical and EEG features of the disease can improve following bone marrow transplantation (50).

12. GLOBOID LEUKODYSTROPHY (KRABBE DISEASE)

Krabbe disease results from a deficiency of the lysosomal enzyme galactosylceramidase. Severe loss of myelin occurs, and globoid cells are seen in the CNS white matter. Early infantile Krabbe disease accounts for 90% of all cases and presents in the first 6 months of life (51) with irritability and rapidly progressive rigidity and tonic spasms. MRI of the brain shows symmetric signal abnormalities in the periventricular regions of the posterior cerebral hemispheres. Peripheral nerves are also affected, but no visceromegaly is observed. The remaining 10% of patients have late-infantile or juvenile Krabbe disease, which presents with ataxia and later exhibits dystonia and visual failure (52).

EEGs are abnormal in a majority of the early infantile cases, but the opposite is true for late-infantile and juvenile-onset patients. Abnormalities consist of slowing without epileptiform activity in 46%, epileptiform activity without slowing in 15%, and both slowing and epileptiform features in 38% of patients (53). Likewise, BAEPs are abnormal in 88% of the early infantile patients and only 40% of the late-onset cases. The most frequent BAEP abnormality is absence of waves III and V (53).

13. PEROXISOMAL DISORDERS

Peroxisomal disorders are a group of heterogeneous conditions that share dysfunction of peroxisomal function. Peroxisomes are bound by a single membrane and contain a fine granular matrix. They are histologically identified by the presence of catalase. They are present in all human tissues except erythrocytes. They carry out over 40 metabolic functions, including beta-oxidation of very-long-chain fatty acids (VLCFAs) and biosynthesis of plasmalogen and cholesterol. Some of those reactions can occur in other organelles, but many are exclusive to peroxisomes.

14. X-LINKED ADRENOLEUKODYSTROPHY

X-linked adrenoleukodystrophy is the most common of the peroxisomal disorders. It is characterized by accumulation of VLCFAs in the brain and adrenal tissues (54). VLCFAs are also detected in fibroblasts, blood cells, and plasma, allowing for identification of the condition (55). X-linked adrenoleukodystrophy affects the CNS or adrenal glands and can have diverse presentations. The cerebral form presents between 4 and 8 years of age with symptoms mimicking those of attention-deficit/hyperactivity disorder (ADHD). Psychomotor regression and cortical blindness follow and seizures are observed late into the disease course. MRI shows lesions of the parieto-occipital white matter with contrast enhancement at the leading edge (56). The mean interval between the first symptom and an apparent vegetative state is 2.4 years (48). Adrenomyeloneuropathy is a variant that affects primarily the spinal cord and does not present until the third decade. Since X-linked adrenoleukodystrophy is an X-linked condition, it presents earlier and with greater severity in males, but heterozygous women can be symptomatic.

During early stages of the disease, EEGs are normal in about half of patients and show posterior slowing in the remainder. The location of the slowing corresponds to the region of MRI abnormalities (48). As the disease progresses, the slowing becomes more widespread and paroxysmal discharges are observed (48). In one reported case, the ictal EEG during a tonic seizure revealed an electrodecrement of the background activity (48).

15. ZELLWEGER SYNDROME

Zellweger syndrome, also known as cerebrohepatorenal syndrome, results from deficiencies of VLCFA beta-oxidation, phytanic acid oxidation, and plasmalogen synthesis. As a result, plasma levels of VLCFAs and phytanic acid are high, whereas erythrocyte concentrations of plasmalogen are reduced. Zellweger syndrome presents in infancy with craniofacial dysmorphism (high forehead, large anterior fontanelle, separated cranial sutures, hypoplastic supraorbital ridges, and epicanthal folds) and hepatomegaly (57). Neurological findings include hypotonia with absent reflexes, profound developmental delays, seizures, and impaired vision and hearing (57). MRI reveals both cortical (polymicrogyria and pachygyria) and white matter (delayed myelination) abnormalities (58).

Interictal EEGs in Zellweger syndrome patients show bilateral independent multifocal spike-waves, predominantly in the frontal motor cortex (59). Continuous negative vertex sharp- and spike-waves are commonly observed. They were found in 9 of 11 patients in one study (60) and seen in a single case in a separate report (61). This finding, observed during wakefulness and sleep, is pathognomonic for Zellweger syndrome (61). BAEPs and VEPs can have absent or delayed responses (60).

16. NEONATAL ADRENOLEUKODYSTROPHY

Neonatal adrenoleukodystrophy is a disorder of peroxisomal biosynthesis resulting from impaired ATPases that are necessary for importing proteins into peroxisomes. It presents at birth with facial dysmorphism (midface hypoplasia) (57). Hepatomegaly and adrenal cortical atrophy can also be observed. Neurologically, patients present with hypotonia, optic nerve atrophy, and seizures (62). Psychomotor regression occurs in early childhood. MRI reveals a severe deficiency of white matter in addition to heterotopias and polymicrogyria.

Interictal EEGs show high-voltage slow waves and bilateral independent multifocal spike-waves. Later in the disease course, background suppression can be observed (59).

17. MITOCHONDRIAL DISORDERS

Mitochondrial diseases are a heterogeneous group of conditions that result from dysfunction of the mitochondrial respiratory chain. The mitochondria's main function is generating ATP to power the cells they reside in. Because mitochondria are present in every cell type, with the sole exception of erythrocytes, mitochondrial dysfunction can have wide-ranging effects. The mitochondrial genome contains 37 genes, of which 13 encode structural proteins for the respiratory chain. The remaining 3,000 or so genes are required to make a mitochondrion reside in the nuclear DNA. Inheritance patterns are therefore varied, with both maternal and Mendelian patterns observed.

18. LEIGH SYNDROME

In 1951, Leigh described a case of subacute necrotizing encephalomyelopathy in a 7-month-old infant. The patient had symmetric lesions of the thalamus, midbrain, pons, medulla, and posterior columns of the spinal cord (63). Leigh syndrome results from defects in cytochrome oxidase or the pyruvate dehydrogenase complex. Inheritance patterns can be maternal, X-linked, or autosomal recessive. Patients presenting prior to 12 months are likely to exhibit psychomotor retardation, vomiting, weight loss, and weakness. In patients presenting after 18 months, symptoms include coma, ophthalmoparesis, or nystagmus (64). Neuroimaging reveals abnormal signal in the basal ganglia and brainstem with sparing of the mammillary bodies. There is a strong predilection for the putamen; absence of putaminal involvement should call the diagnosis into question (65).

The interictal EEG can reveal focal or multifocal epileptiform activity, which becomes more frequent during sleep. During partial seizures, the ictal EEG reveals posterior or hemispheric background attenuation or ictal fast activity (66).

19. MELAS SYNDROME (MITOCHONDRIAL MYOPATHY, ENCEPHALOPATHY, LACTIC ACIDOSIS, AND STROKE)

MELAS is characterized by mitochondrial myopathy, encephalopathy, lactic acidosis, and recurrent stroke-like episodes. Many patients also exhibit seizures, migraines, cortical blindness, short stature, or ragged-red fibers on muscle biopsy (67). The mechanism of stroke in this condition remains controversial. Some implicate a mitochondrial angiopathy, resulting in small vessel occlusion, and others postulate that the impairment of oxidative metabolism results in lactic acidosis and brain injury (68). Imaging studies support the later hypothesis (68,69). MRI abnormalities are most pronounced in the parietal–occipital regions (69).

Likewise, interictal EEGs reveal diffuse sharp waves with an occipital predominance. The epileptiform abnormalities can be enhanced with photic stimulation (66). Periodic epileptiform discharges may be prominent, especially over the affected occipital lobe (70). In one report of 11 patients with a syndrome of overlapping MERRF (myoclonus, epilepsy, ragged-red fibers)–MELAS phenotype, EEG abnormalities correlated with the severity of the clinical phenotype. In milder cases, they included disorganization of the background activity and focal or generalized delta–theta waves (Fig. 13.2). More severely affected patients exhibited bursts of generalized spike- or polyspike- and slow-wave complexes (71). MELAS patients can develop epilepsia partialis continua. EEGs at those

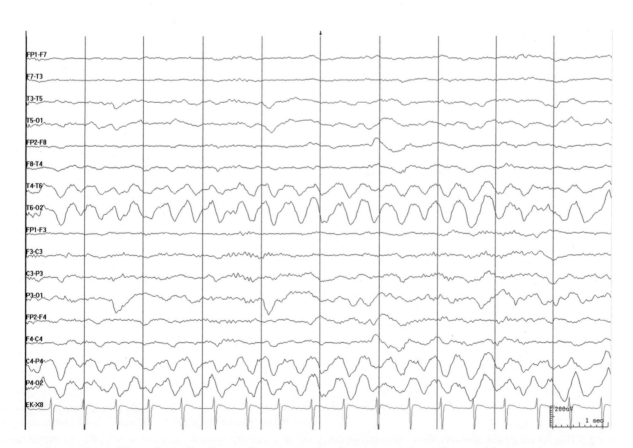

Figure 13.2. EEG in a 13-year-old boy with MELAS syndrome and seizures. Note the continuous semirhythmic right occipital slowing.

times reveal pseudo-periodic spike-waves in the contralateral temporal–occipital regions (71).

20. MERRF SYNDROME

MERRF is characterized by myoclonic epilepsy and myopathy (with ragged-red fibers on muscle biopsy). Dementia, ataxia, and generalized tonic–clonic seizures are also observed. It results from an A-to-G mutation at nucleotide 8344 in the mitochondrial DNA (72). The mutation impairs mitochondrial protein synthesis and thus impairs oxidative phosphorylation. MERRF is transmitted by maternal inheritance, but the clinical phenotype varies, even within the same family.

In one series, EEG abnormalities were seen in six of nine patients. They included slowing of the background activity and generalized epileptiform discharges (15). Polyspike- and spike- and slow-wave complexes are enhanced by photic stimulation and may occur in conjunction with myoclonic jerking (66).

21. ALPERS–HUTTENLOCHER SYNDROME (DIFFUSE DEGENERATION OF CEREBRAL GRAY MATTER WITH HEPATIC CIRRHOSIS)

In 1931, Alpers reported the clinical features and neuropathology of a 4-month-old girl with intractable generalized epilepsy (73). He termed the condition "diffuse progressive degeneration of the gray matter of the cerebrum." The neuropathology is characterized by extensive brain atrophy with loss of cerebral neurons. Psychomotor retardation and intractable epilepsy are universally seen. Liver failure is common but sometimes absent. The syndrome is caused by mutations of the nuclear gene encoding the catalytic subunit of mitochondrial polymerase gamma (POLG). The EEG pattern of rhythmic

high-amplitude delta with superimposed spikes/polyspikes (RHADS) has become associated with POLG mutations, with occipital predominance typically seen (74) (Fig. 13.3).

22. MITOCHONDRIAL DNA DEPLETION SYNDROME

The EEG reveals slow or absent posteriorly dominant rhythms (75). Interictal discharges can be focal, multifocal, or generalized, but the occipital regions are most commonly involved (75). Periodic (approximately 1 Hz) epileptiform discharges can be seen (76), and high-amplitude slowing with polyspikes is characteristic for the condition (77).

23. PROGRESSIVE MYOCLONUS EPILEPSIES

The progressive myoclonus epilepsies are a group of unrelated disorders that share a progressive course with myoclonic seizures and subcortical myoclonus. Generalized tonic–clonic, atypical absence, and focal onset seizures can be seen. They are generally refractory to medical management and worsen over time. Cognitive impairment and ataxia are common among these conditions. MERRF is usually included among the progressive myoclonus epilepsies but is discussed in the section above on mitochondrial disorders.

24. LAFORA DISEASE

Lafora disease generally presents between 12 and 17 years of age (78). Generalized tonic–clonic seizures are the presenting symptom in 71% of cases (15). Cognitive decline, visual impairment,

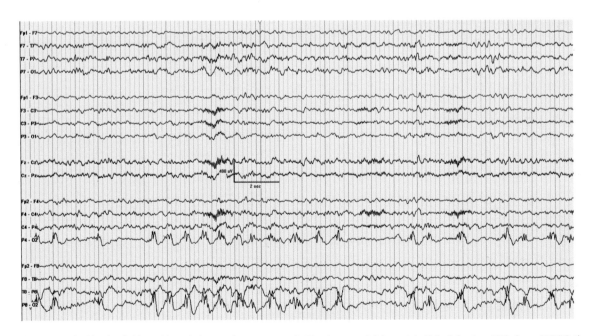

Figure 13.3. This 11-month-old girl with Alpers–Huttenlocher syndrome presented with seizures and right occipital lobe infarction. EEG shows RHADS; the patient had compound heterozygosity for pathogenic POLG-1 mutations p.Lys934Aspfs and p.Arg1096Cys.

occipital seizures, and myoclonic seizures are also observed. The occipital seizures can cause transient blindness, visual hallucinations, or a photoconvulsive response. Myoclonus worsens as the disease progresses. Continuous generalized myoclonus can result in early wheelchair dependency. Most patients die from neurological complications within 10 years of disease onset (78). It is inherited in an autosomal recessive fashion. The pathologic hallmark is the presence of Lafora bodies in neurons, liver, and muscle. Lafora bodies stain positive with periodic-acid Schiff and have a dense core with a less dense periphery. EEGs in Lafora disease reveal background slowing in 97.4% of patients and generalized epileptiform discharges in 84.2% (15). Focal and multifocal discharges can be observed. Photosensitivity with a fast stimulus frequency is seen in 25%. EEG changes can precede clinical symptoms by up to 6 years (79). As the disease progresses, the background rhythm slows and the alpha rhythm and sleep morphologies are lost (78). Generalized irregular spike-wave discharges with an occipital predominance dominate the background activity. Unlike many primary generalized epilepsies, epileptiform discharges diminish during sleep in Lafora disease. In one case series, giant SSEPs were seen in 24 of 31 patients and VEPs revealed prolonged or absent waveforms in 12 of 31 patients (15) (Fig. 13.4).

25. UNVERRICHT–LUNDBERG DISEASE

Unverricht–Lundberg disease presents between 6 and 15 years of age with stimulus-sensitive myoclonus or generalized tonic–clonic seizures (80). The myoclonus may be focal, multifocal, or generalized. It progresses over the course of the illness and can be disabling. Tonic–clonic, absence, and complex partial seizures can also increase over the course of the disease. These symptoms are accompanied by ataxia, tremor, and dysarthria. Cognitive dysfunction and visual impairment are absent or mild (15). Although the condition clinically resembles Lafora disease, Lafora bodies are not seen. Unverricht–Lundberg disease is inherited in an autosomal recessive fashion and results

from an unstable expansion of a 12-nucleotide repeat within the cystatin B (CSTB) gene on chromosome 21q22.3 (81).

The EEG reveals generalized epileptiform discharges (15) with a frequency of 3 to 5/sec. Photic stimulation elicits generalized spikes and polyspikes. As the disease progresses, so does the frequency of the epileptic discharges (80).

26. SEVERE MYOCLONIC EPILEPSY OF INFANCY (DRAVET SYNDROME)

Severe myoclonic epilepsy of infancy presents in the first year of life with febrile seizures (82). The seizures are generalized or focal. Status epilepticus in the setting of fever is common (82). The early age of onset helps distinguish it from other forms of progressive myoclonic epilepsy. It is characterized by generalized tonic, clonic, tonic–clonic, absence, or myoclonic seizures, which are often refractory to medications. A ketogenic diet provides benefit in some patients (82). Ataxia and psychomotor regression are common, although cognitive development is normal prior to 1 year. The condition results from a mutation of the sodium channel gene, SCN1A, which also causes generalized epilepsy with febrile seizures plus (GEFS+) syndrome (83). Severe myoclonic epilepsy of infancy may therefore represent a variant of GEFS+.

During the first 2 years of life, EEGs are normal (82). After the second year, generalized spike- and polyspike-waves are observed (82). The discharges increase in frequency during sleep. Photic stimulation elicits discharges in about one fourth of patients (82).

27. AMINOACIDEMIAS AND ORGANIC ACIDEMIAS

Amino and organic acidemias are conditions that cause an abnormal buildup of amino acids in the blood. Aminoacidemias occur when there are elevated blood levels of any amino acid,

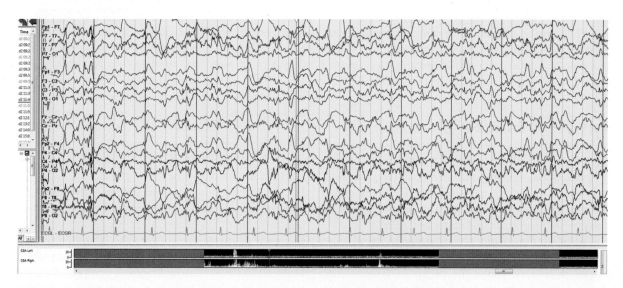

Figure 13.4. EEG in a 17-year-old girl with Lafora body disease shows diffuse background disorganization and slowing with superimposed multifocal sharp and spike discharges.

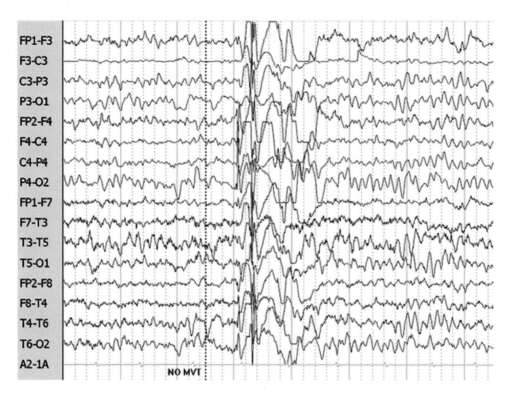

Figure 13.5. EEG in a 3-year-old girl with the organic aciduria SSADH deficiency shows irregular paroxysms of generalized spike-wave activity; hemispheric predominance is variable. Sensitivity 15 mcV/mm, high-frequency filter 70 Hz, low-frequency filter 15 Hz. *Reproduced with permission from Pearl PL, Jakobs C, Gibson KM. Disorders of GABA metabolic and epilepsy. In: PL Pearl, ed. Inherited Metabolic Epilepsies. New York: Demos Medical Publishers; 2013:167–178.*

whereas organic acidemias refer specifically to elevated levels of branched chain amino acids. These conditions are generally diagnosed in infancy. They present with acute metabolic decompensation, during which somnolence, hypotonia, vomiting, and seizures are observed. Multisystemic involvement is common. Untreated, these conditions can result in coma and death. Treatment can include hemofiltration, dietary restriction of particular nutrients or a class of nutrients, and specific supplements designed to remove toxic metabolites. Late-onset forms also exist and may present without overt metabolic crisis. These conditions are diagnosed by chromatography or mass spectroscopy. Laboratory investigations are best performed during acute episodes. EEGs in the amino and organic acidopathies may show nonspecific background slowing or disorganization with generalized or multifocal epileptiform abnormalities. Selected disorders will be discussed in further detail below (Fig. 13.5).

28. PHENYLKETONURIA

Phenylketonuria results from deficient activity of phenylalanine hydroxylase, the enzyme that converts phenylalanine to tyrosine. As a result, phenylalanine accumulates and is excreted in the urine in large amounts as phenylketones. Phenylalanine is neurotoxic and untreated patients develop mental retardation. Restricting phenylalanine in the diet can normalize plasma phenylalanine levels and improve outcome. If instituted in infancy, before the patient is symptomatic, mental retardation can be averted. For this reason, newborn screening has been mandatory since the 1960s.

Some infants exhibit EEG abnormalities at the time of diagnosis, consisting of focal or multifocal spike and sharp waves (84). Many of those same patients will have normal EEGs 1 year after initiating dietary restriction of phenylalanine. Overall, patients who begin treatment sooner are more likely to have normal EEGs (85). Some patients with EEG abnormalities in infancy will develop abnormalities later in childhood, even though they remain on a restricted diet. EEG abnormalities in such patients are indicative of higher phenylalanine levels (generally >20 mg/dL) (86). Older patients and those who initiate treatment later in childhood are more likely to exhibit abnormalities on EEG (86). Patients with atypical phenylketonuria (i.e., hyperphenylalaninemia with normal phenylalanine hydroxylase activity) may have disorders of biopterin synthesis or recycling with severe epilepsy. Focal and generalized epileptiform discharges are noted in phenylketonuria and the biopterin synthesis disorders (Fig. 13.6).

29. MAPLE SYRUP URINE DISEASE

In 1954, Menkes described four siblings with feeding difficulty, irregular respirations, hypertonia, and opisthotonos presenting in the first days of life. All of the infants had urine with the smell of maple syrup (87). The condition, now termed maple syrup urine disease, is caused by deficiency of branched chain alpha-ketoacid dehydrogenase complex. This results in an elevation of branched chain amino acids in the blood and urine. Five clinical phenotypes of the condition exist (89). In

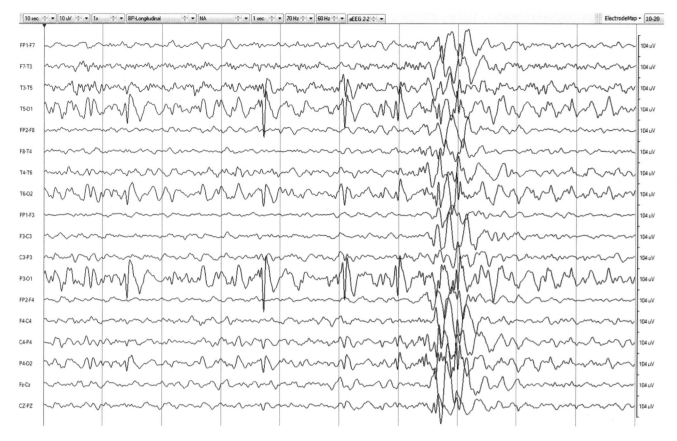

Figure 13.6. EEG in a 7-year-old girl with the biopterin synthesis disorder DHPR (dihydropteridine reductase) deficiency shows focal (maximally left occipital) and diffuse spike-wave discharges.

the classic form, symptoms develop in the first week of life. Seizures are common and coma and death can result if not treated early. Initially, neuroimaging is normal but reveals generalized edema in severe cases (89).

During acute metabolic decompensation, EEG reveals spikes, polyspikes, spike-wave complexes, triphasic waves, severe slowing, and bursts of periodic suppression (90). A characteristic comb-like pattern of rolandic sharp waves is seen on EEG between the second and third weeks and may persist after the acute metabolic decompensation has passed (90). Spike-wave discharges are seen with photic stimuli in just over half of patients (90) (Fig. 13.7).

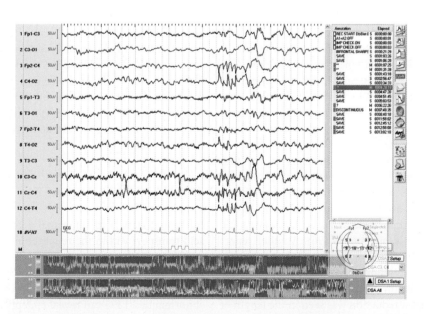

Figure 13.7. EEG in a 2-week-old term neonate with maple syrup urine disease shows the central comb-like rhythm.

30. HOMOCYSTINURIA

Homocystinuria is a metabolic disorder caused by a cystathionine [beta]-synthase gene deficiency, resulting in increased serum levels of homocysteine and methionine. Patients have skeletal changes resembling those of Marfan syndrome. Cognitive delays, psychiatric disturbances, strokes, and extrapyramidal findings can result. Seizures occur in 21% of patients and are usually generalized tonic–clonic (91).

Del Giudice et al. (92) reported EEG findings in 19 patients. Ten of those patients had abnormalities, which generally consisted of background slowing. Midtemporal paroxysmal activity was seen in two patients. Centrotemporal spikes, increasing in drowsiness and sleep, can occur and may mimic benign childhood epilepsy with centrotemporal spikes (93).

31. PROPIONIC ACIDEMIA

Propionic acidemia results from a deficiency of the mitochondrial enzyme propionyl-CoA carboxylase, which converts propionyl-CoA to D-methylmalonyl CoA. Biotin is a co-factor for this reaction. Most patients present as neonates with an acute metabolic crisis with hypotonia, lethargy, or seizures. The seizures may result from NMDA receptor-mediated mechanisms. Later-onset patients present with developmental delays without metabolic decompensation, acute encephalopathy, or episodic ketoacidosis (94). Acute metabolic crises can be treated with total protein restriction and hemofiltration (peritoneal dialysis and exchange transfusion). Carnitine supplementation and antibiotics (to reduce intestinal production of propionic acid by normal gut flora) are also used. Sass et al. (94) reported EEG findings in 32 patients. Of those, 9 showed moderate abnormalities and 6 were clearly abnormal; the remaining 17 patients had normal EEGs. A separate case report (95) revealed disorganized background activity at the time of acute metabolic decompensation.

32. METHYLMALONIC ACIDEMIA

Methylmalonic acidemia is a heterogeneous group of conditions characterized by accumulation of methylmalonic acid and its byproducts. It results from impairments of methylmalonate or cobalamin (vitamin B12) metabolism. Hence, some patients respond to cobalamin supplementation and others do not. Patients with defects of cobalamin metabolism have simultaneous homocystinuria.

Methylmalonic acidemia typically presents in the first weeks of life with vomiting, lethargy, hypotonia, and seizures. Later-onset cases also exist and may present with hypoglycemia, myopathy, or thrombosis (due to homocystinuria). In one case report of an infant with methylmalonic acidemia and tonic seizures, EEG showed polyspike bursts (96). Another report described sharp transients superimposed on a low-voltage and discontinuous tracing with long flat periods. Following treatment with hydroxycobalamin (vitamin B12), blood homocysteine levels declined and a reduction was seen in the length of the interburst periods (97).

33. ISOVALERIC ACIDEMIA

Isovaleric acidemia is caused by a deficiency of the mitochondrial enzyme isovaleryl-CoA dehydrogenase, resulting in accumulation of isovaleryl-CoA derivatives. It generally presents in infancy with poor feeding, vomiting, obtundation, and seizures. The affected infants have a characteristic odor that resembles "dirty socks" and is best appreciated in sweat and cerumen. Patients presenting after the newborn period exhibit failure to thrive, developmental delays, or mental retardation. The initial therapeutic approach is to decrease leucine intake and promote an anabolic state with increased calories. EEG may reveal low-voltage activity (<20 μV) with bursts of delta slowing or sharp waves (98). In an experimental animal model, infusion of isovaleric acid caused slowing on EEG, which worsened as the concentration increased (99).

34. GLYCINE ENCEPHALOPATHY (NONKETOTIC HYPERGLYCINEMIA)

Glycine encephalopathy is caused by dysfunction of the multimeric glycine cleavage enzyme system, resulting in accumulation of glycine in all body tissues, including the brain. The disorder presents in the first week of life with apnea, lethargy, hypotonia, myoclonus, seizures, and feeding difficulty (100). Brain imaging is normal in half of cases. When abnormalities are seen, they include agenesis of the corpus callosum, progressive atrophy, or delayed myelination (100). Diagnosis is confirmed by the detection of elevated levels of glycine in the cerebrospinal fluid (CSF) and an elevation of the CSF-to-plasma glycine ratio (101). Classic neonatal-onset patients have ratios >0.2, but atypical, later-onset cases also exist and have ratios of ~0.09 (101). Atypical presentations can include seizures, developmental delays, and movement disorders outside of the neonatal period. In classical neonatal presentations, EEG demonstrates a burst suppression pattern or hypsarrhythmia (100). In later-onset variants, the EEG can reveal generalized spike and slow waves (102). Since glycine can stimulate NMDA glutamate receptors, treatment with NMDA antagonists (dextromethorphan and ketamine) has been tried. Sodium benzoate decreases CSF glycine levels and can further improve seizure control and alertness (103). In one case, clinical and electrophysiological improvements were seen with a combined regimen of dextromethorphan and sodium benzoate (103).

35. HARTNUP DISEASE

Hartnup disease is an autosomal dominant disorder of amino acid transport within the renal tubules and intestinal tract. It results in malabsorption of neutral monoamino monocarboxylic amino acids and aminoaciduria. Symptoms include pellagroid dermatitis, photosensitivity, ataxia, and neuropsychiatric abnormalities. EEG can reveal epileptiform features (104) but is normal in most cases.

36. LOWE SYNDROME (OCULOCEREBRORENAL SYNDROME)

Lowe syndrome was originally described in 1952 by Lowe et al. (105), who reported the histories of three unrelated male infants with congenital cataracts, glaucoma, developmental retardation, hyporeflexia with low musculature, osteopenia, decreased ammonia production, and a "peculiar, high-pitched, irritating cry." Affected children also exhibit hyperactivity, pseudotumor cerebri, ophthalmoplegia, or hypoglycemia. The condition is X-linked and is caused by mutations of the OCRL1 gene on chromosome Xq26. OCRL1 encodes a protein product that plays a role in cytoskeletal remodeling and cellular trafficking. Lowe syndrome has a high mortality rate in the first months from metabolic derangements and metabolic acidosis. Most patients will survive into the second or third decade but will develop chronic renal disease. MRI reveals small cyst-like changes in the periventricular white matter, and proton magnetic resonance spectroscopy (H-MRS) demonstrates prominent myoinositol peaks indicating gliosis (106,107). EEG shows an irregular, poorly sustained posteriorly dominant rhythm and bursts of high-voltage slowing. Independent bitemporal spike- and slow-wave discharges are seen (108). Generalized tonic–clonic, tonic, atonic, and complex partial seizures have been described. In one report of a patient with atonic seizures, the ictal EEG revealed secondarily generalized epileptiform discharges (109).

37. INBORN ERRORS OF UREA SYNTHESIS

Urea cycle disorders occur when there is deficiency of one of the enzymes in the cycle that converts nitrogen to urea. There are six enzymes involved: carbamyl phosphate synthetase I (CPSI), ornithine transcarbamylase (OTC), arginosuccinate synthetase (ASS), argininosuccinate lyase (ASL), N-acetyl glutamate synthetase (NAGS), and arginase. Dysfunction of any of the enzymes, with the exception of arginase, results in hyperammonemia and metabolic decompensation in infancy. Newborns appear well in the first 24 to 48 hours of life. After the infant begins taking protein from formula or breast milk, vomiting, lethargy, irritability, and poor feeding develop (110). Cerebral edema results in hyperventilation and metabolic alkalosis (111). Half of the affected patients have seizures.

Patients with partial enzyme deficiencies have later-onset presentations. This occurs most commonly in female carriers of OTC, since OTC is an X-linked condition. Late-onset patients exhibit developmental delays, seizures, psychiatric disorders, and chronic vomiting (112). Following high protein loads or catabolic stress, headache, vomiting, and ataxia develop. The diagnosis is suspected when an elevated plasma ammonia level is seen in conjunction with a normal blood glucose level and a normal anion gap. The diagnosis is confirmed by performing enzyme analysis from liver, fibroblasts, or red blood cells.

In one study of four infants with urea cycle disorders (113), all of the patients demonstrated abnormalities on at least one EEG. The most common findings included multifocal spike-and spike- and slow-wave discharges. Clancy and Chung (114) reported burst suppression in cases of neonatal citrullinemia. They observed that the length of the EEG interburst interval correlated with serum levels of ammonia, suggesting that hyperammonemia may directly contribute to encephalopathy. Nagata et al. (115) noted that EEG abnormalities were more often observed in patients with computed tomography (CT) abnormalities, and that patients with a normal CT were less likely to exhibit EEG findings. In the case of arginase deficiency, seizures may correlate with levels of the compound guanidinoacetoacetate (GAA), an intermediate in creatine synthesis for which arginine is a precursor, instead of elevated ammonia levels (116). As is typical of metabolic disorders, patients may have generalized or nonspecific seizures such as epileptic spasms and drop attacks (Figs. 13.8 and 13.9).

38. DISORDERS OF HEAVY METAL ACCUMULATION

38.1. Neurodegeneration with Brain Iron Accumulation

Neurodegeneration with brain iron accumulation is a collection of phenotypically similar conditions that have in common

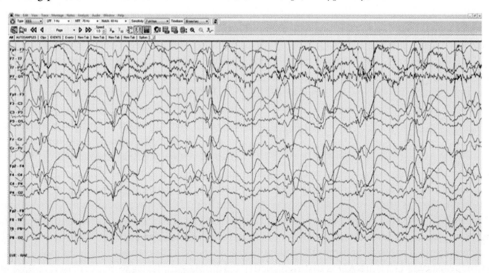

Figure 13.8. EEG in an 18-year-old boy with the urea cycle disorder arginase deficiency. Interictal background shows generalized slow spike-wave pattern.

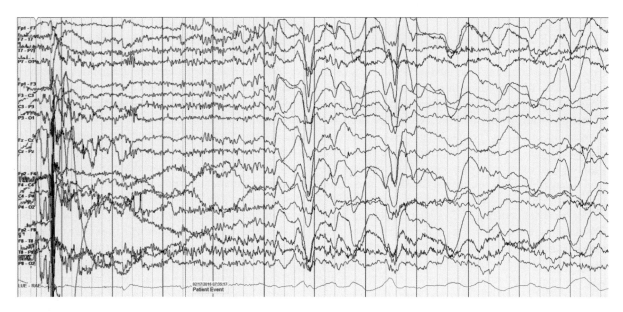

Figure 13.9. Ictal EEG in an 18-year-old boy with arginase deficiency during a drop event, showing diffuse background attenuation with superimposed fast activity, followed by high-amplitude spike-wave discharges and then postictal slowing. Event was also shown in video.

brain iron deposition. Included within this heading are pantothenate kinase-associated neurodegeneration (PKAN), infantile neuroaxonal dystrophy, neuroferritinopathy, and aceruloplasminemia. Patients present with posture and gait abnormalities, bradykinesia, and rigidity (116). MRI distinguishes these disorders, but all share a hypointense globus pallidus on T2 sequencing (117). More definitive confirmation can be accomplished through genetic testing.

PKAN is caused by a mutation of the pantothenate kinase 2 gene (PANK2). It is phenotypically classified into classical and atypical forms. Classical PKAN presents around age 3 with clumsiness and gait abnormalities. Dystonia begins in the lower extremities. Dysarthria, spasticity, visual impairment, and behavioral problems follow. Pigmentary retinopathy is common (117). MRI reveals T2 hyperintense signal surrounded by a rim of hypointensity in the globus pallidus, creating the "eye-of-the-tiger" sign, which is pathognomonic for the condition (118). Atypical presentations have a later onset and are characterized by psychiatric symptoms and movement disorders. The EEG in PKAN is normal in some cases (119,120). Observed abnormalities can include low-voltage slowing and fast activity (120). Swaiman et al. (121) reported a single patient with seizures and bursts of generalized slowing and sharp waves on EEG. Bilateral multifocal spikes and excessive posterior slowing were also noted.

38.2. Infantile Neuroaxonal Dystrophy (Seitelberger Disease)

Infantile neuroaxonal dystrophy (INAD) is characterized pathologically by axonal swelling and spheroid bodies in the CNS. Onset is between 6 months and 2 years. Patients present with neuromotor delay including lack of head control, inability to sit or walk, and poor eye contact. Myoclonic seizures occur. Dysmorphism (micrognathia, a prominent forehead, and low-set ears) is sometimes observed (122). INAD is distinguished from PKAN by the earlier age of onset and greater pyramidal

signs (spasticity and hyperreflexia) (123). Like PKAN, however, INAD is associated with high iron levels in the globus pallidus on MRI (124). Cerebellar atrophy is also observed. The two conditions are genetically distinct; INAD is caused by mutations of the PLA2G6 gene. Death usually occurs by age 10.

Interictal EEG reveals high-voltage fast rhythms (16–22 Hz) in sleep and wakefulness. Diffuse slow spike-wave complexes are also observed (125). In a 4-year-old boy with tonic spasms, the ictal EEG revealed diffuse, high-voltage, irregular sharp and slow-wave complexes followed by desynchronization (125). VEPs are abnormal and EMG demonstrates chronic degeneration.

38.3. Wilson Disease (Hepatolenticular Degeneration)

In Wilson disease, a defect of copper transport and excretion leads to copper accumulation in the liver. As cirrhosis develops, copper leaks into plasma and accumulates in the brain, kidneys, and cornea, where it results in injury. The earliest pathology in Wilson disease occurs in the liver; the initial deposition of hepatic copper is clinically silent.

There is wide variability in the age of disease onset, but the mean is 16 years (126). Younger patients tend to present with hepatic disease and older patients are more likely to exhibit neuropsychiatric symptoms at presentation (127). In one review of 282 patients (126), 69.1% presented with neurological symptoms. Of those, the predominant features were Parkinsonism (62.3%), dystonia (35.4%), cerebellar dysfunction (28%), pyramidal signs (16%), chorea (9%), athetosis (2.2%), myoclonus (3.4%), and behavioral abnormalities (16%). All of the patients with neurological symptoms had Kayser–Fleischer rings on ophthalmologic assessment. Serum ceruloplasmin levels were decreased in 93% and 24-hour copper excretion was increased in 70%. MRI reveals bilateral T2

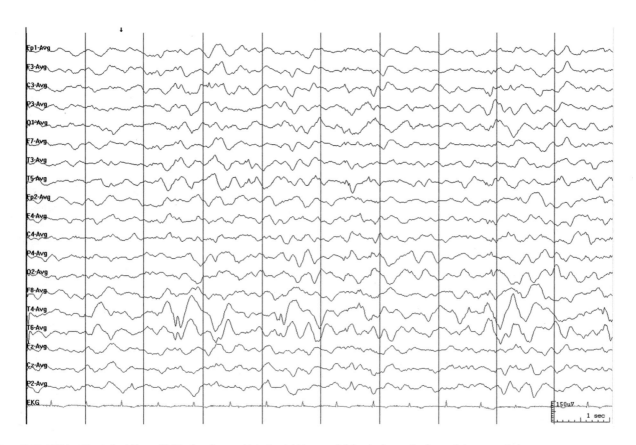

Figure 13.10. EEG in a 9-month-old boy with Menkes disease. Note the right temporal delta slowing and spike- and slow-wave discharges.

hyperintensities within the basal ganglia and thalamus as well as mild to moderate atrophy.

EEG changes in Wilson disease include a reduction in alpha frequency (17.6%), and increased beta (14.7%), theta (20.5%), or delta (2.9%) activity. Focal epileptiform discharges are seen in 11.7% of patients. In one series of 23 patients, only 3 exhibited EEG abnormalities (128), while in a literature review of 80 patients, over half showed EEG abnormalities (129). In general, the degree of EEG abnormality parallels the severity of clinical involvement. The EEG may improve during or after treatment (129). Prolonged latencies and abnormal waveforms are observed with visual and auditory evoked potentials.

38.4. Menkes Disease (Kinky Hair Disease)

Menkes disease is a fatal X-linked condition caused by a mutation of the copper-transport gene ATP7A, which is necessary for copper excretion from enterocytes. Copper deficiency results in impaired function of copper-dependent enzymes. The neurological symptoms result mainly from deficiency of cytochrome c oxidase. The clinical features can therefore resemble those in Leigh disease. Dysfunction of lysyl oxidase leads to connective tissue abnormalities and predisposes patients to arterial aneurysms and intracranial hemorrhage. Tyrosinase deficiency accounts for hypopigmentation of hair and skin. Patients typically present at 2 to 3 months of age with loss of developmental milestones, truncal hypotonia, failure to thrive, temperature instability, and epilepsy. The physical examination is notable for abnormally kinky hair, which is

shorter and sparser over the sides and back. Skin and hair are hypopigmented. Minor dysmorphology, including sagging cheeks, a depressed nasal bridge, and high-arched palate, is noted. MRI reveals intracranial vessel tortuosity, white matter changes, and ischemic lesions of the deep gray matter (130). Treatment with copper replacement may improve clinical outcomes if started early in the course of the disease (131).

Bahi-Buisson et al. (132) classified three stages of Menkes disease based on seizure types and EEG findings. In early disease, patients develop focal clonic status epilepticus, which is accompanied on EEG by slow spike-waves in the posterior head regions. Interictal EEG reveals multifocal polymorphic slow waves. During the intermediate stage of the disease, infantile spasms occur and a modified hypsarrhythmic pattern is seen on EEG. In late-stage disease, patients exhibit multifocal seizures, tonic spasms, and myoclonus. EEG reveals multifocal high-amplitude activity mixed with irregular slow waves (132). The degree of EEG abnormality relates in part to serum copper levels (133) (Fig. 13.10).

39. OTHER METABOLIC CONDITIONS

39.1. Glucose Transporter-1 Deficiency Syndrome (De Vivo Syndrome)

Glucose transporter-1 (GLUT1) is expressed on vascular endothelial cells and is the major transporter of glucose into the central nervous system. Dysfunction of GLUT1 results in low CSF glucose levels in the absence of hypoglycemia. Patients present in infancy with progressive microcephaly, developmental delays, and seizures (134). Patients with atypical forms exhibit ataxia or mental retardation without epilepsy.

Seizure types include generalized tonic, clonic, myoclonic, atonic, and atypical absence. In infancy, the EEG reveals multifocal spike-wave discharges, which localize to the temporal and occipital regions. With maturation, generalized 2.5- to 4-Hz spike- and slow-wave discharges are observed (134). The seizures can worsen with phenobarbital, since it inhibits GLUT1 function. The ketogenic diet is the only effective therapy since it allows the brain to utilize ketone bodies as a fuel source.

39.2. Pyridoxine-Dependent Seizures

Pyridoxine-dependent seizures are a rare autosomal recessive condition, presenting with neonatal epilepsy. A variety of seizure types, including infantile spasms, is observed. The seizures are resistant to traditional anticonvulsants but are well controlled by a daily pharmacological dose of pyridoxine (vitamin B6). Patients with pyridoxine-dependent seizures require pyridoxine supplementation throughout life. In a related condition, pyridoxine-responsive seizures, patients can be weaned off pyridoxine without seizure recurrence. Pyridoxine-dependent seizures are caused by deficiency of the enzyme α-aminoadipic semialdehyde (α-AASA) dehydrogenase, which is encoded by the antiquitin gene (ALDH7A1). α-AASA acts within the lysine catabolism pathway (135). Elevated levels of α-AASA and pipecolic acid result and can serve as biomarkers for the condition.

In pyridoxine-dependent seizures, the interictal EEG is abnormal in both the awake and asleep states. The background is discontinuous with a suppression burst-like pattern. Spike- and polyspike-waves are seen over the central and temporal regions. Continuous high-voltage rhythmic delta slowing occurs (136). Administration of pyridoxine (100–500 mg intravenously) results in rapid normalization of the EEG but should be given under close supervision since it may result in apnea and bradycardia. Folinic acid supplementation and lysine restriction may also play a role in treatment.

39.3. Folinic Acid-Responsive Seizures

Folinic acid-responsive seizures present with myoclonic, clonic, or subtle (apnea and irritability) seizures in infancy. The condition is confirmed by two characteristic peaks of CSF monoamine metabolic analysis. The identity of the peaks remains unknown. MRI reveals white matter abnormalities and atrophy. EEG demonstrates a discontinuous background pattern with multifocal spike or sharp waves (137). In one report of two patients with folinic acid-responsive seizures, both were found to have increased CSF levels of α-AASA and pipecolic acid (138). Those patients were subsequently found to have mutations of the ALDH7A1 gene, indicating that folinic acid-responsive seizures and pyridoxine-dependent seizures may be the same condition.

39.4. Pyridoxal-5-Phosphate Dependency

There is a separate group of patients who are deficient in the enzyme PNPO [pyridox(am)ine 5′-phosphate oxidase], which

converts pyridoxine phosphate and pyridoxamine phosphate to the biologically active form of vitamin B6, pyridoxine 5′ phosphate. EEGs may show high-voltage paroxysms of diffuse spike-wave and patients usually require pyridoxine 5′ phosphate for seizure control and improved outcome (139).

40. CEREBELLAR DISORDERS

40.1. Spinocerebellar Ataxias

Spinocerebellar ataxias (SCAs) are a heterogeneous group of progressive cerebellar syndromes with varying combinations of ataxia, dysmetria, and oculomotor deficits (140). Additional clinical findings include pigmentary retinopathy, extrapyramidal movement disorders (Parkinsonism, dystonia, and chorea), pyramidal signs, dementia, seizures, and peripheral neuropathy (140). MRI reveals cerebellar, olivopontocerebellar, or global brain atrophy. SCAs are genetically heterogeneous autosomal dominant conditions. A gene-based classification scheme is used in which the numbering system represents the order of gene discovery (SCA 1–8, SCA 10–23, and SCA 25). Genes for fibroblast growth factor 14 (FGF14) and dentatorubral-pallidoluysian atrophy (DRPLA) are also included within the family of SCAs. Many forms result from trinucleotide repeat disorders. Anticipation, progressively worsening phenotypes of subsequent generations within the same family, is observed. The age of onset and response to symptomatic treatment differ among the various types of SCA (140).

EEG findings in SCA vary among the different types. Variants that are commonly associated with epilepsy are more likely to reveal EEG abnormalities. In one report of 18 patients with SCA, temporal theta and delta intrusions were noted (141). Epilepsy is common in SCA 10, and a case series of 18 patients found EEG abnormalities in all 18 (142). The most common finding was slow and disorganized background activity. A case report of a father and son with complex partial seizures and SCA 2 noted temporal epileptiform discharges and slowing in both patients (143). Patients with DRPLA also develop epilepsy and may experience complex partial, myoclonic, atypical absence, and generalized tonic–clonic seizures. In 63.6% of patients with DRPLA, the EEG shows epileptiform features. Photosensitivity was observed in 27.3%, and those patients with a photoparoxysmal response also had progressive myoclonic epilepsy (144).

40.2. Friedreich Ataxia

Friedreich ataxia (FRDA1) is an autosomal recessive trinucleotide repeat disorder of the frataxin gene on chromosome 9p. The frataxin gene acts to regulate mitochondrial iron content. Iron overload results in damage to respiratory chain complexes I, II, and III through generation of oxygen free radicals (145). FRDA1 therefore has features of a mitochondrial disorder. It presents prior to adolescence with progressive cerebellar dysfunction and hypoactive knee and ankle reflexes. Patients also exhibit dysarthria, nystagmus, impaired position and vibratory sensation, and a Babinski sign. Cardiac dysfunction (subaortic stenosis and hypertrophic cardiomyopathy) and diabetes are common medical complications, and half of patients die of heart failure (146).

No qualitative EEG pattern is seen in FRDA1 (147). EEG also fails to provide prognostic information, since there is no relationship between the degree of EEG abnormality and the severity of the disease.

41. EEG IN NEUROCUTANEOUS SYNDROMES

41.1. Introduction

Neurocutaneous syndromes, or phakomatoses, are a broad group of disorders affecting both the skin and nervous system. Depending on the specific type, any level of the neuroaxis can be affected, including brain, spinal cord, or peripheral nerves. Because the skin and brain have common embryonic origins, there are many conditions that affect both systems. The manifestations are variable, depending on the specific nature of the neurological impairment. Some, such as tuberous sclerosis complex and neurofibromatosis, are associated with a disruption of cell growth and are therefore associated with tumor development. Others, including incontinentia pigmenti and Sturge–Weber syndrome, involve vascular disruptions that result in cerebral ischemia. The neurological manifestations therefore are broad and can include CNS tumors, intellectual impairment, autism, or epilepsy.

41.2. Tuberous Sclerosis Complex

Tuberous sclerosis complex (TSC) is a dominantly inherited, multisystem condition. It has a high rate of spontaneous mutations and approximately half of all patients do not have an affected parent. Two genes have been cloned for TSC, both of which result in similar clinical features. The TSC1 gene, located on chromosome 9q34, codes for a protein called hamartin. It indirectly links the cell membrane to the cytoskeleton (148). TSC2, located at chromosome 16p13.3, encodes for the protein tuberin. It functions in cellular signaling pathways (148). Hamartin and tuberin interact together as part of a larger protein complex (148) that functions to negatively regulate the mammalian target of rapamycin (mTOR) (149,150). When tuberin or hamartin is nonfunctional, mTOR is active, resulting in increased cell growth and proliferation. Rapamycin acts as an mTOR inhibitor and has shown efficacy in the treatment of subependymal giant cell astrocytomas in patients with TSC (151).

The clinical diagnosis of TSC is divided into three subheadings—definite, probable, and suspect—based on the type and number of abnormalities (152). Clinical expression is based on the location and severity of organ involvement. The primary targets are the skin, kidneys, heart, and CNS. Hypopigmented macules are the most common skin lesions and are present in as many as 90% of affected patients. Adenoma sebaceum, an angiofibromatous lesion occurring in a butterfly distribution about the nose and cheeks, is seen in 50%. Other skin lesions include the shagreen patch (over the lumbosacral or gluteal region), café-au-lait spots, and subungual fibromas. Tumors can occur in multiple organs, such as renal angiomyolipomas, cardiac rhabdomyomas, and retinal hamartomas.

In the brain, the characteristic features include cortical hamartomas (cortical tubers), subependymal hamartomas (subependymal nodules), and giant cell astrocytomas. Cortical tubers are named after potato tubers due to their firm and nodular consistency. On MRI, cortical tubers appear as enlarged, atypically shaped gyri with abnormal signal intensity in the subcortical white matter (153). Microscopically, they resemble focal cortical dysplasia (154), with disorganized lamination and balloon neurons (155). Subependymal nodules along the ventricular surface are at risk of transforming into subependymal giant cell astrocytomas (156).

Cortical tubers often result in epilepsy. In one large case series, epilepsy occurred in 85% of TSC patients (157). In the majority of patients, epilepsy develops in the first year of life. Infantile spasms are particularly common, occurring in just over one third of patients (157). Vigabatrin is a particularly effective treatment for infantile spasms in TSC patients (158) and is widely considered to be first-line therapy in this setting. Infantile spasms are a risk factor for both refractory epilepsy and Lennox–Gastaut syndrome. Poor cognitive outcomes are seen in patients with a history of infantile spasms, early age at seizure onset, and refractory epilepsy. Overall, close to two thirds of patients develop refractory epilepsy (157). Later in life, generalized tonic–clonic seizures predominate, but simple and complex-partial seizures are also common.

The presence of epilepsy is a predictor of cognitive impairment—this is particularly true when seizures develop before age 2 years or when infantile spasms occur. Cognitive impairment can also be predicted by the burden of cortical tubers, with more tubers correlating with greater impairment (159). Autism is common in patients with TSC. It is more likely to develop in those with temporal tubers, seizure onset before age 3, or a history of infantile spasms (160). Attention, language, and behavioral problems are also seen. Most of these patients have epilepsy as well. In general, TSC patients who are cognitively appropriate are seizure-free, and vice versa.

In infants, EEG may predict epilepsy even before seizures are clinically evident. In 2013, Domańska-Pakieła et al. (161) reported on five patients diagnosed with TSC prenatally or perinatally who were regularly monitored with EEG before the onset of epilepsy. In all of the patients, epileptiform discharges preceded the epilepsy onset. The time interval between abnormality detection on EEG and the epilepsy onset varied from 1 to 8 days. In all of the children, epilepsy started with focal motor seizures. Similarly, Ikeno et al. (162) reported clinically silent seizures in a neonate with tuberous sclerosis. Routine EEG revealed ictal changes associated with a subtle increase in heart rate and a brief increase in chin electromyogram. These changes were difficult to identify clinically. The patient later developed focal seizures and epileptic spasms with severe psychomotor delay.

In a larger series, Wu et al. (163) prospectively enrolled infants with TSC in an observational study that included regularly scheduled 1-hour video-EEGs. The infants were younger than 7 months at enrollment, were seizure-free, and had not been treated with vigabatrin or inhibitors of mTOR. The first emergence of epileptiform abnormalities on EEG occurred

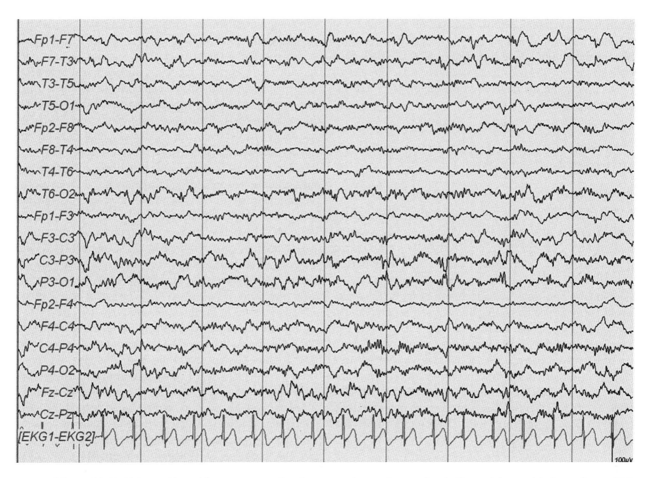

Figure 13.11. A 5-year-old girl with intractable partial-onset symptomatic epilepsy secondary to tuberous sclerosis. Slow and sharp activity is seen from multiple foci including the left anterior temporal and left parietal regions.

at an average age of 4.2 months, preceding seizure onset by a median of 1.9 months. All children with epileptiform discharges eventually developed epilepsy (Fig. 13.11).

Taken together, these reports indicate that EEG has value in predicting the clinical outcome of neonatal patients, even before clinical seizure activity is observed. Early identification of epilepsy is particularly important because earlier seizure onset leads to more significant neuropsychiatric sequelae (164).

Epilepsy in TSC does not consistently correspond with the imaging characteristics. Gallagher et al. (165) evaluated EEG and MRI data from 69 TSC patients. They reported that cyst-like tubers had the highest correlation to epileptiform activity in the same region. MRI findings that did not relate to interictal epileptiform activity included tuber burden, tuber size, and calcified tubers. Interestingly, quadrants without tubers co-registered with interictal epileptiform discharges in two patients, suggesting that epileptic foci may arise in areas free of tubers.

The EEG–MRI correlation is particularly important when planning epilepsy surgery in TSC patients. Correct localization of the epileptogenic region is necessary for good surgical outcome. In the presurgical evaluation of patients, nuclear medicine aids in detection of epileptic foci. When assessing TSC patients on a positron emission tomography (PET) scan, the tracer alpha[11C]methyl-L-tryptophan (AMT) allows for more accurate differentiation from nonepileptogenic tubers. In the interictal state, the lobar sensitivity of AMT PET for seizure onset is

lower, but its specificity is higher than FDG PET. Subdural electrodes adjacent to the area of increased AMT are often involved in seizure onset, and increased AMT uptake corresponds histologically to cortical developmental malformations (166). Such differentiation is necessary with planning epilepsy surgery.

For TSC patients undergoing surgery, proper recognition of intracranial ictal and interictal patterns is essential. Tuber-related ictal rhythms most commonly begin with low-voltage fast activity, later recruiting to rhythmic spiking. This is followed by diffuse slowing or bursts of ripple range fast activity (167) the ictal onset involves only the tuber in 57% and tubers with perituberal cortex in 31%. Fast ripples are confined to tubers only in 73% and involve perituberal cortex in 27%. Interictally, trains of periodic sharp waves on an attenuated background are observed in epileptogenic tubers (167). Microscopically, epileptogenic perituberal tissue contains abnormal cell types, including giant cells and cytomegalic neurons surrounded by morphologically abnormal astrocytes (168).

Arya et al. (169) studied 37 patients with TSC who underwent resective surgery. After a mean follow-up of over 5 years, 56.8% achieved complete seizure freedom and 86.5% had International League Against Epilepsy (ILAE) class 4 outcomes or better. The full-scale IQ on follow-up was significantly higher in patients with ILAE class 1 outcome compared with those with ILAE class 2 or worse. In a separate meta-analysis of surgical outcomes in TSC patients, similar outcomes were reported. ILAE class I outcomes were seen in 56% of patients and class 2 in 13% following epilepsy surgery (170). An absence of generalized seizure semiology, no or mild developmental delays, unifocal ictal scalp EEG abnormalities, and EEG/MRI concordance were all associated with better postoperative seizure outcomes (170). Surgical resection is also more successful when a single epileptogenic area is identified (171).

42. NEUROFIBROMATOSIS TYPE I

Neurofibromatosis type I (NF1) is a disorder of oncogene regulation and tumor formation. Patients with NF1 have an increased volume of gray and white matter, suggesting that brain overgrowth is an intrinsic component of the disease (172). NF1 is an autosomal dominant, single gene defect involving multiple organ systems. The diagnosis is based on National Institute of Health consensus criteria (Table 13.3) and requires two or more of the following:

Six or more café-au-lait spots (0.5 mm or larger in prepubertal and 1.5 mm or larger in postpubertal individuals)

Two or more neurofibromas of any type or one plexiform neurofibroma

Axillary or groin freckling

Two or more Lisch nodules

Optic nerve glioma

Dysplasia of the sphenoid bone or long bone cortex

A first-degree relative with NF1.

Café-au-lait spots are easily recognized and are often the presenting feature of the disease. These hyperpigmented macules increase in size and number with age. Approximately 50% of patients with NF1 lack a family history, likely representing new mutations (173). The gene for NF1 localizes to chromosome 17q11.2 and encodes the protein product neurofibromin. The incidence ranges between 1 in 3,000 and 1 in 4,000.

TABLE 13.3. Clinical Criteria for Neurofibromatosis 1 Diagnosis

Two or more of the following:
Six or more café-au-lait spots (0.5 mm or larger in prepubertal and 1.5 mm or larger in postpubertal individuals)
Two or more neurofibromas
One or more plexiform neurofibromas
Axillary or groin freckling
Two or more Lisch nodules
Optic nerve glioma
Dysplasia of the sphenoid bone or long bone cortex
First-degree relative with neurofibromatosis 1

In childhood, cognitive impairment is the most common complication. A broad range of effects are seen, including low IQ, behavioral problems, and learning disabilities. IQ scores in NF1 patients have a bimodal distribution; some children have intellectual impairment whereas others do not. This separation may have its basis in the white matter T2 hyperintensities, also known as unidentified bright objects, common to NF1 patients. They represent dysplastic glial proliferation and aberrant myelination in the underdeveloped brain. When compared to children without T2 hyperintensities, those with the lesions have significantly lower mean values for IQ and language scores and significantly impaired visuomotor integration and coordination (174). T2 hyperintensities in childhood are also a predictor of cognitive dysfunction in adulthood (175). A study showing a correlation between increased white matter volume and visual-perceptual deficits suggests that brain overgrowth may also be a factor in the associated cognitive deficits (176).

Another consequence of brain overgrowth are tumors, which are common in NF1 and are a major cause of morbidity. Neurofibromas, the tumors for which the disorder takes its name, are benign peripheral nerve sheath tumors that typically develop in adolescence. Although they are unlikely to cause neurological deficit, spinal neurofibromas arising from the dorsal nerve roots can lead to severe pain. Plexiform neurofibromas, on the other hand, are more likely to be present at birth. They can be found anywhere within the body and cause a variety of presenting symptoms depending on their location. Serious complications include pain, spinal cord compression, and spread to the orbit, with resulting sphenoid wing dysplasia and pulsating exophthalmos. Plexiform neurofibromas can undergo transformation to malignant peripheral nerve sheath tumors. Optic nerve gliomas involve the optic nerve, chiasm, or tract. They usually develop prior to age 7 and can be insidious in their onset.

Seizures are another common complication of NF1. Korf et al. (177) characterized the clinical features of seizures in 22 patients with NF1. Their seizure types included infantile spasms, generalized seizures associated with a febrile illness, complex partial seizures, and primary generalized seizures. In none of the individuals with seizures in this study was a structural lesion in the brain visible by neuroimaging. They concluded that seizures were relatively uncommon in NF1 patients. Kulkrantrakorn et al. (178) reported the prevalence of epileptic seizures in NF1 patients to be 4.2%. Seizures in NF1 correspond strongly to tumors, but not to the number or location of unidentified bright objects (179).

EEG findings are as diverse as the seizure types in NF1. Ostendorf et al. (180) reported the findings of 64 EEGs recorded from 35 individuals with NF1. Forty-four percent of those studies were interpreted as normal. The remaining abnormalities were evenly divided between slowing and epileptiform findings. Abnormalities were focal in 27%, generalized in 19%, and multifocal in 5%. A combination of the above abnormalities was seen in 11%.

Likewise, evoked potentials frequently demonstrate abnormalities in patients with NF1. Yerdelen et al. (181) performed brainstem visual, auditory, and somatosensory evoked potentials in 39 patients. Of those, 20 (51.3%) showed abnormal VEPs, 14 (35.9%) showed abnormal SEPs, and 6 (15.4%) showed abnormal

BAEPs. These electrophysiological findings occurred even in the absence of any clinical sign related to the affected system.

As is the case in TSC, epilepsy surgery can be considered for NF1. Barba et al. (182) studied 12 patients with NF1 who underwent epilepsy surgery. MRI abnormalities were present in all patients but one. One year after surgery eight patients were seizure-free, one had worthwhile improvement, and the remaining three had experienced no benefit. Histology revealed dysembryoplastic neuroepithelial tumor in five patients, hippocampal sclerosis in four, mixed pathology in one, and polymicrogyria in one.

43. NEUROFIBROMATOSIS TYPE II

Like NF1, neurofibromatosis type II (NF2) is an autosomal dominant, single gene deficit, which, in NF2, localizes to chromosome 22. The gene product, merlin, also has tumor suppressor function. Tumors and malignancies are, therefore, common in both conditions. Beyond that, few similarities exist. Café-au-lait spots are rarely seen in NF2 and neurofibromas are uncommon. NF2 is much less common than NF1, with an incidence of only 1:30,000 to 1:40,000.

Common tumors in NF2 include schwannomas (which are usually multiple), meningiomas, ependymomas, and gliomas. Vestibulocochlear schwannomas are particularly common and sometimes bilateral (in which case the diagnosis of NF2 is certain). Roughly half of NF2 patients present because of hearing loss, tinnitus, and vertigo resulting from a vestibulocochlear schwannoma.

Epilepsy is rare in NF2. A single case report of status epilepticus exists, but there have not been systematic studies regarding EEG findings in the condition (183).

44. HYPOMELANOSIS OF ITO

The brain malformations of hypomelanosis of Ito include abnormalities of neuronal differentiation such as cortical dysplasia and hemimegalencephaly. Malformations characteristic of later stages of brain development (heterotopia, polymicrogyria) are also seen, suggesting heterogeneity within the disorder. The skin lesions consist of whorls and streaks of decreased pigmentation, which follow the lines of Blaschko. There are no preceding inflammatory or vesicular eruptions as in incontinentia pigmenti and the palms, soles, and mucous membranes are spared. The skin lesions are more prominent over the ventral surface of the torso and on the flexor surface of the extremities. They may be unilateral, in which case they exhibit a midline cutoff. In patients with hypomelanosis of Ito and hemimegalencephaly, the skin lesions are contralateral to the brain abnormality. Systemic manifestations include ophthalmologic, cardiac, musculoskeletal, and genital anomalies. The etiology of hypomelanosis of Ito is likely to be heterogeneous; several different chromosomal abnormalities have been associated with it, and most patients are chromosomal mosaics.

The neurological manifestations include epilepsy and cognitive impairment. Epilepsy occurs in approximately half of patients (184). Generalized tonic–clonic seizures are the most common,

but infantile spasms and focal and myoclonic seizures are also observed. In patients with infantile spasms, asymmetric hypsarrhythmia can be seen on EEG (185). In patients with cognitive impairment but not epilepsy, the EEG may be normal (186).

45. INCONTINENTIA PIGMENTI

Incontinentia pigmenti is a rare, X-linked, dominant, neurocutaneous disorder with the onset of skin changes in the first 6 weeks of life. The cutaneous disorder follows a characteristic evolution from vesicular to verrucous to hyperpigmented and finally atrophic changes. The vesicles and bullae from the original eruption in infancy later give rise to the characteristic swirling pattern of hyperpigmentation. Hair, nail, dental, and ophthalmologic abnormalities are also observed. Neurologically, these infants may develop epilepsy, mental retardation, microcephaly, spasticity, or ataxia. A case report demonstrating periventricular hemorrhagic infarctions in infancy suggests microangiopathy as the cause of the neurological changes (186). The gene for incontinentia pigmenti is NEMO (NF-kappaB essential modulator)/IKKgamma (IkappaB kinase-gamma) and is located on Xq28. NEMO is important for immune, inflammatory, and apoptotic pathways (187). The disorder is lethal in most males, accounting for its 20:1 female-to-male predominance. Males with incontinentia pigmenti have been described but commonly have features of the condition in a limited distribution. Somatic mosaicism is a likely mechanism in such cases (188).

In one infant with extensive cerebral infarction on MRI, EEG showed multifocal epileptiform discharges (189). In a separate case report, infantile spasms with hypsarrhythmia on EEG were described (190).

46. STURGE–WEBER SYNDROME

Sturge–Weber syndrome is characterized by angiomas of the leptomeninges and skin. The cutaneous lesion, also known as a port-wine stain, typically involves the ophthalmic and maxillary distributions of the trigeminal nerve. The leptomeningeal angiomas may be either unilateral or bilateral, but unilateral lesions are more common. The specific neurological effects depend on the location of the lesion, which is most commonly parietal or occipital. Neurological impairment results from a vascular steal phenomenon. Laminar cortical necrosis occurs. Histology reveals neuronal loss, gliosis, cerebral atrophy, and calcifications. The calcifications take on a train-track appearance on plain films and CT. MRI, if done, should be performed with gadolinium to allow for appreciation of the angiomas.

The clinical manifestations include hemiparesis, stroke-like episodes, cognitive impairment, epilepsy, and headaches. Epilepsy is present in 75% to 90% of patients, and the seizures are typically focal. Many patients have refractory epilepsy, in which case cortical resection and possibly hemispherectomy are considered.

Because the leptomeningeal angiomas are typically unilateral, the most consistent EEG finding is unilateral reduction of background amplitude in the waking record (191). Responses to hyperventilation and photic driving are also decreased on the involved side. Epileptiform activity is limited to the involved hemisphere (192). The EEG findings evolve over time, becoming more abnormal with increasing age. Slowing is more common at younger ages, whereas focal spike-waves are seen in older children (192). Ictal EEGs in Sturge–Weber syndrome may demonstrate slowing over the contralateral hemisphere due to ischemic changes resulting from a steal phenomenon (193).

On intracranial EEG, activity is depressed over the affected hemisphere on the interictal study (194). Invasive ictal EEG reveals rhythmic activity within the delta to theta ranges. Seizures occur over the central area of the leptomeningeal angiomas, and not in the periphery of the lesions (194).

47. EEG IN AUTISM SPECTRUM DISORDERS AND INTELLECTUAL IMPAIRMENT

47.1. Autism Spectrum Disorder

Autism spectrum disorder (ASD) is a neurodevelopmental disability characterized by deficits in social-emotional reciprocity, impaired communication, and restricted patterns of behavior, interests, and activities. For autism to be diagnosed, these features first develop in early childhood. The clinical characteristics are outlined by the American Psychiatric Association in the *Diagnostic and Statistical Manual of Mental Disorders*, Fifth Edition (195).

Since ASD is based on clinical symptoms, the diagnosis itself does not reveal specific biological causes. Clinical symptoms alone may not guide prognosis or treatment considerations. At present, genetic testing offers the greatest hope of identifying the biological underpinnings of the condition. Genetics may provide earlier detection, identify medical comorbidities, or assist with prognosis (196). A genetic cause is identified in up to 25% of cases, but in the majority of patients, the underlying causes are still unknown. Hundreds of genes are implicated in autism, many of which are also related to intellectual impairment and epilepsy. Possible genetic abnormalities include chromosomal derangements, copy number variants, and single nucleotide mutations (197).

In comorbid epilepsy and autism, an imbalance of excitation to inhibition exists, selectively increasing excitation and promoting over-connectivity. Such hyperexcitability is mediated by genes that regulate neuronal and synaptic homeostasis (198). Cortical interneurons play a role in excitation/inhibition and are involved in both conditions. Cortical interneurons exert an inhibitory influence via the release of γ-aminobutyric acid (GABA). Disruptions of cortical interneurons alter the balance of excitation to inhibition, favoring increased excitation. Reduced numbers of cortical interneurons have been observed in both autism (199) and epilepsy (200), indicating a shared mechanism between both conditions.

Increased cortical excitability likely accounts for the increased incidence of comorbid ASD and epilepsy. The prevalence of epilepsy in ASD is just over 20% in patients with intellectual disability and 8% in patients without intellectual disability (201,202). Complex partial seizures are the most frequent seizure type observed in ASD patients, and epileptiform

discharges are localized to the frontal area in approximately half of patients (203). Children with autism also have higher rates of epileptic discharges than the general population: 20% to 60% of children with ASD have epileptiform abnormalities on EEG (204,205). Even when excluding children with epilepsy, epileptiform discharges are still seen in 8% to 20% of ASD patients (204). Epileptiform discharges are particularly associated with autistic regression (206), although it remains unknown whether the discharges themselves have a causative role in developmental regression.

47.2. Intellectual Disability

Intellectual disability is characterized by limitations in intellectual functioning and adaptive behavior. Considerable overlap exists between intellectual disability and ASD: approximately two thirds of individuals with ASD have co-occurring intellectual disability (207). Epilepsy and epileptic discharges are also more common in ASD and intellectual disability than in the general population (208). In many cases, ASD, intellectual disability, and epilepsy have the same underlying genetic etiologies. Four common causes of all three include Down syndrome, Fragile X, Angelman syndrome, and Rett syndrome.

47.3. Down Syndrome

Down syndrome is the leading genetic cause of intellectual disability. Some patients with Down syndrome have a pattern of language and social delays that resembles ASD (209). The prevalence of ASD in individuals with Down syndrome is as high as 18% and is even greater in children with more pronounced intellectual impairment (210). Similarly, epilepsy is also common in Down syndrome. The prevalence of epilepsy in patients with Down syndrome ranges between 0% and 13%, with a median of 5.5% (211). In Down syndrome patients who develop epilepsy, seizure onset occurs within the first year of life in 40% (212). Many of those patients present with infantile spasms between 6 and 8 months of age. Infantile spasms in children with Down syndrome may occur secondary to brain injury or structural lesions, as occurs in patients with hypoxic-ischemic encephalopathy and stroke due to congenital heart disease, or they may be cryptogenic and have no identifiable cause (213). EEG helps distinguish symptomatic versus cryptogenic infantile spasms in Down syndrome patients. In patients with cryptogenic spasms there is symmetric hypsarrhythmia, no focus is uncovered by intravenous diazepam, and there are single rather than clustered spasms on ictal EEG. In symptomatic patients, the EEG reveals no interictal paroxysmal activity between consecutive spasms or focal discharges at the onset of electrographic seizures (214).

Lennox–Gastaut syndrome has also been reported in Down syndrome, but surprisingly, in one case series, none of the patients with Lennox–Gastaut syndrome had a prior history of infantile spasms (215). A high rate of reflex seizures, precipitated by sudden unexpected sensory stimulation, is seen in Down syndrome patients with Lennox–Gastaut syndrome. Other seizure types that are commonly seen in Down syndrome include partial and generalized tonic–clonic seizures (212). Even apart from patients with epilepsy, a high frequency of epileptic discharges is seen in Down syndrome patients, although no distinctive pattern is seen (216).

47.4. Fragile X Syndrome

Fragile X syndrome is the most commonly observed genetic cause of ASD. It is a monogenetic disorder caused by a CGG expansion repeat of the FMR1 gene, which encodes the Fragile X mental retardation protein (217). The protein is involved in regulating mRNA transport and protein synthesis both pre- and post-synaptically. Disruption leads to elongated dendritic spines, increased synthesis of metabotropic glutamate receptors, increase in long-term depression, and reduced synaptic maturation (217,218).

The alteration of synapse development and enhanced excitation likely play a role in the high prevalence of ASD in Fragile X patients. As many as 90% of Fragile X patients have some features of ASD (219). The same mechanisms also explain the high rates of seizures and epilepsy. Seizures occur in 10% to 20% of Fragile X patients who have full mutations (220). Their EEGs commonly exhibit features of benign childhood epilepsy with centrotemporal spikes. Even in children without clinical seizures, centrotemporal spikes can be seen in roughly 23% of patients (220). The seizures in Fragile X often resolve in adolescence, indicating a further similarity to benign childhood epilepsy with centrotemporal spikes.

47.5. Angelman Syndrome

Angelman syndrome clinically consists of dysmorphic facial features, absence of speech, paroxysms of laughter, an ataxic puppet-like gait, and epileptic seizures. It is caused by a lack of expression of the UBE3A gene resulting from abnormalities of chromosome 15q11–q13. Approximately 70% of Angelman syndrome cases result from a de novo 15q11–q13 deletion of the maternal chromosome. Five percent to 10% of cases result from a mutation of the maternal UBE3A gene. Three percent to 5% have an abnormality of DNA methylation in the maternal copy of the gene. Two percent to 3% of patients inherited both copies of chromosome 15 from the father and none from the mother and, therefore, have no functional copy of UBE3A from the mother (221). Abnormalities of the same region on 15q11–q13 also result in Prader–Willi syndrome. The phenotype is determined by the parental origin of the chromosome 15 defect, with maternal abnormalities resulting in Angelman syndrome and paternal abnormalities leading to Prader–Willi. Hence, these conditions illustrate the phenomenon of genomic imprinting.

EEG abnormalities develop prior to 1 year of age and are seen in 80% of patients. There are three main findings that are characteristic of the condition (222):

1. Rhythmic 4- to 6-Hz generalized theta activity, exceeding 200 μV

2. Rhythmic 2- to 3-Hz delta slowing with superimposed epileptiform discharges most prominently seen in the anterior regions, with amplitudes ranging between 200 and 500 mv (Fig. 13.12)

3. Spike and sharp wave discharges intermixed with 3- to 4-Hz high-amplitude slowing, with amplitudes exceeding 200 μV.

A genotype–phenotype correlation exists in the EEG patterns of Angelman syndrome. Patients with large chromosome deletions of 15q11–13 have a slow and disorganized background rhythm in combination with bursts of slow (2–3 Hz) triphasic waves or spike-waves (223). On the other hand, up to 72.2% of patients with uniparental disomy, methylation imprinting abnormalities, or UBE3A mutations have a normal awake EEG background (223). The EEG findings in Angelman syndrome evolve with age (224). Bursts of very slow 1- to 3-Hz activity are most evident in patients under 4 years of age. School-aged children not yet at puberty are more likely to display 4- to 6-Hz activity over the posterior regions with mixed spike-and-wave activity. In adulthood, the background rhythm is slow for age with intermixed multifocal spike-waves.

The slow activity with superimposed epileptiform discharges seen in Angelman syndrome resembles the slow spike-and-wave complexes observed in Lennox–Gastaut syndrome. In Lennox–Gastaut syndrome, the spike and slow waves are well defined and demonstrate sleep activation. Conversely, in Angelman syndrome, there is no sleep activation of epileptiform activity (225).

47.6. Rett Syndrome

Rett syndrome is in the differential diagnosis of Angelman syndrome since the two conditions have considerable phenotypic overlap (226). The clinical features of Rett syndrome were defined by a consensus panel held in 2001 (227). Necessary criteria for the diagnosis include female sex, normal development through the first 6 months, deceleration of head growth, psychomotor regression, loss of purposeful hand movements, and hand-wringing stereotypies. Pathologically, Rett syndrome is characterized by reduced dendritic arborization. Seventy percent of patients who meet clinical criteria carry a mutation of the X-linked methyl CpG-binding protein (MECP2) gene (228), which is critical for postnatal neuronal maturation. The X-linked cyclin-dependent kinase-like 5 (CDKL5) gene can also result in a Rett syndrome–like phenotype. Patients with CDKL5 mutations are less likely to exhibit normal development in the first year and more likely to have early-onset intractable epilepsy, infantile spasms, and severe hypotonia (229).

The clinical deterioration of Rett syndrome has been separated into four stages (230). Stage 1, termed the early-onset stagnation stage, involves a developmental arrest with altered communication, diminished interest in playing, hand-washing movements, and a deceleration of skull growth. In stage 2, the rapid destructive stage, developmental deterioration becomes more evident. Patients become ataxic and clumsy. They demonstrate features of autism and dementia. Seizures first develop during this stage. In stage 3, the pseudo-stationary stage, patients continue to have epilepsy and severe hand apraxia, but they seem more attentive and their autistic features may appear less severe. By stage 4, the late motor deterioration stage, patients lose mobility and often become wheelchair-bound. They may become cachectic. Seizures, however, improve.

The EEG findings of Rett syndrome are so consistent that, in the appropriate clinical setting, they are nearly diagnostic (Fig. 13.13). The waking record shows a progressive deterioration with decreasing voltage, whereas sleep contains

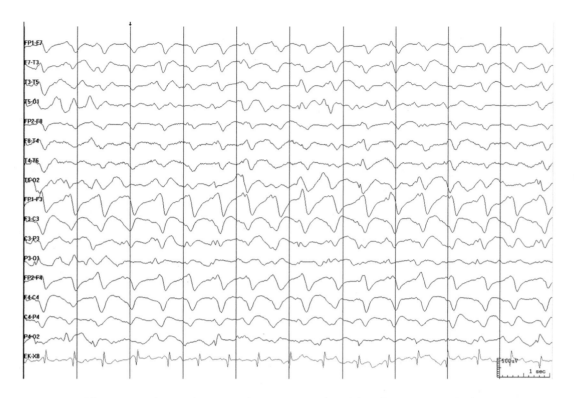

Figure 13.12. *EEG in a 3-year-old boy with Angelman syndrome. Note the continuous, rhythmic, bifrontally predominant delta slowing with intermixed sharp features.*

high-amplitude paroxysmal activity (231). These abnormalities generally precede the development of clinical seizures (232). Epileptiform spikes occur most frequently over the parasagittal regions during all sleep stages but are higher in non-REM sleep than REM sleep. Spikes are also greatest in frequency during the second half of the night (233). Spike-and-wave discharges are elicited by repetitive tactile stimulation.

The progression of EEG abnormalities follows the clinical staging outlined by Hagberg and Wit-Engerstrism (Table 13.4) (230). The EEG is often normal in stage 1. Deterioration of background with mildly excessive slow activity and frequent spike-and-waves, maximal centrally, occurs in stage 2. By stage 3, there is further deterioration of background activity with more abundant and multifocal spikes, and delta waves in both wakefulness and sleep. Stage 4 is characterized on EEG by poorly formed low-voltage background activity (234).

47.7. Cerebral Palsy

Cerebral palsy is a descriptive diagnosis applied to children with impairment in movement and posture resulting from a nonprogressive injury to the developing brain. As a descriptive term, the diagnosis of cerebral palsy does not denote when during development the injury occurred or the predisposing factor (Table 13.5). The prevalence of cerebral palsy is often estimated between 3 and 6 per 1,000 (235), with a recent prevalence estimate of cerebral palsy per 1,000 8-year-old children in the United States demonstrating a drop from 3.5 (95% confidence interval [CI] 3.2–3.9) in 2006 to 2.9 (95% CI 2.6–3.2) in 2010 (236).

Findings on the neurological examination may include spasticity, hypotonia, weakness, balance abnormalities, abnormal movements, and difficulty walking. Although resulting from a static lesion, neurological findings and the extent of disability may progress with age and secondary musculoskeletal abnormalities may develop.

The clinical pattern has frequently been used to divide cerebral palsy into various forms (Table 13.6). The timing of the injury is frequently the factor in determining the site of the injury and, thus, the form of cerebral palsy. For example, the spastic diplegic form is most frequently associated with preterm birth with the injury occurring between 26 and 32 weeks gestational age, which results in periventricular leukomalacia and damage to the descending leg fibers of cortical spinal tracts. In contrast, hemiplegic cerebral palsy most often occurs as the result of a perinatal lesion such as a neonatal stroke of the left middle cerebral artery resulting in right upper extremity spasticity and paresis.

As emphasized at the 2004 International Workshop of Definition and Classification of Cerebral Palsy (237), the motor and balance impairment does not occur in isolation, as many of these children also have comorbid disturbances that can impact cognition, communication, behavior, and sensation. In addition, there is often comorbid epilepsy, frequently with seizures of focal onset (238). As reviewed by Russman and Ashwal (239), the average prevalence of epilepsy in children with cerebral palsy across a combination of 13 prospective and retrospective studies was 43%, with a range of 35% (240) to 62% (241).

The frequency of seizures in this population varies by the type of cerebral palsy and degree of motor disability. Children with spastic quadriplegia (242–246) are at greatest risk, and approximately two thirds of this group will develop epilepsy. However, children with spastic diplegia and the extrapyramidal forms of cerebral palsy have a lower risk of seizures and epilepsy

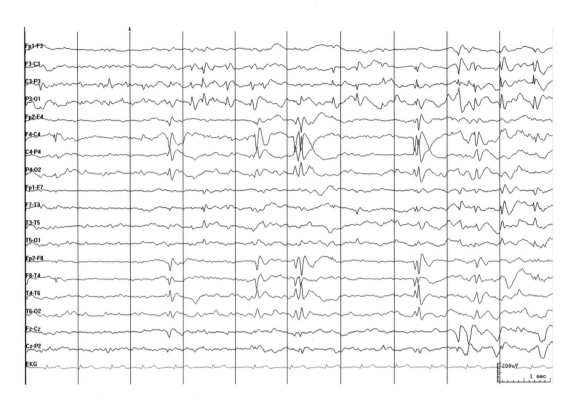

Figure 13.13. EEG in a 3-year-old girl with Rett syndrome. Note the bilateral central spike-waves.

(245,247). Independent of type, epilepsy is far more common in children with cerebral palsy who are not ambulatory (Gross Motor Function Classification System IV and V) versus those who are ambulatory (245,248,249). Additionally, it has been estimated that approximately 15% of children with cerebral palsy may develop epileptic spasms (West syndrome), with children with spastic quadriplegia being at highest risk (247).

Compared to other children with epilepsy, those with cerebral palsy are more likely to require multiple medications and less likely to have prolonged periods of seizure freedom (247,250,251). However, seizure-free periods may occur. Favorable prognostic factors for seizure-free periods lasting 1 year or longer include normal intelligence, spastic diplegia, single seizure type, and monotherapy (248).

For children whose epilepsy remains resistant to antiseizure medications, alternative treatments are considered, such as epilepsy surgery, neurostimulation, and the ketogenic diet. Epilepsy surgery is an option for children whose epilepsy is

TABLE 13.4. EEG Evolution in Rett Syndrome

Stage 1	EEG background often normal
Stage 2	Deterioration of background with mildly excessive slow activity and frequent spike-and-waves, maximal centrally
Stage 3	Further deterioration of background activity
	Abundant and multifocal spikes
	Delta waves in both wakefulness and sleep
Stage 4	Poorly formed low-voltage background activity

TABLE 13.5. Predisposing Factors for Cerebral Palsy*

Prenatal
Genetic and chromosomal disorders
Congenital infection
Cerebral malformations
Multiple gestation
Teratogens/toxins
Vascular abnormalities/Intracranial hemorrhage
Perinatal/Postnatal
Perinatal sepsis or CNS infection
Asphyxia/Hypoxic-ischemic encephalopathy
Placental abruption
Hyperbilirubinemia
Nonaccidental trauma/Head injury
Rhesus incompatibility
Prolonged labor
Stroke

* In a significant minority of children with cerebral palsy, a predisposing factor is not identified.

TABLE 13.6. Types of Cerebral Palsy

TYPE	FINDINGS ON NEUROLOGICAL EXAMINATION	COMORBID EPILEPSY?
Spastic		
Hemiplegia	Unilateral spasticity and paresis	Common
Diplegia	Lower-extremity spasticity	Uncommon
Quadriplegia	Spasticity of all extremities	Common
Dyskinetic		
Athetoid	Chorea, athetosis	Uncommon
Dystonic	Hypertonia, rigid posturing	Uncommon
Ataxic	Ataxia, unsteady gait	Rare

refractory to antiseizure medications. In a recent report, Olsson et al. (252) reviewed their experience in 32 children with cerebral palsy who required epilepsy surgery. A hemispherectomy was performed in 11 cases, with the other children having either a frontal lobe resection (*n* = 7), callosotomy (*n* = 7), or multilobar resections (*n* = 5). Two-year outcome was characterized as seizure-free for 13 of the 32 and a >75% reduction for an additional 8 children.

Due to differential perfusion of the cortex, which favors the apex over the depth of the sulci, perinatal hypoxic-ischemic events can result in greater injury in the depth of the sulci. This differential injury results in mushroom-shaped gyri (ulegyria), which are frequently isolated to watershed zones. Several small case series suggest that the epilepsy associated with ulegyria is amenable to epilepsy surgery (253,254).

In children whose epilepsy is not medically resistant, a wean is attempted after 2 years of seizure freedom, but the risk of relapse is high. In a study of 65 children with cerebral palsy in whom medications were weaned after 2 years of seizure freedom, 27 patients (41.5%) relapsed; the highest rate (61.5%) occurred in those with spastic hemiparesis and the lowest relapse rate (14.3%) was in those with spastic diplegia (255).

As recently noted in the report from the Quality Standards Subcommittee of the American Academy of Neurology and the Practice Committee of the Child Neurology Society, an EEG should not be obtained to determine the etiology of the cerebral palsy but should be obtained when a diagnosis of epilepsy is being considered (256). When reviewing the EEG record of a child with cerebral palsy, it is imperative to note that paroxysmal activity (e.g., spikes) has been observed in children with epilepsy as well as those without (256–258).

Still, in one of the most comprehensive studies of EEG in children with cerebral palsy—that carried out by Meyer Perlstein, Erna Gibbs, and Frederic Gibbs (256,259–262)—great attempts were made to characterize the EEG findings based on the type of cerebral palsy and to correlate with clinical aspects of cerebral palsy. In their work, the most common abnormality observed was multifocal spikes. In addition to this EEG finding, generalized slowing, focal slowing, and asymmetries were also noted more frequently in those older than

2 years. In the younger age group, in those without West syndrome, the abnormalities were often isolated to the absence of normal sleep architecture and voltage depression during sleep.

SCORE EEG SOFTWARE

Further examples related to the topics addressed in this chapter can be found in the interactive online Niedermeyer Educational Platform. EEG recordings with illustrative examples can be opened and browsed. Features are marked and described using the SCORE EEG software. The users can see the features marked by experts, they can score these features themselves, and then compare them with the scorings of the experts.

The Niedermeyer Educational Platform can be accessed at: www.scoreEEG.com/academy

REFERENCES

1. Fukumizu M, Yoshikawa H, Takashima S, et al. Tay Sachs disease: progression of changes on neuroimaging in four cases. Neuroradiology. 1992;34:483–486.
2. Pampiglione G, Harden A. Neurophysiological investigations in GM1 and GM2 gangliosidoses. Neuropediatrics. 1984;15:74–84.
3. Alduligan MS and Pearl PL: Electroencephalography in the metabolic epilepsies. In: PL Pearl, ed. Inherited Metabolic Epilepsies. New York: Demos Medical Publishers, 2013:39–67.
4. Cooperhaver RM, Goodman G. The electroretinogram in infantile, late infantile, and juvenile amaurotic familial infancy. Arch Ophthalmol. 1960;63:559–566.
5. Sakuraba H, Itoh K, Shimmoto M, et al. GM2 gangliosidosis AB variant: clinical and biochemical studies of a Japanese patient. Neurology. 1999;52:372.
6. Zaroff CM, Neudorfer O, Morrison C, et al. Neuropsychological assessment of patients with late onset GM2 gangliosidosis. Neurology. 2004;62:2283.
7. Harden A, Martinovic Z, Pampiglione G. Neurophysiological studies in GM1 gangliosidosis. Ital J Neurol Sci. 1982;3:201–206.
8. Cooper JD. Progress towards understanding the neurobiology of Batten disease or neuronal ceroid lipofuscinosis. Curr Opin Neurol. 2003;16:121.
9. Vinken PJ, Bruyn GW, eds. Handbook of Neurology. Vol 10. Amsterdam: North Holland Publishers; 1970:588–679.
10. Wisniewski K. Neuronal ceroid-lipofuscinoses. Gene Rev. 2006:1–26.
11. Groebel HH, Mole SE, Lake BD, eds. The Neuronal Ceroid Lipofuscinoses (Batten Disease). Amsterdam: IOS Press; 1999:16–36.
12. Santavuori P, Lauronen L, Kirveskari E, et al. Neuronal ceroid lipofuscinoses in childhood. J Neurol Sci. 2000;21:s35–s41.
13. Groebel HH, Mole SE, Lake BD, eds. The Neuronal Ceroid Lipofuscinoses (Batten Disease). Amsterdam: IOS Press; 1999:37–54.
14. Goebel H, Wisniewski KE. Current state of clinical and morphological features of human NCL. Brain Pathol. 2004;14:61–69.
15. Sinha S, Satishchandra P, Gayathri N, et al. Progressive myoclonic epilepsy: a clinical, electrophysiological and pathological study from South India. J Neurol Sci. 2007;252:16–23.
16. Muenzer J. The mucopolysaccharidoses: a heterogeneous group of disorders with variable pediatric presentations. J Pediatr. 2004;144:s27–s34.
17. Ruijter GJG, Valstar MJ, van de Kamp JM, et al. Clinical and genetic spectrum of Sanfilippo type C (MPS IIIC) disease in the Netherlands. Mol Genet Metab. 2008;93:104–111.
18. Husain AM, Escolar ML, Kurtzberg J. Neurological assessment of mucopolysaccharidosis III. Clin Neurophysiol. 2006;117:2059–2063.
19. Kriel RL, Hauser WA, Sung JH, et al. Neuroanatomical and electroencephalographic correlations in Sanfilippo syndrome, type A. Arch Neurol. 1978;35:838–843.
20. Tolar J, Gewal SS, Bjoraker KJ, et al. Combination of enzyme replacement and hematopoietic stem cell transplantation as therapy for Hurler syndrome. Bone Marrow Transplant. 2008;41:531–535.
21. Wrait JE, Clarke LA, Beck M, et al. Enzyme replacement therapy for mucopolysaccharidosis I: a randomized, double-blinded, placebo-controlled, multinational study of recombinant human alpha-L-iduronidase (laronidase). J Pediatr. 2004;144:581–588.

22. Lowden JA, O'Brien JS. Sialidosis: a review of human neuraminidase deficiency. Am J Hum Genet. 1979;31:1–18.
23. Thomas PK, Abrams JD, Swallow D, et al. Sialidosis type I: cherry-red spot myoclonus syndrome with sialidase deficiency and altered electrophoretic mobilities of some enzymes known to be glycoproteins. J Neurol Neurosurg Psychiat. 1979;42:873–880.
24. Swallow DM, Evans L, Stewart G, et al. Sialidosis type I: cherry red spot-myoclonus syndrome with sialidase deficiency and altered electrophoretic mobility of some enzymes known to be glycoproteins. Ann Hum Genet. 1979;43:27–35.
25. Kelly TE, Graetz G. Isolated acid neuraminidase deficiency: a distinct lysosomal storage disease. Am J Med Genet. 1977;1:31–46.
26. Palmeri S, Villanova M, Malandrini A, et al. Type I sialidosis: a clinical, biochemical, and neuroradiological study. Eur Neurol. 2000;43:88–94.
27. Engel J, Rapin I, Giblin DR. Electrophysiological studies in two patients with cherry red spot-myoclonus syndrome. Epilepsia. 1977;18:73–87.
28. Louboutin JP, Nogues B, Caillaud C, et al. Multimodality evoked potentials and EEG in a case of cherry red spot-myoclonus syndrome and alpha-neuraminidase deficiency (sialidosis type I). Eur Neurol. 1995;35:175–177.
29. Tobimatsu S, Fukui R, Shibasaki H, et al. Electrophysiological studies of myoclonus in sialidosis type 2. Electroencephalogr Clin Neurophysiol. 1985;60:16–22.
30. Wasserstein MP, Aron A, Brodie SE, et al. Acid sphingomyelinase deficiency: prevalence and characterization of an intermediate phenotype of Niemann–Pick disease. J Pediatr. 2006;149:554–559.
31. Kolodney EH. Niemann–Pick disease. Curr Opin Hematol. 2000;7:48.
32. Vanier MT, Millat G. Niemann–Pick disease type C. Clin Genet. 2003;64:269–281.
33. Vankova J, Stepanova I, Jech R, et al. Sleep disturbances and hypocretin deficiency in Niemann–Pick disease type C. Sleep. 2003;15:427–430.
34. Greer WL, Riddell DC, Murty S, et al. Linkage disequilibrium mapping of the Nova Scotia variant of Niemann–Pick disease. Clin Genet. 1999;55:248–255.
35. Sevin M, Lesca G, Baumann N, et al. The adult form of Niemann–Pick disease type C. Brain. 2007;130:120–133.
36. Canafoglia L, Bugiani M, Uziel G, et al. Rhythmic cortical myoclonus in Niemann–Pick disease type C. Mov Disord. 2006;21:1453–1436.
37. Chen M, Wang J. Gaucher disease: review of the literature. Arch Pathol Lab Med. 2008;132:851–853.
38. Zhao H, Grabowski GA. Gaucher disease: perspectives on a prototype lysosomal disease. Cell Mol Life Sci. 2002;59:694–707.
39. Brady RO. Enzyme replacement for lysosomal diseases. Annu Rev Med. 2006;57:283–296.
40. Chang YC, Huang CC, Chen CY, et al. MRI in acute neuropathic Gaucher's disease. Neuroradiology. 2000;42:48–50.
41. Miyata R, Watanabe A, Hasegawa T, et al. Neurophysiological analysis in an 18-month-old girl with Gaucher's disease type 2. No To Hattatsu. 2006;38:289–293.
42. Nishimura R, Omos-Lau N, Ajmone-Marsan C, et al. Electroencephalographic findings in Gaucher disease. Neurology. 1980;30:152–159.
43. Zarate YA, Hopkin RJ. Fabry's disease. Lancet. 2008;372:1427–1435.
44. Eng CM, Guffon N, Wilcox WR. Safety and efficacy of recombinant human alpha-galactosidase A-replacement therapy in Fabry's disease. N Engl J Med. 2001;345:9–16.
45. Low M, Nicholls K, Turbridy N, et al. Neurology of Fabry's disease. Int Med J. 2007;37:436–447.
46. Lou HOC, Reske-Nielsen E. The central nervous system in Fabry's disease. Arch Neurol. 1971;25:351–359.
47. Gieselmann V, Franken S, Klein D, et al. Metachromatic leukodystrophy: consequences of sulphatide accumulation. Acta Paediatr Suppl. 2003;443:74–79.
48. Wang PJ, Hwu WL, Shen YZ. Epileptic seizures and electroencephalographic evolution in genetic leukodystrophies. J Clin Neurophysiol. 2001;18:25–32.
49. Eggers C, Lederer H, Scheffner D. EEG changes in the course of progressive cerebral disorders in children. Monatsschr Kinderheilkd. 1977;125:8–15.
50. Solders G, Celsing G, Hagenfeldt L, et al. Improved peripheral nerve conduction, EEG, and verbal IQ after bone marrow transplantation for adult metachromatic leukodystrophy. Bone Marrow Transplant. 1998;22:1119–1122.
51. Scriver CR, Beaudet AL, Sly WS, et al., eds. The Metabolic and Molecular Bases of Inherited Disease. 8th ed. New York: McGraw-Hill; 2001;3669–3693.
52. Lyon F, Hagberg B, Evrand P, et al. Symptomatology of late onset Krabbe's leukodystrophy: the European experience. Dev Neurosci. 1991;13:240.
53. Husain AM, Altuwaijri M, Aldosari M. Krabbe disease: neurophysiologic studies and MRI correlations. Neurology. 204;63:4.
54. Igarashi M, Schaumburg HH, Powers J, et al. Fatty acid abnormality in adrenoleukodystrophy. J Neurochem. 1976;26:851–860.
55. Moser HW, Moser AB, Frayer KK, et al. Adrenoleukodystrophy: increased plasma content of saturated very long chain fatty acids. Neurology. 1981;31:1241–1249.
56. Kumar AJ, Rosenbaum AE, Naidu S, et al. Adrenoleukodystrophy: correlating MR imaging with CT. Radiology. 1987;165:496.
57. Percy AK, Rutledge SL. Adrenoleukodystrophy and related disorders. Ment Retard Dev Disabil Res Rev. 2001;7:179–189.
58. Barkovich AJ, Peck WW. MR of Zellweger syndrome. Am J Neuroradiol. 1997;18:1163–1170.
59. Takahashi Y, Suzuki Y, Kumazaki K, et al. Epilepsy in peroxisomal diseases. Epilepsia. 1997;38:182–188.
60. Govaerts L, Colon E, Rottevell J, et al. A neurophysiological study of children with the cerebro-hepato-renal syndrome of Zellweger. Neuropediatrics. 1985;16:185–190.
61. Panjan DP, Meglic NP, Neubauer D. A case of Zellweger syndrome with extensive MRI abnormalities and unusual EEG findings. Clin Electroencephalogr. 2001;32:28–31.
62. Chang YC, Huang CC, Huang SC, et al. Neonatal adrenoleukodystrophy presenting with seizure at birth: a case report and review of the literature. Pediatr Neurol. 2008;38:137–139.
63. Leigh D. Subacute necrotizing encephalomyelopathy in an infant. J Neurol Neurosurg Psychiatry. 1951;14:216–221.
64. Pincus JH. Subacute necrotizing encephalomyelopathy (Leigh's disease): a consideration for clinical features and etiology. Dev Med Child Neurol. 1971;14:78–87.
65. Medina L, Chi TL, DeVivo DC, et al. MR findings in patients with subacute necrotizing encephalopathy (Leigh syndrome). Am J Neuroradiol. 1989;11:379–384.
66. Canafoglia L, Franceschetti S, Antozzi C, et al. Epileptic phenotypes associated with mitochondrial disorders. Neurology. 2001;56:1340–1346.
67. Pavlakis SG, Phillips PC, DiMauro S, et al. Mitochondrial myopathy, encephalopathy, lactic acidosis, and strokelike episodes: a distinctive clinical syndrome. Ann Neurol. 1984;16:481–488.
68. Stoquart-ElSankari S, Lehmann P, Perin B, et al. MRI and diffusion-weighted imaging follow-up of a stroke-like event in a patient with MELAS. J Neurol. 2008;255:1593–1595.
69. Ito H, Mori K, Harada M, et al. Serial brain imaging analysis of stroke-like episodes in MELAS. Brain Dev. 2008;30:483–488.
70. Demarest ST, Whitehead MT, Turnacioglu S, et al. Phenotypic analysis of epilepsy in the mitochondrial encephalomyopathy, lactic acidosis, and stroke-like episodes-associated mitochondrial DNA A3243G mutation. J Child Neurol. 2014;29:1249–1256. Serra G, Piccinnu R, Tondi M, et al. Clinical and EEG findings in eleven patients affected by mitochondrial encephalomyopathy with MERRF–MELAS overlap. Brain Dev. 1996;18:185–191.
71. Ribacoba R, Salas-Puig J, Gonzalez C, et al. Characteristics of status epilepticus in MELAS. Analysis of four cases. Neurologia. 2006;21:1–11.
72. Shoffner JM, Wallace DC. Mitochondrial genetics: principles and practice [editorial]. Am J Hum Genet. 1992;51:1179–1186.
73. Alpers BJ. Diffuse progressive degeneration of gray matter of cerebrum. Arch Neurol Psychiatry. 1931;25:469–505.
74. Hunter M, Mackay MT, Peters H, et al. Alper's syndrome with POLG mutations: clinical, EEG, and radiological features. J Clin Neurosci. 2008;15:341.
75. Wolf N, Rahman S, Schmitt B, et al. Status epilepticus in children with Alpers' disease caused by POLG1 mutations: EEG and MRI features. Epilepsia. 2009;50:1596–607.
76. Joshi CN, Greenberg CR, Mhanni AA, et al. Ketogenic diet in Alpers–Huttenlocher syndrome. Pediatr Neurol. 2009;40:314–316.
77. Boyd SG, Harden A, Egger J, et al. Progressive neuronal degeneration of childhood with liver disease ("Alpers' disease"): characteristic neurophysiological features. Neuropediatrics. 1986;17:75–80.
78. Minassian BA. Lafora's disease: towards a clinical, pathologic, and molecular synthesis. Pediatr Neurol. 2001;25:21–29.
79. Acharya JN, Satishchandra P, Shankar SK. Familial progressive myoclonus epilepsy: clinical and electrophysiologic observations. Epilepsia. 1995;36:429–434.
80. Koskiniemi M, Donner M, Majuri H, et al. Progressive myoclonus epilepsy. A clinical and histopathological study. Acta Neurol Scand. 1974;50:307–332.
81. Pennacchio LA, Lehesjoki AE, Stone NE, et al. Mutations in the gene encoding cystatin B in progressive myoclonus epilepsy (EPM1). Science. 1996;271:1731–1734.
82. Caraballo RH, Fejerman N. Dravet syndrome: a study of 53 patients. Epilepsy Res. 2006;70s:S231–S238.
83. Del-Favero CL, Ceulemans J, Ceulemans B, et al. De novo mutations in the sodium-channel gene SCN1A cause severe myoclonic epilepsy of infancy. Am J Hum Genet. 2001;68:1327–1332.
84. Blaskovics M, Engel R, Podosin RL, et al. EEG pattern in phenylketonuria under early initiated dietary treatment. Arch Pediatr Adolesc Med. 1981;135:802–808.

85. Mina I, Hirotaka Y, Misao O. EEG pattern in phenylketonuria. J Jpn Pediatr Soc. 2004;108:1366–1371.
86. Gross PT, Berlow S, Schuett VE, et al. EEG in phenylketonuria. Arch Neurol. 1981;38:122–126.
87. Menkes JH, Hurst PL, Craig JM. A new syndrome: progressive familial infantile cerebral dysfunction associated with an unusual urinary substance. Pediatrics. 1954;14:462.
88. Scriver CR, Beaudet AL, Sly WS, et al., eds. The Metabolic and Molecular Bases of Inherited Disease. Vol II. New York: McGraw-Hill; 2001.
89. Brismar J, Aqeel A, Brismar G, et al. Maple syrup urine disease: findings on CT and MR scans of the brain in 10 infants. Am J Neurorad. 1990;11:1219.
90. Korein J, Sansaricq C, Kalmijn M, et al. Maple syrup urine disease: clinical, EEG, and plasma amino acid correlations with a theoretical mechanism of acute neurotoxicity. Int J Neurosci. 1994;79:21–45.
91. Mudd SH, Skovby F, Levy HL, et al. The natural history of homocystinuria due to cystathionine beta-synthase deficiency. Am J Hum Genet. 1985;37:1–3.
92. Del Giudice E, Striano S, Andria G. Electroencephalographic abnormalities in homocystinuria due to cystathionine synthase deficiency. Clin Neurol Neurosurg. 1983;85:165–168.
93. Buoni S, diBartolo RM, Molinelli M, et al. Atypical BECTS and homocystinuria. Neurology. 2003;61:1129–1131.
94. Sass JO, Hofmann M, Skladal D, et al. Proprionic acidemia revisited: a workshop report. Clin Pediatr. 2004;43:837–843.
95. Akman I, Imamoglu S, Demirkol M, et al. Neonatal onset proprionic acidemia without acidosis: a case report. Turk J Pediatr. 2002;44:339–342.
96. Aikoha H, Sasakia M, Sugaia K, et al. Effective immunoglobulin therapy for brief tonic seizures in methylmalonic acidemia. Brain Dev. 1997;19:502–505.
97. Bellieni CV, Ferrari F, DeFelice C, et al. EEG in assessing hydroxycobalamin therapy in neonatal methylmalonic aciduria with homocystinuria. Biol Neonate. 2000;78:327–330.
98. Gilbert-Barness E, Barness LA. Isovaleric acidemia with promyelocytic myeloproliferative syndrome. Pediatr Dev Pathol. 1999;2:286–291.
99. Teychenne PF, Walters I, Claveria LE, et al. The encephalopathic action of five-carbon-atom fatty acids in the rabbit. Clin Sci Mol Med. 1976;50:463–472.
100. Hoover-Fong JE, Shah S, Van Hove JL, et al. Natural history of nonketotic hyperglycinemia in 65 patients. Neurology. 2004;63:1847.
101. Applegarth DA, Toone JR. Nonketotic hyperglycinemia (glycine encephalopathy): laboratory diagnosis. Mol Genet Metab. 2001;74:139–146.
102. Flusser H, Kormann SH, Sato K, et al. Mild glycine encephalopathy (NKH) in a large kindred due to a silent exonic GLDC splice mutation. Neurology. 2005;64:1426–1430.
103. Hamosh A, McDonald JW, Valle D, et al. Dextromethorphan and high-dose benzoate therapy for nonketotic hyperglycinemia in an infant. J Pediatr. 1992;121:131–135.
104. Amladi TS, Kohil M. Hartnup disease. Indian J Dermatol Venereol Leprol. 1994;60:105–107.
105. Lowe CU, Terrey M, MacLachan EA. Organic aciduria, decreased renal ammonia production, hydrophthalamos, and mental retardation: a clinical entity. Am J Dis Child. 1952; 83:164–184.
106. Schneider JF, Boltshauser E, Neuhaus TJ, et al. MRI and proton spectroscopy in Lowe syndrome. Neuropediatrics. 2001;32:45–48.
107. Sener RN. Lowe syndrome: proton MR spectroscopy and diffusion MR imaging. J Neuroradiol. 2004;31:238–240.
108. Ono J, Harada K, Mano T, et al. MRI findings and neurologic manifestation in Lowe oculocerebrorenal syndrome. Pediatr Neurol. 1996;14:162–164.
109. Erdogan F, Ismailogullari S, Soyuer I, et al. Different seizure types and skin lesions in oculocerebrorenal syndrome of Lowe. J Child Neurol. 2007;22:427–431.
110. Leonard JV, Morris AA. Urea cycle disorders. Semin Neonatol. 2002;7:27.
111. Butterworth RF. Effects of hyperammonaemia on brain function. J Inherit Metab Dis. 1998;21(suppl 1):6.
112. Maestri NE, Lord C, Glynn M, et al. The phenotype of ostensibly healthy women who are carriers for ornithine transcarbamylase deficiency. Medicine (Baltimore). 1998;77:389.
113. Verma NP, Hart ZH, Kooi KA. Electroencephalographic findings in urea-cycle disorders. Electroencephalogr Clin Neurophysiol. 1984;57:105–112.
114. Clancy RR, Chung HJ. EEG changes during recovery from acute severe neonatal citrullinemia. Electroencephalogr Clin Neurophysiol. 1991;78:222–227.
115. Nagata N, Matsuda I, Matsuura T, et al. Retrospective survey of urea cycle disorders: part 2. Neurological outcome in forty-nine Japanese patients with urea cycle enzymopathies. Am J Med Genet. 1991;40:477–481.
116. Heumer M, Carvalho DR, Brum JM, et al. Clinical phenotype, biochemical profile, and treatment in 19 patients with arginase 1 deficiency. J Inherit Metab Dis. 2016;39:331–40.
117. Hayflick SJ. Neurodegeneration with brain iron accumulation: from genes to pathogenesis. Semin Pediatr Neurol. 2006;13:182–185.
118. McNeill A, Birchall D, Hayflick SJ, et al. T2 and FSE MRI distinguishes four subtypes of neurodegeneration with brain iron accumulation. Neurology. 2008;70:1614.
119. Cossu G, Melis M, Floris G, et al. Hallervorden Spatz syndrome (pantothenate kinase associated neurodegeneration) in two Sardinian brothers with homozygous mutation in PANK 2 gene. J Neurol. 2002;249:1599–1600.
120. Remond A, ed. Handbook of Electroencephalography and Clinical Neurophysiology. Vol 15A. Amsterdam: Elsevier; 162–191.
121. Swaiman K, Smith SA, Trock GL, et al. Sea blue histiocytes, lymphocytic cytosomes, movement disorder. 59Fe uptake in basal ganglia: Hallervorden-Spatz disease or ceroid storage disease with abnormal isotope scan? Neurology. 1983;33:301–305.
122. Seven M, Ozkilic A, Yuksel A. Dysmorphic face in two siblings with infantile neuroaxonal dystrophy. Genet Counsel. 2002;13:465–473
123. Hortnagel K, Nardocci N, Zorzi G, et al. Infantile neuroaxonal dystrophy and pantothenate kinase-associated neurodegeneration: locus heterogeneity. Neurology. 2004;63:922–924.
124. Morgan NV, Westaway SK, Morton JEV, et al. PLA2G6, encoding a phospholipase A2, is mutated in neurodegenerative disorders with high brain iron. Nat Genet. 2006;38:752–754.
125. Wakai S, Asanuma H, Hayasaka H, et al. Ictal video-EEG analysis of infantile neuroaxonal dystrophy. Epilepsia. 1994;35:823–826.
126. Taly AB, Meenakshi-Sundaram S, Sinha S, et al. Wilson disease: description of 282 patients evaluated over 3 decades. Medicine (Baltimore). 2007;86:112–121.
127. Saito T. Presenting symptoms and natural history of Wilson disease. Eur J Pediatr. 1987;146:261–265.
128. Giagheddu M, Tamburini G, Piga M, et al. Comparison of MRI, EEG, EPs, and ECD-SPECT in Wilson's disease. Acta Neurol Scand. 2001;103:71–81.
129. Heller GL, Kooi KA. The electroencephalogram in hepatolenticular degeneration (Wilson's disease). Electroencephalogr Clinical Neurophysiol. 1962;14:520–526.
130. Hsich GE, Robertson RL, Irons M, et al. Cerebral infarction in Menkes disease. Pediatr Neurol. 2000;23:425–428.
131. Kaler SG, Holmes CS, Goldstein DS, et al. Neonatal diagnosis and treatment of Menkes disease. N Engl J Med. 2008;358:605–614.
132. Bahi-Buisson N, Kaminska A, Nabbout R, et al. Epilepsy in Menkes disease: analysis of clinical stages. Epilepsia. 2006;47:380–386.
133. White SR, Reese K, Sato S, et al. Spectrum of EEG findings in Menkes disease. Electroencephalogr Clin Neurophysiol. 1993;87:57–61.
134. Wang D, Pascual JM, Yang H, et al. GLUT-1 deficiency syndrome: clinical, genetic, and therapeutic aspects. Ann Neurol. 2005; 57(1):111–118.
135. Bennett CL, Chen Y, Hahn S, et al. Prevalence of ALDH7A1 mutations in 18 North American pyridoxine-dependent seizure (PDS) patients. Epilepsia. 2009;50:1167–1175.
136. Nabbout R, Soufflet C, Plouin P, et al. Pyridoxine dependent epilepsy: a suggestive electroclinical pattern. Arch Dis Child Fetal Neonatal Ed. 1999;81:F125–F129.
137. Torres OA, Miller VS, Buist NMR, et al. Folinic acid-responsive neonatal seizures. J Child Neurol. 1999;14:529–532.
138. Gallagher RC, Van Hove JL, Scharer G, et al. Folinic acid-responsive seizures are identical to pyridoxine-dependent epilepsy. Ann Neurol. 2009;65:550–556.
139. Mills PB, Camuzeaux SS, Footitt EJ, et al. Epilepsy due to PNPO mutations: genotype, environment and treatment affect presentation and outcome. Brain 2014;137:1350–60.
140. Manto MU. The wide spectrum of spinocerebellar ataxia (SCAs). Cerebellum. 2005;4:2–6.
141. Sack G, Gruss B, Lossner J, et al. EEG studies of spinocerebellar ataxia. Psychiatr Neurol Med Psychol (Leipz). 1977;29:521–528.
142. Rasmussen A, Matsuura T, Ruano L, et al. Clinical and genetic analysis of four Mexican families with spinocerebellar ataxia type 10. Ann Neurol. 2001;50:234–239.
143. Tan NCK, Zhou Y, Tan ASC, et al. Spinocerebellar ataxia type 2 with focal epilepsy—an unusual association. Ann Acad Med Singapore. 2004;33:103–106.
144. Inazuki G, Baba K, Naito H. Electroencephalographic findings of hereditary dentatorubral-pallidoluysian atrophy (DRPLA). Jpn J Psychiatry Neurol. 1989;43:213–220.
145. Rötig A, de Lonlay P, Chretien D, et al. Aconitase and mitochondrial iron–sulphur protein deficiency in Friedreich ataxia. Nat Genet. 1997;17:215–217.
146. Hewer RL. Study of fatal cases of Friedreich's ataxia. Br Med J. 1968;3:649–652.
147. Bourchard RW, Bouchard JP, Bouchard R, et al. Electroencephalographic findings in Friedreich's ataxia and autosomal recessive spastic ataxia of Charlevoix-Saguenay (ARSACS). Can J Neurol Sci. 1979; 6:191–194.

148. Narayanan V. Tuberous sclerosis complex: genetics to pathogenesis. Pediatr Neurol. 2003;29(5):404–409.
149. Gao X, Zhang Y, Arrazola P, et al. Tsc tumour suppressor proteins antagonize amino-acid#150;TOR signalling. Nat Cell Biol. 2002;4:699–704.
150. Potter CJ, Huang H, Xu T. Drosophila Tsc1 functions with Tsc2 to antagonize insulin signaling in regulating cell growth, cell proliferation, and organ size. Cell. 2001;105:357–368.
151. Franz DN, Leonard J, Tudor C, et al. Rapamycin causes regression of astrocytomas in tuberous sclerosis complex. Ann Neurol. 2006;59:490–498.
152. Roach ES, Smith M, Huttenlocher P, et al. Diagnostic criteria: tuberous sclerosis complex. Report of the Diagnostic Criteria Committee of the National Tuberous Sclerosis Association. J Child Neurol. 1992;7(2):221–224.
153. Barkovich AJ. Pediatric Neuroimaging. New York: Raven Press; 1995:668.
154. Taylor DC, Falconer MA, Bruton CJ, Corsellis JAN. Focal dysplasia of the cerebral cortex in epilepsy. J Neurol Neurosurg Psychiatry. 1971;34:369–387.
155. Crino PB, Eberwine J. Cellular and molecular basis of cerebral dysgenesis. J Neurosci Res. 1997;50:907–916.
156. Kwiatkowski DJ, Zhang H, Bandura JL, et al. A mouse model of TSC1 reveals sex-dependent lethality from liver hemangiomas, and up-regulation of p70S6 kinase activity in Tsc1 null cells. Hum Mol Genet. 2002; 11:525–534.
157. Chu-Shore CJ, Major P, Camposano S, et al. The natural history of epilepsy in tuberous sclerosis complex. Epilepsia. 2010;51(7):1236–1241.
158. Elterman RD, Shields WD, Mansfield KA, Nakagawa J; US Infantile Spasms Vigabatrin Study Group. Randomized trial of vigabatrin in patients with infantile spasms. Neurology. 2001;57:1416–1421.
159. O'Callaghan FJ, Harris T, Joinson C, et al. The relation of infantile spasms, tubers, and intelligence in tuberous sclerosis complex. Arch Dis Child. 2004;89:530–533.
160. Bolton PF, Park RJ, Higgins JN, et al. Neuro-epileptic determinants of autism spectrum disorders in tuberous sclerosis complex. Brain. 2002; 125(Pt 6):1247–1255.
161. Domańska-Pakieła D, Kaczorowska M, Jurkiewicz E, et al. EEG abnormalities preceding the epilepsy onset in tuberous sclerosis complex patients—a prospective study of 5 patients. Eur J Paediatr Neurol. 2014;18:458–468.
162. Ikeno M, Okumura A, Abe S, et al. Clinically silent seizures in a neonate with tuberous sclerosis. Pediatr Int. 2016;58:58–61.
163. Wu JY, Peters JM, Goyal M, et al. Clinical electroencephalographic biomarker for impending epilepsy in asymptomatic tuberous sclerosis complex infants. Pediatr Neurol. 2016;54:29–34.
164. Curatolo P, Moavero R, Roberto D, Graziola F. Genotype/phenotype correlations in tuberous sclerosis complex. Semin Pediatr Neurol. 2015;22:259–273.
165. Gallagher A, Chu-Shore CJ, Montenegro MA, et al. Associations between electroencephalographic and magnetic resonance imaging findings in tuberous sclerosis complex. Epilepsy Res. 2009; 87:197–202.
166. Juhász C, Chugani DC, Muzik O, et al. Alpha-methyl-L-tryptophan PET detects epileptogenic cortex in children with intractable epilepsy. Neurology. 2003; 25;60:960–968.
167. Mohamed AR, Bailey CA, Freeman JL, et al. Intrinsic epileptogenicity of cortical tubers revealed by intracranial EEG monitoring. Neurology. 2012;79:2249–2257.
168. Sosunov AA, McGovern RA, Mikell CB, et al. Epileptogenic but MRI-normal perituberal tissue in tuberous sclerosis complex contains tuber-specific abnormalities. Acta Neuropathol Commun. 2015;3:17.
169. Arya R, Tenney JR, Horn PS, et al. Long-term outcomes of resective epilepsy surgery after invasive presurgical evaluation in children with tuberous sclerosis complex and bilateral multiple lesions. J Neurosurg Pediatr. 2015;15:26–33.
170. Fallah A, Guyatt GH, Snead OC, et al. Predictors of seizure outcomes in children with tuberous sclerosis complex and intractable epilepsy undergoing resective epilepsy surgery: an individual participant data meta-analysis. PLoS One. 2013;8(2):e53565.
171. Guerreiro MM, Andermann F, Andermann E, et al. Surgical treatment of epilepsy in tuberous sclerosis: strategies and results in 18 patients. Neurology. 1998; 51: 1263–1269.
172. Greenwood R, Whit K, Tupler L, et al. Brain volume and cognition in children with neurofibromatosis type 1. Ann Neurol. 2004;56:S93.
173. Lynch TM, Gutmann DH. Neurofibromatosis 1. Neurol Clin. 2002; 20:841–865.
174. North K, Yuille D, Cocks N, Hutchins P. Cognitive function and academic performance in children with neurofibromatosis type 1. Dev Med Child Neurol.1995;37:427–436.
175. Hyman SL, Gill DS, Shores EA, et al. Natural history of cognitive deficits and their relationship to MRI T2-hyperintensities in NF1. Neurology. 2003;60:1139–1145.
176. Greenwood R, Whit K, Tupler L, et al. Brain volume and congniton in children with neurofibromatosis type 1. Ann Neurol. 2004;56:S93.
177. Korf BR1, Carrazana E, Holmes GL. Patterns of seizures observed in association with neurofibromatosis 1. Epilepsia. 1993;34(4):616–620.
178. Kulkantrakorn K1, Geller TJ. Seizures in neurofibromatosis 1. Pediatr Neurol. 1998;19:347–350.
179. Hsieh HY, Fung HC, Wang CJ, et al. Epileptic seizures in neurofibromatosis type 1 are related to intracranial tumors but not to neurofibromatosis bright objects. Seizure. 2011;20:606–611.
180. Ostendorf AP, Gutmann DH, Weisenberg JLZ. Epilepsy in individuals with neurofibromatosis type 1. Epilepsia. 2013;54:1810–1814.
181. Yerdelen D, Koc F, Durdu M, Karakas M. Electrophysiological findings in neurofibromatosis type 1. J Neurol Sci. 2011;306:42–48.
182. Barba C, Jacques T, Kahane P, et al. Epilepsy surgery in neurofibromatosis type 1. Epilepsy Res. 2013;105(3):384–395.
183. DiFrancesco JC, Sestini R, Cossu F, et al. Novel neurofibromatosis type 2 mutation presenting with status epilepticus. Epileptic Disord. 2014;16:132–137.
184. Pascual-Castroviejo I, Roche C, Martinez-Bermejo A, et al. Hypomelanosis of ITO. A study of 76 infantile cases. Brain Dev. 1998;20(1):36–43.
185. Ogino T, Hata H, Minakuchi E, et al. Neurophysiologic dysfunction in hypomelanosis of Ito: EEG and evoked potential studies. Brain Dev. 1994;16:407–412.
186. Hennel SJ, Ekert PG, Volpe JJ, Inder TE. Insights into the pathogenesis of cerebral lesions in incontinentia pigmenti. Pediatr Neurol. 2003;29:148–150.
187. Smahi A, Courtois G, Vabres P, et al. Genomic rearrangement in NEMO impairs NF-kappaB activation and is a cause of incontinentia pigmenti. The International Incontinentia Pigmenti (IP) Consortium. Nature. 2000;405(6785):466–472.
188. Pacheco TR, Levy M, Collyer JC, et al. Incontinentia pigmenti in male patients. J Am Acad Dermatol. 2006;55(2):251–255.
189. Ojha R, Villarreal D, Coughtrey H. Neonatal presentation of incontinentia pigmenti with a family history extending over four generations—a case report. J Neonatal Perinatal Med. 2014;7:151–155.
190. Fujino O, Hashimoto K, Fujita T, et al. Clinico-neuropathological study of incontinentia pigmenti achromians: an autopsy case. Brain Dev. 1995;17:425–427.
191. Brenner RP, Sharbrough FW. Electroencephalographic evaluation in Sturge-Weber syndrome. Neurology. 1976;26(7):629–632.
192. Kossoff EH, Bachur CD, Quain AM, et al. EEG evolution in Sturge-Weber syndrome. Epilepsy Res. 2014;108(4):816–819.
193. Limotai C, Go CY, Baba S, et al. Steal phenomenon in Sturge-Weber syndrome imitating an ictal electroencephalography change in the contralateral hemisphere: report of 2 cases. J Neurosurg Pediatr. 2015;16:212–216.
194. Iimura Y, Sugano H, Nakajima M, et al. Analysis of epileptic discharges from implanted subdural electrodes in patients with Sturge-Weber syndrome. PLoS One. 2016; 11:e0152992.
195. American Psychiatric Association. Diagnostic and Statistical Manual of Mental Disorders. 5th ed. Arlington, VA: American Psychiatric Association; 2013.
196. Johnson HM, Gaitanis J MD, Morrow EM. Genetics in autism diagnosis: adding molecular subtypes to neurobehavioral diagnoses. Med Health R I. 2011;94(5):124–126.
197. Betancur C. Etiological heterogeneity in autism spectrum disorders: more than 100 genetic and genomic disorders and still counting. Brain Res. 2011;1380:42–77.
198. Huguet G, Ey E, Bourgeron T. The genetic landscapes of autism spectrum disorders. Annu Rev Genomics Hum Genet. 2013;14:191–213.
199. Hashemi E, Ariza J, Rogers H, Noctor SC, Martínez-Cerdeño V. The number of parvalbumin-expressing interneurons is decreased in the medial prefrontal cortex in autism. Cereb Cortex. 2016 Feb 27, epub ahead of print.
200. Sessolo M, Marcon I, Bovetti S, et al. Parvalbumin-positive inhibitory interneurons oppose propagation but favor generation of focal epileptiform activity. J Neurosci. 2015;35(26):9544–9557.
201. Amiet C, Gourfinkel-An I, Bouzamondo A, et al. Epilepsy in autism is associated with intellectual disability and gender: evidence from a meta-analysis. Biol Psychiatry. 2008;64:577–582.
202. Woolfenden S, Sarkozy V, Ridley G, et al. A systematic review of two outcomes in autism spectrum disorder—Epilepsy and mortality. Dev Med Child Neurol. 2012;54:306–312.
203. Matsuo M, Maeda T, Sasaki K, et al. Frequent association of autism spectrum disorder in patients with childhood-onset epilepsy. Brain Dev. 2010;32:759–763.
204. Tuchman R. Autism and social cognition in epilepsy: implications for comprehensive epilepsy care. Curr Opin Neurol. 2013;26:214–218.
205. Hughes JR, Melyn M. EEG and seizures in autistic children and adolescents: Further findings with therapeutic implications. Clin EEG Neurosci. 2005;36:15–20.

206. Ballaban-Gil K, Tuchman R. Epilepsy and epileptiform EEG: association with autism and language disorders. Ment Retard Dev Disabil Res Rev. 2000;6:300–308.
207. Dykens EM, Lense M. Intellectual disabilities and autism spectrum disorder: a cautionary note. In Amaral D., Dawson G., Geschwind D, eds. Autism Spectrum Disorders. New York: Oxford University Press; 2011:261–269.
208. Tuchman R. Autism and social cognition in epilepsy: implications for comprehensive epilepsy care. Curr Opin Neurol. 2013;26:214–218.
209. Chapman RS, Hesketh LJ. Behavioral phenotype of individuals with Down syndrome. Ment Retard Dev Disabil Res Rev. 2000;6(2):84–95.
210. DiGuiseppi C, Hepburn S, Davis JM, et al. Screening for autism spectrum disorders in children with Down syndrome: population prevalence and screening test characteristics. J Dev Behav Pediatr. 2010;31:181–191.
211. Stafstrom CE. Epilepsy in Down syndrome: clinical aspects and possible mechanisms. Am J Ment Retard. 1993;98(Suppl):12–26.
212. Menendez M. Down syndrome, Alzheimer's disease and seizures. Brain Dev. 2005;27:246–252.
213. Arya R, Kabra M, Gulati S. Epilepsy in children with Down syndrome. Epileptic Disord. 2011;13(1):1–7.
214. Silva ML, Cieuta C, Guerrini R, et al. Early clinical and EEG features of infantile spasms in Down syndrome. Epilepsia. 1996;37:977–982.
215. Ferlazzo E, Adjien CK, Guerrini R, et al. Lennox-Gastaut syndrome with late-onset and prominent reflex seizures in trisomy 21 patients. Epilepsia. 2009;50:1587–1595.
216. Ellingson RJ, Eisen JD, Ottersberg G. Clinical electroencephalographic observations on institutionalized mongoloids confirmed by karyotype. Electroencephalogr Clin Neurophysiol. 1973;34:193–196.
217. Mc Devitt N, Gallagher L, Reilly RB. Autism spectrum disorder (ASD) and Fragile X syndrome (FXS): two overlapping disorders reviewed through electroencephalography—What can be interpreted from the available information? Brain Sci. 2015;5(2):92–117.
218. Comery TA, Harris JB, Willems PJ, et al. Abnormal dendritic spines in Fragile X knockout mice: maturation and pruning deficits. Proc Natl Acad Sci USA. 1997;94:5401–5404.
219. Bailey DB Jr, Hatton DD, Mesibov G, et al. Early development, temperament, and functional impairment in autism and fragile X syndrome. J Autism Dev Disord. 2000;30(1):49–59.
220. Berry-Kravis E. Epilepsy in fragile X syndrome. Dev Med Child Neurol. 2002;44:724–728.
221. Valente KD, Andrade JQ, Grossmann RM, et al. Angelman syndrome: difficulties in EEG pattern recognition and possible misinterpretations. Epilepsia. 2003;44:1051–1063.
222. Laan LA, Vein AA. Angelman syndrome: is there a characteristic EEG? Brain Dev. 2005;27(2):80–87.
223. Minassian BA, DeLorey TM, Olsen RW, et al. Angelman syndrome: correlations between epilepsy phenotypes and genotypes. Ann Neurol. 1998;43:485–493.
224. Laan LAEM, Renier WO, Arts WFM, Buntinx IM, et al. Evolution of epilepsy and EEG findings in Angelman syndrome. Epilepsia. 1997; 38: 195–199
225. Viani F, Romeo A, Viri M, et al. Seizure and EEG patterns in Angelman's syndrome. J Child Neurol. 1995;10:467–471.
226. Laan LAEM, Vein AA. A Rett patient with a typical Angelman EEG. Epilepsia. 2002;43:1590–1592.
227. Percy A, Lane J. Rett syndrome: clinical and molecular update. Curr Opin Pediatr. 2004;16:670–677.
228. Bahi-Buisson N, Nectoux J, Rosas-Vargas H, et al. Key clinical features to identify girls with CDKL5 mutations. Brain. 2008;131:2647–2661.
229. Glaze DG, Frost JD Jr, Zoghbi HY, et al. Rett's syndrome: correlation of electroencephalographic characteristic with clinical staging. Arch Neurol. 1987;44:1053–1056.
230. Hagberg B, Witt-Engerstrism I. Rett syndrome: a suggested staging system for describing impairment profile with increasing age towards adolescence. Am J Med Genet. 1986;24:47–59.
231. Hagberg B, Aicardi J, Dias K, Ramos O. A progressive syndrome of autism, dementia, ataxia, and loss of purposeful hand use in girls: Rett's syndrome: report of 35 cases. Ann Neurol. 1983;14:471–479.
232. Garofalo EA, Drury I, Goldstein GW. EEG abnormalities aid diagnosis of Rett syndrome. Pediatr Neurol. 1988;4:350–353.
233. Aldrich MS, Garofalo EA, Drury I. Epileptiform abnormalities during sleep in Rett syndrome. Electroencephalogr Clin Neurophysiol. 1990;75:365–370.
234. Robertson R, Langill L, Wong PK, Ho HH. Rett syndrome: EEG presentation. Electroencephalogr Clin Neurophysiol. 1988;70:388–395.
235. Wallace SJ. Epilepsy in cerebral palsy. Dev Med Child Neurol. 2001;43:713–717.

236. Durkin MS, Benedict RE, Christensen D, et al. Prevalence of cerebral palsy among 8-year-old children in 2010 and preliminary evidence of trends in its relationship to low birthweight. Paediatr Perinat Epidemiol. 2016;30(5):496–510.
237. Rosenbaum P, Paneth N, Leviton A, et al. A report: the definition and classification of cerebral palsy April 2006. Dev Med Child Neurol Suppl. 2007;109:8–14.
238. Delgado MR, Riela AR, Mills J, et al. Discontinuation of antiepileptic drug treatment after two seizure-free years in children with cerebral palsy. Pediatrics. 1996;97(2):192–197.
239. Russman BS, Ashwal S. Evaluation of the child with cerebral palsy. Semin Pediatr Neurol. 2004;11:47–57.
240. Cioni G, Sales B, Paolicelli PB, et al. MRI and clinical characteristics of children with hemiplegic cerebral palsy. Neuropediatrics. 1999;30:249–255.
241. Bruck I, Antoniuk SA, Spessatto A, et al. Epilepsy in children with cerebral palsy. Arq Neuropsiquiatr. 2001;59:35–39.
242. Carlsson M, Hagberg G, Olsson I. Clinical and aetiological aspects of epilepsy in children with cerebral palsy. Dev Med Child Neurol. 2003;45:371–376.
243. Kułak W, Sobaniec W. Risk factors and prognosis of epilepsy in children with cerebral palsy in north-eastern Poland. Brain Dev. 2003;25:499–506.
244. Kwong KL, Wong SN, So KT. Epilepsy in children with cerebral palsy. Pediatr Neurol. 1998;19:31–36.
245. Shevell MI, Dagenais L, Hall N; REPACQ Consortium. Comorbidities in cerebral palsy and their relationship to neurologic subtype and GMFCS level. Neurology. 2009;72:2090–2096.
246. Zelnik N, Konopnicki M, Bennett-Back O, et al. Risk factors for epilepsy in children with cerebral palsy. Eur J Paediatr Neurol. 2010;14:67–72.
247. Hadjipanayis A, Hadjichristodoulou C, Youroukos S. Epilepsy in patients with cerebral palsy. Dev Med Child Neurol. 1997;39:659–663.
248. Kirby RS, Wingate MS, Van Naarden Braun K, et al. Prevalence and functioning of children with cerebral palsy in four areas of the United States in 2006: a report from the Autism and Developmental Disabilities Monitoring Network. Res Dev Disabil. 2011;32:462–469.
249. Sellier E, Uldall P, Calado E, et al. Epilepsy and cerebral palsy: characteristics and trends in children born in 1976-1998. Eur J Paediatr Neurol. 2012;16:48–55.
250. Gururaj AK, Sztriha L, Bener A, et al. Epilepsy in children with cerebral palsy. Seizure. 2003;12(2):110–114.
251. Zafeiriou DI, Kontopoulos EE, Tsikoulas I. Characteristics and prognosis of epilepsy in children with cerebral palsy. J Child Neurol. 1999;14:289–294.
252. Olsson I, Danielsson S, Hedstrom A, et al. Epilepsy surgery in children with accompanying impairments. Eur J Paediatr Neurol. 2013;17:645–650.
253. Gil-Nagel A, Garcia Morales I, Jimenez Huete A, et al. Occipital lobe epilepsy secondary to ulegyria. J Neurol. 2005;252:1178–1185.
254. Usui N, Mihara T, Baba K, et al. Posterior cortex epilepsy secondary to ulegyria: is it a surgically remediable syndrome. Epilepsia. 2008;49:1998–2007.
255. Delgado MR, Riela AR, Mills J, et al. Discontinuation of antiepileptic drug treatment after two seizure-free years in children with cerebral palsy. Pediatrics. 1996;97(2):192–197.
256. Perlstein MA, Gibbs EL, Gibbs FA. The electroencephalogram in infantile cerebral palsy. Am J Phys Med. 1955;34:477–496.
257. Ito M, Okuno T, Takao T, et al. Electroencephalographic and cranial computed tomographic findings in children with hemiplegic cerebral palsy. Eur Neurol. 1981;20:312–318.
258. Senbil N, Sonel B, Aydin OF, Gurer YK. Epileptic and non-epileptic cerebral palsy: EEG and cranial imaging findings. Brain Dev. 2002;24:166–169.
259. Perlstein MA, Gibbs EL, Gibbs FA. The electroencephalogram in infantile cerebral palsy. In Lennox WG, Merritt HH, Bamford TE, eds. Epilepsy (Proceedings of the Association for Research in Nervous and Mental Disease, Research Publications, vol. 26). Baltimore: Williams & Wilkins; 1947:377–384.
260. Perlstein MA, Gibbs FA. Clinical significance of electroencephalography in cases of cerebral paralysis. Arch Neurol Psychiatry. 1949;62:682–685.
261. Gibbs FA, Gibbs EL, Perlstein MA, Rich CL. Electroencephalographic prediction of epilepsy as a complication of cerebral palsy. Neurology. 1963;13:143–145.
262. Gibbs FA, Gibbs EL, Perlstein MA, Rich CL. Electroencephalographic and clinical aspects of cerebral palsy. Pediatrics. 1963;32:73–84.

14 | BRAIN TUMORS AND OTHER SPACE-OCCUPYING LESIONS

ADAM L. HARTMAN, MD AND RONALD P. LESSER, MD

ABSTRACT: Brain tumors are a leading cause for new-onset seizures in adults, and many patients still present with seizures as their first manifestation of a tumor. Although at one time electroencephalography (EEG) was important for diagnosing brain tumors and other space-occupying lesions, this is now more commonly done using imaging studies, such as computed tomography and magnetic resonance imaging. However, clinical neurophysiology still is important in managing these patients. This can include the use of electrocorticography during testing to identify the seizure onset zone and eloquent cortex during resection surgeries, application of evoked potentials in assessing the location of sensorimotor cortex or the extent of tumor involvement, and the application of magnetoencephalography for both magnetic source imaging (e.g., in localizing spike-generating zones) and functional mapping. These topics will be discussed in this chapter.

KEYWORDS: electroencephalography, EEG, brain tumor, seizures, space-occupying lesions

PRINCIPAL REFERENCES

1. Klass, D.W. and D.D. Daly, *Electroencephalography in patients with brain tumor.* Med Clin North Am, 1960. **44**: p. 1041–1051.
2. Bickford, R.G., *Electroencephalographic diagnosis of brain tumors.* Am J Surg, 1957. **93**(6): p. 946–951.
3. Daly, D., et al., *The electroencephalogram in cases of tumors of the posterior fossa and third ventricle.* Electroencephalogr Clin Neurophysiol, 1953. **5**(2): p. 203–216.
4. Harvey, A.S. and J.L. Freeman, *Epilepsy in hypothalamic hamartoma: clinical and EEG features.* Semin Pediatr Neurol, 2007. **14**(2): p. 60–64.
5. Cascino, G.D., et al., *Long-term follow-up of stereotactic lesionectomy in partial epilepsy: predictive factors and electroencephalographic results.* Epilepsia, 1992. **33**(4): p. 639–644.
6. Duffau, H., *Acute functional reorganisation of the human motor cortex during resection of central lesions: a study using intraoperative brain mapping.* J Neurol Neurosurg Psychiatry, 2001. **70**(4): p. 506–513.
7. Michel, B., J.L. Gastaut, and L. Bianchi, *Electroencephalographic cranial computerized tomographic correlations in brain abscess.* Electroencephalogr Clin Neurophysiol, 1979. **46**(3): p. 256–273
8. Westmoreland, B.F., *Periodic lateralized epileptiform discharges after evacuation of subdural hematomas.* J Clin Neurophysiol, 2001. **18**(1): p. 20–24.
9. Van Ness, P., *Pros and cons of lesionectomy as treatment for partial epilepsy,* in *The Epilepsies: Etiologies and Prevention,* P. Kotagal and H. Lüders, Editors. 1999, Academic Press: San Diego. p. 391–397.

1. INTRODUCTION

Brain tumors are a leading cause for new-onset seizures in adults, and many patients still present with seizures as their first manifestation of a tumor (Fig. 14.1). Although at one time electroencephalography (EEG) was important for diagnosing brain tumors and other space-occupying lesions, this is now more commonly done using imaging studies, such as computed tomography and magnetic resonance imaging (MRI)

(Fig. 14.2). Clinical neurophysiology still is important in managing these patients, including the use of electrocorticography during testing to identify the seizure onset zone and eloquent cortex during resection surgeries, application of evoked potentials in assessing the location of sensorimotor cortex or the extent of tumor involvement, and the application of magnetoencephalography for both magnetic source imaging (e.g., in localizing spike-generating zones) and functional mapping. These topics will be discussed in this chapter.

The EEG findings discussed below are not specific for tumor type and also can occur with other space-occupying lesions (hence their inclusion in this chapter). In a series of classical experiments, Gloor et al. [1] found that focal delta-range slowing was seen over well-circumscribed lesions in the white matter (with no apparent change in faster-frequency activity) or after a focal thalamic lesion, while diffuse hemispheric slowing was seen after larger thalamic and/or hypothalamic lesions or lesions causing cerebral edema; generalized slowing was seen after lesions were made in the midbrain tegmental area. Solid tumors generally are not epileptogenic in themselves; it is the infiltrated or surrounding nontumor tissue that causes the seizures [2]. Notable exceptions include developmental tumors (discussed below). EEG findings in most nondevelopmental tumors likely are caused by displacement of normal tissue (either by the mass itself or by altered flow of cerebrospinal fluid), physical disruption of normal neuronal circuitry, ischemia, or hemosiderin deposition [3,4], gap-junction proteins [5], and alterations in neurotransmitter pathophysiology, such as increased local glutamate production [6], vesicular glutamate transporters [7], both ionotropic and metabotropic glutamate receptor subunits [8], and GABA receptors [9]. Data on patients with brain tumors provide some of the most convincing arguments for secondary epileptogenesis (wherein an epileptogenic region gives rise to a secondary epileptogenic focus via strong connectivity between the two regions) [10].

2. EPIDEMIOLOGY

The prevalence of seizures depends in part on the type of tumor: for example, anywhere from 66% to 90% of patients with low-grade astrocytomas have seizures at some point [11]. Seizures are more common in patients with low-grade (vs. high-grade) tumors [12]. Seizures are the presenting symptom in up to 76% of children with benign astrocytic

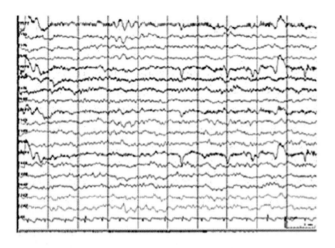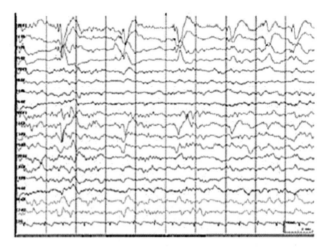

Figure 14.1. EEG from a 4-year-old male who presented to a pediatric epilepsy clinic with a 2-month history of episodes of staring and fumbling with the fingers that lasted about 30 seconds. The EEG showed a burst of slowing in the left hemisphere (left, fourth second) and runs of periodically repeating high-voltage rhythmic sharp activity over the left hemisphere region during sleep (right). A longitudinal bipolar montage is shown.

and oligodendrocytic tumors of the cerebral hemispheres [13]. Seizures occurred in 40% of children with hemispheric brain tumors (with the temporal lobe being most commonly involved), while none with thalamic tumors had seizures [14]. There was a focal component to the majority of the seizures in that series, although nearly 25% of the patients had only generalized seizures. Seizures can occur in children with supratentorial or infratentorial tumors, although they are more commonly the presenting sign in hemispheric tumors [15].

3. HISTORICAL PERSPECTIVES ON THE UTILITY OF EEG

Before the advent of modern imaging, EEG was a critical component in the evaluation of patients with suspected masses, along with pneumoencephalography, ventriculography, and angiography. Postoperative EEGs were used to monitor tumor recurrence, which was heralded by focal arrhythmic slow activity at the former tumor site; a recent study found that EEG slowing

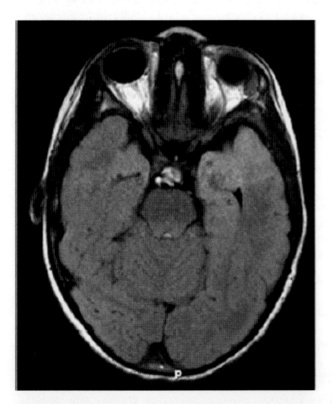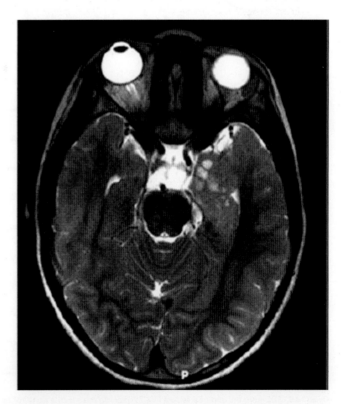

Figure 14.2. MRI of the patient from Figure 14.1. Axial sections (FLAIR and T2-weighted sequences) at the level of the temporal lobes show cystic changes, swelling, and infiltration of normal brain parenchyma in the left anterior mesial temporal lobe. The patient had an MRI soon after his clinic appointment, underwent a near-total resection of a WHO grade II astrocytoma, and has remained seizure-free since surgery.

indicated that postoperative seizure control was less likely [16]. Much of the literature on EEG in tumors and other space-occupying lesions is older and studies were performed without the modern standards of statistical rigor. The classification of tumors also has evolved over time, so we attempted to be as nonspecific as possible in describing tumor type in older studies, while using current tumor nomenclature for more recent studies. One final caveat is that many observers have noted that the routine EEG can be normal or even misleading in terms of lateralization [14,15,17,18], thus limiting the utility of this test in some instances. In fact, normal-frequency activity may be seen ipsilateral to a tumor [17]. A more recent observation is that continuous EEG monitoring can detect nonconvulsive status epilepticus, which may have prognostic significance for survival [19].

4. LOCALIZATION-RELATED ISSUES

4.1. Hemispheric Tumors

Cortical tumors produce abnormal EEGs >96% of the time, including focal delta activity (correctly localized) (see Figs. 14.1 and 14.2); a minority cause focal dysrhythmia, but EEGs can be falsely localizing (Figs. 14.3 and 14.4) [20]. EEGs are abnormal in up to 87% of children with benign astrocytic and oligodendrocytic tumors of the cerebral hemispheres [13]. EEG findings are generally related to location of the tumor and rapidity of growth. Most [3,21] but not all [22] studies associate rapidly growing tumors with very slow delta-range activity, and more slowly growing tumors with arrhythmic theta-range activity with occasional intermixed epileptiform spikes and sharp waves. Some have found epileptogenic activity in the homologous region of the contralateral hemisphere, which may give rise to some confusion in localization [10]. Meningiomas and other slow-growing or midline tumors may be difficult to localize, although hyperventilation may reveal a focus of slowing not seen otherwise [20,23]. Focal theta-range activity can occur with any type of tumor and one series noted it in 75% of patients with hemispheric tumors [17]. In that study, focal delta-range activity was most common in patients with glioblastoma, although it also occurred with meningeal tumors. These researchers also found that activity in the delta range was less frequent with (slow-growing) astrocytomas, where focal sharp activity was more common. Similarly, Newmark et al. found that epileptiform activity was unrelated to focal

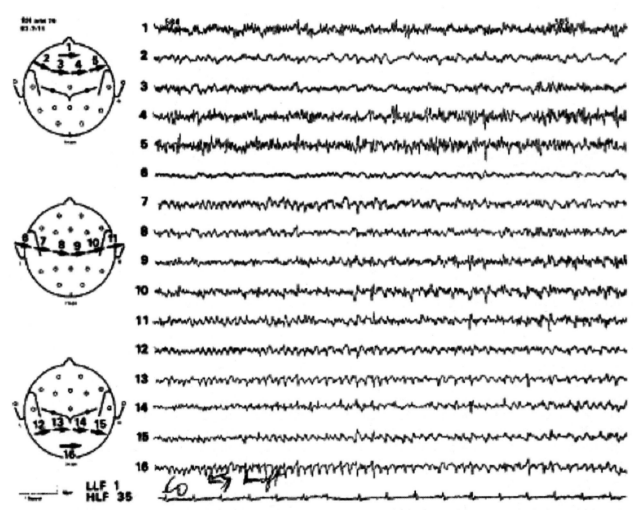

Figure 14.3. EEG from the end of a seizure in a 79-year-old male with a right frontal astrocytoma. Phase reversals are present in the right frontal, temporal, and parietal leads. Also, there is a prominent phase reversal in the left parietal region (channels 12, 13). However, with the transverse montage used, the channels with the most prominent activity indicate only where the differences between the recording electrodes are the greatest; these are not necessarily were the actual amplitudes are greatest.

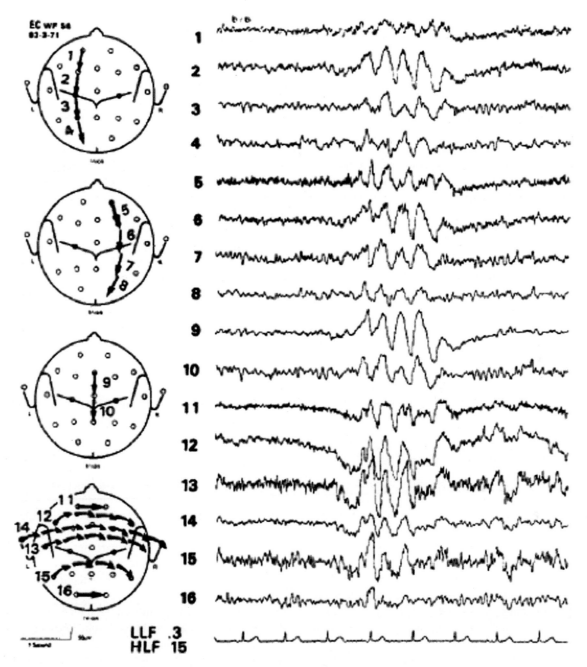

Figure 14.4. EEG from a 56-year-old female with a burst of high-voltage sharply contoured delta-range activity that was bilateral (longitudinal bipolar recordings, channels 1–8) but maximal over the left hemisphere (channels 11–16). Her underlying pathology was a left parietal astrocytoma.

slowing in patients with gliomas [22]. Focal epileptiform activity on the EEG appeared to be correlated generally with clinical seizures in patients with astrocytomas, but clinical seizures were not as common among patients with meningeal tumors; even though they also had a fair amount of focal epileptiform activity on EEG, seizures were not as common. Patients with multiple metastases also may have a good deal of epileptiform activity in their EEGs; over 90% of patients with metastatic disease have abnormal EEGs including epileptiform activity [3], delta-range activity, and dysrhythmias [20].

Focal delta- and theta-range activity correlates with white matter involvement of tumors [1,22]. This includes tumors involving both gray and white matter as well as those involving white matter only. Rhythmic delta activity may indicate

involvement of the thalamus or deep frontal white matter, although involvement of deep frontal white matter may produce similar findings [22].

Attenuation of background activity occurs in patients with high-grade gliomas that have thalamic involvement [22] but also may be seen in regions with extensive peritumoral edema [24], although this is a nonspecific finding. Irregular delta-range activity is unrelated to peritumoral edema [22], and the degree of EEG abnormality does not appear to correlate with degree of edema [24].

Frontal tumors tend to produce the slow patterns noted previously, including at times frontal intermittent rhythmic discharges (FIRDA). It is not clear from the literature whether the frontal rhythmic discharges in patients with frontal tumors have the same appearance as FIRDA occurring in patients with diffuse brain abnormalities. Parietal and occipital tumors may affect the posterior basic rhythm but also may show abnormalities in more anterior regions, possibly leading to false localization (see Fig. 14.4). Temporal tumors can show a unilateral abnormality up to 89% of the time [25] (see Fig. 14.1). Focal delta activity or sharp waves occurred in half of these patients. In >90% of temporal gliomas, slowing was continuous [25]. A more recent series (which included prolonged video-EEG monitoring) noted temporal epileptiform discharges and focal temporal slowing as the most common finding with temporal lobe tumors, although a few patients also showed bilateral, generalized, or false localization [26].

4.2. Posterior Fossa and "Deep" Tumors

Because most tumors in children over 1 year of age are infratentorial, it is important to consider posterior fossa and so-called deep (e.g., sellar, chiasmal, diencephalic) tumors separately. Although most of these patients have had an imaging study, the presenting symptoms can be so nonspecific (e.g., altered mental status) that an EEG might be obtained for other reasons in the course of a patient's treatment (e.g., to rule out nonconvulsive status epilepticus). Therefore, it is important to understand EEG findings in this context so that an appropriate interpretation of EEG patterns can be made. One study found that >75% of records were abnormal in children with posterior fossa tumors, with the likelihood of abnormality decreasing with age (from below 10 to over 50 years) [23]. Location within the posterior fossa may be important: EEGs were abnormal in only 30% of patients with brainstem tumors, while >80% of EEGs were abnormal in those with cerebellar or 4th-ventricle tumors [18]. In that series, 27% had posterior rhythmic delta waves, 32% had generalized bilateral bursts of rhythmic slowing, 51% had posterior arrhythmic delta waves, and 11% had rhythmic theta or delta waves on vertex or anterior quadrants.

Both Bickford and Martinius et al. noted the suppression of abnormal rhythmic delta-range activity upon arousal in patients with deep tumors [18,20]. Because these patterns may be produced by tumors distant from where the abnormal EEG patterns are recorded, they are sometimes referred to as "projected" rhythms. EEG may not lateralize, or may falsely lateralize, posterior fossa tumors [18]. EEG abnormalities (posterior slow activity) were more common in patients with posterior fossa tumors and evidence of increased intracranial pressure (i.e., evidence of 3rd-ventricle dilation) [18]. Arrhythmic delta activity is more common in patients with more rapid progression of symptoms, possibly due to rapid expansion of tumor size [18]. Nearly half the EEGs of patients with tumors of the cerebellopontine angle were normal in one series [23].

4.3. Sellar Tumors

EEG abnormalities in tumors of the sellar region include temporal lobe abnormalities, unilateral delta-range activity, and bitemporal dysrhythmia. It is important to remember this in the differential diagnosis of temporal lobe abnormalities. In tumors that compressed the 3rd ventricle, generalized slowing

was noted, and the degree of compression was the only factor that correlated with abnormalities in the EEG [27]. In that series, EEG abnormalities did not predict tumor type [28].

4.4. Hypothalamic Hamartoma

Hypothalamic hamartoma is a developmental malformation that frequently presents with seizures, including infantile spasms. Other associated conditions may include precocious puberty and behavioral problems. Excellent reviews of the topic are available [29–31]. In children, gelastic seizures are most typical at onset, although this may not be the case in adults, who tend to present with partial-onset seizures [32]. The other main cause of gelastic epilepsy is temporal or frontal lobe epilepsy [33]. The EEG in hypothalamic hamartoma initially may be normal, similar to other deep-seated masses, although over time the EEG may demonstrate focal slowing, then focal epileptiform activity, and then generalized epileptiform activity, consistent with the clinical semiology [31,34]. Eventually, a pattern consisting of generalized slow spike-wave, paroxysmal fast, and electrodecremental patterns can occur, reminiscent of the EEG in Lennox–Gastaut syndrome [35]. There may be associated autonomic features [36].

There is a possibility that the hamartoma in some way generates abnormal activity that propagates through the cortex, leading to the various seizure types noted in hypothalamic hamartoma [31, 37]. In four patients with hypothalamic hamartoma presenting with epileptic manifestations and displaying interictal spikes over the frontal and temporal areas, EEG source analysis, based on scalp recordings (32 electrodes), was able to estimate that the epileptiform spikes have deep sources in the neighborhood of the hamartoma, with later spread to cortical areas [38]. A subsequent study from the same group of a patients with hypothalamic hamartoma and gelastic epilepsy, using simultaneous EEG and functional MRI recordings of several seizures, indicated that the epileptic activity appeared to originate in the area around the tumor and propagate through the left fornix to the temporal lobe, and later through the cingulate fasciculus to the left frontal lobe [39]. Depth electrode studies have confirmed the hypothalamic hamartoma as the source of epileptiform activity in some patients [37,40–42].

5. ELECTROPHYSIOLOGY IN SURGICAL NEURO-ONCOLOGY

Electrophysiology retains a vital role in the surgical management of tumors and other space-occupying lesions because it can identify epileptogenic regions at the perimeter of the lesion that need to be resected (i.e., in addition to the lesion itself) to achieve optimal seizure control. This holds true not only for classical resection surgeries that require an open craniotomy but also for less invasive resections (i.e., MRI-guided laser thermal therapy) [43,44]. One of the most challenging surgical decisions is balancing the desire to resect as much tumor as possible with the desire to leave tissues intact that are important to motor, sensory, or language-related functions. Certain masses, particularly tumors with a tendency to infiltrate otherwise normal tissue (e.g., glioblastoma), but also more slowly growing tumors, pose a real dilemma for the surgery and oncology teams, requiring decisions that may leave the patient either with more residual tumor or without functions critical to optimal daily living [45]. Neurophysiology can offer guidance in defining two important regions: the peritumoral epileptogenic zone and functional cortex (i.e., areas that typically are critical to motor, sensory, or language function and whose resection would lead to significant deficits). Simple lesionectomies also are appropriate in the setting of certain well-defined lesions (e.g., cavernomas) or those near noneloquent cortex. Data from some series [46,47] suggest lesionectomies may be adequate in some cases, although selection of candidates for this approach has not been thoroughly studied. The impact on seizure control of adjacent epileptogenic cortex in developmental tumors has been debated [48]. One series showed that for gangliogliomas (a developmental tumor frequently associated with adjacent epileptogenic tissue), resection of temporal neocortical and extratemporal lesions alone may be sufficient for seizure control, whereas mesial temporal lesions may require invasive monitoring to determine the extent of the epileptogenic zone [49]. Success in selected cases of other tumor types suggests that disruption of an epileptogenic network may suffice to suppress seizure activity [50].

One application of electrophysiology in the operating room is in the resection of tumors that are associated with epilepsy, such as certain astrocytomas, dysembryoplastic neuroepithelial tumors, gangliogliomas, and gangliocytomas. These tumors are associated with epileptogenic tissue at their margins, and although the tumors themselves are not typically aggressive, there can be epileptogenic tissue adjacent to the tumor [51]. Intraoperative electrocorticography (ECoG) using standard individually placed carbon-tipped electrodes or using an electrode grid, with the electrodes in a fixed array, can help define the extent of the epileptogenic zone, even beyond the tumor margin [51]. In this series, seizure control was achieved in one patient after epileptogenic cortex was resected, even though not all the tumor was removed, although this may have been an exceptional case. Additionally, the authors point out this strategy may be more useful in children than adults. Given tumor recurrence rates in some series [52], some suggest that monitoring be done routinely in cases involving tissue near motor, sensory, or language areas. Extraoperative recordings from patients with subdural electrodes show that epileptiform activity can be intermittent and so might be missed during the limited recording time available in the operating room. This was consistent with the findings in a recent meta-analysis showing that the use of intraoperative ECoG did not change seizure outcomes in patients with gangliogliomas or dysembryoplastic neuroepithelial tumors [53]. Possibly extraoperative recording should be performed in some of these patients (but see below).

Cortical mapping of motor, sensory, or language cortex can be done intraoperatively [54] or outside the operating room [55], depending on the goals of the surgery. Each technique has its advantages and applications. Intraoperative mapping may reduce the risks of inserting and maintaining subdural electrodes (e.g., infection and bleeding) and is less expensive, but extraoperative mapping allows for more time to better define

the regions important for specific functions, while minimizing operative time when tissue is removed and minimizing the chances of a stimulation-induced intraoperative seizure [50]. If seizures are not a significant concern, then intraoperative mapping is more straightforward, since only EEG slowing or suppression need be sought. If intractable epilepsy is the major concern, extraoperative EEG recording and mapping should be considered, although good results have been reported with intraoperative mapping alone [54,56,57]. Mapping using evoked potentials is discussed later. The technical aspects of extraoperative mapping are discussed in Chapter 46.

Invasive recordings from patients with tumors have reinforced some findings from scalp recordings but also have identified a number of additional interesting phenomena. Patients with bilateral interictal findings can have unilateral ictal onsets and good postoperative outcomes [26]. In one series, ECoG during resection of gangliogliomas showed high-voltage slowing in the area of the tumor [58]. Another series using stereo-EEG in patients with low-grade tumors showed activity of less than 10 microvolts in white matter that was infiltrated with tumor or only affected by edema in some cases, while high-voltage slowing was noted in others with similarly affected gray matter, or with peritumoral gliosis. Still other patients had normal EEG activity [2]. Solid tumors always showed electrical depression. Intraoperative mapping has demonstrated acute changes in local motor maps right after tumor resection [56].

6. EVOKED POTENTIALS IN THE MANAGEMENT OF BRAIN TUMORS

Electrophysiological techniques such as evoked potentials were once used to help diagnose and locate mass lesions. This has largely been replaced by imaging. However, electrophysiology, used as a test of function, retains an important role in the management of mass lesions, particularly in the operating room. The techniques are not specific to the management of tumors, but instead have been developed to help ensure that surgical procedures are performed as safely as possible.

6.1. Cortical and Subcortical

Preoperative evoked potentials can be used to document whether sensory pathways are intact prior to, or at the start of, surgery. During surgery, changes in response can signal to the surgeon that the surgery might be impinging on the monitored pathway. The surgeon can then modify the surgical approach and extent of surgical resection. However, a change in responses may be irreversible once seen. Moreover, on occasion there can be postoperative deficits even though intraoperative evoked potentials did not change [59].

Phase reversal of somatosensory evoked potentials (SEPs) across the rolandic sulcus helps the surgeon locate, and therefore avoid, the primary sensorimotor cortex [60,61]. Motor cortex stimulation and recording of evoked electromyographic changes peripherally is another way to locate motor cortex [61]. Responses to motor cortex stimulation are sensitive to anesthesia, however, and this restricts its use in some circumstances.

6.2. Posterior Fossa Surgery

Electrophysiology is no longer a primary method for locating posterior fossa tumors but can help to determine the relationship of the mass to auditory pathways [62]. Auditory brainstem responses (ABRs) frequently are lost with cerebellopontine angle tumors, due to the effects on the peripheral or brainstem portions of the auditory pathway [63,64]. Possible changes include decreased amplitude and increased latency [62–65]. As would be expected, ABRs are not as sensitive as MRI in patients with small cerebellopontine angle tumors [66] or tumors that do not impinge on the auditory pathway [67,68]. Six of 40 patients with acoustic neuromas and normal ABRs using standard testing methods [69] had abnormalities when the clicks were given at high stimulus rates.

Brainstem auditory evoked potentials (BAEPs) can be used alone or together with other modalities to assess the effects of tumors on the brainstem, or to monitor during surgery [62]. For example, some have used recordings of the blink or masseter reflex [64,70]. During posterior fossa surgery, other cranial nerves, including III, IV, V, VI, VII, IX, X, XI, and XII, have been monitored, along with muscles innervated by these nerves, and along with SEPs [62, 71]. BAEPs along with electromyelographic monitoring can help ensure safe microvascular decompression procedures in the posterior fossa. When SEPs are used to monitor during posterior fossa surgery, it should be kept in mind that the usually recorded SEP responses to peripheral nerves are generated above and below, but not within, the brainstem [72].

6.3. Magnetoencephalography

Nakasoto et al. [73] evaluated cortical auditory function in 14 patients with temporal lobe tumors using an MRI-linked whole-head magnetoencephalography (MEG) system. The authors suggested that the MEG system could be used to evaluate cortical auditory function noninvasively before and after surgical treatment of temporal lobe tumors. An example of the usefulness of MEG in the preoperative evaluation of tumors using somatosensory evoked fields is presented in Chapter 35 and Figure 32.21.

6.4. Event-Related Potentials

Moore et al. [74] evaluated 33 survivors of childhood cancer with P300, motor reaction time, and neuropsychiatric testing. There were abnormalities in P300 and in neuropsychiatric scores of patients who had received cranial radiation therapy. The authors suggested that cognitive changes in this group might be due to white matter damage. As with other evoked potentials, changes in P300 are nonspecific with respect to etiology but may correlate with overall cognitive status.

7. EEG COHERENCE

EEG coherence, a measure of the association between signals in a specified frequency band from different brain regions, has been used in both surface and invasive recordings. One study that used surface recordings found decreased coherence between the cortical region containing a brain lesion and other portions of the same hemisphere [75]. Another study examined the use of coherence to help locate the central sulcus and sensorimotor area during tumor resections in 10 patients [76]. The central sulcus was a region of low coherence, whereas high coherence was noted in the region of the brain tumor. In contrast, coherence measures were not helpful in the temporal lobe. Both increases and decreases in functional connectivity as well as alterations in small-world network topology have been reported in patients with gliomas and meningiomas [77]. Further work would be needed to resolve the discrepancies between these results.

8. EEG IN BRAIN ABSCESS

Despite the hope expressed in prior editions of this text that brain abscess would become a rare diagnosis, patients with acquired immune deficiency syndrome, increased numbers of patients on immunomodulators or immunosuppression after organ transplant or the diagnosis of autoimmune disease, and increased recognition of congenital immunodeficiencies have led to a resurgence of this condition (Chapter 15). More recent case reports and series of patients with brain abscesses mention both epileptiform activity [78, 79] and periodic lateralized epileptiform discharges [80]. One series showed that 14 of 45 patients had focal EEG abnormalities (not specified further), while an additional 21 had either regional or hemispheric disturbances; of three normal EEGs, two patients had cerebellar abscesses [81].

Michel et al. [82] studied 13 patients with brain abscess and found slowing of background activity in the hemisphere with the abscess in 6 cases and bilateral generalized slowing in another 4 (3 were normal); continuous and nonreactive polymorphic delta-range activity in 12 patients with frontal intermittent delta-range activity in 5 patients; and pseudo-periodic sharp waves in 2 patients. The EEG localized the abscess in 61.5% of their cases. Focal arrhythmic delta-range activity was the most consistent finding in another series of 13 patients [83]. Importantly, although EEG was localizing in most cases, it was falsely localizing in one patient with a cerebellar abscess, perhaps due to connections between each cerebellar hemisphere and the contralateral cerebral hemisphere. Epileptiform activity occurred in four cases. Asymmetry in the distribution of beta-range activity helped lateralize the hemisphere with the abscess in seven cases.

In summary, EEG may be useful in localizing cortical abscesses in many cases but may be misleading or even normal in others.

9. EEG IN SUBDURAL HEMATOMA

Just as in tumors, the typical first diagnostic study obtained in most patients with intracranial hemorrhages is either a computed tomography scan or, less commonly, an MRI. Nonetheless, persistent altered mental status after evacuation or management of a hemorrhage may be due to nonconvulsive status epilepticus or to a postictal state; in either case, an EEG may be obtained. Intracranial hemorrhages may include epidural hematomas (a true neurosurgical emergency), subdural hematomas (both acute and chronic), intraparenchymal hemorrhages, and intraventricular hemorrhages. As with tumors, EEG findings depend heavily on the location, extent, and chronicity of the hemorrhage.

9.1. Acute Subdural Hematoma

Slowing (including slow posterior basic rhythm and paroxysmal slow activity), frontal intermittent rhythmic delta activity, and epileptiform discharges (including at the midline) have been noted in patients with acute subdural hematomas [84–88] (Fig. 14.5). Periodic lateralized epileptiform discharges also have been noted [88,89], although they have been seen after subdural hematomas have been evacuated as well [90]. EEG abnormalities may not be related to the size of the hematoma, among other factors [85]. Acute and subacute hematomas may be associated with changes in EEG amplitude; chronic hematomas may be associated with changes in frequency (i.e., increased slow activity) [88,91].

9.2. Chronic Subdural Hematoma

In a study of patients with unilateral chronic subdural hematomas and herniation who underwent xenon-enhanced computed tomography (to assess cerebral blood flow) and EEG, increased flow was noted in areas where alpha- and beta-range activity predominated, while blood flow was decreased in areas where slower frequencies predominated [92]. Furthermore, electrical activity correlated with thalamic (rather than cortical) blood flow, leading the authors to conclude that thalamus is the source of the abnormal EEG activity in this population. Patients with chronic subdural hematomas also can have normal EEGs; this was the case for eight of nine patients recorded 8 months to nearly 4 years after the initial insult [93].

10. EEG IN NORMAL-PRESSURE HYDROCEPHALUS

The EEG in patients with normal-pressure hydrocephalus (i.e., idiopathic) can be normal or can show unilateral or bilateral intermittent slowing [94]. In one series of 14 patients with normal-pressure hydrocephalus, half had EEGs with bursts of bilateral monorhythmic slow activity. This activity became more

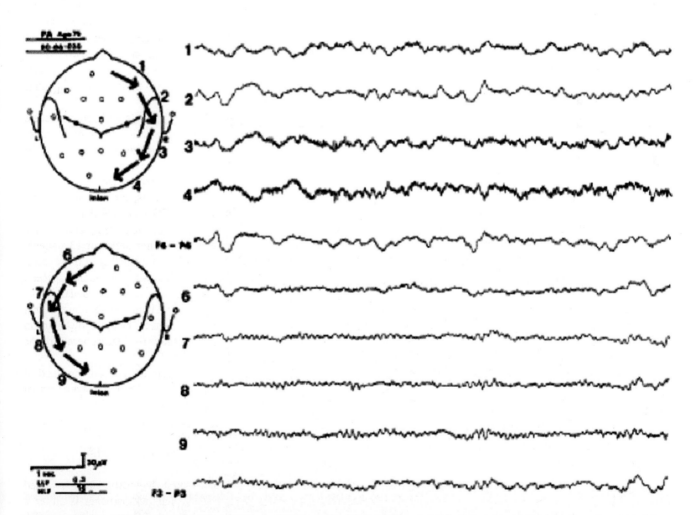

Figure 14.5. EEG from a 76-year-old male showing delta-range slowing over the right hemisphere. A right frontotemporoparietal subdural hematoma and a left temporofrontal hygroma were evacuated at surgery.

noticeable in four of five patients who had serial EEGs, while a similar number had improvements in the EEG after shunting operations [95]. This suggests that EEG changes may be useful for tracking progression of illness in some patients with normal-pressure hydrocephalus, but another paper suggested that patients with normal-pressure hydrocephalus do not have specific patterns on their EEG [95]. Quantitative EEG, or the analysis of different frequency bands, has been applied to patients with normal-pressure hydrocephalus. A number of reports conclude that such methods may be useful in understanding or treating these patients [96,97]. Further investigation and confirmation of findings may lead the way to new strategies of using the EEG to understand normal-pressure hydrocephalus and its treatment.

11. EEG CHANGES DUE TO ONCOLOGICAL AGENTS

Central nervous system toxicity has been associated with many chemotherapy agents. EEG changes include slowing, epileptiform activity, and voltage suppression. One difficulty in interpreting these findings is that patients often are receiving multiple agents, plus radiotherapy. Also, more than one finding can occur in a given patient. Finally, these are patients who often are systemically ill both from their primary illness and from treatments. Therefore, it is difficult to determine whether a given medication represents a primary or secondary cause of the EEG changes. A table outlining changes associated with various chemotherapy agents and a more extensive discussion of this topic can be found in the prior edition of this chapter [98].

12. CONCLUSIONS

Despite a decreasing role in the diagnosis of tumors and space-occupying masses, clinical neurophysiology methods are finding increased use in monitoring functional parameters and helping to define surgical resection margins. Quantitative methods are undergoing further refinement to better meet the needs of clinicians managing patients with space-occupying lesions.

SCORE EEG SOFTWARE

Further examples related to the topics addressed in this chapter can be found in the interactive online Niedermeyer Educational Platform. EEG recordings with illustrative examples can be opened and browsed. Features are marked and described using the SCORE EEG software. The users can see the features marked by experts, they can score these features themselves, and then compare them with the scorings of the experts.

The Niedermeyer Educational Platform can be accessed at: www.scoreEEG.com/academy

REFERENCES

1. Gloor, P., G. Ball, and N. Schaul, *Brain lesions that produce delta waves in the EEG.* Neurology, 1977. **27**(4): p. 326–333.

2. Munari, C., et al., *Correlation between stereo-EEG, CT-scan and stereotactic biopsy data in epileptic patients with low-grade gliomas.* Appl Neurophysiol, 1985. **48**(1–6): p. 448–453.

3. Klass, D.W. and D.D. Daly, *Electroencephalography in patients with brain tumor.* Med Clin North Am, 1960. **44**: p. 1041–1051.

4. Fish, D., *How do tumors cause epilepsy?*, in *The Epilepsies: Etiologies and Prevention*, P. Kotagal and H. Lüders, Editors. 1999, Academic Press: San Diego. p. 301–314.

5. Aronica, E., et al., *Expression of connexin 43 and connexin 32 gap-junction proteins in epilepsy-associated brain tumors and in the perilesional epileptic cortex.* Acta Neuropathol, 2001. **101**(5): p. 449–459.

6. Buckingham, S.C., et al., *Glutamate release by primary brain tumors induces epileptic activity.* Nat Med, 2011. **17**(10): p. 1269–1274.

7. Alonso-Nanclares, L. and J. De Felipe, *Vesicular glutamate transporter 1 immunostaining in the normal and epileptic human cerebral cortex.* Neuroscience, 2005. **134**(1): p. 59–68.

8. Aronica, E., et al., *Ionotropic and metabotropic glutamate receptor protein expression in glioneuronal tumours from patients with intractable epilepsy.* Neuropathol Appl Neurobiol, 2001. **27**(3): p. 223–237.

9. Richardson, M.P., et al., *Benzodiazepine-GABA(A) receptor binding is very low in dysembryoplastic neuroepithelial tumor: a PET study.* Epilepsia, 2001. **42**(10): p. 1327–1334.

10. Morrell, F. and L. de Toledo-Morrell, *Secondary epileptogenesis and brain tumors*, in *The Epilepsies: Etiologies and Prevention*, P. Kotagal and H. Lüders, Editors. 1999, Academic Press: San Diego. p. 357–363.

11. Laws, E.R., Jr., et al., *Neurosurgical management of low-grade astrocytoma of the cerebral hemispheres.* J Neurosurg, 1984. **61**(4): p. 665–673.

12. Lynam, L.M., et al., *Frequency of seizures in patients with newly diagnosed brain tumors: a retrospective review.* Clin Neurol Neurosurg, 2007. **109**(7): p. 634–638.

13. Hirsch, J.F., et al., *Benign astrocytic and oligodendrocytic tumors of the cerebral hemispheres in children.* J Neurosurg, 1989. **70**(4): p. 568–572.

14. Low, N.L., J.W. Correll, and J.F. Hammill, *Tumors of the cerebral hemispheres in children.* Arch Neurol, 1965. **13**(5): p. 547–554.

15. Backus, R.E. and J.G. Millichap, *The seizure as a manifestation of intracranial tumor in childhood.* Pediatrics, 1962. **29**: p. 978–984.

16. Khan, R.B., et al., *Seizures in children with primary brain tumors: incidence and long-term outcome.* Epilepsy Res, 2005. **64**(3): p. 85–91.

17. Kershman, J., A. Conde, and W.C. Gibson, *Electroencephalography in differential diagnosis of supratentorial tumors.* Arch Neurol Psychiatry, 1949. **62**(3): p. 255–268.

18. Martinius, J., A. Matthes, and C.T. Lombroso, *Electroencephalographic features in posterior fossa tumors in children.* Electroencephalogr Clin Neurophysiol, 1968. **25**(2): p. 128–139.

19. Marcuse, L.V., et al., *Nonconvulsive status epilepticus in patients with brain tumors.* Seizure, 2014. **23**(7): p. 542–547.

20. Bickford, R.G., *Electroencephalographic diagnosis of brain tumors.* Am J Surg, 1957. **93**(6): p. 946–951.

21. Kirstein, L., *The occurrence of sharp waves, spikes and fast activity in supratentorial tumours.* Electroencephalogr Clin Neurophysiol, 1953. **5**(1): p. 33–40.

22. Newmark, M.E., et al., *EEG, transmission computed tomography, and positron emission tomography with fluorodeoxyglucose 18F. Their use in adults with gliomas.* Arch Neurol, 1983. **40**(10): p. 607–610.

23. Daly, D., et al., *The electroencephalogram in cases of tumors of the posterior fossa and third ventricle.* Electroencephalogr Clin Neurophysiol, 1953. **5**(2): p. 203–216.

24. Gastaut, J.L. and B. Michel, *The impact of cranial computerized tomography on electroencephalography.* Electroencephalogr Clin Neurophysiol Suppl, 1978(34): p. 123–132.

25. Fischer-Williams, M. and G. Dike, *Brain tumors and other space-occupying lesions*, in *Electroencephalography: Basic Principles, Clinical Applications, and Related Fields*, E. Niedermeyer and F. Lopes da Silva, Editors. 2005, Lippincott Williams & Wilkins: Philadelphia. p. 305–321.

26. Zaatreh, M.M., et al., *Temporal lobe tumoral epilepsy: characteristics and predictors of surgical outcome.* Neurology, 2003. **61**(5): p. 636–641.

27. Nau, H.E., W.J. Bock, and H.E. Clar, *Electroencephalographic investigations in sellar tumours, with special regard to different methods of operative treatment.* Acta Neurochir (Wien), 1978. **44**(3-4): p. 207–214.

28. Allary, M., et al., *[Technics for the study of a total leukocyte dialysate and its fractions].* Rev Fr Transfus Immunohematol, 1977. **20**(3): p. 487–491.

29. Mittal, S., et al., *Hypothalamic hamartomas. Part 1. Clinical, neuroimaging, and neurophysiological characteristics.* Neurosurg Focus, 2013. **34**(6): p. E6.

30. Mittal, S., et al., *Hypothalamic hamartomas. Part 2. Surgical considerations and outcome.* Neurosurg Focus, 2013. **34**(6): p. E7.

31. Harvey, A.S. and J.L. Freeman, *Epilepsy in hypothalamic hamartoma: clinical and EEG features.* Semin Pediatr Neurol, 2007. **14**(2): p. 60–64.

32. Mullatti, N., et al., *The clinical spectrum of epilepsy in children and adults with hypothalamic hamartoma.* Epilepsia, 2003. **44**(10): p. 1310–1319.

33. Arroyo, S., et al., *Mirth, laughter and gelastic seizures.* Brain, 1993. **116** (Pt 4): p. 757–780.

34. Troester, M., et al., *EEG and video-EEG seizure monitoring has limited utility in patients with hypothalamic hamartoma and epilepsy.* Epilepsia, 2011. **52**(6): p. 1137–1143.

35. Berkovic, S.F., et al., *Hypothalamic hamartomas and ictal laughter: evolution of a characteristic epileptic syndrome and diagnostic value of magnetic resonance imaging.* Ann Neurol, 1988. **23**(5): p. 429–439.

36. Cerullo, A., et al., *Autonomic and hormonal ictal changes in gelastic seizures from hypothalamic hamartomas.* Electroencephalogr Clin Neurophysiol, 1998. **107**(5): p. 317–322.

37. Kuzniecky, R., et al., *Intrinsic epileptogenesis of hypothalamic hamartomas in gelastic epilepsy.* Ann Neurol, 1997. **42**(1): p. 60–67.

38. Leal, A.J., et al., *Interictal spike EEG source analysis in hypothalamic hamartoma epilepsy.* Clin Neurophysiol, 2002. **113**(12): p. 1961–1969.

39. Leal, A.J., et al., *Functional brain mapping of ictal activity in gelastic epilepsy associated with hypothalamic hamartoma: a case report.* Epilepsia, 2009. **50**(6): p. 1624–1631.

40. Munari, C., et al., *Role of the hypothalamic hamartoma in the genesis of gelastic fits (a video-stereo-EEG study).* Electroencephalogr Clin Neurophysiol, 1995. **95**(3): p. 154–160.

41. Palmini, A., et al., *Resection of the lesion in patients with hypothalamic hamartomas and catastrophic epilepsy.* Neurology, 2002. **58**(9): p. 1338–1347.

42. Kahane, P., et al., *From hypothalamic hamartoma to cortex: what can be learnt from depth recordings and stimulation?* Epileptic Disord, 2003. **5**(4): p. 205–217.

43. Carpentier, A., et al., *Real-time magnetic resonance-guided laser thermal therapy for focal metastatic brain tumors.* Neurosurgery, 2008. **63**(1 Suppl 1): p. ONS21–28; discussion ONS28–29.

44. Jethwa, P.R., et al., *Treatment of a supratentorial primitive neuroectodermal tumor using magnetic resonance-guided laser-induced thermal therapy.* J Neurosurg Pediatr, 2011. **8**(5): p. 468–475.

45. Englot, D.J., et al., *Extent of surgical resection predicts seizure freedom in low-grade temporal lobe brain tumors.* Neurosurgery, 2012. **70**(4): p. 921–928; discussion 928.

46. Cascino, G.D., et al., *Long-term follow-up of stereotactic lesionectomy in partial epilepsy: predictive factors and electroencephalographic results.* Epilepsia, 1992. **33**(4): p. 639–644.

47. Packer, R.J., et al., *Seizure control following tumor surgery for childhood cortical low-grade gliomas.* J Neurosurg, 1994. **80**(6): p. 998–1003.

48. Palmini, A., E. Paglioli, and V.D. Silva, *Developmental tumors and adjacent cortical dysplasia: single or dual pathology?* Epilepsia, 2013. **54**(Suppl 9): p. 18–24.

49. Giulioni, M., et al., *Lesionectomy in epileptogenic gangliogliomas: seizure outcome and surgical results.* J Clin Neurosci, 2006. **13**(5): p. 529–535.

50. Van Ness, P., *Pros and cons of lesionectomy as treatment for partial epilepsy,* in *The Epilepsies: Etiologies and Prevention,* P. Kotagal and H. Lüders, Editors. 1999, Academic Press: San Diego. p. 391–397.

51. Berger, M.S., et al., *Seizure outcome in children with hemispheric tumors and associated intractable epilepsy: the role of tumor removal combined with seizure foci resection.* Pediatr Neurosurg, 1991. **17**(4): p. 185–191.

52. Ebeling, U., M. Fischer, and K. Kothbauer, *Surgery of astrocytomas in the motor and premotor cortex under local anesthesia: report of 11 cases.* Minim Invasive Neurosurg, 1995. **38**(2): p. 51–59.

53. Englot, D.J., et al., *Factors associated with seizure freedom in the surgical resection of glioneuronal tumors.* Epilepsia, 2012. **53**(1): p. 51–57.

54. Berger, M.S. and G.A. Ojemann, *Intraoperative brain mapping techniques in neuro-oncology.* Stereotact Funct Neurosurg, 1992. **58**(1–4): p. 153–161.

55. Goldring, S., *A method for surgical management of focal epilepsy, especially as it relates to children.* J Neurosurg, 1978. **49**(3): p. 344–356.

56. Duffau, H., *Acute functional reorganisation of the human motor cortex during resection of central lesions: a study using intraoperative brain mapping.* J Neurol Neurosurg Psychiatry, 2001. **70**(4): p. 506–513.

57. Duffau, H., et al., *Intraoperative subcortical stimulation mapping of language pathways in a consecutive series of 115 patients with grade II glioma in the left dominant hemisphere.* J Neurosurg, 2008. **109**(3): p. 461–471.

58. Pilcher, W.H., et al., *Intraoperative electrocorticography during tumor resection: impact on seizure outcome in patients with gangliogliomas.* J Neurosurg, 1993. **78**(6): p. 891–902.

59. Lesser, R.P., et al., *Postoperative neurological deficits may occur despite unchanged intraoperative somatosensory evoked potentials.* Ann Neurol, 1986. **19**(1): p. 22–25.

60. Lueders, H., et al., *Cortical somatosensory evoked potentials in response to hand stimulation.* J Neurosurg, 1983. **58**(6): p. 885–894.

61. Cedzich, C., et al., *Somatosensory evoked potential phase reversal and direct motor cortex stimulation during surgery in and around the central region.* Neurosurgery, 1996. **38**(5): p. 962–970.

62. Cheek, J.C., *Posterior fossa intraoperative monitoring.* J Clin Neurophysiol, 1993. **10**(4): p. 412–424.

63. Nurlu, G., et al., *Brainstem auditory evoked potentials and blink reflexes in patients with pontocerebellar angle tumors.* Neurosurg Rev, 1994. **17**(4): p. 253–260.

64. Csecsei, G.I., et al., *Multimodality electroneurophysiological findings in intra-axial and extra-axial lesions of the brain stem.* Acta Neurochir (Wien), 1995. **137**(1-2): p. 48–53.

65. Stanton, S.G. and M.Z. Cashman, *Auditory brainstem response. A comparison of different interpretation strategies for detection of cerebellopontine angle tumors.* Scand Audiol, 1996. **25**(2): p. 109–120.

66. Naessens, B., et al., *Re-evaluation of the ABR in the diagnosis of CPA tumors in the MRI-era.* Acta Otorhinolaryngol Belg, 1996. **50**(2): p. 99–102.

67. Khatib, Z.A., et al., *Predominance of pilocytic histology in dorsally exophytic brain stem tumors.* Pediatr Neurosurg, 1994. **20**(1): p. 2–10.

68. Baran, J.A., K.P. Catherwood, and F.E. Musiek, *"Negative" ABR findings in an individual with a large brainstem tumor: hit or miss?* J Am Acad Audiol, 1995. **6**(3): p. 211–216.

69. Tanaka, H., A. Komatsuzaki, and H. Hentona, *Usefulness of auditory brainstem responses at high stimulus rates in the diagnosis of acoustic neuroma.* ORL J Otorhinolaryngol Relat Spec, 1996. **58**(4): p. 224–228.

70. Broggi, G., et al., *Neurophysiological monitoring of cranial nerves during posterior fossa surgery.* Acta Neurochir Suppl, 1995. **64**: p. 35–39.

71. Eisner, W., et al., *The mapping and continuous monitoring of the intrinsic motor nuclei during brain stem surgery.* Neurosurgery, 1995. **37**(2): p. 255–265.

72. Lesser, R.P., et al., *Early somatosensory potentials evoked by median nerve stimulation: intraoperative monitoring.* Neurology, 1981. **31**(12): p. 1519–1523.

73. Nakasato, N., et al., *Neuromagnetic evaluation of cortical auditory function in patients with temporal lobe tumors.* J Neurosurg, 1997. **86**(4): p. 610–618.

74. Moore, B.D., 3rd, et al., *Neurophysiological basis of cognitive deficits in long-term survivors of childhood cancer.* Arch Neurol, 1992. **49**(8): p. 809–817.

75. Harmony, T., et al., *EEG coherences in patients with brain lesions.* Int J Neurosci, 1994. **74**(1-4): p. 203–226.

76. Towle, V.L., et al., *Identification of the sensory/motor area and pathologic regions using ECoG coherence.* Electroencephalogr Clin Neurophysiol, 1998. **106**(1): p. 30–39.

77. Derks, J., J.C. Reijneveld, and L. Douw, *Neural network alterations underlie cognitive deficits in brain tumor patients.* Curr Opin Oncol, 2014. **26**(6): p. 627–633.

78. Aebi, C., F. Kaufmann, and U.B. Schaad, *Brain abscess in childhood—long-term experiences.* Eur J Pediatr, 1991. **150**(4): p. 282–286.

79. Ma, J.S., et al., *Brain abscess caused by* Salmonella enterica *subspecies houtenae in a patient with chronic granulomatous disease.* J Microbiol Immunol Infect, 2003. **36**(4): p. 282–284.

80. Gurer, G., et al., *Structural lesions in periodic lateralized epileptiform discharges (PLEDs).* Clin EEG Neurosci, 2004. **35**(2): p. 88–93.

81. Beller, A.J., A. Sahar, and I. Praiss, *Brain abscess. Review of 89 cases over a period of 30 years.* J Neurol Neurosurg Psychiatry, 1973. **36**(5): p. 757–768.

82. Michel, B., J.L. Gastaut, and L. Bianchi, *Electroencephalographic cranial computerized tomographic correlations in brain abscess.* Electroencephalogr Clin Neurophysiol, 1979. **46**(3): p. 256–273.

83. Vignadndra, V., L.T. Ghee, and J. Chawla, *EEG in brain abscess: its value in localization compared to other diagnostic tests.* Electroencephalogr Clin Neurophysiol, 1975. **38**(6): p. 611–622.

84. Gutierrez-Luque, A.G., C.S. MacCarty, and D.W. Klass, *Head injury with suspected subdural hematoma. Effect on EEG.* Arch Neurol, 1966. **15**(4): p. 437–443.

85. Jaffe, R., I.E. Librot, and M.B. Bender, *Serial EEG studies in unoperated subdural hematoma.* Arch Neurol, 1968. **19**(3): p. 325–330.

86. Poole, E.W., *Some aspects of electroencephalographic disturbances following head injury.* J Clin Pathol Suppl (R Coll Pathol), 1970. **4**: p. 187–201.

87. Jones, S.C., et al., *Multiple forms of epileptic attack secondary to a small chronic subdural haematoma.* BMJ, 1989. **299**(6696): p. 439–441.

88. Rudzinski, L.A., et al., *Electroencephalographic findings in acute subdural hematoma.* J Clin Neurophysiol, 2011. **28**(6): p. 633–641.

89. Chu, N.S., *Acute subdural hematoma and the periodic lateralized epileptiform discharges.* Clin Electroencephalogr, 1979. **10**(3): p. 145–150.

90. Westmoreland, B.F., *Periodic lateralized epileptiform discharges after evacuation of subdural hematomas.* J Clin Neurophysiol, 2001. **18**(1): p. 20–24.

91. Ibrahim, M.M. and M. Elian, *A reappraisal of the value of the EEG in subdural haematoma. A report on 86 patients, with a follow-up study.* J Neurol, 1974. **207**(2): p. 117–128.

92. Tanaka, A., et al., *Quantitative electroencephalographic correlates of cerebral blood flow in patients with chronic subdural hematomas.* Surg Neurol, 1998. **50**(3): p. 235–240.

93. Lusins, J., R. Jaffe, and M.B. Bender, *Unoperated subdural hematomas. Long-term follow-up study by brain scan and electroencephalography.* J Neurosurg, 1976. **44**(5): p. 601–607.

94. Brown, D.G. and E.S. Goldensohn, *The electroencephalogram in normal pressure hydrocephalus.* Arch Neurol, 1973. **29**(1): p. 70–71.

95. Hashi, K., et al., *The EEG in normal pressure hydrocephalus.* Acta Neurochir (Wien), 1976. **33**(1-2): p. 23–35.

96. Sand, T., G. Bovim, and R. Gimse, *Quantitative electroencephalography in idiopathic normal pressure hydrocephalus: relationship to CSF outflow resistance and the CSF tap-test.* Acta Neurol Scand, 1994. **89**(5): p. 317–322.

97. Seo, J.G., et al., *Idiopathic normal pressure hydrocephalus, quantitative EEG findings, and the cerebrospinal fluid tap test: a pilot study.* J Clin Neurophysiol, 2014. **31**(6): p. 594–599.

98. Hartman, A.L. and R.P. Lesser, *Tumors and space-occupying lesions,* in *Niedermeyer's Electroencephalography: Basic Principles, Clinical Applications, and Related Fields*, D.L. Schomer and F.H. Lopes da Silva, Editors. 2011, Lippincott Williams & Wilkins: Philadelphia. p. 321–330.

15 | EEG IN INFLAMMATORY DISORDERS, CEREBROVASCULAR DISEASES, TRAUMA, AND MIGRAINE

MARIAN GALOVIC, MD, BETTINA SCHMITZ, MD, AND BARBARA TETTENBORN, MD

ABSTRACT: This chapter describes electroencephalographic (EEG) abnormalities in inflammatory and cerebrovascular diseases, traumatic brain injury, and headache. It focuses on a practical and clinical approach and covers the most important diseases from this extensive field. Particular attention has been paid to viral and autoimmune encephalitis, prion disease, ischemic stroke, posttraumatic coma, and migraine. Several signature patterns are discussed that facilitate early and accurate diagnosis. The use of EEG in guiding treatment decisions and predicting prognosis is reviewed.

KEYWORDS: electroencephalogram, EEG, inflammation, cerebrovascular, stroke, traumatic brain injury, coma, headache, migraine

PRINCIPAL REFERENCES

1. Wieser H-G, Schwarz U, Blättler T, Bernoulli C, Sitzler M, Stoeck K, et al. Serial EEG findings in sporadic and iatrogenic Creutzfeldt–Jakob disease. Clinical Neurophysiology. 2004;115(11):2467–2478.
2. Schmitt SE, Pargeon K, Frechette ES, Hirsch LJ, Dalmau J, Friedman D. Extreme delta brush: a unique EEG pattern in adults with anti-NMDA receptor encephalitis. Neurology. 2012;79(11):1094–1100.
3. Irani SR, Michell AW, Lang B, Pettingill P, Waters P, Johnson MR, et al. Faciobrachial dystonic seizures precede Lgi1 antibody limbic encephalitis. Ann Neurol. 2011;69(5):892–900.
4. Carrera E, Michel P, Despland P-A, Maeder-Ingvar M, Ruffieux C, Debatisse D, et al. Continuous assessment of electrical epileptic activity in acute stroke. Neurology. 2006;67(1):99–104.
5. Claassen J, Jetté N, Chum F, Green R, Schmidt M, Choi H, et al. Electrographic seizures and periodic discharges after intracerebral hemorrhage. Neurology. 2007;69(13):1356–1365.
6. Claassen J, Hirsch LJ, Kreiter KT, Du EY, Connolly ES, Emerson RG, et al. Quantitative continuous EEG for detecting delayed cerebral ischemia in patients with poor-grade subarachnoid hemorrhage. Clin Neurophysiol. 2004;115(12):2699–2710.
7. Vespa PM, Miller C, McArthur D, Eliseo M, Etchepare M, Hirt D, et al. Nonconvulsive electrographic seizures after traumatic brain injury result in a delayed, prolonged increase in intracranial pressure and metabolic crisis. Critical Care Medicine. 2007;35(12):2830–2836.
8. Gronseth GS, Greenberg MK. The utility of the electroencephalogram in the evaluation of patients presenting with headache: a review of the literature. Neurology. 1995;45(7):1263–1267.

1. INFLAMMATORY DISORDERS

The range of electroencephalographic (EEG) abnormalities in inflammatory and infectious disorders was the subject of great interest in the 1950s and 1960s. The following decades saw an improvement in diagnostic imaging modalities, and the resultant recognition of the limitations of the use of EEG in the diagnosis, treatment, and follow-up of most of those conditions, with a few notable exceptions. However, there has been a renewed surge of interest in the past few years. This was mainly due to the recognition of several autoimmune encephalopathies that are associated with seizures and epilepsy. EEG can provide important hints about the diagnosis and response to treatment in these conditions.

Inflammatory disorders can be subdivided into infection-related and immune-mediated central nervous system (CNS) diseases. This distinction is somewhat artificial, since every infection is also mediated by the immune system. The range of EEG abnormalities associated with these conditions is exceptionally diverse. The EEG of an inflamed brain can be completely normal, can reveal minor generalized or lateralized abnormalities, or may show severe focal or global slowing, and may also contain a variety of potentially epileptogenic abnormalities or frank electrographic seizures of focal, lateralized, or generalized onset. The majority of these EEG changes represent the "final common pathway" of the electrographic activity of the inflamed cortex in either primary or secondary inflammation. Hence, many believe that most of those EEG abnormalities are nonspecific, and of low to moderate diagnostic and prognostic value.

Nevertheless, several "signature" EEG patterns corresponding to specific conditions and even to specific pathogens have been recognized (e.g., herpes simplex virus encephalitis, Creutzfeld–Jakob disease, Rasmussen encephalitis, limbic encephalitis). In these conditions, the EEG not only aids the diagnosis but might also guide therapeutic and prognostic decisions.

1.1. Infectious Encephalitis

Encephalitis results from inflammation of the brain due to direct infiltration by an infectious agent. Clinically, it is commonly associated with alterations of consciousness, focal neurological deficits, and seizures. Three neurological infections have a pathognomonic EEG pattern: herpes simplex encephalitis, most common variants of prion disease, and subacute sclerosing panencephalitis (SSPE), although the latter is a very rare diagnostic entity in the Western world, where measles vaccination is a norm.

1.1.1. HERPES SIMPLEX TYPE 1 (HSV-1) ENCEPHALITIS
This catastrophic CNS infection can affect people of all ages, but it is most common in patients above the age of 50 years.

HSV-1 has a predilection for the temporal and orbitofrontal areas. Early diagnosis is crucial to provide immediate treatment and an initial overdiagnosis is preferable. Early EEG abnormalities consist of polymorphic delta slowing, often more prominent over the most involved temporal lobe, with focal sharp complexes appearing and rapidly evolving into pseudo-periodic to periodic epileptiform discharges (periodic lateralized epileptiform discharges or lateralized periodic discharges [LPDs]), 0.3 to 1 Hz in frequency, and diphasic or triphasic broad or tight giant sharp waves (1). These may be bilateral, bifrontal, bitemporal, or even generalized periodic discharges.

On occasion, LPDs are focal with a small field in a specific location, such as the anterior temporal region (Fig. 15.1). At times, LPDs and/or focal sharp complexes reveal themselves within days to a week after the onset of symptoms, but they may persist for several weeks into the illness, and may be correlated with the response to treatment. Because the most common reason for LPDs is a vascular insult, dual etiology needs to be considered as part of the differential diagnosis. The coexistence of HSV-1 encephalitis and ischemic stroke or a hemorrhage is possible, and radiologic correlation is crucial. When clinical motor seizures do occur, the frequency of clonic limb

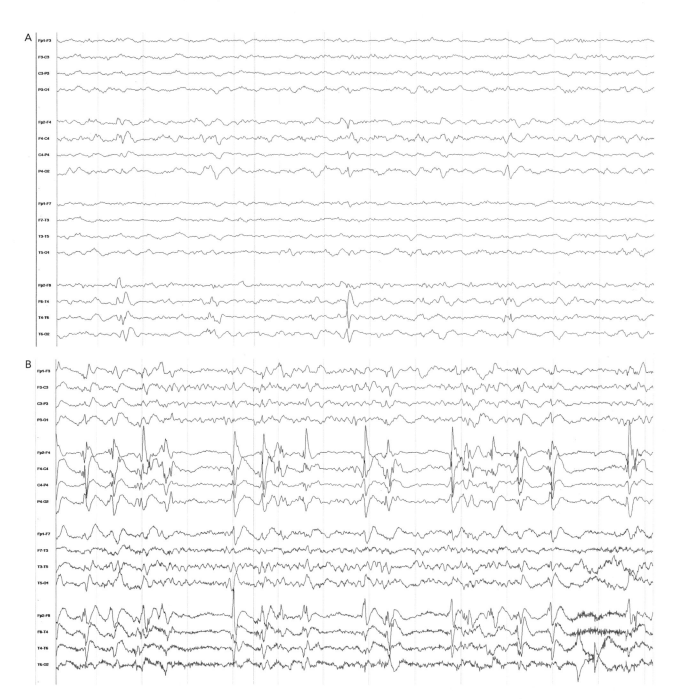

Figure 15.1. EEG from a 62-year-old man with CSF-positive HSV encephalitis and MRI abnormalities maximal in the right frontotemporal head region reveals initially right temporal slowing and isolated sharp waves and spikes (A). With symptomatic progression of the disease, pseudo-periodic lateralized epileptiform discharges followed by suppression over the entire right hemisphere (B).

activity may not match the frequency of LPDs, which may be significantly slower than the clonus (2).

In refractory or fatal cases, a burst-suppression pattern may be seen with generalized EEG attenuation following a burst of LPDs or polyspikes, which indicates a grim prognosis. In nonfatal HSV encephalitis, the strikingly abnormal EEG recovers slowly to almost normal on serial examinations. The LPDs become infrequent and intermittent and are replaced by lateralized slow-wave abnormalities. Clinical improvement often precedes electrographic normalization.

Other, seemingly atypical patterns are frequently seen in HSV encephalitis, including generalized triphasic waves or atypical triphasics, with posterior-to-anterior phase shift, multifocal sharp waves, and severe polymorphic delta slowing. These changes possibly arise due to the associated severe encephalopathy.

1.1.2. Prion Disease

The common pathogen of prion disease is an abnormally folding protein, which causes rapidly progressive dementia associated with psychiatric abnormalities and movement disorders. Creutzfeld–Jakob disease (CJD), variant CJD, Gerstmann–Straussler–Scheinker disease, and the exceedingly rare fatal familial insomnia are four well-described prion disorders, which can be familial, sporadic, or infectious in etiology. The initial EEG abnormalities in typical CJD are nonspecific and mild, usually consisting of generalized slowing and disorganization of the background (3). However, nonconvulsive status epilepticus and epilepsia partialis continua have been repeatedly described as the initial presenting finding (4).

The hallmark of CJD is the periodic sharp-wave complexes. They typically consist of continuous generalized, bisynchronous periodic stereotypic sharp waves (Fig. 15.2). A triphasic appearance with an aftercoming slow component is common. These discharges are sharper and shorter (200–400 msec) than triphasic waves occurring in metabolic encephalopathies. They are typically periodic, with relatively regular intervals of 0.5 to 1 second. Unlike epileptic sharp waves, the discharges in CJD are usually reactive and tend to disappear in sleep. Atypical patterns may be seen, with bifrontal sharp waves that are pseudo-periodic, or even with multifocal spike-wave discharges (Fig. 15.3). Periodic sharp-wave complexes are uncommon in early CJD and are pathognomonic for the clinically developed stage of the disease. Initially, the abnormalities are lateralized; however, they consistently become generalized as disease progresses (3). In advanced CJD, periodic sharp-wave complexes might eventually disappear.

Myoclonic jerks maximal in the upper body may occur in close temporal association with generalized sharp-wave complexes, or they may have no EEG correlate. Startle myoclonus or provoked myoclonus can also be observed. Occasionally, external stimuli can drive the rate of both the myoclonus and the corresponding sharp-wave discharges.

A well-recognized presentation of CJD is the Heidenheim variant, beginning with progressive visual disturbances and eventually leading to blindness (5). These patients exhibit predominant occipital abnormalities of the EEG. In contrast, atypical prion disease variants in younger populations or related to raw meat consumption have been described where the pathognomonic CJD pattern on the EEG is absent.

1.1.3. Subacute Sclerosing Panencephalitis

SSPE occurs in young adults following childhood measles and causes progressive neurological deterioration, seizures, and movement disorders. The EEG presents with periodic giant complexes, with the frequent clinical accompaniment of jerks or whole-body spasms. The pattern, initially described by Radermecker and Poser (6), consists of high-voltage repetitive polyphasic and sharp- and slow-wave complexes 0.5 to 2 seconds in duration. Typical is a long intercomplex interval, ranging from 4 to 20 seconds (Fig. 15.4). This pathognomonic pattern correlates with historical and clinical findings and is definitive for the diagnosis. However, multiple typical and atypical electrographic presentations of SSPE have been described (7). These can involve status epilepticus, bifrontal spikes, or other generalized abnormalities.

1.1.4. HIV-Related Encephalitis

Clinically or electrographically, AIDS-related encephalitis is not different from other viral encephalitides; however, there is evidence of early CNS involvement and poor prognosis in some studies (8,9). HIV, "the great imitator," may present with meningoencephalitis at the early, middle, or late stages of the disease, without the evidence for secondary opportunistic CNS infection (10). No disease-related or diagnostic EEG pattern specific for HIV meningoencephalitis has been reported, though multiple studies confirmed that a variety of generalized and focal abnormalities in the EEG may be seen, which are different for the acute and chronic phases of the disease (8,9). In the early acute phase, the EEG may be normal or may show the nonspecific pattern of diffuse slowing, while in the late stages, severe delta slowing and even suppression can be seen. Encephalitides caused by opportunistic infections in AIDS, such as *Toxoplasma gondii*, cytomegalovirus, and candida, are discussed above and may show focal EEG abnormalities corresponding to the underlying lesions, as well as generalized slowing (10).

1.1.5. Other Types of Encephalitis

Encephalitides associated with common pathogens such as coxsackie virus, adenovirus, mycoplasma, rickettsia, mumps, rubella, measles, and influenza A and B, do not have an EEG pattern of significant diagnostic value. Serial EEG recordings provide a good basis for prognosis (11). Of note is that even a severely abnormal EEG may recover in days or weeks, and the EEG recovery is often correlated with the clinical outcome. Bacterial, viral, tuberculous, spirochetal, parasitic, or fungal encephalitis typically shows generalized severe polymorphic slowing in the delta range on the EEG, but focal slowing is also possible in granulomatous or parasitic disease.

Viral encephalitides caused by enteroviridae, arboviridae, and echoviridae result in EEG abnormalities ranging from mild to severe slowing to electrocerebral silence, and from lateralized potentially epileptogenic discharges to seizures and status epilepticus with burst-suppression pattern or with constant seizures (Fig. 15.5). The acute EEG is rarely highly

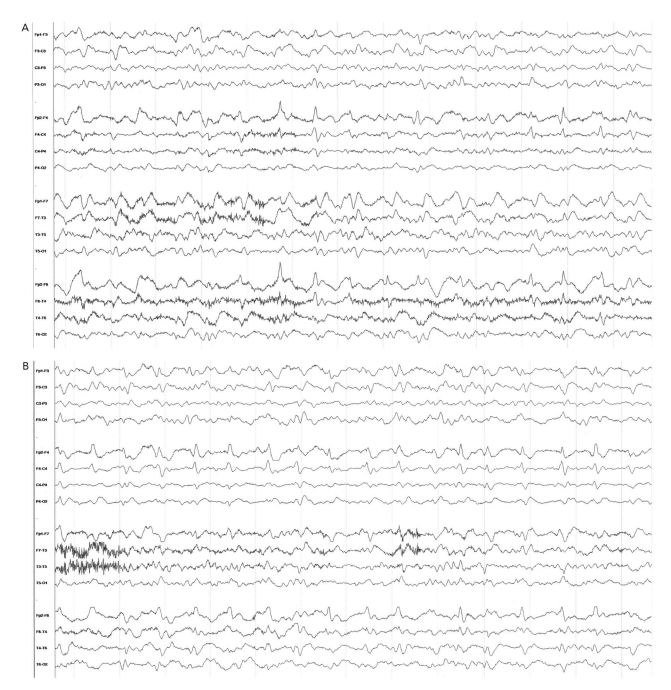

Figure 15.2. EEG of a 61-year-old woman with tremor and confusion, with MRI findings suggesting CJD (abnormal T2 signal in the caudate and lentiform nuclei), reveals a progression over 2 weeks from disorganization and slowing with occasional pseudo-periodic sharp waves (**A**) to continuous periodic sharp-wave discharges that are lateralized with a wide field (**B**), without a clinical correlate.

prognostic unless it contains a pattern of burst-suppression, which is always ominous, and the long-term prognosis, even though fair for survival, puts the patient at lifelong risk of intractable multifocal seizures.

Borrelia burgdorferi–related encephalitis has gotten some recent attention (12,13), although it is not different than other secondary autoimmune CNS inflammatory processes (Fig. 15.6). West Nile encephalitis generally presents with widespread electrographic abnormalities similar to other viral meningoencephalitides (14), though anterior or temporal predominant slowing has been reported (15). The range of EEG abnormalities is wide, from none to status epilepticus

and/or a burst-suppression pattern that is always ominous (Fig. 15.7) (16).

1.2. Infectious Meningitis

Infection and inflammation of the meninges can have bacterial, fungal, parasitic, autoimmune, and malignancy-related pathogenesis, or it can be secondary to a brain abscess or empyema with contiguous spread of infection. In the latter case, lateralizing EEG findings can be anticipated. In the rest of the conditions, the EEG may range from completely normal to severely abnormal, including focal- or generalized-onset seizures and

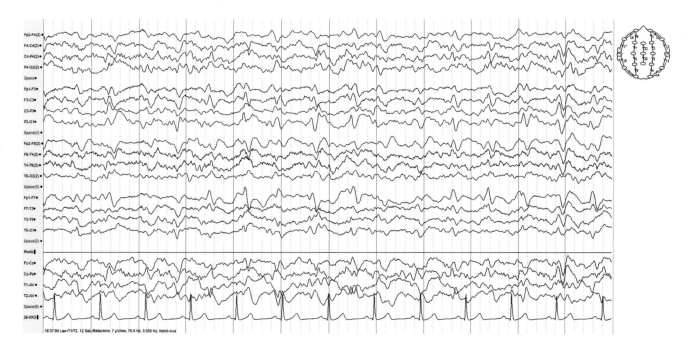

Figure 15.3. EEG of a 75-year old man presenting with rapid cognitive decline, mutism, and myoclonic jerks demonstrates diffuse slowing with bilateral periodic bi- and triphasic sharp and slow waves occurring at a pace of ~1 to 1.5 Hz (CJD).

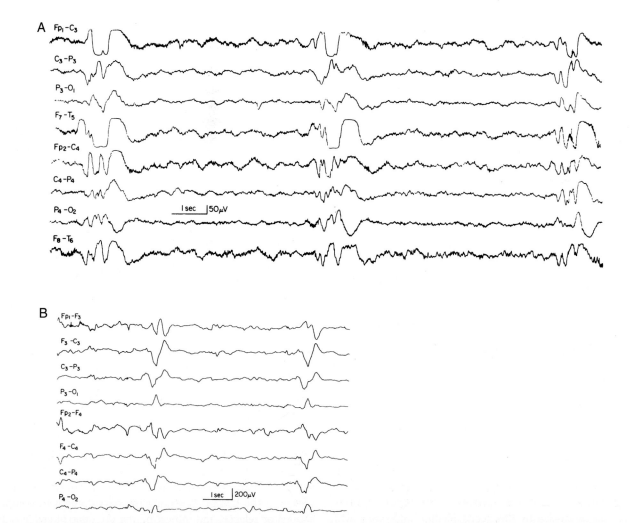

Figure 15.4. Periodic discharges in SSPE. **A:** At an earlier state with some preservation of other activities. **B:** At a more advanced state (recorded from two different patients, ages 8 and 9 years).

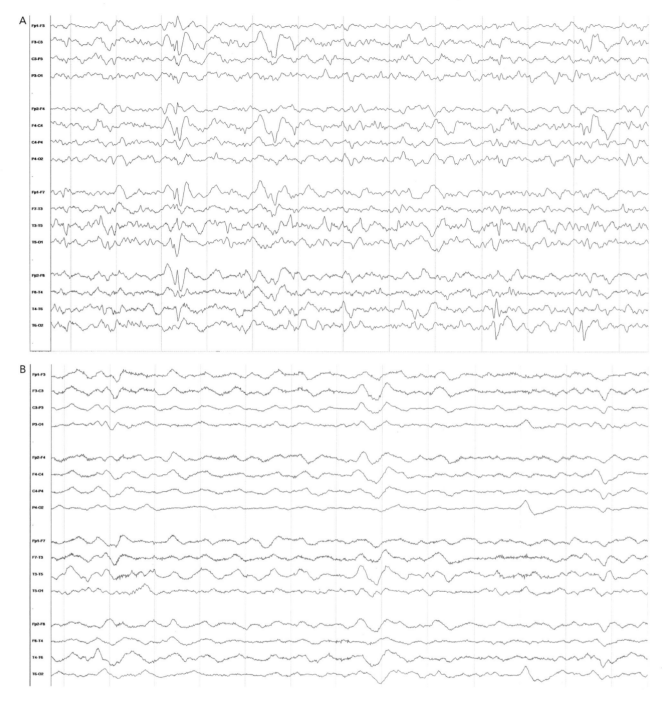

Figure 15.5. **A:** *A typical nonspecific EEG pattern in a 25-year-old woman with encephalitis not otherwise specified without a known pathogen, contracted during a summer vacation. It shows generalized severe slowing and multifocal spikes, some with a narrow field, and some nearly generalized.* **B:** *Another typical nonspecific EEG pattern is from a 17-year-old male with CSF-negative, presumably tick-borne encephalitis with a devastating initial course of coma, choreiform movements, status myoclonus, and wasting. The EEG during clinically comatose state demonstrates generalized moderately severe delta slowing and suppression.*

potentially epileptogenic discharges. However, in the majority of these conditions, only diffuse slow-wave abnormalities of variable severity will be seen.

EEG changes associated with meningitis are a sign of direct or indirect cerebral involvement. Meninges themselves do not generate electrical activity; hence, any changes observed on the EEG are related to disturbances of the cerebral cortex. These can be caused by direct encephalitic infiltration with an infectious agent. More likely, focal or generalized EEG abnormalities are due to indirect encephalopathic involvement by spread of the toxic inflammatory reaction (e.g., cytokines) or due to associated complications (e.g., hydrocephalus or cerebral vasculitis). Although the EEG findings are not essential for making the specific diagnosis of meningitis, the EEG and particularly serial recordings are helpful in following the course of the disease, detecting the development of complications or relapse, and indicating the presence of sequelae of residual brain damage.

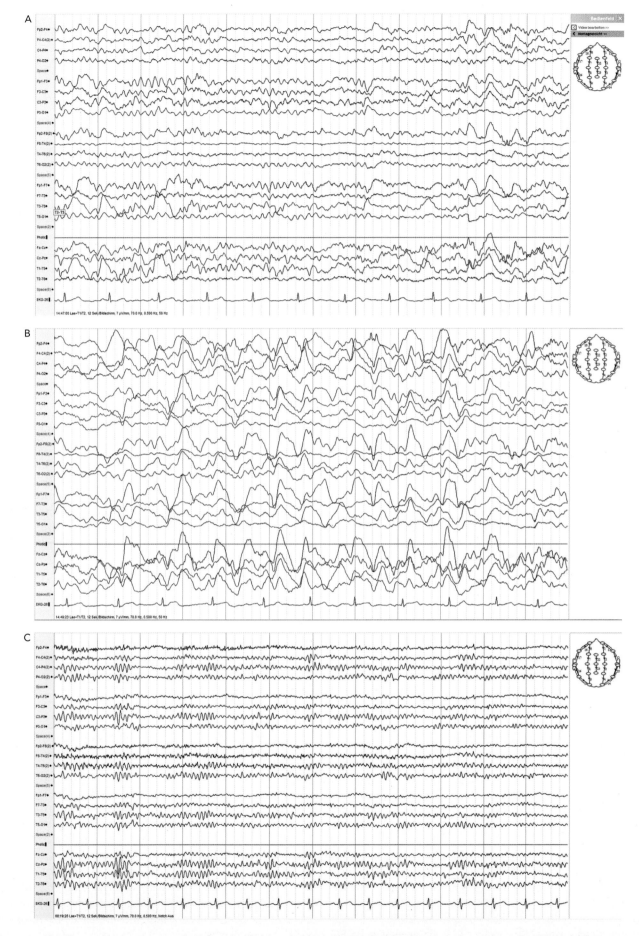

Figure 15.6. This 27-year-old woman presented with fever, headache, and general weakness. Five days later she had somnolence. On MRI, dural enhancement was marked on the left side but there was no sign of encephalitis. CSF was positive for acute tick-borne encephalitis. **A:** EEG on admission shows diffuse slowing with intermittent severe regional slowing on the left, predominantly temporal, and intermittent groups of rhythmic delta activity (IRDA or GRDA = generalized rhythmic delta activity). **B:** One week later, there is improvement with faster background activity. **C:** Three months later, background activity is normal with no focal slowing.

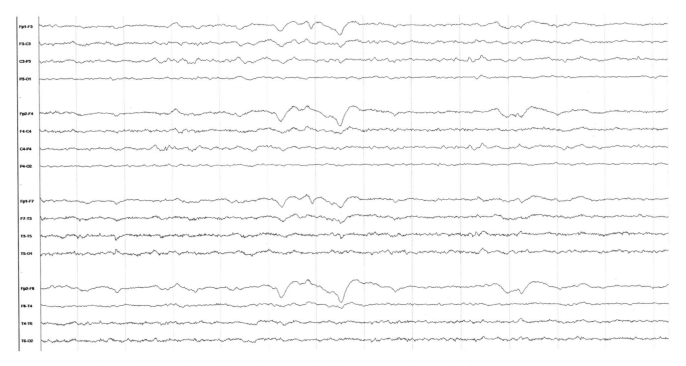

Figure 15.7. *This awake-state EEG from a 60-year-old man with neuroborreliosis demonstrates mostly generalized suppression.*

1.2.1. BACTERIAL MENINGITIS

Approximately three quarters of community-acquired cases are produced by meningococcal, pneumococcal, or *Haemophilus influenzae* infection. Posttraumatic or iatrogenic cases are commonly caused by *Staphylococcus aureus*, group A streptococci, and *Escherichia coli*. Diffuse moderate to very severe and nonspecific slow-wave abnormalities are typical for the EEG in those conditions (Fig. 15.8). The slowing is frequently prominent bifrontally, resembling frontal intermittent rhythmic delta activity (FIRDA), possibly associated with increased intracranial pressure (Fig. 15.9). Studies of the initial EEG evaluation of patients with purulent bacterial meningitis suggest that about half of the patients have slow-wave abnormalities or electrographic seizures. An attempt to predict the bacterial or viral nature of the pathogen from the EEG abnormalities suggests that moderately severe slowing in the delta range is much more likely in bacterial meningitis (17) (Fig. 15.10).

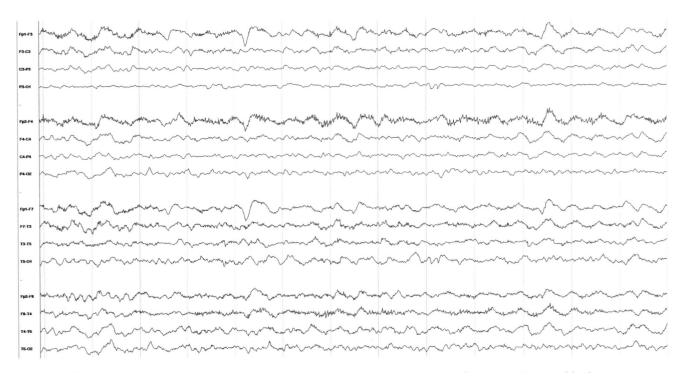

Figure 15.8. *This awake EEG of a 70-year-old man with community-acquired staphylococcal meningitis shows diffuse moderately severe delta slowing.*

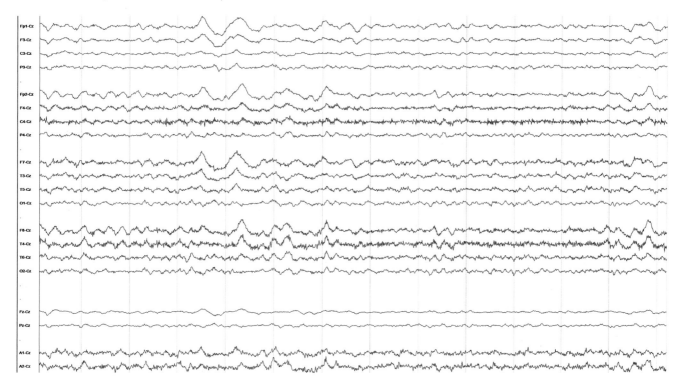

Figure 15.9. This EEG in an obtunded 63-year-old man with cervical methicillin-resistant Staphylococcus aureus (MRSA) abscess and secondary meningitis shows rhythmic bifrontal slowing consistent with FIRDA.

If only community-acquired disease is considered, about 20% of the patients will have clinical seizures, and a small number of those have clinical and electrographic status epilepticus (18). The patients with seizures have mortality of almost three times higher than those without seizures. In neonates with meningitis, with group B streptococcus and *E. coli* being the most common pathogens, the presence of EEG abnormalities and/or electrographic and clinical seizures is directly correlated with prognosis and is associated with a poor outcome (Fig. 15.11).

Brain abscess and subdural empyema can represent either the cause or sequelae of bacterial meningitis. The EEG findings

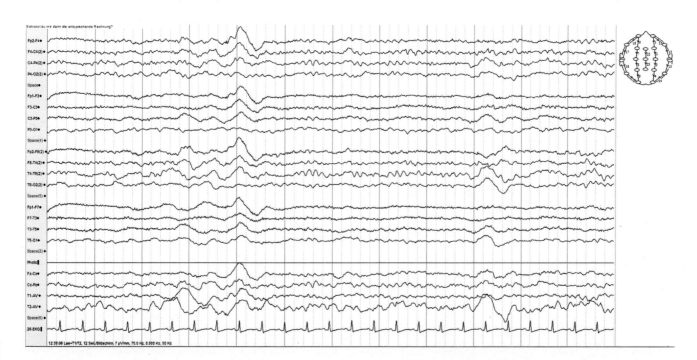

Figure 15.10. This 52-year-old man developed aphasia and right hemiparesis after a febrile infection. MRI showed no sign of acute stroke. CSF showed acute pneumococcal infection. EEG was nonspecific, with diffuse slowing and intermittent groups of generalized delta activity (IRDAs).

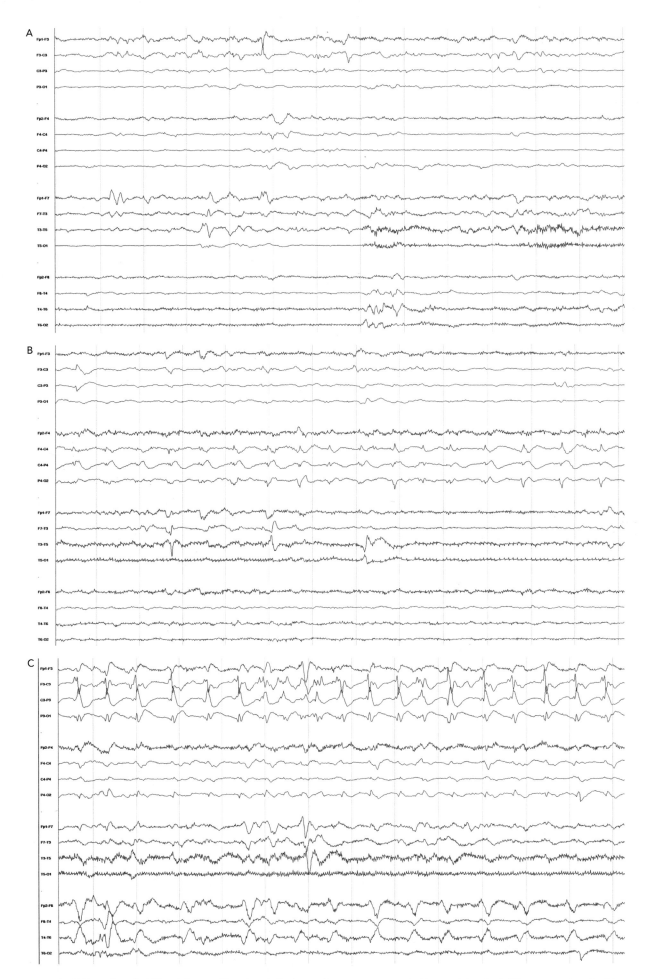

Figure 15.11. This EEG in a 7-week-old female born at 32 weeks, who had group B streptococcus meningitis, reveals interictal diffuse suppression of activity with intermittent focal sharp waves (**A**) and independent left- and right-sided periodic lateralized epileptic discharges (**B** and **C**) with no clinical accompaniment. Electrographic seizures with the subtle correlate of contralateral eye deviation were also seen.

in such cases often reflect a focal lesion—with moderately severe slowing, potentially epileptogenic abnormalities, and clinical and/or electrographic seizures. The focal findings may manifest as polymorphic delta slowing, suppression of activity over the area of suppuration, or, infrequently, lateralized polyphasic potentially epileptogenic abnormalities such as sharp waves or periodic lateralized epileptiform discharges (LPDs).

1.2.2. BASAL MENINGITIS
Basal meningitis affecting the base of the brain is usually caused by tuberculosis, *Listeria*, or spirochetes (syphilis and borreliosis). Because of the association of those pathogens with cerebral vasculitis, it is rare to see a normal EEG in those patients. In one series of 19 patients, 11 had EEG abnormalities. In another series, tuberculous meningitis was associated with similar EEG abnormalities in 24 out of 32 patients.

In addition to varied degrees of generalized slowing, hemispheric asymmetries and sharp paroxysmal activity can be observed. Triphasic waves are not uncommon (19), as well as FIRDA (20), which may reflect the underlying increase in intracranial pressure. Focal epileptic discharges and electrographic seizures are also common in tuberculous meningitis (21), particularly in children, and reflect the patchy focal manner of meningeal inflammation.

1.2.3. FUNGAL AND PARASITIC MENINGITIS
These pathogens most commonly affect immunosuppressed patients, causing cryptococcal, cystericercal, and candidal meningitis. The patients are typically very ill, and their EEG pattern is that of a severe encephalopathy, with polymorphic slowing. Slow-wave abnormalities, focal seizures, and status epilepticus are common, again reflecting the patchy nature of meningeal pathology.

1.2.4. VIRAL MENINGITIS
Viral, otherwise known as "aseptic," meningitis might not result in any EEG changes. In one series of 62 patients, 52% had abnormal EEGs with slow-wave abnormalities (22). Other investigators found that only 28% out of 82 patients (23), or in yet other studies, one third of patients with cerebrospinal fluid (CSF)-confirmed aseptic meningitis, had EEG abnormalities. Thus, a normal EEG with inflammatory CSF findings strongly suggests the viral nature of the pathogen—or early stage of CNS involvement.

Mollaret meningitis is a recurrent, lymphocytic inflammation of the meninges thought to be caused by herpes simplex type 2 virus. The EEG is usually normal; however, diffuse moderately severe slowing can be seen, correlated with the clinical symptoms of headache and confusion. Seizures are unusual.

1.2.5. CARCINOMATOUS MENINGITIS
Involvement of the meninges in the neoplastic process is a not uncommon terminal manifestation of systemic cancer. The EEG in these patients is practically never normal, with moderate or very severe slowing that correlates with the clinical severity of the encephalopathic state. Focal abnormalities such as LPDs, sharp waves, and spikes are also common. Generalized triphasic periodic waves have also been described.

1.3. Immune-Mediated Inflammatory Conditions

In the conditions discussed above, the brain is the primary or secondary target of attack by an infection or a presumed infection. In immune-mediated conditions, no CNS infection can be identified, and other organ systems may be the principal site of the inflammation. In cerebral demyelinating disorders and Rasmussen encephalitis, the principal site of the inflammation appears to be the brain. In immune-mediated conditions, the EEG abnormalities may be diffuse or lesion-specific. In lupus and antiphospholipid antibody diseases, cerebral inflammation is partly secondary to systemic activation of pro-inflammatory cytokines, but the effects on vasculature may also result in ischemia that then accounts for the focal nature of some EEG abnormalities observed clinically. In paraneoplastic CNS injury, although the tumor may be the primary site of immune-mediated attack, the brain is the site of the most damage. Some of the same immunogenic CNS antigens also may be attacked in the absence of a neoplasm, and result in similar damage.

1.3.1. LIMBIC ENCEPHALITIS
The classic syndrome of limbic encephalitis includes subacute memory impairment with behavioral changes, hallucination, sleep disturbance, and temporal lobe seizures. This relatively frequent disorder is associated with an immune reaction to neuronal surface antigens that may respond to immunotherapy. Anti-NMDA-receptor encephalitis is commonly associated with ovarian tumors; however, an increasing number of non-paraneoplastic cases are being described. Almost all of these patients present with an abnormal EEG. the most frequent is a diffuse slowing of the background, which can be severe in one third. Sixty percent of patients had seizures during continuous EEG (cEEG) monitoring. A unique electrographic pattern, termed "extreme delta brush," was recognized in approximately one third of all patients with anti-NMDA-receptor encephalitis (24,25). It is characterized by rhythmic delta activity at 1 to 3 Hz with bursts of rhythmic 20- to 30-Hz beta frequency superimposed over each delta wave (Fig. 15.12). This pattern is nearly continuous and is typically present from the earliest acquired EEG. The activity is nearly symmetrical and synchronous with a broad field across the whole scalp. It is not affected by the sleep/wake cycle and is not reactive to stimulation or arousal. The presence of extreme delta brush was associated with a more prolonged and more severe illness. Some authors found an association with status epilepticus (24). Extreme delta brush is an early finding that can be present despite unremarkable CSF and magnetic resonance imaging (MRI) results (26). Hence, early recognition of this pattern could guide diagnostic testing for NMDA-receptor antibodies.

Typical findings were also recognized in encephalitis with voltage-gated potassium channel (VGKC)-complex/Lgi1 antibodies. These patients commonly exhibit faciobrachial dystonic seizures early in the course of the disease, before developing the full clinical phenotype of limbic encephalitis (27,28). These seizures are characterized by frequent, brief

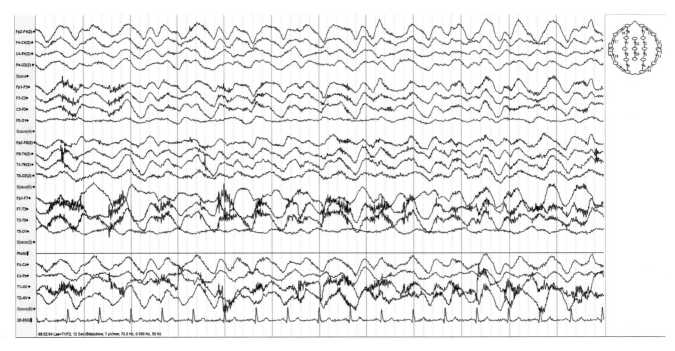

Figure 15.12. This EEG of a 39-year-old women with confirmed anti-NMDA-receptor encephalitis and ovarian teratoma shows generalized 1- to 2-Hz delta waves superimposed with bursts of fast 30-Hz beta frequencies. This pattern is termed extreme delta brush. Clinically she presented with permanent buccolingual dyskinesias.

dystonic posturing of the arm and ipsilateral face. The EEG shows ictal epileptiform activity with a frontal or temporal focus only in a fourth of patients. The seizures did not respond to treatment with anticonvulsants but improved after immunosuppressants were instituted.

There is some controversy as to whether rhythmic delta activity in limbic encephalitis represents limbic status epilepticus. The notching, the evolution of frequency and morphology, and occasional response to treatment were interpreted as clues to the ictal nature of the pattern. Although this might not apply to all patients, a few cases suggestive of status epilepticus were described (29,30). These individuals could benefit from early and appropriately dosed anticonvulsive treatment (Fig. 15.13).

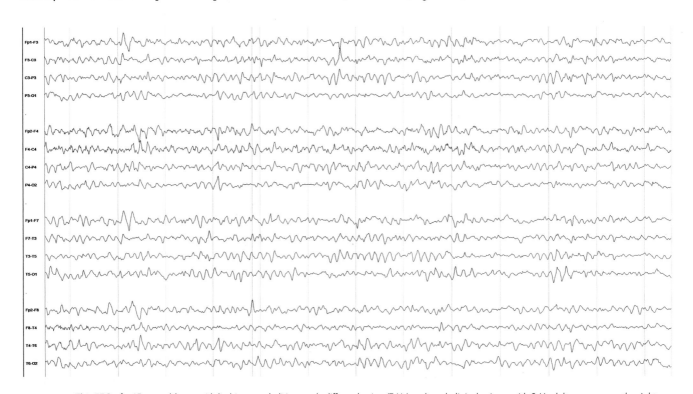

Figure 15.13. This EEG of a 65-year-old man with limbic encephalitis reveals diffuse slowing (7 Hz) and a subclinical seizure with 3-Hz delta waves over the right mesiotemporal region (T2, T4) over nearly 8 seconds.

1.3.2. Systemic Lupus Erythematosus

Abnormal electrographic findings are a frequent finding in patients with systemic lupus erythematosus (31). These are mostly nonspecific generalized slowing in theta and delta ranges. Paroxysmal focal changes and abnormalities in the background are the most common findings. Abnormalities in the EEG suggest CNS involvement, even if patients have no neurological deficits (32). Patients with EEG abnormalities were reported to have significantly lower complement factor C4, more pronounced thrombocytopenia, and a significantly higher titer of anticardiolipin IgG than those with a normal EEG. However, there is no significant association between EEG abnormalities and cerebral atrophy or with neuropsychological deficits (32).

Unilateral and bilateral, focal and more widespread abnormalities including delta and theta slowing and sharp waves have been reported. These frequently affect the left hemisphere, particularly the left temporal leads (31). Routine and quantitative EEG analyses also show theta and delta slowing predominantly affecting the left hemisphere in patients with neuropsychiatric manifestations.

Epileptic seizures occur in one quarter of cases. Seizures occur early after the onset of systemic lupus erythematosus and are related to stroke and the presence of antiphospholipid antibodies. Most patients with a single epileptic seizure have normal EEG findings. Those with recurrent seizures generally have abnormal EEGs, with interictal epileptiform abnormalities predominant in the temporal lobes. Generalized tonic–clonic and complex partial seizures are the most common type of seizures. Other seizure types include simple partial and secondary generalized. Complex partial status epilepticus has been reported with a prolonged period of confusion, and EEG revealed continuous rhythmic slow waves and triphasic waves; resolution of the EEG abnormalities and improvement of clinical findings were noted after a benzodiazepine injection.

1.3.3. Antiphospholipid Syndrome

The antiphospholipid syndrome is defined by the presence of laboratory markers such as antiphospholipid antibody and circulating anticoagulant and clinical manifestations such as recurrent thrombosis and abortions. The main EEG abnormalities are bursts of bitemporal irregular slowing, consisting of a mixture of theta and delta waves, often with accentuation on the left during wakefulness. Epileptogenic potentials such as temporal sharp waves and generalized epileptiform abnormalities can also be seen (33). EEG abnormalities are common in patients with neuropsychiatric symptoms and correlate with the presence of antiphospholipid antibody even in the absence of brain abnormalities on the MRI. Patients with an abnormal EEG were more likely to report memory problems (33).

A relationship between antiphospholipid antibodies and seizures has been suggested. Some studies reported the presence of antiphospholipid antibodies in patients with recurrent seizures and focal epilepsy (34,35), whereas others did not find an association (36). The biggest study to date did not find an overall association, but patients with a long duration of epilepsy and a high frequency of seizures were more likely to have anticardiolipin and antinuclear antibodies compared to those with a short disease duration and few seizures (37). This may reflect the influence of seizures on the immune system (38).

1.3.4. Behcet Disease

Behcet disease is a multisystem disease of unknown etiopathogenesis characterized by recurrent oral and genital aphthous ulcers and uveitis with various clinical manifestations due to CNS involvement. Neurological involvement has been classified into two major forms: (i) intra-axial neuro-Behcet syndrome (inflammation of the small veins of the CNS parenchyma) and (ii) extra-axial neuro-Behcet syndrome (thrombosis of the cerebral venous sinus).

The EEG findings in Behcet disease are nonspecific and range from normal to severely abnormal. The most common finding is a mild to moderate diffuse slowing (39–42). Focal slowing can also be seen, most prominently over the frontal, temporal, or frontotemporal regions (39). This is usually associated with pathologic abnormalities on imaging studies. Only a few patients show epileptic activity in these areas (39). Although periodic lateralized activity is an uncommon finding in Behcet disease, it has been described in two published cases (43,44).

Abnormal EEG findings are found in up to 80% of patients with neurological involvement but also in up to one third of patients without any neurological symptoms (41,42). EEG findings are likely to reflect clinical fluctuations (45). It is unknown whether EEG can be used to monitor disease activity. The reported frequency of seizures varies from 0% to 27%. Epileptic seizures can occur as the initial presentation or as the sole neurological manifestation (39). They also occur during exacerbations and the chronic course of Behcet disease. Seizures have been reported to be provoked by fever, medications (INH, penicillin, and interferon), or withdrawal of antiepileptic medications.

The main risk factor for seizures in Behcet disease is cerebral venous thrombosis, and the prognosis is usually good in these patients. However, seizures are a predictor of poor outcome in patients with brainstem involvement (46).

1.3.5. Rasmussen Encephalitis

Rasmussen encephalitis is a progressive epileptic encephalopathy typically involving one hemisphere. Although the pathogenesis remains uncertain, a major role of immune-mediated CNS inflammation was proposed.

EEG abnormalities initially consist of strictly unilateral slowing, followed in months to years by the emergence of potentially epileptogenic spikes and sharp-wave discharges. These are often associated with clinical and electrographic seizures evolving into the syndrome of epilepsia partialis continua. Focal electrical status epilepticus undetectable on standard scalp EEG has been demonstrated in Rasmussen encephalitis (47).

Late EEG findings reveal frequent unilateral seizures with a wide field, and bilaterally abnormal background (Fig. 15.14). Immune suppression as a therapy in Rasmussen encephalitis may slow the progression of cerebral degeneration and functional decline but has limited, and transient, effects on the clinical or electrographic seizures, or on the progression and evolvement of EEG abnormalities (48).

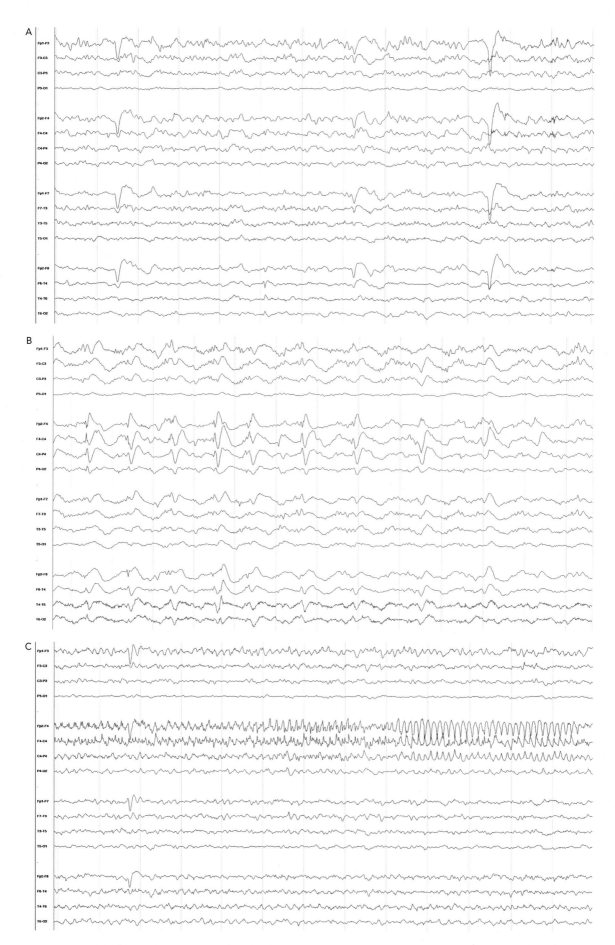

Figure 15.14. These EEG tracings from a 24-year-old man with late sequelae of Rasmussen encephalitis and epilepsia partialis continua illustrate the variety of interictal and ictal abnormalities observed at any time of sampling the EEG. Interictally (**A**), only a moderately severe slowing and a lack of normal background are noted; a periodic lateralized epileptic discharge–like pattern without a clinical correlate is also common (**B**). Epilepsia partialis continua in Rasmussen syndrome may present as morphologically different seizure patterns that may have no clinical accompaniment (**C**) or may be accompanied by rhythmic movements (**D**).

1.3.6. Steroid-Responsive Encephalopathy Associated with Autoimmune Thyroiditis

Steroid-responsive encephalopathy associated with autoimmune thyroiditis, also known as Hashimoto encephalopathy, usually presents with a subacute or abrupt onset of confusional state or alteration of the level of consciousness and is frequently accompanied by the development of focal or generalized seizures. EEG abnormalities can be seen in up to 90% of patients. The most common finding is mild to severe generalized slowing that corresponds to the severity of the clinical encephalopathy. Focal or lateralized slowing and epileptiform discharges (Fig. 15.15) are also frequent (49,50). Occasionally triphasic waves can be observed (51). When follow-up EEGs have been reported, the EEG findings improved or disappeared with steroid treatment.

1.3.7. Primary Angiitis of the CNS

Primary angiitis of the CNS is a rare multisystem vasculitis that primarily involves the CNS. EEG is a highly sensitive test in the diagnosis (52–54). Abnormal findings can be found in at least three quarters of all patients (54); two studies even found a 100% sensitivity of EEG (52,53).

EEG changes tend to present early in the course of the disease, often being the sole laboratory abnormality in the initial evaluation (52). However, the lack of specificity of these changes compromises EEG's usefulness in confirming the diagnosis. The most common abnormality is diffuse slowing. At times it may be focal or bitemporal and is commonly accompanied by runs of dysrhythmic activity (53,54). Epileptic activity is uncommon and was observed in 1 of 10 cases (54).

Seizures have been noted in 10% to 25% of cases (52,54). Clear electrographic seizures are uncommon (54). Partial motor seizures can be related to focal cerebral vasculitis in the temporal and parietal lobes, progressing to generalized tonic–clonic seizures that responded to steroid treatment.

1.3.8. Rheumatoid Arthritis

Cerebral involvement associated with rheumatoid arthritis is rare but well documented. This includes vasculitis, cerebral pachymeningitis, leptomeningitis caused by fibrinoid infiltration and rheumatoid nodule, choroid plexus infiltration, or cerebral complications induced by hyperviscosity associated with high titers of rheumatoid factors presenting as encephalopathy or seizures and responding to immunomodulatory treatment.

The morning symptoms of pain, weakness, and fatigue in rheumatoid arthritis may relate to a nonrestorative sleep disorder associated with a prominent alpha-rhythm EEG anomaly, a presumed arousal state occurring within sleep, during non-REM sleep stages 2, 3, and 4 (55).

In juvenile rheumatoid arthritis, various EEG abnormalities are seen, including slowing of activity that may be continuous or episodic, abundant beta activity, focal-asymmetrical disturbances that could be either paroxysmal or nonparoxysmal, and bilateral paroxysmal disturbances, including photic-induced paroxysm. Patients with positive antinuclear antibodies or visceral symptoms like pericarditis and/or myocarditis have fewer pathologic EEG changes than those suffering from a form of the disease with symptoms only in the joints. There is no clear correlation between EEG changes and the duration of the

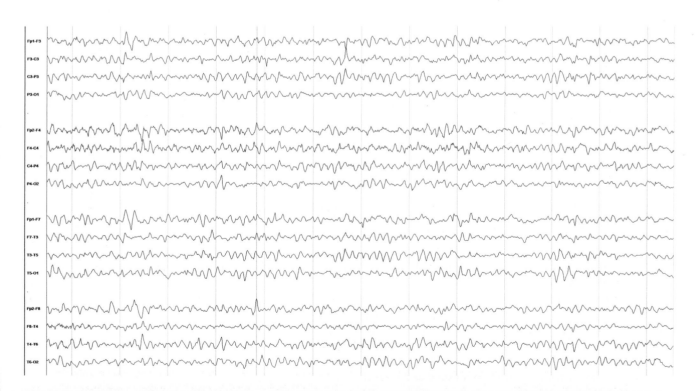

Figure 15.15. This EEG shows interictal slowing and sharp waves in a patient with Hashimoto thyroiditis and subacute encephalopathy. She had C lymphocytosis and increased protein, as well as dramatically elevated thyroid peroxidase and thyroglobulin antibodies. She improved dramatically with a short course of high-dose methylprednisolone (Solu-Medrol). Several years later she relapsed and had similar findings and course.

disease or age at onset (56). The pathologic EEG abnormalities are presumed to be caused by a primary cerebral process connected with the disease itself, probably vasculitis.

1.3.9. Demyelinating Disorders

Although white matter is primarily affected in these conditions, the inflammation may affect both normal cortical function and neuronal excitability and result in EEG abnormalities that are varied and nonspecific, with both diffuse and focal delta slowing typical for deep white matter lesions (57). There may also be focal potentially epileptogenic discharges in tumefactive multiple sclerosis and acute disseminated encephalomyelitis (58). With recovery the EEG usually normalizes, somewhat proportional to the extent of recovery from the initial event.

In chronic and late-stage multiple sclerosis, the EEG is usually abnormal. Diffuse slowing usually reflects the degree of encephalopathy, but without a clear correlation to radiographic plaque load (59). Although overall only 6.5% of multiple sclerosis patients in a recent study had epilepsy, the percentage was significantly higher in those with progressive multiple sclerosis. The interictal EEG of multiple sclerosis patients with epilepsy may reveal epileptiform abnormalities in up to two third of these patients (60).

1.3.10. Sydenham Chorea

Three types of EEG abnormalities were described in 17 of 20 children 10 to 16 years of age with rheumatic chorea (61). Seven patients had an increased amount of posterior slowing, five patients had disruption of the alpha rhythm and diffuse, monomorphic slowing, and five patients had bursts of 2- to 4-Hz posterior delta. No correlation between the EEG abnormalities and the severity of the chorea, or between the localization of the EEG abnormalities and the distribution of movements, was found. Others have found EEG slowing proportional to the severity of the movement disorder (62), and rarely epileptiform abnormalities have been observed. Lateralized suppression of sleep spindles without improvement with the disease regression has also been reported (63). Others report that the EEG may improve with the clinical state or show a delayed response (64).

2. CEREBROVASCULAR DISEASE

Computed tomography (CT) and MRI are the major diagnostic tools in cerebrovascular disease to investigate the morphology of the vascular lesion. The major role of EEG is the evaluation of functional disturbances caused by cerebrovascular disease, mainly the detection of epileptogenic foci. Cerebrovascular events are acute, often catastrophic events that naturally have strong influences on the EEG. The tempo of evolution is an important factor. Acute vascular slow foci may be much more impressive than focal slowing caused by a slowly growing neoplasm. On the other hand, small deep vascular lesions are often too far distant from the cortex and may escape EEG detection, whereas deep vascular lesions in the brainstem and cerebellum reveal themselves only as secondary phenomena in the cerebral hemispheres. In an acute stroke, a massive and highly impressive EEG focus may be present before a CT scan can

demonstrate the lesion (65). The EEG is an indicator of abnormal physiologic function; the function of the involved CNS tissue breaks down before the structure shows its suffering. It has been shown experimentally (66) as well as clinically with the use of CT scans (67) that edema alone does not account for delta activity in the EEG. An experienced electroencephalographer might be able to provide valuable information about the regional and general functional or dysfunctional state in a stroke. An imaginative approach to the EEG evaluation of strokes has been proposed by Velho-Groneberg (68). Accordingly, the EEG reflects dynamic processes that occur in the wake of a stroke.

2.1. Ischemic Stroke

2.1.1. Acute Hemispheric Stroke

The EEG is a sensitive index for functional changes in the acute phase. These changes can be present even before CT scans show any abnormalities. A massive hemispheric infarct due to carotid occlusion causes marked EEG abnormalities (69,70):

- Widespread arrhythmic delta activity occurs over the involved hemisphere, most prominently in temporal or frontotemporal regions (Fig. 15.16).

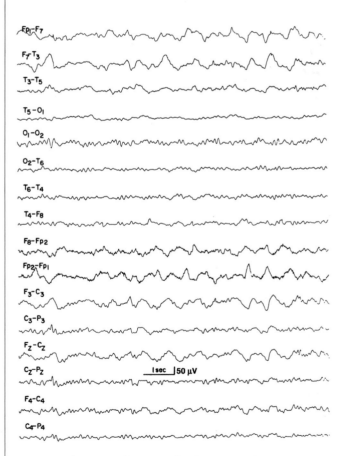

Figure 15.16. This 57-year-old patient suffered an acute cerebrovascular event on the day before this record was obtained. There is marked left frontotemporal polymorphic delta activity. Also note alpha depression and loss of detail over left posterior quadrant. The right hemisphere and especially the right frontal area show some degree of delta activity.

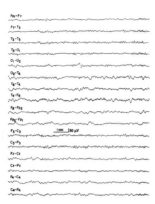

Figure 15.17. *This 64-year-old patient suffered acute cerebrovascular ischemia 3 days earlier due to right MCA thrombosis and good CT scan evidence of infarction in the corresponding territory. Acute left hemiplegia is present. The patient is awake; right-sided alpha is diminished and a large zone of mixed 3–6/sec activity involves most of the right hemisphere.*

- An ipsilateral alpha rhythm may be absent or of lower amplitude and slower frequency. The reactivity of alpha rhythm may diminish or disappear (Fig. 15.17). Rolandic beta activity and sleep spindles may also disappear.

- Extensive infarcts may markedly decrease or "suppress" electrocerebral activity, normal and abnormal, over the affected hemisphere during the first few days.

- In patients with smaller hemispheric infarcts, EEG from the uninvolved hemisphere usually remains normal. With extensive infarcts causing cerebral edema and displacement of midline structures, variable degrees of slow activity appear in contralateral hemicranium, often with bilateral intermittent rhythmic 2 to 3/sec delta activity (IRDA) (Fig. 15.18), which may be marked in the frontal region (FIRDA). In children, this rhythmic delta activity may be most marked occipitally (OIRDA).

During the first days after infarction, EEG abnormalities are most prominent, with the extent and voltage of slow activity progressively declining. Few prospective studies have evaluated EEGs serially in a carefully defined population. Kayser-Gatchalian and Neuendörfer (71) did EEGs on 79 patients with infarcts in the carotid distribution. Initial EEGs were done within 48 hours after infarction and again on days 5, 10, and 22. They visually classified EEG abnormalities into "background slowing" and "focal changes," with each group being divided by defined criteria into the following categories: "none," "mild," "moderate," or "severe." In the initial EEGs, "background slowing" reliably predicted state of consciousness: only 1 of 14 patients with severe or moderate slowing was alert, whereas 33 of 44 patients without slowing were alert. Focal changes paralleled motor deficits: 39 of 51 patients with

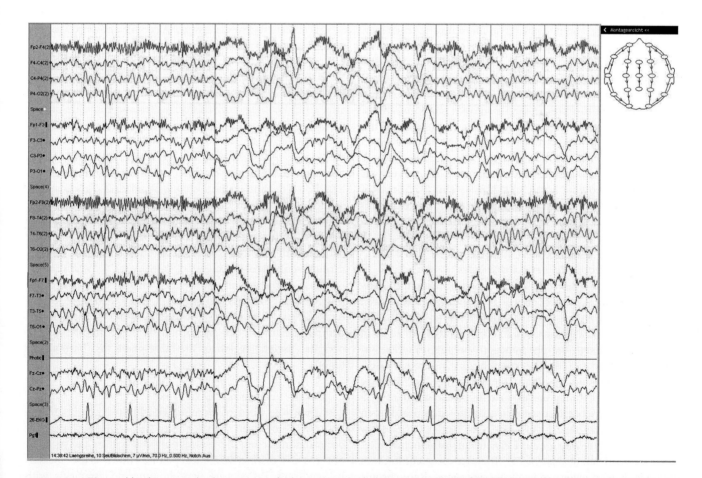

Figure 15.18. *A 79-year-old male presented with acute onset of aphasia, right-sided hemiparesis, and gait instability. CT scan 3 hours after onset of symptoms showed no evidence of acute infarction. EEG showed posterior 9/sec alpha rhythm on the right, suppressed on the left. There was generalized intermittent temporoparietal polymorphic theta/delta slowing (IRDA).*

CHAPTER 15 EEG IN INFLAMMATORY DISORDERS, CEREBROVASCULAR DISEASES, TRAUMA, AND MIGRAINE | 387

moderate or severe focal changes had severe paresis or hemiplegia, whereas only 7 of 17 patients without focal changes had severe weakness. In a smaller series of 15 patients, Sainio et al. (72) compared visual with spectral analysis. Results of visual analysis equaled spectral analysis, except for a lower incidence of focal abnormalities; in general, their findings paralleled the findings of Kayser-Gatchalian and Neuendörfer (71).

Infarction due to occlusion of the anterior cerebral artery is rare. EEG findings consist of (i) ipsilateral frontal delta activity (either arrhythmic or rhythmic, or both) and (ii) depression of anterior beta activity. Occlusion of the posterior cerebral artery may result in (i) infarction of the mesial temporal lobe with arrhythmic delta activity over the posterior head region and (ii) marked disorganization or absence of alpha rhythm. Microangiopathy leading to subcortical infarctions can lead to generalized intermittent delta activity on EEG recording (Fig. 15.19). More commonly, patients with mild subcortical strokes can have a normal EEG. The accuracy of EEG scalp recordings, however, may be limited by adequate sampling of the electrical field. Accurate description of the spatial distribution of the stroke-related EEG might only be achieved with 64- and 128-channel EEG (73).

2.1.2. EPILEPTIC ACTIVITY IN ACUTE STROKE

Routine EEG performed within the first 7 days after stroke onset only rarely shows epileptiform abnormalities. In a cohort of >300 patients, epileptic discharges were seen in only 3% of all patients (74). The odds of recording epileptic discharges were increased by threefold in individuals with seizures after stroke. In another study, there was an increase to almost 30% in patients who suffered acute seizures and those who developed remote symptomatic seizures (75).

The chances to record epileptic activity can be improved with the use of cEEG monitoring (76). In a study of 100 patients, epileptic discharges were recorded in 17. Most common were sharp waves, followed by spikes and periodic lateralized epileptic discharges (LPDs). Subclinical electrical seizures occurred in two monitored individuals. The likelihood of recording epileptic discharges was increased in patients with more severe strokes and, to a lesser extent, in those with cortical infarctions.

2.1.3. PERIODIC EPILEPTIC DISCHARGES

LPDs are a relatively uncommon EEG pattern characterized by lateralized or focal periodic or near-periodic spike, spike-wave, or sharp-wave complexes present throughout most or all of the recording (Fig. 15.20). Chatrian introduced the term *LPDs* in 1964 (77), although the phenomenon was first described in 1952 by Echlin et al. (78). They occur against a slow and disorganized background of rather moderate voltage. The periodic discharges are rhythmic or quasi-rhythmical at a rate of ~0.5 to 2/sec. The discharges may become quite widespread, even reaching into the other hemisphere. Occasionally, they show a superior frontal maximum. LPDs occur infrequently after acute hemispheric stroke (74,76). They are more common in individuals with extensive hemispheric lesions. Rare chronic LPDs, persisting for a period of 3 months to more than 20 years, have been reported in patients with chronic brain lesions and

associated partial seizure disorders. Bilateral, independently occurring LPDs were recognized by Chatrian in 1964 (77) and formally characterized in 1981 by de la Paz and Brenner (79). They are seen in the setting of multifocal or diffuse cerebral injury, such as anoxia, and herald a less favorable prognosis with higher mortality. A clear association with seizure activity has been recognized. Approximately 80% to 90% of patients with LPDs experience clinical seizures. Most commonly, LPDs appear within 1 to 4 days after focal motor seizures. In 40% LPDs were associated with precipitating status epilepticus. The persistence of LPDs in the absence of clinical seizures has led encephalographers to describe them as an interictal pattern. However, it is important to consider that they are firmly associated with an increased disposition for seizures. In one study, all patients with LPDs on the initial EEG later developed seizures (80).

In many cases, rhythmic discharges occurring in status epilepticus can resemble LPDs. A careful evaluation of the clinical picture for focal seizure activity is pivotal to distinguish these two entities and to initiate appropriate treatment. This differentiation might be difficult in ventilated patients in the intensive care unit (ICU) or in unconscious individuals with suspected nonconvulsive status. In these cases the encephalographer should closely examine the reactivity and modulation of the EEG pattern. Status epilepticus is more likely if periodic discharges have a high frequency (>2 Hz) and if there is clear-cut variability of the electric field, amplitude, and frequency (>1 Hz variability) of discharges. Also, fast and steep components are more likely seen in status epilepticus.

2.1.4. WATERSHED ISCHEMIA

Ischemic states usually pertain to the territory of the involved artery, but another mechanism has become clinically important. This is the concept of "extraterritorial ischemia" that gives rise to "watershed infarctions" ("boundary infarctions") along the borders of the major arterial territories, between middle, posterior, and anterior cerebral arteries. This mechanism is based on a decline in the systemic circulation. This is a drop in blood pressure or cardiac output, usually combined with a diseased and plaque-ridden cerebral vasculature. Acute watershed-type ischemia is most commonly found in elderly patients with a history of cerebral arteriosclerosis and chronic cardiovascular problems.

The EEG is typically slow with a mixed delta–theta-range frequency and severely disorganized. These changes are essentially diffuse with consistent lateralization to the affected hemisphere. LPDs can be seen over the posterotemporal–occipital–parietal region of the hemisphere that harbors the lesion.

2.1.5. VERTEBROBASILAR STROKE

Less than one third of patients with limited infarcts to the brainstem show even slightly altered EEGs (81). Basilar artery occlusion infarcting the ventral pons but sparing the tegmentum causes a distinctive clinical picture known as the "locked-in" syndrome. Patients are alert but mute and tetraplegic, with the only preserved motor acts being blinks and vertical eye movements. In these patients, EEG is normal (82); the alpha

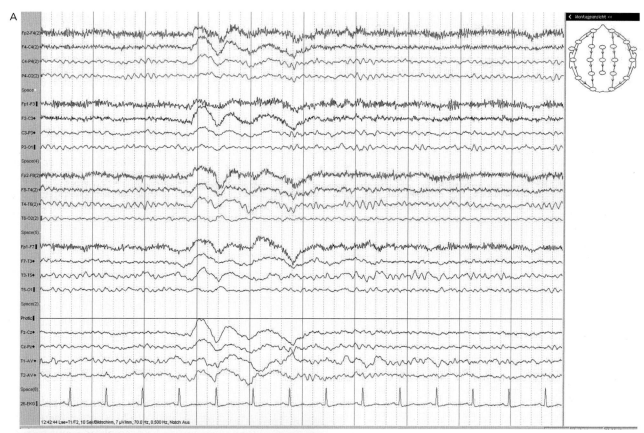

A

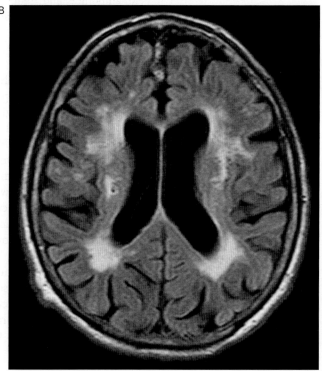

B

Figure 15.19. A 76-year-old female presented with fluctuating aphasia, hemianopia, and right hemiataxia. Symptoms lasted only a few hours. MRI revealed no acute infarction but signs of a chronic microangiopathic encephalopathy with multiple subcortical infarctions. EEG showed intermittent theta slowing in the left temporal region and FIRDA.

rhythm reacts to various stimuli, including intermittent photic stimulation that produces photic responses. Patients with bilateral pontine infarcts involving tegmentum show striking dissociation between clinical and EEG findings (77,83).

Despite coma and extensive bilateral motor deficits, EEGs may show activity of alpha frequency. However, this alpha activity fails to react to various stimuli such as intermittent photic stimulation; hence, it is abnormal. Because of the association

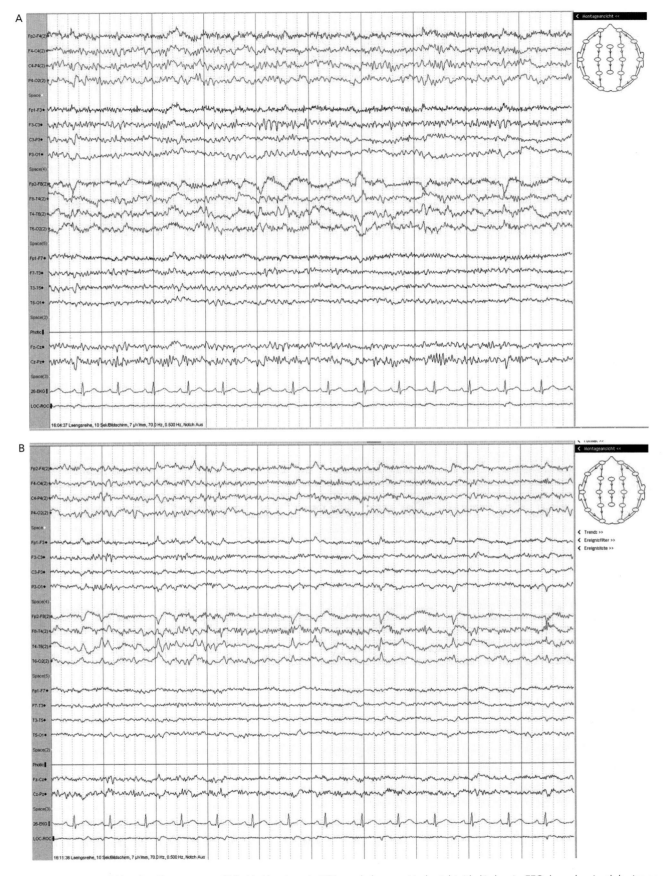

Figure 15.20. A 71-year-old female with acute onset of left-sided hemiparesis. MRI revealed paraventricular right-sided ischemia. EEG showed regional slowing on the right side, predominantly temporal. Here also periodic lateralized epileptiform discharges (LPDs) with maximum over T4 are noticed.

of coma and alpha activity, the term "alpha coma" has been applied to such patients (84). A similar association also occurs in patients rendered comatose by cardiopulmonary arrest (85) or drug overdose (86).

At more rostral level, infarcts of midbrain and diencephalon cause not only coma but also EEG alterations. Bilaterally synchronous and symmetrical theta–delta activity, sometimes maximal over frontal regions, replaces normal rhythms. Nevertheless, these relatively mild changes, compared with the depth of coma and extent of neurological deficits, should alert EEG readers to an intrinsic brainstem lesion. Thrombosis of the rostral portion of the basilar artery can also cause infarcts of occipital lobes. EEGs show posterior arrhythmic delta activity with loss of alpha rhythm, unilaterally or bilaterally.

2.1.6. Transient Ischemic Attacks

In some patients, a transient ischemic attack (TIA) presents with the symptomatology of limb shaking with brief, arrhythmic flailing or jerking movements of the arm or leg, which can be easily misdiagnosed as a seizure disorder. This is most common in those with watershed infarction. EEG testing is often ordered in a patient with limb-shaking TIA because of suspicion of seizures. Taghavy and Hamer (87) reviewed the records of patients with suspected TIAs over a period of 6 years. In 79 patients with clinical TIA, an EEG was performed, in 44.3% demonstrating focal abnormal electrical activity after recovery from TIA corresponding to the affected hemisphere. Only 17.7% of these patients also had an appropriate hypodensity in cranial CT scan. Failure to consider cerebral hypoperfusion as a potential cause of focal delta EEG slowing in the presence of normal structural imaging studies may contribute to delay in correct diagnosis.

Additionally, specific and nonspecific postictal EEG abnormalities were observed in the majority of inhibitory seizure patients, whereas the EEG was normal in more than 90% of TIA patients. Diffuse slowing and intermittent rhythmic delta activities were observed only in patients with seizures, not in TIA patients.

Early EEG should always be performed in patients with a transient episode of focal neurological disturbance, as abnormalities can indicate the possibility of a seizure, whereas in TIA a normal EEG should be expected (88).

2.1.7. Prognosis of Ischemic Stroke

Some authors believe that preservation of faster background activities, especially in subacute forms of middle cerebral artery (MCA) ischemia, is indicative of considerable neuronal survival in the infarcted zone and hence indicative of a good prognosis. Burghaus et al. (89) investigated the value of EEG within 24 hours after the onset of stroke in 25 patients suffering a large MCA infarction. Their findings indicated that the absence of delta activity and the presence of theta and fast beta frequencies within the focus predict a benign course, whereas diffuse generalized slowing and slow delta activity in the ischemic hemisphere may point toward a malignant course. Persistent focal changes paralleled persistent severe hemiparesis or hemiplegia (71). Therefore, EEG can deliver useful information to select those patients who develop malignant edema.

2.1.8. Prediction of Remote Seizures After Ischemic Stroke

Remote symptomatic seizures are defined as those occurring at least 7 days after stroke onset. The recurrence rate of remote seizures due to cerebral infarction is >60%, and many clinicians consider administering anticonvulsive treatment after the first remote seizure. The incidence of remote seizures after stroke of ~6% and the difficulties in reliably predicting these patients complicate the development of antiepileptogenic treatments.

Abnormalities on early EEG within the first 7 days after stroke facilitate the prediction of individuals likely to suffer late seizures. An abnormal EEG was the best predictor of remote seizures, even after correction for stroke severity and location (74). These patients commonly show nonspecific moderate to severe focal slowing on the initial EEG.

Epileptic discharges are uncommon in the overall group of stroke patients. However, if epileptic discharges and especially LPDs are recorded on the initial EEG, the vast majority of these individuals will suffer remote seizures (80). On the other hand, absence of epileptic discharges does not exclude the possibility of remote seizures. Three quarters of patients with poststroke epilepsy do not exhibit epileptic discharges in the acute phase, probably due to the slow process of epileptogenesis.

2.1.9. Sleep EEG After Hemispheric Stroke

Changes in sleep EEG patterns after hemispheric stroke have been described in studies for the last three decades (90,91). Müller et al. (91) found a lower sleep efficacy as well as lower amounts of slow-wave sleep and REM sleep in patients with acute hemispheric stroke. Gottselig et al. (90) documented a reduced spindle activity on the side of the lesion in patients with extrathalamic stroke. Sleep efficiency, preserved spindle activity, and amount of REM sleep in the acute phase of stroke have been shown to be associated with a favorable outcome (92,93).

The frequency of hypersomnia after stroke is essentially unknown but may be as high as 20% to 40% (94). The semiologic spectrum is wide and varies according to stroke topography (95). In deep (subcortical) hemispheric and particularly paramedian thalamic lesions, hypersomnia may correspond to a so-called presleep behavior, during which patients yawn, stretch, close their eyes, curl up, and assume a normal sleeping posture, while complaining of a constant sleep urge. Some of these patients can control this behavior when stimulated or given explicit, active tasks to perform. In some patients with deep frontal, thalamic, or midbrain lesions, hypersomnia evolves to extreme apathy with lack of spontaneity and initiative and poverty of movement, a condition for which the term "akinetic mutism" was coined. A continuum exists between hypersomnia, athymhormia, akinetic mutism, and fatigue. In some patients, episodes of hypersomnia, mutism, and akinesia alternate with episodes of insomnia, psychomotor agitation, or confusional state.

The most striking example of increased sleep is seen in patients with bilateral paramedian thalamic stroke. Arpa et al. (96) described a 44-year-old man with right lateral-tegmental pontine hematoma and severe hypersomnia, in whom long-term EEG monitoring showed increased amounts of sleep ranging from 11 to 15 hours per day during the first 3 months after stroke. The relative amounts of slow-wave sleep (4–11% of total sleep time) and REM sleep (8–10%) were slightly above normal values. Bastiju et al. (97) described a patient with severe hypersomnia due to bilateral thalamomesencephalic stroke with an initial sleep behavior over 18 hours per day. Eight months after stroke, hypersomnia had regressed clinically to about 12 hours per day. By EEG criteria, sleep was similarly present over about 12 hours per day, with an increase in both slow-wave sleep (30% of total sleep) and REM sleep (22%).

2.1.10. POSTSTROKE RECOVERY AND EEG MAPPING

Brain mapping techniques have proven to be vital in understanding the molecular, cellular, and functional mechanisms of recovery after stroke (98). Magnetoencephalography (MEG) and EEG techniques work in a completely different manner than the image of blood flow–based brain mapping methods. MEG and EEG detect signals that arise predominantly from the dendritic fields of cortical pyramidal neurons. They detect these signals from a large area on the order of several square centimeters. With EEG, the tissue between the scalp electrode and the cortex attenuates the strength of the signal and the signal strength decreases with the square of the distance between them. Because tissues do not affect the MEG signal, MEG typically enables better signal source localization than EEG, but the magnetic fluctuations drop off as the cube of the distance between the source and the detector increases. EEG and MEG techniques may use an event-based approach to identify the characteristics of brain activity in response to specific behaviors. Strens et al. (99) found that the degree of signal synchrony was greater between medial and lateral motor areas in stroke patients than in healthy subjects but reduced with recovery. In another study, the degree of reduction in delta-wave signals from perilesional brain tissue correlated with the amount of language recovery following rehabilitation (100). The drawback of the EEG method clearly is the lack of anatomical information.

A number of recent studies report that quantitative EEG measures of cerebral pathophysiology in acute or subacute stroke might augment future prognoses regarding patient outcomes (101,102). Finnigan et al. (102) reported that quantitative EEG (qEEG) delta power measures in acute stroke and delta/alpha power ratio measures in subacute stroke are both highly correlated with ischemic stroke patients' outcomes assessed via the National Institute of Health Stroke Scale (NIHSS). qEEG measures were averaged over all scalp electrodes, and further a significant correlation between subacute delta/alpha power ratio and outcome measures was obtained when the former was computed from a standard, 19-channel array. Moreover, multinomial logistic regression analyses revealed that this qEEG per se enhanced the sensitivity and specificity of outcome prediction beyond that afforded by subacute lesion volume defined via perfusion-weighted MRI. These outcomes are consistent with qEEG and observations by other authors acquired from acute ischemic stroke patients, including those who died in the ensuing days. There seems to be a prognostic value of poststroke shift of scalp delta power maxima from the ipsilateral to the contralateral hemisphere indicating substantial worsening of cerebral pathophysiology (101). A standard 19-electrode array appears adequate for the detection of this marker, and routine use of a standard electrode assay with fewer electrodes renders bedside EEG monitoring more feasible than does a high-density array. The potential limitations of such EEG monitoring are possible contamination of qEEG indices by artifacts such as those due to patient movement and/or by sleep- or drowsiness-related EEG activity. qEEG measures, computed promptly, perhaps automatically, might help guide future clinical therapeutic decisions. In patients with large MCA infarctions, where decompressive surgery is being contemplated, such qEEG observations, in concert with other investigations like MRI, may assist in more timely decisions to operate.

Recovery from stroke can vary greatly among patients even though they may have identical clinical symptoms. Several attempts have been made to determine neuroplastic changes on the basis of EEGs, which are readily available in clinical settings. In many studies, movement-related potentials (MRPs) were studied in connection with stroke rehabilitation. MRPs constitute a waveform that is obtained by taking the "average" EEG, in terms of onset of movement or myoelectrical activity of the prime mover (103). Many studies demonstrated topographical alterations of some MRP components during the recovery period after a stroke (104,105). The analysis of MRP, however, presents methodological difficulties because of its low signal-to-noise ratio. Adequate recording of MRP requires careful repetition of many trials in which the electromyographic envelope of the investigated prime mover is similar, and subjects need to be trained to perform similar movements. These practical issues led Eder et al. (106) to consider more stable EEG phenomena as criteria to mark stroke recovery. Some prior findings indicate that event-related desynchronization (ERD) might achieve this purpose. The ERD of the central mu-rhythm was studied extensively in normal subjects (107). Subsequent normative studies have outlined that the symmetry of the mu-rhythm amplitude had, in comparison with ERD, a greater power to discriminate between normal subjects and stroke patients (108). Results of more recent studies point to the existence of two relatively independent ERD generating systems within the central region of each hemisphere with beta rebound following movement, also referred to as postmovement beta event–related synchronization (PMBS) (109). These beta oscillations are dominant on the contralateral side of movement and are found in the first second after termination of movement. Several studies showed that lateralization of PMBS depended on factors such as handedness, age, and pathologic conditions (e.g., Parkinson's disease (110)). Eder et al. (106) introduced a paradigm for detecting and mapping PMBS for loosely defined movements of the upper extremities on a drawing board, which was tested in eight acute stroke patients with mild hemiparesis and eight normal subjects. Follow-up testing was conducted 3 months after the initial recordings. Their results confirmed reproducibility of PMBS patterns in normal subjects since the replication of the recording has only a negligible effect on the lateralization. The side of hemiparesis in acute stroke patients could be distinguished on the basis of quantitative measure of lateralization. The follow-up testing in three recovered stroke patients revealed a trend of changes in the lateralization toward the contralateral side of movement, an indication that this technique is an option for evaluating therapy-induced changes in cortical movement organization (106).

2.2. Hemorrhagic Stroke

2.2.1. INTRACRANIAL BLEEDING
It is likely that subclinical seizures occur after intracranial hemorrhage. Subclinical seizure activity has gained attention from an increased understanding of the potential harmful effects of clinical seizure activity (111). Claassen et al. (112) performed a retrospective study on 102 consecutive patients with intracerebral hemorrhage who underwent cEEG monitoring. Convulsive seizures occurred in 19%, another 13% of patients had subclinical, purely EEG seizures, and 5% had both EEG and clinical seizures. They found an increased risk of seizures if the hemorrhage reached the cortex or if it expanded by 30% in the first 24 hours. Periodic epileptiform discharges were more frequently seen in hemorrhages closer to the cortex. Midline shift and poor outcome were not more frequent in patients with seizures when compared with those without seizures. By contrast, periodic discharges were independently associated with poor outcome. There was a trend toward worse outcome for patients with EEG seizures, but seizures did not remain a predictor in multivariate analysis. Among those who had seizures during monitoring, 94% of seizures were detected within the first 72 hours. This implies that routinely providing cEEG monitoring for 3 days would frequently detect subclinical seizures; however, the retrospective nature of this study limited it to those 13% of all intracranial hemorrhage admissions for whom cEEG was requested (111). There may have been a selection bias toward those in whom there was some reason to suspect seizure activity. In another prospective study, seizures occurred in 28% of patients after intracerebral hemorrhage, suggesting that they are frequent (113). The true incidence of subclinical seizures after intracerebral hemorrhage awaits a prospective consecutive case series of cEEG monitoring. It could be clinically important to find subclinical seizures if they increase mortality or cause neuronal injury, but Claassen et al. (112) have not found seizures to be associated with poor outcome.

2.2.2. THALAMIC AND BRAINSTEM HEMORRHAGE
Thalamic bleeding usually causes temporary loss of consciousness. Larger hemorrhages may give rise to ipsilateral delta activity (Fig. 15.21). According to Jasper and Van Buren (114), there is a reduction of alpha rhythm in the case of anteroventral thalamic damage. Alpha enhancement may be noted in patients with posterior thalamic lesions. Lack of sleep spindles has also been reported (115).

Mesencephalic bleeding without extension into the pons is most likely to give rise to Parinaud syndrome, a dorsal midbrain syndrome associated with vertical gaze palsy, pupillary signs, and nystagmus. The EEG often shows diffuse activity in the upper theta range.

Patients with lower brainstem hemorrhage may show the striking finding of a well-preserved posterior alpha rhythm that cannot be blocked by various modalities of stimuli (116), but in exceptional cases, the reactivity of the alpha rhythm may persist (117). Other patients show diffuse low-voltage tracings as seen in cases of lower brainstem infarction.

2.2.3. CEREBELLAR HEMORRHAGE
Acute cerebellar hemorrhage rapidly leads to coma after a few minutes of headaches, dizziness, or vertigo. Cerebellar edema rapidly produces a pressure cone (tonsillar herniation) with fatal outcome. The rapidity of the evolution usually precludes EEG studies. A remarkable study of 22 cases was carried out by Rasheva et al. (118); it demonstrated high-voltage delta activity, more over the contralateral cerebral hemisphere. In patients with cerebellar stroke, movement-related cortical potentials were found to be depressed (119).

2.2.4. SUBARACHNOID HEMORRHAGE
The EEG shows diffuse changes, disorganization, disruption of the posterior alpha rhythm, and excessive slow activity. Occasionally, lateralization of slow activity may be indicative of the primarily involved hemisphere (120,121). With total dependence on arteriographic demonstration of the causative lesion and partial dependence on refined CT scan methods, there is no practical need for an EEG in the search for the correct localization. The EEG, however, remains a valuable indicator of the general state of cerebral functioning (122,123).

Subarachnoid hemorrhage is commonly followed by vasospasms. These can cause delayed cerebral ischemia as a severe complication of subarachnoid bleeding. Early identification of ischemia could trigger treatments to increase blood flow and to reduce cerebral damage. cEEG monitoring in the ICU was used to detect vasospasms. However, typically changes associated with vasospasm are only mild, consisting of a decrease in the relative variability of the alpha rhythm (124). Only massive vasospasm would cause marked delta foci.

These slight changes can be reliably identified with quantitative cEEG monitoring. Claassen et al. showed that a decrease in the alpha/delta ratio can consistently predict vasospasms (125). These changes might be demonstrated even before clinical deterioration occurs, facilitating early therapeutic interventions (122). The accuracy can be further improved when intracortical EEG recordings are used (126). In survivors of subarachnoid hemorrhages from aneurysms, epileptic seizures have been found in 12.5% (127); marked EEG changes with spikes can also be found. Scott and Cabral (128) stressed the frequent occurrence of epileptic seizures following intracranial aneurysm surgery (clipping, wrapping). Arteriovenous malformations are the cause of subarachnoid hemorrhages that are much less severe and life-threatening than is bleeding from a ruptured aneurysm. These malformations may also give rise to focal seizures. The EEG of these patients has been consistently described as abnormal (129). However, the interpretation of the abnormalities is beset with difficulties because a sizable number of cases may show a lateralization to the contralateral hemisphere (130–132).

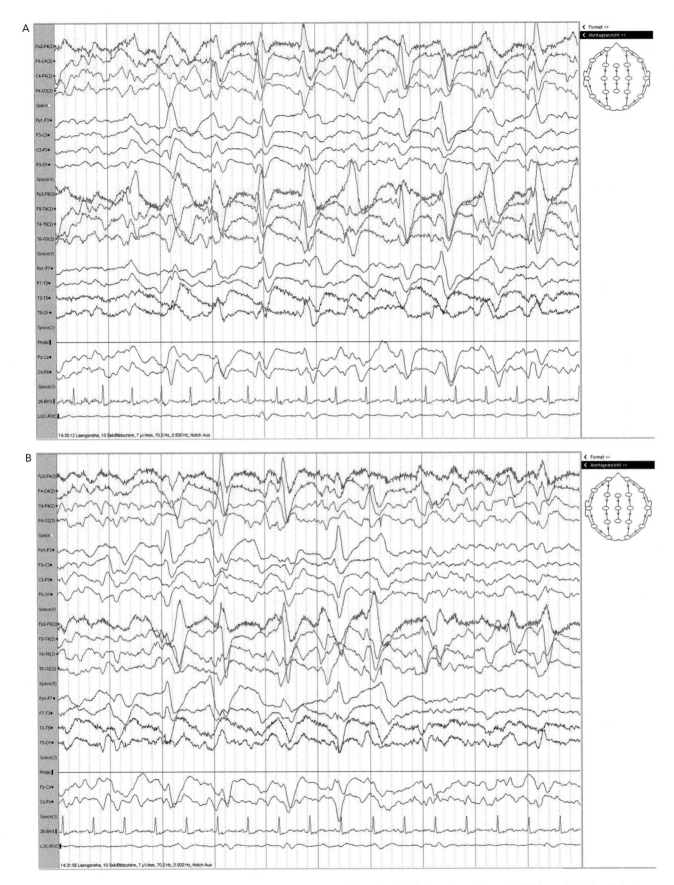

Figure 15.21. A 71-year-old female with acute loss of consciousness. CT scan revealed a right-sided thalamic hemorrhage. **A:** EEG showed right hemispheric rhythmic bi- and triphasic waves also showing on the left, but not synchronously. **B:** After 4 days there was only slight improvement of EEG changes.

2.3. Other Types of Vascular Disease

2.3.1. CEREBRAL VENOUS THROMBOSIS

Cerebral venous thrombosis is an uncommon stroke syndrome accounting for <1% of all strokes. Obstruction of a cerebral sinus or vein can lead to hemorrhage or venous ischemia and is associated with intracranial hypertension, headache, and epileptic seizures. Rapid diagnosis is important to establish effective treatment, since anticoagulation might reduce the risk of poor outcome and disability (133).

At least two thirds of patients with cerebral venous thrombosis will have an abnormal EEG (134). EEG changes might be even more common in children and neonates (135). Abnormal findings are more common in patients with focal signs (70%) than in those with isolated intracranial hypertension (50%). The most common finding is diffuse slowing that can be present despite focal signs. The slowing can be very pronounced with widespread prominent delta activity. These patients are not necessarily in a state of impaired consciousness but show marked changes of higher cortical functions, such as aphasia, mutism, or apraxia. Focal slowing is less common and might be superimposed on the diffuse changes. Epileptic activity can be observed in a third of patients with slow activity.

2.3.2. HYPERTENSIVE ENCEPHALOPATHY

In this condition, severe arterial hypertension gives rise to cerebral edematous changes and hence to signs of intracranial hypertension. The EEG may show surprisingly little in this serious disorder. There is reason to presume that the neuronal oxygenation does not reach critically low values despite the fact that the cerebral blood flow is diminished in this condition. In the case of epileptic convulsions, EEG changes are usually limited to the period immediately before, during, and after the attacks. This is similar to the acute encephalopathy of eclampsia gravidarum, where EEG abnormalities are barely detectable in the preeclamptic state and are practically limited to the grand mal convulsions themselves.

However, there have been reports of very pronounced EEG abnormalities in hypertensive encephalopathy. Aguglia et al. (136) described severe parieto-occipital changes with prominent paroxysmal features. After acute onset of hypertensive encephalopathy (blood pressure 300/140 and age 70), Benna et al. (137) observed generalized spikes and polyspikes followed by a slow wave. With gradual improvement of hypertension, the paroxysmal pattern lingered.

2.3.3. MOYAMOYA DISEASE

According to Aoki et al. (138), a reappearance of the hyperventilation-induced buildup of slow activity ~20 to 60 sec after the activation is a typical finding in Moyamoya disease. This phenomenon has been studied more extensively by Ohyama et al. (139). Hyperventilation as a routine procedure in clinical EEG can activate otherwise latent EEG abnormalities in patients with cerebrovascular disorders. It is probably the hypoxic effect of hyperventilation that produces these changes.

2.3.4. ACQUIRED HEART DISEASE

CNS complications of acute or subacute bacterial endocarditis are essentially infectious diseases and are discussed under that heading. In cardiac decompensation, a variety of causes and mechanisms eventually leads to cerebral hypoxia with slowing and terminal flattening of the EEG (140). EEG abnormalities are common in chronic bronchopneumopathy with cor pulmonale. These changes may (141) or may not parallel the degree of impaired consciousness (142). Paroxysmal tachycardia may be associated with transient EEG abnormalities (143,144), especially when the attack leads to impairment of consciousness. The Adams–Stokes syndrome is usually associated with a permanent heart block and a very slow pulse rate. The electroencephalographer is advised to use electrocardiographic monitoring throughout the recording. During the attack, slow activity appears after a few seconds of asystolia with progressive amplitude of delta waves.

2.3.5. SYNCOPE

Syncope is defined as transient loss of consciousness and of postural control due to transient cerebral hypoperfusion. Clinically, it can be difficult to differentiate syncope from an epileptic seizure. In rare cases, there is an interaction between syncopal and epileptic mechanisms within a single attack. In certain forms of epileptic seizures, especially in complex partial seizures of temporal lobe origin, cardiac arrhythmias can arise, which can then lead to syncope. Conversely, on rare occasions epileptic seizures can emerge from syncope. If the medical history suggests epileptic and syncopal phenomena within the same attack, the diagnosis can only be made by means of ictal EEG and electrocardiographic recordings. Commonly, patients with a syncope demonstrate a few clonic movements, known as convulsive syncope, not to be mistaken for an epileptic seizure.

The EEG during syncope shows generalized high-amplitude slow-wave activity at the onset of unconsciousness, followed by flattening of the EEG, and subsequently slow waves again before the normal background activity returns. This sequence is independent of the mechanism of syncope and of the clinical presentation as convulsive or nonconvulsive syncope as it represents the common final path in terms of global cerebral hypoxia.

The significance of EEG in the diagnosis of syncope is often overestimated. It could be shown that in unselected patients with syncope, the recording of a postictal EEG was not helpful. Epileptiform patterns in an interictal EEG recording can indeed corroborate a diagnosis of epilepsy. However, additional syncopal attacks are not excluded. On the other hand, even in chronic epilepsy epileptiform patterns can be absent during interictal EEG recordings, thus also preventing a definite classification of the attacks. Also, episodic seizures induced by alcohol or benzodiazepine withdrawal are usually not associated with epileptiform patterns in the interictal EEG. Therefore, EEG recordings are not really helpful in differentiating syncope from an epileptic seizure and are not recommended as standard tests after syncope; rather, they should be reserved for patients with a positive history for epileptic seizures.

3. TRAUMATIC BRAIN INJURY

Craniocerebral trauma raises the important question of the degree of cerebral disturbance and its prognosis. This issue is particularly relevant after moderate to severe brain injury with prolonged unconsciousness and signs of brainstem dysfunction. The clinical parameter of the grade of disintegration of brain function and impairment of the brainstem is demonstrated through neurological examination by the development of an acute secondary midbrain and bulbar brain syndrome. In addition, brain imaging easily identifies space-occupying lesions and sometimes demonstrates the displacement of the brainstem. These methods, however, fail to give any information about cerebral activity. Therefore, the EEG is important in the diagnosis of traumatic cerebral lesions, especially in the assessment of the degree of cortical activity, which shows reasonably good correlation with the depth of posttraumatic coma (145–148). An EEG evaluation also gives information about the prognosis of cerebral dysfunction.

Chronic stages of traumatic brain injury demonstrate a diminished correlation between the EEG and neurological findings (149). However, there is an approximate correlation between the EEG and clinical improvement, especially in patients who have had systematic follow-up studies of EEG and clinical examination (150,151). Occasionally, the EEG may return to normal when neurological or psychiatric abnormalities persist, a disparity that indicates a bad prognosis (152). By contrast, in some patients with normal clinical findings, an abnormal EEG may be the forerunner of an intracranial complication such as posttraumatic epilepsy.

3.1. Mild Traumatic Brain Injury

In mild diffuse traumatic brain injury, there may be no or only mild disturbances of consciousness (Glasgow Coma Scale [GCS] score of 13–15), with no persisting signs of primary or secondary brainstem dysfunction (Table 15.1). The vast majority of patients fall under this category.

Typically, the EEG shows only mild and transient abnormalities, and these are more common if the recordings are performed shortly after the injury. EEGs obtained within 30 minutes of the trauma commonly demonstrate diffuse slowing or slight disorganization of the background (153,154). Epileptic activity can be recorded only rarely and is mostly transient (155). This is supported by animal studies showing that epileptic abnormalities subsided within 30 seconds of the injury (156).

TABLE 15.1. Severity of Traumatic Brain Injury

	GLASGOW COMA SCALE	POSTTRAUMATIC AMNESIA	LOSS OF CONSCIOUSNESS
Mild	13–15	<1 day	0–30 minutes
Moderate	9–12	>1 to <7 days	>30 minutes to <24 hours
Severe	3–8	>7 days	>24 hours

In clinical practice, most of the EEGs in mild traumatic brain injury are recorded at least several hours or days after the injury. Recordings done within the first 24 hours are likely to be normal in the vast majority of cases (153,157,158). Some slight abnormalities can be found; a generalized slowing of the alpha rhythm is most common (159). This is particularly frequent in individuals with prolonged loss of consciousness of at least 2 minutes (160).

The decrease in background frequency can be so discrete (only 1–2 Hz) that it would still fall into the alpha range and would not be detected on single EEG recordings. Such minor abnormalities can only be noted in comparison with retrospective or subsequent EEGs. qEEG can be helpful if only a single record is available. An increased theta–alpha ratio of 0.8 in the initial phase after the trauma has been demonstrated (161,162).

Serial EEG studies have consistently shown that EEG abnormalities after mild trauma are highly dynamic and mostly transient. Whereas 82% of EEGs were abnormal within the first 24 hours, only 50% were abnormal 3 weeks after injury, and only 32% were abnormal 8 weeks after injury (162). The theta–alpha ratio on qEEG improves after only 10 days, with complete normalization by 6 weeks (161). This is accompanied by an increase of the mean alpha frequency from 9.3 Hz to 10 Hz within the first 2 months (162).

The mildest disturbance of consciousness seen after craniocerebral trauma is drowsiness and hypersomnia, which are accompanied by the EEG findings of normal sleep (163). There are usually generalized slowing of all frequencies and altered sleep patterns in patients with barely existent periods of wakefulness. Sensory stimulation will block the slowing and sleep.

The vast majority of patients with an abnormal neurological examination will also have an abnormal EEG (164). On the other hand, only 58% of individuals with EEG abnormalities will demonstrate an abnormal clinical status (165). In some cases, there can be marked discrepancies between EEG patterns and clinical findings. A normal neurological status in a patient with no or little complaint may be accompanied by impressively abnormal EEGs (Figs. 15.22 and 15.23). These findings indicate that the EEG might be more sensitive to subtle functional changes than clinical examination alone (155). Nevertheless, these abnormalities are nonspecific and do not correlate well with long-term symptoms (166).

Particularly pronounced discrepancies between electrical cortical activity and the clinical state may be found in children (167,168). Children may show high-amplitude generalized delta activity for weeks or months even in the presence of normal consciousness after a mild brain trauma (163). Immaturity might enhance functional posttraumatic disturbances and produce focal or generalized EEG abnormalities. On the other hand, focal changes have been thought to be a sign of significant brain damage (169).

3.2. Moderate to Severe Traumatic Brain Injury

Moderate traumatic brain injury is usually associated with loss of consciousness for 30 minutes to 24 hours, posttraumatic

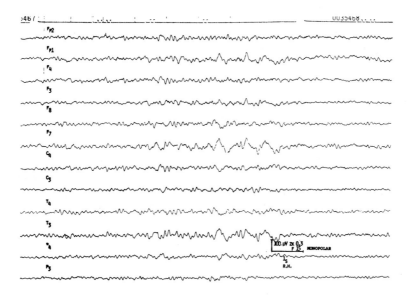

Figure 15.22. EEG from a 35-year-old man reporting vertigo after mild cerebral contusion. At the time of EEG recording he had normal neurological status and a normal CT scan. Intermittent slow activity (theta and delta) in left frontotemporal region was seen.

amnesia for at least 1 day, and a GCS score of 9 to 12 (see Table 15.1). Severe traumatic brain injury is defined as loss of consciousness for at least 24 hours, posttraumatic amnesia for at least 7 days, and a GCS of 3 to 8. EEG abnormalities are much more common in moderate to severe traumatic brain injury. These consist of a variable amount of generalized slowing, focal slowing, and epileptic abnormalities. Generalized slowing is associated with the degree of brainstem injury. Brainstem injuries can be divided into direct (caused by the trauma itself) and indirect (secondary to brainstem compression due to cerebral swelling). Direct brainstem lesions can affect the EEG instantaneously, whereas indirect brainstem injuries demonstrate a typical delayed deterioration. The degree of slowing can range from mild slowing to an isoelectric EEG, depending on the depth of coma.

Focal slowing is usually caused by circumscribed cerebral injuries. Most common are intracranial hematomas that demonstrate slowing in the delta range. The EEG can be abnormal even in the absence of clinical signs. On the other hand, these focal changes might not be evident if there is pronounced generalized slowing. However, they become more prominent when generalized slowing improves.

3.3. Posttraumatic Coma

3.3.1. CLASSIFICATION OF COMA

Loss of consciousness implies that the patient has suffered widespread dysfunction of either both cerebral hemispheres or the brainstem. A diffuse swelling of the brain or bilateral hemispheric lesions lead to a symmetric displacement through

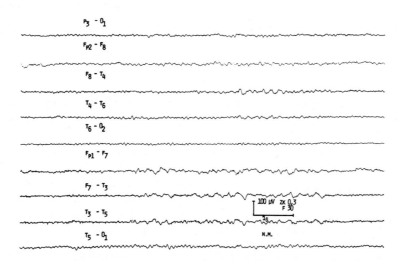

Figure 15.23. EEG from a 45-year-old woman after mild cerebral contusion without signs of brainstem impairment. She had some complaints of vertigo. At the time of EEG recording, she had normal neurological and CT scan findings. Intermittent left temporal theta focus. The recovery of EEG abnormalities follows the same pattern as in adults (23). In children with transient cortical blindness following mild head trauma, posterior slowing with subsequent fast normalization can be observed (124). Lateralized signs consist mainly of focal slow waves in the theta and delta range (17,19,23,32), whereas the other cerebral regions show only minor changes (125). A close correlation with neurological deficits is seen within the first months (17,19,20,126).

the tentorial notch (central tentorial herniation). If downward displacement continues, the contents of the posterior fossa will finally be pressed through the foramen magnum. This brain shift evokes a characteristic sequence of clinical signs (Table 15.2). According to Gerstenbrand and Lücking (170), these signs can be broken down into six stages—four stages of midbrain syndrome (MBS) and two stages of bulbar brain syndrome (BBS). MBS 1 and MBS 2 correspond to the early diencephalic stage, MBS 3 corresponds to the late diencephalic stage, and MBS 4 corresponds to the midbrain-upper pons stage. BBS 1 corresponds to the lower pontine-upper medullary stage and BBS 2 to the medullary stage.

In cases with expanding lesions in the lateral middle fossa or temporal lobe, the medial edges of the uncus and hippocampal gyrus are commonly pushed toward the midline and over the free lateral edge of the tentorium, compressing the third cranial nerve (early uncal herniation). During uncal herniation, a unilateral dilated pupil is the most consistent finding (171).

Neurological signs different from this expected rostrocaudal deterioration are found in cases of primary brainstem injury (172)—in other words, the relatively intact oculomotor functions are in contrast to decerebrate posturing and respiratory abnormalities. Brain imaging is diagnostic in these cases.

3.3.2. EEG and Stages of Coma

According to the clinical deterioration (see Table 15.2), the EEG also exhibits a typical pattern that can be divided into five grades (146):

- Grade 1: predominant alpha and little theta activity
- Grade 2: predominant theta and little delta activity
- Grade 3: predominant high-voltage rhythmic and arrhythmic delta and subdelta activity
- Grade 4: diffuse, mostly low-voltage delta and subdelta activity and low-voltage activity only recognizable with increased amplification (3.5 V/mm)
- Grade 5: isoelectric record.

As a rule, progressive stages of coma exhibit an increasing amount of background slowing. Alpha and theta rhythms gradually disappear in MBS 1 and MBS 2, whereas MBS 3 and MBS 4 and BBS 1 contain almost exclusively delta and subdelta activity. The EEG in BBS 2 is isoelectric (146). With increasing coma stage, the number of different EEG patterns is reduced. MBS 2 exhibits the highest variety, whereas BBS 1 and BBS 2 show the lowest variety (Fig. 15.24).

In accordance with the mild cortical disturbance, the EEG is only moderately abnormal in MBS 1. The background rhythm can display anything from alpha waves to diffuse delta activity. Stimuli to diencephalic or rostromesencephalic structures may induce delta bursts or short runs of delta waves. Local slow activity can be seen only in an otherwise mildly abnormal EEG, while increasing diffuse slowing may overwhelm local abnormalities (173). Borderline EEG patterns occur at MBS 1 but not in deeper stages of MBS.

In MBS 2, the amount of slow activity increases. This increasing abnormality may be due to a direct cortical disturbance or to a more remote effect from deeper structures (174). However, typical sleep potentials indicate a relatively intact cortex (Figs. 15.25 and 15.26) (145). Increasing rostrocaudal deterioration is further characterized by the increased change of typical or atypical sleep potentials (145) and the shift of superimposed fast activity, diffusely spread in lighter stages of MBS, to the frontal regions (175).

In MBS 3, a clear reduction in the number of EEG patterns is noted. A decrease of spontaneous alternating patterns and typical sleep potentials has been thought to indicate an

TABLE 15.2. Clinical Signs in Posttraumatic Patients at the Different Stages of the Midbrain Syndrome (MBS) and Bulbar Brain Syndrome (BBS)

	MBS 1	MBS 2	MBS 3	MBS 4	BBS 1	BBS 2
Spontaneous limb postures	Nonstereotyped movements in the arms and legs	Nonstereotyped movements in arms and legs Extension of the legs	Decorticate posturing (upper extremities flexed, lower extremities extended)	Decerebrate posturing (upper and lower extremities extended)	Flaccidity	Flaccidity
Motor response to pain	Nonstereotyped withdrawal of the limbs	Nonstereotyped withdrawal of the arms	Decorticate response Extensor response of the legs	Decerebrate response	Decerebrate response No response	
Eye position	Roving movements	Roving, more irregular	Immobile, straight ahead	Immobile, divergent	Immobile, divergent	Immobile, divergent
Pupil size	Normal	Normal or Small	Small	Enlarged	Large	Large
Pupil reaction	Reacting	Reacting	Small range of contraction	Small range of contraction	Unreacting	Unreacting
Respiration pattern	Normal	Cheyne-Stokes	Cheyne-Stokes Rapid regular hyperventilation	Regular hyperventilation	Ataxic	No respiration

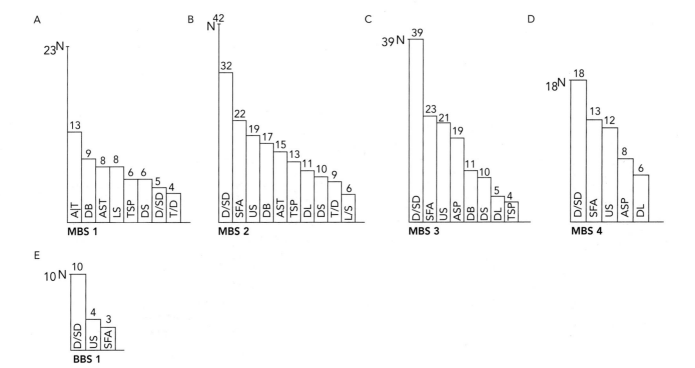

Figure 15.24. *EEG patterns at different stages of acute traumatic secondary midbrain and bulbar brain syndrome. Note the reduction in the variety of EEG patterns in the course of increasing rostrocaudal deterioration. At bulbar brain syndrome stage 2, the EEG is isoelectric. The records were listed under one or more of the following categories: A/T, predominant alpha and little theta activity; T/D, predominant theta and little delta activity; D/SD, predominant diffuse rhythmic and arrhythmic delta and subdelta activity; DB, delta bursts; DS, short runs of delta; DL, long runs of delta; TSP, typical sleep potentials; ASP, atypical sleep potentials; S, spindles; LS, local slowing; US, unilateral predominant slowing; SFA, superimposed fast activity; MBS, midbrain syndrome; BBS, bulbar brain syndrome; N, number of records. (From Rumpl E. Elektro-neurologische Korrelationen in den frühen Phasen des posttraumatischen Komas. I. Das EEG in den verschiedenen Phasen des akuten traumatischen sekundären. Mittelhirn und Bulbärhirnsyndroms. Z. EEG-EMG. 1979;10:148–157; and Rumpl E, Lorenzi E, Hackl JM, et al. The EEG at different stages of acute secondary traumatic mid-brain and bulbar brain syndromes. Electroencephalogr Clin Neurophysiol. 1979;46:487–497, somewhat modified.)*

increasing disturbance of the diencephalic and mesencephalic systems (147).

The EEG patterns are still more simplified in MBS 4 and BBS 1. The absence, reduction, and deterioration of sleep potentials or alternating patterns are suggestive of marked damage at the diencephalic level (176). In BBS 1, low-voltage delta and sub-delta activity appears, followed by low-voltage cerebral activity, often recognizable only with increased amplification.

No electrical cerebral activity can be observed in patients with BBS 2 (146). Patients with an isoelectric EEG or an EEG with repeated isoelectric periods have a very poor prognosis and high mortality (177).

3.3.3. Other EEG Patterns in Posttraumatic Coma

The reaction to external stimuli further characterizes the depth of coma. In MBS 1, sensory stimulation may briefly block the slow activity; sleep, easily recognizable at this stage, may have a similar effect (Fig. 15.27) (163). In further stages of MBS, reactivity consists of widespread delta activity, alternating patterns, and typical or atypical sleep potentials (Fig. 15.28). In BBS 1 and BBS 2, no reactivity can be observed. Reactivity may be immediate or delayed. Delayed reactivity is a slow EEG response inducing a new pattern under the influence of repetitive stimulation. Fischgold and Mathis (178) emphasize the usefulness of auditory and painful stimuli in contrast to

the insignificant effect of visual stimulation. In lighter stages of coma, stimulation may also provoke extracerebral changes such as muscle activity and respiratory artifacts.

Unreactive alpha activity or "alpha-like" rhythms, also termed alpha-coma, are usually seen in patients with extended anoxic damage to both cerebral hemispheres and are associated with a poor prognosis (179). These patterns are infrequent after traumatic supratentorial lesions causing secondary brain-stem involvement. On the other hand, patients with caudal posttraumatic brainstem lesions may have nonreactive alpha activity even in an unresponsive decerebrate state (77). Sleep spindles, vertex sharp waves, and K-complexes suggest in these cases that the lesion is below the still-intact thalamocortical system (114). Rhythmic coma in children, especially in the alpha frequency range, generally has a better prognosis than in adults (180).

Generalized burst-suppression occurs in posttraumatic coma only when cerebral anoxia was sustained with the trauma (163,175). Intersuppression activity between bursts frequently shows delta waves and intermittent spikes. This type of activity carries a poor prognosis because it indicates a diffuse anoxic encephalopathy that interferes with the original traumatic brain damage. In contrast, an overdose of soporific drugs tends to produce uniform intersuppression activity and has a good prognosis (163).

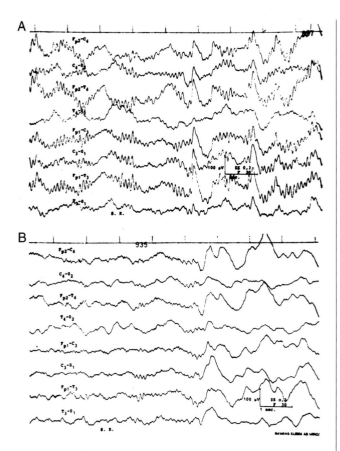

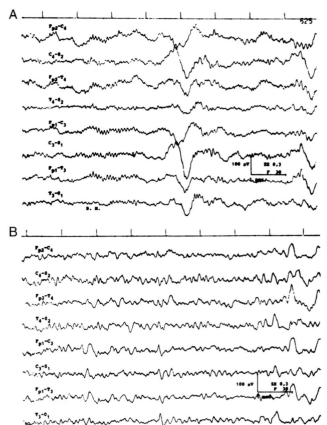

Figure 15.25. *A: EEG from a 23-year-old man in acute coma due to secondary brainstem dysfunction (classical midbrain syndrome stage 2 without lateralization). Easily recognizable typical spindles, symmetrical over both hemispheres, are accompanied by K-complexes and diffuse slowing. CT scan shows moderate brain edema with scattered contusional areas in left frontoparietal and right temporal regions. There are no signs of compression at the tentorial level. There is blood within the interhemispheric fissure. B: EEG from the same patient in prolonged coma. No spindles, superimposed fast activity, and change to high-voltage short- and long-delta runs (alternating pattern). There are no lateralizing signs in the EEG. Outcome was good recovery. (From Rumpl E, Prugger M, Bauer G, et al. Incidence and prognostic value of spindles in post-traumatic coma. Electroencephalogr Clin Neurophysiol. 1983;56(5):420–429.)*

Figure 15.26. *A: EEG from a 20-year-old man in acute coma due to primary brainstem injury. Neurological signs of atypical midbrain syndrome stage 4 (decerebrate posture). Typical spindles, delta bursts, and superimposed fast activity accompanied by diffuse slowing. CT scan was normal. B: EEG from the same patient in prolonged coma. Predominant alpha/theta activity, several delta waves, reactivity in form of blocking slow waves, and no lateralizing EEG signs. Characteristic EEG pattern for pontine lesions. Outcome was good recovery. (From Rumpl E, Prugger M, Bauer G, et al. Incidence and prognostic value of spindles in post-traumatic coma. Electroencephalogr Clin Neurophysiol. 1983;56:420–429.)*

LPDs are rare events in posttraumatic coma; they are usually seen in cases of subdural hematoma (181). More frequent LPDs are seen in patients with acute unilateral lesions of vascular origin (182,183). Triphasic waves may also be produced by subdural hematoma, but they are more characteristic of metabolic disturbances (184), especially when no asymmetry can be detected.

3.3.4. EEG and Outcome of Coma

Favorable prognosis is associated with preserved reactivity, typical sleep potentials, and absence of seizures. Reactivity is usually assessed with auditory and painful stimuli and can exhibit an activating (occurrence of slow waves) or blocking (flattening of EEG) pattern. More than 90% of patients with intact reactivity have a good prognosis and will regain consciousness within 1.5 years (185). Reactivity might be suppressed by sedatives, so absent reactivity does not necessarily imply poor prognosis. However, certain nonreactive EEG

patterns (i.e., alpha-coma and theta-coma) are associated with anoxic brain damage or direct brainstem damage and have a poor prognosis.

Typical sleep spindles are more common in patients with good recovery. The emergence of atypical or asymmetric spindles correlates with worse outcome (see Figs. 15.25 and 15.26). The observation of spindles largely depends on the time of the EEG recording. Variations of the timing of EEG recordings account for the incidence of spindles varying between 14% and 67% in different reports (186). Within 2 days after brain injury, the vast majority of EEGs showed spindles (186).

The appearance of EEG sleep patterns and circadian EEG variations is a favorable prognostic sign (187). Completely organized sleep patterns or increasing organization of nocturnal sleep in successive recordings indicates a more favorable outcome than the absence of such patterns. The occurrence of REM sleep is especially significant in this regard. This finding may be supported by reports of the reappearance of slow-wave sleep with continued absence of the REM phase in patients who never regained consciousness after brainstem vascular

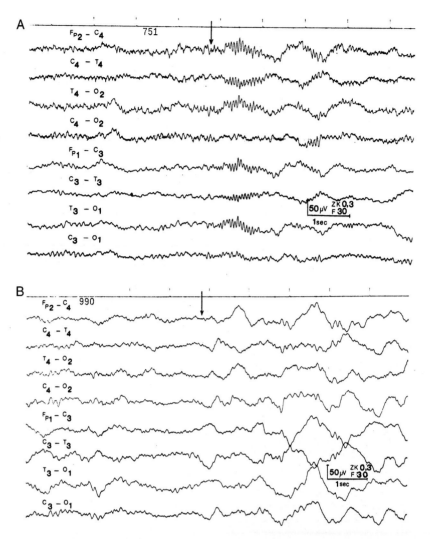

Figure 15.27. **A:** *EEG from a 24-year-old woman in acute midbrain syndrome stage 3 without clinical signs of lateralization. After acoustic stimulus (arrow), appearance of spindles followed by delta and subdelta activity of higher amplitude. Note the symmetry of reaction.* **B:** *EEG from the same patient in the transition stage to the apallic syndrome 4 days after first recording. Uniform delta and subdelta activity; loss of spindles. After acoustic stimulus (arrow), long run of delta. Note the symmetry of reaction.*

accidents (83). In rare cases, positive sharp waves in the occipital regions are seen during sleep.

One study described "benign" and "malignant" EEG patterns (188). Benign EEG patterns included reactive theta and alpha activity, delta activity with sleep spindles, and high-amplitude rhythmic frontal delta in theta–delta background. All patients with these patterns regained consciousness within 5 months. Malignant patterns included nonreactive slow delta with high-frequency bursts <1 sec, nonreactive theta or delta with high-frequency bursts >1 second, and nonreactive alpha or theta pattern; only 30% of these patients regained consciousness.

Posttraumatic seizures are also associated with poor prognosis. The negative influence on outcome is most pronounced for status epilepticus (189). However, nonconvulsive seizures can also negatively influence prognosis by increasing intracranial pressure (190).

There is no doubt that the prognostic EEG patterns are widely suppressed by sedative therapy. Consequently, any prognostic value of the EEG might be lost. Therefore, obtaining EEG recordings without sedatives is essential to make inferences about the patient's prognosis.

3.4. Seizures After Traumatic Brain Injury

Around 8% of adults have clinically apparent seizures within the first week after trauma (191). This figure is even higher in adolescents (20%) and children (31%). However, seizures might be particularly difficult to spot in patients with altered mental status. Routine EEG is usually not sufficient to monitor for subtle or subclinical seizures (Fig. 15.29) (192).

cEEG monitoring is being increasingly used in the ICU. Studies applying cEEG demonstrated that a quarter to a third of all patients with moderate to severe traumatic brain injury suffer from nonconvulsive seizures (189,193). This also implies that at least half of all seizures would be missed on clinical evaluation or routine EEG. Nonconvulsive seizures were associated with increased intracranial pressure and risk of hippocampal atrophy (190,194). The delay to diagnosis of nonconvulsive seizures and their duration correlated with

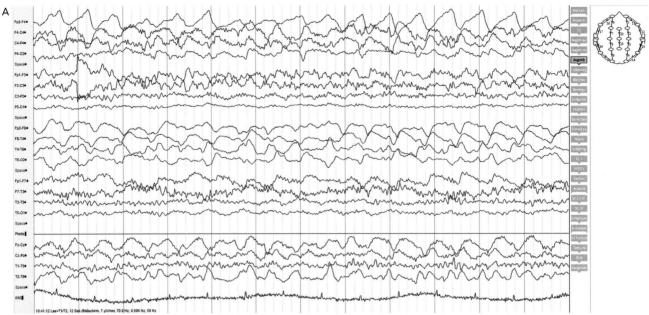

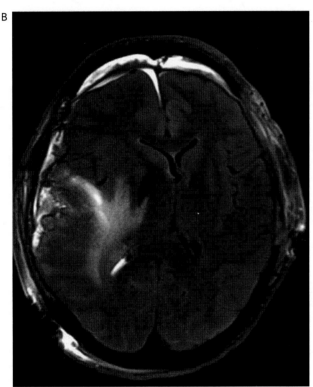

Figure 15.28. A 53-year-old woman after traumatic brain injury with right and left craniectomy. Clinically MBS 3. **A:** EEG demonstrates severe regional slowing with high-voltage delta activity; on the left side still slow-voltage alpha and beta activity and regional slowing over the frontal region. **B:** Posttraumatic MRI.

higher mortality (195). Status epilepticus is also common in these patients, presenting in 7% to 8% (189,193). The mortality is markedly increased in patients with status epilepticus. In one study, all of these patients died, whereas the mortality rate was 24% in the nonseizure group (189).

These results underline the importance of detecting posttraumatic seizures to guide early anticonvulsive treatment. They have led several intensive care societies to recommend the use of cEEG in patients with traumatic brain injury. The Neurocritical Care Society suggests the use of cEEG in patients

with altered mental status or intracranial hemorrhage and the European Society of Intensive Care Medicine in all patients with a GCS of less than 8 (196,197).

Epileptiform activities are more frequently seen in children than in adults (Fig. 15.30). These are isolated spikes or spike-waves, sharp waves, and spike-wave complexes, localized or generalized. In children, posttraumatic status epilepticus is associated with a far less ominous prognosis than in adults (198). The 14 and 6/sec positive spikes can occasionally be found after head injury in children. However, the significance

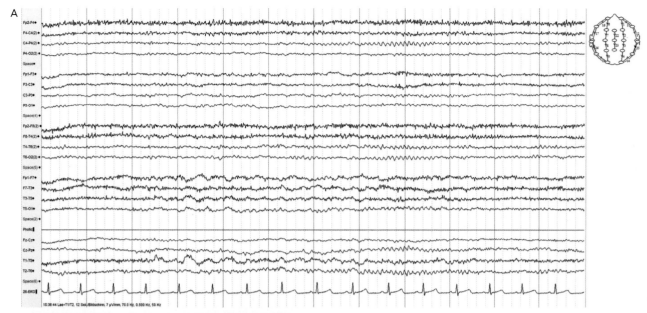

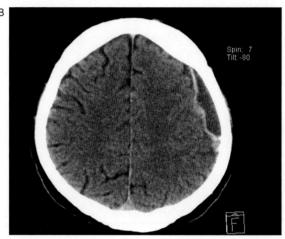

Figure 15.29. This 50-year old man had a focal seizure, with paresthesias over the right arm spreading up to the right face; 2 months ago he had a stumbling fall. **A:** EEG with normal background activity with signs of sleepiness. Regional slowing over the left temporal region. **B:** CT shows left frontoparietal subdural hematoma.

of this pattern is debatable, as it may also be seen in healthy children (199).

3.5. Head Injury in Sports

A generalized reduction in amplitude and slow irregular theta activity has been observed in boxers within 15 to 30 minutes after fighting, with a significant increase of these findings in boxers who had sustained a knockout blow (200). In long-term observations a correlation between the frequency of abnormal EEGs and the number of fights was found, as well as a correlation between EEG abnormalities and short time intervals between fights (201). Repeated fights within a short period have particularly ill effects on the brain, and the extent and degree of EEG abnormalities increased after each fight (201). Usually the EEG of young boxers shows more serious changes than that of older ones. No severe abnormalities were found in amateur boxers either with many or few matches.

There is a chronic progressive traumatic encephalopathy in boxers, especially in those with a history of repeated knockout defeats. A significant increase of EEG abnormalities in boxers who suffered from this encephalopathy in comparison to the EEG of more successful boxers was found (202). However, no correlation between the degree of boxer's encephalopathy and the EEG was eventually seen (202,203). Therefore, the EEG may be useful in determining the severity of trauma after a fight, but it is a less sensitive indicator of boxer's encephalopathy during and beyond the active career.

Similarly, a significantly increased incidence of focal theta activity was found in soccer players at the end of their careers, probably as the result of a cumulative effect due to repeated heading (204). Slightly abnormal to abnormal EEGs were found in 35% of active and in 32% of former soccer players. Interestingly enough, there were fewer abnormal EEG changes among the typical "headers" than among the "nonheaders" (205).

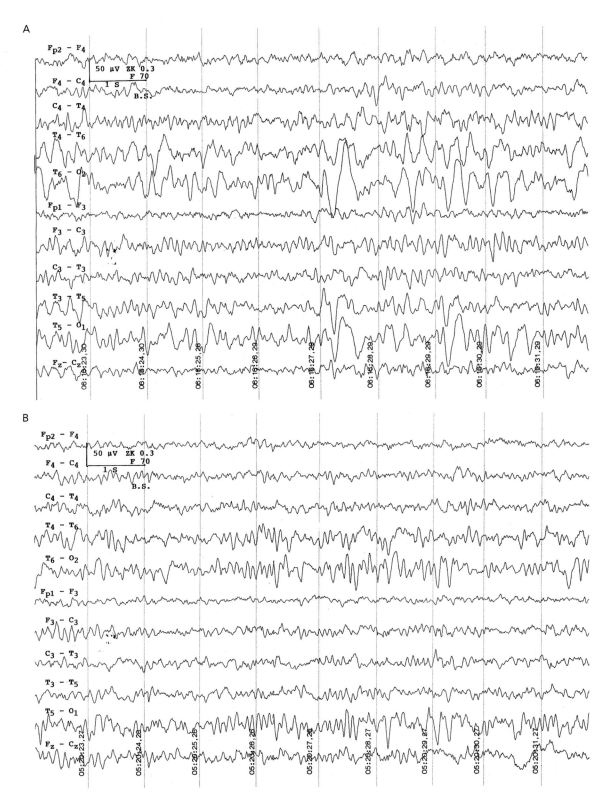

Figure 15.30. **A:** *EEG from a 6-year-old girl who fell on the back of her head after an unexpected push while playing. She had a period of blurred vision, delayed answers to questions, disorientation, drowsiness, and stereotyped finger movements, which lasted about 1 hour. The CT and MRI scans were normal. At the time of the EEG recording 2 days after the accident, the patient was alert with no neurological or mental deficit. The EEG showed high-voltage occipital delta activity intermingled with sharp transients.* **B:** *EEG from the same patient 3 days later within the range of normal.*

4. MIGRAINE AND HEADACHE

EEG abnormalities in headache patients are not uncommon. Due to the low specificity of these findings, these patients are usually referred to the EEG laboratory to rule out underlying cerebral pathology, rather than for a clarification of the type of headache. This type of referral has become less frequent with the greater availability of modern neuroimaging.

Studies did not show that the EEG is an effective screen for structural causes of headache, nor does the EEG effectively distinguish different types of headaches (206). This has led the American Academy of Neurology to advise against performing EEG in headache (207). They argue that brain imaging should be preferred to rule out structural headache causes. Mild to moderate abnormalities, commonly observed in certain primary headaches, may prompt unnecessary procedures and treatments.

Nevertheless, certain well-defined indications for EEG remain in the evaluation of headache. The most important is to differentiate between migraine accompagnée and occipital lobe epilepsy. The second is to distinguish between the epileptic and migrainous nature of an atypical aura that is not followed by headache.

4.1. Migraine

Migraine is a highly prevalent headache disorder with familial clustering that commonly begins in adolescence or early adulthood. The clinical symptomatology consists of largely unilateral, often pulsatile headache associated with nausea, vomiting, irritability, and photophobia. In the classical form, visual symptoms herald the attack, typically flickering uncolored zigzag lines leaving a scotoma.

4.1.1. EEG Recordings Between Migraine Attacks

The literature on EEG recordings in the interval between migraine attacks is conflicting, because almost equal numbers of reports stress the predominance of normal and abnormal tracings. As a rule, it is not unusual to obtain an abnormal recording in a migraine patient, but these abnormalities are typically mild (Fig. 15.31).

The predominance of normal interval EEG records was stressed by several authors (208–210). Others place the emphasis on a variety of mild abnormalities. Heyck (211) found mainly "hypersynchronous bursts" and occasional focal slowing. Weil (212) noted pronounced delta responses to hyperventilation. Multifaceted types of abnormalities were noted by Dow and Whitty (213) and Selby and Lance (214). A high incidence of abnormal EEG records was also emphasized by Barolin (215) and Gschwend (216). Almost equal numbers of normal and abnormal records (with about 45% abnormal tracings) were reported in the extensive work of Smyth and Winter (217). The reported abnormalities, however, were predominantly mild to moderate, with some bursts, slowing, or sharp transients. With the use of computer frequency analysis, Jonkman and Lelieveld (218) demonstrated abnormal interval EEG findings in 55% of migrainous patients.

Intermittent photic stimulation often shows an occipital driving response extending into the range above 30 flashes/second. This was termed the "H response" by Golla and Winter (219). Some authors found the H response to be specific to migraine (220), and further substantiation (221) came with the use of spectral analysis during photic stimulation (Fig. 15.32). On the other hand, the H response was found to be less effective than clinical criteria in distinguishing patients with headaches from individuals without headaches and in distinguishing migraine from other headache types (206).

4.1.2. EEG Recordings During the Attack

EEG findings during the migraine attack range from normal to mildly abnormal (alpha depression) in the initiating ophthalmic phase; even severely abnormal findings have been reported in special cases (222). Based on his large material, Heyck (223) found normal tracings in the ophthalmic-aura as well as in the headache-nausea phase. Schoenen et al. (224) found reduced alpha activity over one occipital region in 19 out of 22 patients recorded during an attack of common migraine. In the light of these observations, the statement that "EEGs have almost always been normal in migraineurs during attacks" (225) might be slightly exaggerated, but EEG abnormalities should be viewed as exceptions.

When the migraine attack is complicated by mild hemiparetic or dysphasic deficits (migraine accompagnée), the EEG may remain normal. In cases with pronounced hemiplegia and aphasia, there is good evidence of delta and theta activity over the affected hemisphere (226,227). The delta activity over the affected hemisphere may be very impressive. The neurological deficit subsides within days (sometimes within weeks), and the focal or lateralized slowing may also linger for some time. Cases of familial hemiplegic migraine have been reported by Whitty (228), Rosenbaum (226), and Bradshaw and Parsons (229). EEG studies in familial hemiplegia show a varying degree of slowing over the brain's affected side (226,229).

4.1.3. Relationship Between Migraine and Epileptic Disorders

The association of migraine with epilepsy has been discussed for a long time. Some authors suggested the rare combination of seizures triggered by migraine, termed "migralepsy" (215,230); however, this disorder is highly debatable (231–233). Although there is good reason why epileptic seizures could be susceptible to triggering through cortical changes induced by migraine (234), this would be a rare event.

More commonly, headache attacks can follow or accompany epileptic seizures. This is frequent in occipital lobe epilepsy (235). These patients report initial visual hallucinations consisting of multiple, brightly colored, small circular spots, circles, or balls moving horizontally through the visual field. They usually last for several seconds and can recur frequently. The subsequent headache can be indistinguishable from migraine. These symptoms commonly progress to extraoccipital manifestations or convulsions, which should prompt evaluation with EEG. In these cases, predominantly occipital epileptic discharges on EEG would support the diagnosis of occipital epilepsy.

4.2. Atypical Forms of Migraine

4.2.1. Childhood Migraine

In childhood migraine, normal EEG recordings are the rule (89%), but "benign" focal spikes, mostly rolandic, were found

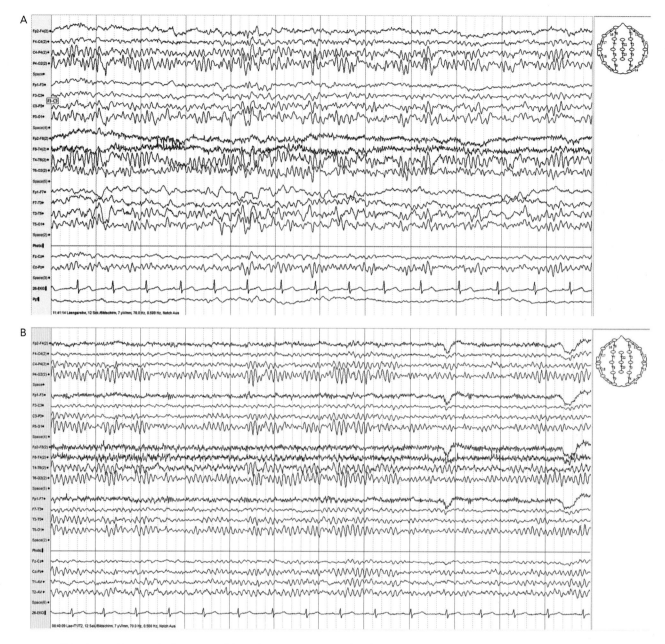

Figure 15.31. *This 26-year-old woman had migraine with hemiplegic aura.* **A:** *EEG on day of migraine demonstrates slow theta and delta activity on the left side, especially over the temporal region.* **B:** *EEG 1 week later is normal.*

in 9% (236). Kellaway et al. (237) stressed the high incidence of 14 and 6/sec positive spikes in the sleep records of these children.

There has been some controversy on the nature of epileptic abnormalities in childhood headache and abdominal pain attacks. Some authors reported a high incidence of paroxysmal EEG changes in these children (238,239). In our view, epileptic discharges are highly atypical for childhood migraine; it is likely that these reports included patients with recently described epilepsy syndromes (i.e., idiopathic occipital lobe epilepsy of Gastaut and Panayiotopoulos syndrome (240)). This would explain the frequent abnormalities found in these studies. Epileptic discharges in children with atypical headache or abdominal pain should prompt the physician to consider an epileptic etiology.

4.2.2. BASILAR MIGRAINE

Basilar migraine represents a syndrome described by Bickerstaff (241) consisting of a sudden transient blurring of vision or blindness, vertigo, gait ataxia, dysarthria, acroparesthesias, and pulsatile occipital headache with vomiting. Even syncopal states and loss of consciousness may occur (242).

The EEG literature is meager in this domain; a case recorded by Slatter (220) during a presumed attack showed diffuse 1.5 to 4/sec activity with subsequent normalization. Lapkin et al. (243) reported two cases (ages 12 and 10) with diffuse and chiefly posterior slowing in the 1.5 to 2/sec and 3 to 4/sec ranges, respectively, during the attack. This activity vanished with serial recordings. Another form with predominant beta activity during the attack was delineated by Parain and Samson-Dollfus (244).

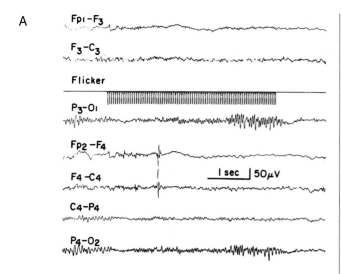

A

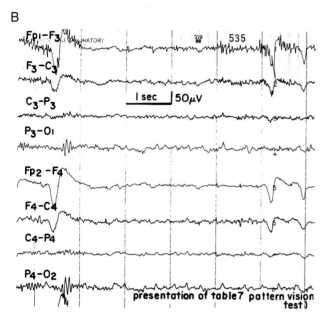

B

Figure 15.32. This 31-year-old woman had a history of classical migraine (flashing lights and some left-sided numbness). A: EEG obtained in interval. Note good occipital photic driving response to a flash rate of 22/sec ("H response"). The right frontal spiky discharge is artifactual. B: Very good occipital lambda activation presentation of pattern vision test tables.

According to Ramelli et al. (245), the EEG of children (11–13 years) with basilar migraine showed diffuse subdelta–delta activity during the attack and occipital delta– theta activity hours afterward. The authors warn against concepts of structural lesions (infarction, inflammation) and presume a temporary dysfunction.

4.3. Other Types of Headache

Cluster headache is a well-defined entity but has no special EEG correlate. Hyperventilation-related headache associated with EEG slowing has been reported by Sbrascini and Bassi (246). Hypnic headache has been related to REM sleep; the EEG is normal (247). It was found that EEG studies done with spectral analysis in patients with tension headaches did not differ from healthy persons (and were also not significantly different from the EEG of migrainous patients) (248).

In general, patients with habitual headaches and no organic disease may show EEG patterns that are believed to reveal some degree of "neuronal hyperexcitability"; this is a vague term without any precise scientific foundation, but with some merit in the domain of medical practice. Rolandic mu rhythm is quite often found in patients referred for headaches without demonstrable organic cause. Other patients show mildly paroxysmal flicker responses; still others show 14 and 6/sec positive spikes or even categorical EEG abnormalities such as psychomotor variant pattern and 6/sec spike waves.

SCORE EEG SOFTWARE

Further examples related to the topics addressed in this chapter can be found in the interactive online Niedermeyer Educational Platform. EEG recordings with illustrative examples can be opened and browsed. Features are marked and described using the SCORE EEG software. The users can see the features marked by experts, they can score these features themselves, and then compare them with the scorings of the experts.

The Niedermeyer Educational Platform can be accessed at: www.scoreEEG.com/academy

REFERENCES

1. Upton A, Gumpert J. Electroencephalography in diagnosis of herpes-simplex encephalitis. Lancet. 1970 Mar 28;1(7648):650–652.
2. Illis LS, Taylor FM. The electroencephalogram in herpes-simplex encephalitis. Lancet. 1972 Apr 1;1(7753):718–721.
3. Wieser H-G, Schwarz U, Blättler T, Bernoulli C, Sitzler M, Stoeck K, et al. Serial EEG findings in sporadic and iatrogenic Creutzfeldt–Jakob disease. Clin Neurophysiol. 2004 Nov;115(11):2467–2478.
4. Shapiro JM, Shujaat A, Wang J, Chen X. Creutzfeldt–Jakob disease presenting as refractory nonconvulsive status epilepticus. J Intensive Care Med. 2004 Nov 1;19(6):345–348.
5. Keyrouz SG, Labib BT, Sethi R. MRI and EEG findings in Heidenhain variant of Creutzfeldt-Jakob disease. Neurology. 2006 Jul 25;67(2):333–3.
6. Radermecker J, Poser CM. The significance of repetitive paroxysmal electroencephalographic patterns. Their specificity in subacute sclerosing leukoencephalitis. World Neurol. 1960 Nov;1:422–433.
7. Westmoreland BF, Sharbrough FW, Donat JR. Stimulus-induced EEG complexes and motor spasms in subacute sclerosing panencephalitis. Neurology. 1979 Aug 1;29(8):1154–4.
8. Tinuper P, De Carolis P, Galeotti M, Baldrati A, Gritti FM, Sacquegna T. Electroencephalogram and HIV infection: a prospective study in 100 patients. Clin Electroencephalogr. 1990 Jul;21(3):145–150.
9. Bernad PG. The neurological and electroencephalographic changes in AIDS. Clin Electroencephalogr. 1991 Apr;22(2):65–70.
10. del Saz SV, Sued O, Falco V, Agüero F, Crespo M, Pumarola T, et al. Acute meningoencephalitis due to human immunodeficiency virus type 1 infection in 13 patients: clinical description and follow-up. J Neurovirol. 2009 Jul 10;14(6):474–479.
11. Misra UK, Kalita J. Seizures in encephalitis: Predictors and outcome. Seizure. 2009 Oct;18(8):583–587.
12. Kerling F, Blumcke I, Stefan H. Pitfalls in diagnosing limbic encephalitis—a case report. Acta Neurol Scand. 2008 Nov 1;118(5):339–342.
13. Eriksson B, Wictor L. EEG with triphasic waves in *Borrelia burgdorferi* meningoencephalitis. Acta Neurol Scand. 2007 Aug 1;116(2):133–136.
14. Klein C, Kimiagar I, Pollak L, Gandelman-Marton R, Itzhaki A, Milo R, et al. Neurological features of West Nile Virus infection during the 2000 outbreak in a regional hospital in Israel. J Neurol Sci. 2002 Aug;200(1-2):63–66.
15. Gandelman-Marton R, Kimiagar I, Itzhaki A, Klein C, Theitler J, Rabey JM. Electroencephalography findings in adult patients with West Nile

virus-associated meningitis and meningoencephalitis. Clin Infect Dis. 2003 Dec 1;37(11):1573–1578.

16. Rodriguez AJ, Westmoreland BF. Electroencephalographic characteristics of patients infected with West Nile virus. J Clin Neurophysiol. 2007 Oct 1;24(5):386–389.

17. Bartel P, Schutte CM, Becker P, van der Meyden C. Discrimination between viral and nonviral meningitis by visually analyzed and quantitative electroencephalography. Clin Electroencephalogr. 1999 Apr;30(2):35–38.

18. Zoons E, Weisfelt M, De Gans J, Spanjaard L, Koelman JHTM, Reitsma JB, et al. Seizures in adults with bacterial meningitis. Neurology. 2008 May 27;70(22 Pt 2):2109–2115.

19. Konno S, Sugimoto H, Nemoto H, Kitazono H, Murata M, Toda T, et al. Triphasic waves in a patient with tuberculous meningitis. J Neurol Sci. 2010 Apr;291(1-2):114–117.

20. Kalita J, Misra UK, Das BK. SPECT changes and their correlation with EEG changes in tuberculous meningitis. Electromyogr Clin Neurophysiol. 2002 Jan;42(1):39–44.

21. Patwari AK, Aneja S, Ravi RNM, Singhal PK, Arora SK. Convulsions in tuberculous meningitis. J Trop Pediatr. 1996 Apr 1;42(2):91–97.

22. Wang R-J, Wang D-X, Wang J-W, Feng Z-J. [Analysis of 62 adult patients with viral meningitis]. Zhonghua Shi Yan He Lin Chuang Bing Du Xue Za Zhi. 2009 Jun;23(3):218–220.

23. Pollak L, Klein C, Schiffer J, Flechter S, Rabey JM. Electroencephalographic abnormalities in aseptic meningitis and noninfectious headache. A comparative study. Headache. 2001 Jan 1;41(1):79–83.

24. Veciana M, Becerra JL, Fossas P, Muriana D, Sansa G, Santamarina E, et al. EEG extreme delta brush: an ictal pattern in patients with anti-NMDA receptor encephalitis. Epilepsy Behav. 2015 Aug;49:280–285.

25. Schmitt SE, Pargeon K, Frechette ES, Hirsch LJ, Dalmau J, Friedman D. Extreme delta brush: a unique EEG pattern in adults with anti-NMDA receptor encephalitis. Neurology. 2012 Sep 11;79(11):1094–1100.

26. Wang J, Wang K, Wu D, Liang H, Zheng X, Luo B. Extreme delta brush guides to the diagnosis of anti-NMDAR encephalitis. J Neurol Sci. 2015;353(1-2):81–83.

27. Irani SR, Michell AW, Lang B, Pettingill P, Waters P, Johnson MR, et al. Faciobrachial dystonic seizures precede Lgi1 antibody limbic encephalitis. Ann Neurol. 2011 May;69(5):892–900.

28. Andrade DM, Tai P, Dalmau J, Wennberg R. Tonic seizures: a diagnostic clue of anti-LGI1 encephalitis? Neurology. 2011 Apr 12;76(15):1355–1357.

29. Kaplan PW, Rossetti AO, Kaplan EH, Wieser H-G. Proposition: limbic encephalitis may represent limbic status epilepticus. A review of clinical and EEG characteristics. Epilepsy Behav. 2012 May;24(1):1–6.

30. Kirkpatrick MP, Clarke CD, Sonmezturk HH, Abou-Khalil B. Rhythmic delta activity represents a form of nonconvulsive status epilepticus in anti-NMDA receptor antibody encephalitis. Epilepsy Behav. 2011 Feb;20(2):392–394.

31. Johnson RT, Richardson EP. The neurological manifestations of systemic lupus erythematosus. Medicine (Baltimore). 1968 Jul;47(4):337–369.

32. Waterloo K, Omdal R, Jacobsen EA, Kløw NE, Husby G, Torbergsen T, et al. Cerebral computed tomography and electroencephalography compared with neuropsychological findings in systemic lupus erythematosus. J Neurol. 1999;246(8):706–711.

33. Lampropoulos CE, Koutroumanidis M, Reynolds PPM, Manidakis I, Hughes GRV, D'Cruz DP. Electroencephalography in the assessment of neuropsychiatric manifestations in antiphospholipid syndrome and systemic lupus erythematosus. Arthritis Rheum. 2005 Mar;52(3):841–846.

34. Sokol DK, McIntyre JA, Wagenknecht DR, Dropcho EJ, Patel H, Salanova V, et al. Antiphospholipid and glutamic acid decarboxylase antibodies in patients with focal epilepsy. Neurology. 2004 Feb 10;62(3):517–518.

35. Verrot D, San-Marco M, Dravet C, Genton P, Disdier P, Bolla G, et al. Prevalence and signification of antinuclear and anticardiolipin antibodies in patients with epilepsy. Am J Med. 1997 Jul;103(1):33–37.

36. Debourdeau P, Gérome P, Zammit C, Saillol A, Aletti M, Bargues L, et al. Frequency of anticardiolipin, antinuclear and anti beta2GP1 antibodies is not increased in unselected epileptic patients: a case-control study. Seizure. 2004 Jun;13(4):205–207.

37. Ranua J, Luoma K, Peltola J, Haapala AM, Raitanen J, Auvinen A, et al. Anticardiolipin and antinuclear antibodies in epilepsy—a population-based cross-sectional study. Epilepsy Res. 2004 Jan;58(1):13–18.

38. Cimaz R, Meroni PL, Shoenfeld Y. Epilepsy as part of systemic lupus erythematosus and systemic antiphospholipid syndrome (Hughes syndrome). Lupus. 2006;15(4):191–197.

39. Aykutlu E, Baykan B, Serdaroglu P, Gökyigit A, Akman-Demir G. Epileptic seizures in Behçet disease. Epilepsia. 2002 Aug;43(8):832–835.

40. Borhani Haghighi A, Pourmand R, Nikseresht A-R. Neuro-Behçet disease. A review. Neurologist. 2005 Mar;11(2):80–89.

41. Midorikawa T, Totsuka S, Arakawa N, Matsumoto Y. A study on the electroencephalograms of neuro-Behçet's syndrome. Clin Neurol. 1969;9:143–155.

42. Midorikawa T. [Electroencephalographic studies on Behçet's disease—with special reference to the electroencephalogram of neuro-Behçet's disease]. Rinsho Shinkeigaku. 1975 Nov;15(11):860–869.

43. Benetó Pascual A, Blasco Olcina R, Ameave Y. [Meningoencephalitis in a case of Behçet's disease. Electroencephalographic findings (author's transl)]. Med Clin (Barc). 1981 May 10;76(9):417–419.

44. Pourmand R, Markand ON, Cook JA. Periodic lateralized EEG abnormality in a case of neuro-Behcet syndrome. Clin Electroencephalogr. 1984 Apr;15(2):122–124.

45. Matsumoto K. [Clinico-electroencephalographical correlation to the underlying neuropathology in neuro-Behçet's syndrome (author's transl)]. Seishin Shinkeigaku Zasshi. 1978 May;80(5):223–235.

46. Kutlu G, Semercioglu S, Ucler S, Erdal A, Inan LE. Epileptic seizures in neuro-Behcet disease: why some patients develop seizure and others not? Seizure. 2015 Mar;26:32–35.

47. Fattouch J, Di Bonaventura C, Di Gennaro G, Quarato PP, Petrucci S, Manfredi M, et al. Electrical status epilepticus "invisible" to surface EEG in late-onset Rasmussen encephalitis. Epileptic Disord. 2008 Sep 1;10(3):219–222.

48. Bien CG, Schramm J. Treatment of Rasmussen encephalitis half a century after its initial description: promising prospects and a dilemma. Epilepsy Res. 2009 Oct;86(2-3):101–112.

49. Sporiš D, Habek M, Mubrin Z, Poljakovic Z, Hajnšek S, Bence-Žigman Z. Psychosis and EEG abnormalities as manifestations of Hashimoto encephalopathy. Cogn Behav Neurol. 2007 Jun 1;20(2):138–140.

50. Rodriguez AJ, Jicha GA, Steeves TDL, Benarroch EE, Westmoreland BF. EEG changes in a patient with steroid-responsive encephalopathy associated with antibodies to thyroperoxidase (SREAT, Hashimoto's encephalopathy). J Clin Neurophysiol. 2006 Aug 1;23(4):371–373.

51. Schäuble B, Castillo PR, Boeve BF, Westmoreland BF. EEG findings in steroid-responsive encephalopathy associated with autoimmune thyroiditis. Clin Neurophysiol. 2003 Jan;114(1):32–37.

52. Oon S, Roberts C, Gorelik A, Wicks I, Brand C. Primary angiitis of the central nervous system: experience of a Victorian tertiary-referral hospital. Intern Med J. 2013 Jun;43(6):685–692.

53. Scolding NJ, Joseph F, Kirby PA, Mazanti I, Gray F, Mikol J, et al. Abeta-related angiitis: primary angiitis of the central nervous system associated with cerebral amyloid angiopathy. Brain. 2005 Mar;128(Pt 3):500–515.

54. Salvarani C, Brown RD, Calamia KT, Christianson TJH, Weigand SD, Miller DV, et al. Primary central nervous system vasculitis: analysis of 101 patients. Ann Neurol. 2007 Nov;62(5):442–451.

55. Hirsch M, Carlander B, Vergé M, Tafti M, Anaya JM, Billiard M, et al. Objective and subjective sleep disturbances in patients with rheumatoid arthritis. A reappraisal. Arthritis Rheum. 1994 Jan;37(1):41–49.

56. Lang H, Anttila R, Svékus A, Laaksonen AL. EEG findings in juvenile rheumatoid arthritis and other connective tissue diseases in children. Acta Paediatr Scand. 1974 May;63(3):373–380.

57. Chabolla DR, Layne Moore J, Westmoreland BF. Periodic lateralized epileptiform discharges in multiple sclerosis. Electroencephalogr Clin Neurophysiol. 1996 Jan;98(1):5–8.

58. Lević ZM. Electroencephalographic studies in multiple sclerosis. Specific changes in benign multiple sclerosis. Electroencephalogr Clin Neurophysiol. 1978 Apr;44(4):471–478.

59. Striano P, Orefice G, Brescia Morra V, Boccella P, Sarappa C, Lanzillo R, et al. Epileptic seizures in multiple sclerosis: clinical and EEG correlations. Neurol Sci. 2003 Dec;24(5):322–328.

60. Martínez-Juárez IE, López-Meza E, González-Aragón MDCF, Ramírez-Bermúdez J, Corona T. Epilepsy and multiple sclerosis: Increased risk among progressive forms. Epilepsy Res. 2009 Apr;84(2-3):250–253.

61. Terzano MG, Camillo Manzoni G, Mancia D, Montanari E, Lechi A. [Evaluation of the EEG aspects of rheumatic chorea as related to the clinico-evolutive parameters of the disease]. Riv Neurol. 1979 Nov;49(6):451–470.

62. Johnson DA, Klass DW, Millichap JG. Electroencephalogram in Sydenham's chorea. Arch Neurol. 1964 Jan 1;10(1):21–27.

63. Ganji S, Duncan MC, Frazier E. Sydenham's chorea: clinical, EEG, CT scan, and evoked potential studies. Clin Electroencephalogr. 1988 Jul;19(3):114–122.

64. Lavy S, Lavy R, Brand A. Neurological and electroencephalographic abnormalities in rheumatic fever. Acta Neurol Scand. 1964 Mar 1;40(1):76–88.

65. Keilson MJ, Miller AE. Early EEG and CTT scanning in stroke—a comparative study. Electroencephalogr Clin Neurophysiol. 1985;61:21.

66. Gloor P, Ball G, Schaul N. Brain lesions that produce delta waves in the EEG. Neurology. 1977 Apr 1;27(4):326–6.

67. Gastaut JL, Michel B, Sabet Hassan S, Cerda M, Bianchi L, Gastaut H. Electroencephalography in brain edema (127 cases of brain tumor investigated by cranial computerized tomography). Electroencephalogr Clin Neurophysiol. 1979 Mar;46(3):239–255.
68. Velho-Groneberg P. The EEG: an important (and often underrated) tool in the diagnosis of strokes. Am J EEG Technology. 2015 Feb 10 [published online].
69. Van der Drift JH, Magnus O. The EEG in cerebral ischemic lesions: correlations with clinical and pathological findings. In Gastaut H, Stirling Meyer J, eds. Cerebral Anoxia and the Electroencephalogram; The Proceedings of the Marseille Colloquium, sponsored by the Reunion Europeenne d'Information Eleectroencephalographique, January 1, 1961, pp. 180–196.
70. Paddison RM, Ferriss GS. The electroencephalogram in cerebral vascular disease. Electroencephalogr Clin Neurophysiol. 1961;13:99–110.
71. Kayser-Gatchalian MC, Neundörfer B. The prognostic value of EEG in ischaemic cerebral insults. Electroencephalogr Clin Neurophysiol. 1980 Sep;49(5-6):608–617.
72. Sainio K, Stenberg D, Keskimäki I, Muuronen A, Kaste M. Visual and spectral EEG analysis in the evaluation of the outcome in patients with ischemic brain infarction. Electroencephalogr Clin Neurophysiol. 1983 Aug;56(2):117–124.
73. Luu P, Tucker DM, Englander R, Lockfeld A, Lutsep H, Oken B. Localizing acute stroke-related EEG changes: assessing the effects of spatial undersampling. J Clin Neurophysiol. 2001 Jul 1;18(4):302.
74. Galovic M, Erdelyi B, Wagner F, Döhler N, Hakman P, Flügel D, et al. Early EEG predicts seizures after ischaemic stroke. J Neurol. 2013 Jun;260 Suppl 1:S193.
75. Holmes GL. The electroencephalogram as a predictor of seizures following cerebral infarction. Clin Electroencephalogr. 1980 Apr;11(2):83–86.
76. Carrera E, Michel P, Despland P-A, Maeder-Ingvar M, Ruffieux C, Debatisse D, et al. Continuous assessment of electrical epileptic activity in acute stroke. Neurology. 2006 Jul 11;67(1):99–104.
77. Chatrian GE, White LE, Shaw C-M. EEG pattern resembling wakefulness in unresponsive decerebrate state following traumatic brain-stem infarct. Electroencephalogr Clin Neurophysiol. 1964;16(3):285–289.
78. Echlin FA, Arnett V, Zoll J. Paroxysmal high voltage discharges from isolated and partially isolated human and animal cerebral cortex. Electroencephalogr Clin Neurophysiol. 1952 May;4(2):147–164.
79. la Paz de D, Brenner RP. Bilateral independent periodic lateralized epileptiform discharges: clinical significance. Arch Neurol. 1981 Nov 1;38(11):713–715.
80. Holmes GL. The electroencephalogram as a predictor of seizures following cerebral infarction. Clin EEG Neurosci. 1980 Apr 1;11(2):83–86.
81. Friedlander WJ. Electroencephalographic changes in acute brain stem vascular lesions. Neurology. 1959 Jan 1;9(1):24–4.
82. Hawkes CH, Bryan-Smyth L. The electroencephalogram in the "locked-in" syndrome. Neurology. 1974 Nov 1;24(11):1015–5.
83. Chase TN, Moretti L, Prensky AL. Clinical and electroencephalographic manifestations of vascular lesions of the pons. Neurology. 1968 Apr 1;18(4):357–7.
84. Westmoreland BF, Klass DW, Sharbrough FW, Reagan TJ. Alpha-coma: electroencephalographic, clinical, pathologic, and etiologic correlations. Arch Neurol. 1975 Nov 1;32(11):713–718.
85. Vignaendra V, Wilkus RJ, Copass MK, Chatrian GE. Electroencephalographic rhythms of alpha frequency in comatose patients after cardiopulmonary arrest. Neurology. 1974 Jun 1;24(6):582–2.
86. Carroll WM, Mastaglia FL. Alpha and beta coma in drug intoxication uncomplicated by cerebral hypoxia. Electroencephalogr Clin Neurophysiol. 1979 Jan;46(1):95–105.
87. Taghavy A, Hamer H. Parenchymal "damage" in transient ischemic attacks (TIAs) and prolonged reversible ischemic neurologic deficits (PRINDs): the role of cranial CT and EEG. Int J Neurosci. 1992 Oct;66(3-4):251–261.
88. De Reuck J, Van Maele G. Transient ischemic attacks and inhibitory seizures in elderly patients. Eur Neurol. 2009;62(6):344–348.
89. Burghaus L, Hilker R, Dohmen C, Bosche B, Winhuisen L, Galldiks N, et al. Early electroencephalography in acute ischemic stroke: prediction of a malignant course? Clin Neurol Neurosurg. 2007 Jan;109(1):45–49.
90. Gottselig JM, Bassetti CL, Achermann P. Power and coherence of sleep spindle frequency activity following hemispheric stroke. Brain. 2002 Feb 1;125(2):373–383.
91. Müller C, Achermann P, Bischof M, Nirkko AC, Roth C, Bassetti CL. Visual and spectral analysis of sleep EEG in acute hemispheric stroke. Eur Neurol. 2002 Oct 4;48(3):164–171.
92. Vock J, Achermann P, Bischof M, Milanova M, Müller C, Nirkko A, et al. Evolution of sleep and sleep EEG after hemispheric stroke. J Sleep Res. 2002 Dec 1;11(4):331–338.
93. Giubilei F, Iannilli M, Vitale A, Pierallini A, Sacchetti ML, Antonini G, et al. Sleep patterns in acute ischemic stroke. Acta Neurol Scand. 1992 Dec 1;86(6):567–571.
94. Bassetti CL. Sleep and stroke. Semin Neurol. 2005 Mar;25(1):19–32.
95. Bassetti CL, Valko P. Poststroke hypersomnia. Sleep Med Clinics. 2006 Mar;1(1):139–155.
96. Arpa J, Rodriguez-Albarino A, Izal E, Sarriá J, Lara M, Barreiro P. Hypersomnia after tegmental pontine hematoma: case report. Neurologia. 1995 Mar;10(3):140–144.
97. Bastuji H, Nighoghossian N, Salord F. Mesodiencephalic infarct with hypersomnia: sleep recording in two cases. J Sleep Res; 1994;3:16.
98. Eliassen JC, Boespflug EL, Lamy M, Allendorfer J, Chu W-J, Szaflarski JP. Brain-mapping techniques for evaluating poststroke recovery and rehabilitation: a review. Top Stroke Rehabil. 2015 Jan 9;15(5):427–450.
99. Strens LHA, Asselman P, Pogosyan A, Loukas C, Thompson AJ, Brown P. Corticocortical coupling in chronic stroke: its relevance to recovery. Neurology. 2004 Aug 10;63(3):475–484.
100. Meinzer M, Elbert T, Wienbruch C, Djundja D, Barthel G, Rockstroh B. Intensive language training enhances brain plasticity in chronic aphasia. BMC Biology. 2004 Aug 25;2(1):1.
101. Finnigan SP, Rose SE, Chalk JB. Contralateral hemisphere delta EEG in acute stroke precedes worsening of symptoms and death. Clin Neurophysiol. 2008 July;119(7):1690–1694.
102. Finnigan SP, Rose SE, Chalk JB. Rapid EEG changes indicate reperfusion after tissue plasminogen activator injection in acute ischaemic stroke. Clin Neurophysiol. 2006 Oct;117(10):2338–2339.
103. Gilden L, Vaughan HG Jr., Costa LD. Summated human EEG potentials with voluntary movement. Electroencephalogr Clin Neurophysiol. 1966 May;20(5):433–438.
104. Platz T, Kim IH, Pintschovius H, Winter T, Kieselbach A, Villringer K, et al. Multimodal EEG analysis in man suggests impairment-specific changes in movement-related electric brain activity after stroke. Brain. 2000 Dec 1;123(12):2475–2490.
105. Green JB, Bialy Y, Sora E, Ricamato A. High-resolution EEG in poststroke hemiparesis can identify ipsilateral generators during motor tasks. Stroke. 1999 Dec;30(12):2659–2665.
106. Eder CF, Sokić D, Čovičković Šternić N, Mijajlović M, Savic M, Sinkjær T, et al. Symmetry of post-movement beta-ERS and motor recovery from stroke: a low-resolution EEG pilot study. Eur J Neurol. 2006 Dec 1;13(12):1312–1323.
107. Pfurtscheller G, Aranibar A. Changes in central EEG activity in relation to voluntary movement. I. Normal subjects. Prog Brain Res. 1980;54:225–231.
108. Köpruner V, Pfurtscheller G. Multiparametric asymmetry score (MAS)—distinction between normal and ischaemic brains. Electroencephalogr Clin Neurophysiol. 1984 Apr;57(4):343–346.
109. Andrew C, Pfurtscheller G. Lack of bilateral coherence of post-movement central beta oscillations in the human electroencephalogram. Neurosci Lett. 1999 Oct 1;273(2):89–92.
110. Pfurtscheller G, Pichler-Zalaudek K, Ortmayr B, Diez J, Reisecker F. Postmovement beta synchronization in patients with Parkinson's disease. J Clin Neurophysiol. 1998 May;15(3):243–250.
111. Fountain NB. Is it time for routine EEG monitoring after intracerebral hemorrhage? Neurology. 2007 Sep 25;69(13):1312–1313.
112. Claassen J, Jetté N, Chum F, Green R, Schmidt M, Choi H, et al. Electrographic seizures and periodic discharges after intracerebral hemorrhage. Neurology. 2007 Sep 25;69(13):1356–1365.
113. Vespa PM, O'Phelan K, Shah M, Mirabelli J, Starkman S, Kidwell C, et al. Acute seizures after intracerebral hemorrhage: a factor in progressive midline shift and outcome. Neurology. 2003 May 13;60(9):1441–1446.
114. Jasper H, van Buren J. Interrelationship between cortex and subcortical structures: clinical electroencephalographic studies. Electroencephalogr Clin Neurophysiol Suppl. 1955;Suppl. 4:168–188.
115. Hirose G, Saeki M, Kosoegawa H, Takado M, Yamamoto T, Tada A. Delta waves in the EEGs of patients with intracerebral hemorrhage. Arch Neurol. 1981 Mar;38(3):170–175.
116. Loeb C, Rosadini G, Poggio GF. Electroencephalograms during coma; normal and borderline records in 5 patients. Neurology. 1959 Sep;9:610–618.
117. Radermecker J. Severe acute necrosis of the pons with long survival. Electro-clinical symptoms and absence of cerebral lesions. Electroencephalogr Clin Neurophysiol. 1967 Sep;23(3):281–282.
118. Rasheva M, Stamenov E, Todorova P. Dynamic of electrical activity of the brain in cerebellar hemorrhage. Electroencephalogr Clin Neurophysiol. 1981;52:78.
119. Gerloff C, Altenmuller E, Dichgans J. Disintegration and reorganization of cortical motor processing in two patients with cerebellar stroke. Electroencephalogr Clin Neurophysiol. 1996 Jan;98(1):59–68.

120. Daly DD, Markand ON. Focal brain lesions. Current practice of clinical electroencephalography. New York: Raven Press, 1990, pp. 335–370.

121. Roseman E, Bloor BM, Schmidt RP. The electroencephalogram in intracranial aneurysms. Neurology. 1951 Jan;1(1):25–38.

122. Labar DR, Fisch BJ, Pedley TA, Fink ME, Solomon RA. Quantitative EEG monitoring for patients with subarachnoid hemorrhage. Electroencephalogr Clin Neurophysiol. 1991 May;78(5):325–332.

123. Logar C, Enge S, Körner EM, Ladurner G, Sager WD, Lechner H. [The value of EEG in subarachnoidal haemorrhagia]. EEG EMG Z Elektroenzephalogr Elektromyogr Verwandte Geb. 1982 Jun;13(2):68–72.

124. Vespa PM, Nuwer MR, Juhász C, Alexander M, Nenov V, Martin N, et al. Early detection of vasospasm after acute subarachnoid hemorrhage using continuous EEG ICU monitoring. Electroencephalogr Clin Neurophysiol. 1997 Dec;103(6):607–615.

125. Claassen J, Hirsch LJ, Kreiter KT, Du EY, Connolly ES, Emerson RG, et al. Quantitative continuous EEG for detecting delayed cerebral ischemia in patients with poor-grade subarachnoid hemorrhage. Clin Neurophysiol. 2004 Dec;115(12):2699–2710.

126. Stuart RM, Waziri A, Weintraub D, Schmidt MJ, Fernandez L, Helbok R, et al. Intracortical EEG for the detection of vasospasm in patients with poor-grade subarachnoid hemorrhage. Neurocrit Care. 2010 Dec;13(3):355–358.

127. Walton JN. The electroencephalographic sequelae of spontaneous subarachnoid haemorrhage. Electroencephalogr Clin Neurophysiol. 1953 Feb;5(1):41–52.

128. Sundt TM, Kobayashi S, Fode NC, Whisnant JP. Results and complications of surgical management of 809 intracranial aneurysms in 722 cases. Related and unrelated to grade of patient, type of aneurysm, and timing of surgery. J Neurosurg. 1982 Jun;56(6):753–765.

129. Husby J, Norlen G, Petersen I. Electroencephalographic findings in intracranial, arterial and arterio-venous aneurysms and subarachnoid haemorrhages. Acta Psychiatr Neurol Scand. 1953;28(3-4):387–400.

130. Yeh HS, Tew JM, Gartner M. Seizure control after surgery on cerebral arteriovenous malformations. J Neurosurg. 1993 Jan;78(1):12–18.

131. Mosmans PC, Jonkman EJ. The significance of the collateral vascular system of the brain in shunt and steal syndromes. Clin Neurol Neurosurg. 1980;82(3):145–156.

132. Groethuysen UC, Bickford RG, Svien HJ. The electroencephalogram in arteriovenous anomalies of the brain. AMA Arch Neurol Psychiatry. 1955 Nov;74(5):506–513.

133. Masuhr F, Mehraein S, Einhäupl K. Cerebral venous and sinus thrombosis. J Neurol. 2004 Jan;251(1):11–23.

134. Bousser MG, Chiras J, Bories J, Castaigne P. Cerebral venous thrombosis—a review of 38 cases. Stroke. 1985 Mar;16(2):199–213.

135. Barron TF, Gusnard DA, Zimmerman RA, Clancy RR. Cerebral venous thrombosis in neonates and children. Pediatr Neurol. 1992 Mar;8(2):112–116.

136. Aguglia U, Tinuper P, Farnarier G, Quattrone A. Electroencephalographic and anatomo-clinical evidences of posterior cerebral damage in hypertensive encephalopathy. Clin Electroencephalogr. 1984 Jan;15(1):53–60.

137. Benna P, Bergamini L, Tarenzi L, Troni W, Pinessi L. Hypertensive encephalopathy: association with unusual EEG changes. Electroencephalogr Clin Neurophysiol. 1984;58(3):P74–4.

138. Aoki Y, Hiraga H, Ichijo S. EEG of Moyamoya disease. Electroencephalogr Clin Neurophysiol. 1977;43(4):490–0.

139. Ohyama H, Niizuma H, Kinjo T, Yonemitsu T, Fujiwara S, Suzuki J, et al. Changes of EEG, tissue pCO2 and tissue pO2 with hyperventilation in children with moyamoya disease. Electroencephalogr Clin Neurophysiol. 1983;56(5):P55–5.

140. Obrist WD, Bissell LF. The electroencephalogram of aged patients with cardiac and cerebral vascular disease. J Gerontol. 1955 Jul;10(3):315–330.

141. Davidson LA, Jefferson JM. Electroencephalographic studies in respiratory failure. Br Med J. 1959 Sep 12;2(5149):396–400.

142. Goulon M, Pocidalo JJ, Christophe M, Margairaz A, Nouialhat F. Clinical, electroencephalographic and biologic correlations in 34 cases of chronic broncho-pneumopathy with asphyxia. In: Cerebral Anoxia and the Electroencephalogram. Springfield, IL: Charles C. Thomas, 1961. pp. 565–577.

143. Tucker JS, Yoe RH. Simultaneous EEG-EKG recording: study of a case with complete heart block and paroxysmal ventricular tachycardia. Electroencephalogr Clin Neurophysiol. 1956 Feb;8(1):129–132.

144. Subbotnik SI, Feinberg YS, Spielberg PI. Electroencephalography in paroxysmal tachycardia. Electroencephalogr Clin Neurophysiol. 1955 Nov;7(4):577–584.

145. Siverman D. Retrospective study of the EEG in coma. Electroencephalogr Clin Neurophysiol. 1963 Jun;15:486–503.

146. Rumpl E, Lorenzi E, Hackl JM, Gerstenbrand F, Hengl W. The EEG at different stages of acute secondary traumatic midbrain and bulbar brain syndromes. Electroencephalogr Clin Neurophysiol. 1979 May;46(5):487–497.

147. Chatrian GE, White LE, Daly D. Electroencephalographic patterns resembling those of sleep in certain comatose states after injuries to the head. Electroencephalogr Clin Neurophysiol. 1963 Apr;15:272–280.

148. Bricolo A, Turella G. Electroencephalographic patterns of acute traumatic coma: diagnostic and prognostic value. J Neurosurg Sci. 1973;17:278–285.

149. Radermecker J. Das EEG bei gedeckten Hirnschaden und seine Beziehungen zu den subjektiven Beschwerden. Munch Med Wschr. 1964;106:1315–1322.

150. Koufen H, Hagel KH. Systematic EEG follow-up study of traumatic psychosis. Eur Arch Psychiatry Neurol Sci. 1987;237(1):2–7.

151. Jabbari B, Vengrow MI, Salazar AM, Harper MG, Smutok MA, Amin D. Clinical and radiological correlates of EEG in the late phase of head injury: a study of 515 Vietnam veterans. Electroencephalogr Clin Neurophysiol. 1986 Oct;64(4):285–293.

152. Strnad P, Strnadová V. Long-term follow-up EEG studies in patients with traumatic apallic syndrome. Eur Neurol. 1987;26(2):84–89.

153. Dow RS, Ulett G, Raaf J. Electroencephalographic studies immediately following head injury. Am J Psychiatry. 1944;101(2):174–183.

154. Kaplan HA, Browder J. Observations on the clinical and brain wave patterns of professional boxers. J Am Med Assoc. 1954 Nov 20;156(12):1138–1144.

155. Schmitt S, Dichter MA. Electrophysiologic recordings in traumatic brain injury. Handb Clin Neurol. 2015;127:319–339.

156. Walker AE. The physiological basis of concussion: 50 years later. J Neurosurg. 1994 Sep;81(3):493–494.

157. Scherzer E. Wert der Electroenzephalographie beim Schädeltrauma. Wien Klin Wschr. 1965;77:543–547.

158. Williams D. The electro-encephalogram in acute head injuries. J Neurol Psychiatry. 1941 Apr;4(2):107–130.

159. Koufen H, Dichgans J. Häufigkeit und Ablauf von traumatischen EEG-Veränderungen und ihre klinischen Korrelationen: systematische verlaufsuntersuchungen bei 344 Erwachsenen. Fortschr Neurol Psychiatr. 1978;46:165–177.

160. Geets W, Louette N. [EEG and brain-stem evoked potentials in 125 recent concussions]. Rev Electroencephalogr Neurophysiol Clin. 1983 Dec;13(3):253–258.

161. Watson MR, Fenton GW, McClelland RJ, Lumsden J, Headley M, Rutherford WH. The post-concussional state: neurophysiological aspects. Br J Psychiatry. 1995 Oct;167(4):514–521.

162. Bierbrauer von A, Weissenborn K, Hinrichs H, Scholz M, Künkel H. [Automatic (computer-assisted) EEG analysis in comparison with visual EEG analysis in patients following minor cranio-cerebral trauma (a follow-up study)]. EEG EMG Z Elektroenzephalogr Elektromyogr Verwandte Geb. 1992 Sep;23(3):151–157.

163. Stockard JJ, Bickford RG, Aung MH. The electroencephalogram in traumatic brain injury. Handb Clin Neurol. 1975;23(part I):217–367.

164. Koufen H, Dichgans J. [Frequency and course of posttraumatic EEG-abnormalities and their correlations with clinical symptoms: a systematic follow up study in 344 adults (author's transl)]. Fortschr Neurol Psychiatr Grenzgeb. 1978 Apr;46(4):165–177.

165. Dichgans J, Koufen H, Kehrle G, Sauer M, Klieser J. [Neurological and EEG-follow-up studies in head-injured adults: criteria for the clinical diagnosis concussion and contusion (author's transl)]. Fortschr Neurol Psychiatr Grenzgeb. 1978 Mar;46(3):144–155.

166. Korinthenberg R, Schreck J, Weser J, Lehmkuhl G. Post-traumatic syndrome after minor head injury cannot be predicted by neurological investigations. Brain Devel. 2004 Mar;26(2):113–117.

167. Lenard HG. EEG-Veränderungen bei frischen Schädeltraumen im Kindesalter. Muench Med Wochenschr. 1965;38:1820–1827.

168. Melin KA. Electroencephalography following head injuries in children. Acta Paediatrica. 1949;38(s75):152–174.

169. Christian W. Klinische Elektroenzephalographie: Lehrbuch und Atlas. Thieme; 1982.

170. Gerstenbrand F, Lücking CH. Die akuten traumatischen Hirnstammschäden. Archiv für Psychiatrie und Nervenkrankheiten. 1970;213(3):264–281.

171. Plum F, Posner JB. Plum and Posner's Diagnosis of Stupor and Coma (3rd ed.). Philadelphia, PA: FA Davis, 1980.

172. Maciver IN, Lassman LP, Thomson CW, McLeod I. Treatment of severe head injuries. Lancet. 1958 Sep 13;2(7046):544–550.

173. Hess R. Sleep and sleep disturbances in the electroencephalogram. Prog Brain Res. 1965;18:127–139.

174. Luecking C. Sleep-like patterns and abnormal arousal reactions in brain stem lesions. Electroencephalogr Clin Neurophysiol. 1970;28(2):214.

175. Rumpl E. Elektro-neurologische Korrelationen in den frühen Phasen des posttraumatischen Komas. II. Das EEG im Übergang zum und im Vollbild des traumatischen apallischen Syndroms. EEG EMG Z Elektroenzephalogr Elektromyogr Verwandte Geb. 1980;11(01):43–50.

176. Bricolo A, Gentilomo A, Rosadini G, Rossi GF. Akinetic mutism following cranio-cerebral trauma. Physiopathological considerations based on sleep studies. Acta Neurochir (Wien). 1968;18(1):68–77.

177. Hutchinson DO, Frith RW, Shaw NA, Judson JA, Cant BR. A comparison between electroencephalography and somatosensory evoked potentials for outcome prediction following severe head injury. Electroencephalogr Clin Neurophysiol. 1991 Mar;78(3):228–233.

178. Fischgold H, Mathis P. Obnubilations, comas et stupeurs, etudes electroencephalographiques. Electroencephalogr Clin Neurophysiol. 1959;11 (suppl):27–68.

179. Chokroverty S. "Alpha-like" rhythms in electroencephalograms in coma after cardiac arrest. Neurology. 1975 Jul;25(7):655–663.

180. Horton EJ, Goldie WD, Baram TZ. Rhythmic coma in children. J Child Neurol. 1990 Jul;5(3):242–247.

181. Toyonaga K, Schlagenhauff RE, Smith BH. Periodic lateralized epileptiform discharges in subdural hematoma: case-reports and review of literature. Clin EEG Neurosci. 1974;5(3):113–118.

182. Markand ON, Daly DD. Pseudoperiodic lateralized paroxysmal discharges in electroencephalogram. Neurology. 1971 Oct;21(10):975–981.

183. Chatrian GE, Shaw C-M, Leffman H. The significance of periodic lateralized epileptiform discharges in EEG: an electrographic, clinical and pathological study. Electroencephalogr Clin Neurophysiol. 1964 Aug;17(2):177–193.

184. Bickford RG, Butt HR. Hepatic coma: the electroencephalographic pattern. J Clin Invest. 1955 Jun;34(6):790–799.

185. Gütling E, Gonser A, Imhof HG, Landis T. EEG reactivity in the prognosis of severe head injury. Neurology. 1995 May;45(5):915–918.

186. Steudel WI, Krüger J, Grau H. Zur alpha-und spindel-aktivität bei komatösen patienten nach einer schädel-Hirn-Verletzung unter besonderer berücksichtigung der computertomographie. Z EEG EMG. 1979;10:143–147.

187. Bergamasco B, Bergamini L, Doriguzzi T, Fabiani D. EEG sleep patterns as a prognostic criterion in post-traumatic coma. Electroencephalogr Clin Neurophysiol. 1968 Apr;24(4):374–377.

188. Logi F, Pasqualetti P, Tomaiuolo F. Predict recovery of consciousness in post-acute severe brain injury: the role of EEG reactivity. Brain Inj. 2011;25(10):972–979.

189. Vespa PM, Nuwer MR, Nenov V, Ronne-Engström E, Hovda DA, Bergsneider M, et al. Increased incidence and impact of nonconvulsive and convulsive seizures after traumatic brain injury as detected by continuous electroencephalographic monitoring. J Neurosurg. 1999 Nov;91(5):750–760.

190. Vespa PM, Miller C, McArthur D, Eliseo M, Etchepare M, Hirt D, et al. Nonconvulsive electrographic seizures after traumatic brain injury result in a delayed, prolonged increase in intracranial pressure and metabolic crisis. Crit Care Med. 2007 Dec;35(12):2830–2836.

191. Asikainen I, Kaste M, Sarna S. Early and late posttraumatic seizures in traumatic brain injury rehabilitation patients: brain injury factors causing late seizures and influence of seizures on long-term outcome. Epilepsia. 1999 May;40(5):584–589.

192. Beni L, Constantini S, Matoth I, Pomeranz S. Subclinical status epilepticus in a child after closed head injury. J Trauma. 1996 Mar;40(3):449–451.

193. Claassen J, Mayer SA, Kowalski RG, Emerson RG, Hirsch LJ. Detection of electrographic seizures with continuous EEG monitoring in critically ill patients. Neurology. 2004 May 25;62(10):1743–1748.

194. Vespa PM, McArthur DL, Xu Y, Eliseo M, Etchepare M, Dinov I, et al. Nonconvulsive seizures after traumatic brain injury are associated with hippocampal atrophy. Neurology. 2010 Aug 31;75(9):792–798.

195. Young GB, Jordan KG, Doig GS. An assessment of nonconvulsive seizures in the intensive care unit using continuous EEG monitoring: an investigation of variables associated with mortality. Neurology. 1996 Jul;47(1):83–89.

196. Brophy GM, Bell R, Claassen J, Alldredge B, Bleck TP, Glauser T, et al. Guidelines for the evaluation and management of status epilepticus. Neurocrit Care. 2012 Aug;17(1):3–23.

197. Claassen J, Taccone FS, Horn P, Holtkamp M, Stocchetti N, Oddo M, et al. Recommendations on the use of EEG monitoring in critically ill patients: consensus statement from the neurointensive care section of the ESICM. Intensive Care Med. 2013 Aug;39(8):1337–1351.

198. Grand W. The significance of post-traumatic status epilepticus in childhood. J Neurol Neurosurg Psychiatry. 1974 Feb;37(2):178–180.

199. Niedermeyer E, Knott JT. Über die Bedeutung der 14 und 6/sec-positiven Spitzen im EEG. Archiv für Psychiatrie und Nervenkrankheiten. 1961;202(3):266–280.

200. Ross RJ, Cole M, Thompson JS, Kim KH. Boxers—computed tomography, EEG, and neurological evaluation. JAMA. 1983 Jan 14;249(2):211–213.

201. Pampus F, Grote W. Elektrencephalographische und klinische Befunde bei Boxern und ihre Bedeutung für die Pathophysiologie der traumatischen Hirnschädigung. Archiv für Psychiatrie und Nervenkrankheiten. 1956;194(2):152–178.

202. Critchley M. Medical aspects of boxing, particularly from a neurological standpoint. Br Med J. 1957 Feb 16;1(5015):357–362.

203. Mawdsley C, Ferguson FR. Neurological disease in boxers. Lancet. 1963 Oct 19;2(7312):795–801.

204. Tysvaer AT, Storli OV, Bachen NI. Soccer injuries to the brain. A neurologic and electroencephalographic study of former players. Acta Neurol Scand. 1989 Aug;80(2):151–156.

205. Tysvaer AT. Head and neck injuries in soccer. Impact of minor trauma. Sports Med. 1992 Sep;14(3):200–213.

206. Gronseth GS, Greenberg MK. The utility of the electroencephalogram in the evaluation of patients presenting with headache: a review of the literature. Neurology. 1995 Jul;45(7):1263–1267.

207. Langer-Gould AM, Anderson WE, Armstrong MJ, Cohen AB, Eccher MA, Iverson DJ, et al. The American Academy of Neurology's top five Choosing Wisely recommendations. Neurology. 2013 Sep 10;81(11):1004–1011.

208. Bille BO. Migraine in school children. Acta Paediatrica. 1962;51(5):614–616.

209. Krischek J. Elektrencephalographische Befunde bei Migräne. J Neurol. 1956;175(1):43–49.

210. Ulett GA, Evans D, O'Leary JL. Survey of EEG findings in 1,000 patients with chief complaint of headache. Electroencephalogr Clin Neurophysiol. 1952 Nov;4(4):463–470.

211. Heyck H. Der Kopfschmerz. G. Thieme; 1964.

212. Weil AA. Observations on "dysrhythmic" migraine. J Nerv Ment Dis. 1962 Mar;134:277–281.

213. Dow DJ, Whitty CWM. Electroencephalographic changes in migraine; review of 51 cases. Lancet. 1947 Jul 12;2(6463):52–54.

214. Selby G, Lance JW. Observations on 500 cases of migraine and allied vascular headache. J Neurol Neurosurg Psychiatr. 1960 Feb;23(1):23–32.

215. Barolin GS. Migraines and epilepsies—a relationship? Epilepsia. 1966 Mar;7(1):53–66.

216. Gschwend J. EEG-Befunde und ihre Interpretation bei einfacher Migräne. Zeitschrift für Neurologie. 1972;201(3):279–292.

217. Smyth VO, Winter AL. The EEG in migraine. Electroencephalogr Clin Neurophysiol. 1964 Jan;16:194–202.

218. Jonkman EJ, Lelieveld MH. EEG computer analysis in patients with migraine. Electroencephalogr Clin Neurophysiol. 1981 Dec;52(6):652–655.

219. Golla FL, Winter AL. Analysis of cerebral responses to flicker in patients complaining of episodic headache. Electroencephalogr Clin Neurophysiol. 1959 Aug;11(3):539–549.

220. Slatter KH. Some clinical and EEG findings in patients with migraine. Brain. 1968 Mar;91(1):85–98.

221. Simon RH, Zimmerman AW, Tasman A, Hale MS. Spectral analysis of photic stimulation in migraine. Electroencephalogr Clin Neurophysiol. 1982 Mar;53(3):270–276.

222. Scollo-Lavizzari G. Das Elektroenzephalogramm bei der Migräne. Neurology. 1975;64:234–237.

223. Heyck H. Neue Beiträge zur Klinik und Pathogenese der Migräne. Georg Thieme; 1956.

224. Schoenen J, Jamart B, De Pasqua V, Delwaide PJ. Mapping of EEG and auditory event-potentials in migraine. Electroencephalogr Clin Neurophysiol. 1990;75:S135.

225. Bazil CW, Herman ST, Pedley TA, Ebersole J, Pedley T. Focal electroencephalographic abnormalities. Current Practice of Clinical Electroencephalography, 3rd ed Philadelphia, PA: Lippincott Williams & Wilkins, 2003, pp. 303–347.

226. Rosenbaum HE. Familial hemiplegic migraine. Neurology. 1960 Feb;10:164–170.

227. Heron JR. Migraine and cerebrovascular disease. Neurology. 1966 Nov;16(11):1097–1104.

228. Whitty CW. Familial hemiplegic migraine. J Neurol Neurosurg Psychiatr. 1953 Aug;16(3):172–177.

229. Bradshaw P, Parsons M. Hemiplegic migraine, a clinical study. Q J Med. 1965 Jan;34:65–85.

230. Alvarez WC. Migraine plus epilepsy. Neurology. 1959 Jul;9(7):487–491.

231. Sances G, Guaschino E, Perucca P, Allena M, Ghiotto N, Manni R. Migralepsy: a call for a revision of the definition. Epilepsia. 2009 Nov;50(11):2487–2496.

232. Verrotti A, Coppola G, Di Fonzo A, Tozzi E, Spalice A, Aloisi P, et al. Should "migralepsy" be considered an obsolete concept? A multicenter retrospective clinical/EEG study and review of the literature. Epilepsy Behav. 2011 May;21(1):52–59.

233. Panayiotopoulos CP. "Migralepsy" and the significance of differentiating occipital seizures from migraine. Epilepsia. 2006 Apr;47(4):806–808.

234. Camfield PR, Metrakos K, Andermann F. Basilar migraine, seizures, and severe epileptiform EEG abnormalities. Neurology. 1978 Jun;28(6):584–588.

235. Panayiotopoulos CP. Elementary visual hallucinations, blindness, and headache in idiopathic occipital epilepsy: differentiation from migraine. J Neurol Neurosurg Psychiatr. 1999 Apr;66(4):536–540.

236. Kinast M, Lueders H, Rothner AD, Erenberg G. Benign focal epileptiform discharges in childhood migraine (BFEDC). Neurology. 1982 Nov;32(11):1309–1311.

237. Kellaway P, Crawley JW, Kagawa N. Paroxysmal pain and autonomic disturbances of cerebral origin: a specific electro-clinical syndrome. Epilepsia. 1959;1(1-5):466–483.

238. Moore MT. Paroxysmal abdominal pain; a form of focal symptomatic epilepsy. JAMA. 1945 Dec 29;129:1233–1240.

239. Ahmed I. Contingent negative variation in migraine: effect of beta blocker therapy. Clin Electroencephalogr. 1999 Jan;30(1):21–23.

240. Panayiotopoulos CP, Michael M, Sanders S, Valeta T, Koutroumanidis M. Benign childhood focal epilepsies: assessment of established and newly recognized syndromes. Brain. 2008 Sep;131(Pt 9):2264–2286.

241. Bickerstaff E. Basilar artery migraine. Lancet. 1961;277(7167):15–17.

242. Bickerstaff ER. Impairment of consciousness in migraine. Lancet. 1961 Nov 11;2(7211):1057–1059.

243. Lapkin ML, French JH, Golden GS, Rowan AJ. The electroencephalogram in childhood basilar artery migraine. Neurology. 1977 Jun;27(6):580–583.

244. Parain D, Samson-Dollfus D. Electroencephalograms in basilar artery migraine. Electroencephalogr Clin Neurophysiol. 1984 Nov;58(5):392–399.

245. Ramelli GP, Sturzenegger M, Donati F, Karbowski K. EEG findings during basilar migraine attacks in children. Electroencephalogr Clin Neurophysiol. 1998 Nov;107(5):374–378.

246. Sbrascini S, Bassi P. Headache and slow hypersynchronization of the EEG during hyperventilation. Electroencephalogr Clin Neurophysiol. 1983;55(1):P3–P3.

247. Evers S, Goadsby PJ. Hypnic headache: clinical features, pathophysiology, and treatment. Neurology. 2003 Mar 25;60(6):905–909.

248. Drake ME, Huber SJ, Pakalnis A, Denio LC. Computerized EEG spectral analysis in migraine and tension headaches. J Clin Neurophysiol. 1987;4(3):301.

16 | EEG IN DEMENTING DISORDERS

CLAUDIO BABILONI, PHD, CLAUDIO DEL PERCIO, PHD, AND ANA BUJÁN, PHD

ABSTRACT: This chapter reviews the most relevant literature on qualitative and quantitative abnormalities in resting-state eyes-closed electroencephalographic (rsEEG) rhythms recorded in patients with dementing disorders due to Alzheimer's disease, frontotemporal lobar degeneration, vascular disease, Parkinson's disease, Lewy body disease, human immunodeficiency virus infection, and prion disease, mainly Creutzfeldt–Jakob disease. This condition of quiet wakefulness is the most used in clinical practice, as it involves a simple, innocuous, quick, noninvasive, and cost-effective procedure that can be repeated many times without effects of stress, learning, or habituation. While rsEEG has a limited diagnostic value (not reflecting peculiar pathophysiological processes directly), delta, theta, and alpha rhythms might be promising candidates as "topographical markers" for the prognosis and monitoring of disease evolution and therapy response, at least for the most diffuse dementing disorders. More research is needed before those topographical biomarkers can be proposed for routine clinical applications.

KEYWORDS: electroencephalography, rsEEG, dementia, Alzheimer's disease, frontotemporal lobar degeneration, vascular disease, Parkinson's disease, Lewy body disease, human immunodeficiency virus, HIV

PRINCIPAL REFERENCES

1. Babiloni C, Lizio R, Marzano N, Capotosto P, Soricelli A, Triggiani AI, et al. Brain neural synchronization and functional coupling in Alzheimer's disease as revealed by resting state EEG rhythms. Int J Psychophysiol. 2016; 103:88–102
2. D'Amelio M, Rossini PM. Brain excitability and connectivity of neuronal assemblies in Alzheimer's disease: from animal models to human findings. Prog Neurobiol. 2012;99(1):42–60.
3. Dauwels J, Vialatte F, Cichocki A. Diagnosis of Alzheimer's disease from EEG signals: where are we standing? Curr Alzheimer Res. 2010;7(6):487–505.
4. Drago V, Babiloni C, Bartrés-Faz D, Caroli A, Bosch B, Hensch T, et al. Disease tracking markers for Alzheimer's disease at the prodromal (MCI) stage. J Alzheimers Dis. 2011;26(s3):159–199.
5. Jelic V, Kowalski J. Evidence-based evaluation of diagnostic accuracy of resting EEG in dementia and mild cognitive impairment. Clin EEG Neurosci. 2009;40(2):129–142.
6. Babiloni C, Triggiani AI, Lizio R, Cordone S, Tattoli G, Bevilacqua V, et al. Classification of single normal and Alzheimer's disease individuals from cortical sources of resting state EEG rhythms. Front Neurosci. 2016;23:10–47.
7. Dubois B, Feldman HH, Jacova C, Hampel H, Molinuevo JL, Blennow K, et al. Advancing research diagnostic criteria for Alzheimer's disease: the IWG-2 criteria. Lancet Neurol. 2014;13(6):614–629.
8. Engedal K, Snaedal J, Hoegh P, Jelic V, Bo Andersen B, Naik M, et al. Quantitative EEG applying the statistical recognition pattern method: a useful tool in dementia diagnostic workup. Dement Geriatr Cogn Disord 2015;40(1-2):1–12.
9. Hsiao F, Wang Y, Yan S, Chen W, Lin Y. Altered oscillation and synchronization of default-mode network activity in mild Alzheimer's disease compared to mild cognitive impairment: an electrophysiological study. PloS One 2013;8(7): e68792.
10. Snaedal J, Johannesson GH, Gudmundsson TE, Blin NP, Emilsdottir AL, Einarsson B, et al. Diagnostic accuracy of statistical pattern recognition of electroencephalogram registration in evaluation of cognitive impairment and dementia. Dement Geriatr Cogn Disord 2012;34(1):51–60.

1. INTRODUCTION

Dementia is a syndrome characterized by a significant decline in one or more cognitive domains from a previous level, with the loss of independence in everyday activities. It often interacts with physiological aging and is associated with emotional, motivational, and behavioral symptoms.

Epidemiologically, dementing disorders are a major burden, especially in the aged Western population. In 2015, 47 million people suffered from dementia worldwide. This number will reach 75 million in 2030 and 135 million in 2050. The estimated cost of dementia worldwide is around US $818 billion in 2015, including direct and indirect costs.

Dementia is caused by several different etiologies. In the American Psychiatric Association's *Diagnostic and Statistical Manual of Mental Disorders* (5th ed.; DSM-5), the term "dementia" is replaced by the gentler "major neurocognitive disorder." However, one can still use dementia due to Alzheimer's disease (ADD), vascular disease (VaD), frontotemporal lobar degeneration (FTD), Parkinson's disease (PDD), Lewy body disease (DLB), HIV infection (HAD), or Creutzfeldt–Jakob disease (CJD).

2. ELECTROENCEPHALOGRAPHY AND DEMENTING DISORDERS

In the clinical environment, resting-state eyes-closed electroencephalographic (rsEEG) activity is recorded typically from 19 scalp electrodes placed according to the 10-20 montage system. This quiet wakefulness is achieved through specific instructions. Subjects are asked to let their mind wander freely, without any sort of oriented mental operation including focused attention, memory recall, planning, and so forth. They are also asked to avoid voluntary or involuntary movements, drowsiness, and falling asleep.

Can rsEEG biomarkers be useful for the diagnosis, prognosis, and monitoring of the dementing disorders? Jelic and Kowalski (1) used high-quality criteria to select qualified 1980–2009 papers regarding the diagnostic accuracy of rsEEG in dementing disorders. They concluded that although several studies reported that the classification accuracy of patients with these disorders exceeded 80%, the evidence of practical diagnostic utility is not yet sufficient to suggest the routine use of rsEEG biomarkers in memory clinics. Along this line, in 2007 the European Federation of the Neurological Societies (EFNS) established a Level B (i.e., suboptimal) recommendation for the use of rsEEG in the diagnosis of patients with suspected CJD or transient epileptic amnesia and only an enrichment value in ADD (2). They also recommended rsEEG as a good practice in differential diagnosis of atypical clinical presentations of ADD but not in the initial assessment of all patients suspected of having dementing disorders (3,4). Other guidelines on AD did not mention rsEEG as a diagnostic, prognostic, or monitoring biomarker (5-7).

3. THE AIM OF THE CHAPTER

In this chapter, we review the relevant literature using Jelic and Kowalski's high-quality criteria ((1), pp. 135 and 136) with the broad aim of determining "whether and how" rsEEG biomarkers might help to characterize abnormal neurophysiological features associated with cognitive impairment in dementing disorders. From a theoretical point of view, we posit that the potential role of the rsEEG measures can be derived from the second paper by the International Working Group (IWG-2) for New Research Criteria for the Diagnosis of AD (5), even if it does not deal with EEG biomarkers. This IWG-2 paper defined two distinct classes of biomarkers for the assessment of AD:

1. The *diagnostic biomarkers* of AD were those measuring directly or indirectly the pathophysiological hallmarks of the disease. They include the following:
   a. The dosing of amyloid beta1-42 (Aβ1-42, the main compound of the senile plaques), total-tau (as a marker for neuronal degeneration) or phospho-tau (as a marker for hyperphosphorylation of tau protein and possibly for the formation of neurofibrillary tangles) in cerebrospinal fluid (CSF).
   b. Indexes of abnormal Aβ1-42 and tau accumulation in brain maps of ligand positron emission tomography (PET).

2. The *topographical biomarkers* were those providing indexes of brain structural, molecular, and functional integrity. Although they reveal abnormalities not necessarily specific for AD (e.g., cortical atrophy is common to two or more dementing disorders), this information is expected to be very useful for the assessment and monitoring of the global brain status during the evolution of the disease. The following topographical biomarkers are included in the IWG-2 criteria:
   a. FDG-PET biomarkers of posterior brain hypometabolism in the resting state condition, possibly reflecting synaptic dysfunction.
   b. Magnetic resonance imaging (MRI) biomarkers of hippocampus/cortical atrophy, probably indicating neurodegenerative neural loss.

Keeping in mind the above theoretical premises, here we posit that different features of the rsEEG might be considered as topographical biomarkers for dementing disorders as opposed to the status of diagnostic biomarker. Among the other topographical biomarkers, the peculiar contribution of the rsEEG biomarker may be to probe the efficiency/frailty of the neurophysiological mechanisms of cortical neural synchronization/desynchronization and oscillatory functional connectivity among cortical regions regulating brain arousal in quiet wakefulness for different dementing disorders. These mechanisms are the biological underpinning of vigilance, which is a prerequisite of many cognitive functions (e.g., attention, consciousness, declarative memory) and might be an important feature of dementing disorders. In these mechanisms, cortical neural synchronization depends on an efficient functional connectivity and signal transmission within both local and long-distance neural networks in the brain spanning cerebral cortex, ascending neurotransmitter systems of the basal forebrain, and subcortical structures, with a pivotal role of the thalamus. In the following, we use the term "rsEEG biomarkers" even if it requires a full validation in future research before routine clinical applications.

The aim of the chapter subtends the following two working hypotheses:

1. The rsEEG topographical biomarkers unveil abnormal neurophysiological mechanisms underlying impaired cognition in pathological aging at both group and individual levels, even if they might be not sufficiently sensitive and specific for routine diagnostic purposes at the individual level. At the group level, the evaluation of these neurophysiological mechanisms might enlighten the interaction between the pathophysiological mechanisms of the diseases and brain circuits generating rsEEG in the quiet wakefulness. At the individual level, that evaluation might provide an index of neurophysiological frailty-robustness as a dimension of the individual cerebral reserve.

2. These rsEEG biomarkers can capture the impairment of neurophysiological mechanisms underlying the disease progression or the beneficial effects of a successful treatment at both group and individual levels. They might be used as neurophysiological endpoints in intervention clinical trials at the group level, and useful indications to confirm or change the therapy at the individual level.

4. FEATURES OF THE RSEEG TOPOGRAPHICAL BIOMARKERS IN DEMENTING DISORDERS

Three classes of rsEEG features are of interest for the chapter aim. The first class, named *waveforms*, refers to the description, through visual analysis at scalp electrodes, of well-known graphic elements (graphoelements) observed on rsEEG traces recorded in some dementing disorders. These graphoelements are supposed to reflect a rapid abnormal change of synchrony of the activity of a local cortical neural population whose summed local field potentials can be detected from scalp electrodes.

The second and third classes are derived from the quantitative analysis of the rsEEG rhythms. The second class was named *synchronization*. As for the waveforms, these features are supposed to reflect the time evolution of the synchronized activity of local cortical neural populations at a spatial scale of few centimeters, which subtends a fluctuating balance of cortical neural synchronization and desynchronization over time (8). In the synchronization class, we include all linear and nonlinear features of the rsEEG rhythms recordable at a given scalp electrode or underlying cortical area (spectral analysis, topographical analysis, complexity measures).

The third class, named *connectivity*, is supposed to reflect the interrelatedness or coupling[1] of the activity of two or more local neural populations at mesoscopic scale whose activity generates recordable rsEEG rhythms at two or more scalp electrodes (8). In the *connectivity* class we included several linear and nonlinear features of rsEEG rhythms (correlational methods, synchronization measures, graph analysis, estimates of causality).

For a comprehensive description of theory and methodological approaches used in EEG analyses, see the Chapter 44 (in this book) and the reviews by Dauwels et al. (9) and Stam et al. (10).

5. RSEEG RHYTHMS IN THE ADULT BRAIN AND PHYSIOLOGICAL AGING

Some reviews have described rsEEG rhythms in the adult brain (Chapter 8) and along with physiological aging (11–13). Visual inspection of rsEEG waveforms shows the following changes over time:

1. A slowing to 7 to 8 Hz in frequency

2. A short time of evident alpha waves

3. Small reactivity of these waves to eyes opening

4. Benign rhythmic subharmonic variants of the delta or theta frequencies (see (13) for a review; (14)).

However, there is no international consensus about what features and thresholds allow discriminating gradual changes of the rsEEG rhythms due to physiological aging from pathological processes in individual seniors. Even "statistically normal" rsEEG rhythms might underlie subclinical pathological aging. Keeping in mind this lack of an international consensus, the following features of the rsEEG waveforms merit some attention and more exams to exclude underlying pathological aging:

1. A posterior alpha rhythm <7 to 8 Hz

2. Slowing of the alpha peak frequency of 1 Hz over 1 year

3. Abnormal focal delta–theta rhythms (<7 Hz) in the anterior temporal areas, especially in the left hemisphere in subjects over 60 years old.

In the rsEEG waveforms, the intermittent delta activity in temporal areas might be considered nonpathological, namely the benign temporal delta transients of the elderly (BTDTE), when nine specified criteria of Klass and Brenner ((13), p. 119) are fulfilled. If these nine typical characteristics are not met, those temporal rsEEG rhythms may indicate vascular or neurodegenerative pathology in temporal cortex (13). In this vein, the association between focal abnormalities in temporal areas and objective mild cognitive impairment (MCI) in a large cohort of memory clinic patients would support this view (15). However, Klass and Brenner's criteria for BTDTE are somewhat complicated to apply in the clinical routine, and no information is available on their intra- and inter-rater reliability and the relation to cognitive dysfunction.

Computerized quantitative spectral analysis of rsEEG rhythms would show some changes of synchronization and connectivity features with physiological aging; however, caution is mandatory due to methodological differences in the reviewed studies regarding power density measures, frequency bands, age ranges of the samples, neuroimaging assessment, and so forth.

Concerning the rsEEG synchronization, most of the studies point to a reduction in the posterior alpha power density in seniors compared with young adults (16–18). This effect seems to be true for both alpha-1 (i.e., low frequency at ~8–10 Hz) and alpha-2 (i.e., high frequency at ~10–12 Hz) sub-bands (16), even in the cortical source space (19). With respect to the other rsEEG frequencies, the results are more controversial. Concerning the delta rhythms (<4 Hz), different studies have shown a decrease (19), an increase (16), or no differences at all (20). In the theta rhythms (4–7 Hz), Finnigan and Robertson (21) found that frontal normalized theta power density correlated positively with cognitive function in healthy seniors. In contrast, Roca-Stappung et al. (22) found a negative correlation between absolute theta power density at frontal sites and working memory measures, but a positive correlation between theta power at temporal and occipital sites and perceptual organization and processing speed measures.

Concerning the rsEEG connectivity, most of the studies report a less efficient communication between brain regions with physiological aging. Vysata et al. (23) reported a tendency toward an age-related decline in global theta and alpha coherence but a global increase in beta coherence. Zhu et al. (24) found that the asymmetry of cortical interactive networks—as measured by partial directed coherence—declines with aging, resulting in a greater loss of connectivity in the left frontal and central areas. Smit et al. (25), assessing lifespan changes in rsEEG connectivity, found a significant decrease in that connectivity at theta, alpha, and beta rhythms (as revealed by rsEEG synchronization likelihood [SL]) in normal elderly (Nold) subjects. In addition, they found that the topology of the graph networks in older adults is characterized by a significant decrement in the path length (i.e., average of the distance of connections between

---

[1] The present feature, connectivity, can be considered as part of the concept of synchronization. Nevertheless, here we propose that in the generation of rsEEG rhythms, synchronization and connectivity are predominantly associated with vertical thalamocortical and horizontal cortical neural interactions, respectively (even with a large overlap in the respective neurophysiological processes). Indeed, coherence, or functional connectivity/coupling of rsEEG rhythms in different cortical sites, is related to some synchronization of distant cortical neural populations. Furthermore, vertical thalamocortical and horizontal cortical neural interactions are typically interrelated in the global topology of the functional human brain connectome.

each node to all the other nodes) in the theta rhythm. Other evidence showed an increase in path length at delta and theta rhythms, and a decrease in alpha rhythm (26). Although both studies point to more random and non-ordered networks with physiological aging, the results of these studies are difficult to compare as the methodologies used differ in many aspects. An important source of variance is the lack of an accurate clinical and neuroimaging assessment of Nold groups to exclude individuals with preclinical dementing disorders.

6. DEMENTIA DUE TO ALZHEIMER'S DISEASE

AD is characterized by deposition of Aβ protein in senile plaques, axonal neurofibrillary tangles composed of abnormally phosphorylated tau protein, neuronal loss, and brain atrophy (27). According to the most recent guidelines (5,7), AD can be diagnosed preclinically, based on pathophysiological diagnostic markers revealed by CSF and positron emission tomography (PET) dosing of Aβ1-42 and tau. In the same line, AD can be diagnosed in the prodromal stage of MCI (AD-MCI) or dementia (ADD). In precedence, "amnestic" MCI (aMCI) was presumably related to AD merely on clinical basis, while non-amnestic MCI was attributed to other causes of dementia (28).

6.1. rsEEG Waveforms in AD

A typical waveform from one ADD patient can be seen in Figure 16.1. In the earliest phase of the disease, the visual inspection cannot reveal gross abnormalities of the rsEEG waveforms (13). In the latest phase, normal EEG waveforms over the whole scalp argue against a diagnosis of AD (15). Focal rsEEG abnormalities are not typical and may be related to the frequent occurrence of vascular pathology in AD. Nevertheless, de Waal et al. (29) found that focal and diffuse rsEEG abnormalities are more prevalent in early than late-onset ADD patients.

6.2. rsEEG Synchronization in AD

Compared with Nold subjects, ADD patients are typically characterized by the following (see (1,30,31) for reviews):

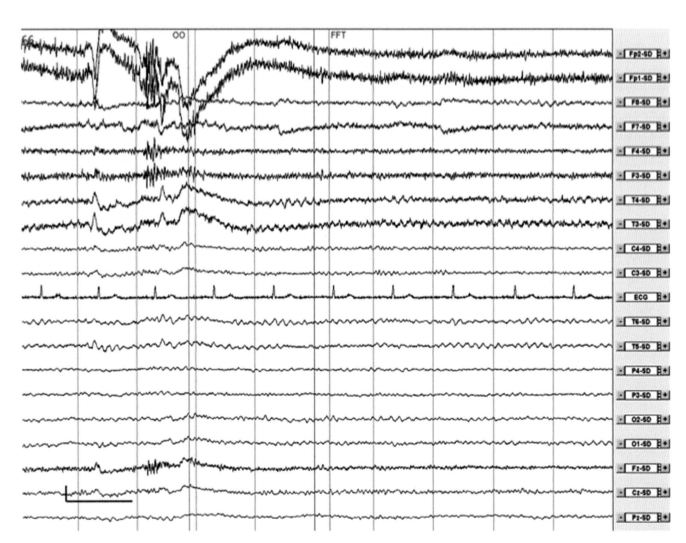

Figure 16.1. Male, 87 years, with Alzheimer's disease. Irregular, mildly slowed alpha rhythm, more pronounced at posterior temporal areas and diminished reactivity to eye closure. Calibration mark: vertical, 50 μV; horizontal, 1 sec. Filter settings: time constant 1 sec. Low-pass filter, 35 Hz. Source derivation.

1. A widespread decrease in posterior power density in the alpha and beta rhythms

2. A widespread increase in theta and delta power density

3. Reduction of the alpha peak frequency

4. Low reactivity of the alpha power density to eye opening.

Babiloni et al. and other independent groups showed topographical details on cortical sources of the rsEEG rhythms in ADD patients (see (32) for a review). Converging evidence points to reduced parieto-occipital dominant alpha and increased low-frequency (delta/theta) source activity in occipital, parietal, and temporal areas in ADD patients compared with Nold individuals as a function of ApoE ε4, cognitive impairment, and structural brain impairment. A similar spatial-frequency pattern with attenuated amplitude of the rsEEG rhythms was observed in patients with aMCI (see (32) for a review; (33)). Furthermore, it was shown (34) that the occipital theta and the frontal delta sources have greater activity in aMCI subjects compared with people with subjective (but not objective) memory complaints and non-amnestic MCI. Finally, nonlinear measures of cortical synchronization showed a loss of complexity of brain dynamics in ADD (see (9) for a review; (35)).

6.3. rsEEG Connectivity in AD

Different measures of rsEEG connectivity point to abnormal functional interactions between brain regions in AD (see (32,36) for reviews), in line with the vision of AD as a brain disconnection syndrome. Compared with Nold subjects, ADD patients are typically characterized by a decrease in the resting-state alpha coherence between electrode pairs, with main effects in temporo-parieto-occipital regions (see (1,9,32) for reviews). In contrast to the alpha rhythm, the low-frequency (delta and theta) rsEEG rhythms show mixed results (37–40), maybe due to a complex topographical pattern (41).

Due to the intrinsic low spatial resolution of the EEG approach, Babiloni et al. (42) limited the connectivity (e.g., linear lagged connectivity) analysis to cortical lobes using the "exact" variant of eLORETA freeware (http://www.uzh.ch/keyinst/loreta.htm). Compared to the Nold group, the ADD group showed higher delta inter- and intra-hemispherical connectivity, mainly among posterior regions. Furthermore, there was a topographically widespread lower alpha connectivity between all pairs of regions (frontal, central, parietal, temporal, occipital, and limbic).

Interesting evidence is derived from an autoregressive measure such as directed transfer function (DTF), the value and direction of the flow of information between EEG signals derived by Granger causality (see for details Chapter 44). The DTF displays a reduction in alpha and beta from parietal to frontal electrodes, and also in full-frequency DTF (a variation of DTF with a global normalization in frequency), in ADD and aMCI patients compared with Nold subjects (43–46). Regarding phase synchronization, Canuet et al. (33) reported a decrease in alpha-2 lagged phase synchronization between temporal and parietal electrodes in ADD patients compared

with Nold subjects, and an increase in low-frequency rsEEG, specifically in the theta band, between and within hemispheres. Nevertheless, in aMCI compared to Nold subjects, the opposite result is found—that is, decreased phase lag index in the delta and theta rhythms within the frontal and between the frontal and temporal/parietal areas, with more pronounced effects 1 year later (47).

The graph theory provides further measures of rsEEG connectivity in the comparison between groups of ADD/aMCI patients and Nold subjects ((48); see also (49) for a review). Compared with Nold subjects, ADD patients are characterized by a more random pattern of rsEEG connectivity, possibly due to a loss of critical communication lines (reviewed in (49)). However, the results are inconsistent, showing both increases and decreases in local connectivity, especially in the alpha-1 band (50,51).

Keeping in mind the above results, the decrease in connectivity of the alpha rhythms might be considered as a consistent hallmark in patients with ADD and aMCI, as an interesting neurophysiological facet of the underlying disconnection syndrome. On the other hand, it is not yet clear what may be the most consistent topographical pattern and mathematical measure to model this abnormality (see (9) for a discussion). More research is needed in this promising direction.

6.4. rsEEG Features of Disease Progression in AD

ADD patients showing abnormal rsEEG waveforms in initial stages may have a worse prognosis with more severe neurological abnormalities, severe cognitive and functional decline, and poor prognosis (see (1)). This evidence well represents the concept of "neurophysiological frailty" that abnormal rsEEG topographical markers might reflect. Along the same line, the following spectral rsEEG features might predict a substantial cognitive decline in aMCI subjects at about 6 to 24 months (see (52) for a review):

1. Combined alpha–theta power density and mean frequency from left temporal-occipital regions (53)

2. Anterior localization of alpha sources (54)

3. High temporal delta sources (55)

4. High theta power density (56)

5. Low posterior alpha power density (57).

At those baseline rsEEG recordings, several EEG features differ between the groups of aMCI subjects progressing to ADD from stable ones:

1. Decreased global alpha power density and anterior localization of theta, alpha, and beta sources (54)

2. Unselective greater activity across delta, theta, and alpha sources (55)

3. Reduced posterior alpha rhythms (57,58)

4. Increased global alpha-3/alpha-2 ratio (59).

Furthermore, several longitudinal studies showed the following changes of the rsEEG features across time (e.g.,~12–24 months) in aMCI subjects and ADD patients (see (52) for a review):

1. Increased delta–theta and increased alpha–beta power density at parieto-occipital electrodes (60)

2. Increased theta power density, decreased beta power density, and decreased mean frequency at the temporal and temporo-occipital electrodes (53,61,62)

3. Increased delta and increased alpha-1 in parieto-occipital sources (63, 64)

4. Reduced cortical connectivity as revealed by graph theory indexes (65).

6.5. rsEEG Features and Severity of AD

The relationship between clinical/cognitive status and rsEEG power density at a group level was investigated by cross-sectional studies. Rodríguez et al. (66) showed that the most severe ADD stages are characterized by the increase of low-frequency rsEEG bands (e.g. delta and theta), with the disappearance of the alpha frequency peak. Along the same line, Jelic et al. (53) reported that compared with the aMCI group, the ADD group has a higher theta power density at temporal, occipital, and centro-parietal electrodes, as well as lower temporoparietal coherence.

Babiloni et al. used LORETA methodology for the estimation and comparison of rsEEG cortical sources between ADD and aMCI patients (see (32) for a review). The aMCI group is characterized by intermediate values of source activity at low-frequency alpha in occipital, temporal, limbic, and parietal regions (intermediate = halfway between ADD patients and Nold subjects). Hsiao et al. (67) confirmed the abnormal activity of posterior cortical sources of rsEEG rhythms with an independent approach (depth-weighted minimum-norm estimation) in mild ADD patients compared with aMCI subjects. Namely, there is a reduction in alpha and beta source activity in the posterior cingulate, precuneus, and parietal regions as well as an enhancement of delta or theta sources in the medial temporal, inferior parietal, posterior cingulate, and precuneus (67).

Concerning the comparison of rsEEG connectivity in cross-sectional studies, Hsiao et al. showed abnormal source coherence in ADD patients in the regions of the default mode and the sensorimotor networks (67,68). In general, the delta and theta source coherence was higher in the ADD than the aMCI group in both networks, while the opposite was true for alpha source coherence in the default mode network. Those findings represent an insightful view of the effects of AD in the rsEEG source space, thus extending previous evidence based on the study of rsEEG connectivity between scalp electrode pairs. Specifically, frontoparietal theta, alpha, and beta connectivity at scalp electrode level, as measured through DTF, shows higher values in Nold subjects, intermediate values in aMCI subjects, and lower values in ADD patients (43,44). Further evidence of cross-sectional studies comes from the use of graph analysis. In a group of aMCI subjects, the topology of the EEG connectivity, as measured by a small-worldness parameter (i.e., balance between local and global connections), pointed to an intermediate value between a group of Nold subjects and a group of ADD patients (48,51).

The relationship between clinical/cognitive status and rsEEG features was further investigated by correlational studies. In ADD patients, the severity of the clinical symptoms positively correlates with an anterior shift of alpha and beta source activity and the stronger source activity in the low-frequency bands (69,70). The global cognitive status (e.g., Mini Mental Status Exam [MMSE] score) is negatively correlated with delta sources but is positively correlated with alpha sources (71,72) and multiscale entropy at the temporal, parietal, and occipital electrodes (73). Furthermore, the global cognitive status is positively correlated with global field synchronization (74) but negatively correlated with temporal theta sources (33) and theta power density at the posterior electrodes (41). Along the same line, neuropsychological measures of memory and executive functioning are positively correlated with alpha source activity (75) and are negatively associated with the theta power density (56). Concerning the EEG connectivity, alpha and beta coherence (76,77) between all electrode pairs shows lower values in patients with ADD compared to Nold subjects, these values being positively correlated with scores of neuropsychological tests or global cognition as revealed by the MMSE score (76,77).

6.6. Abnormal rsEEG Features in Individual AD Subjects

The above rsEEG features were shown to be of great interest to better understand the neurophysiological underpinning and the progression of AD at a group level. However, their practical use in clinical settings would require an accurate classification between Nold and AD individuals based on rsEEG features. Again, we remark that the rsEEG features should be tested in ADD individuals already diagnosed by the measurement of amyloid or tau accumulation in the brain, according to the actual international guidelines (5). In line with the present view, rsEEG features that can classify ADD individuals should be used to evaluate the frailty/integrity of neurophysiological mechanisms of the disease at an individual level rather than as a unique diagnostic biomarker.

Two main papers systematically reviewed the literature on the accuracy of the classification between ADD and Nold individuals by rsEEG features, mainly through the analysis of spectral power density and coherence. On the one hand, Jonkman et al. (78) reviewed 16 studies published from 1983 to 1995, reporting a classification accuracy ranging from 54% to 100% (median 81%). As mentioned above, Jelic and Kowalski (1) reviewed 46 studies published from 1980 to 2008. They reported a classification accuracy with a sensitivity between 40% and 90% and a specificity between 70% and 100% for patients with ADD or MCI and individuals with or without other forms of dementia. Several groups report a comparable classification accuracy of 70% to 84% by both the visually assessed EEG waveforms and the spectral EEG features (see (1), Table 2).

More recently, Moretti et al. (59) reported that increased global theta/gamma and alpha-3/alpha-2 power density ratios predict the conversion from MCI to ADD or non-ADD with an accuracy of 88%. Babiloni et al. reported that the occipital alpha or the ratio between posterior delta and alpha source activity exhibits an accuracy ranging from 75% to 82% in the classification between different groups of ADD and Nold individuals (42,71,79). Trambaiolli et al. (80) reported that the temporal modulation of the energy in the delta, theta, alpha, beta, and gamma rhythms gives an accuracy of 91% for the classification of ADD and Nold individuals using a neural network classifier. In the study by Engedal et al. (81), 20 rsEEG features, including the alpha frequency peak, total power density, and between-electrode coherence, were used as inputs for the so-called statistical pattern recognition method to separate the individuals with ADD from those without or with other forms of dementia (e.g., PDD, DLB). Results showed an accuracy of 90% for the classification of ADD versus Nold individuals and ADD patients versus subjects with other dementing disorders. Concerning the connectivity features, Dauwels et al. (45) compared the classification accuracy of Nold and ADD subjects by many linear and nonlinear markers with a classification accuracy of ~70%, confirmed at the level of rsEEG cortical source space by eLORETA estimates (42). Finally, a novel approach used spatiotemporal rsEEG voltages as an input for a nonlinear auto-associative artificial neural network trained to reproduce those input voltages (82,83). The connection weights of that neural network were used for the binary classification, displaying an accuracy of 85% to 94% for the classification of ADD versus Nold individuals, ADD versus MCI individuals, and stable versus progressing MCI individuals (82,83).

Overall, the above findings suggest that the rsEEG features can support an inexpensive and noninvasive valid assessment of the neurophysiological frailty/integrity in AD individuals at different stages of the disease. More research is needed for a systematic comparison and standardization of those rsEEG features and classifiers for an optimal classification accuracy.

7. DEMENTIA DUE TO FRONTOTEMPORAL LOBAR DEGENERATION

FTD is considered as clinically and pathologically heterogeneous. The recent revised international criteria establish four main FTD variants: a behavioral variant, characterized by prominent early personality or behavioral changes (84), and three types of primary progressive aphasia syndromes (semantic variant, nonfluent/agrammatic variant, and logopenic variant) (85). There is also a consensus on the existence of five major pathological subtypes of frontotemporal lobar degeneration, but most of them are characterized by cellular inclusion bodies composed of either tau or TDP-43, mainly in frontal and medial temporal lobes (86).

7.1. rsEEG Waveforms in FTD

Contrary to the results in ADD, several studies reported normal or only mildly disturbed EEG waveforms in FTD through visual analysis. These waveforms commonly show preserved dominant posterior alpha rhythms and no differences in rsEEG reactivity to eye opening. Nevertheless, the waveforms deteriorate with the severity of the disease (1).

7.2. rsEEG Synchronization in FTD

Compared to ADD patients, those with FTD show well-preserved posterior alpha power and no increases in rsEEG low frequencies (see (1)). FTD patients also show higher activity in posterior alpha-2 and beta sources and lower delta source activity (87,88) while frontal and temporal alpha-1 source activity is lower in FTD than Nold subjects (88). Furthermore, mild FTD patients present with abnormal frontal microstates (i.e., short periods of stable rsEEG voltage topography) compared with both Nold and mild ADD subjects (89).

7.3. rsEEG Connectivity in FTD

Most studies showed normal rsEEG connectivity in FTD patients, mainly assessed through coherence and SL (reviewed in (1)). Normal topological graph features are also found (50).

7.4. Abnormal rsEEG Features in Individual FTD Subjects

Jelic and Kowalski ((1), Table 2) reported 70% to 81% sensitivity and 88% to 90% specificity for the discrimination between ADD and FTD patients. Caso et al. (87) performed a classification analysis based on calculation of z-scores from rsEEG spectral power and source activity. Results show a sensitivity of 48.7% in the detection of ADD patients and a specificity of 85% in the detection of FTD patients. Nishida et al. (88) classified them by computing receiving operating characteristic (ROC) curves from global field power. Results for beta rhythms show a sensitivity of 74% in the detection of ADD patients and a specificity of 63% in the detection of FTD patients. While the above rsEEG differences between ADD and FTD subjects are interesting for a neurophysiological modeling of neurodegenerative diseases, further research is needed to cross-validate these rsEEG features for practical clinical applications.

8. DEMENTIA DUE TO VASCULAR DISEASE

VaD is the second most common dementing disorder after AD, responsible for 10% to 20% of cases of dementia in North America and Europe (90). At present the NINDS-AIREN criteria represent the primary reference for the VaD diagnosis (91). They emphasize the typical irregular evolution of the clinical symptoms and the important role of neuroimaging biomarkers to reveal the vascular brain lesions. Unfortunately, those criteria have a sensitivity of just 43%, associated with a specificity of 95% (92). This low sensitivity is probably due to the vast heterogeneity of the causes of VaD (93), such as multiple cortical infarcts (causing multi-infarct dementia [MID]), lacunar white matter lesions (leading to subcortical ischemic vascular disease [SIVD]), strategic infarct dementia, hypoperfusion dementia caused by watershed infarcts, hemorrhagic dementia, cerebral autosomal dominant arteriopathy with subcortical infarcts and leukoencephalopathy (CADASIL), and AD with cardiovascular disease in the presence of a mixture of vascular and degenerative changes especially affecting the mesial temporal lobe (so-called mixed dementia) (94). The earlier literature had identified VaD with MID, thus missing all other causes of VaD. However, the more recent literature tends to identify VaD with SIVD, certainly the most frequent cause of VaD today. As a further consequence of this heterogeneity, patients diagnosed with VaD present a considerable variability in their cognitive impairment, further complicating the diagnosis and treatment. For diagnostic purposes, the American Heart Association and the American Stroke Association introduced the term *vascular cognitive impairment*, including MCI of probable vascular etiology and VaD (95). In this framework, biomarkers of VaD are highly desirable.

8.1. rsEEG Waveforms in VaD

In VaD patients, rsEEG waveforms typically show a focal slowing, but several studies failed to disentangle patients with ADD, MID, probable VaD, and mixed dementia (reviewed in (1)). This outcome is probably due to the presence of focal and diffuse rsEEG abnormalities in both VaD and ADD patients (15).

8.2. rsEEG Synchronization in VaD

Compared with Nold subjects, subcortical VaD patients show higher delta–theta (96,97) and lower alpha–beta power density (97). In relation to ADD patients, both MID and SIVD patients exhibit higher alpha power density (96,98), lower delta and higher alpha/theta ratio power density (96), as well as lower frequency of the alpha peak and lower alpha-3 power density (98). Furthermore, VaD patients are characterized by theta source activity that is abnormally high in widespread cortical regions compared to mild ADD patients (99).

Nonlinear rsEEG features show further differences between groups of patients with ADD and VaD, including those with large-vessel stroke, multiple subcortical lacunar infarcts, and extensive white matter lesions as revealed by MRI (100). Compared with both Nold and ADD patients, VaD patients show higher rsEEG complexity (100). More research is needed to better understand and cross-validate these findings.

8.3. rsEEG Connectivity in VaD

Brain lesions in VaD are typically diffuse and involve subcortical white matter bundles, so impaired brain functional connectivity is expected. In this vein, when compared to patients with ADD, MID patients show a substantial reduction in the rsEEG coherence in pre- and post-rolandic areas at wide frequency bands (reviewed in (1)). These findings indicate an abnormal coupling in broad cortico-subcortical and cortico-cortical networks in MID patients, especially vulnerable to widespread subcortical vascular damage as revealed by periventricular white matter hyperintensities (101). Nevertheless, a prediction of that neural

model is that the differences in the rsEEG coherence between ADD and cortical MID patients are expected to be modest due to frequent prominent cortical vascular lesions in both groups. Indeed, some results show that both groups of patients with reduced regional cortical blood flow (measured through single photon emission computed tomography [SPECT]) do not differ in terms of rsEEG coherence (102). However, other connectivity measures such as SL point to differences between ADD and VaD patients. In this vein, Babiloni et al. (103) reported that the most distinguished feature in mild ADD with respect to subcortical VaD patients with similar cognitive deficits is a prominent reduction of fronto-parietal SL in alpha-1.

8.4. rsEEG Features and Severity in VaD

In contrast to ADD, VaD patients manifest a less predictable clinical evolution, so there is a keen interest in the quest for biomarkers accounting for the VaD severity and progression from the MCI stage to dementia. In this line, Gawel et al. (104) performed a cross-sectional study comparing several rsEEG features in subcortical VaD patients with mild and moderate dementia. Although the visual analysis of the rsEEG waveform does not show any difference between mild and moderate subcortical VaD, the rsEEG mean frequency and alpha/theta and alpha/delta power density ratios are lower in the subgroup with moderate VaD compared with mild VaD. Concerning MCI patients with prodromal VaD, the severity of the vascular damage as revealed by MRI white matter hyperintensities is associated with increased global delta and decreased global alpha-2 power density (105). Interestingly, subcortical white matter vascular lesions and AD cortical neurodegeneration do interact in the determination of brain functioning and the patient's cognitive status. In this framework, a general view is that the rsEEG features are more sensitive to AD cortical neurodegeneration than subcortical white matter vascular lesions are. Therefore, it is expected that these rsEEG features are quite abnormal in MCI subjects with predominant AD cortical neurodegeneration. In this vein, Babiloni et al. (43,106) investigated the rsEEG sources in MCI subjects with mixed prodromal dementing disorders, namely AD and subcortical VaD. Compared with the group of MCI subjects having lower white matter vascular lesions (and prominent AD neurodegeneration explaining cognitive deficits), the MCI group with higher white matter vascular lesions (and prominent VaD explaining cognitive deficits) showed greater activity of posterior alpha-1 sources (106) and higher frontoparietal SL in the theta, alpha, and beta rhythms (43). Interestingly, a different picture emerged in the MCI subjects who suffered only from prodromal subcortical VaD and executive function deficits. These MCI patients exhibited smaller frontoparietal low-frequency coherence when compared to MCI patients with prodromal AD and episodic memory deficits.

8.5. Abnormal rsEEG Features in Individual VaD Subjects

In the previous sections, we reported different patterns of the rsEEG features in the groups of ADD and VaD patients. Those findings motivated further investigations testing the discriminative value of the rsEEG features at an individual level. In the review by Jelic and Kowalski ((1), Table 2), the classification between ADD and MID patients reached 50% to 69% sensitivity in the detection of ADD patients and 96% to 100% specificity in the detection of MID patients. Recently, Snaedal et al. (107) developed a classification procedure using 20 rsEEG features in seven groups of subjects:

1. Nold

2. ADD with an MMSE score >23

3. VaD

4. MCI stable for >24 months

5. DLB and PDD

6. FTD

7. Depression mimicking mild dementia.

They trained mathematical classifiers for all possible pair combinations of the above groups using a procedure called *statistical pattern recognition*. The classifiers used the area under the ROC curve to determine the classification accuracy. This advanced methodology reached an accuracy of 75% for the classification of ADD and VaD individuals, the latter showing a considerable heterogeneity.

Finally, Sheorajpanday et al. (108) found statistically significant correlations between the rsEEG feature called *pairwise derived brain symmetry index*, as quantitative EEG spectral power asymmetry along homologous channel pairs from a right and left channel (e.g., C3 and C4; P3 and P4 in the frequency range 1–25 Hz), and neuropsychological scores in MCI patients with prodromal subcortical VaD. Verbal fluency and delta plus theta/alpha plus beta ratio emerged as independent diagnostic predictors for these patients from multiple-domain aMCI subjects with an overall classification accuracy of 95%.

The findings regarding the classification between ADD and VaD individuals seem more promising than those obtained in FTD patients. Nevertheless, despite several encouraging studies (i.e., using populations with more accurate diagnostic entities), it remains unclear whether rsEEG features may have additional value compared to neuroimaging biomarkers and clinical impact. Indeed, the contribution of the rsEEG features in the assessment of VaD patients is quite limited at present.

9. DEMENTIA DUE TO PARKINSON'S AND LEWY BODIES DISEASES

After AD, PD is the most prevalent neurodegenerative disorder. Its main pathological characteristic is cell death in the substantia nigra with a dysfunction of five major circuits involving other brain areas along with the basal ganglia, namely the motor, oculomotor, associative, limbic, and orbitofrontal circuits. The microscopic anatomy (histopathology) discloses neuronal loss and Lewy bodies in many damaged nerve cells. From a clinical point of view, PD is characterized by motor symptoms such as akinesia, rigidity, tremor, and postural instability. Mild executive cognitive dysfunction can occur early in the disease, while full-blown dementia (PDD) is a frequent complication in the later stages.

DLB is another progressive neurodegenerative dementia closely related to PD. Its main pathological characteristic is the death of cholinergic neurons, possibly accounting for the cognitive impairment (similarly to AD), and the death of dopaminergic neurons in basal ganglia, responsible for Parkinsonian motor symptoms. The histopathology reveals Lewy bodies in many nerve cells. From a clinical point of view, DLB's primary symptom is cognitive decline with a marked fluctuation across the day in terms of attention, alertness, memory, planning, and abstract thinking. While the prevalence of PDD and DLB is relatively high (10–15%), making the differential diagnosis of DLB over PDD and ADD is tricky and requires new biomarkers.

9.1. rsEEG Waveforms in PDD and DLB

Visual inspection of the rsEEG waveforms in DLB patients revealed an extensive "EEG slowing," but it is still an open issue if this feature allows a clear distinction between DLB and ADD patients (109,110). Some authors reported that the slowing of the rsEEG background activity is more severe in DLB than in ADD (reviewed in (1)). For this reason, rsEEG abnormalities are considered as supportive/suggestive features to enrich the diagnosis of DLB (111). In this line, Liedorp et al. (15) posited that normal rsEEG waveforms or only focal abnormalities argue against a diagnosis of DLB, whereas the presence of both focal *and* diffuse rsEEG abnormalities suggests a diagnosis of DLB. But this result is not specific for a diagnostic claim, as this pattern is also observed for ADD and VaD patients. Among the rsEEG abnormalities, frontal intermittent rhythmic activity (FIRDA) may occur frequently in DLB but not in ADD (see (1)). Specifically, Lee et al. (112) reported the presence of FIRDA in 1.8% of patients with ADD and 17.2% of those with DLB.

9.2. rsEEG Synchronization in PDD and DLB

Compared with Nold subjects, PD patients show higher delta and theta power density in several scalp regions, more evident in association with a progressive cognitive impairment (see (113) for a review). These features appear to be specific, as delta and theta power density is higher in PDD patients than ADD, PD, and Nold subjects (114). In parallel to low-frequency rsEEG abnormalities, low values of frontal alpha power density are observed in PD patients with impairment in executive functions when compared with PD patients without executive impairment (115). Interestingly, the alpha power density partially recovers in PDD patients after a treatment with an acetylcholinesterase inhibitor (rivastigmine) for 12 weeks (116). Concerning the spatial details of the rsEEG slowing, Babiloni et al. (117) reported that compared with Nold and ADD subjects, PPD patients are characterized by higher values of rolandic delta and parieto-occipital theta, besides lower values of parietal-occipital-temporal beta-1 sources. Furthermore, although the parieto-occipital alpha-1 source activity is lower both in ADD and PDD groups when compared with the Nold group, this decrease is greater in the ADD group than the PDD group. Concerning the distinction between DLB and ADD status, global delta–theta power density and variability are higher in patients with DLB than ADD (118,119). Furthermore, treatment with an acetylcholinesterase inhibitor (donepezil) partially normalizes delta and theta power density in DLB but not in ADD (119). The quest for peculiar rsEEG features in DLB does target a characteristic clinical aspect of the disease, namely the fluctuation of vigilance and attention even in short periods of a few minutes. The rsEEG dominant frequencies and global delta power density do fluctuate more in DLB patients than in ADD subjects within 1 hour (118). Furthermore, Bonanni et al. (120) showed that the variability (fluctuation) over a few minutes of the posterior rsEEG dominant frequency is higher in DLB patients than in ADD and PPD patients, being already evident at the MCI stage (121).

9.3. rsEEG Connectivity in PDD and DLB

Fonseca et al. (114) reported that interhemispheric frontal alpha and beta, and intrahemispheric fronto-occipital beta coherence, are higher in PDD than ADD patients. In contrast to PDD patients, DLB patients show a widespread derangement of rsEEG connectivity. Kai et al. (119) reported that intrahemispheric fronto-temporo-central delta and theta and temporo-centro-parieto-occipital beta coherence are higher in DLB than ADD patients. Along the same line, global alpha coherence over the whole scalp is lower in DLB than ADD patients, while global delta coherence exhibits the opposite pattern (118).

9.4. rsEEG Features of Disease Progression in PDD and DLB

In a longitudinal study, Klassen et al. (122) showed which rsEEG features can predict the progression of cognitive symptoms over time in a sample of PD patients. Specifically, the risk of developing dementia is high in PD patients with rsEEG background characterized by low-frequency alpha peak (<8.5 Hz) and high global theta power density.

Concerning DLB, Bonanni et al. (121) followed MCI subjects for 3 years. All MCI patients who converted to DLB showed abnormal rsEEG features when they stayed at the prodromal stage, including dominant rsEEG frequency <8 Hz and dominant frequency variability >1.5 Hz over the few minutes of the recording.

9.5. Abnormal rsEEG Features in Individual PDD and DLB Subjects

Jelic and Kowalski ((1), Table 2) reported that some rsEEG topographical biomarkers show a moderate classification accuracy between PDD/DLB and AD patients. More recently, a semiquantitative visual analysis of the rsEEG waveforms including FIRDA as a main pathological marker (i.e., grand total EEG index with a cutoff of 6.5) discriminates DLB and

ADD individuals with a sensitivity of 79% and a specificity of 76% (112). Using spectral rsEEG features, Snaedal et al. (107) used 20 rsEEG features as an input to a series of trained classifiers (statistical pattern recognition) to discriminate with serial binary classifications patients with ADD, DLB/PDD (collectively named DLBP), and other pathological conditions (see the previous section on VaD for more details). The discrimination values were quite good; specifically, the separation of ADD patients from those with DLBP and FTD was 91% and 88%, respectively, with a discrimination accuracy of DLBP patients from FTD of 93%. Using the same basic methodology, Engedal et al. (81) repeated the classification trial for cross-validation purposes. Results confirmed an accuracy of 92%, a sensitivity of 85%, and a specificity of 87% in the differentiation of DLB/PDD individuals from ADD patients.

10. DEMENTIA DUE TO HUMAN IMMUNODEFICIENCY VIRUS INFECTION

About 2.2 million European people suffered from human immunodeficiency virus (HIV) in 2009 (http://www.avert. org/hiv-aids-europe.htm). One third of these subjects developed the acquired immunodeficiency syndrome (AIDS). HIV passes the brain–blood barrier, triggers neuroinflammation/ immune reactivity, and interferes with synaptic neurotransmission with an impact on cognition ranging from MCI to dementia (HIV-associated dementia; (123)).

Combination antiretroviral therapy (cART) prevents AIDS and extends the lifespan of HIV-positive subjects of about 30 years. Despite this good news, about 45% of asymptomatic HIV-positive individuals show mild to moderate cognitive deficits while only 2% of HIV-positive individuals present with HIV-associated dementia (124). The progression of the HIV infection can be related to brain dysfunction partially due to opportunistic infections (125). This event makes the identification of biomarkers of brain function highly desirable in the field of HIV.

10.1. rsEEG Waveforms in HIV Infection

Visual inspection of the rsEEG waveforms show nonspecific abnormalities in ~50% of HIV-positive subjects. A "slowing" of the rsEEG waveforms is reported, especially in HIV-positive subjects with substantial immunosuppression, opportunistic infections, or some forms of epileptic activity (125). HIV-associated dementia is often related to continuous or intermittent rsEEG "slowing" at <6 Hz, especially in the frontal areas (125,126). Less frequently (10%), an exaggerated fast background EEG rhythm (>20 Hz) is observed (125).

10.2. rsEEG Synchronization in HIV Infection

It was reported that alpha power density decreases in HIV-positive subjects compared with seronegative subjects (127,128), showing a diffuse distribution in cortical sources (129). As an exception, ~20% to 30% of HIV-positive subjects present a paradoxical increase in alpha power density at the scalp electrodes, possibly associated with their psychiatric status or serological characteristics of the infection (127,130). Abnormalities of the spectral rsEEG features are also found at low frequencies. AIDS patients present a pathological increase in delta and theta power density, already observed in HIV-positive subjects with subclinical symptoms (131), especially at central and parietal sources (129). The observed topographical differences are less pronounced in a group of HIV-positive patients who have received prolonged chronic treatment with cART (132).

10.3. rsEEG Features of Disease Progression in HIV Infection

Babiloni et al. (133) performed a longitudinal study in treatment-naïve HIV-positive subjects who received cART for 5 months. Compared with the baseline pretreatment rsEEG activity, HIV-positive subjects showed a significant normalization of the activity in cortical sources of both delta (i.e., decrement) and alpha (i.e., increment) rhythms after receiving cART. These findings have extended previous evidence showing that low-frequency rsEEG rhythms increase in power density at a follow-up of 28 months, while they remain unchanged in the HIV-positive subjects receiving cART (130). Overall, the results indicate that cART partially restores the neurophysiological mechanisms regulating brain arousal and vigilance in HIV-positive subjects.

10.4. rsEEG Features and Severity of HIV Infection

In general, the proportion of AIDS patients (characterized by severe immune system depression) showing rsEEG waveform abnormalities, especially due to excessive rsEEG slowing, is higher than that of HIV-positive patients (25–29% vs. 7–8%), along with more signs of neurological and cognitive dysfunctions (134,135). Continuous or intermittent "slowing" at <6 Hz, focal or sharp rsEEG "slowing," dementia, or opportunistic brain infections are found in 67% of AIDS patients and 36% patients with AIDS-related complex (126).

10.5. Abnormal rsEEG Features in Individual HIV Subjects

A simple statistical procedure was used to identify treatment-naïve HIV-positive individuals with statistically abnormal rsEEG activity compared to a control healthy group (136). That procedure computes the z-score of the ratio between the activity of parietal delta and alpha 3 (~10–12 Hz) sources, showing a relatively high percentage (~40–50%) of treatment-naïve HIV individuals with abnormal rsEEG activity. This procedure might assess HIV infection's effect on brain function at the individual level, but the research in this field is in its infancy for an immediate clinical application.

11. DEMENTIA DUE TO PRION DISEASES

Prion diseases, also called transmissible spongiform encephalopathies (TSEs), are formed by a group of rare progressive neurodegenerative disorders. TSEs are supposed to be caused by transmissible pathogenic agents termed "prions." Human prion diseases are classified as sporadic, genetic, and acquired. In this framework, sporadic CJD is the most common prion disease. The genetic forms are divided into genetic CJD, Gerstmann-Sträussler-Scheinker syndrome, and fatal familial insomnia. The acquired forms include Kuru, iatrogenic CJD, and variant CJD disease. CJD is a rare cause of dementia with a rapid progression. From a clinical point of view, sporadic CJD is highly variable and, in most cases, the onset is subacute. Initial symptoms are cognitive, such as memory problems, executive dysfunction, and language impairment. Extrapyramidal (Parkinsonism, dystonia, myoclonus, and chorea) and pyramidal symptoms are not common initial symptoms but are more frequently seen as the disease progresses. The most used diagnostic criteria guideline for sporadic CJD is that of the World Health Organization, but recently two other guidelines have been developed considering MRI markers. Of note, the three guidelines include abnormalities in the rsEEG rhythms as an essential support for the sporadic CJD diagnosis (see (137) for a review).

11.1. rsEEG Waveforms in CJD

Most of the rsEEG studies in CJD patients focused on the waveform abnormalities commonly encountered in this disease (Fig. 16.2). At early stages of sporadic CJD, the only rsEEG finding is a nonspecific diffuse background slowing with generalized irregular theta and delta waves, and intermittent high-amplitude rhythmic delta activities. Later stages show periodic sharp wave complexes (PSWCs), often biphasic or triphasic (negative, positive, negative) waves, occurring about once every second (see (1)). The PSWCs occur in ~64% of patients with sporadic CJD, usually after serial EEGs and in middle or later stages of the disease (138). These rsEEG complexes are rarely observed before 3 weeks after the onset of the disease. In most cases, they appear at around 8 to 12 weeks, in a few cases even later. Topographically, PSWCs commonly present a bilateral distribution with a maximum over the fronto-precentral midline electrodes (see (139) for a review). According to Steinhoff et al. (140), PSWCs should meet the following criteria:

1. Periodic cerebral potentials with a typical 100- to 600-msec duration and an intercomplex interval of 500 to 2,000 msec

2. Generalization or lateralization

3. At least five repetitive intervals with a duration difference <500 msec to rule out semi-periodic activity.

Unfortunately, no completely satisfactory explanation of PSWCs exists in CJD. Some evidence suggests that these complexes might reflect pathological, highly nonlinear oscillations in corticothalamic neural networks. The short intervals of the PSWCs in CJD suggest that the subcortical-cortical neural networks remain intact. However, the wide and symmetric distribution of the PSWCs suggests the existence of an underlying midline pacemaker, likely thalamic (138).

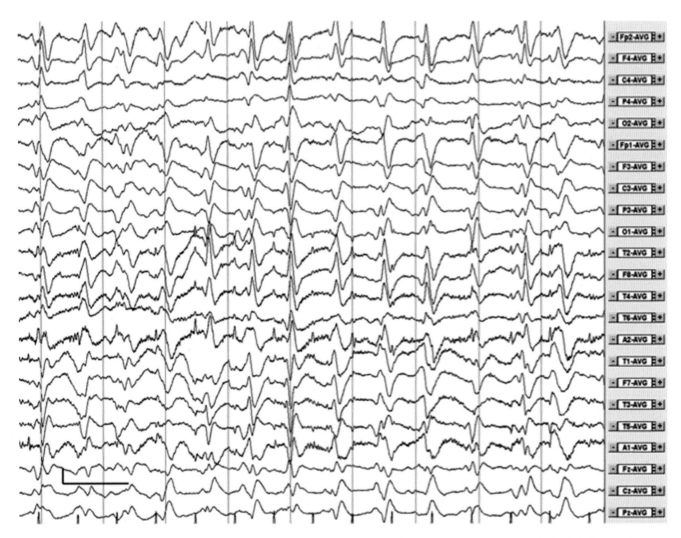

Figure 16.2. Female, 61 years, with progressive cognitive disturbances, myoclonus, and impaired consciousness. Diagnosis: Creutzfeldt–Jakob disease. The EEG shows generalized periodic sharp wave complexes (PSWCs) with a repetition frequency of slightly above 1/sec. Calibration mark: vertical, 50 μV; horizontal, 1 sec. Filter settings: time constant 1 sec. Low-pass filter, 35 Hz. Average reference.

11.2. Abnormal rsEEG Features in Individual CJD Subjects

Steinhoff et al. (138) reported quite good classification values for patients with sporadic CJD using PSWCs, when the strict criteria for this pattern were met. They reported a sensitivity of 64%, a specificity of 91%, a positive predictive value of 95%, and a negative predictive value of 49% (138). Zerr et al. (141) also reported moderate classification values taking into account PSWCs, namely a specificity of 74%, a positive predictive value of 93%, and a sensitivity of 66%. In general, autopsy-confirmed studies indicate that PSWCs have a high specificity but a rather low sensitivity for CJD. In an autopsy series of 201 patients with suspected sporadic CJD, van Everbroeck et al. (142) found PSWCs in 52% of autopsy-confirmed CJD cases. The percentages of false positives (CJD) based on PSWCs are close to zero for ADD, DLB, and VaD. A possible explanation of this low sensitivity is that PSWCs develop later in the disease or may not appear at all in a substantial percentage of CJD patients.

12. CONCLUSIONS

In this chapter we extend Dubois et al.'s view (5) on the "topographic biomarkers of AD," based on MRI and FDG-PET markers, to rsEEG features and all dementing disorders. As explained in the introductory section, "topographical biomarkers" are not supposed to provide specific information on pathophysiological features underlying the dementing processes, for example the extracellular accumulation of Aβ1-42 in the AD brain or the intracellular accumulation of α-synuclein in the Lewy bodies observed in the DLB cerebral cortex. Rather, they may highlight relevant spatial aspects of the patient's global brain structure and functioning, which may be very informative as to the general level of abnormalities in the patient's brain, even if they are not exclusively related to the primary neuropathy underlying a given dementing disorder (e.g., when parallel neuropathological processes do underpin psychiatric and neurological symptoms).

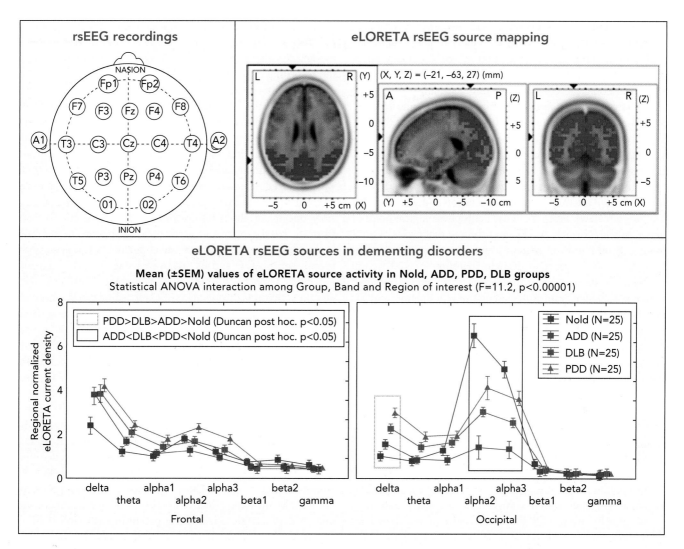

Figure 16.3. *Top left: Diagram showing the placement of the 19 scalp electrodes used for the rsEEG recordings. These electrodes are positioned according to the International 10-20 System (Fp1, Fp2, F7, F3, Fz, F4, F8, T3, C3, Cz, C4, T4, T5, P3, Pz, P4, T6, O1 and O2). In the figure, A1 and A2 indicate the position of linked earlobe reference electrodes. Top right: Example of eLORETA maps modeling source activity of rsEEG rhythms. Bottom: Mean values (± standard error mean) of eLORETA source activity of rsEEG rhythms for the following factors of an ANOVA design (p < .05): group (cognitively normal elderly, Nold; Alzheimer's disease dementia, ADD; Parkinson's disease dementia, PDD; dementia with Lewy Body, DLB), band (delta, theta, alpha-1, alpha-2, beta-1, beta-2, gamma), and region of interest (frontal, occipital). The four groups were perfectly matched for age, gender, and education; the three groups with dementing disorders were also perfectly matched for MMSE score. (Data source: Nold and ADD: University of Rome "La Sapienza," University of Genoa, IRCCS San Giovanni di Dio "Fatebenefratelli," Brescia, Italy; DLB: University of Chieti, Italy; PDD: European PDWAIVE Consortium. Data unpublished.)*

12.1. rsEEG Topographical Biomarkers Reveal Neurophysiological Abnormalities

Concerning physiological aging, visual inspection and quantitative analysis of rsEEG activity point to a reduction in frequency, amplitude, and interrelatedness of dominant rsEEG rhythms at alpha frequencies (8–12 Hz) in Nold people, especially in the parietal and occipital regions of the scalp or cortical sources. This evidence suggests that physiological aging is associated with a less efficient cortical neural synchronization and functional brain connectivity at alpha frequencies in the condition of quiet wakefulness with eyes closed (low vigilance). It can be speculated that such a reduced neural efficiency would be associated with a lower level of activity in the cortico-thalamo-cortical loops that modulate cortical alpha rhythms (143–146). This effect might be associated with disturbances in the regulation of attentional and memory processes.

In dementing disorders, characteristic abnormalities of rsEEG alpha rhythms at the group level would be mainly located in parieto-occipital areas in ADD (marginally in VaD, PDD, and DLB; Fig. 16.3), frontotemporal areas in FTD, and frontocentral areas in PDD. Furthermore, they were topographically diffuse in HIV-positive patients with cognitive deficits (with some exceptions showing paradoxically exaggerated alpha rhythms), and CJD. The reduction in the background posterior alpha rhythms was particularly pronounced in AD, even in the prodromal stage of aMCI, in conjunction with the deterioration of the long anterior-posterior functional brain connectivity.

Overall, these data suggest a peculiar worsening in the cortical neural synchronization and functional brain connectivity at background alpha frequencies in the dementing disorders. Furthermore, they point to the multiple ways by which neurodegenerative, cerebrovascular, and infection-transmissible dementing disorders can derange the neurophysiological mechanisms underpinning the generation of the dominant alpha rhythms in quiet wakefulness and low vigilance.

In physiological conditions, these mechanisms produce repeated cycles of excitation and inhibition in thalamic and cortical neurons. It can be speculated that these cycles gate the flow of visuospatial, auditory, and somatomotor information from thalamus to the cerebral cortex, and vice versa. Furthermore, they might underpin the inhibition and timing of neural activation in those loops that are closely linked to two fundamental functions of attention such as suppression and selection (see (147) for a review). From a cellular neurophysiological point of view, Crunelli, Lörincz, and Hughes showed that cycles of excitation and inhibition in thalamic and cortical neurons might frame perceptual events in discrete snapshots of ~70 to 100 msec during visual and somatosensory information processing, mainly as a result of brain glutamatergic and cholinergic neurons modulating thalamocortical high-threshold neurons that react by oscillating at alpha frequencies (144–146). These thalamocortical neurons would produce intrinsic pacemaker-like oscillations at alpha frequencies for thalamic inhibitory GABAergic interneurons modulating the discharge of thalamocortical relay-mode neurons that respond by sending synchronizing signals at the alpha frequency to cortical pyramidal neurons (144–146). Also, neuromodulatory inputs to the cerebral cortex may regulate coupling constants between cortical pyramidal and GABAergic interneuron cells with substantial effects in the generation of cortical alpha rhythms (reviewed in (8)), the traffic of information in thalamocortical system being constituted by bidirectional nested loops in cortico-thalamo-cortical pathways.

Keeping in mind the above neurophysiological mechanisms, it can be speculated that patients with dementing disorders might present a progressive alteration in this interplay of glutamatergic and cholinergic neurons, thalamocortical high-threshold, GABAergic interneurons, thalamocortical relay-mode, and cortical pyramidal neurons as a primary mechanism contributing to an abnormal cortical arousal and vigilance in quiet wakefulness. Of course, other pathological mechanisms might involve additional neuromodulatory and corticocortical loops underpinning cortical alpha rhythms in quiet wakefulness. All these abnormalities in the synchronizing neurotransmission at the alpha frequency, especially within thalamocortical circuits, might explain the impairment in vigilance, attention, primary consciousness, and other cognitive functions in dementing disorders. More intracerebral rsEEG research on animal models and human subjects undergoing presurgical intracerebral monitoring (e.g., thalamus, cortex) for epilepsy is needed to elucidate the basic neurophysiological thalamocortical mechanisms generating the alpha rhythms as a knowledge platform for productive speculations about the pathophysiological mechanisms generating abnormal rsEEG rhythms at the alpha frequency in dementing disorders.

In the present literature review, the studies also showed an increment in the amplitude of cortical rsEEG rhythms at delta (<4 Hz) and theta (4–7 Hz) frequency bands in many dementing disorders (ADD, VaD, PDD, DLB, and HIV infection with cognitive deficits). In the visual inspection of the rsEEG

waveforms, this electrophysiological phenomenon predicted a progression of the dementing disorders, especially when it was topographically diffuse over the scalp and continuous during the recording (typically lasting 5–10 minutes).

A quantitative analysis of the rsEEG rhythms showed that the abnormalities in the delta and theta rhythms were quite widespread over the scalp or cortical sources, especially in VaD. However, some topographical features were associated with some peculiar underlying neuropathology, at least at the group level. The maximal abnormality in the delta and theta rhythms was localized frontally in FTD and centrally (i.e., rolandic area) in PDD and HIV infection with cognitive deficits, possibly due to an abnormal ascending functional connectivity from the basal ganglia and periventricular regions to the cerebral cortex. Instead, such maximal abnormality was posteriorly prominent in ADD and its prodromal stage of aMCI. Finally, a peculiar temporal fluctuation of widespread posterior delta and theta rhythms during the rsEEG recording can be observed in DLB and PPD (see Fig. 16.3). Keeping in mind those data, we can speculate that in quiet wakefulness, cortical neural synchronization pathologically increases in many dementing disorders (ADD, VaD, PDD, DLB, and HIV infection) at delta and theta rhythms, with some peculiar spatial features even if this evidence is insufficient to support the use of rsEEG indexes as diagnostic markers of those disorders. Such a pathological mechanism might be related to a derangement in the functional brain connectivity, especially thalamocortical, due to neuropathological brain lesions (e.g., neurodegenerative, microvascular) or neuroinflammatory processes (148,149). Abnormalities might include neurophysiological processes commonly involving selective circuits of relay thalamocortical and corticothalamic neurons engaged in intensive information processing in wakefulness (150). More research is needed to create a model explaining the pathological neurophysiological mechanisms generating the abnormal rsEEG rhythms at delta and theta frequencies in dementing disorders.

Table 16.1 reports the most relevant findings of the revised rsEEG studies in patients with dementing disorders after 2009 (for a review of the results previous to 2009, see Table 1 in (1)). It also indicates the most sensitive rsEEG topographical biomarkers in those studies to provide a comparative overview.

12.2. rsEEG Topographical Biomarkers Track Neurophysiological Abnormalities

Few longitudinal studies showed consistent changes in the rsEEG topographical biomarkers at the group level during the progression of the dementing disorders and in response to pharmacological therapy. These studies mainly reflect the deterioration of the neurophysiological mechanisms of cortical neural synchronization in groups of ADD and PDD patients. The rsEEG frequency bands of interest typically range from delta to alpha. Sparser findings reported changes in rsEEG topographical biomarkers during disease progression in groups of VaD, DLB, and HIV-positive patients, especially in delta and theta bands. More abundant were the cross-sectional and correlational rsEEG studies, mostly including ADD patients. Several cross-sectional studies reveal interesting differences in

TABLE 16.1. Most Relevant rsEEG Topographical Biomarkers and Consistent Results Regarding the Neurophysiological Mechanisms Underlying Dementing Disorders

DEMENTING DISORDER	EEG FEATURE	SAMPLE COMPARISONS	EEG TOPOGRAPHICAL BIOMARKERS	MAIN FINDINGS	RELATED REFERENCES
ADD	Synchronization	ADD/aMCI vs. Nold	Delta, theta, alpha and beta power and distributed sources	– Widespread power density decrease of alpha, especially in low alpha at posterior regions, and/or beta rhythms – Widespread power density increase of delta and theta rhythms	30–34
			rsEEG dynamics complexity	Loss of complexity of brain dynamics in ADD	9, 35
	Connectivity	ADD/aMCI vs. Nold	Alpha connectivity	– Decrease of connectivity in the alpha band, mainly in posterior regions – Decrease of parietal to frontal information flux at alpha band, especially at parietal electrodes – Weaker small-world network, more random brain networks	6, 9, 32, 33, 36, 42–45, 48, 49, 51
FTD	Synchronization	FTD vs. Nold/ADD	Delta, alpha, and beta power and distributed sources	– Decrease in power density of alpha-1 band in the orbital frontal and temporal lobe in FDT compared to Nold – Preserved delta, alpha, and beta power compared to ADD	87, 88
	Connectivity	FTD vs. Nold/ADD	-	Preserved connectivity compared to Nold	50
VaD	Synchronization	VaD vs. Nold/ADD	Delta, theta, alpha, beta power and distributed sources	– Higher theta/delta power, lower alpha/beta power compared to Nold – Widespread increase in theta power compared to controls – Higher alpha power compared to ADD	96–99
			rsEEG dynamics complexity	Increase of complexity of brain dynamics compared to Nold and ADD	100
	Connectivity	VaD vs. ADD	Alpha connectivity	– Decrease in coherence in pre- and post-rolandic regions compared to ADD – Increase in frontoparietal SL in the alpha-1 compared to ADD	101, 103
PDD	Synchronization	PDD vs. Nold/ADD	Delta and theta power and distributed sources	– Increase in delta and theta power density compared to Nold and ADD – Increase in rolandic delta and posterior theta and beta sources in PDD compared to Nold and ADD	114, 117
	Connectivity	PDD vs. ADD	Alpha and beta connectivity	Increase in alpha and beta coherence compared to ADD	114
DLB	Synchronization	DLB vs. ADD	Delta and theta power	– Increase in power density in delta and theta bands compared to ADD – Increase in global delta power time variability	118–120
	Connectivity	DLB vs. ADD	Delta, theta, alpha, and beta connectivity	Increase in delta coherence compared to ADD	118, 119
HIV	Synchronization	HIV, age-matched controls	Delta, theta, alpha, and beta power distributed sources	– Widespread decrease in alpha power density – Increase in delta and theta power at central and parietal sources – Higher occipital and temporal alpha-1 sources in treated-HIV compared to non-treated	127–129, 132

For a review of most of the results previous to 2009 see Table 1 in reference 1.

TABLE 16.2. Most relevant rsEEG topographical biomarkers and results regarding neurophysiological abnormalities across the progression of the dementing disorders

DEMENTING DISORDER	STUDY DESIGN	SAMPLE COMPARISONS	EEG TOPOGRAPHICAL BIOMARKERS	MAIN RESULTS	MAIN REFERENCES
ADD	Longitudinal	ADD, aMCI	Delta, theta, alpha, beta power density and sources EEG mean frequency Gamma coherence Network topology	• *Predictors of conversion:* alpha/theta power ratio; delta, theta and alpha power; mean frequency; more anterior alpha sources; midline gamma coherence; alpha 3/alpha-2 power ratio • *Baseline-follow ups:* increase of theta and delta power, decrease of alpha and beta power, decrease of mean frequency at the temporo-occipital electrodes; reduced connectivity	Selected reviews: 52 Selected articles: 53–62, 65
	Cross-sectional	ADD vs aMCI ADD in different severity stages	Delta, theta, alpha, beta power density, sources and connectivity	• *ADD vs aMCI:* widespread higher theta power ; posterior lower alpha and beta power; higher delta and theta coherence in the default-mode and sensoriomotor networks; lower alpha coherence in the default-mode network; lower fronto-parietal connectivity in theta, alpha and beta • Higher delta an theta power and no alpha peak in more severe stages of ADD	Selected reviews: 32 Selected articles: 43, 44, 53, 66–68
	Correlational	ADD, aMCI	Delta, theta, alpha and beta power density and sources Alpha and beta coherence	Correlation with worse clinical/cognitive status: • Anterior sources of alpha and beta • Higher power of theta and delta sources • Lower power of alpha sources • Lower coherence in alpha and beta bands	Selected reviews: 32 Selected articles: 33, 41, 56, 69–72, 75–77
VaD	Cross-sectional	VaD vs VaNCI Mild VaD vs moderate VaD	Alpha/low frequency bands power ratio EEG mean frequency	• *VaD vs VaMCI:* increase global delta power and decrease global alpha-2 power • Moderate VaD vs mild VaD: lower mean frequency, alpha/theta and alpha/theta power ratios	Selected articles: 104, 105
PDD	Longitudinal	PD vs PDD	Alpha and theta power density	*Predictors of conversion:* lower alpha frequency, higher theta power.	Selected articles: 122
DLB	Longitudinal	DLB vs MCI	EEG mean frequency Frequency variability	*Predictors of conversion:* dominant EEG frequency lower than 8 Hz and dominant frequency variability higher than 1.5 Hz	Selected articles: 120
HIV	Longitudinal	HIV patients pre-post antiretroviral therapy	Delta and alpha power sources	Decrease in delta sources and increase in alpha sources after treatment	Selected articles: 133

the rsEEG topographical biomarkers between groups of ADD patients with different severity (e.g., prodromal forms of MCI vs. dementia, mild vs. moderate dementia). In the correlational studies, rsEEG topographical biomarkers (mainly belonging to the synchronization class) are successfully related to clinical/neuropsychological variables. Sparser findings derive from rsEEG studies carried out in groups of VaD and PDD patients, while no data are available for most of the other dementing disorders.

Overall, the reviewed studies encourage the future experimental use of rsEEG topographical biomarkers derived from spectral analysis in clinical longitudinal studies, especially in patients with ADD, PDD, and HIV infection with cognitive impairment. On one hand, those studies will have to confirm if the mentioned neurophysiological mechanisms generating delta, theta, and alpha rhythms in quiet wakefulness are sensitive to the disease progression in a highly repeatable and noninvasive condition as resting state. On the other hand, the availability of new experimental evidence would allow some final conclusions to be made on the effective utility of these candidate rsEEG topographical biomarkers in patient management and pharmacological trials. This future experimental cross-validation will be necessary to obtain consensus on the use of those rsEEG topographical biomarkers. Table 16.2 gives an overview of the most relevant findings in the longitudinal, cross-sectional, and correlational rsEEG studies in patients with dementing disorders.

12.3. rsEEG Topographical Biomarkers Capture Neurophysiological Abnormalities in Single Individuals with Dementing Disorders

Few classification studies show a consistent ability of mathematical classifiers to discriminate single patients with different dementing disorders and individual control subjects based on the rsEEG topographical biomarkers (with successful applications of both linear and nonlinear measurements). Again, most of these studies were performed in patients with ADD or aMCI when compared to healthy control subjects.

In general, the mean classification accuracy of the rsEEG biomarkers in the discrimination of cases and controls ranged from 70% to 85%. The above findings encourage more systematic and well-controlled research on the experimental use of the rsEEG topographical biomarkers in the clinical management of individual patients with dementing disorders. Ideally, those studies will have to compare several rsEEG topographical biomarkers (linear, nonlinear, graphoelements of the waveforms) in order to cross-validate the available results and to identify the most sensitive rsEEG topographical biomarkers for applications.

12.4. Concluding Remarks: From rsEEG Rhythms to Global Cerebral Reserve

Abnormalities in the rsEEG rhythms at delta–theta and alpha frequencies provide fascinating information for a better understanding of the effects of dementing disorders on the neurophysiological mechanisms underpinning brain arousal and vigilance in quiet wakefulness. This information can be captured in a complementary way by the rsEEG topographical biomarkers derived from the traditional visual analysis (e.g., the shapes of the waveform graphoelements) and the quantitative analysis (synchronization and connectivity). Compared with the traditional visual analysis and expert clinical judgment of rsEEG waveforms, quantitative analysis of the rsEEG rhythms may ensure the maximum standardization of the procedures and results in the perspective of future multicentric studies. Along this line, the quantitative rsEEG topographical biomarkers of brain synchronization (i.e., mainly power density) and connectivity (i.e., especially coherence, partial directed coherence, directed transfer function, SL, and regression measurements) at the delta, theta, and alpha frequencies provide useful insights

on the neurophysiological mechanisms reflecting the disease status in ADD/aMCI, VaD, and PDD patients at the group and individual level. Furthermore, the rsEEG topographical biomarkers of brain synchronization at the same frequencies offer insights on the neurophysiology reflecting disease progression, especially in groups of ADD/aMCI, PDD, and DLB patients. Finally, the rsEEG topographical biomarkers of brain synchronization at the alpha frequency are especially sensitive to the prodromal and mild stages of the dementing disorders, while those at delta and theta frequencies reflect later disease stages.

It can be speculated that the rsEEG topographical biomarkers represent an index of the efficiency/frailty of the neurophysiological mechanisms underpinning brain arousal and vigilance in quiet wakefulness. In this sense, these markers would constitute one of the components of the global cerebral reserve, defined as the residual structural, molecular, and functional integrity of the brain, along with other parts of the cerebral reserve such as the neural reserve, the cognitive reserve, and the stress coping reserve (151). This global cerebral reserve would predict the residual capacity of the brain and adaptive cognitive/behavioral functions to resist neuropathological processes inducing dementing disorders. Along this line, the above neural, cognitive, and stress coping reserves being equal, an ADD patient with the additional feature of neurophysiological frailty (i.e., EEG positive) may have a worse prognosis than an ADD patient with neurophysiological resilience (i.e., EEG negative) and should receive more therapeutic resources and clinical attention.

Overall, the findings reviewed in this chapter encourage international public–private investments and clinical work for the development of controlled multicentric longitudinal rsEEG studies in vast cohorts of patients with different dementing disorders from prodromal to dementia stages. These studies will have to cross-validate the rsEEG topographical biomarkers in ADD and are particularly urgent for non-AD dementing diseases.

SCORE EEG SOFTWARE

Further examples related to the topics addressed in this chapter can be found in the interactive online Niedermeyer Educational Platform. EEG recordings with illustrative examples can be opened and browsed. Features are marked and described using the SCORE EEG software. The users can see the features marked by experts, they can score these features themselves, and then compare them with the scorings of the experts.

The Niedermeyer Educational Platform can be accessed at: www.scoreEEG.com/academy

REFERENCES

1. Jelic V, Kowalski J. Evidence-based evaluation of diagnostic accuracy of resting EEG in dementia and mild cognitive impairment. Clin EEG Neurosci. 2009;40(2):129–142.
2. Waldemar G, Dubois B, Emre M, et al. Recommendations for the diagnosis and management of Alzheimer's disease and other disorders associated with dementia: EFNS guideline. Eur J Neurol. 2007;14:e1–e26.
3. Hort J, O'Brien JT, Gainotti G, Pirttila T, Popescu BO, Rektorova I, et al. EFNS guidelines for the diagnosis and management of Alzheimer's disease. Eur J Neurol. 2010;17(10):1236–1248.

4. Sorbi S, Hort J, Erkinjuntti T, Fladby T, Gainotti G, Gurvit H, et al. EFNS-ENS guidelines on the diagnosis and management of disorders associated with dementia. Eur J Neurol. 2012;19(9):1159–1179.

5. Dubois B, Feldman HH, Jacova C, Hampel H, Molinuevo JL, Blennow K, et al. Advancing research diagnostic criteria for Alzheimer's disease: the IWG-2 criteria. Lancet Neurol. 2014;13(6):614–629.

6. Hyman BT, Growdon JH, Albers MW, Buckner RL, Chhatwal J, Gomez-Isla MT, et al. Massachusetts Alzheimer's Disease Research Center: progress and challenges. Alzheimers Dement. 2015;11(10):1241–1245.

7. McKhann GM, Knopman DS, Chertkow H, Hyman BT, Jack CR, Kawas CH, et al. The diagnosis of dementia due to Alzheimer's disease: Recommendations from the National Institute on Aging/Alzheimer's Association workgroups on diagnostic guidelines for Alzheimer's disease. Alzheimers Dement. 2011;7(3):263–269.

8. Pfurtscheller G, Da Silva FL. Event-related EEG/MEG synchronization and desynchronization: basic principles. Clin Neurophysiol. 1999;110(11):1842–1857.

9. Dauwels J, Vialatte F, Cichocki A. Diagnosis of Alzheimer's disease from EEG signals: where are we standing? Curr Alzheimer Res. 2010;7(6):487–505.

10. Stam CJ, Nolte G, Daffertshofer A. Phase lag index: assessment of functional connectivity from multichannel EEG and MEG with diminished bias from common sources. Hum Brain Mapp. 2007;28(11):1178–1193.

11. Babiloni C, Lizio R, Frisoni GB, Ferri R, Rodriguez G, Rossini PM. Resting state cortical electroencephalographic rhythms in Alzheimer's disease. Open Nucl Med J. 2010;2:63–70.

12. Babiloni C, Lizio R, Ferri R, Rodriguez G, Marzano N, et al. Resting state cortical rhythms in mild cognitive impairment and Alzheimer's disease: electroencephalographic evidence. J Alzheimers Dis. 2011;26(s3):201–214.

13. Klass DW, Brenner RP. Electroencephalography of the elderly. J Clin Neurophysiol. 1995;12(2):116–131.

14. Peltz CB, Kim HL, Kawas CH. Abnormal EEGs in cognitively and physically healthy oldest old: findings from the 90+ study. J Clin Neurophysiol. 2010;27(4):292–295.

15. Liedorp M, van der Flier WM, Hoogervorst EL, Scheltens P, Stam CJ. Associations between patterns of EEG abnormalities and diagnosis in a large memory clinic cohort. Dement Geriatr Cogn Disord. 2009;27(1):18–23.

16. Gaal ZA, Boha R, Stam CJ, Molnár M. Age-dependent features of EEG-reactivity—Spectral, complexity, and network characteristics. Neurosci Lett. 2010;479(1):79–84.

17. Klimesch W. EEG alpha and theta oscillations reflect cognitive and memory performance: a review and analysis. Brain Res Rev. 1999;29(2):169–195.

18. Müller V, Lindenberger U. Lifespan differences in nonlinear dynamics during rest and auditory oddball performance. Dev Sci. 2012;15(4):540–556.

19. Babiloni C, Binetti G, Cassarino A, Dal Forno G, Del Percio C, Ferreri F, et al. Sources of cortical rhythms in adults during physiological aging: a multicentric EEG study. Hum Brain Mapp. 2006;27(2):162–172.

20. Caplan JB, Bottomley M, Kang P, Dixon RA. Distinguishing rhythmic from non-rhythmic brain activity during rest in healthy neurocognitive aging. Neuroimage. 2015;112:341–352.

21. Finnigan S, Robertson IH. Resting EEG theta power correlates with cognitive performance in healthy older adults. Psychophysiology. 2011;48(8):1083–1087.

22. Roca-Stappung M, Fernández T, Becerra J, Mendoza-Montoya O, Espino M, Harmony T. Healthy aging: relationship between quantitative electroencephalogram and cognition. Neurosci Lett. 2012;510(2):115–120.

23. Vysata O, Kukal J, Prochazka A, Pazdera L, Simko J, Valis M. Age-related changes in EEG coherence. Neurol Neurochir Pol. 2014;48(1):35–38.

24. Zhu C, Guo X, Jin Z, Sun J, Qiu Y, Zhu Y, et al. Influences of brain development and ageing on cortical interactive networks. Clin Neurophysiol. 2011;122(2):278–283.

25. Smit DJ, Boersma M, Schnack HG, Micheloyannis S, Boomsma DI, Pol HEH, et al. The brain matures with stronger functional connectivity and decreased randomness of its network. PLoS One. 2012;7(5):e36896.

26. Vecchio F, Miraglia F, Bramanti P, Rossini PM. Human brain networks in physiological aging: a graph theoretical analysis of cortical connectivity from EEG data. J Alzheimers Dis. 2014;41(4):1239–1249.

27. Bhat S, Acharya UR, Dadmehr N, Adeli H. Clinical neurophysiological and automated EEG-based diagnosis of Alzheimer's disease. Eur Neurol. 2015;74(3-4):202–210.

28. Petersen RC, Roberts RO, Knopman DS, Boeve BF, Geda YE, Ivnik RJ, et al. Mild cognitive impairment: ten years later. Arch Neurol. 2009;66(12):1447–1455.

29. de Waal H, Stam CJ, Blankenstein MA, Pijnenburg YA, Scheltens P, van der Flier WM. EEG abnormalities in early and late onset Alzheimer's disease: understanding heterogeneity. J Neurol Neurosurg Psychiatry. 2011;82(1):67–71.

30. Hamm V, Héraud C, Cassel JC, Mathis C, Goutagny, R. Precocious alterations of brain oscillatory activity in Alzheimer's disease: a window of opportunity for early diagnosis and treatment. Front Cell Neurosci. 2015;21(9):491.

31. Tsolaki A, Kazis D, Kompatsiaris I, Kosmidou V, Tsolaki M. Electroencephalogram and Alzheimer's disease: clinical and research approaches. Int J Alzheimers Dis. 2014;2014:349249.

32. Babiloni C, Lizio R, Marzano N, Capotosto P, Soricelli A, Triggiani AI, et al. Brain neural synchronization and functional coupling in Alzheimer's disease as revealed by resting state EEG rhythms. Int J Psychophysiol. 2016;103:88–102.

33. Canuet L, Tellado I, Couceiro V, Fraile C, Fernandez-Novoa L, Ishii R, et al. Resting-state network disruption and APOE genotype in Alzheimer's disease: a lagged functional connectivity study. PLoS One. 2012;7(9):e46289.

34. Babiloni C, Visser PJ, Frisoni G, De Deyn PP, Bresciani L, Jelic V, et al. Cortical sources of resting EEG rhythms in mild cognitive impairment and subjective memory complaint. Neurobiol Aging. 2010;31(10):1787–1798.

35. Zhang C, Wang H, Wu M. EEG-based expert system using complexity measures and probability density function control in alpha sub-band. Integr Comput Aided Eng. 2013;20(4):391–405.

36. D'Amelio M, Rossini PM. Brain excitability and connectivity of neuronal assemblies in Alzheimer's disease: from animal models to human findings. Prog Neurobiol. 2012;99(1):42–60.

37. Adler G, Brassen S, Jajcevic A. EEG coherence in Alzheimer's dementia. J Neural Transm. 2003;110(9):1051–1058.

38. Knott V, Mohr E, Mahoney C, Ilivitsky V. Electroencephalographic coherence in Alzheimer's disease: comparisons with a control group and population norms. J Geriatr Psychiatry Neurol. 2000;13(1):1–8.

39. Locatelli T, Cursi M, Liberati D, Franceschi M, Comi G. EEG coherence in Alzheimer's disease. Electroencephalogr Clin Neurophysiol. 1998;106(3):229–237.

40. Babiloni C, Frisoni GB, F, Pievani M, Geroldi C, De Carli C, et al. Global functional coupling of resting EEG rhythms is related to white-matter lesions along the cholinergic tracts in subjects with amnesic mild cognitive impairment. J Alzheimers Dis. 2010;19(3):859–871.

41. Sankari Z, Adeli H, Adeli A. Intrahemispheric, interhemispheric, and distal EEG coherence in Alzheimer's disease. Clin Neurophysiol. 2011;122(5):897–906.

42. Babiloni C, Triggiani AI, Lizio R, Cordone S, Tattoli G, Bevilacqua V, et al. Classification of single normal and Alzheimer's disease individuals from cortical sources of resting state EEG rhythms. Front Neurosci. 2016;10:47.

43. Babiloni C, Frisoni GB, Pievani M, Infarinato F, Geroldi C, et al. White matter vascular lesions are related to parietal-to-frontal coupling of EEG rhythms in mild cognitive impairment. Hum Brain Mapp. 2008;29(12):1355–1367.

44. Babiloni C, Ferri R, Binetti G, Frisoni GB, Lanuzza B, et al. Directionality of EEG synchronization in Alzheimer's disease subjects. Neurobiol Aging. 2009;30(1):93–102.

45. Dauwels J, Vialatte F, Musha T, Cichocki A. A comparative study of synchrony measures for the early diagnosis of Alzheimer's disease based on EEG. Neuroimage. 2010;49(1):668–693.

46. Dauwels J, Vialatte F, Latchoumane C, Jeong J, Cichocki A. EEG synchrony analysis for early diagnosis of Alzheimer's disease: a study with several synchrony measures and EEG data sets. Conf Proc IEEE Eng Med Biol Soc. 2009:2224–2227.

47. Tóth B, File B, Boha R, Kardos Z, Hidasi Z, Gaál ZA, et al. EEG network connectivity changes in mild cognitive impairment-Preliminary results. Int J Psychophysiol. 2014;92(1):1–7.

48. Miraglia F, Bramanti P, Rossini PM. EEG characteristics in "eyes-open" versus "eyes-closed" conditions: small-world network architecture in healthy aging and age-related brain degeneration. Clin Neurophysiol. 2016;127(2):1261–1268.

49. Tijms BM, Wink AM, de Haan W, van der Flier WM, Stam CJ, Scheltens P, Barkhof F. Alzheimer's disease: connecting findings from graph theoretical studies of brain networks. Neurobiol Aging. 2013;34(8):2023–2036.

50. de Haan W, Pijnenburg YA, Strijers RL, van der Made Y, van der Flier WM, Scheltens P, et al. Functional neural network analysis in frontotemporal dementia and Alzheimer's disease using EEG and graph theory. BMC Neurosci. 2009;10:101.

51. Vecchio F, Miraglia F, Marra C, Quaranta D, Vita MG, Bramanti P, et al. Human brain networks in cognitive decline: a graph theoretical analysis of cortical connectivity from EEG data. J Alzheimers Dis. 2014;41(1):113–127.

52. Drago V, Babiloni C, Bartrés-Faz D, Caroli A, Bosch B, Hensch T, et al. Disease tracking markers for Alzheimer's disease at the prodromal (MCI) stage. J Alzheimers Dis. 2011;26(s3):159–199.

53. Jelic V, Johansson S, Almkvist O, Shigeta M, Julin P, Nordberg A, et al. Quantitative electroencephalography in mild cognitive impairment: longitudinal changes and possible prediction of Alzheimer's disease. Neurobiol Aging. 2000;21(4):533–540.

54. Huang C, Wahlund L, Dierks T, Julin P, Winblad B, Jelic V. Discrimination of Alzheimer's disease and mild cognitive impairment by equivalent EEG sources: a cross-sectional and longitudinal study. Clin Neurophysiol. 2000;111(11):1961–1967.

55. Rossini PM, Del Percio C, Pasqualetti P, Cassetta E, Binetti G, Dal Forno G, et al. Conversion from mild cognitive impairment to Alzheimer's disease is predicted by sources and coherence of brain electroencephalography rhythms. Neuroscience. 2006;143(3):793–803.

56. van der Hiele K, Bollen EL, Vein AA, Reijntjes RH, Westendorp RG, van Buchem MA, et al. EEG markers of future cognitive performance in the elderly. J Clin Neurophysiol. 2008;25(2):83–89.

57. Luckhaus C, Grass-Kapanke B, Blaeser I, Ihl R, Supprian T, Winterer G, et al. Quantitative EEG in progressing vs stable mild cognitive impairment (MCI): results of a 1-year follow-up study. Int J Geriatr Psychiatry. 2008;23(11):1148–1155.

58. Babiloni C, Frisoni GB, Vecchio F, Lizio R, Pievani M, Cristina G, et al. Stability of clinical condition in mild cognitive impairment is related to cortical sources of alpha rhythms: an electroencephalographic study. Hum Brain Mapp. 2011;32(11):1916–1931.

59. Moretti D, Frisoni G, Fracassi C, Pievani M, Geroldi C, Binetti G, et al. MCI patients' EEGs show group differences between those who progress and those who do not progress to AD. Neurobiol Aging. 2011;32(4):563–571.

60. Coben LA, Danziger W, Storandt M. A longitudinal EEG study of mild senile dementia of Alzheimer type: changes at 1 year and at 2.5 years. Electroencephalogr Clin Neurophysiol. 1985;61(2):101–112.

61. Soininen H, Partanen J, Laulumaa V, Helkala E, Laakso M, Riekkinen P. Longitudinal EEG spectral analysis in early stage of Alzheimer's disease. Electroencephalogr Clin Neurophysiol. 1989;72(4):290–297.

62. Soininen H, Partanen J, Pääkkonen A, Koivisto E, Riekkinen P. Changes in absolute power values of EEG spectra in the follow-up of Alzheimer's disease. Acta Neurol Scand. 1991;83(2):133–136.

63. Babiloni C, Lizio R, Del Percio C, Marzano N, Soricelli A, Salvatore E, et al. Cortical sources of resting state EEG rhythms are sensitive to the progression of early stage Alzheimer's disease. J Alzheimers Dis. 2013;34(4):1015–1035.

64. Babiloni C, Del Percio C, Lizio R, Marzano N, Infarinato F, Soricelli A, et al. Cortical sources of resting state electroencephalographic alpha rhythms deteriorate across time in subjects with amnesic mild cognitive impairment. Neurobiol Aging. 2014;35(1):130–142.

65. Morabito FC, Campolo M, Labate D, Morabito G, Bonanno L, Bramanti A, et al. A longitudinal EEG study of Alzheimer's disease progression based on a complex network approach. Int J Neural Syst. 2015;25(02):1550005.

66. Rodriguez G, Copello F, Vitali P, Perego G, Nobili F. EEG spectral profile to stage Alzheimer's disease. Clin Neurophysiol. 1999;110(10):1831–1837.

67. Hsiao F, Wang Y, Yan S, Chen W, Lin Y. Altered oscillation and synchronization of default-mode network activity in mild Alzheimer's disease compared to mild cognitive impairment: an electrophysiological study. PLoS One. 2013;8(7):e68792.

68. Hsiao F, Chen W, Wang Y, Yan S, Lin Y. Altered source-based EEG coherence of resting-state sensorimotor network in early-stage Alzheimer's disease compared to mild cognitive impairment. Neurosci Lett. 2014;558:47–52.

69. Babiloni C, Frisoni GB, Del Percio C, Zanetti O, Bonomini C, Cassetta E, et al. Ibuprofen treatment modifies cortical sources of EEG rhythms in mild Alzheimer's disease. Clin Neurophysiol. 2009;120(4):709–718.

70. Dierks T, Ihl R, Frölich L, Maurer K. Dementia of the Alzheimer type: effects on the spontaneous EEG described by dipole sources. Psychiatry Res. 1993;50(3):151–162.

71. Babiloni C, Del Percio C, Boccardi M, Lizio R, Lopez S, Carducci F, et al. Occipital sources of resting-state alpha rhythms are related to local gray matter density in subjects with amnesic mild cognitive impairment and Alzheimer's disease. Neurobiol Aging. 2015;36(2):556–570.

72. Gianotti LR, Künig G, Lehmann D, Faber PL, Pascual-Marqui RD, Kochi K, et al. Correlation between disease severity and brain electric LORETA tomography in Alzheimer's disease. Clin Neurophysiol. 2007;118(1):186–196.

73. Yang AC, Huang C, Yeh H, Liu M, Hong C, Tu P, et al. Complexity of spontaneous BOLD activity in default mode network is correlated with cognitive function in normal male elderly: a multiscale entropy analysis. Neurobiol Aging. 2013;34(2):428–438.

74. Park Y, Che H, Im C, Jung H, Bae S, Lee S. Decreased EEG synchronization and its correlation with symptom severity in Alzheimer's disease. Neurosci Res. 2008;62(2):112–117.

75. Babiloni C, Lizio R, Vecchio F, Frisoni GB, Pievani M, Geroldi C, et al. Reactivity of cortical alpha rhythms to eye opening in mild cognitive impairment and Alzheimer's disease: an EEG study. J Alzheimers Dis. 2010;22(4):1047–1064.

76. Dunkin JJ, Osato S, Leuchter AF. Relationships between EEG coherence and neuropsychological tests in dementia. Clin Electroencephalogr. 1995;26(1):47–59.

77. Jelic V, Shigeta M, Julin P, Almkvist O, Winblad B, Wahlund L. Quantitative electroencephalography power and coherence in Alzheimer's disease and mild cognitive impairment. Dement Geriatr Cogn Disord. 1996;7(6):314–323.

78. Jonkman E. The role of the electroencephalogram in the diagnosis of dementia of the Alzheimer type: an attempt at technology assessment. Neurophysiologie Clinique/Clin Neurophysiol. 1997;27(3):211–219.

79. Lizio R, Del Percio C, Marzano N, Soricelli A, Yener GG, Başar E, et al. Neurophysiological assessment of Alzheimer's disease individuals by a single electroencephalographic marker. J Alzheimers Dis. 2015;49(1):159–177

80. Trambaiolli LR, Falk TH, Fraga FJ, Anghinah R, Lorena AC. EEG spectro-temporal modulation energy: a new feature for automated diagnosis of Alzheimer's disease. Conf Proc IEEE Eng Med Biol Soc. 2011;2011:3828–3831.

81. Engedal K, Snaedal J, Hoegh P, Jelic V, Bo Andersen B, Naik M, et al. Quantitative EEG applying the statistical recognition pattern method: a useful tool in dementia diagnostic workup. Dement Geriatr Cogn Disord. 2015;40(1-2):1–12.

82. Buscema M, Capriotti M, Bergami F, Babiloni C, Rossini P, Grossi E. The implicit function as squashing time model: a novel parallel nonlinear EEG analysis technique distinguishing mild cognitive impairment and Alzheimer's disease subjects with high degree of accuracy. Comput Intell Neurosci. 2007;35021.

83. Buscema M, Grossi E, Capriotti M, Babiloni C, Rossini P. The IFAST model allows the prediction of conversion to Alzheimer disease in patients with mild cognitive impairment with high degree of accuracy. Curr Alzheimer Res. 2010;7(2):173–187.

84. Rascovsky K, Hodges JR, Knopman D, Mendez MF, Kramer JH, Neuhaus J, et al. Sensitivity of revised diagnostic criteria for the behavioural variant of frontotemporal dementia. Brain. 2011;134(Pt 9):2456–2477.

85. Gorno-Tempini ML, Hillis AE, Weintraub S, Kertesz A, Mendez M, Cappa SF, et al. Classification of primary progressive aphasia and its variants. Neurology. 2011;76(11):1006–1014.

86. Mackenzie IR, Neumann M, Bigio EH, Cairns NJ, Alafuzoff I, Kril J, et al. Nomenclature and nosology for neuropathologic subtypes of frontotemporal lobar degeneration: an update. Acta Neuropathol. 2010;119(1):1–4.

87. Caso F, Cursi M, Magnani G, Fanelli G, Falautano M, Comi G, et al. Quantitative EEG and LORETA: valuable tools in discerning FTD from AD? Neurobiol Aging. 2012;33(10):2343–2356.

88. Nishida K, Yoshimura M, Isotani T, Yoshida T, Kitaura Y, Saito A, et al. Differences in quantitative EEG between frontotemporal dementia and Alzheimer's disease as revealed by LORETA. Clin Neurophysiol. 2011;122(9):1718–1725.

89. Nishida K, Morishima Y, Yoshimura M, Isotani T, Irisawa S, Jann K, et al. EEG microstates associated with salience and frontoparietal networks in frontotemporal dementia, schizophrenia and Alzheimer's disease. Clin Neurophysiol. 2013;124(6):1106–1114.

90. Wu L, Wu L, Chen Y, Zhou J. A promising method to distinguish vascular dementia from Alzheimer's disease with standardized low-resolution brain electromagnetic tomography and quantitative EEG. Clin EEG Neurosci. 2014;45(3):152–157.

91. Roman GC, Tatemichi TK, Erkinjuntti T, Cummings JL, Masdeu JC, Garcia JH, et al. Vascular dementia: diagnostic criteria for research studies. Report of the NINDS-AIREN International Workshop. Neurology. 1993;43(2):250–260.

92. Holmes C, Cairns N, Lantos P, Mann A. Validity of current clinical criteria for Alzheimer's disease, vascular dementia and dementia with Lewy bodies. Br J Psychiatry. 1999;174:45–50.

93. O'Brien JT, Thomas A. Vascular dementia. Lancet. 2015; 386(10004): 1698–1706.

94. Bennett D. Public health importance of vascular dementia and Alzheimer's disease with cerebrovascular disease. Int J Clin Pract Suppl. 2001;120:41–48.

95. Gorelick PB, Scuteri A, Black SE, DeCarli C, Greenberg SM, Iadecola C, et al. Vascular contributions to cognitive impairment and dementia a statement for healthcare professionals from the American Heart Association/American Stroke Association. Stroke. 2011;42(9):2672–2713.

96. Sloan EP, Fenton GW. EEG power spectra and cognitive change in geriatric psychiatry: a longitudinal study. Electroencephalogr Clin Neurophysiol. 1993;86(6):361–367.

97. van Straaten EC, de Haan W, de Waal H, Scheltens P, van der Flier, Wiesje M, Barkhof F, et al. Disturbed oscillatory brain dynamics in subcortical ischemic vascular dementia. BMC Neurosci. 2012;13(1):1.

98. Moretti DV, Babiloni C, Binetti G, Cassetta E, Dal Forno G, Ferreric F, et al. Individual analysis of EEG frequency and band power in mild Alzheimer's disease. Clin Neurophysiol. 2004;115(2):299–308.

99. Babiloni C, Binetti G, Cassetta E, Cerboneschi D, Dal Forno G, Del Percio C, et al. Mapping distributed sources of cortical rhythms in mild Alzheimer's disease. A multicentric EEG study. Neuroimage. 2004;22(1):57–67.

100. Jeong J, Chae J, Kim SY, Han S. Nonlinear dynamic analysis of the EEG in patients with Alzheimer's disease and vascular dementia. J Clin Neurophysiol. 2001;18(1):58–67.

101. Leuchter AF, Dunkin JJ, Lufkin RB, Anzai Y, Cook IA, Newton TF. Effect of white matter disease on functional connections in the aging brain. J Neurol Neurosurg Psychiatry. 1994;57(11):1347–1354.

102. Sloan EP, Fenton GW, Kennedy NS, MacLennan JM. Neurophysiology and SPECT cerebral blood flow patterns in dementia. Electroencephalogr Clin Neurophysiol. 1994;91(3):163–170.

103. Babiloni C, Ferri R, Moretti DV, Strambi A, Binetti G, Dal Forno G, et al. Abnormal fronto-parietal coupling of brain rhythms in mild Alzheimer's disease: a multicentric EEG study. Eur J Neurosci. 2004;19(9):2583–2590.

104. Gawel M, Zalewska E, Szmidt-Sałkowska E, Kowalski J. Does EEG (visual and quantitative) reflect mental impairment in subcortical vascular dementia? J Neurol Sci. 2007;257(1):11–16.

105. Moretti D, Miniussi C, Frisoni G, Zanetti O, Binetti G, Geroldi C, et al. Vascular damage and EEG markers in subjects with mild cognitive impairment. Clin Neurophysiol. 2007;118(8):1866–1876.

106. Babiloni C, Frisoni GB, Pievani M, Toscano L, Del Percio C, Geroldi C, et al. White-matter vascular lesions correlate with alpha EEG sources in mild cognitive impairment. Neuropsychologia. 2008;46(6):1707–1720.

107. Snaedal J, Johannesson GH, Gudmundsson TE, Blin NP, Emilsdottir AL, Einarsson B, et al. Diagnostic accuracy of statistical pattern recognition of electroencephalogram registration in evaluation of cognitive impairment and dementia. Dement Geriatr Cogn Disord. 2012;34(1):51–60.

108. Sheorajpanday RV, Marien P, Nagels G, Weeren AJ, Saerens J, van Putten MJ, et al. Subcortical vascular cognitive impairment, no dementia: EEG global power independently predicts vascular impairment and brain symmetry index reflects severity of cognitive decline. J Clin Neurophysiol. 2014;31(5):422–428.

109. Barber P, Varma A, Lloyd J, Haworth B, Haworth J, Neary D. The electroencephalogram in dementia with Lewy bodies. Acta Neurol Scand. 2000;101(1):53–56.

110. Londos E, Passant U, Brun A, Rosén I, Risberg J, Gustafson L. Regional cerebral blood flow and EEG in clinically diagnosed dementia with Lewy bodies and Alzheimer's disease. Arch Gerontol Geriatr. 2003;36(3):231–245.

111. McKeith IG, Dickson DW, Lowe J, Emre M, O'Brien JT, Feldman H, et al. Diagnosis and management of dementia with Lewy bodies: third report of the DLB Consortium. Neurology. 2005;65(12):1863–1872.

112. Lee H, Brekelmans GJ, Roks G. The EEG as a diagnostic tool in distinguishing between dementia with Lewy bodies and Alzheimer's disease. Clin Neurophysiol. 2015;126(9):1735–1739.

113. Caviness JN, Lue L, Adler CH, Walker DG. Parkinson's disease dementia and potential therapeutic strategies. CNS Neurosci Ther. 2011;17(1):32–44.

114. Fonseca LC, Tedrus GM, Carvas PN, Machado EC. Comparison of quantitative EEG between patients with Alzheimer's disease and those with Parkinson's disease dementia. Clin Neurophysiol. 2013;124(10):1970–1974.

115. Kamei S, Morita A, Serizawa K, Mizutani T, Hirayanagi K. Quantitative EEG analysis of executive dysfunction in Parkinson disease. J Clin Neurophysiol. 2010;27(3):193–197.

116. Fogelson N, Kogan E, Korczyn A, Giladi N, Shabtai H, Neufeld M. Effects of rivastigmine on the quantitative EEG in demented Parkinsonian patients. Acta Neurol Scand. 2003;107(4):252–255.

117. Babiloni C, De Pandis MF, Vecchio F, Buffo P, Sorpresi F, Frisoni GB, et al. Cortical sources of resting state electroencephalographic rhythms in Parkinson's disease related dementia and Alzheimer's disease. Clin Neurophysiol. 2011;122(12):2355–2364.

118. Andersson M, Hansson O, Minthon L, Rosen I, Londos E. Electroencephalogram variability in dementia with lewy bodies, Alzheimer's disease and controls. Dement Geriatr Cogn Disord. 2008;26(3):284–290.

119. Kai T, Asai Y, Sakuma K, Koeda T, Nakashima K. Quantitative electroencephalogram analysis in dementia with Lewy bodies and Alzheimer's disease. J Neurol Sci. 2005;237(1):89–95.

120. Bonanni L, Thomas A, Tiraboschi P, Perfetti B, Varanese S, Onofrj M. EEG comparisons in early Alzheimer's disease, dementia with Lewy bodies and Parkinson's disease with dementia patients with a 2-year follow-up. Brain. 2008;131(3):690–705.

121. Bonanni L, Perfetti B, Bifolchetti S, Taylor J, Franciotti R, Parnetti L, et al. Quantitative electroencephalogram utility in predicting conversion of mild cognitive impairment to dementia with Lewy bodies. Neurobiol Aging. 2015;36(1):434–445.

122. Klassen BT, Hentz JG, Shill HA, Driver-Dunckley E, Evidente VG, Sabbagh MN, et al. Quantitative EEG as a predictive biomarker for Parkinson disease dementia. Neurology. 2011;77(2):118–124.

123. Anthony I, Bell PJ. The neuropathology of HIV/AIDS. Int Rev Psychiatry. 2008;20(1):15–24.

124. Antinori A, Arendt G, Becker JT, Brew BJ, Byrd DA, Cherner M, et al. Updated research nosology for HIV-associated neurocognitive disorders. Neurology. 2007;69(18):1789–1799.

125. Sinha S, Satishchandra P. Nervous system involvement in asymptomatic HIV seropositive individuals: a cognitive and electrophysiological study. Neurol India. 2003;51(4):466–469.

126. Gabuzda DH, Levy SR, Chiappa KH. Electroencephalography in AIDS and AIDS-related complex. Clin Electroencephalogr. 1988;19(1):1–6.

127. Baldeweg T, Gruzelier J. Alpha EEG activity and subcortical pathology in HIV infection. Int J Psychophysiol. 1997;26(1-3):431–442.

128. Polich J, Ilan A, Poceta JS, Mitler MM, Darko DF. Neuroelectric assessment of HIV: EEG, ERP, and viral load. Int J Psychophysiol. 2000;38(1):97–108.

129. Babiloni C, Vecchio F, Buffo P, Onorati P, Muratori C, Ferracuti S, et al. Cortical sources of resting-state EEG rhythms are abnormal in naïve HIV subjects. Clin Neurophysiol. 2012;123(11):2163–2171.

130. Baldeweg T, Riccio M, Gruzelier J, Hawkins D, Burgess A, Irving G, et al. Neurophysiological evaluation of zidovudine in asymptomatic HIV-1 infection: a longitudinal placebo-controlled study. J Neurol Sci. 1995;132(2):162–169.

131. Itil TM, Ferracuti S, Freedman AM, Sherer C, Mehta P, Itil KZ. Computer-analyzed EEG (CEEG) and dynamic brain mapping in AIDS and HIV related syndrome: a pilot study. Clin Electroencephalogr. 1990;21(3):140–144.

132. Babiloni C, Buffo P, Vecchio F, Onorati P, Muratori C, Ferracuti S, et al. Cortical sources of resting-state EEG rhythms in "experienced" HIV subjects under antiretroviral therapy. Clin Neurophysiol. 2014;125(9):1792–1802.

133. Babiloni C, Pennica A, Vecchio F, Onorati P, Muratori C, Ferracuti S, et al. Antiretroviral therapy effects on sources of cortical rhythms in HIV subjects: responders vs. mild responders. Clin Neurophysiol. 2015;126(1):68–81.

134. Harrison MJ, Newman SP, Hall-Craggs MA, Fowler CJ, Miller R, Kendall BE, et al. Evidence of CNS impairment in HIV infection: clinical, neuropsychological, EEG, and MRI/MRS study. J Neurol Neurosurg Psychiatry. 1998;65(3):301–307.

135. Newton TF, Leuchter AF, Miller EN, Weiner H. Quantitative EEG in patients with AIDS and asymptomatic HIV infection. Clin Electroencephalogr. 1994;25(1):18–25.

136. Babiloni C, Pennica A, Del Percio C, Noce G, Cordone S, Muratori C, et al. Abnormal cortical sources of resting state electroencephalographic rhythms in single treatment-naïve HIV individuals: A statistical z-score index. Clin Neurophysiol. 2016;127(3):1803–1812.

137. Geschwind MD. Prion diseases. Continuum (Minneap Minn) 2015;21(6):1612–1638.

138. Steinhoff BJ, Zerr I, Glatting M, Schulz-Schaeffer W, Poser S, Kretzschmar HA. Diagnostic value of periodic complexes in Creutzfeldt–Jakob disease. Ann Neurol. 2004;56(5):702–708.

139. Wieser HG, Schindler K, Zumsteg D. EEG in Creutzfeldt–Jakob disease. Clin Neurophysiol. 2006;117(5):935–951.

140. Steinhoff BJ, Racker S, Herrendorf G, Poser S, Grosche S, Zerr I, et al. Accuracy and reliability of periodic sharp wave complexes in Creutzfeldt-Jakob disease. Arch Neurol. 1996;53(2):162–166.

141. Zerr I, Poser S. Clinical diagnosis and differential diagnosis of CJD and vCJD. APMIS. 2002;110(1):88–98.

142. Van Everbroeck B, Dobbeleir I, De Waele M, De Deyn P, Martin J, Cras P. Differential diagnosis of 201 possible Creutzfeldt-Jakob disease patients. J Neurol. 2004;251(3):298–304.

143. Lopes da Silva, FL. EEG and MEG: relevance to neuroscience. Neuron. 2013;80(5):1112–1128.

144. Hughes SW, Crunelli V. Thalamic mechanisms of EEG alpha rhythms and their pathological implications. Neuroscientist. 2005;11(4):357–372.

145. Lörincz ML, Crunelli V, Hughes SW. Cellular dynamics of cholinergically induced alpha (8–13 Hz) rhythms in sensory thalamic nuclei in vitro. J Neurosci. 2008;28(3):660–671.

146. Lörincz ML, Kékesi KA, Juhász G, Crunelli V, Hughes SW. Temporal framing of thalamic relay-mode firing by phasic inhibition during the alpha rhythm. Neuron. 2009;63(5):683–696.

147. Klimesch W. α-band oscillations, attention, and controlled access to stored information. Trends Cogn Sci. 2012;16(12):606–617.

148. Sutter R, Kaplan PW. Clinical and electroencephalographic correlates of acute encephalopathy. J Clin Neurophysiol. 2013;30(5):443–453.

149. Sutter R, Stevens RD, Kaplan PW. Clinical and imaging correlates of EEG patterns in hospitalized patients with encephalopathy. J Neurol. 2013;260(4):1087–1098.

150. Taylor H, Schmiedt JT, Carcak N, Onat F, Di Giovanni G, Lambert R, et al. Investigating local and long-range neuronal network dynamics by simultaneous optogenetics, reverse microdialysis and silicon probe recordings in vivo. J Neurosci Methods. 2014;235:83–91.

151. Stern Y. Cognitive reserve in ageing and Alzheimer's disease. Lancet Neurol. 2012;11(11):1006–1012.

17 | EEG IN METABOLIC DISORDERS, INTOXICATIONS, AND EPILEPTIC ENCEPHALOPATHIES

RAOUL SUTTER, MD, PD, TRUDY PANG, MD, AND PETER W. KAPLAN, MB, BS, FRCP

ABSTRACT: This chapter provides a systematic overview of the diagnostic and prognostic value of electroencephalography (EEG) in adult patients with different types of encephalopathies in association with metabolic, toxic, and epileptic disorders. Most encephalopathies present with a fluctuating course characterized by typical but not pathognomonic symptoms such as cognitive impairment, altered mental status or confusion, lethargy, decreased or rarely increased motor activity, and disturbed sleep/wake cycles. EEG enables rapid, bedside electrophysiological monitoring, providing dynamic real-time information on the integrity of neocortical brain activity. Hence, EEG complements clinical and neuroimaging assessments of encephalopathic patients. Progressive slowing of EEG background activity with increasing cerebral dysfunction, emergence of intermittent transients, electrographic seizures, and impaired background reactivity to external stimuli all provide important diagnostic and prognostic information to guide medical management.

KEYWORDS: electroencephalography, EEG, encephalopathy, altered mental status, cognitive impairment, seizures

PRINCIPAL REFERENCES

1. Sutter R, Stevens RD, Kaplan PW. Clinical and imaging correlates of EEG patterns in hospitalized patients with encephalopathy. *J Neurol* 2013;260(4):1087–1098.
2. Accolla EA, Kaplan PW, Maeder-Ingvar M, et al. Clinical correlates of frontal intermittent rhythmic delta activity (FIRDA). *Clin Neurophysiol* 2011;122(1):27–31.
3. Kaplan P, Schlattman DK. Typical versus atypical triphasic waves. *J Clin Neurophysiol* 2013;30(2):211.
4. Sutter R, Stevens RD, Kaplan PW. Significance of triphasic waves in patients with acute encephalopathy: a nine-year cohort study. *Clin Neurophysiol* 2014;124(10):1952–1958.
5. Castilla-Guerra L, del Carmen Fernandez-Moreno M, Lopez-Chozas JM, et al. Electrolytes disturbances and seizures. *Epilepsia* 2006;47(12):1990–1998.
6. Condon JV, Becka DR, Gibbs FA. Electroencephalographic abnormalities in endocrine disease. *N Engl J Med* 1954;251(16):638–641.
7. Sloan TB. Anesthetic effects on electrophysiologic recordings. *J Clin Neurophysiol* 1998;15(3):217–226.
8. Sutter R, Barnes B, Leyva A, et al. Electroencephalographic sleep elements and outcome in acute encephalopathic patients: a 4-year cohort study. *Eur J Neurol* 2014;21(10):1268–1275.

1. INTRODUCTION

Encephalopathy, also known as delirium, is a term often used by neurophysiologists, neurologists, psychiatrists, and intensivists to describe altered mental status or confusional states. It typically involves lethargy, cognitive impairment, decreased (rarely increased) motor activity, memory, mental processing, and disrupted sleep–wake cycles. Encephalopathy frequently occurs in the elderly and is encountered in intensive care units (ICUs), postoperatively, and on the psychiatric, general medical, and surgical units, constituting a significant cause of morbidity and mortality.

Encephalopathy is a clinical syndrome resulting from disturbed neuronal electrogenesis, which depends on metabolic homeostasis. Nutritive and energy-providing metabolic systems that are essential for the integrity of neurofunctional processes, networks, and the functionality of glial structures can be altered by metabolic, toxic, infectious, or epileptic derangements, frequently in the context of structural brain alterations (1–3). The clinician is often presented with the challenges of determining the cause of confusion (e.g., encephalopathy, seizure, stroke or dementia) and establishing a course of management and prognosis.

Despite the all-too-frequent tendency to obtain neuroimaging studies (3), the electroencephalogram (EEG) is the only examination providing dynamic real-time information regarding neocortical brain activity and cerebral dysfunction. Hence, EEG is essential in rapidly establishing a diagnosis of encephalopathy, excluding other causes of confusion or language disturbance, and guiding the physician toward underlying disorders. However, most EEG patterns are nonspecific, making the distinction between acute encephalopathy and neurodegenerative disorders difficult; moreover, both conditions frequently coexist. Even so, several studies have added further credence to the body of evidence that some EEG patterns may help differentiating between encephalopathy and dementia (4,5) and among several different causes of encephalopathy (1,2,6–14). On quantitative EEG, a specific prolonged EEG background activation pattern (activation with a 3-minute eyes-open period) significantly improved the ability to distinguish between delirious patients with or without underlying dementia by EEG (4). In another study, delirium in dementia was characterized by slower alpha peak frequency, loss of alpha power, and increased theta and delta frequency ranges. These changes correlated with the severity of delirium and cognitive disturbances (5). Other studies revealed associations between EEG background frequency ranges and specific metabolic, toxic, infectious, or structural disorders (2,9,10). Aside from analyses of the basic EEG rhythm, studies revealed associations between particular episodic transients, particularly triphasic waves (TWs) and intermittent generalized rhythmic delta activity with frontal predominance, and metabolic and structural cerebral abnormalities, with neurofunctional outcome following encephalopathy (1,6–9,11,12,14).

Acquisition and interpretation of the EEGs in encephalopathic patients can be limited by a several factors, including electrical interference from other medical devices, especially in patients treated in ICUs, problems of electrode placement, sweating, and movement from agitated patients (15).

In this chapter, the prognostic and diagnostic use of EEG in evaluating encephalopathy in the context of various metabolic, toxic, infectious, and epileptic disorders is discussed. The use of EEG in inherited metabolic, autoimmune, and paraneoplastic diseases and in hypoxic-ischemic encephalopathy is presented elsewhere.

2. THE HISTORY OF EEG IN ENCEPHALOPATHY

The history of the use of EEG for the diagnosis and prognosis in encephalopathy started in the 1920s with the first description of the existence of human electrical brain signals by Hans Berger, a German neuropsychiatrist (16). This examination was followed by investigations in the 1930s of human EEG patterns in hypoxic brain injury and epilepsy and studies evaluating changes in EEG signals with cognitive activities. A relation between EEG slowing and disturbed arousal in encephalopathy was observed in the 1940s (17).

In the 1950s, EEG studies increased worldwide with new discoveries of the use of EEG to identify specific brain regions involved in the genesis of encephalopathic and epileptic activity, the discovery of cerebral recruiting responses, and the description of inhibitory effects of the reticular formation in the brainstem. Major progress was made when the work of Foley, and Bickford and Butt on hepatic coma showed pronounced slowing of the basic EEG activity and formation of TWs (14,18). The contributions of Condon, Cadilhac, and Glaser have provided further important information on the EEG correlates of metabolic encephalopathies (19–21).

In the 1960s, several studies reported generalized slowing in the theta and delta ranges and increases in voltage of the basic EEG rhythm with metabolic abnormalities (22,23). These studies were followed by investigations in the 1970s that revealed progressive slowing of the basic EEG rhythm with increasing depths of anesthesia, clinically worsening of encephalopathy, and deepening levels of coma (24). Figure 17.1 presents different EEG patterns in encephalopathic patients and their correlation with different levels of sedation. Simultaneously, the study group of Gloor described focal EEG changes in animal models with cortical, subcortical, and combined lesions (25), further delineating the diagnostic yield of EEG regarding the differentiation between focal and diffuse brain dysfunction.

In the 1980s and 1990s, observations using time-synchronized video-EEG monitoring led to the conclusions that certain EEG patterns accompanied clinical signs of brain dysfunction in a number of diseases. The EEG patterns most studied were delta patterns, diffuse severe suppression, intermittent rhythmic delta activity (27,28), TWs (12,29–32), unreactive diffuse alpha frequency patterns (33–35), and spindle-like sleep patterns (36,37) (Fig. 17.2).

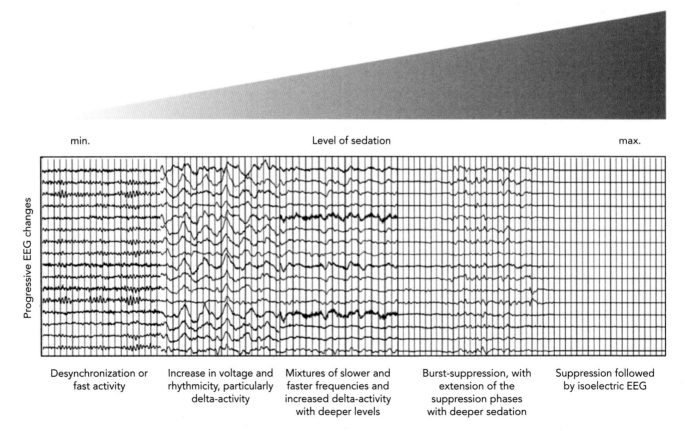

min.   Level of sedation   max.

Progressive EEG changes

| Desynchronization or fast activity | Increase in voltage and rhythmicity, particularly delta-activity | Mixtures of slower and faster frequencies and increased delta-activity with deeper levels | Burst-suppression, with extension of the suppression phases with deeper sedation | Suppression followed by isoelectric EEG |

Figure 17.1. Progressive EEG frequency slowing with deepening anesthesia. Adapted from (26).

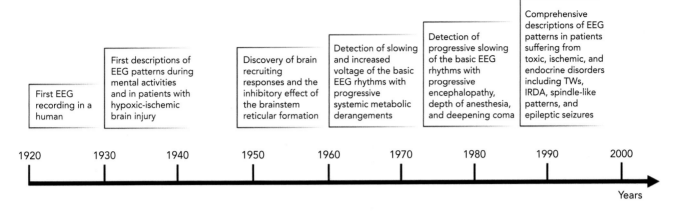

Figure 17.2. Cornerstones in the history of the diagnostic and prognostic use of EEG.

However, the early promises of the diagnostic specificity of EEG in encephalopathy were not confirmed in later studies. Today, despite the long experience of EEG in encephalopathy, systematic investigations of the diagnostic and prognostic value of particular EEG patterns are scarce and limited to a few specific conditions. The lack of evidence could be explained by a need for complex study designs, such as the comparison of EEG patterns between healthy with non-healthy, encephalopathic with non-encephalopathic patients, or comparisons among populations with different underlying etiologies of encephalopathy with controls.

3. EEG IN METABOLIC ENCEPHALOPATHIES

3.1. Hyperammonemic and Hepatic Encephalopathy

3.1.1. PATHOPHYSIOLOGY

Liver dysfunction may lead to variable degrees of EEG changes, from mild slowing of the basic rhythm to an isoelectric EEG. These EEG abnormalities depend on the complex pathophysiological mechanisms involved.

Portal-systemic hepatic encephalopathies are based on a portocaval anastomosis with a consecutive bypass (shunt) of proteins from the hepatic metabolism, a condition typically found in patients with chronic liver cirrhosis with significant portal-systemic venous shunts. In contrast, fulminant acute hepatic failure results in sudden hepatocellular breakdown and dysfunction. In both pathologic conditions, astrocytic swelling resulting from an accumulation of metabolites, especially nitrogenous substances, is considered a major contributor. The exact biochemical and neuropathologic mechanisms of hepatic encephalopathy, however, are not fully understood. The neurotoxic effect of ammonia results from the purported toxic effect of ammonia (or other compounds that coexist with ammonia), a product of the amino acid metabolism (38). Ammonia may accumulate with its impaired degradation in the liver or by its overproduction in pathologic conditions including multiple myeloma, urease-producing bacteria, or drugs (e.g., valproic acid) that inhibit metabolic pathways (38). Increased glutamine production during ammonium clearance, changes in osmolarity and death of astrocytes with consecutive brain edema, as well as an increased GABA tone may be the causes of encephalopathy (38). Hyperammonemia leads to an increased astrocytic pH that results in calcium-dependent release of glutamate, which subsequently contributes to activation of N-methyl D-aspartate (NMDA) receptors and excitotoxicity (39).

In patients with chronic liver disease, hyperammonemia decreases glutamate stores of astrocytes, resulting in inactivation of the glutamate transporter and decreased postsynaptic glutamate receptors on neurons and astrocytes, thereby contributing to increased cerebral inhibition.

3.1.2. EEG

The EEG abnormalities of hepatic encephalopathy are well described since the early investigation by Foley et al. and Bickford and Butt (14,18). The degree of slowing often parallels the level of blood ammonia. Similarly, the degree of EEG slowing correlates with the severity of liver disease (40,41). In an EEG study of patients with hepatic encephalopathy, changes in the basic EEG rhythm were associated with the degree of liver cirrhosis, including low-frequency alpha background rhythms with sudden intermittent random theta waves superimposed in a temporal, frontal, or generalized distribution (41). In line with these findings, another observation described that EEGs of patients with liver cirrhosis showed reduced frequency in the posterior derivations and an increase in interhemispheric parietal relative coherence within the theta band as compared to controls (40). These features were more prominent in patients with liver cirrhosis Child class C and in patients with a history of overt hepatic encephalopathy. As the clinical presentation worsened, the EEGs progressively showed more disorganization with diffuse and asynchronous bihemispheric theta and delta slowing. With deep coma, the background activity decreased in amplitude and frequency and eventually became isoelectric (41,42). In another study of encephalopathic patients with different EEG patterns, serum ammonia levels inversely correlated with the frequency range of the basic EEG rhythms and the emergence of episodic transients such as TWs and intermittent generalized rhythmic delta activity with frontal predominance (formerly known as FIRDA) (2) (Figs. 17.3 and 17.4).

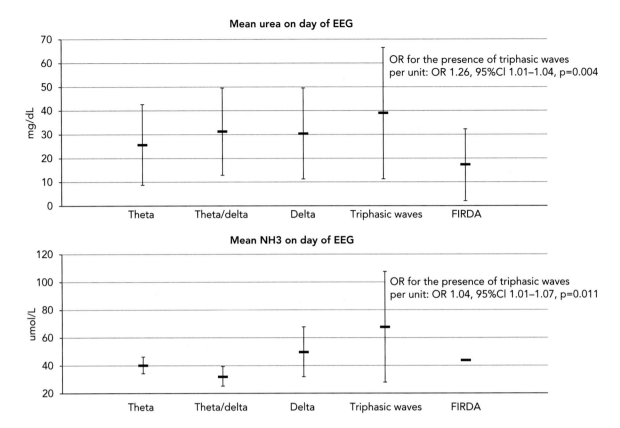

Figure 17.3. Differences of mean serum levels of urea and ammonia (NH₃) in patients with one of the five EEG patterns. Reprinted with kind permission from Springer Science and Business Media (2).

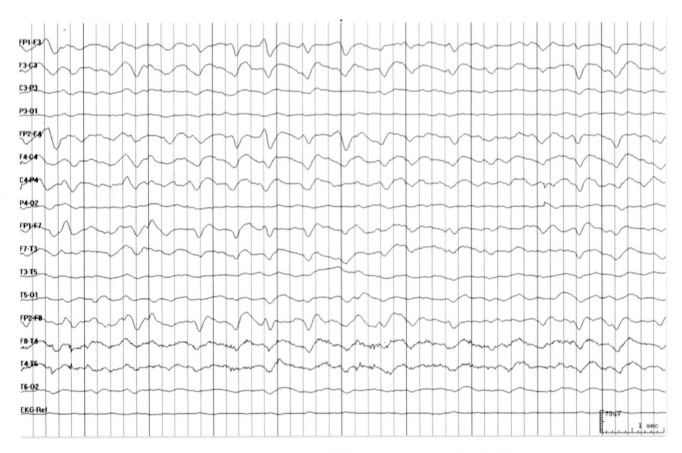

Figure 17.4. Generalized rhythmic delta activity with frontal predominance and TWs in a patient with hepatic failure; the TWs become more prominent with stimulation.

The exact EEG definition and behavior of TWs is outlined in Section 6.2.2. The incidence of TWs in hepatic encephalopathy is approximately 25% (43). Although TWs were initially considered pathognomonic for hepatic encephalopathy and coma (18,44), TWs may be interpreted as an ictal pattern, especially if they have sharper components and temporal evolution that can be difficult to differentiate from nonconvulsive status epilepticus (SE) (45). Despite the paroxysmal appearance of TWs, clinically overt epileptic manifestations are not very common with hepatic encephalopathy and occur much less frequently than in renal encephalopathies (46). Besides TWs, EEGs of patients with hepatic encephalopathy can reveal spikes, focal sharp waves, and generalized spike-waves - episodic transients that are sometimes difficult to differentiate from TWs (47). In a study of a fully automated spectral EEG analysis, different EEG hepatic encephalopathy classification systems were used to evaluate their correlation with neuropsychiatric test results, the severity of liver disease, biochemical markers of liver function, and risk of death (48). The highest correlation with the clinical findings was seen with automatic quantification systems. Spectral EEG analysis has also been used to identify mild hepatic encephalopathy features, including an increase in theta power in the posterior EEG traces and less commonly a decrease in mean dominant frequency and increase in relative delta power (42). In analyses of the prognostic impact of EEG in patients after liver transplantation, the EEGs of patients who did not survive demonstrated a greater incidence of epileptiform abnormalities than survivors (48). In another study with multichannel EEG in cirrhotic patients with various grades of hepatic encephalopathy and healthy volunteers, spectral and dynamic EEG indices were quantified by continuous wavelet analysis (49). In addition, the psychometric hepatic encephalopathy score, continuous reaction time, and biochemical profiles were assessed. EEG analysis, based on continuous wavelet transform, provided quantifiable information on static as well as dynamic EEG features and abnormalities that correlated with psychometric test performance, thereby providing valuable neurophysiological information for surveillance, prognostication and treatment.

In conclusion, semi-quantitative or quantitative spectral analysis of EEGs may help to identify the initial changes associated with minimal hepatic encephalopathy, and the EEG may assist with prognostication and evaluation of the treatment response to liver transplantation. However, a recent study on the agreement and predictive validity of different indices in 132 cirrhotic patients concluded that the most reliable diagnosis of covert hepatic encephalopathy probably requires a combination of clinical, neurophysiological, and neuropsychological indices (50).

In acquired chronic hepatocerebral degeneration, symptoms include dysarthria, ataxia, intention tremor, and choreoathetosis mainly affecting the cranial muscles (51). This clinical entity is considered to occur much more frequently than the familial form (Wilson disease) (51). The acquired form may develop in various chronic liver diseases and often leads to the above-described picture of hepatic encephalopathy, which is less common in Wilson disease. EEG studies so far are restricted to pediatric cohorts (52).

3.2. Uremic Encephalopathy

3.2.1. Pathophysiology

Before dialysis and renal transplantation, uremic encephalopathy was common. Today, the early treatment and correction of biochemical abnormalities in patients with known acute or chronic renal disease often prevents the development of severe encephalopathy. In clinical practice, uremic encephalopathy remains on the differential diagnosis of patients with critical illnesses causing multiple organ failure.

Despite extensive investigations, the pathophysiology of uremic encephalopathy is unknown. Reversible ischemic changes, disorders of cerebral metabolism, and the direct effect of uremic toxins on intracerebral vascular autoregulation have been implicated (53). In acute uremic encephalopathy, frequently described symptoms are confusion, agitation, tremor, fasciculations, myoclonus, and coma. In chronic uremia, patients may experience lethargy, cognitive impairment, irritability, agitation (54), and alterations of sleep, with a decrease in deep restorative sleep, rapid eye movements (REM) sleep, and total sleep times, resulting in difficulty differentiating sleep stages (55). Seizures are usually due to water–electrolyte imbalance (56,57), although they may also occur in the setting of medication side effects, infection, malignant hypertension, or dialysis disequilibrium (58,59).

3.2.2. EEG

Various gradations of EEG abnormalities have been reported in both acute and chronic renal failure and may potentially be reversible with renal replacement therapy or transplantation. According to a recent EEG study of 154 encephalopathic patients, the EEG in acute uremic encephalopathy may demonstrate irregular low-voltage activity with progressive slowing of the posterior basic rhythm, and the odds ratio for the presence of TWs is 1.26 ($p = .004$) for every unit increase in serum urea (Figs. 17.3 and 17.5) (2). In some cases, bilateral spike discharges may or may not be associated with widespread myoclonic jerks. Up to 30% of patients with renal insufficiency develop epileptic seizures (58,59), with mostly partial and generalized convulsive seizures as well as infrequent nonconvulsive SE (NCSE) (60).

In chronic uremic encephalopathy, early studies revealed a slow and disorganized basic EEG rhythm, with more pronounced slowing associated with worsening uremia (54,61–64). Sometimes, theta discharges, sharp waves, and polyspike and wave complexes were detected (62), and photic stimulation may result in photomyoclonic or photoparoxysmal responses (62). In a more recent analysis of quantitative EEG in patients with chronic renal failure and healthy controls, electrical power was most prominent in delta, theta, and alpha frequencies in the temporal and central brain areas. Explorative statistical comparison of the two datasets with respect to these brain areas revealed that the increases in electrical power in delta, theta, and alpha frequency bands were significantly different from controls (65).

In stage 2 sleep, bursts of high-voltage 12- to 13-Hz waves with enhanced vertex sharp-waves in drowsiness, lack of spindles (14 Hz), and prolonged high-voltage slow bursts

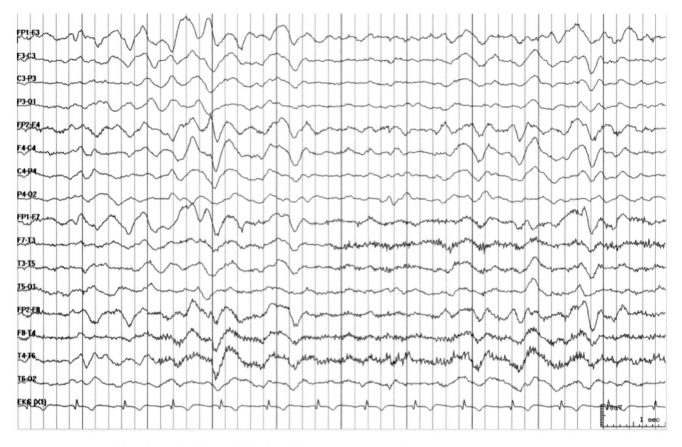

Figure 17.5. *Intermittent, blunted TWs with rhythmic and arrhythmic delta activity in a patient with uremia.*

with awakening have been reported (66). In REM sleep, ocular movements are enhanced; they may even be continuous and associated with blinking and brief myoclonic movements. With hemodialysis, deeper stages of sleep can emerge (55). Although dialysis helps to maintain normal metabolic states in patients with chronic renal failure, it temporarily may worsen EEG patterns, with an increase in background slowing, bursts of frontal slow waves, and rarely spike and wave complexes, and seizures (54,61,67,68). Repeated dialysis may increase EEG background frequency (63). Occasionally, dialysis disequilibrium syndrome occurs at the onset of dialysis therapy or with a rapid and highly effective treatment. This is characterized by irritability, nausea, headache, blurred vision, hallucinations, asterixis, confusion, posterior reversible encephalopathy, and generalized convulsions within the first 24 hours after dialysis (58,69). These symptoms are possibly caused by faster systemic clearance of urea compared to slower clearance in the brain, leading to cerebral edema. The risk for dialysis disequilibrium can be reduced with the use of aluminum-free dialysate; however, with chronic dialysis treatment, dialysis-related encephalopathy may also occur, mainly characterized by speech and memory difficulties, psychiatric symptoms, involuntary movements, epileptic seizures, and death (54). The EEG frequently reveals a slow and disorganized basic EEG rhythm, intermittent generalized rhythmic delta activity with frontal predominance (formerly FIRDA), or paroxysmal frontocentral spike and wave discharges (see Fig. 17.3) (2,54,62). Fortunately, renal transplantation may reverse the EEG background slowing in

the first two postsurgical weeks (64). While there have been various reports of post-renal transplant seizures, more recent studies suggest an incidence of 2.3% (70).

In conclusion, EEGs may reveal altered brain activity in patients with acute or chronic uremic encephalopathy, and may assist with the evaluation of patients and their response to treatment with dialysis and renal transplantation.

3.3. Eclampsia Gravidarum–Related Encephalopathy

3.3.1. PATHOPHYSIOLOGY

Eclampsia gravidarum is an acute and life-threatening complication of pregnancy characterized by generalized convulsions and/or coma in pregnant or postpartum patients with preeclampsia but in the absence of other neurological conditions (71). Preeclampsia is a syndrome occurring after week 20 of gestation and is characterized by hypertension and proteinuria. A number of target organs are affected, including the brain, liver, kidney, and placenta (72). Factors in the complex pathogenesis of preeclampsia involve maternal, fetal, and placental factors. Abnormal development of placental vasculature early in pregnancy is thought to release angiogenic factors into the systemic circulation, causing maternal endothelial dysfunction and thereby systemic vasoconstriction (73,74) as well as cerebral vasoconstriction (75). The latter, together with loss of cerebral autoregulation, is considered the main cause of focal necrosis, hemorrhage, vasogenic edema, and convulsions (76,77).

3.3.2. EEG

There are only a few reports and smaller studies on EEGs in eclampsia. In preeclampsia and the acute stage of eclampsia the preferential location of the main pathologic processes seems to be the occipital lobes, which may lead to observed episodes of cortical blindness (78). In a study of patients with eclampsia, interictal EEG was abnormal in 80%, including diffuse slowing (56%), focal slowing (26%), spike discharges (14%), alpha coma (1%), and electrical silence (3%) (79). In a study comparing cerebral magnetic resonance imaging (MRI) and interictal EEG findings in preeclamptic and eclamptic women, EEG abnormalities were significantly more frequent in eclamptic versus preeclamptic patients, including diffuse slowing, focal or hemispheric slowing, and focal discharges (80). Nevertheless, in patients with mild preeclampsia, 20% demonstrated similar EEG abnormalities. In the eclamptic group, the percentage of patients showing EEG abnormalities was significantly higher at 83%, and the abnormalities included diffuse slowing, focal slowing, focal spike discharges, and multifocal spike discharges. Although most MRI abnormalities were focal, the EEG abnormalities tended to be more diffuse. Of the patients with abnormal EEGs, 94% demonstrated resolution of these abnormalities at 1-month follow-up.

Magnesium sulfate is frequently administered during labor and in the first 12 to 24 hours postpartum in eclamptic patients to prevent vasospasm (81). Although a clinical benefit has been shown with treatment in this setting, magnesium infusion does not influence the EEG abnormalities before, during, or after the infusion (82).

In conclusion, the abnormalities detected by EEG correlate with the pathologic intracerebral processes and help in the diagnosis of eclampsia. However, the prognostic value and its use for treatment monitoring has not been shown.

3.4. Electrolyte Disturbance–Related Encephalopathies

3.4.1. HYPERNATREMIC ENCEPHALOPATHY
3.4.1.1. PATHOPHYSIOLOGY

While hyponatremia is likely to be the underlying etiology of seizures (see below), hypernatremia is more likely to result as a consequence of seizures (83). Hypernatremia is frequently used therapeutically in neurological ICUs in the management of cerebral edema and increased intracranial pressure in order to allow water to shift from the intracellular space to the extracellular space. Seizures are not typically seen in these cases.

3.4.1.2. EEG

Overall, the EEG demonstrates mild diffuse slowing (84). Most reports and case series are focused on pediatric patients. Currently, there is no evidence that EEG monitoring of hypernatremic patients improves diagnosis, course, or clinical outcome. However, patients are frequently on continuous EEG monitoring for the management of their underlying neurological disease.

3.4.2. HYPONATREMIC ENCEPHALOPATHY
3.4.2.1. PATHOPHYSIOLOGY

Decreased serum osmolality, primarily from acute hyponatremia, promotes water shift from the extracellular into the intracellular compartment. This shift results in a cerebral edema that may lead to severe brain dysfunction and increase in interstitial pressure causing an extracellular fluid shift from the brain tissue into the cerebrospinal fluid. Subsequently, the glial cells and neurons lose solutes, promoting an osmotic movement of water from the intracellular to the extracellular space (85). As a consequence, there is disruption of the blood–brain barrier and loss of oligodendroglia in the *basis pontis*. The rapid correction/change of serum sodium levels may cause central pontine myelinolysis, which can be diffuse and involve extrapontine regions of the central nervous system (CNS). However, the exact pathophysiological mechanisms that underlie the demyelination induced by rapid changes of serum sodium levels are not fully understood.

Hyponatremia and acute water intoxication lead to severe brain dysfunction with or without epileptic seizures. The rate or sodium change over time in patients with hyponatremic states is more important than the absolute degree of hyponatremia as the determining factor in the development of mental status changes, EEG abnormalities, and seizures. Initial symptoms include nausea, headache, confusion, and agitation, and as sodium levels decrease further, seizures, coma, respiratory arrest, and death ensue (86).

3.4.2.2. EEG

Hyponatremia and acute water intoxication lead to severe EEG abnormalities with pronounced generalized slowing. In a case of acute compulsive water intake resulting in a serum sodium level of 116 mg/dL, convulsive SE, papilledema, and an EEG with diffuse 0.5- to 2-Hz activity were described (87). Despite rapid electrolyte normalization, EEG normalization was slow. This case description was followed with another report of a patient with convulsive SE induced by polydipsia, with generalized delta waves and spike-wave complexes on EEG (88). In contrast to the first case, the EEG improved quickly with correction of hyponatremia. Other abnormalities have been described, such as periodic delta waves (89), TWs (90) and periodic lateralized epileptiform discharges (91), repetitive seizures (92), and absence SE (93). Several different EEG features have been described in patients presenting with *de novo* NCSE due to hyponatremia and usually consist of generalized epileptiform activity (94). Follow-up EEG after recovery from NCSE may reveal unilateral focal spikes (93).

In conclusion, EEG findings in hyponatremic encephalopathy are nonspecific. However, EEG monitoring is helpful in those who develop seizures, especially if they are nonconvulsive.

3.4.3. HYPERCALCEMIC ENCEPHALOPATHY
3.4.3.1. PATHOPHYSIOLOGY

Blood calcium is regulated within a narrow range for proper cellular processes. Serum calcium exists in three states: bound to proteins, bound to anions, and in an unbound ionized state, which is the only physiologically active form. Hypercalcemia may be due to excessive skeletal calcium release, increased intestinal calcium absorption, or decreased renal calcium excretion. The underlying diseases can be excessive parathyroid activity caused by renal failure, hyperplasia or neoplasm of the parathyroid glands, skeletal decalcification, vitamin A and

D intoxication, paraneoplastic syndromes, or bone metastases from malignancies. Increased serum calcium levels are associated with CNS depression. Clinical symptoms include irritability, lethargy, and malaise with mild elevations of serum calcium concentrations. With increase of serum calcium levels, symptoms may worsen and result in coma (95).

3.4.3.2. EEG
Most EEG changes, accompanied by neurological deficits and mental impairment, appear at a serum calcium level of >12 mg/dL (96,97). According to early case series, the EEG typically shows slowing of the basic EEG rhythm, which may be interrupted by high-voltage anterior delta bursts over 1 to 4 seconds, sometimes intermixed with TWs (98). When blood calcium is restored to physiological concentrations the clinical symptoms disappear within several days to weeks and EEG abnormalities disappear within weeks to months. Epileptiform discharges are usually not detected. However, cases with spike activity independently in both the right and left occipital regions and generalized epileptic seizures have been described (99). Other cases show spike–slow wave complexes and epileptic seizures in association with vasospasm in the posterior circulation system (100).

In conclusion, EEGs in hypercalcemia may show slowing of the basic EEG rhythm with TWs, epileptic discharges, or seizures, while the clinical symptoms may be nonspecific.

3.4.4. HYPOCALCEMIC ENCEPHALOPATHY
3.4.4.1. PATHOPHYSIOLOGY
Common causes of hypocalcemia include hypoparathyroidism, vitamin D deficiency, and chronic renal disease. CNS hyperexcitability may lead to seizures. The occasionally observed tetany is of peripheral origin manifested by carpopedal spasm.

3.4.4.2. EEG
Epileptic manifestations develop at serum calcium levels <6 mg/dL. Epileptic seizures are mostly generalized, although partial seizures may occur and typically respond poorly to antiseizure monotherapy. Although some seizures can be controlled with antiseizure polytherapy, improvement is mostly achieved with restoration of normal serum calcium levels (101). In the interictal phase, the EEG typically consists of high-amplitude delta activity sometimes accompanied by focal spikes and spike-wave discharges, all of which may be enhanced by hyperventilation (101). Surprisingly, in patients with pseudohypoparathyroidism, EEG abnormalities are very similar to cases of hypocalcemia (102).

Of note, the normal EEG in tetanic spasms indicates that these spasms are of peripheral origin rather than cerebral origin. In the CNS, hypocalcemia is highly epileptogenic, producing marked EEG changes with slowing and generalized bursts of spikes. As antiseizure treatment is challenging during prolonged episodes of hypocalcemic encephalopathy, EEGs may assist in monitoring response to treatment.

3.4.5. HYPOMAGNESEMIC ENCEPHALOPATHY
3.4.5.1. PATHOPHYSIOLOGY
Hypomagnesemia can be caused by inadequate intake, malnutrition, increased consumption with stress, sports, or pregnancy,

malabsorption resulting from bowel diseases, excessive diuretic use, or wasting in renal diseases. As magnesium acts as a membrane stabilizer, hypomagnesemia can cause cardiac arrhythmias and hyperexcitability of the peripheral and central nervous systems, especially with serum magnesium levels <1.2 mg/dL (103). The latter typically leads to altered mental status, focal neurological deficits (104), and epileptic seizures (105). As magnesium is essential for the inhibition of secretion and action of the parathyroid hormone, it is typically associated with secondary hypocalcemia (106). Furthermore, the effects of hypomagnesemia are thought to be potentiated by hypokalemia (106).

3.4.5.2. EEG
Although some cases of hypomagnesemic encephalopathy and seizures have been published (105), detailed EEG information is mostly not presented and formal EEG studies with hypomagnesemia are lacking.

3.5. Vitamin Deficiency–Related Encephalopathies
Evidence for the diagnostic yield and prognostic value of particular EEG patterns in vitamin deficiency–related encephalopathies is weak as formal studies are lacking. In Wernicke's encephalopathy, however, the EEG may be particularly useful for the detection of subclinical seizures.

3.5.1. VITAMIN B1 (THIAMINE) DEFICIENCY–RELATED ENCEPHALOPATHY (WERNICKE'S ENCEPHALOPATHY)
3.5.1.1. PATHOPHYSIOLOGY
Wernicke's encephalopathy is caused by thiamine deficiency and is seen in alcohol abuse, inadequate intake, malabsorption, malnutrition, increased metabolism, or its iatrogenic elimination from hemodialysis. The phosphate derivatives of thiamine are involved in many intracellular processes. The best-characterized form is thiamine pyrophosphate, a coenzyme in the catabolism of sugars and amino acids. Vitamin B1 is necessary for the biosynthesis of the neurotransmitter acetylcholine and gamma-aminobutyric acid. In addition, thiamine pyrophosphate is essential for alcoholic fermentation. Vitamin B1 deficiency can further cause an osmotic imbalance with perineural edema and neuronal swelling. Cerebral periventricular lesions may be explained by high rates of vitamin B1-dependent metabolism in these brain regions (107).

There are two forms of thiamine-related clinical syndromes: (1) the encephalopathy consisting of a sensorimotor neuropathy and Wernicke-Korsakoff syndrome and (2) the clinical syndrome consisting of edema and congestive heart failure without significant CNS alteration. Wernicke's encephalopathy, with or without the Korsakoff syndrome, is characterized by predominant oculomotor and cerebellar symptoms (107) and is frequently encountered in alcoholics, although it can emerge in many different critical medical conditions, such as hyperemesis, dialysis, post-gastrointestinal surgery, and with brain metastasis (108).

3.5.1.2. EEG
There is a wide variety of EEG patterns that reflect the severity of the neurofunctional impairment related to vitamin B1

deficiency. Shortly after syndrome onset, the basic EEG rhythm gradually slows down until delta frequency ranges are reached (109). In later and more severe stages of the disease, the delta frequency range activity is intermixed with sharp and slow wave complexes (110). In a group of adult patients, one third of patients with neurological manifestations demonstrated epileptiform activity on their EEGs (111). In a few cases, epileptic seizures were reported and limited to non-alcoholic Wernicke's encephalopathy (112).

In cases of Wernicke's encephalopathy, the EEG may be useful for the detection of seizures in patients with altered mental status.

3.5.2. VITAMIN B3 (NIACIN) DEFICIENCY–RELATED ENCEPHALOPATHY
3.5.2.1. PATHOPHYSIOLOGY
Vitamin B3 acts as part of the two coenzymes nicotinamide adenine dinucleotide and nicotinamide adenine dinucleotide phosphate that are involved in several metabolic reactions in humans. Among many important chemical interactions, niacin plays a key role in glycolysis, in fatty acid synthesis, and in the deamination of amino acids. Thus, niacin is a vital precursor for the coenzymes supplying energy to body cells. Vitamin B3 deficiency may result in pellagra, characterized clinically by dermatitis, diarrhea, depression, and dementia.

3.5.2.2. EEG
EEG studies of patients with pellagra are lacking, and the only published case series of 29 patients revealed nonspecific diffuse slowing of the basic EEG rhythm within the theta and delta frequency ranges that speed up into normal alpha frequency ranges with sufficient niacin supplementation (113).

3.5.3. VITAMIN B6 (PYRIDOXINE) DEFICIENCY–RELATED ENCEPHALOPATHY
3.5.3.1. PATHOPHYSIOLOGY
The active form of vitamin B6, pyridoxal 5′-phosphate, serves as a cofactor in many enzyme reactions in amino acid, glucose, and lipid metabolism. Pyridoxine deficiency has been recognized as a rare etiology of severe and even fatal convulsions mainly in neonates and infants, but cases in adults are described (114).

3.5.3.2. EEG
Typically, the EEG reveals generalized spike activity and epileptic seizures, which typically respond rapidly to treatment with pyridoxine. In a study of eight healthy women with a defined formula diet nearly devoid of vitamin B6, 25% showed abnormal EEG patterns within two weeks, including focal slowing and focal sharp waves that resolved with vitamin B6 repletion. However, epileptic seizures were not seen (114).

Overall, with the exception of this small study, there are no formal studies of the use of EEG in patients with vitamin B6 deficiency.

3.5.4. VITAMIN B12 (COBALAMIN) DEFICIENCY–RELATED ENCEPHALOPATHY
3.5.4.1. PATHOPHYSIOLOGY
Vitamin B12 is essential for normal development and function of the brain. It plays an important role in the generation of myelin, ensuring proper nerve-impulse transmission. Vitamin B12 deficiency can potentially cause severe and irreversible damage to the brain and nervous system, although the mechanisms by which myelin damage occurs remain unclear. Patients may present with neuropathy of the large fibers of the peripheral nervous system and may exhibit CNS dysfunction, including mental status changes, such as delirium or dementia, and hyperreflexia.

3.5.4.2. EEG
Slowing of basic EEG rhythms can occur with or without temporal spike and sharp wave activity (115). However, studies of B12 deficiency were performed in animal models or in pediatric cohorts and EEG changes were found to be nonspecific and did not necessarily parallel clinical symptoms. Formal investigations in adults are lacking.

Overall, in vitamin B12 deficiency, nonspecific changes of the basic EEG rhythm and focal epileptiform activity may be seen.

3.6. Endocrine Disorders–Related Encephalopathies
3.6.1. HYPERGLYCEMIC ENCEPHALOPATHY
3.6.1.1. PATHOPHYSIOLOGY
Hyperglycemia typically occurs in uncontrolled diabetes mellitus and leads to osmotic derangements mainly affecting the subthalamic area, the putamen, and the caudate nucleus (116). The most frequently associated symptoms are movement disorders, seizures, and SE (117). The focal seizures may involve visual hallucinations, forced head and eye deviation, and aphasia (118). Rapid correction of the hyperglycemic state with insulin controls the epileptic seizures more than the administration of antiseizure drugs.

3.6.1.2. EEG
Although EEG manifestations in different states of hyperglycemia are much less specific and predictable than they are in states of hypoglycemia, a study in 1940 on the modification of the cortical frequency spectrum by changes in CO_2, blood sugar, and oxygen found activities in the slow and fast frequency ranges and with some intermingled spiking in patients with serum sugar levels >400 mg/100 mL (119). Occasionally, epileptogenic lesions may result from comatose states (120). However, such complications are more likely in hypoglycemic states. Despite effective treatment, these EEG abnormalities may persist for several days (19).

In non-ketotic hyperglycemia, focal epileptic motor seizures with rolandic EEG spike foci and contralateral clonic motions (121), which can be induced by movements (i.e., reflex epilepsy), are common. In addition, seizures from the occipital cortex are described (122).

In ketotic hyperglycemia, SE with (123) or without (124) visual seizures and a temporal epileptogenic focus on EEG are described.

In conclusion, EEG is helpful in diagnosing seizures and SE in patients with hyperglycemia and altered mental status.

3.6.2. HYPOGLYCEMIC ENCEPHALOPATHY

3.6.2.1. PATHOPHYSIOLOGY

Contrary to hyperglycemic encephalopathy, acute decreases of serum glucose levels usually arise from hypoglycemia-inducing drugs or exogenous or endogenous insulin. This may release aspartate after a fall in the cell membrane ATPase pump activity. Hypoglycemia can manifest with autonomic symptoms such as diaphoresis, tachycardia, tremulousness, and generalized weakness, focal neurological deficits, and different degrees of altered mental status depending on the degree and course of the hypoglycemic state (125).

3.6.2.2. EEG

Early experimental studies revealed that hypoglycemia induces EEG changes and that cortical activity disappears earlier than that of subcortical structures (119,120,126). These experiments found no correlation among EEG changes, levels of awareness, and blood sugar levels (126). These findings were followed by investigations revealing very low blood sugar levels with a normal EEG and wakefulness in some patients (127). However, in most studies mentioned above, an impressive degree of slowing of the basic EEG rhythm in the theta and delta frequencies was seen with increasing hypoglycemia (Fig. 17.6). Later studies revealed that this effect is most pronounced in the frontal cerebral region (128,129). In some patients, hypoglycemia may promote epileptiform discharges that can result in seizures, especially in patients with epilepsy (130).

Spontaneous episodes of hypoglycemia may mimic complex partial seizures, due to the concomitant impaired neuropsychiatric state. Usually, the prolonged nature of these attacks, the atypical semiology, the unresponsiveness to antiseizure drugs, and the provocation by fasting are helpful in differentiating between the two conditions. EEG may help in clarifying the diagnosis or excluding epileptic seizures or SE in patients with hypoglycemic states.

In more recent studies analyzing EEG signals under insulin-induced hypoglycemia in type 1 diabetic patients, the EEG signal changes in response to hypoglycemia were detected beginning at a blood glucose level of <3.3 mmol/L (131) and irrespective of the sleep stages (132). Another study revealed that automated detection of hypoglycemia-induced EEG changes reliably identified hypoglycemia below the threshold of 3.3 mmol/L in subjects with type 1 diabetes (133). This study was followed by an investigation of hypoglycemia-related EEG changes in patients with type 1 diabetes and normal hypoglycemia awareness or unawareness using quantitative EEG (134). Analysis showed that the absolute amplitude of the theta band and alpha–theta band doubled during hypoglycemia, with no difference between the two groups. In the recovery period, the increased theta amplitudes persisted. Another study assessing hypoglycemia-related EEG changes using multi-scale entropy revealed a decrease in the complexity of EEG patterns when a state of hypoglycemia was entered, because of a degradation of the EEG long-range temporal correlations (135). Rapid glucose administration, however, can result in EEG normalization.

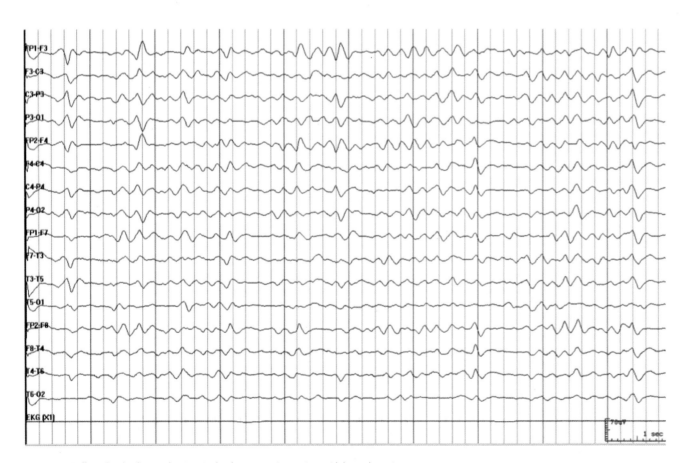

Figure 17.6. Diffuse slow background activity in the theta range in a patient with hypoglycemia.

In conclusion, the EEG changes seen with increasing hypoglycemia in awake or sleeping patients suggest that continuous EEG monitoring and automated real-time analysis may be potentially used as an alarm in patients at risk for hypoglycemic crises. Further studies are need to evaluate the impact of EEG monitoring in overall treatment and outcomes of diabetic patients.

3.6.3. Adrenocortical Insufficiency (Addison's Disease), Hyperfunction (Cushing's Disease) and Pheochromocytoma-Related Encephalopathies

3.6.3.1. Pathophysiology

Adrenocortical insufficiency is the clinical manifestation of deficient production or action of glucocorticoids, with or without concurrent deficiency in mineralocorticoids and adrenal androgens (136). Primary adrenocortical insufficiency (i.e., Addison's disease) occurs when the production of the adrenal hormone cortisol and sometimes aldosterone by the adrenal glands is reduced or lacking. Secondary adrenocortical insufficiency occurs when the pituitary gland does not produce adequate adrenocorticotropin, a hormone stimulating the adrenal glands to produce cortisol. If adrenocorticotropin output is too low, cortisol production decreases. Among many nonspecific symptoms, the most common clinical signs are chronic fatigue, diffuse muscle weakness, loss of appetite, weight loss, and abdominal pain. The EEG abnormalities are thought to be linked to impaired glucose metabolism, as treatment with steroids with consecutive increases in blood glucose levels can significantly improve the clinical symptoms accompanied by normalization of the EEG morphology.

In contrast to adrenocortical insufficiency, adrenocortical hyperfunction is a condition where there is an overproduction of hormones from the adrenal cortex. Among a wide variety of symptoms, the typical clinical features include rapid weight gain of the trunk and face with sparing of the limbs, growth of fat pads along the collarbone, on the back of the neck and face, excess sweating, dilation of capillaries, thinning of the skin, purple or red striae mainly on the trunk, proximal muscle weakness, and hirsutism (137). Pheochromocytoma, a neuroendocrine tumor of the medulla of the adrenal glands, may cause high blood pressures resulting from a high an increased secretion rate of catecholamines.

3.6.3.2. EEG

With mild adrenocortical insufficiency, the EEG may show little or no abnormality. In patients with severe disease, the EEG typically reveals slow background rhythms in the theta and delta frequency ranges (138,139). Less frequently, the EEG background loses reactivity (140) and may show increased sensitivity to hyperventilation and decreased beta activity (141). However, it is unclear whether these EEG changes are solely due to the lack of corticosteroids, since hypocortisolism is frequently accompanied by concomitant metabolic abnormalities, such as hypoglycemia and hyponatremia (142).

In patients with adrenocortical hyperfunction, EEG abnormalities are less prominent. While the EEG may remain entirely normal in many patients (143), some studies reveal nonspecific slowing or acceleration of the basic EEG rhythm with increasing serum cortisol levels (144). Improvement of the EEG is not temporally linked to treatment with adrenocorticotropic hormones or steroids, but treatment-related enhanced seizure susceptibility is reported (143). This seizure susceptibility is mirrored by reports of adult epileptics with abnormal EEG tracings, with increased EEG changes following intravenous administration of cortisone (145). In a study of EEG sleep architecture in Cushing's disease, patients with adrenocortical hyperfunction demonstrated poorer sleep continuity, shortened REM period latency, and increased first REM period density as compared to healthy subjects (146). The sleep architecture is usually restored after treatment (147).

Pheochromocytomas may cause extremely high blood pressures, but the EEG may remain normal (148) unless hypertension-related posterior reversible encephalopathy syndrome (PRES) develops, which leads to slowing of the basic EEG rhythm.

In conclusion, EEG abnormalities are well described in both adrenal insufficiency and hyperfunction. The increased seizure susceptibility in patients treated with steroids calls for the use of EEG in patients with altered level of consciousness or seizure-like symptoms.

3.6.4. Postpartum Anterior Lobe Necrosis of the Pituitary Gland (Sheehan's Syndrome)

3.6.4.1. Pathophysiology

Postpartum necrosis of the anterior lobe of the pituitary gland is a common cause of severe hypopituitarism. In this critical condition, decreased functioning of the pituitary gland is caused by ischemic necrosis secondary to blood loss and hypovolemic shock during and after childbirth. The most common early symptoms are agalactorrhea and/or difficulties with lactation, a slowed heart rate, and low blood pressure.

3.6.4.2. EEG

Despite the high incidence of postpartum necrosis of the anterior lobe of the pituitary gland, there are very few reports of EEG abnormalities in this context and most EEG findings are nonspecific, mainly consisting of diffuse intermittent or continuous theta and delta activity (149). These EEG abnormalities are temporally linked to impaired consciousness, possibly reflecting secondary depression of the adrenocortical gland.

In summary, EEG may be judicially used in the evaluation of patients with postpartum necrosis of the anterior lobe of the pituitary gland.

3.6.5. Hyperthyroidism-Related Encephalopathy

3.6.5.1. Pathophysiology

Hyperthyroidism is a condition in which the thyroid gland produces and secretes excessive amounts of the free, non–protein-bound thyroid hormones triiodothyronine and/or thyroxine. The continuum of neurological symptoms associated with various degrees of hyperthyroidism ranges from subtle impairment of cognitive function, insomnia, emotional liability and anxiety, to severe and potentially life-threatening manifestations, such as severe encephalopathy, seizures, and coma (142).

3.6.5.2. EEG
Observations of a higher alpha rhythm frequency in hyperthyroidism were first reported in the 1930s (150). These observations were followed by reports of enhanced fast EEG activity and an augmented rolandic mu rhythm (20). Most frequently, EEG abnormalities in temporal relation to the administration of thyroid hormones in healthy females emerge predominantly in the premenopausal period and typically show high-voltage and prolonged EEG responses to photic stimulation (151). Hyperthyroidism lowers the seizure threshold in patients with preexisting epilepsy (151). Although several reports describe paroxysmal bursts, complex partial seizures, focal motor seizures, and generalized seizures (152), a study of 3,382 patients with hyperthyroidism revealed that seizures in hyperthyroidism are rare and occur in only 0.2% (153). Furthermore, there is no clear correlation between the degree of EEG abnormality and serum thyroid hormone levels (154). As seizures in patients with thyroid dysfunction typically respond poorly to antiseizure drugs and may result in SE (155), treatment of the underlying endocrine disturbance is essential (152). In a study of 20 patients with hyperthyroidism followed with repeated EEG measurements before and during treatment, one week of therapy with propranolol produced a slight EEG synchronizing effect, and serum triiodo-L-thyronine values were noted to be decreased (154). After four weeks, all patients were euthyroid, but EEG abnormalities persisted in 12 patients to a lesser degree.

In conclusion, in patients with hyperthyroidism and epileptic complications, EEG may be used for diagnosing seizures and monitoring treatment, but there is no clear correlation between EEG abnormality and serum thyroid levels.

3.6.6. HYPOTHYROIDISM-RELATED ENCEPHALOPATHY
3.6.6.1. PATHOPHYSIOLOGY
Hypothyroidism is a common endocrine disorder in which the thyroid gland does not produce enough thyroid hormone. Patients with hypothyroidism may present with a variety of clinical conditionals such as tiredness, weight gain, and myxedema coma (86).

3.6.6.2. EEG
The EEG in adults may be entirely normal, but in severe cases, a slow posterior basic rhythm may emerge (156), as well as low-voltage activity predominantly in the theta and delta frequency range in pronounced cases and myxedema coma (157) with poor or absent EEG background reactivity to noxious stimuli (158). In patients with myxedema coma, epileptic seizures may precede coma (159). In elderly patients with myxedema coma, TWs (160) and generalized periodic sharp waves resembling Creutzfeldt–Jakob disease have been described (157,161). Less frequently, intermittent generalized rhythmic delta activity with frontal predominance (formerly named FIRDA) can be found in patients with hypothyroidism-related encephalopathy (162).

Overall, there are several EEG abnormalities in patients with different stages of hypothyroidism. As in myxedema coma, EEG findings may resemble other diseases, such as Creutzfeldt–Jakob disease, EEG-based diagnosis alone can be misleading. Therefore, comprehensive laboratory analyses including serum thyroid hormone levels should be performed in the context of these EEG findings.

3.6.7. OTHER ENDOCRINE DISTURBANCES–RELATED ENCEPHALOPATHIES
It is likely that EEG changes may be seen in other less frequent endocrine disorders. However, as very few case reports exist with no formal studies, these disorders are not discussed in this section.

4. EEG IN INTOXICATION-RELATED ENCEPHALOPATHIES

4.1. Drug-Related Encephalopathies

With the exception of clear EEG correlations seen with various depths of anesthesia, data regarding the diagnostic yield and prognostic value of particular EEG patterns in patients with drug-related encephalopathies are limited to case series and small studies. Although most EEG patterns that emerge during drug intoxication are nonspecific and do not allow any conclusions to be made regarding the offending drugs, and the evidence for EEG changes in relation to serum drug levels is lacking, TWs and paroxysmal abnormalities in patients treated with lithium or neuroleptics are likely the expression of drug intoxication, especially if other plausible causes for these EEG changes have been excluded.

The EEG changes associated with administration of benzodiazepine and its antidote are well described and can help clinicians to diagnose overdose and monitor treatment in these patients. In addition, current data indicate that EEG is an important tool in the diagnosis of epileptic seizures or SE in patients with intoxication or withdrawal of baclofen and use of certain antibiotic drugs.

4.1.1. ANESTHETICS-RELATED ENCEPHALOPATHY
4.1.1.1. PATHOPHYSIOLOGY
Although the cellular mechanisms of many anesthetic drugs are not fully understood and the role of intracellular signal procedures by second messengers remains uncertain, experimental and clinical research indicates that most anesthetics act directly on proteins rather than on lipids and selectively bind to only a small number of targets in the CNS (163). However, the question of how diverse anesthetic agents alter and disrupt consciousness has persisted over the last few centuries. Anesthetics interact with neuronal ion channels, neurotransmitter receptors, and protein sites. In general, different anesthetic substances induce specific effects that depend on specific target binding sites. Most substances induce amnesia, euphoria, analgesia, excitation, and hyperreflexia in the early phase. With increasing depth of anesthesia, motor and autonomous responses to noxious stimuli diminish.

4.1.1.2. EEG
Early studies by Stockard and Bickford revealed progressive slowing of the basic EEG background frequency with progressive depth of anesthesia, and deepening levels of

encephalopathy and coma (24). Figure 17.1 illustrates EEG changes in encephalopathic patients that resemble the EEG patterns found in different levels of sedation (164). The initial phase in anesthesia is dominated by a fast activity over the frontal lobes. This activity gradually generalizes until the alpha rhythm diminishes in frequency and amplitude (165). When the phase of excitation is reached, epileptiform activities emerge with different anesthetic drugs (166). With deepening anesthesia, the frequency of the basic EEG rhythm decreases and the amplitudes increase and sometimes transform into a burst-suppression pattern. In deepest anesthesia, EEG can become isoelectric (26).

4.1.2. Lithium-Related Encephalopathy
4.1.2.1. Pathophysiology
Lithium is used as a mood-stabilizing drug, primarily in the treatment of bipolar disorder, where it has a role in the treatment of depression and particularly of mania. In the CNS, lithium interacts with a number of neurotransmitters and receptors, decreasing norepinephrine release and increasing serotonin synthesis (167). The exact neurobiochemical mechanisms of lithium in mania are not fully understood.

Acute lithium intoxication can be life-threatening, although the initial symptoms are rather mild and nonspecific, such as fatigue, muscle weakness, or tremor. At serum concentrations >2 mEq/L, systemic toxic effects become more severe and include renal insufficiency, high fever, oculomotor disturbances (168), peripheral neuropathies (169), and encephalopathy encompassing a large variety of neurological symptoms related to cortical and subcortical dysfunction (170). Aside from intermittent brain dysfunction that may be accompanied by TWs or waxing and waning epileptic activity constituting NCSE, irreversible lithium-related brain dysfunction has been described.

4.1.2.2. EEG
Changes in patients treated with lithium are frequent and variable, including diffuse slowing, widening of the frequency spectrum, potentiation and disorganization of background rhythm, increased sensitivity to hyperventilation, and paroxysmal bilaterally synchronous delta activity (171). In a study of 12 patients receiving lithium treatment for >4 months, the effects of lithium on the EEG were analyzed by power spectral analysis controlled for vigilance (172). There was an increase in relative power in both delta and theta bands that was related to the lithium serum level, a decrease in relative alpha power especially in the occipital leads, and a reduction of the dominant alpha frequency. The changes in relative power were more pronounced in the right hemisphere, which is in contrast to the hypothesis of a site-specific localization of lithium effects only in left anterior regions as suggested in an earlier study quantified by spectrum analyses in healthy volunteers treated with lithium (173). In general, these EEG abnormalities are paralleled by increasing serum lithium levels and are reversible with lithium withdrawal.

In contrast to the individual variability of EEG findings under standard lithium therapy, pathologic EEG findings are the rule in the case of intoxication, showing diffuse slowing and paroxysmal abnormalities including spikes and TWs (174). Lithium intoxication causing neurotoxic symptoms can be associated with marked EEG changes despite moderate or even "therapeutic" serum lithium levels (175). Mainly in elderly patients, encephalopathy is accompanied by asynchronous, multifocal TWs (Fig. 17.7), often with a prominent negative phase 1 component. In some cases the EEG patterns have been misleadingly called lithium-induced Creutzfeldt–Jakob syndrome (174), as the clinical and EEG constellation can resemble patterns of acute and rapidly progressive dementia. Some cases of NCSE have been described (176), but the epileptic or encephalopathic nature of these states is sometimes a matter of debate (177).

In conclusion, EEG is an important tool in patients with altered mental status receiving lithium therapy to uncover signs of encephalopathy or seizures. In this context, several reports show a closer relationship between neurotoxic symptoms with EEG abnormalities than with specific serum levels of lithium.

4.1.3. Antipsychotics-Related Encephalopathy
4.1.3.1. Pathophysiology
Aside from conventional older antipsychotic drugs, there is a growing list of newer antipsychotic drugs that are used in clinical practice (including clozapine, amisulpride, olanzapine, quetiapine, risperidone, sertindole, ziprasidone, zotepine, aripiprazole). The newer drugs have been less extensively studied with quantitative EEG methods than have the classic antipsychotic drugs.

Clozapine is classified as an atypical antipsychotic drug because it binds to serotonin as well as dopamine and alpha-adrenergic receptors. A systematic meta-analysis of 31 studies revealed that clozapine was the only drug that exhibited fewer extrapyramidal symptoms and a higher antipsychotic effect as compared to the older conventional drugs (178).

4.1.3.2. EEG
Investigations of the relationship between clozapine dose, clozapine serum levels and EEG changes, revealed a strong relationship between increasing clozapine dose and serum levels and the occurrence of clozapine-induced EEG abnormalities (179). In patients treated with clozapine, EEG power spectra showed an increase in delta, theta, and >21-Hz beta activities. The EEG became abnormal in more than half of the patients as a function of clozapine serum levels (180). Increased slowing in the theta and delta frequency range was prominent over the frontal, central, and parietal lobes (181). Another study of quantitative EEG in schizophrenic patients revealed that chronic treatment with clozapine resulted in EEG slowing as shown by decreases in relative alpha power, mean beta/total spectrum frequency, and widespread increases in absolute total and delta/theta power (182). In a prospective study of EEG findings and occurrence of seizures in patients with refractory schizophrenia treated with clozapine (300 mg/day), EEG abnormalities were seen in 64% and included generalized slowing and epileptic activity (183). Seizure with clozapine emerge in up to 4% of patients (184), especially with doses of >600 mg/day (185) and serum levels of >1,300 ug/L (186,187),

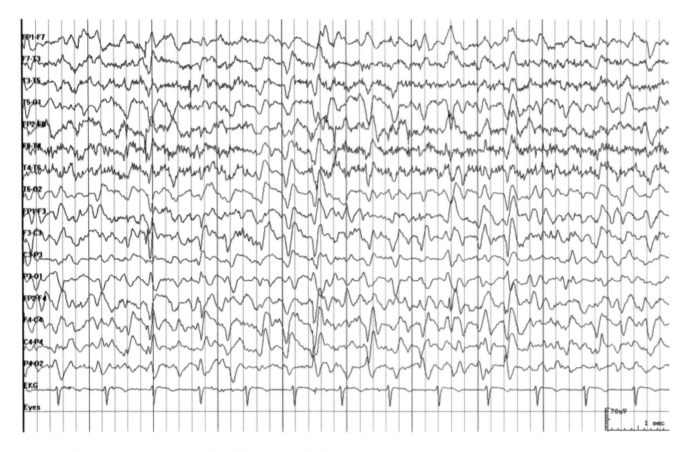

Figure 17.7. Atypical, often asynchronous, multifocal TWs in a patient with lithium intoxication.

and seems to be greater than with other typical and atypical antipsychotic drugs. Another study of quantitative EEG of schizophrenic patients treated with clozapine revealed an augmentation of delta, theta, and frontal EEG alpha power (188).

In conclusion, there is a strong relationship between clozapine dose and level and the occurrence of clozapine-induced EEG abnormalities and seizures. EEG changes with other new antipsychotic drugs are less well investigated. The seizure risk extracted from approval reports is 0.9% for olanzapine, 0.8% for quetiapine, and 0.4% for ziprasidone and aripiprazole (185).

4.1.4. NEUROLEPTIC MALIGNANT SYNDROME
4.1.4.1. PATHOPHYSIOLOGY
Neuroleptic malignant syndrome (NMS) is a life-threatening neurological disorder that is most often, but not exclusively, caused by an adverse reaction to antipsychotic or neuroleptic drugs (189). Typical symptoms include autonomic dysregulation, muscle rigidity, tremor, fever, altered level of consciousness, and leukocytosis (190). These symptoms are usually rapidly progressive and accompanied by elevated levels of plasma creatine phosphokinase (189). The incidence of NMS has decreased since it was first described in the 1960s due to changes in prescribing habits. The mechanism is thought to depend on decreased levels of dopamine activity due to dopamine receptor blockade and genetically reduced function of the dopamine receptor D2 (191). However, these mechanisms do not fully explain the clinical picture and the occurrence of NMS with atypical antipsychotic drugs that do not mainly

target D2 receptors, leading to the hypothesis of sympatho-adrenal hyperactivity (192). The breakdown of normal muscle activity and hyperthermia is likely to be caused by an increased release of calcium from the sarcoplasmic reticulum with antipsychotic usage. Other studies suggest that withdrawal of drugs supplying dopamine can lead to a symptom complex resembling NMS (189).

4.1.4.2. EEG
Reports on the EEG findings in patients with NMS are scarce and formal studies are lacking. In some cases of NMS with myoclonus, the EEG revealed TWs (193), and three other reports describe intermittent periodic bilateral spike-wave discharges with frontal dominance consistent with NCSE (194).

Although the literature of EEG abnormalities in NMS is very limited, reports of NCSE in this context indicate that EEG is important in the overall management of these patients.

4.1.5. ANTIDEPRESSANTS-RELATED ENCEPHALOPATHY
4.1.5.1. PATHOPHYSIOLOGY
Since the first-generation tricyclic antidepressants (e.g., imipramine, amitriptyline, doxepin, desipramine, nortriptyline, and protriptyline), new classes of antidepressant drugs have been introduced. New antidepressants can be classified according to their mode of action into selective serotonin reuptake inhibitors (e.g., fluoxetine, fluvoxamine, paroxetine, citalopram, and sertraline), dual serotoninergics (reuptake inhibitors plus receptor antagonism; e.g., nefazodone),

selective serotonin and noradrenaline reuptake inhibitors (e.g., venlafaxine), noradrenergic and specific serotonergic drugs (e.g., mirtazapine), selective noradrenaline reuptake inhibitors (e.g., reboxetine), and reversible specific monoamine oxidase inhibitors (e.g., moclobemide). Some antidepressants, especially amitriptyline, a tricyclic antidepressant, are also effective in the treatment of neuropathic pain (195). While epileptic seizures may be triggered with tricyclic antidepressants, especially in patients with known epilepsy, there is no high-quality evidence to inform the choice of antidepressant drug or class of drug in treating depression in people with epilepsy, as there are insufficient comparative data on antidepressant classes and their safety in relation to seizures, according to a recent systematic review (196).

4.1.5.2. EEG

The administration of therapeutic doses of tricyclic antidepressants can increase fast and slow activities. Tricyclic antidepressants may lead to inconsistent frequencies and amplitudes of the basic EEG rhythm along with the emergence of paroxysmal slow waves, spikes, and polyspikes (197). While in patients with known epilepsy, therapeutic doses may increase the seizure frequency, seizures in patients without a history of epilepsy are reported only in association with high doses (198). Several cases of absence SE (94,199) have been thought to be due to treatment with tricyclic agents.

Seizures have also been reported with different propensities among the newer antidepressants. With maprotiline and bupropion, the seizure risk is high (1.5%); with trazodone, nefazodone, mirtazapine, and the selective serotonin reuptake inhibitors, the seizure risk seems to be low (185,200,201). In a recent case-control study, seizure duration was significantly longer in patients taking serotonin reuptake inhibitors versus epilepsy patients not taking serotonin reuptake inhibitors (202).

Overall, seizures and SE may be triggered by antidepressants. However, reports describing the exact EEG changes in relation to serum drug levels are lacking and the EEG signs provided in few reports are nonspecific and have not been linked to clinical phenomenology.

4.1.6. SEROTONIN SYNDROME
4.1.6.1. PATHOPHYSIOLOGY

Serotonin syndrome is a life-threatening adverse drug reaction associated with drug–drug interactions (203). Drugs with an increased risk for inducing the serotonin syndrome are selective serotonin reuptake inhibitors, other antidepressant drugs, and monoamine oxidase inhibitors. Excessive levels of serotonin produce a spectrum of clinical manifestations ranging from barely perceptible to lethal. Major symptoms include altered mental status, autonomic hyperactivity, and neuromuscular abnormalities.

4.1.6.2. EEG

Abnormalities with diffuse slowing of the basic EEG rhythm (204,205), spikes, and TWs (206,207) are described in case reports. With discontinuation of the serotonin syndrome-inducing medication, clinical symptoms are reversible and

paralleled by EEG normalization (205). These pathologic patterns are nonspecific and formal studies regarding the diagnostic and prognostic yield of EEG in this context are lacking.

Although the EEG patterns are nonspecific, case reports indicate that EEG monitoring can add important information that may direct treatment in patients with serotonin syndrome.

4.1.7. ANXIOLYTIC DRUG–RELATED ENCEPHALOPATHY
4.1.7.1. PATHOPHYSIOLOGY

As EEG studies in anxiolytic drugs others than benzodiazepines are scarce, this section will focus on benzodiazepine-associated EEG changes. Benzodiazepines are the most frequently used anxiolytic drugs. As a class of psychoactive drugs, they enhance the effect of the neurotransmitter gamma-aminobutyric acid (GABA) at the $GABA_A$ receptor, resulting in sedative, hypnotic, anxiolytic, antiseizure, and muscle relaxant properties (208). At higher doses, they may also cause anterograde amnesia and dissociation. The intracerebral distribution and changing compositions of subunits of the $GABA_A$ receptors contribute to differences in the efficacy of the numerous different benzodiazepines (209). In addition, pharmacokinetic characteristics such as dynamic of absorption, half-life, binding to fat deposits, and activities of metabolites determine the type of action of these substances. All benzodiazepines share the same side effects, such as cognitive impairment, anterograde amnesia, low-dose dependency, rebound anxiety, rebound insomnia, and paradoxical effects including behavioral disinhibition and agitation (210). Discontinuation of long-term treatment with benzodiazepines may cause withdrawal syndromes including seizures (210).

In intoxication, the symptoms are nonspecific, resembling the clinical signs of overdose with other drugs with CNS depressant effects. The prognosis is usually good, except in patients with decreased respiratory function.

4.1.7.2. EEG

A study in the 1970s revealed that benzodiazepines reduce generalized spikes but have no effect on interictal focal spikes (211) except for discharges in rolandic epilepsy (212). This study was followed by observations with quantitative EEG spectral analysis revealing that the administration of benzodiazepine derivatives led to an increase of beta activity that persist for up to two weeks (213). Similar to the effects of barbiturates, benzodiazepine-related increase in cortical fast activities is reduced in the areas of brain lesions (213). Furthermore, the increase of beta activity is paralleled by a generalized decrease of amplitude and alpha activity and an increase of the basic EEG rhythm in the theta frequency range. The effect of benzodiazepines on the EEG sleep architecture has been studied in 46 patients (15 patients with insomnia and benzodiazepine intake, 15 patients with insomnia without benzodiazepines, and 16 patients without sleep disorders) (214). Power spectral analyses revealed no significant differences between drug-free insomnia sufferers and good sleepers. However, benzodiazepine users exhibited significantly less delta and theta activity during sleep than did good sleepers. When compared to drug-free insomnia sufferers, benzodiazepine users had less delta and theta activity within sleep cycle

2. Regarding high-frequency bands, benzodiazepine users had more beta activity within cycle 3 than did good sleepers and more than both drug-free insomnia sufferers and good sleepers within cycle 4.

Because of these observations and the results from a large study comparing different treatment regimens in patients with generalized convulsive SE showing that lorazepam was superior to other antiseizure drugs, benzodiazepines are recommended as first-line antiseizure treatment in patients with SE (215,216). Besides their antiepileptic effects, abrupt withdrawal of benzodiazepines has been considered an etiologic factor of *de novo* absence SE of late onset (94) and first-time seizures (217).

Intoxication with benzodiazepines is linked to prominent fast and unreactive EEG activity. With larger doses, coma patterns can be recorded with a rapid response to flumazenil injection (218).

In conclusion, the EEG changes upon benzodiazepine administration and during the administration of the antidote are well described and help clinicians to diagnose exposure and to monitor treatment in intoxicated patients.

4.1.8. BACLOFEN-RELATED ENCEPHALOPATHY

4.1.8.1. PATHOPHYSIOLOGY

Baclofen, also known as chlorophenibut, is a derivative of GABA. Hence, it is a selective $GABA_B$ receptor agonist used to treat spasticity in many pathologic conditions (219). Its antispastic effect results from actions at spinal and supraspinal sites. Oral and intrathecal administration of baclofen (220) and baclofen withdrawal (221,222) have been associated with epileptic seizures or SE.

4.1.8.2. EEG

After intrathecal baclofen overdose, the EEG can show coma patterns with generalized periodic discharges (223). In patients with abrupt baclofen withdrawal, the EEG may reveal SE with diffuse theta and delta activity interrupted by waxing and waning periodic lateralized discharges with occasional rhythmic delta activity over the frontal lobes. Prolonged episodes of dystonia and dyskinesia resembling SE following intrathecal baclofen withdrawal are described where the EEG shows the nonepileptic nature of the symptoms (224). In other cases, the EEG shows sharply contoured, high-voltage and asymmetric biphasic and triphasic waves with poorly sustained background activity (Fig. 17.8). The triphasic morphology can have somewhat atypically prominent and high-voltage negative phase 1 components.

In summary, current data indicate that EEG is an important tool in the diagnosis of epileptic seizures or SE in patients with intoxication or withdrawal of baclofen. It can also help to differentiate between epileptic and nonepileptic symptoms in these settings.

4.1.9. ANTIBIOTICS-RELATED ENCEPHALOPATHY (ESPECIALLY CEPHALOSPIRINS)

4.1.9.1. PATHOPHYSIOLOGY

Antibiotic drugs, especially unsubstituted penicillins, fourth-generation cephalosporins, imipenem, and ciprofloxacin, in combination with particular clinical conditions may increase patients' risk for epileptic seizures or SE. In contrast to a large number of animal models, evidence from human studies is limited (225).

In an early small prospective study analyzing the effectiveness of high-dose penicillin G (20–80 mega units per day) therapy in patients with infections caused by gram-negative bacteria, epileptic seizures emerged in patients with renal insufficiency or preexisting CNS diseases. In a large series of medical inpatients from various hospitals, seizures occurred in 0.3% of patients receiving penicillin G or oxacillin (226). Similar to case reports and case series on penicillin G or oxacillin-related seizures (227), all patients received high doses of penicillin and had renal insufficiency and no other ictogenic factors could be identified. In addition, cases of piperacillin/tazobactam-induced seizures (228) or SE (229) have been reported.

Cephalosporin use in patients with renal insufficiency has been linked to CNS toxicity with decreased seizure threshold by competitive antagonism at the $GABA_A$ receptor (230). In renal failure, the accumulation of organic acids competes with the exotransportation of cephalosporins from the cerebrospinal fluid to the blood, thus increasing cephalosporin concentrations in the CNS and leading to epileptic seizures or SE (231-233). According to a systematic review, cefazoline is the antibiotic most frequently associated with epileptic seizures among the cephalosporins (225). However, epileptic adverse events have been reported with all four generations of cephalosporins, such as cefotiam, cefixime, ceftriaxone, ceftazidime, and especially cefepime (225).

Early after its clinical introduction, imipenem was noted to have a seizure-inducing propensity, but reports of imipenem-related SE are lacking. Among the carbapenems, however, imipenem seems to be more ictogenic than meropenem (234), with seizures following the administration of imipenem even without additional predisposing or contributing factors (235). The exact origins of the more potent CNS adverse reactions are unknown. A large observational study of patients receiving imipenem revealed epileptic seizures in 3% (236). In another study, 5.3% of patients treated with imipenem had seizures (237). Remarkably, 58 patients had conditions possibly causing breakdown of the blood–brain barrier and consecutive increase of intracerebral imipenem levels. Recognition of several predisposing factors, including renal failure, metabolic derangements, anoxia, and phenytoin discontinuation, has substantially reduced seizure risk with carbapenems (237).

Ciprofloxacin, a widely prescribed fluoroquinolone antibiotic, has been associated with delirium, hallucinations, and epileptic seizures (238). Evidence for epileptic adverse events is limited to case reports describing patients with additional predisposing factors, such as renal insufficiency, brain lesions, and co-administered theophylline (238–240).

4.1.9.2. EEG

In patients with penicillin-related encephalopathy, the EEG reveals poorly formed alpha activity intermixed with intermediate slow activity and diffuse slow waves without presence of focal brain lesions (241,242). In patients with SE, the EEG

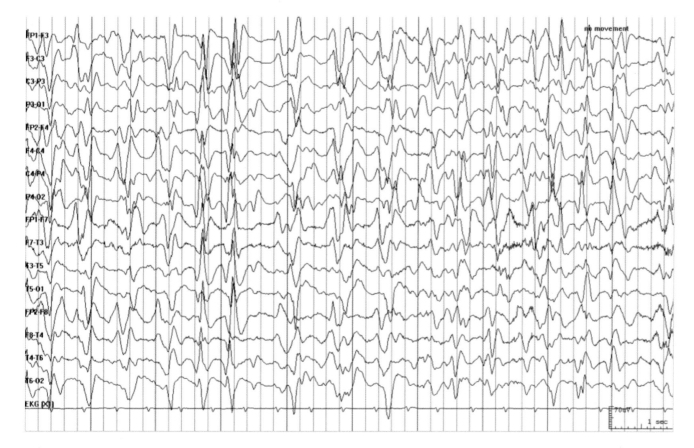

Figure 17.8. Sharply contoured, high-voltage biphasic and triphasic waves seen asymmetrically, bilaterally, with poorly sustained background activity in a patient with baclofen intoxication. The triphasic morphology has somewhat atypically prominent and high-voltage negative phase 1 components.

typically reveals waxing and waning, diffuse dysrhythmia and paroxysmal sharp and spike-wave activity (243).

Almost 60 adverse events with cefepime-associated NCSE have been reported to the U.S. Food and Drug Administration, and SE was suspected to play a major role in at least one of the deaths (244). Beyond epileptic seizures related to cefepime neurotoxicity, encephalopathic EEG changes have been reported, such as lateralized periodic discharges and TWs (245,246). EEG descriptions of patients with carbapenems and fluoroquinolones are scarce.

In conclusion, EEG provides important information in encephalopathic patients receiving antibiotic treatment, especially as seizures and SE are often nonconvulsive. However, EEG patterns are nonspecific and do not allow a straightforward diagnosis of antibiotics related encephalopathy.

4.1.10. Immunosuppressants-Related Encephalopathy (Especially Cyclosporine)
4.1.10.1. Pathophysiology

Cyclosporine, a lipophilic cyclic undecapeptide, is an immunosuppressant drug widely used in organ transplantation to prevent rejection and in the treatment of rheumatic and other autoimmune diseases. Neurotoxicity occurs in 40% to 60% of patients receiving cyclosporine (246,247); these patients mainly present with encephalopathies (frequently restricted to brain regions belonging to the posterior circulation system (248)), seizures, and stroke-like symptoms. The exact pathophysiological mechanisms are unknown; but

hypocholesterolemia has been suggested to explain the neurotoxicity of cyclosporine (249).

4.1.10.2. EEG

In patients with cyclosporine-induced brain dysfunction, the EEG reveals diffuse and focal slowing and epileptiform discharges (250). In patients with posterior reversible encephalopathy syndrome (PRES), the EEG in the acute phase shows continuous focal rhythmic activity mainly in the occipital lobes. These EEG abnormalities normalize after the clinical manifestations had disappeared (251).

Overall, EEG is useful in patients with cephalosporin-induced brain dysfunction, especially for the diagnosis and follow-up of PRES and seizures.

4.1.11. Levodopa-Related Encephalopathy
4.1.11.1. Pathophysiology

Levodopa is the main drug used to treat symptoms of Parkinson disease. Reports on EEG changes in this context are sparse.

4.1.11.2. EEG

Assuming that a change in EEG power spectrum after levodopa intake may be related to dopaminergic mechanisms, the findings of a study of patients with Parkinson's disease are consistent with the hypothesis that dopaminergic defective networks are implicated in cortical oscillatory abnormalities at rest in non-demented Parkinson's disease patients (252). The EEGs of patients receiving levodopa showed a significant increase in alpha and beta rhythms on centro-parietal scalp derivations. In a case series of patients with confusional states following an increase in the dose of levodopa, the EEG revealed periodic generalized TWs (253).

In conclusion, EEG may reveal increases of alpha and beta rhythms over the centro-parietal brain regions. Formal studies of the diagnostic and prognostic yield of EEG in levodopa-related encephalopathy are lacking.

4.1.12. Opioids-Related Encephalopathy
4.1.12.1. Pathophysiology
Opioids resemble morphine in terms of their pharmacological effects by binding to opioid receptors, which are mainly located in the peripheral and central nervous system and the gastrointestinal tract. Besides the analgesic effects, opioids may lead to adverse reactions such as altered consciousness, respiratory depression, constipation, and euphoria. Less frequent neurological effects include confusion, hallucinations, delirium, orthostatic dysregulation, headache, myoclonus, and epileptic seizures.

4.1.12.2. EEG
Morphine and other opiates have only discrete EEG effects, with slowing of the basic EEG alpha rhythm, and sometimes emergence of paroxysmal changes. In a study of the relationship between epileptiform activity and doses of opioids in 20 patients undergoing coronary artery revascularization, 10 subjects were given fentanyl and 10 sufentanil, at 100 micrograms/kg and 10 micrograms/kg, respectively, in four divided doses, three minutes apart (254). Within three minutes of the first opioid dose, 19 of 20 patients developed epileptiform activity, characterized by generalized single and multiphasic, low- to moderate-voltage spike discharges, similar in appearance to benign epileptiform transients of sleep (BETS). Despite continuously increasing serum concentrations of opioid, the number of spike discharges initially increased during the first and second dose intervals and then declined during the third and fourth dose intervals. Immediate cessation of this activity after administration of benzodiazepines reflects an epileptogenic mechanism of the opioid-induced activity. In another study of 13 opioid-dependent patients, local and remote cortical functional connectivity was significantly enhanced for both alpha- and beta-frequency oscillations during opioid withdrawal. A statistical relationship between functional connectivity and the severity of opioid withdrawal has been found (255). Few studies have been performed on the effects of opioids on EEG sleep architecture. In a study using EEG bisector analysis, tape recordings of sleep were analyzed for two beta, three alpha, three theta, and two delta EEG patterns, as well as for detections of sleep spindles, K-complexes, eye movements, body movements, average electromyogram, and calculation of seven sleep/waking stages (256). All three opioids produce a dose-related arousal: they increase electromyelographic and EEG measures of muscle activity, as well as body movements and EEG alpha, while decreasing EEG theta and spindling. These opioids also increase measures of waking state and decrease measures of spindle sleep and REM sleep. Tramadol is the opioid most frequently reported to be associated with epileptic

seizures, which are mostly generalized tonic-clonic and recurrent in cases of intoxication (257).

In conclusion, EEG reveals changes of brain activity during sleep or awake rest. There are insufficient data regarding the correlation of EEG changes and specific opioids or serum concentrations for the recommendation of EEG for diagnosis or monitoring of patients receiving these drugs.

4.2. Psychotogenic (Illicit) Drugs–Related Encephalopathies

Although there is evidence for the neurophysiological effects of lysergic acid diethylamide (LSD), current data on EEG abnormalities in individuals with LSD-related encephalopathy are scarce and do not allow any conclusions to be made regarding the value of EEG for diagnosis and prognosis in this context. In patients with cannabis consumption, EEG findings are nonspecific and do not allow diagnosis of cannabis exposure. EEG changes in alcohol exposure are also nonspecific; however, subacute alcohol-related encephalopathy may lead to epileptic seizures, transient focal cortical deficits, and lateralized periodic discharges in the EEG. Although evidence for a significant association is lacking and the links between alcohol intoxication and symptomatic epileptic seizures are questioned, new-onset seizures and activation of lateralized periodic discharges as well as SE without any other cause are described. In patients with cocaine-related encephalopathy, the use of EEG is limited to diagnosis and treatment monitoring in patients with SE.

4.2.1. LSD-Related Encephalopathy
4.2.1.1. Pathophysiology
LSD is one of the strongest hallucinogenic drugs. It disrupts neuronal interactions mediated by the neurotransmitter serotonin throughout the brain and spinal cord (258).

4.2.1.2. EEG
There are very few EEG studies in patients consuming LSD. In the psychotic state LSD causes a decrease of amplitudes and a depression of slow waves as well as acceleration of the dominant frequencies during the drug-induced psychotic state (259).

4.2.2. Marijuana (Cannabis)-Related Encephalopathy
4.2.2.1. Pathophysiology
In general, cannabis exerts its effects on the CNS through the CB1 cannabinoid receptor (260), leading to a disruption of psychomotor behavior, memory function, appetite induction, and nociceptive and emetic actions. Neuropsychological alteration can last several years following frequent cannabis consumption (261). The risk of cannabis-related psychosis after cannabis intake has stopped is increased (262). Despite these risks, cannabis is increasingly used in the treatment of neuropathic pain and spasticity.

4.2.2.2. EEG
In patients smoking cannabis, EEG is usually normal. The spectral analyses of chronic cannabis users, however, reveal

reduced power in the alpha and beta bands over the occipital lobes (263), and EEG changes may continue for a month after cannabis intake has been stopped.

Overall, EEG changes in patients with cannabis consumption are nonspecific and do not allow the diagnosis of cannabis exposure. Persistent EEG changes after cannabis exposure mirror the prolonged biochemical effects of this drug.

4.2.3. ALCOHOL-RELATED ENCEPHALOPATHY
4.2.3.1. PATHOPHYSIOLOGY

Despite the high incidence of alcohol intoxication, reports describing neuroclinical manifestations in patients with alcohol ingestion are scarce, including for epileptic events. In contrast to EEG studies in patients with alcohol intoxication, several studies on the neurophysiological consequences of alcohol withdrawal have investigated clinical and electrophysiological correlates of alcohol withdrawal and have identified hallucinosis, delirium tremens, and epileptic seizures as signs of withdrawal following alcohol dependence and habituation. In patients with alcohol withdrawal, epileptic seizures and spikes reflect reduced neurotransmission in the inhibitory GABA and NMDA pathways (264). The persistence of these EEG abnormalities in alcoholics with seizures suggests epilepsy or symptomatic seizures unrelated to alcohol (265). A multicenter case-control study of 293 patients with first seizures symptomatic of head trauma, stroke, or brain tumor, matched to 444 hospital controls, did not reveal evidence of an association between alcohol use or alcoholism, and a first symptomatic epileptic seizure (266). However, in a case series of patients with subacute encephalopathy with seizures in alcoholics (SESA), the analyses of the clinical, EEG, and neuroimaging data of these cases led to the conclusion that SESA syndrome may represent a subtype of partial or localization-related NCSE (267).

Wernicke's encephalopathy, Korsakoff syndrome (see also Section 3.5.1), retrobulbar neuritis, polyneuropathy, and cerebral pellagra are additional syndromes related to alcohol-induced malnutrition, mainly with vitamin B1 deficiency.

4.2.3.2. EEG

In studies of EEG changes in alcohol ingestion with subjects being examined during rising serum alcohol levels, and in states without relevant serum alcohol levels, a significant increase in EEG amplitude occurred in the alpha, theta, and beta frequency range in the frontal EEG regions, and an increase in alpha frequency ranges in the central and posterior regions was measured as compared to states without relevant serum alcohol levels (268). In a study of spectral EEG analysis of patients with alcohol consumption and placebo, similar results were found in the anterior and posterior brain regions (269). Subacute alcohol-related encephalopathy may lead to epileptic seizures, transient focal cortical deficits, and lateralized periodic discharges in the EEG. Although evidence for a significant association is lacking and the link between alcohol intoxication and symptomatic epileptic seizures is questioned (266), some reports describe new-onset seizures and activation of lateralized periodic discharges (270) as well as SE (271)

associated with alcohol intoxication and subacute alcohol-induced encephalopathy.

In the first 48 hours of alcohol withdrawal, EEG activity is desynchronized, amplitudes of the basic EEG rhythm are low, and generalized spikes may emerge (272).

In patients with Wernicke's encephalopathy the EEG can show a large variety of abnormalities (see Section 3.5.1).

Overall, EEG is important in the examination of patients with alcohol intoxication, alcohol withdrawal, or subacute alcohol-induced encephalopathy.

4.2.4. COCAINE-RELATED ENCEPHALOPATHY
4.2.4.1. PATHOPHYSIOLOGY

Cocaine is a tropane alkaloid drug that binds strongly to the dopamine reuptake transporter and blocks such reuptake after normal neuronal activity, increasing dopamine concentrations at the synapses and producing the characteristic "cocaine high" (273). As with most illicit drugs, the exact mechanisms of action are not fully understood. Several studies revealed that cocaine acts as a serotonin–norepinephrine–dopamine reuptake inhibitor (i.e., triple reuptake inhibitor). Long-term neuronal synaptic plasticity, especially in the cerebral mesolimbic structures involved in the reward system, seems to play a major role in the addictive potential of cocaine (274). A meta-analysis of several international studies revealed that variants of the dopamine receptor D2 gene have been associated with cocaine addiction (275).

Besides EEG changes during encephalopathy and epileptic events, cocaine use is associated with high mortality and causes many severe neurocritical illnesses, including acute ischemic stroke (276), orbital ischemia (277), oculomotor nerve palsies (278), ocular surface damage through corneal sensitivity impairment (279), subarachnoid and intracerebral hemorrhages (280,281), intracerebral vasculitis of the small vessels (282), severe dyskinesia (283,284), and vascular syndromes of the spine and medulla (276).

4.2.4.2. EEG

In an EEG study of 50 subjects, cocaine led to an increase in beta power that correlated with the area under the cocaine plasma-versus-time curve (285). This study was followed by a study of patients with several years of cocaine use that revealed a reduced absolute EEG theta and beta power in the posterior brain regions (286). These EEG changes were also found in patients after several weeks of cocaine abstinence, indicating that chronic cocaine use is associated with EEG changes that may reflect persisting brain electrophysiological abnormalities during cocaine abstinence (287). In a study of patients with cocaine-associated seizures, 98% of the patients experienced a single tonic-clonic seizure and only one patient developed SE (288). Complex partial SE has also been rarely reported (289).

In conclusion, EEG studies are important for increasing our neurophysiological understanding of the cerebral effects of cocaine. EEG may also play an important role in clinical practice in the diagnosis and treatment monitoring in patients with SE.

4.3. Toxins-Related Encephalopathies

EEG changes in other toxic encephalopathies, including intoxication with lead, mercury, aluminum, thallium, and organophosphates, are nonspecific, with slowing of the basic EEG rhythm; data regarding the diagnostic yield and prognostic value are lacking. After carbon monoxide intoxication, EEG changes depend on the severity of intoxication, and recovery to normal EEG patterns may occur in mild cases or after immediate treatment with hyperbaric oxygen. In patients with manganese intoxication, the basic EEG rhythm may show fast activities and generalized paroxysmal discharges. In acute encephalopathy with severe intoxication with ethylene glycol, the EEG may reveal coma patterns. Intoxication with organophosphates can be linked to nonspecific slowing of the basic EEG rhythm and paroxysmal discharges. However, unlike other acute intoxications, fast rhythmic activities can be recorded in a first stage of deep coma.

4.3.1. CARBON MONOXIDE–RELATED ENCEPHALOPATHY

4.3.1.1. PATHOPHYSIOLOGY

Intoxication with carbon monoxide is a frequent and unfortunately still the leading cause of death by poisoning in the United States. The strong affinity of carbon monoxide for hemoglobin impedes the binding and transport of oxygen, which is necessary for myocardial contraction and intracellular mitochondrial cytochrome oxidase function. Subsequently, the decrease in oxygen transported by the blood leads to chest pain, arrhythmias, hypoperfusion, myocardial ischemia, and hypoxic-ischemic brain damage. In mild cases, the symptoms are subtle and nonspecific, in contrast to severe intoxication, which results in a large and irreversible brain injury with a high mortality. In survivors, however, full recovery is rare and hypoxic-ischemic encephalopathy, vegetative states, focal brain dysfunction, and extrapyramidal syndromes may persist. Some cases with a delayed encephalopathy following a symptom-free period are reported (290).

4.3.1.2. EEG

Studies in patients with carbon monoxide intoxication are limited. Changes in brain activity depend on the duration of exposure, unconsciousness, and the phase of clinical recovery. In less severe cases, the EEG may show a moderate generalized slowing with or without intermixed diffuse sharp waves (291). Focal or lateralized periodic discharges are rare. However, diffuse or focal sharp waves and focal epileptic seizures in acute and protracted encephalopathies (292,293) are reported. Improvement of the occipital basic EEG rhythm can be observed in patients treated with hyperbaric oxygen (294). Overall, EEG changes after carbon monoxide intoxication depend on the severity of intoxication, and recovery to normal EEG patterns may occur in mild cases or after immediate and sufficient treatment with hyperbaric oxygen. However, formal studies on the prognostic value of EEG in this context are lacking.

4.3.2. LEAD-RELATED ENCEPHALOPATHY

4.3.2.1. PATHOPHYSIOLOGY

Lead is an element that interferes with numerous biochemical processes, leading to toxic effects in many tissues, including the heart, bones, intestines, kidneys, reproductive organs, and nervous systems. Consequently, symptoms include abdominal pain, confusion, headache, anemia, agitation, diffuse brain dysfunction, epileptic seizures, coma, and finally death. While acute intoxication has become rare in the last decade, the elevated environmental lead burden is thought to play a causal role in hypertension. Lead may also be linked with neuropsychological disorders in children and possibly even chronic renal failure (295).

4.3.2.2. EEG

Studies and reports of EEG changes in lead-poisoned patients are almost exclusively restricted to children. An EEG study of 20 adults exposed to lead showed no abnormalities, although electrophysiological workup revealed decreased motor conduction velocities of the median and the posterior tibial nerves as compared to unexposed workers (296). This study was followed by quantitative EEG analyses of 60 workers who were exposed to lead, revealing that the alpha and beta activities were more abundant in subjects with higher long-term exposure to lead (297).

In conclusion, the EEG in patients exposed to lead shows nonspecific signs of diffuse encephalopathies, and studies of EEG changes in acute lead intoxication are lacking.

4.3.3. MERCURY-RELATED ENCEPHALOPATHY

4.3.3.1. PATHOPHYSIOLOGY

Mercury, the only metallic element that is liquid at standard conditions for temperature and pressure, can cause severe damage to the nervous system. Exposure to high doses of methyl mercury can lead to altered motor function and severe impairment of the visual, auditory, and somatosensory systems (298). Chronic exposure at lower concentrations can mainly affect renal function.

4.3.3.2. EEG

Abnormalities may consist of diffuse slowing of the basic EEG rhythm (299). In studies of workers exposed to mercury vapors, quantitative EEG revealed significantly increased photic driving as compared to healthy controls (300). Whether the intergroup differences in photic driving were mercury-related could not be determined; the enhanced photic driving might reflect cerebral hyperexcitability.

4.3.4. MANGANESE-RELATED ENCEPHALOPATHY

4.3.4.1. PATHOPHYSIOLOGY

Manganese is a metal mainly used for industrial metal alloys. Poisoning with manganese typically leads to Parkinsonism (301). With chronic exposure additional CNS networks are affected, resulting in spasticity, epileptic seizures, and dementia (302).

4.3.4.2. EEG

Neurophysiological studies in patients with manganese intoxication are scarce and mostly describe nonspecific changes of the basic EEG rhythm; increasing fast activities (303) and generalized paroxysmal discharges (304) were the most common EEG abnormalities.

4.3.5. ALUMINUM-RELATED ENCEPHALOPATHY
4.3.5.1. PATHOPHYSIOLOGY
Aluminum is remarkable for its low density and for its ability to resist corrosion. Hence, it is used frequently in medicine, mainly for hemodialysis. Therefore, the toxic effects of aluminum in humans have almost exclusively been recognized in association with hemodialysis treatment of patients with chronic renal failure.

4.3.5.2. EEG
The EEG in the dialysis encephalopathy syndrome shows diffuse slow activities and spikes (305,306), abnormalities that improve together with clinical recovery a few weeks after interruption of aluminum intake (306).

In conclusion, in aluminum-related encephalopathy the EEG reveals nonspecific changes in the basic rhythm and may detect epileptic activity. However, with improvement in dialysis techniques, hemodialysis-related encephalopathy has almost disappeared in recent years.

4.3.6. THALLIUM-RELATED ENCEPHALOPATHY
4.3.6.1. PATHOPHYSIOLOGY
Thallium sulfide's electrical conductivity changes with the influence of infrared light, so it is useful in photoresistors. Thallium has also been widely used as a rat poison. Thallium exposure or ingestion typically occurs with murderous or suicidal intention, as thallium is almost tasteless, colorless, and odorless and is rapidly absorbed through the skin. Part of the reason for thallium's toxic effects is that, when present in aqueous solution, it exhibits some similarities particularly with potassium. Thallium has a strong affinity for sulfur ligands; thus, this substitution disrupts many cellular processes. Symptoms of thallium intoxication are loss of hair, skin color changes (307), liver dysfunction, and damage to the peripheral (308) and central nervous system (309), leading to severe pain in the limbs, confusion, altered levels of consciousness, and epileptic seizures. However, in high doses, thallium poisoning kills before these symptoms can be recognized.

4.3.6.2. EEG
As thallium intoxication is rare and usually kills rapidly, EEG studies in this setting are lacking. However, EEG abnormalities are nonspecific, including diffuse theta activity and epileptic seizures indicating a widespread cortical dysfunction (309). With rapid and successful treatment, the EEG becomes normal, together with clinical neurological improvement (309).

Overall, there is not enough evidence to draw conclusions regarding the diagnostic and prognostic yield of EEG in patients with thallium intoxication.

4.3.7. ETHYLENE GLYCOL–RELATED ENCEPHALOPATHY
4.3.7.1. PATHOPHYSIOLOGY
Ethylene glycol is frequently used as raw material in the manufacture of polyester fibers, in polyethylene terephthalate resins (PET), and in antifreeze. Intoxications may occur if ethylene glycol is added to drugs, if it is used for suicide or poisoning, and if the substance is added to wine. Intoxication causes rapid renal failure with consecutive encephalopathy, peripheral nerve palsies, and death (310–312).

4.3.7.2. EEG
EEG studies in patients with ethylene glycol intoxication are lacking. However, case reports of comatose patients with acute intoxication describe a burst-suppression pattern that may change into or alternate with ongoing isoelectric periods (313). With successful treatment EEG can normalize and full neurofunctional recovery is possible.

Overall, the EEG may reveal coma patterns in severe intoxication. However, as only EEG normalizes after patients have recovered completely, EEG cannot be used for prognosis in this context. Further, there are too few case reports and formal studies to draw conclusions regarding the diagnostic yield of EEG.

4.3.8. ORGANOPHOSPHATE-RELATED ENCEPHALOPATHY
4.3.8.1. PATHOPHYSIOLOGY
Organophosphates are the basis of many nerve agents, insecticides, herbicides, sprays, and shampoos. In the nervous system, organophosphates inhibit cholinesterase activity; that's why they were also used as sarin in terrorist attacks. Symptoms include muscle weakness, respiratory failure, massive salivation and bronchorrhea, epileptic seizures, SE, coma, and death.

4.3.8.2. EEG
In patients intoxicated with organophosphates, EEG changes are described as nonspecific, with a slowing of the basic rhythm and paroxysmal discharges. Unlike most other acute intoxications, in a first stage of deep coma, fast rhythmic activities were recorded (314). Paroxysmal discharges were found to be exceptional, although massive myoclonic jerks and other convulsive manifestations occurred. In a study of 77 industrial workers with documented sarin exposure, EEGs several months after exposure revealed slowing of the basic rhythm in the theta and delta frequency ranges with superimposed beta activity (315). During sleep there was an increase of REM sleep as compared to healthy workers.

Overall, there are no formal studies on cohorts with organophosphate intoxication and very few reports of patients with exposure several months prior to EEG. Abnormal cortical activity on EEG months after exposure indicates that brain dysfunction from organophosphates can be long-lasting.

5. EPILEPTIC ENCEPHALOPATHIES

5.1. Categorization and Pathophysiology

The International League Against Epilepsy uses the term *epileptic encephalopathy* to encompass a group of childhood epileptic disorders in which "the epileptiform abnormalities are believed to contribute to progressive cerebral dysfunction" (316). These include early myoclonic encephalopathy, early infantile epileptic encephalopathy (Ohtahara syndrome), infantile spasm (West syndrome), severe myoclonic epileptic in infancy (Dravet syndrome), migrating partial seizures in infancy, myoclonic status in nonprogressive encephalopathies, Landau–Kleffner syndrome, epilepsy with continuous spike-waves during slow-wave sleep, and Lennox–Gastaut syndrome (LGS). This is a heterogeneous group of disorders that have variable etiologies and a wide spectrum of clinical features, EEG patterns, and clinical/developmental outcomes. In this section, LGS is discussed with a focus on evolution and long-term outcomes in adult patients. For a detailed discussion of LGS in the pediatric population as well as the other epileptic encephalopathies, please refer to Chapters 13 and 18.

Lennox–Gastaut syndrome, a term introduced by Niedermeyer (317), is one of the most resistant epilepsies and is considered one of the epileptic encephalopathy syndromes. The onset of LGS is usually before age 8, with a peak between three and five years; adult onset is rare. It is commonly associated with mental retardation (318). It is characterized by frequent seizures of multiple seizure types, the most common being tonic seizures, causing falls and drop attacks, and is required for the diagnosis of LGS. Tonic seizures can occur multiple times per day, particularly during sleep. Other common seizure types include atypical absence and generalized tonic-clonic seizures, followed by myoclonic, atonic, and partial seizures. LGS may be symptomatic or cryptogenic, and some patients may evolve from West syndrome (319) or unspecified epilepsies (generalized convulsions, hemiconvulsions, versive seizures, or myoclonic seizures) (320,321). Symptomatic LGS can be related to a variety of pathologies, such as prenatal and perinatal hypoxic-ischemic injury, tumors, meningitis/encephalitis, brain malformations and migration disorders, and genetic syndromes. Still, in up to 25% of patients, the exact cause is unknown (318,319,322). Since many patients do not respond to standard antiseizure medications, alternative treatments may include ketogenic diet, corpus callostomy, and implantation of vagus nerve stimulator.

5.2. EEG

The hallmark feature is diffuse, frontally predominant slow spike-wave discharges at 1 to 2.5 Hz, frequently seen as an interictal pattern, and occasionally these slow spike waves may have lateralization. These discharges are enhanced in non-REM sleep and occur in prolonged runs. Another hallmark feature is runs of fast rhythms, typically at 10 to 20 Hz, which are frequent and repetitive, occurring often in non-REM sleep and also with tonic seizures. Multifocal epileptiform discharges may also be seen. The background rhythm is often slow and disorganized, although some patients may show a normal alpha rhythm. Not surprisingly, the severity of the disease correlates with the degree of background disruption.

The types of seizures occurring in LGS are outlined in Table 17.1. The tonic seizures are usually short, typically lasting 5 to 20 seconds, and are clinically characterized by extension of the axial musculature with opisthotonos and flexion of the arms, and this may be followed by extension. Tonic seizures are common in non-REM sleep and may be very subtle clinically. Electrographically, tonic seizures are characterized by diffuse high-voltage slow wave, followed by generalized low- to medium-voltage fast activity at 15 to 25 Hz with frontal accentuation, often followed by an electrodecrement. A diffuse slow ictal pattern has been mentioned by Gastaut and Broughton, who consider it extremely rare.

TABLE 17.1. Types of Seizures Occurring in Lennox-Gastaut Syndrome

SEIZURE TYPES	INCIDENCE IN LENNOX-GASTAUT SYNDROME
Seizures occurring in other seizure disorders	
• Generalized tonic-clonic	+
• Complex partial	+
• Myoclonic	++
• Focal	+
Seizures occurring almost exclusively in Lennox-Gastaut Syndrome	
• Tonic	+++
• Atonic	+++
• Clonic	+

The atypical absence seizures characterized by staring, with or without blinking, correlate with bursts of generalized frontally predominant and synchronous slow spike-wave activity at 1 to 2.5 Hz. The exact onset and offset of these seizures are occasionally unclear. These slow spike-wave discharges are enhanced during sleep and may be quite prolonged.

5.3. Evolution and Long-Term Outcomes

Studies investigating the long-term evolution and outcome of LGS found that these clinical and EEG features are persistent in approximately one third to one half of patients (318,320,323). In many adults, the runs of slow spike-wave discharges may gradually disappear in wakefulness first, typically after age 16, but repetitive multiple spike-and-wave complexes and runs of fast spikes persist in sleep (320,324). Additionally, focal spikes can develop in the temporal regions, and this sometimes coincides with development of complex partial seizures. This process has been described as "secondary temporalization" and can be seen in up to 78% of patients (324). The background may be slow or normalize in up to 44% of patients as the epileptiform activity in wakefulness decreases (323,324).

Over time in adulthood, daytime tonic and absence seizures may decrease in frequency (323), but tonic seizures appear to be the most persistent seizure type, particularly during sleep, and tend to persist in almost all patients, even after surgical treatment with anterior corpus callosotomy. In a 10-year follow-up study of LGS patients by Yagi, only 8% of patients were reported to be seizure-free (320). Thus, long-term EEG monitoring including sleep recording is important for assessing adult patients with LGS and response to treatment. The presence of atypical absence seizures and frequent epileptiform discharges has been found in a long-term study by Ogawa to be a strong predictor of poor seizure and cognitive outcome (325). Although a study by Oguni found that outcome is poorer and severe mental retardation is more frequent in patients with symptomatic LGS (76%) than in patients with cryptogenic LGS (43%) (326), several other studies found no significant differences between cryptogenic and symptomatic LGS patients over time with respect to several measures: seizure frequency, seizure types, EEG patterns, cognitive outcomes, and response to treatment (319,320,323). The only predictor of better cognitive outcome is later age of onset, which has been attributed to the fact that older patients who have gone through more critical stages of developmental, such as apoptosis and synaptogenesis, may manifest less cognitive impairment (319).

6. DIAGNOSTIC AND PROGNOSTIC YIELD OF EEG IN THE ETIOLOGICAL WORKUP OF ENCEPHALOPATHY

Prognosis in encephalopathic patients is mainly determined by the underlying etiology, since EEG patterns in many types of encephalopathy are often nonspecific. However, in clinical practice, the cause and type of encephalopathy are often unknown at the onset of brain dysfunction. In this setting, information regarding the diagnostic and prognostic yield of EEG is important. Recent studies provided some evidence for the diagnostic and prognostic use of particular EEG patterns in more heterogeneous cohorts of encephalopathic patients.

6.1. Slowing Basic EEG Rhythm

In the following sections, data from several studies are discussed that have uncovered the prognostic impact of different grades of slowing basic EEG rhythm, such as generalized alpha, theta, theta–delta, and delta pattern (Fig. 17.9).

6.1.1. CLINICAL ASSOCIATIONS OF GENERALIZED THETA PATTERN

In a cohort study of patients with different types of encephalopathy categorized according to particular EEG patterns, predominant generalized theta activity with preserved EEG background reactivity was associated with brain atrophy on neuroimaging in multivariable analysis (327). Metabolic derangements were seen in 54% of patients and structural abnormalities in 80% (56% of patients had two or more pathologic conditions).

Another type of encephalopathy with predominant generalized theta activity (i.e., theta coma) is associated with a poor prognosis; it typically appears "invariable" or "invariant" and is mostly unreactive. This pattern is typically seen after hypoxic brain injury and will not be further discussed in this section.

6.1.2. CLINICAL ASSOCIATIONS OF GENERALIZED THETA–DELTA PATTERN

Predominant generalized theta–delta EEG activity has been shown in patients with combined large cortical and subcortical structural abnormalities in a case series of a heterogeneous group of encephalopathic patients (10). In patients with metabolic derangements, generalized theta–delta activity may be interrupted by TWs (2,10). In a study of patients with encephalopathy of different etiologies, intracerebral hemorrhage was the only pathologic condition associated with this EEG pattern in the multivariable analysis (327).

6.1.3. CLINICAL ASSOCIATIONS OF GENERALIZED DELTA PATTERN

Predominant generalized delta activity is mostly seen in late stages of encephalopathy and in deep coma, although the reaction of this slow basic EEG rhythm to noxious stimuli is often preserved. Early studies in patients with encephalopathy identified metabolic disorders in association with generalized delta activity (328,329), and focal or unilateral delta activity in association with focal subcortical brain lesions. More recent studies suggest that predominant generalized delta activity may be the result of widespread subcortical alterations (10). In a study of a heterogeneous encephalopathic cohort, multivariable analysis regarding the association between predefined EEG patterns and underlying pathologies revealed that generalized delta activity was associated with PRES and alcohol or drug abuse (327). Aside from these major associations, several patients also had concurrent pathologies such as metabolic

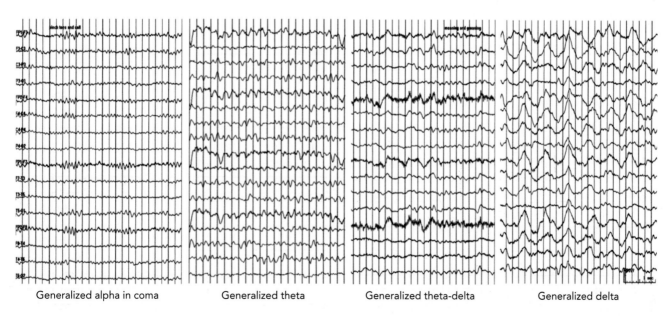

| Generalized alpha in coma | Generalized theta | Generalized theta-delta | Generalized delta |

Figure 17.9. Different grades of slowing basic EEG rhythm in encephalopathy.

disorders and infections, although these were not statistically significant.

6.1.4. CLINICAL ASSOCIATIONS OF GENERALIZED BURST-SUPPRESSION PATTERN

A generalized burst-suppression pattern consists of synchronous bursts of high voltage with irregular activity of different frequencies interrupted by periods of suppression of EEG activity (Fig. 17.10). Both bursts and periods of suppression may be variable in duration.

Hypoxic-ischemic brain injury, hypothermia, intoxication with sedative drugs, and anesthetics are the major underlying causes of the burst-suppression pattern that determine outcome (330). It remains unclear whether a burst-suppression pattern that is reactive to external stimuli (i.e., an interruption by stimulation) is linked to a better outcome as compared to an unreactive burst-suppression.

6.1.5. PREDICTIVE VALUE OF DIFFERENT GRADES OF SLOW BASIC EEG RHYTHM

The only condition in which alpha activity is pathologic is alpha coma. In this EEG pattern, the alpha activity, which is predominantly seen in the anterior EEG traces, usually emerges after anoxia or head trauma, occasionally with drug overdoses, and typically is unreactive to noxious stimuli. After anoxia it has a poor prognosis, but following drugs alone, it portends recovery in 90% of the patients (35,331).

Aside from the more "benign" generalized theta patterns with preserved background reactivity in patients with cortical dysfunction, such as in dementia or mild to moderate encephalopathy (10), unreactive diffuse theta activity can be seen in comatose patients with hypoxic-ischemic brain injury, which carries a poor prognosis (332). However, the typical reactive alpha coma pattern seen in patients with drug overdoses is usually reversible (35,331). Intoxication is usually caused by anesthetic and anxiolytic drugs (333), and if the offending drug is discontinued, neurofunctional outcome is good in most cases (35).

Generalized delta activity is usually associated with poor outcome (333). However, in a study of patients with different types of encephalopathy categorized according to their predominant EEG pattern, generalized high-voltage delta activity was not associated with poor outcome in the multivariable analysis (327). This may be explained by the fact that generalized high-voltage delta activity was associated with potentially reversible pathologic conditions (e.g., PRES, drug abuse).

Other studies of the predictive value of slowing basic EEG rhythms have been limited to cohorts with hypoxic-ischemic encephalopathy and will not be discussed in this section.

6.2. Episodic Nonepileptic Transients in Encephalopathy

6.2.1. CLINICAL ASSOCIATIONS OF INTERMITTENT GENERALIZED RHYTHMIC DELTA ACTIVITY WITH FRONTAL PREDOMINANCE

Intermittent generalized rhythmic delta activity (GRDA) with frontal predominance (formerly FIRDA) is defined as a repetitive appearance of 2 to 4 seconds of frontal rhythmic slow wave

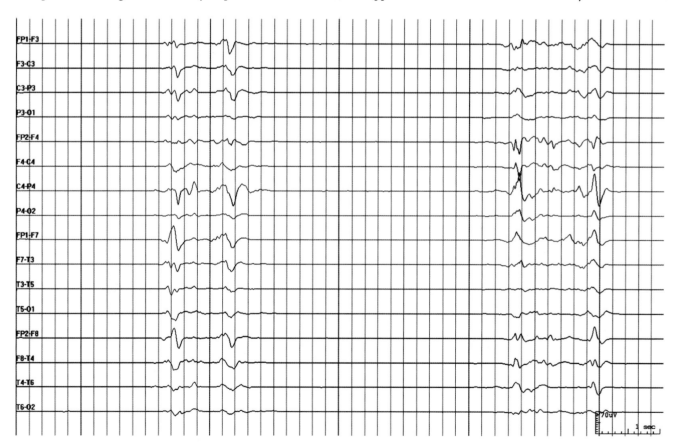

Figure 17.10. Generalized burst-suppression pattern in encephalopathy.

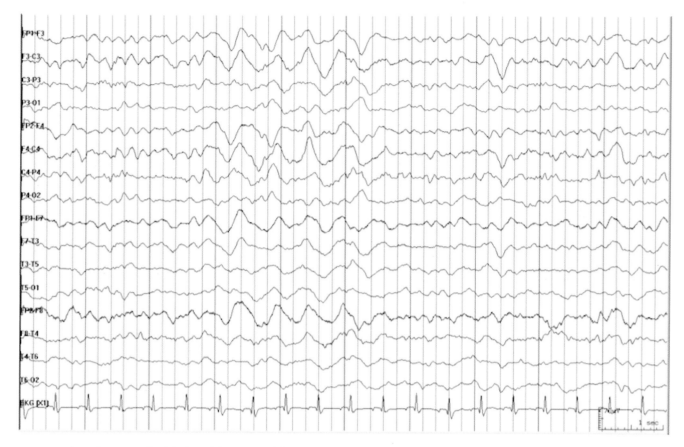

Figure 17.11. Intermittent generalized rhythmic delta activity with frontal predominance in encephalopathy.

activity at <4 Hz (Fig. 17.11) (7,28,334). In contrast to frontal seizures, intermittent GRDA with frontal predominance exhibits no phase reversals and largely retains reactive alpha background activity (327). Intermittent GRDA with frontal predominance is usually reactive to external stimuli (27,335).

Early studies suggested that intermittent GRDA with frontal predominance is associated with high intracranial pressure and lesions in the deep cerebral midline (334), brain tumors (336), and subcortical lesions (337). However, these reports were followed by a study comparing several encephalopathic patients with intermittent GRDA with frontal predominance with other EEG patterns and identified a wider range of brain lesions in association with intermittent GRDA with frontal predominance, indicating its nonspecific nature (7). In another study of encephalopathic patients presenting with slowing of background activity with and without intermittent GRDA with frontal predominance, multivariable analysis revealed an association of remote cerebrovascular accidents with intermittent GRDA with frontal predominance (327). However, as in the prior studies, several patients also had white matter lesions, atrophy, and intracranial hemorrhage. The presence of intermittent GRDA with frontal predominance was associated with favorable outcomes in the multivariable analyses (327).

6.2.2. Clinical Associations of Triphasic Waves
Triphasic waves usually have maximal amplitudes of >70 μV and consist of three waves: a positive sharp transient that is preceded and followed by negative waves of lower amplitude.

They are usually seen bilaterally and synchronously, but with a frontocentral predominance, an anterior-posterior or posterior-anterior time lag, and a frequency range of 1.5 to 2.5 Hz (Fig. 17.12). The typical background activity seen in patients with TWs is in the theta–delta frequency range, but also delta activity can be predominant (327).

When TWs appear asymmetrically they may resemble ictal discharges and can be distinguished from epileptiform activity by their longer complex duration (>80 msec), the lower amplitudes of the initial negative phases, and the long duration between the beginning of the second phase and the end of the vertical portion of the ascending part of the third phase (8,11). The maximal amplitude is seen in the central-frontal rather than the anterior-frontal EEG derivations, a difference that may also help to differentiate them from epileptic discharges (8,11). Furthermore, in contrast to epileptic discharges, TWs usually increase (and sometimes decrease) with arousal or noxious stimuli. Typically there is a decrease of TWs immediately after the administration of benzodiazepines, but without clinical improvement (338).

TWs are believed to reflect altered brain activity within the thalamo-cortical circuits (11,12) and have been associated with liver and multiple-organ dysfunction (327). Most encephalopathic patients with TWs have additional pathologic conditions, such as cerebral structural abnormalities, infections, and metabolic problems. The latter were also described in a large number of different medical conditions. In the 1980s, TWs were described in numerous pathologic conditions, including

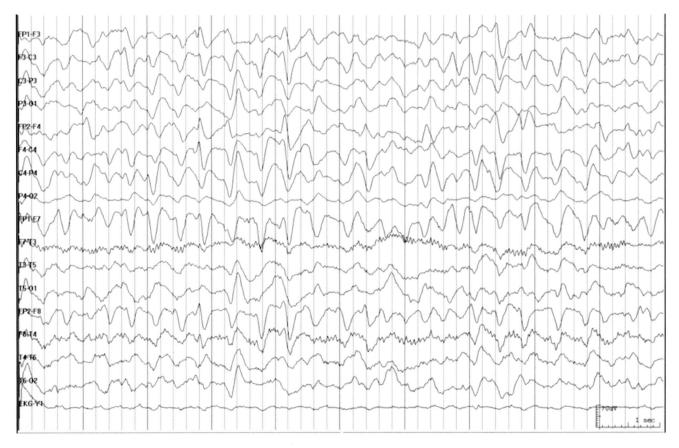

Figure 17.12. TWs in encephalopathy.

ischemic stroke, hypertensive encephalopathy, hyper- or hypo-natremia, hypercalcemia, hypoglycemia, encephalitis, cerebral abscesses, septic shock, dementia, lithium toxicity, and post-ictal states (30). No EEG characteristic of TWs was reliably linked to specific etiologies (30). These results were mirrored by observations of TWs in patients with ischemic strokes, brain tumors, Binswanger's subcortical encephalopathy, and lithium-treated aged psychiatric patients (339). Since then, the range of pathologic conditions in which TWs were detected has further expanded to include renal failure (2,12), hyperos-molarity (12), hypoglycemia (12), bilateral paramedian tha-lamic strokes (340), CNS Lyme disease (341), anoxia (12), postictal stupor (32), sepsis-associated encephalopathy (342), steroid-responsive encephalopathy associated with autoim-mune (Hashimoto) thyroiditis (343), toxic encephalopathies (344), and brainstem infarction (345). In addition, a recent case series described an association between TWs and cere-bral white matter lesions with and without toxic, metabolic, or infectious conditions (10). This observation was confirmed in a study of 205 patients with TWs revealing two or more pathologic conditions in 78% of patients, such as infections, renal or liver insufficiency, and neurostructural abnormalities (i.e., white matter changes, atrophy, ischemic stroke, intracra-nial hemorrhage, brain tumors, signs of traumatic brain injury, encephalitis) (Fig. 17.13) (6).

These findings indicate that these discharges are the result of diffuse brain dysfunction resulting from a complex inter-play of different pathologic conditions. A case-control study uncovered clinical and radiological associations of TWs in encephalopathy in patients with TWs that were matched by Glasgow Coma Scale (GCS) score and the frequency range of EEG background activity with encephalopathic patients with-out TWs (controls) (1). Multivariable analysis revealed higher

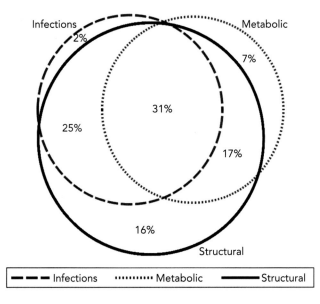

Figure 17.13. Proportional distribution of infections, metabolic derangements, and structural brain abnormalities in 205 encephalopathic patients with TWs. Reprinted with kind permission from Elsevier (6).

odds for liver insufficiency, alcohol abuse, subcortical brain atrophy, and respiratory tract infections in patients with TWs. Despite the nonspecificity for the underlying cause of encephalopathy of TWs, a recent study of encephalopathic patients with different causes of encephalopathy and several EEG patterns revealed that the odds for the presence of TWs increased with every unit of ammonia increase, regardless of the underlying pathologic condition (see Fig. 17.03) (2).

In addition, several studies revealed the prognostic value of TWs. Early studies found that patients with TWs experienced mortalities ranging from 30% with renal encephalopathy, 60% with hepatic encephalopathy, to 100% with anoxia (12,31). However, these studies were performed over 20 years ago and advances in medicine may have lowered the mortality rates associated with these conditions. In a recent study of 154 encephalopathic patients with different EEG patterns, TWs were associated with higher odds for death (by a factor of 4.5) as compared to other EEG patterns (2). This study was followed by an investigation by the same authors analyzing the diagnostic and prognostic value of specific characteristics of TWs, revealing a mortality of 20%. However, the same study showed, in a study of semi-quantitative analyses of TWs, that none of the EEG characteristics of TWs, such as frequencies, amplitudes, localizations, or time lags of TWs, were predictive for outcome, while patients with absent EEG background reactivity to noxious stimuli had higher odds for death (by a factor of 3.7) compared to patients with preserved EEG reactivity (6).

6.2.3. CLINICAL ASSOCIATIONS OF LATERALIZED PERIODIC DISCHARGES

Lateralized periodic discharges (LPDs) are stereotyped discharges that appear at an almost constant frequency and at consistent intervals. Sometimes they resemble epileptic discharges such as sharply contoured slow waves, sharp waves, spikes, polyspikes, or a mixture of spikes and slow waves. Therefore, a clear distinction between nonepileptic LPDs and discharges of epileptic nature is difficult. In these cases, some EEG characteristics enable the differentiation between these two entities. In contrast to nonepileptic LPDs, epileptic discharges have a very short duration, lasting <80 msec, and may be followed by slow waves in the delta frequency range (i.e., spike-waves). In addition, they clearly stand out from the basic EEG rhythm and can evolve in trains (i.e., polyspikes) that occur at up to 20 Hz. Nonepileptic LPDs are typically slower, lasting >80 msec, have a more blunted shape, are not necessarily followed by broader waves, and do not occur in trains at higher frequencies. However, the differentiation between LPDs and sharp waves is more challenging. In contrast to sharp waves, LPDs are followed by much broader slow waves with a frequency range of 1 to 7 Hz. These complexes may appear mono-, bi-, or triphasic and are typically of high amplitudes, with 100 to 300 µV, and occur at intervals of 0.3 seconds up to several seconds. In contrast to "real" TWs, triphasic LPDs rarely have an anterior-posterior or posterior-anterior time lag as described above (see Section 6.2.2). The distinction between epileptic discharges and encephalopathic discharges at the end

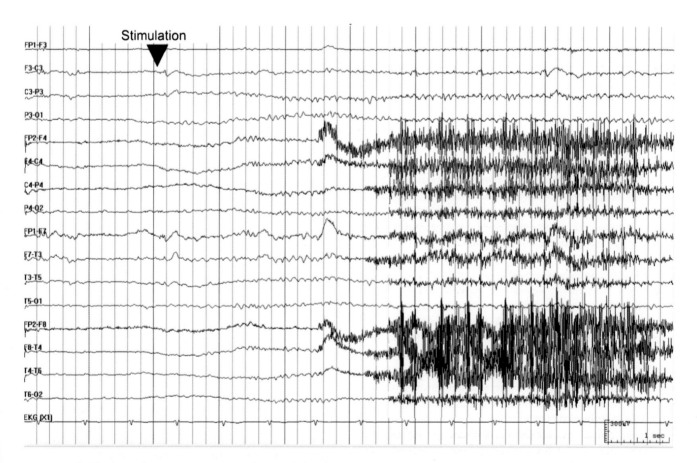

Figure 17.14. EEG background reactivity to noxious stimuli in encephalopathy.

of epileptic seizures, or at the beginning of postictal states, is problematic. This transformation from epileptic seizures to a state of postictal brain dysfunction (also called "postictal encephalopathic state") can be prolonged, with some postictal states lasting several hours or days, especially in patients with prolonged seizures. In this "ictal–interictal continuum," epileptic seizures and postictal encephalopathic states cannot be clearly separated and EEG waveforms during seizures and the clinical response to antiseizure drugs can vary (45). Since the term "ictal–interictal continuum" has been coined, discussions are ongoing, and a clear distinction is not always possible.

6.3. Predictive Value of EEG Background Reactivity in Encephalopathy

The predictive value of the reactivity of the basic EEG rhythm to noxious stimuli (Fig. 17.14) has been well examined in hypoxic-ischemic encephalopathy following cardiac arrest. Recent studies indicate that the predictive value of EEG reactivity is not restricted to patients with hypoxic-ischemic encephalopathies but also has predictive power in non-hypoxic encephalopathies (6).

Alpha coma patterns, which typically show preserved reactive basic EEG rhythm to stimuli, usually emerge after drug overdoses and lead to recovery in most patients (35,331). In contrast, unreactive low-voltage delta coma is associated with severe cerebral dysfunction and a poor outcome (10).

6.4. Predictive Value of EEG Sleep Elements in Encephalopathy

Although sleep alteration is described in up to 80% of patients with hepatic encephalopathy (346) and chronic renal failure (347), the exact neurophysiological mechanisms of sleep disturbances in encephalopathy remain unclear. Healthy sleep-deprived subjects frequently suffer from adverse effects on metabolism, inflammatory reactions, and immune and cardiac function, generating the hypothesis that sleep disturbances may interfere with neuroregeneration and that preserved physiological sleep may predict a favorable outcome. In a study designed to determine the prognostic value of EEG elements of sleep in encephalopathic patients, including detection of vertex sharp-waves, sleep spindles, and K-complexes (348), K-complexes were associated with good outcome, even after adjusting for possible confounders and without significant effect modification across subgroups.

7. NEW PARADIGM FOR OUTCOME PREDICTION IN ENCEPHALOPATHIES

Based on our current knowledge regarding the value of clinical and EEG features for predicting outcomes in patients with non-hypoxic encephalopathies, new scoring systems should be evaluated in future studies to further improve prognostication in the setting of non-hypoxic encephalopathy. Figure 17.15 proposes a new—but not yet validated—paradigm for predicting outcome, compiling the current evidence in this context

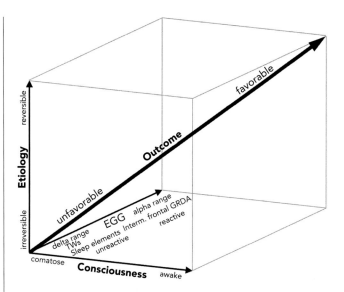

Figure 17.15. Proposed paradigm for prognostication of outcome in encephalopathy. Reprinted with kind permission from Wolters Kluwer Health (349).

(349). In this paradigm, future studies would need to generate and validate new scoring systems for prognostication. The interplay of clinical and EEG-related outcome predictors may increase the reliability of outcome prediction.

SCORE EEG SOFTWARE

Further examples related to the topics addressed in this chapter can be found in the interactive online Niedermeyer Educational Platform. EEG recordings with illustrative examples can be opened and browsed. Features are marked and described using the SCORE EEG software. The users can see the features marked by experts, they can score these features themselves, and then compare them with the scorings of the experts.

The Niedermeyer Educational Platform can be accessed at: www.scoreEEG.com/academy

REFERENCES

1. Sutter R, Kaplan PW. Uncovering clinical and radiological associations of triphasic waves in acute encephalopathy: a case-control study. *Eur J Neurol* 2014;21(4):660–666.
2. Sutter R, Stevens RD, Kaplan PW. Clinical and imaging correlates of EEG patterns in hospitalized patients with encephalopathy. *J Neurol* 2013;260(4):1087–1098.
3. Sutter R, Kaplan PW. What to see when you are looking at confusion: a review of the neuroimaging of acute encephalopathy. *J Neurol Neurosurg Psychiatry* 2015;86:446–459.
4. Thomas C, Hestermann U, Walther S, et al. Prolonged activation EEG differentiates dementia with and without delirium in frail elderly patients. *J Neurol Neurosurg Psychiatry* 2008;79(2):119–125.
5. Thomas C, Hestermann U, Kopitz J, et al. Serum anticholinergic activity and cerebral cholinergic dysfunction: an EEG study in frail elderly with and without delirium. *BMC Neurosci* 2008;9:86.
6. Sutter R, Stevens RD, Kaplan PW. Significance of triphasic waves in patients with acute encephalopathy: a nine-year cohort study. *Clin Neurophysiol* 2014;124(10):1952–1958.

7. Accolla EA, Kaplan PW, Maeder-Ingvar M, et al. Clinical correlates of frontal intermittent rhythmic delta activity (FIRDA). *Clin Neurophysiol* 2011;122(1):27–31.

8. Kaplan PW, Schlattman DK. Comparison of triphasic waves and epileptic discharges in one patient with genetic epilepsy. *J Clin Neurophysiol* 2012;29(5):458–461.

9. Kaplan P, Schlattman DK. Typical versus atypical triphasic waves. *J Clin Neurophysiol* 2013;30(2):211.

10. Kaplan PW, Rossetti AO. EEG patterns and imaging correlations in encephalopathy: encephalopathy part II. *J Clin Neurophysiol* 2011;28(3):233–251.

11. Kwon OY, Jung KY, Park KJ, et al. Source localization of triphasic waves: implications for the pathophysiological mechanism. *Clin EEG Neurosci* 2007;38(3):161–167.

12. Karnaze DS, Bickford RG. Triphasic waves: a reassessment of their significance. *Electroencephalogr Clin Neurophysiol* 1984;57(3):193–198.

13. Newman SE. The EEG manifestations of chronic ethanol abuse: relation to cerebral cortical atrophy. *Ann Neurol* 1978;3(4):299–304.

14. Foley JM, Watson CW, Adams RD. Significance of the electroencephalographic changes in hepatic coma. *Trans Am Neurol Assoc* 1950;51:161–165.

15. Kaplan PW. EEG monitoring in the intensive care unit. *Am J Electroneurodiagnostic Technol* 2006;46(2):81–97.

16. Berger H. Über das Elektrenkephalogramm des Menschen. Erster Bericht. *Arch Psychiatr Nervenkr* 1929;87:527–580.

17. Romano J, Engel GL. Delirium: I. Electroencephalographic data. *Arch Neurol Psychiatry* 1944;5`:356–377.

18. Bickford RG, Butt HR. Hepatic coma: the electroencephalographic pattern. *J Clin Invest* 1955;34(6):790–799.

19. Cadilhac J, Ribstein M. The EEG in metabolic disorders. *World Neurol* 1961;2:296–308.

20. Condon JV, Becka DR, Gibbs FA. Electroencephalographic abnormalities in endocrine disease. *N Engl J Med* 1954;251(16):638–641.

21. Glaser GH. Metabolic encephalopathy in hepatic, renal and pulmonary disorders. *Postgrad Med* 1960;27:611–619.

22. Creutzfeldt OD, Meisch JJ. Changes of cortical neuronal activity and EEG during hypoglycemia. *Electroencephalogr Clin Neurophysiol* 1963;Suppl 24:158–170.

23. Arjundas G, Ramamurthi B, Subramanian R. Electroencephalographic changes in nine cases of hepatic coma. *Neurol India* 1965;13(4):158–161.

24. Stockard JJ, Bickford RG. The neurophysiology of anesthesia. In: Gordon E, ed. *A basis and practice of neuroanesthesia*. Amsterdam: Excerpta Medica; 1975, pp. 3–46.

25. Gloor P, Ball G, Schaul N. Brain lesions that produce delta waves in the EEG. *Neurology* 1977;27(4):326–333.

26. Sutter R, Kaplan PW. Electroencephalographic patterns in coma: when things slow down. *Epileptologie* 2012;29:201–209.

27. Fariello RG, Orrison W, Blanco G, et al. Neuroradiological correlates of frontally predominant intermittent rhythmic delta activity (FIRDA). *Electroencephalogr Clin Neurophysiol* 1982;54(2):194–202.

28. Hooshmand H. The clinical significance of frontal intermittent rhythmic delta activity (FIRDA). *Clin Electroencephalogr* 1983;14(3):135–137.

29. Sundaram MB, Blume WT. Triphasic waves: clinical correlates and morphology. *Can J Neurol Sci* 1987;14(2):136–140.

30. Fisch BJ, Klass DW. The diagnostic specificity of triphasic wave patterns. *Electroencephalogr Clin Neurophysiol* 1988;70(1):1–8.

31. Bahamon-Dussan JE, Celesia GG, Grigg-Damberger MM. Prognostic significance of EEG triphasic waves in patients with altered state of consciousness. *J Clin Neurophysiol* 1989;6(4):313–319.

32. Ogunyemi A. Triphasic waves during post-ictal stupor. *Can J Neurol Sci* 1996;23(3):208–212.

33. Hrachovy RA. Drug-induced alpha coma. *Neurology* 1982;32(11):1319.

34. Iragui VJ, McCutchen CB. Physiologic and prognostic significance of "alpha coma." *J Neurol Neurosurg Psychiatry* 1983;46(7):632–638.

35. Kaplan PW, Genoud D, Ho TW, et al. Etiology, neurologic correlations, and prognosis in alpha coma. *Clin Neurophysiol* 1999;110(2):205–213.

36. Britt CW, Jr., Raso E, Gerson LP. Spindle coma, secondary to primary traumatic midbrain hemorrhage. *Electroencephalogr Clin Neurophysiol* 1980;49(3-4):406–408.

37. Pulst SM, Lombroso CT. External ophthalmoplegia, alpha and spindle coma in imipramine overdose: case report and review of the literature. *Ann Neurol* 1983;14(5):587–590.

38. Rimar D, Bitterman H. Hyperammonemic coma: beyond hepatic encephalopathy. *South Med J* 2008;101(5):467–468.

39. Shawcross D, Jalan R. The pathophysiologic basis of hepatic encephalopathy: central role for ammonia and inflammation. *Cell Mol Life Sci* 2005;62(19-20):2295–2304.

40. Marchetti P, D'Avanzo C, Orsato R, et al. Electroencephalography in patients with cirrhosis. *Gastroenterology* 2011;141(5):1680–1689.

41. Amodio P, Del Piccolo F, Petteno E, et al. Prevalence and prognostic value of quantified electroencephalogram (EEG) alterations in cirrhotic patients. *J Hepatol* 2001;35(1):37–45.

42. Amodio P, Gatta A. Neurophysiological investigation of hepatic encephalopathy. *Metab Brain Dis* 2005;20(4):369–379.

43. Silverman D. Some observations on the EEG in hepatic coma. *Electroencephalogr Clin Neurophysiol* 1962;14:53–59.

44. MacGillivray B, Kennedy JK. The "triphasic waves" of hepatic encephalopathy. *Electroencephalogr Clin Neurophysiol* 1970;28(4):428.

45. Kaplan PW. Nonconvulsive status epilepticus in the emergency room. *Epilepsia* 1996;37(7):643–650.

46. Bauer G, Niedermeyer E. Acute convulsions. *Clin Electroencephalogr* 1979;10(3):127–144.

47. Ficker DM, Westmoreland BF, Sharbrough FW. Epileptiform abnormalities in hepatic encephalopathy. *J Clin Neurophysiol* 1997;14(3):230–234.

48. Amodio P, Pellegrini A, Ubiali E, et al. The EEG assessment of low-grade hepatic encephalopathy: comparison of an artificial neural network-expert system (ANNES) based evaluation with visual EEG readings and EEG spectral analysis. *Clin Neurophysiol* 2006;117(10):2243–2251.

49. Olesen SS, Graversen C, Hansen TM, et al. Spectral and dynamic electroencephalogram abnormalities are correlated to psychometric test performance in hepatic encephalopathy. *Scand J Gastroenterol* 2011;46(7-8):988–996.

50. Montagnese S, Balistreri E, Schiff S, et al. Covert hepatic encephalopathy: agreement and predictive validity of different indices. *World J Gastroenterol* 2014;20(42):15756–15762.

51. Victor M. Victor M. Neurologic changes in liver disease. In: Plum F, ed. *Brain dysfunction in metabolic disorders*. New York: Raven Press; 1974, pp. 1–12.

52. Nevsimalova S, Marecek Z, Roth B. An EEG study of Wilson's disease. Findings in patients and heterozygous relatives. *Electroencephalogr Clin Neurophysiol* 1986;64(3):191–198.

53. Park JH, Kim HJ, Kim SM. Acute chorea with bilateral basal ganglia lesions in diabetic uremia. *Can J Neurol Sci* 2007;34(2):248–250.

54. Hughes JR. Correlations between EEG and chemical changes in uremia. *Electroencephalogr Clin Neurophysiol* 1980;48(5):583–594.

55. Reichenmiller HE, Reinhard U, Durr F. Sleep EEG and uraemia. *Electroencephalogr Clin Neurophysiol* 1971;30(3):263–264.

56. Zuckermann EG, Glaser GH. Urea-induced myoclonic seizures. An experimental study of site of action and mechanism. *Arch Neurol* 1972;27(1):14–28.

57. Posner JB, Plum F, Saper CB. *Plum and Posner's diagnosis of stupor and coma*. New York: Oxford University Press; 2007.

58. Lacerda G, Krummel T, Sabourdy C, et al. Optimizing therapy of seizures in patients with renal or hepatic dysfunction. *Neurology* 2006;67(12 Suppl 4):S28–S33.

59. Boggs JG. Seizures in medically complex patients. *Epilepsia* 1997;38(Suppl 4):S55–S59.

60. Chuang CL, Chen KP, Kwan SY, et al. Creutzfeldt-Jakob-like EEG in a patient with end-stage renal failure. *Nephrol Dial Transplant* 2004;19(1):252–254.

61. Lavy S, Aviram A. EEG changes in uraemic patients undergoing regular haemodialysis. *Electroencephalogr Clin Neurophysiol* 1969;27(2):217.

62. Markand ON. Electroencephalography in diffuse encephalopathies. *J Clin Neurophysiol* 1984;1(4):357–407.

63. Bourne JR, Ward JW, Teschan PE, et al. Quantitative assessment of the electroencephalogram in renal disease. *Electroencephalogr Clin Neurophysiol* 1975;39(4):377–388.

64. Kiley JE, Woodruff MW, Pratt KI. Evaluation of encephalopathy by EEG frequency analysis in chronic dialysis patients. *Clin Nephrol* 1976;5(6):245–250.

65. Rohl JE, Harms L, Pommer W. Quantitative EEG findings in patients with chronic renal failure. *Eur J Med Res* 2007;12(4):173–178.

66. Jacob JC, Gloor P, Elwan OH, et al. Electroencephalographic changes in chronic renal failure. *Neurology* 1965;15:419–429.

67. Scorza FA, Albuquerque M, Arida RM, et al. Seizure occurrence in patients with chronic renal insufficiency in regular hemodialysis program. *Arq Neuropsiquiatr* 2005;63(3B):757–760.

68. Kerr DN, Osselton JW. The EEG as a monitor of cerebral disturbance during fast and slow haemodialysis of patients in chronic renal failure. *Electroencephalogr Clin Neurophysiol* 1967;23(5):488.

69. Soomro A, Al Bahri R, Alhassan N, et al. Posterior reversible encephalopathy syndrome with tactile hallucinations secondary to dialysis disequilibrium syndrome. *Saudi J Kidney Dis Transpl* 2014;25(3):625–629.

70. Yardimci N, Colak T, Sevmis S, et al. Neurologic complications after renal transplant. *Exp Clin Transplant* 2008;6(3):224–228.

71. Sibai BM. Diagnosis, prevention, and management of eclampsia. *Obstet Gynecol* 2005;105(2):402–410.

72. Lain KY, Roberts JM. Contemporary concepts of the pathogenesis and management of preeclampsia. *JAMA* 2002;287(24):3183–3186.

73. Roberts JM, Taylor RN, Goldfien A. Clinical and biochemical evidence of endothelial cell dysfunction in the pregnancy syndrome preeclampsia. *Am J Hypertens* 1991;4(8):700–708.

74. Ferris TF. Pregnancy, preeclampsia, and the endothelial cell. *N Engl J Med* 1991;325(20):1439–1440.

75. Will AD, Lewis KL, Hinshaw DB, Jr., et al. Cerebral vasoconstriction in toxemia. *Neurology* 1987;37(9):1555–1557.

76. Dahmus MA, Barton JR, Sibai BM. Cerebral imaging in eclampsia: magnetic resonance imaging versus computed tomography. *Am J Obstet Gynecol* 1992;167(4 Pt 1):935–941.

77. Senzolo M, Amodio P, D'Aloiso MC, et al. Neuropsychological and neurophysiological evaluation in cirrhotic patients with minimal hepatic encephalopathy undergoing liver transplantation. *Transplant Proc* 2005;37(2):1104–1107.

78. Hiller KM, Honigman B. Cortical blindness in preeclampsia. *Am J Emerg Med* 2004;22(7):631–632.

79. Thomas SV, Somanathan N, Radhakumari R. Interictal EEG changes in eclampsia. *Electroencephalogr Clin Neurophysiol* 1995;94(4):271–275.

80. Osmanagaoglu MA, Dinc G, Osmanagaoglu S, et al. Comparison of cerebral magnetic resonance and electroencephalogram findings in pre-eclamptic and eclamptic women. *Aust N Z J Obstet Gynaecol* 2005;45(5):384–390.

81. Sibai BM. Diagnosis and management of gestational hypertension and preeclampsia. *Obstet Gynecol* 2003;102(1):181–192.

82. Sibai BM, Spinnato JA, Watson DL, et al. Effect of magnesium sulfate on electroencephalographic findings in preeclampsia-eclampsia. *Obstet Gynecol* 1984;64(2):261–266.

83. Castilla-Guerra L, del Carmen Fernandez-Moreno M, Lopez-Chozas JM, et al. Electrolytes disturbances and seizures. *Epilepsia* 2006;47(12):1990–1998.

84. van der Helm-van Mil AH, van Vugt JP, Lammers GJ, et al. Hypernatremia from a hunger strike as a cause of osmotic myelinolysis. *Neurology* 2005;64(3):574–575.

85. Strange K, Jackson PS. Swelling-activated organic osmolyte efflux: a new role for anion channels. *Kidney Int* 1995;48(4):994–1003.

86. Casaletto JJ. Is salt, vitamin, or endocrinopathy causing this encephalopathy? A review of endocrine and metabolic causes of altered level of consciousness. *Emerg Med Clin North Am* 2010;28(3):633–662.

87. Zwang HJ, Cohn D. Electroencephalographic changes in acute water intoxication. *Clin Electroencephalogr* 1981;12(1):35–40.

88. Okura M, Okada K, Nagamine I, et al. Electroencephalographic changes during and after water intoxication. *Jpn J Psychiatry Neurol* 1990;44(4):729–734.

89. Nakayama Y, Tanaka A, Naritomi K, et al. Hyponatremia-induced metabolic encephalopathy caused by Rathke's cleft cyst: a case report. *Clin Neurol Neurosurg* 1999;101(2):114–117.

90. Maruyama T, Tabata K, Nakagawa S, et al. [A case of acute water intoxication showing triphasic waves on EEG]. *Rinsho Shinkeigaku* 1991;31(5):523–527.

91. Itoh N, Matsui N, Matsui S. Periodic lateralized epileptiform discharges in EEG during recovery from hyponatremia: a case report. *Clin Electroencephalogr* 1994;25(4):164–169.

92. Naha K, Vivek G, Dasari S, et al. An unusual cause for hyponatremia with seizures. *BMJ Case Rep* Mar 20 2012. doi: 10.1136/bcr.09.2011.4784.

93. Azuma H, Akechi T, Furukawa TA. Absence status associated with focal activity and polydipsia-induced hyponatremia. *Neuropsychiatr Dis Treat* 2008;4(2):495–498.

94. Thomas P, Beaumanoir A, Genton P, et al. 'De novo' absence status of late onset: report of 11 cases. *Neurology* 1992;42(1):104–110.

95. Ben-Asuly S, Horne T, Goldschmidt Z, et al. Coma due to hypercalcemia in a patient with Paget's disease and multiple parathyroid adenomata. *Am J Med Sci* 1975;269(2):267–275.

96. Cohn R, Sode J. The EEG in hypercalcemia. *Neurology* 1971;21(2):154–161.

97. Spatz R, Kugler J, Angstwurm H. [The EEG in hypercalcemia (author's transl)]. *EEG EMG Z Elektroenzephalogr Elektromyogr Verwandte Geb* 1977;8(2):70–76.

98. Allen EM, Singer FR, Melamed D. Electroencephalographic abnormalities in hypercalcemia. *Neurology* 1970;20(1):15–22.

99. Huott AD, Madison DS, Niedermeyer E. Occipital lobe epilepsy. A clinical and electroencephalographic study. *Eur Neurol* 1974;11(6):325–339.

100. Chen TH, Huang CC, Chang YY, et al. Vasoconstriction as the etiology of hypercalcemia-induced seizures. *Epilepsia* 2004;45(5):551–554.

101. Glaser GH, Levy L. Seizures and idiopathic hypoparathyroidism. A clinical-electroencephalographic study. *Epilepsia* 1960;1:454–465.

102. Swash M, Rowan AJ. Electroencephalographic criteria of hypocalcemia and hypercalcemia. *Arch Neurol* 1972;26(3):218–228.

103. Riggs JE. Neurologic manifestations of electrolyte disturbances. *Neurol Clin* 2002;20(1):227–239, vii.

104. Leicher CR, Mezoff AG, Hyams JS. Focal cerebral deficits in severe hypomagnesemia. *Pediatr Neurol* 1991;7(5):380–381.

105. Pande SD, Wee CK, Maw NN. Unusual case of hypomagnesaemia induced seizures. *BMJ Case Rep* 2009. doi: 10.1136/bcr.06.2009.1933.

106. Shils ME. Magnesium, calcium, and parathyroid hormone interactions. *Ann N Y Acad Sci* 1980;355:165–180.

107. Victor M, Adams RD, Collins GH. The Wernicke-Korsakoff syndrome. A clinical and pathological study of 245 patients, 82 with post-mortem examinations. *Contemp Neurol Ser* 1971;7:1–206.

108. Scalzo SJ, Bowden SC, Ambrose ML, et al. Wernicke-Korsakoff syndrome not related to alcohol use: a systematic review. *J Neurol Neurosurg Psychiatry* 2015;86(12):1362–1368.

109. Frantzen E. Wernicke's encephalopathy. 3 cases occurring in connection with severe malnutrition. *Acta Neurol Scand* 1966;42(4):426–441.

110. Fournet A, Lanternier J. [Electroencephalographic manifestations of 17 cases of Gayet-Wernicke encephalopathy]. *Rev Neurol (Paris)* 1956;94(5):644–645.

111. Keyser A, De Bruijn SF. Epileptic manifestations and vitamin B1 deficiency. *Eur Neurol* 1991;31(3):121–125.

112. Gregory J, Philbrick K, Chopra A. Wernicke encephalopathy in a non-alcoholic patient with metastatic CNS lymphoma and new-onset occipital lobe seizures. *J Neuropsychiatry Clin Neurosci* 2012;24(4):E53.

113. Srikantia SG, Reddy MV, Krishnaswamy K. Electroencephalographic patterns in pellagra. *Electroencephalogr Clin Neurophysiol* 1968;25(4):386–388.

114. Kretsch MJ, Sauberlich HE, Newbrun E. Electroencephalographic changes and periodontal status during short-term vitamin B-6 depletion of young, nonpregnant women. *Am J Clin Nutr* 1991;53(5):1266–1274.

115. Diefenbach WC, Beyers MR, Meyer LM. The encephalographic and psychologic changes in pernicious anemia. *Acta Haematol* 1953;9(4):201–208.

116. Lai PH, Tien RD, Chang MH, et al. Chorea-ballismus with nonketotic hyperglycemia in primary diabetes mellitus. *AJNR Am J Neuroradiol* 1996;17(6):1057–1064.

117. Maccario M, Messis CP, Vastola EF. Focal seizures as a manifestation of hyperglycemia without ketoacidosis. A report of seven cases with review of the literature. *Neurology* 1965;15:195–206.

118. Arieff AI, Carroll HJ. Nonketotic hyperosmolar coma with hyperglycemia: clinical features, pathophysiology, renal function, acid-base balance, plasma-cerebrospinal fluid equilibria and the effects of therapy in 37 cases. *Medicine (Baltimore)* 1972;51(2):73–94.

119. Gibbs FA, Williams D, Gibbs EL. Modification of the cortical frequency spectrum by changes in CO_2, blood sugar and oxygen. *J Neurophysiol* 1940;3:49–58.

120. Engel R, Halberg F, Tichy FY, et al. Electrocerebral activity and epileptic attacks at various blood sugar levels; with a case report. *Acta Neuroveg (Wien)* 1954;9(1–4):147–167.

121. Aquino A, Gabor AJ. Movement-induced seizures in nonketotic hyperglycemia. *Neurology* 1980;30(6):600–604.

122. Harden CL, Rosenbaum DH, Daras M. Hyperglycemia presenting with occipital seizures. *Epilepsia* 1991;32(2):215–220.

123. Martinez-Fernandez R, Gelabert A, Pablo MJ, et al. Status epilepticus with visual seizures in ketotic hyperglycemia. *Epilepsy Behav* 2009;16(4):660–662.

124. Placidi F, Floris R, Bozzao A, et al. Ketotic hyperglycemia and epilepsia partialis continua. *Neurology* 2001;57(3):534–537.

125. Virally ML, Guillausseau PJ. Hypoglycemia in adults. *Diabetes Metab* 1999;25(6):477–490.

126. Gellhorn E, Kessler M. The effect of hypoglycemia on the electroencephalogram at varying degrees of oxygenation of the blood. *Am J Physiol* 1942;136:1–6.

127. Zeigler DK, Presthus J. Normal electroencephalogram at deep levels of hypoglycemia. *Electroencephalogr Clin Neurophysiol* 1957;9:523–526.

128. Tribl G, Howorka K, Heger G, et al. EEG topography during insulin-induced hypoglycemia in patients with insulin-dependent diabetes mellitus. *Eur Neurol* 1996;36(5):303–309.

129. Tamburrano G, Lala A, Locuratolo N, et al. Electroencephalography and visually evoked potentials during moderate hypoglycemia. *J Clin Endocrinol Metab* 1988;66(6):1301–1306.

130. Sperling MR. Hypoglycemic activation of focal abnormalities in the EEG of patients considered for temporal lobectomy. *Electroencephalogr Clin Neurophysiol* 1984;58(6):506–512.

131. Nguyen LB, Nguyen AV, Ling SH, et al. Analyzing EEG signals under insulin-induced hypoglycemia in type 1 diabetes patients. *Conf Proc IEEE Eng Med Biol Soc* 2013;2013:1980–1983.

132. Snogdal LS, Folkestad L, Elsborg R, et al. Detection of hypoglycemia associated EEG changes during sleep in type 1 diabetes mellitus. *Diabetes Res Clin Pract* 2012;98(1):91–97.

133. Juhl CB, Hojlund K, Elsborg R, et al. Automated detection of hypoglycemia-induced EEG changes recorded by subcutaneous electrodes in subjects with type 1 diabetes—the brain as a biosensor. *Diabetes Res Clin Pract* 2010;88(1):22–28.

134. Sejling AS, Kjaer TW, Pedersen-Bjergaard U, et al. Hypoglycemia-associated changes in the electroencephalogram in patients with type 1 diabetes and normal hypoglycemia awareness or unawareness. *Diabetes* 2015;64(5):1760–1769.

135. Fabris C, Sparacino G, Sejling AS, et al. Hypoglycemia-related electroencephalogram changes assessed by multiscale entropy. *Diabetes Technol Ther* 2014;16(10):688–694.

136. Charmandari E, Nicolaides NC, Chrousos GP. Adrenal insufficiency. *Lancet* 2014;383(9935):2152–2167.

137. Carroll TB, Findling JW. The diagnosis of Cushing's syndrome. *Rev Endocr Metab Disord* 2010;11(2):147–153.

138. Hoffman WC, Lewis R, Thorn GW. The electroencephalogram in Addison's disease. *Bull Johns Hopkins Hosp* 1942;70:335–361.

139. Mera A. EEG in Addison's disease. *Electroencephalogr Clin Neurophysiol* 1967;23(6):588.

140. Kollmannsberger A, Hochheuser W, Schwarz K, et al. Addison's encephalopathy. *Electroencephalogr Clin Neurophysiol* 1969;26(4):448.

141. Vas GA, Cracco JB. Diffuse encephalopathies. In: Daly DD, Pedley TA, eds. *Current practice of clinical electroencephalography*. 2 ed. New York: Raven Press; 1990, pp. 371–399.

142. Faigle R, Sutter R, Kaplan PW. Electroencephalography of encephalopathy in patients with endocrine and metabolic disorders. *J Clin Neurophysiol* 2013;30(5):505–516.

143. Pine I, Engel FL, Schwartz TB. The electroencephalogram in ACTH and cortisone treated patients. *Electroencephalogr Clin Neurophysiol* 1951;3(3):301–310.

144. Tucker RP, Weinstein HE, Schteingart DE, et al. EEG changes and serum cortisol levels in Cushing's syndrome. *Clin Electroencephalogr* 1978;9(1):32–37.

145. Glaser GH, Komfeld DS, Knight RP. Intravenous hydrocortisone, corticotropin and the electroencephalograms. *Arch Neurol Psychiatry* 1955;73:338–344.

146. Shipley JE, Schteingart DE, Tandon R, et al. EEG sleep in Cushing's disease and Cushing's syndrome: comparison with patients with major depressive disorder. *Biol Psychiatry* 1992;32(2):146–155.

147. Krieger DT, Gewirtz GP. Recovery of hypothalamic-pituitary-adrenal function, growth hormone responsiveness and sleep EEG pattern in a patient following removal of an adrenal cortical adenoma. *J Clin Endocrinol Metab* 1974;38(6):1075–1082.

148. Raab W, Smithwick RH. Pheochromocytoma with hypothalamic manifestations and excessive hypermetabolism; a case report. *J Clin Endocrinol Metab* 1949;9(8):782–790.

149. Kennedy JM, Thomson AP, Whitfield IC. Coma and electroencephalographic changes in hypopituitarism. *Lancet* 1955;269(6896):907–908.

150. Ross DA, Schwab RJ. The cortical alpha rhythm in thyroid disorders. *Endocrinology* 1939;25:75–79.

151. Wilson WP, Johnson JE, Feist FW. Thyroid hormone and brain function. II. Changes in photically elicited EEG responses following the administration of triiodothyronine to normal subjects. *Electroencephalogr Clin Neurophysiol* 1964;16:329–331.

152. Jabbari B, Huott AD. Seizures in thyrotoxicosis. *Epilepsia* 1980;21(1):91–96.

153. Song TJ, Kim SJ, Kim GS, et al. The prevalence of thyrotoxicosis-related seizures. *Thyroid* 2010;20(9):955–958.

154. Leubuscher HJ, Herrmann F, Hambsch K, et al. EEG changes in untreated hyperthyroidism and under the conditions of thyreostatic treatment. *Exp Clin Endocrinol* 1988;92(1):85–90.

155. Safe AF, Griffiths KD, Maxwell RT. Thyrotoxic crisis presenting as status epilepticus. *Postgrad Med J* 1990;66(772):150–152.

156. Hermann HT, Quarton GC. Changes in alpha frequency with change in thyroid hormone level. *Electroencephalogr Clin Neurophysiol* 1964;16:515–518.

157. Nieman EA. The electroencephalogram in myxoedema coma: clinical and electroencephalographic study of three cases. *Br Med J* 1959;1(5131):1204–1208.

158. Scarpalezos S, Lygidakis C, Papageorgiou C, et al. Neural and muscular manifestations of hypothyroidism. *Arch Neurol* 1973;29(3):140–144.

159. Forester CF. Coma in myxedema. Report of a case and review of the world literature. *Arch Intern Med* 1963;111:734–743.

160. River Y, Zelig O. Triphasic waves in myxedema coma. *Clin Electroencephalogr* 1993;24(3):146–150.

161. Lansing RW, Trunnell JB. Electroencephalographic changes accompanying thyroid deficiency in man. *J Clin Endocrinol Metab* 1963;23:470–480.

162. Schaul N, Lueders H, Sachdev K. Generalized, bilaterally synchronous bursts of slow waves in the EEG. *Arch Neurol* 1981;38(11):690–692.

163. Franks NP, Lieb WR. Molecular and cellular mechanisms of general anaesthesia. *Nature* 1994;367(6464):607–614.

164. Sutter R, Kaplan PW. Clinical and electroencephalographic correlates of acute encephalopathy. *J Clin Neurophysiol* 2013;30(5):443–453.

165. Sloan TB. Anesthetic effects on electrophysiologic recordings. *J Clin Neurophysiol* 1998;15(3):217–226.

166. Chatrian GE. Intraoperative electrocorticography. In: Ebersole JS, Pedley TA, eds. *Current practice in clinical electroencephalography*. 3 ed. Philadelphia: Lippincott Williams & Wilkins; 2003, pp. 681–712.

167. Oruch R, Elderbi MA, Khattab HA, et al. Lithium: a review of pharmacology, clinical uses, and toxicity. *Eur J Pharmacol* 2014;740:464–473.

168. Lee MS, Lessell S. Lithium-induced periodic alternating nystagmus. *Neurology* 2003;60(2):344.

169. Ivkovic A, Stern TA. Lithium-induced neurotoxicity: clinical presentations, pathophysiology, and treatment. *Psychosomatics* 2014;55(3):296–302.

170. Sansone ME, Ziegler DK. Lithium toxicity: a review of neurologic complications. *Clin Neuropharmacol* 1985;8(3):242–248.

171. Fetzer J, Kader G, Danahy S. Lithium encephalopathy: a clinical, psychiatric, and EEG evaluation. *Am J Psychiatry* 1981;138(12):1622–1623.

172. Schulz C, Mavrogiorgou P, Schroter A, et al. Lithium-induced EEG changes in patients with affective disorders. *Neuropsychobiology* 2000;42(Suppl 1):33–37.

173. Thau K, Rappelsberger P, Lovrek A, et al. Effect of lithium on the EEG of healthy males and females. A probability mapping study. *Neuropsychobiology* 1989;20(3):158–163.

174. Casanova B, de Entrambasaguas M, Perla C, et al. Lithium-induced Creutzfeldt-Jakob syndrome. *Clin Neuropharmacol* 1996;19(4):356–359.

175. Gallinat J, Boetsch T, Padberg F, et al. Is the EEG helpful in diagnosing and monitoring lithium intoxication? A case report and review of the literature. *Pharmacopsychiatry* 2000;33(5):169–173.

176. Lee SI. Nonconvulsive status epilepticus. Ictal confusion in later life. *Arch Neurol* 1985;42(8):778–781.

177. Kaplan PW, Birbeck G. Lithium-induced confusional states: nonconvulsive status epilepticus or triphasic encephalopathy? *Epilepsia* 2006;47(12):2071–2074.

178. Leucht S, Wahlbeck K, Hamann J, et al. New-generation antipsychotics versus low-potency conventional antipsychotics: a systematic review and meta-analysis. *Lancet* 2003;361(9369):1581–1589.

179. Varma S, Bishara D, Besag FM, et al. Clozapine-related EEG changes and seizures: dose and plasma-level relationships. *Ther Adv Psychopharmacol* 2011;1(2):47–66.

180. Freudenreich O, Weiner RD, McEvoy JP. Clozapine-induced electroencephalogram changes as a function of clozapine serum levels. *Biol Psychiatry* 1997;42(2):132–137.

181. Joutsiniemi SL, Gross A, Appelberg B. Marked clozapine-induced slowing of EEG background over frontal, central, and parietal scalp areas in schizophrenic patients. *J Clin Neurophysiol* 2001;18(1):9–13.

182. Knott V, Labelle A, Jones B, et al. Quantitative EEG in schizophrenia and in response to acute and chronic clozapine treatment. *Schizophr Res* 2001;50(1-2):41–53.

183. Treves IA, Neufeld MY. EEG abnormalities in clozapine-treated schizophrenic patients. *Eur Neuropsychopharmacol* 1996;6(2):93–94.

184. Baldessarini RJ, Frankenburg FR. Clozapine. A novel antipsychotic agent. *N Engl J Med* 1991;324(11):746–754.

185. Alper K, Schwartz KA, Kolts RL, et al. Seizure incidence in psychopharmacological clinical trials: an analysis of Food and Drug Administration (FDA) summary basis of approval reports. *Biol Psychiatry* 2007;62(4):345–354.

186. Dumortier G, Mahe V, Pons D, et al. Clonic seizure associated with high clozapine plasma level. *J Neuropsychiatry Clin Neurosci* 2001;13(2):302–303.

187. Simpson GM, Cooper TA. Clozapine plasma levels and convulsions. *Am J Psychiatry* 1978;135(1):99–100.

188. Maccrimmon D, Brunet D, Criollo M, et al. Clozapine augments delta, theta, and right frontal EEG alpha power in schizophrenic patients. *ISRN Psychiatry* 2012;2012:596486.

189. Strawn JR, Keck PE, Jr., Caroff SN. Neuroleptic malignant syndrome. *Am J Psychiatry* 2007;164(6):870–876.

190. Lang FU, Lang S, Becker T, et al. Neuroleptic malignant syndrome or catatonia? Trying to solve the catatonic dilemma. *Psychopharmacology (Berl)* 2015;232(1):1–5.

191. Mihara K, Kondo T, Suzuki A, et al. Relationship between functional dopamine D2 and D3 receptors gene polymorphisms and neuroleptic malignant syndrome. *Am J Med Genet B Neuropsychiatr Genet* 2003;117B(1):57–60.

192. Gurrera RJ. Sympathoadrenal hyperactivity and the etiology of neuroleptic malignant syndrome. *Am J Psychiatry* 1999;156(2):169–180.

193. Kramer LD, Locke GE. A case of neuroleptic malignant syndrome with myoclonus and triphasic EEG waves. *J Clin Psychopharmacol* 1987;7(5):354–356.

194. Yoshino A, Yoshimasu H. Nonconvulsive status epilepticus complicating neuroleptic malignant syndrome improved by intravenous diazepam. *J Clin Psychopharmacol* 2000;20(3):389–390.

195. Sindrup SH, Jensen TS. Pharmacologic treatment of pain in polyneuropathy. *Neurology* 2000;55(7):915–920.

196. Maguire MJ, Weston J, Singh J, et al. Antidepressants for people with epilepsy and depression. *Cochrane Database Syst Rev* 2014;12:CD010682.

197. Kugler J, Lorenzi E, Spatz R, et al. Drug-induced paroxysmal EEG-activities. *Pharmakopsychiatr Neuropsychopharmakol* 1979;12(2):165–172.

198. Ducharlet K, Seneviratne U, Sedal L, et al. Seizures during high-dose antidepressant therapy: a case series with clinical and video-electroencephalography characteristics. *Intern Med J* 2013;43(9):1039–1042.

199. Rumpl E, Hinterhuber H. Unusual 'spike-wave stupor' in a patient with manic-depressive psychosis treated with amitriptyline. *J Neurol* 1981;226(2):131–135.

200. Frazer A. Pharmacology of antidepressants. *J Clin Psychopharmacol* 1997;17(Suppl 1):2S–18S.

201. Schmitz B. Antidepressant drugs: indications and guidelines for use in epilepsy. *Epilepsia* 2002;43(Suppl 2):14–18.

202. Dobesberger J, Ristic AJ, Walser G, et al. Selective serotonin reuptake inhibitors prolong seizures—preliminary results from an observational study. *Clin Neurol Neurosurg* 2014;120:89–92.

203. Boyer EW, Shannon M. The serotonin syndrome. *N Engl J Med* 2005;352(11):1112–1120.

204. Cheng PL, Hung SW, Lin LW, et al. Amantadine-induced serotonin syndrome in a patient with renal failure. *Am J Emerg Med* 2008;26(1):112 e115–e116.

205. Perry NK. Venlafaxine-induced serotonin syndrome with relapse following amitriptyline. *Postgrad Med J* 2000;76(894):254–256.

206. Dike GL. Triphasic waves in serotonin syndrome. *J Neurol Neurosurg Psychiatry* 1997;62(2):200.

207. Mittino D, Mula M, Monaco F. Serotonin syndrome associated with tramadol-sertraline coadministration. *Clin Neuropharmacol* 2004;27(3):150–151.

208. Gardner CR, Tully WR, Hedgecock CJ. The rapidly expanding range of neuronal benzodiazepine receptor ligands. *Prog Neurobiol* 1993;40(1):1–61.

209. Doble A, Martin IL. Multiple benzodiazepine receptors: no reason for anxiety. *Trends Pharmacol Sci* 1992;13(2):76–81.

210. Robin C, Trieger N. Paradoxical reactions to benzodiazepines in intravenous sedation: a report of 2 cases and review of the literature. *Anesth Prog* 2002;49(4):128–132.

211. Niedermeyer E. Electroencephalographic studies on the anticonvulsive action of intravenous diazepam. *Eur Neurol* 1970;3(2):88–96.

212. Mitsudome A, Ohfu M, Yasumoto S, et al. The effectiveness of clonazepam on the rolandic discharges. *Brain Dev* 1997;19(4):274–278.

213. Gotman J, Gloor P, Quesney LF, et al. Correlations between EEG changes induced by diazepam and the localization of epileptic spikes and seizures. *Electroencephalogr Clin Neurophysiol* 1982;54(6):614–621.

214. Bastien CH, LeBlanc M, Carrier J, et al. Sleep EEG power spectra, insomnia, and chronic use of benzodiazepines. *Sleep* 2003;26(3):313–317.

215. Brophy GM, Bell R, Claassen J, et al. Guidelines for the evaluation and management of status epilepticus. *Neurocrit Care* 2012;17(1):3–23.

216. Sutter R, Rüegg S. Predicting outcome in adults with status epilepticus. *Zeitschrift für Epileptologie* 2013;26:79–84.

217. Martinez-Cano H, Vela-Bueno A, de Iceta M, et al. Benzodiazepine withdrawal syndrome seizures. *Pharmacopsychiatry* 1995;28(6):257–262.

218. Gijsenbergh FP, Pillen EJ, Delooz HH. Differential diagnostic value and influence on EEG of Anexate (flumazenil, Ro 15-1788) in benzodiazepine-intoxication. A case report. *Acta Anaesthesiol Belg* 1989;40(2):127–129.

219. Sun H, Wu SH. The physiological role of pre- and postsynaptic GABA(B) receptors in membrane excitability and synaptic transmission of neurons in the rat's dorsal cortex of the inferior colliculus. *Neuroscience* 2009;160(1):198–211.

220. Schuele SU, Kellinghaus C, Shook SJ, et al. Incidence of seizures in patients with multiple sclerosis treated with intrathecal baclofen. *Neurology* 2005;64(6):1086–1087.

221. Kofler M, Arturo Leis A. Prolonged seizure activity after baclofen withdrawal. *Neurology* 1992;42(3 Pt 1):697–698.

222. Hyser CL, Drake ME, Jr. Status epilepticus after baclofen withdrawal. *J Natl Med Assoc* 1984;76(5):533, 537–538.

223. Fakhoury T, Abou-Khalil B, Blumenkopf B. EEG changes in intrathecal baclofen overdose: a case report and review of the literature. *Electroencephalogr Clin Neurophysiol* 1998;107(5):339–342.

224. Specchio N, Carotenuto A, Trivisano M, et al. Prolonged episode of dystonia and dyskinesia resembling status epilepticus following acute intrathecal baclofen withdrawal. *Epilepsy Behav* 2011;21(3):321–323.

225. Sutter R, Ruegg S, Tschudin-Sutter S. Seizures as adverse events of antibiotic drugs: a systematic review. *Neurology* 2015;85(15):1332–1341.

226. Boston Collaborative Drug Surveillance Program. Drug-induced convulsions. *Lancet* 1972;2(7779):677–679.

227. Kurtzman NA, Rogers PW, Harter HR. Neurotoxic reaction to penicillin and carbenicillin. *JAMA* 1970;214(7):1320–1321.

228. Lin CS, Cheng CJ, Chou CH, et al. Piperacillin/tazobactam-induced seizure rapidly reversed by high flux hemodialysis in a patient on peritoneal dialysis. *Am J Med Sci* 2007;333(3):181–184.

229. Fernandez-Torre JL, Santos-Sanchez C, Pelayo AL. De novo generalised non-convulsive status epilepticus triggered by piperacillin/tazobactam. *Seizure* 2010;19(8):529–530.

230. Sugimoto M, Uchida I, Mashimo T, et al. Evidence for the involvement of GABA(A) receptor blockade in convulsions induced by cephalosporins. *Neuropharmacology* 2003;45(3):304–314.

231. Yost RL, Lee JD, O'Leary JP. Convulsions associated with sodium cefazolin: a case report. *Am Surg* 1977;43(6):417–420.

232. Bechtel TP, Slaughter RL, Moore TD. Seizures associated with high cerebrospinal fluid concentrations of cefazolin. *Am J Hosp Pharm* 1980;37(2):271–273.

233. Ozturk S, Kocabay G, Topcular B, et al. Non-convulsive status epilepticus following antibiotic therapy as a cause of unexplained loss of consciousness in patients with renal failure. *Clin Exp Nephrol* 2009;13(2):138–144.

234. Norrby SR. Neurotoxicity of carbapenem antibacterials. *Drug Saf* 1996;15(2):87–90.

235. Hunter WJ. Imipenem-induced seizure: a case of inappropriate, excessive, and prolonged surgical prophylaxis. *Hosp Pharm* 1993;28(10):986–988.

236. Calandra G, Lydick E, Carrigan J, et al. Factors predisposing to seizures in seriously ill infected patients receiving antibiotics: experience with imipenem/cilastatin. *Am J Med* 1988;84(5):911–918.

237. Koppel BS, Hauser WA, Politis C, et al. Seizures in the critically ill: the role of imipenem. *Epilepsia* 2001;42(12):1590–1593.

238. Semel JD, Allen N. Seizures in patients simultaneously receiving theophylline and imipenem or ciprofloxacin or metronidazole. *South Med J* 1991;84(4):465–468.

239. Isaacson SH, Carr J, Rowan AJ. Ciprofloxacin-induced complex partial status epilepticus manifesting as an acute confusional state. *Neurology* 1993;43(8):1619–1621.

240. Agbaht K, Bitik B, Piskinpasa S, et al. Ciprofloxacin-associated seizures in a patient with underlying thyrotoxicosis: case report and literature review. *Int J Clin Pharmacol Ther* 2009;47(5):303–310.

241. Conway N, Beck E, Somerville J. Penicillin encephalopathy. *Postgrad Med J* 1968;44(518):891–897.

242. Bloomer HA, Barton LJ, Maddock RK, Jr. Penicillin-induced encephalopathy in uremic patients. *JAMA* 1967;200(2):121–123.

243. Lavy S, Stein H. Convulsions in septicemic patients treated by penicillin. The value of electroencephalograph examination. *Arch Surg* 1970;100(3):225–228.

244. FDA. Drug Safety Communication: Cefepime and risk of seizure in patients not receiving dosage adjustments for kidney impairment. FDA; 2013 [cited 29.04.2015]; Available from: http://www.fda.gov/Drugs/DrugSafety/ucm309661.htm.

245. Naeije G, Lorent S, Vincent JL, et al. Continuous epileptiform discharges in patients treated with cefepime or meropenem. *Arch Neurol* 2011;68(10):1303–1307.

246. Jallon P, Fankhauser L, Du Pasquier R, et al. Severe but reversible encephalopathy associated with cefepime. *Neurophysiol Clin* 2000;30(6):383–386.

247. Gijtenbeek JM, van den Bent MJ, Vecht CJ. Cyclosporine neurotoxicity: a review. *J Neurol* 1999;246(5):339–346.

248. Dzudie A, Boissonnat P, Roussoulieres A, et al. Cyclosporine-related posterior reversible encephalopathy syndrome after heart transplantation: should we withdraw or reduce cyclosporine?: case reports. *Transplant Proc* 2009;41(2):716–720.

249. de Groen PC, Aksamit AJ, Rakela J, et al. Central nervous system toxicity after liver transplantation. The role of cyclosporine and cholesterol. *N Engl J Med* 1987;317(14):861–866.

250. Serkova NJ, Christians U, Benet LZ. Biochemical mechanisms of cyclosporine neurotoxicity. *Mol Interv* 2004;4(2):97–107.

251. Natsume J, Sofue A, Yamada A, et al. Electroencephalographic (EEG) findings in posterior reversible encephalopathy associated with immunosuppressants. *J Child Neurol* 2006;21(7):620–623.

252. Melgari JM, Curcio G, Mastrolilli F, et al. Alpha and beta EEG power reflects L-dopa acute administration in parkinsonian patients. *Front Aging Neurosci* 2014;6:302.

253. Neufeld MY. Periodic triphasic waves in levodopa-induced encephalopathy. *Neurology* 1992;42(2):444–446.

254. Kearse LA, Jr., Koski G, Husain MV, et al. Epileptiform activity during opioid anesthesia. *Electroencephalogr Clin Neurophysiol* 1993;87(6):374–379.

255. Fingelkurts AA, Fingelkurts AA, Kivisaari R, et al. Opioid withdrawal results in an increased local and remote functional connectivity at EEG alpha and beta frequency bands. *Neurosci Res* 2007;58(1):40–49.

256. Kay DC, Pickworth WB, Neidert GL, et al. Opioid effects on computer-derived sleep and EEG parameters in nondependent human addicts. *Sleep* 1979;2(2):175–191.

257. Shadnia S, Brent J, Mousavi-Fatemi K, et al. Recurrent seizures in tramadol intoxication: implications for therapy based on 100 patients. *Basic Clin Pharmacol Toxicol* 2012;111(2):133–136.

258. Schmid Y, Enzler F, Gasser P, et al. Acute effects of lysergic acid diethylamide in healthy subjects. *Biol Psychiatry* 2015;78(8):544–553.

259. Brown BB. Subjective and EEG responses to LSD in visualizer and non-visualizer subjects. *Electroencephalogr Clin Neurophysiol* 1968;25(4):372–379.

260. Iversen L. Cannabis and the brain. *Brain* 2003;126(Pt 6):1252–1270.

261. Messinis L, Kyprianidou A, Malefaki S, et al. Neuropsychological deficits in long-term frequent cannabis users. *Neurology* 2006;66(5):737–739.

262. Nordentoft M, Hjorthoj C. Cannabis use and risk of psychosis in later life. *Lancet* 2007;370(9584):293–294.

263. Herning RI, Better W, Cadet JL. EEG of chronic marijuana users during abstinence: relationship to years of marijuana use, cerebral blood flow and thyroid function. *Clin Neurophysiol* 2008;119(2):321–331.

264. Davis KM, Wu JY. Role of glutamatergic and GABAergic systems in alcoholism. *J Biomed Sci* 2001;8(1):7–19.

265. Sand T, Brathen G, Michler R, et al. Clinical utility of EEG in alcohol-related seizures. *Acta Neurol Scand* 2002;105(1):18–24.

266. Leone M, Tonini C, Bogliun G, et al. Chronic alcohol use and first symptomatic epileptic seizures. *J Neurol Neurosurg Psychiatry* 2002;73(5):495–499.

267. Fernandez-Torre JL, Kaplan PW. Subacute encephalopathy with seizures in alcoholics (SESA syndrome) revisited. *Seizure* 2014;23(5):393–396.

268. Lukas SE, Mendelson JH, Woods BT, et al. Topographic distribution of EEG alpha activity during ethanol-induced intoxication in women. *J Stud Alcohol* 1989;50(2):176–185.

269. Ehlers CL, Wall TL, Schuckit MA. EEG spectral characteristics following ethanol administration in young men. *Electroencephalogr Clin Neurophysiol* 1989;73(3):179–187.

270. Mani J, Sitajayalakshmi S, Borgohain R, et al. Subacute encephalopathy with seizures in alcoholism. *Seizure* 2003;12(2):126–129.

271. Fujiwara T, Watanabe M, Matsuda K, et al. Complex partial status epilepticus provoked by ingestion of alcohol: a case report. *Epilepsia* 1991;32(5):650–656.

272. Krauss GL, Niedermeyer E. Electroencephalogram and seizures in chronic alcoholism. *Electroencephalogr Clin Neurophysiol* 1991;78(2):97–104.

273. Leshner AI. Molecular mechanisms of cocaine addiction. *N Engl J Med* 1996;335(2):128–129.

274. Luscher C, Bellone C. Cocaine-evoked synaptic plasticity: a key to addiction? *Nat Neurosci* 2008;11(7):737–738.

275. Noble EP. D2 dopamine receptor gene in psychiatric and neurologic disorders and its phenotypes. *Am J Med Genet B Neuropsychiatr Genet* 2003;116B(1):103–125.

276. Mody CK, Miller BL, McIntyre HB, et al. Neurologic complications of cocaine abuse. *Neurology* 1988;38(8):1189–1193.

277. Van Stavern GP, Gorman M. Orbital infarction after cocaine use. *Neurology* 2002;59(4):642–643.

278. Migita DS, Devereaux MW, Tomsak RL. Cocaine and pupillary-sparing oculomotor nerve paresis. *Neurology* 1997;49(5):1466–1467.

279. Mantelli F, Lambiase A, Sacchetti M, et al. Cocaine snorting may induce ocular surface damage through corneal sensitivity impairment. *Graefes Arch Clin Exp Ophthalmol* 2015;253(5):765–772.

280. Chang TR, Kowalski RG, Caserta F, et al. Impact of acute cocaine use on aneurysmal subarachnoid hemorrhage. *Stroke* 2013;44(7):1825–1829.

281. Shvartsbeyn M, Phillips DG, Markey MA, et al. Cocaine-induced intracerebral hemorrhage in a patient with cerebral amyloid angiopathy. *J Forensic Sci* 2010;55(5):1389–1392.

282. Krendel DA, Ditter SM, Frankel MR, et al. Biopsy-proven cerebral vasculitis associated with cocaine abuse. *Neurology* 1990;40(7):1092–1094.

283. Frucht S. Cocaine-induced persistent dyskinesias. *Neurology* 2001;57(8):1525.

284. Weiner WJ, Rabinstein A, Levin B, et al. Cocaine-induced persistent dyskinesias. *Neurology* 2001;56(7):964–965.

285. Herning RI, Jones RT, Hooker WD, et al. Cocaine increases EEG beta: a replication and extension of Hans Berger's historic experiments. *Electroencephalogr Clin Neurophysiol* 1985;60(6):470–477.

286. Copersino ML, Herning RI, Better W, et al. EEG and cerebral blood flow velocity abnormalities in chronic cocaine users. *Clin EEG Neurosci* 2009;40(1):39–42.

287. Levin KH, Herning RI, Better WE, et al. EEG absolute power during extended cocaine abstinence. *J Addict Med* 2007;1(3):139–144.

288. Majlesi N, Shih R, Fiesseler FW, et al. Cocaine-associated seizures and incidence of status epilepticus. *West J Emerg Med* 2010;11(2):157–160.

289. Ogunyemi AO, Locke GE, Kramer LD, et al. Complex partial status epilepticus provoked by "crack" cocaine. *Ann Neurol* 1989;26(6):785–786.

290. Kim JH, Chang KH, Song IC, et al. Delayed encephalopathy of acute carbon monoxide intoxication: diffusivity of cerebral white matter lesions. *AJNR Am J Neuroradiol* 2003;24(8):1592–1597.

291. Quinn DK, McGahee SM, Politte LC, et al. Complications of carbon monoxide poisoning: a case discussion and review of the literature. *Prim Care Companion J Clin Psychiatry* 2009;11(2):74–79.

292. Madison D, Niedermeyer E. Epileptic seizures resulting from acute cerebral anoxia. *J Neurol Neurosurg Psychiatry* 1970;33(3):381–386.

293. Neufeld MY, Swanson JW, Klass DW. Localized EEG abnormalities in acute carbon monoxide poisoning. *Arch Neurol* 1981;38(8):524–527.

294. Murata M, Suzuki M, Hasegawa Y, et al. Improvement of occipital alpha activity by repetitive hyperbaric oxygen therapy in patients with carbon monoxide poisoning: a possible indicator for treatment efficacy. *J Neurol Sci* 2005;235(1-2):69–74.

295. Nowack R, Ritz E. Lead intoxication: new insights into an old problem. *Pediatr Nephrol* 1992;6(3):287–291.

296. Jeyaratnam J, Devathasan G, Ong CN, et al. Neurophysiological studies on workers exposed to lead. *Br J Industr Med* 1985;42(3):173–177.

297. Kovala T, Matikainen E, Mannelin T, et al. Effects of low level exposure to lead on neurophysiological functions among lead battery workers. *Occup Environ Med* 1997;54(7):487–493.

298. Mahaffey KR. Methylmercury: a new look at the risks. *Public Health Rep* 1999;114(5):396–399, 402–313.

299. Brenner RP, Snyder RD. Late EEG findings and clinical status after organic mercury poisoning. *Arch Neurol* 1980;37(5):282–284.

300. Urban P, Nerudova J, Cabelkova Z, et al. EEG photic driving in workers exposed to mercury vapors. *Neurotoxicology* 2003;24(1):23–33.

301. Ky SQ, Deng HS, Xie PY, et al. A report of two cases of chronic serious manganese poisoning treated with sodium para-aminosalicylic acid. *Br J Industr Med* 1992;49(1):66–69.

302. Lee JW. Manganese intoxication. *Arch Neurol* 2000;57(4):597–599.

303. Nabys E-D, Kayed KS, Aref MA. EEG induced fast activity in chronic manganese poisoning. *Acta Neurol Scand* 1964;40:259–268.

304. Sinczuk-Walczak H, Jakubowski M, Matczak W. Neurological and neurophysiological examinations of workers occupationally exposed to manganese. *Int J Occup Med Environ Health* 2001;14(4):329–337.

305. Alfrey AC, LeGendre GR, Kaehny WD. The dialysis encephalopathy syndrome. Possible aluminum intoxication. *N Engl J Med* 1976;294(4):184–188.

306. Poisson M, Mashaly R, Lebkiri B. Dialysis encephalopathy: recovery after interruption of aluminium intake. *Br Med J* 1978;2(6152):1610–1611.

307. Aasly JO. Thallium intoxication with metallic skin discoloration. *Neurology* 2007;68(21):1869.

308. Zhao G, Ding M, Zhang B, et al. Clinical manifestations and management of acute thallium poisoning. *Eur Neurol* 2008;60(6):292–297.

309. Tsai YT, Huang CC, Kuo HC, et al. Central nervous system effects in acute thallium poisoning. *Neurotoxicology* 2006;27(2):291–295.

310. Hanif M, Mobarak MR, Ronan A, et al. Fatal renal failure caused by diethylene glycol in paracetamol elixir: the Bangladesh epidemic. *BMJ* 1995;311(6997):88–91.

311. Rollins YD, Filley CM, McNutt JT, et al. Fulminant ascending paralysis as a delayed sequela of diethylene glycol (Sterno) ingestion. *Neurology* 2002;59(9):1460–1463.

312. Zhou L, Zabad R, Lewis RA. Ethylene glycol intoxication: electrophysiological studies suggest a polyradiculopathy. *Neurology* 2002;59(11):1809–1810.

313. Steinke W, Arendt G, Mull M, et al. Good recovery after sublethal ethylene glycol intoxication: serial EEG and CT findings. *J Neurol* 1989;236(3):170–173.

314. Kurtz D. The EEG in acute and chronic drug intoxications. In: Glaser GH, ed. *Metabolic, endocrine and toxic diseases/Handbook of electroencephalography and clinical neurophysiology.* Amsterdam: Elsevier; 1976, pp. 88–104.

315. Duffy FH, Burchfiel JL, Bartels PH, et al. Long-term effects of an organophosphate upon the human electroencephalogram. *Toxicol Appl Pharmacol* 1979;47(1):161–176.

316. Blume WT, Luders HO, Mizrahi E, et al. Glossary of descriptive terminology for ictal semiology: report of the ILAE task force on classification and terminology. *Epilepsia* 2001;42(9):1212–1218.

317. Niedermeyer E. The Lennox-Gastaut syndrome: a severe type of childhood epilepsy. *Dtsch Z Nervenheilkd* 1969;195(4):263–282.

318. Arzimanoglou A, French J, Blume WT, et al. Lennox-Gastaut syndrome: a consensus approach on diagnosis, assessment, management, and trial methodology. *Lancet Neurol* 2009;8(1):82–93.

319. Goldsmith IL, Zupanc ML, Buchhalter JR. Long-term seizure outcome in 74 patients with Lennox-Gastaut syndrome: effects of incorporating MRI head imaging in defining the cryptogenic subgroup. *Epilepsia* 2000;41(4):395–399.

320. Yagi K. Evolution of Lennox-Gastaut syndrome: a long-term longitudinal study. *Epilepsia* 1996;37(Suppl 3):48–51.

321. Olmos-Garcia de Alba G, Valdez JM, Crespo FV. West syndrome evolving into the Lennox-Gastaut syndrome. *Clin Electroencephalogr* 1984;15(1):61–68.

322. Widdess-Walsh P, Dlugos D, Fahlstrom R, et al. Lennox-Gastaut syndrome of unknown cause: phenotypic characteristics of patients in the Epilepsy Phenome/Genome Project. *Epilepsia* 2013;54(11):1898–1904.

323. Ferlazzo E, Nikanorova M, Italiano D, et al. Lennox-Gastaut syndrome in adulthood: clinical and EEG features. *Epilepsy Res* 2010;89(2-3):271–277.

324. Hughes JR, Patil VK. Long-term electro-clinical changes in the Lennox-Gastaut syndrome before, during, and after the slow spike-wave pattern. *Clin Electroencephalogr* 2002;33(1):1–7.

325. Ogawa K, Kanemoto K, Ishii Y, et al. Long-term follow-up study of Lennox-Gastaut syndrome in patients with severe motor and intellectual disabilities: with special reference to the problem of dysphagia. *Seizure* 2001;10(3):197–202.

326. Oguni H, Hayashi K, Osawa M. Long-term prognosis of Lennox-Gastaut syndrome. *Epilepsia* 1996;37 Suppl 3:44–47.

327. Sutter R, Stevens RD, Kaplan WP. Clinical and imaging correlates of EEG patterns in hospitalized patients with encephalopathy. *J Neurol* 2013;260(4):1087–1098.

328. Chatrian GE. Coma, other states of altered responsiveness, and brain death. In: Daly DD, Pedley TA, eds. *Current practice of clinical electroencephalography.* 2 ed. New York: Raven Press; 1990, pp. 425–487.

329. Husain AM. Electroencephalographic assessment of coma. *J Clin Neurophysiol* 2006;23(3):208–220.

330. Besch G, Liu N, Samain E, et al. Occurrence of and risk factors for electroencephalogram burst suppression during propofol-remifentanil anaesthesia. *Br J Anaesth* 2011;107(5):749–756.

331. Deleu D, Ebinger G. Alpha coma with sedative overdose. *Neurology* 1989;39(1):156–157.

332. Berkhoff M, Donati F, Bassetti C. Postanoxic alpha (theta) coma: a reappraisal of its prognostic significance. *Clin Neurophysiol* 2000;111(2):297–304.

333. Chatrian G-E, Turella GS. Electrophysiological evaluation of coma, other altered states of diminished responsiveness and brain death. In: Ebersole JS, Pedley TA, eds. *Current practice of clinical electroencephalography.* Philadelphia: Raven Press; 2003, pp. 405–462.

334. Cordeau JP. Monorhythmic frontal delta activity in the human electroencephalogram: a study of 100 cases. *Electroencephalogr Clin Neurophysiol* 1959;11:733–746.

335. Cobb WA. Rhythmic slow discharges in the electroencephalogram. *J Neurol Neurosurg Psychiatry* 1945;8:65–78.

336. Faure J, Droogleever-Fortuyn J, Gastaut H, et al. [Genesis and significance of rhythms recorded at a distance in cases of cerebral tumors]. *Electroencephalogr Clin Neurophysiol* 1951;3(4):429–434.

337. Jasper H, Van Buren J. Interrelationship between cortex and subcortical structures: clinical electroencephalographic studies. *Electroencephalogr Clin Neurophysiol* 1955;Suppl. 4:168–188.

338. Boulanger JM, Deacon C, Lecuyer D, et al. Triphasic waves versus nonconvulsive status epilepticus: EEG distinction. *Can J Neurol Sci* 2006;33(2):175–180.

339. Blatt I, Brenner RP. Triphasic waves in a psychiatric population: a retrospective study. *J Clin Neurophysiol* 1996;13(4):324–329.

340. Kenangil G, Orken DN, Yalcin D, et al. Triphasic EEG pattern in bilateral paramedian thalamic infarction. *Clin EEG Neurosci* 2008;39(4):185–190.

341. Eriksson G, Wictor L. EEG with triphasic waves in *Borrelia burgdorferi* meningoencephalitis. *Acta Neurol Scand* 2007;116(2):133–136.

342. Young GB, Bolton CF, Archibald YM, et al. The electroencephalogram in sepsis-associated encephalopathy. *J Clin Neurophysiol* 1992;9(1):145–152.

343. Schauble B, Castillo PR, Boeve BF, et al. EEG findings in steroid-responsive encephalopathy associated with autoimmune thyroiditis. *Clin Neurophysiol* 2003;114(1):32–37.

344. Lee S. Pregabalin intoxication-induced encephalopathy with triphasic waves. *Epilepsy Behav* 2012;25(2):170–173.

345. Townsend JB, Drury I. Triphasic waves in coma from brainstem infarction. *Eur Neurol* 1991;31(1):47–49.

346. Samanta J, Dhiman RK, Khatri A, et al. Correlation between degree and quality of sleep disturbance and the level of neuropsychiatric impairment in patients with liver cirrhosis. *Metab Brain Dis* 2013;28(2):249–259.

347. Merlino G, Gigli GL, Valente M. Sleep disturbances in dialysis patients. *J Nephrol* 2008;21(Suppl 13):S66–S70.

348. Sutter R, Barnes B, Leyva A, et al. Electroencephalographic sleep elements and outcome in acute encephalopathic patients: a 4-year cohort study. *Eur J Neurol* 2014;21(10):1268–1275.

349. Kaplan PW, Sutter R. Seeing more clearly through the fog of encephalopathy. *J Clin Neurophysiol* 2013;30(5):431–434.

PART IV | CLINICAL EEG IN THE EVALUATION OF SEIZURES, EPILEPSY, ACUTE BRAIN INSULTS, AND RELATED DISORDERS

18 | SEIZURES AND EPILEPSY IN PRETERM AND TERM NEONATES, INFANTS, CHILDREN, AND ADOLESCENTS

JULES C. BEAL, MD, MONIKA EISERMANN, MD, SUNITA MISRA, MD, PHD, PHILLIP L. PEARL, MD, PERRINE PLOUIN, MD, ELI M. MIZRAHI, MD, AND SOLOMON L. MOSHE, MD

ABSTRACT: Children are often affected by seizure types and epilepsy syndromes that are specific to their age group and distinct from those seen in adults. At the same time, certain epilepsy syndromes affecting the adult population, such as Lennox–Gastaut syndrome and juvenile myoclonic epilepsy, often begin during childhood, as do seizures related to genetic abnormalities. The use of electroencephalography (EEG) and prolonged EEG monitoring has allowed for further insight and greater specificity in identifying and understanding seizures and epilepsy syndromes in children. This chapter reviews the role of EEG in pediatric seizures and the pediatric epilepsies, including electrographic findings in the ictal state and in the interictal period, as well as the correlation with clinical seizure semiology as it contributes to the diagnosis of epileptic phenomena. The chapter discusses EEG patterns, seizure types, and epilepsy syndromes specific to neonates, infants, children, and adolescents.

KEYWORDS: EEG, electroencephalography, epilepsy, seizures, pediatric

PRINCIPAL REFERENCES

1. Glauser TA, Cnaan A, Shinnar S, et al. Ethosuximide, valproic acid, and lamotrigine in childhood absence epilepsy: initial monotherapy outcomes at 12 months. *Epilepsia.* 2013; 54: 141–155.
2. Berg AT, Berkovic SF, Brodie MJ, Buchhalter J, et al. Revised terminology and concepts for organization of seizures and epilepsies: report of the ILAE Commission on Classification and Terminology, 2005–2009. *Epilepsia.* 2010; 51: 676–685.
3. Shinnar S, Bello JA, Chan S, et al. MRI abnormalities following febrile status epilepticus in children: the FEBSTAT Study. *Neurology.* 2012; 79: 871–877.
4. Sadleir LG, Farrell K, Smith S. Electroclinical features of absence seizures in childhood absence epilepsy. *Neurology.* 2006; 67: 413–418.
5. Mizrahi EM, Kellaway P. Characterization and classification of neonatal seizures. *Neurology.* 1987; 37(12): 1837–1844.
6. Arzimanoglou A, French J, Blume WT, et al. Lennox-Gastaut syndrome: a consensus approach on diagnosis, assessment, management, and trial methodology. *Lancet Neurol.* 2009; 8: 82–93.
7. Pellock JM, Hrachovy R, Shinnar S, et al. Infantile spasms: a U.S. consensus report. *Epilepsia.* 2010; 51(10): 2175–2189.
8. Yamatogi Y, Ohtahara S. Early-infantile epileptic encephalopathy with suppression-bursts, Ohtahara syndrome; its overview referring to our 16 cases. *Brain Devel.* 2002; 24(1): 13–23.
9. Gibbs FA, Gibbs EL. *Atlas of Electroencephalography.* Reading, MA: Addison-Wesley; 1952.
10. Bureau M, Genton P, Dravet C, Delgado-Escueta A, Tassinari CA, Thomas P, Wolf P, eds. *Epileptic Syndromes in Infancy, Childhood and Adolescence.* John Libbey Eurotext Ltd; 2012: 125–156.

1. INTRODUCTION

Seizures are among the most common neurological conditions occurring in the pediatric population. Children are often affected by seizure types and epilepsy syndromes that are specific to their age group and distinct from those seen in adult patients. At the same time certain epilepsy syndromes affecting the adult population, such as Lennox–Gastaut syndrome (LGS) or juvenile myoclonic epilepsy, often begin during childhood, as do seizures related to genetic abnormalities. The use of electroencephalography (EEG) and prolonged EEG monitoring has allowed for further insight and greater specificity in identifying and understanding seizures and epilepsy syndromes in the pediatric population.

In this chapter we review the role of EEG in pediatric seizures and the pediatric epilepsies, including electrographic findings both in the ictal state and in the interictal period, as well as the correlation with clinical seizure semiology as it contributes to the diagnosis of epileptic phenomena. Specific EEG patterns as they relate to the pediatric population as well as seizure types and epilepsy syndromes specific to neonates, infants, children, and adolescents are discussed.

2. EEG PATTERNS IN PEDIATRIC PATIENTS

2.1. Focal Interictal Epileptiform Discharges

Spikes and sharp waves are neurophysiologically closely related phenomena; both are typical epileptiform discharges and highly suggestive of an epileptic seizure disorder, although either may occur in patients without a history of a seizure disorder. At times, the terms *spikes* and *sharp waves* have been appropriately used synonymously when discussing the clinical significance of a focal transient.

2.1.1. SPIKES

According to the International Federation of Societies for Electroencephalogram and Clinical Neurophysiology, a spike is an electrographic transient, clearly distinguished from the background activity, with a pointed peak at conventional paper speed and a duration from 20 to <70 msec, with its main component generally negative in polarity with variable amplitude (1). While there are common characteristics among spikes, there are also remarkable variations in the appearance of spikes in individual patients and even between one spike and the next in the same lead (2). A sequence of a minor positive, a major

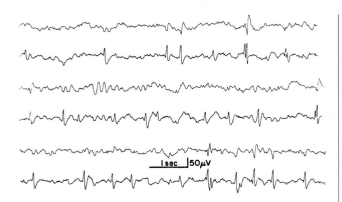

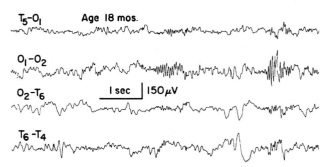

Figure 18.1. *Two-channel recording of various wave morphologies of spikes recorded from the same patient (age 6 years). Tracing 1, T3-T5; Tracing 2, T5-O1. Each lead is continued in successive individual tracings (Tracing 3, T3-T5; Tracing 4, T5-O1; Tracing 5, T3-T5; Tracing 6, T5-O1). Note the multiphasic character of spikes with predominance of the negative phase and occasional formation of double spikes. (With permission from Nordli DR, Riviello JJ, Niedermeyer E. Seizures and epilepsy in infants to adolescents. In Schomer DL, Lopes deSilva FH, eds. Niedermeyer's Electroencephalography, 6th ed. Philadelphia: Lippincott Williams & Wilkins, Fig. 26.1.)*

Figure 18.2. *Distinguishing polyspikes from drug-induced fast activity may be difficult. There is a run of beta activity in the center of the figure and to the right a burst-like run of activity, which represents polyspike activity. A definitive statement depends on the impressions derived from the entire record. (With permission from Nordli DR, Riviello JJ, Niedermeyer E. Seizures and epilepsy in infants to adolescents. In Schomer DL, Lopes deSilva FH, eds. Niedermeyer's Electroencephalography, 6th ed. Philadelphia: Lippincott Williams & Wilkins, Fig. 26.6.)*

negative, and a second minor positive component (Fig. 18.1) may be typical in many instances, although some spikes may appear multiphasic. In other spikes, a slow negative component may trail the spike discharge and often attain about the same amplitude as the negative main component of the spike. Single spikes recorded on the scalp with predominant positive component are rare (3) and when found raise the possibility of defective superficial cortical laminae. However, with dipole formation (especially in benign epilepsy with centrotemporal spikes), a positive spike discharge may be found a moderate distance from the negative spike focus (4).

2.1.2. Sharp Waves

According to the International Federation of Societies for Electroencephalogram and Clinical Neurophysiology (1), a sharp wave is a transient, clearly distinguished from background activity, with a pointed peak at conventional paper speed and a duration of 70 to 200 msec. The main component is generally negative relative to the other components. The term is restricted to epileptiform discharges and does not apply to distinctive physiological waveforms, such as vertex sharp transients, lambda waves, and positive occipital sharp transients of sleep. Jasper (5) pointed out that the rising phase of the sharp wave is of the same order of magnitude as in spikes, but the descending phase is prolonged.

2.1.3. Multiple Spike Complex or Polyspike Complex

This discharge type represents a complex of spikes and may also be called a *polyspike complex* or *multiple spike complex* (1). It has been defined as a complex paroxysmal EEG pattern with close association of two or more diphasic spikes occurring more or less rhythmically in bursts of variable duration, generally with large amplitudes (6) (Fig. 18.2).

2.1.4. Runs of Rapid Spikes

This pattern has been described as "grand mal discharge" (7), "fast paroxysmal rhythms" (8), "rhythmic spikes" (9), and

"generalized paroxysmal fast activity" (10). It is seen primarily in sleep in older children, adolescents, and younger adults (Fig. 18.3). The repetition rate is in most cases somewhat irregular. The bursts last for ~2 to 10 sec; bursts of >5 sec in duration are usually associated with clinical seizures and thus represent an ictal pattern. Although focal, the finding has been associated with LGS (9). According to Niedermeyer it is hardly ever found outside this clinical entity (11), although may occur in all so-called imitators of LGS (12). Little is known about the underlying neurophysiological mechanisms of this pattern. It most likely arises from the frontal lobe, and the associated tonic seizures probably arise from the premotor and supplementary motor portions of the frontal lobes.

2.2. Generalized Interictal Epileptiform Discharges

2.2.1. Spike-and-Slow-Wave Complex (Classical 3-Hz Spike-Wave)

Classical 3-Hz spike-wave complexes are widely known even outside the community of electroencephalographers. It is officially termed *spike-and-slow-wave complex* (1) and is defined as "a pattern consisting of a spike followed by a slow wave," abridged as *3-Hz spike wave*. Older terms such as *spike-and-dome complex, wave-and-spike complex,* and *dart-and-dome complex* are historical terms and no longer used. Spike-wave complexes of the classical variety (3 Hz) have been described as the EEG pattern of absence seizures and have been equated with the disorder. While this was reinforced by the early term *petit mal discharge* (7), Niedermeyer cautioned against the use of this term since such spike-wave discharge as an interictal event correlates with the occurrence of absence epilepsy only in a moderate percentage of patients (~16%) (13,14).

The distinction between classical (3 Hz), slow (1–2.5 Hz), and fast (4–5 Hz) spike-wave complexes can, in part, be made on the basis of different clinical correlates of each spike-wave type. The classical 3-Hz spike-wave discharge is most typical and most pronounced in children with absence seizures. Clinical absences are usually present when the burst duration

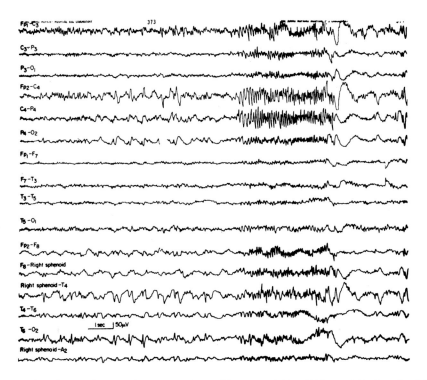

Figure 18.3. *A run of rapid spikes in the right central-temporal region in a 19-year-old patient with LGS. (With permission from Nordli DR, Riviello JJ, Niedermeyer E. Seizures and epilepsy in infants to adolescents. In Schomer DL, Lopes deSilva FH, eds. Niedermeyer's Electroencephalography, 6th ed. Philadelphia: Lippincott Williams & Wilkins, Fig. 26.7.)*

is >3 to 5 sec; shorter bursts are usually subclinical. The classical spike-wave complex is, in most cases, easily activated by hyperventilation, whereas the slow and the fast forms of this discharge show little or no enhancement.

A classical 3-Hz spike-wave burst does not run exactly at a rate of 3 Hz. The complexes are faster at the onset of the burst (mostly ~4 Hz), then slow to 3.5 and 3 Hz for the main portion, and eventually slow to 2.5 Hz at the end of the burst. During a burst, the spike discharges become gradually smaller, often shrinking to insignificance (Fig. 18.4) as in drowsiness and sleep.

2.2.2. SPIKE-WAVE COMPLEX (SLOW, 1–2.5 Hz)

After the demonstration of the 3-Hz spike-wave complex and its relationship to the absence seizure, the occurrence of slow spike-wave complexes was observed in a much different type of patient with seizures other than typical absence. Initially, the classical 3-Hz spike-wave complex was termed *petit mal discharge* and, subsequently, the slow spike-wave complex was termed *petit mal variant discharge*. The wave morphology of the slow spike-wave pattern varies considerably. In the majority, the complex consists of a rather slow spike (according to the definition, a sharp wave, lasting 70 msec or longer) and a

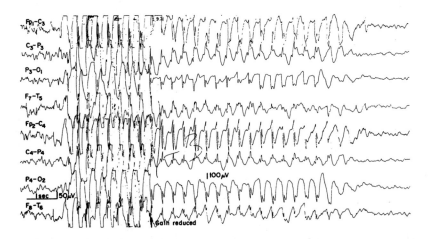

Figure 18.4. *Absence seizure associated with 3-Hz generalized spike-wave complexes. The high amplitude of the complexes at onset prompted lowering of the sensitivity gain. Voltage is maximum anterior and there is a gradual decline of the spike component toward the end of the discharge associated with a gradual slowing of the frequency to ~2.5 Hz. (With permission from Nordli DR, Riviello JJ, Niedermeyer E. Seizures and epilepsy in infants to adolescents. In Schomer DL, Lopes deSilva FH, eds. Niedermeyer's Electroencephalography, 6th ed. Philadelphia: Lippincott Williams & Wilkins, Fig. 26.8.)*

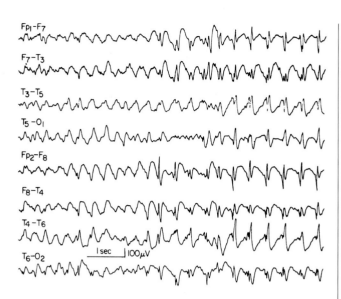

Figure 18.5. Generalized slow spike and slow wave complexes (~2 Hz) in a child with LGS. (With permission from Nordli DR, Riviello JJ, Niedermeyer E. Seizures and epilepsy in infants to adolescents. In Schomer DL, Lopes deSilva FH, eds. Niedermeyer's Electroencephalography, 6th ed. Philadelphia: Lippincott Williams & Wilkins, Fig. 26.9)

slow wave, although in some cases true spikes (60 msec or less in duration) are followed by a slow wave (Fig. 18.5).

The distinction between slow (1–2.5 Hz) and classical (3 Hz) spike-waves is clinically significant. However, many children or adolescents with slow spike waves can also show series of 3-Hz or even 4-Hz spike-wave complexes; the presence of the faster spike-wave discharges has less clinical significance than the slow type. On the other hand, patients with classical 3-Hz spike-wave complexes and a usually benign type of seizure disorder usually do not show slow spike-waves except when the frequency of a 3-Hz or 4-Hz spike-wave burst may slow down to 2.5 Hz at the end.

2.2.3. SPIKE-WAVE COMPLEX (FAST 4 Hz, 4–5 Hz)

This pattern is closely related to the classical 3-Hz spike-wave complex and often both discharge types are grouped together. However, Gastaut (15) described the distinctive features between the 3-Hz and the 4-Hz (or 4–5 Hz) spike-wave discharge: the fast spike-wave burst is usually of shorter duration (1–3 sec), it occurs in patients older than 15 years, the bursts are always subclinical, and the associated seizure disorder is usually characterized by myoclonic jerking, generalized tonic-clonic seizures, or a combination of both seizure types, whereas absence seizures are uncommon. Paroxysmal photic stimulation responses are common in such patients.

2.3. Significance and Natural History of Focal or Generalized Interictal Epileptiform Discharges in Children

Focal or generalized paroxysmal interictal discharges may occur in apparently healthy individuals in all age ranges. These findings may be termed as "false positives," but the EEG abnormalities are real and such spikes are evidence of an underlying

epileptic pathophysiology that may or may not subsequently become manifest clinically. The EEG evaluation of comparatively large healthy populations usually shows a certain percentage of abnormalities. Thorner (16) showed paroxysmal discharges in 0.3% of 1,100 flying cadets; Gibbs and colleagues (17) found epileptic abnormalities in 0.9% of normal adult controls; Harty and associates (18) observed such abnormalities in 3% of candidates for medical service. A study of 682 Air Force applicants showed paroxysmal changes in 2.6%; about one fourth were focal and the rest were of nonfocal character (19).

Kellaway (20) noted that of spike foci present in children, ~40% were temporal, 29% occipital, 23% central, and 8% frontal. Zivin and Ajmone Marsan (21) and Chatrian (22) have contemplated the clinical significance of spikes. In children between 3 and 12 years of age, the occurrence of central-midtemporal (also parietal) spikes was associated with overt seizures in only 50% to 70% of the cases. In occipital spikes (mainly age 3–5 years), the epileptogenicity is even lower. Kellaway (20) noted that spike foci are rare in normal healthy children but are present in about 35% of children age 5 through 11 years who have seizures: of those, ~90% of children with temporal spike foci, 75% with frontal spike foci, <54% with occipital and central spikes, and 76% of children with multifocal spikes had clinical seizures. In general, "benign" focal spikes (such as seen in benign rolandic epilepsy) outnumber generalized synchronous bursts of spikes or spike-waves by a slight to considerable margin.

Cavazzuti and coworkers (23) studied 3,726 children from 6 to 13 years of age without evidence of seizure or neurological deficits. Paroxysmal discharges were found in 131 cases (3.52%). Generalized, mainly polyspike, wave discharges were found in 41 cases, midtemporal spikes in 50, centroparietal spikes in 27, occipital spikes in two, and bilateral (midtemporal or parietal) spikes in 11 children. Changes in spike location and shifts from focal to generalized discharges were rare. The follow-up period was for up to 9 years. The abnormalities disappeared in most, usually during elementary school age or in early adolescence. Only seven children developed clinical epileptic seizures; five had generalized discharges, one had midtemporal, and one had centroparietal spikes. In two subjects there was evidence of epileptic seizures in the family, while six children had siblings with spikes, either generalized or rolandic. Kellaway (20) noted that 50% to 60% of foci in children are no longer evident 1 to 2 years after they were first demonstrated, with <10% persisting on longer follow-up.

3. FEBRILE SEIZURES

The National Institutes of Health Consensus Development Conference on the Management of Febrile Seizures in 1981 (27) defined febrile seizure as a clinical seizure that may occur associated with fever and without evidence of intracranial infection or other definable causes in infants and children between the ages of 3 months and 5 years. The International League Against Epilepsy (ILAE) classified febrile seizures as a "condition with epileptic seizures that are traditionally not diagnosed as a form of epilepsy per se" (24). There are detailed reviews of this topic describing the full range of clinical concerns (25). Febrile seizures occur in 2% to 4% of children in studies conducted in the United States and Europe (26–28) and 8% to 14% in studies from Asia and Pacific regions (29). Peak incidence is between 18 months and 2 years, with 4% occurring in children under 6 months of age, 90% within the first 3 years, and 6% after age 3 (28).

There is a familial predisposition. If one parent is affected, there is a 22% occurrence in offspring, and if both parents are affected, that increases to 56% (30). There is a 7% to 8% concordance in siblings, and a 40% concordance in monozygotic twins (31). Inheritance is thought to be autosomal dominant with incomplete penetrance. Six genetic loci have been mapped: FEB 1 (8q13-q21), FEB 2 (19p13.3), FEB 3 (2q23-q24), FEB 4 (5q14-q15), FEB 5 (6q22-q24), and FEB 6 (18p11.2) (32).

Febrile seizures are characterized as either simple or complex (26). A simple febrile seizure is defined as a short (<15 minutes) generalized tonic-clonic seizure without focality, in a child with a nonfocal neurological examination and without a family history of epilepsy. A febrile seizure is considered complex if the following features are present: its duration is >15 minutes, more than one seizure occurs in a 24-hour period, the seizure has focal features, or the child has an abnormal neurological examination.

Approximately a third of children with a first febrile seizure may experience additional events (26). Risk factors for experiencing more than one event include the following: <1 year of age at onset, a history of febrile seizures in first-degree relatives, fever on presentation for evaluation, and a brief interval between fever onset and seizure presentation. The presence of multiple risk factors increases the likelihood of febrile seizure recurrence (33).

Approximately 1.5% to 4.6% of those with febrile seizures may develop afebrile seizures (34). The risk factors for developing subsequent epilepsy include family history of epilepsy, preexisting neurological abnormalities, or a complex febrile seizure. The likelihood of occurrence increases with the number of risk factors: 2% with one risk factor and 10% with two or three risk factors (35).

Most febrile seizures are self-limited, although some may be prolonged and some can be classified as febrile status epilepticus (FSE). The prolonged events represent an important group of complex febrile seizures, as they may be associated with subsequent epilepsy (36). FSE has been reported to occur in 5% to 9% of children with a first febrile seizure (37). The association of prolonged febrile seizures and the development of temporal lobe epilepsy associated with mesial temporal lobe sclerosis has been investigated through the FEBSTAT study (38,39). In this multicenter trial, 199 children were enrolled after experiencing FSE (seizure duration >30 minutes). Seventeen children had definite magnetic resonance imaging (MRI) abnormalities with increased T2 signal in the hippocampus and five had equivocal findings, compared to none in 96 control subjects with simple febrile seizures. There is also evidence that a transient delay in white matter development may occur after prolonged febrile seizures (40). In addition, developmental abnormalities and memory impairments have

been found to be more common following prolonged febrile seizures (37,41).

The ideal application of the EEG in children with febrile seizures is to predict seizure recurrence and the emergence of epilepsy. Depending upon the category of febrile seizures, this goal has not been routinely achieved. For simple febrile seizures the conventional wisdom regarding the EEG is that the interictal EEG is normal, whereas in a child with epilepsy, the interictal EEG may be abnormal with associated epileptiform features. The recent practice parameters by the American Academy of Pediatrics do not recommend an EEG in the evaluation of neurologically healthy children with simple febrile seizures (42), indicating that there is no evidence that EEG interpretations performed either at the time of presentation after a simple febrile seizure or within the following month are predictive of recurrence of febrile seizures, the development of afebrile seizures, or the development of afebrile seizures/epilepsy within the next 2 years (43). The guidelines discussion notes that there is no evidence that interventions based on EEG would alter outcome.

Some investigators have described EEG findings in children with simple febrile seizures. Gibbs and Gibbs (44) noted that short spike-wave–like bursts in drowsiness and sleep may occur (so-called pseudo petit mal discharges). Des Terres and colleagues (45) found 31 children with spike foci among 500 patients with febrile convulsions. The most common site was the occipital lobe and, in 88%, the spike focus disappeared within 3 years. Kuturec and colleagues (46) reported that the presence of epileptiform discharges on EEG was associated with a higher rate of afebrile seizures. Alvarez (47) described hypnagogic paroxysmal spike-wave activity (minimal epileptiform features, sharp waves embedded into hyperventilation or hypnagogic hypersynchrony) occurring with a higher incidence with febrile seizures.

Japanese child neurologists rely more on EEG and have introduced the concept of epileptic versus nonepileptic febrile convulsions (48). However, children with epileptic febrile convulsions treated with antiepileptic drugs (AEDs) had the same recurrence rate as those not treated with AEDs. Yamatogi and colleagues (49) have stressed the good prognosis of children with febrile convulsions and normal EEGs. Yamatogi and Ohtahara (50) have placed emphasis on the clinical value of follow-up EEG studies. Accorded to Des Terres (45), the prognosis for these children is mostly favorable. The FEBSTAT study also recorded EEG in enrolled children in the period following prolonged febrile seizures (>30 minutes) and found focal slow activity, focal attenuation of activity, or both in 30.2%. These EEG findings were also associated with hippocampal T2 signal abnormality on MRI, suggestive of acute hippocampal injury (51).

4. NEONATAL SEIZURES

Seizures are the most frequent neurological event in newborns and their incidence appears greater than at any other period of human life (52). Seizures occur in 1.8 to 5.5 per 1,000 newborns and are most common in the first week of life (53,54).

They occur in both term and preterm neonates and reflect a large variety of pre-, peri-, and postnatal central nervous system (CNS) disorders ranging from benign self-limited to severe life-threatening disorders. Mortality is ~20% to 42% (55). A newborn with seizures requires rapid diagnosis, etiological workup, and therapeutic plans, as a delayed recognition of a treatable cause can have a significant impact on the child's subsequent neurological outcome (56). Video-EEG monitoring is valuable to make the initial diagnosis and to assess treatment response. In this section we will discuss reactive (provoked) seizures in the neonate as well as epilepsy syndromes specific to the neonatal period.

4.1. Historical Aspects

Early investigators attempting to characterize neonatal seizures relied on clinical observation supplemented by interictal EEG recordings (57). Later, bedside EEG combined with cinematography improved correlation of clinical phenomena with electrographic activity (58,59). These investigators observed that seizures in the neonate had unique clinical features compared to seizures generated by more mature brains. For example, generalized tonic-clonic seizures were found not to occur (59). The more common focal clonic seizures were often asynchronous if they occurred bilaterally, and did not spread in typical Jacksonian sequence (58,59).

Additionally, paroxysmal phenomena with minimal motor manifestations began to be classified as clinical seizures. These included ocular and oro-buccal-lingual movements, repetitive limb movements, changes of skin color, and respiration and other autonomic changes (58,59). Many of these so-called subtle seizures were subsequently found not to be associated with electrographic discharges. This was also observed to be true for other seizures, such as those characterized by generalized tonic posturing. Over the years, this has led to controversy over their pathophysiology. Observing that these events were similar to certain reflex behaviors, Mizrahi and Kellaway (60) postulated that these were primitive brainstem reflexes "released" by forebrain depression, rather than true epileptic events.

These observations and controversies have led to the evolution of current classification systems of neonatal seizures, which are primarily based on semiology, EEG features, and presumed pathophysiology. They have also led to several issues regarding diagnosis and management of neonatal seizures, especially those unaccompanied by prominent clinical manifestations. At present, an ILAE task force is critically reviewing current neonatal seizures and developing new concepts for seizure description and classification in the newborn.

4.2. Terminology

A term newborn is defined as a baby delivered between 37 and 42 weeks of gestation, and a preterm birth as a delivery before 37 completed weeks of gestation. The neonatal period is defined as the first 28 days of life. In the preterm infant, this period extends to the 44 completed weeks conceptional age. It is a period of increased vulnerability to anoxic and metabolic stress, and most seizures during this period are acute reactive (provoked) seizures, as opposed to manifestations of neonatal epilepsy—although the latter may occur with early neonatal seizures being the first of a chronic condition (61). However, the term "epileptic" is used in current classification systems to denote presumed underlying pathophysiology—seizures generated by hypersynchronous cortical neuronal discharges as demonstrated by temporally related EEG changes. This is in contrast to "non-epileptic" paroxysmal events, which occur without any EEG correlate (60). Seizures recorded in the absence of clinical activity are termed "electrical only" or "electrographic seizures." This raises two important issues in neonatal seizures: a possible overestimation of seizures based on clinical phenomena without EEG correlate and a possible underestimation of electrographic seizures without clinical correlate (62).

4.3. Pathophysiology

There are various factors that may underlie the increased susceptibility to reactive (provoked) seizures in the neonatal period, based primarily on relatively enhanced excitation in the immature brain (63–66). For example, in the immature brain, potassium tends to accumulate in the extracellular space, secondary to decreased Na+, K-ATPase activity and immature enzyme systems. This leads to the development of a hyperexcitable state and decreased seizure threshold (63). Excitation may also be enhanced by a relative increase in the density of glutamate receptors and NMDA-gated channels. On the other hand, synapses and receptors for inhibitory neurotransmitters may be less abundant in the developing brain. Also, GABA, the main inhibitory neurotransmitter in the CNS, may have depolarizing effects early on, leading at times to "excitatory" events (67,68). In animal models, the substantia nigra pars reticulata, which in adults is involved in the control of seizures, has been shown to amplify seizures in immature animals (69). These and other factors not only lower the overall seizure threshold but likely also allow seizures to spread more readily (55,64,66,69).

Long-term consequences of neonatal seizures on brain development are unclear and likely affected by multiple factors, such as seizure burden, age of the infant when seizures occur, and underlying etiology. Despite the increased susceptibility to seizures, studies using animal models/rodents provide evidence to suggest that the immature brain is more resistant to seizure-induced hippocampal injury (70). However, in rats with a preexisting lesion, the risk of status epilepticus (SE)–induced injury is significantly elevated (71). Also severe recurrent seizures can lead to impaired synaptogenesis, myelination, and brain growth. Galanopoulou has shown that three episodes of SE in P4-6 rat pups may upregulate the expression of the chloride cotransporter KCC2 in immature neurons with still-depolarizing $GABA_A$ receptor responses, which may prevent the maintenance of the GABA-mediated effects on cell maturation (72). This effect differs from those described in adults and may therefore underlie and partially explain the age-specific consequences of SE. There are also studies that suggest that exposure to currently available AEDs used to control seizures during this period may have similar detrimental effects, causing increased apoptosis or even on occasion promoting seizures (73).

4.4. Differential Diagnosis

The differential diagnosis of neonatal seizures includes physiological and nonphysiological events that may be abnormal or a variation of normal neonatal behavior. Infants withdrawing from in utero drug exposure or those who have suffered anoxic or acute metabolic insults can have tremulous or jittery movements, as well as exaggerated clonus. Unlike seizures, these movements are very stimulus sensitive and can be suppressed by repositioning or restraint. Benign neonatal sleep myoclonus is a common sleep phenomenon often mistaken for seizures that is characterized by focal or bilateral synchronous fast rhythmic myoclonic jerks, primarily involving the extremities, occurring during quiet sleep and stopping with awakening.

Infants with hyperekplexia, a condition caused by a mutation in genes encoding for inhibitory glycine receptor, also tend to have prominent myoclonus in sleep or upon arousal. In addition, they have an excessive startle response triggered by minimal tactile or auditory stimulus, as well as episodes of generalized tonic stiffening with possible severe apnea (74). The Vigevano maneuver, a smooth active flexion of the trunk, can abort these episodes (75).

Subtle sudden or repetitive mouth or limb movements can raise the suspicion for seizures but can be part of the normal neonatal behavioral repertoire. Apnea or changes in autonomic functions are rarely epileptic in origin when they occur in the absence of other autonomic or motor manifestations (76).

4.5. Overall Treatments

Seizures are often the first sign of neurological dysfunction in the newborn. Although determining etiology should not delay the treatment of seizures, in certain circumstances etiology-specific therapy is necessary to control seizures, as with seizures secondary to metabolic disturbances. Similarly, antibiotics and antiviral agents are used empirically when infectious causes are suspected, until ruled out by cerebrospinal fluid (CSF) and blood cultures (77).

When initiating antiseizure therapy, physiological factors unique to the neonate may influence medication choice, route of administration, and dosing. The oral route of administration for initiation of therapy is inappropriate, as absorption of medication is decreased due to immaturity of the gastrointestinal system and variations in gastric pH (78). Intramuscular absorption of medications is also inconsistent due to increased water content and smaller muscle mass in the newborn. These factors also lead to a higher risk of local injury and muscle necrosis (79). Therefore, the most dependable route for administering medications remains intravascular, and establishing access is critical early on.

The half-lives and free drug concentrations of many medications are increased in the neonate due to various factors, including a greater proportion of total body water, decreased albumin concentration and plasma binding of drugs, decreased drug metabolism, and excretion from immature hepatic and renal systems (61). This scenario makes anticonvulsant drug levels highly variable, especially when the infant is receiving other medications. Close monitoring of drug levels is necessary, especially early in the course of treatment. Dosages often need adjustment over time, as the infant's physiological systems mature.

The two medications most frequently used as first-line agents are phenobarbital and phenytoin/fosphenytoin. Studies have shown them to be equally effective in controlling seizures, although overall effectiveness only reaches 50% (80). Phenobarbital is more widely used as a first-line agent. Apparent half-life after 5 to 7 days is 100 hours, or greater in premature infants and in those with impaired hepatic and renal function. Phenytoin or fosphenytoin is often used after phenobarbital. The pro-drug form, fosphenytoin, is generally the preferred agent due to its better side effect profile. Because of highly variable metabolism and oral absorption, half-life ranges from 40 to 100 hours. Due to nonlinear kinetics, small dose changes near maximal therapeutic levels can lead to acute toxicity; therefore, close monitoring is necessary (81). More recently, there has been increasing support for the use of levetiracetam as third- or even second-line therapy in neonates with seizures (82). Depending on the etiology, treatment after the initial period may be discontinued after several months to a year, or continued if a specific diagnosis of epilepsy is established.

4.6. Clinical and EEG Features of Neonatal Seizures

4.6.1. Characterization and Classification of Neonatal Seizures

Accurate differentiation between seizures and non-seizure movements in neonates using clinical evaluation alone can be difficult. Up to 50% of electrographic seizures in this age group have been reported to be without clinical symptoms (83), and clinical seizure phenomena may also occur without an electrical correlate (84), leading to either under- or over-diagnosis. Therefore video-EEG plays an important part in the evaluation of paroxysmal movements to differentiate epileptic seizures from nonepileptic events.

Traditional classification schemes for seizures have been difficult to apply to neonatal seizures, which are generally fleeting events occurring in infants with a limited repertoire of normal behavior to begin with. Neonatal seizures can be classified semiologically as clonic, tonic, myoclonic, and subtle (62), or based on EEG findings as epileptic, nonepileptic, or electrical only (60,85). More than one seizure type can occur in a particular infant. The types of seizures found to be most consistently associated with EEG changes include focal clonic, focal tonic, some myoclonic seizures, and spasms. Seizures not consistently associated with an electrographic signature include generalized tonic, some myoclonic, and motor automatisms.

4.6.1.1. Focal Clonic

These seizures consist of rhythmic, usually slow (approximately one to three jerks per second) repetitive movements of the face, proximal or distal arm or leg muscles, or axial structures. The movements may be confined to one part of the body, hemiconvulsive, or multifocal. Clonic seizures that involve both sides of the body simultaneously are usually asynchronous, unlike true generalized clonic seizures in older individuals. Seizures may alternate between sites within a particular seizure, or may migrate from one site to another, not necessarily spreading in traditional Jacksonian sequence. Focal clonic seizures are usually associated with focal brain lesions such as cerebral infarctions but can also occur with more diffuse neuropathological processes. They are the type of seizures most consistently associated with electrographic correlate.

4.6.1.2. FOCAL TONIC
Sustained posturing of a limb or unilateral flexion of the trunk characterizes these seizures, which can also be accompanied by sustained conjugate deviation to one side. Like focal clonic seizures, tonic seizures are usually associated with synchronized EEG discharges. They occur less frequently than focal clonic seizures.

4.6.1.3. GENERALIZED TONIC
These seizures are characterized by sustained bilateral extension or flexion of the limbs or trunk, resembling decerebrate or decorticate posturing. Unlike their more focal counterpart, these "seizures" are often not associated with EEG correlate and can be classified as nonepileptic. Because they tend to occur in association with other automatic behavior in obtunded infants with diffuse central nervous pathological processes, Mizrahi and Kellaway (60) proposed that such "seizures" are "brainstem release phenomenon" from disinhibition of forebrain structures in clinically depressed infants.

4.6.1.4. MYOCLONIC
These irregular, brief, single or multiple contractions of muscles involving the face, limbs, hands, fingers, or trunk are termed myoclonus. They can be either epileptic or nonepileptic. Myoclonic movements associated with EEG changes are called "cortical myoclonus," while myoclonus with no EEG correlate is termed "sub-cortical myoclonus." The latter term implies that more caudal structures in the brainstem or spinal cord are responsible for generating the movements. Myoclonias can be focal, multifocal, or "generalized." "Generalized" myoclonus consists of bilateral symmetric jerks of the limbs or of massive jerks of the trunk. Multifocal or "fragmentary" myoclonus is characterized by brief asynchronous twitching of different muscle groups. The term "erratic" is used when myoclonias shift from one part of the body to another in a random asynchronous way. Fragmentary or erratic myoclonus is the type least associated with EEG changes, while generalized myoclonus is usually accompanied by EEG correlate.

4.6.1.5. SPASMS
Spasms consist of flexor, extensor, or mixed flexion and extension of limb, head, and truncal muscles. These can be bilateral or asymmetric or focal and are longer than a myoclonic jerk but less sustained than a tonic seizure, both of which are in the differential (Box 18.1). Like spasms in older infants, they can be accompanied by ocular phenomena such as eye revulsion, oculoclonias, or eye deviation, can occur in clusters, isolated or in close relationship to focal seizures, and can be more frequent upon awakening. On EEG, they are associated with a high-voltage slow wave, an attenuation of the background, fast

rhythms, or a combination of these, which can be generalized, asymmetric, or focal (86).

4.6.1.6. MOTOR AUTOMATISMS
Also called "subtle seizures," these are paroxysmal changes in behavior or autonomic function with minimal motor manifestations occurring in the newborn. These consist of various irregular and disconjugate ocular movements, eyelid blinking or fluttering, eye opening, fixation of gaze, nystagmus, oral-buccal-lingual movements such as sucking, smacking, chewing or tongue protrusion, and peculiar extremity progression movements such as pedaling, stepping, rowing, boxing, or swimming movements. These may be associated with simultaneous abnormal EEG discharges (87) or may be classified as nonepileptic (60). In older individuals, paroxysmal automatic behaviors are known to occur without surface EEG correlate as seizure manifestations or postictal behavior (88). Studies in neonatal animals have also shown that epileptiform discharges can occur in deep limbic structures with minimal or no propagation to the cortical surface (66). These observations raise the possibility that subtle seizures in neonates may be true epileptic events with generators in deeper limbic structures, though some of these events are likely reflex behaviors.

4.6.1.7. AUTONOMIC SIGNS
A variety of paroxysmal changes in autonomic activity such as alterations in breathing, heart rate, blood pressure, salivation, sweating, and color changes have also been described as manifestations of subtle seizures (89). However, in isolation, they rarely occur as epileptic phenomena (60). When they are accompanied by ictal EEG correlates, they occur in association with other clinical behavioral or motor manifestations. Apneic seizures with EEG correlate may exhibit other subtle

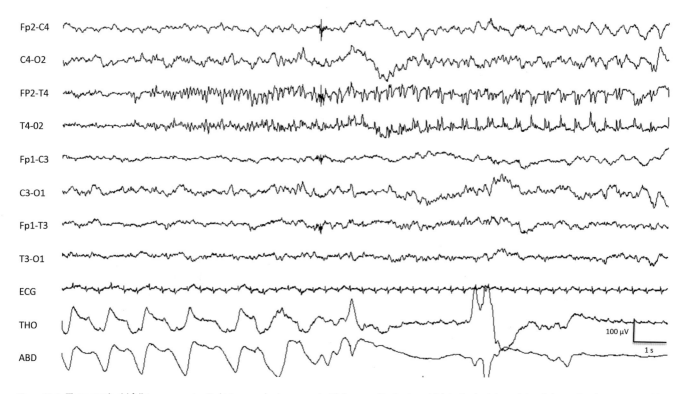

Figure 18.6. Three-week-old full-term neonate. Right temporal seizure onset with low-amplitude sinusoidal rhythmic alpha activity of decreasing frequency evolving into repetitive spikes. Notice apnea recorded on thoracic and abdominal respiration lead.

phenomena such as eye opening, "staring," deviation of the eyes, and mouth movements. The ictal discharge in these seizures frequently originates from the temporal area (76) (Fig. 18.6).

4.6.1.8. Interictal EEG

Assessment of the interictal EEG background can suggest possible etiologies for seizures and helps in determining an infant's degree of cerebral dysfunction, the risk for persistent seizures, and the prognosis for long-term outcome. Unlike in adults, the finding of sharp-wave transients on the interictal record in the neonate does not aid in the diagnosis of seizures or predict epileptogenicity. Transient sharp waves are frequently found in the temporal regions and are a nonspecific finding in term and preterm infants (Fig. 18.7A) (53,90). Positive sharp waves in the rolandic areas (see Fig. 18.7B), however, have been shown to be closely associated with periventricular leukomalacia (91) (see Chapter 7).

EEG findings correlating with diffuse cerebral dysfunction include a depressed undifferentiated background, a suppression burst pattern (Fig. 18.8), multifocal sharp transients, and, in the full-term neonate, asynchrony or dysmaturity (Fig. 18.9). These abnormalities, although mostly nonspecific, can suggest etiologies that result in generalized or multifocal brain injury such as hypoxia, acute metabolic disturbances, inborn errors of metabolism (Fig. 18.10), infection, and bilateral brain hemorrhage. On the other hand, persistent asymmetries of the background and persistently lateralized sharp transients may indicate focal structural brain abnormalities such as focal cerebral infarction (Fig. 18.11) or areas of dysgenesis (Fig. 18.12) as underlying etiologies. The absence of focal features, however, does not rule out a focal structural pathology (55).

Prospective studies in neonates presenting with seizures have found that the background EEG can be used for prognostic purposes. A normal EEG can predict normal neurological development in >80% of infants, while the presence and persistence of background abnormalities suggests a poor outcome (55,92–94). The presence of interictal epileptiform activity, however, is not consistently related to outcome (95). EEG background may also predict persistence of seizures. A normal or immature background has been associated with the absence of electrographic seizures on subsequent video-EEG monitoring, while epileptiform discharges have been associated with the occurrence of electrographic seizures (96). Another study found that post-neonatal epilepsy occurred in 68% of patients with moderately or markedly abnormal EEG backgrounds but in only 25% of those without (97). Ortibus and colleagues, however, did not find background abnormalities to be a strong predictor of seizures past the neonatal period (92).

4.6.2. Ictal EEG

It has been proposed that in the neonate an electrical seizure can be considered when there is rhythmic activity of at least 10 sec in duration (98), more often reported in full-term than in preterm infants, but there are limited data to support this. With increasing conceptional age, seizure discharges tend to increase in duration (54). Onset is usually focal, involving the central and temporal regions more commonly than the frontal and occipital regions. Seizures can be confined to one area but can also arise from multiple areas, propagating asynchronously from different foci. Seizures may remain localized, slowly spread to involve contiguous regions, abruptly involve one hemisphere, or migrate to the other hemisphere (55).

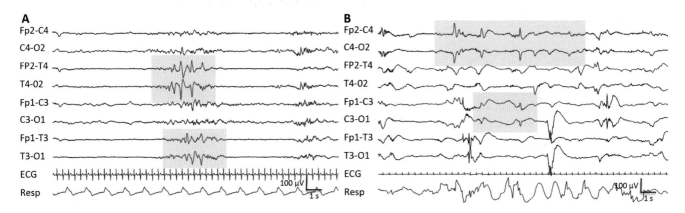

Figure 18.7. **A:** *4-day-old full-term neonate. Background activity is discontinuous (on sedative drugs), with bilateral (right predominating) positive temporal sharp waves.* **B:** *8-day-old premature neonate (31 weeks conceptional age) with bilateral (right predominating) positive rolandic sharp waves.*

Frequency, morphology, and voltage of the discharges may vary within the same seizure, or from one seizure to the next in a given infant. The seizure discharge can consist of repetitive spikes, sharp or slow waves, or a combination of different waveforms (Fig. 18.13).

Electrographic seizures in the absence of clinical activity commonly occur in severely encephalopathic neonates with depressed and undifferentiated background EEG activity (see Fig. 18.13D). Some are lower in voltage and longer in duration and show little tendency to spread or change.

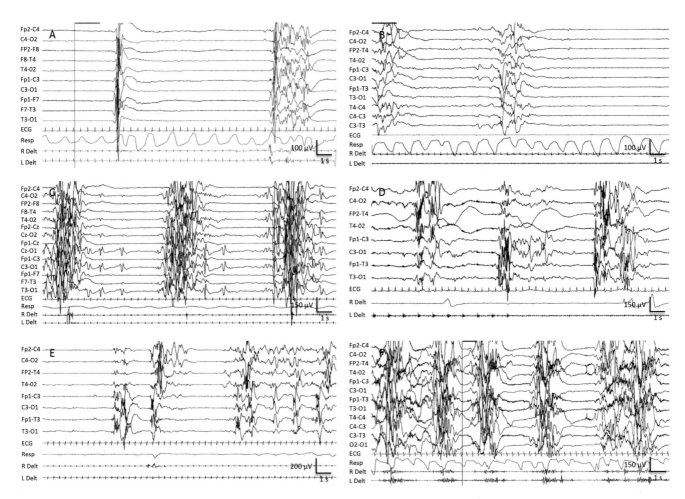

Figure 18.8. *Different aspects of suppression-burst patterns in full-term neonates. "Suppression burst" is defined as a nonreactive invariant pattern consisting of abnormal bursts separated by prolonged and abnormal low-voltage interburst intervals (IBI), defined as IBI voltage <5 μV peak to peak, allowing, however, sparse activity up to 15 μV for one electrode or transient activity up to 15 μV during <2 sec.* **A:** *Early myoclonic encephalopathy.* **B:** *Ohtahara syndrome.* **C:** *Ohtahara syndrome. Notice left occipital focal sharp waves between bursts.* **D:** *Syndrome not classified. Asynchrony of bursts.* **E:** *Syndrome not classified. Asynchrony of bursts.* **F:** *Early myoclonic encephalopathy. Bursts accompanied by a series of asynchronous myoclonic jerks involving the limbs and head recorded on EMG leads.*

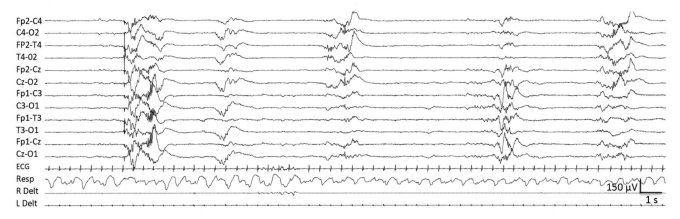

Figure 18.9. *Two-day-old full-term neonate with nonketotic hyperglycinemia. The EEG shows discontinuous, intermittently asynchronous background activity with dysmature features.*

These have been referred to as "seizure discharges of the depressed brain" (53). Alpha seizure discharges are characterized as paroxysmal 8- to 12-Hz alpha activity in the central or temporal regions in encephalopathic newborns and suggest a poor prognosis (76). When neonates are treated for seizures with AEDs, persistent electrical seizure activity can be found long after clinical seizures have stopped, a phenomenon referred to as "decoupling" of electrical from clinical activity (60).

4.6.3. STATUS EPILEPTICUS IN THE NEWBORN

Neonatal SE is not well defined. Some use the traditional definition of SE for children and adults: continuous seizure activity during at least 30 minutes, or recurrent seizures lasting a total of 30 minutes without definitive return to baseline between seizures (99). However, because of the difficulty evaluating the neurological status of the newborn and the high incidence of coexisting encephalopathy, some authors proposed to diagnose SE when the summed duration of seizures represents at least 50% of the recording time (54). Other definitions have specified continuous seizure activity during at least 15, 20, or 30 minutes or 1 hour (54,100), or continuous seizures interrupted only by short periods with frequent sharp waves or spikes during 4 hours (101). The duration of seizures and their responsiveness to medications determine prognosis, as prolonged seizures (56,92) and difficult-to-control seizures (94) have been associated with the worst prognosis. The impact of the number of seizures, however, is less clear, with some

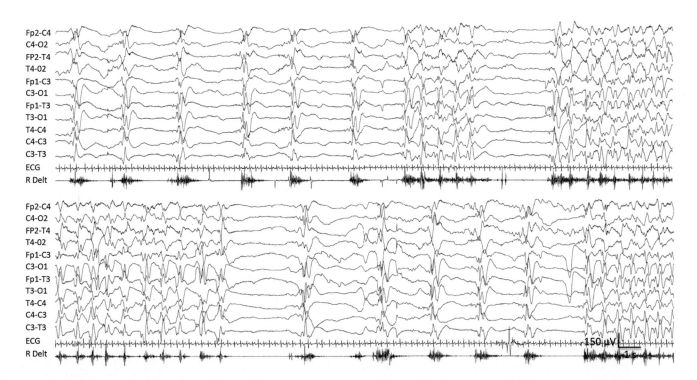

Figure 18.10. *Ten-day-old full-term neonate with pyridoxine deficiency. There is continuous seizure activity with periodic spasm-like jerks, alternating with asynchronous irregular clonic manifestations involving limbs and head. EEG correlate consists of diffuse high-voltage bi- or polyphasic slow complexes followed by electrodecrement.*

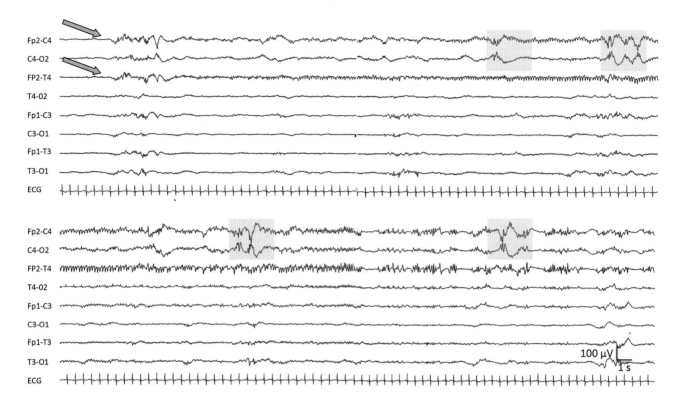

Figure 18.11. Two-day-old neonate with right intracerebral hemorrhage. Right frontal seizure with fast activity at onset (arrows), followed by pseudo-periodic slow waves of positive polarity on C4 (rectangles).

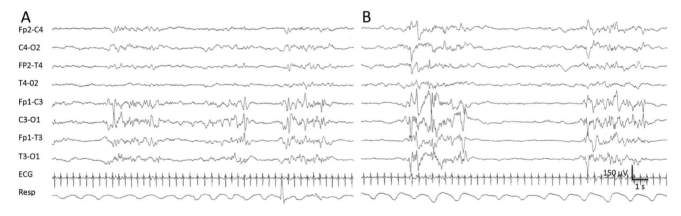

Figure 18.12. Six-week-old infant with hemimegalencephaly. A: Awake state: marked asymmetry with left-sided discontinuous background activity and left hemispheric spikes, sharp waves, and fast rhythms predominating over central area. B: Sleep: left hemi-suppression-burst.

studies showing that frequent seizures predict poorer outcome (102), and other studies showing no correlation (94).

4.7. Causes of Reactive (Provoked) Seizures

4.7.1. Neonatal Encephalopathy and Hypoxic-Ischemic Encephalopathy

Perinatal hypoxic-ischemic injury remains a major cause of neurodevelopment disability and is thought to affect 5 to 10 per 1,000 live births (54,103). The term "neonatal encephalopathy" has gained favor in the literature over "hypoxic-ischemic encephalopathy," as often a direct causal relationship between hypoxia and encephalopathy is hard to establish. When infectious, metabolic, and structural causes of seizures are excluded, neonatal encephalopathy secondary to hypoxic injury is often implicated, especially if accompanied by other systemic signs of anoxia such as persistently low Apgar scores, systemic acidosis, and multiple-organ involvement. Criteria used to diagnose neonatal encephalopathy vary, and it is difficult to assess the true proportion due to asphyxia (104).

Seizures following a perinatal hypoxic-ischemic event occur after a delay of several hours, with a median time reported at about 17 hours and a maximum seizure burden at about 22 hours (105). Semiology is not specific; they may be tonic or clonic, often multifocal, or exhibit only subtle motor

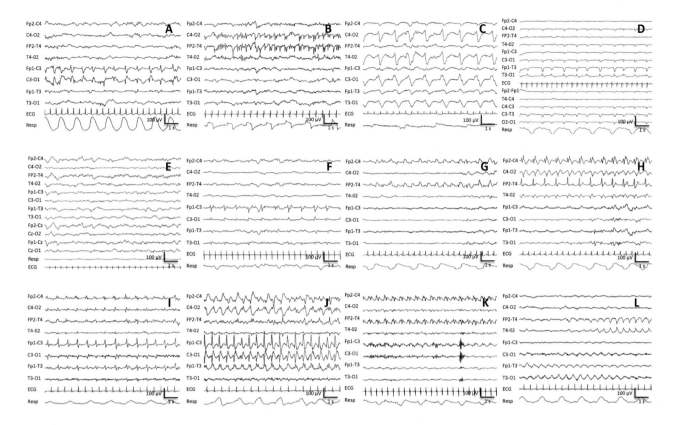

*Figure 18.13. Different aspects of ictal discharges in the full-term neonate. **A:** 5-day-old full-term neonate with intracranial hemorrhage due to alloimmune thrombocytopenia. Periodic medium-voltage spike and sharp wave activity in the left central region. **B:** 3-week-old full-term neonate with bitemporal intracranial hemorrhage. Irregular spike activity evolving from alpha rhythms in the right temporo-occipital region. **C:** 1-day-old full-term neonate with hypoxic-ischemic encephalopathy. Right occipital periodic sharp waves spreading to the left. **D:** 3-day-old full-term neonate with sulfite oxidase deficiency. Diffuse low-voltage rhythmic slow sharp waves predominating on the left hemisphere on depressed and undifferentiated background. **E:** 2-week-old full-term neonate with right posterior intracranial hemorrhage. Subclinical right temporal alpha discharge. **F:** 4-day-old full-term neonate with hypoxic-ischemic encephalopathy. Diffuse low-voltage periodic sharp waves with left central predominance on depressed and undifferentiated background. **G:** 2-day-old full-term neonate with hypoxic-ischemic encephalopathy. Right frontal rhythmic theta/delta activity with some spikes. **H:** Same baby as G. Rhythmic high-amplitude spikes with frontocentral predominance. **I:** 2-day-old full-term neonate with hypoxic-ischemic encephalopathy. Diffuse medium-voltage rhythmic spikes with right frontal predominance. **J:** Same baby as I. Left frontocentral rhythmic high-amplitude spikes and right central rhythmic sharp waves. **K:** Same baby as I. Rhythmic medium-voltage polyphasic sharp waves in the right frontal region. **L:** Same baby as I, 4 days old. Left posterior and right temporal rhythmic medium-voltage slow waves.*

manifestations or autonomic symptoms. Ictal EEG is likewise nonspecific and depends on the seizure.

4.7.2. INTRACRANIAL HEMORRHAGE AND INFARCTIONS

Perinatal stroke is an acute cerebrovascular (including ischemic and hemorrhagic) injury occurring between 20 weeks of gestation and 28 days of postnatal life due to arterial ischemic stroke, cerebral venous thrombosis, or primary intracerebral hemorrhage. It occurs in ~1 in 4,000 full-term births (106) and is a common cause of acute neonatal encephalopathy. Stroke is the second most frequent cause of neonatal seizures, and seizures are the most common first clinical sign observed in babies suffering with arterial ischemic stroke (93).

Seizures in ischemic stroke are frequently focal and stereotyped, often with clonic manifestations. The ictal EEG consists of rhythmic contralateral spikes, often in the central area. Interictal EEG is normal on the unaffected hemisphere and only mildly disturbed with rare focal anomalies on the affected hemisphere. Diagnosis is confirmed by neuroimaging. Prognosis after perinatal stroke is variable, with 40% of infants

neurologically normal and 57% showing neurological or cognitive abnormalities (106).

4.7.3. INFECTIOUS CNS DISORDERS

Infectious CNS disorders can be secondary to postnatally acquired bacterial and viral agents, or congenital, in utero infections, and are responsible for 5% to 10% of seizures in the neonate (103). The most common bacterial causes are group B streptococcus and *Escherichia coli*. Meningoencephalitis secondary to intrauterine infections is caused by toxoplasmosis, herpes simplex, Coxsackievirus, or cytomegalovirus (107). Especially in neonatal sepsis, the mortality (and morbidity) rate remains very high at 3% to 52%, with higher mortality in late-onset sepsis compared to early-onset sepsis (108). No specific EEG signature or seizure type has been described, but constant focal anomalies can be suggestive of brain abscess.

4.7.4. METABOLIC DISTURBANCES

Metabolic disturbances causing seizures are important to identify as many acute conditions are potentially treatable. These include electrolyte abnormalities such as hypocalcemia, hypomagnesemia, and hypoglycemia. Rare inborn errors of metabolism can cause neonatal seizures refractory to AED treatment (Box 18.2). These usually require dietary manipulation or vitamin substitution to control.

The prognosis in isolated hypocalcaemia is excellent. The outcome of seizures due to hypoglycemia depends on etiology and the metabolic context, with a relatively favorable prognosis in isolated hypoglycemia in newborns from diabetic mothers but a less favorable outcome in congenital disorders of glucose metabolism, fatty acid beta oxidation, or hyperinsulinism. Pyridoxine-dependent seizures can produce severe seizures, including spasms, often associated with an impressive hyperexcitability that may respond to pyridoxine or pyridoxine-phosphate. Some conditions may show highly suggestive EEG and clinical seizure patterns, such as myoclonias and focal seizures in pyridoxine-dependent epilepsies (see Fig. 18.10) (109), suppression-burst EEG with immature features and myoclonic seizures in nonketotic hyperglycinemia (see Fig. 18.9) (110), and a rolandic comb-like pattern in maple syrup urine disease (Fig. 18.14) (111).

4.7.5. DRUG WITHDRAWAL

Drug withdrawal or intoxication is another cause of transient seizures in the newborn. History of maternal drug use or of administration of medications during delivery is suggestive of the diagnosis. The affected neonate can appear depressed and exhibit symptoms such as jitteriness that can be difficult to distinguish from seizures.

4.7.6. PARTICULAR FEATURES IN THE PREMATURE NEONATE

Seizures in very preterm babies are rarely reported, but the incidence is likely underestimated. Incidence varies widely between 4% (54) and 48% (112). Seay and Bray (113) studied a population of low-birthweight (<2,500 g) neonates with a mean gestational age of 30 weeks; seizures occurred in 31 of 153 babies (20%) starting within the first 72 hours of life in 72%. Intraventricular hemorrhage was the main underlying cause (87%), followed by infection (two patients), hypocalcemia (one

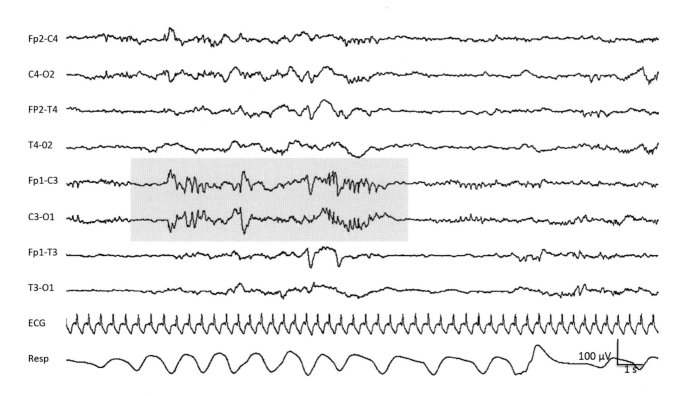

Figure 18.14. Eleven-day-old full-term neonate with maple syrup urine disease. The EEG demonstrates a left central comb-like pattern (rectangle).

patient), and drug withdrawal (one patient). The occurrence of seizures seems to be related to an unfavorable outcome (56,94). During the first 72 hours they are associated with an increased risk of intraventricular hemorrhage, white matter injury, and death, and poorer early language development (112).

4.7.7. PARTICULAR FEATURES IN SURGERY OF CONGENITAL HEART DISEASES

Surgery for congenital heart disease in the neonatal period is a procedure that carries an increased risk for seizures. Electrographic seizures were found in 11% of 183 infants after surgery using cardiopulmonary bypass (114). Seizures are mostly clinically silent, beginning between 4 and 36 hours after surgery, and mainly involve the frontal and central regions (115). The relationship between postoperative seizures and outcome is unclear, but their occurrence may be correlated with neurological and developmental sequelae (115).

4.8. Epilepsies Starting in the Neonatal Period Attributed to a Structural Abnormality

Stereotyped seizures in the neonatal period in the absence of metabolic or infectious disturbances may be related to an underlying structural anomaly such as focal cortical dysplasia, hemimegalencephaly, or lissencephaly. The presence of a brain lesion can be suggested by focal seizures, electrographically arising from the same region (Fig. 18.15), or from asymmetries in voltage or frequency of the background. The interictal EEG can be normal or can show various degrees of pathology, even hemispheric suppression-burst in extended cortical malformation or hemimegalencephaly (see Fig. 18.12). The EEG can be highly suggestive of a specific structural anomaly. For example, periodic focal abnormalities may be present in focal cortical dysplasia or cortical tubers (Fig. 18.16), or characteristic high-voltage monomorphous theta or delta activity may be present in lissencephaly (Fig. 18.17), but diagnosis relies on neuroimaging. Epilepsy related to congenital brain malformations is discussed in more detail in Chapter 13.

5. ELECTROCLINICAL SYNDROMES WITH ONSET IN THE NEONATAL PERIOD

5.1. Benign Familial Neonatal Epilepsy

Previously named benign familial neonatal seizures, benign familial neonatal epilepsy (BFNE) is an autosomal dominant epileptic syndrome with seizure onset in the neonatal period and a benign course. Seizures in affected infants begin by 2 to 8 days of life, with 80% appearing on the second or third day (61). The onset of seizures can be delayed up to 3.5 months, especially in premature infants when they begin when they reach full term (94,116). The seizures are brief, typically 1 to 2

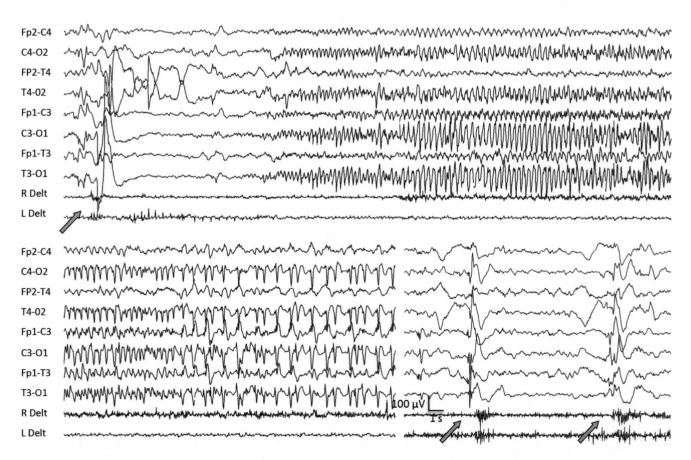

Figure 18.15. Five-week-old infant with left occipital cortical dysplasia and Ohtahara syndrome. There is a left posterior seizure preceded by an epileptic spasm and followed by a cluster of epileptic spasms. Spasms (arrows) are clinically and on EEG asymmetric with sharp slow wave complex predominating in the left posterior region.

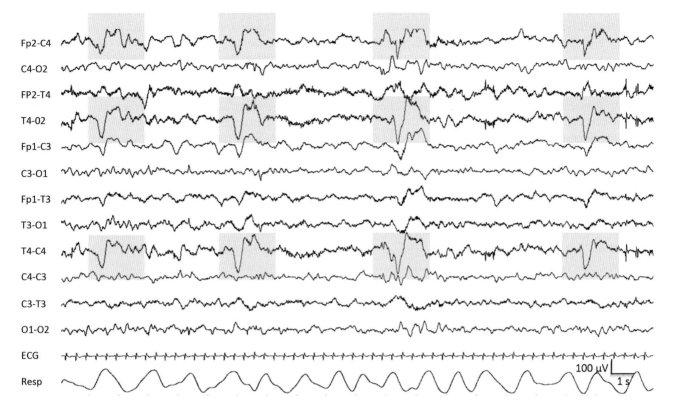

Figure 18.16. Two-month-old infant with tuberous sclerosis complex. The EEG in the awake state shows pseudo-periodic biphasic slow-wave complexes, localized on C4 and O2, with spread to the left.

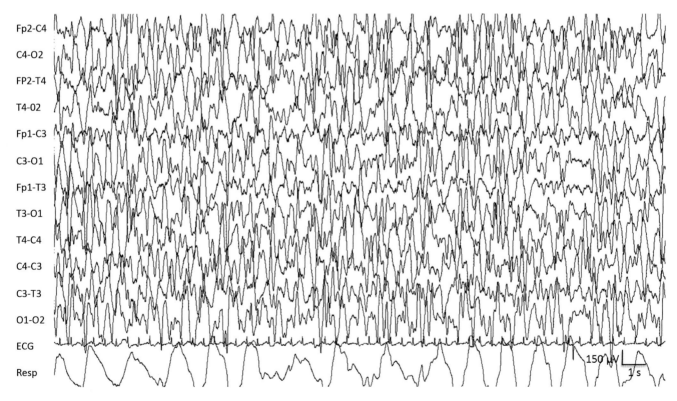

Figure 18.17. Two-month-old infant with LIS1-associated lissencephaly. The EEG in the awake state shows no physiological pattern, with diffuse very-high-voltage slow theta and delta waves with rare diffuse spikes.

minutes, and can occur isolated or in clusters, multiple times a day, possibly evolving into status epilepticus; most seizures remitting by 16 months of life (94,117). The diagnosis is suspected when typical seizures occur without obvious precipitants in an otherwise normal newborn with a family history of similar seizures in the neonatal period, but it requires exclusion of other causes of seizures (118).

Clinical seizures are very suggestive of the diagnosis, presenting with asymmetric tonic posturing and head rotation associated with apnea and possibly other autonomic features or vocalizations, often progressing to focal or generalized clonic movements, involving the oculofacial muscles and then the limbs, and motor automatisms, possibly changing the side from seizure to seizure in a given infant. Myoclonic seizures, generalized tonic-clonic seizures, or spasms are not seen in this condition.

The interictal EEG is nonspecific and may be normal or abnormal. Some abnormalities reported in the literature include interictal sharp transients and the "theta pointu alternant" pattern (119). The latter is a dominant 4- to 7-Hz theta activity and can be alternating or discontinuous, is nonreactive, and is intermixed with sharp activity and frequent interhemispheric asynchrony (Fig. 18.18). It can be present during active and quiet sleep, but also in wakefulness (120). Centrotemporal spikes have also been reported in one patient who later developed one clinical rolandic seizure at age 4 (121). The ictal EEG pattern is characterized by generalized suppression of amplitude at onset (116,122) simultaneously with the tonic motor activity and apnea, and followed by high-voltage slow complexes in the frontocentral areas (122) or lateralized (Fig. 18.19). Bye (123) recorded focal-onset seizures with and without secondary generalization in one neonate, and Plouin

and Anderson (118) also suggest that the electroclinical presentation is closer to that of focal epilepsies.

BFNE is a central nervous system channelopathy caused by mutations in two potassium subunit channel genes, *KCNQ2* on chromosome 20q and *KCNQ3* on chromosome 8q (124,125). BFNE is a rare disorder that may be underrecognized. Its prevalence is unknown. Eighty families have been described (126), with a number of affected generations of one to five. Ronen and colleagues found five familial cases out of 34,615 live births in their population-based study of neonatal seizures in Newfoundland (94).

The prognosis is generally good, with resolution of seizures by 1 to 6 months and a normal neurological outcome in the majority of cases (117). However, 11% to 16% of individuals with BFNE will experience one or more seizures later in life, often provoked by stress (116) or fever (118). Seizures are often treated with AEDs because of their frequency even though they are generally self-limited. Phenobarbital is most commonly used, although phenytoin and valproate have been used in refractory cases (118).

5.2. Benign Idiopathic Neonatal Convulsions

Because of the tendency of the seizures to occur on the fourth or fifth day of life (80% of the cases, ranging from the fourth to the seventh day of life), the term "fifth-day fits" has been commonly used for this condition, which is characterized by nonfamilial self-limited seizures of unknown etiology and a benign course. This condition is not always considered a distinct entity, and the ILAE has not recognized it as a designated epilepsy syndrome (24). Typical seizures in affected infants consist of focal clonic activity typically lasting 1 to 3 minutes.

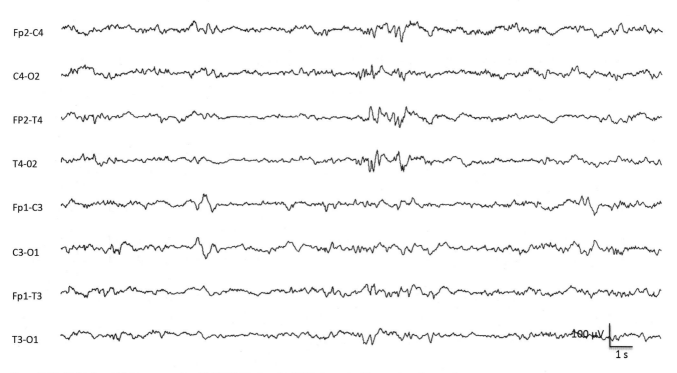

Figure 18.18. Eight-day-old full-term neonate with BFNE. The interictal EEG shows the "theta pointu alternant" pattern.

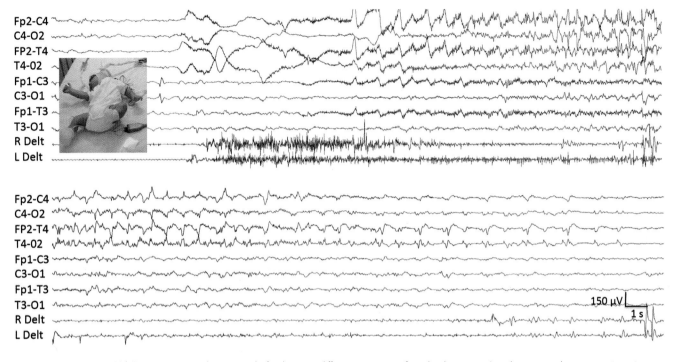

Figure 18.19. Eight-day-old full-term neonate with BFNE. Right focal seizure: diffuse suppression of amplitude at onset (simultaneous to the asymmetric tonic posturing with head rotation, see deltoid muscles) followed by high-voltage slow complexes predominating in the right frontal area and discharge ending in the temporal area.

Multiple clusters of seizures can occur in one day and can lead to status epilepticus with an average duration of 20 hours (from 2 hours up to 3 days) (118). These may or may not be associated with apnea.

The interictal EEG is normal in 10% (118), but 60% of cases may demonstrate the characteristic but nonspecific "theta pointu alternant" pattern as described above (see Fig. 18.18). This pattern can persist for days after cessation of clinical seizures. Other abnormal patterns that have been described include centrotemporal sharp waves, discontinuous patterns, and focal or multifocal nonspecific abnormalities. Ictal EEG patterns are nonspecific and can be focal with secondary generalization or immediately generalized, characterized by rhythmic spikes or rhythmic slow waves; no alpha-like activity has been reported. The seizure discharge can arise from any area but is most commonly seen in the rolandic region (118).

Although the exact incidence is unknown, benign idiopathic neonatal convulsions are suggested to represent 2% to 7% of seizures in the neonate (118), though cases have declined significantly in recent years. Affected infants are usually born at or near term and are products of uneventful pregnancies and deliveries. Boys are more often affected than girls (118). The etiology and pathogenesis of the seizures are unknown. One study found rotavirus in the stool of 95% of affected patients, compared to 40% in the control group (127). Another study found low levels of zinc in the CSF of affected infants (89). In four cases, a mutation in the gene encoding for KCNQ2 (a mutation frequently found in the familial form of benign neonatal convulsions) was identified (125).

Like BFNE, the diagnosis of benign idiopathic neonatal convulsions requires exclusion of other transient causes for seizures (118). Plouin proposed the following diagnostic clinical criteria:

1. Apgar score >7 at 1 minute

2. Typical interval between birth and seizures onset (4–6 days)

3. Normal neurological examination before seizures and interictally

4. Normal laboratory findings (metabolic studies, neuroimaging, and CSF analysis),

5. No family history of neonatal seizures or post-neonatal epilepsy (128). The final criterion distinguishes this syndrome from the familial form.

Seizures usually remit by 48 hours of onset (129). Some argue against treating these self-limited seizures, but many clinicians treat them with AEDs, usually phenobarbital and phenytoin. Mild psychomotor retardation has been described in some survivors; however, the prognosis for neurodevelopmental outcome is considered to be generally favorable (118).

5.3. Early Infantile Epileptic Encephalopathy

Also known as Ohtahara syndrome, early infantile epileptic encephalopathy is an epileptic encephalopathy with suppression-burst EEG beginning in the neonatal period. Seizures begin very soon after birth, usually within the first month of life (130), though intrauterine onset has been suggested in some cases (131). The most characteristic seizures in this syndrome are epileptic spasms and tonic seizures, isolated or in clusters, which can occur up to 300 times a day (132). They can be lateralized, generalized, or asymmetric. Other seizure types, such as focal motor seizures and hemiconvulsions, occur in about one third of patients (130). Although generalized tonic-clonic seizures and rare myoclonic seizures can develop later, the erratic myoclonus that characterizes early myoclonic encephalopathy does not occur in this syndrome (133).

The EEG is characterized by a suppression-burst pattern (see Fig. 18.8), which is an interictal pattern, although some have observed clinical seizures to correlate with the bursts (134). The pattern consist of bursts of high-voltage (150–350 uV) slow waves intermingled with spikes and polyspikes, alternating with periods of suppression of electrical activity. The bursts of spikes and polyspikes can last 1 to 6 sec, while the periods of suppression are usually 2 to 5 sec long (130,135), although they can last up to 18 sec (136). The pattern can involve only one hemisphere or can be more widespread, involving both hemispheres symmetrically or asymmetrically. Asynchrony is possible but not common (130). Focal epileptiform discharges have also been described during the periods of suppression (137). The suppression-burst pattern in Ohtahara syndrome is classically consistent in both waking and sleeping states (132).

The suppression-burst pattern can evolve into hypsarrhythmia between 3 and 6 months of age, coincident with the development of more typical epileptic spasms. This evolution toward West syndrome occurs in up to 75% of patients with Ohtahara syndrome. Later transition into slow-spike and wave morphology (characteristic of LGS) may also occur in a smaller percentage (130).

The EEG during "tonic" spasms principally shows desynchronization with or without evident rapid activity (130). Using video-EEG with surface electromyographic recordings from deltoid muscles, Fusco and coworkers found each burst of the suppression-burst pattern to be associated with tonic contractions of variable duration (134). They also recorded focal seizures clinically consisting of tonic eye deviation, unilateral clonic contractions, or subtle or subclinical phenomena. Yamatogi and Ohtahara described focal seizures arising from a fixed focus and followed by "tonic" spasms in series (130).

Both congenital and acquired structural brain lesions may be present in affected infants. Hemimegalencephaly has been frequently described (133–134). Other associated brain malformations include cerebral dysgenesis, Aicardi syndrome, lissencephaly, porencephaly, hydrocephalus, subacute diffuse encephalopathy, dentato-olivary dysplasia, and polymicrogyria (132,133). Brainstem abnormalities have frequently been reported on autopsy in patients with Ohtahara syndrome (138).

Metabolic causes are rare, but cases of Leigh encephalopathy (139), nonketotic hyperglycinemia (136), cytochrome c oxidase deficiency (140), pyridoxine dependency, and carnitine palmitoyltransferase deficiency (134) have been reported, as have mitochondrial diseases (141). In recent years numerous gene mutations have been described, including mutations in *STXBP1, KCNQ2, ARX, SLC25A22,* and *SCN2A* (142–144).

Seizures are typically refractory to conventional anticonvulsant medications, and affected infants generally do poorly.

ACTH and the ketogenic diet have been inconsistently effective in a small number of cases (132,136). Cases responding to vitamin B6 (134), clonazepam and acetazolamide (132), zonisamide (130), and vigabatrin (145) have been described. Surgical treatment with hemispheric disconnection or focal resection of lesions has been reported to improve seizures and cognitive outcome in patients with underlying structural anomalies (146). Treatment of the seizures does not appear to prevent neurological deterioration. Subsequent brain atrophy is frequently found on imaging studies. Nearly all survivors have profound cognitive disability and are physically handicapped (130).

5.4. Early Myoclonic Encephalopathy

This syndrome, like Ohtahara syndrome, is another neonatal-onset epileptic encephalopathy with a suppression-burst EEG pattern. It is characterized clinically by erratic and fragmentary myoclonic seizures that occur early, often within the first few days or month of life. Myoclonic movements can affect the face, or proximal or distal limb muscles. The jerks can be restricted to a few muscles or can affect multiple muscles asynchronously, shifting erratically from one area to another. Generalized massive myoclonus is less common. The frequency of seizures is variable, but they can be almost continuous. Focal seizures follow the appearance of the erratic myoclonus. These seizures can be characterized by focal clonic movements of a limb, or subtle eye deviation with respiratory changes. Tonic spasms are the last type of seizures to appear, usually between 3 and 4 months, although earlier onset has been described.

The EEG is characterized by a suppression-burst pattern similar to that seen in Ohtahara syndrome (see Fig. 18.8). This burst-suppression pattern is more pronounced in sleep, as opposed to Ohtahara syndrome, in which it may be present in both sleep and wakefulness. It can evolve into hypsarrhythmia in some cases. The EEG can be normal at the onset of the seizures, and repetitive EEGs may be necessary for the diagnosis. Focal seizures are often accompanied by electrographic seizure activity, but the erratic myoclonus may not have a clear EEG correlate.

The neurological examination is abnormal from the onset and affected infants are often lethargic and hypotonic and have psychomotor delays. Developmental regression has also been described (147). The mortality rate is high (up to 50%), and many die within the first 2 years of life (135).

Early myoclonic encephalopathy is thought to be a rare disorder, although the exact incidence is unknown. Various etiologies have been associated with this syndrome, suggesting that it may represent a broad spectrum of clinical entities (138,148,149). Inborn errors of metabolism are commonly reported. Cases associated with nonketotic hyperglycinemia, methylmalonic acidemia, proprionic acidemia, molybdenum co-factor deficiency, and pyridoxine dependency have been reported. Possible but very rare etiologies are methylmalonic acidemia, sulfite oxidase deficiency, Menkes disease, and Zellweger syndrome (135,148,150,151). Structural brain abnormalities have also been described but are less common (131,138).

No treatments have shown to be consistently effective in treating early myoclonic encephalopathy, including AEDs, corticosteroids or ACTH, pyridoxine, or the ketogenic diet. Correction of underlying metabolic disorders may help to improve seizures in the acute setting but does not seem to affect the long-term outcome (152).

Both early myoclonic encephalopathy and early infantile epileptic encephalopathy are quite similar in terms of age of onset, EEG finding of suppression burst, and overlapping seizure types, and therefore their distinction is often difficult, sometimes impossible, at the beginning of the disease (133,138,149). Djukic and colleagues (138) proposed that the conditions may be considered as a continuum, explaining the differentiation between the two syndromes as an epiphenomenon depending on the degree of progressive brainstem injury.

5.5. KNCQ2-Related Neonatal Epileptic Encephalopathy

Recently *KCNQ2* mutations, which are typically associated with benign neonatal epilepsies such as BFNE or less frequently benign idiopathic neonatal convulsions, have been increasingly associated with a more severe phenotype in some patients (153). In these cases seizures occur early, during the first week of life (153). As in BFNE the neonates present with mainly tonic seizures associated with autonomic symptoms, but these are much more difficult to control. The EEG shows a characteristic age-dependent pattern with suppression burst in the beginning followed by multifocal epileptiform discharges. Muscular hypotonia is present and developmental delay soon becomes apparent. In contrast to most early-onset epileptic encephalopathies, seizures diminish gradually during the first year of life and most children become seizure-free by the age of 3 years (153). MRI reveals a characteristic finding with hyperintensities in the basal ganglia and thalamus becoming more subtle later in life, small frontal lobes, thin corpus callosum, and reduced posterior white matter volume (153).

6. EPILEPSY SYNDROMES OF INFANCY

6.1. Benign Infantile Seizures

Benign infantile seizures are divided into familial forms with a characteristic autosomal dominant inheritance trait and an earlier age of onset between 4 and 7 months, and nonfamilial forms with an onset usually later, between 3 and 20 months (154,155). Seizures are focal, typically occurring in clusters. Interictal EEG is normal, though low- or medium-voltage vertex spikes or sharp waves with a dome-like morphology (156) have been described in one form. In the beginning it might be difficult to diagnose infantile seizures as benign, especially in the absence of a family history. Up to 30% of patients diagnosed with "benign" infantile seizures may not have a benign evolution of their condition (157).

6.1.1. BENIGN (NONFAMILIAL) INFANTILE EPILEPSY
Seizures in this condition start between 3 and 20 months of age and present with a focal semiology with motion arrest,

decreased responsiveness, and staring, often with automatisms and mild motor manifestations such as eye deviation or head rotation, and clonic movements involving the head, face, eyelids, or limbs. Seizures last 1 to 4 minutes and occur in clusters 1 to 10 times per day. Interictal EEG is normal in wakefulness and sleep. Ictal EEG shows focal discharges mostly in the temporal areas. Watanabe and colleagues (155) distinguished pure focal forms from secondarily generalized ones, with the latter form showing an onset of the ictal discharge in central, parietal, or occipital areas. The interictal EEG is generally normal. Treatment response to either carbamazepine or phenobarbital is excellent. The infants usually grow to be developmentally normal, with remission of the seizures before age 1 to 3 years (155).

6.1.2. BENIGN FAMILIAL INFANTILE EPILEPSY
Seizures in benign familial infantile epilepsy start between 4 and 7 months and occur mainly in clusters lasting one to several minutes consisting of psychomotor arrest, slow deviation of head and eyes to one side (possibly changing from seizure to seizure), diffuse hypertonia, cyanosis, and unilateral limb jerks. The seizures may be secondarily bilateral, synchronous, or asynchronous, without clear automatisms. Interictal EEG is normal in the awake and asleep states when recorded outside a cluster; however, slow waves and spikes in the parieto-occipital areas can be seen when recorded during a cluster. Ictal EEG consists of recruiting rhythms of increasing amplitude beginning in the centro-occipital areas on either side, spreading to the hemisphere and then to the entire brain. Inheritance is autosomal dominant. In 82% of affected families heterozygous mutations in *PRRT2* have been identified (158); this gene is mainly associated with paroxysmal kinesigenic dyskinesia, familial hemiplegic migraine, and episodic ataxia. Development and outcome are normal.

6.1.3. BENIGN FAMILIAL NEONATAL-INFANTILE EPILEPSY
This may represent a separate entity that lies between the prior two conditions. Onset varies within families, from the neonatal period to 6 months, with most cases occurring around 2 to 3 months of age. Semiology is described as subtle seizures with eye blinking and lip smacking and focal clonic movements of the leg and arm associated with contralateral head rotation. The interictal EEG is mostly normal, though occasional central or posterior spikes have been reported. The ictal EEG shows discharge onset in the posterior quadrants. Molecular studies have revealed mutations in the sodium channel subunit gene *SCN2A* (159).

6.1.4. BENIGN INFANTILE FOCAL EPILEPSY WITH MIDLINE SPIKES AND WAVES DURING SLEEP
Bureau and colleagues (160) and Capovilla and Beccaria (156) described a separate benign condition differing from the previously reported benign infantile seizures because of later onset (between 13 and 30 months), less frequent seizures occurring rarely in clusters, and the lack of ictal automatisms. Seizure semiology is described as loss of contact, motion arrest and staring, with possible eye revulsion, hypotonia, and perioral cyanosis. The interictal EEG during sleep demonstrates

isolated or grouped spikes and waves located on the midline (Fig. 18.20). These may be difficult to see because they can be mixed with spindles or K-complexes. There is usually a family history of epilepsy.

6.1.5. BENIGN FAMILIAL INFANTILE EPILEPSY ASSOCIATED WITH OTHER NEUROLOGICAL CONDITIONS

In 1997 Szepetowski and coworkers (161) described four families with affected individuals presenting with benign familial infantile epilepsy or paroxysmal choreoathetosis or both, termed the infantile convulsions and paroxysmal choreoathetosis syndrome (ICCA syndrome). Linkage to chromosome 16 and dominant inheritance were identified. More recently mutations in *PRRT2* (158) and *SCN8A* (162) have been reported in these conditions. Association of familial hemiplegic migraine with benign familial infantile epilepsy has also been described (163). These different conditions with coexistence of movement disorders, migraine, and epilepsy demonstrate the overlap in their clinical features and etiologic pathways.

6.2. Myoclonic Epilepsy in Infancy

Myoclonic epilepsy in infancy is an electroclinical syndrome recognized in the ILAE classification in 1989 as benign myoclonic epilepsy in infancy among the idiopathic generalized epilepsies (164). The initial term "benign" was given in order to distinguish it from "severe myoclonic epilepsy in infancy" or Dravet disease, but as the evolution is now known to be unfavorable in some children, the term "benign" has been removed from the original name (165). It is characterized by the occurrence of myoclonic seizures in otherwise normal children beginning between 4 months and 3 years of age. Preceding febrile seizures are described in 20% of the children (166).

The seizures consist of myoclonic jerks mostly of the head and proximal arms, occurring in isolation or in brief runs of rhythmic or irregular jerks, varying in frequency and intensity. A slow forward movement of the trunk and an upward and outward movement of arms as well as an upward movement of the eyes can be associated. These seizures occur several times a day, mainly during wakefulness and drowsiness (167), but also in non-REM sleep. Massive myoclonus predominating in the lower limbs causing sudden drop attacks has been reported in 21% of patients (168). Neither atonic seizures nor negative myoclonias have been described (168). Several authors have reported myoclonic seizures triggered by somatosensory stimulation (167), by auditory stimulation (169), and by intermittent photic stimulation (170). These children showed an earlier mean age at onset, 7 months, compared to the patients with spontaneous myoclonias, beginning at 23 months (167). Children can present with spontaneous or reflex myoclonic seizures, or both. Photosensitivity, clinically and electrically, is described in 20% (166).

The interictal EEG is generally normal. In some cases spike-wave bursts have been described, both in the awake state and in sleep (167). The ictal EEG shows, concomitant with the myoclonias, a burst of generalized or diffuse spike-wave activity or polyspikes, mostly described as fast (>3 Hz) but also at slower frequencies of ~1.5 Hz. However, focal discharges, especially in the rolandic and vertex regions, may mimic focal epilepsy (167). Polygraphic video-EEG with surface EMG

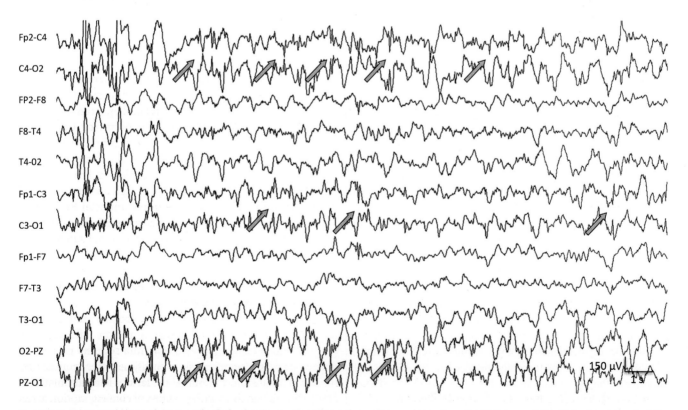

Figure 18.20. Two-year-old boy with benign infantile focal epilepsy with midline spikes and waves during sleep. The EEG demonstrates bilateral central and midline spikes.

recording is useful to identify and characterize the motor manifestation. EEG abnormalities may persist for many years, usually without myoclonic seizures (168).

The etiology is unknown, but a genetic origin is probable. There is a family history of febrile seizures in 50% to 55% of the patients (167). Prognosis is in most cases favorable with normal cognitive outcome and cessation of seizures, mostly within 1 year (166). However cognitive impairment, ranging from mild to severe, has been reported in about 15% of children (166,167,171). Moreover, long-term follow-up studies and case reports have shown that some children, after a seizure-free interval, may develop febrile seizures (171), photic-induced myoclonic or generalized tonic-clonic seizures (167), or other epileptic phenotypes such as CAE (172), myoclonic atonic epilepsy (173), or juvenile myoclonic epilepsy (171).

6.3. Dravet Syndrome

Dravet syndrome, also called severe myoclonic epilepsy in infancy, is characterized by multiple seizure types, prolonged convulsive seizures, and frequent status epilepticus, often fever-induced. It is considered an epileptic encephalopathy, but there is increasing evidence that the cognitive decline is not exclusively the consequence of the epilepsy (174).

Seizures begin in the first year of life (typically around 6 months of age) in a previously normal infant who develops generalized or unilateral clonic seizures, possibly varying from seizure to seizure, typically triggered by fever, illness, or vaccination. They are often prolonged, occur in clusters, and may evolve into status epilepticus. Between 1 and 4 years of age other seizure types may develop, such as focal dyscognitive seizures with staring episodes often accompanied by pallor, oral automatisms, and head and eye deviation, atypical absence seizures that rarely evolve into absence status, or occasionally atonic and tonic seizures (175). Myoclonic seizures occur in many but not all children. Tonic seizures are unusual. One of the main features in Dravet is the low epileptic threshold to external and internal stimuli: in addition to slight body temperature variations and infections, seizures may also be triggered by hot baths, vaccination, physical exercise, emotions, a noisy environment, and photic and pattern stimuli.

The interictal EEG is mostly normal during the first year of life despite the frequent episodes of status epilepticus. Epileptiform abnormalities develop during the second year of life with generalized spikes, polyspikes, and spike-wave activity or focal or multifocal abnormalities, which may be sleep-activated. Progressive background slowing often develops. Children with Dravet after the age of 7 years may have frontal biphasic or triphasic spikes present in the awake state, or subclinical discharges of 5- to 9-Hz spikes activated by sleep lasting 5 to 10 sec (Fig. 18.21) (176).

Photosensitivity is reported in over 40% of children (175) in response to intermittent photic stimulation, bright light, and contrast, but seems to be age-dependent. An increase of photoparoxysmal response from 9% to 41% was reported during the first 2 years after onset (177). However, photosensibility and pattern sensitivity seem to disappear with age (178). Occipital seizures induced by intermittent photic stimulation

have been reported in young children (177). Sleep organization remains mainly normal throughout the disease.

Obtundation status or minor status occurs in 40% of the patients. This is characterized by a variable degree of impaired consciousness accompanied by fragmentary and segmental, erratic myoclonias, involving limbs and face, associated sometimes with hypersalivation. The EEG during these periods consists of diffuse high-voltage slow waves intermingled with focal and diffuse spikes, sharp waves, or spike-waves without constant correlation between spikes and myoclonic jerks (175).

Incidence is reported to be between 1 in 20,000 and 1 in 40,000. Prevalence among infants with seizures beginning in the first year of life is estimated at 3% to 8%. There is a family history of epilepsy or febrile seizures in 23% to 38% (177,178). In about 75% of the patients with Dravet, mutations in the SCN1A gene encoding the alpha-1 subunit of the sodium channel can be identified (179). The presence or absence of an identified mutation does not seem to affect disease presentation. Recently significant age-related differences in duration, focal or generalized aspect, and vigilance state at seizure onset have been demonstrated: patients younger than 5 years were more likely to have provoked, prolonged, focal seizures during wakefulness, whereas adolescents were more likely to have short, generalized-onset seizures occurring during sleep (180).

The seizures are typically treatment-resistant. Valproate, benzodiazepines, and stiripentol may decrease seizure frequency. Topiramate and the ketogenic diet may also be beneficial. Worsening effects have been identified with the use of lamotrigine, carbamazepine, and vigabatrin (181). The long-term outcome is unfavorable. Seizures persist in all patients. Although development remains normal in the first year of life, it slows during the second year of life, and motor impairment, behavioral disturbances, and cognitive dysfunction, which is often severe, may develop. The mortality rate is amongst the highest in the epilepsy population and is reported to be between 5.75% and 17.5%, mainly related to status epilepticus, sudden unexpected death in epilepsy, and accidents (175).

6.4. Epilepsy of Infancy with Migrating Focal Seizures

Migrating partial seizures of infancy, more recently termed "epilepsy of infancy with migrating focal seizures," is a rare early infantile epileptic encephalopathy with a poor prognosis. The hallmarks are as follows: seizure onset before 6 months with the occurrence of almost continuous focal seizures of varying semiology, with migrating random multifocal ictal EEG discharges, and with progressive deterioration of psychomotor development and acquired microcephaly. There appear to be three phases: The first phase, with a mean onset at 3 months (range, first week of life up to 7 months), is characterized by sporadic seizures. During the second phase, the "stormy" phase (ranging from 3 to 10 months), the seizure frequency increases significantly, with clusters of 5 to 30 several times a day or almost continuous seizures for days or weeks (182). During the third phase, with variable age of onset, seizures are significantly reduced but intercurrent diseases may trigger clusters of seizures or status epilepticus.

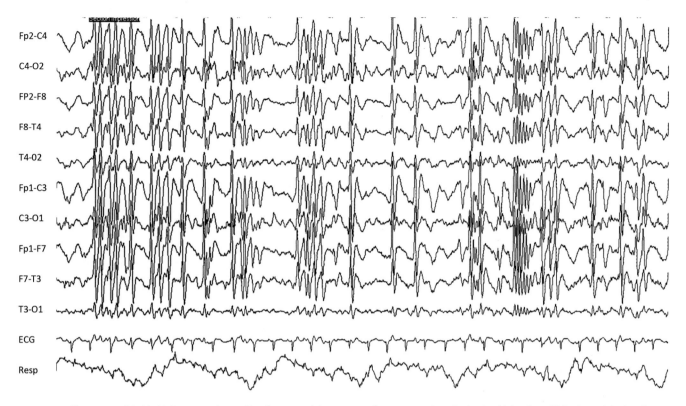

Figure 18.21. Eleven-year-old girl with Dravet syndrome. The sleep record demonstrates frontotemporal predominating high-voltage biphasic or triphasic spikes.

The seizure semiology may include focal motor seizures, lateral head and eye deviation, and eyelid and ocular myoclonia with possible secondary generalization, often with associated autonomic manifestations. Motor manifestations can migrate from one side of the body to the other. Many seizures can be subtle. Spasms are unusual but may occur (182,183).

Early on, the interictal EEG is usually normal. Over time, the background activity becomes progressively slower with possible temporary asymmetries, with multifocal spikes and sharp waves. The ictal EEG is characterized by monomorphic focal rhythmic theta or alpha activity, or focal spikes, which may remain localized or progressively involve a larger area, often moving from one area to another (thus the term migrating) but without the usual propagation patterns. Further seizures can start independently in different areas within the same or contralateral hemisphere before the end of the previous event (Fig. 18.22). Seizures usually last 1 to 4 minutes. With increasing age the ictal pattern tends to increase in amplitude and becomes more prominent in frontal areas (184).

Multiple genes have now been reported in association with this condition. Information about these genes, their mode of inheritance, the encoded protein, the protein function, and the effect on protein function is detailed in a recent study (185). Neuroimaging studies are generally normal in the beginning. Later, nonspecific abnormalities have been reported, including diffuse cerebral atrophy, delayed myelination with white matter hyperintensity, basal ganglia atrophy, thin corpus callosum (186), mesial temporal sclerosis (187) and in one child a dual pathology of the left temporal lobe (atrophy, hippocampal sclerosis, cortical/subcortical blurring) (188).

The long-term prognosis is unfavorable. Between 20% and 57% of patients may die in childhood (183). There is acquired microcephaly, loss of acquired milestones, cognitive disability, axial and peripheral hypotonia, and pyramidal and extrapyramidal signs with athetotic movements (184). The majority of patients are refractory to medications. However, some patients have shown response to bromide, rufinamide, vigabatrin, levetiracetam, adrenocorticotrophin, the ketogenic diet, or different combinations (183,187).

6.5. Hemiconvulsion-Hemiplegia-Epilepsy Syndrome

The hemiconvulsion-hemiplegia-epilepsy syndrome is characterized by prolonged focal status epilepticus, usually occurring during or closely after a febrile illness, followed by transient or permanent hemiplegia ipsilateral to the seizures. Infants under the age of 2 years, but always before the age of 4 years (189), develop convulsive status epilepticus during or soon after a nonspecific febrile illness. Seizures are unilateral or predominating on one side, are mainly clonic, and last several hours and sometimes >24 hours. Impairment of consciousness is variable. The seizures can be associated with autonomic phenomena such as hypersalivation and respiratory manifestations with cyanosis (190).

The ictal EEG shows high-amplitude 2- to 3-Hz delta waves of higher voltage over the affected hemisphere, mixed with low-amplitude fast rhythms at 10 Hz predominating over the posterior areas. Also, pseudo-rhythmic spike-waves contralateral to the convulsions with a periodic electrodecremental pattern lasting 1 to 2 sec have been described. Polygraphic

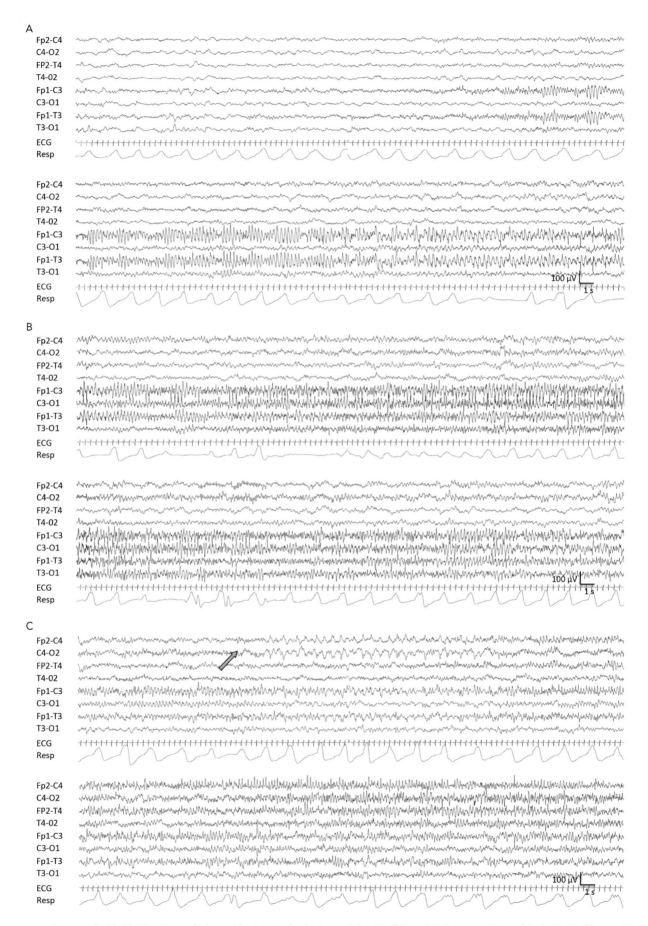

Figure 18.22. Four-month-old girl with epilepsy of infancy with migrating focal seizures. **A:** Part I: Left frontal discharge consisting of rhythmic alpha/theta activity. **B:** Part II: Initial left frontal discharge diffusing on the entire left hemisphere, and onset of right central discharge. **C:** Part III: Migrating discharges independent over different cortical areas; see right central rhythmic slow waves concomitant to clonic movements of the left hand (arrow). **D:** Part IV: Independent discharges of different aspect over different cortical areas. **E:** Part V: Independent discharges of different aspect over different cortical areas, here predominating over the right occipital area. **F:** Part VI: Independent discharges over different cortical areas, here predominating over the left posterior area, and then again migrating to the right frontocentral area.

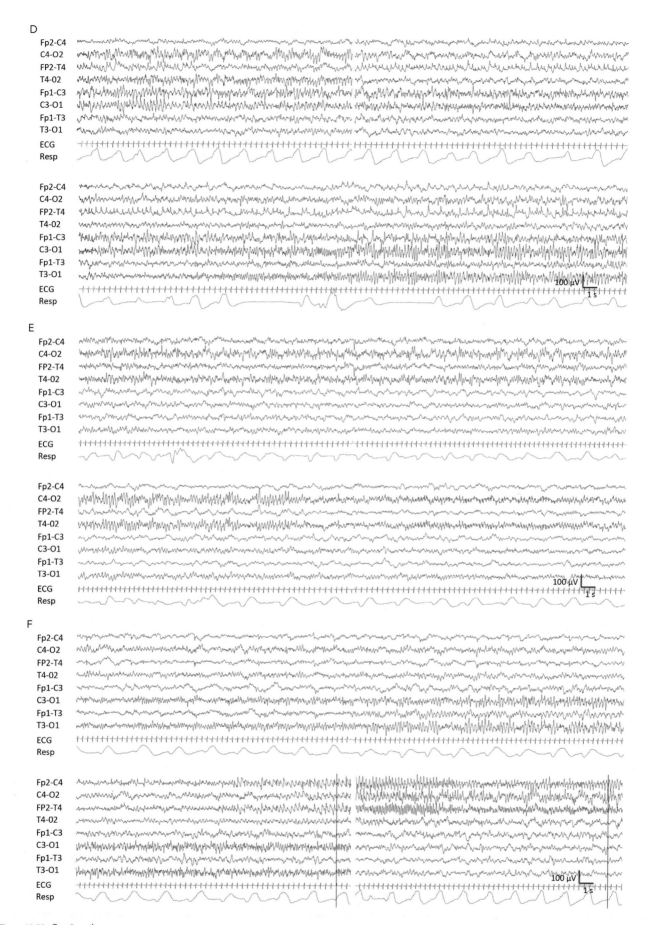

Figure 18.22. Continued

recordings show that correlation between the motor manifestations and the EEG discharges is not constant (190).

As the seizures subside, flaccid hemiplegia is noted that becomes progressively spastic. Complete resolution of hemiplegia is reported in 20% of the patients within the 12 months following the status epilepticus (189). Other associated deficits such as motor aphasia or hemianopsia (191) have been described. A minimum duration of the hemiplegia of at least 1 week (192) has been proposed as a differentiation criterion from deficit after febrile focal seizures (Todd's paresis). Intractable epilepsy develops in two thirds of patients (191) after a seizure-free interval of variable duration ranging from months up to 15 to 20 years (189). Epilepsy is characterized by focal seizures with mainly temporal lobe semiology, though rarely clonic seizures resembling the initial seizures or generalized seizures may be present.

MRI in the acute phase shows unilateral cerebral hemisphere swelling, with sulcal effacement and diffuse cortical and white matter hyperintensities on T2-weighted images, and increased signal on diffusion-weighted images indicating restricted diffusion due to cytotoxic edema. Basal ganglia, ipsi- and contralateral hippocampus, and contralateral posterior brain regions may also be affected (186). Mass effect on the contralateral hemisphere and ipsilateral temporal lobe herniation have been reported (193). In the chronic phase, cerebral atrophy and gliosis develop in the affected hemisphere.

Etiology and pathophysiology remain unknown. It may be symptomatic, observed in children with a preexisting disorders such as tuberous sclerosis complex, Sturge–Weber syndrome, or corpus callosum agenesis, or with other predisposing factors such as head trauma, intracranial infection, and cerebral vascular disease; however, many cases are considered to be idiopathic. As fever is present in most cases in the acute phase, it may be suggested that the hemiconvulsion-hemiplegia-epilepsy syndrome is a severe variant of complicated febrile convulsions. Some authors suggest a primary, presumed viral infection with resulting inflammatory cytokine damage, among which measles (194) and herpes virus 7 (195) have been reported. Others believe that the prolonged ictal activity is responsible for the lesions by impairing the neuronal energy metabolism. Vascular disturbances and relationship to familial migraine disorders with *CACNA1A* gene involvement have been discussed (196). In general, clinical features and animal studies point to inflammation and maturation as probable key factors. Therefore, a concept of age-dependent acute encephalopathies with inflammation-mediated status epilepticus has recently been proposed including idiopathic hemiconvulsion-hemiplegia-epilepsy in infancy and early childhood, febrile infection-related epilepsy syndrome in childhood and adolescence, and new-onset refractory status epilepticus in adulthood (192,197).

Early and aggressive treatment of status epilepticus is essential. In cases of prolonged seizures that do not respond to conventional medical treatment, the ketogenic diet may be an option. Surgical treatment for intractable epilepsy in the chronic phase has been shown to be effective (198). Long-term cognitive outcome is likely unfavorable. Aicardi and colleagues (191) described intellectual disability in 60 out of 72 patients. More recent reports have described poor cognitive outcome in four of five children and seven of eight children with hemiconvulsion-hemiplegia-epilepsy syndrome (194,199).

6.6. West Syndrome

West syndrome is an electroclinical syndrome classically characterized by the triad of epileptic spasms, EEG finding of hypsarrhythmia, and psychomotor arrest or regression. It is an epileptic encephalopathy, defined as a disorder where the epileptic activity itself may contribute to cognitive and behavioral impairments above and beyond what might be expected from the underlying etiology alone (24). The term "infantile spasms" is often used synonymously with West syndrome but leads to confusion because it names a seizure type and a syndrome at the same time. The current international classification (24) recommends using "West syndrome" for the electroclinical syndrome and "epileptic spasms" for the seizure type.

Epileptic spasms consist of flexor, extensor, or mixed flexion and extension contractions of limbs, head, and trunk; they can be bilaterally symmetric or asymmetric or focal. They are longer than a myoclonic jerk and less sustained than a tonic seizure. They can be accompanied by ocular phenomena such as eye revulsion, oculoclonias, and eye deviation, or by a motion arrest. These subtle symptoms can even replace the typical motor phenomenon and can be the only ictal manifestation. The spasms can occur as isolated seizures or in clusters, typically with progressively increasing intensity of the motor component. Spasms can be more frequent upon arousal. Asymmetrical spasms strongly suggest an underlying structural abnormality (200).

The most characteristic interictal EEG aspect in West syndrome is hypsarrhythmia (Fig. 18.23), although it is not observed in all patients, especially in the beginning of the disease. It may be absent in the awake state, underlining the importance of a sleep recording. The classical hypsarrhythmic pattern was described by Gibbs and Gibbs (7): "random high-voltage slow waves and spikes. These spikes vary from moment to moment, both in duration and in location. At times they appear to be focal, and a few seconds later they seem to originate from multiple foci. Occasionally the spike discharge becomes generalized, but it never appears as rhythmically repetitive and highly organized." High amplitude is mostly considered as EEG activity greater than 200 to 300 µV. Hypsarrhythmia varies according to state, generally of higher voltage and showing electrodecremental episodes in non-REM sleep (see Fig. 18.23) and usually markedly reduced or completely absent during REM sleep. The hypsarrhythmic pattern mostly disappears during a cluster of spasms. A positive correlation between the preservation of hypsarrhythmia during a cluster of spasms and favorable outcome has been reported (200,201). In some instances hypsarrhythmia may be accompanied by interictal high frequency (40–140 Hz) oscillations (202).

Variants of hypsarrhythmia have been proposed, also called "atypical hypsarrhythmia" or "modified hypsarrhythmia,"

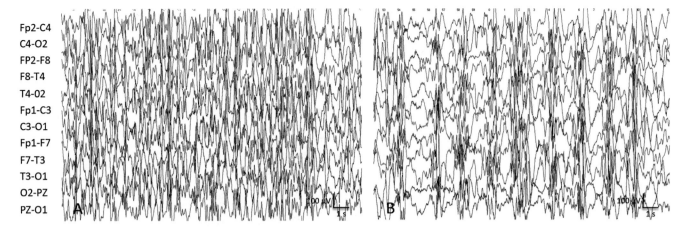

Figure 18.23. Six-month-old infant with West syndrome. **A:** Hypsarrhythmia in the awake state. No physiological pattern, diffuse and generalized asynchronous slow waves, spikes and spike-waves. **B:** Hypsarrhythmia in non-REM sleep showing fragmentation of the spike and spike-wave activity.

though these terms are not well defined. Hrachovy and Frost Jr. (203) described the five following variants:

Hypsarrhythmia with increased interhemispheric synchronization

Asymmetric hypsarrhythmia

Hypsarrhythmia with a consistent focus of abnormal discharge

Hypsarrhythmia with episodes of voltage attenuation

Hypsarrhythmia comprising primarily high-voltage slow activity with little sharp-wave or spike activity.

Hypsarrhythmia is not specific for West syndrome and can occur without epileptic spasms and in different conditions. Vice versa, the absence of hypsarrhythmia does not exclude the presence of epileptic spasms (204). Hypsarrhythmia may be an age-related phenomenon, rarely observed after the age of 5 years (205), and showing decreasing amplitudes with increasing age (206).

The ictal EEG of an epileptic spasm is variable (Fig. 18.24) and associated with a high-voltage slow wave, an attenuation of the background or electrodecremental response, fast rhythms, high-voltage spikes (7), polyspikes and slow waves (86), or various combination of these (Fig. 18.25) (86). The high-voltage slow-wave transient seems to be the most common initial ictal feature of epileptic spasms (206), often followed by fast rhythms, or electrodecremental responses. More recently fast gamma activities concomitant with spasms recorded on scalp EEG have been described (207). These ictal patterns can show significant asymmetry or focal predominance, often associated with clinically asymmetric spasms (Fig. 18.24) (208). On surface EMG recordings, the motor phenomenon of epileptic spasms shows a diamond-shaped aspect with a velocity of the contraction faster than a tonic seizure but slower than a myoclonus (Fig. 18.26). Because of lack of evidence of their generalized or focal origin, epileptic spasms are often classified in their own group, outside of the focal-versus-generalized dichotomy (24).

The incidence of West syndrome is reported at 2 to 4.3 per 10,000 live births (209,210). The peak onset of West syndrome is between 4 and 7 months and it mostly occurs before 12 months of age, though it can evolve or begin at other ages (211,212). When the spasms begin after the age of 1 year they are called late-onset epileptic spasms. Electroclinical features do not differ from those previously described during the first year of life. However, diagnosis is often delayed. Incidence is reported at 2.5% (211) to 9% (213) of all children referred for epileptic spasms.

Causes of West syndrome may be prenatal, perinatal, and postnatal, and include CNS malformations, intrauterine insults, metabolic and genetic diseases, hypoxic-ischemic insults, trauma, hemorrhage, cerebral infections, and tumors. In some cases the cause may be unknown (24). Cerebral malformations described in the setting of West syndrome include focal cortical dysplasia, heterotopias, schizencephaly, hemimegalencephaly, agyria/pachygyria, cerebral midline anomalies such as agenesis of the corpus callosum (i.e., in Aicardi syndrome associated with chorioretinal lacunae) and holoprosencephaly, as well as malformations with a recognized genetic origin such as tuberous sclerosis complex. The presence of epileptic spasms and focal seizures associated with interictal EEG anomalies of focal periodic spikes or bursts of fast rhythms without hypsarrhythmia is highly suggestive of tuberous sclerosis complex or focal cortical dysplasia (see Fig. 18.16). Occipital lesions are described to be associated with the earliest onset of spasms and frontal lesions with late onset, in close relationship with the normal sequence of brain maturation (214). Known chromosomal abnormalities include trisomy 21 (Down syndrome), deletion 1p36 syndrome, deletion 7q11.23 (Williams syndrome plus), tetrasomy 12p (Pallister–Killian syndrome), maternal duplication 15q11q13 (duplication 15q syndrome), and deletion 17p13 (Miller–Dieker syndrome, associated with diffuse cortical malformation and lissencephaly). Multiple specific gene mutations have also been associated with West syndrome (215) (Box 18.3).

The objective of treatment is both cessation of spasms and resolution of hypsarrhythmia. The most recommended first-line treatments are ACTH, oral corticosteroids, and vigabatrin

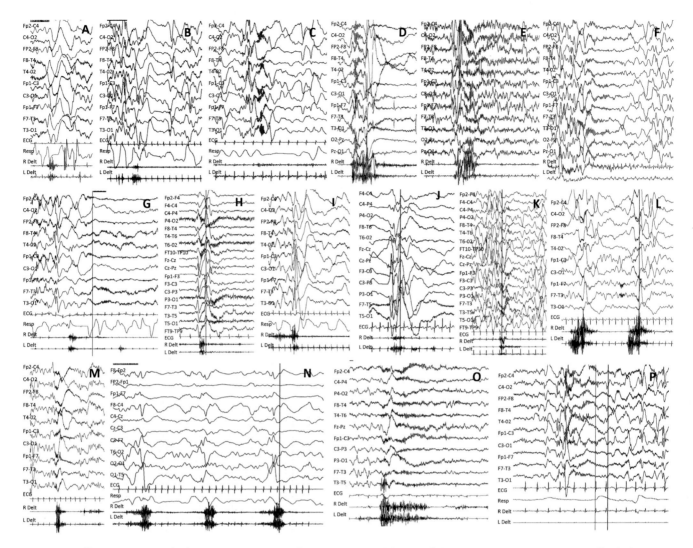

Figure 18.24. *Different EEG aspects of epileptic spasms.* **A:** *1-year-old boy with a congenital disorder of glycosylation (ALG6-CDG—CDG 1c). Diffuse high-voltage slow complex.* **B:** *9-month-old girl with a congenital disorder of glycosylation (ALG1-CDG—CDG lk). Diffuse high-voltage slow complex followed by electrodecrement.* **C:** *7-month-old boy with West syndrome (unknown etiology). Diffuse low-amplitude fast rhythms associated with slow component.* **D:** *2-year-old boy with 1p36 deletion syndrome. Diffuse medium-voltage fast rhythms followed by electrodecrement.* **E:** *3-year-old girl with cryptogenic late-onset epileptic spasms. Frontal predominating high-voltage sharp waves followed by fast rhythms.* **F:** *6-month-old girl with West syndrome, evolution from Ohtahara syndrome (unknown etiology). Diffuse high-voltage slow wave with fast rhythms followed by electrodecrement.* **G:** *6-month-old infant with West syndrome and trisomy 21. Diffuse medium-voltage slow wave and electrodecrement.* **H:** *14-year-old girl with late-onset epileptic spasms of unknown origin. Asymmetric epileptic spasm predominating on right deltoid with diffuse sharp slow-wave complex predominating on left hemisphere.* **I:** *1-year-old boy with a congenital disorder of glycosylation (ALG6-CDG—CDG 1c). Diffuse sharp wave followed by slow complex and electrodecrement.* **J:** *6-week-old infant with left hemimegalencephaly. Sharp slow-wave complex predominating on left hemisphere.* **K:** *18-month-old girl with left posterior cortical malformation. Asymmetric epileptic spasm predominating on right hemibody. Burst of fast rhythms with underlying slow element followed by electrodecrement predominating over left posterior region.* **L:** *4-year-old girl with right hemimegalencephaly. Asynchronous epileptic spasm beginning on left hemibody.* **M:** *2-year-old girl with pharmacoresistant West syndrome of unknown origin. Diffuse fast rhythms.* **N:** *9-month-old boy with tuberous sclerosis complex. Cluster of epileptic spasm with left right hemispheric predominance.* **O:** *6-year-old boy with cryptogenic late-onset epileptic spasms. Epileptic spasm with a more sustained tonic phase.* **P:** *18-month-old girl with mosaic trisomy 13. Diffuse slow wave followed by fast rhythms and electrodecrement. Subclinical.*

(216). ACTH and oral prednisone may have better efficacy than vigabatrin (217). ACTH and vigabatrin are the only AEDs for which there is evidence of efficacy and hypsarrhythmia control (218). Vigabatrin may be especially effective when spasms are caused by tuberous sclerosis and focal cortical dysplasia (219). However, vigabatrin has been associated with irreversible retinal dysfunction and visual field defects. Benzodiazepines, valproic acid, and newer AEDs such as lamotrigine, topiramate, zonisamide, felbamate, and levetiracetam have been used, as well as the ketogenic diet, with variable results. Epileptic spasms may recur after initial response. Children refractory

to medical treatment should undergo evaluation for epilepsy surgery, especially in the presence of a focal lesion on MRI, or positive PET localization (220,221).

Prognosis is mainly determined by the etiology and severity of the underlying disease. However there is evidence that delay of effective treatment will worsen the cognitive and seizure outcome (222,223). There is a reported remission rate of 25% within 1 year of onset in children not treated with hormonal therapy (224), and spasms tend to cease after the fifth year of life (218). Transition to LGS is reported in 20% to 30% of cases (225).

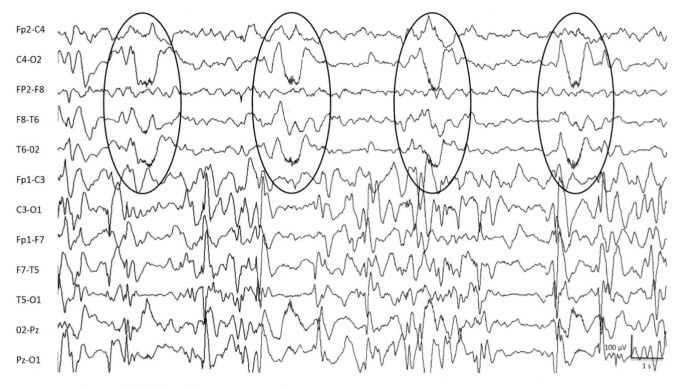

Figure 18.25. Two-month-old girl with Aicardi syndrome. Cluster of asymmetrical (right hemispheric) epileptic spasms.

7. CHILDHOOD EPILEPSY SYNDROMES

7.1. Childhood Absence Epilepsy

Childhood absence epilepsy (CAE) is a generalized epilepsy syndrome affecting school-age children. It is characterized by frequent absence seizures and generalized spike-wave discharges at a frequency of ~3 Hz on EEG.

The onset is typically between 4 and 10 years of age, with a peak from 6 to 7 years (24). Absence seizures consist of abrupt impairment of consciousness accompanied by staring. Motor automatisms include eye blinking, lip licking, swallowing, and perseverative automatisms in which the individual continues actions that were already begun prior to seizure onset. The

seizures last an average of 9 sec, though longer episodes may occur (226). Generalized tonic-clonic seizures may occur in around 12% of patients, typically late in the course of the condition. Patients who experience early treatment failure may be at increased risk for developing generalized tonic-clonic seizures (227).

Interictally, the EEG shows brief (<3 sec) bursts of generalized spike-wave discharges at a frequency of 2.5 to 4.5 Hz (228); these may have a frontal predominance in some cases. Fragments of generalized spike-wave activity may be seen as well, both in wakefulness and more frequently in drowsiness and sleep (226). During non-REM sleep these discharges may also become briefer and more irregular. The underlying

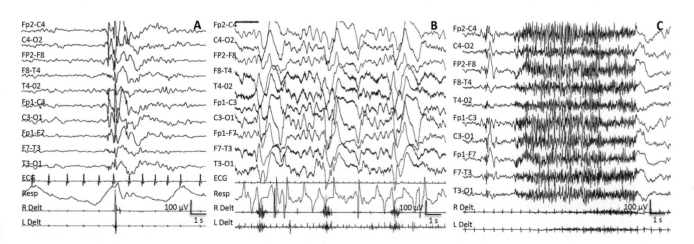

Figure 18.26. Distinction of myoclonus, epileptic spasm, and tonic seizure on polygraphic recording. A: Myoclonic jerk. B: Cluster of epileptic spasms. C: Tonic seizure.

background EEG is usually normal, although occipital intermittent rhythmic delta activity can be seen in up to 30% of CAE patients, occurring at a frequency of 2.5 to 4 Hz (226,229).

The characteristic ictal EEG finding in CAE consists of generalized symmetric spike-wave discharges at a frequency of >2.5 Hz, typically 3 to 4.5 Hz (228) (Figs. 18.4 and 18.27). While >80% of patients display single spike-wave discharges, polyspike and wave discharges may be present at seizure onset in a subset of patients (226,229). The discharges may be maximal in amplitude over the frontal or frontocentral regions. In the majority of patients the discharges are regular, with a consistent relationship between the spike and the slow-wave components throughout the seizure. Some patients may display a more evolving ictal pattern with faster 4-Hz spike-wave discharges at the beginning of the seizure, which then slow to a 3-Hz pattern (Fig. 18.27) (228). Less frequently the seizures may begin with slower activity that then leads into the more typical 3-Hz pattern. In as many of half of patients the seizure may begin with a period of focal slowing or focal spikes lasting an average of 0.5 sec before becoming a generalized discharge. As the seizure develops, the generalized discharges may break down in a subset of patients, becoming irregular and/or focal toward the end of the seizure. Postictal slowing is occasionally present (226).

Atypical EEG findings have been reported, including frontal intermittent rhythmic delta activity, focal sharp waves distinct from the generalized spike-wave activity, and focal slowing (229). Focal epileptiform discharges, when present, occur most commonly in the central regions but may be seen in the frontal, temporal, and parietal areas as well (226). It should be noted that persistent focal slowing or focal spikes occurring over one area may suggest a focal lesion and would warrant further evaluation. Interictal polyspikes may be seen as well, particularly in drowsiness and sleep (226).

The seizures in CAE occur frequently. Greater than 90% of untreated patients have been demonstrated to have at least one

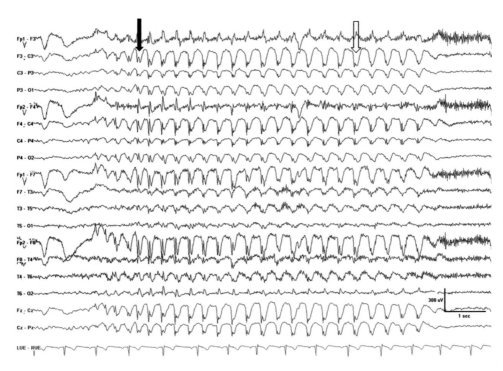

Figure 18.27. An absence seizure in a 10-year-old girl, lasting ~8 sec. The ictal pattern consists of generalized spike-wave discharges with a frontal predominance. At the beginning of the seizure the discharges occur slightly faster, at ~4 Hz (solid arrow). As the seizure continues, the discharges slow to 3 Hz (hollow arrow).

electrographic seizure during a routine 30-minute EEG study with hyperventilation (229). Thus, a diagnosis of absence epilepsy is easily made on a routine EEG for the vast majority of patients. Hyperventilation is the most consistent provoking factor, activating seizures in >90% of untreated patients (226,228). The seizures may also be provoked by hypoglycemia, sleep, and in some cases photic stimulation.

Detailed neuropsychological testing may potentially demonstrate impaired function during spike-wave bursts of any duration in CAE. It has been shown that >90% of discharges that last >3 sec are associated with clinical manifestations on careful testing. Thus, bursts of 3 sec or longer are generally considered to be electrographic seizure patterns even in the absence of gross clinical changes (229,230).

Although children with absence epilepsy often have normal development and grossly normal intellectual functioning at diagnosis, subtle neuropsychological deficits are common. Difficulties with verbal and speech language abilities as well as psychosocial functioning have been demonstrated. Psychiatric diagnoses, especially anxiety and attention-deficit/hyperactivity disorder, are reported in more than half of children with absence epilepsy, and up to a third may have behavioral or social dysfunction (231,232).

CAE is genetically linked, and it is common to have a positive family history. However, no single causative genetic abnormality has been identified. Mutations in genes encoding GABA receptors have been associated with CAE, including *GABRA1, GABRB3,* and *GABARG2* (233,234). Mutations affecting T-type calcium channels, specifically involving *CACNA1H* and *CACNG3,* have also been reported (235,236). The exact pathophysiological link between these mutations and the clinical presentation is not well understood.

First-line therapy for absence epilepsy includes ethosuximide, valproate, and lamotrigine, either alone or in combination. Of these, ethosuximide and valproate have been shown to have superior effectiveness in controlling absence seizures as compared to lamotrigine. A higher incidence of adverse events has been associated with valproate, suggesting that ethosuximide may be the preferred initial treatment agent (230). Carbamazepine and oxcarbazepine are not recommended as they may worsen absence seizures.

7.2. Eyelid Myoclonia with Absences

Also referred to as Jeavons syndrome, this condition is characterized by absence seizures similar to those seen in childhood absence seizures as well as myoclonia of the eyelids, which may occur independently. The interictal EEG consists of brief bursts of generalized spike-wave or polyspike-wave activity at a frequency of ~3 Hz, usually superimposed on an otherwise normal background. These discharges are often frontally predominant, though as many as a third to half of patients may demonstrate occipital predominance at times as well (237,238).

The ictal EEG similarly consists of brief runs of bilateral spike-wave activity at a frequency of 2.5 to 5 Hz that may have a frontal, or in some cases occipital, predominance (237,239). Clinically the seizures consist of eyelid myoclonia, also at a frequency of ~3 Hz, with or without an associated absence

seizures. The seizures can often be elicited by photic stimulation or by eye closure (fixation-off sensitivity). Hyperventilation may also trigger seizures in some patients (238).

In some patients, the generalized spike-wave or polyspike-wave discharges may be preceded by runs of focal spikes over either the frontal or occipital regions. Focal interictal spikes have also been reported over the frontal region, posterior quadrant, and less commonly temporal regions (237–239). A subset of patients may also display rhythmic "spiky" occipital discharges on the interictal EEG; these are intermixed with the normal posterior alpha activity but are higher in frequency and higher in amplitude than the patient's baseline alpha rhythm (237,238).

There is a family history of seizures and epilepsy in >80% of patients, including febrile seizures, CAE, juvenile myoclonic epilepsy, and generalized epilepsy with febrile seizures plus (240). Eyelid myoclonia with absence is now classified by the ILAE as an absence seizure with special features, as opposed to an independent epilepsy syndrome (24).

7.3. Epilepsy with Myoclonic Absences

The myoclonic absence seizures that are characteristic of this syndrome consist of rhythmic bilateral myoclonic jerks associated with variable degrees of impairment of consciousness. Other seizure types may occur also in as many as two thirds of cases; these include generalized tonic-clonic seizures (45%), atonic seizures (33%), and simple absence seizures (4%) (241). The interictal EEG background is typically normal. Generalized spike-wave discharges can be seen interictally in about one third of cases (241). These can have a frontal predominance and at times may display focal asymmetries. As with CAE, there may be fragmentation of the interictal spike-wave activity during sleep. The discharges during sleep may be associated with myoclonus.

The ictal EEG during myoclonic absence seizures is characterized by bilateral synchronous spike-wave or polyspike-wave discharges at a frequency of ~3 Hz, similar to that seen in CAE. The onset and offset are typically abrupt, though at times the ictal pattern may end with evolving frontal delta activity, which can be asymmetric in some cases. The seizures occur multiple times per day and may last up to a minute. As with CAE, they can be provoked by hyperventilation. In up to 14% of patients they may also be elicited by photic stimulation (241). The seizures do not occur during REM or slow-wave sleep but may be present during light sleep with a shorter duration and less prominent myoclonus.

EMG recordings during the seizures demonstrate rhythmic myoclonus that occurs at the same frequency as the spike-wave activity. The myoclonus can be unilateral or asymmetric and generally involves the muscles of the shoulders, arms, and legs. There is often an associated tonic component, leading to progressive elevation of the arms during the seizure (242). Involvement of the facial muscles is less common, and eyelid involvement is rare. The impairment of consciousness is variable and in some cases may not be as dramatic as in CAE.

This onset of this condition is typically between 1 and 12 years of age, with a mean of 7 years (242). As many as 45% of patients may demonstrate cognitive impairments prior to diagnosis. Predisposing factors such as structural brain injury and chromosomal anomalies have been reported in up to a third of patients (241). The mainstay of treatment is sodium valproate and ethosuximide, often in combination (243). Addition of lamotrigine or topiramate may provide additional control (242,244), though lamotrigine has also been shown to worsen myoclonic seizures in some patients (245). Carbamazepine, oxcarbazepine, and phenytoin may worsen the seizures.

7.4. Epilepsy with Myoclonic-Atonic Seizures

Also called myoclonic astatic epilepsy or Doose syndrome, this condition is characterized by multiple seizure types including myoclonic-atonic, absence, myoclonic, tonic, and atonic seizures as well as generalized tonic-clonic seizures. Nonconvulsive status epilepticus is common. The background EEG may be normal initially. Interictal generalized spike-wave discharges and polyspike-wave discharges at a slow frequency of 2 to 3 Hz are typical. These tend to be polymorphic and irregular, and can occur singly or in bursts. They may appear lateralized with shifting asymmetries, but typically there is no persistent focality (246) (Fig. 18.28). The discharges tend to increase during sleep. They may also be activated by photic stimulation. Other common abnormalities in the interictal background include the presence of 4- to 7-Hz rhythmic theta activity that is most prominent over the parietal areas. An occipital 4-Hz delta rhythm that abates with eye opening may be present as well (247).

During a myoclonic-atonic seizure, the EEG shows bursts of bilaterally synchronous spike-wave or polyspike-wave discharges. These build in amplitude and slow in frequency from 3 to 4 Hz to 1.5 to 2 Hz over a period of 2 to 6 sec. They may end with a high-amplitude diffuse slow wave (see Fig. 18.28B). Clinically the seizures consist of brief symmetric myoclonic jerks involving the neck, shoulders, and extremities causing the arms to abduct and the knees to flex. This is followed by a loss of muscle tone, often resulting in a fall. Both the EEG discharges and the muscle jerks occur synchronously from both sides of the body, suggesting a primary generalized process (246).

Patients can also have isolated myoclonic or isolated atonic seizures. The atonic seizures can at times be very brief, characterized only by a momentary head drop without falling and with preserved consciousness. Atypical absence seizures and generalized tonic-clonic seizures may also be present. Vibratory tonic seizures have been described, characterized by the sudden appearance of generalized spike-wave discharges similar to those described above, followed quickly by diffuse fast activity; the EEG is then obscured by muscle artifact as the patient has tonic extension of the arms with vibratory movements (247).

Absence status epilepticus can occur and can last for extended periods. During periods of absence status epilepticus the EEG shows long runs of irregular slow waves or slow spike-wave complexes. Periods of myoclonic status have also been reported, which are likewise characterized by prolonged runs of slow spike-wave discharges. In both instances, the discharges are accompanied by generalized disorganization and loss of the physiological background rhythms. These patterns can wax and wane over a period of hours or even days.

The onset of myoclonic astatic epilepsy is typically between 7 months and 6 years of age, often in previously healthy children. Although development is generally normal prior to diagnosis, the clinical course is variable. The seizures subside within 3 years in more than half of patients, while others develop intractable epilepsy. Similarly, cognitive outcome is normal in about half of patients, while others develop some degree of mental retardation or behavioral abnormality (247,248). Poor prognostic factors include absence status epilepticus, younger age at seizure onset, and the presence of focal spikes (248,249).

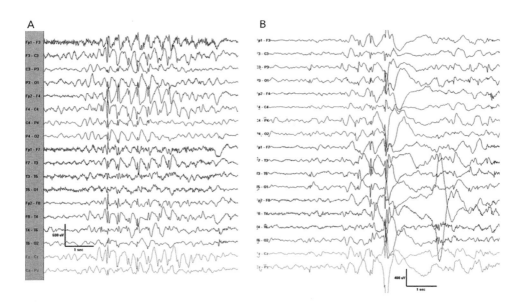

Figure 18.28. A 3-year-old boy with myoclonic astatic epilepsy. **A:** The interictal EEG demonstrates runs of generalized spike-wave discharges at a frequency of ~2.5 Hz. **B:** The ictal discharge during a myoclonic seizure consists of bursts of bilaterally synchronous spike- and polyspike-wave discharges that increase in amplitude and decrease in frequency over a period of seconds, terminating with a high-amplitude slow wave.

Individuals with myoclonic astatic epilepsy often have a family history of epilepsy, suggesting that some cases may be genetic. However, no specific associated gene has been identified, and the inheritance patterns are likely multifactorial. Mutations in the *SCN1A, SCN1B,* and *GABRG2* genes have been reported (250). Myoclonic astatic epilepsy has also been associated with mutations of the GABA transporter gene *SLC6A1* (251), as well as mutations of *SCL2A1,* which is associated with glucose transporter 1 (GLUT1) deficiency (252).

AEDs used for myoclonic astatic epilepsy are primarily valproic acid and benzodiazepines. Ethosuximide may be useful in treating absence seizures. The ketogenic diet is often very effective and in some instances has been demonstrated to be superior to medications in controlling the seizures (247). In particular, patients with GLUT1 deficiency may improve substantially with the ketogenic diet (252). Carbamazepine, oxcarbazepine, and phenytoin may worsen the seizures in this condition.

7.5. Self-Limited Epilepsy with Centrotemporal Spikes

Also called benign epilepsy with centrotemporal spikes or rolandic epilepsy, this childhood epilepsy syndrome is marked by brief nocturnal motor seizures and centrotemporal spikes with a horizontal dipole appearance on EEG that increase during sleep. Seizures arise out of sleep or shortly after awakening, and most commonly involve hemifacial twitching, at times with associated clonic activity of the ipsilateral hand or arm, and less frequently with involvement of the lower extremity.

This may be accompanied by unilateral numbness around the mouth, tongue, or lips. Speech arrest is common, as is hypersalivation. Oropharyngeal symptoms involving "guttural" or "gargling" sounds are reported in more than half of patients (253).

The characteristic spikes are stereotyped, are generally of high amplitude, and are followed by a prominent slow wave. They become more frequent during non-REM sleep, increasing as much as fivefold, and at times they may become quasirhythmic or periodic (Fig. 18.29). In some patients the spikes occur only during sleep (254). During REM sleep, on the other hand, spike frequency may decrease. An important aspect of the spikes in this condition is the presence of a horizontal dipole. This classically involves a maximum negative pole over the central or centrotemporal region with a positive pole bifrontally (see Fig. 18.29C). Gregory and Wong (255) proposed a hypothesis that these discharges arise from a generator oriented tangentially to the surface of the brain, located in the lower rolandic region between the frontal positivity and centrotemporal negativity. The presence of this horizontal dipole is considered to be important in identifying the syndrome. It has been demonstrated that children with centrotemporal spikes without a horizontal dipole may be more likely to have frequent seizures and neurodevelopmental abnormalities, and therefore may be better classified as a separate entity (255).

Although called centrotemporal, the negativity of the spikes can often be maximal over the central regions, either in the high central (EEG leads C3 and C4) or low central (C5 and C6) regions (254). The spikes can be unilateral or can occur bilaterally. Bilateral spikes can be either synchronous or asynchronous. The laterality and symmetry of the spikes may

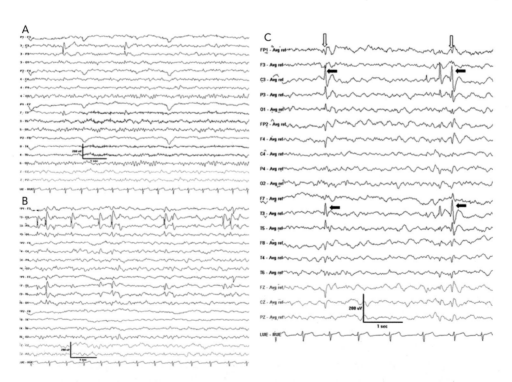

Figure 18.29. A 9-year-old girl with rolandic epilepsy. **A:** The interictal record in the longitudinal bipolar montage demonstrates high-amplitude spikes over the left central and temporal regions. **B:** During sleep the spikes become more frequent. **C:** In the average reference, the horizontal dipole is apparent: a maximum negativity is seen over the central and temporal regions (C3 and T3, solid arrows), with a relative positivity over the frontal regions at Fp1 (hollow arrows).

change over time in the same patient. There does not seem to be a correlation between the frequency or location of spikes and the severity of the seizures. While treatment may decrease the frequency of spike discharges, this is of unclear prognostic significance (256).

The seizures are infrequent, and a subset of patients will have only one lifetime seizure. They tend to be brief, lasting ~1 to 2 minutes. Secondary generalization can occur. Status epilepticus is rare. Because the seizures are infrequent, ictal EEGs are not commonly obtained. The available descriptions are of focal seizure onset arising over the centrotemporal region on one side, at times with secondary spread. The initial EEG findings are variable and may consist of rhythmic spikes, focal fast activity, or focal rhythmic slowing (257). The activity may then spread from the centrotemporal region to involve the ipsilateral hemisphere and subsequently the contralateral side as well. At times the focal discharges may be preceded by focal attenuation of electrical activity (257).

Less common EEG abnormalities may include apparent focal slowing in the same distribution as the spikes, especially when the spikes become frequent (256,258). This may be a result of the slow-wave discharges accompanying the spikes rather than a true focal slowing of the EEG background. Focal spikes outside of the centrotemporal regions are rare (254). Generalized spike-wave activity at 3 to 5 Hz has been reported, though this is considered an atypical finding and is not consistently seen (254,256).

The onset of epilepsy in this condition is between the ages of 2 and 13 years, with the majority of cases starting between ages 5 and 10. The seizures typically resolve during or before adolescence, though a very small number of patients may continue to have seizures during adulthood (253). Patients are often grossly neurologically and intellectually intact at diagnosis. However, neuropsychological testing has increasingly demonstrated attention difficulties, visual-spatial deficits, and impairments in auditory processing and language and reading skills (259,260). These impairments may be recognizable at diagnosis on careful testing and may worsen over time (261). They may or may not be reversible as the condition resolves.

This syndrome is a familial condition, generally thought to be an autosomal dominant trait with variable penetrance, although no single causative gene has been identified. Abnormalities involving chromosome 15q14, *GRIN2A*, *KCNQ2*, and chromosome 11p13 involving elongator protein complex 4 (ELP4) have been reported (262–265).

As the seizures are often infrequent, brief, and expected to remit by adolescence, treatment with medications is not always required. If treatment is indicated, valproic acid, carbamazepine, oxcarbazepine, and levetiracetam can all be useful in controlling the seizures (266). Benzodiazepines may be particularly effective in eliminating the spikes (258). Clobazam at night for patients with nocturnal seizures can be very effective and was better tolerated than carbamazepine in one study (267).

Not all children with spikes over the centrotemporal region have this condition. Rolandic spikes can, for example, occur in normal children who may never go on to develop seizures (253). Central or centrotemporal spikes can be seen commonly in both Rett syndrome and Fragile X syndrome (268,269).

Epileptic aphasia (Landau–Kleffner syndrome) and epileptic encephalopathy with continuous spike-and-wave during sleep can also present with midtemporal or centrotemporal spikes that become abundant during sleep. Structural lesions involving the rolandic area may also rarely result in spikes in a similar distribution to that seen in self-limited epilepsy with centrotemporal spikes. Identification of a typical horizontal dipole may help to differentiate self-limited epilepsy from other causes of centrotemporal spikes (255). An appropriate clinical setting is essential to make the diagnosis.

7.6. Panayiotopoulos Syndrome

Children with Panayiotopoulos syndrome have infrequent, largely autonomic seizures. They often arise out of sleep and can be quite prolonged. The seizures typically begin with symptoms such as nausea, retching, and vomiting. Other autonomic features may include pallor, cyanosis, mydriasis, and thermoregulatory changes. Unilateral eye deviation or head deviation is common. Consciousness is often intact at the beginning of the seizure but becomes impaired as the seizure progresses (270). Autonomic status epilepticus may occur. Syncope-like seizures, marked by complete unresponsiveness and flaccidity, occur in as many as half of patients (271). The age of onset can be between 1 and 14 years, with a mean age between 5 and 6 years (272). The syndrome occurs in otherwise neurologically intact patients with no family history of epilepsy. Brain imaging is normal. The majority of patients will have less than five lifetime events, and many will have only one. Remission commonly occurs 1 to 2 years after onset, though periods of >7 years have been reported.

The interical EEG classically shows posterior spikes, with approximately two thirds of patients demonstrating occipital spikes on at least one EEG (Fig. 18.30) (272,273). The spikes are frequently of high amplitude and may appear morphologically similar to the centrotemporal spikes seen in rolandic epilepsy (278). They vary in frequency and can be rare. The spikes may demonstrate a dipolar field, often with a parieto-occipital distribution (274). Multifocal spikes and spike-wave complexes can also occur independently over other regions of the brain with shifting foci. These interictal discharges are usually superimposed on an otherwise normal interictal background. The initial interictal EEG is normal in ~10% of patients (270).

Serial EEGs have shown that the spike focus may shift over time from a posterior predominance to a centrotemporal or, less commonly, frontal predominance. At times there may be frontal spikes that appear synchronous with the occipital spikes, although in fact the occipital spikes precede the frontal ones by a few milliseconds. This is therefore thought to represent propagation in which frontal spikes are activated by occipital foci (274).

More rarely, variations in morphology such as small subtle spikes or spikes with a positive polarity may occur (273). Brief bursts of generalized spike and slow-wave complexes can occasionally be present. In some cases generalized spikes may be the only abnormal finding, or they may be intermixed with focal spikes. The spikes are often activated by sleep. In some cases they are eliminated by opening the eyes.

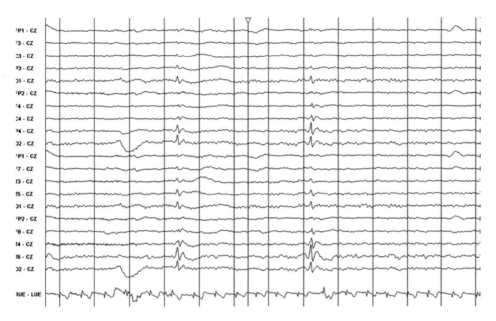

Figure 18.30. A 7-year-old boy with Panayiotopoulos syndrome and one lifetime seizure. The interictal EEG shows high-amplitude spikes over the right greater than left posterior quadrants. Sensitivity 10 uV/mm; time base 30 mm/sec.

The ictal EEG is characterized by rhythmic slow activity, generally in the delta or sometimes theta ranges, which may be intermixed with spikes. The seizures are typically focal in onset and often begin over the posterior head regions, although they may begin more anteriorly as well. The electrographic seizure activity may precede the onset of clinical symptoms, sometimes by as much as 10 minutes or longer. As the seizure evolves the focal rhythmic slowing may change in frequency and may generalize. The seizures can be quite prolonged, typically lasting >5 minutes and in some cases lasting several hours. More than 40% of patients experience autonomic status epilepticus with symptoms lasting >30 minutes and in some cases up to several hours (272).

As the seizures are usually infrequent and often resolve spontaneously, treatment is not always necessary. Treatment should be considered when the seizures interfere with the child's functioning. In these cases no single medication has been demonstrated to be superior. Carbamazepine is often used, and oxcarbazepine, valproate, levetiracetam, phenytoin, and lamotrigine may all be effective. Cases of autonomic status epilepticus must be acutely assessed and treated. Benzodiazepines are often used, but care should be taken with aggressive intravenous benzodiazepine use in autonomic status epilepticus as there is potential for worsening respiratory depression, hypotension, and cardiopulmonary arrest (275).

7.7. Late-Onset Childhood Occipital Epilepsy (Gastaut Type)

This syndrome is also referred to as idiopathic childhood occipital epilepsy of Gastaut and childhood epilepsy with occipital paroxysms. The seizures primarily consist of simple visual hallucinations and/or blindness, and they are often followed by a headache. The seizures are often frequent, occurring up to several times per day in untreated patients. The characteristic visual hallucinations usually consist of shapes and colors that develop rapidly and may appear to multiply or move as the seizure progresses, lasting seconds to minutes. They usually have a stereotyped appearance and progression (270). Ictal blindness is abrupt in onset and usually total, often lasting several minutes with preserved consciousness (276). Less than 10% of patients also have complex visual hallucinations including faces and objects or visual distortions such as micropsia and palinopsia (277). Motor symptoms including eye deviation, eyelid fluttering, and head deviation may also occur, usually following the visual symptoms. The seizures may progress to complex focal seizures, hemiconvulsions, or generalized convulsions (270,276). Postictal headache occurs in about half of patients (276,277). The headache may occur immediately after the seizure or may be delayed by several minutes. Associated symptoms, such as nausea, vomiting, photophobia, and phonophobia, may occur, making this postictal headache indistinguishable from migraine. This condition usually affects children in late childhood and early adolescence, with a peak onset at age 8 to 9 years (277).

The interictal EEG demonstrates occipital or posterior temporal spikes, often with an otherwise normal background (270,277). The spikes are high in amplitude, up to 200 to 300 microvolts. They can be unilateral or bilateral, though even when bilateral they are often asymmetric. The frequency with which the discharges occur can vary, with some patients demonstrating spikes only in sleep and some having a consistently normal interictal EEG (276). Generalized spike-wave or polyspike-wave discharges, centrotemporal spikes, or other focal spikes may also occur in a subset of patients (277).

The occipital spikes often demonstrate fixation-off sensitivity, wherein they can be induced by eliminating visual fixation, as in darkness or closing the eyes. Conversely, the spikes may be eliminated by eye opening or visual fixation, even in darkness. Less commonly, hyperventilation or photic stimulation may also activate the occipital discharges (278).

During a seizure, the interictal spikes disappear and rhythmic fast activity appears over the occipital region, sometimes intermixed with low-amplitude occipital spikes (279). Eyelid movement and oculomotor involvement have been associated with the development of slow spike-wave discharges as the seizure evolves. Head deviation has been associated with the development of rhythmic activity in the theta frequency range. Eye deviation may be preceded by a rapid rhythmic spiking (279). During ictal blindness the EEG shows pseudo-periodic slow waves and spikes (279). The seizure may propagate and spread, leading to hemiconvulsions or generalized tonic-clonic seizures.

As with self-limited rolandic epilepsy, it is important to bear in mind that the characteristic spikes are not necessarily pathognomonic for this syndrome. Occipital spikes may be seen in structural lesions involving the occipital regions, in patients with visual impairments, and in a small number of normal children (276). Other epilepsy syndromes, including absence epilepsy, Panayiotopolous syndrome, and photosensitive reflex epilepsy, may all demonstrate occipital spikes as well.

7.8. Epileptic Encephalopathy with Continuous Spike and Waves During Sleep

Epileptic encephalopathy with continuous spike and waves during sleep (CSWS) is an electroclinical syndrome characterized by developmental regression and an EEG demonstrating continuous epileptiform discharges during sleep. The terms "continuous spike and waves during slow-wave sleep" and "electrical status epilepticus in sleep" are often used interchangeably. However, some use the former to refer to the syndrome itself and the latter to refer to the electrographic findings, which can be present in other syndromes as well (280).

The syndrome occurs in school-aged children who generally have preexisting neurocognitive deficits. The hallmark is developmental regression, which may follow the onset of seizures by up to 1 to 2 years. This is often a generalized decline, marked by diminished IQ, deterioration in language, temporospatial disorientation, and behavioral changes. Decreased attention span, aggression, hyperactivity, and rarely psychosis have all been described as the condition progresses (281). The pattern of regression may vary by individual. This is in contrast to acquired epileptic aphasia, or Landau–Kleffner syndrome, in which the regression is predominantly in the language domain.

The distinguishing electrographic feature involves the presence of continuous spike-wave discharges during non-REM sleep. These discharges appear suddenly at the onset of sleep and persist throughout all stages of sleep except REM sleep. They are typically bilateral and diffuse, occurring at a frequency of 1.5 to 2 or 2.5 Hz (Fig. 18.31). Atypical morphologies, including repetitive spikes without the slow wave, sharp waves, and asymmetric discharges, may be present as well (281). In the classical description by Patry and colleagues (282), the spikes occupied between 87% and 100% of the sleep record, and a spike index of >85% during sleep is often considered necessary to make the diagnosis (283). During REM sleep

there is fragmentation of the discharges and the EEG pattern may resemble that of the awake record. The discharges often resolve abruptly upon awakening.

The background EEG during the awake state may be normal or there may be interictal epileptiform discharges, which can vary from person to person. Generalized spike-wave discharges may be present, either singly or in bursts at a frequency of 2 to 3 Hz, either with or without clinical correlate (see Fig. 18.31A) (283). Focal spikes are also described, particularly over the frontal, frontotemporal, or centrotemporal regions. Multifocal spikes are less common (281,282).

The mechanism by which electrical status epilepticus in sleep leads to neuropsychological dysfunction and regression is not fully understood. It is thought that the continuous epileptiform discharges, even without apparent clinical manifestations, may interfere with specific cerebral processes and lead to derangements in language and other developmental domains (284).

Clinical seizures can be of varying types, including focal seizures, primary or secondarily generalized tonic-clonic seizures, and absences. The seizures initially tend to be rare, but as the condition progresses they may become more frequent or may change in semiology (281). Treatments include benzodiazepines, steroids, and conventional AEDs including phenytoin, carbamazepine, and valproate. Surgical options, including multiple subpial transection, hemispheric surgery, and corpus callosotomy, have been successful as well. A recent pooled analysis reported improvement in EEG and/or cognition in 49% of patients treated with AEDs (excluding benzodiazepines), 68% of those treated with benzodiazepines, 81% of those treated with steroids, and 90% of those who underwent surgery (285).

7.9. Landau–Kleffner Syndrome

Acquired epileptic aphasia, or Landau–Kleffner syndrome (LKS), is a rare epileptic encephalopathy of childhood. It consists of language regression in the setting of an abnormal EEG demonstrating epileptiform discharges and usually develops in previously neurologically normal children between the ages of 3 and 7 years.

Clinically, patients develop either abrupt or gradual loss of language abilities, including a profound impairment of oral language and a loss of ability to decode auditory speech. The latter, often referred to as "auditory agnosia," is the dominant feature of the condition (286). The initial symptom is commonly inability to understand spoken words, or "word deafness," which then progresses to a paucity of spoken language as well. Written language and signing may be less affected. The language interruption may precede, coincide with, or follow the onset of seizures and/or an abnormal EEG (287). Multiple seizure types can occur, including focal motor seizures, atypical absences, generalized tonic-clonic seizures, and rarely tonic seizures. The seizures are typically infrequent and easily controlled with medication. They often decrease in frequency as the child ages (288).

There is not a defining EEG pattern; frequently the interictal record shows spikes, sharp waves, or spike-wave activity

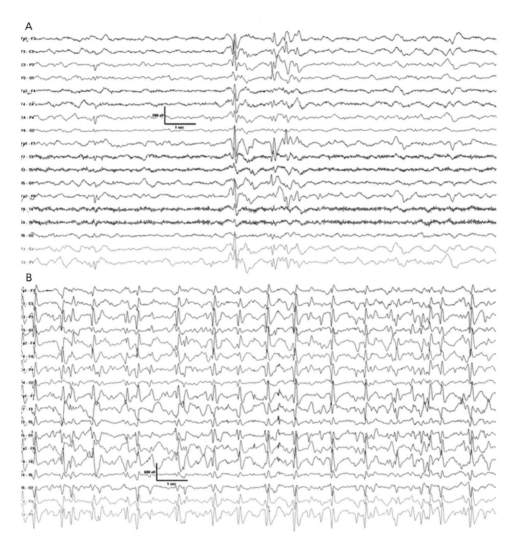

Figure 18.31. *An 11-year-old boy with autism and language regression diagnosed with CSWS. A: The interictal EEG shows occasional generalized spikes or spike-wave discharges. B: During slow-wave sleep there are diffuse spikes and spike-wave discharges, occurring nearly continuously at a frequency of ~1.5 to 2 Hz.*

that occurs primarily over the temporal or parietal regions (289). The spikes are often bilateral and repetitive. They may occur more focally in the rolandic regions, frontal regions, or parietal-occipital regions. They may also be multifocal or generalized. These discharges are activated by sleep, often dramatically. At times the abnormalities may only be present during sleep, so obtaining a sleep EEG is important in the evaluation of this condition.

LKS is highly associated with electrical status epilepticus during sleep. In these cases, nearly continuous spikes or spike-wave discharges emerge during sleep, usually at a frequency of 1.5 to 2.5 Hz. These discharges occupy 85% or more of the sleep record and are usually generalized, though they can be unilateral or focal as well (281). Many if not most children with LKS will develop electrical status epilepticus during sleep at some point (290), but it is not required to make the diagnosis of LKS.

There is considerable clinical and electrographic overlap between LKS and CSWS, though there are distinguishing characteristics. LKS tends to occur in previously normal children, while preexisting neuropsychological deficits may be present

in children who develop CSWS. The regression in LKS is primarily related to language, while more generalized behavioral and cognitive regression may occur in CSWS. The EEG finding of electrical status epilepticus during sleep is required for the diagnosis of CSWS, while it may or may not be present in LKS (288,290). The two conditions are often grouped together, though they remain classified as separate electroclinical syndromes (24).

7.10. Genetic Epilepsy with Febrile Seizures Plus

Also termed "generalized epilepsy with febrile seizures plus," or GEFS+, this is a familial epilepsy syndrome with heterogeneous phenotypes and a predisposition to febrile seizures. Patients may have typical febrile seizures, or they may have febrile seizures that persist beyond the age of 5 or 6 years, termed febrile seizures plus. Seizures in the absence of fever may also occur, either concurrently with the febrile seizures or after they have resolved. A spectrum of afebrile seizure types can be present, including absences, myoclonic seizures, and atonic seizures (291). Focal seizures, particularly temporal lobe seizures, may be present as well (292). The seizures often resolve by adolescence (291,292). Although there is usually a strong family history of epilepsy, individuals within the same family often present with varying phenotypes (293).

There is no typical electrographic pattern associated with GEFS+. EEG abnormalities are determined by the type of seizure a given individual may have. It has been speculated that some patients with other epilepsy syndromes, including Dravet syndrome, LGS, and myoclonic atonic epilepsy (Doose syndrome), may fall under the umbrella of GEFS+ (292). In such cases the typical EEG findings would be those of the electroclinical syndrome.

GEFS+ is a familial condition, following either an autosomal dominant pattern or complex inheritance patterns. Several different genes may be involved. The most commonly identified mutations are those involving the alpha-1 subunit gene of the neuronal sodium channel, *SCN1A*, on chromosome 2q24-33 (294). Mutations of the beta-1 subunit gene, *SCN1B* on chromosome 19q13, are also common, and in fact this was the first gene to be associated with GEFS+ (295). The GABA$_A$ receptor gamma2 subunit gene, *GABRG2* (5q34), has also been strongly implicated (296), and other genetic abnormalities have been associated with the condition as well (Box 18.4).

7.11. Lennox–Gastaut Syndrome

LGS is a severe intractable epilepsy syndrome that consists of a mixture of multiple seizure types with associated mental retardation; there are characteristic slow spike-wave discharges and paroxysmal fast activity on EEG. Onset is usually between 1 and 8 years, with a peak incidence between 3 and 5 years; onset after 10 years of age is rare. The seizures are often very frequent and may occur hundreds of times per day (9). Tonic seizures are the most common seizure type, followed by atypical absences and atonic seizures. Other seizure types, including myoclonic seizures, generalized tonic-clonic seizures, and focal seizures, occur frequently as well. Approximately 50% to 75% of LGS patients develop nonconvulsive status epilepticus (225). Symptoms can occur without any apparent cause, or the syndrome can occur in conjunction with a known brain injury or an underlying condition such as anoxic encephalopathy, trauma, infection, degenerative disorders, or genetic etiology. Approximately 20% to 30% of patients who develop LGS have a history of infantile spasms or West syndrome (9,225).

The interictal slow spike-wave discharges occur at a frequency of 1.5 to 2.5 Hz and are typically generalized and synchronous, though lateralization can occur. There is frequently

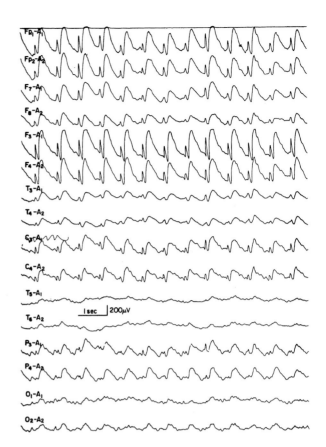

Figure 18.32. An 11-year-old patient with LGS. The EEG shows pronounced slow (~1.5 Hz) spike-wave complexes in generalized synchrony with a frontal maximum. The patient was awake at the time of this recording; there were no clinical ictal manifestation. (With permission from Nordli DR, Riviello JJ, Niedermeyer E. Seizures and epilepsy in infants to adolescents. In: Schomer DL, Lopes deSilva FH, eds. Niedermeyer's Electroencephalography, 6th ed. Philadelphia: Lippincott Williams & Wilkins. Fig. 26.32B)

a frontal predominance (246) (Figs. 18.5 and 18.32). The morphology and frequency may vary from burst to burst or even within a single burst (Fig. 18.33). The discharges are often abundant but may wax and wane significantly (225). Occasionally, rapid spike-and-wave discharges at 3 Hz or even 4 Hz may occur in combination with the slow spike-and-wave activity (9). Photic stimulation has no effect on the spikes (225).

The interictal EEG background is often slow and disorganized, though in some cases it can be less abnormal. During non-REM sleep, the spike-wave discharges are enhanced and polyspikes may emerge. Runs of lower-voltage fast activity at a frequency of ~10 Hz are present in non-REM sleep as well. This paroxysmal fast activity is also considered to be a defining feature of LGS. The runs may occur without clinical correlate or may be associated with subtle seizures or tonic seizures. They typically last a few seconds at a time and tend to occur at frequent intervals (225). During REM sleep the spikes and fast discharges become more frontally predominant and decrease in frequency.

The ictal EEG in LGS varies depending on the seizure type. During tonic seizures the EEG typically shows bilateral rhythmic activity at 10 to 20 Hz, lasting 5 to 15 sec (Fig. 18.34). The amplitude may be maximal at onset or may progressively increase over the course of the seizure. This is often followed

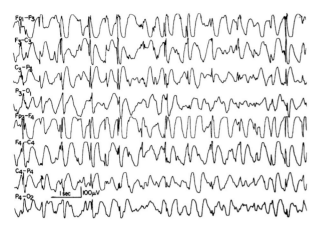

Figure 18.33. The EEG tracing of an 8-year-old boy with LGS showing irregular slow (1.5–2.5 Hz) spike-wave complexes. (With permission from Nordli DR, Riviello JJ, Niedermeyer E. Seizures and epilepsy in infants to adolescents. In: Schomer DL, Lopes deSilva FH, eds. Niedermeyer's Electroencephalography, 6th ed. Philadelphia: Lippincott Williams & Wilkins. Fig. 26.32A)

by high-amplitude slow activity in the delta range. Atypical absences are generally associated with runs of slow spike-wave activity at a frequency of <2.5 Hz. These are often irregular and can be frontally predominant or asymmetric. They may be difficult to differentiate from interictal discharges. In atonic seizures, the EEG may show high-amplitude activity at ~10 Hz or bursts of slow spike-wave discharges. This can be preceded by a fast recruiting rhythm. Myoclonic seizures are associated with bursts of irregular spike- or polyspike-waves that are often frontal in onset (246).

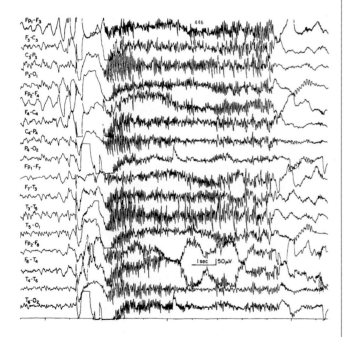

Figure 18.34. A tonic seizure in light sleep in a 20-year-old patient with LGS. A generalized run of rapid spikes is preceded by a few large slow waves mixed with spikes. (With permission from Nordli DR, Riviello JJ, Niedermeyer E. Seizures and epilepsy in infants to adolescents. In: Schomer DL, Lopes deSilva FH, eds. Niedermeyer's Electroencephalography, 6th ed. Philadelphia: Lippincott Williams & Wilkins. Fig. 26.34)

In patients previously affected by West syndrome, the evolution of the EEG is from hypsarrhythmia to multifocal interictal spikes to generalized spike discharges to the typical slow spike-and-wave discharges of LGS. As patients with LGS age, the defining slow spike-waves and runs of fast activity in sleep may fragment or disappear entirely. In as many as 78% of cases focal spikes involving the temporal regions may emerge, which may be associated with the onset of focal temporal lobe seizures. This process is often referred to as "secondary temporalization" (297).

Patients with LGS have significant slowing or arrest of psychomotor development. This may be more pronounced in individuals who present at a younger age (9). Behavioral abnormalities, including hyperactivity, autistic features, aggressiveness, emotional instability, or hypersexuality, can occur. Prognosis is generally poor. Most patients will have progressive deterioration of intellectual abilities with intractable seizures (225). Even when the seizures are controlled cognitive impairment tends to persist (298).

LGS is a notoriously pharmacoresistant epilepsy syndrome. No clear optimal approach has been established. Most patients require multiple AEDs, and additional treatments are often used as adjuncts, including devices such as the vagus nerve stimulator, surgical interventions including corpus callosotomy, and specialized diets such as the ketogenic diet. Vagus nerve stimulation and corpus callosotomy may be particularly effective at treating atonic and tonic seizures but less effective at treating the other seizure types (299).

8. EPILEPSY SYNDROMES OF OLDER CHILDREN AND ADOLESCENTS

8.1. Juvenile Absence Epilepsy

The typical seizure type in juvenile absence epilepsy (JAE) is absence seizures, similar to those seen in CAE. Onset is usually around puberty. The absence seizures in JAE are less frequent and tend to be more prolonged than those in CAE. Absence status epilepticus may also be more frequent in JAE. Generalized tonic-clonic seizures are common, often occurring on awakening, and myoclonic seizures may be present as well.

The interictal EEG is characterized by generalized spike-wave or polyspike-wave discharges superimposed on an otherwise normal background. These discharges, however, are generally faster than those in CAE, occurring at a frequency of 3 to 4 Hz. They may be faster still, up to 4 to 5 Hz, at the onset of the burst. There may be a frontal predominance. The spike-wave discharge is generally more fragmented and disorganized than in CAE. Focal features, including focal slowing, focal spikes, or asymmetry of the spike-wave discharges, have been reported (300). Intermittent rhythmic delta activity over the temporal regions may be seen in ~13% of patients with JAE. This is usually around 3 Hz and may be activated by drowsiness or by hyperventilation (301).

The ictal discharges in JAE typically consist of generalized spike-wave or polyspike-wave discharges at a frequency of 3.5 to 4 Hz. These often have a frontal predominance. As with the interictal discharges, they may be more fragmented and occur in longer runs in comparison to the discharges seen in CAE.

The outcome of JAE is variable. Cognitive abnormalities and academic problems may be present early at onset. The seizures resolve in 15% to 40% of patients, but for others it can be a lifelong condition (302). The presence of generalized tonic-clonic seizures appears be associated with a decreased likelihood of remission. Valproate and ethosuximide have been shown to be more effective than lamotrigine at controlling the seizures (230). Valproate is often considered the first-line medication in JAE as it also controls the generalized tonic-clonic seizures associated with this syndrome. Lamotrigine may be considered in women of childbearing potential in whom teratogenicity is a concern, but lamotrigine may also worsen myoclonus (245). Carbamazepine and oxcarbazepine may worsen absence seizures.

8.2. Juvenile Myoclonic Epilepsy

Juvenile myoclonic epilepsy is an epilepsy syndrome characterized by myoclonic, generalized tonic-clonic, and absence seizures. Onset is typically around puberty. It occurs in previously neurologically intact individuals. Myoclonic seizures are the hallmark of the condition and are necessary to make the diagnosis. They typically occur after awakening and are aggravated by fatigue, sleep deprivation, or alcohol. They are generally bilateral and mild to moderate in intensity. They may involve the entire extremity rather than isolated muscles, often involving the upper limbs and neck more than the lower limbs (303). The patient may drop objects or fall. Myoclonic status epilepticus can occur in a subset of patients but is not common. Generalized tonic-clonic seizures are frequent, occurring in nearly all patients (303,304). Myoclonic jerks usually precede the generalized tonic-clonic seizures and may become progressively more frequent until they evolve into a

generalized tonic-clonic seizure. Like the myoclonic seizures, generalized tonic-clonic seizures usually occur shortly after awakening (303). Typical absence seizures also occur in 20% or more of patients (304).

The interictal EEG is characterized by bursts of rapid generalized spike-wave or polyspike-wave discharges occurring at a frequency of 3.5 to 6 Hz (Fig. 18.35). At times slower-frequency spike-wave activity may occur as well (305). There may be an anterior predominance. Focal EEG abnormalities, including focal spikes or focal slow waves, may be present (304). Interictal abnormalities are often more common during sleep, especially non-REM sleep. Sleep deprivation may activate the epileptiform activity. The interictal EEG is normal in a small number of patients (305).

During a myoclonic seizure, the EEG is characterized by rapid spike and slow- wave complexes that are synchronous and symmetric, occurring at a frequency of 10 to 16 Hz. The spikes are often maximal in the front of the head and may increase in amplitude over the course of the burst. These EEG discharges immediately precede the myoclonic jerk. There are often irregular slow waves at a frequency of 3 to 4 Hz following, or sometimes preceding, the discharges. Photosensitivity is common, and photic stimulation may evoke the epileptiform discharges or may provoke a seizure (303).

Juvenile myoclonic epilepsy has a strong genetic component: 50% of patients have first- and second-degree relatives with epilepsy. A single genetic cause, however, has not been identified. Mutations involving the alpha-1 subunit of the GABA receptor subtype A (*GABRA1*), as well as the *EFHC1* or myoclonin gene, are most consistently linked to juvenile myoclonic epilepsy (306,307). Other genetic abnormalities have been identified less consistently, including those involving chromosome 15q and the short arm of chromosome 6 (308,309).

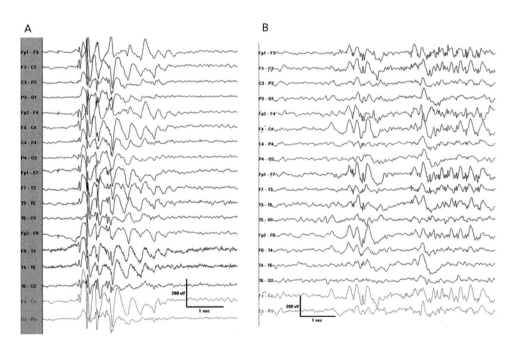

Figure 18.35. An 18-year-old girl with juvenile myoclonic epilepsy. **A:** During wakefulness there are runs of generalized spike- and polyspike-wave discharges with a frontal predominance at a frequency of 4 to 5 Hz. **B:** During non-REM sleep the discharges are less regular and more fragmented, with a more prominent polyspike component.

The seizures can often be controlled with medication, but patients may require lifelong treatment. Valproate is generally considered to be first-line treatment, and levetiracetam or lamotrigine is often used in female patients in whom teratogenicity is a concern. Topiramate, zonisamide, barbiturates, and benzodiazepines all may be effective (303).

8.3. Epilepsy with Generalized Tonic-Clonic Seizures on Awakening

In this disorder, also called epilepsy with grand mal on awakening, generalized tonic-clonic seizures occur exclusively or predominantly shortly after awakening (310). The EEG shows fast spike and wave bursts, similar to that seen in juvenile myoclonic epilepsy. These bursts are relatively short and dominated by 4-Hz or 4- to 5-Hz spike-wave complexes that are, contrary to the classical 3-Hz or 3- to 4-Hz spike waves, not readily activated by hyperventilation. Photosensitivity is common, occurring in about 13% of cases (310). The onset is usually in the second decade of life. Absence or myoclonic seizures may also occur in addition to the generalized tonic-clonic seizures. The seizures can be triggered by sleep deprivation. A family history of epilepsy is often present.

9. EPILEPSY RELATED TO SPECIFIC GENETIC ABNORMALITIES

9.1. Epilepsy Related to Chromosomal Anomalies

9.1.1. ANGELMAN SYNDROME

Angelman syndrome, a severe neurodevelopmental disorder of a heterogeneous genetic origin, is characterized by severe developmental delay, speech impairment with no or minimal use of words and better receptive and nonverbal communication, ataxia and tremulous movements of limbs, hand flapping, and unique behaviors including hyperactivity and frequent and inappropriate laughter. It is associated frequently with postnatal microcephaly and seizures and in some children (20–80%) with peculiar facial traits, wide-spaced teeth, brachycephaly, and sleep disorders (311). Epilepsy is present in 70% to 80% of patients (312). Seizures tend to decrease in adolescence and adulthood. Onset of epilepsy usually precedes the diagnosis. Seizure types are atypical absences, possibly detectable only on EEG (313), myoclonic seizures, generalized tonic-clonic seizures, and focal clonic seizures. Epileptic spasms are exceptional. More than half of the patients develop nonconvulsive status epilepticus, corresponding clinically to episodes of regression with worsening of the ataxia.

Interictal EEG abnormalities may, like seizure onset, precede the diagnosis. Boyd and colleagues in 1988 described three EEG patterns suggestive of Angelman syndrome, present in 98% of the patients:

1. Generalized high-voltage (reaching 200 μV or more) rhythmic 4- to 6-Hz activity not influenced by eye closure (Fig. 18.36A–G)

2. Very-high-amplitude (>200 μV) rhythmic delta activity at 2 to 3 Hz, often prominent over anterior regions and sometimes associated with spikes forming an "ill-defined spike-wave complex" (later named "notched delta") (see Fig. 18.36H, I)

3. Spike and sharp waves mixed with 3- to 4-Hz components of amplitude >200 μV, mainly posterior, occasionally asymmetric, and triggered by eye closure.

Interictal focal or multifocal epileptiform discharges are described in 46% of the patients (313). The notched delta waves show posterior predominance at a young age and anterior predominance at an older age (314,315).

Episodes of myoclonic status epilepticus may be observed, mainly in younger children and never in children older than 6 years. This falls into the category of myoclonic encephalopathy in nonprogressive disorders, an electroclinical syndrome in infancy characterized by continuous diffuse high-voltage spike and wave complexes or delta waves associated with synchronous or asynchronous myoclonic jerks or negative motor phenomena, which correlate with transient or recurrent motor, behavioral, and cognitive disturbances (316,317). Myoclonic encephalopathy in nonprogressive disorders can be divided into three groups, with a main subgroup (49–62%) occurring predominantly in genetic etiologies such as Angelman, Prader–Willi, Wolf–Hirschhorn, and Rett syndromes. Because of the preexisting intellectual deficit and the common presence of abnormal movements, this condition may be difficult to recognize clinically, but it can be easily identified on video-EEG recording. Myoclonic manifestations may be correlated with spikes, but in many patients myoclonic jerks remain erratic and without obvious correlation with EEG anomalies (Fig. 18.37).

The prevalence of Angelman syndrome is indicated as 1 in 10,000 to 1 in 40,000. Genetic mechanisms are multiple, confirmed in 85% to 90% of the patients, and involve the proximal portion of the long arm of the maternally derived chromosome 15 (15q11-q13) with deletion (75%), UBE3A mutations (5–10%), imprinting center abnormalities (3%), and uniparental paternal disomy (1–2%) causing loss of UBE3A gene function (318). In the remaining patients where no genetic anomaly has been detected, diagnosis is made on clinical presentation and EEG. The occurrence of myoclonic encephalopathy in nonprogressive disorders in Angelman syndrome has been specifically related to chromosome 15q11-q13 deletions and UBE3A mutations, but the condition has also been described in uniparental paternal disomy (319).

9.1.2. DOWN SYNDROME (TRISOMY 21)

Trisomy 21 or Down syndrome, one of the most frequent chromosomal disorders, is characterized by well-known dysmorphic features including brachycephaly, flattened nasal bridge, upward-slanted eyes, epicanthal folds, small ears, and simian crease. It is associated with intellectual disability, muscular hypotonia, growth retardation, and hypogonadism. Patients have an increased risk of cardiac malformations, leukemia, and epilepsy. It is the most common genetic cause of intellectual disability, with an incidence of 1 per 600 to 1,000 live births.

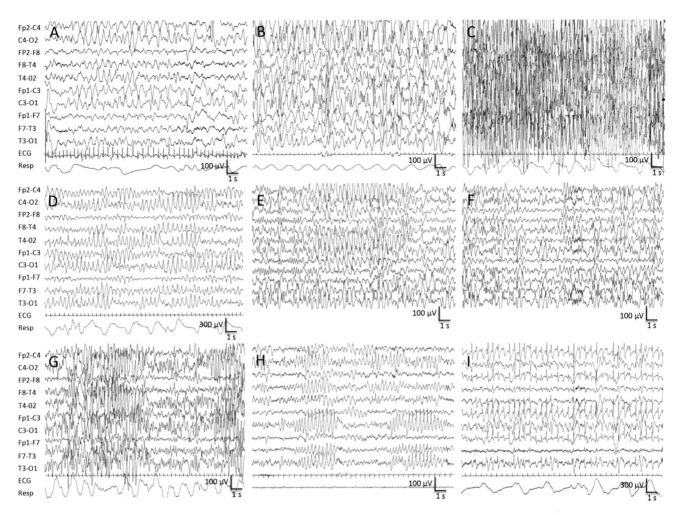

Figure 18.36. *Different EEG characteristics in Angelman syndrome. A: 5-month-old infant. The EEG in the awake state shows a background that is slow for the child's age. B: Same infant as A. The sleep record shows high-voltage slow waves and absence of normal physiological sleep figures. C and D: 16-month-old child. The EEG in the awake state with eyes open shows very-high-voltage monomorphous 3- to 4-Hz activity predominating over posterior areas. C is at 10 μV/mm and D at 30 μV/mm. E and F: 18-month-old infant. Awake state and sleep. See presence of sleep spindles. G: 16-month-old boy. Very-high-voltage 4- to 6-Hz activity can be seen with rare spikes predominating over posterior areas. H: 4-year-old girl. High-voltage 3- to 4-Hz activity with notched appearance predominates over posterior areas. I: 6-year-old boy. High-voltage 3- to 4-Hz activity with notched appearance predominates over anterior areas.*

Although EEG abnormalities have been demonstrated in 20% to 25% of patients with Down syndrome, even in the absence of seizures, no distinctive EEG pattern has been recognized. The prevalence of epilepsy is reported at 0% to 13% with a mean of 5.5% (320), which is higher than that in the general population but lower than that of other patients with intellectual disability. Seizure onset shows an age-dependent, trimodal distribution with peaks in infancy, in early adulthood, and after the age of 50 to 55 years. Forty percent of the epileptic patients with Down syndrome present during the first year of life and another 40% after the age of 30 years. The mechanism underlying this increased seizure susceptibility is not known. In some cases epilepsy can be attributed to medical complications such as hypoxic-ischemic events, cardiovascular disease, and recurrent infections. Other cases are thought to be due to inherent neuronal structural or functional anomalies (320).

West syndrome is the most frequent epileptic syndrome in Down syndrome. Epileptic spasms are marked by typical electroclinical features including hypsarrhythmia and the electrodecremental response (see Figs. 18.23 and 18.24). There is a generally favorable response to treatment with ACTH.

Seizures are often overlooked, as epileptic spasms may be misinterpreted as behavioral. Such a delay in diagnosis and therefore delay of effective treatment may worsen cognitive outcome, and response to treatment may become poor (223). Reflex seizures have been reported in Down syndrome with clinical expression as massive myoclonias, tonic spasms, and falls (321). LGS may be present, showing late seizure onset without preceding West syndrome and the presence of reflex seizures (322). In adults with Down syndrome, myoclonic epilepsy associated with Alzheimer's disease is described, showing an evolution in three stages:

1. Onset with dementia, diffuse EEG anomalies in sleep, and cerebellar anomalies on neuroimaging

2. Myoclonic epilepsy

3. Nonepileptic myoclonias, cerebellar signs, and severe dementia

This condition has been termed "senile myoclonic epilepsy" or "late-onset myoclonic epilepsy in Down syndrome."

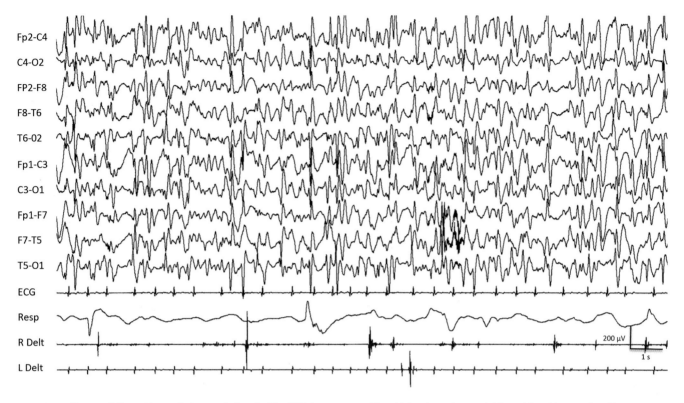

Figure 18.37. Six-year-old boy with myoclonic encephalopathy. The EEG demonstrates diffuse high-voltage theta and delta activity with rare spikes. Erratic myoclonic jerks recorded on surface deltoid muscles are not correlated with the spikes.

9.1.3. FRAGILE X SYNDROME (MARTIN–BELL SYNDROME)

Fragile X syndrome is a genetic trinucleotide repeat disorder characterized by mild to profound intellectual disability, autism spectrum disorders, attention-deficit/hyperactivity disorder, and muscular hypotonia, often with dysmorphic features such as large ears, long face, macrocephaly and macroorchidism, and seizures. Prevalence is reported at 1 per 4,000 males and 1 per 5,000 to 8,000 females.

Epilepsy is present in Fragile X in 4% of girls and 16% of boys (323), beginning between 4 and 10 years of age with mostly focal seizures, usually at low frequency and responsive to treatment. Differential diagnosis with nonepileptic events may be difficult, as episodes of staring or behavioral arrest are very frequent in patients with Fragile X. Therefore, ictal EEG recording is needed to confirm or rule out their epileptic origin.

EEG background slowing is reported in half of patients and interictal epileptiform abnormalities in 77% of patients with seizures and in 23% without seizures. These consist of bi- or triphasic spikes of medium or high amplitude over the central or centrotemporal areas, which may be isolated or in brief sequences, showing a similar appearance to those in self-limited epilepsy with centrotemporal spikes (rolandic epilepsy) (323,324). Cortical hyperexcitability has been described, indicated by the presence of spikes evoked during EEG recording by finger tapping and the presence of giant somatosensory evoked potentials (324).

9.1.4. WOLF–HIRSCHHORN SYNDROME (DELETION 4p)

Wolf–Hirschhorn syndrome is a severe neurodevelopmental disorder caused by variable partial deletions of the most terminal portion of the short arm of chromosome 4. Incidence is estimated at 1 per 50,000 live births, with a female predilection of 2:1. Clinical phenotype is characterized by typical craniofacial features consisting of the "Greek warrior helmet appearance" caused by a high nasal bridge, high forehead, prominent glabella, and widely spaced eyes, as well as epicanthus, highly arched eyebrows, short philtrum, downturned mouth, micrognathia, and poorly formed ears. Microcephaly, pre- and postnatal growth deficiency, and muscular hypotonia are present in >80% of these individuals. Developmental delay is present in all patients to a variable degree.

Epilepsy is a major finding and is present in >90% of patients (325). Seizures usually start before the age of 3 years with a peak incidence at around 6 to 12 months (325). The main seizure type (74%) is generalized tonic-clonic; this is the only seizure type in 40% of Wolf–Hirschhorn patients with epilepsy. Otherwise tonic spasms, complex partial seizures, and clonic seizures occur, possibly in clusters lasting >15 minutes. In 50% of patients unilateral or generalized clonic or tonic-clonic status epilepticus occurs during the first 3 years of life. Up to 33% of children develop, by 1 to 6 years of age, atypical absences often accompanied by myoclonias involving the eyelids and hands. Epilepsy often improves with age.

Distinctive EEG findings have been described in 90% of patients with Wolf–Hirschhorn (325), showing some overlap with those reported in Angelman syndrome. These include diffuse high-amplitude sharp waves or spike-wave complexes at a frequency of 2 to 3.5 Hz occurring in long bursts and activated in slow sleep (also seen in patients without seizures), and frequent high-amplitude spike- and polyspike-wave complexes at

4 to 6 Hz over the posterior third of the head, triggered by eye closure. The background is often slow for age.

9.1.5. Ring Chromosome Syndromes

Ring chromosomes result from breaks at the end of the chromosome arms and subsequent fusion. They have been reported for all human chromosomes. Associated phenotypes are highly variable.

Ring chromosome 20 (R20) syndrome is a rare disorder, affecting 1 per 30,000 to 60,000 live births. It is characterized by highly refractory epilepsy often associated with a suggestive EEG pattern. Further features such as intellectual deficiency and behavioral disorders are variable. Diagnosis is often delayed because of the lack of a consistent pattern of dysmorphic features. Seizure onset usually occurs in childhood with episodes of loss of contact or confusional states, often prolonged as in nonconvulsive status epilepticus, the hallmark of the condition.

The interictal EEG may be normal or may show high-voltage theta or delta waves with occasional spikes or sharp waves occurring continuously or in runs, predominantly over the frontal areas (Fig. 18.38). Sleep EEG is characterized by the presence of high-amplitude delta activity with a sharply contoured or notched appearance prevalent over the frontal regions, and by a progressive deterioration with the loss of physiological non-REM sleep architecture (spindles, K-complexes) and the loss of recognizable non-REM sleep stages (326).

The ictal EEG during the periods of nonconvulsive status epilepticus shows high-amplitude monomorphous theta or delta waves with occasional spikes or periodic spike-wave complexes predominantly in the frontal areas. These episodes last 10 to 50 minutes, rarely exceeding 1 hour (327). Clouding of the consciousness may be fluctuating and not so severe as to cause complete unresponsiveness. Other ictal manifestations include automatisms, wandering, terror, or hallucinations, especially at an older age, that could wrongly be attributed to psychiatric disorders. Nocturnal frontal lobe seizures seem to occur in all patients; the manifestations are difficult to distinguish from physiological arousal behavior such as subtle stretching, turning, or rubbing movements. The ictal EEG during these events consists of bursts of diffuse or frontally maximal high-voltage beta activity evolving into bi-frontal high-voltage subdelta waves (see Fig. 18.38) (328).

Seizures are usually pharmacoresistant. Vagus nerve stimulation may be a treatment option. Prognosis is generally poor. Seizures tend to become progressively more frequent and more difficult to treat. Cognitive development stagnates or declines from the beginning of the epilepsy, and considering this entity an epileptic encephalopathy is a matter of discussion. Most patients have chromosomal abnormalities in the form of a mosaic, and there is evidence that early seizure onset and more severe cognitive impairment are correlated with a higher percentage of affected cells (329).

9.1.6. Epilepsy Related to Specific Gene Mutations

In recent years significant progress has been made in identifying single gene disorders that underlie specific epilepsy syndromes. Many of these monogenic epilepsy syndromes have clinical and neurophysiological features that increase suspicion for these disorders but are insufficient to make the diagnosis without specific gene testing. Here we review several of these monogenic epilepsy syndromes.

9.1.6.1. Glut1 Deficiency (Glucose type I transporter encoded by SLC2A1 at chromosome 1p34.2, MIM#606777)

Clinical features of this syndrome include normoglycemia with hypoglycorrhachia (CSF glucose <40 mg/dL), episodic

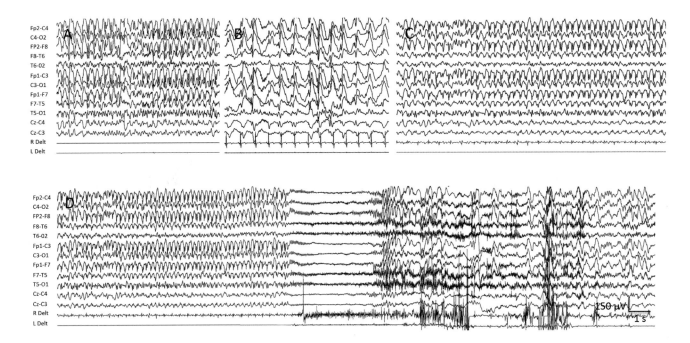

Figure 18.38. Twelve-year-old girl with ring chromosome 20. **A:** Awake state. **B:** Non-REM sleep. **C:** Clinical absence. **D:** Tonic seizure.

movement disorders, acquired microcephaly, and epilepsy refractory to common AEDs (330). The disorder is unique in its responsiveness to the ketogenic diet, which can often ameliorate these symptoms and may improve neurodevelopmental outcomes if initiated early in the disease process (330).

Seizure onset is typically within the first year of life, with a mean age of 8 months. There are a variety of seizure types—in descending order of frequency, generalized tonic-clonic, absence, focal dyscognitive (complex partial), focal or generalized myoclonic, drop attacks, focal or generalized tonic, simple focal, infantile spasms, and epileptic spasms (331). In some case series, a normal EEG is the most common finding (330). The most common abnormalities on EEG are generalized spike waves, generalized slowing, mixed generalized and focal slowing, mixed generalized and focal spike waves, and focal or multifocal slowing (331). Seizures captured on EEG were predominantly generalized in onset but could rarely have focal or multifocal onsets. Frequently EEG abnormalities are improved after initiation of the ketogenic diet (331).

Thus, in patients with early-onset epilepsy that is refractory to common AEDs, acquired microcephaly, and movement disorders, diagnostic testing with serum and CSF glucose should be considered. Gene testing can be done if the CSF glucose level is <40 mg/dL. EEG is included in the diagnostic workup but its findings are not specific enough to make the diagnosis. Once the diagnosis is confirmed, the ketogenic diet should be started.

9.1.6.2. PCDH19 (Protocadherin 19 at chromosome Xq22.3, MIM#300460, Early Infantile Epileptic Encephalopathy 9)

PCDH belongs to the cadherin superfamily of cell-adhesion proteins that are predominantly expressed in the developing nervous system. In 2008, mutations in PCDH19 were identified as causing epilepsy and intellectual deficits in females in a few large families (332). As more cases have been identified, the heterogeneity in clinical features, including age of seizure onset, seizure types, epilepsy severity, and degree of intellectual disability, has become apparent. Large-scale studies looking for monogenic disorders have recently shown PCDH19 to be the second most important gene (following SCN1A), and often patients with this disorder have features similar to those of Dravet syndrome (332).

Seizure onset is typically in late infancy or early childhood, with a mean of 12.9 months. Frequently febrile seizures are the initial presentation, and throughout the disease course seizures remain sensitive to fever in ~90% of patients (332). Status epilepticus can also be the initial seizure presentation. The most frequent types of seizures include generalized tonic, generalized clonic, generalized tonic-clonic, and/or focal seizures with or without secondary generalization. Less commonly atypical absence, atonic, and myoclonic seizures may be observed (332). The hallmark of this disorder is the presence of brief seizure clusters lasting 1 to 5 minutes up to 10 times a day. Frequently the seizures are refractory to typical AEDs. The severity of the epilepsy often decreases over time beginning after puberty (332).

The EEG background activity is commonly normal and slow in ~15% of cases. Focal unilateral spike and slow wave complexes or multifocal spike and slow wave discharges are present in more than half of the patients (332). About one third of patients also have generalized spike and slow wave discharges on EEG. Focal seizures arising from the centro-parieto-occipital and frontotemporal regions were captured more commonly than atypical absence and generalized tonic-clonic seizures (333).

Thus, in female patients with early-onset epilepsy that is refractory to common AEDs, with seizures provoked by fever and occurring in brief clusters up to 10 times a day, PCHD19 gene testing should be performed. EEG is included in the diagnostic workup but its findings are not specific enough to make the diagnosis.

9.1.6.3. DEPDC5 (DEP domain-containing protein 5 at chromosome 22q12.2-12.3, MIM#604364)

Recently brain somatic, germline, and germline mosaic DEPDC5 mutations have been associated with epilepsy. The function of DEPDC5 is not yet well known, but it has been associated with intracellular signal transduction. In the majority of cases the epilepsy is related to a focal cortical dysplasia that is thought to arise from the function of DEPDC5 as an upstream negative regulator of mammalian target of rapamycin (mTOR) complex 1 (334). Mutations in DEPDC5 are thought to account for up to one third of inherited focal epilepsies, particularly familial focal epilepsy with variable foci, familial temporal lobe epilepsy, and autosomal dominant nocturnal frontal lobe epilepsy (334). More rarely, children with these mutations may have unclassified focal childhood epilepsy, benign epilepsy with centrotemporal spikes, a bottom of the sulcus focal cortical dysplasia, and focal band heterotopia (334).

Seizure onset is usually in infancy or early childhood, with a mean age of 18 months. The seizures are often medically intractable and patients have a high seizure burden. Brain MRI often reveals a frontocentral lesion consistent with a focal cortical dysplasia type II. In some patients nocturnal or sleep-related epilepsy may increase suspicion for this disorder (334).

The EEGs of these patients typically show focal sharp waves and spikes in the frontal or frontocentral regions and may show bilateral posterior slowing (335). Stereo-EEGs from several patients have identified epileptogenic zones in the frontopolar and frontal regions extending back to the primary motor cortex. In some cases, stereo-EEG has shown continuous rhythmic spikes with subclinical ictal discharges (334). These patients should be considered for resective epilepsy surgery as that may be curative in some cases (334).

Thus, in patients with early-onset epilepsy, refractory to anticonvulsants, with focal seizures by clinical semiology and ictal or interictal EEG findings, the workup should include a brain MRI. If a focal cortical dysplasia is identified, strong consideration for DEPDC5 mutation should be given. If no focal cortical dysplasia is identified, DEPDC5 mutation may still be the underlying cause if clinical features are supportive.

9.2. Sodium Channelopathies

Epilepsy can be caused by mutations in a number of voltage-gated sodium channels, including SCN1A (Na$_V$1.1), SCN2A

(Na$_V$1.2), *SCN3A* (Na$_V$1.3), *SCN8A* (Na$_V$1.6), and *SCN1B*, an accessory sodium channel subunit (336). These various genes are associated with a broad range of epilepsy phenotypes that have been discussed earlier in this chapter, ranging in severity from mild (e.g., benign familial neonatal infantile seizures) to very severe (e.g., Ohtahara syndrome). Mutations in *SCN1A* are the most common single gene involved in epilepsy and are associated with Dravet syndrome and GEFS+. Mutations in *SCN2A* are associated with severe epilepsy phenotypes (e.g., early onset epileptic encephalopathies, Ohtahara syndrome, Dravet syndrome) and less severe epilepsy phenotypes (e.g., GEFS+, benign familial neonatal infantile seizures). Rarely mutations in *SCN3A* have been identified in patients with focal epilepsy of unknown etiology (336). Rarely mutations in *SCN8A* have been identified in children with epileptic encephalopathies with varying degrees of intellectual disability and possible cardiac arrhythmias (337). Mutations in *SCN1B* are associated with GEFS+ and Dravet syndrome (336).

Most of these epilepsy phenotypes have early onset of seizures. The EEG findings in sodium channelopathies are typically nonspecific and have features similar to the clinical syndrome the patient has. In general, sodium channelopathies are not treated with sodium channel blocking medications; these may exacerbate seizures, since most mutations are theorized to be pathogenic due to loss of channel function (336). In contrast, recent studies have shown that many of the patients with *SCN8A* mutations may improve with sodium channel blocking agents because some of these are gain of channel function mutations (337). Thus, the overall prognosis depends largely on which sodium channel mutation and which epilepsy syndrome fit the clinical details.

9.3. Potassium Channelopathies

Several different potassium channels have been implicated in epilepsy. Typically mutations in *KCNA1*, which encodes K$_V$1.1, cause episodic ataxia type 1, though these patients are 10-fold more likely to develop focal dyscognitive or tonic-clonic seizures. In one large family, mutations of *KCNMA1*, encoding K$_{Ca}$1.1, cause generalized epilepsy and paroxysmal dyskinesias (338). The most common epilepsy-associated mutations of potassium channels involve *KCNQ2*, encoding K$_V$7.2, and *KCNQ3*, encoding K$_V$7.3. Usually these mutations are associated with the mild epilepsy benign familial neonatal seizures (described above), but they have also been reported in other neonatal seizures and benign epilepsy with centrotemporal spikes (338).

More recently mutations in *KCNQ2* have been identified in up to 10% of patients with severe sporadic infantile epileptic encephalopathy. The more severely affected patients often have frequent tonic seizures that are highly resistant to AEDs. The interictal EEG usually shows burst suppression or multifocal spikes. Often the seizure burden improves as children near school age, but moderate to severe cognitive impairment persists (338). This disorder is thought to result when pathogenic mutations cause loss of function with a strong dominant negative effect. Recent studies have shown some response to the potassium channel opener retigabine or with carbamazepine, but further studies are required (338).

Thus, potassium channelopathies are a heterogeneous group of disorders. The prognosis depends on whether the clinical features fit a benign epilepsy or a more severe epileptic encephalopathy, as does the response to pharmacotherapy.

SCORE EEG SOFTWARE

Further examples related to the topics addressed in this chapter can be found in the interactive online Niedermeyer Educational Platform. EEG recordings with illustrative examples can be opened and browsed. Features are marked and described using the SCORE EEG software. The users can see the features marked by experts, they can score these features themselves, and then compare them with the scorings of the experts.

The Niedermeyer Educational Platform can be accessed at: www.scoreEEG.com/academy

REFERENCES

1. IFSECN. A glossary of terms commonly used by electroencephalographers. *Electroencephalogr Clin Neurophysiol.* 1974; 37: 538–548.
2. Kiloh LG, McComas AJ, Osselton JW. *Clinical Electroencephalography.* 3rd ed. London: Butterworth; 1972.
3. Matsuo F, Knott JR. Focal positive spikes in electroencephalography. *Electroencephalogr Clin Neurophysiol.* 1977; 42: 15–25.
4. Gregory DL, Wong PK. Topographical analysis of the centrotemporal discharges in benign rolandic epilepsy of childhood. *Epilepsia.* 1984; 25: 705–711.
5. Jasper HH. Epilepsy. In: Penfield W, Erickson TC, eds. *Epilepsy and Cerebral Localization.* Springfield, IL: Charles C. Thomas;1941: 380–454.
6. Duterette F. Catalogue of the main EEG patterns. In: Remond A, ed-in-chief. *Handbook of Electroencephalography and Clinical Neurophysiology.* Vol. 1A. Amsterdam: Elsevier; 1977:40–79.
7. Gibbs FA, Gibbs EL. *Atlas of Electroencephalography.* Vol. 2. Reading, MA: Addison-Wesley; 1952.
8. Jasper HH, Kershman J. Classification of the EEG in epilepsy. *Electroencephalogr Clin Neurophysiol.* 1949; 2(suppl): 123–131.
9. Gastaut H, Roger J, Soulayrol R, et al. Childhood epileptic encephalopathy with diffuse slow spike-waves (otherwise known as "petit mal variant") or Lennox syndrome. *Epilepsia.* 1966; 7(2): 139–179.
10. Brenner RP, Atkinson R. Generalized paroxysmal fast activity: electroencephalographic and clinical features. *Ann Neurol.* 1982; 11: 386–390.
11. Niedermeyer E. *Compendium of the Epilepsies.* Springfield, IL: Charles C. Thomas; 1972.
12. Niedermeyer E. The electroencephalogram in the differential diagnosis of the Lennox-Gastaut syndrome. In: Niedermeyer E, Degen R. eds. *The Lennox-Gastaut Syndrome.* New York: Alan R. Liss; 1988: 177–220.
13. Silverman D. Clinical correlates of the spike-wave complexes. *Electroencephalogr Clin Neurophysiol.* 1954; 6: 663–669.
14. Clark EC, Knott JR. Paroxysmal wave and spike activity and diagnostic subclassification. *Electroencephalogr Clinc Neurophysiol.* 1955; 7: 161–164.
15. Gastaut H. Clinical and electroencephalographic correlates of generalized spike and wave bursts occurring spontaneously in man. *Epilepsia.* 1968; 9: 179–184.
16. Thorner MW. Procurement of electroencephalograph tracings in 1000 flying cadets for evaluating the Gibbs technique in relation to flying ability. *USAD School of Aviation Medical Research Report, No. 7 -1;* 1942.
17. Gibbs FA, Gibbs EL, Lennox WG. Electroencephalographic classification of epileptic patients and control subjects. *Arch Neurol Psychiatry.* 1943; 50: 111–128.
18. Harty JE, Gibbs EG, Gibbs FA. Electroencephalographic study of two hundred and seventy-five candidates for military service. *War Med.* 1942; 2: 923–930.
19. Buchthal F, Lennox M. The EEG effect of Metrazol and photic stimulation in 682 normal subjects. *Electroencephalogr Clinc Neurophysiol.* 1953; 5: 545–558.

20. Kellaway P. The incidence, significance and natural history of spike foci in children. In: Henry CE, ed. *Current Clinical Neurophysiology*. Amsterdam: Elsevier; 1981: 151–176.
21. Zivin L, Ajmone Marsan C. Incidence and prognostic significance of "epileptiform" activity in the EEG of nonepileptic subjects. *Brain* 1968; 91: 751–777.
22. Chatrian GE. Paroxysmal pattern in "normal" subjects. In: Remond A, ed-in-chief. *Handbook of Electroencephalography and Clinical Neurophysiology*. Vol. 6A. Amsterdam: Elsevier; 1976: 114–123.
23. Cavazzuti G, Cappella L, Nalin A. Longitudinal study of epileptiform EEG patterns in normal children. *Epilepsia*. 1980; 21: 43–55.
24. Berg AT, Berkovic SF, Brodie MJ, Buchhalter J, et al. Revised terminology and concepts for organization of seizures and epilepsies: report of the ILAE Commission on Classification and Terminology, 2005-2009. *Epilepsia*. 2010; 51: 676–685.
25. Seinfield Duchowny MC. Febrile seizures. In: Wyllie E, ed. *Wyllie's Treatment of Epilepsy: Principles and Practice*. Philadelphia, PA: Wolters Kluwer; 2015: 426–430.
26. Nelson KB, Ellenberg JH. Predictors of epilepsy in children who have experienced febrile seizures. *N Engl J Med*. 1976; 295(19): 1029–1033
27. National Institutes of Health. Consensus Development Conference on febrile seizures. Proceedings. *Epilepsia*. 1981; 22: 377–381.
28. Verity CM, Butler NR, Golding J. Febrile convulsions in a national cohort followed up from birth. I. Prevalence and recurrence in the first five years of life. *Br Med J*. 1985; 290: 1307–1310.
29. Tsuboi T. Epidemiology of febrile and afebrile convulsions in children in Japan. *Neurology*. 1984; 34: 175–181.
30. Hauser WA, Annegers JF, Anderson VE, Kurland LT. The risk of seizure disorders among relatives of children with febrile convulsions. *Neurology*. 1985; 35: 1268–1273.
31. Berkovic SF, Howell RA, Hay DA, Hopper JL. Epilepsies in twins: genetics of the major epilepsy syndromes. *Ann Neurol*. 1998; 43: 435–445.
32. Nakayama J, Arinami T. Molecular genetics of febrile seizures. *Epilepsy Res*. 2006; 70S: S190–198.
33. Berg AT, Shinnar S, Darefsy AS, et al. Predictors of recurrent febrile seizures. A prospective cohort study. *Arch Pediatr Adolesc Med*. 1997; 151:371–378.
34. Hauser WA, Kurland LT. The epidemiology of epilepsy in Rochester, Minnesota, 1935 to 1967. *Epilepsia*. 1975; 16: 1–66.
35. Nelson KB, Ellenberg JH. Prognosis in children with febrile seizures. *Pediatrics*. 1978; 61: 720–727.
36. Shinnar S. Febrile seizures and mesial temporal sclerosis. *Epilepsy Curr*. 2003; 3: 115–118.
37. Hesdorffer DC, Benn EK, Bagiella E, et al. Distribution of febrile seizure duration and associations with development. *Ann Neurol*. 2011; 70: 93–100.
38. Shinnar S, Bello JA, Chan S, et al. MRI abnormalities following febrile status epilepticus in children: The FEBSTAT Study. *Neurology*. 2012; 79: 871–877.
39. Lewis DV, Shinnar S, Hesdorffer DC, et al. Hippocampal sclerosis after febrile status epilepticus: the FEBSTAST study. *Ann Neurol*. 2014; 75(2): 178–185.
40. Yoong M, Seunarine K, Martinos M, Chin RF, Clark CA, Scott RC. Prolonged febrile seizures cause reversible reductions in white matter integrity. *Neuroimage Clin*. 2013; 3: 515–521.
41. Martinos MM, Yoong M, Patil S, et al. Recognition memory is impaired in children after prolonged febrile seizures. *Brain*. 2012; 135(Pt 10): 3153–3164.
42. Subcommittee on Febrile Seizures, American Academy of Pediatrics. Neurodiagnostic evaluation of the child with a simple febrile seizure. *Pediatrics*. 2011; 127(2): 389–394.
43. Thorn I. The significance of electroencephalography in febrile convulsions. In: Akimoto H, Kazamatsuri H, Seino M, Ward A eds. *Advances in Epileptology: XIIIth International Epilepsy Symposium*. New York: Raven Press; 1982: 93–95
44. Gibbs FA, Gibbs EL. *Atlas of Electroencephalography*. Vol. 3. Reading, MA: Addison-Wesley; 1964.
45. Des Terres H, Mises J, Plouin P, Lerique A, Guyot D. The "spike focus" during the evolution of febrile convulsions: an electrophysiological and clinical study of 35 patients. *Electroencephalogr Clin Neurophysiol*. 1978; 45: 370.
46. Kuturec M, Emoto SE, Sofijanov N, et al. Febrile seizures: is the EEG a useful predictor of recurrence? *Clin Pediatr (Phila)*. 1997; 36(1): 31–36.
47. Alvarez N, Lombroso CT, Medina C, Cantlon B. Paroxysmal spike and wave activity in drowsiness in your children: its relationship to febrile convulsions. *Electroencephalogr Clin Neurophysiol*. 1983; 56: 406–413.
48. Okumura A, Ishiguro Y, Sofue A, et al. Treatment and outcome in patients with febrile convulsions associated with epileptiform discharges on electroencephalography. *Brain Dev*. 2004; 26: 241–244.
49. Yamatogi Y, Ishida S, Terasaki T, et al. An electroencephalographic study of febrile convulsions. *Electroencephalogr Clin Neurophysiol*. 1982; 54: 27P–28P.
50. Yamatogi Y, Ohtahara S. EEG in febrile convulsions. *Am J EEG Technol*. 1990; 30: 267–280.
51. Nordli DR, Moshe SL, Shinnar S, et al. Acute EEG findings in children with febrile status epilepticus: Results of the FEBSTAT Study. *Neurology*. 2012; 79: 1–7.
52. Rose AL, Lombroso CT. A study of clinical, pathological, and electroencephalographic features in 137 full-term babies with a long-term follow-up. *Pediatrics*. 1970; 45(3): 404–425.
53. Kellaway P, Hrachovy RA. Status epilepticus in newborns: A perspective on neonatal seizures. In: Delgado-Escueta AV, Wasterlain CG, Treiman DM, Porter RJ, eds. *Advances in Neurology*. Vol. 34. New York: Raven Press; 1983: 93.
54. Scher MS, Aso K, Beggarly ME, Hamid MY, et al. Electrographic seizures in preterm and full-term neonates: Clinical correlates, associated brain lesions, and risk for neurologic sequelae. *Pediatrics*. 1993; 91(1): 128–134.
55. Mizrahi EM, Kellaway P. *Diagnosis and Management of Neonatal Seizures*. Philadelphia: Lippincott-Raven; 1998: 91.
56. Pisani F, Cerminara C, Fusco C, Sisti L. Neonatal status epilepticus vs recurrent neonatal seizures: Clinical findings and outcome. *Neurology*. 2007; 69(23): 2177–2185.
57. Massa T, Niedermeyer E. Convulsive disorders during the first three months of life. *Epilepsia*. 1968; 9(1): 1–9.
58. Passouant P, Cadilhac J. EEG and clinical study of epilepsy during maturation in man. *Epilepsia*. 1962; 3: 14–43.
59. Dreyfus-Brisac C, Monod N. Electroclinical studies of status epilepticus and convulsions in the newborn. In: Kellaway P, Petersen I, eds. *Neurological and Electroencephalographic Correlative Studies in Infancy*. New York: Grune and Stratton; 1964: 250–272.
60. Mizrahi EM, Kellaway P. Characterization and classification of neonatal seizures. *Neurology*. 1987; 37(12): 1837–1844.
61. LaJoie J, Moshe SL. Neonatal seizures and neonatal epilepsy syndromes. In: Devinsky O, Westbrook LE, eds. *Epilepsy and Developmental Disabilities*. Boston: Butterworth-Heinemann; 2002.
62. Volpe JJ. Neonatal seizures: Current concepts and revised classification. *Pediatrics*. 1989; 84(3): 422–428.
63. Swann JW, Moshe SL. Developmental issues in animal models. In: Engel J, Pedley TA, eds. *Epilepsy: A Comprehensive Textbook*. 2nd ed. New York: Raven Press; 1997: 467–480.
64. Moshe SL, Sperber EF, Velisek L. Critical issues of developmental seizure disorders. *Physiol Res*. 1993; 42(3): 145–154.
65. Moshe SL. Epileptogenesis and the immature brain. *Epilepsia*. 1987; 28(Suppl 1): S3–15.
66. Moshe SL, Albala BJ, Ackermann RF, Engel J,Jr. Increased seizure susceptibility of the immature brain. *Brain Res*. 1983; 283(1): 81–85.
67. Galanopoulou AS. Developmental patterns in the regulation of chloride homeostasis and GABA(A) receptor signaling by seizures. *Epilepsia*. 2007; 48(Suppl 5): 14–18.
68. Briggs SW, Galanopoulou AS. Altered GABA signaling in early life epilepsies. *Neural Plast*. 2011; 2011: 527–605.
69. Giorgi FS, Galanopoulou AS, Moshé SL. Sex dimorphism in seizure-controlling networks. *Neurobiol Dis*. 2014; 72(Pt B): 144–152.
70. Sperber EF, Moshe SL. The effects of seizures on the hippocampus of the immature brain. In: Engel J, Morrell F, eds. *Brain Plasticity and Epilepsy: The Legacy of Frank Morell*. San Diego: Academic Press; 2001.
71. Scantlebury MH, Ouellet PL, Psarropoulou C, Carmant L. Freeze lesion-induced focal cortical dysplasia predisposes to atypical hyperthermic seizures in the immature rat. *Epilepsia*. 2004; 45(6): 592–600.
72. Galanopoulou AS. Dissociated gender-specific effects of recurrent seizures on GABA signaling in CA1 pyramidal neurons: role of GABA(A) receptors. *J Neurosci*. 2008; 28(7): 1557–1567.
73. Kaushal S, Tamer Z, Opoku F, Forcelli PA. Anticonvulsant drug-induced cell death in the developing white matter of the rodent brain. *Epilepsia*. 2016; 57(5): 727–734.
74. Bakker MJ, van Dijk JG, van den Maagdenberg AM, Tijssen MA. Startle syndromes. *Lancet Neurol*. 2006; 5(6): 513–524.
75. Eisermann M, Lardeux C, Nicloux M, et al. Not all myoclonic jerking and tonic posturing in the neonate is epilepsy. *J Pediatr*. 2014; 164(3): 664.
76. Watanabe K, Hara K, Miyazaki S, Hakamada S, Kuroyanagi M. Apneic seizures in the newborn. *Am J Dis Child*. 1982; 136(11): 980–984.
77. Co JP, Elia M, Engel J, Jr, et al. Proposal of an algorithm for diagnosis and treatment of neonatal seizures in developing countries. *Epilepsia*. 2007; 48(6): 1158–1164.

78. Heimann G. Enteral absorption and bioavailability in children in relation to age. *Eur J Clin Pharmacol.* 1980; 18(1): 43–50.
79. Guillet R, Morselli PL. Pharmacokinetics of anticonvulsants in the neonate. In: Wasterlain CG, Vert P, eds. *Neonatal Seizures.* New York: Raven Press, Ltd; 1990: 257–267.
80. Painter MJ, Scher MS, Stein AD, et al. Phenobarbital compared with phenytoin for the treatment of neonatal seizures. *N Engl J Med.* 1999; 341(7): 485–489.
81. Bourgeouis BF, Dodson WE. Phenytoin elimination in newborns. *Neurology.* 1983; 33(2): 173–178.
82. Abend NS, Gutierrez-Colina AM, Monk HM, et al. Levetiracetam for treatment of neonatal seizures. *J Child Neurol.* 2011; 26(4): 465–470.
83. Scher MS, Painter MJ, Bergman I, Barmada MA, Brunberg J. EEG diagnoses of neonatal seizures: clinical correlations and outcome. *Pediatr Neurol.* 1989; 5(1): 17–24.
84. Weiner SP, Painter MJ, Geva D, Guthrie RD, Scher MS. Neonatal seizures: electroclinical dissociation. *Pediatr Neurol.* 1991; 7(5): 363–368.
85. Mizrahi EM. Electroencephalographic/polygraphic/video monitoring in childhood epilepsy. *J Pediatr.* 1984; 105(1): 1–9.
86. Kellaway P, Hrachovy RA, Frost JD Jr, Zion T. Precise characterization and quantification of infantile spasms. *Ann Neurol.* 1979; 6(3): 214–218.
87. Watanabe K. Neurophysiological aspects of neonatal seizures. *Brain Dev.* 2014; 36(5): 363–371.
88. Biraben A, Taussig D, Thomas P, et al. Fear as the main feature of epileptic seizures. *J Neurol Neurosurg Psychiatry.* 2001; 70(2): 186–191.
89. Goldberg HJ, Sheehy EM. Fifth day fits: An acute zinc deficiency syndrome? *Arch Dis Child.* 1982; 57(8): 633–635.
90. Mizrahi EM, Hrachovy RA, Kellaway P. *Atlas of Neonatal Electroencephalography.* 3rd ed. Philadelphia: Lippincott Williams & Wilkins; 2003.
91. Novotny EJ, Jr, Tharp BR, Coen RW, Bejar R, Enzmann D, Vaucher YE. Positive rolandic sharp waves in the EEG of the premature infant. *Neurology.* 1987; 37(9): 1481–1486.
92. Ortibus EL, Sum JM, Hahn JS. Predictive value of EEG for outcome and epilepsy following neonatal seizures. *Electroencephalogr Clin Neurophysiol.* 1996; 98(3): 175–185.
93. Tekgul H, Gauvreau K, Soul J, et al. The current etiologic profile and neurodevelopmental outcome of seizures in term newborn infants. *Pediatrics.* 2006; 117(4): 1270–1280.
94. Ronen GM, Buckley D, Penney S, Streiner DL. Long-term prognosis in children with neonatal seizures: A population-based study. *Neurology.* 2007; 69(19): 1816–1822.
95. Rowe JC, Holmes GL, Hafford J, et al. Prognostic value of the electroencephalogram in term and preterm infants following neonatal seizures. *Electroencephalogr Clin Neurophysiol.* 1985; 60(3): 183–196.
96. Laroia N, Guillet R, Burchfiel J, McBride MC. EEG background as predictor of electrographic seizures in high-risk neonates. *Epilepsia.* 1998; 39(5): 545–551.
97. Clancy RR, Legido A. Postnatal epilepsy after EEG-confirmed neonatal seizures. *Epilepsia.* 1991; 32(1): 69–76.
98. Clancy RR, Legido A. The exact ictal and interictal duration of electroencephalographic neonatal seizures. *Epilepsia.* 1987; 28(5): 537–541.
99. Pavlidis E, Spagnoli C, Pelosi A, Mazzotta S, Pisani F. Neonatal status epilepticus: differences between preterm and term newborns. *Eur J Paediatr Neurol.* 2015; 19(3): 314–319.
100. Yamamoto H, Aihara M, Niijima S, Yamanouchi H. Treatments with midazolam and lidocaine for status epilepticus in neonates. *Brain Dev.* 2007; 29(9): 559–564.
101. Wertheim D, Mercuri E, Faundez JC, Rutherford M, Acolet D, Dubowitz L. Prognostic value of continuous electroencephalographic recording in full term infants with hypoxic ischaemic encephalopathy. *Arch Dis Child.* 1994; 71(2): F97–102.
102. Legido A, Clancy RR, Berman PH. Neurologic outcome after electroencephalographically proven neonatal seizures. *Pediatrics.* 1991; 88(3): 583–596.
103. Volpe JJ. *Neurology of the Newborn.* Philadelphia: W.B. Saunders; 2008.
104. Perlman JM. Summary proceedings from the neurology group on hypoxic-ischemic encephalopathy. *Pediatrics.* 2006; 117(3 Pt 2): S28–33.
105. Lynch NE, Stevenson NJ, Livingstone V, Murphy BP, Rennie JM, Boylan GB. The temporal evolution of electrographic seizure burden in neonatal hypoxic ischemic encephalopathy: temporal evolution-EEG seizures in HIE. *Epilepsia.* 2012; 53: 549–557.
106. Nelson KB, Lynch JK. Stroke in newborn infants. *Lancet Neurol.* 2004; 3(3): 150–158.
107. Lee KY, Oh KW, Weon YC, Choi SH. Neonatal seizures accompanied by diffuse cerebral white matter lesions on diffusion-weighted imaging

108. are associated with rotavirus infection. *Eur J Paediatr Neurol.* 2014; 18: 624–631.
108. Cortese F, Scicchitano P, Gesualdo M, et al. Early and late infections in newborns: where do we stand? A review. *Pediatr Neonatol.* 2016; 57(4): 265–273.
109. Nabbout R, Soufflet C, Plouin P, Dulac O. Pyridoxine-dependent epilepsy: a suggestive electroclinical pattern. *Arch Dis Child Fetal Neonatal Ed.* 1999; 81: F125–129.
110. Mises J, Moussali-Salefranque F, Plouin P, Temam G, Saudubray JM. [The E.E.G. in non-ketotic hyperglycinaemia (author's transl)]. *Rev Electroencephalogr Neurophysiol Clin.* 1978; 8(1): 102–106.
111. Tharp BR. Unique EEG pattern (comb-like rhythm) in neonatal maple syrup urine disease. *Pediatr Neurol.* 1992; 8(1): 65–68.
112. Vesoulis ZA, Inder TE, Woodward LJ, Buse B, Vavasseur C, Mathur AM. Early electrographic seizures, brain injury, and neurodevelopmental risk in the very preterm infant. *Pediatr Res.* 2014; 75(4): 564–569.
113. Seay AR, Bray PF. Significance of seizures in infants weighing less than 2,500 grams. *Arch Neurol.* 1977; 34(6): 381–382.
114. Clancy RR, Sharif U, Ichord R, et al. Electrographic neonatal seizures after infant heart surgery. *Epilepsia.* 2005; 46(1): 84–90.
115. Rappaport LA, Wypij D, Bellinger DC, et al. Relation of seizures after cardiac surgery in early infancy to neurodevelopmental outcome. Boston Circulatory Arrest Study Group. *Circulation.* 1998; 97(8): 773–779.
116. Ronen GM, Rosales TO, Connolly M, Anderson VE, Leppert M. Seizure characteristics in chromosome 20 benign familial neonatal convulsions. *Neurology.* 1993; 43(7): 1355–1360.
117. Zonana J, Silvey K, Strimling B. Familial neonatal and infantile seizures: An autosomal-dominant disorder. *Am J Med Genet.* 1984; 18(3): 455–459.
118. Plouin P, Anderson VE. Benign familial and nonfamilial neonatal seizures. In: Roger J, Bureau M, Dravet C, Genton P, Tassinari CA, Wolf P, eds. *Epileptic Syndromes in Infancy, Childhood and Adolescence.* 4th ed. John Libbey Eurotext Ltd; 2005: 3–15.
119. Camfield PR, Dooley J, Gordon K, Orlik P. Benign familial neonatal convulsions are epileptic. *J Child Neurol.* 1991; 6(4): 340–342.
120. Dehan M, Quillerou D, Navelet Y, et al. Convulsions in the fifth day of life: a new syndrome? *Arch Fr Pediatr.* 1977; 34(8): 730–742.
121. Maihara T, Tsuji M, Higuchi Y, Hattori H. Benign familial neonatal convulsions followed by benign epilepsy with centrotemporal spikes in two siblings. *Epilepsia.* 1999; 40(1): 110–113.
122. Hirsch E, Velez A, Sellal F, et al. Electroclinical signs of benign neonatal familial convulsions. *Ann Neurol.* 1993; 34(6): 835–841.
123. Bye AM. Neonate with benign familial neonatal convulsions: Recorded generalized and focal seizures. *Pediatr Neurol.* 1994; 10(2): 164–165.
124. Leppert M, Singh N. Benign familial neonatal epilepsy with mutations in two potassium channel genes. *Curr Opin Neurol.* 1999; 12(2): 143–147.
125. Claes LR, Ceulemans B, Audenaert D, et al. De novo KCNQ2 mutations in patients with benign neonatal seizures. *Neurology.* 2004; 63(11): 2155–2158.
126. Orphanet. The Portal for rare diseases and orphan drugs. http://www.orpha.net/orphacom/cahiers/docs/GB/Prevalence_of_rare_diseases_by_alphabetical_list.pdf. Published March 2016. Accessed June 1, 2016.
127. Herrmann B, Lawrenz-Wolf B, Seewald C, Selb B, Wehinger H. 5th day convulsions of the newborn infant in rotavirus infections. *Monatsschr Kinderheilkd.* 1993; 141(2): 120–123.
128. Plouin P. Benign familial neonatal seizures and benign idiopathic neonatal seizures. In: Engel J, Pedley TA, eds. *Epilepsy: A Comprehensive Textbook.* New York: Lippincott-Raven Publishers; 1997: 2247–2255.
129. Pryor DS, Don N, Macourt DC. Fifth day fits: A syndrome of neonatal convulsions. *Arch Dis Child.* 1981; 56(10): 753–758.
130. Yamatogi Y, Ohtahara S. Early-infantile epileptic encephalopathy with suppression-bursts, Ohtahara syndrome; its overview referring to our 16 cases. *Brain Devel.* 2002; 24(1): 13–23.
131. du Plessis AJ, Kaufmann WE, Kupsky WJ. Intrauterine-onset myoclonic encephalopathy associated with cerebral cortical dysgenesis. *J Child Neurol.* 1993; 8(2): 164–170.
132. Ohtahara S, Yamatogi Y. Ohtahara syndrome: With special reference to its developmental aspects for differentiating from early myoclonic encephalopathy. *Epilepsy Res.* 2006; 70(Suppl 1): S58–67.
133. Schlumberger E, Dulac O, Plouin P. Early-infantile epileptic syndrome(s) with suppression-burst: Nosological considerations. In: Roger J, Bureau M, Dravet C, Genton P, Tassinari CA, Wolf P, eds. *Epileptic Syndromes in Infancy, Childhood and Adolescence.* John Libbey & Company Ltd; 1992: 35–42.
134. Fusco L, Pachatz C, Di Capua M, Vigevano F. Video/EEG aspects of early-infantile epileptic encephalopathy with suppression-bursts (Ohtahara syndrome). *Brain Dev.* 2001; 23(7): 708–714.

135. Aicardi J, Ohtahara S. Severe neonatal epilepsies with suppression-burst pattern. In: Roger J, Bureau M, Dravet C, Genton P, Tassinari CA, Wolf P, eds. *Epileptic Syndromes in Infancy, Childhood and Adolescence*. 4th ed. John Libbey Eurotext Ltd; 2005: 39–50.

136. Clarke M, Gill J, Noronha M, McKinlay I. Early infantile epileptic encephalopathy with suppression burst: Ohtahara syndrome. *Dev Med Child Neurol*. 1987; 29(4): 520–528.

137. Al-Futaisi A, Banwell B, Ochi A, et al. Hidden focal EEG seizures during prolonged suppressions and high-amplitude bursts in early infantile epileptic encephalopathy. *Clin Neurophysiol*. 2005; 116(5): 1113–1117.

138. Djukic A, Lado FA, Shinnar S, Moshé SL. Are early myoclonic encephalopathy (EME) and the Ohtahara syndrome (EIEE) independent of each other? *Epilepsy Res*. 2006; 70(Suppl 1): 68–76.

139. Tatsuno M, Hayashi M, Iwamoto H, Sasaki Y, Hara M. Autopsy case of leigh's encephalopathy with wide lesions in central nervous system and early infantile epileptic encephalopathy with burst suppression. *No To Hattatsu*. 1984; 16(1): 68–75.

140. Williams AN, Gray RG, Poulton K, Ramani P, Whitehouse WP. A case of Ohtahara syndrome with cytochrome oxidase deficiency. *Dev Med Child Neurol*. 1998; 40(8): 568–570.

141. Molinari F. Mitochondria and neonatal epileptic encephalopathies with suppression burst. *J Bioenerg Biomembr*. 2010; 42(6): 467–471.

142. Pavone P, Spalice A, Polizzi A, Parisi P, Ruggieri M. Ohtahara syndrome with emphasis on recent genetic discovery. *Brain Dev*. 2012; 34(6): 459–468.

143. Saitsu H, Kato M, Koide A, et al. Whole exome sequencing identifies KCNQ2 mutations in Ohtahara syndrome. *Ann Neurol*. 2012; 72(2): 298–300.

144. Nakamura K, Kato M, Osaka H, et al. Clinical spectrum of SCN2A mutations expanding to Ohtahara syndrome. *Neurology*. 2013; 81(11): 992–998.

145. Baxter PS, Gardner-Medwin D, Barwick DD, et al. Vigabatrin monotherapy in resistant neonatal seizures. *Seizure*. 1995; 4(1): 57–59.

146. Bulteau C, Otsuki T, Delalande O. Epilepsy surgery for hemispheric syndromes in infants: Hemimegalencephaly and hemispheric cortical dysplasia. *Brain Dev*. 2013; 35: 742–747.

147. Dalla Bernardina B, Dulac O, Fejerman N, Dravet C, et al. Early myoclonic epileptic encephalopathy (E.M.E.E.). *Eur J Pediatr*. 1983; 140(3): 248–252.

148. Wang PJ, Lee WT, Hwu WL, Young C, Yau KI, Shen YZ. The controversy regarding diagnostic criteria for early myoclonic encephalopathy. *Brain Dev*. 1998; 20(7): 530–535.

149. Beal JC, Cherian K, Moshe SL. Early-onset epileptic encephalopathies: Ohtahara syndrome and early myoclonic encephalopathy. *Pediatr Neurol*. 2012; 47: 317–323.

150. Lombroso CT. Early myoclonic encephalopathy, early infantile epileptic encephalopathy, and benign and severe infantile myoclonic epilepsies: A critical review and personal contributions. *J Clin Neurophysiol*. 1990; 7(3): 380–408.

151. Aukett A, Bennett MJ, Hosking GP. Molybdenum co-factor deficiency: An easily missed inborn error of metabolism. *Dev Med Child Neurol*. 1988; 30(4): 531–535.

152. Rossi S, Daniele I, Bastrenta P, Mastrangelo M, Lista G. Early myoclonic encephalopathy and nonketotic hyperglycinemia. *Pediatr Neurol*. 2009; 41: 371–374.

153. Weckhuysen S, Mandelstam S, Suls A, et al. KCNQ2 encephalopathy: emerging phenotype of a neonatal epileptic encephalopathy. *Ann Neurol*. 2012; 71(1): 15–25.

154. Specchio N, Vigevano F. The spectrum of benign infantile seizures. *Epilepsy Res*. 2006; 70(Suppl 1): 156–167.

155. Watanabe K, Negoro T, Aso K. Benign partial epilepsy with secondarily generalized seizures in infancy. *Epilepsia*. 1993; 34(4): 635–638.

156. Capovilla G, Beccaria F. Benign partial epilepsy in infancy and early childhood with vertex spikes and waves during sleep: a new epileptic form. *Brain Dev*. 2000; 22: 93–98.

157. Kikuchi K, Hamano S, Higurashi N, et al. Difficulty of early diagnosis and requirement of long-term follow-up in benign infantile seizures. *Pediatr Neurol*. 2015; 53(2): 157–162.

158. Heron SE, Grinton BE, Kivity S, Afawi Z, et al. PRRT2 mutations cause benign familial infantile epilepsy and infantile convulsions with choreoathetosis syndrome. *Am J Hum Genet*. 2012; 90(1): 152–160.

159. Heron SE, Crossland KM, Andermann E, et al. Sodium-channel defects in benign familial neonatal-infantile seizures. *Lancet*. 2002; 360(9336): 851–852.

160. Bureau M, Kaleli O, Maton B, Dravet C. EEG correlates of benign focal epilepsy in early childhood. *Epilepsia*. 1998; Suppl 2: 91–92.

161. Szepetowski P, Rochette J, Berquin P, et al. Familial infantile convulsions and paroxysmal choreoathetosis: a new neurological syndrome linked to the pericentromeric region of human chromosome 16. *Am J Hum Genet*. 1997; 61(4): 889–898.

162. Gardella E, Becker F, Møller RS, et al. Benign infantile seizures and paroxysmal dyskinesia caused by an SCN8A mutation. *Ann Neurol*. 2016; 79(3): 428–436.

163. Terwindt GM, Ophoff RA, Lindhout D, et al. Partial cosegregation of familial hemiplegic migraine and a benign familial infantile epileptic syndrome. *Epilepsia*. 1997; 38(8): 915–921.

164. Commission on Classification and Terminology of the International League Against Epilepsy. Proposal for revised classification of epilepsies and epileptic syndromes. *Epilepsia*. 1989; 30(4): 389–399.

165. Engel J Jr. Report of the ILAE classification core group. *Epilepsia*. 2006; 47(9): 1558–1568.

166. Dravet C, Bureau M. Benign myoclonic epilepsy in infancy. *Adv Neurol*. 2005; 95: 127–137.

167. Darra F, Fiorini E, Zoccante L, et al. Benign myoclonic epilepsy in infancy (BMEI): a longitudinal electroclinical study of 22 cases. *Epilepsia*. 2006;47(Suppl 5): 31–35.

168. Caraballo RH, Flesler S, Pasteris MC, Lopez Avaria MF, Fortini S, Vilte C. Myoclonic epilepsy in infancy: an electroclinical study and long-term follow-up of 38 patients. *Epilepsia*. 2013; 54(9): 1605–1612.

169. Zafeiriou D, Vargiami E, Kontopoulos E. Reflex myoclonic epilepsy in infancy: a benign age-dependent idiopathic startle epilepsy. *Epileptic Disord*. 2003; 5(2): 121–122.

170. Capovilla G, Beccaria F, Gambardella A, Montagnini A, Avantaggiato P, Seri S. Photosensitive benign myoclonic epilepsy in infancy. *Epilepsia*. 2007; 48(1): 96–100.

171. Auvin S, Pandit F, De Bellecize J, et al. Benign myoclonic epilepsy in infancy: Electroclinical features and long-term follow-up of 34 patients. *Epilepsia*. 2006; 47: 387–393.

172. Mangano S, Fontana A, Spitaleri C, et al. Benign myoclonic epilepsy in infancy followed by childhood absence epilepsy. *Seizure*. 2011; 20(9): 727–730.

173. Auvin S, Lamblin MD, Cuvellier JC, Vallée L. A patient with myoclonic epilepsy in infancy followed by myoclonic astatic epilepsy. *Seizure*. 2012; 21(4): 300–303.

174. Nabbout R, Chemaly N, Chipaux M, et al. Encephalopathy in children with Dravet syndrome is not a pure consequence of epilepsy. *Orphanet J Rare Dis*. 2013; 8: 176.

175. Dravet C, Bureau M, Oguni H, Cokar O, Guerrini R. Dravet syndrome (severe myoclonic epilepsy in infancy). In: Bureau M, Genton P, Dravet C, Delgado-Escueta A, Tassinari CA, Thomas P, & Wolf P, eds. *Epileptic Syndromes in Infancy, Childhood and Adolescence*. 5th ed. John Libbey Eurotext Ltd; 2012: 125–156.

176. Nabbout R, Desguerre I, Sabbagh S, et al. An unexpected EEG course in Dravet syndrome. *Epilepsy Res*. 2008; 81(1): 90–95.

177. Specchio N, Balestri M, Trivisano M, et al. Electroencephalographic features in Dravet syndrome: five-year follow-up study in 22 patients. *J Child Neurol*. 2012; 27(4): 439–444.

178. Akiyama M, Kobayashi K, Yoshinaga H, Ohtsuka Y. A long-term follow-up study of Dravet syndrome up to adulthood. *Epilepsia*. 2010; 51(6): 1043–1052.

179. Depienne C, Trouillard O, Saint-Martin C, et al. Spectrum of SCN1A gene mutations associated with Dravet syndrome: analysis of 333 patients. *J Med Genet*. 2009; 46(3): 183–191.

180. Kim SH, Nordli DR Jr, Berg AT, Koh S, Laux L. Ictal ontogeny in Dravet syndrome. *Clin Neurophysiol*. 2015; 126(3): 446–455.

181. Chiron C, Dulac O. The pharmacologic treatment of Dravet syndrome. *Epilepsia*. 2011; 52(Suppl 2): 72–75.

182. Coppola G. Malignant migrating partial seizures in infancy: an epilepsy syndrome of unknown etiology. *Epilepsia*. 2009; 50(Suppl 5): 49–51.

183. McTague A, Appleton R, Avula S, et al. Migrating partial seizures of infancy: expansion of the electroclinical, radiological and pathological disease spectrum. *Brain*. 2013; 136(5): 1578–1591.

184. Dulac O. Malignant migrating partial seizures in infancy. In: Roger J, Bureau M, Dravet C, Genton P, Tassinari CA, Wolf P eds. *Epileptic Syndromes in Infancy, Childhood and Adolescence*. 4th ed. John Libbey Eurotext Ltd; 2005: 73–76.

185. Stödberg T, McTague A, Ruiz AJ, et al. Mutations in SLC12A5 in epilepsy of infancy with migrating focal seizures. *Nat Commun*. 2015; 6: 8038.

186. Barcia G, Desguerre I, Carmona O, et al. Hemiconvulsion-hemiplegia syndrome revisited: longitudinal MRI findings in 10 children. *Dev Med Child Neurol*. 2013; 55(12): 1150–1158.

187. Caraballo RH, Fontana E, Darra F, et al. Migrating focal seizures in infancy: analysis of the electroclinical patterns in 17 patients. *J Child Neurol.* 2008; 23(5): 497–506.

188. Coppola G, Operto FF, Auricchio G, D'Amico A, Fortunato D, Pascotto A. Temporal lobe dual pathology in malignant migrating partial seizures in infancy. *Epileptic Disord.* 2007; 9(2): 145–148.

189. Gastaut H, Poirier F, Payan H, et al. H.H.E. syndrome; hemiconvulsions, hemiplegia, epilepsy. *Epilepsia.* 1960; 1: 418–447.

190. Chauvel P, Dravet C. HHE syndrome (hemiconvulsions, hemiplegia, epilepsy). In: Roger J, Bureau M, Dravet C, Genton P, Tassinari CA, Wolf P, eds. *Epileptic syndromes in infancy, childhood and adolescence.* 4th ed. John Libbey Eurotext Ltd; 2005: 277–294.

191. Aicardi J, Amsili J, Chevrie JJ. Acute hemiplegia in infancy and childhood. *Dev Med Child Neurol.* 1969; 11(2): 162–173.

192. Nabbout R. FIRES and IHHE: Delineation of the syndromes. *Epilepsia.* 2013; 54(Suppl 6): 54–56.

193. Berhouma M, Chekili R, Brini I, et al. Decompressive hemicraniectomy in a space-occupying presentation of hemiconvulsion-hemiplegia-epilepsy syndrome. *Clin Neurol Neurosurg.* 2007; 109(10): 914–917.

194. van Toorn R, Janse van Rensburg P, Solomons R, Ndondo AP, Schoeman JF. Hemiconvulsion-hemiplegia-epilepsy syndrome in South African children: insights from a retrospective case series. *Eur J Paediatr Neurol.* 2012; 16(2): 142–148.

195. Kawada J, Kimura H, Yoshikawa T, et al. Hemiconvulsion-hemiplegia syndrome and primary human herpesvirus 7 infection. *Brain Dev.* 2004; 26(6): 412–414.

196. Yamazaki S, Ikeno K, Abe T, Tohyama J, Adachi Y. Hemiconvulsion-hemiplegia-epilepsy syndrome associated with CACNA1A S218L mutation. *Pediatr Neurol.* 2011; 45(3): 193–196.

197. Nabbout R, Vezzani A, Dulac O, Chiron C. Acute encephalopathy with inflammation-mediated status epilepticus. *Lancet Neurol.* 2011; 10(1): 99–108.

198. Kim DW, Kim KK, Chu K, Chung CK, Lee SK. Surgical treatment of delayed epilepsy in hemiconvulsion-hemiplegia-epilepsy syndrome. *Neurology.* 2008; 70(22 Pt 2): 2116–2122.

199. Mirsattari SM, Wilde NJ, Pigott SE. Long-term cognitive outcome of hemiconvulsion-hemiplegia-epilepsy syndrome affecting the left cerebral hemisphere. *Epilepsy Behav.* 2008; 13(4): 678–680.

200. Fusco L, Vigevano F. Ictal clinical electroencephalographic findings of spasms in West syndrome. *Epilepsia.* 1993; 34(4): 671–678.

201. Dulac O, Plouin P, Jambaqué I. Predicting favorable outcome in idiopathic West syndrome. *Epilepsia.* 1993; 34(4): 747–756.

202. Kobayashi K, Akiyama T, Oka M, Endoh F, Yoshinaga H. A storm of fast (40–150Hz) oscillations during hypsarrhythmia in West syndrome. *Ann Neurol.* 2015; 77(1): 58–67.

203. Hrachovy RA, Frost JD Jr. Infantile epileptic encephalopathy with hypsarrhythmia (infantile spasms/West syndrome). *J Clin Neurophysiol.* 2003; 20(6): 408–425.

204. Caraballo RH, Fejerman N, Bernardina BD, et al. Epileptic spasms in clusters without hypsarrhythmia in infancy. *Epileptic Disord.* 2003; 5(2): 109–113.

205. Gibbs EL, Fleming MM, Gibbs FA. Diagnosis and prognosis of hypsarrhythmia and infantile spasms. *Pediatrics.* 1954; 13(1): 66–73.

206. Lee YJ, Berg AT, Nordli DR Jr. Clinical spectrum of epileptic spasms in children. *Brain Dev.* 2015; 37(1) :37–48

207. Nariai H, Beal J, Galanopoulou AS, Bickel S, Sogawa Y, Jehle R, Shinnar S, Moshe SL. Scalp EEG ictal gamma activity in the centroparietal channels indicates focal cortical onsets of epileptic spasms in West Syndrome. Presented at: Annual Meeting of the American Epilepsy Society; December 5, 2015; Philadelphia, PA.

208. Gaily EK, Shewmon DA, Chugani HT, Curran JG. Asymmetric and asynchronous infantile spasms. *Epilepsia.* 1995; 36(9): 873–882.

209. Cowan LD, Hudson LS. The epidemiology and natural history of infantile spasms. *J Child Neurol.* 1991; 6(4): 355–364.

210. Riikonen R. Epidemiological data of West syndrome in Finland. *Brain Dev.* 2001; 23(7): 539–541.

211. Bednarek N, Motte J, Soufflet C, Plouin P, Dulac O. Evidence of late-onset infantile spasms. *Epilepsia.* 1998; 39(1): 55–60.

212. Eisermann MM, Ville D, Soufflet C, et al. Cryptogenic late-onset epileptic spasms: an overlooked syndrome of early childhood? *Epilepsia.* 2006; 47(6): 1035–1042.

213. Auvin S, Lamblin MD, Pandit F, Vallée L, Bouvet-Mourcia A. Infantile epileptic encephalopathy with late-onset spasms: report of 19 patients. *Epilepsia.* 2010; 51(7): 1290–1296.

214. Koo B, Hwang P. Localization of focal cortical lesions influences age of onset of infantile spasms. *Epilepsia.* 1996; 37(11): 1068–1071.

215. Pavone P, Striano P, Falsaperla R, Pavone L, Ruggieri M. Infantile spasms syndrome, West syndrome and related phenotypes: what we know in 2013. *Brain Dev.* 2014; 36(9): 739–751.

216. Wilmshurst JM, Gaillard WD, Vinayan KP, et al. Summary of recommendations for the management of infantile seizures: Task Force Report for the ILAE Commission of Pediatrics. *Epilepsia.* 2015; 56(8): 1185–1197.

217. Lux AL. Is hypsarrhythmia a form of non-convulsive status epilepticus in infants? *Acta Neurol Scand.* 2007; 115(4 Suppl): 37–44.

218. Pellock JM, Hrachovy R, Shinnar S, et al. Infantile spasms: a U.S. consensus report. *Epilepsia.* 2010; 51(10): 2175–2189.

219. Chiron C, Dumas C, Jambaqué I, Mumford J, Dulac O. Randomized trial comparing vigabatrin and hydrocortisone in infantile spasms due to tuberous sclerosis. *Epilepsy Res.* 1997; 26(2): 389–395.

220. Caraballo RH, Reyes G, Falsaperla R, et al. Epileptic spasms in clusters with focal EEG paroxysms: A study of 12 patients. *Seizure.* 2016; 35: 88–92.

221. Chugani HT, Ilyas M, Kumar A, et al. Surgical treatment for refractory epileptic spasms: The Detroit series. *Epilepsia.* 2015; 56(12): 1941–1949.

222. Riikonen R. Long-term outcome of West syndrome: a study of adults with a history of infantile spasms. *Epilepsia.* 1996; 37(4): 367–372.

223. Eisermann MM, DeLaRaillère A, Dellatolas G, Tozzi E, Nabbout R, Dulac O, Chiron C. Infantile spasms in Down syndrome—effects of delayed anticonvulsive treatment. *Epilepsy Res.* 2003; 55(1-2): 21–27.

224. Hrachovy RA, Glaze DG, Frost JD Jr. A retrospective study of spontaneous remission and long-term outcome in patients with infantile spasms. *Epilepsia.* 1991; 32(2): 212–214.

225. Arzimanoglou A, French J, Blume WT, et al. Lennox-Gastaut Syndrome: a consensus approach on diagnosis, assessment, management, and trial methodology. *Lancet Neurol.* 2009; 8: 82–93.

226. Sadleir LG, Farrell K, Smith S. Electroclinical features of absence seizures in childhood absence epilepsy. *Neurology.* 2006; 67: 413–418.

227. Shinnar S, Cnaan A, Hu F, et al. Long-term outcomes of generalized tonic-clonic seizures in a childhood absence epilepsy trial. *Neurology.* 2015; 85(13): 1108–1114.

228. Panayiotopoulos CP. Typical absence seizures and related epileptic syndromes: assessment of current state and directions for future research. *Epilepsia.* 2008; 49(12): 2131–2139.

229. Dlugos D, Shinnar S, Cnaan A, et al. Pretreatment EEG in childhood absence epilepsy: associations with attention and treatment outcome. *Neurology.* 2013; 81: 150–156.

230. Glauser TA, Cnaan A, Shinnar S, et al. Ethosuximide, valproic acid, and lamotrigine in childhood absence epilepsy: initial monotherapy outcomes at 12 months. *Epilepsia.* 2013; 54: 141–155.

231. Caplan R, Siddarth P, Stahl L, et al. Childhood absence epilepsy: behavioral, cognitive, and linguistic comorbidities. *Epilepsia.* 2008; 49: 1838–1846.

232. Masur D, Shinnar S, Cnaan A, et al. Pretreatment cognitive deficits and treatment effects on attention in childhood absence epilepsy. *Neurology.* 2013; 81(18): 1572–1580.

233. Marini C, Harkin LA, Wallace RH, Mulley JC, Scheffer IE, Berkovic SF. Childhood absence epilepsy and febrile seizures: a family with a GABA(A) receptor mutation. *Brain.* 2003; 126: 230–240.

234. Yalçin O. Genes and molecular mechanisms involved in the epileptogenesis of idiopathic absence epilepsies. *Seizure.* 2012; 21(2): 79–86.

235. Chen Y, Lu J, Pan H, et al. Association between genetic variation of CACNA1H and childhood absence epilepsy. *Ann Neurol.* 2003; 54(2): 239–243.

236. Everett KV, Chioza B, Aicardi J, et al. Linkage and association analysis of CACNG3 in childhood absence epilepsy. *Eur J Hum Genet.* 2007; 15(4): 463–472.

237. Viravan S, Go C, Ochi A, et al. Jeavons syndrome existing as occipital cortex initiating generalized epilepsy. *Epilepsia.* 2011; 52: 1273–1279.

238. Wang XL, Bao JX, Liang-Shi, et al. Jeavons syndrome in China. *Epilepsy Behav.* 2014; 32: 64–71.

239. Takahashi S, Yamamoto S, Tanaka R, et al. Focal frontal epileptiform discharges in a patient with eyelid myoclonia and absence seizures. *Epilepsy Behav Case Rep.* 2015; 4: 35–37.

240. Sadleir LG, Vears D, Regan B, Redshaw N, Bleasel A, Scheffer IE. Family studies of individuals with eyelid myoclonia with absences. *Epilepsia.* 2012; 53(12): 2141–2148.

241. Bureau M, Tassinari CA. Epilepsy with myoclonic absences. *Brain Dev.* 2005; 27: 178–184.

242. Manonmani V, Wallace SJ. Epilepsy with myoclonic absences. *Arch Dis Child.* 1994; 70: 288–290.

243. Ikeda H, Fujiwara T, Shigematsu H, et al. Symptoms and clinical course of epilepsy with myoclonic absences. *No To Hattatsu.* 2011; 43(1): 14–18.

244. Cherian A, Jabeen SA, Kandadai RM, et al. Epilepsy with myoclonic absences in siblings. *Brain Dev.* 2014; 36(10): 892–898.

245. Crespel A, Genton P, Berramdane M, et al. Lamotrigine associated with exacerbation or de novo myoclonus in idiopathic generalized epilepsies. *Neurology.* 2005; 65: 762–764.

246. Bonanni P, Parmeggiani L, Guerrini R. Different neurophysiological patterns of myoclonus characterize Lennox-Gastaut Syndrome and myoclonic-astatic epilepsy. *Epilepsia.* 2002; 43: 609–615.

247. Oguni H, Tanaka T, Hayashi K, et al. Treatment and long-term prognosis of myoclonic-astatic epilepsy of early childhood. *Neuropediatrics.* 2002; 33(3): 122–132.

248. Trivisano M, Specchio N, Cappelletti S, et al. Myoclonic astatic epilepsy: an age-dependent epileptic syndrome with favorable seizure outcome but variable cognitive evolution. *Epilepsy Res.* 2011; 97(1-2): 133–141.

249. Inoue T, Ihara Y, Tomonoh Y, et al. Early onset and focal spike discharges as indicators of poor prognosis for myoclonic-astatic epilepsy. *Brain Dev.* 2014; 36(7): 613–619.

250. Tang S, Pal DK. Dissecting the genetic basis of myoclonic-astatic epilepsy. *Epilepsia.* 2012; 53(8): 1303–1313.

251. Carvill GL, McMahon JM, Schneider A, et al. Mutations in the GABA transporter SLC6A1 cause epilepsy with myoclonic-atonic seizures. *Am J Hum Genet.* 2015; 96(5): 808–815.

252. Mullen SA, Marini C, Suls A, et al. Glucose transporter 1 deficiency as a treatable cause of myoclonic astatic epilepsy. *Arch Neurol.* 2011; 68(9): 1152–1155.

253. Beaussart M. Benign epilepsy of children with rolandic (centrotemporal) paroxysmal foci. A clinical entity. Study of 221 cases. *Epilepsia.* 1972; 13: 795–811.

254. Berroya AM, Bleasel AF, Stevermuer TL, Lawson J, Bye AM. Spike morphology, location, and frequency in benign epilepsy with centrotemporal spikes. *J Child Neurol.* 2005; 20(3): 188–194.

255. Gregory DL, Wong PK. Topographical analysis of centrotemporal discharges in benign rolandic epilepsy of childhood. *Epilepsia.* 1984; 25: 705–711.

256. Nicolai J, van der Linden I, Arends JB, et al. EEG characteristics related to educational impairments in children with benign childhood epilepsy with centrotemporal spikes. *Epilepsia.* 2007; 48(11): 2093–2100.

257. Capovilla G, Beccaria F, Bianchi A, et al. Ictal EEG patterns in epilepsy with centro-temporal spikes. *Brain Dev.* 2011; 33(4): 301–309.

258. Mitsudome A, Ohfu M, Yasumoto S, Ogawa A. Rhythmic slow activity in benign childhood epilepsy with centrotemporal spikes. *Clin Electroencephalogr.* 1997; 28(1): 44–48.

259. Bedoin N, Ciumas C, Lopez C, et al. Disengagement and inhibition of visual-spatial attention are differently impaired in children with rolandic epilepsy and Panayiotopoulos syndrome. *Epilepsy Behav.* 2012; 25(1): 81–91.

260. Boscariol M, Casali RL, Amaral MI, et al. Language and central temporal auditory processing in childhood epilepsies. *Epilepsy Behav.* 2015; 53: 180–183.

261. Garcia-Ramos C, Jackson DC, Lin JJ, et al. Cognition and brain development in children with benign epilepsy with centrotemporal spikes. *Epilepsia.* 2015; 56(10): 1615–1622.

262. Neubauer BA, Fiedler B, Himmelein B, et al. Centrotemporal spikes in families with rolandic epilepsy: linkage to chromosome 15q14. *Neurology.* 1998; 51(6): 1608–1612.

263. Strug LJ, Clarke T, Chiang T, et al. Centrotemporal sharp wave EEG trait in rolandic epilepsy maps to Elongator Protein Complex 4 (ELP4). *Eur J Hum Genetics.* 2009; 17: 1171–1181.

264. Lemke JR, Lal D, Reinthaler EM, et al. Mutations in GRIN2A cause idiopathic focal epilepsy with rolandic spikes. *Nat Genet.* 2013; 45(9): 1067–1072.

265. Ishii A, Miyajima T, Kurahashi H, et al. KCNQ2 abnormality in BECTS: benign childhood epilepsy with centrotemporal spikes following benign neonatal seizures resulting from a mutation of KCNQ2. *Epilepsy Res.* 2012; 102(1-2): 122–125.

266. Coppola G, Franzoni E, Verrotti A, et al. Levetiracetam or oxcarbazepine as monotherapy in newly diagnosed benign epilepsy of childhood with centrotemporal spikes (BECTS): an open-label, parallel group trial. *Brain Dev.* 2007; 29(5): 281–284.

267. Andrade R, García-Espinosa A, Machado-Rojas A, García-González ME, et al. A prospective, open, controlled and randomised study of clobazam versus carbamazepine in patients with frequent episodes of Rolandic epilepsy. *Rev Neurol.* 2009; 49(11): 581–586.

268. Niedermeyer E, Naidu S. Further EEG observations in children with the Rett syndrome. *Brain Dev.* 1990; 12: 53–54.

269. Musumeci SA, Colognaola RM, Ferri R, et al. Fragile X syndrome: A particular epileptogenic EEG pattern. *Epilepsia.* 1988; 29: 41–47.

270. Michael M, Tsatsou K, Ferrie CD. Panayiotopoulos syndrome: an important childhood autonomic epilepsy to be differentiated from occipital epilepsy and acute non-epileptic disorders. *Brain Dev.* 2010; 32(1): 4–9.

271. Koutroumanidis M, Ferrie CD, Valeta T, Sanders S, Michael M, Panayiotopoulos CP. Syncope-like epileptic seizures in Panayiotopoulos syndrome. *Neurology.* 2012; 79(5): 463–467.

272. Lada C, Skiadas K, Theodorou V, Loli N, Covanis A. A study of 43 patients with Panayiotopoulos syndrome, a common and benign childhood seizure susceptibility. *Epilepsia.* 2003; 44(1): 81–88.

273. Panayiotopoulos CP. *Panayiotopoulos Syndrome: A Common and Benign Childhood Epilepsy Syndrome.* London: John Libbey & Company; 2002.

274. Yoshinaga H, Kobayashi K, Ohtsuka Y. Characteristics of the synchronous occipital and frontopolar spike phenomenon in Panayiotopoulos syndrome. *Brain Dev.* 2010; 32(8): 603–608.

275. Lacroix L, Fluss J, Gervaix A, Korff CM. Benzodiazepines in the acute management of seizures with autonomic manifestations: anticipate complications! *Epilepsia.* 2011; 52(10): e156–159.

276. Caraballo R, Koutroumanidis M, Panayiotopoulos CP, Fejerman N. Idiopathic childhood occipital epilepsy of Gastaut: a review and differentiation from migraine and other epilepsies. *J Child Neurol.* 2009; 24(12): 1536–1542.

277. Gastaut H, Zifkin BG. Benign epilepsy of childhood with occipital spike and wave complexes. In: Andermann F, Lugaresi E, eds. *Migraine and Epilepsy.* Boston: Butterworths; 1987: 47–81.

278. Panayiotopoulos CP. Benign childhood epilepsy with occipital paroxysms: A 15-year prospective study. *Ann Neurol.* 1989; 26: 51–56.

279. Beaumanoir A. Semiology of occipital seizures in infants and children. In: Andermann F, Beaumanoir A, Mira L, Roger J, Tassinari CA, eds. *Occipital Seizures and Epilepsies in Children.* London: John Libbey; 1993: 71–86.

280. Fernández IS, Chapman KE, Peters JM, et al. The tower of Babel: survey on concepts and terminology in electrical status epilepticus in sleep and continuous spikes and waves during sleep in North America. *Epilepsia.* 2013; 54(4): 741–750.

281. Tassinari CA, Rubboli G, Volpi L, et al. Encephalopathy with electrical status epilepticus during slow sleep or ESES syndrome including the acquired aphasia. *Clin Neurophysiol.* 2000; 111(Suppl 2): S94–S102.

282. Patry G, Lyagoubi S, Tassinari CA. Subclinical "electrical status epilepticus" induced by sleep in children. *Arch Neurol.* 1971; 24: 242–252.

283. Beaumanoir A. EEG data. In: Beaumanoir A, Bureau M, Deonna T, Mira L, Tassinari CA, eds. *Continuous Spikes and Waves During Slow Sleep.* London: John Libbey; 1995: 217–223.

284. Ballaban-Gil K, Goldberg R, Moshe SL, Shinnar S. EEG evaluation and treatment of children with language regression. *Epilepsia.* 1998; 39(Suppl 6):156.

285. van den Munckhof B, van Dee V, Sagi L, et al. Treatment of electrical status epilepticus in sleep: A pooled analysis of 575 cases. *Epilepsia.* 2015; 56(11): 1738–1746.

286. Rapin I, Mattis S, Rowan AJ, Golden GG. Verbal auditory agnosia in children. *Dev Med Child Neurol.* 1977; 19(2): 197–207.

287. van Bogaert P, King MD, Paquier P, et al. Acquired auditory agnosia in childhood and normal sleep electroencephalography subsequently diagnosed as Landau Kleffner syndrome: report of three cases. *Dev Med Child Neurol.* 2013; 55(6): 575–579.

288. Galanopoulou AS, Bojko A, Lado F, Moshé SL. The spectrum of neuropsychiatric abnormalities associated with electrical status epilepticus in sleep. *Brain Dev.* 2000; 22(5): 279–295.

289. Landau WM, Kleffner FR. Syndrome of acquired aphasia with convulsive disorder in children. *Neurology.* 1957; 7: 523–530.

290. Hirsch E, Marescaux C, Maquet P, et al: Landau-Kleffner syndrome: A clinical and EEG study of five cases. *Epilepsia.* 1990; 31: 756–767.

291. Scheffer IE, Berkovic SF. Generalized epilepsy with febrile seizures plus: A genetic disorder with heterogeneous clinical phenotypes. *Brain.* 1997; 120: 479–490.

292. Singh R, Scheffer IE, Crossland K, Berkovic SF. Generalized epilepsy with febrile seizures plus: A common childhood-onset genetic epilepsy syndrome. *Ann Neurol.* 1999; 45: 75–81.

293. Xu XJ, Zhang YH, Sun HH, Liu XY, Wu HS, Wu XR. Phenotype and SCN1A gene mutation screening in 39 families with generalized epilepsy with febrile seizures plus. *Zhonghua Er Ke Za Zhi.* 2012; 50(8): 580–586.

294. Marini C, Mei D, Temudo T, et al. Idiopathic epilepsies with seizures precipitated by fever and SCN1A abnormalities. *Epilepsia.* 2007; 48(9): 1678–1685.

295. Wallace RH, Wang DW, Singh R, et al. Febrile seizures and generalized epilepsy associated with a mutation in the Na+ -channel beta1 subunit gene SCN1B. *Nat Genet.* 1998; 19(4): 366–370.

296. Baulac S, Huberfeld G, Gourfinkel-An I, et al. First genetic evidence of GABA(A) receptor dysfunction in epilepsy: a mutation in the gamma2-subunit gene. *Nat Genet.* 2001; 28(1): 46–48.

297. Hughes JR, Patil VK. Long-term electro-clinical changes in the Lennox-Gastaut syndrome before, during, and after the slow spike-wave pattern. *Clin Electroencephalogr.* 2002; 33(1): 1–7.

298. Filippini M, Boni A, Dazzani G, Guerra A, Gobbi G. Neuropsychological findings: myoclonic astatic epilepsy and Lennox-Gastaut syndrome. *Epilepsia.* 2006; 47(S2): 56–59.

299. Kostov K, Kostov H, Taubøll E. Long-term vagus nerve stimulation in the treatment of Lennox-Gastaut syndrome. *Epilepsy Behav.* 2009; 16(2): 321–324.

300. Tezar FI, Sahin G, Ciger A, Saygi S. Focal EEG findings in juvenile absence syndrome and the effect of antiepileptic drugs. *Clin EEG Neurosci.* 2008; 39: 33–38.

301. Gelisse P, Serafini A, Velizarova R, Genton P, Crespel A. Temporal intermittent delta activity: a marker of juvenile absence epilepsy? *Seizure.* 2011; 20: 38–41.

302. Danhofer P, Brazdil M, Oslejskova H, Kuba R. Long-term seizure outcome in patients with juvenile absence epilepsy; a retrospective study in a tertiary referral center. *Seizure.* 2014; 23(6): 443–447.

303. Kasteleijn-Nolst Trenité DG, Schmitz B, Janz D, et al. Consensus on diagnosis and management of JME: From founder's observations to current trends. *Epilepsy Behav.* 2013; 28(Suppl 1): S87–90.

304. Jayalakshmi SS, Srinivasa Rao B, Sailaja S. Focal clinical and electroencephalographic features in patients with juvenile myoclonic epilepsy. *Acta Neurol Scand.* 2010; 122(2): 115–123.

305. Montalenti E, Imperiale D, Rovera A, Bergamasco B, Benna P. Clinical features, EEG findings, and diagnostic pitfalls in juvenile myoclonic epilepsy: a series of 63 patients. *J Neurol Sci.* 2001; 184: 65–70.

306. Cossette P. Channelopathies and juvenile myoclonic epilepsy. *Epilepsia.* 2010; 51(Suppl 1): 30–32.

307. de Nijs L, Wolkoff N, Coumans B, Delgado-Escueta AV, Grisar T, Lakaye B. Mutations of EFHC1, linked to juvenile myoclonic epilepsy, disrupt radial and tangential migrations during brain development. *Hum Mol Genet.* 2012; 21(23): 5106–5117.

308. Durner M, Janz D, Zingsem J, Greenberg DA. Possible association of juvenile myoclonic epilepsy with HLA-DRw6. *Epilepsia.* 1992; 33: 814–816.

309. Elmslie FV, Rees M, Williamson MP, et al. Genetic mapping of a major susceptibility locus for juvenile myoclonic epilepsy on chromosome 15q. *Hum Mol Genet.* 1997; 6: 1329–1334.

310. Janz D, Wolf P. Epilepsy with grand mal on awakening. In: Engel J, Pedley TA, eds. *Epilepsy: A Comprehensive Textbook.* Philadelphia: Lippincott-Raven, 1997: 2347.

311. Williams CA, Beaudet AL, Clayton-Smith J, et al. Angelman syndrome 2005: updated consensus for diagnostic criteria. *Am J Med Genet A.* 2006; 140(5): 413–418.

312. Zuberi SM. Chromosome disorders associated with epilepsy. *Handb Clin Neurol.* 2013; 111: 543–548.

313. Valente KD, Andrade JQ, Grossmann RM, et al. Angelman syndrome: difficulties in EEG pattern recognition and possible misinterpretations. *Epilepsia.* 2003; 44(8): 1051–1063.

314. Korff CM, Kelley KR, Nordli DR Jr. Notched delta, phenotype, and Angelman syndrome. *J Clin Neurophysiol.* 2005; 22(4): 238–243.

315. Yum MS, Lee EH, Kim JH, Ko TS, Yoo HW. Implications of slow waves and shifting epileptiform discharges in Angelman syndrome. *Brain Dev.* 2013; 35(3): 245–251.

316. Dalla Bernardina B, Fontana E, Darra F. Myoclonic status in nonprogressive encephalopathies (MSNPE). In: Bureau M, Genton P, Dravet C, Delgado-Escueta A, Tassinari CA, Thomas P, Wolf P, eds. *Epileptic Syndromes in Infancy, Childhood and Adolescence.* 5th ed. John Libbey Eurotext Ltd; 2012: 157–173.

317. Caraballo RH, Cersosimo RO, Espeche A, Arroyo HA, Fejerman N. Myoclonic status in nonprogressive encephalopathies: study of 29 cases. *Epilepsia.* 2007; 48: 107–113.

318. Buiting K, Clayton-Smith J, Driscoll DJ, et al. Clinical utility gene card for: Angelman Syndrome. *Eur J Hum Genet.* 2015; 23(2).

319. Nicita F, Garone G, Papetti L, et al. Myoclonic status and central fever in Angelman syndrome due to paternal uniparental disomy. *J Neurogenet.* 2015; 29(4): 178–182.

320. Stafstrom CE, Patxot OF, Gilmore HE, Wisniewski KE. Seizures in children with Down syndrome: etiology, characteristics and outcome. *Dev Med Child Neurol.* 1991; 33(3): 191–200.

321. Guerrini R, Genton P, Bureau M, Dravet C, Roger J. Reflex seizures are frequent in patients with Down syndrome and epilepsy. *Epilepsia.* 1990; 31(4): 406–417.

322. Ferlazzo E, Adjien CK, Guerrini R, et al. Lennox-Gastaut syndrome with late-onset and prominent reflex seizures in trisomy 21 patients. *Epilepsia.* 2009; 50(6): 1587–1595.

323. Berry-Kravis E, Raspa M, Loggin-Hester L, Bishop E, Holiday D, Bailey DB. Seizures in fragile X syndrome: characteristics and comorbid diagnoses. *Am J Intellect Dev Disabil.* 2010; 115(6): 461–472.

324. Musumeci SA, Hagerman RJ, Ferri R, et al. Epilepsy and EEG findings in males with fragile X syndrome. *Epilepsia.* 1999; 40(8): 1092–1099.

325. Battaglia A, Filippi T, Carey JC. Update on the clinical features and natural history of Wolf-Hirschhorn (4p-) syndrome: experience with 87 patients and recommendations for routine health supervision. *Am J Med Genet C Semin Med Genet.* 2008; 148C(4): 246–251.

326. Zambrelli E, Vignoli A, Nobili L, et al. Sleep in ring chromosome 20 syndrome: a peculiar electroencephalographic pattern. *Funct Neurol.* 2013; 28(1): 47–53.

327. Inoue Y, Fujiwara T, Matsuda K, et al. Ring chromosome 20 and nonconvulsive status epilepticus. A new epileptic syndrome. *Brain.* 1997; 120(6): 939–953.

328. Augustijn PB, Parra J, Wouters CH, Joosten P, Lindhout D, van Emde Boas W. Ring chromosome 20 epilepsy syndrome in children: electroclinical features. *Neurology.* 2001; 57(6): 1108–1111.

329. Nishiwaki T, Hirano M, Kumazawa M, Ueno S. Mosaicism and phenotype in ring chromosome 20 syndrome. *Acta Neurol Scand.* 2005; 111(3): 205–208.

330. Leary LD, Wang D, Nordli Jr DR, Engelstad K, De Vivo DC. Seizure characterization and electroencephalographic features in Glut-1 deficiency. *Epilepsia.* 2003; 44: 701–707.

331. Pong AW, Geary BR, Engelstad KM, Natarajan A, Yang H, De Vivo DC. Glucose transporter type I deficiency syndrome: epilepsy phenotypes and outcomes. *Epilepsia.* 2012; 53: 1503–1510.

332. Depienne C, LeGuern E. PCDH19-related infantile epileptic encephalopathy: an unusual X-linked inheritance disorder. *Hum Mutat.* 2012; 33(4): 627–634.

333. Marini C, Mei D, Parmeggiani L, et al. Protocadherin 19 mutations in girls with infantile-onset epilepsy. *Neurology.* 2010; 75: 646–653.

334. Baulac S, Ishida S, Marsan E, et al. Familial focal epilepsy with focal cortical dysplasia due to DEPDC5 mutations. *Ann Neurol.* 2015; 77: 675–683.

335. Scheffer IE, Heron SE, Regan BM, et al. Mutations in mammalian target of rapamycin regulator DEPDC5 cause focal epilepsy with brain malformations. *Ann Neurol.* 2014; 75: 782–787.

336. Brunklaus A, Ellis R, Reavey E, Semsarian C, Zubari SM. Genotype phenotype associations across the voltage-gated sodium channel family. *J Med Genet.* 2014; 51: 650–658.

337. Poduri A. The expanding SCN8A-related epilepsy phenotype. *Epilepsy Curr.* 2015; 15(6): 333–334.

338. Maljevic S, Lerche H. Potassium channel genes and benign familial neonatal epilepsy. *Prog Brain Res.* 2014; 213: 17–53.

19 | THE APPLICATION OF EEG TO EPILEPSY IN ADULTS AND THE ELDERLY

VAISHNAV KRISHNAN, MD, PHD, BERNARD S. CHANG, MD, MMSC, AND DONALD L. SCHOMER, MD

ABSTRACT: Surface or scalp electroencephalography (EEG) has become an indispensable tool for the diagnosis, classification, and care of patients with epilepsy across the age spectrum. This chapter provides an overview of interictal and corresponding ictal scalp EEG patterns observed in adults with certain classical epilepsy syndromes. In patients with one or more new-onset seizures, the value of EEG testing begins with a close examination of the interictal record. The morphology, frequency, and topography of interictal epileptiform discharges (when present) are typically sufficient to broadly distinguish between the propensity to develop "generalized seizures" (those that rapidly engage a distributed epileptogenic network) or "focal seizures" (which have a stereotyped onset within a clearly lateralized focal region or network). Epileptiform discharges may also be seen in patients without epilepsy who are affected by certain acute (e.g., severe metabolic encephalopathies) or chronic neuropsychiatric syndromes (e.g., autism spectrum disorder). An examination of the ictal recording is of crucial importance in patients with medication-refractory focal onset seizures as it serves to guide patient selection and ancillary testing for the possibility of resective surgery for epilepsy. This chapter also highlights the limited anatomical sensitivity of EEG for seizures that lack an associated impairment in consciousness ("simple partial seizures") or those that remain confined to mesial, deep or inferior cortical regions.

KEYWORDS: electroencephalography, EEG, seizures, epilepsy, interictal epileptiform discharges

PRINCIPLE REFERENCES

1. Gibbs, F.A., et al. *The electroencephalogram in epilepsy and in conditions of impaired consciousness.* Arch Neurol Psychiatry, 1935. **34**(6): p. 1133–1148.
2. Gibbs, F.A., et al. *Electroencephalographic classification of epileptic patients and control subjects.* Arch Neurol Psychiatry (Chicago), 1943. **50**: p. 111–128.
3. Seneviratne, U., et al. *The electroencephalogram of idiopathic generalized epilepsy.* Epilepsia, 2012. **53**(2): p. 234–248.
4. Berg, A.T., et al. *Revised terminology and concepts for organization of seizures and epilepsies: report of the ILAE Commission on Classification and Terminology, 2005–2009.* Epilepsia, 2010. **51**(4): p. 676–685.
5. El Achkar, C.M. and S.J. Spence. *Clinical characteristics of children and young adults with co-occurring autism spectrum disorder and epilepsy.* Epilepsy Behav, 2015. **47**: p. 183–190.
6. Bourgeois, B.F., et al. *Lennox-Gastaut syndrome: a consensus approach to differential diagnosis.* Epilepsia, 2014. **55**(Suppl 4): p. 4–9.
7. Devinsky, O., et al. *Clinical and electroencephalographic features of simple partial seizures.* Neurology, 1988. **38**(9): p. 1347–1352.
8. Ebersole, J.S. and S. V. Pacia. *Localization of temporal lobe foci by ictal EEG patterns.* Epilepsia, 1996. **37**(4): p. 386–399.
9. Pacia, S.V. and J.S. Ebersole. *Intracranial EEG substrates of scalp ictal patterns from temporal lobe foci.* Epilepsia, 1997. **38**(6): p. 642–654.
10. Brigo, F. *Intermittent rhythmic delta activity patterns.* Epilepsy Behav, 2011. **20**(2): p. 254–256.

1. INTRODUCTION AND HISTORICAL PERSPECTIVE

The availability of electroencephalography (EEG) in all its various forms has been vital to the practice of modern epileptology. The two fields have been closely intertwined since a seminal 1935 study by Gibbs, Davis, and Lennox at Harvard Medical School in which a string galvanometer-based EEG was used to record the very first ictal EEG patterns [1]. A single channel of EEG was obtained using two hypodermic needle electrodes, one inserted into the scalp at the vertex and another inserted into the earlobe of the left ear (ground). To record "grand mal" seizures, a "crown" electrode was used as the ground, "made of wire and wrapped with cotton soaked with salt solution." After summarizing their own formulations of normal EEG patterns during wakefulness and sleep, they reported the EEG findings obtained from 12 patients with "petit mal epilepsy":

> . . . in all cases during the seizure an outburst of waves of great amplitude, amounting from 100 to 300 microvolts at a frequency of 3 per second. These waves may be very smooth and approximately sinusoidal in shape but usually include a sharp negative spike breaking into the record near the positive crest of the main wave.

In this paper the researchers also coined the term "larval" seizures, which were briefer runs of 3-Hz discharges that "fade out again instead of developing the characteristic picture" (interictal discharges). This paper also described the electrographic signature of "grand mal" seizures, where gradual alterations in EEG frequency were seen "before any other evidence of the seizure appears."

Just two years later (1937), thanks in large part to the EEG machines built by Albert and Ellen Grass, Lennox and the Gibbses (see Chapter 1) summarized their interpretation of EEG data obtained from over 400 patients with epilepsy in "approximately 60 miles (96 kilometers) of records" [2]. In this review, epilepsy was for the first time asserted to be a "paroxysmal cerebral dysrhythmia," with the explanation that "Grand mal epilepsy is characterized by extreme acceleration of the electrical activity of the cortex; psychomotor attacks, by extreme slowing of this activity, and petit mal, by alternation of fast and slow activity."

Outside of Harvard, several other pioneering groups must be also cited for their tremendous contributions to the application of EEG to the study *and* treatment of patients with epilepsy. These include a large group of neurologist/neurophysiologists from France led by Henri Gastaut [3,4] and Jean Aicardi [5,6], the "Johns Hopkins group" including William Grey Walter and Ernst Niedermeyer [7,8], as well as the "Montreal group" championed by Herbert Jasper [9,10], Pierre Gloor [11], Wilder Penfield [12,13], and Theodore Rasmussen [14,15] (see Chapter 1).

This chapter serves to define and describe various scalp EEG abnormalities associated with epilepsy. These can be broadly distinguished into two groups: those that occur at the time of seizures (*ictal seizure patterns*) and those that occur between seizures (*interictal epileptiform discharges* [IEDs]). An emphasis will be placed on demonstrating clinical–EEG correlations between (i) interictal discharges, (ii) corresponding ictal EEG onset patterns, and (iii) corresponding seizure semiology. A few points of clarification are made at the outset.

First and foremost, the presence of an IED is all too often interpreted as a confirmation of the presence of epilepsy. In reality, assigning an epileptiform value to any element of the EEG represents only an electroencephalographer's impression about whether such discharges are typically associated with epilepsy or an epilepsy syndrome. This is a Catch-22: as we discuss below, a number of other conditions are also associated with a high incidence of IEDs of unclear clinical relevance. Thus, the occurrence of IEDs only serves to support a diagnosis of epilepsy when the clinical history provides evidence that is consistent with one or several prior epileptic seizures. The absence of interictal epileptiform discharges also does not preclude a diagnosis of epilepsy: only 40% to 60% of patients with epilepsy display clear epileptiform abnormalities on their first "screening" routine scalp EEG [16]. In those patients with a clear history of seizures and without IEDs on routine scalp EEGs, one can infer either that (i) their epilepsy is *not* associated with IEDs that are frequent enough to be discovered on routine testing, or that (ii) their IEDs possess a dipole that is oriented unfavorably for standard scalp EEG technique (see Chapter 5 for a further discussion).

Ironically, despite decades of EEG-based epilepsy research, there remains confusion and lack of consensus about how to precisely define "seizure." Not all epileptic seizures have a clear corresponding representation on scalp EEG, and the International League Against Epilepsy (ILAE) does not impose an EEG-based definition for an epileptic seizure ("a transient occurrence of signs and/or symptoms due to excess or synchronous neuronal activity in the brain" [17]). Similarly, in a variety of clinical scenarios, a clearly "seizure-like" EEG pattern may be present without an obvious or overt clinical correlate. These have been variously termed "electrographic seizures" or "subclinical seizures" [18]. Accordingly, such seizures have been defined by electrographic criteria: unequivocal electrographic seizures display "generalized spike-wave discharges at 3/s or faster, or clearly evolving discharges of any type that reach a frequency of >4/s, whether focal or generalized" [19]. For the majority of epileptic seizures, these two definitions are largely congruent. Intermediate EEG patterns (e.g., evolving patterns

of rhythmic activity that do not meet these frequency criteria) "may or may not be ictal" [19] but nevertheless represent correlates of excess synchronous neuronal activity [17] for which at least a consideration of treatment is warranted.

With the increasing application of continuous video-EEG for the care of patients with epilepsy and other disorders of consciousness, there is now a greater appreciation for EEG patterns that are truly intermediate between "ictal" and "interictal." These EEG patterns that constitute what is now known as the "ictal–interictal continuum" [20] (including lateralized periodic discharges) are described in Chapter 22.

In a similar vein, "interictal" epileptiform discharges are classified as such precisely because they are not associated with a clear seizure. However, with real-time neuropsychological testing, it has become increasingly clear that focal or generalized IEDs may be associated with a transient cognitive impairment [21–23], once again blurring the classical distinction between ictal and interictal epileptiform changes (i.e., symptomatic vs. asymptomatic discharges).

2. INTERICTAL EPILEPTIFORM DISCHARGES

2.1. *Sharp Waves and Spikes*

Sharp waves are defined by the International Federation of Societies for EEG and Clinical Neurophysiology (IFSECN) as "a transient, clearly distinguished from background activity, with pointed peak and duration of 70-200ms." Sharp waves are often distinguished from spikes, which may be morphologically or anatomically similar but of a shorter duration (20–70 msec), reflecting a greater degree of neuronal synchrony. The terms "sharp wave" and "spike" should be restricted to the description of epileptiform findings. Therefore, it is not appropriate to describe vertex waves as "sharp waves." As such, any "sharp-appearing" biphasic paroxysm that is clearly *not* epileptiform is often referred to by many electroencephalographers as a "sharp transient," a term not recognized by the IFSECN [18]. On scalp EEG, sharp waves and spikes are typically electronegative with respect to surrounding regions, reflecting the local extracellular field negativity of perpendicularly oriented pyramidal neurons that receive a massive influx of extracellular sodium ions. In contrast, truly epileptiform "surface-positive" spikes or sharp waves are seen frequently in intracranial EEG and may also be seen within a breach rhythm. Surface positive sharp waves also represent a graphoelement of the normal neonatal EEG (see Chapter 7) and do not necessarily portend any association with epilepsy or seizures.

Ultimately, since sharp waves and spikes do not differ in clinical valence, attempting to impose a clear duration-based distinction between sharp waves and spikes is probably unnecessary as it does not convey any additional diagnostic or prognostic information. Regardless of duration, an epileptiform discharge must be "clearly distinguished from background activity," thereby "standing out" and disrupting the normal background activity. Thus, identifying the presence of epileptiform discharges in atypical background patterns (such as those with excessive slowing or high amplitudes) may be challenging, and this is one of several factors that contributes to the poor interrater reliability of IED detection [24]. Some of this interrater reliability problem may be helped by applying a combination of automated EEG waveform identification (see Chapter 27) with standardized EEG report generation (see Chapter 26).

From studies that have combined intracranial and scalp EEG, we know that the likelihood of observing a scalp-detected spike or sharp wave depends on several factors. Spikes originating from deeper structures such as mesial temporal or mesial frontal structures are often absent on scalp EEG and require some form of *averaging* so as to be reliably visualized [25,26]. Further, surface spikes are also likely to be identified when underlying cortical (or deep) generators display greater synchrony and/or a greater coordinated surface area of depolarization. The requirement for sufficient source area and synchrony also applies to ictal discharges [27].

2.2. Sharp or Spike and Slow Wave Complexes and Polyspikes

Isolated spikes and sharp waves may often be "adorned" by additional features that add to the complexity and diversity of IEDs. In and of themselves, the presence of these additional features/adornments does not perfectly correlate with the apparent malignancy or refractoriness of an epileptogenic lesion. Instead, they should be appreciated merely as the temporal summation of local field potentials that are in and of themselves not perfectly synchronous so as to create a single "isolated" spike or sharp wave.

Spike-slow wave or sharp-slow wave discharges refer to the presence of a slow wave following the initial spike or sharp wave. These slow waves ultimately represent a slow cycle of repolarization and hyperpolarization following the initial train of local action potentials that constitute the spike. Slow waves that are an element of spike-slow wave complexes may be obscured by excessive background slowing of the same frequency. The ratio of the amplitude of the spike to the slow wave (when a slow wave is present) tends to be larger in patients with generalized epilepsies [28].

Polyspikes refer to the occurrence of spikes in very rapid succession without intervening "background" activity, which may or may not be followed by a slow wave.

3. CLASSIFICATION OF SEIZURES

The most recent iteration of the ILAE's guidelines on seizure classification (2010) principally differs from previous versions by the prominent exclusion of the modifiers "simple" and "complex" for partial or focal seizures. These terms, designed to comment on the presence or absence of impaired consciousness, were often misused or misunderstood [29]. The term "secondarily generalized" has also been removed based on our more current understanding that truly "generalized" epileptic seizures (such as those seen in primary or symptomatic generalized epilepsies) likely all originate at some "focal" region within rapidly engaging bilaterally distributed networks. Thus,

"generalized" seizures that form a part of primary or symptomatic generalized epilepsy syndromes may also themselves be "secondarily generalized," albeit with a far more rapid time course of diffuse spread. In contrast, focal epileptic seizures can be conceptualized as originating within networks limited to one hemisphere. Under the revised classification scheme, there exist only two main seizure types, each with several subtypes:

Generalized Seizures

Tonic-clonic (in any combination)

Absence (typical, atypical, myoclonic absence, or eyelid myoclonia)

Myoclonic (myoclonic, myoclonic atonic, myoclonic tonic)

Clonic

Tonic

Atonic

Focal Seizures

Without impairment of consciousness

With observable motor or autonomic components

Involving subjective psychic or sensory phenomena only

With dyscognitive features

Evolving into bilateral convulsive seizures

To a large extent, this schema is sufficient to classify all epileptic seizures (defined clinically) across the age spectrum. Epileptic spasms, however, are a notable exception in that it remains unclear whether mechanisms underlying the expression of epileptic spasms are more consistent with a focal or a generalized mechanism of seizure onset (see Chapter 18).

4. INTERICTAL EPILEPTIFORM DISCHARGES IN PATIENTS WITHOUT EPILEPSY

As we pointed out above, the term *interictal epileptiform discharge* is ultimately a misnomer. Epileptiform discharges do occur, albeit at vastly lower rates, in patients who are seemingly healthy as well as in patients with specific neuropsychiatric syndromes of which electroencephalographers must be aware. Gibbs, Gibbs, and Lennox in 1943 published one of the first large comparisons of 20-minute EEGs from 1,000 healthy subjects and 1,260 patients with epilepsy. "Paroxysmal" or epileptiform EEG changes occurred in only 0.9% of healthy individuals and in 29.3% of patients with epilepsy [30]. Quantitatively similar results (~1–3%) have been obtained in other studies of subjects without a history of epilepsy, often air force or military cadets [31–34] (reviewed extensively in

[35]). These results demonstrate that the presence of IEDs on an interictal EEG confers high specificity and positive predictive value for the diagnosis of epilepsy, but relatively low sensitivity and negative predictive value. In other words, EEG is (far) better at "ruling in" rather than "ruling out" epilepsy. In either case, the identification of IEDs in neurologically normal patients *without* a history consistent with one or more prior seizures is of questionable clinical relevance and likely an incidental finding. Such IEDs may relate to the future risk of developing provoked or unprovoked seizures, though longitudinal studies designed to quantify and stratify this risk are yet to be performed. Extrapolating seizure risk from the presence or frequency of IEDs is complex. From our experience in patients with epilepsy who are admitted to seizure monitoring units, IED frequency often (but not always) increases with anticonvulsant medication withdrawal. However, various anticonvulsant medications suppress IEDs to varying extents [36–38]. In addition, many medically or surgically treated patients with epilepsy whose seizures are well controlled continue to display IEDs, suggesting that IEDs may relate more with the presence of an underlying epileptogenic lesion, or the residua of an epileptic network in postsurgical cases, rather than as a true direct biomarker of an individual's predisposition to imminent or future seizures.

Outside of neurologically "healthy" individuals, an increased prevalence of IEDs has been reported in patients with a variety of neuropsychiatric syndromes. The occurrence of such IEDs most prominently impacts (and complicates) the clinical management of those conditions that both (i) involve a high incidence of paroxysmal behavioral changes (concerning for seizures) and (ii) display a strong epidemiological association with epilepsy. A classic example of this scenario is the increased prevalence of IEDs in patients with autism spectrum disorder; such discharges are reported to occur in up to 5% to 60% of autistic patients [39,40]. While the true incidence of epilepsy in autism patients is significantly lower [41] (but nevertheless exaggerated compared with control populations [41]), there remains no clear consensus about the pathological significance of such IEDs and in particular whether aggressive treatment with antiseizure medications may improve indices of autistic disability or prevent autistic regression [41–43]. Another comparable example is the occurrence of epileptiform abnormalities in patients with Alzheimer's or mixed dementia [44], where the development of epilepsy is associated with an accelerated decline in function [45]. Cerebral palsy [46] and attention-deficit/hyperactivity disorder (47]) are two other noteworthy examples. Across all of these syndromes, what is clearly required are more long-term studies that subdivide patients based on specific disease features and that employ longer durations of EEG recording. Unfortunately, precisely because of the behavioral symptoms associated with such syndromes, longer epochs of EEG recording are often difficult to obtain.

Finally, epileptiform discharges, electroclinical seizures, and pure electrographic seizures may occur in patients without epilepsy in the context of moderate to severe toxic-metabolic encephalopathies [48], the presence of which has popularized the field of continuous EEG monitoring. This is discussed further in Chapters 15, 17, 21, and 22 on toxic, metabolic, infectious, and postinfectious conditions and on EEG in the intensive care unit.

5. INTERICTAL AND ICTAL EEG FINDINGS IN PATIENTS WITH "GENERALIZED" SEIZURES

Typical IEDs associated with generalized seizures as a part of generalized epilepsy syndromes most commonly display a frontocentrally maximal electronegativity. Spikes or spike-wave complexes are common (in relation to most typical focal epilepsy syndromes), and an increase in IED frequency during sleep is not unexpected. While most generalized IEDs appear to have a bilaterally synchronous appearance, on occasion one may observe that IEDs display a shifting hemispheric predominance, with maxima alternating between left and right frontal regions. This phenomenon is not an artifact and is a reflection of the rapidly engaging bilaterally distributed networks [29] implicated in the pathophysiology of "generalized" seizures. As an example, in patients with juvenile myoclonic epilepsy (JME, a prototypical generalized epilepsy syndrome), studies that have combined scalp EEG with dipole analysis and source localization demonstrate that typical IEDs (within the same patient) may have several focal "sources" distributed within orbitofrontal, medial frontal, and basal temporal regions in either hemisphere [49]. The frontal or frontocentral predominance of typical generalized IEDs has been confirmed by others using similar approaches including magnetoencephalography, where lateral [50] and medial frontal [51] sources have also been identified.

In contrast, frontally maximal IEDs that have a consistent localized maximum should raise the suspicion instead for possible frontal epilepsy that may or may not be associated with a mesial or deep frontal lesion. Patient history and event semiology may be helpful in distinguishing these two possibilities but may be of limited value in a patient with nocturnal convulsive events that are poorly described or unwitnessed. In these cases, the results of anatomical (magnetic resonance imaging) and functional (positron emission tomography or single photon emission computed tomography) neuroimaging may be complemented with the use of high-density EEG to capture both interictal and ictal findings (see Chapters 6, 35, and 46).

5.1. Three-Per-Second Spike-Wave Complexes

Classical bursts of 3-Hz spike-wave complexes (Fig. 19.1), such as those first described by Gibbs and Lennox, are widely known outside the community of electroencephalographers. The spatial distribution of these bursts is very characteristic: the maximum almost always lies over frontal midline regions, whereas the minimum is found over temporal and occipital areas. These bursts do not run exactly at a rate of 3/sec, often demonstrating faster frequencies at the onset of the burst (~4/sec) and then slowing down to 3 to 3.5/sec for the main portion, only to eventually slow further to 2.5/sec at the end of the burst.

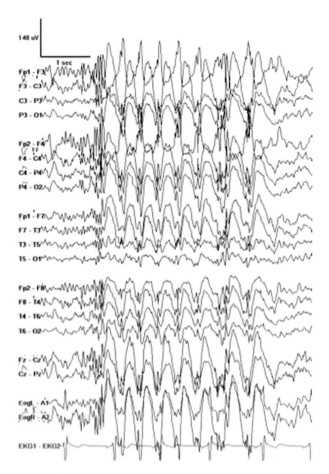

Such 3/s spike-wave complexes are the signature of absence seizures, which constitute one symptom of several epilepsy syndromes, including childhood absence epilepsy (CAE), juvenile absence epilepsy (JAE), JME, and Lennox–Gastaut syndrome (LGS). Absence seizures that are part of pure CAE have been termed "typical" absence seizures: electrographically, typical absence seizures display a burst frequency quite close to 3 Hz, have a generally rapid offset, and return to previous background activity, which itself is typically normal (Fig. 19.2). Clinically, absence seizures involve a behavioral arrest with staring and occasional automatisms, and those events that are appreciated by caregivers are typically 9 to 10 sec long; however, individual variations do exist. Rarely, patients with CAE or JAE may also suffer from generalized tonic-clonic seizures (Fig. 19.3, see section below on fast generalized discharges).

In contrast, atypical absence seizures seen in other non-CAE syndromes (almost by definition) tend to be longer in duration, hemispherically asymmetric at times, and more variable and irregular in frequency (typically slower, at ~2.5 Hz) but have similar clinical manifestations, suggesting that typical and atypical absences may simply represent two ends of a continuum of absence ictal patterns [52–54]. Absence seizures may rarely be associated with myoclonus of the eyelid, a condition that has been termed Jeavons syndrome. Here, eyelid myoclonus and upward eye deviation occur together with generalized spike-wave discharges [55]. These eyelid movements should be distinguished from eyelid automatisms or eye fluttering and their associated EEG artifacts, which can occur as an aspect of seizure semiology or as a nonspecific interictal finding. Common to all forms of absence seizures is that they

Figure 19.1. A brief 2- to 3-sec-long burst of diffuse frontocentrally predominant 3-Hz spike-wave discharges in the EEG of an adult patient with idiopathic generalized epilepsy.

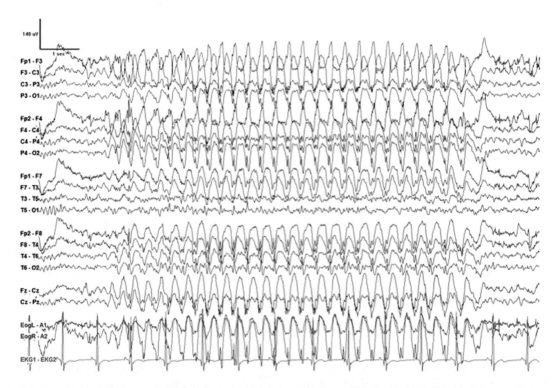

Figure 19.2. A ~7- to 8-sec-long typical absence seizure from the same patient depicted in Figure 19.1. Electrographically, typical absence seizures associated with childhood absence epilepsy or juvenile myoclonic epilepsy demonstrate a regular discharge frequency that is quite close to 3 Hz and with fairly symmetric features. Note the relatively rapid return to baseline and lack of true postictal slowing.

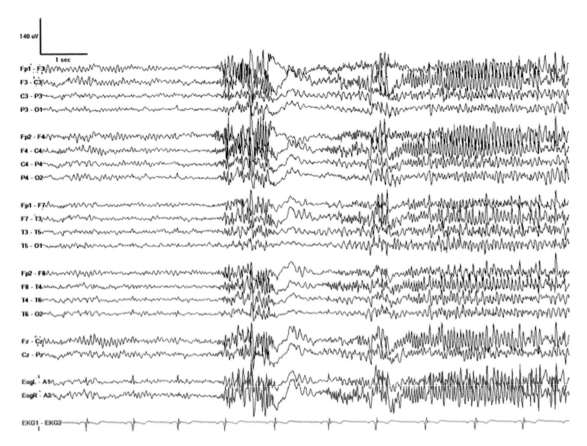

Figure 19.3. Electrographic onset of a generalized tonic-clonic seizure emerging out of sleep, beginning with a burst of diffuse but frontocentrally predominant fast repetitive spikes. After a brief pause, fast activity is seen to build up prior to the development of the tonic phase, during which EMG activity typically dominates the EEG.

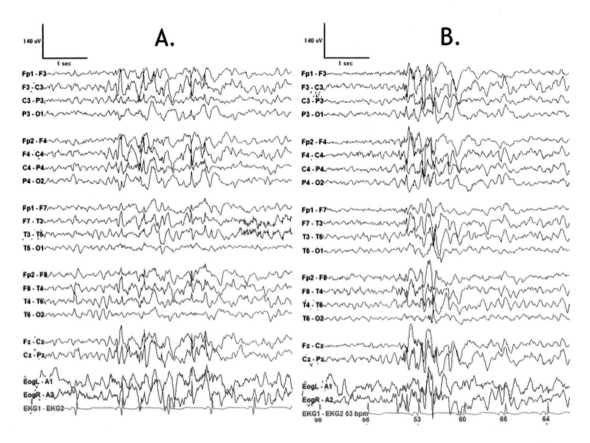

Figure 19.4. Two examples of interictal slow spike-wave discharges, with the characteristic 1- to 2-Hz discharge frequency that is less regular in frequency and often occurring in the context of generalized background slowing.

can be provoked by hyperventilation and photic stimulation (see Chapter 18 for a more detailed discussion).

5.2. "Slow" Spike-Wave Complexes

Interictal generalized spike-wave complexes that are generally slower than 3 Hz have been broadly labeled as "slow" spike-wave complexes. In contrast with classic 3-Hz spike-wave bursts that are correlated with absence seizures and CAE, slow spike-wave complexes (Fig. 19.4) are often less rhythmic and do not produce regular monomorphic bursts. Often, patients with slow spike-wave complexes also display abnormally slowed and disorganized background activity during wakefulness, which may or may not contain distinct and separate focal epileptiform discharges in a variety of locations [56]. These features are a reflection of the encephalopathy associated with the underlying insult in slow spike-wave syndromes (which can be quite varied) and multifocal cortical irritability. The canonical example of an epilepsy syndrome associated with slow spike-wave complexes is LGS [57], which is an etiologically nonspecific triad of intellectual disability, multiple seizure types, and an abnormal EEG containing slow spike-wave complexes. In addition to generalized tonic-clonic and absence seizures, patients with LGS and related syndromes may also display myoclonic, tonic, or atonic seizures. See Chapter 18 for a more complete discussion of this syndrome.

Myoclonic seizures (Fig. 19.5) refer specifically to the occurrence of myoclonus of an epileptic etiology. Myoclonus, defined as the sudden involuntary contraction of a muscle or group of muscles, need not necessarily have an epileptic origin and can occur in certain neurodegenerative conditions (e.g., Creutzfeldt–Jakob disease), metabolic derangements (e.g., uremia), and anoxic brain injury. The presence of epileptic myoclonus or myoclonic seizures can be confirmed by concurrent EEG, typically revealing frontally maximal generalized polyspikes or polyspike-wave discharges that precede myoclonic movements by 20 to 40 msec [58]. See Chapter 37 for a full discussion of myoclonus and its clinical and neurophysiological correlates.

5.3. "Fast" Spikes or Spike-Wave Discharges

Interictal generalized spike-wave discharges in the 4- to 6-Hz range, typically with polyspike components, constitute a classical interictal EEG signature of JME (Fig. 19.6), characterized by a triad of epileptic myoclonic jerks, absence seizures, and generalized tonic-clonic seizures. Background activity is typically normal, and ictal EEG findings during these various seizure types are no different from their counterparts in other pure epilepsy syndromes (e.g., CAE). Higher-frequency generalized spiking, usually in the alpha or beta range, has been referred to variously as "grand mal discharges" [59], "fast paroxysmal rhythms," "generalized paroxysmal fast activity," or "generalized repetitive fast discharges" (GRFD [60]). Interictally, such discharges occur almost exclusively in LGS (Fig. 19.7). High-frequency spiking also constitutes an important early component of the ictal EEG pattern of both generalized tonic-clonic seizures (see Fig. 19.3) and clonic seizures (Fig. 19.8).

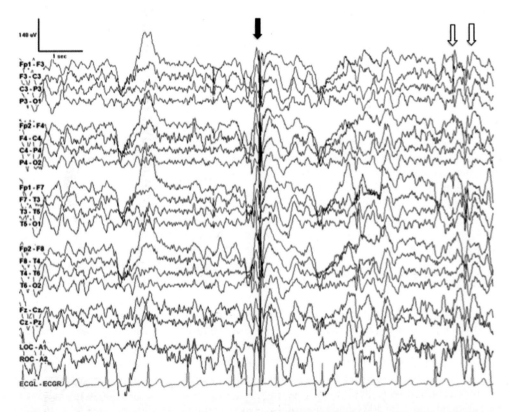

Figure 19.5. *In a patient with a symptomatic generalized epilepsy syndrome, an isolated diffuse myoclonic jerk associated with a polyspike-wave discharge (black arrow) is captured as a single high-amplitude diffuse muscle spike that is temporally related to a polyspike-wave discharge. This EEG also illustrates the presence of generalized irregular background slowing as well as separate slow-spike wave discharges (white arrows) that are without a clinical correlate.*

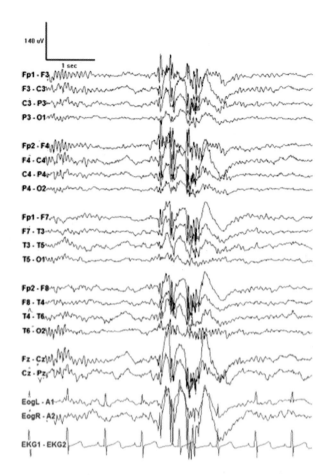

Figure 19.6. Generalized 4- to 5-Hz spike-wave or polyspike-wave discharges constitute the interictal EEG hallmarks of generalized epilepsy syndromes associated with fast spike-wave discharges, such as JME.

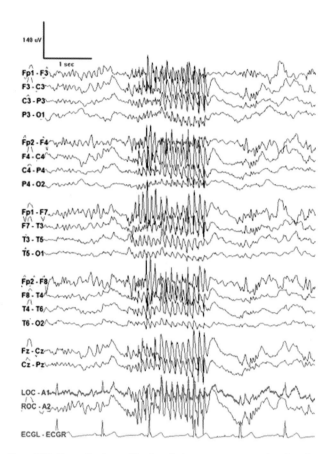

Figure 19.7. Generalized repetitive fast discharges were previously referred to as grand mal discharges. Such interictal high-frequency frontally predominant discharges are rarely seen outside of LGS.

Atonic seizures, which require simultaneous electromyography (typically a chin EMG lead) to make a formal diagnosis, are a fairly rare seizure type in adult populations and can have a variety of ictal EEG patterns, including an electrodecremental response with diffuse desynchronization, with or without spike-wave discharges and paroxysmal fast activity (Fig. 19.9) [61]. Tonic seizures, characterized clinically by a brief and sudden diffuse increase in muscle tone, also feature paroxysmal fast activity on simultaneous EEG recordings. When they emerge out of sleep, such fast repetitive generalized spikes are easier to visualize prior to the onset of diffuse myogenic artifact (Figs. 19.10 and 19.11). Tonic seizures may also be represented as a brief diffuse electrodecremental response, similar to that shown in Figure 19.9.

6. INTERICTAL AND ICTAL EEG FINDINGS IN PATIENTS WITH FOCAL SEIZURES

In contrast to generalized epileptiform discharges and seizures, where a rapidly activated distributed epileptogenic network fairly consistently produces frontocentrally maximal electrographic correlates, interictal and ictal EEG findings in focal epilepsies often reflect the focality of the corresponding epileptogenic lesion, but may be absent altogether or paradoxically mislateralized to the contralateral hemisphere (see sections below). Obtaining a fairly precise appreciation of the "true" neuroanatomical source of ictal and interictal discharges is of paramount importance to patients with medication-refractory focal seizures that may be amenable to surgical resection or responsive neurostimulation (discussed in Chapter 38).

6.1. Interictal and Ictal EEG Findings in Patients with Focal Seizures Without Impairment of Consciousness

Such seizures were previously referred to as "simple partial seizures" and when they involve only a pure sensory perception are often referred to as "auras" (and not seizures) by some patients. On scalp EEG, ictal epileptiform correlates are present in only 15% to 30% of focal seizures that are not associated with an impairment of consciousness [62]. Those seizures with a clear motor component tend to have a higher likelihood of demonstrating a clear ictal correlate, and rates may be enhanced further with the use of additional scalp electrodes [63] (see Chapter 6). Such low rates of detection reflect the poor anatomical sensitivity of the classical 10-20 montage scalp EEG to relatively small focal regions of ictal synchronous activity that give rise to such focal seizures. Complementing scalp EEG with high-density EEG and/ or magnetoencephalography (MEG) may provide higher

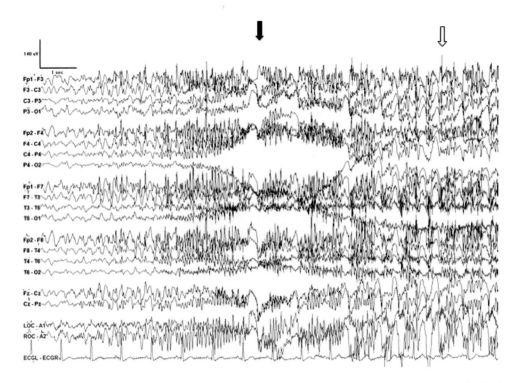

Figure 19.8. *Pure clonic seizures are one of several seizure types seen in LGS and other related epilepsy syndromes. In this patient with LGS, frontally predominant fast spike-wave discharges build up in frequency, resulting in a head raise (correlating with electrode movement artifact, black arrow) followed by rhythmic spike-wave discharges (white arrow) that are synchronous with diffuse clonic movements of the upper extremities.*

yields, although these techniques have more limited portability. The absence of an impairment or loss of consciousness is also related to the seizure's lack of spread to brain regions involved in maintaining consciousness, which remains an active area of research [64–66]. Ultimately, in concert with seizure semiology and the results of neuroimaging studies, invasive/intracerebral EEG may be necessary to identify and confirm the location of the epileptogenic zone. For example, in patients with medication-refractory focal clonic seizures, polyspike-wave discharges can be appreciated in subdural electrodes appropriately placed over the contralateral primary motor cortex [67].

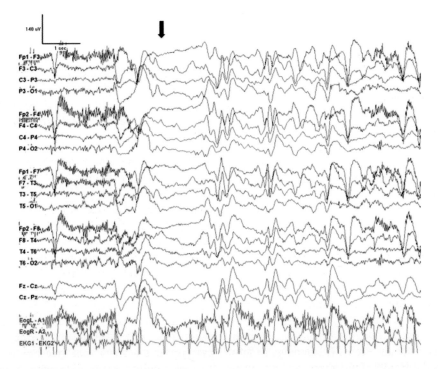

Figure 19.9. *A brief burst of generalized low-amplitude fast activity ("electrodecrement") is seen during this atonic seizure. Notice the abrupt and temporary reduction in background EMG activity (black arrow) correlating with diffuse atonia and head drop.*

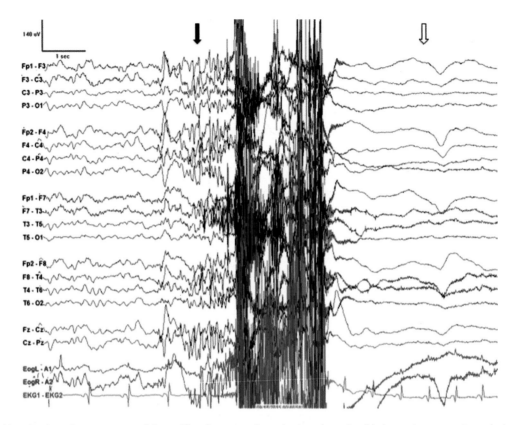

Figure 19.10. In this tonic seizure that emerges out of sleep, diffuse frontocentrally predominant fast spikes (black arrow) are seen prior to the burst of EMG activity associated with diffuse tonic contraction. Postictally, generalized voltage suppression is seen (white arrow).

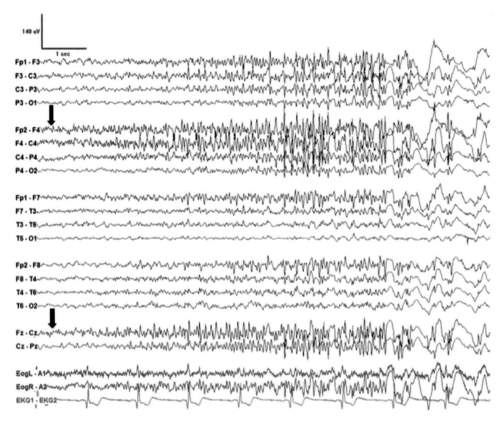

Figure 19.11. In this tonic seizure with a focal onset, a preponderance of fast activity emerges over the right frontal and central regions (black arrows), evolving quickly into repetitive spikes and spike-wave discharges.

6.2. Interictal and Ictal EEG Findings in Patients with Temporal Lobe Seizures

Temporal lobe epilepsy (TLE) is a major contributor to cases of medication-refractory partial-onset epilepsies in adult populations [68,69]. Given the very real possibility of a timely surgical cure through a conventional anterior temporal lobectomy or other related techniques [70,71], there exists a vast body of literature devoted to the application of EEG to ictal and interictal EEG findings in TLE. This section will only provide a brief introduction to relevant EEG findings/patterns and their relations to a suspected epileptogenic zone: we refer our readers elsewhere [72–75] (and Chapter 29) for a more comprehensive discussion of the role of EEG in the surgical evaluation of patients with temporal and extratemporal epilepsies.

Scalp-detected IEDs that correlate with the presence of temporal lobe seizures can be broadly divided into those that display maximal electronegativity at either the anterior temporal/inferior frontal regions (Fig. 19.12A, corresponding to F7/F8 or T1/T2 electrodes) or the posterior/midtemporal regions (see Fig. 19.12B, C, corresponding to T3/T4 or T5/T6 electrodes). Like IEDs associated with "generalized" seizures, many patients display temporal IEDs almost exclusively during sleep (typically non-rapid eye movement sleep) [76], and sleep-activated temporal IEDs may provide greater localizing value [77]. As shown in Figure 19.12C, a significant proportion of patients with TLE may display independent left *and* right temporal IEDs [78]. Bitemporal IEDs clearly signify more broad hyperexcitability: the presence of independent bitemporal IEDs is associated with independent bitemporal seizures [79] as well as a poorer prognosis following unilateral TLE surgery [75,80,81]. In contrast, strictly unitemporal IEDs (in particular, when concordant with the location of mesial temporal sclerosis or hippocampal atrophy) suggest a greater likelihood of postoperative seizure remission [82–85].

Important insights have been gained from studies of limited groups of patients who have been implanted with simultaneous scalp *and* intracranial EEG electrodes, thus permitting a direct correlation of scalp and depth or electrocorticographic recordings with perfect temporal precision. However, there are two main caveats to this type of analysis. First, for any given patient, the locations of implanted intracranial EEG electrodes (either strips, grids, or depth electrodes) are precisely tailored to various patient characteristics, including clinical semiology, the presence of a discrete lesion, and/or the location of scalp-detected ictal and interictal discharges. Such a tailored approach imposes limits on standardization and can only comment on IEDs that are captured at intracranial sites that are "covered" by subdural or depth electrodes. Second, the presence of a craniotomy often (but not always) results in a breach artifact [86], offering the possibility of anatomical distortion (in addition to frequency distortions). Nevertheless, in such studies of patients with TLE, anterior and mid/posterior temporal IEDs are *both* generated by neocortical sources corresponding to the anterolateral temporal neocortex and lateral posterior/mid-temporal neocortex respectively [26,87]. IEDs that are confined to mesial temporal structures (including the hippocampus) almost always produce no observable scalp correlate unless there is intrinsic distortion of the local anatomy. Similarly, ictal rhythms that remain confined to the hippocampus (measured with depth electrodes) also typically do not have a clear scalp representation [88] given the "closed loop" configuration of the intact hippocampus.

Aside from temporal sharp waves or spikes, bursts of rhythmic activity in the temporal regions may also be seen in patients with TLE and have been termed *temporal intermittent rhythmic delta activity* (TIRDA, Fig. 19.13) [89]. TIRDA may have a "sawtooth" or sinusoidal appearance and vary in frequency between 1 and 4 Hz. The occurrence of TIRDA is strongly correlated with other clinical and electrographic biomarkers of ipsilateral TLE

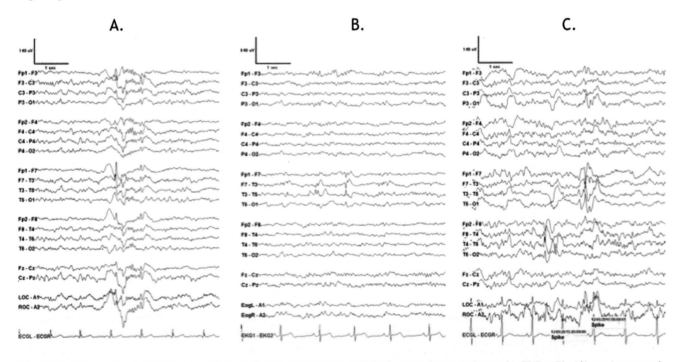

Figure 19.12. IEDs associated with TLE can be broadly divided into those that have an (A) anterior predominance (maximal at F7/8) or (B) mid/posterior temporal predominance (maximal at T3/4 or T5/6). Independent bitemporal interictal epileptiform discharges can also be seen at times (C).

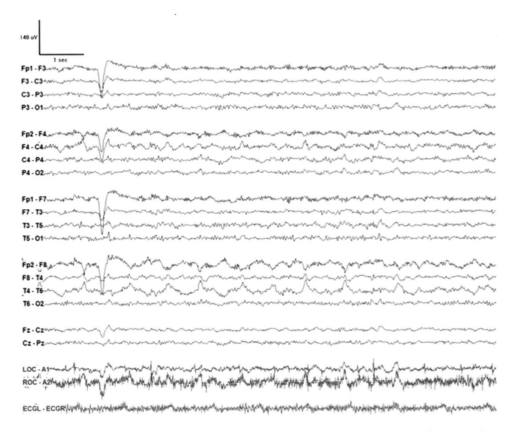

Figure 19.13. TIRDA can display a saw-tooth or sinusoidal appearance (as shown here). In a patient with TLE, TIRDA is typically associated with synchronous rhythmic spiking in temporal structures and represents an interictal phenomenon.

[90–92] but has also been identified in patients with JAE and in the EEGs of healthy nonagenarians [93,94]. Thus, one must be cautious in assigning an epileptiform value to TIRDA. In the presurgical evaluation of a patient with other definite electro-clinical features of TLE, the lateralization of TIRDA may serve to effectively substitute for IEDs that may be absent or bilateral. In patients implanted with subdural electrodes, electrocortico-graphic equivalents of TIRDA can be seen in basal and anterolat-eral temporal neocortex and less frequently in mesial, posterior temporal, or extratemporal regions and are closely anatomically related to the cortical location of IEDs and ictal onset zones [95].

Three main clinical seizure types are observed in TLE: focal seizures without impairments in consciousness ("simple partial"), focal seizures with dyscognitive features ("complex partial"), and focal seizures that evolve into bilateral convulsive seizures ("sec-ondarily generalized"). Patients with TLE can experience a wide variety of ictal symptoms without impairments in consciousness ("auras"), ranging from abdominal rising sensations, pure olfac-tory/gustatory or somatosensory symptoms, autonomic changes (e.g., tachycardia or flushing), emotional or psychic symptoms (e.g., *déjà vu*), or combinations of these various symptoms. As we alluded to earlier, scalp EEG has a very limited sensitivity to detect such simple partial seizures [62]. Sphenoidal electrodes or fora-men ovale electrodes, both designed to capture field potentials at the temporal pole, are more sensitive for the detection of such sei-zures [96] and, through computational techniques, may guide the design of seizure-detection algorithms for scalp-negative seizures [97]. The occurrence of impaired consciousness ultimately relates to seizure propagation to broad cortical regions required for the preservation of consciousness. Thus, on intracranial EEG, sei-zures with impaired consciousness typically involve some degree of spread to bilateral frontal and parietal cortices where 1- to 2-Hz delta frequency slowing can be appreciated [98,99].

As expected, the main contributors to epilepsy-related dis-ability in TLE are focal seizures with dyscognitive features that either evolve or have the potential to evolve into bilateral con-vulsive seizures. The scalp EEG onset patterns of such seizures can be as dramatically varied as their semiology [100]. By reviewing the scalp and intracranial EEG patterns of patients with TLE, a scalp EEG-based electrographic classification scheme was proposed first by Ebersole and Pacia [88,101]:

Type I seizures are defined by the presence of 5- to 9-Hz rhythmic activity in the temporal/subtemporal regions or vertex/parasagittal regions (Fig. 19.14). This pattern is most specific for hippocampal-onset seizures that rapidly recruit adjacent inferolateral temporal neocortical regions.

Type II seizures, in contrast, are characterized by initial background flattening followed by lateralized but less anatomically defined polymorphic 2- to 5-Hz activity (Fig. 19.15). This type corresponds to a temporal neocortical onset (inferolateral or lateral temporal).

Type III seizures have no clear lateralized EEG discharge and at most reveal widespread background slowing or attenuation. On intracranial EEG, a type III seizure pattern is correlated with the presence of ictal activity that either (i) remains confined to the hippocampus, (ii)

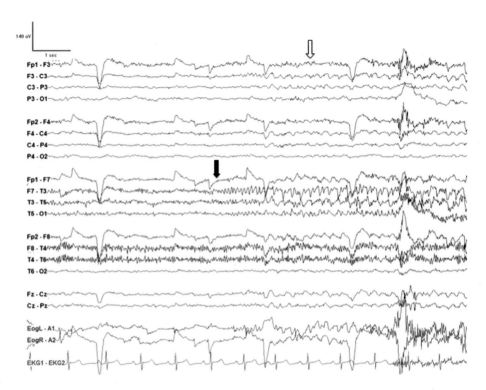

Figure 19.14. According to a classification scheme proposed by Ebersole and Pacia, type I seizures are characterized by a 5- to 9-Hz inferotemporal rhythm (black arrow) with or without a similar vertex/parasagittal positive rhythm (white arrow). This pattern is quite specific for hippocampal-onset seizures.

quickly propagates to the contralateral temporal lobe, or (iii) does not achieve widespread cortical synchrony.

The relationships between scalp and intracranial EEG proposed in this classification scheme have been confirmed by studies of dipole source localization [102].

The existence of severe unilateral hippocampal atrophy has been associated with a paradoxical contralateral scalp ictal onset pattern: this is thought to relate to the atypical spread of ictal discharges to the contralateral temporal lobe. Importantly, such patients also benefit from a temporal resection on the atrophic side [103].

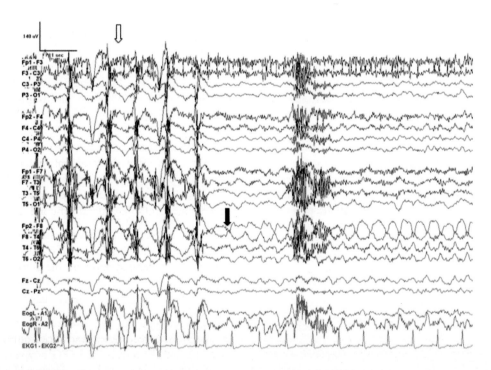

Figure 19.15. In contrast to type I seizures, temporal seizures of a neocortical origin often display lateralized 2- to 5-Hz rhythmic activity (black arrow). This EEG also demonstrates the presence of chewing artifact (white arrow) corresponding to ictal oral automatisms occurring prior to the electrographic onset of the seizure.

6.3. Ictal and Interictal Findings in Patients with Extratemporal Seizures

In several clinical situations, the presence of an extratemporal focus may be obvious, either by way of semiology (e.g., visual auras for occipital seizures or hypermotor nocturnal events in frontal lobe seizures) or by the presence of a discrete focal lesion that is concordant with the described semiology. In contrast, when seizure semiology may not clearly point to one lobe of origin involvement and/or when the MRI is "nonlesional," scalp EEG may or may not be helpful. Interictally, IEDs may or may not be present, and when present, may either mislateralize or appear as generalized discharges, as in the case of mesial frontal lobe epilepsies [104,105]. Similarly, ictal EEG patterns may be absent entirely or represented only as diffuse rhythmic slowing. Thus, for patients with extratemporal nonlesional medication-refractory epilepsy, the consideration for epilepsy surgery requires an even greater emphasis on concordance between various EEG and non-EEG modalities (including neuropsychological testing, MEG, and markers of ictal and interictal metabolism changes, such as positron emission tomography or single photon emission computed tomography). The success rates for epilepsy surgeries designed for this specific population are expectedly lower [106].

SCORE EEG SOFTWARE

Further examples related to the topics addressed in this chapter can be found in the interactive online Niedermeyer Educational Platform. EEG recordings with illustrative examples can be opened and browsed. Features are marked and described using the SCORE EEG software. The users can see the features marked by experts, they can score these features themselves, and then compare them with the scorings of the experts.

The Niedermeyer Educational Platform can be accessed at: www.scoreEEG.com/academy

REFERENCES

1. Gibbs, F.A., H. Davis, and W.G. Lennox, *The electroencephalogram in epilepsy and in conditions of impaired consciousness.* Arch Neurol Psychiatry, 1935. **34**(6): p. 1133–1148.
2. Gibbs, F.A., E.L. Gibbs, and W.G. Lennox, *Cerebral dysrhythmias of epilepsy: measures for their control.* Arch Neurol Psychiatry (Chicago), 1938. **39**: p. 289–314.
3. Gastaut, H., et al., *[Electrographic studies in man and in animal in so-called psychomotor epilepsy].* Rev Neurol (Paris), 1953. **88**(5): p. 310–354.
4. Cornil, L., A. Cremieux, and H. Gastaut, *Importance sémiologique de l'électroencéphalographie dans ie diagnostic des crises épileptiqués de l'enfant.* Sem Hop, 1948. **24**(50): p. 1609–1613.
5. Aicardi, J., et al., *General conclusions concerning familial factors in epilepsy.* Epilepsia, 1969. **10**(1): p. 65–68.
6. Aicardi, J. and J.J. Chevrie, *Myoclonic epilepsies of childhood.* Neuropadiatrie, 1971. **3**(2): p. 177–190.
7. Niedermeyer, E., *Dipole theory and electroencephalography.* Clin Electroencephalogr, 1996. **27**(3): p. 121–131.
8. Niedermeyer, E., *Primary (idiopathic) generalized epilepsy and underlying mechanisms.* Clin Electroencephalogr, 1996. **27**(1): p. 1–21.
9. Jasper, H.H., *Physiopathological mechanisms of post-traumatic epilepsy.* Epilepsia, 1970. **11**(1): p. 73–80.
10. Jasper, H.H., *Some physiological mechanisms involved in epileptic automatisms.* Epilepsia, 1964. **5**: p. 1–20.
11. Gloor, P., *Contributions of electroencephalography and electrocorticography to the neurosurgical treatment of the epilepsies.* Adv Neurol, 1975. **8**: p. 59–105.
12. Penfield, W., *Classification of the epilepsies.* Arch Neurol Psychiatry, 1948. **60**(2): p. 107–118.
13. Penfield, W., *Epilepsy and the cerebral lesions of birth and infancy.* Can Med Assoc J, 1939. **41**(6): p. 527–534.
14. Aguilar, M.J. and T. Rasmussen, *Role of encephalitis in pathogenesis of epilepsy.* Arch Neurol, 1960. **2**: p. 663–676.
15. Rasmussen, T. and H. Gossman, *Epilepsy due to gross destructive brain lesions. Results of surgical therapy.* Neurology, 1963. **13**: p. 659–669.
16. King, M.A., et al., *Epileptology of the first-seizure presentation: a clinical, electroencephalographic, and magnetic resonance imaging study of 300 consecutive patients.* Lancet, 1998. **352**(9133): p. 1007–1011.
17. Fisher, R.S., et al., *ILAE official report: a practical clinical definition of epilepsy.* Epilepsia, 2014. **55**(4): p. 475–482.
18. Noachtar, S., et al., *A glossary of terms most commonly used by clinical electroencephalographers and proposal for the report form for the EEG findings. The International Federation of Clinical Neurophysiology.* Electroencephalogr Clin Neurophysiol Suppl, 1999. **52**: p. 21–41.
19. Hirsch, L.J., et al., *American Clinical Neurophysiology Society's Standardized Critical Care EEG Terminology: 2012 version.* J Clin Neurophysiol, 2013. **30**(1): p. 1–27.
20. Rodriguez, V., M.F. Rodden, and S.M. LaRoche, *Ictal-interictal continuum: A proposed treatment algorithm.* Clin Neurophysiol, 2016. **127**(4): p. 2056–2064.
21. Aldenkamp, A.P. and J. Arends, *Effects of epileptiform EEG discharges on cognitive function: is the concept of "transient cognitive impairment" still valid?* Epilepsy Behav, 2004. **5**(Suppl 1): p. S25–34.
22. Kleen, J.K., et al., *Hippocampal interictal epileptiform activity disrupts cognition in humans.* Neurology, 2013. **81**(1): p. 18–24.
23. Seneviratne, U., M. Cook, and W. D'Souza, *The electroencephalogram of idiopathic generalized epilepsy.* Epilepsia, 2012. **53**(2): p. 234–248.
24. Grant, A.C., et al., *EEG interpretation reliability and interpreter confidence: a large single-center study.* Epilepsy Behav, 2014. **32**: p. 102–107.
25. Ramantani, G., et al., *Simultaneous subdural and scalp EEG correlates of frontal lobe epileptic sources.* Epilepsia, 2014. **55**(2): p. 278–288.
26. Wennberg, R., T. Valiante, and D. Cheyne, *EEG and MEG in mesial temporal lobe epilepsy: where do the spikes really come from?* Clin Neurophysiol, 2011. **122**(7): p. 1295–1313.
27. Tao, J.X., et al., *The impact of cerebral source area and synchrony on recording scalp electroencephalography ictal patterns.* Epilepsia, 2007. **48**(11): p. 2167–2176.
28. Terney, D., et al., *The slow-wave component of the interictal epileptiform EEG discharges.* Epilepsy Res, 2010. **90**(3): p. 228–233.
29. Berg, A.T., et al., *Revised terminology and concepts for organization of seizures and epilepsies: report of the ILAE Commission on Classification and Terminology, 2005-2009.* Epilepsia, 2010. **51**(4): p. 676–685.
30. Gibbs, F.A., E.L. Gibbs, and W.G. Lennox, *Electroencephalographic classification of epileptic patients and control subjects.* Arch Neurol Psychiatry, 1943. **50**(2): p. 111–128.
31. Thorner, M.W., *Procurement of Electroencephalograph Tracings in 1000 Flying Cadets for Evaluating the Gibbs Technique in Relation to Flying Ability* USAD School of Aviation Medical Research Report, 1942(No. 7-1).
32. Williams, D., *The nature of transient outbursts in the electroencephalogram of epileptics.* Brain, 1944. **67**: p. 10–37.
33. Harty, J.E., E.L. Gibbs, and F.A. Gibbs, *Electroencephalographic study of 275 candidates for military service.* War Med., 1952. **2**: p. 923–930.
34. Buchthal, F. and M. Lennox, *The EEG effect of Metrazol and photic stimulation in 682 normal subjects.* Electroencephalogr Clin Neurophysiol, 1953. **5**: p. 545–558.
35. So, E.L., *Interictal epileptiform discharges in persons without a history of seizures: what do they mean?* J Clin Neurophysiol, 2010. **27**(4): p. 229–238.
36. Guida, M., et al., *Effects of antiepileptic drugs on interictal epileptiform discharges in focal epilepsies: an update on current evidence.* Expert Rev Neurother, 2015. **15**(8): p. 947–959.
37. Stodieck, S., et al., *Effect of levetiracetam in patients with epilepsy and interictal epileptiform discharges.* Seizure, 2001. **10**(8): p. 583–587.
38. Libenson, M.H. and B. Caravale, *Do antiepileptic drugs differ in suppressing interictal epileptiform activity in children?* Pediatr Neurol, 2001. **24**(3): p. 214–218.
39. El Achkar, C.M. and S.J. Spence, *Clinical characteristics of children and young adults with co-occurring autism spectrum disorder and epilepsy.* Epilepsy Behav, 2015. **47**: p. 183–190.
40. Spence, S.J. and M.T. Schneider, *The role of epilepsy and epileptiform EEGs in autism spectrum disorders.* Pediatr Res, 2009. **65**(6): p. 599–606.
41. Tuchman, R., D. Hirtz, and L.A. Mamounas, *NINDS epilepsy and autism spectrum disorders workshop report.* Neurology, 2013. **81**(18): p. 1630–1636.
42. Buckley, A.W. and G.L. Holmes, *Epilepsy and autism.* Cold Spring Harb Perspect Med, 2016. **6**(4): p. a022749.

43. Berg, A.T. and S. Plioplys, *Epilepsy and autism: is there a special relationship?* Epilepsy Behav, 2012. **23**(3): p. 193–198.

44. Horvath, A., et al., *Epileptic seizures in Alzheimer disease: a review.* Alzheimer Dis Assoc Disord, 2016. **30**(2): p. 186–192.

45. Vossel, K.A., et al., *Seizures and epileptiform activity in the early stages of Alzheimer disease.* JAMA Neurol, 2013. **70**(9): p. 1158–1166.

46. Jaseja, H., *Treatment of interictal epileptiform discharges in cerebral palsy patients without clinical epilepsy: hope for a better outcome in prognosis.* Clin Neurol Neurosurg, 2007. **109**(3): p. 221–224.

47. Swatzyna, R.J., et al., *The utility of EEG in attention deficit hyperactivity disorder: a replication study.* Clin EEG Neurosci, 2016. [March 27; Epub before print]

48. Schmitt, S.E., *The utility of clinical features for the diagnosis of seizures in the intensive care unit.* J Clin Neurophysiol, 2017. **34**(2): p. 158–161.

49. Holmes, M.D., J. Quiring, and D.M. Tucker, *Evidence that juvenile myoclonic epilepsy is a disorder of frontotemporal corticothalamic networks.* Neuroimage, 2010. **49**(1): p. 80–93.

50. Tenney, J.R., et al., *Focal corticothalamic sources during generalized absence seizures: a MEG study.* Epilepsy Res, 2013. **106**(1-2): p. 113–122.

51. da Silva Braga, A.M., E.K. Fujisao, and L.E. Betting, *Analysis of generalized interictal discharges using quantitative EEG.* Epilepsy Res, 2014. **108**(10): p. 1740–1747.

52. Sadleir, L.G., et al., *Electroclinical features of absence seizures in childhood absence epilepsy.* Neurology, 2006. **67**(3): p. 413–418.

53. Hughes, J.R., *Absence seizures: a review of recent reports with new concepts.* Epilepsy Behav, 2009. **15**(4): p. 404–412.

54. Holmes, G.L., M. McKeever, and M. Adamson, *Absence seizures in children: clinical and electroencephalographic features.* Ann Neurol, 1987. **21**(3): p. 268–273.

55. Appleton, R.E., et al., *Eyelid myoclonia with typical absences: an epilepsy syndrome.* J Neurol Neurosurg Psychiatry, 1993. **56**(12): p. 1312–1316.

56. Markand, O.N., *Slow spike-wave activity in EEG and associated clinical features: often called 'Lennox' or "Lennox-Gastaut" syndrome.* Neurology, 1977. **27**(8): p. 746–757.

57. Bourgeois, B.F., L.M. Douglass, and R. Sankar, *Lennox-Gastaut syndrome: a consensus approach to differential diagnosis.* Epilepsia, 2014. **55** (Suppl 4): p. 4–9.

58. Kojovic, M., C. Cordivari, and K. Bhatia, *Myoclonic disorders: a practical approach for diagnosis and treatment.* Ther Adv Neurol Disord, 2011. **4**(1): p. 47–62.

59. Rodin, E., N. Smid, and K. Mason, *The grand mal pattern of Gibbs, Gibbs and Lennox.* Electroencephalogr Clin Neurophysiol, 1976. **40**(4): p. 401–406.

60. Koubeissi, M.Z. and E.L. So, *EEG in adult epilepsy*, in *Current Practice of Clinical Electroencephalography*, J. Ebersole, Editor. 2014, Wolters Kluwer Health: Philadelphia, PA.

61. Baraldi, S., et al., *Drop attacks, falls and atonic seizures in the Video-EEG monitoring unit.* Seizure, 2015. **32**: p. 4–8.

62. Devinsky, O., et al., *Clinical and electroencephalographic features of simple partial seizures.* Neurology, 1988. **38**(9): p. 1347–1352.

63. Bare, M.A., et al., *Electroencephalographic changes during simple partial seizures.* Epilepsia, 1994. **35**(4): p. 715–720.

64. Cavanna, A.E., H. Rickards, and F. Ali, *What makes a simple partial seizure complex?* Epilepsy Behav, 2011. **22**(4): p. 651–658.

65. Sedigh-Sarvestani, M., et al., *Seizures and brain regulatory systems: consciousness, sleep, and autonomic systems.* J Clin Neurophysiol, 2015. **32**(3): p. 188–193.

66. Detyniecki, K. and H. Blumenfeld, *Consciousness of seizures and consciousness during seizures: are they related?* Epilepsy Behav, 2014. **30**: p. 6–9.

67. Hamer, H.M., et al., *Electrophysiology of focal clonic seizures in humans: a study using subdural and depth electrodes.* Brain, 2003. **126**(Pt 3): p. 547–555.

68. Semah, F., et al., *Is the underlying cause of epilepsy a major prognostic factor for recurrence?* Neurology, 1998. **51**(5): p. 1256–1262.

69. Tellez-Zenteno, J.F. and L. Hernandez-Ronquillo, *A review of the epidemiology of temporal lobe epilepsy.* Epilepsy Res Treat, 2012. **2012**: p. 630853.

70. Wiebe, S., et al., *A randomized, controlled trial of surgery for temporal-lobe epilepsy.* N Engl J Med, 2001. **345**(5): p. 311–318.

71. Chang, E.F., D.J. Englot, and S. Vadera, *Minimally invasive surgical approaches for temporal lobe epilepsy.* Epilepsy Behav, 2015. **47**: p. 24–33.

72. Jette, N. and S. Wiebe, *Update on the surgical treatment of epilepsy.* Curr Opin Neurol, 2013. **26**(2): p. 201–207.

73. Miller, J.W. and S. Hakimian, *Surgical treatment of epilepsy.* Continuum (Minneap Minn), 2013. **19**(3 Epilepsy): p. 730–742.

74. Kilpatrick, C., et al., *Preoperative evaluation for temporal lobe surgery.* J Clin Neurosci, 2003. **10**(5): p. 535–539.

75. Schulz, R., et al., *Interictal EEG and ictal scalp EEG propagation are highly predictive of surgical outcome in mesial temporal lobe epilepsy.* Epilepsia, 2000. **41**(5): p. 564–570.

76. Malow, B.A., et al., *Lateralizing value of interictal spikes on overnight sleep-EEG studies in temporal lobe epilepsy.* Epilepsia, 1999. **40**(11): p. 1587–1592.

77. Adachi, N., et al., *Predictive value of interictal epileptiform discharges during non-REM sleep on scalp EEG recordings for the lateralization of epileptogenesis.* Epilepsia, 1998. **39**(6): p. 628–632.

78. Ergene, E., et al., *Frequency of bitemporal independent interictal epileptiform discharges in temporal lobe epilepsy.* Epilepsia, 2000. **41**(2): p. 213–218.

79. Didato, G., et al., *Bitemporal epilepsy: A specific anatomo-electro-clinical phenotype in the temporal lobe epilepsy spectrum.* Seizure, 2015. **31**: p. 112–119.

80. Janszky, J., et al., *Clinical differences in patients with unilateral hippocampal sclerosis and unitemporal or bitemporal epileptiform discharges.* Seizure, 2003. **12**(8): p. 550–554.

81. Holmes, M.D., et al., *Identifying potential surgical candidates in patients with evidence of bitemporal epilepsy.* Epilepsia, 2003. **44**(8): p. 1075–1079.

82. Sylaja, P.N., et al., *Seizure outcome after anterior temporal lobectomy and its predictors in patients with apparent temporal lobe epilepsy and normal MRI.* Epilepsia, 2004. **45**(7): p. 803–808.

83. Gilliam, F., et al., *Association of combined MRI, interictal EEG, and ictal EEG results with outcome and pathology after temporal lobectomy.* Epilepsia, 1997. **38**(12): p. 1315–1320.

84. Radhakrishnan, K., et al., *Predictors of outcome of anterior temporal lobectomy for intractable epilepsy: a multivariate study.* Neurology, 1998. **51**(2): p. 465–471.

85. Aull-Watschinger, S., et al., *Outcome predictors for surgical treatment of temporal lobe epilepsy with hippocampal sclerosis.* Epilepsia, 2008. **49**(8): p. 1308–1316.

86. Cobb, W.A., R.J. Guiloff, and J. Cast, *Breach rhythm: the EEG related to skull defects.* Electroencephalogr Clin Neurophysiol, 1979. **47**(3): p. 251–271.

87. Javidan, M., *Electroencephalography in mesial temporal lobe epilepsy: a review.* Epilepsy Res Treat, 2012. **2012**: p. 637430.

88. Pacia, S.V. and J.S. Ebersole, *Intracranial EEG substrates of scalp ictal patterns from temporal lobe foci.* Epilepsia, 1997. **38**(6): p. 642–654.

89. Reiher, J., M. Beaudry, and C.P. Leduc, *Temporal intermittent rhythmic delta activity (TIRDA) in the diagnosis of complex partial epilepsy: sensitivity, specificity and predictive value.* Can J Neurol Sci, 1989. **16**(4): p. 398–401.

90. Brigo, F., *Intermittent rhythmic delta activity patterns.* Epilepsy Behav, 2011. **20**(2): p. 254–256.

91. Di Gennaro, G., et al., *Localizing significance of temporal intermittent rhythmic delta activity (TIRDA) in drug-resistant focal epilepsy.* Clin Neurophysiol, 2003. **114**(1): p. 70–78.

92. Geyer, J.D., et al., *Significance of interictal temporal lobe delta activity for localization of the primary epileptogenic region.* Neurology, 1999. **52**(1): p. 202–205.

93. Gelisse, P., et al., *Temporal intermittent delta activity: a marker of juvenile absence epilepsy?* Seizure, 2011. **20**(1): p. 38–41.

94. Peltz, C.B., H.L. Kim, and C.H. Kawas, *Abnormal EEGs in cognitively and physically healthy oldest old: findings from the 90+ study.* J Clin Neurophysiol, 2010. **27**(4): p. 292–295.

95. Tao, J.X., et al., *Interictal regional delta slowing is an EEG marker of epileptic network in temporal lobe epilepsy.* Epilepsia, 2011. **52**(3): p. 467–476.

96. Velasco, T.R., et al., *Foramen ovale electrodes can identify a focal seizure onset when surface EEG fails in mesial temporal lobe epilepsy.* Epilepsia, 2006. **47**(8): p. 1300–1307.

97. Lam, A.D., et al., *Widespread changes in network activity allow non-invasive detection of mesial temporal lobe seizures.* Brain, 2016. **139**(Pt 10): p. 2679–2693.

98. Englot, D.J., et al., *Impaired consciousness in temporal lobe seizures: role of cortical slow activity.* Brain, 2010. **133**(Pt 12): p. 3764–3777.

99. Blumenfeld, H., et al., *Ictal neocortical slowing in temporal lobe epilepsy.* Neurology, 2004. **63**(6): p. 1015–1021.

100. So, N.K., *Temporal lobe epilepsies*, in *Wyllie's Treatment of Epilepsy: Principles and Practice*, E. Wyllie, Editor. 2015, Wolters Kluwer: Philadelphia, PA.

101. Ebersole, J.S. and S.V. Pacia, *Localization of temporal lobe foci by ictal EEG patterns.* Epilepsia, 1996. **37**(4): p. 386–399.

102. Jung, K.Y., et al., *Spatiotemporospectral characteristics of scalp ictal EEG in mesial temporal lobe epilepsy with hippocampal sclerosis.* Brain Res, 2009. **1287**: p. 206–219.

103. Mintzer, S., et al., *Unilateral hippocampal sclerosis with contralateral temporal scalp ictal onset.* Epilepsia, 2004. **45**(7): p. 792–802.

104. Laskowitz, D.T., et al., *The syndrome of frontal lobe epilepsy: characteristics and surgical management.* Neurology, 1995. **45**(4): p. 780–787.

105. Appel, S., et al., *A comparison of occipital and temporal lobe epilepsies.* Acta Neurol Scand, 2015. **132**(4): p. 284–290.

106. Jobst, B.C. and G.D. Cascino, *Resective epilepsy surgery for drug-resistant focal epilepsy: a review.* JAMA, 2015. **313**(3): p. 285–293.

20 | CONVULSIVE STATUS EPILEPTICUS

FRANK W. DRISLANE, MD, SUSAN T. HERMAN, MD, AND PETER W. KAPLAN, MB, BS, FRCP

ABSTRACT: Generalized convulsive status epilepticus (GCSE) is a serious neurologic illness causing unresponsiveness, major physiologic disturbances, risk of injury and, if prolonged enough, neuronal damage. Causes are many, and the outcome often depends as much on the etiology as on the epileptic seizure itself. Several anti-seizure medications are used in treatment of GCSE, but some cases continue electrographically when clinical convulsions cease (nonconvulsive SE), and EEG is essential in their diagnosis. About 20% of cases become refractory to initial treatment, and the EEG becomes even more crucial in diagnosis and management. This chapter also covers other forms of SE with significant motor manifestations including: focal motor status (including *epilepsia partialis continua*); myoclonic status, which includes some relatively benign forms as well as some with a very poor prognosis; and clonic and tonic status. It reviews the many different EEG findings in those forms of status, and the use of EEG in their treatment and management, especially in prolonged cases.

KEYWORDS: EEG, status epilepticus, convulsive status epilepticus, focal status epilepticus, myoclonic status epilepticus, refractory status epilepticus, treatment

PRINCIPAL REFERENCES

1. Brophy GM, Bell R, Claassen J, Alldredge B, Bleck TP, Glauser T, Laroche SM, Riviello JJ Jr, Shutter L, Sperling MR, Treiman DM, Vespa PM. Neurocritical Care Society Status Epilepticus Guideline Writing Committee. Guidelines for the evaluation and management of status epilepticus. Neurocrit Care 2012;17(1):3–23.
2. Chen JW, Naylor DE, Wasterlain CG. Advances in the pathophysiology of status epilepticus. Acta Neurol Scand 2007;115(suppl 4):7–15.
3. Claassen J, Mayer SA, Kowalski RG, Emerson RG, Hirsch LJ. Detection of electrographic seizures with continuous EEG monitoring in critically ill patients. Neurology 2004;62:1743–1748.
4. DeLorenzo RJ, Hauser WA, Towne AR, Boggs JG, Pellock JM, Penberthy L, Garnett L, Fortner CA, Ko D. A prospective, population-based epidemiologic study of status epilepticus in Richmond, Virginia. Neurology 1996;46:1029–1035.
5. Guerrini R, Bonanni P, Rothwell J, Hallett M. Myoclonus and epilepsy. In: Guerrini R, Aicardi J, Andermann F, Hallett M, eds., Epilepsy and movement disorder. Cambridge: Cambridge University Press, 2002:165–210.
6. Rossetti AO, Hurwitz S, Logroscino G, Bromfield EB. Prognosis of status epilepticus: role of aetiology, age, and consciousness impairment at presentation. J Neuro Neurosurg Psychiatry 2006;77:611–615.
7. Shorvon S, Ferlisi M. The treatment of super-refractory status epilepticus: a critical review of available therapies and a clinical treatment protocol. Brain 2011;134:2802–2818.
8. Snodgrass SM, Tsuburaya K, Ajmone-Marsan C. Clinical significance of periodic lateralized epileptiform discharges: Relationship with status epilepticus. J Clin Neurophysiol 1989;6:159–172.
9. Treiman DM, Meyers PD, Walton NY, Collins JF, Colling C, Rowan AJ, Handforth A, Faught E, Calabrese VP, Uthman BM, Ramsay RE, Mamdani MB. A comparison of four treatments for generalized convulsive status epilepticus. N Engl J Med 1998;339:792–798.
10. Trinka E, Cock H, Hesdorffer D, Rossetti AO, Scheffer IE, Shinnar S, Shorvon S, and Lowenstein DH. A definition and classification of status epilepticus—Report of the ILAE Task Force on Classification of Status Epilepticus. Epilepsia 2015;56:1515–1523.

1. HISTORY

Status epilepticus may have been described as early as 600 to 700 BC in cuneiform writings, one of which notes: "If the possessing demon possesses him many times during the middle watch of the night, and at the time of his possession his hands and feet are cold, he is much darkened, keeps opening and shutting his mouth, is brown and yellow as to the eye. It may go on for some time, but he will die" (1,2). Caelius Aurelianus, a scholar from the late Roman empire, noted that "fits can recur . . . even in the same day" (3). In 17th-century England, Thomas Willis wrote, "when as fits are often repeated, and every time grow more cruel, the animal function is quickly debilitated [and] the vital function is by little and little enervated, till at length, the whole body languishing, and the pulse loosened, and at length ceasing, at last the vital flame is extinguished" (4).

Reports of status epilepticus were few through the 18th century, but in the 1800s the study of epilepsy flourished in Paris at the Salpêtrière, which, with 8,000 patients, was Europe's largest asylum. Physicians there, including Charcot, provided extensive clinical descriptions of status epilepticus. The topic was brought to modern attention in the university dissertation of Calmeil in Paris, who reported that the phrase derives from the patients' use of the term: *"C'est ce que les malades appellent entre eux l'état de mal"* (5) ("It's what the patients among themselves called a bad condition [of epilepsy]"). He detailed the illness's severity and a sequence of seizures without pause that forebode a poor outcome. The use in (Latinized) English of *status epilepticus* appeared when Bazire translated the lectures of Trousseau, who wrote, "You, however, have heard of circumstances where fits have lasted two or three days, and ended in death. It is in these cases that one spoke of, at the Salpêtrière or at Bicêtre, of an *état de mal* (status epilepticus)" (6). Rather than simply repeated seizures, status epilepticus was then assumed to be a distinct entity representing the "maximum expression of epilepsy with its own particular characteristics, although restricted at the time to tonic-clonic seizures" (1).

In 1903, Clark and Prout described the clinical and pathologic appearance of status epilepticus (SE) in 38 patients, detailing a fusion of successive convulsions over 2 to 9 days, to the point of coma and exhaustion, along with changes in respiration, temperature and pulse (7). The presentation was "composed of delirium, stupor or coma . . . and a variety of psychic states, which have for their basis cortical discharges." They listed three stages of SE, with the third described as stupor—likely corresponding to the nonconvulsive SE that follows generalized convulsive SE with "electromechanical dissociation" and continued electrochemical seizure activity in the brain after cessation of clinically observable convulsions, sometimes now referred to as "subtle" SE (8).

Whitty and Taylor in 1949 noticed that outcome worsened the longer the SE lasted (9). By 1964, Janz had uncovered that most symptomatic cases arose from frontal foci. In the United Kingdom, a review of the Register General found that one third of deaths in epileptic patients was from SE. Identifiable precipitants of SE were infections and changes in medication regimens.

Convulsive SE can be characterized clinically without electrophysiologic data, but Berger's development of the electroencephalogram (EEG) in 1929 led to valuable understanding of the different forms of SE, especially for nonconvulsive SE (10) (see next chapter).

The first modern meetings on SE, the Marseille Colloquia of 1962 and 1964 (11,12), promulgated better definitions and classification for seizures and SE and suggested that SE was the prolongation of many different types of epileptic seizures. The Xth Marseille Colloquium led to the proposal that SE be defined when duration exceeded 60 minutes (11). Gastaut, the organizer of the meetings, stated that there were "as many forms of status epilepticus as there were types of seizures." Today, most literature recognizes SE's own particular pathophysiology, which is not always identical to that of prolongation of an individual seizure (13). The most recent International League Against Epilepsy (ILAE) definition is from 2015 (14). Since the 1960s, increasing scientific and clinical attention has turned to the physiologic underpinnings, neurochemistry, and pharmacology of SE, most recently with genetic investigations and functional imaging.

In the management of SE, relatively little progress was made until the 20th century. In the 1960s, phenytoin replaced bromides and phenobarbital as the drug of choice for SE (15). The principal therapeutic development was the use of intravenous benzodiazepines (16), with subsequent determination of lorazepam as the appropriate initial treatment for SE (17), although often with clonazepam in Europe. In the last 20 years, with the growing use of EEGs and particularly continuous EEG monitoring in intensive care units (ICUs), more cases were found to become refractory and "super-refractory" SE, almost always in a later, nonconvulsive form (18,19), leading to the increased use of major sedating or "anesthetic" agents such as propofol, midazolam, and pentobarbital. With various treatment regimens moving beyond first-, second-, and third-line medications, newer treatments such as the ketogenic diet, deep brain stimulation, surgery, and others are being explored (20–22).

2. DEFINITIONS

Gastaut defined SE as "an epileptic seizure that is so frequently repeated or so prolonged as to create a fixed and lasting epileptic condition" (12). At first, no duration was specified. The ILAE specified "a single epileptic seizure of > 30-min duration or a series of epileptic seizures during which function is not regained between ictal events in a 30-minute period" (23). Although without a definite scientific basis, 30 minutes has been the standard criterion for duration in most clinical studies until recently (24).

SE is often a series of individual seizures, without recovery between seizures. Alternatively, a single convulsion can be very prolonged, and many convulsive seizures progress to become nonconvulsive status epilepticus (NCSE), in which the EEG can demonstrate ongoing (nonconvulsive) seizure activity. If recovery occurs between individual convulsions, this is considered a clustering of seizures rather than SE.

While experimental studies show plentiful evidence of neurologic damage after 30 minutes of generalized convulsive status epilepticus (GCSE), there is a clinical imperative with human patients to begin treatment of convulsive seizures much sooner. Prospective clinical trials must define SE as diagnosable expeditiously, and urgent treatment is a clinical necessity. Thus, the largest trial of different anti-seizure drugs (ASDs) for the treatment of GCSE (17) considered it mandatory to make the diagnosis and begin treatment within 10 minutes. In 1999, an "operational" definition of GCSE proposed that 5 minutes was the time by which SE should be interrupted to avoid morbidity, mortality, or refractory SE (25). This duration has been accepted generally as appropriate to characterize SE in the case of GCSE and has been used to define GCSE in many recent reports. It may be reasonable to use longer durations (in some cases, 30 minutes) to define other types of SE.

The duration of seizures appropriate to define SE clearly depends on the type of SE being considered. A recent Task Force report from the ILAE focused on physiology, duration of seizure activity, and potential neuropathologic consequences, defining SE as

> a condition resulting either from the failure of the mechanisms responsible for seizure termination or from the initiation of mechanisms which lead to abnormally prolonged seizures (after time point t1). It is a condition which can have long-term consequences (after time t2), including neuronal death, neuronal injury, and alteration of neuronal networks depending on the type and duration of seizures (14).

Time point t1 is considered the time by which seizures are unlikely to stop on their own, so treatment should be initiated, lest the SE continue through time t2 with damaging consequences. That report cited evidence that for GCSE "t1" is 5 minutes, and t2 possibly 30 minutes. The respective t1 and t2 for nonconvulsive SE were considered substantially more speculative.

3. PATHOPHYSIOLOGY OF STATUS EPILEPTICUS

Clinically, episodes of SE often appear to begin in the same way as individual seizures of the same type, but there are many different types of seizures and SE, and it is rare to capture the beginning of SE on a routine EEG. Most individual secondarily generalized convulsions cease on their own in under 2 minutes and the patient recovers thereafter (26). Almost half of seizures lasting from 10 to 29 minutes cease spontaneously, without treatment (27), and a significant subset of patients (~10%) had prolonged seizures that terminate spontaneously (28). The main risk factor for prolonged seizures is a prior history of a prolonged seizure (28).

Video-EEG monitoring studies demonstrate that convulsive seizures usually last <2 minutes and are very unlikely to last >11 minutes (29), while almost all focal seizures with impairment of consciousness (or complex partial seizures) last <7 to 10 minutes, and almost all focal seizures *without* impairment of consciousness cease within 11 minutes (29,30). (This pathophysiology section concerns primarily GCSE.)

Some seizures, however, continue despite the brain's intrinsic capacity to terminate shorter seizures, and they progress to the longer episodes of SE. Seizures in several electrical and chemical models of SE become self-sustaining rapidly, even when the stimulus for seizures is withdrawn (31). The transition from individual seizures to seemingly self-sustaining prolonged seizures or SE appears to depend substantially on the relative balance of excitatory and inhibitory electrochemical function at the time—at intracellular, membrane, extracellular, and interneuronal levels.

There are probably several pathophysiologic mechanisms that facilitate the continuation of seizures, and in some seizures, the balance of electrochemical function appears to shift, unfavorably, toward excessive excitatory activity as seizures progress. To a large extent, SE implies a failure of the typical inhibitory function of the brain in terminating seizures as usual (31).

In experimental animals, one of the primary cellular changes in the transition from prolonged seizures to refractory SE is a marked and progressive impairment of gamma-amino butyric acid (GABA) agonist-mediated inhibitory function, in turn favoring recurrent excitatory circuits (32).

The electrochemical activity of ongoing seizures induces gene transcription and neurotransmitter receptor changes almost immediately and new peptide production after several minutes, leading to the production of numerous molecular factors with excitatory or inhibiting effects on continuing seizures.

Early in SE, there is a marked and maladaptive modification of GABA receptors (even within 45 minutes, showing rapid functional plasticity (33)), with a diminution in the number of GABA-A receptors on neuronal surfaces (34). This occurs in large part due to progressive internalization or endocytosis of those receptors (35), particularly the β2/3 subunit- and the γ2 subunit-containing synaptic GABA-A receptors (36). This likely contributes to the reduced effectiveness of GABA agonists in terminating seizures.

As seizures progress, in both experimental animals and in human studies, they appear to become resistant to many ASDs, especially those acting through the GABA system, such as benzodiazepines and barbiturates (33), and those drugs become less useful in treating SE. For example, GABA-A receptor δ-subunit assemblies with either an α4 or α6

subunit are insensitive to benzodiazepines. These extrasynaptic receptors, however, are sensitive to general anesthetics and to neurosteroids—suggesting potentially useful targets and agents for the treatment of refractory SE (37).

Within minutes of the onset of SE (concomitant with the decay in GABA receptor function), there is increasing excitatory activity of glutamate receptors, especially the N-methyl-D-aspartate (NMDA) and α-amino-3-hydroxy-5-methyl-4-isoxazolepropionic acid (AMPA) receptors, as those receptors move to the synaptic membrane, promoting and prolonging the hyperexcitable state (31,37,39). When glutamate binds to the NMDA receptor, membrane ion flow can still be blocked by magnesium, but with sufficient repetitive depolarization (as occurs during seizures), the magnesium is released and the ion channel opens more completely in a "use-dependent" facilitation of glutamatergic activity (40). NMDA receptor antagonists are not effective in blocking the initiation of SE, but as seizures continue with repetitive depolarization, they appear to become more effective anticonvulsants in the same "use-dependent" manner (41). At that point, glutamate antagonists (such as ketamine) may become more effective treatments (42).

With more prolonged SE, enhanced excitability is maintained by changes in gene transcription occurring over minutes to hours. Increased expression of pro-convulsive neuropeptides (substance P and neurokinin B) and decreased availability of inhibitory neuropeptides (dynophin, galanin, somatostatin, and neuropeptide Y) facilitate ongoing SE (31,29,43).

As seizures continue, stimulation of glutamate (especially NMDA) receptors leads to excessive sodium and calcium entry into neurons, and this may cause cell death. Gene activation during SE may lead to the production of kinases and phosphatases that accelerate the harmful process. Later, inflammation, glial cell changes, and neuronal sprouting or cell loss may contribute to the refractoriness of subsequent seizures (31). The potential neuronal injury from prolonged seizures or SE may depend somewhat on the intensity (or frequency) of the epileptiform discharges (44).

The genetics of SE remain elusive, but some findings may shed light on its pathophysiology (45). One twin study showed a higher proband-wise concordance of SE in monozygotic (0.31) than in dizygotic (0.0) twins, suggesting that genetics plays a role in susceptibility to SE. Although some identified gene mutations (e.g., those causing cortical dysplasias, inborn errors of metabolism, epileptic encephalopathies, and mitochondrial diseases) appear to predispose to SE, there are no "pure" identified genes for SE itself (45). A wide variety of genes involved in cerebral development, cerebral and mitochondrial energy production, membrane and transmitter function, and network defects have been implicated in susceptibility to SE, suggesting that there may be other mechanisms for SE beyond a simple excitatory–inhibitory imbalance (45). These findings contrast strongly with the elucidation of many genetic abnormalities that produce *epilepsy syndromes*, indicating yet another way in which SE is not simply the continuation of the same types of seizures (as suggested by Gastaut long ago) but rather has a pathophysiology (or several pathophysiologies) particular to SE itself and its process of generation.

There is abundant experimental (if much more modest clinical) evidence that neuronal damage results from GCSE, particularly when prolonged. A century ago, this damage was attributed to ischemia, but in the 1970s, Meldrum and colleagues showed that excessive excitatory neuronal activity was the cause of nerve cell damage, at least in experimental animals with prolonged GCSE (46–48). In baboons given bicuculline to induce SE, prolonged convulsions with continued EEG spike discharges for 1 to 5 hours caused neuronal damage in the neocortex, cerebellum, and hippocampus (46–49). By "clamping" blood flow, brain oxygenation, and glucose supply to preserve homeostasis during SE, they showed that hypoperfusion was not crucial in the development of such damage. Neuronal injury still occurred in the hippocampus, and it appeared to be due to excitatory neurotransmitter activity. Thus, the prolonged ongoing cellular electrochemical activity of *SE itself* (rather than concomitant physiologic derangements) was sufficient to cause neuronal injury, although systemic abnormalities contributed. This hippocampal damage may correlate with prolonged memory and other cognitive dysfunction in humans following SE.

It is difficult to prove that SE leads to neuronal damage in humans (as it clearly does in experimental animals exposed to prolonged, intense electrical stimulation), in part because SE is seldom fatal without causation by other severe neurologic illnesses that themselves cause neuropathologic damage independent of the SE. Nevertheless, a disproportionately decreased neuronal cell density was seen in the hippocampus of some patients who died from GCSE (but not NCSE) (50). Forms of SE other than GCSE may not be as harmful and may not require exactly the same treatment, but concern for the possibility of such damage leads to a clear mandate for urgent treatment.

4. EPIDEMIOLOGY AND CAUSES

Studies of the incidence of SE vary tremendously in terms of definitions and different populations studied. The corrected, age-adjusted incidence of SE was 17.1 cases per 100,000 population per year in Germany and 54.5 per 100,000 in subjects older than 60 years; the case-fatality rate was 9.3% (51). This study included all forms of SE. Most were due to remote symptomatic causes such as cerebrovascular disease. The mean age of adult patients was 65 years. SE is more common in children younger than 1 year and in the elderly. In French-speaking Switzerland, the incidence was 10.3 per 100,000 and was greatest for children less than 1 year of age and in the elderly; the case-fatality rate was 7.6% (52). About half of all cases of SE treated in acute care medical centers are GCSE (24,52). The incidence of SE is several times greater in developing countries, particularly in children (53).

The incidence of all forms of SE was 41 cases per 100,000 in Richmond, Virginia, but 20 per 100,000 in the white population, similar to that in Germany (24). The incidence was higher in African-Americans, and also likely higher because of ascertainment in an urban medical setting. Extrapolation from the same database suggests an incidence of up to 50 per 100,000 per year, substantially higher than most estimates (24). In another study, mortality of SE was 19% within the first 30 days

and was highly associated with the acute cause of SE (54). Short-term case fatality is generally 20% to 25% when considering GCSE alone, and in all series it is due primarily to the underlying illness causing SE (24). In another study of patients with afebrile SE, 32% had recurrence of SE within 10 years of follow-up (55). Recurrence is higher in patients with progressive neurologic disorders.

Causes of SE are numerous. They may be grouped into larger categories similar to the causes of seizures and epilepsy syndromes (23):

Symptomatic: a consequence of a known or suspected cerebral dysfunction such as head injury, vascular disease, infection, tumor or other mass lesion, toxic or metabolic disturbances, or following surgery

Idiopathic: such as in the idiopathic generalized epilepsies (IGEs), almost always related to a known or presumed genetic-based syndrome

Cryptogenic: there is a presumed underlying cause, but it cannot be identified.

The IGEs lead to SE relatively infrequently, and the SE is usually nonconvulsive (see next chapter), although GCSE occurs occasionally, including in the unusual case of generalized convulsions upon awakening (56).

The most common cause of SE in most larger series, especially in non-hospitalized patients, is "remote symptomatic" (with the cause present for more than a week), often due to earlier injuries such as stroke, and often with more immediate exacerbation by some systemic problem such as infection, medications, or ASD withdrawal (57,58). The next largest category of causes is probably an exacerbation of earlier epilepsy, also commonly with an acute precipitant such as lowered ASD levels, infection, or metabolic disturbance. In acute care hospitals, most SE patients have "acute symptomatic" causes—that is, due to a recent (within a week) neurologic injury or illness, the most common example of which is a new stroke (59). Most have no history of seizures and are often older adults with acute and severe medical or neurologic illnesses.

In order to discuss diagnosis, management, and outcome, it is important to recognize the tremendous variety of clinical situations that fall under the rubric of SE and to specify exactly which clinical syndrome a patient has. Cases of SE, like seizures, can be organized clinically into those with a focal onset and those with a generalized onset—although many generalized cases cannot be divided easily into those of a primarily generalized nature versus those with a focal onset and secondary generalization (Table 20.1). Many epidemiologic studies do not specify the type of SE covered, but those that do indicate that convulsions with focal onset and secondary generalization are the most common type (~40% of all SE), and that about three quarters of all cases of SE became generalized convulsions by their end (24,60). Forms of SE with prominent motor signs, whether convulsive, myoclonic, or tonic, are covered in this chapter; those with primarily non-motor manifestations are described in the next.

TABLE 20.1. Different Forms of Status Epilepticus

CONVULSIVE	
GENERALIZED	*FOCAL*
Generalized convulsive SE (GCSE)	Focal motor SE
Primary generalized GCSE	*Epilepsia partialis continua* (EPC)
Secondarily generalized GCSE (focal onset)	
Myoclonic (see Table 20.2)	
Tonic (may actually start as focal)	
Clonic (may actually start as focal)	
Atonic (very rare for SE)	
NONCONVULSIVE	
"Classic" absence SE	Complex partial SE, with prolonged
Other primary generalized NCSE	or repeated complex partial seizures.
"Atypical" absence SE	Other focal SE with non-motor features (e.g., aphasic, sensory)
Other generalized NCSE (often secondarily generalized)	
"SE in coma" SE in critically ill patients Electrographic SE	

5. GENERALIZED CONVULSIVE STATUS EPILEPTICUS

5.1. Presentation, Clinical Observations

GCSE is the best described form of SE and has the greatest morbidity, mortality, and clinical urgency for treatment (61). It may begin as primary generalized convulsive seizures or evolve from a focal or complex partial seizure (or "focal onset seizure with dyscognitive features") and progress to generalized convulsions. Most cases of GCSE have some evidence of a focal onset or focal lesion (24) (i.e., ~70–80% of cases are secondarily generalized (57)). Some patients have recurrent seizures without recovery of consciousness between seizures; others evolve from the first convulsion into a more prolonged seizure, with motor manifestations becoming less regular clonic movements and regular or irregular myoclonic jerking activity, in a continuous epileptic ("ictal") state (61). It is uncommon for GCSE to occur in the primary generalized or idiopathic epilepsies (57,62), except when precipitated by ASD discontinuation or as the consequence of using inappropriate ASDs, or with other drugs or systemic illness in patients with idiopathic generalized epilepsies (IGEs) (56).

Clinically, GCSE is readily recognizable by its motor manifestations, which are often dramatic. Typically, convulsive activity consists of paroxysmal or continuous bilateral, usually rhythmic, tonic movements or clonic shaking of the limbs, commonly with facial and truncal manifestations as well, and with loss of consciousness. Convulsions may have some lateralized emphasis, even though the physiologic seizure activity is bilateral or generalized. If the generalized convulsion is primary, the patient may exhibit no movement for a second or two, followed by the tonic phase of a seizure in which muscle contraction occurs throughout the whole body, including a tightening of chest muscles giving rise to the "epileptic cry." The tonic phase typically lasts ~10 sec (63,64) and is interrupted by the clonic phase, with particularly rapid and forceful flexion contractions of the arms. Sometimes movements are more subtle, and there may be a faster quivering, for example in tonic seizures. Typically, there is a progressive lessening of the violence of the convulsions, often within the first minute of SE. Eventually the frequency of clonic contractions lessens, and they cease (63,64). The patient is then flaccid, but there may be a large generalized myoclonic jerk at the end of the motor phase. The tonic, and then clonic, phases of an individual seizure usually last no more than 2 minutes (26). As GCSE progresses, motor manifestations may lessen and include just relatively subtle eyelid or facial or other myoclonic jerking, or motor phenomena may disappear entirely (8). Progression to this "subtle" GCSE (see below) is not characteristic of primary GCSE (56,61). Repeated seizures also diminish in duration and intensity over time (61,65).

Consciousness is lost completely at the beginning of GCSE with the first convulsion, or earlier, and the patient is apneic during the tonic and clonic phase. The eyes are usually open and may show pupillary dilation. Tachycardia, hypertension, and other autonomic changes are common. Following an isolated convulsion, muscle tone and consciousness return gradually, usually with some improvement within minutes, but in SE, recovery does not occur before the next generalized convulsion or progression to more subtle or nonconvulsive SE.

5.2. The EEG of Generalized Convulsive Status Epilepticus

EEG patterns in SE undergo evolution, usually paralleling the clinical manifestations. At the onset, primary generalized convulsions typically show bilaterally symmetric activity (behavioral and on EEG) from the onset, and may progress through a stereotyped sequence of clinical and electrographic manifestations (8,65) (Fig. 20.1). The initial brief interruption in behavior is often accompanied by widespread voltage attenuation with fast frequencies at 20 to 40 Hz, sometimes called "electrodecremental." This may be a widespread desynchronization of the background, but with implanted EEG electrode recording, very rapid (>200 Hz) activity may be evident in the area of seizure onset (very seldom evident on routine, surface EEG), suggesting a role for pathologic organization of networks or circuits of neurons in the generation of seizures (66). Within seconds, as the initial tonic contraction occurs, generalized rhythmic electrographic seizure activity, including rapid spike discharges, increases gradually in voltage and decreases in frequency to ~10 Hz, although the EEG is often obscured by muscle artifact during the tonic phase.

Not all episodes of GCSE begin this way. Some start with early electrographic signs of an IGE that, within seconds,

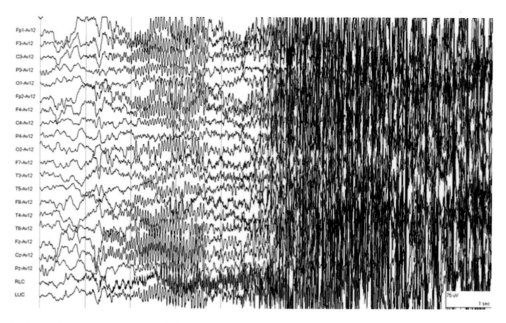

Figure 20.1. A generalized tonic-clonic seizure in a 20-year-old woman with cryptogenic generalized epilepsy. At the onset there is diffuse frontally maximal low- to moderate-voltage beta activity, followed by diffuse muscle artifact as low-amplitude clonus begins.

assumes the clinical and EEG picture of a tonic and then clonic seizure (Fig. 20.2A–D). Still others begin as focal-onset seizures and generalize rapidly. Within seconds, all three can appear very similar clinically and on EEG.

During the clonic phase of the seizure, there is rhythmic slow activity, sometimes with interspersed spikes, for 10 seconds or more (see Fig. 20.2B). Generalized spike and slow waves or polyspike and slow-wave activity correspond to the frequency of the clinical manifestations.

Many of the initial EEG rhythms of GCSE are obscured by the muscle activity of the convulsion, unless the patient has received paralyzing drugs. If GCSE is continuing steadily (as opposed to intermittently recurring seizure activity) the EEG may be nearly or completely obscured by muscle and movement artifact and has little diagnostic value compared to the clinical manifestations. It is often only when the motor manifestations lessen that the EEG becomes interpretable. Sometimes, epileptiform discharges can be seen at the vertex. The superimposed electromyographic activity, however, may exhibit its own characteristic rhythmic appearance, synchronous with the clinical jerking activity, and this muscle activity on the EEG still indicates generalized convulsions (see Fig. 20.2C).

If the seizure ends (or between seizures) the epileptiform discharges give way to a slow, encephalopathic background in all areas, or sometimes a very suppressed background (i.e., a postictal generalized EEG suppression [PGES]), before gradual resumption of a normal drowsy and then waking pattern (see Fig. 20.2D). In GCSE characterized by repetitive seizures with impaired consciousness, the intervening EEG shows diffuse slowing, voltage attenuation, and disorganization, not returning to normal activity before the occurrence of the next clinical seizure. Between seizures, there are often persistent generalized epileptiform discharges with a rhythmic appearance, but slower than during the convulsion (67).

As GCSE becomes prolonged, the EEG becomes more discontinuous, and clinical manifestations become more subtle, often with relatively minimal eyelid or facial or other myoclonic jerking, nystagmoid eye movements, or even absence of all movement, while the EEG continues to show repetitive, rhythmic epileptiform discharges. When the visible motor manifestations of GCSE cease this becomes a form of electromechanical dissociation, sometimes termed "subtle" GCSE (8).

Some have proposed that there is a characteristic sequence of EEG changes during GCSE, based on recordings from animals and humans during various stages of SE (Fig. 20.3) (8):

1. Seizures are initially discrete and followed by background slowing and attenuation until the next seizure begins.

2. The seizures merge gradually, with waxing and waning of voltage and frequency.

3. Eventually, seizures become continuous, although ictal discharges are frequently asymmetric, reflecting the focal onset of many of the seizures.

4. With time, seizures become discontinuous; there are brief (0.5–8 sec) periods of generalized voltage attenuation or flattening.

5. In late SE, generalized periodic (epileptiform) discharges (GPEDs, or GPDs) or bursts of polyspikes with frequencies from 0.5 to 4 Hz arise from a relatively flat background.

"Subtle" SE often corresponds to EEG stages 4 and 5 (8). Patients are typically comatose, with minimal or no motor manifestations at this point (8,67).

Sequential EEG changes, such as the decreased prominence of ictal discharges and increase in intervening background attenuation (in parallel with the diminution of clinical manifestations), represent progressive neuronal dysfunction, possibly due to metabolic depletion (8). As the EEG "deteriorates," motor manifestations become more subtle or disappear entirely. Other investigators have not found the same sequence of EEG changes (18,68,69). While these EEG patterns were seen frequently, they often occurred out of sequence or in only some patients, and in some patients one EEG pattern persists throughout the course of SE. Evolution of the EEG patterns depends on the etiology of SE and the baseline condition of each patient, time from SE onset, type of SE, duration of seizure activity, and treatment. Such variation makes classification of SE based purely on EEG criteria difficult and adds to the controversy regarding which patterns are "ictal"—that is, the electrographic manifestations of an ongoing epileptic seizure. Stage 4 above usually has subtle or no motor manifestations but has very frequent and rhythmic epileptiform discharges and is usually considered to represent NCSE. Stage 5 is far more controversial as to its "ictal" nature.

There is no definite difference in clinical significance if SE is manifested on EEG by recurrent discrete electrographic

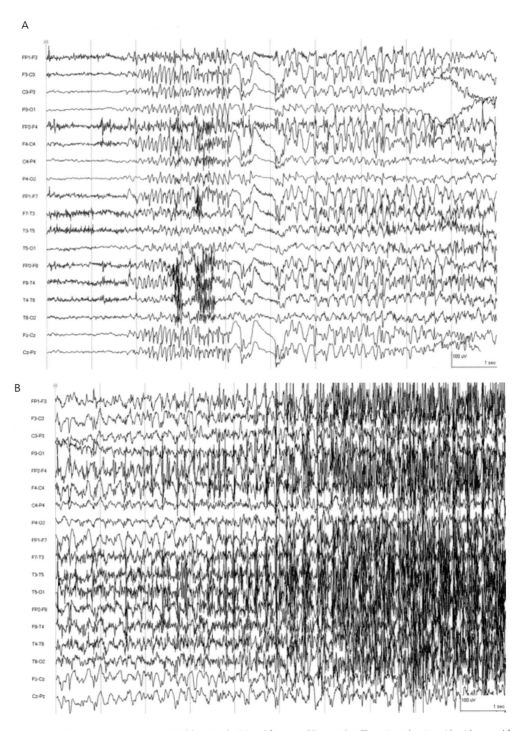

Figure 20.2. **A:** *A generalized tonic-clonic seizure in a 43-year-old man with IGE and frequent SE episodes. The seizure begins with widespread frontally maximal alpha activity, then 5-Hz spike and slow-wave discharges.* **B:** *Continuation of the seizure. Slower rhythmic activity, with admixed spike and wave discharges, gradually becomes obscured by muscle activity.* **C:** *After a period nearly entirely obscured by muscle activity (not shown here), there is evolution into generalized 1.5-Hz bursts of EMG artifact corresponding to the patient's generalized clonic jerking.* **D:** *The seizure ends and is followed by diffuse background-voltage attenuation.*

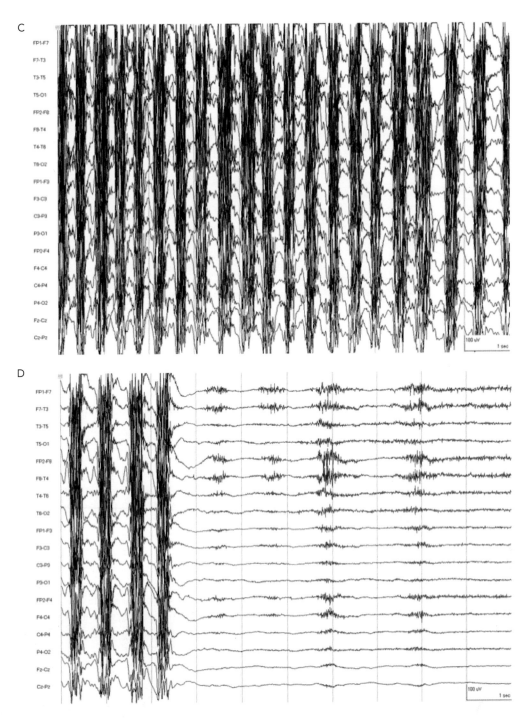

Figure 20.2. Continued

seizures or by continuous epileptiform discharges. In one series of focal SE, there was no significant difference in the etiologies and outcome of patients with either continuous discharges or recurrent discrete seizures on EEG (70). In another series, patients with continuous clinical seizure activity appeared to be more severely ill than those with discrete seizures (71), but the management and outcome do not differ much between the two patterns.

5.3. Complications, Morbidity

GCSE engenders major physiologic changes, several of which may contribute to its significant potential for morbidity and mortality (57,72). At the beginning of GCSE (as with isolated convulsions) heart rate and blood pressure increase rapidly, along with a substantial surge of catecholamines into the bloodstream. Cardiac arrhythmias, including bradyarrhythmias and tachyarrhythmias, are common and sometimes serious; cardiac arrest may occur (73). Blood pressure and glucose concentrations increase early but return to baseline levels after several minutes, and may even decrease further (72,74,75). Hypoperfusion can affect the liver and pancreas. Respiratory rhythm disturbances are common, as is aspiration pneumonia, often leading to fever. Prolonged treatment may be associated with infections or sepsis, thrombophlebitis, and pulmonary emboli.

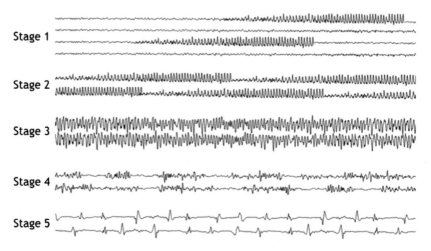

Figure 20.3. Stages of SE, illustrated by single-channel recordings showing EEG evolution (see text for details). Stage 1: Discrete seizures with intervening normal EEG. Stage 2: Merging seizures, with some intervening normal EEG. Stage 3: Continuous seizure activity. Stage 4: Discontinuous seizure activity with intervening periods of a flat background. Stage 5: Somewhat periodic epileptiform discharges on a low-voltage background.

Metabolic complications include electrolyte disturbances such as hyponatremia. Peripheral leukocytosis and cerebrospinal fluid pleocytosis are common. Increased intracranial pressure and cerebral edema may develop, especially in children (76). Disseminated intravascular coagulation can lead to multi-organ failure. Fractures of long bones are common, particularly with falls and trauma, as are vertebral compression fractures. Falls also cause facial, dental, skull, and other injuries.

Violent muscle contractions increase lactate levels, contributing to a systemic acidosis, and systemic temperatures often rise significantly (57). Prolonged muscle contraction can also lead to rhabdomyolysis, and myoglobinuria can cause renal failure (77). Hyperthermia may be due to continued convulsions or to infection, for which the underlying cause must be sought and treated. Hyperthermia due to the SE itself usually resolves with prompt treatment of the SE. Prolonged SE can also increase the likelihood and morbidity of systemic infections (78).

The physiologic consequences of SE may have direct harmful effects on the brain as well—some mediated by excitatory neurotransmitter toxicity and some via inflammation (48,79). Imaging studies, including computed tomography, magnetic resonance imaging, and positron emission tomography (PET) scans, have shown substantial changes in brain tissue with SE, but their clinical implications are often uncertain (80). Many such changes resolve over days or weeks, but others may lead to more permanent changes such gliosis and atrophy (81). There are some well-detailed cases of permanent and severe tissue damage, such as hippocampal atrophy, reasonably attributed to very prolonged SE alone—and accompanied by neuropsychologic deficits (82).

Several studies (most of which are pediatric and retrospective) have found minimal cognitive morbidity following SE. Several found negative consequences, but it is unclear if they were due to the underlying illness or SE itself (83,84). Comprehensive neurologic and neuropsychologic evaluations before and after SE are seldom available; patients with progressive illnesses worsen, whether or not related to the SE; and neurologic deficits may fluctuate with time. It is also difficult to control for the influence of ASDs and other medications.

One group studied 193 children with SE (almost all GCSE) and concluded that "the major neurologic sequelae are usually due to the underlying insult rather than to the prolonged seizure itself" (83). Another group performed thorough neuropsychologic testing on 15 adults with prior epilepsy (without underlying lesions or symptomatic causes) before and after episodes of SE; they found no significant cognitive morbidity accruing from the SE and suggested that the morbidity in other series comes from the underlying etiology, not from the SE itself (85). Long-term cognitive complications of SE appear to be relatively uncommon, occurring primarily in the most prolonged and severe cases.

About 10% of patients with chronic epilepsy present with an episode of SE (86). Conversely, about 30% to 40% of survivors of GCSE develop subsequent epilepsy (87,88), four times the rate following a single acute symptomatic seizure. SE might lead to epilepsy but alternatively, patients more likely to have later epilepsy may present with more severe seizures at the onset—in other words, SE may represent a marker for a more severe epileptic process that has already begun (89). While chronic epilepsy may follow SE, and SE is a risk factor for such epilepsy (90), it does not appear to be causal in most.

5.4. Outcome: Mortality

Mortality in "the status epileptici" (with all forms taken together) is approximately 20% to 25% (24), with most studies focusing primarily on GCSE. The mortality in a given study depends on the type of SE investigated; it is generally much higher for GCSE than for most forms of NCSE. Also, if SE is defined with a shorter temporal duration (e.g., 5 minutes vs. 30 minutes), the incidence of SE will be greater but the mortality lower. Even for GCSE, outcome varies considerably and depends heavily on etiology and possibly on other factors. In one of the largest prospective, population-based studies of SE, case fatality was 3% for children and 26% for adults, using a

30-minute definition and including all types of SE (24). Large databases indicate that in-hospital mortality of SE is ~4% to 9% (91,92); the mortality in single-center studies is about 20% (93). Longer-term mortality, after hospitalization, is likely to be much higher (94). The case-fatality rate for SE occurring for the first time during hospitalization is as high as 60% (95). Almost all studies conclude that most of the morbidity and mortality of SE derives primarily from the illness precipitating the SE rather than from the SE itself (96,97). By one estimate, no more than 2% of fatalities come from the SE itself (98).

Etiology is overwhelmingly the most important prognostic factor. Short-term mortality is highest when SE occurs in the setting of an acute insult, especially stroke and anoxia (24,54,88,89). Patients with multiple medical problems, including sepsis, fare poorly, while those with SE due to tumors, trauma, alcohol abuse, or other drugs have an intermediate or lower mortality (24,57). Generally, the most favorable etiology is epilepsy itself, with some exacerbating factor (e.g., reduced ASDs, fever, sleep deprivation, or an intercurrent illness or other precipitant) prompting the SE (24). Older patients with a symptomatic cause of GCSE have a mortality exceeding 50% (59). Presentation in coma (vs. stupor or confusion) confers a poor prognosis (100), but this may also be related to the severity of the etiology. While etiology is key in most cases, one study found that death following SE appeared unrelated to etiology in about 10% and may have been caused by complications of prolonged ICU stays in coma, or of the treatment (101).

Children with SE have a low mortality but the elderly a much higher one. In one series, SE patients older than age 60 had a mortality of nearly 40%; and it was nearly 60% in those older than 80 (102). Most SE types in the elderly are focal, or focal with secondary generalization (totaling 74%; (102)), reflecting the focal pathology, particularly stroke—the most common cause of SE in the elderly. Younger patients with earlier epilepsy had a much lower mortality (103). Mortality of SE increases with age, but this may be explained largely by the increasing incidence of acute medical illnesses, such as strokes and other concomitant conditions (96,104).

The duration of SE may influence outcome. Experimentally induced seizures in rodents become more refractory to treatment with benzodiazepines after 45 minutes (compared to those lasting 10 minutes) (32). In clinical studies (not always controlled for etiology) patients with 2 or 4 hours of SE had more morbidity than those with shorter episodes (58,105). In the largest epidemiologic study of duration and SE, patients whose SE lasted 1 hour or more had a 32% mortality within one month versus 2.7% for shorter durations, even corrected for other factors by multivariate analysis (106), but there was no definite correlation between duration and mortality *beyond* 1 hour. When controlled for etiology and other factors, duration of SE was not a prognostic factor in at least two studies (54,107), indicating that prolonged SE should not be considered untreatable—unless the etiology is particularly ominous. Patients with shorter SE durations do better, at least in large part because the SE has more benign causes. It has been impossible to separate duration (beyond the first hour) conclusively from the influence of etiology.

Appropriate treatment of SE appears to reduce morbidity and mortality, but it is impossible to carry out a randomized trial of treatment and nontreatment. A study comparing two centers found that poorer-quality treatment (primarily the use of inadequate benzodiazepine doses early in SE) led to worsened outcome (108). Another found that *most* treatment was inadequate and correspondingly ineffective, also suggesting that adequate doses of appropriate ASDs led to better outcomes (109). On the other hand, concern has been raised recently that treatment of refractory SE (both convulsive and nonconvulsive, but excluding anoxic cases) with highly sedating drugs can be associated with worsened outcome, even with an attempt to control for the severity of the SE (110).

A few groups have formulated prognostic models for outcome in SE. The STatus Epilepticus Severity Score (STESS) includes four variables (age, type of SE, level of consciousness before treatment, and history of previous seizures), with a higher score having an excellent negative predictive value (0.97) for mortality (111). The more detailed Epidemiology-based Mortality Score in Status Epilepticus (EMSE) (112) also includes comorbidities and was better at predicting good outcomes but required information that is not always available early, such as the exact etiology.

Overall, the mortality of SE may be declining over the past few decades—often attributed to faster recognition and treatment (94). It is possible, however, that a wider variety of SE types is now being diagnosed, including more benign cases with lower morbidity and mortality, thus increasing the reported incidence of SE and improving the reported outcome. (In part, this may be a consequence of the 5-minute "operational" definition of SE replacing the older 30-minute definition.) One study reported a recent decrease in mortality, at least when myoclonic SE (usually following cardiac arrest and anoxia) was excluded (94).

5.5. Treatment of Generalized Convulsive Status Epilepticus

Clinical management of SE is beyond the scope of a Clinical Neurophysiology chapter but will be alluded to briefly. Although there is a substantial difference between the duration of SE that leads to neuronal damage in experimental animals and the shorter duration of SE now felt to warrant prompt treatment in patients, seizures should be treated long before they last 30 minutes, and certainly by the time of "impending status" (113). The "operational" definition above recommended treatment within 5 minutes to avoid morbidity, mortality, or refractory SE (25). This applies primarily to GCSE, although all forms of SE should be treated expeditiously.

As an emergency condition, GCSE warrants admission and ICU care in most cases, with urgent attention to airway, breathing, circulation, and basic medical care, addressing the underlying cause of SE and the medical illness causing or worsening it (114). There has been just one large randomized controlled trial comparing different intravenous ASDs for GCSE (17). In that series, the treatment success rate in patients with overt GCSE was 56%, but only 15% in those with "subtle" SE. Lorazepam had the greatest success, terminating seizures in

65% of cases of overt GCSE. Phenobarbital (58.2%), diazepam followed by phenytoin (55.8%), and phenytoin alone (43.6%) followed, but these differences were not statistically significant (except for lorazepam vs. phenytoin).

Based primarily on that trial, several other studies, and common practice, treatment recommendations have come from several organizations. Those from the Neurocritical Care Society recommend beginning treatment with sufficient doses of an intravenous benzodiazepines, the most rapidly acting medications (115,116). With its longer duration of action, lorazepam is frequently preferred, usually at a dose of 0.1 mg/kg (16,116,117). Other large randomized trials concluded that emergency treatment (even in the field) could use either intravenous benzodiazepines or intramuscular midazolam (118,119).

This should almost always be followed by an intravenous infusion of a longer-acting ASD such as phenytoin, fosphenytoin, phenobarbital, valproate, lacosamide, or levetiracetam (115–117). If the first agent is unsuccessful in treating SE, a second drug (often one of the other intravenous ASDs) is used frequently (120). Often, adjunctive use is made of enterally administered carbamazepine, topiramate, or other ASDs that are unavailable in intravenous form.

If SE continues after the first ASD, a second ASD succeeds in stopping SE <10% of the time (and even less often with subtle or purely electrographic SE) (17,121). At this point, SE is considered refractory, and most experts move on to more definitive or "aggressive" treatment with continuous intravenous ASDs (115).

Common causes of treatment failure include failure to diagnose the cause or underlying etiology (which must be treated), misdiagnosis in the case of psychogenic nonepileptic seizures, inadequate dosing of the initial ASD (122), and failure to maintain adequate ASD therapy after the initial treatment—leading to a relapse of SE, a common complication and often one signifying or predicting a worsened outcome (123).

5.6. Refractory Status Epilepticus

Most cases of SE respond to appropriate use of ASDs, but some cases become refractory to treatment. The primary causes of refractory status epilepticus (RSE) are similar to those of SE overall, including stroke or central nervous system tumor (20%), epilepsy-related (20%), toxic-metabolic encephalopathy (19%), central nervous system infection (19%), hypoxia-ischemia (12%), and traumatic brain injury (5%) (124). The minimal duration of seizure activity to define RSE has varied from unspecified to 2 hours, but most epileptologists now use the term *refractory* without regard to temporal duration. Rather, RSE is SE that persists despite adequate doses of an initial intravenous benzodiazepine and an adequate loading dose of a second, longer-acting intravenous ASD. It is important to stress that these intravenous ASDs must be administered promptly and in adequate doses (104,117,122).

The prevalence of RSE varies from 10% to >30% of all SE cases, depending on definitions (104,117,124). In the VA Cooperative Study of GCSE treatment, RSE, defined as 10 minutes of seizure activity continuing after two ASDs, occurred in

38% of 384 patients with overt GCSE and 82% of 134 patients with "subtle" GCSE (17). In a retrospective study of all types of SE, RSE (defined as lasting >60 minutes, with failure of two ASDs) occurred in 31% of 83 episodes of SE in 74 patients (104). RSE was more common in patients with nonconvulsive SE (88% vs. 26% with other forms of SE) and focal motor SE. In children, ~40% of SE episodes become RSE, defined as 60 minutes of seizures unresponsive to two ASDs (125). In one series of ICU patients (with SE identified and treated quickly) SE became refractory in 25% and was fatal in 21%; continuous SE had a higher case-fatality rate than intermittent SE (126). A prospective study of SE in adults in a tertiary center found that 23% of SE cases became refractory (127).

Patients with *particularly* prolonged and refractory SE have been labeled as having "malignant" SE (128), or "super-refractory status epilepticus"—that is, SE that continues or recurs 24 hours or more after the onset of "anesthetic" therapy (usually consisting of midazolam, pentobarbital, or propofol), including those cases in which SE recurs upon reduction or withdrawal of "anesthesia" (129). Many cases of super-refractory SE occur in young adults with encephalitis or SE of an unknown cause, usually following GCSE with a continuation clinically or electrographically (128–131). They remain in RSE or relapsing and remitting SE for up to weeks. This "new-onset refractory status epilepticus" (NORSE) (132) overlaps with "febrile infection-related epilepsy syndrome" (FIRES), usually described in children (133). Many cases appear to have an inflammatory or autoimmune etiology, but the precise agent or associated antibody is often impossible to determine (134).

Malignant SE and NORSE (often the same illness) have mortality rates often exceeding 30% (124,135). Even among survivors there is major long-term morbidity such that no more than about one fourth of all patients return to their previous, normal baseline function (136). Similarly, the prognosis for most patients treated with prolonged courses of pentobarbital or other aggressive treatment for RSE is dismal, with the very high mortality usually attributed to the almost invariably severe underlying etiology (123,124,137). Nevertheless, there are several reports of critically ill patients surviving SE (most of the episodes NCSE), lasting over a month (138–141), and recovery can be good, depending on the etiology (138). Postanoxic SE, on the other hand, is a fatal condition in almost all cases; therapeutic hypothermia may help to save some patients, especially if brainstem reflexes, somatosensory evoked potentials, and some reactivity of the EEG background are preserved (142). The persistence of electrographic SE following anoxia predicts an outcome even worse than that from the anoxia alone (143). A longer duration of SE is rarely a good sign, but it is also unwarranted to conclude that the situation is hopeless when SE has continued for hours or days, especially if the cause is relatively more benign (144).

5.7. Treatment of Refractory Status Epilepticus

For patients with RSE, ICU admission and mechanical ventilation are necessary. Treatment usually begins with a benzodiazepine followed by a longer-acting ASD (145), but patients with refractory and super-refractory SE usually require more definitive treatment, typically with continuous intravenous infusions of medications frequently labeled as "coma-inducing" or "anesthetic": midazolam, pentobarbital (or often thiopental in Europe), or propofol (116,128,146,147). In one meta-analysis, pentobarbital had a lower incidence of short-term treatment failure, breakthrough seizures, and need for another drug but a higher incidence of hypotension (124). The study concluded that pentobarbital was more effective in short-term seizure control but was associated with more adverse effects, without improved outcome. "Anesthetic" treatment should generally be continued for days, or at least for 24 hours after seizures stop, and then tapered gradually, with concurrent EEG monitoring (115,116,129).

As noted above, use of these major sedating drugs is associated with poorer outcomes. This is usually attributed to the severe underlying illnesses causing RSE (19,124), but the side effects of the medications and the prolonged ICU courses with which they are also associated may contribute to the morbidity and mortality (101,110). These medications may be necessary in refractory GCSE and its nonconvulsive continuation, but not always for other forms of SE.

A few patients require treatment with inhaled anesthetics, usually isoflurane and desflurane, typically used to produce a burst-suppression pattern (148). There has been increasing interest in the glutamatergic NMDA antagonist ketamine (in part because GABA-inhibiting drugs appear to lose efficacy as SE continues), but experience is limited (149,150). In cases of known or suspected autoimmune etiology, several immunosuppressive treatments are appropriate (134,151,152).

Many cases of RSE are difficult to treat, but most yield eventually to intravenous medications, at times augmented with enteral ASDs. There are also infrequent cases, sometimes of focal RSE from focal cortical lesions (such as cortical maldevelopments), that are amenable to surgical treatment. Typically, the seizure focus is identified by neuroimaging or electrocorticography (153), although this can be difficult. When scans are normal, surgical localization may be guided by ictal single photon emission computed tomography (SPECT) (154). In one series of 10 children with focal RSE (all with focal imaging abnormalities) who failed to respond to at least 2 weeks of high-dose suppressive therapy, SE was terminated by surgery in all, and 7 of 10 became seizure-free (22). Surgery may consist of focal resection of the epileptogenic zone; wider, lobar or even multilobar resections, even to the point of functional or anatomical hemispherectomy; occasional larger operations such as corpus callosotomy (155) and hemispherectomy, the last frequently in cases of devastating epilepsies of childhood, including Rasmussen's encephalitis; and multiple subpial transections (156), with or without focal resections (157).

5.8. EEG Use in Refractory Status Epilepticus

EEG is not necessary to make a diagnosis of GCSE, but if a patient does not awaken quickly following treatment, an explanation must be sought. In the VA Cooperative study, only 17% of patients with overt GCSE (and none with "subtle" GCSE) regained normal alertness within 12 hours of treatment (17). Importantly, failure to recover may be explained by the electrographic persistence of seizure activity (i.e., NCSE—which most epileptologists consider a continuation of GCSE and warranting urgent treatment).

As GCSE progresses, seizure manifestations become subtle or completely absent, and clinical assessment (e.g., cessation of motor activity) is inadequate in determining treatment effect. It is often impossible to distinguish whether GCSE has entered a postictal phase or if the lack of recovery is due to continuing SE. Both are possible.

Electrographic seizures lasting <30 minutes occur in about half of patients after treatment for GCSE (18). For patients with RSE or persistently impaired mental status, EEG alone can distinguish patients who are in drug-induced coma from the 14% to 20% of patients with continued nonconvulsive seizure activity (18). Patients who have received long-acting neuromuscular paralyzing agents also require EEG for accurate diagnosis and management.

Several recent guidelines and consensus statements highlight the critical role of continuous EEG monitoring in the diagnosis of ongoing SE (usually NCSE), particularly in those patients with persistently altered mental status after control of clinically evident GCSE or other seizures (115,158,159). Continuous EEG recording should be initiated as quickly as possible in suspected NCSE, optimally within 1 hour (115).

After diagnosis, and during prolonged intensive treatment with continuous intravenous ASDs, continuous EEG is essential to assess the effectiveness of that treatment and to recognize later seizure activity and manage its retreatment (115,158,159). Continuous EEG is essential to watch for relapse of nonconvulsive seizures or NCSE, which is not rare, especially in the first 24 hours (18). Relapse occurs in up to 69% of patients when continuous intravenous ASDs are tapered (135). In a retrospective study of RSE treatment, nonconvulsive seizures were found in 18% of patients within the first 6 hours of intravenous midazolam infusion, and breakthrough seizures occurred in 56% of patients later; they were clinically undetectable (i.e., purely electrographic) in 89% (135).

Electrographic seizures during continuous EEG predict a relapse of clinical seizures and SE (123) and usually warrant an increase in ASD treatment. Most epileptologists retreat with higher doses of definitive treatment, or for longer at doses that were successful earlier, and then have more ASDs (or higher levels of other ASDs) on board for the next attempt at tapering. This can lead to a long ICU course. Clearly, these seizures cannot be suppressed unless they are detected. Isolated epileptiform discharges, however, do not appear to necessitate more treatment (160).

Continued or recurrent SE should be suppressed for some time, usually 12 to 24 hours (129,158,159) or more (115) (especially during definitive treatment with midazolam, pentobarbital, or propofol) to ensure the absence of electrographic (and, of course, clinical) seizures. Nevertheless, the optimal electroclinical goal of treatment (simple cessation of seizures; both clinical and electrographic seizure control; or a certain degree of suppression of cerebral activity—often a burst-suppression pattern [Fig. 20.4]) has never been studied well prospectively. One retrospective study of patients with RSE found that patients whose EEGs were suppressed with pentobarbital to the

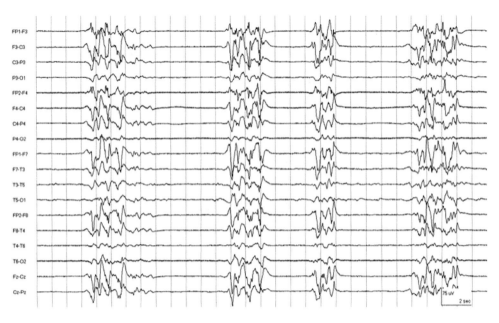

Figure 20.4. Burst-suppression EEG in a 15-year-old boy with RSE, after treatment with pentobarbital.

point of a "flat" background did better than those with a burst-suppression pattern, but three other patients whose EEGs showed simply freedom from seizures also survived (160). The study was retrospective, and patients thought more likely to survive may have been treated more intensively. Another study found no clear difference in outcome depending on the depth of EEG suppression (161).

In a meta-analysis, patients treated with the goal of EEG background suppression (mostly with pentobarbital) had a 4% likelihood of breakthrough seizures versus 53% for patients treated to control clinical and electrographic seizures only (mostly with midazolam or propofol) (124). Patients treated to EEG background suppression had a 76% likelihood of significant hypotension versus 29% for those treated to suppress seizures only. Whatever the depth of suppression, mortality was 48%, always attributed to the severity of the underlying illness causing SE. This controversy in EEG endpoints for SE treatment is reflected in recent guidelines, which do not endorse specific background-suppression goals (115,158,159).

The duration of treatment (and monitoring with continuous EEG) is also inadequately studied. Many investigators have used 12 to 24 hours of seizure or EEG suppression and then a taper of medication, typically over 12 to 24 hours (129), but several trials of midazolam have been shorter (124). One study of patients on pentobarbital raised the possibility that a prolonged period of seizure and EEG suppression could be beneficial (160).

During treatment of RSE, EEG should be reviewed immediately, and then periodically until SE is terminated or a burst-suppression record is induced with continuous intravenous ASDs (115,158,159). Use of further EEG monitoring is dictated by the patient's condition. If seizures are suppressed, less frequent evaluation may be sufficient, while continued or recurrent seizures require more intensive monitoring. Optimally, continuous EEG monitoring should be performed and reviewed from the time aggressive therapy (i.e., general anesthesia) is started, until seizures are stopped and the patient returns to normal consciousness, or until electrographic seizures are controlled for 24 hours (115,158,159). If continuous EEG is not available, EEGs might be repeated every 6 to 12 hours, until seizure activity does not return, but this practice is likely to miss almost all nonconvulsive seizures.

EEG findings can also help to predict outcome after SE. After carotid artery distribution strokes, subarachnoid hemorrhage, meningitis, encephalitis, or closed head injury, a diagnosis of SE increases the mortality rate above that associated with the precipitating event itself (162). There are persistent "ictal" discharges (rhythmic spikes, sharp waves, or spike-wave discharges), lasting 10 seconds to minutes, in 48% of patients after control of GCSE (18). Discharges lasting >30 minutes are associated with higher mortality rates, even after controlling for age and etiology of SE. Delayed epileptiform discharges occurring >30 minutes after SE has been controlled completely, however, did not worsen outcome. Patients with normal EEGs after SE had no significant morbidity or mortality.

Periodic lateralized epileptiform discharges (PLEDs) after SE are associated with an increased mortality, typically attributed to more severe etiologies (69,163). The presence of generalized periodic epileptiform discharges late in SE was associated with poor outcome in one study (69) but not in another (164). Burst-suppression patterns are also associated with worse outcomes, whether pharmacologically induced or due to hypoxia (19,163). In children older than 2 years, lack of background reactivity after SE portended a poorer prognosis (165). In a recent study of 120 consecutive adult patients with SE, only the absence of a posterior dominant rhythm and absent or abnormal sleep patterns were significantly associated with outcome, after correction for known clinical predictors of mortality, including etiology and SE severity (166).

Recording EEGs in the ICU is fraught with numerous difficulties (167) (see also next chapter). Patients are, by definition, critically ill and may need to be moved by nursing staff, producing plentiful artifact during EEG, and electrodes are more likely to become disconnected. Machinery in the ICU, including bed equipment, ventilators, fluid infusion pumps, and other monitors, can interfere with EEG recording by introducing electrical artifact. Also, patients are often sedated with benzodiazepines, barbiturates, general anesthesia, and other medications, with their own effects, often obscuring EEG findings or even suppressing EEG rhythms entirely. Head injury introduces additional challenges, including lacerations, surgical bandages, skull defects, subgaleal fluid collections, and edema, plus dressings, drains, and shunts, all of which can reduce the voltage recorded from the underlying brain and distort waveform morphologies. Continuous EEG lasting days requires significantly more attention from the EEG technologist to maintaining integrity of EEG leads than does routine EEG recording on cooperative patients.

6. FOCAL MOTOR STATUS EPILEPTICUS

6.1. Focal Status Epilepticus

Focal status epilepticus (FSE) has impressively varied manifestations, ranging from readily recognized focal motor seizures to focal sensory and aphasic seizures that remain markedly underdiagnosed. FSE without impairment of consciousness or abnormal movements appears relatively infrequent, but it may remain under-recognized due to the lack of noticeable clinical findings. The clinical manifestations of simple partial status epilepticus reflect ictal involvement of discrete brain regions, such as motor, sensory, special sensory, autonomic, psychic, language, or other cognitive function; its diagnosis requires preserved consciousness (168). The incidence of simple partial status epilepticus has been estimated as no more than 10 cases per million population per year (169). This chapter considers examples of FSE with motor manifestations; those without motor phenomena are considered in the chapter on nonconvulsive status.

There are many causes of FSE. Vascular (e.g., stroke, hemorrhage, or vasculitis) and infectious (e.g., encephalitis) are the most common, but mass lesions, trauma, multiple sclerosis, and, rarely, mitochrondrial or degenerative disorders can be responsible (170,171). Increasingly, with better imaging, focal cortical dysplasias are being recognized as the cause (154). Occasionally, benign idiopathic (genetic-based) focal epilepsies, such as rolandic epilepsy, lead to SE (172). Medication and metabolic changes may precipitate an episode, presumably with an underlying focal lesion.

Many cases of focal SE occur in the setting of acute stroke—in one series causing 41% of all cases of SE, and 61% in the elderly (99). In another series, 5% of stroke patients had new seizures, one fifth of these SE (173). These patients had a high mortality rate, just over 50%. In another series, the most common cause (75%) of FSE was stroke, and most patients had a history of epilepsy; all except for one with aphasic SE had motor-predominant seizures, and about half had *epilepsia partialis continua* (EPC) (174). The median duration of SE was 4 hours, but three patients had EPC continuing for weeks. Duration did not correlate with outcome, which was determined primarily by the underlying cause.

The morbidity and mortality of focal SE are determined largely by etiology. Among 47 FSE patients, acute strokes caused the only poor (fatal) outcome, in four patients (174). Persistent morbidity occurred in another 10 patients, attributed to the underlying lesion (usually stroke) in almost all. One study found a synergistic (for the worse) effect of acute stroke and SE in 83 patients (99). Rarely, FSE becomes extremely refractory and even life-threatening and necessitates surgical treatment (e.g., some cases of FSE due to focal cortical dysplasias) (154).

In a large epidemiologic study, SE with focal features had the same mortality as generalized SE (20–30%) (106), but this database included (relatively benign) absence SE in the generalized group and patients with secondarily generalized convulsive SE in the focal group. For simple partial status epilepticus without motor manifestations, there is no evidence of mortality or long-term morbidity.

6.2. The EEG of Focal Status Epilepticus

In focal seizures, the EEG may be normal or show nonspecific changes such as focal slowing. In other patients, a variety of ictal patterns may occur, such as focal high-frequency discharges, rhythmic waveforms with evolving morphology, and repetitive epileptiform discharges (Fig. 20.5) (70,170,175). Still, only 20% to 35% of simple partial seizures have an ictal electrographic correlate detectable by scalp EEG (176), usually either because a limited volume of brain tissue is involved or because the focus is located in mesial or inferior brain regions.

Focal SE may show discrete electrographic seizures with widespread fields, with regional, multiregional, or hemispheric ictal patterns. Although temporal lobe seizures are most common in chronic focal epilepsy, seizures in focal SE are often extratemporal, perhaps reflecting the varied location of acute brain injuries commonly causing focal SE (177). Seizure activity may be either continuous or discontinuous (53). More than half of focal SE cases are discontinuous, with repetitive discrete seizures showing evolving frequencies of 2 to 6 Hz, lasting 30 to 60 seconds or more (70,177). The background EEG activity between seizures is often slow and disorganized with voltage attenuation and loss of faster frequencies. Periodic discharges, lateralized periodic discharges (LPDs) and generalized periodic discharges (GPDs), are often present, particularly in patients with acute brain injuries (19). Although clinical manifestations of a seizure may be focal, the EEG may show generalized discharges later, and an EEG initiated during the course of SE may be unable to distinguish between focal and generalized SE.

6.3. Epilepsia Partialis Continua

EPC—focal motor SE with very prolonged jerking activity—has been defined as "clonic muscular twitching repeated at fairly regular intervals in one part of the body for a period of days or weeks" (178). It includes continuous or nearly continuous, relatively slow (every 0.5–2 seconds), often somewhat irregular, clonic jerking motions of groups of muscles on one side of the body, often both agonist and antagonist simultaneously, and often affecting the upper body more than the lower

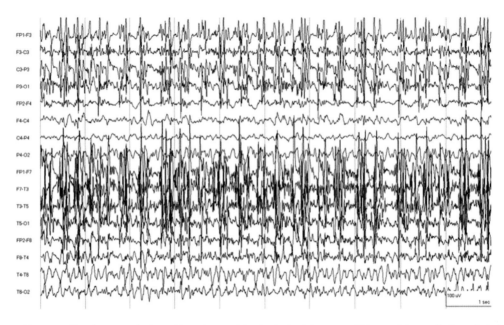

Figure 20.5. *A 78-year-old woman with colon cancer had repetitive seizures originating in the right temporal lobe, evolving gradually to clonic jerking of the left face and neck. These seizures occurred every 5 to 10 minutes for >12 hours, gradually increasing in duration, becoming focal motor SE. This EEG is from a period of 3 hours of continuous seizure activity. Rhythmic epileptiform activity is seen in the right posterior temporal region, with contralateral EMG artifact from the left face, and with neck muscle clonus.*

(178). EPC can be remarkably persistent, with episodes lasting days, weeks, or even years (179). It is readily diagnosed clinically because of its prominent and long-lasting motor manifestations. While EPC has become close to a synonym for focal motor SE, it is this prolonged continuous jerking activity that is EPC, while repetitive isolated discrete seizures are usually termed simply focal motor SE. The prevalence of EPC is estimated to be under one patient per million population in the United Kingdom (180).

EPC was described by Kozhevnikov in 1895 in cases of Russian spring-summer encephalitis, which included spreading focal motor seizures (181). Most cases involved children, often appearing months after a presumed infectious illness and with continuation for years. Similar cases followed other encephalitides. EPC in the modern era is far more often the result of strokes, both hemorrhagic and ischemic, and other vascular lesions (including venous infarcts) in adults (171,178,179). Tumors are a very uncommon cause of new-onset EPC (182). Cortical migration abnormalities, or heterotopias, and other developmental abnormalities, are found increasingly and occasionally lead to refractory focal SE (154). Other causes include focal infections such as tuberculosis, syphilis, toxoplasmosis, and HIV, progressive multifocal leukoencephalopathy, tuberous sclerosis, subacute sclerosing panencephalitis, Sturge–Weber syndrome, perinatal injury, congenital abnormalities including cortical dysplasias, and trauma (180). Unusual causes include multiple sclerosis; mitochondrial disorders including mitochondrial encephalopathy with lactic acid and stroke-like episodes (MELAS) (183); and paraneoplastic syndromes (184). In children, Rasmussen's encephalitis is the characteristic cause of EPC.

In addition to laboratory studies to look for infectious and metabolic causes, all patients with new-onset EPC need to undergo magnetic resonance imaging to look for focal lesions.

There is usually an identifiable brain lesion, although it may be small. Fluid-attenuated inversion-recovery (FLAIR) sequences are often best at demonstrating the lesion (185). A particularly important cause for recognition and treatment is hypernatremia and nonketotic hyperglycemia, which may precipitate EPC especially in a patient with an earlier focal lesion, most often stroke (186). This EPC is usually treatable readily with correction of the serum glucose and volume status. EPC often occurs in patients with chronic neurologic illness and is often relatively stable clinically, and not always in need of urgent intervention.

6.3.1. PATHOPHYSIOLOGY

Most investigators conclude that EPC results from epileptic discharges in focal cortical, pyramidal neurons, often involving a relatively small area of the cortex near the rolandic region or motor strip. Small cortical lesions can produce EPC experimentally (187). Physiologic studies of EPC show cortical dysfunction (179,188,189), with the pathophysiology that of epileptogenic foci in hyperexcitable motor cortex (190). Focal cortical hyperexcitability can be demonstrated by correlation with focally enhanced somatosensory evoked potentials (145,146). Dysfunction in subcortical structures may also contribute (192); thalamic generation of EPC can occur and may act to prolong the EPC. Subcortical lesions may engender hyperexcitability of the overlying cortex, possibly through deafferentation (178,182,193).

EPC can be considered to take two forms (194). Type 1 arises from a focal, nonprogressive lesion (e.g., due to the classic Russian spring-summer encephalitis). Repetitive jerking tends to occur in a restricted group of muscles but can progress to complex partial seizures or generalized convulsions. Type 2 is associated with progressive brain lesions, and there is a greater variety of seizures and, occasionally, of muscle groups involved. Type 2 EPC may have multifocal motor activity and may be associated with other seizure types, more disturbance of the EEG background, and a progressive neurologic deficit, such as the hemiparesis of Rasmussen's syndrome (see below).

6.3.2. TREATMENT AND OUTCOME

The continued focal jerking of EPC is often refractory to ASD treatment (116). Valproate, clonazepam, and levetiracetam are common treatments, as are steroids. One review found that topiramate and levetiracetam were more helpful than were other ASDs (195). Intravenous immunoglobulin (IVIG) and plasma exchange are used increasingly (116). Resective surgery can be curative if the lesion is small enough, but that is not always the case (180). Larger resections and corpus callosotomy can be helpful at times (22,155). Multiple subpial transsections are another possibility when the epileptogenic area is in cortical structures and motor or language function is at risk from hemispherectomy (157,196,197). Occasionally, transcranial magnetic stimulation may help (198). EPC may also resolve without treatment (180). While EPC is often refractory, ASDs may help prevent more dangerous secondarily generalized convulsions.

The long-term prognosis for patients with EPC depends primarily on the underlying lesion or illness. It is often poor. Long-term morbidity of EPC in terms of weakness, sensory and visual loss, and language dysfunction is substantial, and many patients have severe cognitive deficits (180). In one series, nearly half the patients died over a follow-up averaging 3 years, usually because of the lesion causing EPC (179).

6.3.3. EEG

While EPC is a subtype of simple partial status epilepticus characterized by continuous motor seizures, the relationship between clinical manifestations and EEG findings is inconsistent. EPC is often associated with irregular discrete focal spikes, sharp waves, and sharp and slow-wave discharges, LPDs, or slow-wave activity, with a frequency of 0.5 to 3 Hz, centering on ~1 Hz (199) (Fig. 20.6). The discharges may wax and wane, paralleling changes in the intensity of clinical manifestations. Depending on the population studied, epileptiform discharges on scalp recordings contralateral to the motor manifestations may occur in most, or in a minority of, patients (179,180), presumably because the responsible lesions are small or, more likely, because of an "inconvenient" orientation of discharges with respect to the cortical surface. One series reported focal discharges on scalp EEG in only 22% of patients (180), but additional electrodes can show focal discharges in up to 71% (179). Discharges not seen on scalp EEGs may be more evident on corticography or other invasive recordings (189). Back-averaging of EEG time-locked to clinical myoclonus can demonstrate a relationship between scalp-recorded discharges and muscle jerks in 37% to 45% of patients (179,180). PLEDs are seen in 22% to 71% of patients (179,200).

The EEG background rhythm may remain normal in EPC, especially in areas farther from the lesion, but EPC is often associated with structural lesions that produce some focal slowing or attenuation of the EEG background, if not epileptiform discharges. Fewer than 10% of patients have completely normal EEGs (179); another 10% to 30% may show only subtle nonspecific findings (171,179,198). Clinically, the EEG is often surprisingly unrevealing, but it is not always necessary for management.

6.4. Rasmussen's Encephalitis

Rasmussen's encephalitis is itself uncommon, but it is a relatively common cause of EPC. It was first described at the

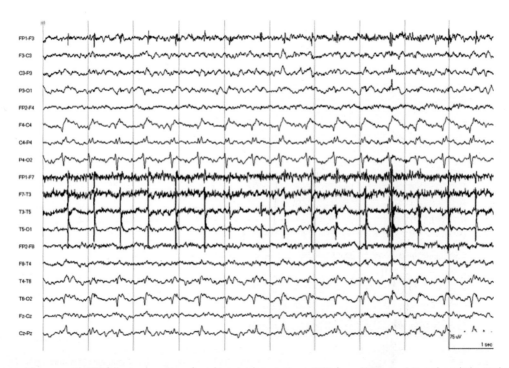

Figure 20.6. A 56-year-old woman with EPC following resection of a right parietal meningioma. EEG shows PLEDs at ~2 Hz in the right hemisphere, more posteriorly, with EMG artifact from rhythmic facial twitching over the left temporal channels.

Montreal Neurologic Institute in 1958, usually occurring in children and adolescents and almost always restricted to one hemisphere (201,202). It often follows some earlier, viral infection (203). It has an inflammatory basis and is posited to represent a persistent and chronic focal encephalitis of infectious or autoimmune basis (204,205). In most patients, Rasmussen's encephalitis is a progressive illness with neurologic deterioration, often with unremitting focal seizures, contralateral hemiparesis, and worsening cognitive function. The neurologic deficit may progress for years and then stabilize, with persistent EPC (Fig. 20.7). For unclear reasons, some cases stop progressing spontaneously, and occasionally the disease is self-limiting (204). On EEG, there is prominent focal slowing, correlating with the underlying and widespread inflammatory or immune lesion (206).

The EPC of Rasmussen's encephalitis includes jerking at 1 to 2 Hz of both agonist and antagonist muscles in the same area of the body. It is typically refractory to treatment with ASDs and persists for years. Benzodiazepines, valproate, and ethosuximide may be useful in treating myoclonic jerks and seizures, but even high doses of ASDs usually fail to suppress all seizures. Because Rasmussen's encephalitis appears related to glutamate receptor antibodies (197), immune therapies such as high-dose corticosteroids and IVIG have been attempted, with variable success in the short-term reduction of seizures, but the hemiparesis persists (208).

Resective surgery becomes necessary in many patients (205) and is usually the best treatment (197), especially for seizure control; sometimes there is improved neurologic function postoperatively. A minority of patients may have seizures

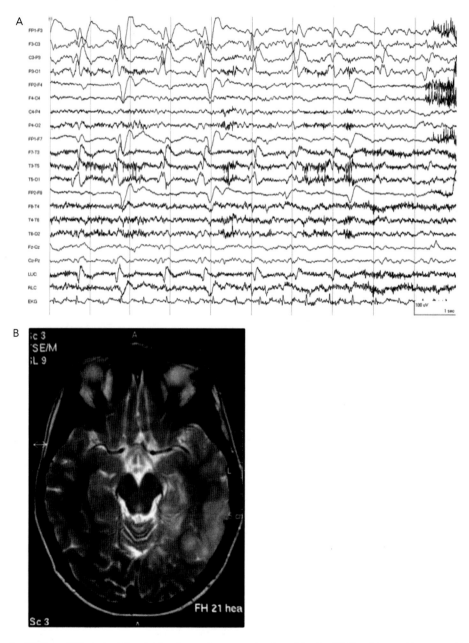

Figure 20.7. A: EEG showing PLEDs, or LPDs, in the left parietal and posterior temporal regions, following FSE in a 26-year-old woman with adult-onset Rasmussen's encephalitis. B: MRI following SE in the same patient with recurrent secondarily generalized seizures shows cortical T2 hyperintensity and focal thickening (edema) of the cortex on the left.

reduced or even eliminated by hemispherectomy, but this may entail major morbidity. Often, a partial hemispherectomy is the only helpful treatment (209). Multiple subpial transections, with or without focal resections, are a possible option (157,196,197).

7. PERIODIC LATERALIZED (EPILEPTIFORM) DISCHARGES

PLEDs were first described by Chatrian as spike or sharp-and-slow wave complexes, with repetition rates of ~1 to 2 Hz (200). They are surface-negative bi-, tri-, or polyphasic discharges consisting of spike, sharp, or polyspike components, with variable following slow-wave complexes lasting 60 to 600 msec (mean 200 msec), of 50 to 150 uV (occasionally up to 300 uV), usually recurring at 0.5 to 2 Hz (ranging from 0.2 to 3 Hz); occasionally, intervals are up to 10 sec (Fig. 20.8). Discharges are broadly distributed over most of one hemisphere and may reflect to the opposite hemisphere as well. Between discharges, the background activity is usually markedly attenuated and slow. EEG waveform morphologies stay fairly constant for a given patient and EEG, but the discharge frequency may decline with time, and most PLEDs resolve within 1 to 2 weeks (200). Rarely, they persist for months or even years (210). The equivalent terminology offered by the American Clinical Neurophysiology Society is "lateralized periodic discharges" (LPDs) an attempt to not specify whether these waveforms are related to clinical epilepsy (211); the terms are interchangeable.

PLEDs, or LPDs, occur most commonly after acute large structural destructive lesions such as stroke (the most common cause), tumor, or infection, but also in chronic seizure disorders and static lesions (210). One series of 147 cases of PLEDs found the etiology to be stroke in 27%, anoxia or old stroke in 12% each, infection 8%, tumor in 7%, and "other" in 34% (212). Patients are often obtunded, with focal neurologic deficits and often focal motor seizures. EPC is common. Clinical seizures occur in at least 80% of patients with PLEDs, often before the EEG is obtained, and electrographic seizures are present in even higher proportions. Many had prior SE (212,213). PLEDs seen on continuous EEG monitoring are associated with clinical seizures in ~30% to 50% of cases (19,214). Half of patients without prior epilepsy who survive the acute illness develop long-term epilepsy (215).

Most electroencephalographers do not consider PLEDs to be "ictal" (i.e., a manifestation of ongoing seizures or SE), at least at the time of the EEG recording (200,215,216). They are often considered "the terminal phase of status epilepticus" (212). Nevertheless, PLEDs are highly associated with clinical seizures and may lie somewhere along an "ictal–interictal continuum" (217). PLEDs may also occur on limited segments of an EEG (e.g., 20–30 minutes) with definite electrographic seizures later in the same recording (218) (Fig. 20.9A, B), indicating that they may not be "ictal" when seen but are recorded in patients who have clear seizures at other times (212). Seizures typically begin with rhythmic fast activity, sometimes with a field distinct from that of underlying PLEDs; the PLEDs may then disappear. Patients with "PLEDs plus," or LPDs+ (with lower-voltage rhythmic epileptiform discharges, or other rhythmic patterns between the higher-voltage periodic sharp waves) (219) (Figs. 20.9 and 20.10), or PLEDs with intermittent electrographic seizures are more likely to have clinically evident epileptic seizures (see Fig. 20.9B) and should be considered for more vigorous treatment with ASDs.

Periodic discharges are generally considered ictal if they occur consistently with stereotyped clinical behavior that

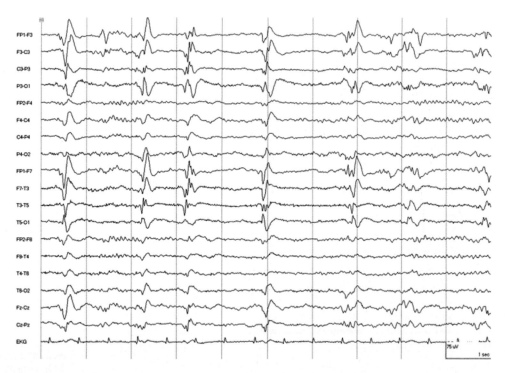

Figure 20.8. Left hemisphere PLEDs in a 72-year-old woman following a left middle cerebral artery territory stroke.

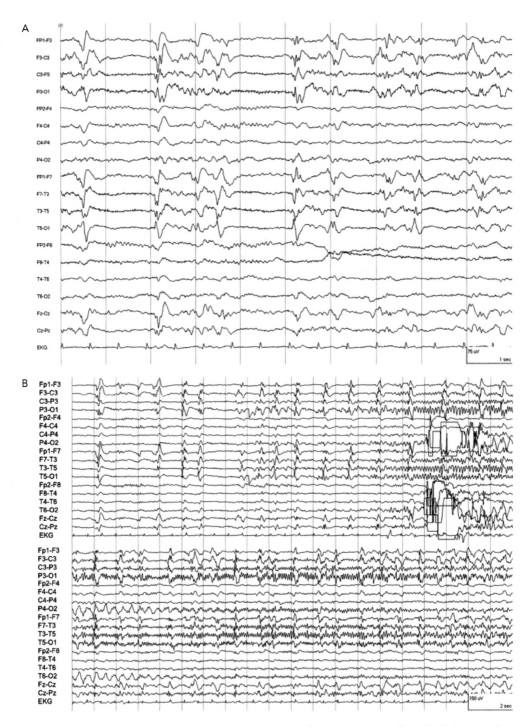

Figure 20.9. A: Same patient as in Figure 20.8. Later EEG shows "PLEDs plus" (or LPDs+), a faster repetition rate of periodic discharges with intervening faster frequency patterns. B: Same patient; periodic discharges evolving into a focal left hemisphere seizure.

appears epileptic. More rapid discharges (at least 1.5 Hz and certainly >2 Hz) would also be interpreted as representing seizures (and, if prolonged enough, SE) by most EEG-ers. In a patient with confusion, PLEDs or bilateral independent pseudoperiodic lateralized epileptiform discharges (BiPLEDs), or BiLPDs (bilateral independent LPDs), are likely to be ictal if the EEG discharges resolve and clinical symptoms improve after benzodiazepine treatment. Also, some studies have found focal hyperperfusion on SPECT scans (220,221) or evidence of focally increased metabolic activity on PET at the time of the

PLEDs (222), suggesting that PLEDs may be ictal (i.e., the sign of ongoing seizures) in those cases.

Sometimes PLEDs are definite signs of seizures. One report of seven patients described recurrent confusional episodes associated with PLEDs (223). There were no structural lesions, and EEG discharge intervals were as long as 4 sec. Clinical deficits resolved, with slowing of EEG discharges, spontaneously or in response to benzodiazepines. Carbamazepine appeared to prevent recurrences, but patients relapsed when it was decreased. The authors considered PLEDs an "unusual status epilepticus of the elderly." Another group recorded PLEDs during clinically well-defined SE, with an EEG evolution in frequency and amplitude terminating in a more typical seizure pattern—with a favorable response to benzodiazepine treatment (224). They concluded that PLEDs was an ictal EEG pattern when there are appropriate clinical signs. PLEDs observed during EPC are certainly a manifestation of clinical seizures (225).

PLEDs may be seen during seizures or SE, and their clinical significance differs in individual cases. EEG findings must be discussed and interpreted in the clinical setting.

Similar discharges, bilateral independent pseudoperiodic lateralized epileptiform discharges (BiPLEDs), occur independently and asynchronously over the two hemispheres (226). Discharges over each hemisphere can have different amplitudes, fields, and repetition rates (Fig. 20.11). Background activity is often severely attenuated bilaterally. BiPLEDs, or BiLPDs, are typically due to anoxia (28%), central nervous system infections (28%), chronic seizure disorders (22%), or vascular causes, and are associated more often with impaired mental status (coma in 72% vs. 24%) and higher mortality rates (61% vs. 29%) than PLEDs, but focal seizures are less common (226). Generalized periodic epileptiform discharges (GPEDs, or GPDs), also considered ictal sometimes and interictal at other times, are discussed further in the next chapter.

8. MYOCLONIC STATUS EPILEPTICUS

Persistent myoclonus may or may not be epileptic in origin. Without evidence of an epileptic cause, it is typically (and probably best) labeled *status myoclonicus*, or sometimes *myoclonus status*. It includes prolonged, but frequently nonrhythmic, myoclonic jerking, usually of large amplitude, often involving the face, trunk, and limbs, but sometimes multifocal or asynchronous. The cause is usually an acute and severe encephalopathy, often anoxia or possibly metabolic disturbances such as renal failure (227). The EEG may show widespread slowing indicative of an encephalopathy and have no spikes or sharp waves correlating with the myoclonic jerks (Fig. 20.12). In more severe encephalopathies, there may be a burst-suppression pattern or periodic discharges.

Continuing myoclonic jerks with an EEG showing persistent rapid and rhythmic epileptiform discharges are persuasive for an epileptic origin, in which case the diagnosis is better termed myoclonic status epilepticus (MSE) (228). MSE is characterized by prolonged myoclonic jerking activity, by usual definition >30 minutes in duration. Myoclonus may be isolated to one particular muscle group or, particularly in the primary "idiopathic" generalized epilepsies, appear bilaterally and symmetrically, particularly in flexor muscle groups in the arms. Myoclonus may be rhythmic, but this is not uniform, even with generalized discharges on the EEG. Pathophysiologically, epileptic myoclonus is of the cortical reflex type (229).

MSE has a remarkable variety of causes, although clinical presentations may be similar from one to the next. The prognosis depends on the etiology (67,228). Although MSE is discussed in the convulsive SE chapter because movements are a prominent component of the SE, some myoclonic jerks are of minimal amplitude, and MSE can appear largely nonconvulsive clinically (230).

An insightful review of the different forms of MSE divides cases into those due to epilepsy itself and those symptomatic of other brain illnesses (231) (Table 20.2). The pure, or epileptic, forms include MSE occurring in the primary "idiopathic"

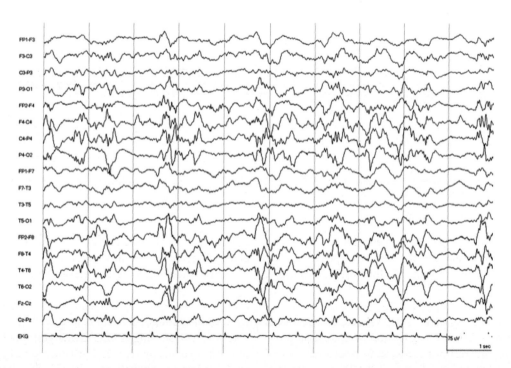

Figure 20.10. Another example of "PLEDs plus" (PLEDs with intervening faster components) in a 56-year-old man with HIV infection and a left temporal ring-enhancing lesion.

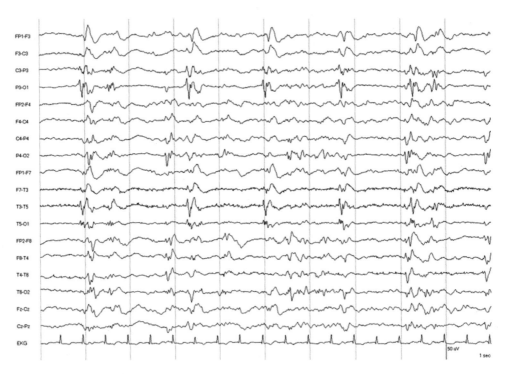

Figure 20.11. *A 68-year-old woman with herpes encephalitis and SE. EEG after control of clinical seizures showed bilateral independent pseudoperiodic lateralized epileptiform discharges (BiPLEDs), with independent and different discharge frequencies over the two hemispheres.*

generalized epilepsies in which myoclonus is a prominent manifestation both ictally and interictally, such as juvenile myoclonic epilepsy (Fig. 20.13), childhood and juvenile absence epilepsy, and grand mal seizures upon awakening (Fig. 20.14) (232,234). Most myoclonic seizures in the IGEs have a thalamocortical origin, stimulating a hyperexcitable cortex (234).

They are usually associated with generalized spike or polyspike discharges (234).

With MSE in the IGE syndromes, episodes may include myoclonic jerking activity up to five times a second (but often less frequently), particularly in proximal muscles, often with bilateral synchrony, and can last for hours—somewhat

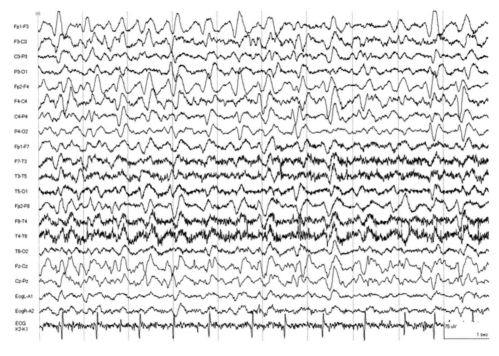

Figure 20.12. *Irregular generalized and multifocal sharp waves in an 87-year-man with acute renal failure, altered mental status, and frequent myoclonic jerking activity. The EEG sharp waves are less rhythmic than would be considered indicative of seizures by most electroencephalographers, and the background indicates an encephalopathy.*

TABLE 20.2. Myoclonic Status Epilepticus

Primary: in generalized epilepsy syndromes such as absence epilepsy, juvenile myoclonic epilepsy, and other myoclonic epilepsies
Secondary: in other epilepsy syndromes:
"Minor" epileptic status (of Brett)
Severe myoclonic epilepsy of infancy
MSE in myoclonic astatic epilepsy, Lennox–Gastaut syndrome
Epilepsy with myoclonic absences
SE with negative myoclonus, and brief atonic episodes
"Symptomatic" of acute neurologic illness (e.g., anoxia, injuries, encephalopathies)

(Adapted from Ohtahara (231))

surprisingly without necessarily affecting consciousness (232). Some patients have frequent prolonged myoclonic seizures with normal consciousness between individual myoclonic jerks (233), even with frequent 3- to 6-Hz epileptiform discharges on the EEG. Myoclonus can also consist primarily of eyelid myoclonia (235). The individual syndrome predicts the frequency of SE (56,236).

In juvenile myoclonic epilepsy, MSE may occur upon awakening and begin with irregular and isolated myoclonus with an accelerating or crescendo pattern, ending in SE. Patients with generalized myoclonic epilepsies (e.g., juvenile myoclonic epilepsy and some other IGEs) may go into MSE when medications are changed (228). Sleep deprivation is another common precipitant, and some ASDs (e.g., phenytoin and carbamazepine) may lead to an exacerbation of epilepsy, sometimes to the point of MSE (see Fig. 20.14A,B) (237,238). Overall, the

IGE syndromes lead to MSE relatively infrequently (with MSE occurring in only 1–2% of juvenile myoclonic epilepsy patients (239)), and the MSE is usually easy to treat and the long-term outcome good (179).

MSE also occurs in epilepsy syndromes other than the IGEs in which myoclonus is a less prominent feature of the interictal baseline (231). In these syndromes, the myoclonic jerks are more often asymmetric and asynchronous than in the IGE syndromes, and they may be of smaller amplitude and less rhythmic (231). These MSE causes include the progressive myoclonus epilepsies caused by storage diseases (Fig. 20.15) such as lipidoses and lipofuscinosis, and Lafora disease, Unverricht–Lundborg disease, and mitochondrial diseases (240). In the progressive myoclonus epilepsies the epilepsy tends to become worse with age and refractory to ASDs, and the likelihood of MSE increases (241). MSE also occurs in infectious illnesses such as encephalitis, and severe childhood epilepsies such as Dravet syndrome (242). MSE is more common in several of these forms of childhood myoclonic epilepsy than in the primary syndromes (231), and they are frequently refractory to ASDs.

Many episodes of MSE occur in very young children with early life genetic or structural deficits or inborn errors of metabolism and severe baseline encephalopathies. These include the Lennox–Gastaut syndrome (LGS), where MSE may be mixed with other forms of SE such as "myoclonic astatic" seizures with irregular facial and limb myoclonus, and epilepsy with myoclonic absences (Fig. 20.16). SE is not rare in LGS, but myoclonus is usually not the dominant feature. MSE in LGS is often associated with the slow spike and wave EEG patterns seen in atypical absence SE (see next chapter). Altered consciousness may be mixed with myoclonic jerking activity—which by itself

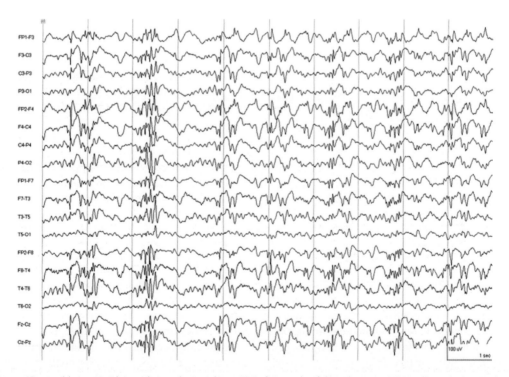

Figure 20.13. MSE in an 18-year-old woman with juvenile myoclonic epilepsy. EEG after a night of sleep deprivation showed irregular bursts of generalized spike-and-wave and polyspike-and-wave discharges for nearly 1 hour. Most bursts were associated with clinical myoclonic jerking activity.

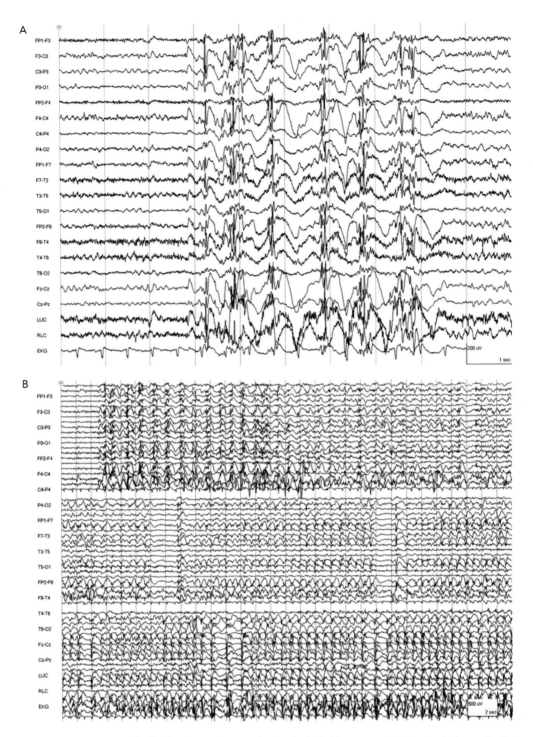

Figure 20.14. A: EEG during MSE in a 15-year-old girl with epilepsy with generalized tonic-clonic seizures on awakening. She had no earlier history of myoclonus but was admitted with nearly continuous myoclonic jerking after being started on carbamazepine. **B:** Same patient. After 20 minutes, the individual generalized myoclonic jerks evolve into rhythmic generalized clonic jerking (clonic status epilepticus).

does not necessarily affect consciousness. MSE also occurs in younger children with infantile spasms and hypsarrhythmia.

Severe myoclonic epilepsy of infancy or Dravet syndrome may include myoclonic jerking activity, but impairment of consciousness ("obtundation status"), sometimes prolonged, is usually the greater clinical problem (242). The irregular myoclonic activity often involves the face or limbs and may persist for hours. It usually presents in infancy but may lead to NCSE around the age of 2 years. The EEG may be normal at first but later includes focal or multifocal epileptiform discharges interictally, with eventual generalized spike-wave discharges on a very disturbed, slow, and irregular background (243). The long-term outcome is often poor, reflective of the underlying illness rather than because of the MSE itself.

MSE may occur as a manifestation of underlying encephalopathies unrelated to an earlier epilepsy syndrome, particularly in severe encephalopathies due to anoxia or metabolic derangements (Fig. 20.17) (227,228,244). The MSE, *per se,*

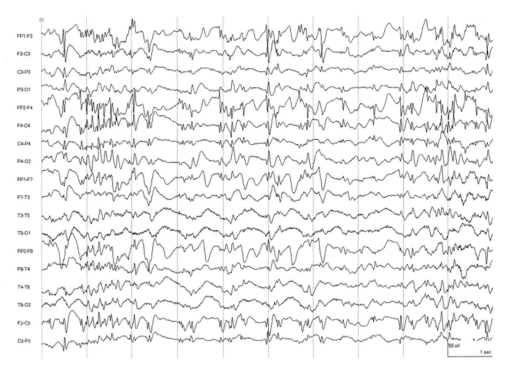

Figure 20.15. *MSE in a 32-year-old man with progressive myoclonus epilepsy due to Unverricht–Lundborg disease. The background activity is slow and disorganized, and EEG shows generalized and multifocal spikes and polyspikes. Clinically, the patient was more confused than at baseline and showed continuous fragmentary myoclonus.*

is usually less important than the devastation caused by the encephalopathy, particularly in the case of anoxia. MSE may be part of an acute postanoxic syndrome following cardiac arrest, often beginning 8 to 24 hours after the insult, with continuous irregular generalized or fragmentary myoclonic jerks (245). This MSE is often refractory to therapy and almost always has a poor outcome (143,228,246–249). Sometimes, the MSE may

be abolished by ASDs, but without improvement in the overall outcome.

MSE can also be caused by drugs, including pregabalin and tiagabine (250,251), even without prior epilepsy.

Chronic postanoxic action myoclonus is the Lance-Adams syndrome (252): segmental or generalized myoclonic jerks typically precipitated by action or stimulation (252,253). EEG

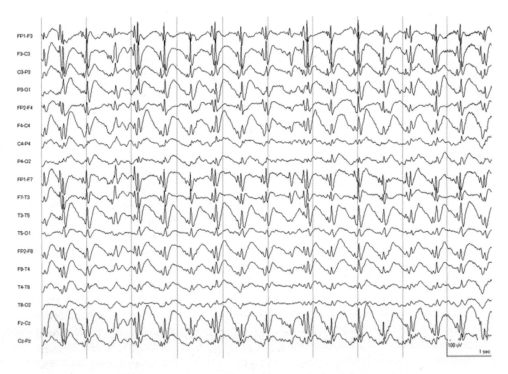

Figure 20.16. *Generalized polyspikes at ~2 Hz during MSE in a 16-year-old boy with Lennox–Gastaut syndrome.*

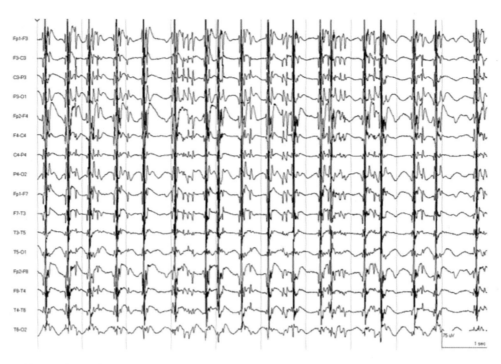

Figure 20.17. *A 50-year-old man with MSE after cardiac arrest. There are both generalized polyspikes and EMG artifact from myoclonic jerks. The EEG between myoclonic jerks shows severe diffuse voltage attenuation.*

patterns vary but often include irregular centrally maximal polyspike-and-wave discharges.

8.1. EEG

The EEG can be extremely helpful in distinguishing among different types and causes of MSE, whether related to a particular epilepsy syndrome (in which the EEG findings are often an important component of the syndrome and its diagnosis) or due to a nonepileptic encephalopathy (see Figs. 20.13–20.17). In the IGE syndromes, the EEG is often definitive and may show frequent generalized, frontally predominant spikes and polyspikes with faster frequencies of 4 Hz or so interictally, on a normal background (see Fig. 20.13). Spike discharges may precede the myoclonic jerking activity immediately (231).

Sometimes (e.g., in juvenile myoclonic epilepsy), frequent myoclonic jerking activity increases before a seizure. The frequency and duration of the EEG discharges may increase gradually over minutes to hours, paralleling the increasing severity and broader distribution of clinical myoclonic jerks, often culminating in a generalized convulsion (56). During seizures, there are generalized, frontally maximal irregular spike-and-wave or polyspike-and-wave discharges, sometimes correlating with clinical myoclonic jerks, occurring singly or in brief clusters (231). In MSE, the EEG often shows intermittent 1- to 2-sec bursts of epileptiform discharges, with an intervening normal background.

In MSE occurring in epilepsy syndromes other than the IGEs, the EEG background is often slow, reflecting the encephalopathy (see Fig. 20.15). Spike-wave discharges may come in irregular bursts, often with a slower, 2- to 2.5-Hz appearance. In both primary and secondary cases, there is often a poor correlation between the epileptiform discharges and the myoclonic

jerking activity. In symptomatic generalized epilepsies with MSE, such as Lennox–Gastaut, there is usually a background encephalopathy and more prolonged irregular spike-and-wave or polyspike-and-wave discharges, but with prominent intervening frontally maximal delta slowing (see Fig. 20.16). In MSE due to encephalopathies, the EEG might have no simple spike-wave discharges but often shows somewhat arrhythmic, slower spikes on a slow background. In postanoxic MSE, the EEG background shows severe voltage attenuation or a burst-suppression pattern, often with superimposed generalized periodic epileptiform discharges (228) (see Fig. 20.17). The characteristic suppressed (often nearly flat) background augurs poorly for prognosis.

8.2. Treatment

MSE in the IGE syndromes usually responds readily to ASDs (56); many episodes are interrupted expeditiously by benzodiazepines (231). Intravenous valproate may also be effective (254), and enteral ethosuximide is another possible treatment. Primary generalized epilepsies with prominent myoclonic components may be aggravated by use of inappropriate ASDs, particularly including sodium channel blocking agents such as carbamazepine and phenytoin, as well as those with putative GABA-ergic mechanisms, including gabapentin, tiagabine, and others (255,256).

Appropriate management of other forms of MSE depends overwhelmingly on etiology and can be very difficult. The MSE is often interruptible, but the prognosis corresponds to that of the underlying syndrome or illness. For MSE in the setting of anoxia, benzodiazepines and valproic acid are among the medications that can diminish the myoclonic jerking, but they seldom if ever alter the ultimate outcome.

8.3. Prognosis and Outcome

The prognosis in status myoclonicus (without evidence of epileptic pathophysiology) follows the etiology. It is particularly ominous after anoxia but also poor in metabolic encephalopathies and infection (227). In one study of 107 patients comatose after cardiac resuscitation, myoclonus status was present in 37% (245). All patients died—although 70% of resuscitated patients without myoclonus status also died. The authors argued that this was a reliable sign that anoxic status myoclonicus had a hopeless prognosis and should not be treated as epilepsy. There have been a few reports of patients recovering from status myoclonicus, but most of those were resuscitated almost immediately after primarily respiratory (rather than cardiac) failure, and several had a subsequent Lance-Adams syndrome, with action myoclonus, but with a reasonably favorable cognitive outcome (253,257,258).

The outcome of MSE is also determined strongly by the etiology. Patients with MSE in the IGE syndromes tend to respond to ASDs well, and the prognosis is usually good. In syndromes such as the myoclonic epilepsies of childhood, episodes can remit and the patient can return to baseline—but those baselines may be quite abnormal. In storage diseases and progressive illness, the SE may stop, but the underlying disease progresses. The prognosis is worst for patients with MSE due to an acute new illness and is particularly poor following anoxia (246). Anoxic MSE following cardiac arrest is nearly always fatal—determined by the anoxic damage, rather than by any epileptic phenomenon (143,247). Fewer than 5% of patients recover reasonably, although hypothermia may improve the prognosis somewhat (142,259).

9. CLONIC AND TONIC STATUS EPILEPTICUS

Clonic status epilepticus is relatively rare in adults. It is seen primarily in infants and children, particularly those with Lennox–Gastaut syndrome (260). Clinical manifestations are similar to those of GCSE but without a tonic phase, or with the tonic phase following the initial generalized clonic jerking. The repetitive clonic jerks usually involve the face and trunk and all limbs but may be asymmetric or irregular.

EEG patterns vary. Some show rhythmic bilateral bursts of high-amplitude delta slowing with intermixed spikes or polyspikes (12) (see Fig. 20.14), often occurring synchronously with the clonic jerking. As in GCSE, the EEG may be largely obscured by muscle and movement artifact.

Generalized tonic status epilepticus occurs predominantly in young patients with major neurologic and cognitive deficits or other severe encephalopathies from birth or early childhood (261), such as in the Ohtahara syndrome or in the Lennox–Gastaut syndrome (262). Tonic status epilepticus is rare in adults in the absence of other seizure types. Infrequently, tonic status epilepticus arises in patients with IGEs (263). Tonic seizures may be precipitated by benzodiazepines in children with Lennox–Gastaut syndrome and atypical absence seizures (264).

In clinically obvious cases of tonic status epilepticus there are usually brief (10–15 sec) tonic contractions of the face and axial musculature and often in proximal limb muscles, or in combinations of these, recurring frequently enough that a tonic posture is maintained, rather than with convulsions (261). Motor activity may be very subtle, showing only

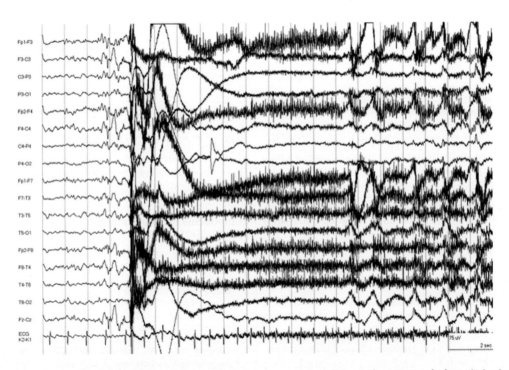

Figure 20.18. Tonic status epilepticus in a 48-year-old man with Lennox–Gastaut syndrome. Forty-eight hours after initiation of rufinamide, he developed recurrent tonic seizures every 5 minutes, without recovery to baseline between seizures. EEG showed a high-voltage generalized slow wave, followed by a generalized "electrodecremental" period with superimposed EMG activity.

mild tonic contractions of paraspinal musculature or upward deviation of the eyes. Tonic seizures usually last <10 sec but can recur hundreds of times in a day. Nocturnal tonic seizures are characteristic of Lennox–Gastaut syndrome (223). Tonic status epilepticus can be difficult to interrupt with ASDs (265); lacosamide may be helpful in some cases (266). Benzodiazepines may precipitate or worsen tonic status epilepticus in some cases (267,268). EEG may be necessary to make the diagnosis of tonic status epilepticus, given the frequently subtle presentations, especially in patients who already have neurologic abnormalities. It often shows widespread symmetric low-voltage, fast (20–30 Hz) activity initially, or very rapid spikes, but may also include periods of sudden background suppression or attenuation, generalized electrodecremental activity (voltage suppression), or brief runs of low-voltage generalized fast activity on a suppressed background (Fig. 20.18). The amplitude of the ictal discharges increases gradually and the frequency decreases to 10 to 20 Hz over the first several seconds of the seizure, sometimes followed by rhythmic generalized spikes (65).

SCORE EEG SOFTWARE

Further examples related to the topics addressed in this chapter can be found in the interactive online Niedermeyer Educational Platform. EEG recordings with illustrative examples can be opened and browsed. Features are marked and described using the SCORE EEG software. The users can see the features marked by experts, they can score these features themselves, and then compare them with the scorings of the experts.

The Niedermeyer Educational Platform can be accessed at: www.scoreEEG.com/academy

REFERENCES

1. Shorvon S. The concept of status epilepticus and its history. In: Shorvon S, ed. Status epilepticus: its clinical features and treatment in children and adults. Cambridge: Cambridge University Press, 1994:1–20.
2. XXV–XXVIth tablet of the Sakkiku cuneiform, 718–612 BC. British Museum; Kinnier Wilson JV, Reynolds EH. Translation and analysis of a cuneiform text forming part of a Babylonian treatise on epilepsy. Med Hist 1990;34:185–198.
3. Temkin O, ed. The falling sickness. Baltimore: Johns Hopkins Press, 1971:149.
4. Willis T. Pathologiae cerebri et nervosi generis specimen. In quo agitur de morbis convulsivis et de scorbuto, 1667, translated by S. Pordage, 1681. London: Dring. Cited in Shorvon S, ed. Status epilepticus: its clinical features and treatment in children and adults. Cambridge: Cambridge University Press, 1994:1–20.
5. Calmeil LF. De l'épilepsie, étudiée sous le rapport de son siege et de son influence sur la production de l'aliénation mentale. Paris: Thèse de Université de Paris, 1824.
6. Trousseau A. Lectures on clinical medicine delivered at the Hôtel Dieu, Paris, 1868 vol. 1, translated by Bazire, PV. London: New Sydenham Society.
7. Clark LP, Prout TP. Status epilepticus: a clinical and pathological study in epilepsy (An article in 3 parts.) Am J Insanity 1903/4; 60:291–306; 60:645–675; 61:81–108.
8. Treiman DM, Walton NY, Kendrick C. A progressive sequence of electroencephalographic changes during generalized convulsive status epilepticus. Epilepsy Res 1990;5:49–60.
9. Whitty CWM, Taylor M. Treatment of status epilepticus. Lancet 1949;254:591–594.
10. Gloor P. The work of Hans Berger. In: Cobb WA, ed., Appraisal and perspective of the functional explorations of the nervous system. Handbook of electroencephalography and clinical neurophysiology. Amsterdam: Elsevier Publishing Co., 1971: IA11–24.
11. Gastaut H. A propos d'une classification symptomatologique des états de mal épileptiques. In: Gastaut H, Roger J, Lob H, editors. Les états de mal épileptiques. Paris: Masson; 1967. p. 1–8.
12. Gastaut H. Classification of status epilepticus. In: Delgado Escueta AV, Wasterlain CG, Treiman DM, Porter RJ, eds. Status epilepticus: mechanisms of brain damage and treatment. Advances in Neurology, vol 34. New York: Raven Press; 1983:15–35.
13. Shorvon S. Definition, classification and frequency of status epilepticus. In: Shorvon S, ed. Status epilepticus: its clinical features and treatment in children and adults. Cambridge: Cambridge University Press, 1994:21–33.
14. Trinka E, Cock H, Hesdorffer D, Rossetti AO, Scheffer IE, Shinnar S, Shorvon S, Lowenstein DH. A definition and classification of status epilepticus. Report of the ILAE Task Force on Classification of Status Epilepticus. Epilepsia 2015;56:1515–1523.
15. Lombroso CT. The treatment of status epilepticus. Pediatrics 197453(4):536–540.
16. Leppik IE, Derivan AT, Homan RW, Ramsay RE, Patrick B. Double-blind study of lorazepam and diazepam in status epilepticus. JAMA 1983;249(11):1452–1454.
17. Treiman DM, Meyers PD, Walton NY, Collins JF, Colling C, Rowan AJ, Handforth A, Faught E, Calabrese VP, Uthman BM, Ramsay RE, Mamdani MB. A comparison of four treatments for generalized convulsive status epilepticus. N Engl J Med 1998;339:792–798.
18. DeLorenzo RJ, Waterhouse EJ, Towne AR, Boggs JG, Ko D, DeLorenzo GA, Brown A, Garnett L. Persistent nonconvulsive status epilepticus after the control of convulsive status epilepticus. Epilepsia 1998;39:833–840.
19. Claassen J, Mayer SA, Kowalski RG, Emerson RG, Hirsch LJ. Detection of electrographic seizures with continuous EEG monitoring in critically ill patients. Neurology 2004;62:1743–1748.
20. Thakur KT, Probasco JC, Hocker SE, Roehl K, Henry B, Kossoff EH, Kaplan PW, Geocadin RG, Hartman AL, Venkatesan A, Cervenka MC. Ketogenic diet for adults in super-refractory status epilepticus. Neurology 2014 (25);82:665–670.
21. Fisher R, Salanova V, Witt T, et al. Electrical stimulation of the anterior nucleus of thalamus for treatment of refractory epilepsy. Epilepsia 2010;51(5):899–908.
22. Alexopoulos A, Lachhwani DK, Gupta A, Kotagal P, Harrison AM. Resective surgery to treat refractory status epilepticus in children with focal epileptogenesis. Neurology 2005;64:567–570.
23. Commission on Epidemiology and Prognosis, International League Against Epilepsy. Guidelines for Epidemiologic Studies on Epilepsy. Epilepsia 1993;34:592–596.
24. DeLorenzo RJ, Hauser WA, Towne AR, Boggs JG, Pellock JM, Penberthy L, Garnett L, Fortner CA, Ko D. A prospective, population-based epidemiologic study of status epilepticus in Richmond, Virginia. Neurology 1996;46:1029–1035.
25. Lowenstein DH, Bleck T, Macdonald RL. It's time to revise the definition of status epilepticus. Epilepsia 1999;40:120–122.
26. Theodore WH, Porter RJ, Albert P, Kelley K, Bromfield E, Devinsky O, Sato S. The secondarily generalized tonic-clonic seizure: a videotape analysis. Neurology 1994;44:1403–1407.
27. DeLorenzo RJ, Garnett LK, Towne AR, Waterhouse EJ, Boggs JG, Morton L, Choudhry MA, Barnes T, Ko D. Comparison of status epilepticus with prolonged seizure episodes lasting from 10 to 29 minutes. Epilepsia 1999;40:164–169.
28. Shinnar S. Who is at risk for prolonged seizures? J Child Neurol 2007;22(suppl 5):14–20S.
29. Jenssen S, Gracely EJ, Sperling MR. How long do most seizures last? A systematic comparison of seizures recorded in the epilepsy monitoring unit. Epilepsia 2006;47(9):1499–1503.
30. Doberberger J, Risti J, Walser G, Kuchukhidze G, Unterberger I, Hofler J, Amann E, Trinka E. Duration of focal complex, secondarily generalized tonic-clonic, and primarily generalized tonic-clonic seizures—a video-EEG analysis. Epilepsy Behav 2015;49:111–117.
31. Chen JW, Naylor DE, Wasterlain CG. Advances in the pathophysiology of status epilepticus. Acta Neurol Scand 2007;115(suppl 4):7–15.
32. Kapur J, Macdonald RL. Rapid seizure-induced reduction of benzodiazepine and Zn 2+ sensitivity of hippocampal dentate granule cell GABA-A receptors. J Neurosci 1997;17:7532–7540.

33. Kapur J. Pathophysiology of nonconvulsive status epilepticus. In: Kaplan PW, Drislane FW, eds., Nonconvulsive status epilepticus. New York: Demos Medical Publishing, 2009:81–94.

34. Naylor DE, Liu H, Wasterlain CG. Trafficking of GABA(A) receptors, loss of inhibition, and a mechanism for pharamacoresistance in status epilepticus. J Neurosci 2005;25:7724–7733.

35. Goodkin HP, Yeh JL, Kapur J. Status epilepticus increases the intracellular accumulation of GABA receptors. J Neurosci 2005;25:5511–5520.

36. Goodkin HP, Joshi S, Mtchedlishvili Z, Brar J, Kapur J. Subunit-specific trafficking of GABA(A) receptors during status epilepticus. J Neurosci 2008;28(10):2527–2538.

37. Broomall E, Natale JE, Grimason M, Goldstein J, Smith CM, Chang C, Kanes S, Rogawski MA, Wainwright MS. Pediatric super-refractory status epilepticus treated with allopregnanolone. Ann Neurol 2014;76(6):911–915.

38. Bertram EH, Lothman EW. NMDA receptor antagonists and limbic status epilepticus: A comparison with standard anticonvulsants. Epilepsy Res 1990;5:177–184.

39. Wasterlain CG, Liu H, Mazarati AM, Baldwin RA, Shirasaka Y, Katsumori H, Thompson KW, Sankar R, Pereira de Vasconselos A, Mehlig A. Self-sustaining status epilepticus: a condition maintained by potentiation of glutamate receptors and by plastic changes in substance P and other peptides neuromodulators. Epilepsia 2000;41:134–143.

40. Fountain NB. Cellular damage and the neuropathology of status epilepticus. In: Drislane FW, ed., Status epilepticus, a clinical perspective. Totowa, NJ: Humana Press, 2005:181–193.

41. Williamson JM, Lothman EW. The effect of MK-801 on kindled seizures: implications for use and limitations as an antiepileptic drug. Ann Neurol 1989;26:85–90.

42. Mazarati AM, Wasterlain CG. N-methyl-D-aspartate receptor antagonists abolish the maintenance phase of self-sustaining status epilepticus in rat. Neurosci Lett 1999;265:187–190.

43. Mazarati A, Lu X. Regulation of limbic status epilepticus by hippocampal galanin type 1 and type 2 receptors. Neuropeptides 2005;39:277–280.

44. Lowenstein DH, Shimosaka S, So YT, Simon RP. The relationship between electrographic seizure activity and neuronal injury. Epilepsy Res 1991;10:49–54.

45. Bhatnagar M, Shorvon S. Genetic mutations associated with status epilepticus. Epilepsy Behav 2015;49:104–110.

46. Meldrum BS, Horton RW. Physiology of status epilepticus in primates. Arch Neurol 1973;28:1–9.

47. Meldrum BS, Brierley JB. Prolonged epileptic seizures in primates. Ischemic cell change and its relation to ictal physiological events. Arch Neurol 1973;28:10–17.

48. Meldrum BS, Vigouroux RA, Brierley JB. Systemic factors and epileptic brain damage. Arch Neurol 1973;29:82–87.

49. Lothman EW, Bertram EH, Bekenstein JW, Perlin JB. Self-sustaining limbic status epilepticus induced by "continuous" hippocampal stimulation: electrographic and behavioral characteristics. Epilepsy Res 1989;3:107–119.

50. DiGiorgio CM, Tomiyasu U, Gott PS, Treiman DM. Hippocampal pyramidal cell loss in human status epilepticus. Epilepsia 1992;33:23–27.

51. Knake S, Rosenow F, Vescovi M, Oertel WH, Mueller H-H, Wirbatz A, Katsarou N, Hamer HM. Incidence of status epilepticus in adults in Germany: a prospective, population-based study. Epilepsia 2001;42:714–718.

52. Coeytaux A, Jallon P, Galobardes B, Morabia A. Incidence of status epilepticus in French-speaking Switzerland. Neurology 2000;55:693–697.

53. Sadarangani M, Seaton C, Scott JAG, Ogutu B, Edwards T, Prins A, Gatakaa H, Idro R, Berkley JA, Peshu N, Neville BG, Newton CR. Incidence and outcome of convulsive status epilepticus in Kenyan children: a cohort study. Lancet Neurol 2008;7:145–150.

54. Logroscino G, Hesdorffer DC, Cascino G, Annegers JF, Hauser WA. Short-term mortality after a first episode of status epilepticus. Epilepsia 1997;38:1344–1349.

55. Hesdorffer DC, Logroscino G, Cascino GD, Hauser WA. Recurrence of afebrile status epilepticus in a population-based study in Rochester, Minnesota. Neurology 2007;69:73–78.

56. Shorvon S, Walker M. Status epilepticus in idiopathic generalized epilepsy. Epilepsia 2005;46:73–79.

57. Aminoff MJ, Simon RP. Status epilepticus: causes, clinical features, and consequences in 98 patients. Am J Med 1980;69:657–666.

58. Lowenstein DH, Alldredge BK. Status epilepticus at an urban public hospital in the 1980's. Neurology 1993;43:483–488.

59. Barry E, Hauser W. Status epilepticus: the interaction of epilepsy and acute brain disease. Neurology 1993;43:1473–1478.

60. Vignatelli L, Rinaldi R, Galeotti M, de Carolis P, D'Alessandro R. Epidemiology of status epilepticus in a rural area of northern Italy: a 2-year population-based study. Eur J Neurol 2005;12:897–902.

61. Treiman DM. Electroclinical features of status epilepticus. J Clin Neurophysiol 1995;12:343–362.

62. Janz D. Conditions and causes of status epilepticus. Epilepsia 1961;2:170–177.

63. Gastaut H, Broughton R. Epileptic seizures: clinical and electrographic features, diagnosis and treatment. Springfield, IL: Charles C. Thomas, 1972.

64. Niedermeyer E. Epileptic seizure disorders. In: Niedermeyer E, Lopes da Silva F., eds., Electroencephalography: basic principles, clinical applications, and related fields. 5th ed. Philadelphia: Lippincott Williams & Wilkins, 2005:505–619.

65. Roger J, Lob H, Tassinari CA. Status epilepticus. In: Vinken P, Bruyn G, eds., Handbook of clinical neurology, Vol. 15: The epilepsies. Amsterdam: North Holland Publishing Co., 1974:145–188.

66. Bragin A, Engel JJr, Wilson CL, Fried I, Mathern GW. Hippocampal and entorhinal cortex high-frequency oscillations (100–500 Hz) in human epileptic brain and in kainic acid-treated rats with chronic seizures. Epilepsia 1999;40:127–137.

67. Drislane FW, Schomer DL. Clinical implications of generalized electrographic status epilepticus. Epilepsy Res 1994;19:111–121.

68. Lowenstein D, Aminoff M. Clinical and EEG features of status epilepticus in comatose patients. Neurology 1992;42:100–104.

69. Nei M, Lee JM, Shanker VL, Sperling MR. The EEG and prognosis in status epilepticus. Epilepsia 1999;40:157–163.

70. Drislane FW, Blum AS, Schomer DL. Focal status epilepticus: clinical features and significance of different EEG patterns. Epilepsia 1999;40:1254–1260.

71. Waterhouse EJ, Garnett LK, Towne AR, Morton LD, Barnes T, Ko D, DeLorenzo RJ. Prospective population-based study of intermittent and continuous convulsive status epilepticus in Richmond, Virginia. Epilepsia 1999;40:752–758.

72. Fountain NB. Status epilepticus: risk factors and complications. Epilepsia 2000;41(suppl 2):23–30.

73. Boggs JG, Painter JA, DeLorenzo RJ. Analysis of electrocardiographic changes in status epilepticus. Epilepsy Res 1993;14:87–94.

74. Lothman E. The biochemical basis and pathophysiology of status epilepticus. Neurology 1990;40(suppl 2):13–23.

75. Simon RP. Physiologic consequences of status epilepticus. Epilepsia 1985;26(suppl 1):S58–66.

76. Brown JK, Husain IHMI. Status epilepticus. I: Pathogenesis. Dev Med Child Neurol 1991;35:3–17.

77. Singhal PC, Chugh KS, Gulati DR. Myoglobinuria and renal failure after status epilepticus. Neurology 1978;28(2):200–201.

78. Sutter R, Tschudin-Sutter S, Grize L, Fuhr P, Bonten MJ, Widmer AF, Marsch S, Rüegg S. Associations between infections and clinical outcome parameters in status epilepticus: a retrospective 5-year cohort study. Epilepsia 2012;53(9):1489–1497.

79. Devinsky O, Vezzani A, Najjar S, DeLanerolle NC, Rogawski MA. Glia and epilepsy: excitability and inflammation. Trends Neurosci 2013;36(3):174–184.

80. Cole AJ. Status epilepticus and periictal imaging. Epilepsia 2004;45(suppl 4):72–77.

81. Cianfoni A, Caulo M, Cerase A, Della Marca G, Falcone C, Di Lella GM, Gaudino S, Edwards J, Colosimo C. Seizure induced brain lesions: a wide spectrum of variably reversible MRI abnormalities. Eur J Radiol 2013;82(11):1964–1972.

82. Pohlmann-Eden B, Gass A, Peters CAN, Wennberg R, Bluemcke I. Evolution of MRI changes and development of bilateral hippocampal sclerosis during long lasting generalised status epilepticus. J Neurol Neurosurg Psychiatry 2004;75:898–900.

83. Maytal J, Shinnar S, Moshe SL, Alvarez LA. Low morbidity and mortality of status epilepticus in children. Pediatrics 1989;83:323–331.

84. Dodrill CB, Wilensky AJ. Intellectual impairment as an outcome of status epilepticus. Neurology 1990;40:(suppl 2):23–27.

85. Adachi N, Kanemoto K, Muramatsu R, Kato M, Akanuma N, Ito M, Kawasaki J, Onuma T. Intellectual prognosis of status epilepticus in adult patients: analysis with Wechsler Adult Intelligence Scale-Revised. Epilepsia 2005;46:1502–1509.

86. Shinnar S, Babb TL, Moshé SL, Wasterlain CG. Long-term sequelae of status epilepticus. In: Engel J, Pedley TA, eds., Epilepsy: a comprehensive textbook. 2nd ed. Philadelphia: Lippincott-Raven Publishers, 2008:751–759.

87. Hesdorffer D, Logroscino G, Cascino G, Annegers J, Hauser W. Incidence of status epilepticus in Rochester, Minnesota, 1965–1984. Neurology 1998;50:735–741.

88. Eriksson KJ, Koivikko MJ. Status epilepticus in children: aetiology, treatment, and outcome. Dev Med Child Neurol 1997;39:652–658.

89. Berg AT, Shinnar S. Do seizures beget seizures? An assessment of the clinical evidence in humans. J Clin Neurophysiol 1997;14:102–110.

90. Hauser WA, Rich SS, Annegers JF, Anderson VE. Seizure recurrence after a 1st unprovoked seizure: an extended follow-up. Neurology 1990;40:1163–1170.
91. Dham BS, Hunter K, Rincon F. The epidemiology of status epilepticus in the United States. Neurocrit Care 2014; 20:476–483.
92. Koubeissi M, Alshekhlee A. In-hospital mortality of generalized convulsive status epilepticus: a large US sample. Neurology 2007;69:886–893.
93. Vignatelli L, Tonon C, D'Alessandro R. Incidence and short-term prognosis of status epilepticus in adults in Bologna, Italy. Epilepsia 2003;44:964–968.
94. Logroscino G, Hesdorffer DC, Cascino G, Annegers JF, Hauser WA. Time trends in incidence, mortality, and case-fatality after first episode of status epilepticus. Epilepsia 2001;42:1031–1035.
95. Delanty N, French JA, Labar DR, Pedley TA, Rowan AJ. Status epilepticus arising de novo in hospitalized patients: an analysis of 41 patients. Seizure 2001;10:116–119.
96. DeLorenzo RJ, Towne AR, Pellock JM, Ko D. Status epilepticus in children, adults and the elderly. Epilepsia 1992;33(suppl 4):15–25.
97. Oxbury JM, Whitty CWM. Causes and consequences of status epilepticus in adults. A study of 86 cases. Brain 1971;94:733–744.
98. Hauser WA. Status epilepticus: epidemiologic considerations. Neurology 1990;40(suppl 2):9–13.
99. Waterhouse EJ, Vaughan JK, Barnes TY, Boggs JG, Towne AR, Kopec-Garnett L, DeLorenzo RJ. Synergistic effect of status epilepticus and ischemic brain injury on mortality. Epilepsy Res 1998;29:175–183.
100. Rossetti AO, Hurwitz S, Logroscino G, Bromfield EB. Prognosis of status epilepticus: role of aetiology, age, and consciousness impairment at presentation. J Neuro Neurosurg Psychiatry 2006;77:611–615.
101. Sokic DV, Jankovic SM, Vojvodic NM, Ristic AJ. Etiology of a short-term mortality in the group of 750 patients with 920 episodes of status epilepticus within a period of 10 years (1988–1997). Seizure 2009;18:215–219.
102. DeLorenzo RJ. Clinical and epidemiologic study of status epilepticus in the elderly. In: Rowan AJ, Ramsay RE, eds., Seizures and epilepsy in the elderly. Boston: Butterworth-Heinemann, 1997:191–205.
103. Logroscino G, Hesdorffer DC, Cascino GD, Annegers JF, Bagiella E, Hauser WA. Long-term mortality after a first episode of status epilepticus. Neurology 2002;58:537–541.
104. Mayer SA, Claassen J, Lokin J, Mendelsohn F, Dennis LJ, Fitzsimmons BF. Refractory status epilepticus. Frequency, risk factors, and impact on outcome. Arch Neurol 2002;59:205–210.
105. Scholtes FB, Renier WO, Meinardi H. Generalized convulsive status epilepticus: causes, therapy, and outcome in 346 patients. Epilepsia 1994;35:1104–1112.
106. Towne AR, Pellock JM, Ko D, DeLorenzo, RJ. Determinants of mortality in status epilepticus. Epilepsia 1994;35:27–34.
107. Drislane FW, Blum AS, Lopez MR, Gautam S, Schomer DL. Duration of refractory status epilepticus and outcome: loss of prognostic utility after several hours. Epilepsia 2009;50:1566–1571.
108. Vignatelli L, Rinaldo R, Baldin E, Tinuper P, Michelucci R, Galeotti M, de Carolis P, D'Alessandro R. Impact of treatment on the short-term prognosis of status epilepticus in two population-based cohorts. J Neurol 2008;255:197–204.
109. Cascino GD, Hesdorffer D, Logroscino G, Hauser WA. Treatment of non-febrile status epilepticus in Rochester, Minn., from 1965 through 1984. Mayo Clin Proc 2001;76:39–41.
110. Sutter R, Marsch S, Fuhr P, Kaplan PW, Rüegg S. Anesthetic drugs in status epilepticus—risk or rescue? Results from a six-year cohort study. Neurology 2014;82:656–664.
111. Rossetti AO, Logroscino G, Bromfield EB. A clinical score for prognosis of status epilepticus in adults. Neurology 2006;66:1736–1738.
112. Leitinger M, Höller Y, Kalss G, Rohrbacher A, Novak HF, Höfler J, Dobesberger J, Kuchukhidze G, Trinka E. Epidemiology-based mortality score in status epilepticus (EMSE). Neurocrit Care 2015;22:273–282.
113. Chen JWY, Wasterlain CG. Status epilepticus: pathophysiology and management in adults. Lancet Neurol 2006;5:246–256.
114. Alvarez V, Westover MB, Drislane FW, Dworetzky BA, Curley D, Lee JW, Rossetti AO. Evaluation of a clinical tool for early etiology identification in status epilepticus. Epilepsia 2014;55(12):2059–2068.
115. Brophy GM, Bell R, Claassen J, Alldredge B, Bleck TP, Glauser T, Laroche SM, Riviello JJ Jr, Shutter L, Sperling MR, Treiman DM, Vespa PM. Neurocritical Care Society Status Epilepticus Guideline Writing Committee. Guidelines for the evaluation and management of status epilepticus. Neurocrit Care 2012;17(1):3–23.
116. Shorvon S, Baulac M, Cross H, Trinka E, Walker M (for the TaskForce on Status Epilepticus of the ILAE Commission for European Affairs). The drug treatment of status epilepticus in Europe: consensus document from a workshop at the first London Colloquium on Status Epilepticus. Epilepsia 2008;49:1277–1284.
117. Lowenstein DH, Alldredge BK. Status epilepticus. N Engl J Med 1998;338:970–976.
118. Silbergleit R, Durkalski V, Lowenstein D, Conwit R, Pancioli A, Palesch Y, Barsan W. Intramuscular versus intravenous therapy for prehospital status epilepticus. N Engl J Med 2012;366(7):591–600.
119. Alldredge BK, Gelb AM, Isaacs SM, Corry MD, Allen F, Ulrich SK, Gottwald MD, O'Neil N, Neuhaus JM, Segal MR, Lowenstein DH. A comparison of lorazepam, diazepam, and placebo for the treatment of out-of-hospital status epilepticus. N Engl J Med 2001;345:631–637.
120. Knake S, Hamer HM, Rosenow F. Status epilepticus: a critical review. Epilepsy Behav 2009;15:1–14.
121. Bleck TP. Critical care of the patient in status epilepticus. In: Wasterlain C, Treiman DT, eds., Status epilepticus. Boston: MIT Press, 2006:607–613.
122. Alvarez V, Lee JW, Drislane FW, Westover MB, Novy J, Dworetzky BA, Rossetti AO. Practice variability and efficacy of clonazepam, lorazepam, and midazolam in status epilepticus: a multicenter comparison. Epilepsia 2015;56(6):933–941.
123. Krishnamurthy KB, Drislane FW. Relapse and survival after barbiturate anesthetic treatment of refractory status epilepticus. Epilepsia 1996;37:863–867.
124. Claassen J, Hirsch LJ, Emerson RG, Mayer SA. Treatment of refractory status epilepticus with pentobarbital, propofol, or midazolam: a systematic review. Epilepsia 2002;43:146–153.
125. Lambrechtsen FACP, Buchhalter JR. Aborted and refractory status epilepticus in children: a comparative analysis. Epilepsia 2008;49:615–625.
126. Legriel S, Mourvillier B, Bele N, Amaro J, Fouet P, Manet P, Hilpert F. Outcomes in 140 critically ill patients with status epilepticus. Intensive Care Med 2008;34:476–480.
127. Novy J, Logroscino G, Rossetti AO. Refractory status epilepticus: a prospective observational study. Epilespia 2010;51(2):251–256.
128. Holtkamp M, Othman J, Buchheim K, Masuhr F, Schielke E, Meierkord H. A "malignant" variant of status epilepticus. Arch Neurol 2005;62:1428–1431.
129. Shorvon S, Ferlisi M. The treatment of super-refractory status epilepticus: a critical review of available therapies and a clinical treatment protocol. Brain 2011;134:2802–2818.
130. Sahin M, Menache CC, Holmes GL, Riviello JJ. Prolonged treatment for acute symptomatic refractory status epilepticus: outcome in children. Neurology 2003;61:398–401.
131. Kalita J, Nair PP, Misra UK. Status epilepticus and encephalitis. A study of clinical findings, magnetic resonance imaging and response to antiepileptic drugs. J Neurovirol 2008;14:412–417.
132. Costello DJ, Kilbride RD, Cole AJ. Cryptogenic new onset refractory status epilepticus (NORSE) in adults—infectious or not? J Neurol Sci 2009;277(1-2):26–31.
133. van Baalen A, Hausler M, Boor R, Rohr A, Sperner J, Kurlemann G, Panzer A, Stephani U, Kluger G. Febrile infection-related epilepsy syndrome (FIRES): a nonencephalitic encephalopathy in childhood. Epilepsia 2010;51(7):1323–1328.
134. Spatola M, Novy J, Pasquier Du R, Dalmau J, Rossetti AO. Status epilepticus of inflammatory etiology: a cohort study. Neurology 2015;85(5):464–470.
135. Claassen J, Hirsch LJ, Emerson RG, Bates JE, Thompson TB, Mayer SA. Continuous EEG monitoring and midazolam infusion for refractory nonconvulsive status epilepticus. Neurology 2001;57:1036–1042.
136. Alvarez V, Drislane FW. Is favorable outcome possible after prolonged refractory status epilepticus? J Clin Neurophysiol 2016;33(1):32–41.
137. Yaffe K, Lowenstein DH. Prognostic factors for pentobarbital therapy for refractory generalized status epilepticus. Neurology 1993;43:895–900.
138. Sahin M, Menache CC, Holmes GL, Riviello JJ. Outcome of severe refractory status epilepticus in children. Epilepsia 2001;42:1461–1467.
139. Krishnamurthy KB, Drislane FW. Phenobarbital and benzodiazepine assisted withdrawal of prolonged pentobarbital treatment for refractory status epilepticus. J Epilepsy 1997;10:211–214.
140. Mirski MA, Williams MA, Hanley DF. Prolonged pentobarbital and phenobarbital coma for refractory generalized status epilepticus. Crit Care Med 1995;23:400–404.
141. Bausell R, Svoronos A, Lennihan L, Hirsch LJ. Recovery after severe refractory status epilepticus and 4 months of coma. Neurology 2011;77,1494–1495.
142. Rossetti AO, Oddo M, Liaudet L, Kaplan PW. Predictors of awakening from postanoxic status epilepticus after therapeutic hypothermia. Neurology 2009;72:744–749.

143. Rossetti AO, Logroscino G, Liaudet L, Ruffieux C, Ribordy V, Schaller MD, Despland PA, Oddo M. Status epilepticus. An independent outcome predictor after cerebral anoxia. Neurology 2007;69:255–260.
144. Cooper AD, Britton JW, Rabinstein AA. Functional and cognitive outcome in prolonged refractory status epilepticus. Arch Neurol 2009;66:1505–1509.
145. Claassen J, Hirsch LJ, Mayer SA. Treatment of status epilepticus: a survey of neurologists. J Neurol Sci 2003;211:37–41.
146. Holtkamp M. The anaesthetic and intensive care of status epilepticus. Curr Opin Neurol 2007;20:188–193.
147. Rashkin MC, Youngs C, Penovich P. Pentobarbital treatment of refractory status epilepticus. Neurology 1987;37:500–503.
148. Mirsattari SM, Sharpe MD, Young GB. Treatment of refractory status epilepticus with inhalational anesthetic agents isoflurane and desflurane. Arch Neurol 2004;61:1254–1259.
149. Sheth RD, Gidal BE. Refractory status epilepticus: response to ketamine. Neurology 1998;51:1765–1766.
150. Gaspard N, Foreman B, Judd LM, Brenton JN, Nathan BR, McCoy BM, Al-Otaibi A, Kilbride R, Fernández IS, Mendoza L, Samuel S, Zakaria A, Kalamangalam GP, Legros B, Szaflarski JP, Loddenkemper T, Hahn CD, Goodkin HP, Claassen J, Hirsch LJ, Laroche SM. Intravenous ketamine for the treatment of refractory status epilepticus: a retrospective multicenter study. Epilepsia 2013;54(8):1498–1503.
151. Davis R, Dalmau J. Autoimmunity, seizures, and status epilepticus. Epilepsia 2013;54(suppl 6):46–49.
152. Johnson N, Henry C, Fessler AJ, Dalmau J. Anti-NMDA receptor encephalitis causing prolonged nonconvulsive status epilepticus. Neurology 2010;75(16):1480–1482.
153. Ng Y, Kim HL, Wheless JW. Successful neurosurgical treatment of childhood complex partial status epilepticus with focal resection. Epilepsia 2003;44:468–471.
154. Desbiens R, Berkovic SF, Dubeau F, Andermann F, Laxer KD, Harvey S, Leproux F, Melanson D, Robitaille Y, Kalnins R, Olivier A, Fabinyi G, Barbaro NM. Life-threatening focal status epilepticus due to occult cortical dysplasia. Arch Neurol 1993;50:695–700.
155. Lhatoo SD, Alexopoulos AV. The surgical treatment of status epilepticus. Epilepsia 2007;48(suppl 8):61–65.
156. D'Giano CH, Garcia MDC, Pomata H, Rabinowicz AL. Treatment of refractory partial status epilepticus with multiple subpial transaction: case report. Seizure 2001;10:382–385.
157. Spencer SS, Schramm J, Wyler A, O'Connor M, Orbacj D, Krauss G, Sperling M, Devinsky O, Elger C, Lesser R, Mulligan L, Westerveld M. Multiple subpial transaction for intractable partial epilepsy: an international meta-analysis. Epilepsia 2002;43:141–145.
158. Claassen J, Taccone FS, Horn P, et al. Recommendations on the use of EEG monitoring in critically ill patients: consensus statement from the neurointensive care section of the ESICM. Intensive Care Med. 2013;39(8):1337–1351.
159. Herman ST, Abend NS, Bleck TP, et al. Consensus statement on continuous EEG in critically ill adults and children, part I: indications. J Clin Neurophysiol 2015;32(2):87–95.
160. Krishnamurthy KB, Drislane FW. Depth of EEG suppression and outcome in barbiturate anesthetic treatment for refractory status epilepticus. Epilepsia 1999;40:759–762.
161. Rossetti AO, Logroscino G, Bromfield EB. Refractory status epilepticus: effect of treatment aggressiveness on prognosis. Arch Neurol 2005;62:1698–1702.
162. Knake S, Rochon J, Fleischer S, Katsarou N, Back T, Vescovi M, Oertel WH, Hamer HM, Rosenow F. Status epilepticus after stroke is associated with increased long-term case fatality. Epilepsia 2006;47:2020–2026.
163. Jaitly R, Sgro JA, Towne AR, Ko D, DeLorenzo RJ. Prognostic value of EEG monitoring after status epilepticus: a prospective adult study. J Clin Neurophysiol 1997;14:326–334.
164. Husain AM, Mebust KA, Radtke RA. Generalized periodic epileptiform discharges: etiologies, relationship to status epilepticus, and prognosis. J Clin Neurophysiol 1999;16:51–58.
165. Jette N, Claassen J, Emerson RG, Hirsch LJ. Frequency and predictors of nonconvulsive seizures during continuous electroencephalographic monitoring in critically ill children. Arch Neurol 2006;63:1750–1755.
166. Alvarez V, Drislane FW, Westover MB, Dworetzky BA, Lee JW. Characteristics and role in outcome prediction of continuous EEG after status epilepticus: a prospective observational cohort. Epilepsia 2015;56(6):933–941.
167. Hirsch LJ. Continuous EEG monitoring in the intensive care unit: an overview. J Clin Neurophysiol 2004;21:332–340.
168. Ferrie CD, Caraballo R, Covanis A, Demirbilek V, Dervent A, Fejerman N, Fusco L, Grunewald RA, Kanazawa O, Koutroumanidis M, Lada C, Livingston JH, Nicotra A, Oguni H, Martinovic Z, Nordli DR Jr, Parisi P, Scott RC, Specchio N, Verrotti A, Vigevano F, Walker MC, Watanabe K, Yoshinaga H, Panayiotopoulos CP. Autonomic status epilepticus in Panayiotopoulos syndrome and other childhood and adult epilepsies: a consensus view. Epilepsia 2007;48:1165–1172.
169. Wieser HG, Chauvel P. Simple partial status epilepticus and epilepsia partialis continua of Kozhevnikov. In: Engel J, Pedley TA, eds., Epilepsy: a comprehensive textbook. 2nd ed. Philadelphia: Lippincott-Raven Publishers, 2008:705–723.
170. Schomer DL. Focal status epilepticus and epilepsia partialis continua in adults and children. Epilepsia 1993;34(suppl 1):S29–36.
171. Sinha S, Satishchandra P. Epilepsia partialis continua over last 14 years: experience from a tertiary care center from South India. Epilepsy Res 2007;74:55–59.
172. Fejerman N, DiBlasi AM. Status epilepticus of benign partial epilepsies in children: Report of two cases. Epilepsia 1987; 28:351–355.
173. Rumbach L, Sablot D, Berger E, Tatu L, Vuillier F, Moulin T. Status epilepticus and stroke. Report on a hospital-based stroke cohort. Neurology 2000;54:350–354.
174. Scholtes FB, Renier WO, Meinardi H. Simple partial status epilepticus: causes, treatment, and outcome in 47 patients. J Neurol Neurosurg Psychiatry 1996;61:90–92.
175. Grand'Maison F, Reiher J, Leduc CP. Retrospective inventory of EEG abnormalities in partial status epilepticus. Electroencephalogr Clin Neurophysiol 1991;79:264–270.
176. Devinsky O, Kelley K, Porter RJ, Theodore WH. Clinical and electroencephalographic features of simple partial seizures. Neurology 1988;38:1347–1352.
177. Gosavi TD, See SJ, Lim SH. Ictal and interictal EEG patterns in patients with nonconvulsive and subtle convulsive status epilepticus. Epilepsy Behav 2015;49:263–267.
178. Juul-Jensen P, Denny-Brown D. Epilepsia partialis continua. A clinical, electroencephalographic, and neuropathological study of nine cases. Arch Neurol 1966;15:563–578.
179. Thomas JE, Reagan TJ, Klass DW. Epilepsia partialis continua. A review of 32 cases. Arch Neurol 1977;34:266–275.
180. Cockerell OC, Rothwell J, Thompson PD, Marsden CD, Shorvon SD. Clinical and physiological features of epilepsia partialis continua. Cases ascertained in the UK. Brain 1996;119(Pt 2):393–407.
181. Kozhevnikov A. Eine besondere Form von corticaler Epilepsie. Neurol Centralbl 1895;14:47–48.
182. Botez MI, Brossard L. Epilepsia partialis continua with well-delimited subcortical frontal tumor. Epilepsia 1974;15:39–43.
183. Feddersen B, Bender A, Arnold S, Klopstock T, Noachtar S. Aggressive confusional state as a clinical manifestation of status epilepticus in MELAS. Neurology 2003;61:1149–1150.
184. Shavit YB, Graus F, Probst A, Rene R, Steck AJ. Epilepsia partialis continua: a new manifestation of anti-Hu-associated paraneoplastic encephalomyelitis. Ann Neurol 1999;45:255–258.
185. Ruggieri PM, Najm I, Bronen R, Campos M, Cendes F, Duncan JS, Wieser HG, Theodore WH. Neuroimaging of the cortical dysplasias. Neurology 2004;62(suppl 3):S27–29.
186. Singh BM, Strobos RJ. Epilepsia partialis continua associated with non-ketotic hyperglycemia: clinical and biochemical profile of 21 patients. Ann Neurol 1980;8:155–160.
187. Lamarche M, Chauvel P. Movement epilepsy in the monkey with an experimental motor focus. Electroencephalogr Clin Neurophysiol 1978;34(suppl):323–328.
188. Kuroiwa Y, Tohgi H, Takahashi A, Kanaya H. Epilepsia partialis continua: active cortical spike discharges and high blood flow in the motor cortex and enhanced transcortical long loop reflex. J Neurol 1985;232:162–166.
189. Wieser HG, Graf HP, Bernoulli C, Siegfried J. Quantitative analysis of intracerebral recordings in epilepsia partialis continua. Electroencephalogr Clin Neurophysiol 1978;44:14–22.
190. Watanabe K, Kuroiwa Y, Toyokura A. Epilepsia partialis continua. Epileptogenic focus in motor cortex and its participation in transcortical reflexes. Arch Neurol 1984;41:1040–1044.
191. Cowan JMA, Rothwell JC, Wise RJS, Marsden CD. Electrophysiological and positron emission studies in a patient with cortical myoclonus, epilepsia partialis continua and motor epilepsy. J Neurol Neurosurg Psychiatr 1986;49:796–807.
192. Guerrini R. Physiology of epilepsia partialis continua and subcortical mechanisms of status epilepticus. Epilepsia 2009;50(Suppl 12):7–9.
193. Kristiansen K, Kaada BR, Henriksen GF. Epilepsia partialis continua. Epilepsia 1971;12:263–267.
194. Bancaud J, Bonis A, Trottier S, Talairach J, Dulac O. L'épilepsie partielle continue: syndrome et maladie. Rev Neurol (Paris) 1982;138:803–814.

195. Mameniskiene R, Bast T, Bentes C, et al., Clinical course and variability of non-Rasmussen, nonstroke motor and sensory epilepsia partialis continua: a European survey and analysis of 65 cases. Epilepsia 2011;52(6):1168–1176.

196. Morrell F, Whisler WW, Bleck TP. Multiple subpial transection: a new approach to the surgical treatment of focal epilepsy. J Neurosurg 1989;32:553–559.

197. Morrell F, Whisler WW, Smith MC. Multiple subpial transection in Rasmussen's encephalitis. In: Andermann F, ed., Chronic encephalitis and epilepsy. Rasmussen's syndrome. Boston: Butterworth-Heinemann, 1991:219–233.

198. Rotenberg A, Bae EH, Takeoka M, Tormos JM, Schachter SC, Pascual-Leone A. Repetitive transcranial magnetic stimulation in the treatment of epilepsia partialis continua. Epilepsy Behav 2009;14:253–257.

199. Pandian JD, Thomas SV, Santoshkumar B, et al. Epilepsia partialis continua—a clinical and electroencephalography study. Seizure 2002;11(7):437–441.

200. Chatrian GE, Shaw CM, Leffman H. The significance of periodic lateralized epileptiform discharges in EEG: An electrographic, clinical and pathological study. Electroenceph Clin Neurophysiol 1964;17:177–193.

201. Rasmussen T, Olszewski J, Lloyd-Smith DL. Focal seizures due to chronic localized encephalitis. Neurology 1958;8:435–445.

202. Varadkar S, Bien C, Kruse C, Jensen F, Bauer J, Pardo C, Vincent A, Mathern G, Cross JH. Rasmussen's encephalitis: clinical features, pathobiology, and treatment advances. Lancet Neurol 2014;13:195–205.

203. Oguni H, Andermann F, Rasmussen TB. The natural history of the syndrome of chronic encephalitis and epilepsy. A study of the MNI series of forty-eight cases. In: Andermann F, ed., Chronic encephalitis and epilepsy. Boston: Butterworth-Heinemann, 1991:7–35.

204. Aguilar MJ, Rasmussen T. Role of encephalitis in pathogenesis of epilepsy. Arch Neurol 1960;2:663–676.

205. Rasmussen T. Further observations on the syndrome of chronic encephalitis and epilepsy. Appl Neurophysiol 1978;41:1–12.

206. So NK, Gloor P. Electroencephalographic and electrocorticographic findings in chronic encephalitis of the Rasmussen type. In: Andermann F, ed., Chronic encephalitis and epilepsy. Boston: Butterworth-Heinemann, 1991:37–46.

207. Rogers SW, Andrews PI, Gahring LC, McNamara J. Autoantibodies to glutamate receptor GluR3 in Rasmussen's encephalitis. Science 1996;46: 242–246.

208. Hart YM, Cortez M, Andermann F, Hwang P, Fish DR, Dulac O, Silver K, Fejerman N, Sherwin A, Caraballo R. Medical treatment of Rasmussen's syndrome (chronic encephalitis and epilepsy): effect of high-dose steroids or immunoglobulins in 19 patients. Neurology 1994;44:1030–1036.

209. Villemure JG, Vernnet O, Delalande O. Hemispheric disconnection: callosotomy and hemispherectomy. Adv Tech Stand Neurosurg 2000;26:25–78.

210. Westmoreland BF, Klass DW, Sharbrough FW. Chronic periodic lateralized epileptiform discharges. Arch Neurol 1986;43:494–496.

211. Hirsch LJ, LaRoche SM, Gaspard N, Gerad E, Svoronos A, Herman ST, Mani R, Arif H, Jette N, Minazad Y, Kerrigan JF, Vespa P, Hantus S, Claassen J, Young GB, So E, Kaplan PW, Nuwer MR, Fountain NB, Drislane FW. American Clinical Neurophysiology Society's standardized critical care EEG terminology: 2012 version. J Clin Neurophysiol 2013;30:1–27.

212. Snodgrass SM, Tsuburaya K, Ajmone-Marsan C. Clinical significance of periodic lateralized epileptiform discharges: relationship with status epilepticus. J Clin Neurophysiol 1989;6:159–172.

213. Baykan B, Kinay D, Gokyigit A, Gurses C. Periodic lateralized epileptiform discharges: association with seizures. Seizure 2000;9:402–406.

214. Westover MB, Shafi MM, Bianchi MT, Moura LM, O'Rourke D, Rosenthal ES, Chu CJ, Donovan S, Hoch DB, Kilbride RD, Cole AJ, Cash SS. The probability of seizures during EEG monitoring in critically ill adults. Clin Neurophysiol 2015;126(3):463–471.

215. Schraeder PL, Singh N. Seizure disorders following periodic lateralized epileptiform discharges. Epilepsia 1980;21:647–653.

216. Schwartz MS, Prior PF, Scott DR. The occurrence and evolution in the EEG of a lateralized periodic phenomenon. Brain 1973;96:613–622.

217. Chong DJ, Hirsch LJ. Which EEG patterns warrant treatment in the critically ill? Reviewing the evidence for treatment of periodic epileptiform discharges and related patterns. J Clin Neurophysiol 2005;22:79–91.

218. Jirsch J, Hirsch LJ. Nonconvulsive seizures: developing a rational approach to the diagnosis and management in the critically ill population. Clin Neurophysiol 2007;118:1660–1670.

219. Reiher J, Rivest J, Grand'Maison F, Leduc CP. Periodic lateralized epileptiform discharges with transitional rhythmic discharges: association with seizures. Electroencephalogr Clin Neurophysiol 1991;78:12–17.

220. Ali II, Pirzada NA, Vaughn BV. Periodic lateralized epileptiform discharges after complex partial status epilepticus associated with increased focal cerebral blood flow. J Clin Neurophysiol 2001;18:565–569.

221. Assal F, Papazyan JP, Slosman DO, Jallon P, Goerres GW. SPECT in periodic lateralized epileptiform discharges (PLEDs): a form of partial status epilepticus? Seizure 2001;10:260–265.

222. Handforth A, Cheng JT, Mandelkern MA, Treiman DM. Markedly increased mesiotemporal lobe metabolism in a case with PLEDs: further evidence that PLEDs are a manifestation of partial status epilepticus. Epilepsia 1994;35:876–881.

223. Terzano MG, Parrino L, Mazzucchi A, Moretti G. Confusional states with periodic lateralized epileptiform discharges (PLEDs): a peculiar epileptic syndrome in the elderly. Epilepsia 1986;27:446–457.

224. Garzon E, Fernandes RMF, Sakamoto AC. Serial EEG during human status epilepticus. Evidence for PLED as an ictal pattern. Neurology 2001;57:1175–1183.

225. Liguori C, Romigi A, Placidi F, Izzi F, Albanese M, Sancesario G, Marciani MG. Pure ictal sensory seizures may represent a clinical manifestation of PLEDs. Epilepsy Behav 2012;23(4):509.

226. de la Paz D, Brenner RP. Bilateral independent periodic lateralized epileptiform discharges. Clinical significance. Arch Neurol 1981;38:713–715.

227. Celesia GG, Grigg MM, Ross E. Generalized status myoclonicus in acute anoxic and toxic-metabolic encephalopathies. Arch Neurol 1988;45:781–784.

228. Jumao-as A, Brenner RP. Myoclonic status epilepticus: a clinical and electroencephalographic study. Neurology 1990;40:1199–1202.

229. Hallett M. Myoclonus: relation to epilepsy. Epilepsia 1985;26(suppl 1):67–77.

230. Wakamoto H, Nagao H, Manabe K, Kobayashi H, Hayashi M. Nonconvulsive status epilepticus in eyelid myoclonia with absences—evidence of provocation unrelated to photosensitivity. Neuropediatrics 1999;30:149–150.

231. Ohtahara S, Ohtsuka Y. Myoclonic status epilepticus. In: Engel J Jr, Pedley TA, eds., Epilepsy: a comprehensive textbook. 2nd ed. Philadelphia: Lippincott-Raven Publishers, 2008:725–729.

232. Asconape J, Penry JK. Some clinical and EEG aspects of benign juvenile myoclonic epilepsy. Epilepsia 1984;25:108–114.

233. Kimura S, Kobayashi T. Two patients with juvenile myoclonic epilepsy and nonconvulsive status epilepticus. Epilepsia 1996;37:275–279.

234. Guerrini R, Bonanni P, Rothwell J, Hallett M. Myoclonus and epilepsy. In: Guerrini R, Aicardi J, Andermann F, Hallett M, eds., Epilepsy and movement disorder. Cambridge: Cambridge University Press, 2002:165–210.

235. Adachi M, Inoue T, Tsuneishi S, Takada S, Nakamura H. Eyelid myoclonia with absences in monozygotic twins. Pediatr Int 2005;47:343–347.

236. Wheless JW. Acute management of seizures in the syndromes of idiopathic generalized epilepsies. Epilepsia 2003;44(suppl 2):22–26.

237. Genton P, Gelisse P, Thomas P, Dravet C. Do carbamazepine and phenytoin aggravate juvenile myoclonic epilepsy? Neurology 2000;55:1106–1109.

238. Thomas P, Valton L, Genton P. Absence and myoclonic status epilepticus precipitated by antiepileptic drugs in idiopathic generalized epilepsy. Brain. 2006;129(Pt 5):1281–1292.

239. Dziewas R, Kellinghaus C, Ludemann P. Nonconvulsion status epilepticus in patients with juvenile myoclonic epilepsy: types and frequencies. Seizure. 2002;11(5):335–339.

240. Berkovic SF, Andermann F, Carpenter S, Wolfe LS. Progressive myoclonus epilepsies: specific causes and diagnosis. N Engl J Med 1986;315:296–305.

241. Miyahara A, Saito Y, Sugai K, Nakagawa E, Sakuma H, Komaki H, et al. Reassessment of phenytoin for treatment of late stage progressive myoclonus epilepsy complicated with status epilepticus. Epilepsy Res 2009;84(2-3):201–209.

242. Dravet C, Bureau M, Oguni H, Fukuyama Y, Cokar O. Severe myoclonic epilepsy in infancy: Dravet syndrome. Adv Neurol 2005;95:71–102.

243. Korff CM, Laux L, Kelley Kr, Goldstein J, Koh S, Nordli DR Jr. Dravet syndrome (severe myoclonic epilepsy in infancy): a retrospective study of 16 patients. J Child Neurol 2007;22:185–194.

244. Simon RP, Aminoff MJ. Electrographic status epilepticus in fatal anoxic coma. Ann Neurol 1986;20:351–355.

245. Wijdicks EF, Young GB. Myoclonus status in comatose patients after cardiac arrest. Lancet 1994;343:1642–1643.

246. Krumholz A, Stern BJ, Weiss HD. Outcome from coma after cardiopulmonary resuscitation. Neurology 1988;38:401–405.

247. Young GB, Gilbert JJ, Zochodne DW. The significance of myoclonic status epilepticus in postanoxic coma. Neurology 1990;40:1843–1848.

248. Fugate JE, Wijdicks EFM, Mandrekar J, Claassen DO, Manno EM, White RD, Bell MR, Rabinstein AA. Predictors of neurologic outcome in hypothermia after cardiac arrest. Ann Neurol 2010;68:907–914.

249. Knight WA, Hart KW, Adeoye OM, Bonomo JB, Keegan SP, Ficker DM, Szaflarski JP, Privitera MD, Lindsell CJ. The incidence of seizures in patients undergoing therapeutic hypothermia after resuscitation from cardiac arrest. Epilepsy Res 2013;106(3):396–402.

250. Knake S, Klein KM, Hattemer K, Wellek A, Oertel WH, Hamer HM, et al. Pregabalin-induced generalized myoclonic status epilepticus in patients with chronic pain. Epilepsy Behav 2007;11(3):471–473.

251. Vollmar C, Noachtar S. Tiagabine-induced myoclonic status epilepticus in a nonepileptic patient. Neurology. 2007;68(4):310.

252. Lance JW, Adams RD. The syndrome of intention or action myoclonus as a sequel to hypoxic encephalopathy. Brain 1963;86:111–136.

253. Brown P, Thompson PD, Rothwell JC, Day BL, Marsden CD. A case of postanoxic encephalopathy with cortical action and brainstem reticular reflex myoclonus. Mov Disord 1991;6:139–144.

254. Sheth RD, Gidal BE. Intravenous valproic acid for myoclonic status epilepticus. Neurology 2000;54:1201.

255. Perucca E, Gram L, Avanzini G, Dulac O. Antiepileptic drugs as a cause of worsening seizures. Epilepsia 1998;39:5–17.

256. Genton P. When antiepileptic drugs aggravate epilepsy. Brain Dev 2000;22:75–80.

257. Arnoldus EPJ, Lammers GJ. Postanoxic coma: good recovery despite myoclonus status. Ann Neurol 1995;38:697.

258. Morris HR, Howard RS, Brown P. Early myoclonic status and outcome after cardiorespiratory arrest. J Neurol Neurosurg Psychiatry 1998;64:267–268.

259. Rossetti AO, Oddo M, Logroscino G, Kaplan PW. Prognostication after cardiac arrest and hypothermia. A prospective study. Ann Neurol 2010;67:301–307.

260. Kaplan PW. The EEG of status epilepticus. J Clin Neurophysiol 2006;23(3):221–229.

261. Gastaut H, Roger J, Ouahchi S, Timsit M, Broughton R. An electroclinical study of generalized epileptic seizures of tonic expression. Epilepsia 1963;4:15–44.

262. Camfield PR. Definition and natural history of Lennox-Gastaut syndrome. Epilepsia 2011;52(suppl 5):3–9.

263. Kobayashi E, Thomas P, Andermann F. Tonic status epilepticus in patients with idiopathic generalized epilepsy. Epileptic Disord 2005;7:327–331.

264. DiMario FJ, Clancy RR. Paradoxical precipitation of tonic seizures by lorazepam in a child with atypical absence seizurers. Pediatr Neurol 1988;4(4):249–251.

265. Somerville ER, Bruni J. Tonic status epilepticus presenting as a confusional state. Ann Neurol 1983;13:549–551.

266. Jain V, Harvey AS. Treatment of refractory tonic status epilepticus with intravenous lacosamide. Epilepsia 2012;53(4):761–762.

267. Tassinari CA, Dravet C, Roger J, Cano JP, Gastaut H. Tonic status epilepticus precipitated by intravenous benzodiazepine in five patients with Lennox-Gastaut syndrome. Epilepsia 1972;13:421–435.

268. Prior PF, Maclaine GN, Scott DF, Laurance BM. Tonic status epilepticus precipitated by intravenous diazepam in a child with petit mal status. Epilepsia 1972;13(3):467–472.

21 | NONCONVULSIVE STATUS EPILEPTICUS

FRANK W. DRISLANE, MD, SUSAN T. HERMAN, MD,

AND PETER W. KAPLAN, MB, BS, FRCP

abstract
ABSTRACT: The clinical presentation and encephalographic (EEG) findings of nonconvulsive status epilepticus (NCSE) can be complicated, making diagnosis difficult. There are generalized (e.g., absence status) and focal (e.g., aphasic status, complex partial status) forms. Some patients are responsive but have cognitive or other neurologic deficits; others are less responsive or even comatose. Increasingly, the diagnosis of NCSE is considered in intensive care unit patients. Here, without clinical signs of seizures such as convulsions, EEG is critical in diagnosis, but there is uncertainty about which EEG patterns represent seizures and which clinical situations and EEG patterns warrant aggressive treatment. Antiseizure medications are tailored to the NCSE type and the clinical condition. Treatment is often easier for NCSE, and the outcome better, than for convulsive SE, but this is not always true for critically ill patients with NCSE in the ICU, for whom continuous EEG monitoring is often crucial for diagnosis and management.

KEYWORDS: nonconvulsive status epilepticus, absence, complex partial, EEG, electroencephalogram, NCSE

PRINCIPAL REFERENCES

bibliography
1. Agathonikou A, Panayiotopoulos CP, Giannakodimos S, Koutroumanidis M. Typical absence status in adults: diagnostic and syndromic considerations. Epilepsia 1998;39:1265–1276.
2. Andermann F, Robb JP. Absence status: a reappraisal following review of thirty-eight patients. Epilepsia 1972;13:177–187.
3. Boulanger JM, Deacon C, Lecuyer D, Gosselin S, Reiher J. Triphasic waves versus nonconvulsive status epilepticus: EEG distinction. Can J Neurol Sci 2006;33:175–180.
4. Butler CR, Graham KS, Hodges JR, Kapur N, Wardlaw JM, Zeman AZJ. The syndrome of transient epileptic amnesia. Ann Neurol 2007;61:587–598.
5. Gloor P, Fariello RG. Generalized epilepsy: some of its cellular mechanisms differ from those of focal epilepsy. Trends Neurosci 1988;11:63–68.
6. Granner MA, Lee SI. Nonconvulsive status epilepticus: EEG analysis in a large series. Epilepsia 1994;35:42–47.
7. Hirsch LJ, Brenner RP, Drislane FW, So E, Kaplan PW, Jordan KG, Herman ST, LaRoche SM, Young GB, Bleck TP, Scheuer ML, Emerson RG. The ACNS subcommittee on research terminology for continuous EEG monitoring: Proposed standardized terminology for rhythmic and periodic EEG patterns encountered in critically ill patients. J Clin Neurophysiol 2005;22:128–135.
8. Sutter R, Kaplan PW. Electroencephalographic criteria for nonconvulsive status epilepticus: Synopsis and comprehensive survey. Epilepsia 2012;53 (suppl 3):1–51.
9. Thomas P, Zifkin B, Migneco O, Lebrun C, Darcourt J, Andermann F. Nonconvulsive status epilepticus of frontal origin. Neurology 1999;52:1174–1183.
10. Towne AR, Waterhouse EJ, Boggs JG, Garnett LK, Brown AJ, Smith JR, Jr., DeLorenzo RJ, Smith JR Jr. Prevalence of nonconvulsive status epilepticus in comatose patients. Neurology 2000;54:340–345.

1. HISTORY

Although generalized convulsive status epilepticus (GCSE) has been recognized for millennia, nonconvulsive status epilepticus (NCSE) is a much more recent concept. Perhaps by association with other forms of epilepsy with altered consciousness, some speculation about the possible existence of NCSE emerged by 1800 or so. Trousseau, at Hotel Dieu in Paris, noted that petit mal seizures might recur with sufficient frequency "that one seizure would become confused with the next, simulating a continuous seizure which might persist for two or three days," thus anticipating a diagnosis of absence status epilepticus [1–3]. Nonconvulsive spells also attracted the attention of Jules Falret (1824–1902), who said that a patient with "*petit mal intellectuel* . . . might leave home or work, with clouded mind . . . [and] . . . complete lapses of memory" [2,4].

Samuel Wilks in London in the late 1800s described a patient who was

in the condition which is popularly called 'lost;' he is scarcely conscious of acts and conversation going on around him, yet he may continue walking in a given direction, showing that his movements must still, in a measure, be guided by his senses . . . in much the same state as a somnambulist. This condition . . . is called the status epilepticus, although the term is more usually applied to [a] patient . . . who, after a succession of fits, lay for hours in a state of lethargy. In the milder forms it is one of great interest from a physiology point-of-view and seems to point to the possibility of a subconscious state, in which the brain is sufficiently active to control the spinal system and yet not awake [for] consciousness. [1,5]

Also in the late 1800s, Charcot and others described cases suggestive of NCSE. Charcot postulated that a state of somnambulism derived from ongoing seizures. He presented a patient with a nonconvulsive form of long-lasting seizures several times in his "*Leçons du Mardi*" at the Saltpêtrière—a delivery man who wandered about Paris and even to the coast, at Brest, being arrested on one occasion and released only on the cognizance of Charcot—who treated him with bromides [6]. In Britain, Gowers speculated that similar states, rather than being ictal, occurred after the seizure: "After epileptic fits of moderate severity, the patient may pass into a condition of mental automatism, in which various acts are performed in an apparently conscious manner, but of which no recollection is afterwards retained" [7].

Charcot's observations fostered speculation about the existence of NCSE, but without an appreciation of the role of electricity in the nervous system (starting to emerge in the

17th century [8]), it would be hard to conceive of a modern understanding of NCSE. Clinical descriptions of confusional states (even with signs of epilepsy such as twitching of facial or limb muscles) were insufficient to prove that NCSE was a proper diagnosis. Encephalopathy, psychogenic unresponsiveness, or postictal behavior might appear very similar.

Berger's invention and development of the electroencephalogram (EEG) in the 1920s made it possible to record the previously suspected electrical activity of the brain [9]. He also began studies correlating EEG activity, as a measure of brain electrical function, with psychologic and behavioral abnormalities and, eventually, epileptic seizures [10]. Thus, earlier historical descriptions of what might have been NCSE were thrust into a provable domain. Just over a decade later, clinical–EEG correlations showed beyond doubt that NCSE was part of epilepsy, and not, as some had suspected, from hysterical or nonepileptic fugue states.

Lennox detailed one of the first cases of "petit mal status" with an electrographic correlate in 1945 [11]. In 1954, Penfield and Jasper described simple partial status epilepticus or *aura continua* in the form of recurrent sensory phenomena, commenting that they were "at least as common as continuing circumscribed movements" [12]. In the first thorough description of complex partial status epilepticus in 1956, Gastaut and Roger described a nurse whose seizures may have lasted months [13].

In the past half-century, there have been numerous reports from centers around the world detailing the electro–clinical correlates and nature of NCSE. Many have addressed the clinical characteristics [14] and EEG correlations of various types of NCSE [15,16] and EEG criteria for the diagnosis of nonconvulsive seizures and NCSE [17–19].

In the past two decades, with the development of continuous EEG (C-EEG) monitoring in intensive care units (ICUs) and elsewhere [20], attention has focused increasingly on NCSE in patients with altered responsiveness and other neurologic deficits, with concomitant medical and other neurologic illnesses. Many NCSE cases have been identified in patients with diminished responsiveness or coma following presumed resolution of convulsive seizures or GCSE [21–23].

The formation of research consortia among academic centers has facilitated the collection of multicenter data on patients with status epilepticus (SE) and their clinical and EEG data, including many patients with different types of NCSE. Treatment for NCSE has improved and is now better tailored to the type of NCSE.

2. DEFINITION

It is difficult to state a definition of NCSE because its clinical manifestations are protean and the EEG findings, even while crucial for diagnosis, are often ambiguous or controversial. The significance of epileptiform waveforms and other abnormalities on the EEG is often unclear, and even the role of clearly epileptiform EEG abnormalities in causing clinical deficits can be uncertain or impossible to determine. Because NCSE is considered an epileptic process without convulsions

(or no more than minimal motor manifestations), almost all definitions insist on EEG evidence of continuing or very frequent epileptiform activity.

The definition of GCSE can be complicated and controversial, but that for NCSE is much more so. The proposed definition of (all forms of) SE from the International League Against Epilepsy (ILAE) is in the previous chapter [24]. That definition is useful practically for clinical diagnosis and decision making for NCSE but does not specify its essence. Earlier, Shorvon proposed that NCSE is a

> range of conditions in which electrographic seizure activity is prolonged and results in nonconvulsive clinical symptoms. [It is . . .] primarily as a form of epileptic cerebral response which is dependent largely on the level of cerebral development and integrity, the presence or absence of encephalopathy, the type of epilepsy syndrome, and the anatomical location of the epileptic activity. [25]

This definition reflects the pleomorphic character of NCSE and alludes to important insights into its biology, but diagnosis of individual cases can remain challenging.

Many definitions include a temporal criterion for the duration of seizure activity, or non-recovery from serial seizures. While most neurologists have adopted the "operational" definition of GCSE as 5 minutes [26], it has been useful "in the field" to consider NCSE as seizures persisting or continuing for 10 to 30 minutes [27]. The latest ILAE proposal for classification of NCSE recommends that "t1" (the time beyond which seizures are abnormally prolonged and unlikely to stop on their own [i.e., become SE]) is 10 minutes for absence SE and for complex partial SE (or "focal SE with impaired consciousness") [24].

3. EPIDEMIOLOGY

Most epidemiologic studies of SE concentrate on GCSE (see previous chapter) [27,28]. Shorvon estimated from the incidence of different types of SE that about 40% of SE cases are NCSE [29], suggesting an incidence of up to 15 cases per 100,000 persons per year in the general population [27,30], but about half of all cases in a German study of SE were nonconvulsive, with that study implying about 6 cases per 100,000 per year [31]. Absence SE alone constitutes about 6% of all SE cases, and complex partial SE represents about one third of SE cases [30,31]. Given different studies' variations in diagnosis, and the recent increase in diagnosis of NCSE in sick, hospitalized patients, these estimates of the incidence of NCSE may be low.

4. CLINICAL PRESENTATION

NCSE has remarkably varied and often very subtle presentations [32,33]. At times, it follows generalized seizures and GCSE—that is, GCSE continues in a more subtle form; the epileptiform discharges of a seizure continue on the EEG after the motor manifestations (convulsions) have ceased. In this case, it is best to consider NCSE as a later stage of GCSE, in terms of its pathophysiology, clinical implications, and mandate for treatment. Any patient who has not recovered from a seizure within 20 to 30 minutes or so should be considered as possibly in NCSE.

NCSE can also occur without clinically evident seizures (i.e., purely nonconvulsive events). Even then, it has pleomorphic presentations. Its behavioral correlates in different types of NCSE arise from, or are at least associated with, different areas of maximal involvement of seizure activity in the brain.

NCSE typically encompasses an ictal impairment of mental status, cognition, or behavior compared with a baseline state; automatisms; or change in sensory perception (e.g., auditory, visual, somatosensory; or psychic) [14]. Anterograde and retrograde memory may be affected; affect can be altered (agitation, sadness, weeping); speech and language may be impaired (with mutism or paraphasic errors); and confusional states occur. There can be psychomotor retardation or behavioral changes, beyond the patient's baseline. Sometimes, there are admixed, but generally minimal, motor manifestations, such as subtle facial or limb jerking, blinking, eye deviation with nystagmus [34], or perioral and eyelid myoclonus—highly suggestive of NCSE in the appropriate clinical setting [35].

5. DIFFERENTIAL DIAGNOSIS

NCSE often occurs in patients with underlying chronic medical and neurologic illnesses (including epilepsy), and also with acute and subacute medical problems such as infections, vascular disease, or metabolic abnormalities. The other illnesses may obscure the diagnosis. Many patients with NCSE have had their compromised cognition attributed to problems such as electrolyte imbalance, hyperglycemia, pneumonia, or earlier seizures [36]. Many others have dementia, mental retardation, or psychiatric disorders, making it difficult for unfamiliar observers, including physicians, to notice a new perturbation in cognition or behavior [14,36–40]. It is often difficult to determine if the patient is "more confused than usual," "confused beyond what might be attributable to an infection or metabolic disturbance," or "inappropriately lethargic after a convulsion."

Altered alertness or behavior may be ascribed to an encephalopathy or a postictal state, delaying diagnosis [14,36]. Patients with chronic psychiatric illness are at risk of delayed diagnosis of NCSE because of their neuroleptic burden and propensity for starting and stopping benzodiazepines, which are triggers for *de novo* NCSE [41]. Especially in the elderly, NCSE may present with confusion, suggesting medication side effects or dementia [42,43]. Many sick, hospitalized patients have altered mental status due to medications, infections, and metabolic encephalopathies from their underlying illnesses, and the same illness may cause or precipitate NCSE [44,45]. Diagnostic clues of NCSE include an earlier history of epilepsy or risk factors for epilepsy.

NCSE is typically discovered in the emergency department, in ICUs, and on Neurology and Psychiatry services, although it can occur on other hospital services and even in ambulatory patients. In the emergency department, the diagnosis of NCSE may be missed when there is lethargy or confusion attributed to a postictal state; ictal confusion mistaken for a metabolic encephalopathy; unresponsiveness and catalepsy presumed to be psychogenic; obtundation thought to be due to alcohol or drug intoxication; hallucinations and agitation mistaken for psychosis or delirium; lethargy presumed due to hyperglycemia; mutism attributed to aphasia; and laughing and crying ascribed to emotional lability [36]. In hospitalized or institutionalized patients, NCSE can present primarily as an impaired level of consciousness or responsiveness.

Drugs precipitating some cases of NCSE include neuroleptics, cephalosporins, radiologic contrast agents [46], and GABA agonists, including baclofen [47], tiagabine and vigabatrin [48,49]. Occasionally, refractory NCSE can be caused by mitochondrial disorders, including mitochondrial encephalomyopathy with lactic acidosis and stroke-like episodes (MELAS) [50]. Unusual forms of NCSE may result from paraneoplastic syndromes, especially those caused by cell surface antibodies [51]. In the anti-NMDA-receptor–associated encephalitis, patients are particularly likely to be young women with ovarian teratomas, presenting with psychiatric or memory disorders, transferred to ICUs with stupor, refractory NCSE, and bizarre orofacial dyskinesias; many respond well to immunosuppressive treatment (and tumor removal) but may take many months to return to normal function [52].

Mimics of NCSE include migraine, transient global amnesia, or sleep disorders, including cataplexy. Others include psychiatric disorders, metabolic derangements, paroxysmal cardiovascular or autonomic dysfunction, endocrine dysfunction, and limbic encephalitis—whether paraneoplastic or other autoantibody syndromes [51], and confusional states induced by many drugs, such as lithium, other psychotropic medications, or alcohol [36,53].

An important mimic of NCSE is psychogenic nonepileptic seizures or pseudoseizures, a conversion disorder, not responsive to antiseizure drugs (ASDs) [54–56]. Psychogenic SE, or "pseudostatus," can mimic NCSE, with prolonged staring, blinking, and unresponsiveness, and even expert clinicians may be unable to distinguish it from SE—although most instances of psychogenic nonepileptic seizures mimic convulsive SE. Often, psychogenic SE can be diagnosed definitively by EEG alone. EEG recording during an attack is by far the best way to make the correct diagnosis—which is crucial to avoid treatment with unnecessary and potentially harmful ASDs or even coma-inducing medications [57]. It is also important to note that some epileptic seizures (many of frontal origin) can mimic psychogenic attacks [58,59].

6. OVERVIEW OF DIAGNOSIS

While generalized convulsions are usually apparent clinically, nonconvulsive seizures (probably the majority in adults) are harder to recognize. Paradoxically, NCSE may be even harder to recognize than individual nonconvulsive seizures because there may be no sudden behavioral change at onset; the patient's condition may fluctuate little over the day; the significance of many EEG patterns is controversial; and the response to ASDs may be subtle or delayed [36].

The diagnosis of NCSE derives from two major elements: an alteration in baseline cognition, behavior, or other neurologic function, and concurrent epileptiform seizure patterns on the EEG [16,18]. Satisfying these criteria is often complicated and difficult. To recognize the clinical features, one must maintain a high index of suspicion. The sign of NCSE is not merely the abnormal behavior, but its change from a baseline state [36].

To diagnose NCSE, epileptologists have required impaired consciousness for 30 to 60 minutes and an EEG with continuous [60] or at least some form of seizure activity [18,19]. EEG waveform morphologies may include rhythmic slowing, sharp waves, spikes, and mixtures of these features [15]. Discharges may be continuous, persistent with brief pauses of a few seconds, or intermittent. Many EEGs are more ambiguous (see section on Diagnosis of NCSE by EEG later in the chapter), with more blunted waveforms slower than 1.5 Hz, sometimes resembling triphasic waves [61]. Over time, NCSE patterns tend to evolve in morphology, voltage, and frequency, and wax or wane. EEG ictal discharges should be continuous or recurrent for more than 30 minutes, without the patient's return to a normal clinical state or resumption of the pre-ictal EEG pattern between seizures. Specific EEG features of several types of NCSE are detailed later in the chapter.

Although the EEG is the most reliable diagnostic test for NCSE, it is not always definitive. In some cases, an ASD challenge is very helpful. Some patients with less "classic" EEG findings show a clinical and electrographic response to benzodiazepines or other ASDs. In the appropriate clinical setting, a rapid response to ASDs can be persuasive for a diagnosis of NCSE. Lorazepam or another (nonsedating) ASD may be given in small sequential doses, while monitoring blood pressure, respiratory rate, and oxygenation and watching for hypoventilation or hypotension [62]. To be diagnostic of ongoing seizure activity there should be prompt improvement in *both* the patient's clinical state and on the EEG, or complete cessation of electrographic seizure activity with return of normal EEG background activity [19] (see Figs. 21.6, 21.14, 21.15, 21.19, and 21.25 later in the chapter). Intravenous benzodiazepines may abolish electrographic seizures, but they can also suppress nonepileptic EEG patterns such as triphasic waves [63], so improvement in the EEG alone upon ASD administration does not prove that a particular EEG pattern was a seizure. A controversial EEG pattern is confirmed as ictal only when marked clinical improvement accompanies the EEG improvement—but often such improvement does not occur. Frequently, the response to ASDs is inconclusive, and the diagnosis must be made on clinical and EEG grounds alone.

Importantly, lack of prompt improvement with ASDs does not refute a diagnosis of NCSE. Even in patients with definite NCSE, a rapid clinical response is uncommon, especially in obtunded or comatose patients [64]. In many, the response is equivocal or substantially delayed [21,36], and sedation from a benzodiazepine may also impair a clinical response. Following a clinical seizure, if the patient improves on EEG but not

clinically, C-EEG monitoring should be considered to look for evidence of subsequent recurrent seizures.

There are a few EEG patterns characteristic of a particular etiology—for instance, those associated with some types of paraneoplastic or immune-based etiologies including limbic encephalitis with autoantibodies, some forms of which include rhythmic slow activity, "extreme delta brush" patterns, and more usual spike-slow wave activity seen unilaterally or bilaterally, often particularly over temporal and parietal regions [18,65,66].

There have also been a few cases of focal NCSE diagnosed clearly by neuroimaging, for example with 18F-fluorodeoxyglucose (FDG)-positron emission tomography (PET) scans [67,68]. Some patients in these reports had clear areas of persistent focal hypermetabolism during clinical episodes of definite aphasia or apparent epileptic amnesia (with an unremarkable EEG, or focal slowing) and an appropriate and quick response to intravenous benzodiazepines. Occasionally, hyperperfusion on ictal single photon emission computed tomography (SPECT) may help to make, or confirm, the diagnosis [69].

7. PATHOPHYSIOLOGY

The pathophysiology of convulsive status epilepticus is discussed in Chapter 20. That of NCSE is substantially less well understood, both in the generation of neural activity that produces and sustains NCSE, and in the possibility of its inducing subsequent neuronal damage and longer-lasting epilepsy on its own.

Most cases of NCSE, at least in adults, represent either complex partial SE or secondary generalized NCSE—with an underlying focal onset, whether evident clinically or not. This NCSE usually begins at the same focus of epileptogenesis as for focal seizures that do not become prolonged to the point of SE. How do these focal seizures reach a self-sustaining state?

In a rodent model of limbic SE produced by repetitive, rapid direct electrical stimulation of the hippocampus for 30 to 90 minutes, seizures progress from self-limited to much more prolonged, and eventually self-sustaining SE, persisting for 12 to 24 hours after the stimulation has ceased [70,71]. The induced seizures appear similar to those of humans with complex partial SE (CPSE)—although it is still unclear whether an analogous process occurs in humans. Seizures beginning in the hippocampus appear to promote the propagation of yet more seizure activity, which is maintained in a circuit of structures including the entorhinal cortex, dentate gyrus, and parts of the hippocampus and subiculum [72,73]. The initiation of SE in these models is similar to that for individual seizures, but inhibitory or terminating mechanisms fail (see previous chapter). Generalized seizures, or seizures with onset in other areas, can also precipitate focal temporolimbic seizures and focal SE by way of secondary involvement of the hippocampus or other mesial temporal structures [74].

The activity of certain neurotransmitters can facilitate or inhibit the activation of complex circuits of limbic neuronal activity, prolonging or interrupting nonconvulsive seizures in a (somewhat similar) model of self-sustaining SE produced by stimulation of the perforant pathway in rats [75]. For example, injection into the hippocampus of galanin (a peptide that inhibits glutamate release presynaptically) attenuates seizure activity [76]. Galanin production can decline during SE, while substance P (which may enhance SE by promoting glutamate release) may increase [77], facilitating the prolongation of seizures. As with GCSE, the balance of excitatory and inhibitory function appears to shift toward excitation as NCSE progresses.

The pathophysiology of absence SE and other forms of primarily generalized SE, however, is starkly different from that of focal-onset NCSE [78]. These generalized forms of NCSE involve excessively prolonged synchronization in widespread thalamocortical circuits as part of the generation, maintenance, and reinforcement of aberrant excitatory electrical rhythms in a neuronal system involving both cortical and subcortical structures [72,79]. These abnormal electrical rhythms are manifested by rhythmic generalized, anteriorly predominant, spike and polyspike and slow-wave discharges on the EEG.

Experimentally, these 3-Hz generalized cortical spike and slow-wave discharges can be produced by electrical stimulation of midline intralaminar nuclei of the thalamus [80], and the same thalamic discharges occur during absence seizures in humans [81]. The discharges are dependent on low-threshold, T-type calcium channel activity [72]. Thalamic injections of GABA-B agonists increase the spike and slow-wave discharges, and this activity can be suppressed by specific ASDs [72].

NCSE in critically ill patients may differ pathophysiologically from NCSE in patients with established epilepsy. Following acute brain injury, there may be local hypoxia, hypoglycemia, or ischemia in injured cortex, local hemorrhage or edema, changes in blood–brain barrier permeability, or systemic electrolyte or glucose abnormalities—whether caused by stroke, tumor, trauma, or infection. A variety of acute factors, including release of excitatory neurotransmitters from injured or dying neurons, may promote excitability and impair normal inhibitory processes, and facilitate prolonged or recurrent seizures.

Little experimental evidence is available on the long-term consequences of NCSE. Models of repetitive limbic seizures and SE have been produced by local tissue damage caused by injections of kainic acid, but chemical and electrical methods of inducing SE may damage neurologic tissue independent of the subsequent seizures, that is, it may be, it may be the local electrical or chemical precipitant or toxin that damages neurons.

There are clinical reports of patients with hippocampal edema during episodes of NCSE, with subsequent hippocampal atrophy in the same area [82,83], but not all studies show this progression to atrophy, possibly depending in part on how prolonged the episodes of NCSE were. These results also contrast with the very minimal clinical morbidity attributable to NCSE directly. Lothman has summarized the many physiologic changes that occur during SE, but most apply primarily to GCSE; some may apply to NCSE [84].

It is very difficult to prove that neurologic damage accrues from many cases of NCSE. Pathologic studies of the effects of GCSE in humans are relatively few, in part because fatal SE cases are often associated with acute, severe brain-injuring illnesses that may cause damage independently. Episodes of

NCSE are less often fatal unless they occur in association with GCSE or other acute, severe neurologic illness—in which case it is difficult to sort out the cause of any neuronal damage. For the most part, pathologic studies of patients with pure forms of NCSE remain unavailable.

The experimental models described in the chapter on GCSE included SE durations of well over 30 minutes (typically 1–2 hours of convulsions and electrical discharging activity) to produce neuronal damage in animals. In one rodent model of SE, neurologic damage in the amygdala and pyriform cortex correlated strongly with prolonged "high frequency" (10 Hz) discharges, but there was no damage following discharges slower than 1 Hz [85]. Damage was directly related to the duration and intensity of electrographic seizure activity. It is not clear that such prolonged intense stimulation, or the resultant 10-Hz spike discharges, are an accurate model of human NCSE. Also, in the NCSE model with continuous hippocampal stimulation, neuronal loss did not occur when the interval between nonconvulsive seizures was increased [86]. Currently, knowledge about the pathologic effects of NCSE in humans is limited. Clinical consequences of NCSE are discussed in later sections.

8. CLASSIFICATION

No classification system for NCSE will be satisfactory to all basic investigators, clinical neurophysiologists (electroencephalographers [EEG-ers]), clinicians, and scholars. Gastaut stated that there were "as many types of status as there are types of epileptic seizures" [87], but the correspondence is not strict. For example, different focal seizures emanate from different brain areas, with different signs and symptoms, but many can go on to generalized convulsions and GCSE, and to subsequent NCSE after convulsions—with many later stages appearing similar despite the different origins.

Others reject a classification of NCSE according to seizure types, pointing out that epilepsy syndromes such as juvenile myoclonic epilepsy consist of more than seizures types alone, and also that NCSE is not always simply the prolongation of individual seizures [88]. Also, different physiologic processes contribute to the initiation, maintenance, and perpetuation of SE that are not involved significantly in isolated, individual seizures (see previous chapter). Different NCSE syndromes include different EEG, clinical, genetic, and developmental aspects, age-specific presentations, varied concomitant structural brain abnormalities or encephalopathies, markedly varied responses to treatment, and different longer-term outcome. There are several classifications of types of NCSE and EEG-based definitions of NCSE [16,18,89].

In 2015, the ILAE Task Force proposed a diagnostic classification system based on four axes: semiology (prominent motor vs. non-motor symptoms), etiology (known and unknown), EEG correlates (pattern, morphology, location, time-related features, modulation, effect of intervention), and age (neonatal, infancy, childhood, adolescent and adulthood, and elderly) [24]. The Task Force focused on seizure duration and its relationship to potentially harmful consequences. For NCSE it referred to abnormally prolonged seizures as after "t1"—thought to be 10 minutes for absence SE and for "focal SE with impaired consciousness" (or complex partial SE). For NCSE, "t2" (the time after which long-term neurologic injury would be an urgent concern and a reason for more aggressive treatment) was thought to be either 60 minutes for focal SE with impaired consciousness, or completely unknown for absence SE [24].

Another organizational system classifies NCSE based primarily on age and the state of cerebral development or maturation, presence or absence of a concomitant encephalopathy, occurrence within an epilepsy syndrome, and (for NCSE of focal origin) understanding by anatomic localization [25] (Box 21.1). This perspective aids in understanding NCSE in the context of the brain's development and prior condition. Many of its syndromes occur in neonates, infants, and young children; some continue into adolescence in individuals, or occur in adults.

This system also describes "boundary syndromes" that do not fit easily into categories. They are mostly syndromes with markedly abnormal baseline neurologic conditions and epileptiform abnormalities on EEG, in which it is difficult or impossible to determine what role the epileptiform discharges have in causing the clinical manifestations. Most are pediatric syndromes that occur within a broad range of illnesses such as the Lennox–Gastaut syndrome (LGS). They include electrical Electrical status epilepticus of sleep (ESES), described more extensively in Chapter 18, and epileptiform EEG patterns of uncertain significance such as periodic discharges (lateralized or generalized), "triphasic" waves, or "subtle SE," as occurs with continued coma, and often myoclonus, after generalized convulsions, where there is substantial uncertainty in differentiating whether the EEG pattern represents seizure activity or not [25,89].

The recent ILAE classification (above) focuses on semiologic and EEG features (i.e., an electroclinical organization). NCSE is thus organized into focal and generalized forms, acknowledging that seizures can progress from a focal onset to generalized clinical and EEG manifestations. NCSE may also be divided into cases in which there is preserved consciousness (i.e., responsiveness) and others constituting "focal SE with impaired consciousness" [24], with impaired ability to respond appropriately to stimuli. Myoclonic, tonic, and clonic SE are detailed further in the previous chapter because of their motor manifestations.

9. EARLY LIFE, AGE-RELATED NCSE SYNDROMES

Many neonatal seizures and NCSE have minimal clinical manifestations and remain underdiagnosed if EEG monitoring is not used [90,91], especially in neonates with severe brain injury [92] and in pharmacologically paralyzed infants. Electrographic patterns of neonatal seizures also differ from those of older patients, often remaining localized to relatively small brain areas, likely due to incomplete myelination and neuronal migration [93]. Multifocal seizures are common, especially with multifocal or diffuse brain injury. Some seizures show evolution in frequency, amplitude, morphology, or spatial distribution, but many do not [93]. Morphologies include sharply contoured, sinusoidal, or rounded waveforms in the alpha, theta, and delta frequency range, but the frequency and morphology may vary within a single seizure and from seizure to seizure. Many neonatal seizures last 2 to 3 minutes but recur frequently; prolonged continuous seizures are less frequent [94]. Conversely, not all abnormal-appearing neonatal movements are seizures [91]; some are nonepileptic movements such as stimulus-sensitive clonus or myoclonus.

Many of the most important pediatric NCSE syndromes associated with underlying developmental delay or regression demonstrate activation of epileptiform abnormalities during

---

BOX 21.1. CLASSIFICATION OF NCSE SYNDROMES

1. *Neonatal and infantile syndromes, including:*
   - West syndrome, Ohtahara syndrome
   - Severe myoclonic epilepsy of infancy (Dravet syndrome)
2. *Childhood syndromes, including:*
   - Genetic-based illnesses such as ring chromosome 20 syndrome; Angelman, Rett syndrome
   - Benign childhood epilepsies without a discrete genetic origin (e.g., Panayiotopoulos syndrome)
   - Childhood epileptic encephalopathies (e.g., Landau–Kleffner syndrome and electrical status epilepticus in slow sleep [ESES])
   - Febrile SE
3. *Childhood and adult forms of NCSE*
   a. *With epileptic encephalopathy*
      - i. e.g., within the Lennox-Gastaut syndrome (LGS), with atypical absence SE or tonic SE, and the continuation of LGS into adulthood
      - ii. other epileptic encephalopathies
   b. *Without epileptic encephalopathy*
      - Typical absence SE of idiopathic generalized epilepsies
      - Focal NCSE, sometimes referred to as *aura continua* with sensory, autonomic, or cognitive symptoms
      - Complex partial SE: limbic, or nonlimbic
      - NCSE that follows the convulsions of generalized seizures or generalized convulsive SE
      - "Subtle" SE with myoclonic SE following convulsions
4. *Later adult NCSE:* including *de novo* absence SE of late onset
5. *"Boundary syndromes"*

   - Some "atypical absence" SE of childhood
   - Epileptic behavioral disturbances or psychosis
   - Other forms of epileptic encephalopathy and coma due to brain injury (e.g., anoxia) with epileptiform discharges, including "subtle" status
   - Drug or metabolic confusional states with epileptiform discharges (generally not considered true NCSE)

(Modified from Shorvon [25].)

sleep [95,96]. ESES implies activation by sleep of persistent epileptiform activity suggestive of SE, but not all children with these EEGs have clinical seizures. The waking EEG usually shows infrequent focal or occasionally generalized epileptiform discharges, with the spike component usually more prominent than the slow wave.

Some children have an associated ESES syndrome, with ESES on the EEG along with progressive cognitive dysfunction, often referred to as an epileptic encephalopathy [97]. One such syndrome, continuous spikes and waves during slow sleep (CSWS), is an age-related pediatric epilepsy syndrome, usually starting late in the first decade of life in children who were neurologically normal before seizures began [98]. Seizures include generalized convulsions and often evolve to become atypical absence and atonic seizures with dangerous falls [95,99]. The EEG during wakefulness and rapid eye movement (REM) sleep shows infrequent focal or generalized epileptiform discharges. Non-REM sleep prompts continuous generalized or bilaterally synchronous (if sometimes asymmetric) spike-and-wave complexes at 1.5 to 3.5 Hz (Fig. 21.1). Continuous spike-wave patterns occupying at least 85% of slow-wave sleep are required for the diagnosis of CSWS [99,100].

Most children with CSWS have focal or generalized seizures, global behavioral problems, and regression of cognitive function, more than in language alone [99,101]. The epilepsy is often severe and can include many seizure types, including prolonged atypical absence SE [95]. CSWS may last for years, but the typical EEG pattern usually occurs between ages 5 and 15 years. The EEG eventually normalizes, including during sleep, and almost all seizures resolve, but cognitive and behavioral problems usually persist [95,99]. In LGS, the CSWS syndrome may include a prominent component of negative myoclonus or asterixis, at times explaining apparent atonic seizures and dangerous falls [39].

The Landau–Kleffner syndrome (LKS) can be considered another "boundary" syndrome and may overlap with CSWS and other "benign" focal epilepsy syndromes. It is characterized by acquired aphasia, seizures, and a behavioral disorder presenting in children with previously normal language development, between the ages of 2 and 4 years [102]. A gradual deterioration, specifically in language and speech output, may begin with apparent word deafness or a form of auditory agnosia [103]. LKS exhibits clinical seizures in most cases, but seldom overt SE. It is unclear whether the deterioration in language function is the result of epileptiform activity or if the language deterioration and epileptic activity (both clinical and EEG) result from a common underlying pathologic condition. Most cases of LKS are of unknown origin; a few cases are due to symptomatic lesions [104]. Corticosteroids are the most common treatment for LKS [105], but most children have persistent language deficits [103,106].

The waking EEG in LKS may be normal or show unilateral or bilateral temporal spike-and-wave discharges. There are sleep-activated bursts of diffuse or multifocal spike-and-wave discharges at 1.5 to 3.5 Hz (ESES) (Fig. 21.2).

LKS and other ESES syndromes are often treated with ASDs, especially benzodiazepines, with a goal of eliminating epileptiform discharges and the speculation that the epileptic process contributes to the cognitive deterioration. Though episodes of ESES may recur frequently, the prognosis for seizure control is good, but CSWS has a poor prognosis for cognitive function. Fortunately, LKS and CSWS are rare syndromes, each accounting for about 0.2% of all pediatric epilepsy patients [107]. Infant and pediatric SE is detailed more extensively in Chapter 18; the rest of this chapter will focus on NCSE in adults.

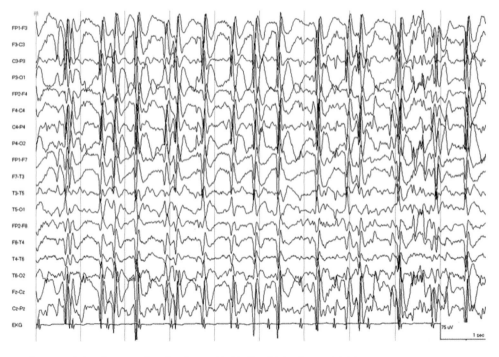

Figure 21.1. Continuous spike-waves during slow-wave sleep in a 9-year-old girl with mild developmental delay.

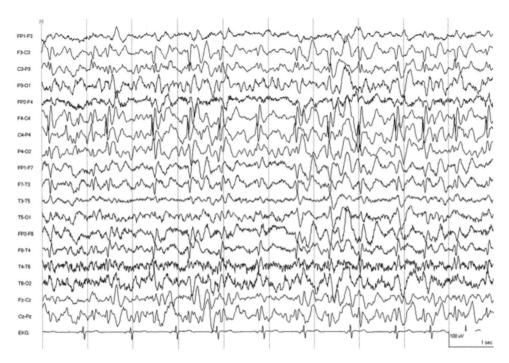

Figure 21.2. A 4-year-old boy with language regression, LKS. EEG during sleep shows bilateral 1-Hz centrotemporal sharp waves, more prominent over the right hemisphere.

While the biology of NCSE in children may be understood best in the context of age and brain development, the descriptions of NCSE in adults in this chapter follow the more familiar seizure types and syndromes, both clinical and electrographic, as confronted by clinicians, focusing on the type of seizure persisting and apparently causing the patient's clinical deficit.

FOCAL NONCONVULSIVE STATUS EPILEPTICUS

As with generalized SE, focal SE may or may not include prominent motor manifestations, whether convulsive, as in focal motor SE or *epilepsia partialis continua*, or tonic or major myoclonic movements, as covered in the previous chapter. Focal SE without major motor manifestations is covered here.

Focal NCSE without impairment of consciousness or other cognitive function has been labeled simple partial SE. Ictal deficits reflect involvement of discrete regions of the brain, such as sensory disturbances (e.g., visual hallucinations or hemianopia) or affective, psychic, or autonomic symptoms [108]. Those patients with changes in awareness or responsiveness have been considered to be in "focal SE with impaired consciousness" or CPSE, the term used here and in most earlier clinical reports.

There are also patients with focal NCSE who can still respond or remain "conscious" but have deficits in some cognitive function such as language, memory, or other areas. They have no "impaired consciousness," but have impaired cognition. They may be referred to as in "focal SE with dyscognitive features," with "aphasic status" perhaps the best example.

Overall, focal onset of SE symptoms and electrographic abnormalities is more common than SE with a generalized onset [27]. Focal NCSE is seen frequently after strokes or other

acute brain injuries, and should be suspected when patients do not stabilize or improve as expected. In some critically ill patients, NCSE consists of brief cyclical electrographic seizures occurring every 5 to 10 minutes over several hours [109]. Focal lesions from vascular causes, trauma, and developmental abnormalities (e.g., heterotopias and other migration abnormalities) and mitochondrial disorders are among many possible causes [110,111].

10. FOCAL SENSORY AND PERCEPTUAL NCSE

Persistent sensory seizures (without motor accompaniment) have been called *aura continua* [112,113]. Infrequently, they may last for hours. Simple partial sensory SE (SPSE) is identical to the prolonged continuation of an isolated *aura continua*. In these cases, local inhibitory function is sufficient to prevent spread of the seizure more broadly in the brain. If, on the other hand, these seizures spread to involve areas of the brain necessary for responsiveness (for a long period), this may become CPSE. Occasionally, benign rolandic epilepsy, in which there is speech arrest, drooling, dysphagia, facial weakness, head deviation, and mild confusion, may be prolonged enough to constitute NCSE [114,115].

Pure sensory SE is generally considered rare, but this may reflect a detection bias, as an EEG may show little at the time of SE [108], and persistent sensory disturbances are often attributed to transient ischemia [116] or other nonepileptic causes. In one report, four patients had focal sensory NCSE lasting up to several days, without motor or behavioral symptoms or alteration in responsiveness [117]. Some were frontal or temporal in origin. They appear to be less common than auras progressing to more obvious seizures, and far less common than CPSE.

Focal lesions in temporal, parietal, and occipital regions may produce SE with persistent cognitive or sensory symptoms, with hallucinations of any sensation, including visual, auditory, olfactory, gustatory, somatosensory, or vertiginous perception [113,118]. Olfactory hallucinations from temporal epilepsy may be the most common. Some cases of (SPSE) consist of auditory sensations alone, with epileptiform discharges confined to Heschl's gyrus [119].

Transient cortical blindness or visual field loss (also referred to as *status epilepticus amauroticus*) can be a manifestation of occipital SPSE [120], although simple visual hallucinations and ictal blindness are usually brief [121]. Occipital seizures can also include macropsia, micropsia, misperception of spatial orientation, hallucinations of faces or animals, or simple patterns of color and light [121] (Figs. 21.3 and 21.4). There may be scotomata or simple visual hallucinations predominating in the central visual field, but complex hallucinations are also possible [122]. Slightly more anteriorly, involvement of the temporo-parieto-occipital junction may produce nystagmus with contraversive eye deviation [34].

The "positive" sensory symptom of pain during SPSE appears even rarer, although shorter painful seizures have been reported [113,123]. Some are parietal in origin, in the somatosensory area. Parietal NCSE can also be manifested solely by persistent paresthesias [68]. Other unpleasant epileptic sensory seizures may include nausea, anorexia, poorly described visceral sensations, and the distress of "abdominal epilepsy" originating in mesial temporal areas, especially involving the amygdala [124,125]. One of the best described is "ictal fear" as a manifestation of NCSE [126,127]. Autonomic symptoms are reported increasingly frequently, particularly in children [128].

Some cases of focal SE involve a larger brain area than a typical simple focus, and could be called "regional." The most common (usually pediatric) form of regional SE is the Panayiotopoulos syndrome, in which an exact focus is often difficult to determine [129]. This syndrome is an age-dependent epileptic susceptibility that is usually idiopathic and benign, although perhaps 15% of cases are due to focal lesions. It affects about 13% of all children ages 3 to 6 with non-febrile seizures. Manifestations are primarily autonomic, with ictal emesis and occasional syncope, usually arising from sleep. Half of the episodes last longer than 30 minutes and thus constitute autonomic SE. Most children have few episodes and typically do better without ASD treatment, and the long-term risk of epilepsy is small [129]. Earlier described in correlation with occipital spikes, this syndrome may have discharges elsewhere or multifocally and is probably better considered a regional (but not quite generalized) form of seizures and SE.

11. AMNESTIC, APHASIC, AND OTHER DYSCOGNITIVE NCSE

Persistent memory dysfunction often follows complex partial seizures in the postictal period. It may also be due to an episode of NCSE [130,131]. Episodes of pure amnesia (with preserved cognitive function in other realms) can be due to individual epileptic seizures, referred to as *transient epileptic amnesia* (TEA) [132,133]. TEA usually occurs in patients with earlier epilepsy and is often associated with additional persistent memory deficits. Seizures preferentially affecting memory may require involvement of medial temporal structures bilaterally, as shown by depth-electrode recording [134]. TEA

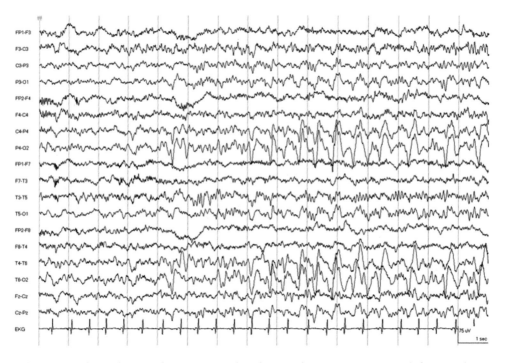

Figure 21.3. An 8-year-old boy with simple partial status epilepticus arising in the right occipital region. Seizures consisted of seeing pulsating green and red circles in the left visual field.

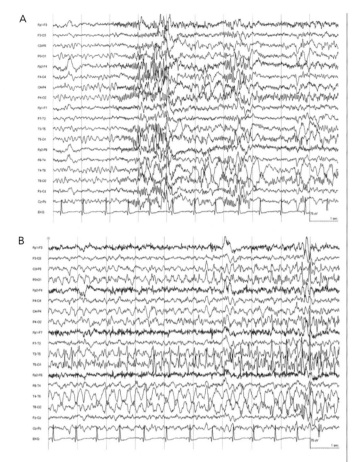

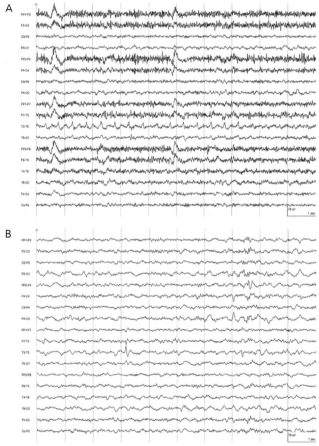

mistaken for other syndromes such as transient ischemia or psychiatric illness.

A wide variety of aphasic NCSE types has been characterized by appropriate and thorough language testing, with preserved responsiveness and other cognition except for the aphasia [144]. Often, the ongoing epileptiform discharges on EEG correspond anatomically to the area associated with a particular aphasia (Fig. 21.5), such as posterotemporal focal discharges in patients with clinically evident Wernicke's-type aphasia [140,142]. Those with more anterior aphasias (some with frontotemporal discharges on EEG) are often unable to speak but may retain verbal memory and respond appropriately to verbal commands, giving evidence of relatively preserved comprehension [138,139]. Some have alexia and reduction in spontaneous speech. Still, the correlation to classical (usually stroke-defined) areas of clinical involvement for different types of aphasia is far from precise [144].

12. DIAGNOSIS OF FOCAL NCSE

Focal NCSE is usually more subtle in presentation than either focal motor SE or generalized forms of SE. SPSE manifested by sensory or cognitive symptoms alone can be very difficult

Figure 21.4. *Focal SE in a 14-year-old girl with right occipito-parietal cortical dysplasia. **A:** Seizure begins with rhythmic beta activity over both occipital regions, more prominent on the right. **B:** Seizure evolves into high-voltage 3- to 4-Hz spikes in the left occipital region, and spikes with slower frequencies in the right occipital region. Seizures recurred every 2 to 3 minutes for several hours before presentation to the emergency department.*

typically occurs in older patients, thus overlapping clinically, and often difficult to distinguish from, (nonepileptic) transient global amnesia. Many episodes of TEA are prolonged beyond 30 minutes, constituting NCSE with amnesia as the sole clinical manifestation [132]. Other amnestic syndromes can be caused by frontal or generalized NCSE [135]; the frontal discharges suggest an inability to access extant memory during the seizures. Some such episodes are frequent or prolonged enough to mimic progressive dementing illnesses [136].

Similarly, a profound hemi-spatial neglect syndrome can be produced by NCSE [137]. In patients without earlier epilepsy (or with different types of seizures) this can appear indistinguishable from an acute middle cerebral artery stroke, even to stroke specialists. Other cognitive deficits, including apraxia and acalculia, can also occur in NCSE, as well as prolonged mood changes, such as depression and panic attacks [138].

Aphasic SE, with preserved responsiveness and a clinical deficit restricted to language dysfunction alone, is a focal or regional NCSE (while complex partial SE implies a disturbance in responsiveness) [139–143]. Careful language testing is necessary to determine that the deficit is truly an aphasia [141,144]; speech arrest alone can result from seizures in many areas. A focal neurologic deficit in speech production may be

Figure 21.5. *A 49-year-old woman with mild developmental delay who presented with an anterior aphasia. She was able to follow commands. **A:** EEG during the aphasia shows repetitive sharp waves in the left temporal region at 2 Hz. **B:** Same patient after 2 mg intravenous lorazepam. EEG shows resolution of ictal activity and a left midtemporal spike. The aphasia resolved.*

to diagnose and can be confused with many other illnesses (as noted above). While not all patients with focal NCSE have diagnostic findings, the EEG can be extremely helpful in establishing a diagnosis. In one report of six patients with prolonged neurocognitive deficits and evidence of focal-onset NCSE, all had rapid rhythmic epileptiform discharges on EEG and eventual resolution of all symptoms with treatment [138].

Surface EEGs, even when recorded during the symptoms, have limited sensitivity for detection of epileptiform discharges in simple partial seizures, at least in part because the seizures may involve a small volume of brain tissue. The EEG may be normal or show nonspecific changes [145]. One report described 87 well-characterized simple partial seizures in 14 patients, and just 20% of seizures had discernible epileptiform abnormalities on scalp EEG [108]. Two thirds of seizures had primarily sensory symptoms, and these showed ictal EEG changes in just 15%. In another study, only 20% to 35% of simple partial seizures had ictal correlates on surface EEG [146]. Sometimes, focal NCSE can remain undiagnosed until invasive EEG monitoring is performed—usually carried out because of (other) refractory seizures [147,148].

When focal SE is visible on EEG, it usually shows an onset with a single topographic EEG maximum, followed by evolution in frequency, voltage, and distribution. Focal fast-frequency discharges, rhythmic waveforms with evolving morphology, repetitive epileptiform discharges, or regional or lateralized alterations in EEG background activity may be seen [145,146]. If SE is discontinuous, the background activity between seizures is typically slow and disorganized near the seizure-onset zone, with occasional focal interictal (sometimes periodic) epileptiform discharges.

Electrographic focal SE is seen in some stuporous or comatose patients with no clear clinical signs of seizure activity [149]. Seizures may be either continuous or repetitive, with EEG patterns similar to those in simple partial seizures and CPSE. Such focal SE is not rare after strokes or other acute brain injuries and should be suspected when patients in those settings do not stabilize or improve as expected. EEG should be performed for any ICU patient in whom mental status changes are unexplained or appear out of proportion to the degree of acute neurologic injury. Patients with suspected focal NCSE also warrant a magnetic resonance imaging (MRI) scan to look for an underlying focal lesion.

13. COMPLEX PARTIAL SE

The first definite case of CPSE was reported by Gastaut and Roger in 1956 [13]. In the 1970s and 1980s, CPSE was considered rare and was the subject of isolated case reports [130,131], and by 1985 only 17 clearly identified cases had been published [150]. With the realization that absence SE is a separate category rather than simply *any* NCSE with generalized discharges, CPSE or "focal SE with impaired consciousness" was eventually recognized as more common [32,33,151]—though it is probably still underdiagnosed [152]. Other, largely antiquated, terms for CPSE include temporal lobe SE (which exists, but

is often an inaccurate localization), prolonged epileptic fugue state, and psychomotor SE [150,153–156].

The definition of SE as a seizure or series of seizures without recovery for 30 minutes [157] allows for the possibility that CPSE can consist of a single very long complex partial seizure or a series of recurrent complex partial seizures without clinical normalization between seizures [131]. CPSE is probably the most common form of NCSE in adults who are ambulatory or not critically ill.

CPSE begins as a focal-onset seizure, progressing to involve more of the brain such that responsiveness is impaired, and then with prolongation or recurrence. CPSE may last hours, days, or even months [32,158]. The most common causes are new acute vascular disease or old strokes with a more recent precipitant such as infection or metabolic derangement [60,159]. Other infections (e.g., encephalitis), tumors, congenital developmental abnormalities, and vascular malformations are possible. The diagnosis of CPSE should be considered in patients who are partially or completely unresponsive, especially those with earlier epilepsy or vascular disease.

While most patients have earlier epilepsy [29], CPSE may arise in patients without prior seizures. CPSE is seldom reported in children, but it may be significantly underrecognized and occur especially in those with substantial developmental delay and neurologic deficits, and even in those with other seizure types [58]. From the incidence of SE in different populations with epilepsy, it has been estimated that CPSE occurs in 35 cases per million population per year, but possibly five times as often in developmentally delayed patients [29].

CPSE may present as abnormal behavior or diminished responsiveness associated with lateralized epileptiform seizure activity. It may begin with a simple partial seizure, or consciousness may be impaired at the onset. Impairment of consciousness, which may cycle or fluctuate, ranges from almost indiscernible clouding of higher cortical function to coma [58,60,109,131]. CPSE may include an "epileptic twilight state" with a lack of responsiveness or confusion, and bizarre, and particularly fluctuating, behavior or paranoia [32,130,131,150,156] (Fig. 21.6). The extensive variety of clinical presentations of CPSE makes EEG essential to distinguish CPSE from other causes of altered mental status.

Lip-smacking, other oro-alimentary automatisms, lateralized limb automatisms and dystonic posturing, eye deviation, and nystagmus are typical of CPSE; myoclonus is rare [60,156,160]. Fear, aggressiveness, irritability, and anxiety, and stereotyped, complex automatisms are more frequent with CPSE than with absence SE [160], but when the automatisms or movements are minimal, CPSE can be difficult to distinguish from absence SE on clinical grounds.

In contrast to SPSE, most patients with CPSE show discernible surface EEG changes. The EEG patterns of CPSE are variable, reflecting differences in the location of ictal onset zones and propagation pathways, but they are often very similar to those seen in isolated complex partial seizures. CPSE may be characterized either by repetitive complex partial seizures, each showing focal onset, with background slowing between seizures, or by continuous epileptiform rhythms, corresponding to cycling or continuous clinical manifestations

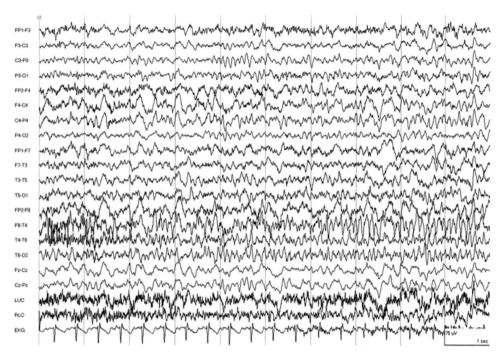

Figure 21.6. "Psychic" SE in a 41-year-old woman with right mesial temporal sclerosis. She presented with mild confusion but could follow most commands. She did not answer questions and had bizarre speech, repeating "you are my Norm, you are my one true love" continuously.

[87,109,150,161,162]. Rarely, ictal patterns arise independently from both hemispheres (Fig. 21.7). Waveform morphologies include repetitive epileptiform spikes, spike-and-slow wave discharges, or rhythmic theta, delta, or alpha frequencies, or rhythmic low-voltage fast activity [15]. Occasionally, the EEG can be normal or obscured by artifact [163].

Often, early EEG abnormalities are focal or lateralized throughout the episode [146]. Focal onset is usually followed by evolution in distribution, voltage, and frequency, in commonly recognized patterns of electrographic seizures [121,164,165]. Epileptiform discharges may merge gradually to produce continuous focal seizure activity. Many have subsequent spread to involve a greater area of the cortex (Fig. 21.8) and result in diffuse or generalized epileptiform discharges difficult to distinguish from those of absence SE [15,33,60]. As CPSE progresses, the epileptiform discharges often increase in voltage, slow in frequency, and broaden in distribution. Later, seizures may become fragmentary, interrupted by brief periods of background attenuation [166]. Between discrete seizures, the background shows focal slowing, focal epileptiform discharges, or periodic lateralized (epileptiform) discharges [166].

14. TEMPORAL VERSUS FRONTAL CPSE

CPSE may arise from many brain regions. Many episodes represent prolonged temporal lobe seizures, as demonstrated clearly by depth-electrode recording [167], but another study of eight patients with depth-electrode–recorded episodes of CPSE all had frontal origins for the seizures [58]. Overall, extratemporal onset of CPSE may be more common, including in children [115]. At least on the scalp EEG, CPSE with

prominent parietal features (clinically) is usually nonlocalizing or falsely localizing [168].

Extratemporal foci may produce visual, auditory, somesthetic, or vestibular hallucinations, a perception of warmth, changes in facial color, nausea, or unilateral arm automatisms or posturing. When seizures spread to involve the amygdala and hippocampus, there may be chewing movements, lip-smacking, and gesticulatory automatisms [131].

Frontal CPSE often has less impairment of consciousness and fewer fluctuations than does temporal lobe CPSE [160]. Frontal CPSE may recur frequently but be misdiagnosed often. Temporal CPSE includes more fear, anxiety, anger, irritability, aggressiveness, agitation, and simple and complex automatisms [160]. Psychomotor slowing is more frequent in frontal than in temporal lobe CPSE, but about the same as in absence SE, and CPSE with a frontal origin may be very difficult to distinguish from absence SE.

15. TEMPORAL CPSE

The clinical manifestations of temporolimbic CPSE are extensive. "Experiential" sensations involving memories of perceptions or experiences, often with an emotional overtone, indicate limbic structure involvement of seizures [169] (Box 21.2). For the seizure to be "experienced," or remembered, there should be involvement of neocortical as well as medial temporal structures [112]. Seizures involving limbic areas of the hippocampus and amygdala interfere with responsiveness and may progress to become temporal lobe CPSE [112]; CPSE may also evolve from *aura continua* [167].

Temporal CPSE may have a sudden or gradual onset [112]. Hippocampal, amygdalar, and amygdalohippocampal CPSE

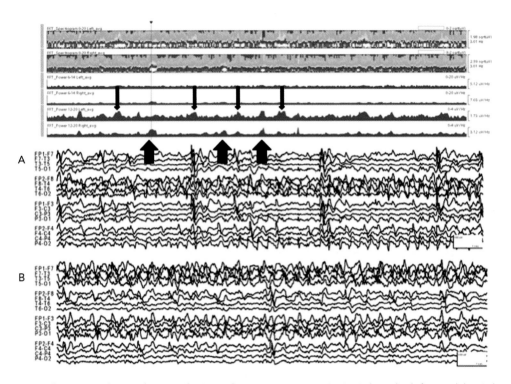

Figure 21.7. Quantitative EEG showing complex partial status epilepticus with recurrent seizures originating independently from each hemisphere, in a 45-year-old woman with multiple sclerosis and malfunction of an intrathecal baclofen pump. The bottom two lines of the compressed spectral array (CSA) show peaks (arrows) of rhythmic activity of alpha and theta frequencies indicative of seizures. The expanded "usual" EEG below shows **A**: right hemisphere seizures, corresponding to the thick arrows on the CSA, and **B**: left hemisphere seizures corresponding to the thin arrows on the CSA above.

often presents with cyclical changes in behavior [109,112,131]. An early report described a "twilight state" with partial responsiveness and intermittent speech arrest [131]. Some patients were completely unresponsive, with motionless staring. Others had oro-alimentary or more complex automatisms, vocalizations, and perseverative gesticulations. A more anterior seizure origin or spread may induce bizarre limb automatisms or wandering, as in a fugue state ("poriomania") [131]. Behavior may

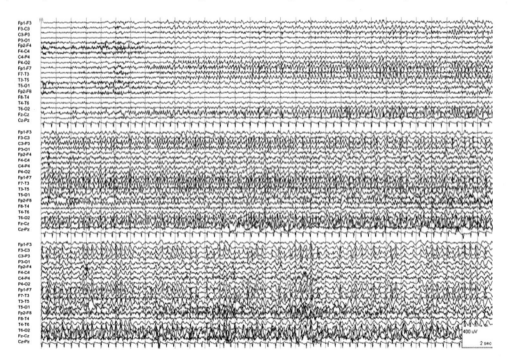

Figure 21.8. Left temporal seizure evolution in a 21-year-old woman with intractable epilepsy admitted with confusion and aphasia. She had complex partial status epilepticus consisting of frequent discrete electrographic and clinical seizures. EEG in three horizontal sections of 18 channels each. Top section: One of frequent discrete electrographic seizures arises in the left frontotemporal region, evolving with higher-voltage, slightly lower-frequency sharp waves in the left temporal region; with spread to the right side [in the middle section], and eventual slowing of discharges and interruption by brief non-discharging periods [in the bottom section]. Just after this, there was generalized, 1.5-Hz slowing for 5 seconds and then a very suppressed background in all areas as the seizure ended.

fluctuate and become very strange. Memory for the event is often impaired or obliterated.

CPSE originating in the temporal lobes may have different manifestations from seizures starting elsewhere and spreading to temporal structures. Opercular, frontal, and occipital origin seizures can all spread secondarily to involve mesial temporal regions. Some seizures with temporal lobe–related manifestations originate in the frontal lobes, with the initial behavioral features representing frontal dysfunction.

CPSE arising from mesial temporal regions usually begins with unilateral temporal 5- to 7-Hz rhythmic activity that appears within 30 seconds of the initial clinical symptoms or signs [164] (Figs. 21.8 and 21.9). Interictally, there may be focal slowing or attenuation on the side of seizure onset. In neocortical temporal seizures, discharges are more widely distributed, sometimes over the entire hemisphere. The EEG changes of neocortical temporal CPSE often begin with slower frequencies, show less stable frequencies and voltages, and appear later after clinical signs than those of medial temporal CPSE [165].

16. FRONTAL CPSE

Thomas and colleagues described two types of frontal lobe NCSE [155]. Type I had continuous mood and behavioral disturbances, with mild hypomania, affective disinhibition (or, conversely, indifference), and subtle impairment of cognition, but no overt confusion. Patients could exhibit a blank facial expression, lack of spontaneous emotion, and decreased verbal fluency. Some could recall events that occurred during the spell and could carry out routine activities, such as eating. There were simple gestural automatisms such as scratching, rubbing, or picking at clothes, but complex bimanual or bipedal automatisms were not observed. Type 1 frontal lobe CPSE led to no morbidity in later cognitive function.

The rarer type 2 frontal lobe CPSE had greater impairment of consciousness, often with cyclic fluctuations. There was marked behavioral disturbance, temporo-spatial disorientation, confusion, and prominent perseveration, and occasional catatonic stupor. Some patients required restraints because of aggressiveness. There was occasional head and eye deviation, and perioral myoclonia. Patients were universally amnestic for the episode.

While the ictal EEG is nonlocalizing or normal in many patients with frontal lobe complex partial seizures [163], scalp EEGs eventually show bilateral sharp-and-slow-wave activity in most cases of frontal lobe CPSE [58] (Fig. 21.10). Some patients have focal rhythmic alpha or beta activity at the onset of seizures originating near scalp electrodes [163], but the scalp EEG often shows no changes until the seizure spreads to medial temporal structures, producing ictal patterns typical for medial temporal seizures. In type 1 frontal lobe CPSE, the EEG showed a unilateral frontal focus; in type 2, there were bilateral asymmetric frontal foci with an abnormal background [155]. Spread of epileptiform activity from a unilateral frontal focus

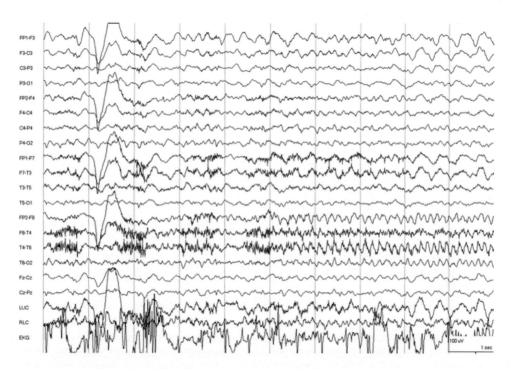

Figure 21.9. Right temporal complex partial seizure in a 32-year-old man with mesial temporal sclerosis, presenting with SE consisting of repetitive seizures. The early EEG before the seizure shows widespread postictal slowing following the previous seizure.

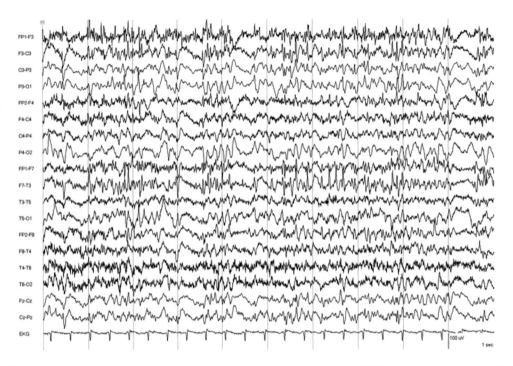

Figure 21.10. *Frontal lobe complex partial SE in a 56-year-old woman with a history of traumatic brain injury. EEG shows irregular 5- to 8-Hz spikes and polyspikes over the left frontal region.*

may lead to bilaterally synchronous or generalized discharges on EEG, indistinguishable from those of absence SE, and often associated with a similar clinical appearance [154,170].

17. FOCAL NCSE: TREATMENT AND OUTCOME

Treatment of NCSE varies markedly depending on the type of NCSE. Focal NCSE (including pure sensory or cognitive deficits) has been difficult to diagnose and thus the subject of relatively small case series. Most patients seemed to respond to modest doses of ASDs used for similar types of seizures and almost never required aggressive treatment such as coma-inducing medications [138,171].

Usually by the time of diagnosis of CPSE, seizures have been present for at least 30 minutes, so treatment should begin promptly with intravenous ASDs. Possibly because of the association with vascular disease and other lesions, and prior focal epilepsy, CPSE is often harder to treat than primary generalized SE and is more likely to recur [32]. Fortunately, patients with CPSE in the setting of earlier epilepsy are very likely to recover and generally warrant a less aggressive approach than do those with GCSE [172]. CPSE is usually treated in the same way as focal-onset GCSE, but somewhat less aggressively if there is an earlier history of epilepsy. CPSE is usually treated more easily than is GCSE [173,174].

The outcome from episodes of CPSE depends primarily on the etiology; morbidity often derives from the unresponsive state and from complications of the underlying illness causing the SE (particularly encephalitis and strokes) rather than from the CPSE itself. In one study, there was no difference in mortality between patients with CPSE (with focal discharges on EEG) and those with GCSE, but the CPSE patients often had secondary generalization of seizures [175]. With CPSE, mostly of frontal origin, patients with episodes of longer duration had no worse an outcome than those with shorter durations [58].

Early reports on CPSE included very few patients. Almost all returned to normal or "baseline cognitive function" [150,155,176], with resolution of all neurologic deficits over time, but this may take weeks or months [130]. In one CPSE series, none of 20 patients had lasting cognitive deterioration, and five had meticulous neuropsychologic assessment [32]. There are reports of prolonged memory and other cognitive deficits lasting weeks or months after NCSE [68,130,131,138,159], but many resolve eventually. In some cases, both clinical and imaging abnormalities can resolve completely over a period as long as a year [32,155].

Long-term clinical effects of CPSE could also include worsened cognitive function or increased subsequent seizure frequency. Most outcome studies, however, are of GCSE—which correlates with worsened seizure control, but this might be attributed to the underlying illness rather than to the episode of SE itself [177].

GENERALIZED NONCONVULSIVE STATUS EPILEPTICUS

18. ABSENCE STATUS EPILEPTICUS

Although *petit mal intellectual* was postulated in the 19th century, Lennox demonstrated in 1945 that altered mental status could be caused by absence seizures. He suspected that a series of such seizures and EEG discharges could persist for much longer than was generally recognized [11]. Absence Status Epilepticus (SE) was described as "status epilepticus in petit mal" by Schwab in

1953 [178], recognizing the same EEG patterns seen in petit mal epilepsy by Lennox earlier. The prolonged confusion and slowed behavior were labeled "spike-wave stupor" by Niedermeyer and Khalifeh [179]. Typical absence SE has also been called petit mal status, minor epileptic status, *absence continué, epilepsia minoris continua*, and status pyknoepilepticus.

Early reports and classification of NCSE (i.e., in the 1970s to 1990s) generally divided NCSE into two types: "absence SE" (which meant all cases of NCSE with generalized epileptiform discharges on the EEG) on the one hand, and others felt to have a focal seizure onset, labeled "complex partial SE." CPSE could have focal EEG discharges or a clear focal onset clinically [60]. This oversimplification of the generalized forms is no longer tenable.

Absence SE is a pure form of primary generalized epilepsy with clinical episodes lasting over 30 minutes. In its classic appearance, it occurs in patients with earlier absence epilepsy or other idiopathic generalized epilepsies (IGEs) [180–182]. Absence epilepsy (see Chapters 18 and 19) begins anywhere from age 3 years until early adulthood, but usually in childhood or adolescence; seizures usually decrease markedly in the third decade. Episodes of absence SE appear later, usually after 10 years of age. Episodes of absence SE represent about 2% to 6% of all SE cases [30, 31]; its overall incidence has been estimated at about one case per million people per year [29]. About 10% of adults who still have absence epilepsy will have at least one episode of absence SE [183].

Absence SE occurs in nearly all IGE syndromes, including juvenile absence epilepsy (Fig. 21.11), juvenile myoclonic epilepsy (JME), perioral myoclonia with absences, eyelid myoclonus and absence, and IGEs with phantom absences [184]—even when those syndromes are usually manifested by other types of seizures (e.g., myoclonus in JME [182]; Box 21.3). NCSE is uncommon in JME [185].

Precipitants include sleep deprivation, alcohol ingestion, metabolic abnormalities, and intercurrent illnesses. Many medications have been implicated in the precipitation of absence SE, especially neuroleptics, tricyclic antidepressants, and lithium, as well as benzodiazepine withdrawal. ASDs such as phenytoin and carbamazepine may precipitate an episode of absence SE [186,187], as may GABA-ergic drugs such as vigabatrin and tiagabine [48,188]. A generalized convulsion may set off an episode of absence SE or end it. In the evaluation of patients with absence SE, MRI scans are almost invariably normal.

Typical absence SE starts abruptly, without warning, and consists of individual seizures in rapid succession without recovery over a long period or, more commonly, a single prolonged episode with continuous epileptiform discharges and impaired consciousness [189]. The clinical presentation can be very subtle, with cognitive deficits discernible only on formal neuropsychologic testing. There may be just a relatively hard-to-diagnose change in responsiveness, with preserved alertness [180]. Cognition may fail when more complex planning is needed. Patients may remain reactive to external stimuli, and some can walk or carry on relatively complex activities without interruption, but usually with slowness and diminished insight and complexity of activities [179,189]. There is more a clouding than an absence of consciousness, often a fluctuating diminution of responsiveness or overt confusion. Language use may be relatively preserved, but with slowness, paucity of speech, and monosyllabic answers [189], and inability to discuss more complex concepts. Language may be reduced to simple phrases or less, and patients may follow only the simplest of

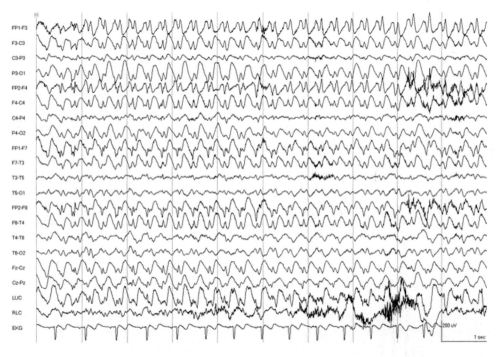

Figure 21.11. Absence SE with generalized, frontally predominant, 3-Hz spike and slow wave discharges.

instructions, or none. Very infrequently, absence SE progresses to complete unresponsiveness [179].

Motor abnormalities are minimal. There may be brief sporadic myoclonic eyelid jerks and eye-blinking, especially in the IGE syndromes [160]. Limb myoclonus is common. Gestural and ambulatory automatisms occur [181,190], but automatisms are usually less complex than in CPSE. Gait tends to be preserved if the patient can stand. Sometimes there are bradykinesia, delayed reactions, and withdrawal [181]. Patients may appear to have diminished initiative or motivation. Perseveration in motor activity or on performance tests is typical.

Patients' descriptions of the event can be vivid. Among the best descriptions are those in the seminal paper by Andermann and Robb [189]. There may be visual hallucinations, a dreamy state, and inappropriate manner. Some patients are aware, themselves, of slowing or difficulty with thought and speech, sometimes noticeable only to those closest to them. Occasionally, patients show hostility and aggression, agitation, and impulsive behavior [189]. Behavior mistaken for psychosis is more likely with CPSE, and confabulation is characteristic of CPSE only [160]. Absence SE often induces relatively little amnesia or postictal confusion [189].

Absence SE may last anywhere from 30 minutes to months [36]. It may cease abruptly—spontaneously or upon treatment with benzodiazepines, with rapid return to normal mentation. Some episodes end with a generalized convulsion. Most reported cases have been isolated, but some recur, and some of those frequently [189]. Some patients have a syndrome in which episodes of absence SE are the primary manifestation of epilepsy, with few other seizures [184]. All these (adult) patients had normal neurologic examinations and imaging and no family history of epilepsy. Episodes of absence SE lasted from 30 minutes to a few weeks, and many recurred several times a year.

Clinically, absence SE may appear remarkably similar to CPSE of frontal or temporal origin, and all of these can be difficult to differentiate from postictal confusion or from nonepileptic causes, including psychiatric conditions such as dissociative states, depression, or hysterical behavior [181,189], or from posttraumatic amnesia or metabolic encephalopathies [36]. Medication side effects can appear very similar to absence SE clinically. Myoclonus, while uncommon in CPSE, is not rare in absence SE [160].

19. ABSENCE STATUS EPILEPTICUS, ELECTROENCEPHALOGRAM

EEG is often required for the accurate diagnosis of absence SE. The characteristic EEG is very similar to that of absence epilepsy: frequently recurrent or prolonged uninterrupted seizures for over 30 minutes, with extremely rhythmic, bilaterally symmetric runs of spike-and-slow-wave discharges; polyspikes may be admixed (Figs. 21.11 and 21.12) [191,192]. Other EEG patterns include generalized rhythmic slowing with intermixed spike-and-slow-wave complexes, irregular sharp-and-slow-wave discharges, or diffuse background slowing with superimposed bursts of fast activity [189]. The epileptiform discharges are bilaterally synchronous and usually of maximal voltage over frontal and central regions. Characteristic-appearing generalized epileptiform discharges may have some asymmetry, but this should not be overinterpreted [154].

Discharge frequencies may reach up to 4 Hz at the onset of the episode but typically slow to the usual 3-Hz pattern within seconds. Discharges are characteristically regular, at 3 to 3.5 Hz. If seizures are prolonged, the discharges may slow to less than 3 Hz and may become irregular [193]. More rapid discharges and polyspikes suggest other IGE syndromes. Discharges are occasionally interrupted by brief bursts of normal EEG background activity. Interictal EEGs may show the same discharges in brief bursts, almost always on a normal background.

20. TREATMENT OF ABSENCE STATUS EPILEPTICUS

Typical absence SE that occurs within absence epilepsy or other IGE syndromes is almost always interrupted readily (clinically and on EEG) by relatively low doses of benzodiazepines or other ASDs, preferably intravenously, but sometimes effective even orally (Fig. 21.13). Interruption by intravenous benzodiazepines is so often effective that it is a useful diagnostic test. Lorazepam doses of less than 0.1 mg/kg will often suffice [180]. Intravenous valproic acid at 20 mg/kg is a reasonable alternative [194] and is also effective in patients with recurrent absence SE, particularly in the IGE syndromes [195]. Lamotrigine is helpful frequently. Typically, the EEG will resume a normal background quickly, and the patient may emerge from the confusion within minutes. Phenytoin and carbamazepine are generally to be avoided as they may exacerbate or even precipitate absence SE [187].

For typical absence SE, the outcome and consequences depend on the etiology—in this case, the epilepsy syndrome, which is benign. Absence SE has produced no mortality and minimal morbidity in reported series, and no significant long-term morbidity can be attributed to it [41,189] or any other NCSE in the IGE syndromes. Nevertheless, this conclusion rests on clinical impressions in moderate-sized series rather than on confirmation by neuropsychologic testing. Still, the prognosis of absence SE is superb.

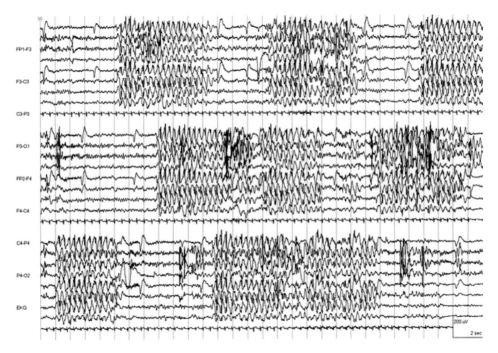

Figure 21.12. *Absence SE in a 17-year-old boy with juvenile absence epilepsy. Brief absence seizures (during an episode of SE) demonstrate generalized frontally maximal spike-wave activity at 3 Hz. Frequent 5- to 10-second absence seizures recurred every 5 to 10 seconds over 20 minutes until administration of intravenous lorazepam. Clinical manifestations were staring, unresponsiveness, eyelid fluttering, and subtle limb automatisms.*

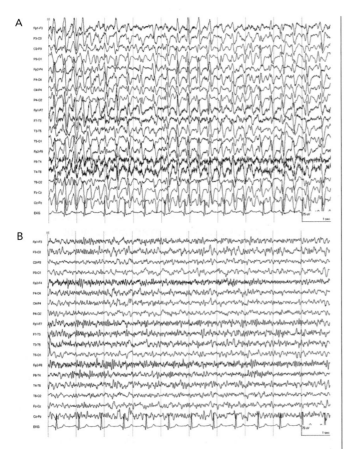

Figure 21.13. *A 75-year-old woman with a history of generalized tonic-clonic seizures (probably a longstanding IGE), now with absence SE causing confusion. **A:** EEG shows semirhythmic high-voltage 3-Hz sharp-and-slow-wave discharges, alternating with periods of diffuse delta activity and slower epileptiform discharges. **B:** In the same patient, complete cessation of epileptiform activity after the administration of intravenous lorazepam, likely causing the widespread faster, beta activity.*

21. *DE NOVO* ABSENCE STATUS EPILEPTICUS

Typical absence SE is unlikely in older patients without an earlier history of an IGE, but occasional episodes have been reported in patients older than 50 years with no prior epilepsy ("*de novo* absence SE of late onset") [41]. Most have moderate impairment of consciousness. The most common setting is that of withdrawal of benzodiazepines used for sleep or psychiatric reasons. Other triggers include toxins or metabolic dysfunction and the use of neuroleptic and other psychotropic medications [196]. It is unclear that all of these cases are truly *de novo*. Some patients may have had primary generalized epilepsies earlier in life without diagnosis, and others may have been misdiagnosed [197]. Fortunately, episodes of *de novo* SE are relatively uncommon and usually easy to interrupt quickly [182]. Especially when precipitated by some identifiable cause such as benzodiazepine withdrawal, most patients do not need maintenance ASDs.

The EEG in *de novo* absence SE tends to be characteristic of absence SE, showing generalized spike-and-wave activity at frequencies from 0.5 to 4 Hz [198] (Fig. 21.14). The spike-and-wave component can be less prominent and more irregular, and recur at a slightly lower frequency than in typical absence SE, but it shows a similar frontal or centrally maximal distribution [41].

22. OTHER FORMS OF PRIMARY GENERALIZED NONCONVULSIVE STATUS EPILEPTICUS

Typical absence SE may occur in 20% to 40% of patients with absence seizures and an IGE [199], but there are also numerous

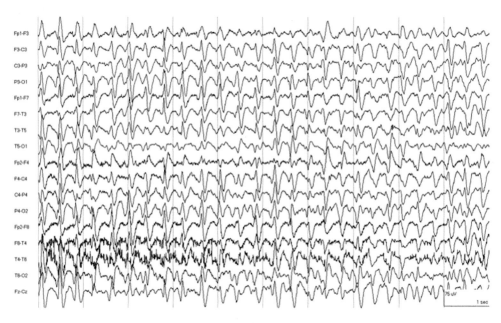

Figure 21.14. *A 58-year-old woman with no history of epilepsy, admitted with confusion. EEG shows generalized 2-Hz spike and slow-wave activity. A few minutes later, after the administration of 2 mg intravenous lorazepam, the EEG showed mild diffuse slowing with plentiful beta activity. The confusion improved concurrently with the EEG improvement, about 4 minutes after the lorazepam administration.*

types of SE generated by other primary generalized or genetic epilepsies, including JME with absence manifestations; eyelid or perioral myoclonia with absences; and IGE with phantom absences. NCSE is uncommon in JME, occurring in 1% to 2% of cases [185,200]. Phantom absences and perioral myoclonia with absences are more common, with almost half of patients having periods of absence-like SE.

Cases of eyelid myoclonia (Jeavons syndrome) with or without absence spells, photosensitivity, or eye-closure paroxysms constitute about 13% of generalized epilepsies [201]. Rarely, they progress to absence SE with eyelid myoclonias lasting minutes to 5 hours—usually treatable with valproate [202] or benzodiazepines. Precipitants are largely situational and include metabolic disturbances and sleep deprivation. The EEG may show spike-waves or polyspike-waves from 2 to 6 Hz.

Some spells of eyelid myoclonia with absence spells have been called fixation-off sensitivity, a term coined by Panayiotopoulos for types of EEG patterns and epilepsies that could be elicited by interfering with fixation and central vision ("scotosensitive") [203]. Paroxysms on the EEG can be triggered by eye closure, and may be photosensitive or scotosensitive. Such spells are often accompanied by focal occipital abnormalities on EEG, but also with generalized epileptic discharges in cryptogenic and symptomatic epilepsies. Cases of SE are rare in this syndrome. They may respond to valproate [201].

23. ATYPICAL ABSENCE STATUS EPILEPTICUS

Atypical absence SE (AASE) is a relatively rare type of SE that occurs primarily in children with cryptogenic and secondarily generalized epilepsy, such as in LGS with substantial neurologic deficits, developmental delay, and severe encephalopathies

[87,204,205]. These patients often have mixed epilepsies, with multiple seizure types and episodes of tonic, atonic, and myoclonic seizures (Fig. 21.15). The incidence of AASE is anywhere from 100 to 200 episodes per million per year [29].

Atypical absence seizures resemble typical absence seizures in their occurrence primarily in young patients, with generalized spike- and slow-wave discharges, and usually the same responses to medications (i.e., exacerbation with ASDs such as carbamazepine, and treatment with ethosuximide and benzodiazepines) [206]. Nevertheless, AASE is more complicated than typical absence SE: it presents at an earlier age, typically before adolescence, with significant background encephalopathies, both clinical and on EEG [204].

The clinical manifestation of AASE is often a further slowing or reduction in cognitive activity, from a poor baseline. Patients are more confused or less responsive than before. They may become mute or immobile, but some children are able to follow simple commands [204]. Consciousness may fluctuate and become markedly impaired. Patients exhibit poor control of movements and frequent falls ("pseudoataxia") and cognitive difficulties with near stupor ("pseudodementia") [39]. AASE can go on for days, without a precise onset or ending. There is typically a gradual onset and resolution of altered behavior in prolonged episodes, but automatisms and other motor activity (such as walking) may continue, even while responsiveness is reduced [207]. Often, there are no overt clinical seizures, and it can be very difficult to distinguish atypical absence SE from the encephalopathic, developmental, or psychiatric behavioral baseline of the (often institutionalized) patients.

LGS is the most common setting for atypical absence SE. With LGS and "myoclonic-astatic" seizures, there may be myoclonus or stupor [205]. When the AASE of LGS continues into adulthood, psychiatric features may predominate,

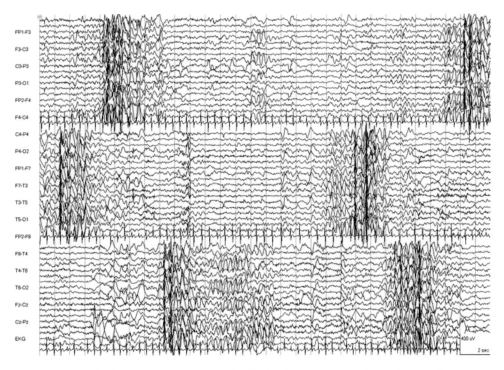

Figure 21.15. Atonic SE in a 12-year-old girl with new-onset epilepsy. Generalized high-voltage slow waves with irregular generalized spikes correlated with atonic episodes of the limbs and trunk. Ninety seconds of EEG show recurrent atonic seizures; a similar pattern persisted for more than 30 minutes.

including "regressive behavior" or stubbornness; episodes of obtundation may point to NCSE [40]. Other etiologies include several genetic syndromes associated with mental retardation [204]. Angelman syndrome can cause atypical absence seizures, with high-voltage bursts of slowing on the EEG, evolving to spike and wave discharges later in childhood [208].

Making the diagnosis of AASE is difficult, primarily because most patients have severe underlying encephalopathies and neurologic deficits, along with a markedly abnormal mental status, even when not in SE. AASE includes impaired responsiveness, prominent epileptiform discharges, and electrographic seizures. To qualify as SE, there should be a clear change from baseline, both clinically and electrographically, but because patients often progress in and out of AASE, electrographic seizures may not correlate well with clinical signs, and it is unclear what role the epileptiform discharges play in the clinical syndrome. It could thus be considered another "boundary syndrome." Radiologic scans are often unremarkable, but some show evidence of cortical dysplasia or hematomas [204].

Episodes of AASE can recur frequently and remain refractory to treatment. Intravenous benzodiazepines may interrupt the EEG discharges without changing behavior substantially, and benzodiazepines may precipitate tonic seizures or tonic SE in these patients [209,210]. The underlying mental retardation and the difficulty of differentiating AASE from an interictal state has often led to less vigorous treatment. When episodes end, the baseline neurologic function is often still significantly impaired. Occasionally, convulsions herald or terminate atypical absence SE. Long-term morbidity is essentially always considered due to the underlying neurologic condition.

The EEG of AASE is characterized by generalized spike or polyspike and slow-wave discharges with a dominant frequency below 3 Hz ("slow-spike-and-wave"), with somewhat less rhythmicity and less perfect symmetry than seen in absence seizures (Figs. 21.16 and 21.17) [207]. Discharge frequencies usually range from 1 to 2.5 Hz and are often irregular, usually superimposed on a slow background. Discharge voltages are usually maximal over the frontal or frontotemporal regions [16]. EEG changes may not correlate well with clinical manifestations. Interictally, the background is usually quite abnormal, including generalized or focal slowing with generalized spike and sharp waves, in isolation or in brief bursts, and admixed low-voltage generalized paroxysmal alpha or beta frequency activity [87, 205].

In a model of AASE with the same response to ASDs as in human AASE, there was a gradual onset of reduced movement, and epileptiform discharges were slower than in absence SE [206]. In typical absence seizures the epileptiform spike and wave discharges appear more restricted to thalamocortical circuitry, but in experimental models of atypical absence, epileptiform discharges also involve the hippocampus and other deep limbic structures [211,212]. Correspondingly, clinical AASE in humans appears to involve more of deeper structures, correlating with the more persistent memory and other cognitive problems in AASE, as opposed to an apparent lack of residua following typical absence SE. The epileptiform discharges of AASE also appear more likely to engender (pathologic) hippocampal synchronization than occurs in typical absence subjects, perhaps because of earlier cerebral damage in patients with LGS or other causes of severe childhood epilepsies [211].

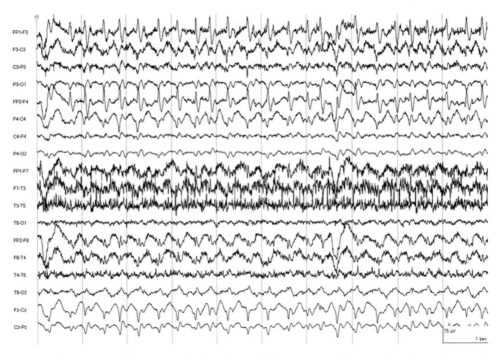

Figure 21.16. AASE in a 49-year-old man with LGS who presented with drooling and lethargy. Interictal EEG shows slow spike and wave activity at 1 Hz. EEG during AASE showed 2- to 2.5-Hz generalized spike-and-wave activity.

24. "NON-CLASSIC" AND SECONDARILY GENERALIZED NONCONVULSIVE STATUS EPILEPTICUS

The forms of NCSE discussed so far, both focal and generalized, constitute the "classic" types of NCSE—absence SE and similar generalized forms of NCSE on the one hand, and CPSE or focal-onset NCSE with dyscognitive features or altered awareness on the other. Most or many cases are related to (and often exacerbations of) prior epilepsy syndromes, sometimes with an acute precipitant. Most cases of NCSE are diagnosed currently, however, are not of these "classic" types but are rather related to acute medical, neurologic, or traumatic illnesses, occasionally superimposed upon epilepsy syndromes but more often arising anew during the acute illness.

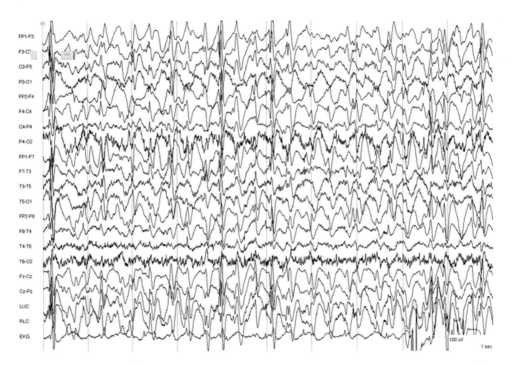

Figure 21.17. AASE in a 26-year-old woman with tuberous sclerosis and LGS. Clinically, there were frequent episodes of staring and blinking lasting 20 to 30 seconds followed by confusion.

In the last two decades, relatively large and increasing numbers of cases of NCSE have been diagnosed in seriously ill patients. Often, those other illnesses contribute to the reduced level of responsiveness and, in turn, make the recognition of NCSE and its clinical significance harder to determine. Consequently, the diagnosis rests heavily on the EEG. These "non-classic" cases are the most common types of NCSE in ICUs.

Generalized NCSE in adults without prior IGE or other epilepsy syndromes is usually not truly "absence" SE, but often secondarily generalized from a focus [27,155], even though the EEG and clinical signs may be generalized at the time of diagnosis. Many are the result of metabolic derangements. Secondarily generalized NCSE is the true diagnosis in many reports of NCSE described earlier as "absence SE," but they have little to do with typical absence epilepsy. They may appear similar clinically (and on EEG) to cases of primary generalized NCSE, and it may be impossible to tell the difference at the time of presentation. True absence SE, for instance in the IGE syndromes, is relatively uncommon, is typically easy to treat, and has an excellent prognosis. "Non-classic" or secondarily generalized NCSE usually has underlying (and sometimes severe) lesions, is much harder to treat, and has the prognosis of the underlying illness.

Many cases of NCSE in ICUs follow the inadequate or unsuccessful treatment of generalized convulsions or GCSE, often found on C-EEG monitoring [20] (see EEG Diagnosis of Nonconvulsive Status Epilepticus, below]. Those patients with minimal movement after GCSE have been called in "subtle generalized convulsive" SE [213]; they are usually stuporous or comatose and often have prominent myoclonus. Many other NCSE patients have had earlier generalized convulsions or GCSE, often in the setting of serious medical illness with cerebrovascular disease, sepsis, hypoxia, or severe metabolic derangements. This NCSE is important to diagnose and treat as clinically significant SE, albeit nonconvulsive.

In these "non-classic" cases of NCSE, the EEG often shows rapid epileptiform discharges on EEG without clinical signs of seizures. Often, generalized NCSE cases cannot be separated easily into those of a primarily generalized nature versus those with focal onset spreading to a broader or even generalized distribution. (Experimentally, generalized epileptiform discharges can result from focal electrical stimulation in frontal regions [214].) Rarely does one capture the onset of SE on EEG except during C-EEG monitoring, and an EEG begun after the onset of NCSE may not allow distinction between focal-onset and generalized forms.

Despite these limitations, the EEG is often helpful in deducing whether there was a focal onset to the seizures. Focal epileptiform discharges, especially with a consistent location, help point to a focal onset. Some episodes of generalized NCSE include prominent focal features on the EEG and clinically [154], possibly because the generalized epileptiform discharges, regular as they appear, are secondarily generalized (Figs. 21.18 and 21.19). Some of these EEGs include discharges with more irregularity or asymmetry than in primarily generalized SE. Also, some apparently generalized epileptiform activity in NCSE evolves toward unilateral discharges with treatment, suggesting a focal onset [15]. Finally, some seizures

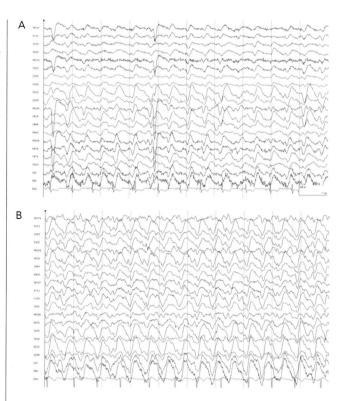

Figure 21.18. A 31-year-old woman with metastatic colon cancer, admitted with catatonia. A: The initial EEG shows rhythmic 1.5-Hz delta activity over the right hemisphere. B: Several hours later, the EEG shows generalized sharp and slow wave discharges at 1.5 Hz, mimicking generalized SE. Ten minutes after 4 mg of intravenous lorazepam was administered, the EEG showed resolution of all rhythmic and sharp activity, and the patient became more responsive clinically.

have minimal or no clinical or EEG features suggesting a focal onset but are associated with known structural lesions and are very likely to have focal origins.

In one review of EEG patterns during NCSE, there were three main groups: (1) epileptiform discharges generalized at the onset; (2) discharges that begin focally, with or without secondary generalization; and (3) patterns with both focal and generalized features, or otherwise poorly classified [15]. In that series of 85 episodes of NCSE in 78 patients, 69% had a generalized pattern of epileptic discharges or other abnormalities, 13% a focal pattern, and 18% a generalized pattern with focal predominance. Among pediatric ICU patients, focal or multifocal NCSE (65%) was more common than generalized SE (35%), often reflecting underlying focal brain lesions [215].

This ongoing electrographic (nonconvulsive, and often secondarily generalized) seizure activity is very common among critically ill ICU patients. Some refer to these patients as in electrographic status epilepticus (ESE) (Fig. 21.20) [45]. Others refer to "status epilepticus in coma," but not all patients with ongoing electrographic seizures are comatose. Some label these patients with severe medical illness as having "epileptic encephalopathies"—indicating that the underlying disease causing the discharges is key, and that the epileptic component is not primary and may not respond to ASDs. This term, however, is probably best reserved for childhood conditions such as those associated with ESES (above).

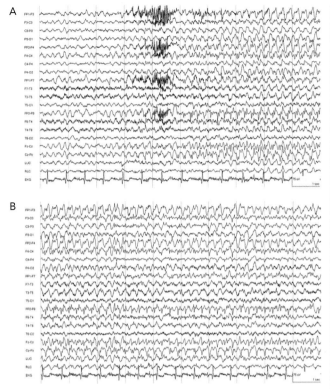

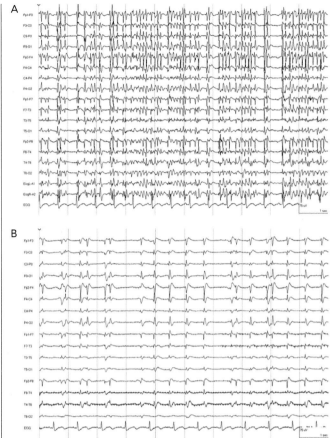

Figure 21.19. A 46-year-old man with a right frontal cavernous malformation, admitted with bizarre behavior. **A:** The EEG during an episode of SE shows initial bilateral frontal (right > left) polyspike and wave activity. **B:** Within 10 seconds of onset, the EEG evolves to show generalized symmetric polyspike and wave activity at 4 Hz, suggestive of primary generalized epilepsy. He had 32 seizures in a 4-hour period.

Figure 21.20. **A:** Electrographic SE in a 50-year-old man with multiple-organ dysfunction after an anoxic insult. The patient was comatose, but there were no other clinical manifestations of seizures. **B:** Same patient after treatment with intravenous levetiracetam, now showing subtle generalized electrographic SE.

The term "subtle" SE often describes the later stages of GCSE, in which initially overt convulsions subside gradually, though the patient remains unresponsive (see previous chapter). The EEG may show discontinuous epileptiform activity with brief bursts of generalized spikes or generalized periodic discharges [45,213]. Some consider these EEG patterns to indicate ongoing SE only if the patient had previous clinical seizures or SE [44]. Many consider this NCSE as a natural progression from GCSE [213]. Most agree that the urgency of treatment continues during the persistent electrographic seizures, at least when preceded by generalized convulsions. Nevertheless, abolition of electrographic seizures does not always lead to clinical improvement, and these patients have high morbidity and mortality [44,213,216,217].

Despite the prominent epileptiform activity on EEG, the diagnosis of NCSE is not always clear (see below). In clinical practice, however, ESE (rhythmic, relatively rapid [>2 Hz] epileptiform discharges, typical for SE on the EEG) without obvious clinical manifestations should be considered SE rather than simply an encephalopathy with epileptiform discharges, even if treatment is unsuccessful in effecting a clinical improvement. The EEGs are very similar to those in many published NCSE studies. Also, patients with ESE upon emergence from pentobarbital or midazolam infusion treatment usually go on to have clinically evident seizures [218,219], indicating that ESE is not just an EEG aberration. Finally, some patients with these EEGs do respond well to ASDs [220].

25. NONCONVULSIVE STATUS EPILEPTICUS IN THE ICU

The diagnosis of NCSE in acutely ill patients with abnormal mental status is often complicated and difficult, and many other conditions mimic NCSE. Among the many reasons for altered behavior and impaired consciousness are severe toxic, metabolic, and infectious encephalopathies, sedating medications, postictal or postoperative encephalopathies (many due to medications), benzodiazepine withdrawal states or toxicity, neuroleptic malignant and serotonin syndromes, and other systemic illnesses. Several of these conditions are accompanied by abnormal EEGs, sometimes even with epileptiform features such as sharp waves.

On the other hand, NCSE is surprisingly common among ICU patients with impaired responsiveness [22,23,220], especially when they have had earlier seizures or clinically evident SE [21,45,219,221]. Of 164 patients who had EEGs after apparent control of clinical SE in one series, 42% had continued seizure discharges, and 14% were considered to be in NCSE [22]. Similarly, 8% of patients with coma of all causes and similar monitoring (without clinical signs of seizures) had NCSE [23]. With C-EEG monitoring for the question of seizures or to evaluate coma, another group found that 19% of patients monitored in a neurologic ICU over a

6-year period had seizures recorded, and 92% of these were strictly nonconvulsive [20].

There are many causes of NCSE in the ICU. Patients with acute neurologic injuries are at particular risk, especially those with intracerebral or subarachnoid hemorrhage, central nervous system infection, brain tumors, severe head trauma, or following neurosurgery: in each of these, 20% to 30% of monitored patients had nonconvulsive seizures in different studies [20,221,223–227].

Coma is a particular risk for NCSE in the ICU, especially if the cause is unclear. In one study, more than half of 97 comatose patients undergoing C-EEG had electrographic seizures [20]. Other risks include recent generalized convulsions, a history of epilepsy, remote symptomatic central nervous system insults (e.g., stroke, neurosurgical intervention, tumor), infection and sepsis, and severe metabolic disturbances [20,35,227].

One group determined that nonconvulsive seizures and NCSE should be suspected in the ICU when (1) a prolonged encephalopathy follows generalized convulsions, an operation, or a neurologic insult; (2) there is acutely impaired or fluctuating consciousness interrupted by normal alertness; (3) there is impaired consciousness with facial myoclonus or nystagmus; (4) staring, aphasia, or automatisms (e.g., limb or facial) occur episodically; or (5) other acutely altered behavior has no obvious cause [216].

The patients at highest risk for unrecognized NCSE are those who were in GCSE and are thought to have been treated successfully—but were not! A prolonged "postictal" state after a convulsion should raise concern for the possibility of ongoing NCSE, and EEG is usually the only way to make the diagnosis [21,22,23,45]. After generalized convulsions, most patients begin to recover responsiveness within 20 to 30 minutes, although there is a broad range. All patients with seizures or SE who do not return to a normal level of consciousness should have EEGs to see if treatment was adequate or if the patient is still seizing.

Correspondingly, the American Clinical Neurophysiology Society (ACNS) Consensus Statement on C-EEG monitoring in critically ill adults and children recommends C-EEG to identify nonconvulsive seizures and NCSE in critically ill patients with (1) persistently abnormal mental status following GCSE or other clinically evident seizures; (2) acute supratentorial brain injury with altered mental status; (3) fluctuating mental status or unexplained alteration of mental status without known acute brain injury; (4) generalized periodic discharges (GPDs), lateralized periodic discharges (LPDs), or bilateral independent periodic discharges (BIPDs) on routine or emergency EEG; (5) requirement for pharmacologic paralysis (e.g., therapeutic hypothermia protocols, extracorporeal membrane oxygenation and risk for seizures); and (6) clinical paroxysmal events suspected to be seizures, to determine if they are epileptic or nonepileptic [228].

How long should C-EEG be continued in the search for nonconvulsive seizures and NCSE? In one study, a routine 30-minute EEG identified electrographic seizures in 11% of 105 critically ill patients, while the subsequent C-EEG (for a median of 2.9 days) found seizures in 27% [229]. In another series, only half of 110 patients with seizures seen eventually on EEG had them during the first hour of recording [20]. In that series, 95% of noncomatose patients had their seizures found in the first 24 hours, versus 80% of comatose patients. After 48 hours, this increased to 98% and 87%, respectively. Among children with seizures, half had the first seizure detected in the first hour of EEG recording, and 80% within 24 hours [230]. These authors concluded that C-EEG monitoring was appropriate for 24 hours in patients without coma and 48 hours in comatose patients, those with periodic discharges, or when ASDs are being withdrawn.

The ACNS Consensus Statement recommends at least 24 hours of recording for critically ill patients with suspected nonconvulsive seizures [228]. Nevertheless, if the first 4 hours of C-EEG show no epileptiform discharges, continued monitoring is unlikely to demonstrate seizures [231]. See also Chapter 22, EEG in the ICU.

26. EEG DIAGNOSIS OF NONCONVULSIVE STATUS EPILEPTICUS

Some unresponsive patients in ICUs (and elsewhere) are having seizures or NCSE, and others are not. It is often impossible to tell the difference solely by clinical examination. EEG is far superior to any other technique in detecting nonconvulsive seizures and is crucial in the assessment of unresponsive patients, particularly those who have had earlier seizures. Nevertheless, seizures can be intermittent, and an individual EEG may miss them, so most modern ICUs utilize C-EEG to detect seizures and other changes in neurophysiologic function.

There are also patients treated for SE with the wrong diagnosis! When clinical manifestations are atypical and appear refractory to first-line ASDs, some diagnoses of SE should be questioned and should be confirmed by EEG prior to more aggressive treatment. It is sometimes necessary to exclude psychogenic nonepileptic SE, a conversion disorder (see Differential Diagnosis, above). The correct diagnosis can prevent inappropriate, aggressive treatment with intravenous ASDs, general anesthesia, and intubation—and their (sometimes very serious) complications [57,232–234].

In psychogenic SE, the EEG background activity is usually normal (Fig. 21.21), but muscle and movement artifact may obscure the EEG [55]. Following epileptic seizures, postictal slowing is the rule, and the presence of a normal alpha rhythm immediately following apparent convulsions (or during brief pauses in motor activity) provides strong evidence for "pseudostatus" (Fig. 21.22).

Seizures captured in their entirety typically show progression from low-voltage high-frequency spikes to high-voltage lower-frequency spike slow-wave activity, before stopping abruptly and being replaced by background slowing or suppression. Usual morphologic features include typical rhythmic, generalized, symmetric spike-and-waves or polyspikes-and-waves at 2 to 3.5 Hz; atypical spike-and-wave with lower frequency and less symmetry; multiple spike-and-wave (repetitive complexes of two or more spikes followed by a slow wave); and high-voltage, repetitive, rhythmic, focal or generalized delta slowing with intermixed spikes, sharp waves, or sharp components (Fig. 21.23) [15,16]. Diagnosis is more difficult when the seizure (or SE) precedes the beginning of the tracing and continues beyond its end. In such cases, rhythmic

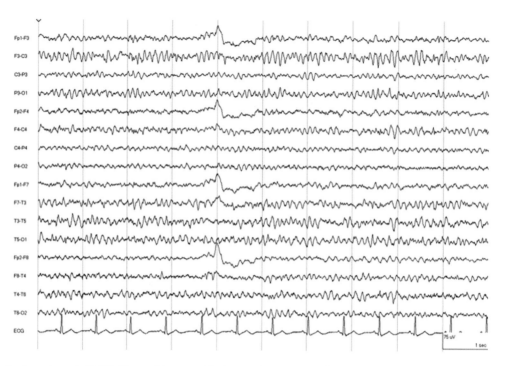

Figure 21.21. *Nonepileptic psychogenic SE. This 51-year-old woman with a history of epilepsy and left temporal lobectomy was admitted with more than 30 episodes per hour characterized by speech arrest, unresponsiveness, and closed eyelids during the episode. EEG shows left hemisphere breach artifact from temporal lobe surgery, but no epileptiform changes.*

sharp features, typically faster than 1 Hz, may be seen, often with variability.

The diagnosis of seizures and NCSE on an EEG relies on the determination by a clinical neurophysiologist that certain patterns are "ictal" in nature (i.e., signifying an ongoing epileptic seizure), but controversy exists regarding which EEG patterns are diagnostic of, or consistent with, NCSE. Sometimes, seizures and NCSE are readily apparent on the EEG, with characteristic or even "classic" features. Other EEGs show disorganized slowing, without rhythmicity or epileptiform abnormalities, more suggestive of encephalopathies than seizures. Very similar EEG findings, however, can be seen in NCSE and in metabolic encephalopathies, and many EEG patterns are neither pathognomonic nor easy to interpret. Even after

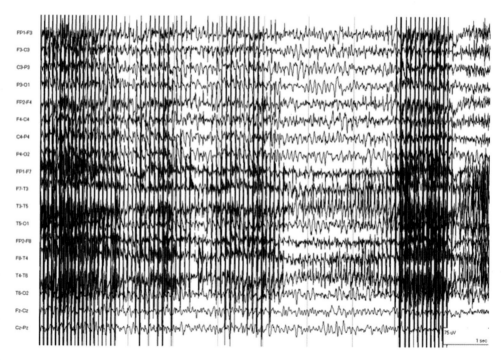

Figure 21.22. *Psychogenic generalized SE. This 22-year-old woman had prolonged episodes of generalized on/off tremulous limb movements. The EEG shows repetitive electromyelographic artifact, with normal background EEG activity evident in the areas between the tremor artifact.*

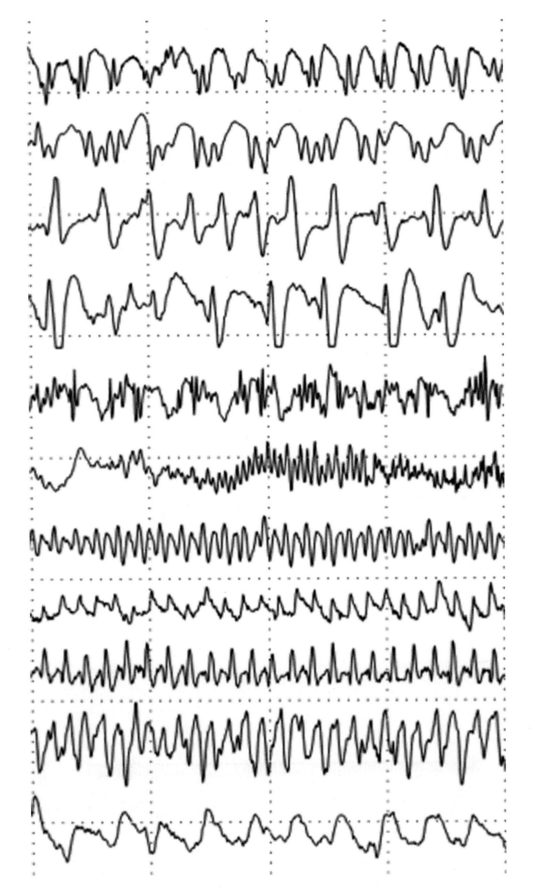

Figure 21.23. *Various EEG waveform morphologies seen in NCSE.*

the diagnosis of NCSE, the clinical significance of the epileptiform discharges can be unclear—that is, the electrographic seizure activity may or may not be the cause of the clinical abnormalities.

The orderly temporal progression of EEG patterns described for GCSE (see the previous chapter) usually does not occur in NCSE [44,235]. In one study of 40 patients, 53% had discrete seizures alone, without any other ictal patterns; 28% had discrete seizures with periodic epileptiform discharges between seizures; and 8% had continuous epileptic activity [235]. Continuous seizures, discrete seizures, or periodic discharges could occur at any time after SE, and no predictable pattern of evolution was identified. EEG evolution probably depends on the etiology and type of SE, baseline condition of the patient, duration of seizure activity, and type and duration of treatment. The variability in evolution adds to the controversy regarding which patterns represent seizures.

There have several proposals for electrographic (EEG) definitions of seizures and NCSE, but there has been a lack of consensus on the terms and descriptors for electrographic seizures and periodic and other abnormal EEG patterns, and on EEG-based definitions of NCSE. To address these problems, a committee of the ACNS recommended standardized terminology for periodic and potentially epileptiform EEG findings in order to facilitate multicenter clinical research [17]. They recommended that EEG findings be described by morphology, location, frequency, and periodicity of waveforms—without using clinical connotations, but with subsequent interpretation in the clinical context. The committee proposed criteria for the EEG diagnosis of seizures [17], as detailed in Box 21.4, and, if persistent enough, NCSE [89,223].

Many investigators follow the ACNS recommendations, noting that seizures are generally indicated by (1) repetitive focal or generalized epileptiform activity or rhythmic waveforms, continuing at a rate faster than 2.5 Hz, lasting longer than 10 seconds or (2) similar discharges slower than 2.5 Hz with (a) unequivocal evolution in frequency, morphology, or field (location); (b) clinical motor manifestations (though often subtle, such as limb or facial twitching); or (c) clear clinical and EEG improvement after administration of rapid-acting intravenous ASDs, typically benzodiazepines [17]. "Evolution" of the electrographic discharges of seizures on the EEG over time includes an increase or decrease in frequency by at least 1 Hz, significant change in waveform morphology, or spread to at least two adjacent EEG electrodes [17] (see Fig. 21.8). Slower discharges are more likely to signify epileptic seizures if they evolve, as above, or follow clinical seizures or SE. This EEG-based diagnosis should be made in a patient with a neurologic deficit that has not resolved or returned to clinical baseline [89].

For patients with a prior "epileptic encephalopathy," criteria include a clear change in prominence or frequency of the features in Box 21.4 when compared to baseline, along with an observable change in clinical state, and an improvement in the clinical and EEG features with intravenous ASDs [16, 89].

Straightforward examples of NCSE on EEG conform to the patterns described above and continue for over 30 minutes. Still, the range of different EEG patterns in NCSE is extensive, as illustrated in one review [16].

BOX 21.4. AMERICAN CLINICAL NEUROPHYSIOLOGY SOCIETY RESEARCH CRITERIA FOR NONCONVULSIVE SEIZURES (AND, IF >30 MINUTES, NONCONVULSIVE STATUS EPILEPTICUS)

1. Repetitive generalized or focal spikes, polyspikes, sharp waves, spike-and-wave or sharp-and-slow-wave complexes, or other rhythmic waveforms at ≥2.5/sec, lasting >10 sec
2. The same waveforms as above, with discharges <2.5/sec, but with:
   a. Clear clinical ictal phenomena, such as facial twitching, nystagmus, or limb myoclonus; or
   b. An unequivocal evolution of the rhythmic pattern, including increase or decrease in frequency (by ≥1 Hz), change in discharge morphology, or change in location (gradual spread of rhythmic activity into or out of a region involving at least two electrodes). Changes in discharge amplitude or "sharpness" alone are not sufficient; or
   c. Rhythmic theta or delta waves at ≥1/sec, with the additional criterion of unequivocal clinical improvement, or improvement on EEG (e.g., resolution of epileptiform discharges and reappearance of previously absent normal background rhythms and reactivity) or both, following quickly after acute administration of rapidly acting ASDs, typically benzodiazepines. (Resolution of discharges leaving a slow background alone, without clinical improvement, would not suffice.)

Adapted from Hirsch and colleagues [17] and Chong and Hirsch [89].

Whatever the generalized or focal pattern, if the patient returns rapidly to a baseline state (after ASD treatment or spontaneously) and the EEG becomes normal, then this very likely was NCSE (Fig. 21.24). Resolution of the epileptiform discharges on EEG and resumption of a posterior alpha frequency background suggestive of wakefulness are also considered diagnostic of a recent seizure.

The ACNS criteria have good specificity for nonconvulsive seizures and NCSE and offer improved certainty in their diagnosis. As such, they are often used clinically. The criteria were designed, however, as guides for research purposes (thus the need for specificity), and sensitivity can be a problem given the wide range of potential findings in patients with clinically confirmed NCSE [15,16]. There are patients whose EEGs do not meet these criteria who are very likely having seizures or are in NCSE [15,223], so clinical judgment is still crucial in diagnosis. For example, in well-established clinical cases of NCSE, stereotypic spike-and-wave activity at 3 Hz or greater was seen in only 7% of patients; discharge frequency was usually 1 to 2.5 Hz [15]. Similar rhythmic and sharp EEG patterns are still strongly suggestive of seizure activity in the appropriate clinical setting, especially following earlier generalized convulsions or GCSE.

Some epileptiform EEG findings generally agreed upon to NOT represent seizures include mid-temporal theta of

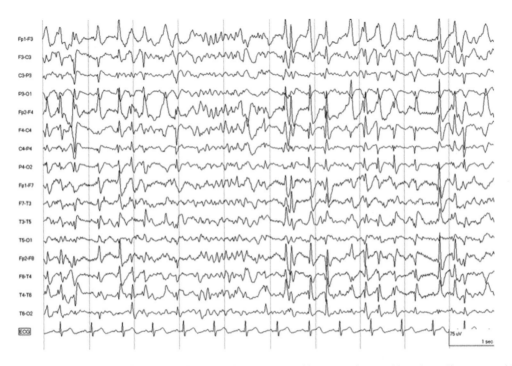

Figure 21.24. Generalized periodic (epileptiform) discharges (GPEDs, or GPDs) in a 62-year-old woman with intractable epilepsy. There is a variable discharge repetition rate, up to 3 Hz, with intervening periods including rhythmic fast activity and variable morphology, which may represent seizure activity. After treatment with intravenous lorazepam, the background showed mild diffuse slowing but no further epileptiform activity. The patient became less confused and was able to answer questions.

drowsiness, rhythmic mid-temporal theta activity, subclinical rhythmic EEG discharges of adults (SREDA), and wicket spikes [223] (see also Chapter 12, Patterns of Unclear Significance). Other patterns generally not considered to represent NCSE include periodic discharges in patients with acute cerebral injuries but without prior clinical seizures, and discharges in patients with epileptic encephalopathies in which the periodic discharges appear similar to those on the baseline EEG [89,236].

Frequently, the EEG determination of seizures is not a blinded exercise. The interpreter may be aware of the patient's staring, facial twitching, or subtle myoclonus and be predisposed to diagnose ambiguous patterns as NCSE. For example, the appearance of periodic discharges at 1 Hz in a patient with occasional focal twitching would favor a diagnosis of seizure over that of an interictal periodic pattern [16]. Often, EEG determination of seizures needs reinterpretation in the clinical setting.

27. CONTROVERSIAL EEG PATTERNS

27.1. Periodic Discharges

Sharp and rhythmic EEG features vary remarkably and range from the "irritative" (postictal, interictal, or pre-ictal) to the "actively seizing" along an "ictal–interictal continuum" [16,89,237]. Periodic discharges have various repetition rates and morphologies and include periodic lateralized (epileptiform) discharges, traditionally labeled PLEDs and more recently LPDs; bilateral independent periodic lateralized (epileptiform) discharges (BiPLEDs or BIPDs); and generalized periodic (epileptiform) discharges (GPEDs or GPDs). Periodic discharges are more likely to be "ictal" (i.e., indicating ongoing epileptic seizure activity) when they are rapid (>2 Hz) (Fig. 21.25), or show clear evolution as described above (see Box 21.4) [89,223]. Periodic discharges with intervening fast and admixed sharp components ("PLEDs-plus" or LPDs+) are also more likely to be ictal than simpler periodic sharp waves (see also Chapter 20, Fig. 20.9A,B) [238]. Finding any of these periodic patterns should prompt consideration of C-EEG monitoring to look for electrographic seizures arising out of that background [239]. Lateralized periodic discharges are discussed further in the preceding chapter.

Generalized periodic (epileptiform) discharges are continuous generalized spikes, polyspikes, sharp-and-slow waves, or sharp waves with triphasic morphology, often with a repetition rate of 1 Hz or greater, typically arising from a diffusely slow or low voltage background (Figs. 21.25, 21.26, 21.27, 21.28) [236]. They are a common finding in C-EEG monitoring in the ICU and highly associated with an abnormal mental status, coma, convulsions, NCSE, and a poor outcome—but given the serious illnesses known to prompt them, GPDs are not *per se* an independent risk factor for the poor outcome [240]. Many are seen following anoxia or other catastrophes, metabolic insults, recent overt seizures, or in the late stages of GCSE [213]. GPDs are highly associated with clinical seizures but not necessarily indicative of seizures proceeding at that time [235,241]. Some consider most GPDs to be definitely ictal and recommend aggressive ASD therapy [242], while others believe that they are the sign of neuronal injury but not actual seizures and do not require aggressive treatment (see Figs. 21.26 and 21.27) [241,243]. One study did not find any features that could

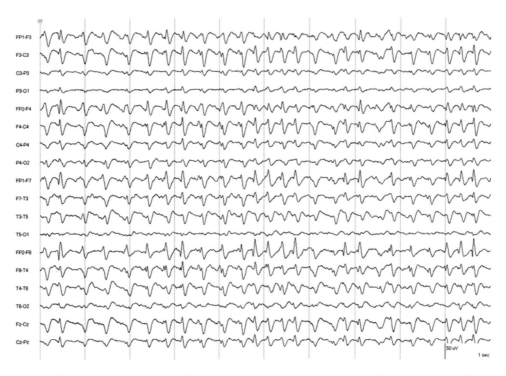

Figure 21.25. EEG of a 72-year-old man following cardiac arrest. On weaning of propofol, continuous electrographic seizures began, with repetitive spike-and-slow-wave discharges at 2.5 to 3 Hz.

distinguish clearly between GPDs after anoxia and GPDs after SE [244], even though those conditions have markedly different implications for treatment. GPDs tend to persist even with aggressive therapy, and it is not known whether patients benefit from ASD treatment for them.

Focal or generalized periodic and quasi-periodic discharges can also be elicited in stuporous or comatose patients upon stimulation—"stimulus-induced rhythmic, periodic, or ictal discharges" (SIRPIDs; see Fig. 21.28) [245]. SIRPIDs usually abate after the stimulus recedes. Whether they represent seizures or an abnormal arousal process is often unclear. Some are definitely seizures [246]. When elicited along with facial or limb jerking (as in a minority of cases), they are more likely to be epileptic phenomena. Many appear to lie along the

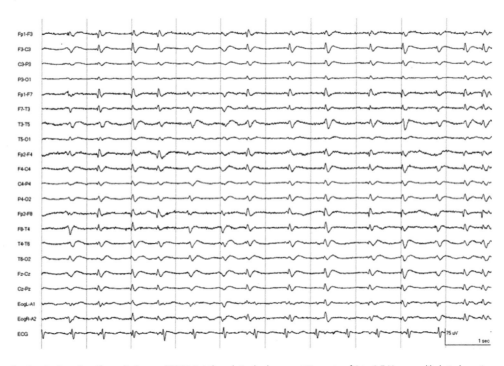

Figure 21.26. Generalized periodic epileptiform discharges (GPEDs) at the relatively slow repetition rate of 1 to 1.5 Hz are unlikely to be seizure activity.

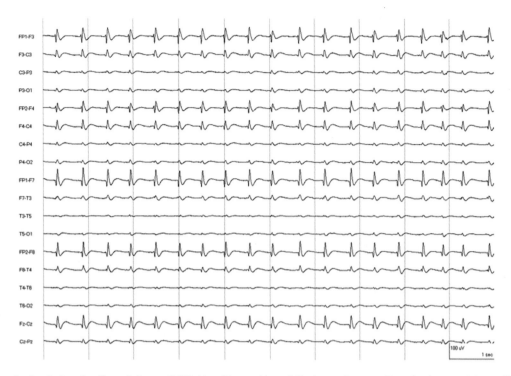

Figure 21.27. Generalized periodic epileptiform discharges (GPEDs) in a 77-year-old man following cardiac arrest. Note the absence of almost all EEG activity other than the discharges.

"ictal–interictal continuum," especially when there is no clinical motor correlate.

27.2. Triphasic Waves

Another controversial area in EEG diagnosis is that of triphasic waves or "GPDs with triphasic morphology"—bursts of moderate- to high-voltage (100–300 uV) rhythmic complexes, often recurring at 1 to 2 Hz (see Fig. 21.24). Triphasic waves are named for their multiphasic morphology, consisting of an initial blunted, low-voltage negative spike-like phase; a second phase consisting of a slowly rising high-voltage positive component; and third phase of a lower-voltage, broad negative slow wave. Triphasic waves are broadly distributed, usually with a

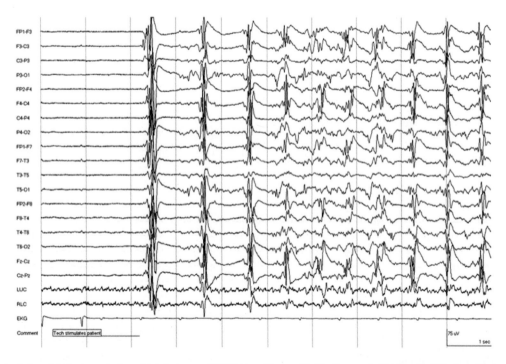

Figure 21.28. Stimulus-induced rhythmic, periodic, or ictal discharges (SIRPIDs) in a 17-year-old girl with encephalitis. Despite high-dose thiopental, she continued to have frequent electrographic seizures, both spontaneously and induced by stimulation, as in this example. Some SIRPIDs were brief and seen only on EEG, but others evolved into clinical generalized convulsions.

frontal voltage maximum. They frequently occur in clusters, but may be continuous at 0.5 to 2 Hz [63]. Triphasic waves are commonly state responsive, increasing with stimulation and attenuating with deeper levels of stupor or coma, and may be abolished or regress after administration of intravenous ASDs or other drugs [63]. Triphasic waves are often associated with diminished levels of consciousness, and occasionally with myoclonus. There is often an underlying toxic or metabolic state, including uremia, hepatic insufficiency, and hypothyroidism; toxicity from lithium, baclofen, ifosfamide, tiagabine, cefapime, neuroleptics, and other medications; or the neuroleptic malignant or serotonin syndromes [53,63,247].

Triphasic waves have long been a source of confusion because of their "epileptiform" appearance on EEG even while they occur in both encephalopathies and NCSE. Typical triphasic waves are generally not considered epileptic by most investigators, but they may be identical to the discharges that occur in definite NCSE, especially when they have a frequency exceeding 1 Hz [248]. "Encephalopathic" triphasic waves are usually of a broader, more blunted appearance than typical epileptiform discharges. Epileptiform discharges in generalized NCSE usually have higher frequencies (mean 2.4 vs. 1.8 Hz), more polyspikes (69% vs. 0%), sharper morphologies, and less concomitant background slowing than triphasic waves associated with encephalopathies [61]. Triphasic waves also have a relative lack of phase reversal, a longer duration, and a lesser slope of incline in the third phase of the waveform. A phase lag from anterior to posterior channels is often seen with triphasic waves (Fig. 21.29A), but not usually with NCSE. Facial or limb myoclonus is more suggestive of SE. Box 21.5 lists characteristics that can help to distinguish NCSE from triphasic waves. Nevertheless, even very experienced EEG-ers have a remarkably poor interrater reliability in distinguishing "epileptic" from encephalopathic triphasic waves [249].

Resolution of triphasic waves in response to administration of benzodiazepines may suggest a diagnosis of NCSE, but benzodiazepines may also abolish typical, even rhythmic, triphasic waves from an underlying encephalopathy, usually without clinical improvement [16,53,63]. Resolution of abnormalities and resumption of a normal alpha waking pattern are more suggestive of NCSE, while resolution of triphasic waves leaving an encephalopathic slow background suggests a nonepileptic encephalopathy. Still, some cases of true NCSE do not respond to ASDs or may also give way to an encephalopathic pattern without clinical improvement. In the end, whether a particular morphology or evolution represents an encephalopathy or NCSE must be determined by an individual, experienced EEG-er. Both conditions may resolve on EEG with benzodiazepines, and there is much that remains unresolved or unproven regarding triphasic waves.

28. TECHNOLOGY

Rapid detection of nonconvulsive seizures, in the ICU or elsewhere, requires near "real-time" review of EEG. Linking continuous digital EEG recordings to a hospital computer network allows EEG technologists and EEG-ers to access ongoing EEG

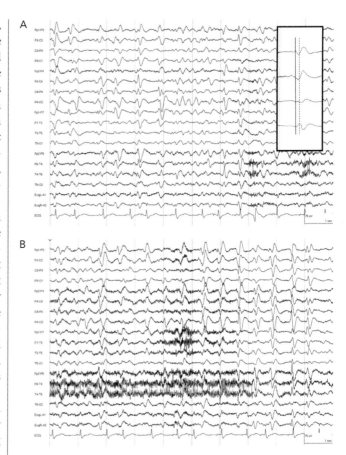

Figure 21.29. A 65-year-old woman with uremia and intermittent episodes of unresponsiveness. *A:* There are occasional 1-Hz frontally maximal triphasic waves. The inset shows the characteristic anterior-to-posterior gradient of triphasic waves—the first negative component in channel 1 (frontal) precedes the negative component in channel 3 (occipital) by about 50 msec. *B:* With stimulation, the triphasic waves increase in amplitude, field, and frequency, mimicking electrographic seizure activity.

from a variety of locations, including offsite over the internet. It also facilitates post-recording adjustment of montages, sensitivity, and filters; acquisition and storage of large amounts of data; quantitative data analysis; and automated spike and seizure detection. For C-EEG to be useful for clinical decisions, records should be reviewed and interpreted by trained personnel several times a day. In one study, only 40% of nonconvulsive seizures were detected visually online at the time of the seizure, with the remainder found at later review [250].

C-EEG produces more data than an individual clinical neurophysiologist can review, at least in its raw form; for example, following an episode of SE, long periods of C-EEG must be reviewed to ensure that breakthrough or recurrent seizures have not occurred. Several digital analysis methods and graphical displays of quantitative EEG are commonly used to condense the enormous quantity of data produced by C-EEG. These methods allow rapid detection of even subtle changes in EEG activity, obviating the need to review thousands of pages or screens of raw EEG data [251]. In a study of ICU EEGs, a display panel of quantitative EEG (Q-EEG) trends shortened the time needed to review 6 hours of EEG, with a seizure identification sensitivity of 51% to 67% and a false-positive rate of one seizure per hour [252]. See also Chapter 22, EEG in the ICU.

Automated detection programs identify EEG segments that include events of interest, such as epileptiform spikes or patterns suggestive of seizures, flagging events for later review by EEG-ers (Fig. 21.30). Several commercially available systems have algorithms designed to identify paroxysmal rhythmic activity with increased voltage or frequency compared to background activity [253,254]. The sensitivity of variables such as frequency (usually 3–20 Hz), field, and voltage can be adjusted to refine detection. Alternatively, artificial neural networks can be trained to detect events by presenting many samples representative of seizures and non-seizures, with the network trained to distinguish between the two patterns [253,255].

A practical concern in using detection algorithms is that nonconvulsive seizures and NCSE exhibit very different electrographic patterns in critically ill patients from those in patients in standard epilepsy monitoring units (EMUs) being evaluated for epilepsy surgery or for a question of seizure versus pseudoseizure [256]. Seizures and NCSE in critically ill patients often have poorer organization, slower frequencies, longer duration, and indistinct onsets and endings. The difference in electrographic seizure morphology makes it harder for standard algorithms to detect seizures in ICUs. Diffuse background slowing, focal slowing or attenuation, and breach artifact may also alter the sensitivity of detection algorithms. Most currently available software has been "trained" and validated primarily on samples from EMUs and ambulatory epilepsy patients [254,257] and is inadequate for detection of ictal patterns in patients with critical neurologic illnesses. New software trained on these patients, and better suited to C-EEG in ICUs, should increase the utility of these algorithms in the ICU [251,253,258].

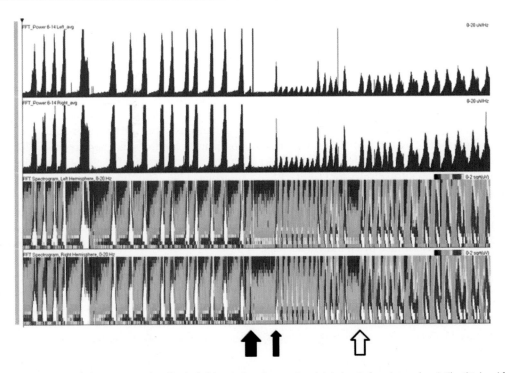

Figure 21.30. CSA shows total power in the 6- to 14-Hz band in the left hemisphere (top row) and right hemisphere (second row). The third and fourth lines show a color density spectrogram in the left and right hemispheres, respectively. Peaks (in blue, top two rows; white, bottom two rows) indicate seizures. Recurrent generalized seizures are eventually controlled by intravenous thiopental (thick arrow) but recur soon as brief seizures (thin arrow), which gradually increase in duration (white arrow).

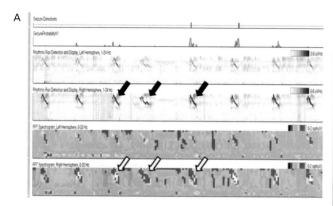

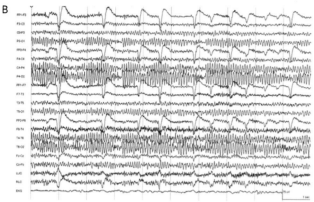

Figure 21.31. A 30-year-old woman with mild mental retardation and intractable epilepsy admitted with lethargy and intermittent head and eye deviation to the right. *A:* Continuous EEG monitoring with automated seizure detection shows frequent right hemisphere seizures over a 2-hour period. Seizures are apparent both on rhythmic run detection and display (black arrows), and color spectrogram (white arrows). EEG showed frequent electrographic seizures beginning with rhythmic beta activity in the right occipital region (seen on traditional EEG display in B). *B:* Individual episode of seizure activity (corresponding to large black arrow on the rhythmic run detection and color spectrogram in A). EEG showed frequent electrographic seizures beginning with rhythmic beta activity in the right occipital region, gradually increasing in amplitude and spreading to the right posterior temporal region and left occipital region.

One commonly employed technique involves creation of graphical displays of Q-EEG data, which uses fast Fourier transformation of digital EEG signals into their component frequencies and amplitudes. Compressed spectral array (CSA) is the most commonly used graphical display for Q-EEG. EEG data for single channels or combinations of channels over each hemisphere, displayed as color graphs of power (e.g., total power; power in certain frequency bands, usually theta and alpha; ratios of power in certain bands to total power) versus time can be used to detect electrographic seizures (Fig. 21.31) [258]. Q-EEG methods can help to select episodes for review by EEG-ers [256]. CSA displays can also assist with an initial, bedside EEG interpretation by ICU personnel and physicians not trained in EEG [258,259], who can then notify EEG technologists or clinical neurophysiologists to review the EEG sections in question.

Still, automatic detection algorithms do not detect all seizures, and they often select artifacts as possible seizures (below); the sensitivity and specificity of these techniques for NCSE in the ICU have not been determined well. Power changes seen on CSA can be caused by seizures, periodic patterns, changes in sleep–wake states, arousal, or artifacts; the specific cause cannot be determined by reviewing the CSA display alone. The associated original, raw EEG data must be available for review to exclude state changes and artifacts altering the Q-EEG, and to confirm that electrographic seizures are not missed (see Fig. 21.31B). Computer analysis can aid in data compression, but it cannot currently replace review by an expert clinical neurophysiologist.

29. ARTIFACTS

C-EEG in the ICU is particularly susceptible to contamination with a variety of artifacts, hindering accurate interpretation [260,261]. Electrode integrity can be difficult to maintain, necessitating use of needle electrodes or disk electrodes affixed with collodion. ICU equipment, bed machinery, hemoperfusion pumps, and ventilators may produce 60-Hz line noise. Artifacts include electrocardiogram, ballistocardiographic, and pacemaker effects. They can also result from skull defects and scalp edema. Nursing care, stimulation, spontaneous arousals, chewing artifact, and chest percussion during physical therapy can all produce artifact. Some artifacts are periodic or rhythmic and mimic epileptiform discharges or electrographic seizures (Figs. 21.32 and 21.33).

ICU patients who are restless or agitated produce substantial movement artifact on EEG. Nonepileptic but rhythmic or paroxysmal movements such as dystonic posturing and (nonepileptic) myoclonus can produce artifacts, as well. Comatose ICU patients may have clinical episodes of twitching, tremors, posturing, or sudden changes of heart rate or blood pressure that may appear to be seizures clinically, and by video. This is not diagnostic unless correlated with simultaneous EEG evidence of seizure activity [246]. The EEG may show some such activity to be very unlikely to be epileptic, and inappropriate to treat as seizures. Accurate interpretation is also facilitated by staff assessment of the patient and recording nursing interventions on the EEG, and by video and audio recording obtained simultaneously with the EEG (which also helps diagnose pseudoseizures). Findings that appear epileptiform may be due to artifact, and others may be seizures when they appear at first to be artifact [246,260]. Video–EEG correlation also aids in clarifying the clinical and behavioral correlates of nonconvulsive seizure activity. Similar behavior might otherwise be ascribed to postictal or interictal confusion or psychosis. Many laboratories use video now even with routine EEG recordings to look for artifacts and their causes.

30. NCSE TREATMENT IN THE ICU

There have been no randomized controlled trials evaluating the treatment of NCSE. Treatment decisions are extrapolated from trials of GCSE treatment or tailored to the perceived urgency and morbidity of the type of NCSE encountered [235,236]. The likelihood of successful treatment is strongly related to the etiology and type of NCSE. Treatment and outcome of absence

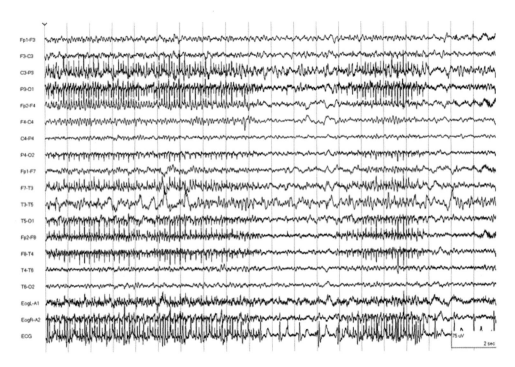

Figure 21.32. Rhythmic artifact from chest percussion obscures much of the EEG.

SE, primary generalized NCSE (i.e., NCSE in absence epilepsy and other IGE syndromes), and CPSE are discussed above in the sections on individual types of NCSE.

As detailed above, absence SE and *de novo* absence SE are usually treated easily and successfully and essentially never require aggressive treatment. AASE is much harder to diagnose and treat. Except for occasional AASE and some more refractory cases of CPSE, however, they are seldom seen in ICUs. The "non-classic" and secondarily generalized NCSE common in ICUs is more often refractory to treatment [36].

Patients with NCSE in the setting of earlier epilepsy are usually treated successfully, often with increased does of their earlier ASDs, or with the addition of other nonsedating ASDs. They generally warrant a less aggressive approach than does GCSE—unless the NCSE is the continuation of GCSE [157]. Treatment is usually similar to that for GCSE (see Treatment of Refractory Status Epilepticus in Chapter 20), but the most aggressive therapies, often those causing respiratory compromise, are usually avoided [173,174] unless NCSE is refractory [262]. Even with NCSE following GCSE, or in the setting of

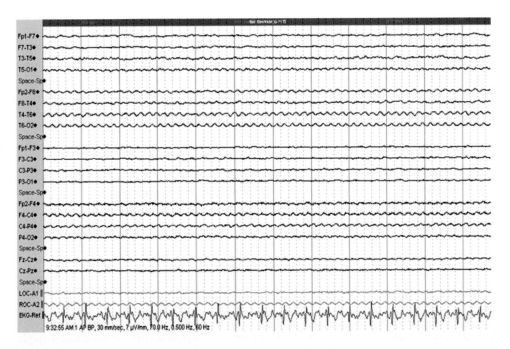

Figure 21.33. Bed percussion artifact.

acute medical illness with severe encephalopathy, much of the diminished level of consciousness and consequent neurologic morbidity stems from the underlying cause of SE rather than from the seizures themselves [220,263].

When the NCSE that follows GCSE becomes refractory, it often necessitates treatment with high doses of sedating ("anesthetic") drugs. It remains unclear, however, whether the best electrographic (EEG) goal of therapy should be seizure suppression alone or greater EEG background suppression to the point of a burst-suppression pattern or even a "flat" EEG [264]. Also, aggressive therapy with midazolam, pentobarbital, or propofol can result in hypotension or prolonged mechanical ventilation and is associated with worsened outcomes—though that is usually attributed to the severe underlying illnesses [20]. One recent study (that included NCSE) raised concern about an association between the use of aggressive management with highly sedating "anesthetic" drugs in ICU patients and poorer outcomes [265]. Nevertheless, it is very difficult to control for the severity of illness and for the refractoriness of the NCSE that prompts the aggressive treatment, and most epileptologists still consider aggressive therapy necessary in the treatment of highly refractory SE in the ICU—definitely including the NCSE or "subtle" GCSE that follows convulsive seizures or GCSE [239,266].

The key to improving outcome in the highly refractory cases may be the expeditious but careful withdrawal of highly sedating medications after control of SE in the ICU, without precipitating relapse of the SE. In this, C-EEG can help guide treatment, tapering of medications, and avoiding under-treatment or overtreatment (see below, and also EEG Use in Refractory Status Epilepticus in Chapter 20).

While risks of overtreatment exist, most patients with NCSE should be treated quickly with ASDs because they are having ongoing seizures with impaired consciousness and other neurologic deficits that are potentially reversible. There is also the attendant morbidity of incidental trauma, aspiration pneumonia, and so on, and many episodes of NCSE begin, and may end, with potentially harmful generalized convulsions.

31. EEG USE IN THE ICU MANAGEMENT OF NCSE

Even after the diagnosis of nonconvulsive seizures or NCSE, most ICU patients need C-EEG monitoring during prolonged treatment. NCSE persists in 14% to 20% of patients after cessation of clinically evident seizure activity [22]. Clinical signs of NCSE are nonspecific, subtle, or nonexistent, and C-EEG is necessary to monitor the response of seizures and NCSE to treatment, including continuous intravenous ASDs for refractory NCSE [228]. EEG also helps to determine if NCSE recurs during treatment. Relapse of NCSE is not rare, especially in the first 24 hours of treatment [22] and also when ASDs are being tapered, but it portends a worsened outcome and should be avoided if possible [267].

Nonconvulsive seizures can be missed if EEG monitoring is intermittent. A given EEG may show a "postictal" encephalopathy, drug effect, isolated or periodic discharges, or a burst-suppression tracing at one point—and nonconvulsive seizures or NCSE may occur shortly thereafter (Figs. 21.34 and 21.35; see also Fig. 20.9A,B in Chapter 20). Without C-EEG, the seizures will not be detected.

If NCSE recurs, it should be treated again while following the EEG, but the best method, intensity, and duration of treatment have not yet been determined. For refractory

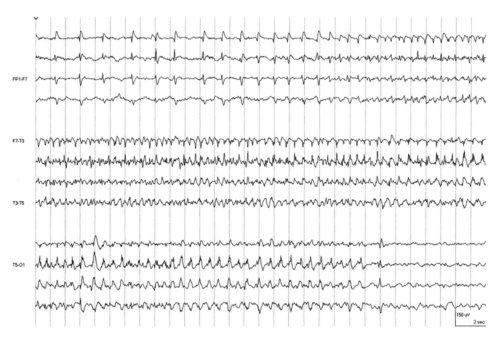

Figure 21.34. Evolution of an electrographic seizure in a comatose 55-year-old woman with a left temporal intracerebral hemorrhage. EEG shows left temporal periodic lateralized epileptiform discharges (PLEDs) evolving into faster-frequency, sharply contoured delta activity. Evolution of the seizure includes spread in the left temporal region, and then the left parasagittal region, and eventual end of the seizure. The patient remained comatose, without clinical manifestation of the seizure.

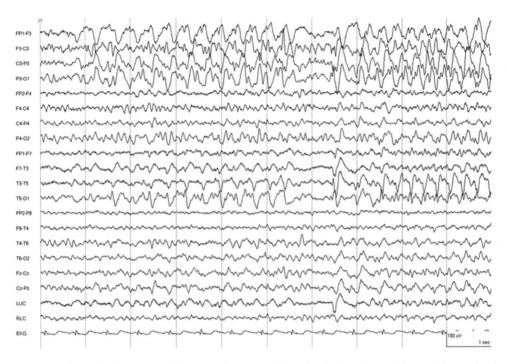

Figure 21.35. A focal seizure arises from the left hemisphere after an EEG showing PLEDs (see Fig. 20.7A in Chapter 20) in the left parietal and posterior temporal regions in a 26-year-old woman with adult-onset Rasmussen's encephalitis and earlier focal SE.

NCSE, many neurologists will use additional standard ASDs and then, if this is unsuccessful, a trial of aggressive treatment (often with midazolam, pentobarbital, or propofol) to at least suppress all electrographic and clinical seizures [268,269].

Often, C-EEG also offers important prognostic information for nonconvulsive seizures and NCSE. Earlier diagnosis and C-EEG–guided ICU treatment may improve the care of patients with SE, but their effect on outcome has not been established conclusively [263,270].

Many patients supported in cardiac ICUs following the return of circulation after cardiorespiratory arrest are treated with therapeutic hypothermia and are paralyzed and sedated, with consequent absence of clinical markers of brain dysfunction. C-EEG has also been used increasingly to monitor for nonconvulsive seizures and NCSE, and to assess EEG reactivity in these patients [271,272].

32. MORBIDITY AND OUTCOME OF NCSE

Outcome for specific NCSE types is discussed above for simple partial SE, absence SE, and well-defined cases of CPSE, but many clinical series describe NCSE without specifying the type. The prognosis for these many different illnesses depends heavily on the type of NCSE, as identified clinically and by EEG, and on their causes and precipitants, and may also be influenced by age and medical comorbidities. Etiology is by far the most important prognostic factor; generally, the most favorable etiology is epilepsy itself with some relatively benign precipitant, such as reduced ASDs. Some types of NCSE have an excellent prognosis, without evidence of morbidity in any case, but others have a high likelihood of a fatal outcome. For example, there is essentially no mortality risk with absence or

simple partial sensory SE [117,181,189], but NCSE in medically ill ICU patients and those in coma has a much poorer prognosis [172].

Longer-term risks of NCSE should consider both experimental and clinical data, but most basic studies on the damage due to SE have used models of GCSE. While GCSE poses a definite threat to health and warrants vigorous treatment, there is little evidence of lasting harm due to NCSE alone [273]. The treatment imperative is less, but not negligible. Overall, NCSE may be potentially "underdiagnosed and overtreated" [152].

In non-ICU patients, clinical reports of NCSE show few long-term sequelae of the NCSE itself [37,38,274], but most have had limited follow-up. Cognitive deficits caused by NCSE, including language dysfunction, can persist for months [68]. One study of 65 NCSE patients found good outcomes in all but one [275]. Another reported neuropsychologic testing on 15 epilepsy patients (without underlying lesions or "symptomatic" causes) before and after episodes of SE (half nonconvulsive) [276] demonstrating that no significant cognitive morbidity accrued from the SE itself. Long-term cognitive complications of NCSE, especially among non-ICU patients, appear relatively uncommon, occurring primarily in the most prolonged and severe cases.

Outcome is not nearly as favorable for patients with "nonclassic" and secondarily generalized NCSE in the setting of serious medical and neurologic illness, especially in the ICU. The physiologic effects of persistent NCSE in critically ill patients can include increased cerebral blood flow, intracranial pressure, and oxygen demands, and changes in the lactate–pyruvate ratio [277,278]. NCSE might exacerbate neuronal damage in patients with acute insults such as traumatic brain injury or stroke [221]. Patients with both intracerebral hemorrhage and nonconvulsive electrographic seizures had a worse outcome in two reports, but it was not possible to determine if this was due to the seizures or (more likely) the underlying illness [224,225]. Among 94 consecutive patients with moderate to severe traumatic brain injury, 22% had electrographic seizures on EEG, and 29% were in NCSE, with higher mortality in these patients than in similar trauma patients without seizures [221]. It remains unclear whether better treatment of nonconvulsive seizures would have changed this [279]. In one series of 49 patients with nonconvulsive seizures, mortality correlated with etiology, age, and length of ICU stay, but only seizure duration and delay to diagnosis were significant predictors upon multivariate analysis [216].

One series of patients with NCSE found that patients with minimal obtundation had a mortality of 7% versus 39% for those with deep lethargy or coma [172]. Patients with anoxia or multiple medical problems, including sepsis, fare poorly, while those with strokes, tumors, trauma, infection, alcohol abuse, or other drugs have intermediate results [27].

In the setting of severe medical or neurologic disease, the morbidity and mortality of NCSE are substantial [172], although it is difficult to dissect out that portion of the long-term harm caused by epileptiform discharges, seizures, or SE from the damage caused by the underlying illness [44,45,220,222]. Little of this morbidity is usually attributed to the NCSE itself, but in one pediatric ICU, the total nonconvulsive seizure "burden" (the percentage of time in nonconvulsive seizures or NCSE) correlated strongly and independently with a greater clinical deterioration, even in patients with the same disease etiologies [280]. This suggests that the nonconvulsive seizures and NCSE themselves contributed significantly to longer-term neurologic dysfunction. Complications of treatment can also contribute to morbidity [263].

SCORE EEG SOFTWARE

Further examples related to the topics addressed in this chapter can be found in the interactive online Niedermeyer Educational Platform. EEG recordings with illustrative examples can be opened and browsed. Features are marked and described using the SCORE EEG software. The users can see the features marked by experts, they can score these features themselves, and then compare them with the scorings of the experts.

The Niedermeyer Educational Platform can be accessed at: www.scoreEEG.com/academy

REFERENCES

1. Temkin O, ed. The falling sickness. Baltimore: The Johns Hopkins Press, 1971.
2. Shorvon S. The concept of status epilepticus and its history. In: Shorvon S, ed., Status epilepticus: its clinical features and treatment in children and adults. Cambridge: Cambridge University Press, 1994:1–20.
3. Trousseau A. Lectures on clinical medicine delivered at the Hôtel Dieu, Paris. vol. 1, translated by Bazire PV. London: New Sydenham Society, 1868.
4. Falret J. "De l'état mental des épileptiques." Archives Générales de Médecine, Fifth Series 1860;16:661–679; 1861;17:461–449.
5. Wilks S. Lectures on diseases of the nervous system. London: Churchill, 1878.
6. Goetz CG. Charcot the clinician: the Tuesday lessons. New York: Raven Press, 1987.
7. Gowers WR. Epilepsy and other chronic convulsive disorders. London: Churchill, 1901.
8. Zimmer C. Soul made flesh. The discovery of the brain—and how it changed the world. New York: Free Press, Simon & Schuster, 2004.
9. Berger H. Über das Elektrenkephalogramm des Menschen. Arch Psychiat Nerv Krankh 1929;87:527.
10. Gloor P. The work of Hans Berger. In: Cobb WA, ed., Appraisal and perspective of the functional explorations of the nervous system. Handbook of electroencephalography and clinical neurophysiology. Amsterdam: Elsevier Publishing Co., 1971: IA11–24.
11. Lennox WG. The treatment of epilepsy. Med Clin North Am 1945;29:1114–1128.
12. Penfield W, Jasper HH. Epilepsy and functional anatomy of the human brain. Boston: Little Brown, 1954.
13. Gastaut H, Roger A. Sur la signification de certain fugues épileptiques: état de mal temporal. Rev Neurol 1956;94:298–301.
14. Kaplan PW. Behavioral manifestations of nonconvulsive status epilepticus. Epilepsy Behav 2002; 3:122–139.
15. Granner MA, Lee SI. Nonconvulsive status epilepticus: EEG analysis in a large series. Epilepsia 1994;35:42–47.
16. Sutter R, Kaplan PW. The neurophysiologic types of nonconvulsive status epilepticus: EEG patterns of different phenotypes. Epilepsia 2013;54(suppl 6):23–27.
17. Hirsch LJ, Brenner RP, Drislane FW, So E, Kaplan PW, Jordan KG, Herman ST, LaRoche SM, Young GB, Bleck TP, Scheuer ML, Emerson RG. The ACNS subcommittee on research terminology for continuous EEG monitoring: Proposed standardized terminology for rhythmic and periodic EEG patterns encountered in critically ill patients. J Clin Neurophysiol 2005;22:128–135.
18. Sutter R, Kaplan PW. Electroencephalographic criteria for nonconvulsive status epilepticus: Synopsis and comprehensive survey. Epilepsia 2012;53(suppl 3):1–51.
19. Kaplan PW. Electroencephalographic criteria for nonconvulsive status epilepticus. Epilepsia 2007;48(suppl 8):39–41.
20. Claassen J, Mayer SA, Kowalski RG, Emerson RG, Hirsch LJ. Detection of electrographic seizures with continuous EEG monitoring in critically ill patients. Neurology 2004;62:1743–1748.
21. Fagan KJ, Lee SI. Prolonged confusion following convulsions due to generalized non-convulsive status epilepticus. Neurology 1990;40:1689–1694.
22. DeLorenzo RJ, Waterhouse EJ, Towne AR, Boggs JG, Ko D, DeLorenzo GA, Brown A, Garnett L. Persistent nonconvulsive status epilepticus after the control of convulsive status epilepticus. Epilepsia 1998;39:833–840.
23. Towne AR, Waterhouse EJ, Boggs JG, Garnett LK, Brown AJ, Smith JR, Jr., DeLorenzo RJ, Smith JR Jr. Prevalence of nonconvulsive status epilepticus in comatose patients. Neurology 2000;54:340–345.
24. Trinka E, Cock H, Hesdorffer D, Rossetti AO, Scheffer IE, Shinnar S, Shorvon S, Lowenstein DH. A definition and classification of status epilepticus—Report of the ILAE Task Force on Classification of Status Epilepticus. Epilepsia 2015;56:1515–1523.
25. Shorvon SD. What is nonconvulsive status epilepticus, and what are its subtypes? Epilepsia 2007;48(suppl 8):35–38.
26. Lowenstein DH, Bleck T, Macdonald RL. It's time to revise the definition of status epilepticus. Epilepsia 1999;40:120–122.
27. DeLorenzo RJ, Hauser WA, Towne AR, Boggs JG, Pellock JM, Penberthy L, Garnett L, Fortner CA, Ko D. A prospective, population-based epidemiologic study of status epilepticus in Richmond, Virginia. Neurology 1996;46:1029–1035.
28. Vignatelli L, Rinaldi R, Galeotti M, de Carolis P, D'Alessandro R. Epidemiology of status epilepticus in a rural area of northern Italy: a 2-year population-based study. Eur J Neurol 2005;12:897–902.
29. Shorvon S. Definition, classification and frequency of status epilepticus. In: Shorvon S, ed., Status epilepticus: its clinical features and treatment in children and adults. Cambridge: Cambridge University Press, 1994:21–33.
30. Coeytaux A, Jallon P, Galobardes B, Morabia A. Incidence of status epilepticus in French-speaking Switzerland. Neurology 2000;55:693–697.
31. Knake S, Rosenow F, Vescovi M, Oertel WH, Mueller H-H, Wirbatz A, Katsarou N, Hamer HM. Incidence of status epilepticus in adults in Germany: a prospective, population-based study. Epilepsia 2001;42:714–718.
32. Cockerell OC, Walker MC, Sander JWAS, Shorvon SD. Complex partial status epilepticus: a recurrent problem. J Neurol Neurosurg Psychiatry 1994;57:835–837.
33. Tomson T, Svanborg E, Wedlund JE. Nonconvulsive status epilepticus: high incidence of complex partial status. Epilepsia 1986;27:276–285.

34. Kaplan PW, Tusa RJ. Neurophysiologic and clinical correlations of epileptic nystagmus. Neurology 1993;43:2508–2514.
35. Husain AM, Horn GJ, Jacobson MP. Non-convulsive status epilepticus: usefulness of clinical features in selecting patients for urgent EEG. J Neurol Neurosurg Psychiatry 2003;74:189–191.
36. Kaplan PW. Nonconvulsive status epilepticus in the emergency room. Epilepsia 1996;37:643–650.
37. Guberman A, Cantu-Reyna G, Stuss D, Broughton R. Nonconvulsive generalized status epilepticus: clinical features, neuropsychological testing, and long-term follow-up. Neurology 1986;36:1284–1291.
38. Dunne JW, Summers QA, Stewart-Wynne EG. Non-convulsive status epilepticus: a prospective study in an adult general hospital. Q J Med 1987;62:117–126.
39. Stores G, Zaiwalla Z, Styles E, Hoshika A. Non-convulsive status epilepticus. Arch Dis Child 1995;73:106–111.
40. Brodtkorb E, Sand T, Kristiansen A, Torbergsen T. Non-convulsive status epilepticus in the adult mentally retarded. Seizure 1993;2:115–123.
41. Thomas P, Beaumanoir A, Genton P, Dolisi C, Chatel M. "De novo" absence status of late onset: report of 11 cases. Neurology 1992;42:104–110.
42. Tatum WO, Ross J, Cole AJ. Epileptic pseudodementia. Neurology 1998;50:1472–1475.
43. Chicarro AV, Kanner AM. Psychiatric manifestations of nonconvulsive status epilepticus. In Kaplan PW, Drislane FW, eds., Nonconvulsive status epilepticus. New York: Demos Medical Publishing, 2009:203–215.
44. Lowenstein D, Aminoff M. Clinical and EEG features of status epilepticus in comatose patients. Neurology 1992;42:100–104.
45. Drislane FW, Schomer DL. Clinical implications of generalized electrographic status epilepticus. Epilepsy Res 1994;19:111–121.
46. Pritchard PB 3d, O'Neal DB. Nonconvulsive status epilepticus following metrizamide myelography. Ann Neurol 1984;16:252–254.
47. Zak R, Solomon G, Petito F, Labar D. Baclofen-induced generalized nonconvulsive status epilepticus. Ann Neurol 1994;36:113–114.
48. Panayiotopoulos CP, Agathonikou A, Sharoqi IA, Parker AP. Vigabatrin aggravates absences and absence status. Neurology 1997;49(5):1467.
49. Shinnar S, Berg AT, Treiman DT, Hauser WA, Hesdorffer DC, Sackellares JC, Leppik I, Sillanpaa M, Sommerville KW. Status epilepticus and tiagabine therapy: review of safety data and epidemiologic comparisons. Epilepsia 2001;42:372–379.
50. Feddersen B, Bender A, Arnold S, Klopstock T, Noachtar S. Aggressive confusional state as a clinical manifestation of status epilepticus in MELAS. Neurology 2003;61:1149–1150.
51. Dalmau J, Rosenfeld MR. Paraneoplastic syndromes of the CNS. Lancet Neurol 2008;7:327–340.
52. Dalmau J, Gleichman AJ, Hughes EG, Rossi JE, Peng X, Lai M, Dessain SK, Rosenfeld MR Balice-Gordon R, Lynch DR. Anti-NMDA-receptor encephalitis: case series and analysis of the effects of antibodies. Lancet Neurol 2008;7:1091–1098.
53. Kaplan PW, Birbeck G. Lithium-induced confusional states: nonconvulsive status epilepticus or triphasic encephalopathy? Epilepsia 2006;47:2071–2074.
54. Dworetzky BA, Bubrick EJ, Szaflarski JP. Nonepileptic psychogenic status: markedly prolonged psychogenic nonepileptic seizures. Epilepsy Behav 2010;19:65–68.
55. Holtkamp M, Othman J, Buchheim K, Meierkord H. Diagnosis of psychogenic nonepileptic status epilepticus in the emergency setting. Neurology 2006;66:1727–1729.
56. Asadi-Pooya AA, Emami Y, Emami M, Sperling MR. Prolonged psychogenic nonepileptic seizures or pseudostatus. Epilepsy Behav 2014;31:304–306.
57. Reuber M, Baker GA, Gill R, Smith DF, Chadwick DW. Failure to recognize psychogenic nonepileptic seizures may cause death. Neurology 2004;62:834–835.
58. Kanner AM, Morris HH, Luders H, Dinner DS, Wyllie E, Medendorp SV, Rowan AJ. Supplementary motor seizures mimicking pseudoseizures: some clinical differences. Neurology 1990;40:1404–1407.
59. Williamson PD, Spencer DD, Spencer SS, Novelly RA, Mattson RH. Complex partial status epilepticus: a depth-electrode study. Ann Neurol 1985;18:647–654.
60. Tomson T, Lindbom U, Nilsson BY. Nonconvulsive status epilepticus in adults: thirty-two consecutive patients from a general hospital population. Epilepsia 1992;33:829–835.
61. Boulanger JM, Deacon C, Lecuyer D, Gosselin S, Reiher J. Triphasic waves versus nonconvulsive status epilepticus: EEG distinction. Can J Neurol Sci 2006;33:175–180.
62. Hirsch LJ, Gaspard N. Status epilepticus. Continuum 2013;19(3 Epilepsy):767–794.
63. Fountain NB, Waldman WA. Effects of benzodiazepines on triphasic waves: implications for nonconvulsive status epilepticus. J Clin Neurophysiol 2001;18:345–352.
64. Treiman DM, Meyers PD, Walton NY, Collins JF, Colling C, Rowan AJ, Handforth A, Faught E, Calabrese VP, Uthman BM, Ramsay RE, Mamdani MB. A comparison of four treatments for generalized convulsive status epilepticus. Veterans Affairs Status Epilepticus Cooperative Study Group. N Engl J Med 1998;339:792–798.
65. Schmitt SE, Pargeon K, Frechette ES, Hirsch LJ, Dalmau J, Friedman D. Extreme delta brush: a unique EEG pattern in adults with anti-NMDA receptor encephalitis. Neurology 2012 11;79(11):1094–1000.
66. Sutter R, Kaplan PW. Electroencephalography of autoimmune limbic encephalopathy. J Clin Neurophysiol 2013;30:490–504.
67. Dong C, Sriram S, Delbeke D, Al-Kaylani M, Arain AM, Singh P, McLean MJ, Abou-Khalil B. Aphasic or amnestic status epilepticus detected on PET but not EEG. Epilepsia 2009;50:251–255.
68. van Paesschen W, Porke K, Fannes K, Vandenberghe R, Palmini A, van Laere K, Dupont P. Cognitive deficits during status epilepticus and time course of recovery: a case report. Epilepsia 2007;48:1979–1983.
69. Kutluay E, Beattie J, Passaro EA, Edwards JC, Minecan D, Milling C, Selwa L, Beydoun A. Diagnostic and localizing value of ictal SPECT in patients with nonconvulsive status epilepticus. Epilepsy Behav 2005;6:212–217.
70. Lothman EW, Bertram EH, Bekenstein JW, Perlin JB. Self-sustaining limbic status epilepticus induced by "continuous" hippocampal stimulation: electrographic and behavioral characteristics. Epilepsy Res 1989;3:107–119
71. van Landingham KE, Lothman EW. Self-sustaining limbic status epilepticus. I. Acute and chronic cerebral metabolic studies: limbic hypermetabolism and neocortical hypometabolism. Neurology 1991;41:1942–1949.
72. Kapur J. Pathophysiology of nonconvulsive status epilepticus. In: Kaplan PW, Drislane FW, eds., Nonconvulsive status epilepticus. New York: Demos Medical Publishing, 2009:81–94.
73. van Landingham KE, Lothman EW. Self-sustaining limbic status epilepticus. II. Role of hippocampal commissures in metabolic responses. Neurology 1991;41:1950–1957.
74. Lothman EW, Bertram EH. Epileptogenic effects of status epilepticus. Epilepsia 1993;34(suppl 1):59–70.
75. Wasterlain CG, Mazarati AM, Naylor D, Niquet J, Liu H, Suchomelova L, Baldwin R, Katsumori H, Shirasaka Y, Shin D, Sankar R. Short-term plasticity of hippocampal neuropeptides and neuronal circuitry in experimental status epilepticus,. Epilepsia 2002;43(suppl 5):20–29.
76. Mazarati AM, Halaszi E, Telegdy G. Anticonvulsant effects of galanin administered into the central nervous system upon the picrotoxin-kindled seizure syndrome in rats. Brain Res 1992;589:164–166.
77. Liu H, Mazarati AM, Katsumori H, Sankar R, Wasterlain CG. Substance P is expressed in hippocampal principal neurons during status epilepticus and plays a critical role in the maintenance of status epilepticus. Proc Natl Acad Sci USA 1999;96:5286–5291.
78. Hughes JR. Absence seizures: a review of recent reports with new concepts. Epilepsy Behav 2009:15:404–412.
79. Gloor P, Fariello RG. Generalized epilepsy: some of its cellular mechanisms differ from those of focal epilepsy. Trends Neurosci 1988;11:63–68.
80. Jasper HH, Droogleever-Fortuyn J. Experimental studies on the functional anatomy of petit mal epilepsy. Res Publ Assoc Nerv Ment Dis. 1947;26: 272–298.
81. Williams D. The thalamus and epilepsy. Brain 1965;88:539–556.
82. Tien RD, Felsberg GJ. The hippocampus in status epilepticus: demonstration of signal intensity and morphologic changes with sequential fast spin-echo MR imaging. Radiology. 1995;194:249–256.
83. Wieshmann UC, Woermann FG, Lemieux L, Free SL, Bartlett PA, Smith SJ, Duncan JS, Stevens JM, Shorvon SD. Development of hippocampal atrophy: a serial magnetic resonance imaging study in a patient who developed epilepsy after generalized status epilepticus. Epilepsia 1997;38:1238–1241.
84. Lothman E. The biochemical basis and pathophysiology of status epilepticus. Neurology 1990;40(suppl 2):13–23.
85. Lowenstein DH, Shimosaka S, So YT, Simon RP. The relationship between electrographic seizure activity and neuronal injury. Epilepsy Res 1991;10:49–54.
86. Bertram EH, Lothman EW, Lenn NJ. The hippocampus in experimental chronic epilepsy: a morphometric analysis. Ann Neurol 1990;27:43–48.
87. Gastaut H. Classification of status epilepticus. Adv Neurol 1983;34:15–35.
88. Shorvon S. The classification of nonconvulsive status epilepticus. In: Kaplan PW, Drislane FW, eds., Nonconvulsive status epilepticus. New York: Demos Medical Publishing, 2009:11–22.
89. Chong DJ, Hirsch LJ. Which EEG patterns warrant treatment in the critically ill? Reviewing the evidence for treatment of periodic epileptiform discharges and related patterns. J Clin Neurophysiol 2005;22(2):79–91.
90. Olmos-Garcia de Alba G, Udaeta Mora E, Malagon Valdez J, Villaneuva Garcia D, Valarezo Crespo F. Neonatal status

epilepticus II: Electroencephalographic aspects. Clin Electroencephalogr 1984;15:197–201.

91. Mizrahi EM, Kellaway P. Characterization and classification of neonatal seizures. Neurology 1987;37:1837–1844.

92. Knauss TA, Carlson CB. Neonatal paroxysmal monorhythmic alpha activity. Arch Neurol 1978;35:104–107.

93. Scher MS. Controversies regarding neonatal seizure recognition. Epileptic Disord 2002;4:139–158.

94. Clancy RR, Legido A. The exact ictal and interictal duration of electroencephalographic neonatal seizures. Epilepsia 1987;28:537–541.

95. Bureau M. "Continuous spikes and waves during slow sleep" (CSWS): definition of the syndrome. In: Beaumanoir A, Bureau M, Deonna T, Mira L, Tassinari CA., eds., Continuous spikes and waves during slow sleep. London: John Libbey and Co., 1995:17–26.

96. Riviello JJ Jr. Status epilepticus in children. In: Drislane FW, ed., Status epilepticus: a clinical perspective. Totowa, NJ: Humana Press, 2005:313–338.

97. Hadjiloizou S, Riviello JJ. Epileptic and epileptiform encephalopathies. Neurology, Emedicine, WebMD, 2006.

98. Patry G, Lyagoubi S, Tassinari CA. Subclinical "electrical status epilepticus" induced by sleep in children. A clinical and electroencephalographic study of six cases. Arch Neurol 1971;24:242–252.

99. Tassinari CA, Bureau M, Dravet C, Dalla Bernardina B, Roger J. Epilepsy with continuous spikes and waves during slow sleep—otherwise described as ESES (epilepsy with electrical status epilepticus during slow sleep). In: Roger J, Bureau M, Dravet C, Dreifuss FE, Perret A, Wolf P, eds., Epileptic syndromes in infancy, childhood, and adolescence (2nd ed). London: John Libbey and Co., 1992:245–256.

100. De Negri M. Electrical status epilepticus during sleep (ESES). Different clinical syndromes: towards a unifying view? Brain Dev 1997;19:447–451.

101. Guilhoto LMFF, Morrell F. Electrophysiological differences between Landau-Kleffner Syndrome and other conditions showing the CSWS electrical pattern [abstract]. Epilepsia 1994;35(suppl. 8):126.

102. Landau WM, Kleffner FR. Syndrome of acquired epileptic aphasia with convulsive disorder in children. Neurology 1957;7:523–530.

103. Bishop DVM. Age of onset and outcome in acquired aphasia with convulsive disorder (Landau-Kleffner syndrome). Dev Med Child Neurol 1985;27:705–712.

104. Riviello JJ Jr. Nonconvulsive status epilepticus in children. In: Kaplan PW, Drislane FW, eds., Nonconvulsive status epilepticus. New York: Demos Medical Publishing, 2009:227–237.

105. Lerman P, Lerman-Sagie T, Kivity S. Effect of early corticosteroid therapy for Landau-Kleffner syndrome. Dev Med Child Neurol 1991;33:257–260.

106. Shinnar S, Rapin I, Arnold S, Tuchman RF, Shulman L, Ballaban-Gil K, Maw M, Deuel RK, Volkmar FR. Language regression in childhood. Pediatr Neurol 2001;24:183–189.

107. Kramer U, Nevo Y, Neufeld MY, Fatal A, Leitner Y, Harel S. Epidemiology of epilepsy in childhood: a cohort of 440 consecutive patients. Pediatr Neurol 1998;18:46–50.

108. Devinsky O, Kelley K, Porter RJ, Theodore WH. Clinical and electroencephalographic features of simple partial seizures. Neurology 1988;38:1347–1352.

109. Friedman DE, Schevon C, Emerson RG, Hirsch LJ. Cyclic electrographic seizures in critically ill patients. Epilepsia 2008;49:281–287.

110. Iizuka T, Sakai F, Suzuki N, Hata T, Tsukahara S, Fukuda M, Takiyama Y. Neuronal hyperexcitability in stroke-like episodes of MELAS syndrome. Neurology 2002;59:816–824.

111. Taylor I, Scheffer IE, Berkovic SF. Occipital epilepsies: identification of specific and newly recognized syndromes. Brain 2003;126:753–769.

112. Wieser HG, Fischer M. Temporal lobe nonconvulsive status epilepticus. In Kaplan PW, Drislane FW, eds., Nonconvulsive status epilepticus. New York: Demos Medical Publishing, 2009:119–137.

113. Seshia SS, McLachlan RS. Aura continua. Epilepsia 2005;46:454–455.

114. Fejerman N, DiBlasi AM. Status epilepticus of benign partial epilepsies in children: Report of two cases. Epilepsia 1987; 28:351–355.

115. Colamaria V, Sgro V, Caraballo R, Simeone M, Zullini E, Fontana E, Zanetti R, Grimau-Merino R, Dalla Bernardina B. Status epilepticus in benign rolandic epilepsy manifesting as anterior operculum syndrome. Epilepsia 1991;32:329–334.

116. Scott JS, Masland RL. Occurrence of "continuous symptoms" in epilepsy patients. Neurology 1953;3:297–301.

117. Manford M, Shorvon SD. Prolonged sensory or visceral symptoms: an under-diagnosed form of non-convulsive focal (simple partial) status epilepticus. J Neurol Neurosurg Psychiatry 1992;55:714–716.

118. Tarnutzer AA, Lee SH, Robinson KA, Kaplan PW, Newman-Toker DE. Clinical and electrographic findings in epileptic vertigo and dizziness: a systematic review. Neurology 2015;84(15):1595–1604.

119. Blair HT. Temporal lobe or psychomotor status epilepticus. A case report. Electroencephalog Clin Neurophysiol 1980;48:558–572.

120. Barry E, Sussman NM, Bosley TM, Harner RN. Ictal blindness and status epilepticus amauroticus. Epilepsia 1985;26:577–584.

121. Salanova V, Andermann F, Olivier A, Rasmussen T, Quesney LF. Occipital lobe epilepsy: electroclinical manifestations, electrocorticography, cortical stimulation and outcome in 42 patients treated between 1930 and 1991. Brain 1992;115:1655–1680.

122. Sowa MV, Pituck S. Prolonged spontaneous complex visual hallucinations and illusions as ictal phenomena. Epilepsia 1989;30:524–526.

123. Young G, Blume WT. Painful epileptic seizures. Brain 1983;106:537–554.

124. Peppercorn M, Herzog AG. The spectrum of abdominal epilepsy in adults. Am J Gastroenterol 1989;84;1294–1296.

125. Eschle D, Siegel AM, Wieser H-G. Epilepsy with severe abdominal pain. Mayo Clin Proc 2002;77:1358–1360.

126. Brigo F, Ferlisi M, Fiaschi A, Bongiovanni LG. Fear as the only clinical expression of affective focal status epilepticus. Epilepsy Behav 2011;20(1):107–110.

127. McLachlan RS, Blume WT. Isolated fear in complex partial status epilepticus. Ann Neurol 1980;8(6):639–641.

128. Kikumoto K, Yoshinaga H, Kobayashi K, Oka M, Ohtsuka Y. Complex partial status epilepticus in children with epilepsy. Brain Devel 2009;31:148–157.

129. Panayiotopoulos CP. Autonomic seizures and autonomic status epilepticus peculiar to childhood: diagnosis and management. Epilepsy Behav 2004;5:286–295.

130. Engel J, Ludwig BI, Fetell M. Prolonged partial complex status epilepticus: EEG and behavioral observations. Neurology 1978;28:863–869.

131. Treiman DM, Delgado-Escueta AV. Complex partial status epilepticus. In: Delgado-Escueta AV, Wasterlain CG, Treiman DM, Porter RJ, eds., Status epilepticus. (Advances in Neurology; vol 34.) New York: Raven Press, 1983:69–81.

132. Butler CR, Graham KS, Hodges JR, Kapur N, Wardlaw JM, Zeman AZJ. The syndrome of transient epileptic amnesia. Ann Neurol 2007;61:587–598.

133. Asadi-Pooya AA. Transient epileptic amnesia: a concise review. Epilepsy Behav 2014;31:243–245.

134. Palmini AL, Gloor P, Jones-Gotman M. Pure amnestic seizures in temporal lobe epilepsy. Definition, clinical symptomatology and functional anatomical considerations. Brain 199;115:749–769.

135. Vuilleumier P, Despland PA, Regli F. Failure to recall (but not to remember): pure transient amnesia during nonconvulsive status epilepticus. Neurology 1996;46:1036–1039.

136. Del Felice A, Broggio E, Valbusa V, Gambina G, Arcaro C, Manganotti P. Transient epileptic amnesia mistaken for mild cognitive impairment? A high-density EEG study. Epilepsy Behav 2014;36:41–46.

137. Schomer AC, Drislane FW. Severe hemispatial neglect as a manifestation of seizures and nonconvulsive status epilepticus: utility of prolonged EEG monitoring. J Clin Neurophysiol 2015;32(2):e4–7.

138. Profitlich T, Hoppe C, Reuber M, Helmstaedter C, Bauer J. Ictal neuropsychological findings in focal nonconvulsive status epilepticus. Epilepsy Behav 2008;12:269–275.

139. Hamilton NG, Matthews T. Aphasia: the sole manifestation of focal status epilepticus. Neurology 1979; 29:745–748.

140. Racy A, Osborn MA, Vern BA, Molinari G. Epileptic aphasia. First onset of prolonged monosymptomatic status epilepticus in adults. Arch Neurol 1980;37:419–422.

141. Gilmore RL, Heilman KM. Speech arrest in partial seizures: evidence of an associated language disorder. Neurology 1981;31:1016–1019.

142. Knight RT, Cooper J. Status epilepticus manifesting as reversible Wernicke's aphasia. Epilepsia 1986;27:301–304.

143. Kirshner HS, Hughes T, Fakhoury T, Abou-Khalil B. Aphasia secondary to partial status epilepticus of the basal temporal language area. Neurology 1995;45:1616–1618.

144. Benatar M. Ictal aphasia. Epilepsy Behav 2002;3:413–419.

145. Schomer DL. Focal status epilepticus and epilepsia partialis continua in adults and children. Epilepsia 1993;34(suppl 1):S29–36.

146. Grand'Maison F, Reiher J, Leduc CP. Retrospective inventory of EEG abnormalities in partial status epilepticus. Electroencephalogr Clin Neurophysiol 1991;79:264–270.

147. Hirsch LJ, Emerson RG, Pedley TA. Prolonged "postictal" aphasia: demonstration of persistent ictal activity with intracranial electrodes. Neurology 2001;56:134–136.

148. Jobst BC, Roberts DW, Williamson PD. Occipital lobe nonconvulsive status epilepticus. In Kaplan PW, Drislane FW, eds., Nonconvulsive status epilepticus. New York: Demos Medical Publishing, 2009:139–150.

149. Drislane FW, Blum AS, Schomer DL. Focal status epilepticus: clinical features and significance of different EEG patterns. Epilepsia 1999;40:1254–1260.

150. Ballenger CE, King DW, Gallagher BB. Partial complex status epilepticus. Neurology 1983;33:1545–1552.

151. Williamson PD. Complex partial status epilepticus. In: Engel JE, Jr, Pedley T, eds., Epilepsy. A comprehensive text (2nd ed). Philadelphia: Lippincott Williams & Wilkins, 2008:677–692.

152. Kaplan PW. Assessing the outcomes in patients with nonconvulsive status epilepticus: nonconvulsive status epilepticus is underdiagnosed, potentially overtreated, and confounded by comorbidity. J Clin Neurophysiol 1999;16:341–352.

153. Mikati MA, Lee WL, DeLong GR. Protracted epileptiform encephalopathy: an unusual form of partial complex status epilepticus. Epilepsia 1985;25:563–571.

154. Niedermeyer E, Fineyre F, Riley T, Uematsu S. Absence status (petit mal status) with focal characteristics. Arch Neurol 1979;36:417–421.

155. Thomas P, Zifkin B, Migneco O, Lebrun C, Darcourt J, Andermann F. Nonconvulsive status epilepticus of frontal origin. Neurology 1999;52:1174–1183.

156. Belafsky MA, Carwille S, Miller P, Waddell G, Boxley-Johnson J, Delgado-Escueta AV. Prolonged epileptic twilight states: continuous recordings with nasopharyngeal electrodes and videotape analysis. Neurology 1978;28:239–245.

157. Commission on Epidemiology and Prognosis, International League Against Epilepsy. Guidelines for epidemiologic studies on epilepsy. Epilepsia 1993;34:592–596.

158. Shorvon S. Clinical forms of status epilepticus. In: Shorvon S, ed., Status epilepticus: its clinical features and treatment in children and adults. Cambridge: Cambridge University Press, 1994:34–138.

159. Krumholz A, Sung GY, Fisher RS, Barry E, Bergey GK, Grattan LM. Complex partial status epilepticus accompanied by serious morbidity and mortality. Neurology 1995;45:1499–1504.

160. Rohr-le-Floch J, Gauthier G, Beaumanoir A. États confusionelles d'origine épileptique: interêt de l'EEG fait en urgence. Rev Neurol (Paris) 1988;144:425–436.

161. Markand ON, Wheeler GL, Pollack SL. Complex partial status epilepticus (psychomotor status). Neurology 1978;28:189–196.

162. Mayeux R, Lueders H. Complex partial status epilepticus: case report and proposal for diagnostic criteria. Neurology 1978;28:957–961.

163. Salanova V, Morris HH, Van Ness P, Kotagal P, Wyllie E, Lüders H. Frontal lobe seizures: electroclinical syndromes. Epilepsia 1995;36:16–24.

164. Williamson PD, French JA, Thadani VM, Kim JH, Novelly RA, Spencer SS, Spencer DD, Mattson RH. Characteristics of medial temporal lobe epilepsy: II. Interictal and ictal scalp electroencephalography, neuropsychological testing, neuroimaging, surgical results, and pathology. Ann Neurol 1993;34:781–787.

165. Foldvary N, Lee N, Thwaites G, Mascha E, Hammel J, Kim H, Friedman AH, Radtke RA. Clinical and electrographic manifestations of lesional neocortical temporal lobe epilepsy. Neurology 1997;49:757–763.

166. Nowack WJ, Shaikh IA. Progression of electroclinical changes in complex partial status epilepticus: filling in the blanks. Clin Electroencephalogr 1999;30:5–8.

167. Wieser HG. Temporal lobe or psychomotor status epilepticus: a case report. Electroencephalogr Clin Neurophysiol 1980;48:558–572.

168. Williamson PD, Boon PA, Thadani VM, Darcey TM, Spencer DD, Spencer SS, Novelly RA, Mattson RH. Parietal lobe epilepsy: diagnostic considerations and results of surgery. Ann Neurol 1992;31:193–201.

169. Gloor P, Olivier A, Quesney LF, Andermann F, Horowitz S. The role of the limbic system in experiential phenomena of temporal lobe epilepsy. Ann Neurol 1982;12:129–144.

170. Kudo T, Sato K, Yagi K, Seino M. Can absence status epilepticus be of frontal lobe origin? Acta Neurol Scand 1995;92:472–477.

171. Ericson EJ, Gerard EE, Macken MP, Schuele SU. Aphasic status epilepticus: electroclinical correlation. Epilepsia 2011;52:1452–1458.

172. Shneker BF, Fountain NB. Assessment of acute morbidity and mortality in nonconvulsive status epilepticus. Neurology 2003;61:1066–1073.

173. Shorvon S, Baulac M, Cross H., Trinka E, Walker M. The drug treatment of status epilepticus in Europe: consensus document from a workshop at the first London Colloquium on Status Epilepticus. Epilepsia 2008;49:1277–1284.

174. Meierkord H, Holtkamp M. Non-convulsive status epilepticus in adults: clinical forms and treatment. Lancet Neurol 2007;6:329–339.

175. Towne AR, Pellock JM, Ko D, DeLorenzo, RJ. Determinants of mortality in status epilepticus. Epilepsia 1994;35:27–34.

176. McBride MC, Dooling EC, Oppenheimer EY. Complex partial status epilepticus in young children. Ann Neurol 1981;9:526–530.

177. Berg AT, Shinnar S. Do seizures beget seizures? An assessment of the clinical evidence in humans. J Clin Neurophysiol 1997;14:102–110.

178. Schwab RS. A case of status epilepticus in petit mal. Electroenceph Clin Neurophysiol 1953;5:441–442.

179. Niedermeyer E, Khalifeh R. Petit-mal status ("spike-wave stupor"). An electro-clinical appraisal. Epilepsia 1965;6:250–262.

180. Wheless JW. Acute management of seizures in the syndromes of idiopathic generalized epilepsies. Epilepsia 2003;44(suppl 2):22–26.

181. Agathonikou A, Panayiotopoulos CP, Giannakodimos S, Koutroumanidis M. Typical absence status in adults: diagnostic and syndromic considerations. Epilepsia 1998;39:1265–1276.

182. Shorvon S, Walker M. Status epilepticus in idiopathic generalized epilepsy. Epilepsia 2005;46:73–79.

183. Thomas P, Snead OC. Absence status epilepticus. In: Engel J, Pedley TA, eds., Epilepsy: a comprehensive textbook (2nd ed). Philadelphia: Lippincott-Raven Publishers, 2008:693–703.

184. Genton P, Ferlazzo E, Thomas P. Absence status epilepsy: delineation of a distinct idiopathic generalized epilepsy syndrome. Epilepsia 2008;49:642–649.

185. Kimura S, Kobayashi T. Two patients with juvenile myoclonic epilepsy and nonconvulsive status epilepticus. Epilepsia 1996;37:275–279.

186. Thomas P, Valton L, Genton P. Absence and myoclonic status epilepticus precipitated by antiepileptic drugs in idiopathic generalized epilepsy. Brain 2006;129:1281–1292.

187. Osorio I, Reed RC, Peltzer JN. Refractory idiopathic status epilepticus: a probable paradoxical effect of phenytoin and carbamazepine. Epilepsia 2000;41:887–894.

188. Knake S, Hamer HM, Schomburg U, Oertel WH, Rosenow F. Tiagabine-induced absence status in idiopathic generalized epilepsy. Seizure 1999;8(5):314–317.

189. Andermann F, Robb JP. Absence status: a reappraisal following review of thirty-eight patients. Epilepsia 1972;13:177–187.

190. Niedermeyer E, Ribeiro M. Considerations of nonconvulsive status epilepticus. Clinical EEG 2000; 31:192–195.

191. Baykan B, Gokyigit A, Gurses C, Eraksoy M. Recurrent absence status epilepticus: clinical and EEG characteristics. Seizure 2002;11:310–319.

192. Berkovic SF, Bladin PF. Absence status in adults. Clin Exp Neurol 1983;19:198–207.

193. Treiman DM. Electroclinical features of status epilepticus. J Clin Neurophysiol 1995;12:343–362.

194. Hovinga CA, Chicella MF, Rose DF, Eades SK, Dalton JT, Phelps SJ. Use of intravenous valproate in three pediatric patients with nonconvulsive or convulsive status epilepticus. Ann Pharmacother 1999;33:579–584.

195. Berkovic SF, Andermann F, Guberman A, Hipola D, Bladin PF. Valproate prevents the recurrence of absence status. Neurology 1989; 39:1294–1297.

196. Fernandez-Torre JL. De novo absence status of late onset following withdrawal of lorazepam: a case report. Seizure 2001;10:433–437.

197. Pro S, Vicenzini E, Randi F, Pulitano P, Mecarelli O. Idiopathic late-onset absence status epilepticus: a case report with an electroclinical 14 years follow-up. Seizure 2011;20(8):655–658.

198. D'Agostino MD, Andermann F, Dubeau F, Fedi M, Bastos A. Exceptionally long absence status: multifactorial etiology, drug interactions and complications. Epileptic Disord 1999;1:229–232.

199. Michelucci R, Rubboli G, Passarelli D, et al. Electroclinical features of idiopathic generalised epilepsy with persisting absences in adult life. J Neurol Neurosurg Psychiatry 1996;61:471–477.

200. Dziewas R, Kellinghaus C, Ludemann P. Nonconvulsive status epilepticus in patients with juvenile myoclonic epilepsy: types and frequencies. Seizure 2002;11:335–339.

201. Giannakodimos S, Panayiotopoulos CP. Eyelid myoclonia with absences in adults: a clinical and video-EEG study. Epilepsia 1996;37:36–44.

202. Yang T, Liu Y, Liu L, Yan B, Zhang Q, Zhou D. Absence status epilepticus in monozygotic twins with Jeavons syndrome. Epileptic Disord 2008;10(3):227–230.

203. Agathonikou A, Koutroumanidis M, Panayiotopoulos CP. Fixation-off-sensitive epilepsy with absences and absence status: video-EEG documentation. Neurology 1997;48(1):231–234.

204. Nolan M, Bergazar M, Chu B, Cortez MA, Snead OC. Clinical and neurophysiologic spectrum associated with atypical absence seizures in children with intractable epilepsy. J Child Neurol 2005;20:404–410.

205. Roger J, Lob H, Tassinari CA. Status epilepticus. In: Vinken P, Bruyn G, eds., Handbook of clinical neurology, Vol. 15: The epilepsies. Amsterdam: North Holland Publishing Co., 1974:145–188.

206. Cortez MA, McKerlie C, Snead OC. A model of atypical absence seizures. EEG, pharmacology, and developmental characterization. Neurology 2001;56:341–349.
207. Holmes GL, McKeever M, Adamson M. Absence seizures in children: clinical and electroencephalographic features. Ann Neurol 1987;21:268–273.
208. Matsumoto A, Kumagai T, Miura K, Miyazaki S, Hayakawa C, Yamanaka T. Epilepsy in Angelman syndrome associated with chromosome 15q deletion. Epilepsia 1992;33:1083–1090.
209. Gastaut H, Roger J, Ouahchi S, Timsit M, Broughton R. An electroclinical study of generalized epileptic seizures of tonic expression. Epilepsia 1963;4:15–44.
210. DiMario FJ, Clancy RR. Paradoxical precipitation of tonic seizures by lorazepam in a child with atypical absence seizures. Pediatr Neurol 1988 4:249–251.
211. Perez Velazquez JL, Huo JZ, Dominguez LG, Leshchenko Y, Snead OC. Typical versus atypical absence seizures: network mechanisms of the spread of paroxysms. Epilepsia 2007;48:1585–1593.
212. Onat FY, van Luijtelaar G, Nehlig A, Snead OC. The involvement of limbic structures in typical and atypical absence epilepsy. Epilepsy Res 2013;103(2–3):111–123.
213. Treiman DM, Walton NY, Kendrick C. A progressive sequence of electroencephalographic changes during generalized convulsive status epilepticus. Epilepsy Res 1990;5:49–60.
214. Bancaud J, Talairach J, Morel P, Bresson M, Bonis A, Geier S, Hemon E, Buser P. "Generalized" epileptic seizures elicited by electrical stimulation of the frontal lobe in man. Electroencephalogr Clin Neurophysiol 1974;37:275–282.
215. Abend NS, Dlugos DJ. Nonconvulsive status epilepticus in a pediatric intensive care unit. Pediatr Neurol 2007;37:165–170.
216. Young GB, Jordan KG, Doig GS. An assessment of nonconvulsive seizures in the intensive care unit using continuous EEG monitoring: an investigation of variables associated with mortality. Neurology 1996;47:83–89.
217. Barry E, Hauser W. Status epilepticus: the interaction of epilepsy and acute brain disease. Neurology 1993;43:1473–1478.
218. Krishnamurthy KB, Drislane FW. Depth of electroencephalogram suppression and outcome in pentobarbital coma for refractory status epilepticus. Epilepsia 1999;40:759–762.
219. Claassen J, Hirsch LJ, Emerson RG, Bates JE, Thompson TB, Mayer SA. Continuous EEG monitoring and midazolam infusion for refractory nonconvulsive status epilepticus. Neurology 2001;57:1036–1042.
220. So EL, Ruggles KH, Ahmann PA, Trudeau SK, Weatherford KJ, Trenerry MR. Clinical significance and outcome of subclinical status epilepticus in adults. J Epilepsy 1995;8:11–15.
221. Vespa PM, Nuwer MR, Nenov V, Ronne-Engstrom E, Hovda DA, Bergsneider M, Kelly DF, Martin NA, Becker DP. Increased incidence and impact of nonconvulsive and convulsive seizures after traumatic brain injury as detected by continuous electroencephalographic monitoring. J Neurosurg 1999;91:750–760.
222. Privitera M, Hoffman M, Moore JL, Jester D. EEG detection of nontonic-clonic status epilepticus in patients with altered consciousness. Epilepsy Res 1994;18:155–166.
223. Jirsch J, Hirsch LJ. Nonconvulsive seizures: developing a rational approach to the diagnosis and management in the critically ill population. Clin Neurophysiol 2007;118:1660–1670.
224. Vespa PM, O'Phelan K, Shah M, Mirabelli J, Starkman S, Kidwell C, Saver J, Nuwer MR, Frazee JG, McArthur DA, Martin NA. Acute seizures after intracerebral hemorrhage: A factor in progressive midline shift and outcome. Neurology 2003;60:1441–1446.
225. Claassen J, Jette N, Chum F, Green R, Schmidt M, Choi H, Jirsch J, Frontera JA, Connolly ES, Emerson RG, Mayer SA, Hirsch LJ. Electrographic seizures and periodic discharges after intracerebral hemorrhage. Neurology 2007;69:1356–1365.
226. Carrera E, Claassen J, Oddo M, Emerson RG, Mayer SA, Hirsch LJ. Continuous electroencephalographic monitoring in critically ill patients with central nervous system infections. Arch Neurol 2008;65(12):1612–1618.
227. Oddo M, Carrera E, Claasssen J, Mayer SA, Hirsch LJ. Continuous electroencephalography in the medical intensive care unit. Crit Care Med 2009;37(6):2051–2056.
228. Herman ST, Abend NS, Bleck TP, Chapman KE, Drislane FW, Emerson RG, et al. Consensus statement on continuous EEG in critically ill adults and children, part I: indications. J Clin Neurophysiol 2015;32(2):87–95.
229. Pandian JD, Cascino GD, So EL, Manno E, Fulgham JR. Digital video-electroencephalographic monitoring in the neurological-neurosurgical intensive care unit: clinical features and outcome. Arch Neurol 2004;61:1090–1094.
230. Jette N, Claassen J, Emerson RG, Hirsch LJ. Frequency and predictors of nonconvulsive seizures during continuous electroencephalographic monitoring in critically ill children. Arch Neurol 2006;63:1750–1755.
231. Shafi MM, Westover MB, Cole AJ, Kilbride RD, Hoch DB, Cash SS. Absence of early epileptiform abnormalities predicts lack of seizures on continuous EEG. Neurology 2012;79(17):1796–1801.
232. Wilner AN, Bream PR. Status epilepticus and pseudostatus epilepticus. Seizure 1993;2:257–260.
233. Howell SJ, Owen L, Chadwick DW. Pseudostatus epilepticus. Q J Med 1989;71:507–519.
234. Duncan R, Oto M, Wainman-Lefley J. Mortality in a cohort of patients with psychogenic non-epileptic seizures. J Neurol Neurosurg Psychiatry 2012;83:761–762.
235. Nei M, Lee JM, Shanker VL, Sperling MR. The EEG and prognosis in status epilepticus. Epilepsia 1999;40:157–163.
236. Brenner RP. Is it status? Epilepsia 2002;43(suppl 3):103–113.
237. Pohlmann-Eden B, Hoch DB, Cochius JI, Chiappa KH. Periodic lateralized epileptiform discharges—a critical review. J Clin Neurophysiol. 1996;13:519–530.
238. Reiher J, Rivest J, Grand'Maison F, Leduc CP. Periodic lateralized epileptiform discharges with transitional rhythmic discharges: association with seizures. Electroencephalogr Clin Neurophysiol 1991;78:12–17.
239. Brophy GM, Bell R, Claassen J, Alldredge B, Bleck TP, Glauser T, Laroche SM, Riviello JJ Jr, Shutter L, Sperling MR, Treiman DM, Vespa PM. Neurocritical Care Society Status Epilepticus Guideline Writing Committee. Guidelines for the evaluation and management of status epilepticus. Neurocrit Care 2012;17(1):3–23.
240. Foreman B, Claassen J, Abou Khaled K, Jirsch J, Alschuler DM, Wittman J, Emerson RG, Hirsch LJ. Generalized periodic discharges in the critically ill: a case-control study of 200 patients. Neurology 2012;79:1951–1960.
241. Brenner RP, Schaul N. Periodic EEG patterns: classification, clinical correlation, and pathophysiology. J Clin Neurophysiol 1990;7:249–267.
242. Treiman DM. Status epilepticus. Baillieres Clin Neurol 1996;5:821–839.
243. Krumholz A. Epidemiology and evidence for morbidity of nonconvulsive status epilepticus. J Clin Neurophysiol 1999;16:314–322.
244. Husain AM, Mebust KA, Radtke RA. Generalized periodic epileptiform discharges: etiologies, relationship to status epilepticus, and prognosis. J Clin Neurophysiol 1999;16:51–58.
245. Hirsch LJ, Claassen J, Mayer SA, Emerson RG. Stimulus-induced rhythmic, periodic, or ictal discharges (SIRPIDs): a common EEG phenomenon in the critically ill. Epilepsia 2004;45:109–123.
246. Hirsch LJ, Pang T, Claassen J, Chang C, Khaled KA, Wittman J, Emerson RG. Focal motor seizures induced by altering stimuli in critically ill patients. Epilepsia 2008;49:968–973.
247. Fisch BJ, Klass DW. The diagnostic specificity of triphasic wave patterns. Electroenceph Clin Neurophysiol 1988;70:1–8.
248. Sheridan PH, Sato S. Triphasic waves of metabolic encephalopathy versus spike-wave stupor. J Neurol Neurosurg Psychiatry 1986;49:108–109.
249. Foreman B, Mahulikar A, Tadi P, Claassen J, Szaflarski J, Halford JJ, Dean BC, Kaplan PW, Hirsch LJ, LaRoche S. Generalized periodic discharges and 'triphasic waves': a blinded evaluation of inter-rater agreement and clinical significance. Clin Neurophysiol 2016;127:1073–1080.
250. Jordan KG. Continuous EEG and evoked potential monitoring in the neuroscience intensive care unit. J Clin Neurophysiol 1993;10:445–475.
251. Scheuer ML, Wilson SB. Data analysis for continuous EEG monitoring in the ICU: seeing the forest and the trees. J Clin Neurophysiol 2004;21:353–378.
252. Haider HA, Esteller R, Hahn CD, Westover MB, Halford JJ, Lee JW, Shafi MM, Gaspard N, Herman ST, Gerard EE, Hirsch LJ, Ehrenberg JA, LaRoche SM and the Critical Care EEG Monitoring Research Consortium. Sensitivity of quantitative EEG for seizure identification in the intensive care unit. Neurology 2016;30;87(9):935–944.
253. Agarwal R, Gotman J. Long-term EEG compression for intensive-care settings. IEEE Eng Med Biol Mag 2001;20:23–29.
254. Gotman J. Automatic detection of seizures and spikes. J Clin Neurophysiol 1999;16:130–140.
255. Wilson SB. Algorithm architectures for patient dependent seizure detection. Clin Neuophysiol 2006;117:1204–1216.
256. Jirsch J, Hirsch LJ. Nonconvulsive status epilepticus in critically ill and comatose patients in the intensive care unit. In: Kaplan PW, Drislane FW, eds., Nonconvulsive status epilepticus. New York: Demos Medical Publishing, 2009:175–186.
257. Wilson SB. A neural network method for automatic and incremental learning applied to patient-dependent seizure detection. Clin Neurophysiol 2005;116:1785–1795.
258. Scheuer ML. Continuous EEG monitoring in the intensive care unit. Epilepsia 2002;43(suppl 3):114–127.

259. Abend NS, Dlugos D, Herman S. Neonatal seizure detection using multi-channel display of envelope trend. Epilepsia 2008;49:349–352.
260. Hirsch LJ. Continuous EEG monitoring in the intensive care unit: an overview. J Clin Neurophysiol 2004;21:332–340.
261. Bleck TP. Intensive care unit management of patients with status epilepticus. Epilepsia 2007;48(suppl 8):59–60.
262. Walker M, Cross H, Smith S, Young C, Aicardi J, Appleton R, Aylett S, Besag F, Cock H, DeLorenzo R, Drislane F, Duncan J, Ferrie C, Fujikawa D, Gray W, Kaplan P, Koutroumanidis M, O'Regan M, Plouin P, Sander J, Scott R, Shorvon S, Treiman D, Wasterlain C, Wieshmann U. Nonconvulsive status epilepticus: Epilepsy Research Foundation Workshop Reports. Epilep Disord 2005;7:253–296.
263. Litt B, Wityk RJ, Hertz SH, Mullen PD, Weiss H, Ryan DD, Henry TR. Nonconvulsive status epilepticus in the critically ill elderly. Epilepsia 1998;39:1194–1202.
264. Rossetti AO, Logroscino G, Bromfield EB. Refractory status epilepticus: effect of treatment aggressiveness on prognosis. Arch Neurol 2005;62(11):1698–1702. Erratum in: Arch Neurol 2006;63(10):1482.
265. Sutter R, Marsch S, Fuhr P, Kaplan PW, Rüegg S. Anesthetic drugs in status epilepticus—risk or rescue? Results from a six-year cohort study. Neurology 2014;82:656–664.
266. Shorvon S, Ferlisi M. The treatment of super-refractory status epilepticus: a critical review of available therapies and a clinical treatment protocol. Brain 2011;134:2802–2818.
267. Krishnamurthy KB, Drislane FW. Relapse and survival after barbiturate anesthetic treatment of refractory status epilepticus. Epilepsia 1996;37:863–867.
268. Walker MC. Diagnosis and treatment of nonconvulsive status epilepticus. CNS Drugs 2001;15:931–939.
269. Claassen J, Hirsch LJ, Emerson RG, Mayer SA. Treatment of refractory status epilepticus with pentobarbital, propofol, or midazolam: a systematic review. Epilepsia 2002;43:146–153.
270. Drislane FW, Lopez MR, Blum AS, Schomer DL. Detection and treatment of refractory status epilepticus in the intensive care unit. J Clin Neurophysiol 2008;25:181–186.
271. Rossetti AO, Oddo M, Liaudet L, Kaplan PW. Predictors of awakening from postanoxic status epilepticus after therapeutic hypothermia. Neurology 2009;72:744–749.
272. Rossetti AO, Oddo M, Logroscino G, Kaplan PW. Prognostication after cardiac arrest and hypothermia—a prospective study. Ann Neurol 2010;67:301–307.
273. Drislane FW. Evidence against permanent neurologic damage from nonconvulsive status epilepticus. J Clin Neurophysiol 1999;16:323–331.
274. Lee SI. Nonconvulsive status epilepticus. Ictal confusion in later life. Arch Neurol 1985;42:778–781.
275. Scholtes FB, Renier WO, Meinardi H. Non-convulsive status epilepticus: causes, treatment, and outcome in 65 patients. J Neurol Neurosurg Psychiatry 1996;61:93–95.
276. Adachi N, Kanemoto K, Muramatsu R, Kato M, Akanuma N, Ito M, Kawasaki J, Onuma T. Intellectual prognosis of status epilepticus in adult patients: analysis with Wechsler Adult Intelligence Scale-Revised. Epilepsia 2005;46:1502–1509.
277. Nevander G, Ingvar M, Auer R, Siesjo BK. Status epilepticus in well-oxygenated rats causes neuronal necrosis. Ann Neurol 1985;18:281–290.
278. Vespa PM, Miller C, McArthur D, Eliseo M, Etchepare M, Hirt D, Glenn TC, Martin N, Hovda D. Nonconvulsive electrographic seizures after traumatic brain injury result in a delayed, prolonged increase in intracranial pressure and metabolic crisis. Crit Care Med 2007;35:2830–2836.
279. Ruegg SJ, Dichter MA. Diagnosis and treatment of nonconvulsive status epilepticus in an intensive care unit setting. Curr Treat Options Neurol 2003;5:93–110.
280. Payne ET, Zhao XY, Frndova H, McBain K, Sharma R, Hutchison JS, Hahn CD. Seizure burden is independently associated with short term outcome in critically ill children. Brain 2014;137:1429–1438.

22 | EEG IN THE INTENSIVE CARE UNIT: ANOXIA, COMA, BRAIN DEATH, AND RELATED DISORDERS

GAMALELDIN M. OSMAN, MD, JAMES J. RIVIELLO, JR., MD,
AND LAWRENCE J. HIRSCH, MD

ABSTRACT: The field of continuous electroencephalographic monitoring (cEEG) in the intensive care unit has dramatically expanded over the past two decades. Expansion of cEEG programs led to recognition of the frequent occurrence of electrographic seizures, and complex rhythmic and periodic patterns in various critically ill populations. The majority of electrographic seizures are of nonconvulsive nature, hence the need for cEEG for their identification. Guidelines on when and how to perform cEEG and standardized nomenclature for description of rhythmic and periodic patterns are now available. Quantitative EEG analysis methods depict EEG data in a compressed (hours on one screen) colorful graphical representation, facilitating early identification of key events, recognition of slow, long-term trends, and timely therapeutic intervention. Integration of EEG with other invasive and noninvasive modalities of monitoring brain function provides critical information about the development of secondary neuronal injury, providing a valuable window of opportunity for intervention before irreversible damage ensues.

KEYWORDS: EEG, continuous EEG monitoring, intensive care unit, seizure, nonconvulsive

PRINCIPAL REFERENCES

1. Claassen J, Mayer SA, Kowalski RG, Emerson RG, Hirsch LJ. Detection of electrographic seizures with continuous EEG monitoring in critically ill patients. *Neurology.* 2004;62(10):1743–1748.
2. Herman ST, Abend NS, Bleck TP, et al. Consensus statement on continuous EEG in critically ill adults and children, part I: indications. *J Clin Neurophysiol.* 2015;32(2):87–95.
3. Leitinger M, Beniczky S, Rohracher A, et al. Salzburg Consensus Criteria for Non-Convulsive Status Epilepticus—approach to clinical application. *Epilepsy Behav.* 2015;49:158–163.
4. Hirsch LJ, LaRoche SM, Gaspard N, et al. American Clinical Neurophysiology Society's standardized critical care EEG terminology: 2012 version. *J Clin Neurophysiol.* 2013;30(1):1–27.
5. Claassen J. How I treat patients with EEG patterns on the ictal–interictal continuum in the neuro ICU. *Neurocritical Care.* 2009;11(3):437–444.
6. Moura LMVR, Shafi MM, Ng M, et al. Spectrogram screening of adult EEGs is sensitive and efficient. *Neurology.* 2014;83(1):56–64.
7. Sivaraju A, Gilmore EJ, Wira CR, et al. Prognostication of post-cardiac arrest coma: early clinical and electroencephalographic predictors of outcome. *Intensive Care Med.* 2015;41(7):1264–1272.
8. Claassen J, Hirsch LJ, Kreiter KT, et al. Quantitative continuous EEG for detecting delayed cerebral ischemia in patients with poor-grade subarachnoid hemorrhage. *Clin Neurophysiol.* 2004;115(12):2699–2710.
9. Claassen J, Perotte A, Albers D, et al. Nonconvulsive seizures after subarachnoid hemorrhage: multimodal detection and outcomes. *Ann Neurol.* 2013;74(1):53–64.
10. Vespa P, Tubi M, Claassen J, et al. Metabolic crisis occurs with seizures and periodic discharges after brain trauma. *Ann Neurol.* 2016;79(4):579–590.

1. INTRODUCTION

Electroencephalography (EEG) represents a unique noninvasive tool for dynamic monitoring of brain function. Technological advances involving EEG data acquisition, storage, and analysis have made it possible to monitor critically ill patients for extended periods of time. Though EEG has long been used for grading encephalopathy in critically ill patients, the primary goal of continuous EEG (cEEG) monitoring today is detecting subclinical seizures. Electrographic seizures are common in critically ill patients, occurring in 6% to 59% of monitored patients, depending on the study population[1-13] (Fig. 22.1). The majority of these seizures (~75% overall) are not associated with clear clinical correlate, and thus cannot be identified without cEEG monitoring. There is accumulating evidence that electrographic seizures as well as rhythmic and periodic discharges are correlated with poor outcome[4,14-16]. However, it is not yet clear when these patterns contribute independently to poor outcome and when they merely represent epiphenomena of structural or functional brain damage. In this chapter, we will review the indications for cEEG monitoring in critically ill individuals and commonly encountered patterns in these patients. We will also summarize available data on impact of seizures and rhythmic and periodic patterns on outcome, advances in quantitative EEG data analysis, and other clinical applications for EEG monitoring, including prognostication in postanoxic patients. We will also discuss the now-infrequent use of EEG as an ancillary test in the diagnosis of brain death.

2. INDICATIONS

cEEG monitoring in the intensive care unit (ICU) has dramatically evolved over the past two decades. The main clinical application today is identifying subclinical seizures. Other clinical applications include monitoring response to therapy in patients with status epilepticus (SE), early detection of delayed cerebral ischemia (DCI) in patients with subarachnoid hemorrhage (SAH), and prognosticating outcome in patients with postanoxic encephalopathy. The American Clinical Neurophysiology Society (ACNS) recently released guidelines on indications for cEEG in critically ill adults and children[17]. Similar recommendations were released by the Neurocritical Care Society in collaboration with the European Society of Intensive Care Medicine (ESICM) as part of a consensus statement on multimodality monitoring in neurocritical care[18]. A summary of both guidelines is presented in Table 22.1. The ACNS has also produced guidelines for cEEG monitoring in

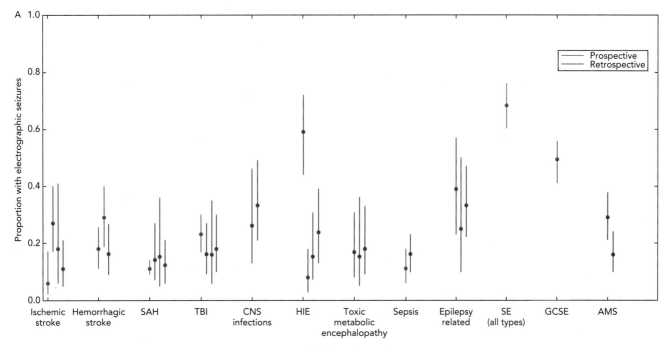

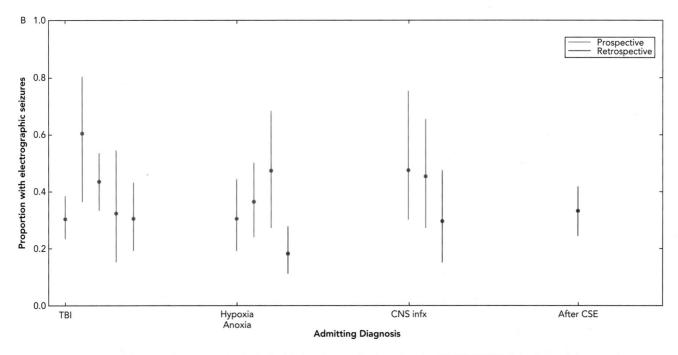

Figure 22.1. *A: Incidence of electrographic seizures in critically ill adults by admitting diagnosis. Data from[1,2,4–11,13,20,166,206,251]. B: Incidence of electrographic seizures in critically ill children by admitting diagnosis. Data from[16,23,24,26,252–255]. The confidence intervals were not reported in the original studies but were calculated based on the number of subjects in each study and the proportion of patients with electrographic seizures.*

neonates[19]. In this section, we will highlight the main clinical applications.

2.1. Diagnosis of Nonconvulsive Seizures

The primary goal for cEEG monitoring is detection of nonconvulsive seizures. Electrographic seizures are common in critically ill patients, occurring in 6% to 59% of monitored patients, depending on the study population[1–13]. Though it may seem quite sensible that electrographic seizures are

commonly encountered in the midst of acute brain injury and following generalized convulsive status epilepticus (GCSE), electrographic seizures are also fairly common in critically ill patients with no evidence of structural brain injury. In one recent prospective study evaluating 100 episodes of sepsis in 98 patients, periodic discharges were detected on EEG in 25 sepsis episodes; 10 of them also had nonconvulsive seizures[20]. In addition, 15% to 18% of patients with toxic metabolic encephalopathy in three retrospective studies had electrographic seizures[1–3].

TABLE 22.1. Indications for cEEG Monitoring in the ICU[17,18]

	INDICATION	ACNS RECOMMENDATIONS	NCC SOCIETY/ESICM RECOMMENDATIONS
A: cEEG monitoring for diagnosis of nonconvulsive seizures	Acute brain injury with alteration in mental state	Yes; acute supratentorial brain injury	Yes; "unexplained and persistent altered consciousness" (strong recommendation, low quality of evidence)
	Fluctuating mental status or unexplained alteration of mental status without acute brain injury	Yes	Yes (weak recommendation, low quality of evidence)
	Persistent alteration of mental state following generalized convulsive status epilepticus	Indicated if there is no clear improvement in consciousness within 10 minutes or persistent impairment of consciousness after 30 minutes of motor activity.	Urgent EEG is recommended in patients not returning to functional baseline within 60 minutes after seizure medication (strong recommendation, low quality of evidence)
	Paroxysmal events to determine ictal nature	Yes	-----
	Pharmacological paralysis indication in patients at high risk for seizures	Yes	-------
B: Ischemia detection	Ischemia detection in patients at high risk for ischemia	Suggested as an adjunct method	Suggested for ischemia detection in subarachnoid hemorrhage patients with unreliable neurological exam (weak recommendation, low quality of evidence)
C: Monitoring of sedation in patients requiring IV sedation or induced coma		Yes	------
D: Assessment of the degree of encephalopathy and prognostication		Populations include: 1. Severe traumatic brain injury 2. Hypoxic-ischemic encephalopathy 3. Subarachnoid hemorrhage	EEG is recommended in postanoxic patients during therapeutic hypothermia and within 24 hours of rewarming to exclude nonconvulsive seizures.

Adapted from Herman S, et al. Consensus Statement on Continuous EEG monitoring in Critically Ill Adults and Children, Part I: Indications. *J Clin Neurophysiol.* 2015;32:87–95; Consensus summary statement of the International Multidisciplinary Consensus Conference on Multimodality Monitoring in Neurocritical Care: a statement for healthcare professionals from the Neurocritical Care Society and the European Society of Intensive Care Medicine. *Intensive Care Med.* 2014;40(9):1189–1209.

The majority of seizures encountered in critically ill patients are purely electrographic and thus cannot be identified without EEG monitoring[1]. Though subtle clinical signs such as nystagmus, hippus, eye deviation, and subtle focal twitching may help in identifying seizures in critically ill patients[21], these signs may be difficult to discern at the bedside, and may also be encountered in patients with no seizures on EEG. On the other hand, the majority of paroxysmal events suspected to be seizures in critically ill patients are of nonepileptic nature. One retrospective study reviewed 52 EEG studies ordered for paroxysmal motor events in the ICU and found that 38 (73%) of these events were nonepileptic. These events included tremor-like movements, multifocal myoclonus with no clear EEG correlate, and slow semi-purposeful movements[22]. Thus, EEG monitoring plays a crucial role not only in identifying subclinical seizures, but also in determining ictal versus nonictal nature of paroxysmal events. The ACNS recommends cEEG monitoring for all patients with acute supratentorial brain lesions with altered mental status and for patients with fluctuating or unexplained mental status disturbance in the absence of known acute brain injury[17]. ACNS also recommends cEEG monitoring for patients at risk for seizures requiring pharmacological paralysis and patients with paroxysmal events suspected to be seizures to determine whether or not they are epileptic[17].

Electrographic seizures are also commonly encountered in critically ill children, occurring in 30% to 60% of monitored children. Patients with non-accidental traumatic brain injury (i.e., abuse or "shaken baby syndrome") appear to be at a particularly increased risk, as 49% to 58% of these patients had electrographic seizures in two prospective studies[23,24]. Yang et al.[25] recently developed a model for predicting electrographic seizures in critically ill children based on a multicenter retrospective database. This model was then validated using a single-center prospectively acquired database. EEG background features were the strongest predictors of electrographic seizures. Burst-suppression pattern and background attenuation in particular were associated with high risk of electrographic seizures[25]. Other predictors included age ≤ 24 months, presence of clinical seizures before monitoring, and interictal epileptiform discharges on EEG[25]. These risk factors may assist in selecting candidates for cEEG monitoring in low-resource settings.

2.2. Monitoring of Therapy for Seizures

Monitoring of therapy for seizures is one of the main indications for cEEG monitoring. One prospective study included 164 patients with convulsive status epilepticus (CSE) undergoing cEEG monitoring after adequate control of clinical seizures and found that 48% of these patients had persistent electrographic seizures during 24 hours of cEEG. The majority of these seizures were purely electrographic, though some patients had subtle convulsive activity. Fourteen percent of all patients met criteria for nonconvulsive status epilepticus[13].

Electrographic seizures after CSE are also commonly encountered in children and young adults. One recent retrospective multicenter study included 96 children and young adults undergoing cEEG monitoring after CSE and found that 33% of patients had electrographic seizures after CSE: 34.4% of these patients had purely electrographic seizures and 46.9% of patients with electrographic seizures met criteria for electrographic SE. Patients with a previous diagnosis of epilepsy as well as those with interictal epileptiform discharges on EEG were more likely to have electrographic seizures[26]. These data highlight the importance of cEEG monitoring in guiding therapy for seizures. Most authorities recommend cEEG monitoring until achieving 24 hours without electrographic seizures[27].

2.3. Ischemia Detection

EEG has now been used for more than four decades to monitor brain ischemia during carotid surgery[28]. EEG signal is primarily generated by graded excitatory and inhibitory postsynaptic potentials at pyramidal neurons in cortical layers 3, 5, and 6[29]. These neurons are particularly sensitive to ischemia[30]. EEG changes occur as early as within three minutes after carotid clamping in patients undergoing carotid endarterectomy[31], well before expected diffusion-weighted imaging (DWI) changes[32].

EEG changes correlate well with changes in regional cerebral blood flow (rCBF). Figure 22.2 illustrates EEG changes correlating with various degrees of CBF decline. As rCBF declines to 25 mL/100 g/min, EEG shows attenuation of fast frequencies in the affected region. Further CBF decline is associated with slowing of background frequencies in the involved region, where 5- to 7-Hz theta frequencies predominate as rCBF reaches 18 to 25 mL/100 g/min and delta frequencies predominate as rCBF reaches 12 to 18 mL/100 g/min. Finally, complete suppression of EEG background rhythm occurs at CBF levels <10 to 12 mL/100 g/min, corresponding to the development of irreversible neuronal injury[33]. However, discordance between EEG and CBF changes is occasionally observed owing to the paradoxical increase in cerebral perfusion of the ischemic penumbra, which is often labeled as "luxury perfusion." EEG provides a more accurate reflection of neuronal function in these cases[34].

The previously described EEG changes in response to ischemia may serve as targets for early therapeutic intervention in ischemic stroke. Regional attenuation without delta (RAWOD) is a distinctive EEG pattern characterized by attenuation of all EEG frequencies without superimposed delta activity (i.e., suppression of all frequencies). In one study involving 18 patients with severe acute ischemic stroke and

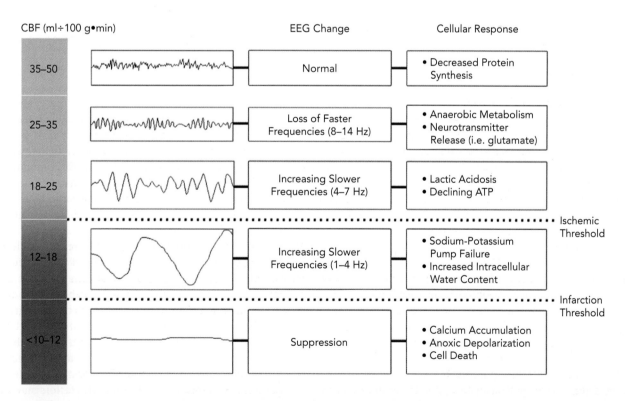

Figure 22.2. *EEG changes associated with cerebral ischemia at different CBF levels. Reproduced with permission from Foreman B, Claassen J. Quantitative EEG for detection of brain ischemia. Critical Care. 2012;16:216.*

RAWOD pattern on EEG, 75% developed massive cerebral edema and 67% died. This pattern potentially represents an early marker of malignant hemispheric infarction, and may serve as an early target for therapeutic interventions targeting massive cerebral edema[35]. One of the other important applications for cEEG monitoring is early detection of DCI in patients with SAH. More details are provided later in this chapter as regards this application.

2.4. Prognostication in Postanoxic Encephalopathy and Other Settings

Prognostication in post–cardiac arrest patients represents one of the most challenging situations facing clinicians worldwide. Cardiac arrest causes >424,000 annual deaths in the United States, >300,00 deaths in Europe, and >3.7 million deaths worldwide[36]. Implementation of therapeutic hypothermia protocols has led to remarkably increased survival in postanoxic patients[37], albeit with added difficulties to the prognostication process. EEG has played a major role in prognostication strategies in postanoxic coma since the 1960s[38]. The American Academy of Neurology (AAN) published guidelines in 2006 on outcome prediction in comatose patients after cardiac arrest and concluded that "burst suppression or generalized epileptiform discharges on EEG predicted poor outcome but with insufficient prognostic accuracy (Level of recommendation C)"[39]. However, these guidelines were published before the widespread implementation of therapeutic hypothermia protocols, and more studies were published recently evaluating the role of EEG in predicting outcome in postanoxic patients in the therapeutic hypothermia era. More details are discussed later in this chapter regarding the utility of different EEG patterns in predicting outcome in postanoxic encephalopathy.

In addition, EEG has been utilized for the sake of outcome prediction in patients with severe traumatic brain injury. EEG reactivity was the strongest predictor of good outcome—better than Glasgow Coma Scale (GCS) score or somatosensory evoked potential (SSEP) central conduction time—in one prospective study involving 50 comatose patients with severe non-missile head injury[40]. Another recent prospective study involving 106 patients with coma due to various etiologies found that the combination of EEG reactivity and the presence of sleep spindles strongly predicted one-month awakening from coma[41].

2.5. Monitoring the Depth of Sedation

cEEG monitoring is also used to assess depth of sedation in various settings. The most common application is monitoring therapeutic response in patients with refractory status epilepticus (RSE) requiring therapeutic coma. The most commonly employed therapeutic target is attaining burst-suppression pattern[27], although we usually target seizure suppression rather than a specific background EEG pattern as long as we have cEEG to monitor the patient closely. Other applications include monitoring depth of sedation in patients with refractory intracranial hypertension necessitating the use of barbiturate-induced coma. Bispectral index (BIS) monitor, a processed EEG measure initially designed to monitor depth of sedation during surgeries, is more frequently utilized today to monitor depth of sedation in critically ill patients. However, there are conflicting data on the reliability of its use for assessing depth of sedation in these patients[42,43], and we advise caution when considering using BIS or other highly focal limited channel EEGs in neurologically abnormal patients; in general, full EEG should be utilized for these cases (see later).

3. PATTERNS ENCOUNTERED DURING CEEG MONITORING

The recognition of the role of EEG in assessment of encephalopathy is almost as old as the advent of EEG itself. Hans Berger[44] in 1929 first described EEG changes occurring with alteration of consciousness. Despite the tremendous recent advances in structural and functional neuroimaging, EEG still plays a central role in assessment of encephalopathy, owing to its unique temporal resolution and noninvasiveness. However, lack of standardization of reporting of EEG background features has been a major limitation to the use of EEG in monitoring and prognosticating various causes of encephalopathy. The ACNS recently published standardized terminology for description of key background features[45]. A summary of this terminology is presented in Table 22.2. The ACNS also proposed standard terminology and categorization of cEEG findings in neonates[46].

The interrater reliability of ACNS background terminology was recently evaluated in patients with postanoxic encephalopathy. One multicenter study included 103 routine EEGs interpreted by four EEG experts of different nationalities and found that the interrater agreement was substantial (kappa 0.71) for highly malignant background patterns and moderate (kappa 0.44) for malignant background patterns, while that for EEG reactivity was only fair (kappa 0.26). "Highly malignant" patterns included background suppression and periodic discharges on a suppressed background, whereas "malignant" background patterns included discontinuous background with suppression periods, low-voltage backgrounds, and reversed anterior–posterior gradient[47]. These data strengthen the utility of EEG as an integral component of postanoxic prognostication strategies (see later).

3.1. Background Frequency

Slowing of EEG background rhythms as a key feature of encephalopathy was first recognized almost a century ago. Hans Berger[44] in 1929 described background slowing in patients with altered awareness. Parsons-Smith et al.[48] in 1957 classified EEG changes in patients with hepatic encephalopathy into five main categories, grades A through E. Grade A was characterized by generalized suppression of the alpha rhythm and its frequent replacement by diffuse beta activity, while grade E was characterized by predominant 2-Hz delta activity. These changes correlated well with degree of disturbance of consciousness as well as serum ammonia levels[48]. Amodio et al.[49] later modified this classification (Table 22.3).

TABLE 22.2. ACNS Nomenclature for Describing Background Features[45]

Symmetry	1. Symmetric
	2. Mild asymmetry (<50% amplitude asymmetry or 0.5- to 1-Hz frequency asymmetry)
	3. Marked asymmetry (≥ 50% amplitude asymmetry or >1-Hz frequency asymmetry
Posterior dominant "alpha" rhythm	Must be demonstrated to attenuate with eye opening.
Predominant frequency	1. Delta
	2. Theta
	3. ≥Alpha
Anterior-posterior (AP) gradient	1. Present
	2. Absent
	3. Reversed
Variability	1. Yes
	2. No
	3. Unknown/Unclear/Not applicable
Reactivity	1. Yes
	2. No
	3. Unknown/Unclear/Not applicable
	4. SIRPIDs only
Voltage	1. Normal
	2. Low (most background activity ≤20 µv)
	3. Suppressed (all background activity <10 µv)
Continuity	1. Continuous
	2. Nearly continuous (periods of attenuation/suppression represent ≤10% of the record):
	a. With attenuation (periods of lower voltage are ≥10 µv but <50% of background voltage)
	b. With suppression (periods of lower voltage are <10 µv)
	Specify if "SI only."
	3. Burst attenuation/burst suppression (50–99% of the record is attenuated or suppressed)
	4. Suppression (all the record is suppressed)
Sleep transients (sleep spindles/K-complexes)	1. Normal
	2. Present but abnormal
	3. Absent

Adapted from Hirsch LJ et al. American Clinical Neurophysiology Society's Standardized Critical Care EEG Terminology: 2012 version. *J Clin Neurophyiol.* 2013;30(1):1–27.

TABLE 22.3. Amodio Grading of EEG Changes in Hepatic Encephalopathy[49]

SCORE	DESCRIPTION
0: Normal EEG	Well-structured EEG with stable and symmetrical posterior basic rhythm >8 Hz and <13 Hz dominant in the posterior regions. Such activity has medium amplitude (30–50 µV) and is reactive to eye opening. No slow activities or irritative signs are present.
1: Normal-limit EEG	Unstable or suppressed alpha rhythm frequently replaced by high prevalence of diffuse beta rhythm. (Corresponding to grade A of Parsons-Smith's classification)
2: Mild signs of encephalopathy	Low-frequency alpha rhythm (8 Hz) disturbed by random waves in the theta range over both hemispheres. (Corresponding to grade B of Parsons-Smith's classification)
3: Distinctive features of encephalopathy	Background activity in the theta range, diffuse over both hemispheres. Random appearance of high waves in the delta range. (Roughly corresponding to grade C of Parsons-Smith's classification)
4: Signs of severe encephalopathy	Severe disorganization of EEG activity without any normal elements. Diffuse asynchronous theta and delta waves over both hemispheres with or without triphasic waves. (Roughly corresponding to grade D–E of Parsons-Smith's classification)

Reproduced from: Amodio P et al. Spectral versus visual EEG analysis in mild hepatic encephalopathy. *Clin Neurophysiol.* 1999;110:1334–1344, with permission from Elsevier Limited.

EEG background changes in progressive degrees of encephalopathy (Fig. 22.3) are quite reminiscent of those seen with incrementing depth of anesthesia. Stockard and Bickford[50] described these changes, classifying them into six main EEG levels. Initial level was characterized by predominance of fast activity followed by increased voltage and rhythmicity of background rhythms with predominance of slow frequencies. EEG background amplitude then gradually declines with increasing sedation until EEG finally becomes isoelectric with maximal doses of anesthetics[50].

Unfortunately, EEG often cannot reliably identify the underlying cause of encephalopathy. Nevertheless, EEG may still provide useful information that may guide further investigations targeted at identifying the underlying cause of encephalopathy. EEG focal abnormalities in the setting of encephalopathy usually indicate the presence of a structural brain lesion[51] (Fig. 22.4). However, focal slowing of background rhythms can occasionally be seen in the absence of structural brain injury. Postictal state[52], hypoglycemia[53], and complicated migraine[54] represent the most frequently encountered examples.

In addition to the role of EEG in unmasking structural brain lesions, EEG may also provide clues about which brain structures are involved. Animal data indicate that pure white matter involvement causes polymorphic delta slowing overlying the affected region, whereas pure cortical lesions cause regional background attenuation without superimposed delta activity[55]. Human studies replicated these findings. For instance, a retrospective study published in 1968 investigated histopathological correlates of EEG changes in 32 patients with diffuse encephalopathy and found that pure cortical gray matter lesions were associated with EEG background disturbance in the form of background slowing or decreased amplitude, whereas pure white matter lesions were primarily associated with diffuse polymorphic delta activity[56]. Nearly two decades later, Schaul et al.[57] studied EEG correlates of hemispheric structural lesions seen on computed tomography (CT) and demonstrated that continuous focal abnormalities correlated with the size of the lesion and the presence of mass effect, whereas background abnormalities contralateral to the side of the lesion correlated with the degree of alteration of consciousness.

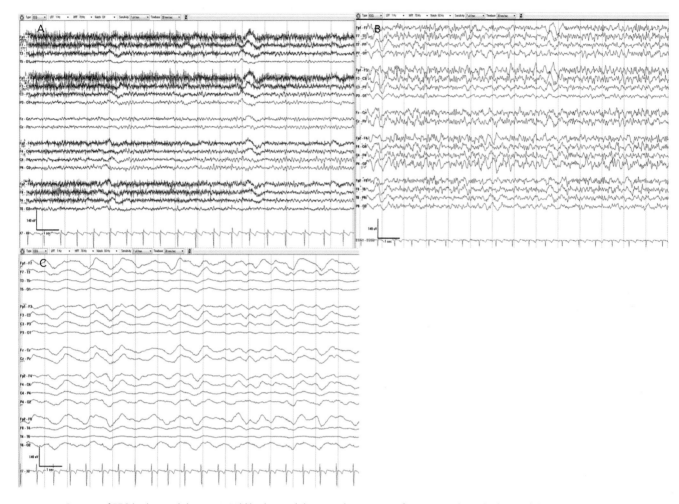

Figure 22.3. Degrees of EEG background slowing. A: Mild background slowing with intact PDR of 8 Hz. B: Moderate background slowing (mixed theta-delta frequencies). C: Severe background slowing (delta frequencies). Filter settings for all three EEG tracings: LFF = 1 Hz, HFF = 70 Hz, Notch on.

A more recent study evaluated imaging correlates of EEG abnormalities in 154 hospitalized patients with altered mental status and found that theta background was associated with brain atrophy, whereas a mixed theta/delta background was associated with intracerebral hemorrhage and pure delta background was more likely to be seen in patients with acute intoxication, HIV-infected patients, and those with posterior encephalopathy[58].

EEG provides a valuable adjunctive toot to clinical examination and laboratory and imaging investigations to distinguish organic from psychogenic unresponsiveness. However, brainstem lesions may present a potential pitfall as patients with brainstem lesions, particularly those involving the lower brainstem, may have little or no EEG background alteration despite significant disturbance of consciousness[59]. The alpha coma pattern caused by lower brainstem lesions is characterized by a posteriorly predominant alpha pattern resembling a normal posterior dominant rhythm. Preservation of EEG reactivity is the rule in "locked-in" states[60] but can also be seen in alpha coma patterns[61]; clinical examination is the key in distinguishing both patterns.

3.2. Background Continuity

Background is classified based on the degree of continuity according to ACNS classification into five main categories[45]:

1. Continuous: Background is not interrupted by any periods of suppression (where the background is <10 μv) or attenuation (≥10 μv but <50% of the background voltage).

2. Nearly continuous: Periods of attenuation/suppression make up ≤10% of the record.

3. Discontinuous: Periods of attenuation/suppression make up 11% to 49% of the record.

4. Burst-suppression/ burst-attenuation: ≥50% of the record is attenuated/suppressed (Fig. 22.5).

5. Background suppression: All the record is suppressed (Fig. 22.6).

Background continuity carries great prognostic significance, particularly in cases with postanoxic encephalopathy. Burst-suppression pattern (see Fig. 22.5) can be seen either as a drug-induced pattern in response to various intravenous (IV) anesthetics or as a spontaneous pattern primarily in the setting of postanoxic coma. The former is used as therapeutic target guiding drug titration while the latter is generally associated with poor outcome. Background-suppression and burst-suppression patterns were invariably associated with poor prognosis in postanoxic coma in three recent studies[62–64],

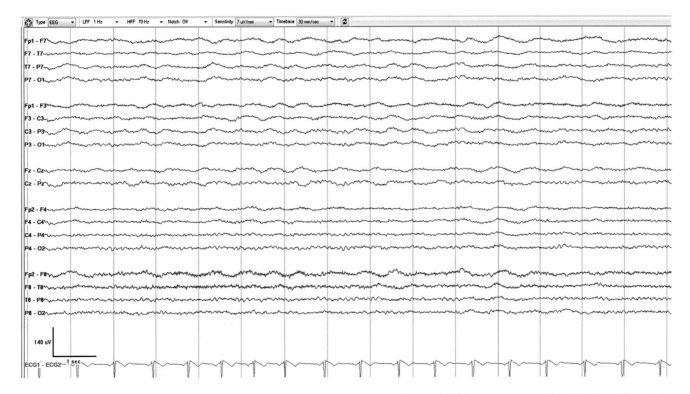

Figure 22.4. Left hemispheric focal slowing and attenuation of faster frequencies in a 53-year-old man with left frontemporoparietal SDH. LFF = 1 Hz, HFF = 70 Hz, Notch off.

although there are limitations to all of these studies, mainly the withdrawal of care and the chance of a self-fulfilling prophecy. Meanwhile, the presence of either burst-suppression pattern or background attenuation strongly predicted the occurrence of electrographic seizures in critically ill children in a recent retrospective multicenter study[25].

"Highly epileptiform bursts"[45] (Fig. 22.7) is a term recently coined by the ACNS taskforce describing the situation where >50% of the bursts contain multiple epileptiform discharges or rhythmic potentially ictal patterns at a rate of ≥1/sec. The presence of highly epileptiform bursts was a strong predictor of seizure recurrence in patients with drug-induced burst suppression in two recent studies[65,66]. Further prospective studies are needed to define the exact prognostic and therapeutic implications of this pattern.

3.3. Reactivity

Reactivity is defined as "change in cerebral EEG activity to stimuli." This includes change in background frequency or amplitude including background attenuation. However, increase in muscle activity or eye-blinking alone is not considered a form of EEG reactivity[45]. In our institution, technologists stimulate patients at least twice daily to assess for reactivity. Absence of EEG reactivity strongly predicts poor outcome in postanoxic encephalopathy and severe traumatic brain injury[67]. Meanwhile, the preservation of EEG reactivity was associated with an increased likelihood of more favorable outcome in one retrospective study including 33 comatose children undergoing EEG within 72 hours of onset of coma[68]. However, lack of standardization of stimulation methods and lack of objectivity

in identifying EEG reactivity both limit its inclusion in prognostication paradigms. A recent prospective study compared the reliability of three different nociceptive stimuli in assessment of EEG reactivity. Bilateral synchronous nipple pinching was the stimulus most likely to produce changes in background activity[69]; we do not utilize this method, but rather use nasal tickling (benign tickling just inside the nostril, but a potent stimulus) and trapezius squeeze. Our protocol for testing for EEG reactivity is highlighted in Box 22.1.

The interrater agreement for identifying EEG reactivity in patients with postanoxic coma was only fair (kappa 0.26) in a recent multicenter study[47]. Recently proposed quantitative algorithms for assessment of EEG reactivity may provide objective methods for identifying and quantifying the degree of reactivity, as opposed to dichotomizing reactivity into its mere presence or absence based on pure visual analysis. Temporal brain symmetry index total (a measure of normalized difference between spectral estimates of all EEG frequencies before and after stimulation) fared the best among 13 quantitative EEG (qEEG) parameters in a recent study[70].

3.4. Sleep Architecture

It has long been recognized that normal-appearing sleep architecture can be identified in certain comatose patients (see later). In addition, the presence of normal sleep transients (typically refers to K-complexes and spindles) is a good prognostic determinant in non-comatose encephalopathic patients as it implies preservation of thalamocortical pathways, which play a key role in maintaining consciousness. In one recent study involving 142 critically ill patients with acute encephalopathy,

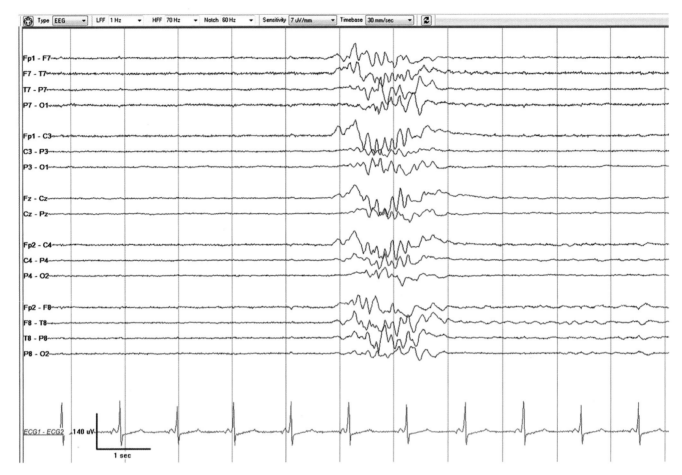

Figure 22.5. Burst-suppression pattern in an 85-year-old man with postanoxic encephalopathy. LFF = 1 Hz, HFF = 70 Hz, Notch on.

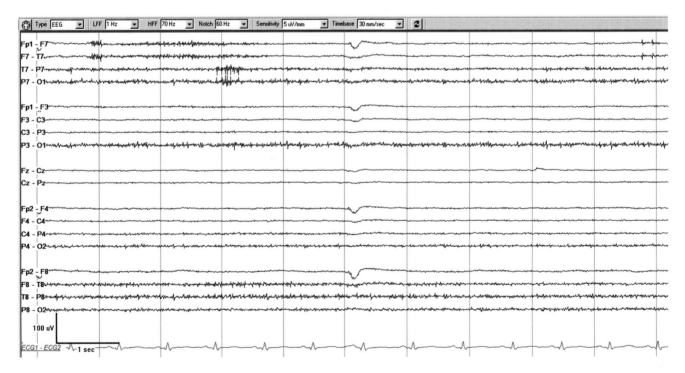

Figure 22.6. Background suppression in a 52-year-old woman with post-hypoglycemic coma. LFF = 1 Hz, HFF = 70 Hz, Notch on.

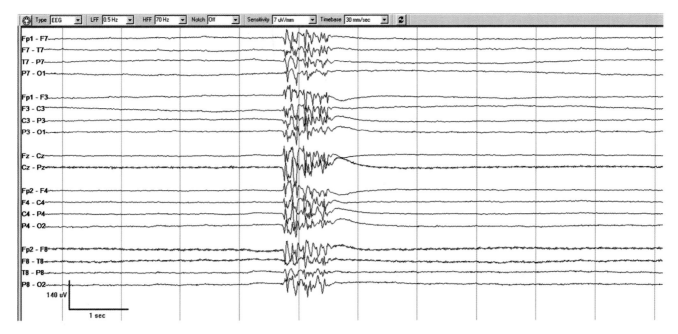

Figure 22.7. Burst suppression with highly epileptiform bursts in a 49-year-old man with postanoxic encephalopathy. LFF = 0.5 Hz, HFF = 70 Hz, Notch off.

the presence of K-complexes was independently associated with good outcome. Though the presence of other normal sleep structures such as sleep spindles and vertex transients was more frequently observed in patients with good outcome, it was not significantly associated with good outcome on multivariate analysis[71]. However, the lack of normal frequency and amplitude spindles per se in the setting of encephalopathy should not be interpreted as a sign of grave prognosis, as there are reports of delayed recovery of sleep spindles up to 150 days in patients who eventually recovered consciousness[72,73].

3.5. Cyclic Alternating Pattern

"Cyclic alternating pattern" (CAP), initially described as a distinct pattern in encephalopathic patients by Bermagasco et al.[74] in 1968, is characterized by the alternation of two distinct background patterns in a cyclic manner. Phase A is characterized by the presence of high-voltage delta activity, whereas phase B is characterized by the presence of low-voltage theta activity. Phase A represents the more aroused state associated with increased heart rate, respiratory rate, muscle activity, and restlessness (a similar pattern often can be elicited by stimulation), whereas phase B represents the less aroused state associated with less autonomic and muscle activity. As the clinical condition improves, phase A is replaced by a sequential run of K-complexes, suggesting that this pattern represents an alteration of the normal arousal phenomena[75,76]. To date, the clinical implications of the presence of CAP, if any, are unknown. Normal individuals have CAP; it is felt to represent a less stable stage of non-rapid eye movement (REM) sleep than non-CAP sleep[77].

3.6. Classical Coma Patterns

3.6.1. ALPHA COMA

The recognition of occurrence of EEG patterns resembling normal wakefulness in certain comatose patients dates back to 1953 when Loeb and Poggio reported the presence of 8- to 9-Hz bifrontally predominant activity in a comatose patient with pontomesencephalic hemorrhage[78]. Westmoreland et al.[79] called this pattern "alpha coma" and classified it into two main

---

BOX 22.1. YALE PROTOCOL FOR ASSESSING EEG REACTIVITY IN THE ICU (ABBREVIATED VERSION)

- EEG reactivity is assessed by stimulating the patient verbally and tactilely. For accuracy, stimulation should be performed in a standardized fashion.
- Stimulation should be performed when the patient has been resting quietly.
- If patient has ICP or blood pressure issues, be sure to monitor closely and abort protocol if there are any concerns. Please document in the EEG recording if and why the stimulation was aborted.
- If the patient is on sedation, please enter the drip rates in the EEG recording. If sedation is held, please indicate the type and time at which sedation was held.

Perform the stimulation protocol as outlined below and document stimulation in EEG recording as "STIM: grade (ACYST)". If the patient is Grade A, there is no need to proceed.

GRADES

- A = already Awake and alert
- C = aroused by Calling name
- Y = aroused by Yelling name and clapping
- S = aroused by gentle Shaking
- T1 = reaction to nostril Tickling
- T2 = reaction to Trapezius squeezing

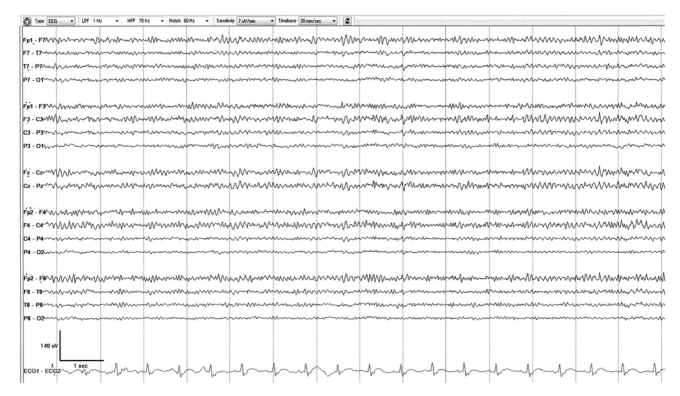

Figure 22.8. Frontally predominant alpha coma in a 20-year-old man with postanoxic encephalopathy in the setting of heroin intoxication. LFF = 1 Hz, HFF = 70 Hz, Notch on.

subtypes. The first subtype is characterized by frontally predominant alpha rhythm (Fig. 22.8) and is most frequently seen in postanoxic coma, while the second subtype is characterized by posteriorly predominant alpha rhythm resembling normal wakefulness and is usually seen in brainstem lesions at or below the pontomesencephalic junction. These lesions seem to spare the upper midbrain and rostral structures thought to be involved in generation of the alpha rhythm[79]. It is important to distinguish such cases from "locked-in state" conditions. The distinction between both conditions on basis of EEG alone may be challenging. The preservation of EEG reactivity is the rule in "locked-in" cases[60] but is also occasionally seen in some cases of alpha coma[80].

Occasionally, alpha frequencies may be mixed with theta frequencies or theta frequencies may predominate. These two patterns are called "alpha-theta coma" and "theta coma," respectively[81]. Though alpha coma was initially thought to be a pattern with invariably dismal prognosis, it now appears more likely that the outcome is primarily dependent on the underlying etiology. Postanoxic alpha coma carries the worst prognosis, whereas drug-induced alpha coma carries the best prognosis. The preservation of EEG reactivity appears to be the strongest EEG predictor of outcome[61].

3.6.2. SPINDLE COMA

It has been mentioned previously that the presence of normal sleep structures serves as an important prognostic determinant in critically ill patients with encephalopathy. In addition, patterns resembling normal sleep may represent the primary background pattern in certain comatose patients. Chatrian et al.[82]

in 1963 reported on 11 patients with severe traumatic brain injury and sleep-like patterns on EEG. These patterns included vertex waves, sleep spindles, and sensory stimulation induced K-complexes and are collectively labeled "spindle coma" (Fig. 22.9). All patients eventually recovered consciousness and were discharged 8 to 26 days after injury[82]. This pattern was later reported in a variety of cases of nontraumatic coma as well[83]. There is conflicting evidence on the prognostic implication of spindle coma; the most compelling evidence indicates that outcome is largely dependent on the underlying etiology. As in alpha coma, intact EEG reactivity strongly predicts better outcome[84].

3.6.3. BETA COMA

Beta coma is characterized by the presence of diffuse, occasionally frontally predominant 12- to 16-Hz beta activity. The most common etiology is drug intoxication or withdrawal, usually involving barbiturates or benzodiazepines. Beta coma can occasionally be seen in other settings such as acute brainstem lesions. Beta coma, particularly in the setting of drug intoxication or withdrawal, generally entails good prognosis as it implies intact cortical response to pharmacological stimulation[85].

3.7. EEG Background Scoring Systems

Several EEG background scoring methods have been proposed, aiming at providing a systematic way of stratifying EEG changes in encephalopathy, correlating these changes with the patient's clinical state, and finally prognosticating outcome in conjunction with other clinical, neurophysiological, and imaging measures. The first systematic classification of EEG

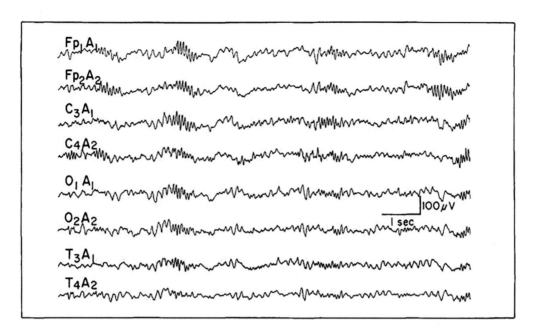

Figure 22.9. *Spindle coma in a comatose patient with subarachnoid hemorrhage. Reproduced from Britt CW. Nontraumatic "spindle coma": Clinical, EEG and prognostic features. Neurology. 1981;31:393–397. With permission from Wolters Kluwer.*

changes in encephalopathy came from Parsons-Smith et al. around 70 years ago; they classified EEG changes in encephalopathy into five main grades (A–E). These changes correlated well with clinical changes as well as serum ammonia levels[48]. A modified version was proposed by Amodio et al.[49] decades later and is shown in Table 22.3.

The first systematic classification of EEG changes in postanoxic encephalopathy came from Hockaday et al.[38] in 1965, based on EEG findings in 39 patients with postanoxic encephalopathy, and included five main grades. Progressive grades of encephalopathy correlated well with outcome, as all patients with grade 1 encephalopathy survived and none of those with grade 5 encephalopathy did. Two major limitations of this classification were that it was primarily centered on background frequency slowing, overlooking other critical elements of the background such as background reactivity, and it did not include uncommon distinct coma patterns such as alpha coma and spindle coma. Given these considerations, Synek[86] (Table 22.4) refined this classification while taking into account EEG changes observed in patients with posttraumatic encephalopathy as well. Young et al.[87] further modified Synek's scale, creating a more simplified classification for EEG grading of coma secondary to various etiologies[87] (Table 22.5). The interrater agreement for classifying EEG of comatose patients on the basis of Young's classification was near perfect (kappa 0.90), while that for classifying EEG on basis of Synek's classification was substantial (kappa 0.75) in one study involving blinded EEG interpretation of 100 EEGs by two interpreters[87].

3.8. Electrographic Seizures and the Ictal-interictal Continuum

The primary goal of cEEG monitoring in the ICU is to identify subclinical seizures. The majority of electrographic seizures are purely electrographic and thus cannot be identified without cEEG monitoring[1]. Identification of nonconvulsive seizures in the ICU setting is often hindered by the presence of a disturbed background, the presence of rhythmic and periodic patterns that are difficult to distinguish from ictal patterns, and the myriad of artifacts mimicking seizures. Young et al.[88] proposed a criteria set in 1996 for defining nonconvulsive seizures. This set of criteria, known as the "Salzburg criteria," underwent

TABLE 22.4. Synek Grading of Encephalopathy

GRADE	SUBGRADE
Grade 1: Alpha predominance, few theta intrusions	
Grade 2: Theta predominance, occasional alpha and delta	i. Reactive ii. Unreactive
Grade 3: Delta predominance, usually reactive	i. Frontally predominant rhythmic delta activity with little theta or alpha ii. Spindle coma iii. Low-amplitude delta activity interrupted by periods of attenuation iv. Diffuse medium-voltage delta (either rhythmic or irregular)
Grade 4: Burst-suppression pattern	i. Presence of epileptiform discharges ii. Alpha coma iii. Theta coma iv. Low-voltage background
Grade 5: Isoelectric EEG	

Adapted from Synek VM. Prognostically important EEG patterns in diffuse anoxic and traumatic encephalopathies in adults. *J Clin Neurophysiol.* 1988;5(2):161–174.

TABLE 22.5. Young Classification of coma

CATEGORY	SUBCATEGORY
I Delta/theta > 50% of record (not theta coma)	A. Reactivity B. No reactivity
II Triphasic waves	
III Burst suppression	A. With epileptiform activity B. Without epileptiform activity
IV Alpha/theta/spindle coma (unreactive)	
V Epileptiform activity (not in burst-suppression pattern)	A. Generalized B. Focal or multifocal
VI Suppression	A. <20 µv but > 10 µv B. <10 µv

Reproduced from Young GB et al. An electroencephalographic classification for coma. *Can J Neurol Sci.* 1997;24:320–325, with permission from Cambridge University Press.

several revisions; the most recent version was released in 2015[89] (Box 22.2). Based on these criteria, the presence of either of the following two features defines electrographic seizures:

1. Presence of >2.5-Hz epileptiform discharges for ≥10 sec

2. Presence of <2.5-Hz epileptiform discharges or >0.5-Hz rhythmic discharges lasting ≥10 sec with one of the following: clear spatiotemporal evolution; subtle clinical correlate; or positive EEG *and* clinical response to an IV antiepileptic drug (AED) trial.

Further conditions for defining nonconvulsive seizures in the setting of epileptic encephalopathy include the presence of a clear change in the following features from baseline and a change in clinical state or a clear EEG and clinical response to IV AEDs. The use of a 2.5-Hz cutoff point for epileptiform discharges lasting >10 sec to be considered ictal represents a minor change from previous criteria, which mostly required a frequency of 3 Hz or greater. In one recent retrospective study involving 50 patients with NCSE and 50 matched controls, three of the four patients with >2.5-Hz epileptiform discharges lasting >10 sec were identified as having NCSE using the 2.5-Hz threshold and would have been missed with the long-used 3-Hz threshold[89]. Moreover, incorporating the ACNS criteria for defining rhythmic patterns (see below) remarkably improved the specificity of the Salzburg criteria for identifying NCSE, with a decrease of the false-positive rate in controls from 28% to 0%[89]. An example of an electrographic seizure is depicted in Figure 22.10.

Despite the availability of several sets of criteria for defining nonconvulsive seizures, the interrater agreement for seizure identification in the critically ill population remains moderate at best in both adult and pediatric populations[90–92]. This is largely due to the plenitude of rhythmic and periodic patterns closely resembling ictal patterns. We believe that dichotomizing rhythmic and periodic patterns in the ICU into definite ictal and nonictal patterns is not only fraught with difficulties, but also often ill advised on the basis of EEG alone. Rhythmic

and periodic patterns that are not definitely ictal but could be, and that may still serve as potential culprits for neuronal damage under certain circumstances, are considered to lie along the "ictal–interictal continuum" (IIC). There is no consensus agreement yet on defining criteria for IIC patterns, but we generally include 1- to 2.5-Hz fluctuating rhythmic or periodic patterns, particularly when having a plus modifier per the ACNS criteria (see later for a thorough explanation of ACNS terminology) under the IIC spectrum. A thorough approach to evaluating these patterns is discussed later in this chapter.

3.9. Rhythmic and Periodic Patterns

The expansion of cEEG monitoring in the ICU setting has led to identification of a variety of rhythmic and periodic patterns. In an attempt to provide common language for use by critical care EEG-ers and researchers worldwide, the ACNS proposed standardized nomenclature for describing these patterns. This nomenclature underwent several modifications since its original proposal in 2005[93] until it was finally released in an official guideline by the ACNS in late 2012[45]. Table 22.6 summarizes the main components of the final version. It is also readily available at http://www.acns.org/practice/guidelines, including related practical educational (training module) and clinical tools (e.g., "pocket version").

Patterns are described in the ACNS nomenclature based on two main defining features, called "main term 1 and 2." Main term 1 describes the location of the pattern, while main term 2 describes its type. Patterns are classified into three main types: rhythmic delta activity (RDA), periodic discharges (PDs), and spike-and-wave or sharp-and-wave discharges (SW). Rhythmic discharges are defined as discharges of relatively uniform morphology and duration occurring in a repetitive manner with no intervening background activity (i.e., no interdischarge interval). On the other hand, periodic discharges (PDs) are defined as discharges of relatively uniform morphology and duration occurring at nearly regular intervals with an interdischarge interval. Finally, the SW pattern includes spikes, polyspikes, or sharp waves attaining a constant relationship with the proceeding slow wave, and with no intervening background between one spike-wave complex and the next. Modifiers are added to describe additional features of the pattern (see Table 22.6 for a brief description).

The interrater agreement for describing rhythmic and periodic patterns using the published 2012 ACNS terminology was near perfect for main terms 1 and 2, while that for most modifiers was moderate/substantial in one recent study[94]. However, the interrater agreement for evolution was only fair, possibly owing to the short duration of epochs provided in the study, which made it difficult for interpreters to appreciate evolution[94]. Interestingly, the interrater agreement was similar across interpreters with different levels of EEG expertise ranging from 1 to 30 years. This could be attributed at least partially to the provision of a web-based tutorial (the ACNS training module) to all interpreters before reviewing EEG epochs of interest. These results corroborate the interrater reliability of the ACNS terminology, allowing for research and clinical use. A database was created by the Critical Care EEG Monitoring Research

BOX 22.2. MODIFIED SALZBURG CRITERIA FOR DIAGNOSIS OF NCSE

EEG changes fulfilling the criteria have to be continuously present for ≥10 sec. Criteria not applicable to physiological graphoelements.

A: Patients without known epileptic encephalopathy (at least ONE of the criteria 1–3 should be fulfilled for diagnosis of NCSE)

   1. EDs > 2.5 Hz (i.e., >25 EDs in "worst" 10-second epoch)

   2. Typical ictal spatiotemporal evolution* of:
  - (2a) EDs OR
  - (2b) Rhythmic activity** (> 0.5 Hz)

   3. Subtle ictal clinical phenomena*** with:
  - (3a) EDs OR
  - (3b) Rhythmic activity** (> 0.5 Hz)

   4. If criteria 1–3 are not fulfilled, but one of the following patterns is present, apply appropriate IV AED(s) after careful consideration of clinical situation and document response****:
  - (4a) EDs ≤ 2.5 Hz with fluctuation***** OR
  - (4b) Rhythmic activity** (> 0.5 Hz) with fluctuation***** OR
  - (4c) Rhythmic activity** (> 0.5 Hz) without fluctuation*****

B: Patients with known epileptic encephalopathy

In addition to the criteria above (A), these patients have to fulfill one of the following:

- Increase in prominence or frequency when compared to baseline *with* observable change in clinical state
- Improvement of clinical and EEG features with IV AEDs (see A.4.)

Explaining remarks and specifications:

EDs = epileptiform discharges (spikes, polyspikes, sharp waves, sharp-and-slow-wave complexes); IV AED: intravenous antiepileptic drug.

Incrementing onset (increase in voltage and change in frequency), or evolution in pattern (change in frequency > 1 Hz and change in location), or decrementing termination (voltage and frequency), AND ACNS criterion for "evolving" (ACNS-evolving): "at least 2 unequivocal, sequential changes in frequency, morphology or location defined as follows: Evolution in frequency is defined as at least 2 consecutive changes in the same direction by at least 0.5/ s, e.g. from 2 to 2.5 to 3/s, or from 3 to 2 to 1.5/s; Evolution in morphology is defined as at least 2 consecutive changes to a novel morphology; Evolution in location is defined as sequentially spreading into or sequentially out of at least two different standard 10–20 electrode locations. In order to qualify as present, a single frequency or location must persist at least 3 cycles (e.g. 1/s for 3 seconds, or 3/s for 1 second)"

**ACNS criterion for rhythmic delta activity (ACNS-RDA): "Rhythmic = repetition of a waveform with relatively uniform morphology and duration, and without an interval between consecutive waveforms. RDA = rhythmic activity < 4 Hz. The duration of one cycle (i.e., the period) of the rhythmic pattern should vary by < 50% from the duration of the subsequent cycle for the majority (> 50%) of cycle pairs to qualify as rhythmic".*

***Minor twitching of mouth, periorbital region, or extremities should appear in close temporal relation to EEG pattern (be cautious concerning nonepileptic involuntary movements as mimics, e.g., parkinsonian tremor, drug-induced myoclonus (e.g., opioids), serotonin syndrome).

****Reactivity to IV AEDs within 10 min after AED fully applied.

Clinical presentation tested: improvement is defined as better performance in one of five domains: (i) *"say your surname"*, (ii) *"repeat 1,2,3"*, (iii) *"raise your arms"* (first tell, if no response demonstrate), (iv) patient opens eyes to i–iii, and (v) patient looks at the examiner in response to i–iii. If no response, repeat procedure after strong tactile stimuli on both sides of the body.

EEG tested: improvement is defined as reduction of the pattern in question to absent, rare or *"occasional"*, i.e., 1–9% of epoch.

Document response:

– No EEG improvement and no clinical improvement

– Only EEG improvement but no clinical improvement

– Only clinical improvement but no EEG improvement

– EEG AND clinical improvements

For clinical practice: the latter two responses (i.e., including clinical improvement) qualify as definite NCSE (based on the clinical setting). EEG improvement alone or no response at all is considered "possible NCSE" (i.e., it does not exclude NCSE clinically).

For research projects: patient qualifies for NCSE if EEG and clinical improvement are documented, provided the clinical context is also in concordance with that.

*****ACNS criterion for fluctuation (ACNS-fluctuation): "> 3 changes, not more than one minute apart, in frequency (by at least 0.5/s), > 3 changes in morphology, or > 3 changes in location (by at least 1 standard interelectrode distance), but not qualifying as evolving. This includes patterns fluctuating from 1 to 1.5 to 1 to 1.5/s; spreading in and out of a single electrode repeatedly; or alternating between 2 morphologies repeatedly"*

Modified from Leitenger M et al. Salzburg Consensus Criteria for Non-Convulsive Status Epilepticus—approach to clinical application. *Epilepsy Behav.* 2015;49:158–163, with permission from Elsevier.

Consortium incorporating key clinical and research variables of critical care EEG reporting. It was validated in a multicenter study and is now available for public download at (https://www.acns.org/research/critical-care-eeg-monitoring-research-consortium-ccemrc). It can be used for multicenter collaborative research as well as for daily clinical EEG reporting.

3.10. LPDs/PLEDs

The first report of periodic EEG patterns dates back to 1950 when Cobb and Hill reported long-interval generalized periodic discharges in five patients with subacute sclerosing panencephalitis (SSPE)[95]. Fourteen years later, Chatrian et al.[96] coined the term "periodic lateralized epileptiform discharges" (PLEDs) to describe repetitive sharp-wave discharges, occurring in a periodic fashion, primarily involving one hemisphere[96]. However, given that these discharges are not always epileptiform in appearance nor is their epileptogenic nature clearly defined, the word "epileptiform" was omitted from the ACNS terminology and this pattern was renamed (to match the naming convention of other terms as well) "lateralized periodic discharges" (LPDs)[45]. These two terms are used interchangeably in this chapter. LPDs may take the form of spikes, sharp waves, sharply contoured or even blunt waveforms (Fig. 22.11), as long as they are lateralized and periodic.

Reiher et al.[97] classified PLEDs into two main subtypes: "PLEDs proper" and "PLEDs plus." The PLEDs plus subtype encompasses PLEDs associated with rhythmic discharges of any frequency (most commonly faster frequencies) and was associated with a remarkably increased risk for seizures compared with the PLEDs proper subtype: 74% of patients with PLEDs plus had electrographic seizures compared to only 6% of patients with PLEDs proper in one retrospective study involving 84 patients with PLEDs[97]. "LPDs plus" was more

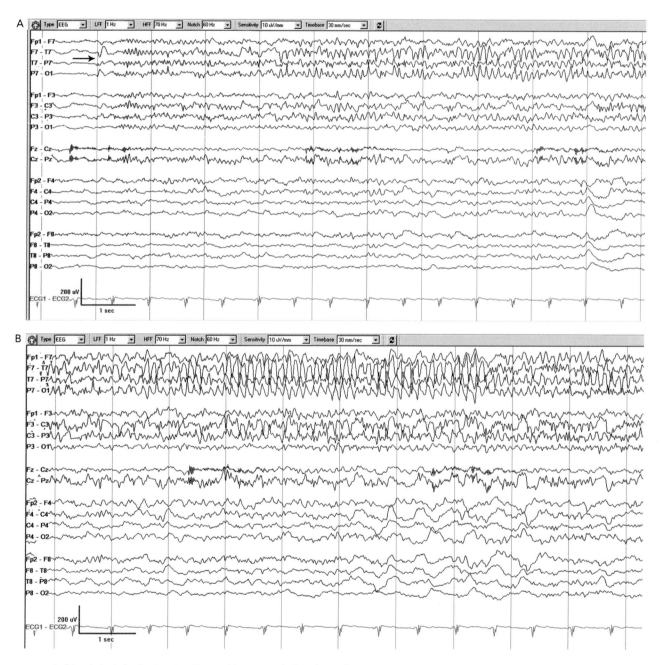

Figure 22.10. Left hemispheric focal seizure in a 25-year-old woman with altered mental status. A: Seizure onset (arrow). Sharply contoured theta-frequency waveform is seen at onset evolving rapidly into beta-frequency activity involving the left hemisphere and midline, which evolve within 4 seconds of onset into sharply contoured rhythmic alpha activity. B: Seizure continued to evolve in the left hemisphere. C: Seizure offset 95 seconds after seizure onset; seizure had spread bilaterally between B and C. Clinically the patient had behavioral arrest and oral automatisms. LFF = 1 Hz, HFF = 70 Hz, Notch on.

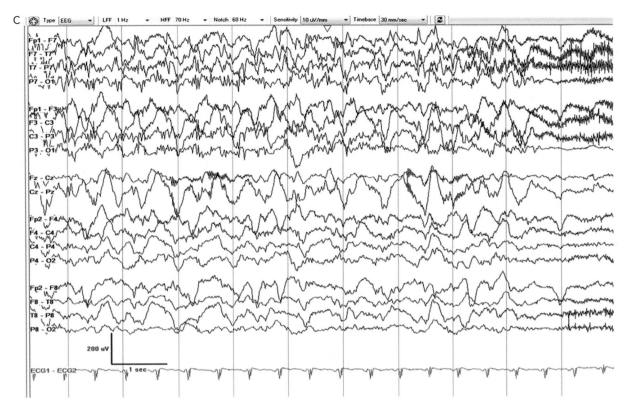

Figure 22.10. Continued

recently subclassified in the ACNS terminology into three main subtypes:

1. "LPDs+R": LPDs associated with rhythmic discharges of any frequency

2. "LPDs+F" (Fig. 22.12): LPDs associated with fast frequency

TABLE 22.6. ACNS Nomenclature for Description of Rhythmic and Periodic Patterns[45]

MAIN TERM # 1	MAIN TERM # 2
Generalized (G)	Periodic discharges (PD)
Lateralized (L)	Rhythmic delta activity (RDA)
Bilateral independent (BI)	Spike-and-wave or sharp-and-wave (SW)
Multifocal (Mf)	

- For L: Reporter can specify whether the discharge is unilateral or bilateral asymmetric and lobe(s) or hemisphere most involved.
- For G: Reporter can specify if the discharge is frontally predominant, occipitally predominant, midline predominant or truly generalized (generalized NOS).
Modifiers are to be specified for each category. Modifiers specify prevalence, frequency, duration, number of phases, sharpness, amplitude, polarity, presence of stimulus induced patterns, presence of evolving or fluctuating patterns, as well as presence of plus modifiers. Plus modifiers include +S (for sharply contoured waveforms or for rhythmic patterns with superimposed sharp waves or spikes), +F (for discharges with superimposed fast frequency activity) and +R (for superimposed rhythmic or quasi-rhythmic delta activity) or a combination of these plus modifiers (+FR or +FS).
Adapted from Hirsch LJ et al. American Clinical Neurophysiology Society's Standardized Critical Care EEG Terminology: 2012 version. *J Clin Neurophyiol.* 2013;30(1):1–27.

3. "LPDs+FR": LPDs associated with both of the aforementioned characteristics[45].

LPDs are primarily seen in the setting of acute structural brain lesions, with acute stroke being the most common underlying etiology[98]. Other etiologies include central nervous system (CNS) infections, CNS tumors, intracranial hemorrhage and less commonly CNS demyelinating disease, and anoxic and toxic-metabolic encephalopathies[98]. LPDs can also rarely be seen as an interictal pattern in patients with long-standing epilepsy[99]. Periodic discharges were initially thought to be caused by disconnection between the cerebral cortex and subcortical structures secondary to subcortical brain lesions[95]. This hypothesis was primarily based on animal studies demonstrating that transecting the brain at any level below the cerebral cortex produced periodic discharges[95]. However, LPDs were reported in both isolated cortical and subcortical lesions in multiple human studies[100,101], challenging this hypothesis. LPDs were most frequently seen in patients with coexistent cortical and subcortical lesions in one retrospective study involving 79 patients with LPDs[100]. LPDs associated with cortical lesions were more likely to be of longer duration and less stereotypic morphology than those associated with subcortical lesions in another retrospective study involving 106 patients with LPDs[101].

There is strong evidence that LPDs portend a markedly increased risk for seizures in the setting of acute neurological insults, where ~57% to 70% of patients with LPDs have seizures during the course of their illness[100,102]. One recent study demonstrated that LPDs, particularly when associated with nonconvulsive seizures, are associated with a long-term

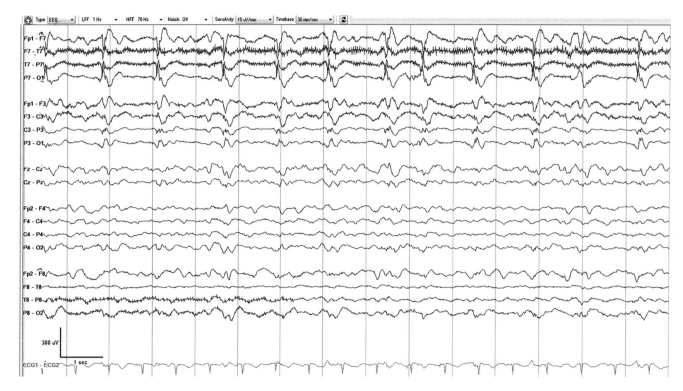

Figure 22.11. 0.75- to 1-Hz left temporal static LPDs in a 65-year-old woman with left temporal intraparenchymal hematoma. LFF = 1 Hz, HFF = 70 Hz, Notch off.

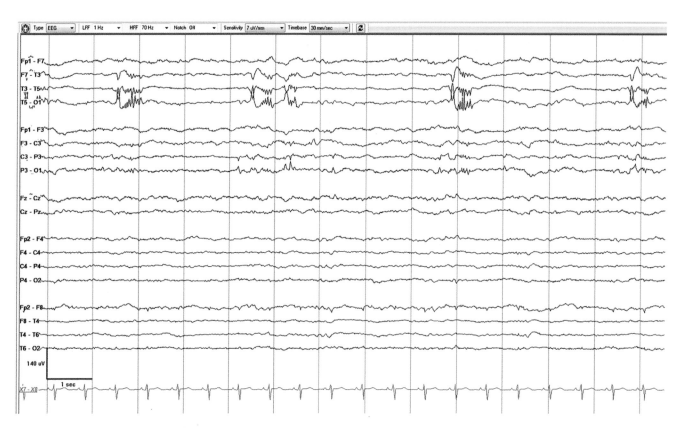

Figure 22.12. 0.25-Hz left posterior temporal LPD+F in a 65-year-old woman with left subdural hematoma (SDH). (If these discharges were mostly longer than 0.5 seconds, these would qualify as bursts, and the pattern would be focal burst suppression with highly epileptiform bursts.)

increased risk of epilepsy as well[103]. However, there has been a longstanding debate on whether LPDs per se represent an ictal pattern, an interictal pattern, or merely a marker of brain injury. Arguments for the ictal nature of LPDs include the following:

1. Motor movements can be seen time-locked to LPDs, particularly those with central EEG localization, raising the possibility that the lack of clinical correlate in most cases is due to involvement of "silent" brain areas[104]. Moreover, negative motor phenomena such as hemiparesis, aphasia, sensory neglect, and homonymous hemianopia were reported in patients with LPDs in the absence of a clear underlying structural cause[105,106]. These symptoms often reversed completely with treatment of LPDs[107].

2. Improvement of consciousness was reported in some cases with LPDs coupled with resolution of the pattern on EEG (positive clinical and EEG response), implying the ictal nature of LPDs at least in these cases[107] (see below).

3. Periodic patterns are occasionally seen as an intervening pattern in SE[108].

4. There are reports of LPDs associated with notable focal changes on structural and functional neuroimaging typically seen in patients with SE. These include restricted diffusion on DWI, increase rCBF on CT or magnetic resonance imaging (MRI) perfusion[109] and single photon emission computed tomography (SPECT) imaging[110], and hypermetabolism on positron emission tomography (PET)

scans[111,112]. These changes often reversed completely with treatment of LPDs, suggesting their ictal nature.[109]

5. LPDs are often associated with markers of neuronal injury such as increased lactate and decreased glucose levels in cerebral microdialysate[113] (see later).

6. Periodic patterns including LPDs are frequently associated with frank electrographic seizures on simultaneous depth-EEG recording.

On the other hand, arguments for LPDs being an interictal pattern include the following:

1. Chronic LPDs have been demonstrated in rare cases with longstanding epilepsy, suggesting that LPDs either represent an interictal pattern or less likely an ictal pattern associated with a relatively benign course[99].

2. Electrographic seizures with a completely different frequency or pattern are often seen emerging from LPDs (Fig. 22.13), similar to their emergence from other interictal patterns commonly seen in the epilepsy monitoring unit (EMU) setting.

Given the state of uncertainty about the ictal nature of many rhythmic and periodic patterns in the critically ill population, these patterns are often considered (including by us) to lie along the IIC. There is no consensus yet on the defining features of IIC patterns, but we generally include 1- to 2.5-Hz rhythmic or periodic patterns, particularly those with fluctuating character and/or a plus modifier, under the IIC umbrella. It

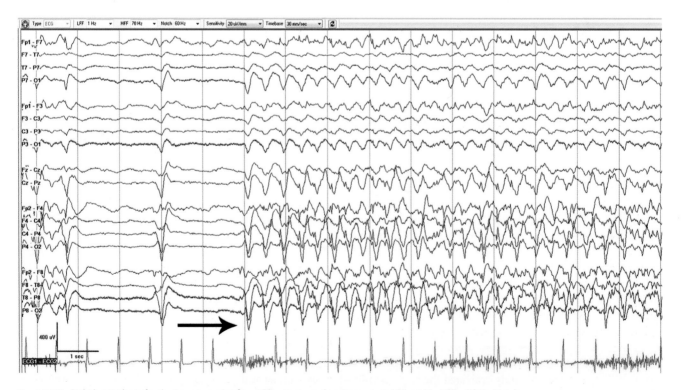

Figure 22.13. Right hemispheric focal seizure emerging from LPDs. Arrow marks seizure onset. LFF = 1 Hz, HFF = 70 Hz, Notch on.

is important to exclude clear ictal and interictal patterns before labeling a pattern as such.

3.11. Approach to IIC Patterns

IIC patterns need to be further evaluated to determine their ictal nature, their contribution to the patient's impaired mental status, and their contribution to neuronal injury; results may help guide the aggressiveness of management. Possible approaches include the following:

1. IV AED trial

2. Correlating EEG patterns with known imaging markers of ongoing ictal activity

3. Correlating EEG patterns with markers of neuronal injury

The first approach to evaluating IIC patterns utilizes a therapeutic drug trial. An IV AED trial is an underutilized test providing a simple, noninvasive means for diagnosing and possibly treating NCSE. The most commonly employed drug is a short-acting benzodiazepine given in sequential very low doses (e.g., 1 mg midazolam) with careful monitoring of the patient's clinical state throughout the test. Neurological assessment and careful EEG review are performed after each dose and the trial is stopped if a positive EEG or clinical response occurs or if a significant adverse effect (e.g., respiratory depression or hypotension) arises, or possibly if a maximal dose is reached.

Resolution of the EEG pattern of interest and either clinical improvement or recovery of previously absent normal EEG background rhythms are required for the result to be deemed a positive response. Improvement of the EEG pattern alone is not considered a positive response as many nonictal patterns may resolve in response to benzodiazepines. This situation (EEG improvement without clinical improvement) is called "possible NCSE"[114]. There is no negative result for this test. The lack of EEG or clinical response doesn't exclude NCSE; it simply doesn't confirm its presence. Interpretation of the test result is often confounded by the sedating effect of benzodiazepines. Thus we often use a loading dose of a nonsedating AED such as fosphenytoin, valproate, levetiracetam, or lacosamide instead. The clinical response to all agents, especially nonsedating AEDs and especially after prolonged NCSE, can be delayed, often up to 24 hours after the drug administration.

Several studies investigated the yield of an IV AED trial to diagnose NCSE. Hopp et al.[115] retrospectively identified 62 patients receiving an IV benzodiazepine trial for suspected NCSE; 53 (85%) of these had complete or partial EEG response. Thirty-five of the 53 patients (66%) with a positive EEG response recovered consciousness before discharge, and 40 (76%) survived. Thus, 35 of the 62 patients (56%) had a positive EEG and clinical response to the IV benzodiazepine trial. Positive EEG response correlated strongly with recovery of consciousness but not with survival, though there was a trend toward increased survival in patients with complete EEG response[115]. A more recent study evaluated the response rates of patients with unexplained encephalopathy and a "triphasic

wave" (TW) pattern—a pattern long thought to be of nonepileptic nature—on EEG to an IV AED trial. Twenty-two of the 64 patients (34.4%) had a definite clinical and EEG response to either IV benzodiazepine or nonsedating AED[116]. These two studies underscore the utility of an AED trial as an inexpensive, noninvasive reliable tool for diagnosing and potentially treating NCSE. An example of resolution of the TW pattern (now known as GPDs with triphasic morphology) following an IV AED trial is shown in Figure 22.14.

The second approach to investigating the ictal nature of these patterns involves correlating EEG patterns with distinct neuroimaging findings typically associated with seizures. However, it is important to distinguish these findings from changes secondary to the underlying etiology. Examples of these findings include restricted diffusion on DWI[109], increased regional perfusion on CT or MRI perfusion[109] or SPECT imaging[110], and hypermetabolism on PET scans[111,112]. Reversal of these changes on successful treatment of the EEG pattern provides further evidence of the ictal nature of these patterns[109].

The third approach involves correlating EEG findings with markers of neuronal injury. These include serial levels of neuron-specific enolase (NSE) and cerebral microdialysis lactate, pyruvate, glutamate, glucose, and glycerol levels[109]. Other than a therapeutic drug trial, these approaches are still investigational and more research is needed to determine their exact role in clinical management.

3.12. BIPDs (BIPLEDs)

LPDs arising independently from both hemispheres are termed bilateral independent periodic discharges (BIPDs; previously called BIPLEDs) (Fig. 22.15). Similar to LPDs, BIPDs are most frequently seen in the setting of structural brain lesions. However, bilateral or diffuse structural abnormalities are more common in patients with BIPDs than in patients with LPDs[100]. In addition, BIPDs are more frequently seen in patients with postanoxic encephalopathy than LPDs[117]. The risk of seizures is high in patients with BIPDs, but there are conflicting data on the relative risk compared to patients with LPDs. 78% of patients with BIPDs had seizures during their acute illness compared to 82% of patients with LPDs in one retrospective study published more than 30 years ago[118]. On the other hand, seizures were detected in 43% of patients with BIPDs compared to 70% of patients with LPDs in a more recent study in 2009[100]. However, patients with LPDs were not matched in any way to their BIPDs counterparts in either of these two studies. BIPDs are generally considered a more malignant pattern than LPDs: BIPDs were associated with 61% mortality compared to 29% mortality with LPDs in one retrospective study[118]. More studies are needed to further define the clinical significance of BIPDs compared to other patterns encountered in the critically ill population.

3.13. GPDs

Generalized periodic discharges (GPDs) are bilateral synchronous symmetric discharges, of relatively uniform morphology, occurring at regular intervals, with an interdischarge interval;

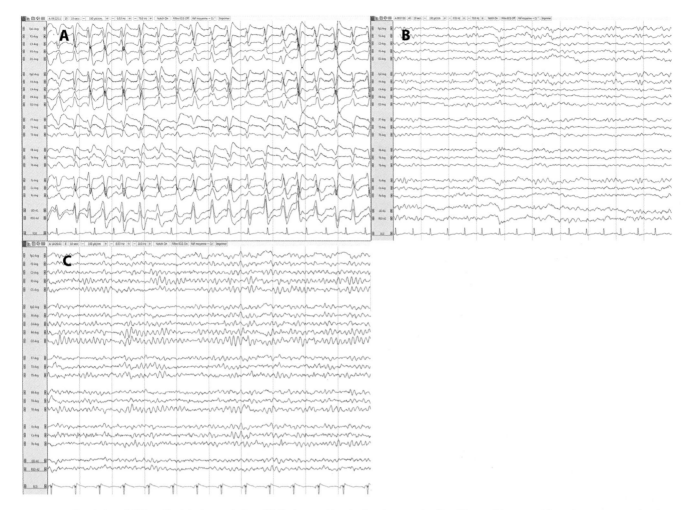

Figure 22.14. *Resolution of GPDs with triphasic morphology (TWs) after receiving 1 g levetiracetam load in a 72-year-old woman with moderate acute-on-chronic renal failure, treated with ceftazidime for skin infection and presenting acutely for sudden alteration of mental status with staring and oral automatisms. This is an example of ictal TW. **A:** EEG before levetiracetam was loaded. **B:** EEG 30 minutes after levetiracetam was loaded. **C:** EEG 12 hours after levetiracetam was loaded showing re-emergence of background. Patient's level of consciousness improved a few hours after levetiracetam load. LFF = 0.53 Hz, HFF = 70 Hz, Notch on. Figure courtesy of Nicolas Gaspard, MD, PhD, Brussels, Belgium.*

they most commonly occur at a rate of 1 to 2/sec. The most common presenting illnesses in patients with GPDs based on a large recent-case control study include, in descending order of frequency: acute brain injury, toxic metabolic encephalopathy, postanoxic encephalopathy, and epilepsy. Among adult patients with acute brain injury, ischemic stroke is the most common underlying etiology[119], whereas encephalitis was the most common cause of GPDs in critically ill children in another study[120]. GPDs are also classically associated with Creutzfeldt–Jakob disease (CJD) (Fig. 22.16) and SSPE[121]. Short-interval GPDs, occurring in 0.5- to 4-sec intervals, are classically seen in CJD (most commonly 1/sec), whereas long-interval, high-amplitude GPDs, occurring in 4- to 20-sec intervals and associated with myoclonus, are typically observed in patients with SSPE[121].

GPDs can also be seen in the setting of various drug intoxications. Common examples include lithium, phencyclidine (PCP), and IV cephalosporins. Lithium intoxication is characterized by the presence of short-interval GPDs resembling those seen in CJD[122], whereas long-interval GPDs resembling those seen in SSPE are classically seen in the setting of PCP

intoxication[123]. Finally, GPDs are rarely seen in patients receiving IV cephalosporin therapy, particularly in older patients with renal dysfunction[124,125]. Cefepime seems to carry the highest risk among cephalosporins, where 1.25% of patients receiving it developed GPDs, often associated with severe encephalopathy in one retrospective study[126].

GPDs are associated with a significantly increased risk for acute seizures in critically ill patients. In a retrospective case-control study involving 200 patients with GPDs and 200 matched controls undergoing cEEG, 46% of patients with GPDs had seizures of any kind (clinical or subclinical) compared to 34% of controls ($p = .014$); 27% of patients with GPDs had nonconvulsive seizures compared to 8% of controls ($p < .001$); and 22% had NCSE compared to 7% of controls ($p < .001$)[119]. As with LPDs, there is controversy on whether GPDs themselves represent an ictal pattern. Similar to LPDs, GPDs are often considered to lie along the IIC, and their potentially ictal nature can be investigated in a similar fashion (see above). We showed that GPDs evolve into electrographic seizures[120].

GPDs with triphasic morphology (TWs) (see Fig. 22.14) are one of the longest-recognized yet most bewildering EEG

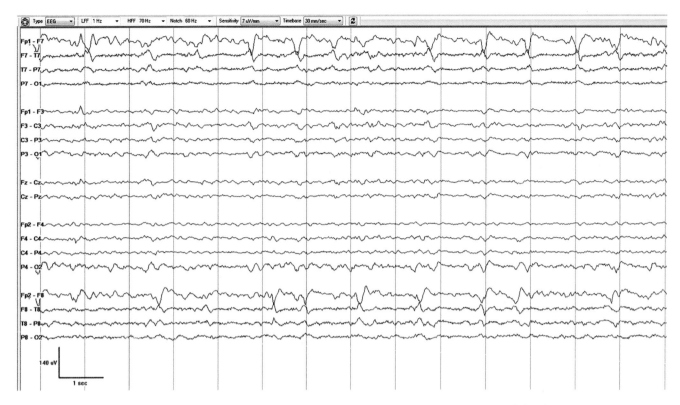

Figure 22.15. BIPDs (independent left and right temporal periodic discharges) in a 64-year-old woman with postanoxic encephalopathy. LFF = 1 Hz, HFF = 70 Hz, Notch on.

patterns in encephalopathy. This pattern was initially termed "blunt spike and wave" by Foley et al. in 1950[127]. Bickford and Butt[128] in 1955 defined the morphological features of this pattern and renamed it TWs. This pattern consists of a surface-positive high-amplitude deflection, preceded and followed by lower-amplitude negative deflections. TWs are typically diffuse with frontal predominance, usually occur at a rate of 1.5 to 2 Hz, and are classically characterized by

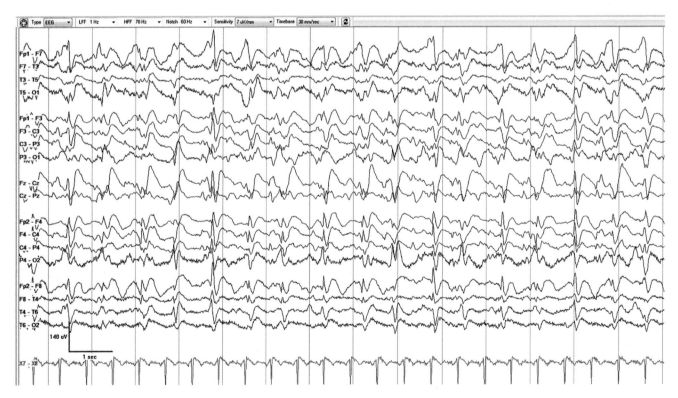

Figure 22.16. 1-Hz GPD+R in a 57-year-old woman with CJD. LFF = 1 Hz, HFF = 70 Hz, Notch on.

frontal-occipital and less frequently occipital-frontal time delay (lag), predominantly involving the positive component of the discharge. This "phase lag" was initially thought to be caused by a traveling wave sweeping the cortex from frontal to occipital regions[128]. However, it is often eliminated on referential montage display, suggesting that it may, at least in part, represent an artifact of phase cancellation in bipolar recordings.

Though initially thought to be a pathognomonic feature of hepatic encephalopathy, it now appears clear that TWs are nonspecific and can be seen in a broad range of structural, metabolic, and epileptic conditions. One recent case-control study evaluated 95 patients with a TW pattern on EEG and matched controls, and found that the following predictors were associated with increased odds for occurrence of TWs: hepatic encephalopathy, alcohol abuse, respiratory failure, and subcortical brain atrophy. Moreover, the odds for occurrence of TWs were tripled if more than one of these predictors was present, underscoring the importance of an interplay of structural and metabolic derangements in the genesis of TWs[129].

The close resemblance of TWs to ictal patterns has been recognized since their first identification by Foley et al. in 1950[127]. One retrospective study found that 40% of EEGs with slow spike-wave complexes also had sporadic TWs[130]. Subsequently, there have been several attempts to identify distinguishing features between TWs and ictal patterns. Proposed distinguishing features include frequency of the discharges, duration of phase 1, amplitude predominance of phase 2, lag of phase 2, effect of stimulation on the discharges, and background frequency[131]. Although it has traditionally been taught that induction by stimulation suggested TWs and metabolic encephalopathy rather than epileptic patterns, it has become apparent that ictal patterns are also commonly induced by stimulation, further complicating the distinction between both patterns[132]. Furthermore, the interrater agreement for identifying TWs was only fair in a recent multicenter study[133], reflecting the difficulty in distinguishing TWs from periodic epileptiform discharges even among ICU EEG experts. That study also found that when EEGs with periodic discharges were read blindly by experts, patients with triphasic morphology were just as likely to have seizures (25%) as those with other periodic discharges (26%), and were no more likely to have metabolic abnormalities (55% vs. 79%, $p < .01$)[133].

There are conflicting data on the effect of AED treatment in encephalopathic patients with TW patterns on EEG. Ten patients receiving a benzodiazepine trial in one study had transient or permanent resolution of TW patterns, yet none of them had noticeable improvement in clinical status[134]. However, a larger, more recent multicenter retrospective study demonstrated positive clinical and EEG response in 10 of 53 (18.9%) patients with TWs receiving a benzodiazepine drug trial and in 19 of 45 (42.3%) patients receiving nonsedating IV AEDs[116], denoting the ictal nature of the TW pattern in these patients. Data derived from multimodality monitoring may provide more insights in the future into the ictal nature of these patterns.

3.14. LRDA

Lateralized rhythmic delta activity (LRDA), a recently described pattern[102], is seen in 4.7% of critically ill patients. As its name implies, it is characterized by rhythmic delta activity predominantly involving one hemisphere (focally, regionally, or diffusely) (Fig. 22.17). One retrospective study found that 63% of critically ill patients with LRDA on EEG had seizures during their acute illness, compared to 57% of patients with LPDs. The co-occurrence of LPDs added substantially to the seizure risk: 84% of patients with both LRDA and LPDs had electrographic seizures on cEEG monitoring. The majority of these seizures were nonconvulsive[102].

3.15. GRDA

Generalized rhythmic delta activity (GRDA) is one of the frequently seen and long-recognized encephalopathic EEG

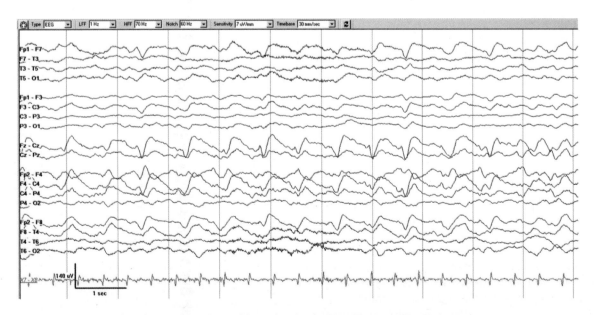

Figure 22.17. *1- to 1.5-Hz static right frontal LRDA+S in a 60-year-old woman with right SDH. LFF = 1 Hz, HFF = 70 Hz, Notch on.*

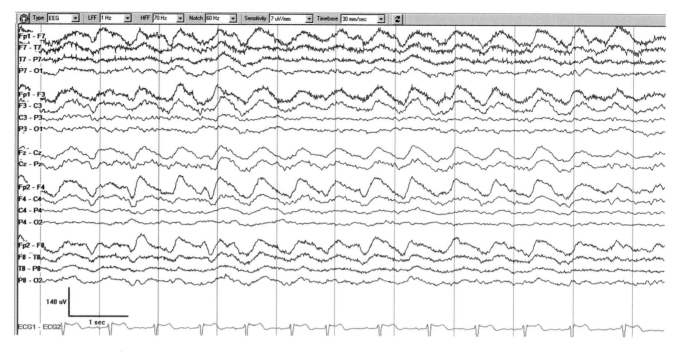

Figure 22.18. *1.5-Hz static frontally predominant GRDA in a 60-year-old man with SAH. LFF = 1 Hz, HFF = 70 Hz, Notch on.*

patterns. It is characterized by the presence of bilateral, symmetric, synchronous rhythmic delta activity (Fig. 22.18). Frontally predominant GRDA (f-GRDA; including the previously termed frontal intermittent rhythmic delta activity [FIRDA]) is the most frequently encountered form. The first recognition of the occurrence of diffuse rhythmic delta activity in encephalopathic patients dates back to 1945, when Cobb et al.[135] reported the occurrence of bilateral 1.5- to 2-Hz rhythmic delta activity in 10 patients with midline tumors and 2 patients with left hemispheric tumors encroaching on midline. Though initially considered a marker of subcortical midline lesions, later studies demonstrated that these lesions represent a small proportion of underlying etiologies, and GRDA is now largely considered a nonspecific marker of encephalopathy[136]. One recent preliminary multicenter retrospective study found that GRDA was not associated with an increased risk for electrographic seizures on cEEG monitoring[137]. Meanwhile, the presence of frontally predominant GRDA was associated with an increased likelihood of favorable outcome in another study[58]. The seizure risk associated with various rhythmic and periodic patterns in illustrated in Figure 22.19.

3.16. SIRPIDs

Stimulus-induced rhythmic, periodic, or ictal discharges (SIRPIDs) (Fig. 22.20), described by Hirsch et al. in 2004, are found in ~22% of critically ill patients undergoing EEG monitoring[132]. SIRPIDs have also been reported in critically ill children[138]. SIRPIDs usually represent purely electrographic phenomena lacking clinical correlate. However, the occasional occurrence of stimulus-induced focal motor seizures in the ICU setting[139] and the reports of improvement of SIRPIDs and neurological functioning following AED administration[140] argue for the ictal nature of these patterns in at least some patients.

On the other hand, there are reports of SPECT-negative SIRPIDs[141,142], possibly indicating the nonictal nature of some of these discharges or at least the lack of usual seizure-associated hyperperfusion. Hence, SIRPIDs are often considered to lie along the IIC and can be further investigated through the aforementioned strategies for evaluating IIC patterns. SIRPIDs are most likely caused by cortical excitability, with arousal causing thalamocortical activation (via normal arousal pathways) that can trigger a seizure or other potentially ictal patterns in the abnormally excitable cortex[132]. One recent multicenter retrospective study demonstrated that SIRPIDs were not independently associated with in-hospital mortality in critically ill

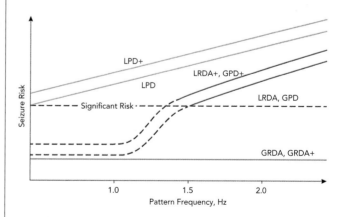

Figure 22.19. *Seizure risk associated with different rhythmic and periodic patterns. Seizure risk is depicted on the y axis and EEG pattern frequency on the x axis. The horizontal dotted line represents the threshold above which seizure risk is significantly increased. GRDA, generalized rhythmic delta activity; LRDA, lateralized rhythmic delta activity; GPD, generalized periodic discharges; LPD, lateralized periodic discharges. Reproduced from Rodriguez A et al. Association of periodic and rhythmic electroencephalographic patterns with seizure in critically ill patients. JAMA Neurol. 2017;74(2):186, with permission from American medical association.*

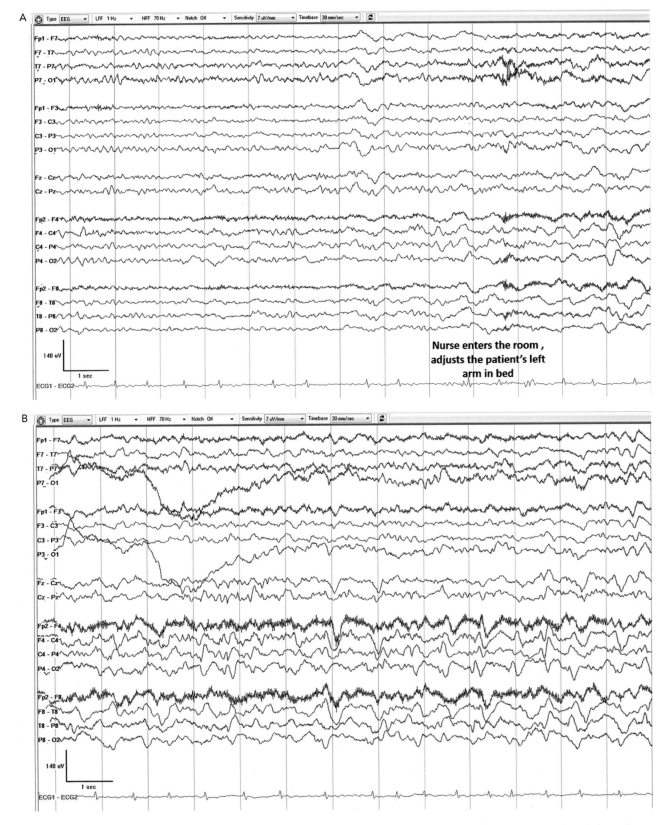

Figure 22.20. SIRPIDs in an 80-year-old woman with left frontoparietal SDH and right thalamic infarction. **A:** Stimulus-induced reactivity in the right hemisphere (nurse entering the room and adjusting patient's left arm in bed). **B:** Contiguous page shows right hemispheric LPDs emerging from reactivity. **C:** 6 minutes later, right hemispheric LPDs continue. They continue for about 25 minutes (much longer than most SIRPIDs), during which time the patient is markedly confused. LFF = 1 Hz, HFF = 70Hz, Notch off.

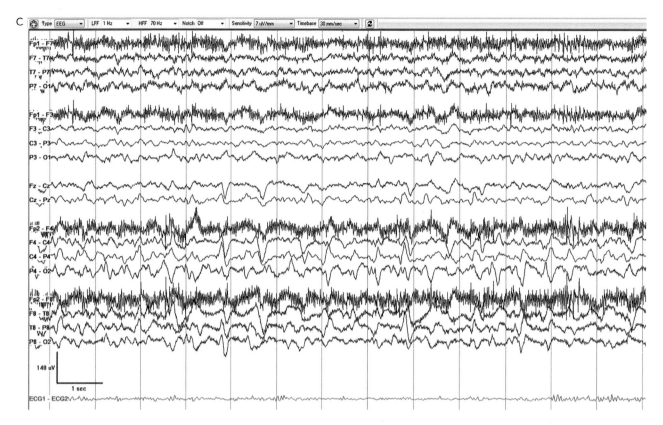

C

Figure 22.20. Continued

patients[143], while another study showed that SIRPIDs were correlated with poor outcome after cardiac arrest[144].

Other than possibly limiting stimulation in these patients, in general we treat stimulus-induced patterns in the same manner as we treat spontaneous patterns as there is no evidence thus far that they are less harmful. In the ACNS nomenclature, any pattern that can be elicited by alerting stimuli (even if it also occurs seemingly spontaneously as well) is considered "stimulus-induced" (SI prefix) and the pattern elicited is stated as SI-GPDs, SI-LRDA, and so forth.

3.17. B(I)RDs

This pattern called "brief potentially ictal rhythmic discharges," previously described in neonates[46], was recently described as a harbinger of seizures in critically ill patients. B(I)RDs consist of rhythmic discharges, whether evolving or not (often too short to tell), occurring at a frequency of >4 Hz and lasting <10 sec (Fig. 22.21). Benign EEG variants and normal rhythms need to be excluded before identifying a pattern as such[145]. The occurrence of B(I)RDs is associated with a substantially increased risk for seizures in critically ill patients: 75% of patients with B(I)RDs had electrographic seizure on EEG monitoring in one recent study[145]. Seizures often arise from the same location and bear similar morphological features. In addition, B(I) RDs often resolve after treatment of seizures, suggesting that B(I) RDs represent truncated seizures. However, their exact prognostic and therapeutic implications remain to be determined. The "(I)" is meant to convey the potentially ictal nature of the pattern, though the parentheses are often omitted.

3.18. Extreme Delta Brush Pattern

Delta brush pattern (also known as "beta-delta complex" or "ripples of prematurity") is one of the hallmark features of EEG background in preterm neonates[146]. It is characterized by the presence of delta-frequency transients with overriding beta-frequency activity. It generally appears at 26 weeks conceptional age and is maximal in the central head region, extending into the temporal and occipital region as the infant matures, and is rarely seen after 48 weeks conceptional age[147]. A similar pattern was recently described in patients with anti-NMDA receptor (NMDAR) encephalitis and was labeled "extreme delta brush" pattern[148] (Fig. 22.22). This pattern is nearly continuous, is usually synchronous and symmetric, and is seen broadly across all head regions, in contrast to the centrally predominant delta brush pattern seen in preterm neonates, predominantly in quiet sleep. Extreme delta brush pattern was found in 30.4% of patients with NMDAR encephalitis in one recent retrospective study and is generally associated with more prolonged hospitalization and a trend toward worse modified Rankin scores[148].

4. ARTIFACTS

The ICU is a relatively hostile environment, with myriad sources of physiological and nonphysiological artifacts hindering adequate EEG interpretation. EEG signals of noncerebral origin are considered artifacts. These artifacts may be confused with cerebral EEG signals and may obscure the underlying

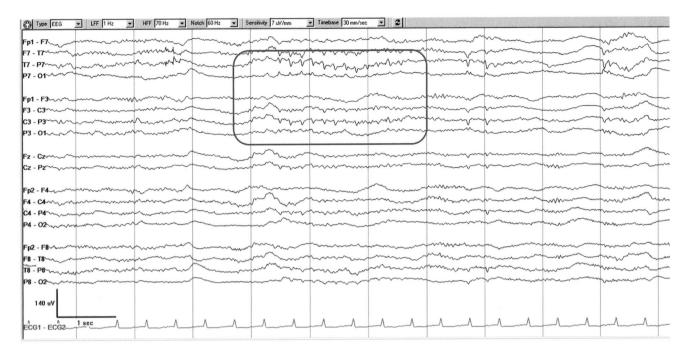

Figure 22.21. *B(I)RD consisting of 4- to 6-Hz sharp rhythmic theta arising from the left posterior quadrant in a 55-year-old woman with epilepsy presenting with sudden unresponsiveness. She later had longer runs of these that evolved and qualified as seizures. LFF = 1 Hz, HFF = 70 Hz, Notch on.*

EEG activity, occasionally to the point of rendering the EEG completely uninterpretable. However, not all artifacts are undesirable; in fact, some artifacts, such as those related to eye movements and muscle activity, may provide useful information about the state of the patient. A summary of common physiological and nonphysiological artifacts in the ICU setting is presented in Table 22.7, and examples of artifacts in the ICU environment are illustrated in Figures 22.23 through 22.33.

Several features may suggest that the questionable EEG activity is an artifact. These include lack of a physiological electrical field, the presence of atypical multiple phase reversals, the solitary involvement of a single electrode, as well as the presence of a highly stereotypic pattern or a periodic pattern with very regular periodicity[149]. However, some of these features may occasionally be observed with cerebral rhythms as well. For example, electrographic seizures in critically ill patients can be confined to a single electrode, particularly in the setting of an overlying skull defect. Simultaneous video recording is often the key in identifying artifacts and distinguishing them from cerebral rhythms. Additional channels monitoring electrocardiographic and respiratory activity as well as eye movements can also provide clues about the noncerebral origin of correlated EEG activity.

When encountering artifacts, many EEG-ers are tempted to use filters to attempt to eliminate them. Examples include using the notch filter to eliminate 60-Hz interference artifact and decreasing the high-frequency filter (HFF) cutoff to 15 Hz to eliminate excessive electromyelographic (EMG) artifact. However, we recommend using these filters judiciously, as the excessive use of the notch filter may mask the presence of inadequately applied electrodes, often leading to false interpretation of electrode artifacts as cerebral rhythms. Meanwhile, decreasing the HFF cutoff alters the shape of EMG

artifact, often leading to their misinterpretation as beta activity or polyspikes. Several artifact-reduction algorithms have been proposed, but most of these algorithms primarily target elimination of physiological artifacts such as those created by blinks, muscle movement, and cardiac activity, with little influence on various nonphysiological artifacts that are particularly common in the ICU[150–153]. Spatial filtering models cerebral activity and artifacts, allowing their separation, followed by artifact elimination with minimal alteration of cerebral rhythms[153]. More research is needed to determine the utility of these filtering models in in the artifact-rich ICU environment.

5. QUANTITATIVE EEG DATA ANALYSIS IN THE ICU

Recent technological advances have led to wide expansion of cEEG monitoring programs over the past two decades. Visual analysis of raw EEG remains the primary method for reviewing EEG in the ICU as in other settings. However, visual analysis is largely subjective time-consuming and requires considerable EEG expertise. Therefore, EEG interpretation in real time 24 hours a day is rarely feasible due to the limited availability of skilled EEG interpreters. In addition, slowly developing background changes are often missed with sole reliance on raw EEG visual analysis. qEEG data analysis tools provide a graphical representation of EEG signals and can be utilized as an EEG screening tool to identify events of interest for further confirmation via raw EEG. In addition, qEEG trends display EEG data in a compressed time scale: 1 to 24 hours of EEG data can be viewed on a single page. This allows a rapid screen of many hours of EEG, facilitates identification of slowly developing background changes, and quantifies events of interest, a

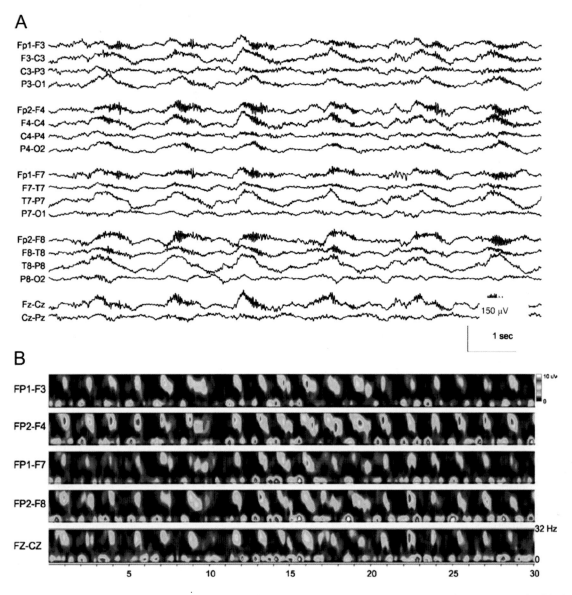

Figure 22.22. Extreme delta brush pattern. EEG in a 23-year-old woman with anti-NMDA receptor encephalitis, seizures, and coma. **A:** Generalized rhythmic or periodic delta waves with superimposed frontally predominant bursts of rhythmic beta-frequency activity. LFF = 0.5 Hz, HFF = 70 Hz, Notch off. **B:** Compressed spectral array over 30 seconds of recording demonstrated increased low-frequency power with rhythmic bursts of 18- to 32-Hz power, which is characteristic of extreme delta brush pattern. Reproduced from Schmitt SE et al. Extreme delta brush: a unique EEG pattern in adults with anti-NMDA receptor encephalitis. Neurology. 2012;79(11):1094–1100, with permission from LWW.

process that may be very tedious when solely relying on raw EEG. qEEG trends can be presented alongside other bedside monitors, and alarms can be set. Alarms (though far from perfect) allow for identification of EEG changes in real time, triggering clinical examination and therapeutic intervention if warranted.

Most quantitative EEG trending tools involve decomposition of the EEG signal into its key components, which are then graphically displayed. There are three main methods of qEEG data analysis: time-domain analysis, frequency-domain analysis, and frequency-time analysis. Time-domain analysis methods depict EEG signal changes over time. The primary example is amplitude integrated EEG (aEEG), largely used in seizure detection and monitoring of encephalopathy in neonates. aEEG involves filtering, rectification, and smoothing of EEG signal, which is then displayed on a semi-logarithmic scale to depict variations in minimum and maximum EEG amplitude[154]. Another time-domain method is envelope trend analysis, which displays the median amplitude of raw EEG signal within a specified frequency range in a chosen time period, thus minimizing the effect of transient changes in EEG signal created by artifacts, which are common in the ICU[155].

Frequency-domain analysis (also known as power spectral analysis), the most widely used qEEG analysis method, involves decomposition of EEG signal into its main frequency components. Most frequency-domain analysis methods employ fast Fourier transform (FFT) algorithms, which calculate the weighted sum of sine waves of different frequencies[154]. Fourier spectrum refers to the plot of frequency versus amplitude. Spectral power can be displayed as the total power of all frequency bands or the relative spectral power of

TABLE 22.7. EEG Artifacts in the ICU

PHYSIOLOGICAL ARTIFACTS	NONPHYSIOLOGICAL ARTIFACTS
Ocular artifacts a. Eye movements (vertical, lateral, and oblique) b. Eye blinks c. Nystagmus d. Ocular flutter e. Electroretinogram (ERG) artifact	Electrical interference (60 Hz in USA, 50 Hz in Europe)
Muscle (EMG) artefact a. Shivering (esp. during hypothermia)	Electrode artifacts
Sweat artefact	Environmental artifacts a. Ventilator artifact b. Bed percussion artifact c. Chest percussion artifact d. Cardiopulmonary resuscitation (CPR) artifacts e. IV drip artifact f. Continuous renal replacement therapy (CRRT) or hemodialysis artifact g. Extracorporeal membrane oxygenation (ECMO) artifact h. Patting artifact (common in neonates)
Cardiovascular artifacts a. EKG artifact b. Pacemaker artifact c. Pulse artifact d. Cardioballistic artifact	Other instrumental artifacts (e.g., capacitive artifacts; electrostatic artifacts)
Movement artifact, such as random body movements and rhythmic movements (e.g., tremors, rigors, posturing, clonus)	

individual frequencies. Power ratios depict the ratio of power in two distinct frequency bands[156]. Alpha-to-delta ratio is often employed for monitoring of ischemia, particularly in the setting of aneurysmal SAH[157] (see later). Spectral edge frequency (SEF) is the frequency under which a certain percentage of the total power of EEG signal resides. SEF95, SEF90, and SEF50 are all reduced with deepening levels of sedation[158] and can be utilized to monitor the depth of sedation during surgical procedures as well as in the ICU.

The main drawback of frequency-domain analysis is that it assumes that EEG signal is stationary and slowly varying, which is obviously an erroneous assumption. One possible solution is dividing EEG signal into short representative epochs where Fourier transform can be computed. However, analyzing short time windows may compromise spectral power resolution. Time-frequency analysis methods such as short-time Fourier transform (STFT) and wavelet transform provide a more efficient alternative and are employed in many qEEG trending tools[159]. Two main types of spectral array displays are available: compressed spectral array (CSA) and density spectral array (DSA). CSA displays power versus frequency versus time data as a pseudo-three-dimensional plot, whereas DSA depicts the same data on either a gray scale or a color-coded scale[159]. The latter display, often called color density spectral array (CDSA), is the most widely used today. CDSA depicts frequencies on the y axis, time scale on the x axis, and power as a color-coded scale on the z axis.

On CDSA, seizures are characterized by an abrupt rise in spectral power followed by a gradual decline, resembling a solid flame (Fig. 22.34)[160]. Seizures need to be differentiated from various artifacts. Muscle artifact is generally seen as descending from the top of the tracing (like stalactites [c for ceiling], rather than seizures, which arise from the bottom like stalagmites [g for ground]) as muscle artifact involves frequencies higher than the displayed frequencies. Rhythmicity spectrogram is a proprietary qEEG tool (Persyst, Inc., Prescott, AZ) that highlights the rhythmic or periodic component of different frequencies. A diagonal pattern is characteristic of seizures as it depicts rapidly evolving rhythmicity across different frequencies, a pattern typically associated with seizures.

qEEG-based tools can also monitor the degree of burst suppression, which can guide the titration of IV anesthetics in patients with RSE as well as other critically ill patients requiring induced coma, such as patients with refractory intracranial

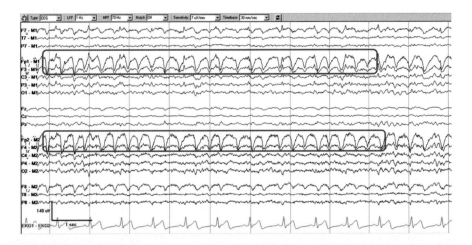

Figure 22.23. Ocular flutter in a 20-year-old woman with history of stroke secondary to Moyamoya disease presenting with new-onset seizures. The frontopolar predominance of these discharges (boxes) with relative sparing of other nearby electrodes points to the ocular origin of these discharges. LFF = 1 Hz, HFF = 70 Hz, Notch off.

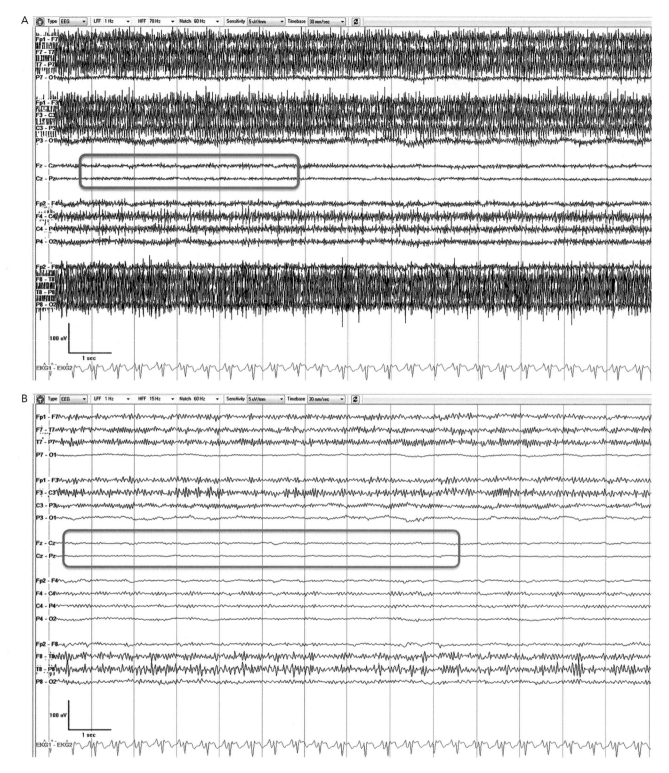

Figure 22.24. A: *Excessive EMG artifact in a 71-year-old man with postanoxic encephalopathy. Note the relative sparing of the midline chains (box). HFF = 70 Hz, LFF = 1 Hz, Notch on.* **B:** *Same epoch with use of 15-Hz HFF shows filtered muscle activity mimicking beta activity. Again note the relative sparing of the midline chains (box). LFF = 1 Hz, HFF = 70 Hz, Notch on.*

hypertension. EEG-based depth of anesthesia monitors such as bispectral index system monitor (BIS monitor™; Medtronic, Inc., Dublin, Ireland), Narcotrend (Narcotrend-gruppe, Inc., Hannover, Germany), and Entropy™ (GE Healthcare, Inc., New York)[161] can be utilized to monitor the depth of sedation during surgical procedures in neurologically normal patients, and less commonly in critically ill patients. High interindividual variability, EMG signal interference, and the paucity of data on the reliability of these monitors for seizure identification limit their utility in those with neurological dysfunction or in critically ill patients[162,163], and confirmation via expert review of raw EEG is always recommended.

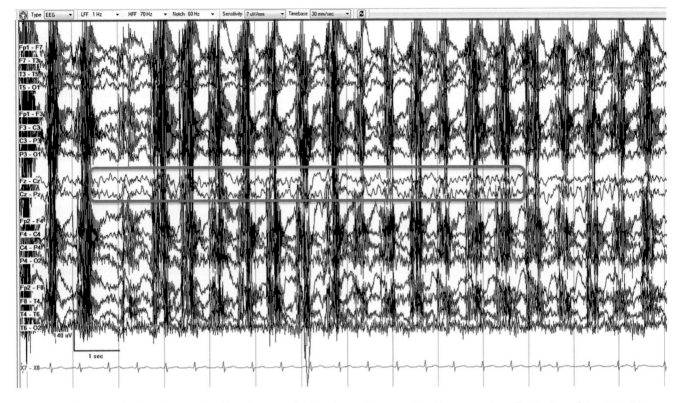

Figure 22.25. Chewing artifact. Repetitive muscle artifact due to chewing in a 58-year-old woman with epilepsy presenting with episodic confusion. LFF = 1 Hz, HFF = 70 Hz, Notch on. Again notice the relative sparing of midline chains (box).

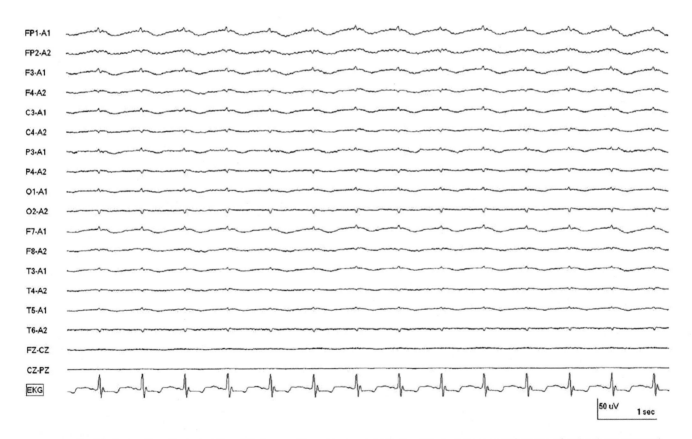

Figure 22.26. Cardioballistic artifact. Rhythmic delta activity is present in a widespread distribution. This represents a cardioballistic artifact (head movement with each pulse) in a 62-year-old man being evaluated for brain death. The slow waves have a fixed relationship to the QRS complex. LFF = 1 Hz, HFF = 70 Hz, Notch off. Reproduced from Hirsch LJ, Brenner RP. Atlas of EEG in Critical Care. Chichester, West Sussex, UK: Wiley-Blackwell: 2010:214[256], with permission from the author.

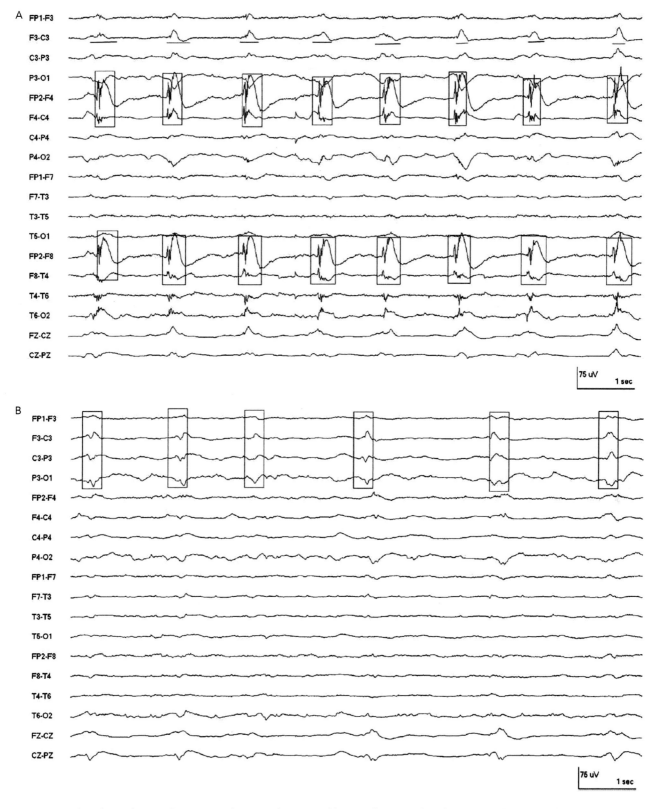

Figure 22.27. Facial twitching atifact mimicking LPDs. **A:** The EEG in this 39-year-old woman shows periodic spike-wave or polyspike-wave-like potentials over the right hemisphere (boxes). Lower-voltage periodic slow waves (blunt LPDs) are present on the left (underlined). LFF = 1 Hz, HFF = 70 Hz, Notch off. **B:** Vecuronium adminstration cleared up the right-sided spikes, leaving the left-sided LPDs (boxes) unchanged, indicating that the left-sided LPDs were genuine whereas the right-sided periodic discharges represented artifacts related to facial twitching. LFF = 1 Hz, HFF = 70 Hz, Notch off. **A** and **B:** Reproduced from Hirsch LJ, Brenner RP. Atlas of EEG in Critical Care. Chichester, West Sussex, UK: Wiley-Blackwell: 2010[256], with permission from the author.

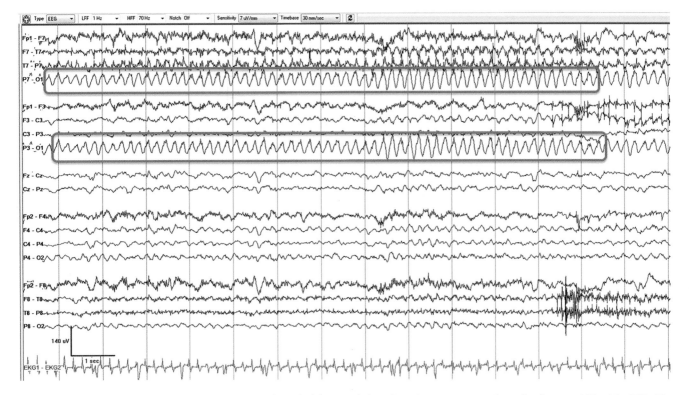

Figure 22.28. Tremor artifact. 4.5-Hz rhythmic theta activity involving the left occipital chains (boxes) is seen corresponding to head tremors. LFF = 1 Hz, HFF = 70 Hz, Notch off.

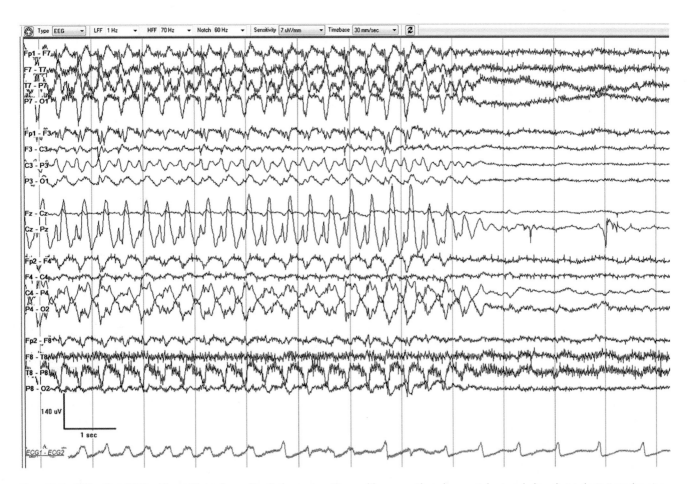

Figure 22.29. CPR artifact. 2.5-Hz diffuse spike-and-wave-like discharges in a 60-year-old woman with cardiac arrest due to pulseless electrical activity undergoing chest compressions. LFF = 1 Hz, HFF = 70 Hz, Notch on.

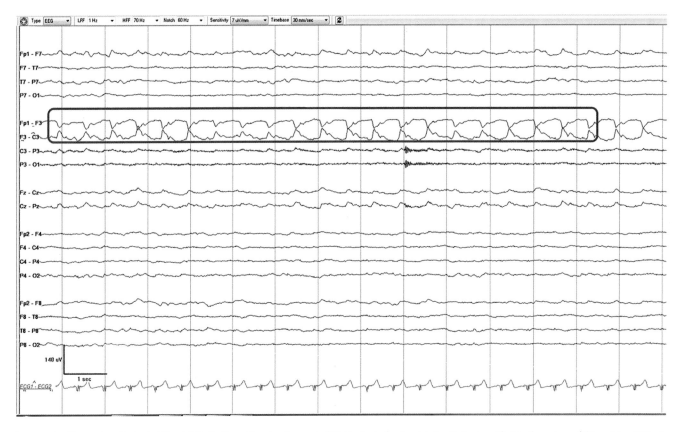

Figure 22.30. *Electrode artifact mimicking LRDA+S. The solitary involvement of F3 electrode (box) points to electrode artifact as the source of this pattern. LFF = 1 Hz, HFF = 70 Hz, Notch on.*

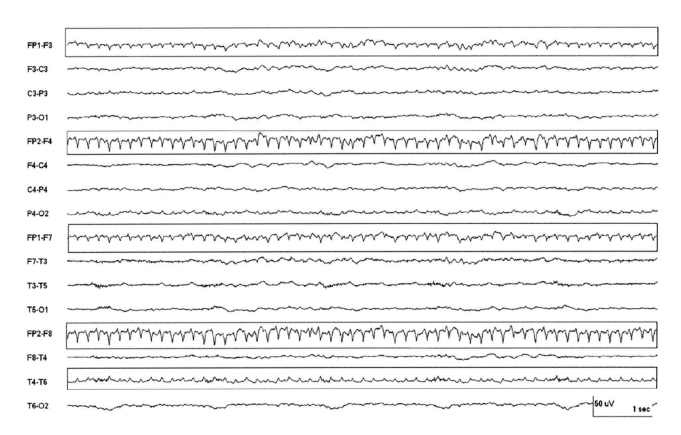

Figure 22.31. *Dialysis artifact. The EEG in this 92-year-old man with mental status changes and renal failure shows rhythmic artifact (boxes), predominantly involving the anterior head regions (electrodes Fp1 and Fp2), more marked on the right. The patient was being dialyzed utilizing slow continuous ultra-filtration, which resulted in this artifact. LFF = 1 Hz, HFF = 70 Hz, Notch off. Reproduced from Hirsch LJ, Brenner RP. Atlas of EEG in Critical Care. Chichester, West Sussex, UK: Wiley-Blackwell: 2010:210[256], with permission from the author.*

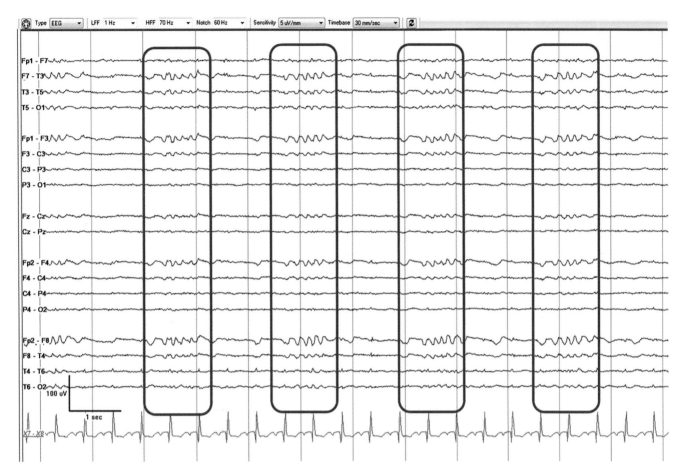

Figure 22.32. *Ventilator artifact. 6- to 7-Hz diffuse rhythmic theta is seen periodically every 2 to 3 seconds (boxes). These discharges were time-locked to the patient's respirations. Ventilator artifact in the setting of a suppressed background can often be confused for a burst-suppression pattern. A distinct faster-frequency artifact can occasionally be seen independent of the patient's respirations due to moving water molecules in the endotracheal tube. Clearance on tube suctioning is the key in identifying this artifact. LFF = 1 Hz, HFF = 70 Hz, Notch on.*

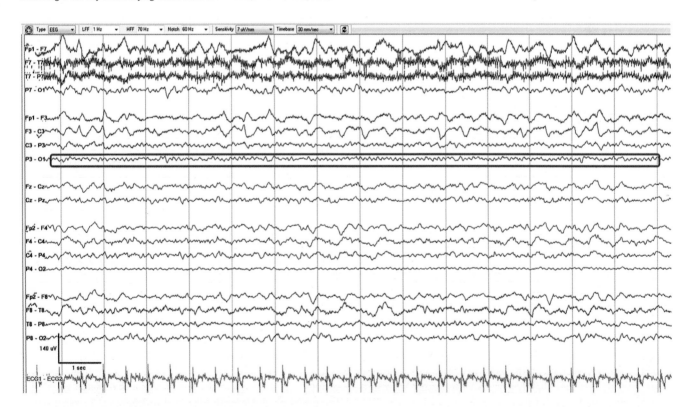

Figure 22.33. *Bed percussion artifact. 9- to 10-Hz "pseudo-alpha" activity is seen predominantly involving the left posterior quadrant channels (box) due to bed percussion. This artifact may be confused for a posterior dominant rhythm. LFF = 1 Hz, HFF = 70 Hz, Notch on.*

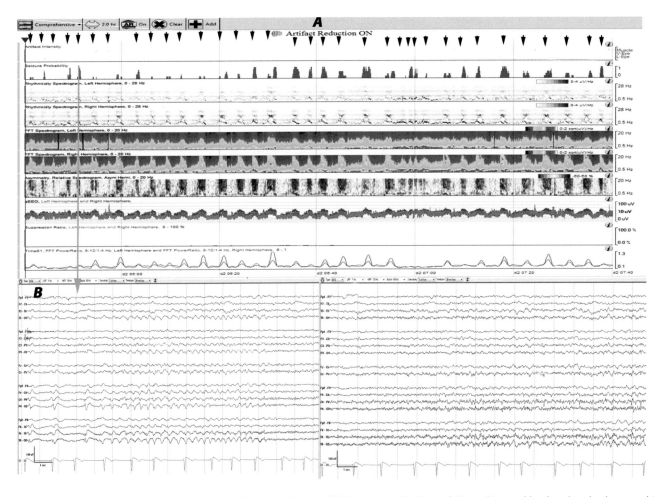

Figure 22.34. Quantitative EEG trends (comprehensive panel view) from Persyst 12™ (Persyst, Inc., San Diego, CA) in an 81-year-old male with cyclic electrographic seizures. The patient was monitored due to prolonged postictal left hemiparesis after an episode of generalized tonic-clonic seizure. **A:** 2-hour qEEG page showing long-term trends. Artifact intensity (first from top): Amount of muscle artifact and vertical and lateral eye movement present (green, blue, and red bands, respectively). The intensity of these artifacts may help determine the state of the patient. Seizure probability (second from top): Red bars display seizure probability on a scale from 0 to 1, as determined by the Persyst seizure detection algorithm. Most seizures in this epoch were detected by the seizure probability algorithm. Rhythmicity spectrogram for left and right hemispheres (third and fourth from top, respectively) illustrates rhythmic components of different frequencies, darker colors being more rhythmic. FFT spectrogram for left and right hemispheres (fifth and sixth from top, respectively) demonstrates power of different frequencies at different time periods. Time is displayed on x axis, frequencies are displayed on y axis, and power of different frequencies is displayed as different colors on z axis (see color scale). Relative asymmetry spectrogram (seventh from top): Comparison of power of different frequencies at homologous electrodes in each hemisphere (blue if higher power on left, red if on right). Suppression ratio (percentage) (eighth from top) displays the percent of the EEG record that is below a determined threshold amplitude (e.g., 10 uV). No EEG suppression is seen in this panel. aEEG (ninth from top; combined left and right hemispheres; left: blue; right: red; overlap: pink): Mean filtered, rectified, and smoothed EEG amplitude (y axis) across time (x axis). FFT power ratio (last from top): alpha/delta ratio across time in both left (blue) and right (red) hemisphere. 35 seizures were detected in this 2-hour page (black arrowheads), evidenced by surges in FFT power and aEEG, as well as evolving rhythmicity on rhythmicity spectral analysis. Most of these seizures were also detected by seizure probability index (red bars on seizure probability index, second panel from top). **B:** Contiguous pages of raw EEG for one of the detected seizures (marked by the gray arrow). Raw EEG shows 2- to 3-z evolving rhythmic delta activity (RDA) in the right posterior quadrant evolving from preexisting LPDs. 9 seconds after seizure onset, RDA evolves into low-voltage fast activity (just prior to the middle of this EEG sample), which eventually slows and increases in amplitude (second half of EEG). This seizure lasted around 1 minute with no clear clinical correlate, as with all the patient's identified seizures. LFF = 1 Hz, HFF = 70 Hz, Notch off.

Several studies investigated the utility of qEEG trend analysis for identifying seizures in the ICU. Stewart et al.[164] evaluated the use of qEEG panels for seizure identification in critically ill children by three qEEG-naïve neurophysiologists after receiving 2 hours of qEEG training and found that the sensitivity of qEEG for seizure identification was 83.3% using CDSA and 81.5% using aEEG. There were some patients in whom all seizures were missed. Strictly focal, low-amplitude, and brief seizures were the most likely to be missed[164]. Another study investigated the reliability of CSA for seizure identification in critically ill adults by qEEG-naïve neurology residents receiving only 2 hours of qEEG training and found that the seizure detection rate was high: 89% of seizures and 100% of periodic discharges were identified. However, there was a high false-positive rate: for every one true seizure identification, 13.8 segments were falsely identified as seizures[165]. A more recent study investigated the use of multiple qEEG panels for seizure identification in critically ill adults by neurophysiologists, ICU nurses, and EEG technologists and found that the overall sensitivity for seizure identification among all reviewer groups was 84% while the specificity was 69%. Interestingly, there was no statistically significant difference in sensitivities between different reviewer groups[166]. These data underscore the reliability of qEEG trend analysis as an initial screening tool to be utilized by both experienced and inexperienced readers, but it is not specific enough to be used without reviewing the underlying EEG to confirm seizures. In one study, qEEG-guided EEG review reduced EEG review time by 78% compared to sole raw EEG review, with minimal loss of sensitivity[167]. Several automated algorithms have been proposed to aid in identifying seizures[168] and rhythmic and periodic patterns[169] in a timely fashion and intervene accordingly.

6. DURATION OF MONITORING

Advances in EEG data acquisition and storage have made it possible to monitor critically ill patients for days or even weeks. cEEG monitoring substantially improves the diagnostic yield of EEG compared to routine EEG recordings. cEEG monitoring detected electrographic seizures in 26% of monitored patients compared to only 11.4% detected by 30-minute routine EEG in one retrospective study involving 105 patients[170]. Another retrospective study including 570 critically ill patients undergoing cEEG monitoring found that 56% of patients with nonconvulsive seizures had their first seizure detected during the first hour of recording, whereas 88% of these patients had their first seizure during the first 24 hours of recording[1]. Similar data were reported in a study of 117 critically ill children: 50% of patients with electrographic seizures had their first seizure detected within the first hour of recording, while 80% occurred during the first 24 hours[171]. ACNS recommends monitoring for at least 24 hours in most clinical settings. Comatose patients, pharmacologically sedated patients, and patients with periodic discharges are more likely to have their first seizure after >24 hours of cEEG; thus, extending the duration of monitoring to 48 hours or more seems rational in these patients before concluding that they are not having nonconvulsive seizures[17]. It has been recently proposed that shorter duration of monitoring may be sufficient in patients with no epileptiform discharges during their initial EEG recording. One recent retrospective study found that the 72-hour likelihood of seizure occurrence declined to <5% in patients with no epileptiform discharges or seizures during the initial 2 hours of monitoring[2]. Further research is need to confirm or refute these conclusions.

7. IMPACT OF ELECTROGRAPHIC SEIZURES AND RHYTHMIC AND PERIODIC DISCHARGES ON OUTCOME

There is considerable evidence derived from both animal and human studies that seizures, including nonconvulsive seizures, can lead to neuronal damage. The seminal study by Meldrum et al.[172] in 1973 demonstrated that bicuculline-induced SE in paralyzed and artificially ventilated baboons was associated with ischemic cell damage involving neocortical, thalamic, and hippocampal neurons[172]. Both convulsive SE and nonconvulsive SE are often associated with increased serum and cerebrospinal levels of NSE—a sensitive but not specific marker of neuronal injury—even in the absence of acute brain insults[173–175]. SE-induced neuronal damage is primarily attributed to a seizure-induced increase in Ca^{++} influx, which in turn activates nitric oxide synthase (NOS) and other proteolytic enzymes, eventually leading to cell death[176]. Even brief seizures cause hippocampal neuronal damage in kindled rats[177], and acute posttraumatic nonconvulsive seizures in humans are associated with an increased risk for long-term hippocampal atrophy[7].

In addition to their intrinsic potential to cause neuronal damage, seizures and periodic and rhythmic discharges in the setting of acute brain injury place an increased metabolic demand on already vulnerable neurons, potentially leading to further worsening of underlying brain injury. Microdialysis studies demonstrated the presence of metabolic crisis—marked by increased lactate/pyruvate ratio and decreased glucose level in brain interstitial fluid as measured by cerebral microdialysis—in association with periodic discharges and nonconvulsive seizures[113]. Increased nonconvulsive seizure burden correlated positively with infarct volume in a focal cerebral ischemia rat model, and successful seizure treatment was associated with reduced infarct volumes and decreased mortality in the same model[178]. In accordance with animal data, the occurrence of electrographic seizures after spontaneous (not traumatic) intracerebral hemorrhage was associated with clinical neurological worsening on the NIH Stroke Scale, increased midline shift, and a trend toward worse short-term outcome in one study of 63 patients[4]. Furthermore, posttraumatic nonconvulsive seizures were associated with episodic and persistent intracranial pressure rise in one study involving 20 patients with moderate to severe TBI[179]. In addition, the occurrence of electrographic seizures and periodic discharges were each independently associated with an increased long-term risk of epilepsy in one recent study[103].

Seizure burden is an important prognostic determinant of electrographic seizures in critically ill patients. Prolonged seizure duration and delay to diagnosis are each associated with increased mortality in NCSE[14]. In addition, increased seizure burden following SAH correlated with poor long-term functional and cognitive outcome in one recent prospective study[15]. Electrographic SE—but not electrographic seizures—was associated with poor short- and long-term functional outcome in critically ill children in two recent prospective studies from a single cohort[180,181], whereas increased seizure burden was independently associated with an increased likelihood of neurological decline in critically ill children[16]. A 20% seizure burden was the threshold above which the probability of neurological decline significantly increased[16].

Though it is quite clear from previous data that seizures are harmful to critically ill patients, it is not yet known whether treatment mitigates seizure-associated harms and how aggressive treatment of NCSE should be. One retrospective study found that 56% of critically ill patients with SE had improvement in level of consciousness following increasing AED therapy[182]. However, three recent studies reported that aggressive treatment of SE was correlated with poor outcome[183–185]. This correlation was more pronounced in patients with complex partial SE in the latter study[185]. However, the retrospective nature of these studies made it nearly impossible—despite considerable effort—to fully account for severity of the underlying illness or refractoriness of SE; thus, it may simply be that SE that is more refractory to treatment is associated with worse outcome. Furthermore, none of these studies evaluated long-term cognitive outcome or the effect of aggressive treatment on long-term risk of epilepsy in survivors. Moreover, these findings were contradicted by another study demonstrating decreased mortality in patients with refractory SE receiving high-dose midazolam infusion compared to patients receiving lower-dose midazolam infusion[186], indicating that aggressive therapy may improve outcome in a significant proportion of patients. Unfortunately, so far there are no published randomized controlled trials investigating the effect of treatment of nonconvulsive seizures in critically ill patients. Most neurologists and intensivists are reluctant to conduct such a trial given the available data on the detrimental effects of seizures; however, randomizing to different levels of aggressiveness may still be feasible. Data from brain multimodality monitoring may in the future help tailor therapy more rationally, based on evidence of ongoing neuronal damage regardless of the specific EEG patterns.

8. SPECIAL CLINICAL APPLICATIONS

8.1. Diagnosis of Brain Death

Historically, death used to be determined solely on the basis of complete cessation of respiration and circulation. However, the introduction of mechanical ventilation and intensive care medicine in the past century made it possible for patients with no real chance of recovery of consciousness to maintain their vital functions for months or even years. Mollaret and Goulon[187] in 1959 coined the term "coma Dépassé" to describe a state of irreversible coma in which spontaneous vegetative functions cannot be maintained and the patient is completely dependent on artificial ventilation for maintenance of breathing[187]. In 1968, an ad hoc committee from Harvard Medical School published a report defining irreversible coma as a new criterion for brain death in comatose patients with no discernible CNS activity[188]. The Unified Determination of Death Act[189], issued by the U.S. President's Commission for Study of Ethical Problems in Medicine, Biomedical and Behavioral Research, defined death as either (1) irreversible cessation of circulatory and respiratory function or (2) irreversible cessation of all functions of the entire brain, including the brainstem. The commission did not discuss the criteria for defining brain death but asserted that "the determination of death must be made in accordance with accepted medical standards"[189]. The AAN published guidelines defining criteria for diagnosing brain death in adults in 1995[190]. The final revision was released in 2010[191]. Prerequisites for considering the diagnosis of brain death include establishing an irreversible and proximate cause of coma while carefully excluding the effect of CNS depressants, the presence of normal or near-normal temperature (>36°C), and a normal systolic blood pressure. The diagnosis is made primarily on the basis of history and clinical examination showing lack of any

BOX 22.3. TECHNICAL REQUIREMENTS FOR USE OF EEG AS AN ANCILLARY TEST FOR DIAGNOSIS OF BRAIN DEATH

- A minimum of 8 scalp electrodes should be used.
- Interelectrode impedance should be between 100 and 10,000 Ω.
- The integrity of the entire recording system should be tested.
- The distance between electrodes should be at least 10 cm.
- The sensitivity should be increased to at least 2 μV for 30 minutes with inclusion of appropriate calibrations.
- The high-frequency filter setting should not be set below 30 Hz, and the low-frequency setting should not be above 1 Hz.
- Electroencephalography should demonstrate a lack of reactivity to intense somatosensory or audiovisual stimuli.

Adapted from Wijdicks EF et al. Evidence-based guidelines update: determining brain death in adults: Report of the Quality standards Subcommittee of the American Academy of Neurology. *Neurology.* 2010;74(23):1911–1918, with permission from LWW.

evidence of responsiveness, absence of brainstem reflexes, and absence of a breathing drive[191].

Ancillary tests can be performed to confirm the diagnosis when the reliability of the clinical examination cannot be ascertained or when apnea testing cannot be performed. These include EEG, cerebral angiography, nuclear scan, transcranial doppler (TCD), computed tomographic angiography, and MRI/magnetic resonance angiography. The technical requirements for the use of EEG for confirming the diagnosis of brain death are listed in Box 22.3.[191] Electrocerebral inactivity, defined as "No EEG activity over 2 μv when recording from scalp electrode pairs 10 cm or more apart with interelectrode impedance under 10,000 ohms but over 100 ohms"[192] marks the diagnosis of brain death. Elimination of EMG artifact via use of neuromuscular blocking agents such as pancuronium bromide or succinyl choline is often needed[192].

Although it was commonly used in the past, we rarely use EEG today for diagnosing brain death. However, EEG may play a critical role in patients lacking an identifiable cause of coma. A normal EEG in these cases may raise the possibility of peripheral causes such as fulminant Guillain–Barré syndrome mimicking brain death[193].

8.2. Role of EEG in Postanoxic Prognostication Strategies

Cardiac arrest causes >424,000 annual deaths in the United States and >300,000 annual deaths in Europe[36]. Withdrawal of life-sustaining therapy is the immediate cause of death in the majority of successfully resuscitated cases[194]. Prognosticating outcome in post–cardiac arrest patients represents one of the most challenging decisions facing clinicians and intensivists worldwide. The introduction of therapeutic hypothermia significantly reduced morbidity and mortality after cardiac arrest[195]. However, delayed recovery is not unusual after hypothermia, complicating prognostication attempts. Most studies examining postanoxic prognostication strategies are subject to the "self-fulfilling prophecy," as treating clinicians are usually unblinded to the results of the tests in question and the decision to withdraw life-sustaining therapy is influenced by the results of these tests, making it impossible to determine whether the patients with deemed poor prognostic indicators could have eventually achieved a good outcome had life-sustaining therapy been extended.

EEG has long played a central role in postanoxic prognostication strategies. EEG signal is primarily generated by graded excitatory and inhibitory postsynaptic potentials of pyramidal neurons[29]. These neurons are sensitive to the effects of hypoxia, making it a relatively reliable tool for assessment of the severity of postanoxic neuronal injury. In addition, EEG signal is minimally altered by the typical levels of mild hypothermia utilized,[196] and cEEG monitoring provides useful information in both hypothermic and normothermic patients. However, the confounding effects of IV sedation should always be considered. In addition, EEG changes often evolve considerably in postanoxic encephalopathy (Fig. 22.35), and the time point at which prognostication based on EEG data should be pursued is not yet established. Nevertheless, EEG still plays a critical role in prognostication strategies in conjunction with clinical history and examination, comorbidities, other electrophysiological modalities such as SSEP, neuroimaging, and serum biomarkers of neuronal injury.

EEG-based prognostic indicators can be categorized into two main categories: background features and epileptiform features, including SE.

8.2.1. BACKGROUND FEATURES AFTER CARDIAC ARREST

Background features are the most important EEG-based prognostic indicators in postanoxic encephalopathy. The first systematized grading of EEG background changes in postanoxic encephalopathy came from Hockaday et al.[38] in 1964, who classified EEG changes in postanoxic encephalopathy in 39 patients into five main grades. All patients with grade I survived while no patients with grade V EEG changes survived. This classification underwent several modifications. Crepeau et al.[12] recently classified EEG abnormalities in postanoxic encephalopathy into three main grades; all 18 patients with grade 3 EEG background on rewarming had poor outcome.

The degree of background continuity, background amplitude, and EEG reactivity represent the most important background features influencing outcome. Malignant background patterns associated with poor outcome include burst suppression at any time during the recording, and an isoelectric or low-voltage background at 24 hours of recording[63]. Burst suppression with identical bursts, defined as "bursts in which the first 500 milliseconds are identical regardless of the amplitude or subsequent duration of the bursts on interburst interval"[197], is a recently described burst-suppression subtype suggested to be more strongly predictive of poor outcome based on a two recent studies from a single cohort[197,198]; this may be because burst suppression with non-identical bursts can be induced by sedating medications, especially barbiturates and propofol, whereas identical bursts seem to occur mainly or only with

severe anoxic injury. Additional studies are needed before this can be relied upon.

Meanwhile, lack of EEG reactivity in normothermic patients was associated with poor outcome in four recent studies[12,63,199,200], whereas the presence of continuous, reactive EEG background is generally associated with good prognosis[12,201]. One study demonstrated that background continuity is negatively correlated with NSE levels. Patients with flat EEG or burst-suppression pattern tended to have the highest NSE levels[202]. In children, a normal EEG or mild background slowing is associated with good outcome, whereas burst-suppression pattern, lack of reactivity, and electrocerebral silence are associated with poor outcome[203]. Absence of reactivity and electrographic seizures are generally associated with a worse EEG background[204].

8.2.2. EPILEPTIFORM FEATURES AND SE

Postanoxic periodic discharges and SE are generally considered poor prognostic indicators. However, recent data indicate that they do not completely preclude good outcome. One recent retrospective study found that 10 of 36 patients with postanoxic periodic discharges survived, though only one of them had good functional outcome and became independent at discharge. Intact EEG reactivity was more common among survivors[205]. A pattern with periodic discharges on a suppressed background in particular is almost invariably associated with poor outcome[64], and SIRPIDs were associated with poor outcome in one recent study[144]. Again, the self-fulfilling prophecy limits the utility of most or all of these studies.

Electrographic seizures are common after cardiac arrest, occurring in 8% to 59% of monitored patients[2,10,11,206]. The majority of these seizures meet criteria for SE. Postanoxic SE (Fig. 22.36) was long considered a marker of invariably dismal outcome, and many clinicians and intensivists are reluctant to treat it aggressively given the perceived futility of treatment. However, there have been multiple recent reports of patients with postanoxic SE, including myoclonic SE, achieving good outcome[207-210]. Seizures tend to occur late in these patients (around 45 hours after cardiac arrest)[208], and evolve from a continuous, reactive background[207-209]. In addition, these patients usually have preserved brain stem reflexes, N20 peaks on SSEPs, and normal or only moderately elevated NSE levels[209], underscoring the importance of integrating clinical examination, neurophysiological investigations, and serum biomarkers and not relying solely on a single tool in prognosticating outcome. There is no clear evidence thus far indicating that treatment of postanoxic SE improves outcome. A multicenter randomized clinical trial is currently under way[211] (NTC02056236, www.telstartrial.nl).

8.3. Role of qEEG in Postanoxic Prognostication

Visual analysis of raw EEG remains the primary method of EEG interpretation in postanoxic encephalopathy as in other clinical settings. However, the lack of objectivity, difficulty in appreciating slowly developing background changes, and the need for considerable EEG expertise are the main drawbacks of sole reliance on visual analysis of raw EEG. Various qEEG methods provide objective measures for dynamic assessment of brain function in postanoxic patients. Several studies investigated the utility of various qEEG parameters in postanoxic prognostication. One study demonstrated that the presence of a continuous aEEG pattern at normothermia strongly predicted recovery of consciousness[212]. Cerebral recovery index (CRI) is a recently introduced qEEG derived index based on a combination of five qEEG features grading EEG patterns in postanoxic encephalopathy. A CRI ≤ 0.29 was always associated with poor outcome, whereas a CRI > 0.69 was associated with good outcome[213].

The AAN published guidelines in 2006 on prognostication after cardiac arrest and concluded that "generalized suppression to ≤ 20 μv, burst suppression pattern with generalized epileptiform activity or generalized periodic complexes on a flat background are strongly but not invariably associated with poor outcome"[39]. However, these guidelines were issued before the widespread implementation of therapeutic hypothermia protocols, bringing into question their validity today. More recently, ESICM and the European Resuscitation Council in 2014 published updated guidelines on prognostication in cardiac arrest comatose survivors and suggested using absence of EEG reactivity and presence of burst-suppression pattern or SE only in combination with each other to predict poor outcome[214].

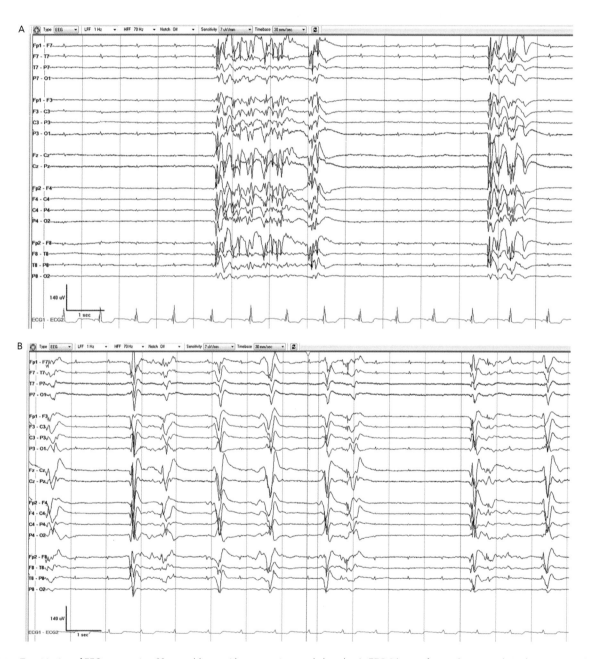

Figure 22.35. *Transitioning of EEG patterns in a 33-year-old man with postanoxic encephalopathy.* **A:** *EEG 9 hours after cardiac arrest shows burst-suppression pattern with highly epileptiform bursts.* **B:** *EEG 24 hours after cardiac arrest shows GPDs on a suppressed background.* **C:** *EEG 48 hours after cardiac arrest shows 1.5-Hz generalized spike-wave discharges.* **D:** *EEG 72 hours after cardiac arrest shows marked decrease in epileptiform discharges coupled with re-emergence of background rhythms.* **E:** *EEG 96 hours after cardiac arrest shows Background suppression. Patient died 12 days later without awakening from coma at any point. LFF = 1 Hz, HFF = 70 Hz, Notch on.*

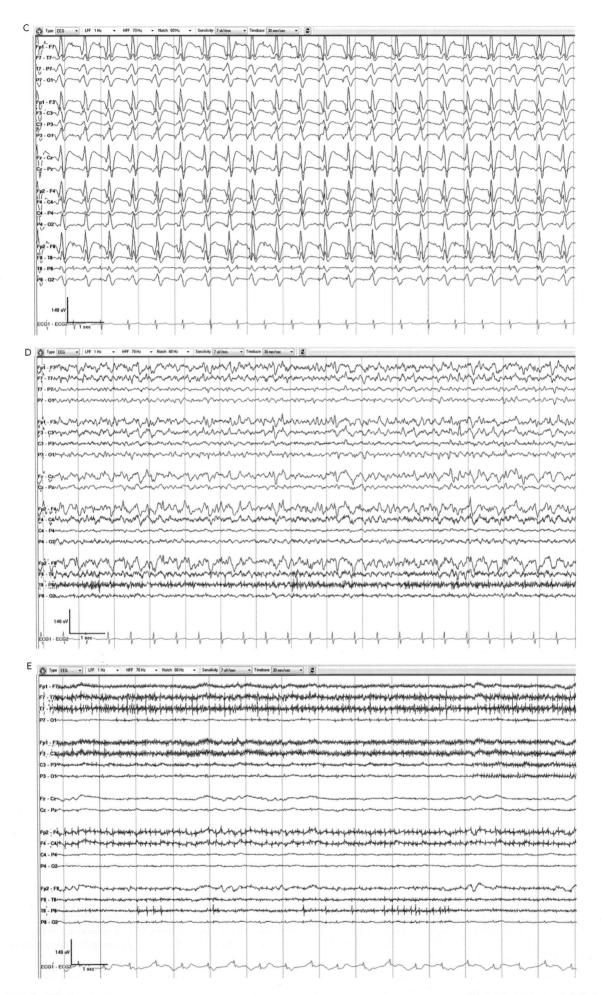

Figure 22.35. Continued

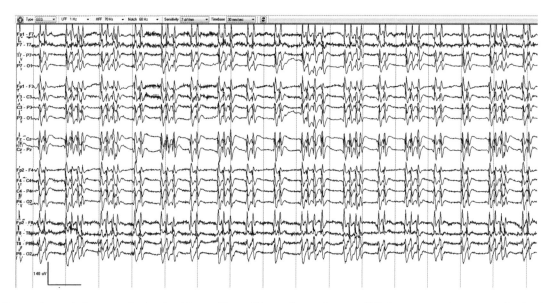

Figure 22.36. Postanoxic myoclonic status epilepticus in a 45-year-old man 48 hours after cardiac arrest. EEG shows near-continuous generalized epileptiform discharges on a suppressed background, occurring at a frequency of up to 5 Hz. These discharges were occasionally associated with whole-body myoclonic jerks. LFF = 1 Hz, HFF =70 Hz, Notch off.

8.4. Role of EEG in Early Detection of Delayed Cerebral Ischemia (DCI) After SAH

EEG's s superior temporal resolution makes it a unique tool for dynamic assessment of brain function. EEG signal is primarily generated by graded excitatory and inhibitory postsynaptic potentials of pyramidal neurons, which are particularly vulnerable to the effects of cerebral ischemia[29]. cEEG monitoring represents a unique, relatively inexpensive, noninvasive tool for ischemia detection, providing a valuable window of opportunity for early therapeutic intervention. One of the most important applications is monitoring DCI in patients with SAH.

DCI is a common complication of SAH, occurring in up to 30% of cases[215]. Several pathophysiological mechanisms are implicated, including microthrombosis, microvascular and macrovascular constriction, inflammation, blood–brain barrier disruption, and cortical spreading depolarization. DCI usually occurs 3 to 14 days after SAH and is a major cause of morbidity and mortality in these patients[216]. DCI is defined as the occurrence of a focal neurological deficit such as hemiparesis, aphasia, or hemianopia, or a 2-point decline of consciousness on the GCS. These changes must not be present at the time of initial presentation and cannot be explained by other causes[217].

Poor clinical status and increased volume of SAH are associated with increased risk for DCI[218]. DCI may be difficult to identify clinically in patients with profound disturbance of consciousness, limiting the reliability of clinical examination. Available methods for detection of DCI include serial TCD scans, CT or MRI scans, angiography, cEEG monitoring, and invasive brain monitoring, including brain tissue oxygenation monitoring ($PbtO_2$) and cerebral microdialysis[215]. TCD ultrasonography is the most widely used imaging modality for monitoring DCI, but its use is limited by its poor sensitivity for detecting ischemia outside the proximal middle cerebral artery territory[219]. The first report of EEG use for this purpose came from Rivierez et al.[220] in 1991, who found that the development of focal or bilateral asymmetric polymorphic delta on day 5 after SAH strongly correlated with the development of angiographic vasospasm. qEEG analysis methods facilitate identification of DCI in a timely manner and may trigger alarms, prompting clinical examination and therapeutic intervention if warranted.

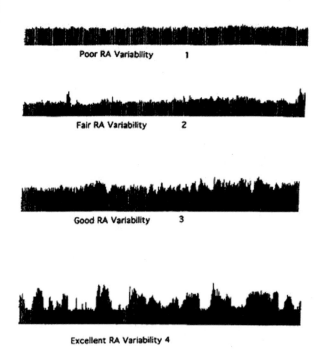

Figure 22.37. Scoring relative alpha variability in four patients with SAH. Relative alpha variability is reflected by the vertical lines, minute by minute in each trend. Each trend here is 8 to 12 hours long[221]. Reproduced from Vespa P et al. Early detection of vasospasm after acute subarachnoid hemorrhage using continuous EEG ICU monitoring. Electroenceph Clin Neurophysiol. 1997;103:607–615, with permission from Elsevier Ltd.

Several qEEG parameters have been utilized, including the following:

1. Relative alpha variability[221] (Fig. 22.37)

2. Alpha-to-delta ratio (ADR)[222,223]

3. Total power[224]

4. Alpha-theta power[225]

5. Composite alpha index: a composite measure of alpha variability and relative alpha power[226]

ADR decline was the strongest predictor of DCI among different qEEG parameters in two prospective studies[222,223]. qEEG clips following stimulation were visually scored in the first study[222]. An ADR decline of >10% from baseline in six consecutive recordings was 100% sensitive and 70% specific for DCI, whereas a decrease of >50% from baseline in any single measurement was 89% sensitive and 84% specific for DCI[222]. An ADR decrease of ≥38% was 100% sensitive and 83.3% specific for DCI in the latter study. qEEG changes preceded clinical and radiological diagnosis of DCI by a median of 7 hours and 44 hours respectively[223].

Rosenthal et al.[227] recently proposed scoring cEEG data for DCI detection based on five main measures (Fig. 22.38):

1. Alpha variability decrease from baseline

2. New ADR decrement or asymmetry

3. New focal slowing

4. New epileptiform discharges

5. New subjective impression of electrographic worsening

Based on these measures, the sensitivity of cEEG for DCI detection was 76% and the positive predictive value was 69%; TCDs had a sensitivity of 48% and a positive predictive value of 38%. EEG changes preceded clinical diagnosis of DCI in 71.4% of patients[227].

These data underscore the utility of EEG as a noninvasive tool for early identification of DCI, potentially providing a window of opportunity for early therapeutic intervention before irreversible injury ensues.

8.5. Use of EEG for Noninvasive Intracranial Pressure Monitoring

Intracranial hypertension is a common, serious complication of a variety of acute neurological and systemic insults. Intracranial hypertension causes neuronal damage via compromising cerebral blood flow or via compression, displacement, and herniation of brain tissue[228]. The Brain Trauma Foundation recommends intracranial pressure (ICP) monitoring in all patients with severe TBI with GCS scores of 3 to 8 and abnormal head CT, or if two or more of the following features were identified: age >40, unilateral or bilateral motor posturing, or systolic blood pressure > 90 mmHg[229]. In addition, ICP monitoring is more often employed today in other clinical settings portending high ICP risk, such as intracerebral hemorrhage, SAH, and

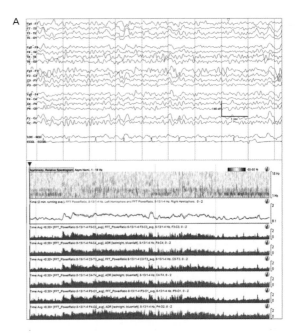

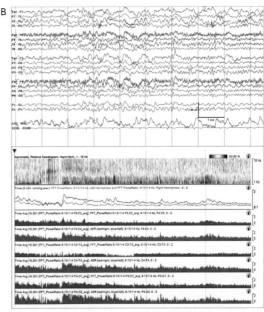

Figure 22.38. Raw EEG and quantitative EEG data from cEEG monitoring in a 61-year-old woman with Hunt & Hess 1, Modified Fisher 3 SAH. **A.** Raw EEG and quantitative trends on day 2 of monitoring. Raw EEG (first panel from top) demonstrates intermittent left hemispheric slowing, which is reflected as light blue shading in the delta frequency band in the relative asymmetry spectrogram (second panel from top). However, ADR trends (third panel from top) are symmetric across both hemispheres, indicated by the superimposition of blue and red lines (which correspond to left and right ADR trends, respectively), and relative alpha variability is scored as 4, "excellent." **B:** Raw EEG and quantitative trends on day 6 of monitoring. Left hemispheric focal slowing is now more prominent on raw EEG tracing, associated with deepening of the blue shading in the relative asymmetry spectrogram, separation of the ADR trends due to decreased left ADR, and decreased relative alpha variability grade from 4, "excellent," to 3, "good." These changes altogether are highly suspicious of ischemia. DCI diagnosis was confirmed on day 7 due to development of new-onset aphasia. Time windows: raw EEG (top panel), 10 seconds; asymmetry spectrogram, ADR, and relative alpha variability panels, 4 hours. Reproduced from Muniz CF et al. Clinical development and implementation of an institutional guideline for prospective EEG monitoring and reporting of delayed cerebral ischemia. In preparation, with kind permission from the authors.

malignant hemispheric infarction. Invasive ICP monitoring via intraventricular catheter or intraparenchymal probes is the primary method used in these settings. Both of these methods carry a significant risk of associated infections (more with the intraventricular catheter use)[230], highlighting the need for reliable noninvasive means for ICP monitoring. Several noninvasive methods have been proposed, including serial CT and MRI, TCD, EEG, and ophthalmological and audiological methods.

Intracranial hypertension compromises cerebral perfusion pressure and CBF, resulting in ischemic injury of brain tissues[228]. Ischemic brain damage causes attenuation of EEG activity[33], which can be reflected as a decrease in spectral power. EEG power spectral analysis may provide indirect reflection of ICP changes. Pressure index, an automatically calculated power spectral analysis derived index, was recently introduced and found to correlate negatively with ICP levels obtained by lumbar puncture in one recent study[231]. Meanwhile, barbiturate coma is often resorted to in patients with refractory intracranial hypertension, and EEG can be used to monitor depth of sedation in these cases. Several qEEG-based depth-of-anesthesia monitors are now available and can be utilized for that purpose (see above), though high interindividual variability and EMG signal interference significantly limit their utility[163].

8.6. Multimodality Brain Monitoring

Scalp EEG is just one of the available tools for monitoring brain function in critically ill patients. Several invasive modalities are now available, including intracranial EEG via intracortical mini-depth electrodes, or subdural strips, ICP monitoring via intraventricular catheters or intraparenchymal probes, brain tissue oxygenation (PbtO$_2$) monitoring via specialized probes, indirect global cerebral oxygenation monitoring via jugular bulb oximetry, continuous CBF monitoring via thermal diffusion probes, and monitoring of brain metabolism via cerebral microdialysis[232–234]. Integration of data from EEG and invasive modalities in conjunction with other noninvasive physiological data provides real-time information that can help identify causes of secondary neuronal injury, including cerebral edema, ischemia, seizures, and systemic insults, allowing for rational, individualized, and timely intervention before the development of irreversible neuronal damage.

Intracortical EEG often identifies electrographic seizures missed by scalp EEG recording. In one study involving 14 patients with acute brain injury undergoing simultaneous scalp and mini-depth EEG recordings, only 2 of 10 patients with electrographic seizures on intracortical EEG had correlated ictal activity on scalp EEG recording (Fig. 22.39)[235]. Another recent study including 48 patients with SAH undergoing invasive multimodality brain monitoring identified intracortical seizures in 38% of monitored patients. Intracortical seizures were associated with increased heart rate, respiratory rate, mean arterial pressure, and minute ventilation. Forty-three percent of intracortical seizures were not detected on scalp EEG, while 19% of seizures were associated with IIC patterns on scalp EEG[236]. The theory is that these comatose patients have multifocal small seizures picked up by intracortical EEG but they are not synchronized sufficiently to create discernible change on scalp EEG; in

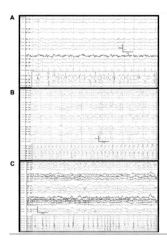

Figure 22.39. Simultaneous scalp and intracortical EEG recording in three patients with SAH demonstrating definite or probable electrographic seizure activity (>2-Hz continuous epileptiform activity with evolution or fluctuation) only demonstrable on intracortical EEG. Filter settings are (A, C) LFF = 1 Hz, HFF = 70 Hz, Notch off and (B) LFF = 1 Hz, HFF off, Notch off[235]. Reproduced from Waziri A et al. Intracortical electroencephalography in acute brain injury. Ann Neurol. 2009;66(3):366–37, with permission from John Wiley and Sons.

order to be seen on scalp, a large area of cortex (~10 cm^2) needs to be firing synchronously, and a very injured brain cannot do this. These multifocal miniseizures may be contributing to the patient's comatose state, and perhaps causing neuronal stress or injury. Simultaneous data from other modalities can help individualize therapy based on the metabolic and hemodynamic effects of these seizures. Seizures and periodic discharges are often, but not always, associated with metabolic crisis, which is characterized by increased cerebral microdialysate lactate/pyruvate ratio and decreased glucose levels, reflecting increased and unmet metabolic demand[237] (Fig. 22.40).

In addition to its crucial role in identifying subclinical seizures, cEEG monitoring in conjunction with intracranial EEG monitoring can identify cortical spreading depolarizations and cortical spreading depression (CSD) in the vicinity of acutely injured brain. Cortical spreading depolarization, described initially by the Brazilian biologist Aristides Leão in 1944[238], is a self-propagating wave of massive neuronal and glial depolarization associated with immense ionic disequilibrium, manifesting as cessation of all spontaneous and induced electrical cortical activity that propagates slowly from the area of onset to surrounding regions at a rate of 3 to 5 mm/minute. This self-propagating cessation of electrical cortical activity is termed CSD[238–240].

Though CSD was long thought to be a relatively benign process primarily associated with migraine[240], there is accumulating evidence from both animal and human studies indicating that it plays a major role in the pathomechanism of secondary neuronal injury after TBI, ischemic and hemorrhagic stroke, and SAH[241–244]. The repolarization process consumes a large amount of cellular energy that cannot always be met in the injured or ischemic brain. An inverse hemodynamic response characterized by spreading oligemia (Fig. 22.41) is often associated with CSD in the vicinity of injured brain tissue, in clear contrast to the spreading hyperemia typically induced by spreading depolarization in healthy brain. Spreading oligemia in the face of an increased metabolic demand in tissue that is already at risk further accentuates

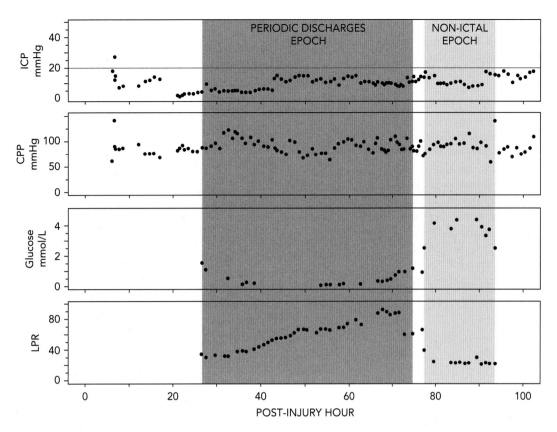

Figure 22.40. Time-aligned graphs of ICP, cerebral perfusion pressure (CPP), cerebral microdialysis glucose (mmol/L), and cerebral microdialysis lactate/pyruvate ratio (LPR) of a patient with severe TBI and periodic discharges on EEG. Cerebral microdialysis increases coupled with decreased cerebral microdialysis glucose during epochs in which periodic discharges were identified (dark gray), followed by decline of LPR and rise of glucose in the postictal phase (light gray).[113] Reproduced from Vespa P et al. Metabolic crisis occurs with seizures and periodic discharges after brain trauma. Ann Neurol. 2016;79(4):570–590, with permission from John Wiley and Sons.

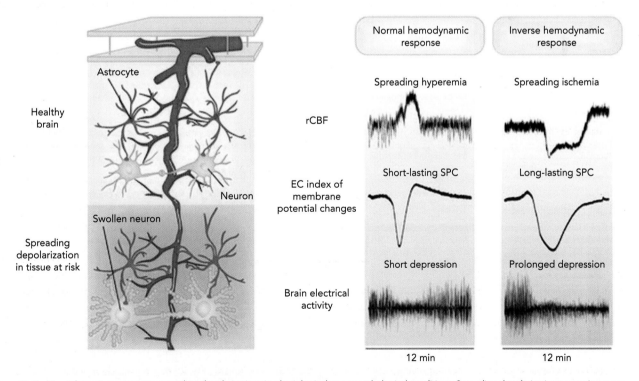

Figure 22.41. Hemodynamic response to spreading depolarizations in physiological versus pathological conditions. Spreading depolarization causes immense ionic disequilibrium and neuronal swelling[257]. Under physiological conditions, this triggers a neurovascular response characterized by vasodilation and increased rCBF leading to a wave of spreading hyperemia, which is best measured by subdural optoelectrodes/laser Doppler flowmetry (right). This process provides adequate perfusion facilitating clearance of excessive metabolites and recovery of energy-dependent membrane pumps, re-establishing ionic homeostasis and leading to short-lasting slow potential changes (SPC) and spreading depression (CSD). In contrast, spreading depolarization under pathological conditions triggers a wave of severe vasoconstriction (spreading oligemia), leading to further prolongation of SPC and spreading depression[258]. Reproduced from Dreier JP. The role of spreading depression, spreading depolarization and spreading ischemia in neurological disease. Nat Med. 2011;17(4):439–447, with permission from Nature Publishing Group.

the supply–demand mismatch, leading to infarct expansion across penumbral tissue[245]. Spreading oligemia associated with CSD may also contribute to the development of DCI after SAH[246]. Simultaneous near-infrared spectroscopy monitoring in one patient with SAH demonstrated increased cerebral blood volume and hyperoxic response associated with CSD events, in contrast to prolonged hypoxic response and decreased cerebral blood volume associated with CSD clusters[247].

In addition, CSD is associated with an MMP9 increase, which in turn leads to alteration of blood–brain barrier permeability, possibly contributing to edema formation in various causes of acute brain injury[248]. Therefore, CSD represents a potential therapeutic target for neuroprotective therapies aiming at preventing secondary neuronal damage after acute brain injury. Seizures often co-occur together with CSD (in a complex bidirectional manner) in patients with acute brain injury[249], and the effect of aggressive seizure management on ameliorating CSD events and subsequent neuronal damage remains to be determined.

SCORE EEG SOFTWARE

Further examples related to the topics addressed in this chapter can be found in the interactive online Niedermeyer Educational Platform. EEG recordings with illustrative examples can be opened and browsed. Features are marked and described using the SCORE EEG software. The users can see the features marked by experts, they can score these features themselves, and then compare them with the scorings of the experts.

The Niedermeyer Educational Platform can be accessed at: www.scoreEEG.com/academy

REFERENCES

1. Claassen J, Mayer SA, Kowalski RG, Emerson RG, Hirsch LJ. Detection of electrographic seizures with continuous EEG monitoring in critically ill patients. *Neurology*. 2004;62(10):1743–1748.
2. Westover MB, Shafi MM, Bianchi MT, et al. The probability of seizures during EEG monitoring in critically ill adults. *Clin Neurophysiol*. 2015;126(3):463–471.
3. Swisher CB, Shah D, Sinha SR, Husain AM. Baseline EEG pattern on continuous ICU EEG monitoring and incidence of seizures. *J Clin Neurophysiol*. 2015;32(2):147–151.
4. Vespa PM, O'Phelan K, Shah M, et al. Acute seizures after intracerebral hemorrhage: a factor in progressive midline shift and outcome. *Neurology*. 2003;60(9):1441–1446.
5. Claassen J, Jette N, Chum F, et al. Electrographic seizures and periodic discharges after intracerebral hemorrhage. *Neurology*. 2007;69(13):1356–1365.
6. O'Connor KL, Westover MB, Phillips MT, et al. High risk for seizures following subarachnoid hemorrhage regardless of referral bias. *Neurocrit Care*. 2014;21(3):476–482.
7. Vespa PM, McArthur DL, Xu Y, et al. Nonconvulsive seizures after traumatic brain injury are associated with hippocampal atrophy. *Neurology*. 2010;75(9):792–798.
8. Oddo M, Carrera E, Claassen J, Mayer SA, Hirsch LJ. Continuous electroencephalography in the medical intensive care unit. *Crit Care Med*. 2009;37(6):2051–2056.
9. Carrera E, Claassen J, Oddo M, Emerson RG, Mayer SA, Hirsch LJ. Continuous electroencephalographic monitoring in critically ill patients with central nervous system infections. *Arch Neurol*. 2008;65(12):1612–1618.
10. Knight WA, Hart KW, Adeoye OM, et al. The incidence of seizures in patients undergoing therapeutic hypothermia after resuscitation from cardiac arrest. *Epilepsy Res*. 2013;106(3):396–402.
11. Mani R, Schmitt SE, Mazer M, Putt ME, Gaieski DF. The frequency and timing of epileptiform activity on continuous electroencephalogram in comatose post-cardiac arrest syndrome patients treated with therapeutic hypothermia. *Resuscitation*. 2012;83(7):840–847.
12. Crepeau AZ, Rabinstein AA, Fugate JE, et al. Continuous EEG in therapeutic hypothermia after cardiac arrest: prognostic and clinical value. *Neurology*. 2013;80.
13. DeLorenzo RJ, Waterhouse EJ, Towne AR, et al. Persistent nonconvulsive status epilepticus after the control of convulsive status epilepticus. *Epilepsia*. 1998;39(8):833–840.
14. Young BG, Jordan KG, Doig GS. An assessment of nonconvulsive seizures in the intensive care unit using continuous EEG monitoring: an investigation of variables associated with mortality. *Neurology*. 1996;47(1):83–89.
15. De Marchis GM, Pugin D, Meyers E, et al. Seizure burden in subarachnoid hemorrhage associated with functional and cognitive outcome. *Neurology*. 2016;86(3):253–260.
16. Payne ET, Zhao XY, Frndova H, et al. Seizure burden is independently associated with short term outcome in critically ill children. *Brain*. 2014;137(Pt 5):1429–1438.
17. Herman ST, Abend NS, Bleck TP, et al. Consensus statement on continuous EEG in critically ill adults and children, part I: indications. *J Clin Neurophysiol*. 2015;32(2):87–95.
18. Le Roux P, Menon DK, Citerio G, et al. Consensus summary statement of the International Multidisciplinary Consensus Conference on Multimodality Monitoring in Neurocritical Care: a statement for healthcare professionals from the Neurocritical Care Society and the European Society of Intensive Care Medicine. *Intensive Care Med*. 2014;40(9):1189–1209.
19. Shellhaas RA, Chang T, Tsuchida T, et al. The American Clinical Neurophysiology Society's guideline on continuous electroencephalography monitoring in neonates. *J Clin Neurophysiol*. 2011;28(6):611–617.
20. Gilmore EJ, Gaspard N, Choi HA, et al. Acute brain failure in severe sepsis: a prospective study in the medical intensive care unit utilizing continuous EEG monitoring. *Intensive Care Med*. 2015;41(4):686–694.
21. Husain AM, Horn GJ, Jacobson MP. Non-convulsive status epilepticus: usefulness of clinical features in selecting patients for urgent EEG. *J Neurol Neurosurg Psychiatry*. 2003;74(2):189–191.
22. Benbadis SR, Chen S, Melo M. What's shaking in the ICU? The differential diagnosis of seizures in the intensive care setting. *Epilepsia*. 2010;51(11):2338–2340.
23. Abend NS, Arndt DH, Carpenter JL, et al. Electrographic seizures in pediatric ICU patients: cohort study of risk factors and mortality. *Neurology*. 2013;81(4):383–391.
24. O'Neill BR, Handler MH, Tong S, Chapman KE. Incidence of seizures on continuous EEG monitoring following traumatic brain injury in children. *J Neurosurg Pediatr*. 2015;16(2):167–176.
25. Yang A, Arndt DH, Berg RA, et al. Development and validation of a seizure prediction model in critically ill children. *Seizure*. 2015;25:104–111.
26. Sanchez Fernandez I, Abend NS, Arndt DH, et al. Electrographic seizures after convulsive status epilepticus in children and young adults: a retrospective multicenter study. *J Pediatr*. 2014;164(2):339–346.e331–332.
27. Brophy G, Bell R, Claassen J, et al. Guidelines for the evaluation and management of status epilepticus. *Neurocrit Care*. 2012;17(1):3–23.
28. Whittemore AD, Kauffman JL, Kohler TR, Mannick JA. Routine electroencephalographic (EEG) monitoring during carotid endarterectomy. *Ann Surg*. 1983;197(6):707–713.
29. Ebersole J. Cortical generators and EEG voltage fields. In: Ebersole J, Husain AM, Nordli DR, eds. *Current practice of clinical electroencephalography*. Philadelphia: Lippincott Williams & Wilkins, 2014:29–44.
30. Deimer NH, Valente E, Bruhn T, Berg M, Jørgensen MB, Johansen FF. Glutamate receptor transmission and ischemic nerve cell damage: evidence for involvement of excitotoxic mechanisms. In: Kogure k, Hossmann KA, Siesjö B, eds. *Neurobiology of ischemic brain damge*. Philadelphia: Elsevier Science Publishers, 1993:105.
31. Sharbrough FW, Messick JM, Jr., Sundt TM, Jr. Correlation of continuous electroencephalograms with cerebral blood flow measurements during carotid endarterectomy. *Stroke*. 1973;4(4):674–683.
32. Moseley ME, Cohen Y, Mintorovitch J, et al. Early detection of regional cerebral ischemia in cats: comparison of diffusion- and T2-weighted MRI and spectroscopy. *Magn Reson Med*. 1990;14(2):330–346.
33. Jordan KG. Emergency EEG and continuous EEG monitoring in acute ischemic stroke. *J Clin Neurophysiol*. 2004;21(5):341–352.
34. Copen WA, Schaefer PW, Wu O. MR perfusion imaging in acute ischemic stroke. *Neuroimag Clin North Am*. 2011;21(2):259–283.
35. Schneider AL, Jordan KG. Regional attenuation without delta (RAWOD): a distinctive EEG pattern that can aid in the diagnosis and management of severe acute ischemic stroke. *Am J Electroneurodiagnostic Technol*. 2005;45(2):102–117.

36. Kudenchuk PJ, Sandroni C, Drinhaus HR, et al. Breakthrough in cardiac arrest: reports from the 4th Paris International Conference. *Ann Intensive Care.* 2015;5:22.

37. Soleimanpour H, Rahmani F, Safari S, Ej Golzari S. Hypothermia after cardiac arrest as a novel approach to increase survival in cardiopulmonary cerebral resuscitation: a review. *Iranian Red Crescent Med J.* 2014;16(7):e17497.

38. Hockaday JM, Potts F, Epstein E, Bonazzi A, Schwab RS. Electroencephalographic changes in acute cerebral anoxia from cardiac or respiratory arrest. *Electroenceph Clin Neurophysiol.* 1965;18(6):575–586.

39. Wijdicks EFM, Hijdra A, Young GB, Bassetti CL, Wiebe S. Practice parameter: prediction of outcome in comatose survivors after cardiopulmonary resuscitation (an evidence-based review): report of the Quality Standards Subcommittee of the American Academy of Neurology. *Neurology.* 2006;67(2):203–210.

40. Gütling E, Gonser A, Imhof H-G, Landis T. EEG reactivity in the prognosis of severe head injury. *Neurology.* 1995;45(5):915–918.

41. Kang X-g, Yang F, Li W, Ma C, Li L, Jiang W. Predictive value of EEG-awakening for behavioral awakening from coma. *Ann Intensive Care.* 2015;5(1):1–8.

42. Nasraway SS, Jr., Wu EC, Kelleher RM, Yasuda CM, Donnelly AM. How reliable is the bispectral index in critically ill patients? A prospective, comparative, single-blinded observer study. *Crit Care Med.* 2002;30(7):1483–1487.

43. Deogaonkar A, Gupta R, DeGeorgia M, et al. Bispectral index monitoring correlates with sedation scales in brain-injured patients. *Crit Care Med.* 2004;32(12):2403–2406.

44. Berger H. Über das Elektrenkephalogramm des Menschen. *Archiv für Psychiatrie und Nervenkrankheiten.* 1929;87(1):527–570.

45. Hirsch LJ, LaRoche SM, Gaspard N, et al. American Clinical Neurophysiology Society's standardized critical care EEG terminology: 2012 version. *J Clin Neurophysiol.* 2013;30(1):1–27.

46. Tsuchida TN, Wusthoff CJ, Shellhaas RA, et al. American Clinical Neurophysiology Society standardized EEG terminology and categorization for the description of continuous EEG monitoring in neonates: report of the American Clinical Neurophysiology Society critical care monitoring committee. *J Clin Neurophysiol.* 2013;30(2):161–173.

47. Westhall E, Rosén I, Rossetti AO, et al. Interrater variability of EEG interpretation in comatose cardiac arrest patients. *Clin Neurophysiol.* 2015;126(12):2397–2404.

48. Parsons-Smith BG, Summerskill WH, Dawson AM, Sherlock S. The electroencephalograph in liver disease. *Lancet.* 1957;273(7001):867–871.

49. Amodio P, Marchetti P, Del Piccolo F, et al. Spectral versus visual EEG analysis in mild hepatic encephalopathy. *Clin Neurophysiol.* 1999;110(8):1334–1344.

50. Stockard J, Bickford R. The neurophysiology of anesthesia. In: Gordon E, ed. *A basis and practice of neuroanesthesia.* Amsterdam, Netherlands: Excerpta Medica, 1973:3–42.

51. Young GB. The EEG in coma. *J Clin Neurophysiol.* 2000;17(5):473.

52. So NK, Blume WT. The postictal EEG. *Epilepsy Behav.* 2010;19(2):121–126.

53. Smith SJM. EEG in neurological conditions other than epilepsy: when does it help, what does it add? *J Neurol Neurosurg Psychiatry.* 2005;76(suppl 2):ii8–ii12.

54. Sand T. EEG in migraine: a review of the literature. *Functional Neurol.* 1991;6(1):7–22.

55. Gloor P, Ball G, Schaul N. Brain lesions that produce delta waves in the EEG. *Neurology.* 1977;27(4):326–333.

56. Gloor P, Kalabay O, Giard N. The electroencephalogram in diffuse encephalopathies: electroencephalographic correlates of grey and white matter lesions. *Brain.* 1968;91(4):779–802.

57. Schaul N, Green L, Peyster R, Gotman J. Structural determinants of electroencephalographic findings in acute hemispheric lesions. *Ann Neurol.* 1986;20(6):703–711.

58. Sutter R, Stevens RD, Kaplan PW. Clinical and imaging correlates of EEG patterns in hospitalized patients with encephalopathy. *J Neurol.* 2013;260(4):1087–1098.

59. Schaul N, Gloor P, Gotman J. The EEG in deep midline lesions. *Neurology.* 1981;31(2):157.

60. Hawkes CH, Bryan-Smyth L. The electroencephalogram in the "locked-in" syndrome. *Neurology.* 1974;24(11):1015.

61. Kaplan PW, Genoud D, Ho TW, Jallon P. Etiology, neurologic correlations, and prognosis in alpha coma. *Clin Neurophysiol.* 1999;110(2):205–213.

62. Rossetti AO, Urbano LA, Delodder F, Kaplan PW, Oddo M. Prognostic value of continuous EEG monitoring during therapeutic hypothermia after cardiac arrest. *Crit Care.* 2010;14(5):R173.

63. Sivaraju A, Gilmore EJ, Wira CR, et al. Prognostication of post-cardiac arrest coma: early clinical and electroencephalographic predictors of outcome. *Intensive Care Med.* 2015;41(7):1264–1272.

64. Westhall E, Rossetti AO, van Rootselaar AF, et al. Standardized EEG interpretation accurately predicts prognosis after cardiac arrest. *Neurology.* 2016;86(16):1482–1490.

65. Thompson SA, Hantus S. Highly epileptiform bursts are associated with seizure recurrence. *J Clin Neurophysiol.* 2016;33(1):66–71.

66. Johnson E, Ritzl EK. EEG characteristics of successful burst suppression for status epilepticus. Poster session presented at 69th annual meeting of the American Epilepsy Society, December 4–8, 2015, Philadelphia, PA.

67. Rossetti AO, Oddo M, Logroscino G, Kaplan PW. Prognostication after cardiac arrest and hypothermia: a prospective study. *Ann Neurol.* 2010;67(3):301–307.

68. RamachandranNair R, Sharma R, Weiss SK, Cortez MA. Reactive EEG patterns in pediatric coma. *Pediatr Neurol.* 2005;33(5):345–349.

69. Tsetsou S, Novy J, Oddo M, Rossetti AO. EEG reactivity to pain in comatose patients: importance of the stimulus type. *Resuscitation.* 2015;97:34–37.

70. Hermans MC, Westover MB, van Putten MJ, Hirsch LJ, Gaspard N. Quantification of EEG reactivity in comatose patients. *Clin Neurophysiol.* 2016;127(1):571–580.

71. Sutter R, Barnes B, Leyva A, Kaplan PW, Geocadin RG. Electroencephalographic sleep elements and outcome in acute encephalopathic patients: a 4-year cohort study. *Eur J Neurol.* 2014;21(10):1268–1275.

72. Rossetti AO, Maeder-Ingvar M, Reichhart MD, Despland PA, Bogousslavsky J. Transitory sleep spindles impairment in deep cerebral venous thrombosis. *Clin Neurophysiol.* 2005;35(1):19–23.

73. Urakami Y. Relationship between, sleep spindles and clinical recovery in patients with traumatic brain injury: a simultaneous EEG and MEG study. *Clin EEG Neurosci.* 2012;43(1):39–47.

74. Bergamasco B, Bergamini L, Doriguzzi T, Fabiani D. EEG sleep patterns as a prognostic criterion in post-traumatic coma. *Electroenceph Clin Neurophysiol.* 1968;24(4):374–377.

75. Terzano MG, Parrino L. The cyclic alternating pattern in human sleep. In: Guilleminault C, ed. *Clinical neurophysiology of sleep disorders.* Amsterdam, Netherlands: Elsevier, 2005:79–90.

76. Kassab MY, Farooq MU, Diaz-Arrastia R, Van Ness PC. The clinical significance of EEG cyclic alternating pattern during coma. *J Clin Neurophysiol.* 2007;24(6):425–428.

77. Parrino L, Ferri R, Bruni O, Terzano MG. Cyclic alternating pattern (CAP): the marker of sleep instability. *Sleep Med Rev.* 2012;16(1):27–45.

78. Loeb C, Poggio G. Electroencephalograms in a case with ponto-mesencephalic haemorrhage. *Electroenceph Clin Neurophysiol.* 1953;5(2):295–296.

79. Westmoreland BF, Klass DW, Sharbrough FW, Reagan TJ. Alpha-coma: electroencephalographic, clinical, pathologic, and etiologic correlations. *Arch Neurol.* 1975;32(11):713–718.

80. Kaplan PW, Genoud D, Ho TW, Jallon P. Etiology, neurologic correlations, and prognosis in alpha coma. *Clin Neurophysiol.* 1999;110(2):205–213.

81. Young GB, Blume WT, Campbell VM, et al. Alpha, theta and alpha-theta coma: a clinical outcome study utilizing serial recordings. *Electroenceph Clin Neurophysiol.* 1994;91(2):93–99.

82. Chatrian GE, White Jr LE, Daly D. Electroencephalographic patterns resembling those of sleep in certain comatose states after injuries to the head. *Electroenceph Clin Neurophysiol.* 1963;15(2):272–280.

83. Britt CW, Jr. Nontraumatic "spindle coma": clinical, EEG, and prognostic features. *Neurology.* 1981;31(4):393–397.

84. Kaplan PW, Genoud D, Ho TW, Jallon P. Clinical correlates and prognosis in early spindle coma. *Clin Neurophysiol.* 2000;111(4):584–590.

85. Otomo E. Beta wave activity in the electroencephalogram in cases of coma due to acute brain-stem lesions. *J Neurol Neurosurg Psychiatry.* 1966;29(5):383–390.

86. Synek VM. Value of a revised EEG coma scale for prognosis after cerebral anoxia and diffuse head injury. *Clin Electroencephalogr.* 1990;21(1):25–30.

87. Young GB, McLachlan RS, Kreeft JH, Demelo JD. An electroencephalographic classification for coma. *Can J Neurol Sci.* 1997;24(4):320–325.

88. Young GB, Jordan KG, Doig GS. An assessment of nonconvulsive seizures in the intensive care unit using continuous EEG monitoring: an investigation of variables associated with mortality. *Neurology.* 1996;47(1):83–89.

89. Leitinger M, Beniczky S, Rohracher A, et al. Salzburg Consensus Criteria for Non-Convulsive Status Epilepticus—approach to clinical application. *Epilepsy Behav.* 2015;49:158–163.

90. Halford JJ, Shiau D, Desrochers JA, et al. Inter-rater agreement on identification of electrographic seizures and periodic discharges in ICU EEG recordings. *Clin Neurophysiol.* 2015;126(9):1661–1669.

91. Ronner HE, Ponten SC, Stam CJ, Uitdehaag BMJ. Inter-observer variability of the EEG diagnosis of seizures in comatose patients. *Seizure.* 2009;18(4):257–263.

92. Abend NS, Gutierrez-Colina A, Zhao H, et al. Interobserver reproducibility of electroencephalogram interpretation in critically ill children. *J Clin Neurophysiol.* 2011;28(1):15–19.

93. Hirsch LJ, Brenner RP, Drislane FW, et al. The ACNS Subcommittee on Research Terminology for Continuous EEG Monitoring: proposed standardized terminology for rhythmic and periodic EEG patterns encountered in critically ill patients. *J Clin Neurophysiol.* 2005;22(2):128–135.

94. Gaspard N, Hirsch LJ, LaRoche SM, Hahn CD, Westover MB, the Critical Care EEGMRC. Interrater agreement for critical care EEG terminology. *Epilepsia.* 2014;55(9):1366–1373.

95. Cobb W, Hill D. Electroencephalogram in subacute progressive encephalitis. *Brain.* 1950;73(3):392–404.

96. Chatrian GE, Shaw CM, Leffman H. The significance of periodic lateralized epileptiform discharges in EEG: an electrographic, clinical and pathological study. *Electroenceph Clin Neurophysiol.* 1964;17:177–193.

97. Reiher J, Rivest J, Grand'Maison F, Leduc CP. Periodic lateralized epileptiform discharges with transitional rhythmic discharges: association with seizures. *Electroenceph Clin Neurophysiol.* 1991;78(1):12–17.

98. Garcia-Morales I, Garcia MT, Galan-Davila L, et al. Periodic lateralized epileptiform discharges: etiology, clinical aspects, seizures, and evolution in 130 patients. *J Clin Neurophysiol.* 2002;19(2):172–177.

99. Westmoreland BF, Klass DW, Sharbrough FW. Chronic periodic lateralized epileptiform discharges. *Arch Neurol.* 1986;43(5):494–496.

100. Orta DS, Chiappa KH, Quiroz AZ, Costello DJ, Cole AJ. Prognostic implications of periodic epileptiform discharges. *Arch Neurol.* 2009;66(8):985–991.

101. Kalamangalam GP, Diehl B, Burgess RC. Neuroimaging and neurophysiology of periodic lateralized epileptiform discharges: observations and hypotheses. *Epilepsia.* 2007;48(7):1396–1405.

102. Gaspard N, Manganas L, Rampal N, Petroff OA, Hirsch LJ. Similarity of lateralized rhythmic delta activity to periodic lateralized epileptiform discharges in critically ill patients. *JAMA Neurology.* 2013;70(10):1288–1295.

103. Punia V, Garcia CG, Hantus S. Incidence of recurrent seizures following hospital discharge in patients with LPDs (PLEDs) and nonconvulsive seizures recorded on continuous EEG in the critical care setting. *Epilepsy Behav.* 2015;49:250–254.

104. Sen-Gupta I, Schuele SU, Macken MP, Kwasny MJ, Gerard EE. "Ictal" lateralized periodic discharges. *Epilepsy Behav.* 2014;36:165–170.

105. Bussiere M, Pelz D, Reid RH, Young GB. Prolonged deficits after focal inhibitory seizures. *Neurocrit Care.* 2005;2(1):29–37.

106. Meador KJ, Moser E. Negative seizures. *J Int Neuropsychol Soc.* 2000;6(6):731–733.

107. Hughes JR. Periodic lateralized epileptiform discharges: do they represent an ictal pattern requiring treatment? *Epilepsy Behav.* 2010;18(3):162–165.

108. Treiman DM, Walton NY, Kendrick C. A progressive sequence of electroencephalographic changes during generalized convulsive status epilepticus. *Epilepsy Res.* 1990;5(1):49–60.

109. Claassen J. How I treat Patients with EEG patterns on the ictal–interictal continuum in the neuro ICU. *Neurocritical Care.* 2009;11(3):437–444.

110. Assal F, Papazyan JP, Slosman DO, Jallon P, Goerres GW. SPECT in periodic lateralized epileptiform discharges (PLEDs): a form of partial status epilepticus? *Seizure.* 2001;10(4):260–265.

111. Handforth A, Cheng JT, Mandelkern MA, Treiman DM. Markedly increased mesiotemporal lobe metabolism in a case with PLEDs: further evidence that PLEDs are a manifestation of partial status epilepticus. *Epilepsia.* 1994;35(4):876–881.

112. Struck AF, Westover MB, Hall LT, Deck GM, Cole AJ, Rosenthal ES. Metabolic correlates of the ictal-interictal continuum: FDG-PET during continuous EEG. *Neurocrit Care.* 2016;24(3):324–331.

113. Vespa P, Tubi M, Claassen J, et al. Metabolic crisis occurs with seizures and periodic discharges after brain trauma. *Ann Neurol.* 2016;79(4):579–590.

114. Beniczky S, Hirsch LJ, Kaplan PW, et al. Unified EEG terminology and criteria for nonconvulsive status epilepticus. *Epilepsia.* 2013;54:28–29.

115. Hopp JL, Sanchez A, Krumholz A, Hart G, Barry E. Nonconvulsive status epilepticus: value of a benzodiazepine trial for predicting outcomes. *Neurologist.* 2011;17(6):325–329.

116. O'Rourke D, Chen PM, Gaspard N, et al. Response rates to anticonvulsant trials in patients with triphasic-wave EEG patterns of uncertain significance. *Neurocrit Care.* 2016;24(2):233–239.

117. San-Juan OD, Chiappa KH, Costello DJ, Cole AJ. Periodic epileptiform discharges in hypoxic encephalopathy: BiPLEDs and GPEDs as a poor prognosis for survival. *Seizure.* 2009;18(5):365–368.

118. de la Paz D, Brenner RP. Bilateral independent periodic lateralized epileptiform discharges. Clinical significance. *Arch Neurol.* 1981;38(11):713–715.

119. Foreman B, Claassen J, Abou Khaled K, et al. Generalized periodic discharges in the critically ill: a case-control study of 200 patients. *Neurology.* 2012;79(19):1951–1960.

120. Akman CI, Abou Khaled KJ, Segal E, Micic V, Riviello JJ. Generalized periodic epileptiform discharges in critically ill children: clinical features, and outcome. *Epilepsy Res.* 2013;106(3):378–385.

121. Chong DJ, Hirsch LJ. Which EEG patterns warrant treatment in the critically ill? Reviewing the evidence for treatment of periodic epileptiform discharges and related patterns. *J Clin Neurophysiol.* 2005;22(2):79–91.

122. Smith SJ, Kocen RS. A Creutzfeldt-Jakob like syndrome due to lithium toxicity. *J Neurol Neurosurg Psychiatry.* 1988;51(1):120–123.

123. Stockard JJ, Werner SS, Aalbers JA, Chiappa KH. Electroencephalographic findings in phencyclidine intoxication. *Arch Neurol.* 1976;33(3):200–203.

124. Martinez-Rodriguez JE, Barriga FJ, Santamaria J, et al. Nonconvulsive status epilepticus associated with cephalosporins in patients with renal failure. *Am J Med.* 2001;111(2):115–119.

125. Jallon P, Fankhauser L, Du Pasquier R, et al. Severe but reversible encephalopathy associated with cefepime. *Clin Neurophysiol.* 2000;30(6):383–386.

126. Naeije G, Lorent S, Vincent JL, Legros B. Continuous epileptiform discharges in patients treated with cefepime or meropenem. *Arch Neurol.* 2011;68(10):1303–1307.

127. Foley J, Watson C, Adams R. Significance of the electroencephalographic changes in hepatic coma. *Trans Am Neurol Assoc.* 1950;75:161–165.

128. Bickford RG, Butt HR. Hepatic coma: the electroencephalographic pattern. *J Clin Invest.* 1955;34(6):790–799.

129. Sutter R, Kaplan PW. Uncovering clinical and radiological associations of triphasic waves in acute encephalopathy: a case-control study. *Eur J Neurol.* 2014;21(4):660–666.

130. Sundaram MB, Blume WT. Triphasic waves: clinical correlates and morphology. *Can J Neurol Sci.* 1987;14(2):136–140.

131. Boulanger JM, Deacon C, Lecuyer D, Gosselin S, Reiher J. Triphasic waves versus nonconvulsive status epilepticus: EEG distinction. *Can J Neurol Sci.* 2006;33(2):175–180.

132. Hirsch LJ, Claassen J, Mayer SA, Emerson RG. Stimulus-induced rhythmic, periodic, or ictal discharges (SIRPIDs): a common EEG phenomenon in the critically ill. *Epilepsia.* 2004;45(2):109–123.

133. Foreman B, Mahulikar A, Tadi P, et al. Generalized periodic discharges and 'triphasic waves': a blinded evaluation of inter-rater agreement and clinical significance. *Clin Neurophysiol.* 2016;127(2):1073–1080.

134. Fountain NB, Waldman WA. Effects of benzodiazepines on triphasic waves: implications for nonconvulsive status epilepticus. *J Clin Neurophysiol.* 2001;18(4):345–352.

135. Cobb WA. Rhythmic slow discharges in the electroencephalogram. *J Neurol Neurosurg Psychiatry.* 1945;8:65–78.

136. Accolla EA, Kaplan PW, Maeder-Ingvar M, Jukopila S, Rossetti AO. Clinical correlates of frontal intermittent rhythmic delta activity (FIRDA). *Clin Neurophysiol.* 2011;122(1):27–31.

137. Rodriguez A, Vlachy J, Lee JW, et al. Association of periodic and rhythmic electroencephalographic patterns with seizures in critically ill patients. *JAMA Neurol.* 2017;74(2):181–188

138. Skjei KL, Kessler SK, Abend NS. SIRPIDs in a 13-year-old following overdose and respiratory arrest. *Pediatr Neurol.* 2011;45(5):350–351.

139. Hirsch LJ, Pang T, Claassen J, et al. Focal motor seizures induced by alerting stimuli in critically ill patients. *Epilepsia.* 2008;49(6):968–973.

140. Kaplan PW, Duckworth J. Confusion and SIRPIDs regress with parenteral lorazepam. *Epileptic Disord.* 2011;13(3):291–294.

141. Smith CC, Tatum WO, Gupta V, Pooley RA, Freeman WD. SPECT-negative SIRPIDs: less aggressive neurointensive care? *J Clin Neurophysiol.* 2014;31(3):e6–e10.

142. Zeiler SR, Turtzo LC, Kaplan PW. SPECT-negative SIRPIDs argues against treatment as seizures. *J Clin Neurophysiol.* 2011;28(5):493–496.

143. Braksick SA, Burkholder DB, Tsetsou S, et al. Associated factors and prognostic implications of stimulus-induced rhythmic, periodic, or ictal discharges. *JAMA Neurol.* 2016;73(5):585–590.

144. Alvarez V, Oddo M, Rossetti AO. Stimulus-induced rhythmic, periodic or ictal discharges (SIRPIDs) in comatose survivors of cardiac arrest: characteristics and prognostic value. *Clin Neurophysiol.* 2013;124(1):204–208.

145. Yoo J, Rampal N, Petroff OA, Hirsch LJ, Gaspard N. Brief potentially ictal rhythmic discharges in critically ill adults. *JAMA Neurol.* 2014;71(4):454–462.

146. Husain AM. Review of neonatal EEG. *Am J Electroneurodiagnostic Technol.* 2005;45(1):12–35.

147. Andre M, Lamblin MD, d'Allest AM, et al. Electroencephalography in premature and full-term infants. Developmental features and glossary. *Clin Neurophysiol.* 2010;40(2):59–124.

148. Schmitt SE, Pargeon K, Frechette ES, Hirsch LJ, Dalmau J, Friedman D. Extreme delta brush: a unique EEG pattern in adults with anti-NMDA receptor encephalitis. *Neurology.* 2012;79(11):1094–1100.

149. Gaspard N, Hirsch LJ. Pitfalls in ictal EEG interpretation: critical care and intracranial recordings. *Neurology.* 2013;80(1 Suppl. 1):S26–S42.

150. Croft RJ, Barry RJ. Removal of ocular artifact from the EEG: a review. *Clin Neurophysiol.* 2000;30(1):5–19.

151. Berg P, Scherg M. A multiple source approach to the correction of eye artifacts. *Electroenceph Clin Neurophysiol.* 1994;90(3):229–241.

152. Nakamura M, Shibasaki H. Elimination of EKG artifacts from EEG records: a new method of non-cephalic referential EEG recording. *Electroenceph Clin Neurophysiol.* 1987;66(1):89–92.

153. Ille N, Berg P, Scherg M. Artifact correction of the ongoing EEG using spatial filters based on artifact and brain signal topographies. *J Clin Neurophysiol.* 2002;19(2):113–124.
154. Sinha SR. Quantitative EEG basic principles. In: LaRoche S, ed. *Handbook of ICU EEG monitoring.* New York: Demos Medical, 2013:221–228.
155. Akman CI, Micic V, Thompson A, Riviello JJ, Jr. Seizure detection using digital trend analysis: factors affecting utility. *Epilepsy Res.* 2011;93(1):66–72.
156. Scheuer ML, Wilson SB. Data analysis for continuous EEG monitoring in the ICU: seeing the forest and the trees. *J Clin Neurophysiol.* 2004;21(5):353–378.
157. Claassen J, Hirsch LJ, Kreiter KT, et al. Quantitative continuous EEG for detecting delayed cerebral ischemia in patients with poor-grade subarachnoid hemorrhage. *Clin Neurophysiol.* 2004;115(12):2699–2710.
158. Schwender D, Daunderer M, Mulzer S, Klasing S, Finsterer U, Peter K. Spectral edge frequency of the electroencephalogram to monitor "depth" of anaesthesia with isoflurane or propofol. *Br J Anaesth.* 1996;77(2):179–184.
159. Al-Nashash H, Sabesan S, Krishnan B, et al. Nonstationarity in EEG and time-frequency analysis. In: Tong S, Thakor NV, eds. *Quantitative EEG analysis methods and clinical applications.* Norwood, MA: Artech House, 2009:63–73.
160. Amorim E, Williamson C, Moura L, et al. A spectogram-based classification system for seizure identification: a pilot study. Poster presentation presented at American Clinical Neurophysiology Society annual meeting, Feb. 10–14, 2016, Orlando, FL.
161. Musialowicz T, Lahtinen P. Current status of EEG-based depth-of-consciousness monitoring during general anesthesia. *Curr Anesthesiol Rep.* 2014;4(3):251–260.
162. Riess ML, Graefe UA, Goeters C, Van Aken H, Bone HG. Sedation assessment in critically ill patients with bispectral index. *Eur J Anaesthesiol.* 2002;19(1):18–22.
163. Roustan JP, Valette S, Aubas P, Rondouin G, Capdevila X. Can electroencephalographic analysis be used to determine sedation levels in critically ill patients? *Anesth Analg.* 2005;101(4):1141–1151.
164. Stewart CP, Otsubo H, Ochi A, Sharma R, Hutchison JS, Hahn CD. Seizure identification in the ICU using quantitative EEG displays. *Neurology.* 2010;75(17):1501–1508.
165. Williamson C, Wahlster S, Shafi M, Westover MB. Sensitivity of compressed spectral arrays for detecting seizures in acutely ill adults. *Neurocritical Care.* 2014;20(1):32–39.
166. Swisher CB, White CR, Mace BE, et al. Diagnostic accuracy of electrographic seizure detection by neurophysiologists and non-neurophysiologists in the adult ICU using a panel of quantitative EEG trends. *J Clin Neurophysiol.* 2015;32(4):324–330.
167. Moura LMVR, Shafi MM, Ng M, et al. Spectrogram screening of adult EEGs is sensitive and efficient. *Neurology.* 2014;83(1):56–64.
168. Sackellares JC, Shiau DS, Halford JJ, LaRoche SM, Kelly KM. Quantitative EEG analysis for automated detection of nonconvulsive seizures in intensive care units. *Epilepsy Behav.* 2011;22(Suppl. 1):S69–73.
169. Fürbass F, Hartmann MM, Halford JJ, et al. Automatic detection of rhythmic and periodic patterns in critical care EEG based on American Clinical Neurophysiology Society (ACNS) standardized terminology. *Clin Neurophysiol.* 2015;45(3):203–213.
170. Pandian JD, Cascino GD, So EL, Manno E, Fulgham JR. Digital video-electroencephalographic monitoring in the neurological-neurosurgical intensive care unit: clinical features and outcome. *Arch Neurol.* 2004;61(7):1090–1094.
171. Jette N, Claassen J, Emerson RG, Hirsch LJ. Frequency and predictors of nonconvulsive seizures during continuous electroencephalographic monitoring in critically ill children. *Arch Neurol.* 2006;63(12):1750–1755.
172. Meldrum BS, Vigouroux RA, Brierley JB. Systemic factors and epileptic brain damage. Prolonged seizures in paralyzed, artificially ventilated baboons. *Arch Neurol.* 1973;29(2):82–87.
173. Rabinowicz AL, Correale JD, Bracht KA, Smith TD, DeGiorgio CM. Neuron-specific enolase is increased after nonconvulsive status epilepticus. *Epilepsia.* 1995;36(5):475–479.
174. DeGiorgio CM, Correale JD, Gott PS, et al. Serum neuron-specific enolase in human status epilepticus. *Neurology.* 1995;45(6):1134–1137.
175. Correale J, Rabinowicz AL, Heck CN, Smith TD, Loskota WJ, DeGiorgio CM. Status epilepticus increases CSF levels of neuron-specific enolase and alters the blood-brain barrier. *Neurology.* 1998;50(5):1388–1391.
176. Holmes GL. Seizure-induced neuronal injury: animal data. *Neurology.* 2002;59(9 Suppl. 5):S3–6.
177. Cavazos JE, Das I, Sutula TP. Neuronal loss induced in limbic pathways by kindling: evidence for induction of hippocampal sclerosis by repeated brief seizures. *J Neurosci.* 1994;14(5 Pt 2):3106–3121.
178. Williams AJ, Tortella FC, Lu XM, Moreton JE, Hartings JA. Antiepileptic drug treatment of nonconvulsive seizures induced by experimental focal brain ischemia. *J Pharmacol Exp Ther.* 2004;311(1):220–227.
179. Vespa PM, Miller C, McArthur D, et al. Nonconvulsive electrographic seizures after traumatic brain injury result in a delayed, prolonged increase in intracranial pressure and metabolic crisis. *Crit Care Med.* 2007;35(12):2830–2836.
180. Topjian AA, Gutierrez-Colina AM, Sanchez SM, et al. Electrographic status epilepticus is associated with mortality and worse short-term outcome in critically ill children. *Crit Care Med.* 2013;41(1):215–223.
181. Wagenman KL, Blake TP, Sanchez SM, et al. Electrographic status epilepticus and long-term outcome in critically ill children. *Neurology.* 2014;82(5):396–404.
182. Drislane FW, Lopez MR, Blum AS, Schomer DL. Detection and treatment of refractory status epilepticus in the intensive care unit. *J Clin Neurophysiol.* 2008;25(4):181–186.
183. Kowalski RG, Ziai WC, Rees RN, et al. Third-line antiepileptic therapy and outcome in status epilepticus: the impact of vasopressor use and prolonged mechanical ventilation. *Crit Care Med.* 2012;40(9):2677–2684.
184. Sutter R, Marsch S, Fuhr P, Kaplan PW, Rüegg S. Anesthetic drugs in status epilepticus: risk or rescue? A 6-year cohort study. *Neurology.* 2014;82(8):656–664.
185. Marchi NA, Novy J, Faouzi M, Stähli C, Burnand B, Rossetti AO. Status epilepticus: impact of therapeutic coma on outcome. *Crit Care Med.* 2015;43(5):1003–1009.
186. Fernandez A, Lantigua H, Lesch C, et al. High-dose midazolam infusion for refractory status epilepticus. *Neurology.* 2014;82(4):359–365.
187. Mollaret P, Goulon M. [The depassed coma (preliminary memoir)]. *Rev Neurol.* 1959;101:3–15.
188. A definition of irreversible coma. Report of the Ad Hoc Committee of the Harvard Medical School to Examine the Definition of Brain Death. *JAMA.* 1968;205(6):337–340.
189. Abram MB, Fox RC, Medearas DN, et al. *Defining death.* Washington, DC: President's Commission for Study of Ethical Problems in Medicine and Biomedical and Behavioral Research, July 9, 1981.
190. Wijdicks EF. Determining brain death in adults. *Neurology.* 1995;45(5):1003–1011.
191. Wijdicks EFM, Varelas PN, Gronseth GS, Greer DM. Evidence-based guideline update: determining brain death in adults: Report of the Quality Standards Subcommittee of the American Academy of Neurology. *Neurology.* 2010;74(23):1911–1918.
192. Guideline 3: Minimum technical standards for EEG recording in suspected cerebral death. *J Clin Neurophysiol.* 2006;23(2):97–104.
193. Bakshi N, Maselli RA, Gospe SM, Jr., Ellis WG, McDonald C, Mandler RN. Fulminant demyelinating neuropathy mimicking cerebral death. *Muscle Nerve.* 1997;20(12):1595–1597.
194. Rittenberger JC, Polderman KH, Smith WS, Weingart SD. Emergency neurological life support: resuscitation following cardiac arrest. *Neurocrit Care.* 2012;17(Suppl 1):S21–28.
195. Mild therapeutic hypothermia to improve the neurologic outcome after cardiac arrest. *N Engl J Med.* 2002;346(8):549–556.
196. Stecker MM, Cheung AT, Pochettino A, et al. Deep hypothermic circulatory arrest: I. Effects of cooling on electroencephalogram and evoked potentials. *Ann Thoracic Surg.* 2001;71(1):14–21.
197. Hofmeijer J, Tjepkema-Cloostermans MC, van Putten MJ. Burst-suppression with identical bursts: a distinct EEG pattern with poor outcome in postanoxic coma. *Clin Neurophysiol.* 2014;125(5):947–954.
198. Hofmeijer J, Beernink TMJ, Bosch FH, Beishuizen A, Tjepkema-Cloostermans MC, van Putten MJAM. Early EEG contributes to multimodal outcome prediction of postanoxic.
199. Rossetti AO, Oddo M, Logroscino G, Kaplan PW. Prognostication after cardiac arrest and hypothermia: a prospective study. *Ann Neurol.* 2010;67(3):301–307.
200. Lamartine Monteiro M, Taccone FS, Depondt C, et al. The prognostic value of 48-h continuous EEG during therapeutic hypothermia after cardiac arrest. *Neurocrit Care.* 2016;24(2):153–162.
201. Rossetti AO, Urbano LA, Delodder F, Kaplan PW, Oddo M. Prognostic value of continuous EEG monitoring during therapeutic hypothermia after cardiac arrest. *Critical Care.* 2010;14(5):R173–R173.
202. Cronberg T, Rundgren M, Westhall E, et al. Neuron-specific enolase correlates with other prognostic markers after cardiac arrest. *Neurology.* 2011;77(7):623–630.
203. Abend NS, Licht DJ. Predicting outcome in children with hypoxic ischemic encephalopathy. *Pediatr Crit Care.* 2008;9(1):32–39.
204. Topjian AA, Sanchez SM, Shults J, Berg RA, Dlugos DJ, Abend NS. Early electroencephalographic background features predict outcomes in children resuscitated from cardiac arrest. *Pediatr Crit Care.* 2016;17(6):547–557.

205. Ribeiro A, Singh R, Brunnhuber F. Clinical outcome of generalized periodic epileptiform discharges on first EEG in patients with hypoxic encephalopathy postcardiac arrest. *Epilepsy Behav.* 2015;49:268–272.

206. Crepeau AZ, Fugate JE, Mandrekar J, et al. Value analysis of continuous EEG in patients during therapeutic hypothermia after cardiac arrest. *Resuscitation.* 2014;85(6):785–789.

207. Rossetti AO, Oddo M, Liaudet L, Kaplan PW. Predictors of awakening from postanoxic status epilepticus after therapeutic hypothermia. *Neurology.* 2009;72(8):744–749.

208. Ruijter BJ, van Putten MJ, Hofmeijer J. Generalized epileptiform discharges in postanoxic encephalopathy: quantitative characterization in relation to outcome. *Epilepsia.* 2015;56(11):1845–1854.

209. Dragancea I, Backman S, Westhall E, Rundgren M, Friberg H, Cronberg T. Outcome following postanoxic status epilepticus in patients with targeted temperature management after cardiac arrest. *Epilepsy Behav.* 2015;49:173–177.

210. Seder DB, Sunde K, Rubertsson S, et al. Neurologic outcomes and postresuscitation care of patients with myoclonus following cardiac arrest. *Critical Care Med.* 2015;43(5):965–972.

211. Ruijter BJ, van Putten MJ, Horn J, et al. Treatment of electroencephalographic status epilepticus after cardiopulmonary resuscitation (TELSTAR): study protocol for a randomized controlled trial. *Trials.* 2014;15:433.

212. Rundgren M, Rosén I, Friberg H. Amplitude-integrated EEG (aEEG) predicts outcome after cardiac arrest and induced hypothermia. *Intensive Care Med.* 2006;32(6):836–842.

213. Tjepkema-Cloostermans MC, van Meulen FB, Meinsma G, van Putten MJ. A Cerebral Recovery Index (CRI) for early prognosis in patients after cardiac arrest. *Critical Care.* 2013;17(5):1–11.

214. Sandroni C, Cariou A, Cavallaro F, Cronberg T, Friberg H, Hoedemaekers C. Prognostication in comatose survivors of cardiac arrest: an advisory statement from the European Resuscitation Council and the European Society of Intensive Care Medicine. *Resuscitation.* 2014;85(12):1779–1789.

215. Macdonald RL. Delayed neurological deterioration after subarachnoid haemorrhage. *Nature Rev Neurol.* 2014;10(1):44–58.

216. Rowland MJ, Hadjipavlou G, Kelly M, Westbrook J, Pattinson KTS. Delayed cerebral ischaemia after subarachnoid haemorrhage: looking beyond vasospasm. *Br J Anaesth.* 2012;109(3):315–329.

217. Vergouwen MDI, Vermeulen M, van Gijn J, et al. Definition of delayed cerebral ischemia after aneurysmal subarachnoid hemorrhage as an outcome event in clinical trials and observational studies: proposal of a multidisciplinary research group. *Stroke.* 2010;41(10):2391–2395.

218. de Oliveira Manoel AL, Jaja BN, Germans MR, et al. The VASOGRADE: a simple grading scale for prediction of delayed cerebral ischemia after subarachnoid hemorrhage. *Stroke.* 2015;46(7):1826–1831.

219. Carrera E, Schmidt JM, Oddo M, et al. Transcranial Doppler for predicting delayed cerebral ischemia after subarachnoid hemorrhage. *Neurosurgery.* 2009;65(2):316–323.

220. Rivierez M, Landau-Ferey J, Grob R, Grosskopf D, Philippon J. Value of electroencephalogram in prediction and diagnosis of vasospasm after intracranial aneurysm rupture. *Acta Neurochir (Wien).* 1991;110(1-2):17–23.

221. Vespa PM, Nuwer MR, Juhász C, et al. Early detection of vasospasm after acute subarachnoid hemorrhage using continuous EEG ICU monitoring. *Electroenceph Clin Neurophysiol.* 1997;103(6):607–615.

222. Claassen J, Hirsch LJ, Kreiter KT, et al. Quantitative continuous EEG for detecting delayed cerebral ischemia in patients with poor-grade subarachnoid hemorrhage. *Clin Neurophysiol.* 2004;115.

223. Rots ML, van Putten MJAM, Hoedemaekers CWE, Horn J. Continuous EEG monitoring for early detection of delayed cerebral ischemia in subarachnoid hemorrhage: a pilot study. *Neurocritical Care.* 2015:1–10.

224. Labar DR, Fisch BJ, Pedley TA, Fink ME, Solomon RA. Quantitative EEG monitoring for patients with subarachnoid hemorrhage. *Electroenceph Clin Neurophysiol.* 1991;78(5):325–332.

225. Gollwitzer S, Groemer T, Rampp S, et al. Early prediction of delayed cerebral ischemia in subarachnoid hemorrhage based on quantitative EEG: a prospective study in adults. *Clin Neurophysiol.* 2015;126(8):1514–1523.

226. Rathakrishnan R, Gotman J, Dubeau F, Angle M. Using continuous electroencephalography in the management of delayed cerebral ischemia following subarachnoid hemorrhage. *Neurocrit Care.* 2011;14(2):152–161.

227. Rosenthal ES, O'Connor KL, Zafar SF, Biswal S, Westover MB. Clinical performance of a prospective continuous electroencephalography (cEEG) ischemia monitoring service for predicting neurologic decline after aneurysmal subarachnoid hemorrhage (SAH). American Clinical Neurophysiology Society annual meeting, 2015, Houston, TX.

228. Mayer SA, Chong JY. Critical care management of increased intracranial pressure. *J Intensive Care Med.* 2002;17(2):55–67.

229. Guidelines for the management of severe traumatic brain injury. *J Neurotrauma.* 2007;24(Suppl 1):S1–106.

230. Bekar A, Doğan Ş, Abaş F, et al. Risk factors and complications of intracranial pressure monitoring with a fiberoptic device. *J Clin Neurosci.* 2009;16(2):236–240.

231. Chen H, Wang J, Mao S, Dong W, Yang H. A new method of intracranial pressure monitoring by EEG power spectrum analysis. *Can J Neurol Sci.* 2012;39(4):483–487.

232. Oddo M, Villa F, Citerio G. Brain multimodality monitoring: an update. *Curr Opin Critical Care.* 2012;18(2):111–118.

233. Miller CM. Update on multimodality monitoring. *Curr Neurol Neurosci Rep.* 2012;12(4):474–480.

234. Ko S-B. Multimodality monitoring in the neurointensive care unit: a special perspective for patients with stroke. *J Stroke.* 2013;15(2):99–108.

235. Waziri A, Claassen J, Stuart RM, et al. Intracortical electroencephalography in acute brain injury. *Ann Neurol.* 2009;66(3):366–377.

236. Claassen J, Perotte A, Albers D, et al. Nonconvulsive seizures after subarachnoid hemorrhage: multimodal detection and outcomes. *Ann Neurol.* 2013;74(1):53–64.

237. Vespa P, Tubi M, Claassen J, et al. Metabolic crisis occurs with seizures and periodic discharges after brain trauma. *Ann Neurol.* 2016;79(4):579–590.

238. Leo AAP. Spreading depression of activity in the cerebral cortex. *J Neurophysiol.* 1944;7(6):359–390.

239. Grafstein B. Mechanism of spreading cortical depression. *J Neurophysiol.* 1956;19(2):154–171.

240. Lauritzen M. Pathophysiology of the migraine aura. The spreading depression theory. *Brain.* 1994;117(1):199–210.

241. Strong AJ, Fabricius M, Boutelle MG, et al. Spreading and synchronous depressions of cortical activity in acutely injured human brain. *Stroke.* 2002;33(12):2738–2743.

242. Hartings JA, Rolli ML, Lu XC, Tortella FC. Delayed secondary phase of peri-infarct depolarizations after focal cerebral ischemia: relation to infarct growth and neuroprotection. *J Neurosci.* 2003;23(37):11602–11610.

243. Hartings JA, Wilson JA, Hinzman JM, et al. Spreading depression in continuous electroencephalography of brain trauma. *Ann Neurol.* 2014;76(5):681–694.

244. Fabricius M. Cortical spreading depression and peri-infarct depolarisation in stroke—a mechanism for secondary deterioration. *Clin Neurophysiol.* 2008;119(Suppl. 1):S19.

245. Busch E, Gyngell ML, Eis M, Hoehn-Berlage M, Hossmann K-A. Potassium-induced cortical spreading depressions during focal cerebral ischemia in rats: contribution to lesion growth assessed by diffusion-weighted NMR and biochemical imaging. *J Cerebral Blood Flow Metab.* 1996;16(6):1090–1099.

246. Dreier JP, Woitzik J, Fabricius M, et al. Delayed ischaemic neurological deficits after subarachnoid haemorrhage are associated with clusters of spreading depolarizations. *Brain.* 2006;129(12):3224.

247. Seule M, Keller E, Unterberg A, Sakowitz O. The hemodynamic response of spreading depolarization observed by near infrared spectroscopy after aneurysmal subarachnoid hemorrhage. *Neurocrit Care.* 2015;23(1):108–112.

248. Gursoy-Ozdemir Y, Qiu J, Matsuoka N, et al. Cortical spreading depression activates and upregulates MMP-9. *J Clin Investig.* 2004;113(10):1447–1455.

249. Fabricius M, Fuhr S, Willumsen L, et al. Association of seizures with cortical spreading depression and peri-infarct depolarisations in the acutely injured human brain. *Clin Neurophysiol.* 2008;119(9):1973–1984.

250. Synek VM. Prognostically important EEG coma patterns in diffuse anoxic and traumatic encephalopathies in adults. *J Clin Neurophysiol.* 1988;5(2):161–174.

251. Alvarez V, Drislane FW, Westover MB, Dworetzky BA, Lee JW. Characteristics and role in outcome prediction of continuous EEG after status epilepticus: A prospective observational cohort. *Epilepsia.* 2015;56(6):933–941.

252. Arndt DH, Lerner JT, Matsumoto JH, et al. Subclinical early posttraumatic seizures detected by continuous EEG monitoring in a consecutive pediatric cohort. *Epilepsia.* 2013;54(10):1780–1788.

253. Topjian AA, Gutierrez-Colina AM, Sanchez SM, et al. Electrographic status epilepticus is associated with mortality and worse short-term outcome in critically ill children. *Critical Care Med.* 2013;41(1):215–223.

254. Schreiber JM, Zelleke T, Gaillard WD, Kaulas H, Dean N, Carpenter JL. Continuous video EEG for patients with acute encephalopathy in a pediatric intensive care unit. *Neurocrit Care.* 2012;17(1):31–38.

255. Abend NS, Topjian A, Ichord R, et al. Electroencephalographic monitoring during hypothermia after pediatric cardiac arrest. *Neurology.* 2009;72(22):1931–1940.

256. Hirsch LJ, Brenner RP. *Atlas of EEG in critical care.* First edition. Chichester, West Sussex, UK: Wiley-Blackwell; 2010.

257. Takano T, Tian G-F, Peng W, et al. Cortical spreading depression causes and coincides with tissue hypoxia. *Nature Neurosci.* 2007;10(6):754–762.

258. Dreier JP. The role of spreading depression, spreading depolarization and spreading ischemia in neurological disease. *Nature Med.* 2011;17(4):439–447.

23 | EEG-BASED ANTICIPATION AND CONTROL OF SEIZURES

STILIYAN KALITZIN, PHD AND FERNANDO H. LOPES DA SILVA, MD, PHD

ABSTRACT: Early seizure-prediction paradigms were based on detecting electroencephalographic (EEG) features, but recent approaches are based on dynamic systems theory. Methods that attempted to detect predictive features during the preictal period proved difficult to validate in practice. Brain systems can display bistability (both normal and epileptic states can coexist), and the transitions between states may be initiated by external or internal dynamic factors. In the former case prediction is impossible, but in the latter case prediction is conceivable, leading to the hypothesis that as seizure onset approaches, the excitability of the underlying neuronal networks tends to increase. This assumption is being explored using not only the ongoing EEG but also active probes, applying appropriate stimuli to brain areas to estimate the excitability of the neuronal populations. Experimental results support this assumption, suggesting that it may be possible to develop paradigms to estimate the risk of an impending transition to an epileptic state.

KEYWORDS: seizures, epilepsy, paradigm, prediction, EEG, bistability, networks

PRINCIPAL REFERENCES

1. K. Gadhoumi, J. M. Lina, F. Mormann and J. Gotman, *Seizure prediction for therapeutic devices: A review*, Journal of Neuroscience Methods 2016;260:270–282.
2. W. W. Lytton, *Computer modelling of epilepsy*, Nature Reviews Neuroscience 2008;9(8):626–637.
3. R. Aschenbrenner-Scheibe, T. Maiwald, M. Winterhalder, H. U. Voss, J. Timmer and A. Schulze-Bonhage, *How well can epileptic seizures be predicted? An evaluation of a nonlinear method*, Brain 2003;126(12):2616–2626.
4. M. J. Cook, T. J. O'Brien, S. F. Berkovic, M. Murphy, A. Morokoff, G. Fabinyi, W. D'Souza, R. Yerra, J. Archer, L. Litewka, S. Hosking, P. Lightfoot, V. Ruedebusch, W. D. Sheffield, D. Snyder, K. Leyde and D. Himes, *Prediction of seizure likelihood with a long-term, implanted seizure advisory system in patients with drug-resistant epilepsy: A first-in-man study*, Lancet Neurology 2013;12(6):563–571.
5. S. Kalitzin, J. Parra, D. N. Velis and F. H. Lopes da Silva, *Enhancement of phase clustering in the eeg/meg gamma frequency band anticipates transitions to paroxysmal epileptiform activity in epileptic patients with known visual sensitivity*, IEEE Transactions on Biomedical Engineering 2002;49(11):1279–1286.
6. K. Lehnertz and C. E. Elger, *Spatio-temporal dynamics of the primary epileptogenic area in temporal lobe epilepsy characterized by neuronal complexity loss*, Electroencephalography and Clinical Neurophysiology 1995;95(2):108–117.
7. F. Lopes da Silva, W. Blanes, S. N. Kalitzin, J. Parra, P. Suffczynski and D. N. Velis, *Epilepsies as dynamical diseases of brain systems: Basic models of the transition between normal and epileptic activity*, Epilepsia 2003;44(Suppl 12):72–83.
8. J. Martinerie, C. Adam, M. Le Van Quyen, M. Baulac, S. Clemenceau, B. Renault and F. J. Varela, *Epileptic seizures can be anticipated by nonlinear analysis*, Nature Medicine 1998;4(10):1173–1176.
9. F. Mormann, R. G. Andrzejak, C. E. Elger and K. Lehnertz, *Seizure prediction: The long and winding road*, Brain 2007;130(2):314–333.
10. V. Navarro, J. Martinerie, M. Le Van Quyen, S. Clemenceau, C. Adam, M. Baulac and F. Varela, *Seizure anticipation in human neocortical partial epilepsy*, Brain 2002;125(3):640–655.

1. INTRODUCTION

In this chapter we deal with the possibility of anticipating seizures based on the analysis of electroencephalogram (EEG) recordings. Some reports state that epileptic patients may feel an approaching seizure, but most of these are based on relatively small patient populations. Nonetheless, we should take this issue into consideration since it may be relevant in order to determine the value of any automatic method based on EEG recordings. Schulze-Bonhage et al. [1] carried out a comprehensive analysis of subjective seizure anticipation reported by 500 consecutively recruited outpatients with focal and generalized epilepsy. The patients were asked to report any premonitory symptoms they experienced at least 30 minutes prior to a seizure. No auras were included. These authors found that 6.2% of patients were able to report anticipating seizures. The median estimated time interval between occurrence of premonitory symptoms and seizure onset was 90 minutes. More recently Scaramelli et al. [2] investigated the existence of premonitory or *prodromal signs* (PS) in a randomly selected population of 100 adult epileptic patients both with focal and generalized epilepsies. Using a semistructured protocol and personal interviews they found evidence for PS (behavioral, cognitive, and mood changes, excluding auras) in 39% of patients, mostly in those having complex partial and generalized tonic-clonic seizures. In this study PS were reported to have an insidious onset and a duration ranging from 30 minutes to several hours prior to seizure onset.

We should note that these results might be relevant, although it is not yet possible to estimate the corresponding sensitivity and specificity with respect to their relevance to estimate a preictal period. The fact that no EEG recordings were generally carried out simultaneously during the period when the patients reported PS also raises the question as to whether EEG signal changes might be associated with the presence of PS. Nonetheless, in assessing the clinical significance of EEG automatic methods of analysis, it is important to keep these results on subjective experiences of epileptic patients in mind.

In their thoughtful account of the "state of seizure prediction," Zaveri et al. [3] considered that three historical phases can be distinguished in this research field over the last decades. In the first phase in the 1970s, a variety of attempts were tried, ranging from measuring epileptiform spike rates to estimating time-varying EEG spectral features. In the second phase, particularly in the late 1980s and beginning 1990s, the question of anticipating epileptic seizures was approached within the framework of mathematical methods derived from the theory of nonlinear dynamical systems. In the third phase, since about 2000, more sophisticated studies are appearing, particularly with respect to theoretical models of seizure dynamics, to statistical methods of evaluating clinical application studies, and to proposals of new strategies. In any case the development of reliable methods to anticipate seizures is the aim of a wide range of researchers. The goal is to be able to control the occurrence of seizures, ideally avoiding their onset.

Considering the relevance of the mathematical approaches, however, we start by presenting a sketch of the analytical tools used in this context. We have divided those tools and approaches into two major categories according to the method of their derivation. The first category consists of the empirically derived, evidence-based signal analysis techniques. This approach was the first to be used, and even today these techniques form a large part of those applied in the context of seizure prediction. More recently a second line of research has gained momentum, based on the development of analytical computational models of brain dynamics. According to this approach, model-based EEG analysis attempts to "reverse engineer" the underlying system generating the EEG signals, leading eventually to making predictions about the system's behavior.

First we introduce the category of empirical techniques. Before dealing with the main question of *anticipation* of epileptic seizures, we consider how mathematical analyses applied to EEG signals were used to characterize the dynamics of neuronal networks *during* seizures. This is useful to better understand the dynamics of the corresponding EEG signals in the course of the transition from the interictal to the ictal or seizure state. Next, we discuss strategies for seizure anticipation and the methodology used for their validation. We dedicate a paragraph to alternative, more general, methods developed to identify the conditions under which neuronal systems generate seizures. The application of such methods can go beyond the framework of seizure anticipation and can be used also for therapeutic outcome assessment. A subclass of these methods consists of the so-called active paradigms, which in general involve the direct electrical or magnetic stimulation of the brain to probe the excitability state of the underlying neuronal networks.

The second part of this chapter is devoted to model-based EEG analysis, especially in relation to theoretical modeling of seizure dynamics. In this context it is interesting to note that the question of predicting seizures is related to similar problems in other fields of science. Recently Scheffer et al. [4] reviewed this issue in a general way and concluded that there may exist generic early warning signals that may indicate for a wide class of systems with multiple attractors if a critical threshold is approaching, such as in the case of an approaching epileptic seizure. The authors assume in this paper, however, that transitions occur when a critical threshold is crossed. In reality, internal or external fluctuations, or "noise," can trigger a transition even far away from the critical threshold in a multiple-attractor system. This implies that in order to define effectively an early warning signal (i.e., a precursor or forerunner of an epileptic seizure), it is necessary to have a specific model of critical transitions.

Finally, we make a brief survey of the possible application of models for developing and testing alternative therapeutic intervention strategies.

2. ANTICIPATING EPILEPTIC SEIZURES BASED ON SPONTANEOUS EEG SIGNALS

First we consider an operational definition of what is meant by *anticipating or predicting* epileptic seizures. *Predictability* may be defined operationally as "the demonstration that there exists a statistically significant association between the outcomes of a set of measurements preceding a seizure, and the time to the first seizure following these measurements." The main point that has to be identified is the kind of measurement that is appropriate for the required association. Here we will review a number of measures that have been proposed and explored.

An early and simple idea was to use as a measure the rate of occurrence of epileptiform spikes—in other words, to check whether there exists any consistent association between variations in the rate of occurrence of epileptiform spikes and the time of seizure onset. While some early reports indicated a possible relationship, in a well-controlled study Gotman and Marciani [5], in 44 patients with focal epilepsy where spiking rates were quantified by an automatic detection method, demonstrated that spiking rates do not change systematically before seizures but may even increase markedly after these. Thus, neither high nor low spiking rates appear to be associated with the occurrence of seizures, and spike rating is not a reliable biomarker to predict seizure onset. Nonetheless, how epileptiform spikes are related to the occurrence of seizures continues to be the object of discussions. Thus, Krishnan et al. [6], proposing a novel algorithm to identify spikes automatically, determined the spiking rates in five patients with temporal lobe epilepsy during a peri-ictal period of 40 minutes (20 minutes before seizure onset and 20 minutes after the seizure) in relation to 94 seizures. The spike rates averaged over all seizures yield mixed results. A refined analysis, separating clinical and subclinical seizures, however, revealed that in clinical seizures the spike rate was significantly larger in the preictal than in the postictal period, while in the subclinical seizures the corresponding difference was not significant. The number of patients studied, however, was relatively small. This issue may remain controversial.

Other statistical properties of the ongoing EEG have been used with the aim of detecting hidden information in the preictal period that might be useful in predicting the impending occurrence of a seizure. Thus, Viglione and Walsh [7], using pattern-recognition analytic procedures of spectral data, reported that EEG changes characteristic of preseizure states could be detected a few seconds before seizure onset. Although this work resulted in a patent application, clinical results were elusive until now [8]. Using linear autoregressive models fitted to ongoing EEG signals in 12 epileptic patients suffering from "absences," Rogowski et al. [9] showed that the location of the poles in the z and s planes, as a function of time, presented a specific pattern linked with the occurrence of the seizure.

These authors noted further that the trajectory of the "most mobile pole" during the preseizure period could aid in the prediction of a seizure by several seconds. Later Salant et al. [10] used multivariate spectral estimation based on parametric modeling (determination of pole trajectories and coherence functions) to detect EEG changes preceding the outbreak of a seizure. Prediction of oncoming primary generalized seizures was based on detecting increased preictal synchronization. Prediction times of 1 to 6 sec were found in several seizures from five patients. These methods, however, had short prediction windows. Furthermore, these techniques were not tested thoroughly in a general clinical setting.

Efforts to solve the problem of anticipation in a more general context received a considerable boost with the application of mathematical concepts developed in the framework of nonlinear complex dynamical systems. Although there is evidence that during epileptic seizures EEG signals display lower complexity, the question remains whether this is also the case before seizure occurrence (i.e., in the preictal period). Quantifying signal complexity has evolved thanks to the seminal contributions of Destexhe and Babloyantz [11], Pijn et al. [12], Iasemidis et al. [13–15], Lehnertz and Elger [16], and Martinerie et al [17]. A tutorial review of nonlinear dynamical EEG analysis is given by Pritchard and Duke [18].

One fundamental approach to explore the complexity of a dynamic system is to estimate the dimensionality of its stable state, or attractor. A seizure onset, in general, represents a transition from a high-dimensional to a low-dimensional state. A practical quantification of the dimensionality is provided by the so-called correlation dimension, D_2, representing the scaling behavior of the number of neighboring points close to a given test point of the system state. High values of D_2 are indicative of a random process; low values indicate deterministic, organized behavior. The estimation of D_2 has to take into consideration a number of critical choices to avoid wrong conclusions, as described by Pijn et al. [19], among others. The question of whether phase transitions from higher to lower dimensions may be detectable already in the preictal period has been further pursued using several techniques. Among the most promising ones were those based on the estimation of the stability properties of the system.

Iasemidis et al. [13–15] analyzed long stretches of EEG signals, starting many hours before a seizure, recorded from subdural and implanted electrodes in the hippocampus of patients with temporal lobe epilepsy. They reconstructed for each EEG epoch the phase space and estimated the corresponding maximum Lyapunov exponent (L_{max}). The values of L_{max} of EEG epochs recorded from different sites in general showed fluctuations over time but started to converge (phase of entrainment) several minutes before a seizure. These authors noted that a critical number of sites should display entrainment over a certain time before a seizure occurs. Based on these data, Iasemidis et al. [20] proposed an adaptive seizure prediction algorithm to analyze continuous EEG signals for the prediction of temporal lobe epilepsy seizures.

Lehnertz and Elger [16] applied the concept of EEG signal "complexity," defined as the variability of a set of consecutive D_2 estimates, in order to determine whether seizure onset could

be anticipated. They found that "complexity" was reduced in EEG epochs recorded close to seizure onset, and proposed that "neuronal complexity loss" could be used to anticipate seizure occurrence.

Martinerie et al. [17] analyzed 19 seizures from a homogeneous group of 11 patients with mesial temporal lobe epilepsy associated with hippocampal sclerosis (using indwelling electrodes) by reconstructing intracranial EEG signals as trajectories in a phase space. They introduced nonlinear indicators to characterize the signal dynamics, taking into account the EEG signals both as functions of time and space, and were able to pinpoint the brain sites where seizure apparently started and showed that in most cases seizure onset could be anticipated within 2 to 6 minutes. Later this group developed alternative methods comparing the dynamical properties of successive epochs of EEG signals to those of a reference window. In this way a new measure was introduced: the "dynamical similarity index," which quantified changes in dynamics relative to the reference window. These authors reported a decrease of the dynamical similarity index several minutes before seizures in intracranial [21–26] (Fig. 23.1) and even in scalp EEG recordings [27]. More recently the same group [28] introduced a method for analyzing multivariate phase synchronization in EEG signals that basically tracks multivariate phase synchronization in space and time-frequency domains; they called it frequency flow analysis. Using this approach, groups of EEG signals were identified as belonging to common frequency flows. This method was applied to simulated signals and real EEG or magnetoencephalographic (MEG) signals recorded before and during epileptic seizures [24]. It appeared to be relevant in tracking transient collective dynamics fluctuating in time, frequency, and space.

The reader may be overwhelmed by the number of methods we have reviewed in this short chapter. They are the result of the very inventive work of several research groups pursuing the still-evasive objective of developing "the" optimal EEG analysis method with respect to detecting relevant dynamical features of EEG signals in the preictal phase. An excellent critical description of the various methods used in this field is given by Mormann et al. [29].

2.1. Assessing the Performance of Algorithms in Anticipating Epileptic Seizures

The early studies, described above, were followed by a series of investigations in which researchers tried a variety of modifications of those approaches and proposed additional algorithms such as the "accumulated energy" algorithm, based on wide frequency band spectral energy [30], and presented critical studies with the aim of evaluating the results obtained by means of different methods in a rigorous way. In the context of a critical evaluation of the performance of the "dynamical similarity index" (referred to above), Navarro et al. [26] analyzed the dynamics of long EEG epochs recorded from patients with indwelling electrodes undergoing monitoring for presurgical evaluation of refractory partial epilepsy at the Montreal Neurological Institute. The similarity index detected preictal changes considered relevant in two thirds of the seizures.

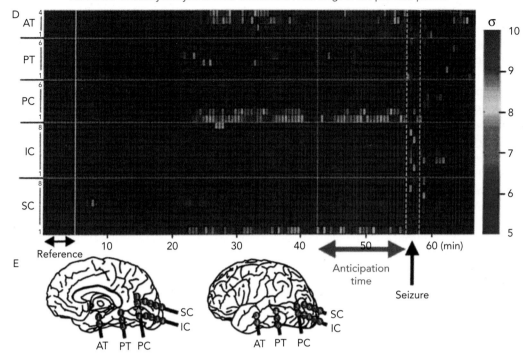

An example of a "passive" paradigm for analysis of prediction:
Non-linear similarity analysis of intra-cranial EEG recordings in the pre-ictal period

Figure 23.1. Nonlinear analysis of an intracranial EEG signal showing changes in the "similarity index" computed between a reference period and successive time windows preceding the seizure (D). The statistical significance is indicated by color code (blue indicates significance levels up to 5 standard deviations). The anticipation time with respect to seizure onset for EEG channel PC1 (precuneus gyrus) is 13.5 min in this case. Channels with and without preictal changes are depicted in red and blue, respectively, on a diagram showing the locations of intracranial electrodes (E). The first channel where seizure onset is detected is indicated by a yellow star. AT = anterior temporal lobe; PT = posterior temporal lobe; PC = precuneus gyrus; IC = infracalcarine; SC = supracalcarine. Adapted with permission from Navarro et al. [25].

These detections preceded a seizure on average by about 12 minutes, but the index could display fluctuations that were not directly followed by seizures. Many of these fluctuations were related to changes of vigilance or behavior. These authors carefully noted that the dynamic changes detected preictally may "represent physiologic changes acting as facilitating factors or pathologic changes reflecting a network dysfunction."

An important assessment study in this context is that by Aschenbrenner-Scheibe et al. [31]. They investigated the sensitivity and specificity of Lehnertz and Elger's method [16, 32, 33] based on estimating a "dimension complexity loss" of sufficient amplitude and duration as indicative of the preictal state. In invasive 24-hour-long EEG recordings from 21 patients with medically refractory partial epilepsies, who underwent invasive presurgical monitoring, they found that only one out of 88 seizures was preceded by a significant preictal "dimension drop." Using another dataset they found that this algorithm resulted in a sensitivity of 38% in hippocampal seizures and 33% in neocortical seizures, considering that a false-positive rate of 0.1/h was allowed. Regarding the clinical applicability of this algorithm, Aschenbrenner-Scheibe et al. [31] concluded with the comment that "used as a pure warning system, a prediction method of this quality would probably be ignored after a short time."

This study produced clear evidence that it is not sufficient to study EEG signals during relatively short periods (namely 1 hour preceding a seizure) in order to estimate the sensitivity and specificity of automatic analysis methods; these estimates

have to be made on long-term EEG recordings lasting many hours, or preferably several days and nights, including the natural variations in wakefulness and sleep state [34, 35]. More refined methods of assessing the statistical validity of algorithms applied in this kind of data have been proposed [36, 37].

Also with respect to other algorithms, subsequent tests under controlled conditions in practice showed that results reported earlier were difficult to reproduce [38]. This was the case for the results obtained using the accumulated energy algorithm of Litt et al. [30], which were not reproduced by Harrison et al. [39]. Maiwald et al. [40] introduced a criterion called the "seizure prediction characteristic" that incorporates the assessment of sensitivity and false-prediction rate to evaluate the performance of seizure prediction algorithms. Applying this criterion, three algorithms were evaluated on a large EEG dataset comprising seizures of 21 patients. The dynamical similarity index [26] yielded 1 to 3.6 false predictions per day and had a sensitivity between 21% and 42%; the accumulated energy algorithm [30] yielded a sensitivity between 18% and 31% for the extended, prospective version; and values between 13% and 30% were found for the effective correlation dimension [33, 41]. Performances at this level preclude clinical applications in a general setting. Similarly, the results obtained using the Lyapunov exponent [15] could not be reproduced by Lai et al. [42] due to finite-time statistical fluctuations and noise. Furthermore, Lai et al. [43] examined in more detail the predictive power of Lyapunov exponents using "control tests" with artificial signals and also applying this method to real electrocorticographic (ECoG) signals. They concluded that the use of Lyapunov exponents for seizure prediction is "practically impossible as the brain dynamical system generating the ECoG signals is more complicated than low-dimensional chaotic systems, and is noisy."

This accumulation of control studies reporting a rather weak performance of the initially proposed algorithms for seizure prediction damped the expanding optimistic mood of this research field into what Mormann et al. [29] called "the rise of skepticism." Nonetheless, the Australian group of Cook et al. [44], the Canadian group of Gadhoumi et al. [45], and a European consortium [46] have made interesting contributions to the field by investigating the long-term monitoring of seizure prediction algorithms in groups of patients.

Cook et al. [44] carried out a feasibility study of the practical usefulness of a seizure advisory system that consisted of creating very long (several months up to more than 1 year in some cases) ECoG recordings in patients with a diversity of partial-onset seizures. The ECoG signals were sent by telemetry to an external device that performed data analysis and provided advisory signals indicating the likelihood (low, moderate, or high) that the patient would have a seizure within a relatively short time window. The algorithm used for the ECoG analysis was patient-specific, based on data collected during a period where at least five seizures were recorded. Although no details of the patient-specific algorithms are given, the sensitivity of the algorithm was calculated for clinically *correlated* seizures (i.e., seizures that were associated with typical clinical manifestations) and also for *equivalent* seizures (i.e., seizures that were electrographically similar to the previous ones but did not display clinical manifestations). The largest high-likelihood sensitivity in the case of correlated seizures reached 100% in two patients (with three seizures each), and the lowest was 18% in another one; in the remaining five patients it varied between 54% and 71%. In general, it was lower, however, if equivalent seizures were also included. The warning times were highly variable. This study may be qualified as yielding the proof-of-concept that it is possible to predict some epileptic seizures in long-term intracranial recordings of some patients, using a patient-specific algorithm, but its clinical usefulness is, as yet, inconclusive.

Gadhoumi et al. [45] investigated the performance of an algorithm that was trained to discriminate between preictal EEG and interictal EEG signals in 17 patients with mesial temporal lobe epilepsy using indwelling electrodes. Scale-free dynamics of the intracerebral EEG were quantified using scaling exponents—the first cumulants—derived from a wavelet leader and bootstrap-based multifractal analysis. These cumulants were investigated for their capacity to discriminate between preictal and interictal epochs. Patient-specific seizure prediction algorithms were thus created and were sequentially tested on long-lasting EEG data. Using the first cumulant in combination with state similarity measures, seizures were predicted above chance with a sensitivity of 80.5% and a specificity of 25.1% of total time under warning for prediction horizons above 25 minutes in up to 13 of 17 patients. These methodologies open novel possibilities for improving seizure prediction performance, but further validation is needed in other clinical settings.

Teixeira et al. [46] conducted a study involving 278 patients recruited from three centers from the European Epilepsy Database [47]. They selected six electrodes from each patient (scalp and intracranial) and computed 22 univariate features for each EEG signal, creating for each patient a training set (the first two or three seizures) and a test set (the remaining seizures). To classify the feature sets, two types of machine-learning techniques were used. In this way, patient-specific predictors of seizures with reasonable performance could anticipate at least 50% of the seizures with a false-alarm rate of less than 1 in 6 h ($<0.15\,h^{-1}$) in 32% of the patients (89 patients). Curiously, the results obtained with scalp electrodes were similar to those obtained with intracranial electrodes. This study presents a comprehensive analysis of many technical aspects that may influence the results.

Using the same EEG database, Bandarabadi et al. [48] tested the contribution of a set of bivariate spectral features. Six EEG channels were used per patient, and five normalized spectral power values within five frequency bands—in other words, 30 normalized spectral power values per EEG epoch. Comparing with other studies the authors stated that their prediction algorithm yielded good results. Nonetheless, more collaborative controlled investigations, making use of data sharing (for practical details see Wagenaar et al. [49]) are necessary. The accumulated evidence to the present indicates that universal predictors that would be applicable in large patient populations have not yet been established. At best, it may be expected that patient-specific EEG predictors that may be practically useful in selected patients will be developed. The lack of a better understanding of the basic mechanisms underlying seizure dynamics remains a substantial impediment.

2.2. Are There Specific Biomarkers of Epilepsy that Also Are Precursors for Impending Seizures?

In addition to applying analytical methods to ongoing EEG signals in general, in the last decade special attention has also been given to particular EEG features that may be considered specific biomarkers of epilepsy, whether or not they are directly related to seizure occurrence. This is the case of the *high-frequency or fast oscillations* (HFOs), which are described in more detail in Chapter 33. HFOs were described in the hippocampus and entorhinal cortex of rats with spontaneous seizures [50], called *fast ripples* (FRs) because they have a higher frequency range (250–500 Hz) than the ripple oscillations (100–200 Hz) described previously in normal brain [51] [52], not only in the limbic cortex but also in the neocortex [53]. It is striking that ripple oscillations do not occur in the dentate gyrus of normal mice [54], such that all fast oscillations above 100 Hz that are recorded in the hippocampal dentate gyrus of pilocarpine-treated epileptic mice are considered biomarkers of the epileptic state and called "pathological HFOs" (pHFOs). Similar FRs were also encountered in the epileptic zones of patients with temporal lobe epilepsy [55]. Furthermore, quite frequently focal seizures begin with HFOs [55, 56]. Nonetheless, not all HFOs are pathological, and basic studies show that different kinds of neuronal mechanisms can account for HFOs [53, 55, 56]. The terminology of the field of gamma oscillations and HFOs is still hazy. A critical challenge is how to obtain experimental evidence to identify the properties of HFOs that may be considered specific biomarkers of epileptic tissue in human. Jacobs et al. [57] found evidence that the occurrence of FRs (250–500 Hz) was associated with the seizure onset zone. The frequency of FRs, however, did not change in a systematic way in the preictal period in seven consecutive patients with mesial temporal lobe epilepsy [58].

The question of how HFOs may be a biomarker of impending seizures has been approached in a computational modeling study [59] that can generate both HFOs and epileptic seizure activities. This model study predicted that only HFOs of bursting type are related to the epileptic condition.

Since the seminal papers mentioned above, a number of studies have been carried out with the precise objective of finding how to discriminate between HFOs occurring under physiological conditions in the normal brain, and pHFOs that may be biomarkers of epileptogenic brain tissue. In particular, the investigation by Matsumoto et al. [60] assumed that HFOs occurring *spontaneously* in epileptic patients may be considered pHFOs, while those *evoked* by specific stimuli may be considered physiological or normal. Compared to normal HFOs (broadband from 50 to 700 Hz), pHFOs had a larger mean spectral amplitude (about double that of normal HFOs), a longer mean duration (mean = 23.1 msec, standard deviation = 19.5), and a lower mean frequency (mean = 188.4 Hz, standard deviation = 104.7). However, this study included only a small group of patients.

Malinowska et al. [61] studied the same phenomenon in a larger population consisting of 45 patients. These authors found that the average rate of pHFOs was higher in the seizure onset zone. Furthermore, these pHFOs presented similar characteristics as those reported by Matsumoto et al. [60]. These authors warn, however, that large numbers of HFOs are necessary to identify a seizure onset zone. This represents a handicap for the practical use of these biomarkers to assess the seizure onset zone in individual patients. In addition, pHFOs did not change in a systematic way in the preictal period and hence do not appear to be indicators of impending seizures—thus, they are not practically useful in the sense of seizure prediction. The question in the heading of this section, for the time being, has to be answered negatively.

The above biomarkers associated with epilepsy are primarily derived from individual-channel EEG recordings and therefore may represent only relatively local properties of the neuronal tissue. Recently introduced alternative approaches dealing with the brain as a highly connected dynamic system [62, 63] are being explored with respect with network dynamics behind the generation of epileptic seizures, but this is still in an exploratory phenomenological phase.

2.3. Active Paradigms for Assessment of the Epileptic Condition Using EEG Signals Triggered by External Stimulation

The study of EEG/MEG signals preceding seizures in photosensitive epileptic patients [64, 65] revealed that the phase clustering of harmonically related frequency components of a subject's MEG/EEG responses evoked by intermittent photic stimulation increases significantly seconds before a seizure occurs. This led to the introduction of a quantity—the phase clustering index (PCI, see [64] for a mathematical description)—by means of which this enhancement can be quantified. This quantity reflects the degree of excitability of the underlying dynamical system and can indicate the presence of nonlinear dynamics. Applying this form of analysis, researchers found that the patients who develop seizures during intermittent photic stimulation present an enhancement of the PCI at the gamma frequency band, compared with that at the driving frequency; this is why the index is called relative PCI (rPCI). The findings obtained in the study of EEG/MEG signals preceding seizures in photosensitive epileptic patients prompted this group to investigate whether rPCI of EEG signals recorded in patients with mesial temporal lobe epilepsy could also predict seizures. In patients with photosensitive epilepsy, a specific visual stimulus (intermittent flickering light) was used, but in patients with mesial temporal lobe epilepsy, it was necessary to resort to deep-brain electrical stimulation using available intracranial electrodes that were implanted for long-term EEG monitoring of seizures. Thus, an *active* electrical direct-stimulation paradigm was developed. With this objective patients were stimulated in the hippocampal formation and neighboring areas by means of indwelling electrodes using short bursts of periodic electrical pulses. These bursts were repeated at intervals of 20 seconds over a long period of hours and even days, at which time the intracranial EEG was sampled in parallel. This stimulation paradigm may be called a carrier frequency modulation probe [66]. The rPCI was computed for all signals and all stimulated epochs of six patients and was found to be larger for the electrode sites near the seizure onset zone compared to those farther away. Even more interesting was the finding that it was possible to forecast the probability of a seizure occurring within a certain time based on the rPCI estimated at a given moment in time (Fig. 23.2). For example, in the patient population analyzed in this study, a value of rPCI above 0.6 predicted that a seizure would occur in less than 2 hours, with an accuracy exceeding 80%.

This study should be considered as a "proof-of-principle" since no further controlled studies have so far been published. Nonetheless, the application of "active probes" opens a novel strategy in the field of seizure anticipation. This led to the conclusion that the rPCI reflects the ability of the neuronal system to generate epileptic discharges. Remarkably, the measurement of rPCI does not involve provoking those discharges, unlike other stimulation-based techniques. Notwithstanding these positive results, the neuronal mechanisms underlying the rPCI remain unexplained. To unravel these mechanisms, combined computational and neurophysiological studies, *in silico, in vitro* and *in vivo*, are necessary [67–70].

The value of using "active" paradigms to test changes in the excitability of neuronal networks that occur in the preictal (or, better, the pro-ictal) period as a seizure approaches has been corroborated by simulations using a computational model of seizure generation. A modeling study by Suffczynski et al. [67] indicated that an active paradigm, combined with appropriate analytical tools such as rPCI, yields more relevant information

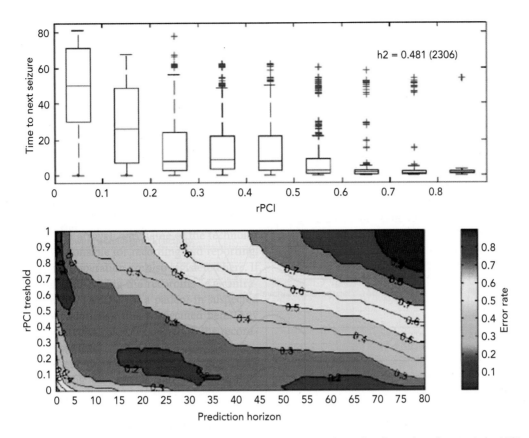

Figure 23.2. Results of the analysis of intracranial EEG signals from patients with temporal lobe epilepsy. The relative phase clustering index (rPCI) was computed for several EEG channels of six patients at various times before seizure onset. Above: Median values and 95% confidence intervals for the six patients are shown along the horizontal axis; along the vertical axis, the time interval to the next seizure is plotted. The rPCI values increase with a decrease in the duration of this interval. Below: Plot of the rPCI value (vertical axis) against the prediction horizon—that is, the time interval to seizure onset. The error rate of the prediction is indicated in color, from a low error (dark blue) to a large error (red, brown). For rPCI values above 0.6 there is a probability of a seizure occurring in less than 2 hours with an accuracy of >80%. Adapted with permission from Kalitzin et al. [66].

about the change in excitability that characterizes the pro-ictal period than do analytical algorithms applied only to the ongoing EEG. Therefore, the development and testing of "active" paradigms with the aim of characterizing excitability changes preceding a seizure deserve further investigation.

The importance of active paradigms also arises in studies of quite different tools. This is the case of the investigation by Badawy et al. [71], who used transcranial magnetic stimulation in patients with different forms of epilepsy (generalized, focal, or focal with secondary generalization) to determine the cortical motor threshold and paired pulse recovery curves (at short [2–15 msec] and long [50–400 msec] interstimulus intervals) at 24 hours before a seizure, and also in the postseizure period. They found decreased motor threshold, increased intracortical facilitation, and decreased intracortical inhibition, indicative of an increase in cortical excitability and/or a decrease in cortical inhibitory processes, at short and long interstimulus intervals, in the 24 hours before a seizure—but the opposite changes in the 24 hours after a seizure. Nonetheless, these results are based on measurements of averages of the transcranial magnetic stimulation responses obtained in experimental sessions that lasted for 60 to 90 minutes. These measurements were not followed for a long time, so it is not known whether these changes co-vary with the progressive approximation of a seizure.

3. ANALYTICAL AND COMPUTATIONAL MODELS AS INSTRUMENTS FOR SYSTEM DYNAMICS RECONSTRUCTION AND CONTROL

In this section we depart from the "evidence-based" EEG signal analysis and focus on the rapidly growing model-based neuronal *system analysis*. These analytical and computational models can not only describe the observed EEG behavior but can also predict critical system properties and even prescribe approaches for corrective interventions leading to the abatement of epileptic activity by reactive direct stimulation of the brain.

3.1. Model-Based EEG Signal Description in Terms of Underlying System Features and Architecture

A basic problem in developing reliable methods of anticipating seizures is that at present relatively little is known about the dynamics of the neuronal processes leading to seizures, as mentioned above. Nonetheless, some theoretical concepts have been formulated that are essential to gain insight into these processes, as well as to put in perspective experimental findings in animals and humans.

In this context, we assume that in the epileptic brain, some neuronal networks possess an abnormal set of parameters that enable the occurrence of different kinds of dynamical states. In other words, these networks may have bi- or multi-stable properties. This means that, in addition to a normal steady state, they also have an abnormal one characterized by widespread synchronous activity, and that the transition between these two states may occur more or less abruptly. This accounts for the two main characteristics of epilepsy: (a) that an epileptic brain can function apparently normally between seizures (i.e., during the interictal state) and (b) that the seizures occur in a paroxysmal way, thereby impairing brain functioning transiently. In this sense, epileptic disorders may be considered special cases of the large class of dynamical diseases, meaning those pathophysiological states characterized as intermittent occurrence of abnormal dynamics, a theoretical concept proposed by Glass and Mackey [72] and Bélair et al. [73], and also extended to the domain of epilepsy[74][75].

The theory of nonlinear dynamics offers the possibility to understand, in formal terms, how the manifestations of dynamical diseases take place. In general we can distinguish [68, 75–77] two basic models that can account for transitions to an epileptic seizure. Above we presented some of the properties of complex nonlinear dynamical systems, but a further element should be added. These systems possess attractors—that is, sets of values to which a dynamical system settles some time after being perturbed, or in mathematical terminology an asymptotically stable manifold in the phase space of the system. Topologically, an attractor can be a point, a curve like a limit cycle, a manifold, or even a complicated set with a fractal structure known as a strange attractor; the latter is typical of a chaotic dynamical system. With respect to

epilepsy in general, we proposed [75, 76] the following general scheme:

Model 1: Bifurcation model—Bi- or multi-stable systems where jumps between two or more coexisting attractors can take place, caused by stochastic fluctuations (noise) of any input. In this case the transition between interictal state and a seizure may occur at random due to some fluctuations in input conditions or in some system's parameters—in other words, seizures can be generated autonomously due to internal instability causing intermittent behavior (Fig. 23.3). An example of this model type 1 is the occurrence of spike-and-wave discharges in the thalamocortical system, typical of absence seizures (see Section 3.4 of Chapter 3).

Model 2: Deformation model—Systems with deformable parameters such that the dynamics may evolve from one attractor that represents the normal, or interictal state, to another attractor or to a series of attractors. An example of model type 2 is the occurrence of partial seizures in mesial temporal lobe epilepsy (see Section 3.3 of Chapter 3). The parametric deformation may be caused by the fact that some parameters may be (biologically) unstable, may be sensitive to some endogenous modulating influences (e.g., chemical neurotransmitters, hormones, composition of extracellular medium, such as $[K^+]_o$, pH, blood glucose levels), or may be induced by an external stimulus (e.g., sensory stimulus, as in reflex epilepsies). An interesting observation in this respect was presented by Baumgartner et al. [78], who performed preictal single photo emission computed tomography (SPECT) scans fortuitously while video-EEG monitoring was being carried out in

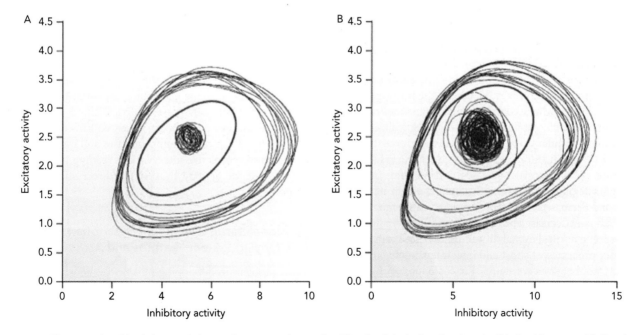

Figure 23.3. Phase portraits of the thalamocortical system in two cases: A: normal and B: epileptic brain. Sample trajectories (thin lines) from normal (left) and epileptic model (right) projected onto a two-dimensional slice of state space. The axes are values of two state variables: cortical excitatory and inhibitory activity. The thick line separates two attractors. Adapted with permission from Lopes da Silva et al. [76] and Lytton [97].

two patients with temporal lobe epilepsy. These authors found in preictal SPECT a significant increase in regional cerebral blood flow in the epileptic temporal lobe that was not associated with significant changes in the ongoing EEG. They interpreted this finding as indicating that the changes in regional cerebral blood flow observed on peri-ictal SPECT may reflect a subtle change in neuronal activity precipitating the transition from the interictal to the ictal state.

In addition, we can also consider systems displaying a *combination of these two processes*—that is, scenarios where the system "deforms" from a single attractor to multi-stable dynamics (bifurcation). One feature of both the bifurcation and deformation models is that they are not, strictly speaking, autonomous. They need external or endogenous inputs in order to enable the transitions to occur, and these may be realized in a multitude of ways. The term "spontaneous seizures" simply expresses our lack of knowledge about those enabling or precipitating factors.

Recently the possibility of a third class of models of epileptic seizure generation has been put forward. In these models the system possesses a feature called dynamic intermittency [79–81], such that transitions to epileptiform activity would occur autonomously, without the intervention of any endogenous or exogenous factor. Although intermittency has been suggested as a possible mechanism for seizure

generation [82], a realistic neuronal model of intermittency expressed in terms of changes in neuronal dynamics has yet to be developed.

Modeling studies throw new light on the issue of how the deformation of certain parameters in a neuronal network can cause its dynamics to evolve to a full-blown seizure. In this respect an important advance was provided by the models of Wendling et al. [83, 84] showing how the deformation of a small number of specific parameters (GABA-ergic synaptic transmission both with slow and fast kinetics) leads to a succession of phases characterized by different EEG patterns (spikes, bursts of HFOs) and ultimately to a seizure. These computational models describe the collective dynamics of large neuronal populations and rely on physiologically realistic properties (Fig. 23.4).

Another class of models that use general mathematical features of the neuronal dynamics have been developed as well. A recent example in this context is the generic model called Epileptor [85], which describes the most predominant kinds of epileptic seizures displaying saddle-node and homoclinic bifurcations to explain seizure onset and termination. In this model a slow permittivity parameter controls these dynamic bifurcations.

Besides their general scientific value, computational models may become indispensable as testing tools for experimenting signal analytical procedures and developing new EEG feature extraction techniques.

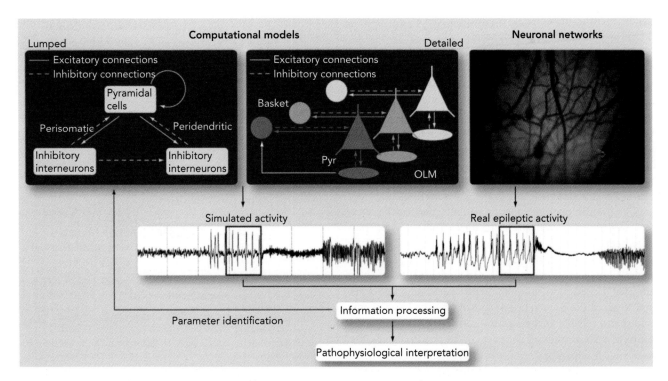

Figure 23.4. *Computational model (left-hand side) based on a lumped approach of a hippocampal network (based on the representation of neuronal subpopulations of pyramidal neurons and two populations of interneurons) and a real neuronal network (right-hand side, based on the explicit representation of cells and interconnections) approach. Simulated activity (local field potentials) can be quantitatively compared to real activity using information-processing techniques. This quantitative analysis allows for identifying the parameter settings for which models best reproduce real data. Performing this identification over a sliding time window can trace the evolution of model parameters, providing information on the mechanisms responsible for the transition between normal and seizure states. Adapted with permission from Wendling [84].*

3.2. Model Prescriptions for EEG-Based Reactive Control of Dynamic Transitions

Another dimension concerning the issue of seizure anticipation is the development of approaches aiming at *seizure control*, which use EEG-based reactive control to avoid seizure occurrence or to abort seizures at a very early stage. Theoretical studies [86, 87] showed that seizures can be aborted with accurately tuned stimulation intervention. Experimentally, this possibility has been demonstrated [88, 89] in animal models of epileptic seizures. Preventive stimulation may even be preferred in order to keep the system constantly away from an epileptic seizure transition. Another model has prescribed a stimulation paradigm aimed at system desynchronization [90]. The prediction ability of this model has been tested and validated in an animal model of epilepsy [91].

4. CONCLUDING REMARKS

A deeper insight into the nature of epileptic seizures and their initiation, termination, and possible anticipation, should include related dynamic phenomena such as the generation of interictal activities and postictal generalized electrographic suppression and also cortical spreading depression [92, 93]. Incorporating all these features into a comprehensive model is a formidable challenge, but such a model may pave the way for the development of novel therapeutic strategies.

The road toward the development of methodologies aiming at the reliable detection of a pro-ictal state has been full of exciting theoretical challenges, clever experimental approaches, and some disappointments. Even though the scientific community has learned a lot about the dynamics of neuronal networks in the context of epileptic seizures in the past two decades, we are still far from having a generally accepted and robust approach for seizure anticipation. A positive development is that the community has set up a number of workshops on seizure prediction (see [8, 94]) and a digital database that can be used to develop and test suitable algorithms in a real collaborative effort. The need for new strategies in this field is becoming even more pressing since the access to deep-brain stimulation techniques for a variety of brain diseases is now also open to epileptic patients, particularly those who have pharmacologically refractory disease and yet have either been rejected for a surgical intervention or have failed to respond to epilepsy surgery. Thus, it would be desirable to have reliable methods capable of seizure anticipation so that a dedicated "closed-loop" stimulation procedure might be developed to avoid the occurrence of seizures on the basis of continuous and reliable analysis of the running EEG record. The success of such procedures depends on the possibility of either foreseeing an impending seizure or detecting its occurrence at the earliest possible stage, and only then applying a counter-stimulus to arrest it. In a recent review, Gadhoumi et al. [95] concluded that the majority of published approaches suggests that seizure prediction may work better in closed-loop seizure-control devices rather than as seizure advisory devices. A few closed-loop approaches are starting to be explored, namely using properties of the measured EEG signal to determine the exact timing of the counter-stimulation or generating an appropriate seizure-suppression stimulation waveform [96]. We may refer to the latter as "state-reactive control." This topic is discussed theoretically in more detail by Kalitzin et al. [77], who provide arguments to justify different scenarios for seizure control depending on different dynamical models of seizure generation.

This challenging field requires the convergence of a variety of disciplines and scientific approaches to achieve results that may have practical usefulness in clinical epilepsy.

REFERENCES

1. A. Schulze-Bonhage, C. Kurth, A. Carius, B. J. Steinhoff and T. Mayer, *Seizure anticipation by patients with focal and generalized epilepsy: A multicentre assessment of premonitory symptoms*, Epilepsy Research 2006;70(1):83–88.
2. A. Scaramelli, P. Braga, A. Avellanal, A. Bogacz, C. Camejo, I. Rega, T. Messano and B. Arciere, *Prodromal symptoms in epileptic patients: Clinical characterization of the pre-ictal phase*, Seizure 2009;18(4):246–250.
3. H. Zaveri, M. Frei and I. Osorio, State of seizure prediction: A report on informal discussions with participation of the 3rd international workshop on seizure prediction. In: B. Schelter, J. Timmer and A. Schulze-Bonhage (Eds.), *Seizure prediction in epilepsy*. Weinheim: John Wiley/VCH Verlag, 2008:325–330.
4. M. Scheffer, J. Bascompte, W. A. Brock, V. Brovkin, S. R. Carpenter, V. Dakos, H. Held, E. H. van Nes, M. Rietkerk and G. Sugihara, *Early-warning signals for critical transitions*, Nature 2009;461(7260):53–59.
5. J. Gotman and M. G. Marciani, *Electroencephalographic spiking activity, drug levels, and seizure occurrence in epileptic patients*, Annals of Neurology 1985;17(6):597–603.
6. B. Krishnan, I. Vlachos, A. Faith, S. Mullane, K. Williams, A. Alexopoulos and L. Iasemidis, *A novel spatiotemporal analysis of peri-ictal spiking to probe the relation of spikes and seizures in epilepsy*, Annals of Biomedical Engineering 2014;42(8):1606–1617.
7. S. S. Viglione and G. O. Walsh, *Proceedings: Epileptic seizure prediction*, Electroencephalography and Clinical Neurophysiology 1975;39(4):435–436.
8. B. J. Gluckman and C. A. Schevon, *Seizure prediction 6: from mechanisms to engineered interventions for epilepsy*, Journal of Clinical Neurophysiology 2015;32 (3): 181–187.
9. Z. Rogowski, I. Gath and E. Bental, *On the prediction of epileptic seizures*, Biological Cybernetics 1981;42(1):9–15.
10. Y. Salant, I. Gath and O. Henriksen, *Prediction of epileptic seizures from two-channel eeg*, Medical & Biological Engineering & Computing 1998;36(5):549–556.
11. A. Babloyantz and A. Destexhe, *Low-dimensional chaos in an instance of epilepsy*, Proceedings of the National Academy of Sciences of the United States of America 1986;83(10):3513–3517.
12. J. P. Pijn, J. Van Neerven, A. Noest and F. H. Lopes da Silva, *Chaos or noise in EEG signals; dependence on state and brain site*, Electroencephalography and clinical neurophysiology 1991;79(5):371–381.
13. L. Iasemidis, J. Principe, J. Czaplewski, R. Gilmore, S. Roper and J. C. RSackellares, Spatiotemporal transitions to epileptic seizures: A nonlinear dynamical analysis of scalp and intracranial EEG recordings. In F. Lopes da Silva, J. Principe and L. Almeida (Eds.), *Spatiotemporal models in biological and artificial systems*. Amsterdam: IOS Press, 1996:81–88.
14. L. D. Iasemidis, L. D. Olson, R. S. Savit and J. C. Sackellares, *Time dependencies in the occurrences of epileptic seizures*, Epilepsy Research 1994;17(1):81–94.
15. L. D. Iasemidis, J. C. Sackellares, H. P. Zaveri and W. J. Williams, *Phase space topography and the Lyapunov exponent of electrocorticograms in partial seizures*, Brain Topography 1990;2(3):187–201.
16. K. Lehnertz and C. E. Elger, *Spatio-temporal dynamics of the primary epileptogenic area in temporal lobe epilepsy characterized by neuronal complexity loss*, Electroencephalography and Clinical Neurophysiology 1995;95(2):108–117.
17. J. Martinerie, C. Adam, M. Le Van Quyen, M. Baulac, S. Clemenceau, B. Renault and F. J. Varela, *Epileptic seizures can be anticipated by non-linear analysis*, Nature Medicine 1998;4(10):1173–1176.

18. W. S. Pritchard and D. W. Duke, *Measuring chaos in the brain: A tutorial review of nonlinear dynamical EEG analysis*, International Journal of Neuroscience 1992;67(1–4):31–80.

19. J. P. Pijn, D. N. Velis, M. J. van der Heyden, J. DeGoede, C. W. van Veelen and F. H. Lopes da Silva, *Nonlinear dynamics of epileptic seizures on basis of intracranial EEG recordings*, Brain Topography 1997;9(4):249–270.

20. L. D. Iasemidis, D. S. Shiau, W. Chaovalitwongse, J. C. Sackellares, P. M. Pardalos, J. C. Principe, P. R. Carney, A. Prasad, B. Veeramani and K. Tsakalis, *Adaptive epileptic seizure prediction system*, IEEE Transactions on Biomedical Engineering 2003;50(5):616–627.

21. M. Le Van Quyen, J. Martinerie, M. Baulac and F. Varela, *Anticipating epileptic seizures in real time by a non-linear analysis of similarity between EEG recordings*, Neuroreport 1999;10(10):2149–2155.

22. M. Le Van Quyen, C. Adam, J. Martinerie, M. Baulac, S. Clemenceau and F. Varela, *Spatio-temporal characterizations of non-linear changes in intracranial activities prior to human temporal lobe seizures*, European Journal of Neuroscience 2000;12(6):2124–2134.

23. M. Le Van Quyen, *Anticipating epileptic seizures: From mathematics to clinical applications*, Comptes Rendus Biologiques 2005;328(2):187–198.

24. M. Le Van Quyen, F. Amor and D. Rudrauf, *Exploring the dynamics of collective synchronizations in large ensembles of brain signals*, Journal of Physiology (Paris) 2006;100(4):194–200.

25. V. Navarro, J. Martinerie, M. Le Van Quyen, S. Clemenceau, C. Adam, M. Baulac and F. Varela, *Seizure anticipation in human neocortical partial epilepsy*, Brain 2002;125(Pt 3):640–655.

26. V. Navarro, J. Martinerie, M. Le Van Quyen, M. Baulac, F. Dubeau and J. Gotman, *Seizure anticipation: Do mathematical measures correlate with video-EEG evaluation?* Epilepsia 2005;46(3):385–396.

27. M. Le Van Quyen, J. Martinerie, V. Navarro, P. Boon, M. D'Have, C. Adam, B. Renault, F. Varela and M. Baulac, *Anticipation of epileptic seizures from standard EEG recordings*, Lancet 2001;357(9251):183–188.

28. D. Rudrauf, A. Douiri, C. Kovach, J. P. Lachaux, D. Cosmelli, M. Chavez, C. Adam, B. Renault, J. Martinerie and M. Le Van Quyen, *Frequency flows and the time-frequency dynamics of multivariate phase synchronization in brain signals*, NeuroImage 2006;31(1):209–227.

29. F. Mormann, R. G. Andrzejak, C. E. Elger and K. Lehnertz, *Seizure prediction: The long and winding road*, Brain 2007;130(Pt 2):314–333.

30. B. Litt, R. Esteller, J. Echauz, M. D'Alessandro, R. Shor, T. Henry, P. Pennell, C. Epstein, R. Bakay, M. Dichter and G. Vachtsevanos, *Epileptic seizures may begin hours in advance of clinical onset: A report of five patients*, Neuron 2001;30(1):51–64.

31. R. Aschenbrenner-Scheibe, T. Maiwald, M. Winterhalder, H. U. Voss, J. Timmer and A. Schulze-Bonhage, *How well can epileptic seizures be predicted? An evaluation of a nonlinear method*, Brain 2003;126(Pt 12):2616–2626.

32. K. Lehnertz, R. G. Andrzejak, J. Arnhold, T. Kreuz, F. Mormann, C. Rieke, Widman and C. E. Elger, *Nonlinear EEG analysis in epilepsy: Its possible use for interictal focus localization, seizure anticipation, and prevention*, Journal of Clinical Neurophysiology 2001;18(3):209–222.

33. C. E. Elger and K. Lehnertz, *Seizure prediction by non-linear time series analysis of brain electrical activity*, European Journal of Neuroscience 1998;10(2):786–789.

34. B. Litt and K. Lehnertz, *Seizure prediction and the preseizure period*, Current Opinion in Neurology 2002;15(2):173–177.

35. B. Litt and J. Echauz, *Prediction of epileptic seizures*, Lancet Neurology 2002;1(1):22–30.

36. B. Schelter, H. Feldwisch-Drentrup, J. Timmer, J. Gotman and A. Schulze-Bonhage, *A common strategy and database to compare the performance of seizure prediction algorithms*, Epilepsy & Behavior 2010;17(2):154–156.

37. B. Schelter, M. Winterhalder, T. Maiwald, A. Brandt, A. Schad, A. Schulze-Bonhage and J. Timmer, *Testing statistical significance of multivariate time series analysis techniques for epileptic seizure prediction*, Chaos 2006;16(1):013108.

38. M. A. Harrison, I. Osorio, M. G. Frei, S. Asuri and Y. C. Lai, *Correlation dimension and integral do not predict epileptic seizures*, Chaos 2005;15(3):33106.

39. M. A. Harrison, M. G. Frei and I. Osorio, *Accumulated energy revisited*, Clinical Neurophysiology 2005;116(3):527–531.

40. T. Maiwald, M. Winterhalder, R. Aschenbrenner-Scheibe, H. Voss, A. Schulze-Bonhage and J. Timmer, *Comparison of three nonlinear seizure prediction methods by means of the seizure prediction characteristic*, Physica D 2004;194(3-4):357–368.

41. B. Weber, K. Lehnertz, C. E. Elger and H. G. Wieser, *Neuronal complexity loss in interictal EEG recorded with foramen ovale electrodes predicts side of primary epileptogenic area in temporal lobe epilepsy: A replication study*, Epilepsia 1998;39(9):922–927.

42. Y. C. Lai, M. A. Harrison, M. G. Frei and I. Osorio, *Inability of Lyapunov exponents to predict epileptic seizures*, Physical Review Letters 2003;91(6):068102.

43. *Controlled test for predictive power of Lyapunov exponents: Their inability to predict epileptic seizures*, Chaos 2004;14(3):630–642.

44. M. J. Cook, T. J. O'Brien, S. F. Berkovic, M. Murphy, A. Morokoff, G. Fabinyi, W. D'Souza, R. Yerra, J. Archer, L. Litewka, S. Hosking, P. Lightfoot, V. Ruedebusch, W. D. Sheffield, D. Snyder, K. Leyde and D. Himes, *Prediction of seizure likelihood with a long-term, implanted seizure advisory system in patients with drug-resistant epilepsy: A first-in-man study*, Lancet Neurology 2013;12(6):563–571.

45. K. Gadhoumi, J. M. Lina and J. Gotman, *Seizure invariance properties of intracerebral EEG improve seizure prediction in Mesial Temporal Lobe Epilepsy*, PLoS ONE 2015;10(4):e0121182:1–23.

46. C. Teixeira, B. Direito, M. Bandarabadi and A. Dourado, *Output regularization of SVM seizure predictors: Kalman filter versus the "firing power" method*, Conference proceedings: Annual International Conference of the IEEE Engineering in Medicine and Biology Society, 2012:6530–6533.

47. J. Klatt, H. Feldwisch-Drentrup, M. Ihle, V. Navarro, M. Neufang, C. Teixeira, C. Adam, M. Valderrama, C. Alvarado-Rojas, A. Witon, M. Le Van Quyen, F. Sales, A. Dourado, J. Timmer, A. Schulze-Bonhage and B. Schelter, *The Epilepsiae database: An extensive electroencephalography database of epilepsy patients*, Epilepsia 2012;53(9):1669–1676.

48. M. Bandarabadi, C. A. Teixeira, J. Rasekhi and A. Dourado, *Epileptic seizure prediction using relative spectral power features*, Clinical Neurophysiology 2015;126(2):237–248.

49. J. B. Wagenaar, G. A. Worrell, Z. Ives, D. Matthias, B. Litt and A. Schulze-Bonhage, *Collaborating and sharing data in epilepsy research*, Journal of Clinical Neurophysiology 2015;32(3):235–239.

50. A. Bragin, C. L. Wilson, R. J. Staba, M. Reddick, I. Fried and J. Engel, Jr., *Interictal high-frequency oscillations (80–500 Hz) in the human epileptic brain: Entorhinal cortex*, Annals of Neurology 2002;52(4):407–415.

51. G. Buzsaki, Z. Horvath, R. Urioste, J. Hetke and K. Wise, *High-frequency network oscillation in the hippocampus*, Science 1992;256(5059):1025–1027.

52. J. Csicsvari, B. Jamieson, K. D. Wise and G. Buzsaki, *Mechanisms of gamma oscillations in the hippocampus of the behaving rat*, Neuron 2003;37(2):311–322.

53. G. Buzsaki and F. Lopes da Silva, *High-frequency oscillations in the intact brain*, Progress in Neurobiology 2012;98(3):241–249.

54. A. Bragin, S. K. Benassi, F. Kheiri and J. Engel, Jr., *Further evidence that pathologic high-frequency oscillations are bursts of population spikes derived from recordings of identified cells in dentate gyrus*, Epilepsia 2011;52(1):45–52.

55. A. Bragin, J. Engel, Jr., C. L. Wilson, I. Fried and G. Buzsaki, *High-frequency oscillations in human brain*, Hippocampus 1999;9(2):137–142.

56. R. D. Traub, A. Draguhn, M. A. Whittington, T. Baldeweg, A. Bibbig, E. H. Buhl and D. Schmitz, *Axonal gap junctions between principal neurons: A novel source of network oscillations, and perhaps epileptogenesis*, Reviews in the Neurosciences 2002;13(1):1–30.

57. J. Jacobs, M. Zijlmans, R. Zelmann, C. E. Chatillon, J. Hall, A. Olivier, F. Dubeau and J. Gotman, *High-frequency electroencephalographic oscillations correlate with outcome of epilepsy surgery*, Annals of Neurology 2010;67(2):209–220.

58. J. Jacobs, R.Zelmann, J. Jirsch, R. Chander, CE Chatillon, F. Dubeau, J. Gotman, High frequency oscillations (80 – 500 Hz) in the preictal period in patients with focal seizures, Epilepsia 2009;50(7):1770–1792.

59. R. M. Helling, M. M. Koppert, G. H. Visser and S. N. Kalitzin, *Gap junctions as common cause of high-frequency oscillations and epileptic seizures in a computational cascade of neuronal mass and compartmental modeling*, International Journal of Neural Systems 2015;25(6):1550021.

60. A. Matsumoto, B. H. Brinkmann, S. Matthew Stead, J. Matsumoto, M. T. Kucewicz, W. R. Marsh, F. Meyer and G. Worrell, *Pathological and physiological high-frequency oscillations in focal human epilepsy*, Journal of Neurophysiology 2013;110(8):1958–1964.

61. U. Malinowska, G. K. Bergey, J. Harezlak and C. C. Jouny, *Identification of seizure onset zone and preictal state based on characteristics of high frequency oscillations*, Clinical Neurophysiology 2015;126(8):1505–1513.

62. C. J. Stam, *Use of magnetoencephalography (MEG) to study functional brain networks in neurodegenerative disorders*, Journal of the Neurological Sciences 2010;289(1-2):128–134.

63. C. J. Stam, *Characterization of anatomical and functional connectivity in the brain: A complex networks perspective*, International Journal of Psychophysiology 2010;77(3):186–194.

64. S. Kalitzin, J. Parra, D. N. Velis and F. H. Lopes da Silva, *Enhancement of phase clustering in the EEG/MEG gamma frequency band anticipates transitions to paroxysmal epileptiform activity in epileptic patients with known visual sensitivity*, IEEE Transactions on Biomedical Engineering 2002;49(11):1279–1286.

65. J. Parra, S. N. Kalitzin, J. Iriarte, W. Blanes, D. N. Velis and F. H. Lopes da Silva, *Gamma-band phase clustering and photosensitivity: Is there an underlying mechanism common to photosensitive epilepsy and visual perception?* Brain 2003;126(Pt 5):1164–1172.

66. S. Kalitzin, D. Velis, P. Suffczynski, J. Parra and F. Lopes da Silva, *Electrical brain-stimulation paradigm for estimating the seizure onset site and the time to ictal transition in temporal lobe epilepsy*, Clinical Neurophysiology 2005;116(3):718–728.

67. P. Suffczynski, S. Kalitzin, F. Lopes da Silva, J. Parra, D. Velis and F. Wendling, *Active paradigms of seizure anticipation: Computer model evidence for necessity of stimulation*, Physical Review E: Statistical, Nonlinear, and Soft Matter Physics 2008;78(5 Pt 1):051917.

68. S. Kalitzin, M. Koppert, G. Petkov, D. Velis and F. Lopes da Silva, *Computational model prospective on the observation of proictal states in epileptic neuronal systems*, Epilepsy & Behavior 2011;22(Suppl 1):S102–109.

69. M. Koppert, S. Kalitzin, D. Velis and F. Lopes da Silva and M. A. Viergever, *Dynamics of collective multi-stability in models of multi-unit neuronal systems*, International Journal of Neural Systems 2014;24(2):1430004.

70. L. Kuhlmann, D. B. Grayden, F. Wendling and S. J. Schiff, *Role of multiple-scale modeling of epilepsy in seizure forecasting*, Journal of Clinical Neurophysiology 2015;32(3):220–226.

71. R. Badawy, R. Macdonell, G. Jackson and S. Berkovic, *The periictal state: Cortical excitability changes within 24 h of a seizure*, Brain 2009;132(Pt 4):1013–1021.

72. L. Glass and M. Mackey, *The rhythms of life*, Princeton, NJ: Princeton University Press, 1988.

73. J. Belair, L. Glass, U. An Der Heiden and J. Milton, *Dynamical disease: Identification, temporal aspects and treatment strategies of human illness*, Chaos 1995;5(1):1–7.

74. R. G. Andrzejak, G. Widman, K. Lehnertz, C. Rieke, P. David and C. E. Elger, *The epileptic process as nonlinear deterministic dynamics in a stochastic environment: An evaluation on mesial temporal lobe epilepsy*, Epilepsy Research 2001;44(2-3):129–140.

75. F. Lopes da Silva, W. Blanes, S. N. Kalitzin, J. Parra, P. Suffczynski and D. N. Velis, *Epilepsies as dynamical diseases of brain systems: Basic models of the transition between normal and epileptic activity*, Epilepsia 2003;44(Suppl 12):72–83.

76. F. H. Lopes da Silva, W. Blanes, S. N. Kalitzin, J. Parra, P. Suffczynski and D. N. Velis, *Dynamical diseases of brain systems: Different routes to epileptic seizures*, IEEE Transactions on Biomedical Engineering 2003;50(5):540–548.

77. S. N. Kalitzin, D. N. Velis and F. H. Lopes da Silva, *Stimulation-based anticipation and control of state transitions in the epileptic brain*, Epilepsy & Behavior 2010;17(3):310–323.

78. C. Baumgartner, W. Serles, F. Leutmezer, E. Pataraia, S. Aull, T. Czech, U. Pietrzyk, A. Relic and I. Podreka, *Preictal SPECT in temporal lobe epilepsy: Regional cerebral blood flow is increased prior to electroencephalography-seizure onset*, Journal of Nuclear Medicine 1998;39(6):978–982.

79. E. Ohayon, H. Kwan, W. Burnham, P. Suffczynski, F. Lopes da Silva and S. Kalitzin, *Adaptable intermittency and autonomous transitions in epilepsy and cognition*, In: R. Wang, E. Shen and F. Gu (Eds.), *Advances in cognitive neurodynamics, ICCN 2007*. Dordrecht: Springer, 2007:485–490.

80. E. L. Ohayon, S. Kalitzin, P. Suffczynski, F. Y. Jin, P. W. Tsang, D. S. Borrett, W. M. Burnham and H. C. Kwan, *Charting epilepsy by searching for intelligence in network space with the help of evolving autonomous agents*, Journal of Physiology (Paris) 2004;98(4-6):507–529.

81. O. C. Zalay and B. L. Bardakjian, *Mapped clock oscillators as ring devices and their application to neuronal electrical rhythms*, IEEE Transactions on Neural Systems and Rehabilitation Engineering 2008;16(3):233–244.

82. J. L. Velazquez, H. Khosravani, A. Lozano, B. L. Bardakjian, P. L. Carlen and R. Wennberg, *Type III intermittency in human partial epilepsy*, European Journal of Neuroscience 1999;11(7):2571–2576.

83. F. Wendling, F. Bartolomei, J. J. Bellanger and P. Chauvel, *Epileptic fast activity can be explained by a model of impaired GABAergic dendritic inhibition*, European Journal of Neuroscience 2002;15(9):1499–1508.

84. F. Wendling, *Computational models of epileptic activity: A bridge between observation and pathophysiological interpretation*, Expert Review of Neurotherapeutics 2008;8(6):889–896.

85. V. K. Jirsa, W. C. Stacey, P. P. Quilichini, A. I. Ivanov and C. Bernard, *On the nature of seizure dynamics*, Brain 2014;137(Pt 8):2210–2230.

86. P. Suffczynski, S. Kalitzin and F. H. Lopes Da Silva, *Dynamics of nonconvulsive epileptic phenomena modeled by a bistable neuronal network*, Neuroscience 2004;126(2):467–484.

87. M. Koppert, S. Kalitzin, D. Velis, F. H. Lopes da Silva and M. A. Viergever, *Reactive control of epileptiform discharges in realistic computational neuronal models with bistability*, International Journal of Neural Systems 2013;23(1):1250032.

88. I. Osorio and M. G. Frei, *Seizure abatement with single DC pulses: Is phase resetting at play?*, International Journal of Neural Systems 2009;19(3):149–156.

89. A. Berenyi, M. Belluscio, D. Mao and G. Buzsaki, *Closed-loop control of epilepsy by transcranial electrical stimulation*, Science 2012;337(6095):735–737.

90. P. A. Tass and C. Hauptmann, *Therapeutic modulation of synaptic connectivity with desynchronizing brain stimulation*, International Journal of Psychophysiology 2007;64(1):53–61.

91. V. R. Cota, D de C. Medeiros, M. R. Vilela, M. C. Doretto and M. F. Moraes, *Distinct patterns of electrical stimulation of the basolateral amygdala influence pentylenetetrazole seizure outcome*, Epilepsy & Behavior 2009;14(Suppl 1):26–31.

92. Y. Wei, G. Ullah and S. J. Schiff, *Unification of neuronal spikes, seizures, and spreading depression*, Journal of Neuroscience 2014;34(35):11733–11743.

93. K. El Houssaini, A. I. Ivanov, C. Bernard and V. K. Jirsa, *Seizures, refractory status epilepticus, and depolarization block as endogenous brain activities*, Physical Review E: Statistical, Nonlinear, and Soft Matter Physics 2015;91(1):010701.

94. M. G. Frei, H. P. Zaveri, S. Arthurs, G. K. Bergey, C. C. Jouny, K. Lehnertz, J. Gotman, I. Osorio, T. I. Netoff, W. J. Freeman, J. Jefferys, G. Worrell, V. Quyen Mle, S. J. Schiff and F. Mormann, *Controversies in epilepsy: Debates held during the fourth international workshop on seizure prediction*, Epilepsy & behavior 2010;19(1):4–16.

95. K. Gadhoumi, J. M. Lina, F. Mormann and J. Gotman, *Seizure prediction for therapeutic devices: A review*, Journal of Neuroscience Methods 2016;260:270–282.

96. G. Ullah and S. J. Schiff, *Tracking and control of neuronal Hodgkin-Huxley dynamics*, Physical Review E: Statistical, Nonlinear, and Soft Matter Physics 2009;79(4 Pt 1):040901.

97. W. W. Lytton, *Computer modelling of epilepsy*, Nature Reviews Neuroscience 2008;9(8):626–637.

24 | NONEPILEPTIC EVENTS

DAVID K. CHEN, MD AND W. CURT LAFRANCE, JR., MD, MPH

ABSTRACT: Nonepileptic events (NEE) represent important differential diagnoses in patients with neurobehavioral paroxysms, especially those with apparent drug-resistant epilepsy. Errant recognition of NEE may not only subject the patient to potential complications of unnecessary epilepsy treatment, but delay the delivery of treatment that properly addresses the underlying pathology. For many patients with NEE, such as those with the conversion disorder psychogenic nonepileptic seizures (PNES) or with physiologic NEE (e.g., cardiac-induced syncope), delays in the provision of proper treatment have been shown to be associated with significant morbidity. This review focuses on clinical evaluations aiming to enhance the recognition of the different etiologies of NEE and distinguish between NEE and epilepsy, as well as between NEE of varying pathologies. Evidence-based treatments and management of NEE, particularly those pertaining to PNES, will also be discussed.

KEYWORDS: differential diagnosis, nonepileptic events, psychogenic nonepileptic seizures, conversion disorder, treatment, epilepsy

PRINCIPAL REFERENCES

1. LaFrance WC Jr, Baker GA, Duncan R, et al. Minimum requirements for the diagnosis of psychogenic nonepileptic seizures: a staged approach: a report from the International League Against Epilepsy Nonepileptic Seizures Task Force. Epilepsia 2013;54(11):2005–2018.
2. Moya A, Sutton R, Ammirati F, et al. Guidelines for the diagnosis and management of syncope (version 2009): the Task Force for the Diagnosis and Management of Syncope of the European Society of Cardiology (ESC). Eur Heart J 2009;30(21):2631–2671.
3. LaFrance WC Jr, Reuber M, Goldstein LH. Management of psychogenic nonepileptic seizures. Epilepsia 2013;54(Suppl 1):53–67.
4. Soteriades ES, Evans JC, Larson MG, et al. Incidence and prognosis of syncope. N Engl J Med 2002;347(12):878–885.
5. Lempert T, Bauer M, Schmidt D. Syncope: a videometric analysis of 56 episodes of transient cerebral hypoxia. Ann Neurol 1994;36(2):233–237.
6. Goldstein LH, Chalder T, Chigwedere C, et al. Cognitive-behavioral therapy for psychogenic nonepileptic seizures: a pilot RCT. Neurology 2010;74(24):1986–1994.
7. LaFrance WC Jr, Baird GL, Barry JJ, et al. Multicenter pilot treatment trial for psychogenic nonepileptic seizures: a randomized clinical trial. JAMA Psychiatry 2014;71(9):997–1005.
8. Reiter J, Andrews D, Reiter C, LaFrance Jr WC. Taking control of your seizures: workbook. New York: Oxford University Press; 2015.
9. Benbadis SR, LaFrance WC Jr. Clinical features and role of video-EEG monitoring. In Schachter SC, LaFrance WCJr. (eds.), Gates and Rowan's nonepileptic seizures (3rd ed.). Cambridge: Cambridge University Press, 2010:38–50.
10. LaFrance Jr WC, Wincze J. Treating nonepileptic seizures: therapist guide. New York: Oxford University Press, 2015.
11. Kalogjera-Sackellares D. Psychodynamics and psychotherapy of pseudoseizures. Wales: Crown House Publishing, 2004:3–42.

1. INTRODUCTION

Nonepileptic events (NEE) are defined as paroxysms of altered sensorimotor function, consciousness, or behavior that are similar to epileptic seizures but are not caused by abnormal electrical discharges in the brain. Within epilepsy centers, about a quarter of referrals for apparent pharmacoresistant epilepsy are found to be misdiagnosed (1). The average time delay to establish the correct diagnosis for such patients ranges between 1 and 7 years (2,3). Consequently, patients with NEE will frequently have sustained more iatrogenic adverse effects and used greater healthcare resources than patients with epilepsy (4). NEE, therefore, represent an important differential consideration in patients presenting with neurobehavioral paroxysms.

NEE are principally categorized as either psychogenic or physiologic in etiology. Psychogenic nonepileptic seizures (PNES) reflect somatic expression of psychological distress and represent a predominant majority (70–88%) of nonepileptic cases that are confirmed with video-electroencephalography (VEEG) monitoring in specialized epilepsy centers (5, 6). In contrast to PNES, physiologic nonepileptic events (PNEE) result from transient systemic alterations or non-neuropathophysiologic disease states that can manifest paroxysmal symptoms (Box 24.1). The evaluations of PNES, and of PNEE, such as syncopal episodes, movement disorders imitating epileptic seizures and pediatric paroxysms of nonepileptic etiologies, will be the main focal points of this review. The remaining differential etiologies of PNEE will be covered in other chapters of this textbook. Management of NEE, particularly as pertaining to PNES, will also be discussed.

2. EVALUATION OF PNES

The symptomatology of PNES has been well described since the 19th century from the seminal works of Briquet, Charcot, and Freud (7). In the past, several terminologies have been utilized to describe this condition. Some terms, such as "pseudoseizures" or hysterical seizures, are perceived to be pejorative by patients, as they connote either disingenuous or gender-biased origins of the seizures, respectively. These terms have largely been abandoned by modern practitioners. Whether to label this condition as psychogenic nonepileptic "events" or "seizures" has been the subject of some debate. Using the term "events" adds clarity to the explanation of the diagnosis to patients, clearly distinguishing the paroxysms of interest from epileptic seizures (8). When the patient fully adopts the term "events" in place of "seizures," then the risk of mismanagement by clinicians who may not necessarily have detailed access to the patient's medical records (e.g., emergency room staff) may likely diminish. However, for some patients and families (particularly those who have a prolonged history of being given a seizure diagnosis), an abrupt retraction of the seizure label may be difficult to accept, may risk estranging the patient, and may hamper future therapeutic alliances with the treatment team (9). For some patients with PNES, the actualization of diagnostic insight may require a more tempered, stepwise approach:

1. The initial concept to establish is that their seizures are nonepileptic in origin (hence, the term "nonepileptic seizures" preferred by some authors to introduce this diagnosis).

2. The subsequent concept is that their seizures have psychological underpinnings. The term PNES may be acceptable for those who appropriately process this intermediate step.

3. The third concept is that the illness experience of their seizures is unique, and not any less consequential than that of epileptic seizures. Upon embracing this last concept, the term "events", rather than seizures, may become more acceptable to patients.

Patients' background experiences are often very similar across developmental histories, but psychological mindedness can differ. Therefore, how empathetically the diagnosis is communicated by the neurologist or other medical provider to the patient is of great importance. Also relevant is whether the clinician conveys an understanding of the patient's account of the illness experience and associated tribulations back to the patient (and family) (10) (see treatment section below).

While the absence of epileptiform activity during an ictus on co-registered EEG confirms that a captured event may be nonepileptic in origin, such a finding does not necessarily distinguish a psychogenic versus physiologic etiology. Consideration of psychogenic etiology requires the demonstration of PNES-consistent ictal semiology, in the context of supportive historical presentation. These supportive clinical contexts can be derived from careful exploration of the following factors: background characteristics, precipitating factors, ictal semiology, temporal course/evolution, and confirmation of conversion disorder criteria.

2.1. Background Characteristics of PNES

Three fourths of patients with PNES are women in civilian population studies, with symptoms typically starting in their 20s and 30s (11). Psychiatric comorbidities are common, with prevalences of 62% for personality disorders, 49% for posttraumatic stress disorder (PTSD), 47% for major depressive disorder, and 47% for anxiety disorders other than PTSD (12). It is also notable that past or concurrent somatoform disorders have been known to be a strong risk factor for other forms of psychosomatic symptoms in the future (13). In addition to emotional traumatic experiences, there is evidence that physical factors (such as traumatic brain injuries) (14), health-related complications (15), and surgical procedures (16) can provoke PNES and may be precipitated by processes that are physiologic, as much as psychological in nature.

2.2. Precipitating Factors of PNES

While emotional stressors are frequently endorsed by patients as triggers to their seizures, they are not pathognomonic for PNES; similar emotional stressors have also been shown to provoke epileptic seizures (17). Some patients with PNES demonstrate a propensity to experience PNES during medical situations, such as when undergoing diagnostic testing (18), attending clinic visits (19) and when recovering from general anesthesia (20). Moreover, the reporting of more pedestrian physical triggers, such as certain foods, high-pitched noises, or certain lighting conditions would be unusual for epilepsy (i.e., reflex epilepsies). Endorsements of such specific triggers should raise suspicion for PNES, especially if they are associated with producing seizures with PNES semiology, as described below.

2.3. Ictal Semiology of PNES

Recognition of PNES entails a two-step characterization process, each of which should be considered separately. The first step involves the determination that ictal features are not consistent with known semiologies of epileptic seizures (Table 24.1, top portion). Knowledge of cortical representation and corresponding symptomatology upon ictal activation can help distinguish epileptic seizures from alternative nonepileptic etiologies. The second decision step involves the identification of ictal features that are supportive of a psychogenic process (Table 24.1, bottom portion). Based on the updated *Diagnostic and Statistical Manual of Mental Disorders* (DSM-5) (21), a diagnosis of PNES (i.e., conversion disorder presenting with seizures) can be established upon demonstration or "inclusion" of clinical findings that are incongruent with known neuroanatomy, neruropathophysiology, or medical/neurological disease. This use of non-neuroanatomic signs on exam as a diagnosis of inclusion is in contrast to the previous edition of DSM, which approached conversion disorder as a "diagnosis of exclusion."

Postictal clinical features are frequently better described or recalled by witnesses than ictal features, due to more ample observational opportunities. Observers may also be

TABLE 24.1. Semiologic and Exam Features that Can Help Distinguish Psychogenic Nonepileptic Seizures from Epileptic Seizures

DISTINGUISHING SEMIOLOGIC OR EXAM FEATURES	PSYCHOGENIC NONEPILEPTIC SEIZURES	EPILEPTIC SEIZURES
Emergence out of EEG-confirmed sleep	Rare	Common
Concurrent tongue-biting (severe, side of tongue) and urinary incontinence	Rare	Common after GTC
Ictal dystonic posture with contralateral automatisms	Not present	Occurs in mesial TLE
Ictal figure-of-4 sign	Not present	Occurs in TLE
Ictal fencing posture	Not present	Occurs in mesial FLE
Ictal grasping (gripping of an object with one hand or both hands)	Rare	Occurs in FLE and TLE
Postictal stertorous breathing	Not present	Common after GTC
Postictal nose rubbing	Not present	Occurs in TLE
Impaired corneal reflex	Not present	Common after GTC
Extensor plantar response	Not present	Common after GTC
Closed eyelid during peak of ictus	Very common	Rare
Gradual onset and prolonged duration	Common	Rare
Undulating motor activity	Common	Very rare
Asynchronous limb movements	Common	Rare
Side-to-side head shaking	Common	Rare
Ictal or postictal whispering/stuttering	Common	Rare
Ictal signs of emotional distress (e.g., grimacing, weeping)	Common	Rare
Pelvic thrusting	Sometimes	Rare
Memory recall for period of unresponsiveness	Sometimes	Rare
Resisted eyelid opening	Common	Very rare
Guarding of hand dropping over face	Common	Rare

GTC, generalized tonic–clonic epileptic seizures; TLE, temporal lobe epilepsy; FLE, frontal lobe epilepsy.
Modified from Benbadis SR, LaFrance WC Jr. Clinical features and role of video-EEG monitoring. In Schachter SC, LaFrance WC Jr. (Eds.), Gates and Rowan's nonepileptic seizures (3rd ed.). Cambridge: Cambridge University Press, 2010:38–50, with permission.

less emotionally charged during the postictal recovery period (allowing for more adequate processing of the events) compared to the moment of ictus. Observer-confirmed stertorous breathing postictally should raise suspicion for epileptic convulsions. In contrast, observer's affirmation of nearly immediate recovery after apparent convulsive activities or some memory recall for details during the period of unresponsiveness can suggest a psychogenic etiology.

While careful patient and witness interviews can uncover important diagnostic clues, there is evidence that patient/witness-reported and VEEG-documented ictal semiologies can be significantly discrepant (22). To assist with more accurate differentiation of epileptic from nonepileptic seizures, the International League Against Epilepsy's Nonepileptic Seizure Task Force proposed four stratified levels of diagnostic certainty for PNES:

Documented (ictus captured and confirmed nonepileptic by Video EEG, [inpatient, ambulatory or outpatient])

Clinically established (observed by an experienced clinician in person or via video review, with non-epileptiform ictus captured on routine or ambulatory EEG without video)

Probable (observed by an experienced clinician in person or via video review, with non-epileptiform interictal EEG)

Possible (based on witness or patient reporting, with non-epileptiform interictal EEG) (23).

The diagnosis of PNES is based on three components: a history consistent with PNES, witnessed semiology consistent with PNES, and EEG with the absence of epileptiform activity.

Another important caveat regarding semiology is that a witness may frequently miss the moment of seizure onset, and instead will depict the middle or recovery phase of the seizure. Notably, the neurobehavioral manifestations during the post-ictal recovery phase of an epileptic seizure can highly resemble the ictal semiology of some PNES. Moreover, no individual semiologic feature is definitively diagnostic of PNES (22), even when interpreting well-documented events from VEEG.

2.4. Temporal Course/Evolution

Beyond overt semiologic manifestations, assessment of the characteristic seizure temporal course/evolution is frequently helpful in distinguishing epileptic seizures from PNES. Ictal vocalization in epileptic seizures is usually primitive in nature and stereotypically restricted to the beginning of the seizure. On the other hand, the vocalization in PNES can not only present in the beginning but can persist or even intensify through the course of the ictus. It is also frequently associated with affective component reflective of emotional distress (e.g., crying, moaning) (24). Generalized tonic-clonic epileptic seizures evolve through an organized fashion, beginning with adduction and external rotation of limbs, followed by limb tonic extension, and then diffuse, clonic jerking movements. As the clonic frequency progressively declines, the jerk amplitude increases until seizure cessation. By contrast, convulsive PNES typically demonstrate less organized or more simplistic evolution, with movements that show variable amplitudes or unchanging frequency throughout the ictus (25). Epileptic seizures frequently emerge with a clear-cut onset, reach peak behavioral manifestations within 70 seconds (26), and are followed by an overt offset usually within a few minutes. Some PNES instead demonstrate poorly discernible ictal onset or offset, sometimes amidst the setting of apparent sleep, during which the EEG discordantly correlates with features indicative of wakefulness or light drowsiness (27). Regarding seizure duration, about 78% of patients with PNES endorsed having had at least one seizure lasting longer than 30 minutes (PNES-status)(28).

2.5. EEG Observations

Routine EEG studies are generally not helpful in the evaluation of PNES due to the low probability of capturing a patient's typical event during these studies' time-limited duration and low sensitivity for diagnosing epilepsy interictally. Beyond the aforementioned low yields of routine EEG, false-positive interpretation of EEG portends a significant patient management dilemma. Unless the actual tracing of the EEG in question is (re-)reviewed (preferably by an epileptologist), no amount of subsequent normal EEGs can invalidate the ostensibly "abnormal" finding. One study found that about one third of patients with VEEG-confirmed PNES have had at least one EEG study that was initially read as having "epileptiform" abnormality. Upon re-inspection, many of the overinterpreted patterns

tended to be normal fluctuations of background activity (e.g., sharply contoured alpha rhythms, hyperventilation-induced slowing, hypnagogic hypersynchrony) and well-described normal variants (e.g., wicket spikes) (29).

Compared to routine EEG, outpatient ambulatory EEG (available with concurrent video recordings) has the advantage of longer study duration, allowing for more opportunity to capture and visualize habitual events of interest. By allowing patients to be exposed to the stressors of and triggers in their indigenous milieu, ambulatory EEG can in some cases yield a greater likelihood of capturing an ictus than EEG recording in hospital settings. However, due to lack of standardized ictal/postictal neurological examination and greater susceptibility to environment-related artifacts, the qualities of the ambulatory EEG and video data outside the epilepsy monitoring unit (EMU) can be quite variable. Moreover, an important caveat is that a scalp-negative EEG should be interpreted in the context of supportive historical, ictal/postictal exam, and ictal semiologic features in order to establish a PNES diagnosis with "documented" (i.e., highest) level of certainty (23). For cases in which supportive semiologic and/or historical contexts are less sufficient, ambulatory EEGs (especially those without corresponding video) should be interpreted with caution.

VEEG in the EMU entails continuous, technician-monitored recording of the patient, allowing for simultaneous video, EEG, and ictal/postictal exam documentation of the habitual seizures of interest. The inpatient setting affords the neurologist sufficient opportunity to comprehensively explore the patient's historical presentation. Upon reaching a concordant impression from each of the above data elements, VEEG offers a diagnostic "gold standard" with high levels of certainty as well as excellent interrater reliability (22).

2.6. Nuances of EEG Interpretation

When an ictus is associated with unconsciousness, a physiologic explanation can be excluded by the concurrent presence of an intact alpha rhythm on the EEG—a neurophysiologic correlate of alertness. On the other hand, for an ictus involving preserved consciousness and rather restricted motor, autonomic, or sensory/psychic components, the absence of EEG epileptiform correlate *does not* necessarily preclude the consideration of focal, simple partial epileptic seizures. Considering that simple partial epileptic seizures can arise from only a small pool of neuronal tissue, only 21% of them have been shown to demonstrate ictal epileptiform correlate on scalp EEG (30). These nuanced concepts underscore the importance of bedside exam for ictal sensorium of patients in the EMU.

The ictal EEG epileptiform correlates of some frontal lobe epileptic seizures can be quite subtle, falsely lateralizing, or undiscernible. These observations derive from the fact that some frontal lobe epileptic seizures arise from deep-seated foci (e.g., orbitofrontal or interhemispheric regions), such that ictal epileptiform discharges are conducted/distributed across a widespread area bilaterally, demonstrate a contralateral maximum, or become obscured by artifacts related to hypermotor activity. Semiologic features are often the primary basis in diagnosing frontal lobe epileptic seizures and include a tendency to be brief (<30 sec), to emerge out of physiologic sleep, to occur in clusters, and to be associated with minimal or brief postictal confusion (31). When evaluating captured events without clear-cut EEG epileptiform correlate, exclusion of frontal lobe epileptic seizures represents a crucial diagnostic consideration.

Due to the frequent amnestic nature of seizures in patients with PNES, any captured events should be confirmed by a witness (who has observed past seizures) to be the typical seizure for the patient. If deemed to be atypical of the usual seizure(s), then the clinical relevance of the captured event(s) is less certain. Some patients with PNES present with two or more semiologically independent event types. For definitive characterization of such cases, a semiologic description of the various types and an occurrence of each type should be recorded, as independent event types may reflect distinct etiologies, such as mixed PNES and epileptic seizures. Otherwise, any EEG noncaptured event type should be diagnosed with a lower level of certainty (23). This caution is warranted by the finding that ~10% of patients with PNES also have an independent diagnosis of epilepsy (32). When comparing PNES semiologies among patients with lone PNES versus mixed epilepsy with PNES, one study showed that ictal autonomic symptoms (e.g., abdominal symptoms, tachycardia, respiratory changes) were significantly more common in patients with lone PNES (33). Furthermore, when comparing the semiologies of PNES versus epileptic seizures among patients with mixed disorders, only some of these patients (36–60%) demonstrate readily distinguishable PNES versus epileptic seizures (34, 35). In other words, for many patients with mixed disorders, the clinical manifestations of their PNES were challengingly similar to their epileptic seizures.

2.7. Psychopathology of PNES

PNES are most commonly conceptualized as a subtype of somatic symptom disorder, conversion disorder (CD), seizure type, in which psychological conflicts are converted into physical symptoms resembling epileptic seizures. In essence, when attention is focused upon outward seizure activities, inner stressors are mitigated from conscious awareness (i.e., a psychological defense mechanism) (36). Among several etiologic models for CD manifesting as PNES, one model proposes two main types of underlying psychological "causes": posttraumatic and developmental (37).

Posttraumatic PNES develop in response to psychological or physical trauma(s) or abuse that the patient struggles to adequately process or integrate. Some authors postulate that PNES reflect an automatic "cutoff phenomenon" in response to spontaneous intrusion into consciousness of such unspeakable memories (38). About three quarters of patients with PNES endorse traumatic antecedent factors, such as abuse, accidents, bereavement, and health-related traumas (15). Sexual abuse, the most common antecedent factor, is endorsed by about one third of patients with PNES with traumatic histories (15). This subgroup with history of sexual abuse has been reported to be significantly more likely to experience severe PNES manifestations (e.g., convulsive or self-injury during seizures) and psychopathologies (e.g., personality disorders or other medically unexplained symptoms) (39).

Developmental PNES derive from difficulties coping with complex life tasks and milestones along the patient's continuum of psychosocial development. The maladaptive development frequently occurs in an environment of emotional privation or neglect. Some patients with PNES have been shown to rely on avoidant coping responses (denial and repression) to perceived threats (40), hence hindering appropriate maturation of psychosocial development. PNES (as well as other forms of CDs) reflect a disorder of communication, where distress is expressed somatically rather than through healthy verbal channels.

Some neurobehavioral paroxysms are considered within the "border zone" of PNES as they are derived from psychological underpinnings but are etiologically distinct from CD described above. Panic attacks, which are paroxysmal manifestations of panic disorder or other conditions associated with anxiety, represent an important consideration within the border zone of PNES. Some symptoms of panic attacks, such as palpitations, shortness of breath, intense fear, tremulousness, and derealization/depersonalization, can parallel the autonomic and psychic features present in some complex partial epileptic seizures or PNES. Compared to epileptic seizures, the temporal evolution of panic attacks demonstrates a slower progression to peak behavioral manifestations and longer overall attack duration, generally lasting between 5 and 30 minutes (41). Careful exploration of the overall presentation should uncover other key features meeting DSM-5 (42) criteria for panic attacks. Patients with panic attacks will also frequently have comorbid anxiety disorders, such as agoraphobia or social phobia.

Similar to panic attacks, some of the behavioral presentations of PTSD can resemble seizure activities. From functional neuroimaging studies, two subtypes of PTSD have been proposed: (1) intrusive attacks involving hyperaroused flashback of trauma and (2) unresponsive dissociative states (43). Some patients with presumed PNES may in fact be exhibiting misdiagnosed PTSD of dissociative subtype. Therefore, upon careful evaluation, should the patient's overall symptomatology be better explained by PTSD according to DSM-5 criteria, then the additional diagnosis of CD (manifesting as PNES) should be avoided.

Not infrequently, patients present with exclusively sensory symptoms (such as paresthesias or numbness) or subjective experiences for which simple partial epileptic seizures are deemed improbable based on suggestible nature, inter-event variability, or widespread or multifocal distribution of symptoms. Most of these cases likely represent anxious misinterpretation of common, nonspecific paroxysmal symptoms of everyday life, including transient dizziness, limb numbness, or head sensations that may briefly disrupt attention. The misinterpretation of benign symptoms as being more pathological may be more common in patients who have had personal experiences with seizures, or who have other neurological or medical conditions. Psychogenic movement disorders with paroxysmal semiology and no alteration in level of consciousness are also in the differential diagnosis for simple partial manifestations of PNES. Another scenario that falls within the border zones of PNES is the purposeless and repetitive behavioral mannerisms ("learned behavior") that can occur in some cognitively impaired patients (44).

3. SYNCOPE

Syncope has been defined as a sudden loss of consciousness due to transient global cerebral hypoperfusion. Syncopal semiology is characterized by rapid onset, short duration, and spontaneous complete recovery (45). Syncope is a prevalent disorder, accounting for 3% of emergency room visits and 6% of hospital admissions per year in the United States (46). In light of this high prevalence, syncope represents the second most common cause of nonepileptic events (physiologic) (after PNES) referred to neurologists (1). The distinction of syncope from other causes of neurobehavioral paroxysms demands careful historical exploration of background characteristics, preictal factors, ictal semiology, and temporal evolution. In cases involving significant cerebral hypoperfusion, syncope-specific EEG changes emerge.

3.1. Background Characteristics of Syncope

Incidence rates of syncope follow a bimodal distribution, with an initial peak during teenage years, followed by a second peak upon reaching senescence. In a survey of young adults (medical students), the cumulative incidence of at least one syncopal event was 47% in females and 24% in males by the age of 24. The median age for the first episode of syncope was 15 years, and syncope was rarely reported before age 10 years (47). Most of these syncopal cases were attributed to vasovagal etiology (see below). In this study, the cumulative incidence rate in women was almost twice that of men. This observed gender difference has been postulated to be related to lower cardiac filling in women (47). Notably, very few women correlated their syncopal events to menstruation. In a large population study of older patients (mean age of 51), a sharp increase in the incidence rate of syncope was observed after age 70 (48). This enhanced susceptibility to syncope with advancing age can be due to age-related physiologic impairments of heart rate and blood pressure regulation, cardiac comorbidities, and polypharmacy (49).

3.2. Preictal Factors of Syncope

Classical descriptions of prodromal symptoms in syncope can be categorized into two main groups. The first group is due to cerebral and retinal hypoperfusion, resulting in concentration difficulty, light-headedness, pallor, hearing loss with "fading of sounds," loss of peripheral vision, or blurring of vision. The second group involves "autonomic activation" from a combination of sympathetic/parasympathetic activity and is associated with diaphoresis, sense of warmth, nausea, epigastric discomfort, sighing and tachypnea, yawning, palpitations, or restlessness. While not all of these symptoms are experienced in every case, the suspicion for syncope is strengthened with a greater number of matching symptoms from these two main groups. By contrast, epileptic auras typically entail a more restricted range of symptoms, considering the limited electrical propagation of simple partial epileptic seizures (premonitory auras). In a study of young adults with vasovagal syncope, the most common precipitating factors included warm environments, prolonged standing, and pain, with each factor being endorsed by ≥25% of patients with syncope (47). Syncopal events also frequently occur contiguously with very specific situations such as abrupt change of posture, onset or offset of physical exertion, shaving, coughing fits, and micturition/defecation. Such specific situational associations would be less common with epileptic seizures.

3.3. Ictal Semiology of Syncope

Apparent "swoon" attacks that strictly involve immobile unresponsiveness are often misconstrued to be the typical semiology of syncope but are more likely to be PNES. On the contrary, involuntary motor accompaniments are quite common in cerebrovascular-related syncope. In a study involving video analysis of 42 episodes of physiologic syncope, 38 (90%) of the episodes were associated with myoclonic activity (50). The most commonly observed myoclonic activity was multifocal, arrhythmic jerks both in proximal and distal muscles, usually lasting only a few seconds. Frequently, superimposition of more generalized myoclonus was also evident. Only rarely was partially preserved consciousness observed in the context of myoclonic activity. Other commonly observed features included eyes being open and showing initial upward deviation, righting movements, head turns, lip-smacking or chewing, and fumbling movements (50). Whereas motor accompaniments were commonly associated with physiologic syncope, significant perisyncopal amnesia beyond the period of unconsciousness was rarely observed (59). By contrast, epileptic seizures have a known predilection to involve the hippocampi, and hence anterograde or retrograde amnesia can be quite dense in many cases of complex partial (focal dyscognitive) epileptic seizures or generalized tonic–clonic epileptic seizures. Compared to motor accompaniments, the presence of significant peri-ictal amnesia may often be more helpful in distinguishing syncope from epileptic seizures.

Ictal manifestation of immobile unresponsiveness (dialeptic seizures) is a common and yet challenging presentation, with broad differential considerations that include syncope, epileptic seizures, and PNES. Ictal semiology involving flaccid behavioral arrest and unresponsiveness would be an unusual presentation for any type of epileptic seizures. Atonic epileptic seizures may cause abrupt falls, but the duration of unresponsiveness and loss of tone is usually very brief (few seconds). The occurrence of atonic epileptic seizures is also fairly exclusive to patients with developmental delay. While tonic, absence, complex partial epileptic, and generalized tonic–clonic epileptic seizures can cause dialeptic symptoms with alteration of awareness, they are not associated with ictal flaccidity. An important caveat is that patients with epileptic seizures can sometimes manifest prolonged motionlessness, flaccidity, and eye closure during the postictal recovery phase of epileptic generalized tonic–clonic seizures. Similarly, the "convulsive" portion of syncope may have been missed by the witness. It is therefore imperative that the observer accounts must confidently encompass the entirety of the event from its onset, and not just the postictal phase.

3.4. Temporal Course/Evolution of Syncope

The average duration of vasovagal syncope (the most common mechanism for syncope; see below) from the moment of event onset to recovery of full consciousness has been shown to range from 23 to 41 sec (51). Paroxysms of swoons that last >1 minute should, therefore, raise suspicion for etiologies other than syncope. The duration of symptoms preceding a syncopal event varies depending on the cause of syncope. Premonitory symptoms in arrhythmia-related cardiac syncope are very brief (seconds), whereas changes in cardiorespiratory dynamics can emerge about 3 minutes before impending vasovagal syncope (52). The time frames of prodromes in syncope are thus not readily distinguishable from those in epileptic seizures. Instead, assessing the temporal evolution of the convulsive elements of syncope may yield more distinguishing clues. The motor symptoms of syncope terminate when the patient assumes a horizontal position, as this position facilitates restoration of cerebral blood flow. On the contrary, generalized convulsive epileptic seizures will complete their expectant clinical course (evolving from the tonic to the clonic phase) regardless of the patient's body position. Table 24.2 summarizes the semiologic features that distinguish syncope from epileptic seizures.

3.5. EEG Observations in Syncope

EEG background activity progresses through a stereotyped pattern of alterations during a syncope event, with each change correlating with the extent of cerebral dysfunction related to blood flow reduction. This EEG pattern typically begins with moderate- to high-amplitude, generalized theta-range (4–5 Hz) slow activity, followed by an even higher-amplitude activity of slower frequency in the delta range (1.5–3 Hz) (51). This progressive slowing of electrographic activity has been postulated to reflect an increasing failure of network activity as synaptic connectivity decreases. Should cerebral blood flow subsequently fall below 0.16 to 0.17 mL/g/min, then diffuse suppression of all EEG background activity ensues, denoting a complete network failure (53). Upon restoration of cerebral blood flow, the EEG background progresses conversely from generalized delta slow activity, to theta slow activity, followed by relatively rapid recovery of the posterior dominant rhythm (i.e., normal awake background rhythms) (51).

Detailed semiologic components of syncope in relation to EEG changes have also been examined (54). In most patients, loss of consciousness, eye opening, and general stiffening developed concomitantly with the delta slow activity, persisted through the suppressed and subsequent delta slow segments, and recovered within seconds after the end of the latter delta slow activity. Myoclonus can occur in two clusters with syncope. The first cluster of myoclonus coincided with the onset of the initial delta slow activity but ended at the onset of EEG suppression. The second cluster of myoclonus occurred either

TABLE 24.2. Comparison of Semiologic Features Between Epileptic Seizures and Syncope

	EPILEPTIC SEIZURES	SYNCOPE
Preictal factors		
Stereotypy	Highly stereotyped	Somewhat stereotyped
Range of symptoms	Restricted range of symptoms	Broader constellation of symptoms—including those derived from (a) cerebral/retinal hypoperfusion and (b) autonomic activation.
Consistent situational triggers	Rare	Situational syncopes are associated with coughing, micturition, defecation, etc.
Precipitation by stress	Possible	Rare
Ictal semiology		
Eyes	Open and rolled up	Open and rolled up
Motor features	Can be GTC, tonic, atonic, clonic, or myoclonic depending on type of epileptic seizure	Usually multifocal, arrhythmic myoclonus
Amnesia	Dense anterograde or retrograde amnesia	Negligible or trace peri-ictal amnesia
Temporal course/evolution		
Duration of preictal aura	Seconds to minutes	Seconds to minutes depending on etiology
Duration of altered mental state	Usually >1 minute in CPS or GTC	<1 minute
Evolution of motor features	Not affected by body position	Abates upon assuming horizontal position

GTC, generalized tonic–clonic convulsions, ES, epileptic seizures; CPS, complex partial seizures.

during or shortly after the subsequent delta slow activity. Moreover, several additional signs, such as spontaneous vocalization, roving eye movements, and stertorous breathing, were observed exclusively during the EEG suppressed segments.

3.6. Nuances of EEG Interpretation for Syncope

While epileptic seizures and syncope are ostensibly distinct and unrelated etiologically, there are rare incidences in which these two entities can co-occur contiguously within the same event. Selective activation of parasympathetic or sympathetic centers via the electrical propagation of epileptic seizures can contribute to cardiac rate changes, with ictal sinus tachycardia being evident in the majority of patients with epilepsy. In a prospective study of patients with epilepsy who were chronically implanted with loop recorders to monitor cardiac rhythms, 2.1% of documented epileptic seizures were associated with ictal bradycardia or asystole (55). When examined specifically for concomitant syncopal symptoms during epileptic seizures, another study identified ictal asystole in 0.27% of VEEG-monitored patients with proven epilepsy. The majority of these patients with ictal asystole had temporal lobe epilepsy, and their ictal semiology showed a sudden loss of postural tone (unusual for temporal lobe epilepsy) an average of 42 sec into the typical clinical course of complex partial epileptic seizures. Cardiac asystole developed an average of 29.9 sec after electrographic ictal onset. The average duration of asystole was 13.2 sec (3.9–33 sec), and all cases were preceded by sinus bradycardia (56).

Some investigators have proposed a lateralization hypothesis whereby seizures with a left-sided focus are preferentially associated with ictal bradyarrhythmias, while right-sided seizures are associated with ictal tachyarrhythmias (57). However, case reports showing the converse association are well documented (58), and the mechanisms underlying ictal cardiac arrhythmias remain uncertain (56). The overall incidence rate of ictal arrhythmias is presumed to be underreported, as diagnosis of this condition requires simultaneous ictal EEG and electrocardiographic recording. In fact, many ictal arrhythmias are detected incidentally in EMUs among patients without known cardiovascular risk factors or baseline electrocardiographic abnormalities (56). This diagnostic elusiveness, in the context of a potentially lethal condition, underscores the importance of clinical vigilance for this condition.

3.7. Etiologies of Syncope

Various etiologies can result in cerebral hypoperfusion and syncope. Determination of underlying etiology not only influences treatment decisions but portends prognosis and morbidity.

Neurally mediated syncope is the most common etiology of syncope, representing 21% of all causes of syncope in the general population (48) and an even higher proportion in other study settings (i.e., emergency department, syncope units) (45). This mechanism applies to a heterogeneous group of conditions in which cardiovascular reflexes that normally maintain proper circulatory perfusion become transiently disrupted as reflected by vasodilation (vasodepressor type) and/or bradycardia (cardioinhibitory type). Cerebral perfusion diminishes as the result of vasodilation, bradycardia, or a combination of both processes. Neurally mediated syncope has been classified by the triggers of the inappropriate reflex responses. *Vasovagal syncope* is triggered by abrupt emotional insult (e.g., fear, pain) or orthostatic stress (e.g., prolonged standing). *Situational syncope* refers to syncope associated with some specific settings that stress the cardiovascular reflexes, such as micturition, defecation, or coughing. In *carotid sinus hypersensitivity*, mechanical manipulation (e.g., from a neck collar) stimulates the carotid sinus baroreceptor to trigger an inappropriate reflex response. The more common presentation, however, is that no mechanical trigger is identified by history, and the diagnosis is confirmed by carotid sinus massage (59). Neurally mediated

syncope is not known to be life-threatening in itself and typically occurs in healthy individuals with normal blood pressure (48). However, this syncopal mechanism can sometimes coexist with other etiologies of syncope (described below), contributing to additional morbidity.

Cardiac disease represents the second most common cause of syncope, especially when uncovered in studies involving emergency departments or specialty syncope clinic settings (45). Arrhythmias and structural diseases are the two main cardiac mechanisms contributing to compromised circulatory perfusion. Regarding cardiac arrhythmias, both bradyarrhythmias (e.g., intrinsic sick sinus, atrioventricular block) and tachyarrhythmias (e.g., supraventricular tachycardia, ventricular tachycardia) can impair cardiac efficiency and diminish cardiac output. Persistently restricted cardiac output can result from structurally obstructive processes within the heart, such as valvular disease, hypertrophic cardiomyopathy, or cardiac masses. Low ejection fraction may also result from prior myocardial infarctions or cardiomyopathies of various causes. An important caveat is that compared to patients without syncope, patients with cardiac-induced syncope have significantly increased risks of myocardial infarction or death from coronary artery disease (hazard ratio = 2.66), nonfatal or fatal stroke (hazard ratio = 2.01), and death from all causes (hazard ratio = 2.01) (48). Clinical vigilance for cardiac syncope is therefore well warranted, particularly in patients with preexisting cardiac disease.

Orthostatic hypotension is a physical sign delineated by a drop in systolic blood pressure of >20 mmHg and in diastolic blood pressure of >10 mmHg within 3 minutes of assuming a standing position (60). When the drop in blood pressure sufficiently compromises cerebral perfusion, then syncope can occur. One cause of orthostasis is autonomic dysfunction in which sympathetic efferent activity to blood vessels is chronically impaired such that compensatory vasoconstriction is deficient when needed (i.e., upon standing). Autonomic dysfunction may result from neurodegenerative conditions (e.g., Shy–Drager syndrome, Parkinson's disease) or acquired autonomic neuropathy related to systemic diseases (e.g., alcoholism, diabetes). In addition, medications that promote peripheral vasodilation (e.g., alpha blockers) may contribute to the impairment of compensatory vasoconstriction response. Moreover, orthostasis can also result from insufficient blood volume, such as from dehydration or blood loss.

In the general population, no definitive etiology can be established in ~37% of patients with syncope despite extensive evaluations (48). Some of these patients with syncope of unknown origin experience intractable events and high rates of health resource utilization. The prevalence of psychogenic syncope among patients with syncope of unknown origin has ranged between 5.5% and 24% (61, 62). Among patients with atypical presentation of syncope (e.g., high frequency, prolonged duration, unusual triggers), some investigators advocate the pursuit of VEEG monitoring with provocative induction, noting that it is the only way to positively demonstrate a psychogenic etiology (63). Considering the present underutilization of VEEG to evaluate syncope of unknown origin, the prevalence of psychogenic syncope may be underestimated

(63). Alternatively, recording EEG concurrently with tilt-table testing is of benefit when assessing neurocardiogenic syncope to differentiate physiologic and psychogenic presentations.

4. MOVEMENT DISORDERS IMITATING EPILEPTIC SEIZURES

Hyperkinetic movement disorders represent another important mimicker of epileptic seizures. In general, the presence of a premonitory aura, ictal involvement of any sensory modality, or ictal progression leading to altered sensorium would be more consistent with epileptic seizures rather than movement disorders. In some cases, however, the distinction between paroxysmal movement disorders and epileptic seizures with predominantly motor symptoms can be difficult. This enigma is accentuated by the observation that the early stages of some movement disorders can manifest only intermittent symptoms. Moreover, paroxysmal exacerbation of involuntary movements by stress, posture, or fatigue is not an unusual presentation in some movement disorders—hence mimicking the episodic nature of epileptic seizures (64). Evaluation with ictal EEG may be necessary in these enigmatic cases to rule out epileptic seizures. Some movement disorders that can closely resemble epileptic seizures are described below.

4.1. Myoclonus

Myoclonus describes the presence of sudden, shock-like jerking from either activation of a muscle or group of muscles (positive myoclonus) or instantaneous cessation of muscle tone (negative myoclonus). Myoclonus may occur alone or in sequence manifesting a regular or irregular pattern of jerk movements. Symptoms can involve isolated muscle groups (focal/segmental), various parts of the body at different times (multifocal), or the entire body (diffuse).

While myoclonus can manifest as part of an epileptic syndrome, other major (nonepileptic) categories of myoclonus include symptomatic, physiologic, and essential etiologies (65). Symptomatic myoclonus can be the result of identifiable metabolic, infectious, or neurodegenerative disturbances. Encephalopathy is usually a prominent feature, with accompanying myoclonic jerks that are usually diffuse or multifocal in distribution. A notable caveat is that some cases of symptomatic myoclonus may demonstrate a cortical origin (i.e., cortical myoclonus) as evident by coinciding spike discharge on EEG or back-averaged EEG. However, cortical myoclonus in such cases is consequent to underlying systemic derangements rather than epilepsy syndromes (64). While pragmatic distinction between epileptic and nonepileptic disorders involving cortical myoclonus can usually be made, a fundamental mechanistic distinction is less clear amidst substantial neurophysiologic complexity (66). Symptomatic myoclonus can also result from acquired spinal cord injuries. In such cases, myoclonus manifests a segmental distribution limited to the myotome(s) innervated by the injured spinal cord region. Physiologic myoclonus includes common muscle jerks, such as hiccups and hypnic jerks, which are considered normal phenomena.

Essential myoclonus is an inherited (autosomal dominant) disorder characterized by an onset of myoclonic jerks in the first two decades of life, with symptoms typically affecting the arms and axial muscles. Essential myoclonus can have a varying presentation depending on the extent of accompanying dystonia and symptomatic response to alcohol (67).

4.2. Dystonia

Dystonia is characterized by sustained or repetitive co-contraction of agonist and antagonist muscles, leading to twisting movements or abnormal postures. Similar to how epileptic seizures manifest with stereotyped semiology, dystonic movements are typically "patterned" in the sense that the same group of muscles is consistently affected. In early stages, the dystonia is frequently "reversible" in that the patient can still actively or passively move the affected body part back to normal posture. Adding to the epileptic seizure–like paroxysmal mannerism is the observation that the timing and intensity of some dystonic movements can be influenced by emotion, relaxation, fatigue, and task-specific motor activity (i.e., action dystonia, such as writer's cramp). Indeed, some patients' dystonic movements may fluctuate drastically: patients may be nearly symptom-free during one occasion but then experience pronounced and disabling symptoms on another occasion (68). To help distinguish dystonia from epileptic seizures, patients with dystonia may endorse that their symptoms are ameliorated by particular sensory tricks (*gestes antagonists*). Touching the cheek is an example of a common sensory maneuver used by patients to correct torticollis (69). Dystonic movements usually abate during sleep, whereas the propensity for epileptic seizures is enhanced during drowsiness and sleep. Moreover, as dystonia advances in its disease course, the symptoms become more persistently fixed and widespread, with additional muscle groups becoming involved (69).

When no etiologic factor or other neurological abnormality can be identified, the dystonia is referred to as primary dystonia, which includes both sporadic and genetic forms. Sporadic forms, the more common type of dystonia, typically present in adulthood with symptoms involving a specific body part, such as task-specific dystonia, torticollis, or blepharospasm. Genetic forms are more diverse in phenomenology, presenting with focal, segmental, or generalized symptoms that can range from mild to severely disabling. When coexisting neurological features are uncovered (such as parkinsonism or corticospinal tract signs), the term "dystonia-plus" may be appropriate. Secondary dystonia is diagnosed when a specific cause for the symptoms has been identified (64).

4.3. Hemifacial Spasm

Due to disproportionately large representation for the face on the motor homunculus, epileptic activity involving the motor cortex has a predilection to be associated with facial symptoms. As such, hemifacial spasm, which is characterized as irregular, clonic contractions of the muscles innervated by the seventh cranial nerve, may be mistaken for focal motor seizures involving the face. Several clinical features can help distinguish hemifacial spasms from epileptic seizures. The onset of hemi-facial spasm is usually at the orbicularis oculi muscle (i.e., upper face) and may spread to other ipsilateral facial muscles over a period of months to years (70). By contrast, facial motor seizures typically involve the perioral area due to the preferentially larger representation of the lower face (when compared to the upper face) on the motor homunculus. Hemifacial spasm is a chronically progressive disorder, and clonic contractions may eventually be replaced by sustained tonic contractions, hence causing forceful eyelid closure. Facial motor epileptic seizures, on the other hand, are "paroxysmal," so patients are free of facial clonic symptoms interictally. Moreover, should facial motor epileptic seizures propagate more widely, other muscle groups beyond the myotome of the seventh cranial nerve can become involved. Examples of such seizure propagation would be early symptomatic involvement of the ipsilateral hand, which also has a relatively large representation on the motor and sensory homunculi.

The majority of cases are classified as primary hemifacial spasms and are presumed to be related to vascular compression of the ipsilateral facial nerve at its root exit zone in the brainstem (70). Thorough brain magnetic resonance imaging/magnetic resonance angiography investigations have shown that ~88% of primary hemifacial spasm cases demonstrate neurovascular compression of the affected facial nerve (71). Hemifacial spasm has also been reported to be secondary to identified causes, such as Bell's palsy or other facial nerve injury, demyelinating disease, and brain vascular insults. A small proportion of patients have hereditary hemifacial spasm with an autosomal dominant inheritance pattern (70).

4.4. Paroxysmal Dyskinesias

Paroxysmal dyskinesias (PD) represent a rare group of movement disorders highlighted by their episodic nature, with symptoms emerging out of a background of normal motor activity and behavior. Symptoms typically manifest within the first two decades of life and are characterized by any combination of hyperkinetic movements, including dystonia, chorea, athetosis, and ballism. PD have been classified based on the nature of clinical conditions known to trigger the dyskinesias (72).

In paroxysmal kinesigenic dyskinesia (PKD), the most common subtype of PD, sudden attacks of involuntary, dyskinetic movements are precipitated by movement. Common triggering movements include sudden change of body position (e.g., standing up quickly) or prolonged physical exercise. Abrupt startles (e.g., from a ringing bell) are another common precipitating factor. Some patients describe a sensory prodrome of paresthesias, muscle tension, or dizziness. Once provoked, the symptoms usually manifest unilaterally but may alternate or even demonstrate bilateral involvement. Consciousness is fully preserved, even with bilateral or diffuse dyskinetic symptoms. Ictal EEG findings are unremarkable (73). Attack duration is typically <1 minute, while attacks can occur very frequently (up to 100 per day). Despite copious attack frequency, neurological function is normal between attacks. The disease course is nonprogressive or may even improve, with

a diminished attack burden during adulthood (74). The gene locus for PKD has been mapped to chromosome 16, and it can be inherited through an autosomal dominant pattern with high penetrance (75). Sporadic cases (without a family history of PKD) have also been well described. More rarely, PKD can also be secondary to other disorders, such as demyelinating disease, cerebrovascular disease, and cerebral palsy (74).

In paroxysmal non-kinesigenic dyskinesia (PNKD), attacks are not precipitated by sudden movement or exertion. Instead, they occur either spontaneously or may be triggered by emotional stress, fatigue, caffeine, or alcohol. Clinical characteristics of the dyskinetic movements are generally similar to those seen in PKD. However, key differences in PNKD are comparatively longer attack duration (lasting minutes to hours) and lower attack frequency (at most a few attacks per day). Moreover, the dyskinesias in PNKD more frequently affect speech function and may be misinterpreted as a change in mental status despite fully preserved consciousness. The gene locus for PNKD has been mapped to chromosome 2 and like PKD is inherited through an autosomal dominant pattern with high penetrance (76). Sporadic cases are reported, as are secondary cases of PNKD, including demyelinating disease, endocrine dysfunction, and HIV infection (74).

4.5. Psychogenic Movement Disorders

As noted above, some paroxysmal psychogenic movement disorders are also mimics for seizures. Just as PNES can present with any seizure semiologic presentation, psychogenic movement disorders can present with presentations of neurological movement disorders, including psychogenic myoclonus, dystonia, dyskinesias, hyper/hypokinetic/akinetic movements, and tremors. Care must be taken to obtain a complete neurological and psychiatric history for establishing the CD/psychogenic movement disorder. As is the case with epileptic and nonepileptic seizures, the semology of the movement disorders can aid in distinguishing neurologic movement disorders from psychogenic movement disorders. While an extensive discussion of psychogenic movement disorders is beyond the scope of this chapter, some signs observed on exam in psychogenic movement disorders include entrainment, distractibility, migration, and suppressibility.

5. PAROXYSMAL DISTURBANCES IN INFANTS AND CHILDREN IMITATING EPILEPTIC SEIZURES

5.1. Breath-Holding Attacks

Breath-holding attacks represent a special form of syncope consisting of involuntary apnea, changes in postural tone, and unconsciousness for a brief period. Similar to convulsive syncope in adults, generalized stiffening and myoclonic activity may accompany more pronounced attacks. Breath-holding attacks are usually triggered by adverse stimuli, such as emotionally upsetting (i.e., frustration, anger, fright) or physically painful events. These attacks occur in ~5% of otherwise healthy children, typically between 6 and 18 months of age

(77). Despite the apparent dramatic nature of the symptoms, these attacks follow a benign clinical course with no evidence that the recurrent loss of consciousness causes brain injury. Attacks remit spontaneously by the age of 6 in 90% of affected children (78).

Breath-holding attacks can be classified into two main forms—cyanotic and pallid. The cyanotic form is the more common of the two types. The attacks are heralded by temper tantrums in response to upsetting stimuli. Following a period of vigorous crying, breathing is interrupted during expiration. The child then develops cyanosis and becomes unconscious. If significant hypoxia occurs, generalized stiffening and myoclonic activity can emerge and may be misinterpreted for an epileptic seizure. Key to the diagnosis is the crying and cyanosis, which consistently occur prior to the convulsive activity (79). Diagnosis becomes more difficult when the onset of the attacks is not well witnessed. The pallid form is usually preceded by a painful experience, such as falling down or being startled. The painful stimulus then quickly activates an exaggerated vagal response that results in significant bradycardia or even asystole (briefly). Consequently, the child develops apnea, becomes pale, and rapidly loses consciousness. Unlike the cyanotic form, there may be very little or no crying that heralds these attacks. Abnormal autonomic regulation of the cardiovascular system is thought to underlie this condition. Autonomic dysfunction is evidenced by the demonstration of exaggerated oculocardiac reflexes (ocular compression triggering bradycardia/asystole) in many patients with the pallid form of breath-holding attacks (77, 80).

5.2. Nonepileptic Staring Spells

Nonepileptic staring spells can occur in some children who are either bored or idle, such as when sitting in a classroom or watching TV. While such spells can occur in some normal children, they more commonly occur in children with intellectual disability, autism, and attention-deficit/hyperactivity disorder (81). They represent an important mimicker of absence or complex partial epileptic seizures, as one study showed that nonepileptic staring spells represented about one third of all VEEG-confirmed nonepileptic events in children (82). Several clinical features can be helpful in distinguishing staring spells from epileptic seizures:

1. Staring spells are readily interruptible by tactile or vocal stimulation, although visual stimuli (i.e., hand-waving) alone may sometimes be insufficient to disrupt these events.

2. They are never accompanied by automatisms, myoclonus, or other motor mannerisms typical of some epileptic seizures.

3. Unlike epileptic seizures, they do not spontaneously emerge out of sleep, and only rarely do they occur in midst of physical activity.

4. Upon redirection of attention, the child can readily respond to questions appropriately and does not show the postictal confusional state characteristic of some epileptic seizures.

5.3. Hyperekplexia

Hyperekplexia (startle disease), a rare disorder that typically begins during infancy, is characterized by an exaggerated and nonhabituating startle reaction to unexpected sensory (auditory, tactile, or visual) stimuli or strong emotions (fright, anguish). Several seconds after the initial startle, the patient experiences tonic spasms that consist of generalized stiffening, lasting for seconds. Consciousness remains fully intact. Beyond the morbidity from abrupt falls, the tonic spasms have been associated with regurgitation, hernias, or even apnea. During sleep, many patients also develop spontaneous or reactive clonic movements of the legs, typically lasting a few minutes (83). As opposed to a normal startle response, which is usually restricted to the upper half of the body and readily habituates, the movements in hyperekplexia show greater amplitude, more widespread involvement, and minimal habituation with repetition. Hyperekplexia must also be distinguished from startle epilepsy, which consists of startle-triggered tonic epileptic seizures that are also brief (<30 sec) and may lead to falls. Startle epilepsy occurs more commonly in patients with significant neurological deficits, such as infantile hemiparesis, diffuse encephalopathy, and symptomatic generalized epilepsy. EEG abnormalities in startle epilepsy usually consist of epileptiform discharges in the supplementary motor area as well as the vicinity of the paracentral lobule (84). Hyperekplexia, on the hand, typically occurs in individuals with normal intelligence, unremarkable EEG, and otherwise no comorbid neurological deficits. It is further distinguished by the presence of brainstem reflexes that are hyperactive and do not habituate with repetitive. Examples include brisk head retraction and palmomental and snout reflexes.

Another key distinction from other conditions associated with startle responses is that hyperekplexia is typically an inherited condition; thus, there is often another affected member. Hyperekplexia derives from an abnormality in the inhibitory glycine receptor (GLYR) and in most cases is inherited through an autosomal dominant pattern, with a high penetrance of >90% (85). More rarely, autosomal recessive and sporadic forms occur. Familial and sporadic cases demonstrate the same clinical phenotype.

5.4. Shuddering Attacks

Shuddering attacks consist of a rapid, fine tremor of the head, shoulder, and trunk that resemble "shuddering" episodes from a chill. Consciousness is fully intact. Each attack lasts only a few seconds, but they can recur copiously—up to hundreds of times per day. Feeding, head movements, and excitement are known precipitating factors. These attacks may begin as early as 4 months of age, or later in childhood. The neurological examination and interictal/ictal EEG yield normal findings. The cause of shuddering attacks is unknown, but an association with a family history of essential tremor has been reported (86).

5.5. Sandifer's Syndrome

Infants with Sandifer's syndrome demonstrate paroxysmal dystonic movements of the head and neck, at times progressing to more generalized opisthotonic posturing. Additional accompanying features of apnea, staring, or subtle limb jerking can further confound the differentiation from epileptic seizures. The EEG is normal during these paroxysms, while an association of symptoms within 30 minutes of feeding has been observed in many cases. As such, manifestations of Sandifer's syndrome may reflect a pain response to the acidic content of gastroesophageal reflux or a mechanism to protect air passages from reflux content (87). This syndrome can occur in otherwise normal children or in children with a predisposition to acid reflux, such as hiatal hernia or tracheomalacia.

5.6. Tics and Stereotypies

Tics are abrupt, brief, and repetitive activation of discrete muscle groups, leading to motor movements (e.g., eye-blinking) or vocalization (e.g., throat-clearing). One hallmark of tics is the premonitory buildup of an urge to "tic" that is relieved by its performance. By comparison, stereotypies are ritualistic, purposeless actions that can range from simple postures (e.g., rocking of the body) to more complex movements (e.g., crossing and uncrossing of legs). However, rather than a conscious relief of an accruing urge by performing the tic, stereotypies appear to be self-stimulating behaviors in response to subconscious tension and anxiety (64). Additional distinguishing features include the following:

1. Stereotypies typically emerge at an earlier age (mean onset, <2 years) than do tics (mean onset, 6–7 years).

2. Phenotypic patterns in stereotypies are fixed, with a generally predictable frequency of occurrence, whereas tics can sometimes shift from one body location to involve another body part and display a larger degree of fluctuation in frequency and severity.

3. Movements in stereotypies are characterized by a fairly continuous and rhythmic nature, as opposed to the brief and abrupt nature of tics (88).

In terms of similarities, both stereotypies and tics can be exacerbated during periods of excitement or stress. Likewise, while both conditions can occur in normal children, they demonstrate a greater prevalence among children with neuropsychiatric disorders, such as autism/mental retardation (for stereotypies) and obsessive-compulsive disorder (for tics in Tourette's syndrome).

6. MANAGEMENT OF PSYCHOGENIC NONEPILEPTIC SEIZURES

The treatment of PNES can be divided into three stages:

1. Establishing and communicating the diagnosis

2. Gaining control of seizures

3. Maintenance management.

6.1. Establishing and Communicating the Diagnosis

For patients with PNES, treatment begins with the seizure-evaluation process. As a group, patients with PNES are more likely to deny emotional factors as the cause of seizures and to endorse an external health-related locus of control than those with epilepsy (89). Physical explanations of symptoms are often vehemently pursued by patients at first, only to be dismissed by many prior emergency department or other medical encounters as "pseudo"-seizures. To address this incongruity, the management of these patients should begin with a comprehensive evaluation (i.e., seizure history, psychosocial assessment, VEEG) that includes a developmental history and review of past trauma and abuse in the *intake* neurological assessment, rather than as an afterthought with a "stat psych consult" just before discharge from the EMU when the diagnosis of PNES is made. Evaluation of PNES through these dedicated efforts during the monitoring conveys to patients that the seizures in PNES are just as legitimate and important as those in epilepsy.

Legitimization of PNES through these efforts can also enhance the patient's acceptance of the subsequent diagnostic explanation. When such a diagnosis is confirmed by VEEG and then appropriately accepted by the patient, it has been reported that up to one third of patients with PNES can become seizure-free during short-term follow-up, often without any additional intervention. Such therapeutic ramification underscores the importance of the communication process by which the diagnosis is explained to the patient and family members. Several communication strategies have been proposed, and the consensus is that the explanation should be communicated to the patient via a tactful, empathetic, positive, non-pejorative, and unequivocal approach (10). Communication with family and other involved clinicians regarding this diagnosis may also augment the uniformity of diagnostic insight in the patient's milieu. Provision of diagnostic letters or supplementary written information may not only facilitate this sharing of diagnostic information but also enhances consolidation (and further legitimizes) the PNES diagnosis.

6.2. Gaining Control of Seizures

While sharing the diagnosis alone may be associated with an initial symptomatic remission for some patients, PNES are likely to relapse without further therapeutic effort aiming to understand the underlying psychological processes in an effort to gain control of seizures (90). Moreover, other somatic and affective symptoms may later evolve if the psychological core issues have not been properly addressed (91). Patients and family should be informed that effective treatment is available to thoroughly address the predisposing, precipitating, and perpetuating factors that contribute to seizure occurrences. Such discussion provides hope to patients, inspires motivation toward self-improvement, and empowers treating clinicians to engage (92).

Among psychotherapeutic approaches for patients with PNES, the most substantial body of data entails the application of core principles and techniques of cognitive-behavioral therapy (CBT), with varying modifications in the therapeutic approach. To date, two CBT-based approaches that have undergone pilot randomized controlled trials for PNES are those used by Goldstein et al. (93) and LaFrance et al. (3).

The CBT evaluated by Goldstein et al. was traditional CBT, based on a fear escape-avoidance model, which views PNES as dissociative responses to cues associated with extremely distressing or life-threatening experiences. These experiences are in turn linked to unbearable feelings of fear and distress. Treatment is delivered across 12 weekly or biweekly manualized sessions, with key topics that include empowering patients to interrupt the behavioral/physiologic/cognitive responses that herald breakthrough seizures, dealing with avoidance behaviors, and addressing negative thoughts as well as illness beliefs that are key to the development and perpetuation of PNES. In the pilot randomized controlled trial, the CBT group experienced significantly less seizure burden than the control group at the end of treatment, and trended toward lower seizure frequency than the control group during follow-up at 6 months after treatment. Also at follow-up, the CBT group trended toward a greater likelihood of having experienced 3 consecutive months of seizure freedom (93).

The therapeutic approach of LaFrance was based on a multimodality, CBT-informed psychotherapy model (CBT-ip) from a therapy that was initially developed to enhance self-control of epileptic seizures (94). This model conceptualizes PNES as the somatic manifestations of maladaptive core beliefs (negative schemas) that have been derived chronically from life experiences as well as acute or recurring traumas. The treatment is delivered as "patient-led, therapist-guided" appointments (95) across 12 weekly manualized sessions; key topics include promoting healthy communication, support seeking, and goal setting; conducting a functional behavioral analysis; identifying seizure warnings/auras; linking triggers, negative states, and target symptoms; practicing relaxation; examining external stressors and internal conflicts; and providing motivation for ongoing health and wellness. In the pilot randomized clinical trial, patients in the CBT-ip intervention showed significant seizure reduction compared to before the intervention. Secondary outcome measures such as depression, anxiety, quality of life, and global functioning measures all showed improvement at the end of treatment compared to before treatment. Notably, the treatment-as-usual (control) group showed no significant difference in seizure frequency or any secondary outcome measures at the end of treatment when compared to before treatment (3).

Despite VEEG confirmation of PNES, some patients may still hesitate to fully embrace a psychiatric diagnosis of CD, in the place of a previously assumed neurological explanation for their seizures. Under such scenarios, psychoeducational approaches have been shown to consolidate the patient's understanding of PNES and promote more open-mindedness toward acceptance of this diagnosis (96, 97). While a pilot randomized controlled trial of a brief group psychoeducational treatment did not result in a significant difference of PNES burden, the intervention group did endorse significantly less impairment in important areas of psychosocial functioning (97). In other words, this group modality may serve as a "stepping stone" from which further therapeutic alliance can build upon or be more readily achieved to transition into individual therapy.

6.3. Maintenance Management

There are several reasons why the working relationship between the neurologist and patient should not abruptly end after a diagnosis of PNES has been established. For some patients who have been chronically misdiagnosed as having epileptic seizure, a "one shot" disclosure may be insufficient to achieve proper understanding of the diagnosis. Instead, iterative and empathetic explanation of the diagnosis across serial visits may gradually foster the patient's acceptance for mental health referrals. Moreover, patients' personal circumstances can change, such that those who were unable to engage in psychological treatment previously may well be able to proceed with treatment at a later time.

While the patient is transitioning into mental health care follow-up, the neurologist's role should include the following:

1. Making sure that the diagnosis of PNES does not change (i.e., back to one of epilepsy)

2. Limiting invasive investigation of other symptoms for which a medical cause has been ruled out

3. Reducing the risk of iatrogenic injury (i.e., supervising the taper of antiepileptic drugs [AEDs]). Early, as opposed to delayed, AED withdrawal (assuming that there is no alternative indication [i.e., documented bipolar disorder, migraine prophylaxis, or neuropathic pain conditions]) is associated with greater benefits on several clinical outcomes (10). For patients with PNES who do not demonstrate epileptiform VEEG findings, the neurologist should follow them for at least 6 months after discontinuing AEDs. This recommendation is consequent to the very small but present possibility of coexisting epilepsy and that the fact the breakthrough epileptic seizures can occur several months after discontinuation of AEDs.

Once the transition to mental health care has been complete, then discussion can commence regarding the patient's discharge from the neurologist's practice. However, the neurologist should continue to follow patients with known interictal or ictal epileptiform abnormalities on their VEEG. Patients with mixed epilepsy with PNES should be treated with the lowest effective AED dose for the epilepsy. They should be counseled that AEDs do not treat PNES, whereas behavioral interventions are the more appropriate treatment for PNES.

7. MANAGEMENT OF PHYSIOLOGIC NONEPILEPTIC EVENTS

Physiologic nonepileptic events result from systemic alterations or disease states that produce an ictus. Since addressing the underlying pathophysiology is the primary treatment of such conditions, achieving an accurate diagnosis has critical therapeutic implications. Whenever feasible, the physiologic nonepileptic diagnoses should be as etiologically specific as possible. For instance, in addition to an overarching diagnosis of syncope, consideration of the etiologic subtype of the syncope (i.e., neurally mediated, orthostasis, primary cardiac disease) can significantly influence the subsequent clinical management.

Detailed management approaches to syncope, movement disorders, and pediatric paroxysms that mimic epileptic seizures are beyond the scope of the present chapter. Readers are referred to the primary literature within each of the respective subspecialties for elaboration of therapeutic approaches.

8. CONCLUSION

In 2014, the National Institutes of Health Epilepsy Benchmarks stipulated as a priority to "Develop effective approaches for earlier and accurate diagnosis and treatment" of nonepileptic seizures (www.ninds.nih.gov/About-NINDS/Strategic-Plans-Evaluations/Strategic-Plans/2014-NINDS-Benchmarks-Epilepsy-Research). This recognition underscores the importance to consider NEE in the differential diagnosis of patients with apparent drug-resistant epilepsy. An erroneous diagnosis of epilepsy not only subjects the patient to the potential complications of unnecessary epilepsy treatment, but delays the delivery of treatment that properly addresses the underlying pathology. These quandaries are compounded by the long delay before establishing a correct diagnosis (2, 3). As such, an important prognostic factor (especially for PNES) is the duration of illness, in which the prognosis can worsen the longer the patient has been mistreated as having epilepsy and does not receive the indicated mental health treatment (98). Indeed, regarding the proper characterization of neurobehavioral paroxysms, correct diagnosis is the first step toward treatment, and as effective treatments are available, patients and providers are now empowered to deliver care to this challenging and once-dismissed population.

REFERENCES

1. Smith D, Defalla BA, Chadwick DW. The misdiagnosis of epilepsy and the management of refractory epilepsy in a specialist clinic. QJM 1999;92(1):15–23.
2. Reuber M, Fernandez G, Bauer J, et al. Diagnosis delay in psychogenic nonepileptic seizures. Neurology 2002;58(3):493–495.
3. LaFrance WC Jr, Baird GL, Barry JJ, et al. Multicenter pilot treatment trial for psychogenic nonepileptic seizures: a randomized clinical trial. JAMA Psychiatry 2014;71(9):997–1005.
4. Reuber M, Baker GA, Gill R, et al. Failure to recognize psychogenic nonepileptic seizures may cause death. Neurology 2004;62(5):834–835.
5. Benbadis SR, O'Neill E, Tatum WO, et al. Outcome of prolonged video-EEG monitoring at a typical referral epilepsy center. Epilepsia 2004;45(9):1150–1153.
6. Salinsky M, Spencer D, Boudreau E, et al. Psychogenic nonepileptic seizures in US veterans. Neurology 2011;77:945–950.
7. Trimble M. Psychogenic nonepileptic seizures: historical review. In Schachter SC, LaFrance WC Jr. (Eds.), Gates and Rowan's nonepileptic seizures (3rd ed.). Cambridge: Cambridge University Press, 2010:17–26.
8. Benbadis SR. Psychogenic nonepileptic "seizures" or "attacks"? It is not just semantics: attacks. Neurology 2010;75:84–86.
9. LaFrance WC Jr. Psychogenic nonepileptic "seizures" or "attacks"? It is not just semantics: seizures. Neurology 2010;75:87–88.

10. LaFrance WC Jr, Reuber M, Goldstein LH. Management of psychogenic nonepileptic seizures. Epilepsia 2013;54(Suppl 1):53–67.
11. Szaflarski JP, Ficker DM, Cahill WT, et al. Four-year incidence of psychogenic nonepileptic seizures in adults in Hamilton County, OH. Neurology 2000;55:1561–1563.
12. Bowman ES, Markand ON. Psychodynamics and psychiatric diagnoses of pseudoseizure subjects. Am J Psychiatry 1996;153(1):57–63.
13. Binzer M, Andersen PM, Kullgren G. Clinical characteristics of patients with motor disability due to conversion disorder: a prospective control group study. J Neurol Neurosurg Psychiatry 1997;63(1):83–88.
14. Westbrook LE, Devinsky O, Geocadin R. Nonepileptic seizures after head injury. Epilepsia 1998;39(9):978–982.
15. Duncan R, Oto M. Predictors of antecedent factors in psychogenic nonepileptic attacks: multivariate analysis. Neurology 2008;71(13):1000–1005.
16. Reuber M, Kral T, Kurthen M, et al. New-onset psychogenic seizures after intracranial neurosurgery. Acta Neurochir (Wien) 2002;144(9):901–907.
17. Frucht MM, Quigg M, Schwaner C, et al. Distribution of seizure precipitants among epilepsy syndromes. Epilepsia 2000;41(12):1534–1539.
18. McGonigal A, Oto M, Russell AJ, et al. Outpatient video EEG recording in the diagnosis of non-epileptic seizures: a randomised controlled trial of simple suggestion techniques. J Neurol Neurosurg Psychiatry 2002;72(4):549–551.
19. Benbadis SR. A spell in the epilepsy clinic and a history of "chronic pain" or "fibromyalgia" independently predict a diagnosis of psychogenic seizures. Epilepsy Behav 2005;6(2):264–265.
20. Lichter I, Goldstein LH, Toone BK, et al. Nonepileptic seizures following general anesthetics: a report of five cases. Epilepsy Behav 2004;5(6):1005–1013.
21. American Psychiatric Association. Diagnostic and statistical manual of mental disorders, 5th ed. (DSM-5). Arlington, VA: American Psychiatric Association, 2013.
22. Syed TU, LaFrance WC Jr, Kahriman ES, et al. Can semiology predict psychogenic nonepileptic seizures? A prospective study. Ann Neurol 2011;69(6):997–1004.
23. LaFrance WC Jr, Baker GA, Duncan R, et al. Minimum requirements for the diagnosis of psychogenic nonepileptic seizures: a staged approach: a report from the International League Against Epilepsy Nonepileptic Seizures Task Force. Epilepsia 2013;54(11):2005–2018.
24. Elzawahry H, Do CS, Lin K, et al. The diagnostic utility of the ictal cry. Epilepsy Behav 2010;18(3):306–307.
25. Vinton A, Carino J, Vogrin S, et al. "Convulsive" nonepileptic seizures have a characteristic pattern of rhythmic artifact distinguishing them from convulsive epileptic seizures. Epilepsia 2004;45(11):1344–1350.
26. Chen DK, Graber KD, Anderson CT, et al. Sensitivity and specificity of video alone versus electroencephalography alone for the diagnosis of partial seizures. Epilepsy Behav 2008;13(1):115–118.
27. Benbadis SR, Lancman ME, King LM, et al. Preictal pseudosleep: a new finding in psychogenic seizures. Neurology 1996;47(1):63–67.
28. Reuber M, Pukrop R, Mitchell AJ, et al. Clinical significance of recurrent psychogenic nonepileptic seizure status. J Neurol 2003;250(11):1355–1362.
29. Benbadis SR, Tatum WO. Overintepretation of EEGs and misdiagnosis of epilepsy. J Clin Neurophysiol 2003;20(1):42–44.
30. Devinsky O, Kelley K, Porter RJ, et al. Clinical and electroencephalographic features of simple partial seizures. Neurology 1988;38(9):1347–1352.
31. Frontera AT Jr. Classification of seizures and epilepsy syndromes. In Husain AM, Tran TT (Eds.), Department of Veterans Affairs epilepsy manual. San Francisco: Epilepsy Centers of Excellence, Department of Veterans Affairs, 2014:2–19.
32. Benbadis SR, Agrawal V, Tatum WO 4th. How many patients with psychogenic nonepileptic seizures also have epilepsy? Neurology 2001;57(5):915–917.
33. Galimberti CA, Ratti MT, Murelli R, et al. Patients with psychogenic nonepileptic seizures, alone or epilepsy-associated, share a psychological profile distinct from that of epilepsy patients. J Neurol 2003;250(3):338–346.
34. Mari F, Di Bonaventura C, Vanacore N, et al. Video-EEG study of psychogenic nonepileptic seizures: differential characteristics in patients with and without epilepsy. Epilepsia 2006;47(Suppl 5):64–67.
35. Reuber M, Qurishi A, Bauer J, et al. Are there physical risk factors for psychogenic non-epileptic seizures in patients with epilepsy? Seizure 2003;12(8):561–567.
36. Bowman ES, Markand ON. Psychodynamics and psychiatric diagnoses of pseudoseizure subjects. Am J Psychiatry 1996;153(1):57–63.
37. Kalogjera-Sackellares D. Psychodynamics and psychotherapy of pseudoseizures. Wales: Crown House Publishing, 2004:3–42.
38. Betts T, Boden S. Diagnosis, management and prognosis of a group of 128 correlates of intractable pseudoseizures. Part II. Previous childhood sexual abuse in the aetiology of these disorders. Seizure 1992;1(1):27–32.

39. Selkirk M, Duncan R, Oto M, et al. Clinical differences between patients with nonepileptic seizures who report antecedent sexual abuse and those who do not. Epilepsia 2008;49(8):1446–1450.

40. Jawad SS, Jamil N, Clarke EJ, et al. Psychiatric morbidity and psychodynamics of patients with convulsive pseudoseizures. Seizure 1995;4(3):201–206.

41. Grady MM, Stahl SM. Panic attacks and panic disorders: The great imitators. In Kaplan PW, Fisher RS (Eds.), Imitators of epilepsy (2nd ed.). New York: Demos Medical Publishing, 2005:277–288.

42. American Psychiatric Association. Diagnostic and statistical manual of mental disorders (5th ed.). Arlington, VA: American Psychiatric Association, 2013.

43. Bowman ES. Posttraumatic stress disorder, abuse, and trauma: relationships to psychogenic nonepileptic seizures. In Schachter SC, LaFrance WC Jr. (Eds.), Gates and Rowan's nonepileptic seizures (3rd ed.). Cambridge: Cambridge University Press, 2010:213–224.

44. Kim SH, Kim H, Lim BC, et al. Paroxysmal nonepileptic events in pediatric patients confirmed by long-term video-EEG monitoring—Single tertiary center review of 143 patients. Epilepsy Behav 2012;24(3):336–340.

45. Moya A, Sutton R, Ammirati F, et al. Guidelines for the diagnosis and management of syncope (version 2009). The Task Force for the Diagnosis and Management of Syncope of the European Society of Cardiology (ESC). Eur Heart J 2009; 30 (21): 2631–2671.

46. Sarasin FP, Louis-Simonet M, Carballo D, et al. Prospective evaluation of patients with syncope: a population-based study. Am J Med 2001;111(3):177–184.

47. Ganzeboom KS, Colman N, Reitsma JB, et al. Prevalence and triggers of syncope in medical students. Am J Cardiol 2003;91(8):1006–1008, A8.

48. Soteriades ES, Evans JC, Larson MG, et al. Incidence and prognosis of syncope. N Engl J Med 2002;347(12):878–885.

49. Kenny RA. Syncope in the elderly: diagnosis, evaluation, and treatment. J Cardiovasc Electrophysiol 2003;14(9 Suppl):S74–S77.

50. Lempert T, Bauer M, Schmidt D. Syncope: a videometric analysis of 56 episodes of transient cerebral hypoxia. Ann Neurol 1994;36(2):233–237.

51. Ammirati F, Colivicchi F, Di Battista G, et al. Electroencephalographic correlates of vasovagal syncope induced by head-up tilt testing. Stroke 1998;29(11):2347–2351.

52. Lipsitz LA, Hayano J, Sakata S, et al. Complex demodulation of cardiorespiratory dynamics preceding vasovagal syncope. Circulation 1998;98(10):977–983.

53. Astrup J, Siesjö BK, Symon L. Thresholds in cerebral ischemia—the ischemic penumbra. Stroke 1981;12(6): 723–725.

54. van Dijk JG, Thijs RD, van Zwet E, et al. The semiology of tilt-induced reflex syncope in relation to electroencephalographic changes. Brain 2014;137(Pt 2):576–585.

55. Rugg-Gunn FJ, Simister RJ, Squirrell et al. Cardiac arrhythmias in focal epilepsy: a prospective long-term study. Lancet 2004;364(9452):2212–2219.

56. Schuele SU, Bermeo AC, Alexopoulos AV, et al. Video-electrographic and clinical features in patients with ictal asystole. Neurology 2007;69(5):434–441.

57. Tinuper P, Bisulli F, Cerullo A, et al. Ictal bradycardia in partial epileptic seizures: autonomic investigation in three cases and literature review. Brain 2001;124(Pt 12):2361–2371.

58. Chu J, Majmudar S, Chen DK. Cardiac asystole associated with seizures of right hemispheric onset. Epilepsy Behav Case Rep 2014;2:127–129.

59. Tea SH, Mansourati J, L'Heveder G, et al. New insights into thepathophysiology of carotid sinus syndrome. Circulation 1996;93(7):1411–1416.

60. Consensus statement on the definition of orthostatic hypotension, pure autonomic failure, and multiple system atrophy. J Neurol Sci 1996;144(1-2):218–219.

61. Petersen ME, Williams TR, Sutton R. Psychogenic syncope diagnosed by prolonged head-up tilt testing. Q J Med 1995;88(3):209–213.

62. Linzer M, Felder A, Hackel A. Psychiatric syncope. Psychosomatics 1990;31(2):181–188.

63. Benbadis SR, Chichkova R. Psychogenic pseudosyncope: an underestimated and provable diagnosis. Epilepsy Behav 2006;9(1):106–110.

64. Helms A, Shulman L. Movement disorders that imitate epilepsy. In Kaplan PW, Fisher RS (Eds.), Imitators of epilepsy (2nd ed.). New York: Demos Medical Publishing, 2005:163–183.

65. Fahn S, Marsden CD, Van Woert MH. Definition and classification of myoclonus. Adv Neurol 1986;43:1–5.

66. Crompton DE, Berkovic SF. The borderland of epilepsy: clinical and molecular features of phenomena that mimic epileptic seizures. Lancet Neurol 2009;8(4):370–381.

67. Gasser T. Inherited myoclonus-dystonia syndrome. Adv Neurol 1998;78:325–334.

68. Jankovic JJ, Fahn S. Dystonic disorders. In Jankovic JJ, Tolosa E (Eds.), Parkinson's disease and movement disorders (4th ed.). Philadelphia: Lippincott Williams & Wilkins, 2002:331–357.

69. Abdo WF, van de Warrenburg BP, Burn DJ, et al. The clinical approach to movement disorders. Nat Rev Neurol 2010;6(1):29–37.

70. Yaltho TC, Jankovic J. The many faces of hemifacial spasm: differential diagnosis of unilateral facial spasms. Mov Disord 2011;26(9):1582–1592.

71. Ho SL, Cheng PW, Wong WC, et al. A case-controlled MRI/MRA study of neurovascular contact in hemifacial spasm. Neurology 1999;53(9):2132–2139.

72. Jankovic J, Demirkiran M. Classification of paroxysmal dyskinesias and ataxias. Adv Neurol 2002;89:387–400.

73. Sadamatsu M, Masui A, Sakai T, et al. Familial paroxysmal kinesigenic choreoathetosis: an electrophysiologic and genotypic analysis. Epilepsia 1999;40(7):942–949.

74. Sethi KD. Paroxysmal dyskinesias. In Jankovic JJ, Tolosa E (Eds.), Parkinson's disease and movement disorders (4th ed.). Philadelphia: Lippincott Williams & Wilkins, 2002:431–437.

75. Bennett LB, Roach ES, Bowcock AM. A locus for paroxysmal kinesigenic dyskinesia maps to human chromosome 16. Neurology 2000;54(1):125–130.

76. Fink JK, Hedera P, Mathay JG, et al. Paroxysmal dystonic choreoathetosis linked to chromosome 2q: clinical analysis and proposed pathophysiology. Neurology 1997;49(1):177–183.

77. Lombroso CT, Lerman P. Breathholding spells (cyanotic and pallid infantile syncope). Pediatrics 1967;39(4):563–581.

78. Evans OB. Breath-holding spells. Pediatr Ann 1997;26(7):410–414.

79. Laux L, Nordli DR. Nonepileptic spells in neonates and infants. In Kaplan PW, Fisher RS (Eds.), Imitators of epilepsy (2nd ed.). New York: Demos Medical Publishing, 2005:79–87.

80. Khurana DS, Valencia I, Kruthiventi S, et al. Usefulness of ocular compression during electroencephalography in distinguishing breath-holding spells and syncope from epileptic seizures. J Child Neurol 2006;21(10):907–910.

81. Hindley D, Ali A, Robson C. Diagnoses made in a secondary care "fits, faints, and funny turns" clinic. Arch Dis Child 2006;91(3):214–218.

82. Bye AM, Kok DJ, Ferenschild FT, et al. Paroxysmal non-epileptic events in children: a retrospective study over a period of 10 years. J Paediatr Child Health 2000;36(3):244–248.

83. Andermann F, Keene DL, Andermann E, et al. Startle disease or hyperekplexia: further delineation of the syndrome. Brain 1980;103(4):985–997.

84. Aguglia U, Tinuper P, Gastaut H. Startle-induced epileptic seizures. Epilepsia 1984;25(6):712–720.

85. Ryan SG, Sherman SL, Terry JC, et al. Startle disease, or hyperekplexia: response to clonazepam and assignment of the gene (STHE) to chromosome 5q by linkage analysis. Ann Neurol 1992;31(6):663–668.

86. Vanasse M, Bedard P, Andermann F. Shuddering attacks in children: an early clinical manifestation of essential tremor. Neurology 1976;26(11):1027–1030.

87. Kabakuş N, Kurt A. Sandifer syndrome: a continuing problem of misdiagnosis. Pediatr Int 2006;48(6):622–625.

88. Mahone EM, Bridges D, Prahme C, et al. Repetitive arm and hand movements (complex motor stereotypies) in children. J Pediatr 2004;145(3):391–395.

89. Stone J, Binzer M, Sharpe M. Illness beliefs and locus of control: a comparison of patients with pseudoseizures and epilepsy. J Psychosom Res 2004;57:541–547.

90. Wilder C, Marquez AV, Farias ST, et al. Abstract 2.469. Long-term follow-up study of patients with psychogenic nonepileptic seizures. Epilepsia 2004;45:349.

91. Nunez-Wallace KR, Murphey DK, Proto D, et al. Health resource utilization among US veterans with psychogenic nonepileptic seizures: a comparison before and after video-EEG monitoring. Epilepsy Res 2015;114:114–121.

92. LaFrance WC Jr, Devinsky O. Treatment of nonepileptic seizures. Epilepsy Behav 2002;3(5 Suppl. 1):S19–23.

93. Goldstein LH, Chalder T, Chigwedere C, et al. Cognitive-behavioral therapy for psychogenic nonepileptic seizures: a pilot RCT. Neurology 2010;74(24):1986–1994.

94. Reiter J, Andrews D, Reiter C, LaFrance WC Jr. Taking control of your seizures: workbook. New York: Oxford University Press, 2015.

95. LaFrance WC Jr, Wincze JP. Treating nonepileptic seizures: therapist guide. New York: Oxford University Press, 2015.

96. Zaroff CM, Myers L, Barr WB, et al. Group psychoeducation as treatment for psychological nonepileptic seizures. Epilepsy Behav 2004;5(4):5875–5892.

97. Chen DK, Maheshwari A, Franks R, et al. Brief group psychoeducation for psychogenic nonepileptic seizures: a neurologist-initiated program in an epilepsy center. Epilepsia 2014;55(1):156–166.

98. Selwa LM, Geyer J, Nikakhtar N, et al. Nonepileptic seizure outcome varies by type of spell and duration of illness. Epilepsia 2000;41(10):1330–1334.

25 | EEG IN PSYCHIATRIC DISORDERS: DOES IT HAVE A ROLE IN THEIR EVALUATION?

ANDRES M. KANNER, MD, FANA, FAES, FAAN AND ADRIANA BERMEO-OVALLE, MD

ABSTRACT: Psychiatric symptoms are not restricted to primary psychiatric disorders and are relatively frequent in medical and neurological disorders. They may represent the clinical manifestations of these disorders, of a comorbid psychiatric disorder, or of iatrogenic complications of pharmacological and/or surgical therapies. Clearly, proper diagnosis is of the essence to provide the correct treatment. Electroencephalographic (EEG) studies are used on a regular basis to identify a potential organic cause of psychiatric symptomatology. This chapter reviews the diagnostic yield of EEG recordings in psychiatric symptomatology associated with primary psychiatric disorders, with neurological and medical conditions, and in particular with epilepsy, and provides suggestions on the optimal use of the different types of EEG recordings in clinical practice.

KEYWORDS: psychiatric symptoms, EEG, electroencephalography, neurology, epilepsy

PRINCIPAL REFERENCES

1. Hesdorffer DC, Ishihara L, Mynepalli L, Webb DJ, Weil J, Hauser WA. Epilepsy, suicidality, and psychiatric disorders: a bidirectional association. Ann Neurol. 2012 Aug;72(2):184–191.
2. Kanner AM. Management of psychiatric and neurological comorbidities in epilepsy. Nat Rev Neurol. 2016 Feb;12(2):106–116.
3. Olbrich S, Arns M. EEG markers in major depressive disorder: discriminative power and prediction of treatment response. Int Rev Psychiatry. 2013;25(5):604–618.
4. Inui K, Motomura E, Okushima R, Kaige H, Inoue K, Nomura J. Electroencephalographic findings in patients with DSM-IV mood disorder, schizophrenia, and other psychotic disorders. Biol Psychiatry. 1998 Jan 1;43(1):69–75.
5. Endres D, Perlov E, Feige B, Fleck M, Bartels S, Altenmüller DM, Tebartz van Elst L. Electroencephalographic findings in schizophreniform and affective disorders. Int J Psychiatry Clin Pract. 2016;20(3):157–164.
6. Varma S, Bishara D, Besag FMC, Taylor D. Clozapine-related EEG changes and related seizures: dose and plasma levels reletionships. Ther Adv Psychopharmacol. 2011;1(2):47–66.
7. Degner D, Nitsche MA, Bias F, Ruther E, Reulbach U. EEG alterations during treatment with olanzapine. Eur Arch Psychiatry Clin Neurosci. 2011;261:483–488.
8. Kanner AM, Soto A, Gross-Kanner H. Prevalence and clinical characteristics of postictal psychiatric symptoms in partial epilepsy. Neurology. 2004;9;62(5):708–713.
9. Chong DJ, Dugan P; EPGP Investigators. Ictal fear: Associations with age, gender, and other experiential phenomena. Epilepsy Behav. 2016 Jul 29;62:153–158.
10. Foff EP, Taplinger D, Suski J, Lopes MB, Quigg M. EEG findings may serve as a potential biomarker for anti-NMDA receptor encephalitis. Clin EEG Neurosci. 2017;48:48–53.
11. Wieser HG, Fischer M. Temporal lobe non-convulsive status epilepticus. In: Nonconvulsive Status Epilepticus. PW Kaplan and FW Drislane, Eds. New York: Demos Medical Publishing, 2009:119–139.
12. Chicharro A, Kanner AM. Psychiatric manifestations of nonconvulsive status epilepticus. In: Nonconvulsive Status Epilepticus. PW Kaplan and FW Drislane, Eds. New York: Demos Medical Publishing, 2009:203–218.

1. INTRODUCTION

The past three decades have witnessed an impressive explosion in our understanding of neurobiological pathogenic mechanisms operant in the primary psychiatric disorders, including mood, anxiety, psychotic, and attention-deficit/hyperactivity (ADHD) disorders. In fact, the majority of research articles published in major scientific journals of psychiatry have been focusing on the investigation of their neuroanatomical, neurochemical, and neurophysiologic changes. For example, in primary major depressive disorders (MDD), neuroimaging studies have demonstrated the existence of bilateral hippocampal atrophy, decreased volume of basal ganglia and thalamus, and decreased cortical thickness in dorsal-lateral prefrontal and orbitofrontal regions, while neuropathological studies have demonstrated neuronal and glial cell loss in various cortical layers of the frontal lobe. Furthermore, a complex relation between psychiatric and neurological disorders has been suggested in epidemiological studies whereby patients with neurological disorders are at increased risk of developing mood, anxiety, psychotic and ADHD, while patients with these conditions are at increased risk of developing epilepsy [1]. Likewise, primary mood disorders have been associated with an increased risk of stroke, migraines, dementias, and Parkinson's disease [2]. Given all of these data, it would be logical to expect abnormalities in electroencephalographic (EEG) recordings.

For two decades, psychiatrists tried to use quantitative EEG (QEEG) as a diagnostic test of primary psychiatric disorders. Unfortunately, the application of QEEG in these conditions was based on unproven principles and faulty methodology and its use in clinical psychiatric practice was discouraged by professional neurological and neurophysiologic societies alike. In recent years, there has been a revival in the interest of QEEG techniques in the investigation of EEG biomarkers of neurobiological pathogenic mechanisms of psychiatric disorders, as a potential diagnostic tool and as a predictor of therapeutic response to pharmacological and somatic (e.g., electroshock therapy) treatments [3]. Yet today QEEG remains a research tool and is not ready to be used for clinical purposes. This chapter reviews the role of EEG studies (routine, prolonged, and video-EEG monitoring) in the evaluation of psychiatric symptomatology in clinical practice.

2. PSYCHIATRIC SYMPTOMATOLOGY: WHAT ARE WE TALKING ABOUT?

Psychiatric symptomatology can represent (i) the expression of primary psychiatric disorders, (ii) the clinical manifestation of the neurological and/or medical disorder, (iii) a comorbid psychiatric disorder whose onset may precede or follow that of associated neurological and/or medical conditions, or (iv) iatrogenic symptoms of pharmacological and surgical treatments of the underlying medical and/or neurological disorders.

Clearly, psychiatric symptomatology is multifaceted and a careful and comprehensive clinical history and physical and neurological examinations are of the essence to generate a diagnostic hypothesis. Yet the following caveats have to be kept in mind. First, the absence of any identifiable signs and symptoms of neurological or medical disease does not necessarily imply a primary psychiatric disorder, since psychiatric symptoms may be their initial and/or prominent clinical manifestations; Table 25.1 lists some examples. Conversely, the presence of a neurological disorder does not exclude the possibility that the psychiatric symptoms in question are the expression of a comorbid "primary" psychiatric disorder, which may have preceded the onset of the neurological disorders and may not play a pathogenic role in the development of the latter. In fact, the lifetime prevalence of comorbid psychiatric disorders is relatively high in patients with the major neurological disorders and has been estimated to range between 30% and 40% in patients with stroke, epilepsy, multiple sclerosis, movement disorders, dementia, headaches, brain tumors, and traumatic brain injury [2].

3. THE ROLE OF EEG IN THE EVALUATION OF PSYCHIATRIC PHENOMENA

In general, neurologists tend to order EEG studies when psychiatric symptomatology is suspected to have an organic cause, though psychiatrists may often order a study in patients with an established primary psychiatric disorder in the hopes of identifying an underlying "organic" trait. The next question is this: What are the specific circumstances in which EEG recordings may yield valuable diagnostic data, and when can they lead to a false-positive diagnosis of a neurological disorder? And if EEG recordings can have a potential diagnostic role in the evaluation of psychiatric symptomatology, which type of EEG study should be considered? Is a routine EEG sufficient or is an ambulatory study a more appropriate option, or should the patient undergo a video-EEG monitoring study? Here are some basic concepts to consider:

1. Routine and prolonged EEG studies are likely to be normal in unmedicated patients with primary psychiatric disorders. For example, in a study of 143 consecutive patients with mood and psychotic disorders, EEG recordings revealed benign variants (e.g., 14 and 6, wicked spikes, small sharp transients of sleep) [4]. While another study reported diffuse slowing of the background activity in up to 6% of recordings obtained in patients with primary mood and psychotic disorders, these data must be interpreted with great caution as the authors failed to control for the presence of psychotropic treatment [5]. Therefore, EEG studies do not add any diagnostic yield in patients with established primary psychiatric disorders in whom there is no suspicion of a potential organic cause.

2. Occasionally, routine EEG studies may identify an organic cause of psychiatric symptomatology that had initially been thought to be the expression of a primary psychiatric disorder and/or unmask an association of these symptoms to an unrecognized neurological disorder. For example, symptoms of inattention and distractibility and behavioral disturbance originally attributed to ADHD may be the expression of and/or associated with unrecognized childhood and/or juvenile absence epilepsy or with benign rolandic focal epilepsy of childhood.

3. Interpretation of EEG recordings in patients taking psychotropic drugs must take into account the potential effects that these drugs may have on electrographic recordings before suggesting a neurological/medical cause. Indeed, psychotropic drugs can cause a variety of EEG abnormalities. Diffuse slowing may occur when drugs are used at high doses (though some drugs can cause slowing of the background activity at therapeutic doses [e.g., neuroleptic drugs, lithium]). Diffusely distributed excessive beta activity has often been associated with benzodiazepines. Two of the second-generation neuroleptic drugs, clozapine and olanzapine, can cause interictal epileptiform activity, and the former can cause myoclonic jerks [6,7]. Of note, the presence of epileptiform activity is not necessarily predictive of an increased risk of seizures, though both drugs have been associated with such risk (clozapine > olanzapine). Table 25.2 summarizes the EEG changes associated with the use of psychotropic drugs.

4. EEG recordings of psychiatric phenomena that are a clinical expression of a neurological disorder and/or the neurological complication of a medical disorder are likely to display abnormal findings corresponding to the underlying neurological pathology (e.g., slowing of the background activity [of variable severity and distribution] in the setting of acute, subacute, and chronic encephalopathic processes). The first part of Table 25.3 summarizes some of the EEG changes identified in patients with common neurological disorders and comorbid psychiatric disorders.

5. Iatrogenic psychiatric symptomatology resulting from a pharmacological therapy may result in abnormal EEG findings if it is the expression of a toxic encephalopathic process. It can consist of diffuse slowing of the background activity of variable severity and at times can include certain patterns such as runs of triphasic waves. On the other hand, EEG recordings are likely to be normal when the psychiatric symptoms (e.g., behavioral, psychotic, anxiety, or depressive symptoms) reflect the effects of intrinsic negative psychotropic properties of

TABLE 25.1. Examples of Medical/Neurological Disorders with Psychiatric Symptomatology

TYPE OF NEUROLOGICAL/ MEDICAL DISORDER	SPECIFIC DISORDER	PSYCHIATRIC SYMPTOMATOLOGY
Metabolic	Uremia and dialysis dementia	Depression, anxiety, hypomanic/manic symptoms
	Porphyria	Anxiety, depression, hallucinations, disorientation, apathy, restlessness
Endocrine	Hypothyroidism	Depression, anxiety, paranoid delusions, hallucinations
	Hyperthyroidism	Depression, anxiety, hallucinations, paranoid delusions, mania, hyperactivity
	Hypoparathyroidism	Depression, anxiety, irritability, apathy, mania, cognitive impairment
	Hyperparathyroidism	Depression, anxiety, irritability, personality changes, hallucinations, paranoid delusions
	Addison's disease	Depression, anxiety, irritability, hallucinations, paranoid delusions, catatonic posturing
	Cushing's disease	Depression, anxiety, emotional lability, paranoia
	Recurrent menstrual psychosis	Sudden onset, short duration, complete remission, depression, mania, stupor, mutism, delusions, hallucinations relative to menstruation
Deficiency states	Vitamin B12/folate	Depression, anxiety, irritability, paranoid delusions, catatonia
	Niacin (pellagra)	Aggression, insomnia, anxiety, delusions
Inflammatory	Systemic lupus erythematosus	Depression, anxiety, hallucinations, paranoid delusions, confusion
	Sarcoidosis	Depression, psychosis
	Antiphospholipid antibody syndrome	Depression, psychosis
Infectious, viral	Rabies	Hyperexcitability, agitation, hallucinations
	HIV encephalopathy	Depression, anxiety, mania, cognitive impairment, hallucinations, delusions, catatonia, sleep disturbances
Infectious, nonviral	Cerebral malaria	Paranoid delusions, manic symptoms
	Central nervous system syphilis	Delusions, hallucinations, depression, anxiety, mania, irritability, emotional lability, catatonia
Degenerative/dementias	Creutzfeldt-Jakob disease	Personality changes, cognitive decline, anxiety, emotional lability, euphoria, insomnia
	Alzheimer's disease	Depression
	Dementia with Lewy bodies	Delusions, visual hallucinations
	Frontotemporal dementia	Delusions, paranoia, disinhibition
Neoplasms	Brain tumors	Apathy, depression, behavioral disturbances
Demyelinating	Multiple sclerosis	Depression, psychosis, manic, hypomanic symptoms
Movement disorders		
	Parkinson's disease	Depression, anxiety
	Huntington's disease	Anxiety, depression, mania, paranoid/grandiose, dementia, delusions, hallucinations
	Sydenham's chorea	Emotional lability, irritability, obsessive-compulsive symptoms
	Wilson's Disease	Personality changes, disinhibition, paranoid delusions, hallucinations, depression
	Idiopathic basal ganglia calcification	Personality changes, agitation

TABLE 25.2. EEG Changes Associated with Psychotropic Drugs at Therapeutic Doses

PSYCHOTROPIC DRUG	IMPACT ON EEG RECORDINGS
Antidepressants	None
Benzodiazepines	Diffuse beta activity
	Diffuse slowing of background activity at high doses
Neuroleptics	Slowing of background activity
	Interictal epileptiform activity associated with clozapine and olanzapine
Lithium	Slowing of background activity

the drug. In addition, iatrogenic psychiatric symptoms may result from neurosurgical procedures, particularly following the resection of temporal and frontal lobe structures. In such cases, the EEG recordings are likely to reveal changes associated with the site and extent of the resection (e.g., focal slowing with a breech rhythm in the area of the resection) and associated complications (e.g., diffuse slowing in the setting of edema with mass effect). The first part of Table 25.3 summarizes the EEG changes associated with iatrogenic psychiatric symptoms in patients with nonepileptic neurological disorders.

6. Psychiatric symptomatology associated with seizure disorders is complex and deserves to be reviewed

TABLE 25.3. A. EEG Findings Identified in Patients with Primary Psychiatric Disorders and with Comorbid Psychiatric Symptomatology Associated with Neurological Disorders

PSYCHIATRIC SYMPTOMS OCCURRING IN THE SETTING OF	MOST COMMON PSYCHIATRIC SYMPTOMS	EEG FINDINGS	EEG ABNORMALITIES RELATED TO PSYCHIATRIC SYMPTOMS?
Primary psychiatric disorders			
Mood disorders		Normal EEG recordings (in the absence of psychotropic drugs)	No
Anxiety disorders			
ADHD			
Psychotic disorders			
Personality disorders			
Alcohol and/or substance abuse		Diffuse slowing	No
		Excessive diffuse beta	
		Periodic pattern with triphasic waves	
Neurological disorders			
Stroke	Depression	Normal EEG	No
	Anxiety	Focal slowing	
		Diffuse slowing	
Multiple sclerosis	Depression	Normal EEG	No
	Anxiety	Focal slowing	
	Manic/hypomanic episodes	Diffuse slowing	
Dementia	Depression	Normal EEG	No
	Anxiety	Diffuse slowing	
	Psychosis		
	Agitation		
Limbic encephalitis	Depression	Diffuse slowing	No
	Anxiety	Bitemporal slowing	
	Psychosis	Extreme delta brushes (see Fig. 25.1)	
	Agitation		

(continued)

TABLE 25.3. Continued

PSYCHIATRIC SYMPTOMS OCCURRING IN THE SETTING OF	MOST COMMON PSYCHIATRIC SYMPTOMS	EEG FINDINGS	EEG ABNORMALITIES RELATED TO PSYCHIATRIC SYMPTOMS?
Parkinson's disease	Depression	Normal	No
	Psychosis	Diffuse slowing	
Huntington's disease	Depression	Normal EEG	No
	Anxiety	Focal slowing	
	Psychosis	Diffuse slowing	
Wilson's disease	Psychosis	Normal	No
		Diffuse slowing	
Headaches	Depression	Normal	No
	Anxiety		
Migraines	Depression	Normal	No
	Anxiety	Epileptiform activity in occipital regions	
Brain tumor	Depression	Normal EEG recordings	No
	Anxiety	Focal slowing	
	Apathy	Diffuse slowing	
	Behavioral disturbances		
Traumatic brain injury	Depression	Normal	No
	Anxiety	Focal slowing	
	Behavioral disturbances	Diffuse slowing	

B. EEG Findings Identified in Patients with Primary Epilepsy and Comorbid Psychiatric Symptomatology

TEMPORAL RELATION OF PSYCHIATRIC SYMPTOMS WITH SEIZURE DISORDER	TYPE OF PSYCHIATRIC SYMPTOMS	EEG FINDINGS	EEG ABNORMALITIES RELATED TO PSYCHIATRIC SYMPTOMS?
Interictal	Depression	Normal EEG recordings	No
	Anxiety	Interictal epileptiform discharges, according to the epileptic syndrome	
	Psychotic	Focal/diffuse slowing, depending on the epileptic syndrome and/or pharmacotherapy with AEDs	
	Irritability/frustration		
	Impulsivity		
	Behavioral disturbance		
Pre-ictal	Depression	Normal EEG recordings	No
	Anxiety	Interictal epileptiform discharges, according to the epileptic syndrome	
	Psychotic	Focal/diffuse slowing, depending on the epileptic syndrome and/or pharmacotherapy with AEDs	
	Irritability/frustration		
	Impulsivity		
	Behavioral disturbance		

TABLE 25.3. Continued

TEMPORAL RELATION OF PSYCHIATRIC SYMPTOMS WITH SEIZURE DISORDER	TYPE OF PSYCHIATRIC SYMPTOMS	EEG FINDINGS	EEG ABNORMALITIES RELATED TO PSYCHIATRIC SYMPTOMS?
Postictal	Depression	Normal EEG recordings	No
	Anxiety	Interictal epileptiform discharges, according to the epileptic syndrome	
	Psychotic	Focal/diffuse slowing, depending on the epileptic syndrome and/or pharmacotherapy with AEDs	
	Irritability/frustration		
	Impulsivity		
	Behavioral disturbance		
Ictal	Depression	Ictal epileptiform activity consistent with seizures of focal or generalized origin (absence status)	Yes (see text)
	Anxiety		
	Psychotic		
Para-ictal	Depression	Normal EEG	No
	Anxiety	Diffuse slowing	
	Psychosis		
	Agitation		
Iatrogenic secondary to AEDs	Depression	Normal EEG recordings	Yes (with encephalopathic process associated with psychotic symptoms)
	Anxiety	Interictal epileptiform discharges, according to the epileptic syndrome	
	Psychosis	Focal/diffuse slowing, depending on the epileptic syndrome and/or pharmacotherapy with AEDs	
		Periodic pattern with triphasic waves	
Iatrogenic secondary to epilepsy surgery	Depression	Normal EEG	No
	Anxiety	Focal slowing	
	Psychosis	Diffuse slowing	

separately to ensure the proper use of EEG recordings in its evaluation. The second part of Table 25.3 includes the EEG findings identified in patients with epilepsy and psychiatric symptomatology. Consideration of the temporal relation between psychiatric symptoms and seizure occurrence (and/or its treatment) is pivotal in the proper diagnosis of any psychiatric symptom in patients with epilepsy. Accordingly, psychiatric symptoms can be the expression of *interictal, peri-ictal, para-ictal*, or *iatrogenic* phenomena [8].

(i) *Interictal* psychiatric symptoms refer to those occurring independently of seizure occurrence and are the most frequently recognized symptoms.

(ii) *Peri-ictal* symptomatology is temporally related to seizure occurrence and is separated into three categories: *pre-ictal, ictal*, and *postictal. Pre-ictal*

symptoms appear during a period ranging between three days and a few hours before the seizure onset. *Ictal* psychiatric symptoms are the expression of the actual seizure. *Postictal* symptoms occur after seizures following a symptom-free period that can range from a few hours to up to seven days. Ictal psychiatric symptoms of panic and depression are relatively frequent and are often misdiagnosed as primary panic disorder and/or depression [9]. Postictal psychiatric symptoms are relatively frequent in patients who have treatment-resistant focal epilepsy, with close to 50% of patients reporting symptoms of depression and/or anxiety and 10% reporting psychotic symptoms [8]. Unfortunately, the existence of peri-ictal psychiatric symptoms is rarely investigated by clinicians and hence is underrecognized.

(iii) *Para-ictal* psychiatric symptoms refer to the development of psychiatric symptoms associated with the sudden remission of ictal activity in patients with chronic treatment-resistant epilepsy. This phenomenon has also been referred as "forced normalization," given the observation that epileptiform activity disappears from interictal recordings with the advent of the psychiatric symptoms. These phenomena have been estimated to occur in ~1% of patients with treatment-resistant epilepsy.

(iv) *Iatrogenic* psychiatric symptoms are relatively frequent and result from the addition of antiepileptic drugs (AEDs) with negative psychotropic properties (e.g., barbiturates, benzodiazepines, levetiracetam, zonisamide, vigabatrin, perampanel) or the discontinuation of AEDs with mood-stabilizing properties in patients with a prior history of a mood disorder that was kept in remission by these drugs. In addition, iatrogenic psychiatric symptoms have resulted from epilepsy surgery of mesial temporal and frontal lobe structures, particularly those involving the limbic circuit.

EEG recordings can play an important role in the evaluation of peri-ictal and para-ictal psychiatric symptoms to ensure that they are not the expression of ictal phenomena. As summarized in the second part of Table 25.3, the EEG findings associated with interictal, pre-ictal, and postictal psychiatric symptoms depend totally on the underlying seizure disorder and/or the impact of the pharmacological treatment on the electrical activity.

Based on these observations, how should EEG studies be used in the evaluation of psychiatric symptoms in patients with epilepsy?

Routine EEG studies may not add any diagnostic yield in patients experiencing interictal psychiatric symptoms, unless there is a question of whether the symptoms in question are the expression of ictal activity (see above). In such cases, the aim of the study should be to capture the target symptoms(s) with EEG recordings; thus, the ideal strategy is the use of ambulatory EEG and/or video-EEG monitoring studies.

Routine EEG studies may yield useful data in patients with interictal psychiatric symptoms in the setting of an encephalopathic process; in fact, in some cases, like n-methyl-D-aspartate (NMDA) receptor encephalitis, EEG recordings can yield a specific pattern (extreme delta brushes [Fig. 25.1]), which can help establish the diagnosis [10].

Given the close temporal relation between pre-ictal and postictal psychiatric symptoms and the actual seizures, EEG recordings are usually ordered to establish whether they may be the expression of ictal activity. In these cases as well, prolonged ambulatory EEG recordings and/or video-EEG monitoring studies should be the preferred approach.

Ictal psychiatric symptoms are the clinical expression of ictal activity involving limbic structures and presenting as focal seizures without loss of consciousness (known as auras) or as focal status without loss of consciousness (aura continua), although the latter may evolve intermittently to ictal activity with dyscognitive features [11]. As stated above, the most frequent ictal psychiatric symptoms include fear (ictal fear or ictal panic), followed by symptoms of depression, euphoric symptoms, sexual emotions, and less frequently formed visual and auditory hallucinations. Penfield referred to these seizures as "experiential" and separated them into

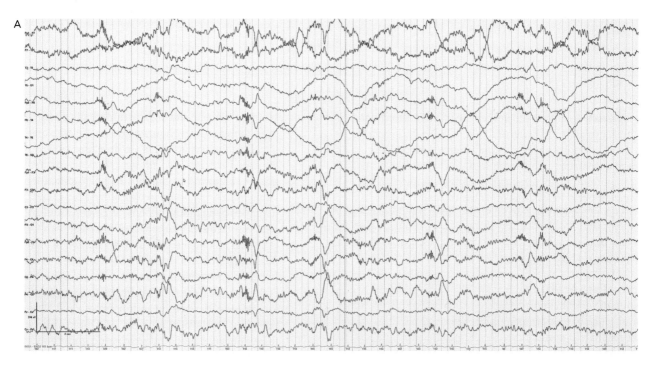

Figure 25.1. Extreme delta brushes in an adolescent girl with NMDA encephalitis.

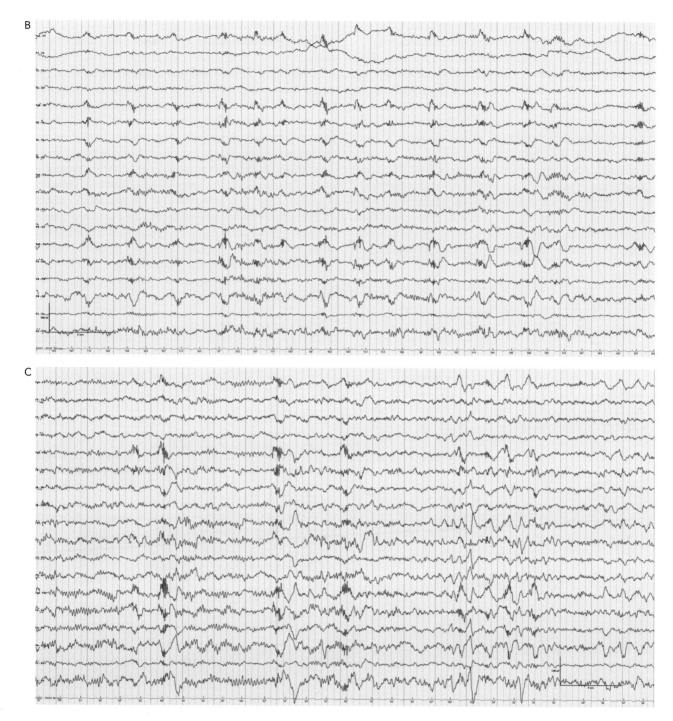

Figure 25.1. Continued

illusions, hallucinations, or both, or described as a dream, a memory, or a flashback. Lennox and Gloor reported that the content of these seizures was related to the patient's personal experiences [11].

Concurrent scalp EEG recordings of psychiatric auras and aura continua often fail to identify any ictal pattern, and confirmation of their diagnosis may require intracranial recordings. The absence of epileptiform discharges on scalp interictal and ictal recordings compounds the diagnostic problem, lest the ictal fear evolve into a focal seizure with loss of consciousness and/or secondarily generalized tonic–clonic seizure. Indeed,

ictal fear is associated with seizures of mesial-temporal origin, in particular the amygdala, a structure known for the generation of epileptiform discharges with a very narrow electric field. In the evaluation of ictal psychiatric symptoms of mesial temporal origin, recordings have to include the use of anterotemporal, basal-temporal, and/or sphenoidal electrodes to increase the diagnostic yield. The diagnosis of ictal fear should be suspected on the basis of the following clinical characteristics: short duration (<30 sec vs. 5–20 minutes in panic attacks); panic feeling that does not reach the level of impending doom (as is typical of panic attacks); associated symptoms suggestive of mesial temporal focal seizures, including epigastric discomfort, *déjà vu, jamais vu,* feelings of derealization and/or depersonalization, and excessive salivation (vs. dry mouth in panic attacks). As alluded to above, failure to recognize ictal fear has resulted in one of the frequent diagnostic errors distinguishing panic disorders and this form of focal epilepsy, leading to an erroneous treatment and compounded by the fact that patients with ictal fear are at increased risk of having interictal panic attacks.

Ictal psychiatric symptoms presenting as bizarre behavior can also be the expression of nonconvulsive status epilepticus with focal seizures associated with loss of consciousness and absence status [12]. The confusional state and intermittent unresponsiveness facilitate the suspicion of an organic process, and the ictal nature of these symptoms is documented with scalp EEG recordings.

4. FUTURE OF EEG IN THE EVALUATION OF PRIMARY PSYCHIATRIC SYMPTOMS

After a failed attempt to bring QEEG into the clinical practice of psychiatric disorders, there has been a move in the past decade to reassess its role in their diagnosis and its use as a predictor of response to various treatments. For example, some studies have suggested that excess theta activity in patients with MDD may be associated with a failure to respond to pharmacotherapy with antidepressant drugs. Some of the QEEG measures under study have included EEG source estimates, left/right asymmetry of the various EEG band ranges, and nonlinear and linear coherence [3]. Whether QEEG will be an accepted diagnostic tool in clinical psychiatry remains to be established at this time.

5. CONCLUDING OBSERVATIONS

Psychiatric symptomatology is relatively common in patients with primary neurological disorders and/or as an expression of neurological complications of underlying medical disorders. Psychiatric disorders have a close and complex relation with several neurological disorders and may share common pathogenic mechanisms, though the former are not the cause of the latter and vice versa. In clinical practice, EEG can play a significant diagnostic role in the evaluation of psychiatric symptomatology in which a careful history and neurological and physical exams suggest a possible association with an underlying neurological/medical disorder, whereas its use in symptoms that are an expression of primary psychiatric disorders is unlikely to yield additional diagnostic data. Prolonged ambulatory and video-EEG monitoring studies may often be necessary to establish objectively the nature of psychiatric symptoms, in particular with patients with known epilepsy, but as discussed above, false-negative findings may not be infrequent in the evaluation of ictal psychiatric symptoms. As with any other diagnostic tool, the optimal diagnostic use of EEG depends on the proper use of the various available types of studies (including the use of additional electrodes) and on an interpretation that factors in a carefully generated diagnostic hypothesis derived from a detailed clinical history and exam.

REFERENCES

1. Hesdorffer DC, Ishihara L, Mynepalli L, Webb DJ, Weil J, Hauser WA. Epilepsy, suicidality, and psychiatric disorders: a bidirectional association. Ann Neurol. 2012 Aug;72(2):184–191.
2. Kanner AM. Management of psychiatric and neurological comorbidities in epilepsy. Nat Rev Neurol. 2016 Feb;12(2):106–116.
3. Olbrich S, Arns M. EEG markers in major depressive disorder: discriminative power and prediction of treatment response. Int Rev Psychiatry. 2013;25(5):604–618.
4. Inui K, Motomura E, Okushima R, Kaige H, Inoue K, Nomura J. Electroencephalographic findings in patients with DSM-IV mood disorder, schizophrenia, and other psychotic disorders. Biol Psychiatry. 1998 Jan 1;43(1):69–75.
5. Endres D, Perlov E, Feige B, Fleck M, Bartels S, Altenmüller DM, Tebartz van Elst L. Electroencephalographic findings in schizophreniform and affective disorders. Int J Psychiatry Clin Pract. 2016;20(3):157–164.
6. Varma S, Bishara D, Besag FMC, Taylor D. Clozapine-related EEG changes and related seizures: dose and plasma levels reletionships. Ther Adv Psychopharmacol. 2011;1(2):47–66.
7. Degner D, Nitsche MA, Bias F, Ruther E, Reulbach U. EEG alterations during treatment with olanzapine. Eur Arch Psychiatry Clin Neurosci. 2011;261:483–488.
8. Kanner AM, Soto A, Gross-Kanner H. Prevalence and clinical characteristics of postictal psychiatric symptoms in partial epilepsy. Neurology. 2004;9;62(5):708–713.
9. Chong DJ, Dugan P; EPGP Investigators. Ictal fear: Associations with age, gender, and other experiential phenomena. Epilepsy Behav. 2016 Jul 29;62:153–158.
10. Foff EP, Taplinger D, Suski J, Lopes MB, Quigg M. EEG findings may serve as a potential biomarker for anti-NMDA receptor encephalitis. Clin EEG Neurosci. 2017;48:48–53.
11. Wieser HG, Fischer M. Temporal lobe non-convulsive status epilepticus. In: Nonconvulsive Status Epilepticus. PW Kaplan and FW Drislane, Eds. New York: Demos Medical Publishing, 2009:119–139.
12. Chicharro A, Kanner AM. Psychiatric manifestations of nonconvulsive status epilepticus. In: Nonconvulsive Status Epilepticus. PW Kaplan and FW Drislane, Eds. New York: Demos Medical Publishing, 2009:203–218.

26 | STANDARDIZING EEG INTERPRETATION AND REPORTING

SÁNDOR BENICZKY, MD, PHD, HARALD AURLIEN, MD, PHD,

JAN BRØGGER, MD, PHD, RONIT PRESSLER, MD, PHD, MRCPCH,

AND LAWRENCE J. HIRSCH, MD

ABSTRACT: This chapter describes how to standardize electroencephalographic (EEG) interpretation and reporting in clinical practice. The Standardized Computer-Based Organized Reporting of EEG (SCORE) software program was developed by an international taskforce under the auspices of the International League Against Epilepsy and the International Federation of Clinical Neurophysiology. Clinically relevant features are scored by choosing predefined terms in the software. This process automatically generates a report and at the same time builds up a database for education, quality assurance, and research. SCORE is the template used for the interactive online educational EEG platform of this textbook.

KEYWORDS: EEG, software, electroencephalography, interpretation, reporting, standardization, SCORE

PRINCIPAL REFERENCES

1. Noachtar S, Binnie C, Ebersole J, et al. A glossary of terms most commonly used by clinical electroencephalographers and proposal for the report for the EEG findings. Electroencephal Clin Neurophysiol 1999;Suppl 52:21–41.
2. Morgan TA, Helibrun ME, Kahn CE Jr. Reporting initiative of the Radiological Society of North America: progress and new directions. Radiology 2014;273:642–645.
3. Ellis DW, Srigley J. Does standardised structured reporting contribute to quality in diagnostic pathology? The importance of evidence-based datasets. Virchows Arch 2016;468:51–59.
4. Bretthauer M, Aabakken L, Dekker E, et al. Reporting systems in gastrointestinal endoscopy: Requirements and standards facilitating quality improvement: European Society of Gastrointestinal Endoscopy position statement. Endoscopy 2016;48:9291–294.
5. Aurlien H, Gjerde IO, Gilhus NE, et al. A new way of building a database of EEG findings. Clin Neurophysiol 1999;110:986–995.
6. Finnerup NB, Fuglsang-Frederiksen A, Røssel P, Jennum P. A computer-based information system for epilepsy and electroencephalography. Int J Med Inform 1999;55:127–134.
7. Aurlien H, Gjerde IO, Aarseth JH, et al. EEG background activity described by a large computerized database. Clin Neurophysiol 2004;115:665–673.
8. Aurlien H, Aarseth JH, Gjerde IO, et al. Focal epileptiform activity described by a large computerised EEG database. Clin Neurophysiol 2007;118:1369–1376.
9. Aurlien H, Gjerde IO, Eide GE, et al. Characteristics of generalised epileptiform activity. Clin Neurophysiol 2009;120:3–10.
10. Beniczky S, Aurlien H, Brøgger JC, et al. Standardized computer-based organized reporting of EEG: SCORE. Epilepsia 2013;54:1112–1124.
11. Hirsch LJ, LaRoche SM, Gaspard N, et al. American Clinical Neurophysiology Society's Standardized Critical Care EEG Terminology: 2012 version. J Clin Neurophysiol 2013;30:1–27.
12. Gaspard N, Hirsch LJ, LaRoche SM, Hahn CD, Westover MB; the Critical Care EEG Monitoring Research Consortium. Interrater agreement for Critical Care EEG Terminology. Epilepsia 2014;55:1366–1373.

1. INTRODUCTION

The clinically relevant features seen in electroencephalographic (EEG) recordings are extremely complex, and a huge number of combinations of these features is possible, allowing one to characterize a particular recording uniquely. This complexity is easily appreciated in reports written in free-text format, which is flexible enough to account for the complexity of EEG. However, the free-text format leads to considerable inter-observer variability, and the extracted features are not stored in a format that would allow systematic search. Although a glossary of terms for reporting EEG has been issued by the International Federation of Clinical Neurophysiology (IFCN)[1], the free-text format still allows the use of terms that are not in the glossary. Furthermore, the same term is used for different phenomena in different centers.

Another important aspect in this context is the goal of the report. The free-text reports are largely based on the tradition originating in the era of analog recordings where paper EEGs could not be stored for long time due to the huge demand for space. That is why reports were extensively descriptive, aiming at reproducing the recordings, but in a condensed manner. The costs of storing digital EEG recordings is today so low that it is really inexpensive to save the original, whole-length recordings. This is obviously the best way of archiving, in an undistorted fashion, the primary data. Therefore, the emphasis in reports today has shifted toward extracting clinically relevant features rather than merely describing the primary data.

Software that gives EEG-ers the option of selecting predefined EEG features while interpreting EEGs has numerous benefits. Based on these selections, the software can automatically generate a report. In the meantime, a database is automatically created with the extracted features. This standardized method of EEG assessment, using the predefined terms for EEG features, contributes to higher inter-observer agreement and is an important educational tool for training young neurophysiologists. The database containing the extracted EEG features has great potential for further research. Similar approaches are under active development for other specialties such as radiology, pathology, and endoscopy[2-4].

Such an approach to EEG assessment and reporting is a semi-automated one. In the absence of clinically validated, reliable algorithms for extracting the clinically relevant EEG features, it is the trained EEG-er who does the feature extraction. However, these features are scored and stored in a standardized way, using software. Standardizing the EEG features and subsequently validating them in clinical practice can be considered the first step toward a fully automated expert system. To create such a system, obviously we need to know precisely which features should be extracted by the algorithms.

There have been several attempts to use software for reporting EEGs in clinical practice. Some of these systems have been published[5,6] and have served as the basis for further studies using the database of extracted EEG features[7-9]. Other systems have been implemented in clinical practice but not published. We mention here a few unpublished examples based on personal communications. At Massachusetts General Hospital, Robert R. Young, Keith H. Chiappa, and their colleagues used a locally developed software for reporting EEG findings in the 1980s. At Johns Hopkins, Ronald Lesser and his colleagues have been using a locally developed form of software ("Reporter") since 1998 for reporting EEG. However, these systems have only been used locally, and there was considerable difference between them.

The International League Against Epilepsy—Commission on European Affairs (ILAE-CEA) and the European Chapter of the International Federation of Clinical Neurophysiology (EC-IFCN) endorsed a taskforce to develop a form of software for EEG reporting. The system was named SCORE (Standardized Computer-Based Organized Reporting of EEG). During the development process, SCORE was tested and adjusted by applying it to real clinical data. The European Consensus Statement on reporting clinical EEGs, and the software based on it (SCORE), has been endorsed by both the ILAE-CEA and the EC-IFCN[10]. This international SCORE process is similar to initiatives in pathology (ICCR), radiology (RADLEX), and endoscopy (GET-C)[2-4]. In 2013, the IFCN appointed a taskforce for developing an international consensus on the standardized structure and terms used in computer-based

reporting of EEGs. This chapter reviews the currently final output from this effort.

Two versions of the software are available: a free version and a premium (commercial) one. The free version is a standalone software program, independent from the EEG-reader software. It completes the scoring of EEG recordings, it automatically generates reports. The commercial version is integrated with the EEG viewer. Items scored in the software are connected to labels in the recording (shown in the viewer). Selecting an item in SCORE automatically moves the recording to the corresponding point (or period) in time in the viewer.

This chapter introduces the reader to using the SCORE system. Besides the items encountered in standard recordings, specific templates have been created for scoring seizures (clinical episodes), rhythmic and periodic patterns in critically ill patients, and neonates.

2. MAIN STRUCTURE OF SCORE

The patient database contains a list of all patients who had their recording scored in that particular hospital/center. Patients can be searched based on their names or personal identification code/social security number. The displayed list can be adjusted using filters—for example, selecting patients only recorded that day, or on a specific date, or restricting the list to the recordings that have not been scored yet (Fig. 26.1).

The database has a hierarchical structure. Each local (hospital) database has many patients, and each patient may have several recordings. Each recording has one currently valid description/report, but in case the reports were revised, the previous versions are also kept in the database. Basic demographic information is saved for each patient (name, gender, handedness, date of birth, social security number). Each recording has the following types of data in SCORE: (1) metadata related to the recording, (2) findings, and (3) report.

The metadata comprise information on the referral and on recording conditions. The "referral" screen stores data on the

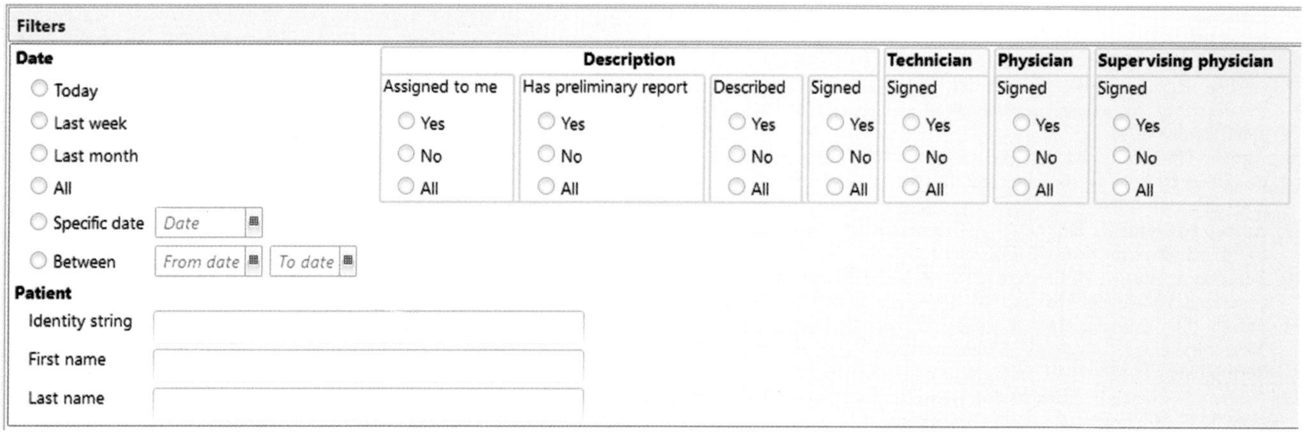

Figure 26.1. Patient database filters help to select the patient or the group of patients.

referring physician/unit, indication for EEG (chosen from a standardized list [Table 26.1]), diagnosis at referral (ICD-10), and information on seizure frequency and/or medication, if appropriate (Fig. 26.2).

Recordings can be "tagged" here—that is, labeled for research projects or teaching database. Departments considering implementing SCORE are advised to implement a standardized referral form, where specific pieces of information are provided by the referring physicians.

The recording conditions screen (Fig. 26.3) stores basic technical information about the recording, such as ID, time and duration, type (e.g., standard EEG, sleep-deprived EEG, long-term monitoring), type of electrode array (e.g., 10-20, 10-10, or other, user-defined arrays), and name of the technologist and physician(s) responsible for recording and reporting. Alertness and degree of cooperation are also registered here. If medication is administered during the recording (e.g., intravenous antiepileptic drugs [AEDs] for a patient in suspected nonconvulsive status epilepticus), this is specified here. Any additional comments or technical notes related to the recording can be typed in as free text.

The findings represent the heart of SCORE (Fig. 26.4). Besides the entries scoring the normal and abnormal EEG

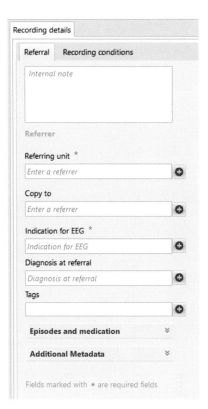

Figure 26.2. Referral information.

features in the recording, the "findings" section also contains information on the type of modulators/procedures and the diagnostic significance in the end. In the free version of SCORE, each new finding is entered by clicking on the corresponding folder (e.g., interictal findings) or by clicking on the icon with the plus sign on the top of the page. Then the entered finding is scored (characterized) in the software. In the premium version, when the neurophysiologist observes a change in the EEG that has to be scored, a label is inserted into the EEG reader. There are three kinds of labels: PDR (posterior dominant rhythm), episode (clinical episodes) and graphoelement (any other finding). Then the inserted item is scored in the software.

The modulators/procedures feature lists the provocation methods used during the recording (hyperventilation, intermittent photic stimulation) and other procedures that could modulate the EEG (e.g., nociceptive stimulation in a patient in coma, or AED administered during the recording to a patient with suspected nonconvulsive status epilepticus (Fig. 26.5). In the premium version, these items are connected to labels in the EEG viewer, corresponding to the time of their appearance.

3. HOW TO USE SCORE

We will now explain how to use the software to score the features observed in a recording. The list of the features is long, since there are many clinically relevant features that can occur in an EEG recording. Nevertheless, the structure of the system is user-friendly—that is, items that are not present in the

TABLE 26.1. Standardized List of Indications for EEG

Epilepsy-related indications	- Clinical suspicion of epilepsy - Reconsider the initial diagnosis of epilepsy - Classification of a patient diagnosed with epilepsy - Changes in seizure pattern - Suspicion of nonconvulsive status epilepticus - Monitoring of status epilepticus - Monitoring of seizure frequency - Monitoring the effect of medication - Considering stopping AED therapy - Presurgical evaluation - Driver's license or flight certificate
Other differential diagnostic questions	- Psychogenic non-epileptic seizures - Loss of consciousness - Disturbance of consciousness - Encephalopathy - Encephalitis - Dementia - Cerebral vascular disease - Paroxysmal behavioral changes - Other psychiatric/behavioral symptoms - Coma - Brain death
Specific pediatric indications	- Genetic syndrome - Metabolic disorder - Regression - Developmental problems
Follow-up EEG	
Assessment of prognosis	
Research project	
Other indication	

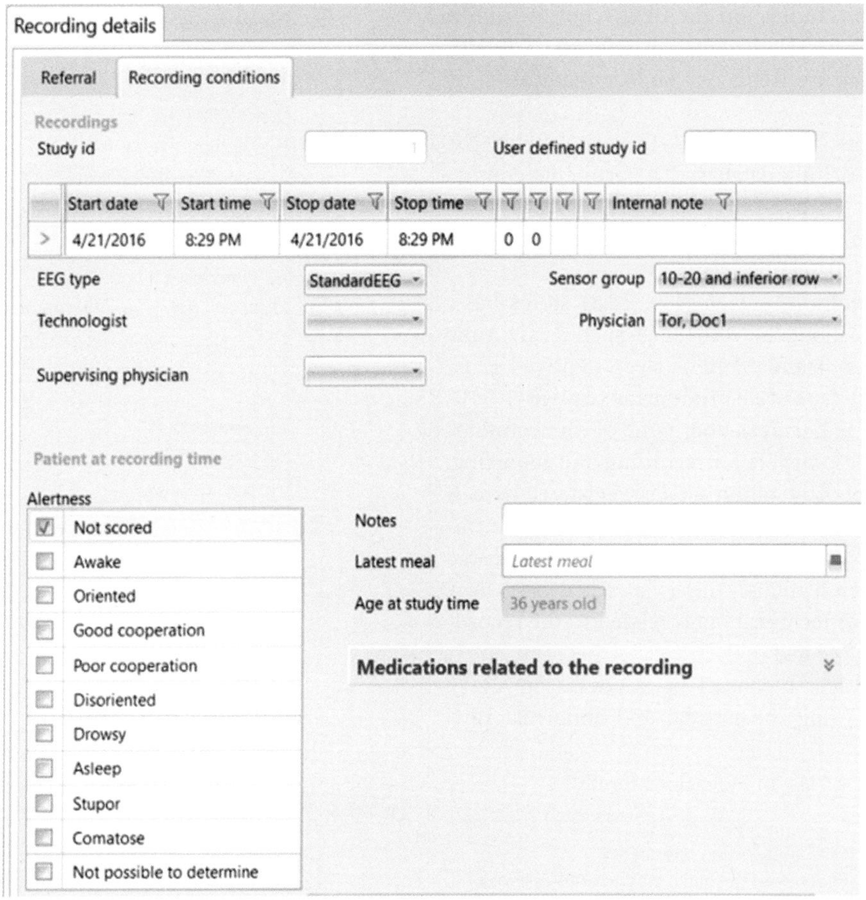

Figure 26.3. Recording conditions.

recording should not be opened and thus do not cause any delay in generating a report. Scoring a normal recording takes <30 sec, but of course the more complex the abnormalities are in a recording, the longer it takes to score them. However, the centers that have implemented SCORE have found that

- Modulators and procedures
- Background activity
- Sleep and drowsiness
- Interictal findings
- Rhythmic and periodic patterns in critical ill patients
- Episodes
- Physiologic patterns
- Patterns of uncertain significance
- Artefacts
- Polygraphic channels
- Unclassified
- Trend analysis
- ▶ Diagnostic significance (1)

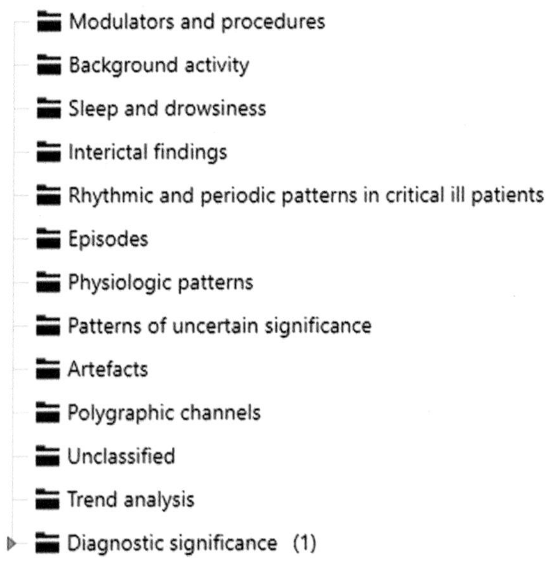

Figure 26.4. The list of findings contains all entities that can be scored for a recording.

using the software takes less time than dictating the report in free-text format and then checking the printed report before signing it.

In the free version of SCORE, clicking on a folder in the findings box automatically adds an "unclassified" item for that folder, which then has to be scored by choosing the relevant terms and properties in selection boxes. In the premium version, a label is inserted into the recording where a feature to be scored is observed. This label is automatically transferred to SCORE for further characterization. While scoring an entry, the selected features/properties are automatically summarized in a text box on top of the selection window. Features and terms in SCORE are defined, and the definition can be opened in a popup box when right-clicking on the term/feature.

3.1. Background Activity

The ongoing activity can be scored as PDR, other organized rhythms, or "special feature" (Fig. 26.6). There is a shortcut key that leads directly to scoring PDR. If PDR is absent, that can be specified here, and the reviewer can account for any possible reason for its absence. Frequency values for PDR are typed in. Amplitude ranges, amplitude and frequency symmetry/asymmetry, and reactivity to eye-opening are selected from predefined lists. The significance (interpretation) of the PDR

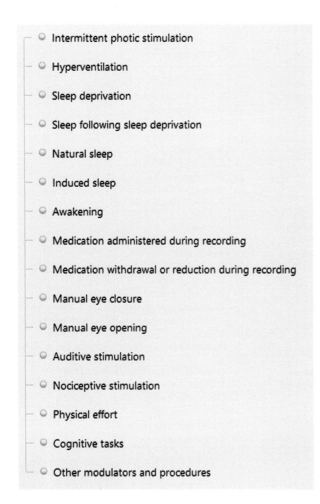

- Intermittent photic stimulation
- Hyperventilation
- Sleep deprivation
- Sleep following sleep deprivation
- Natural sleep
- Induced sleep
- Awakening
- Medication administered during recording
- Medication withdrawal or reduction during recording
- Manual eye closure
- Manual eye opening
- Auditive stimulation
- Nociceptive stimulation
- Physical effort
- Cognitive tasks
- Other modulators and procedures

Figure 26.5. List of modulators and procedures.

is scored as normal, abnormal, no definite abnormality, or not possible to determine.

Any rhythmic activity belonging to the background, but not PDR or mu rhythm, is scored under "other organized rhythms" (Fig. 26.7). This comprises alpha activity, beta activity and low-frequency activity. After choosing the type of rhythm, its location, frequency, and reactivity are scored, along with its extent (percentage of the recording where this rhythm is observed). Finally, its significance is specified, just as for the PDR. Special features (see Fig. 26.7) is used for scoring background activity in critically ill patients: continuous, nearly continuous, discontinuous, burst-attenuation, burst-suppression, suppression, electrocerebral inactivity.

3.2. Sleep and Drowsiness

Sleep and drowsiness are scored to the extent that is relevant for clinical EEG recordings (Fig. 26.8). Sleep during the recording can be classified as normal sleep stages, sleep-onset rapid eye movement (REM), or nonreactive sleep activity. Absence of sleep in the recording can be also specified here ("sleep not recorded"). When hypnagogic or hypnopompic hypersynchrony is observed, it can be documented by choosing this term in the selection box. Abnormal asymmetry or absence of sleep graphoelements can be scored here (e.g., the absence of sleep spindles over one hemisphere). The sleep stages that were reached during the recording are specified by checking them in the selection box (N1, N2, N3, REM).

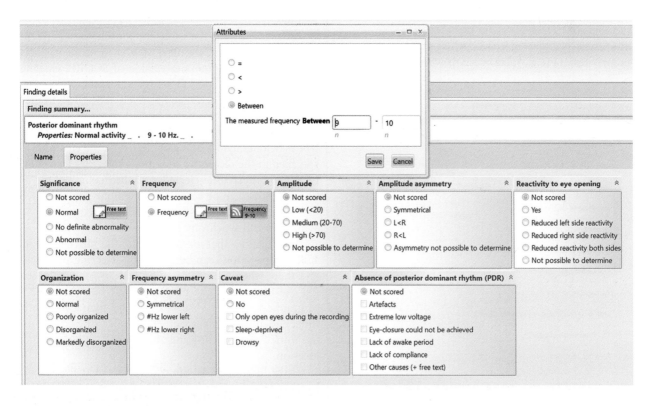

Figure 26.6. Scoring the PDR (posterior dominant rhythm).

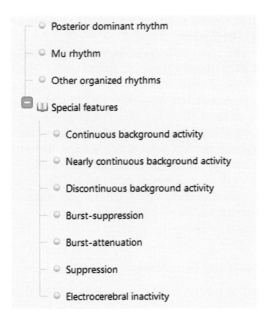

- Posterior dominant rhythm
- Mu rhythm
- Other organized rhythms
- Special features
  - Continuous background activity
  - Nearly continuous background activity
  - Discontinuous background activity
  - Burst-suppression
  - Burst-attenuation
  - Suppression
  - Electrocerebral inactivity

Figure 26.7. The entities that can be scored for background activity.

3.3. Interictal Findings

This is the most commonly used findings folder for scoring abnormal EEGs. The scoring follows the logical thinking of the EEG-er when assessing an abnormal graphoelement.

The first step is to identify the graphoelement by naming it. There are three main categories listed here: epileptiform interictal activity, abnormal rhythmic activity, and "special patterns." In this window, by clicking on the plus sign in front of "special patterns," the list of the names appears: periodic discharges (lateralized, bilateral-independent, generalized, multifocal), extreme delta brushes, burst-suppression, burst-attenuation.

The next step, under "morphology," is to specify the form of the graphoelement (e.g., spike or sharp-wave for epileptiform

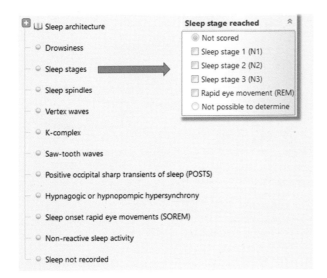

- Sleep architecture
- Drowsiness
- Sleep stages →
- Sleep spindles
- Vertex waves
- K-complex
- Saw-tooth waves
- Positive occipital sharp transients of sleep (POSTS)
- Hypnagogic or hypnopompic hypersynchrony
- Sleep onset rapid eye movements (SOREM)
- Non-reactive sleep activity
- Sleep not recorded

Sleep stage reached ⌃
- Not scored
- Sleep stage 1 (N1)
- Sleep stage 2 (N2)
- Sleep stage 3 (N3)
- Rapid eye movement (REM)
- Not possible to determine

Figure 26.8. Scoring sleep.

TABLE 26.2. Morphology Lists for the Interictal Findings

NAME	MORPHOLOGY
Epileptiform interictal activity	• Spike • Spike-and-slow-wave • Runs of rapid spikes • Polyspike • Polyspike-and-slow-wave • Sharp-wave • Sharp-and-slow-wave • Slow sharp-wave • Hypsarrhythmia—classic • Hypsarrhythmia—modified
Abnormal rhythmic activity	• Delta activity • Theta activity • Alpha activity • Beta activity • Gamma activity • Polymorphic delta • Frontal intermittent rhythmic delta activity (FIRDA) • Occipital intermittent rhythmic delta activity (OIRDA) • Temporal intermittent rhythmic delta activity (TIRDA)
Special patterns	• Lateralized periodic discharges (LPDs) • Bilateral independent periodic discharges (BI-PDs) • Generalized periodic discharges (GPDs) • Extreme delta brushes • Burst-suppression pattern • Burst-attenuation pattern

activity). When several forms of the same category of graphoelement are observed, several items under morphology can be selected, provided that they are seen in the same location(s). Table 26.2 shows the morphology lists for the interictal findings.

After identifying the name and morphology of the interictal graphoelement, the next step is to score its location (Fig. 26.9). In the premium version of SCORE, clicking on the electrodes in the EEG viewer automatically selects the region names. This can then be edited in SCORE. In the free version, the location is noted by first choosing the names of the regions and the laterality. This produces the list of electrodes belonging to that region, based on the electrode array specified in the recording conditions section. Electrodes can be edited (selected/deselected) and the maxima of the negative potentials can be specified. If a graphoelement is scored as "bilateral," additional boxes appear for scoring amplitude symmetry and synchrony.

Propagation that occurs within the discharge (intra-spike propagation) can be scored by selecting propagation, and then, when the new location window opens, by selecting the location of the propagation. When the same type of graphoelement is observed in more than two locations, independently from each other, these can be scored under the same entry by choosing "multifocal" as a descriptor of location.

If the location is determined by source analysis, this can be scored by choosing the sub-lobar region of the source (last

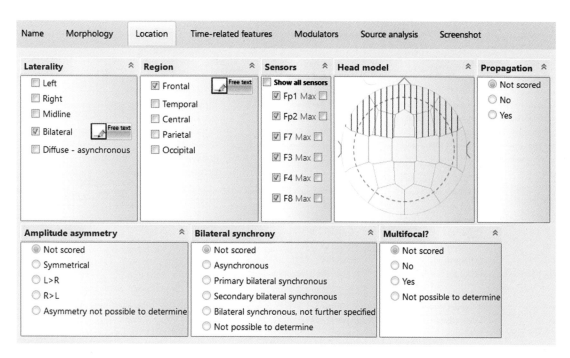

Figure 26.9. Scoring location.

selection window). Time-related features (Fig. 26.10) contain the following: mode of appearance (random/periodic/variable), discharge pattern (single discharges/rhythmic trains or bursts/arrhythmic trains or bursts/fragmented patterns). For periodic patterns, the interval between the discharges is specified here. For trains or bursts, duration can be specified. For rhythmic patterns, the frequency can be further specified. For single discharges, the amount of the discharge in the recording is estimated and scored in the incidence window (number/

time period). For trains or bursts, this is estimated in the prevalence box, expressed as the percentage of the recording covered by this pattern.

Under modulators (Fig. 26.11) the reviewer scores the effect of the various provocation methods or procedures on the described graphoelement (increased/decreased/only during/stopped by/unmodified). For scoring the effect of intermittent photic stimulation, a specific list is available, according to the ILAE recommendation.

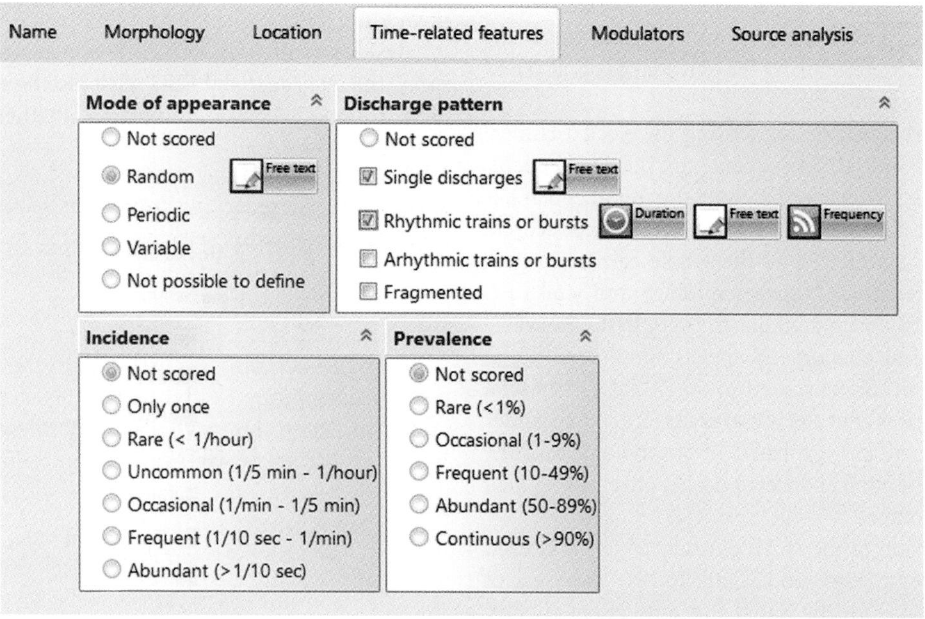

Figure 26.10. Time-related features.

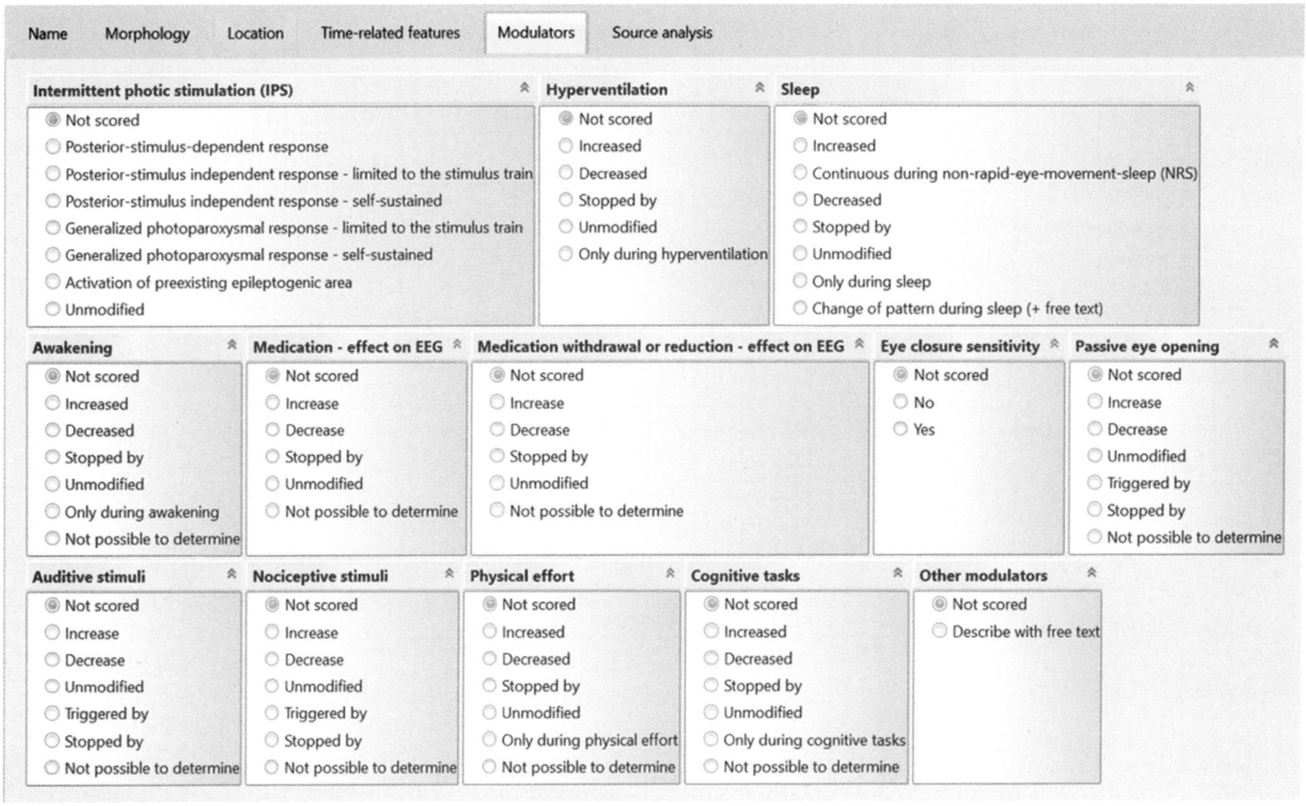

Name
Morphology
Location
Time-related features
Modulators
Source analysis
Intermittent photic stimulation (IPS)
Not scored
Posterior-stimulus-dependent response
Posterior-stimulus independent response - limited to the stimulus train
Posterior-stimulus independent response - self-sustained
Generalized photoparoxysmal response - limited to the stimulus train
Generalized photoparoxysmal response - self-sustained
Activation of preexisting epileptogenic area
Unmodified
Hyperventilation
Not scored
Increased
Decreased
Stopped by
Unmodified
Only during hyperventilation
Sleep
Not scored
Increased
Continuous during non-rapid-eye-movement-sleep (NRS)
Decreased
Stopped by
Unmodified
Only during sleep
Change of pattern during sleep (+ free text)
Awakening
Not scored
Increased
Decreased
Stopped by
Unmodified
Only during awakening
Not possible to determine
Medication - effect on EEG
Not scored
Increase
Decrease
Stopped by
Unmodified
Not possible to determine
Medication withdrawal or reduction - effect on EEG
Not scored
Increase
Decrease
Stopped by
Unmodified
Not possible to determine
Eye closure sensitivity
Not scored
No
Yes
Passive eye opening
Not scored
Increase
Decrease
Unmodified
Triggered by
Stopped by
Not possible to determine
Auditive stimuli
Not scored
Increase
Decrease
Unmodified
Triggered by
Stopped by
Not possible to determine
Nociceptive stimuli
Not scored
Increase
Decrease
Unmodified
Triggered by
Stopped by
Not possible to determine
Physical effort
Not scored
Increased
Decreased
Stopped by
Unmodified
Only during physical effort
Not possible to determine
Cognitive tasks
Not scored
Increased
Decreased
Stopped by
Unmodified
Only during cognitive tasks
Not possible to determine
Other modulators
Not scored
Describe with free text

Figure 26.11. *Scoring the effect of modulators.*

3.4. Episodes

Clinical episodes (e.g., epileptic seizures, syncope, psychogenic seizures) are scored in this folder. Specific sub-folders for ictal EEG and semiology are available for characterizing the intricate electro-clinical correlations during seizures. The conclusion about the type of the episode and its name (classification) are scored, along with its timing and context. If any medication is administered during the episode, its clinical and EEG effects can be scored here.

Three epochs are available for scoring the electro-clinical findings (Fig. 26.12): initial, subsequent, and postictal epochs. For short seizures (e.g., myoclonus), only the initial epoch has to be scored; when the following two epochs are not scored, the initial phase is considered as the whole seizure period. For each of the three phases, both semiology and ictal EEG are scored. The initial epoch contains the very first observable phenomena. If several phenomena appear simultaneously at seizure onset, they all can be scored in the initial epoch. Ictal phenomena that appear after the initial epoch are scored under the subsequent epoch and are listed in chronological order. The time between the clinical onset and EEG onset is specified in the timing and context.

A modified version of the ILAE glossary of terms is used for scoring semiology (Figs. 26.13 and 26.14). Two sets of terms are available: one for the initial and subsequent epochs, and another one for the postictal phase.

After choosing the term for the ictal/postictal semiologic finding, the somatotopic modifier (Fig. 26.15) must be scored by specifying the part of the body where the phenomenon is observed. For some semiologic findings, the name itself specifies its somatotopy (e.g., epigastric aura), while for the others, its location must be scored by the user (e.g., myoclonic jerk).

Besides semiology, for each epoch of the episode (seizure), the ictal/postictal EEG must also be scored (Fig. 26.16). First, a name is chosen, indicating whether an ictal/postictal

Episodes (1)
? Unclassified
Semiology
Initial
Subsequent
Postictal
EEG
Initial
Subsequent
Postictal

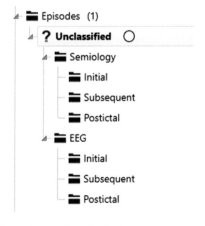

Figure 26.12. *The scoring template of episodes.*

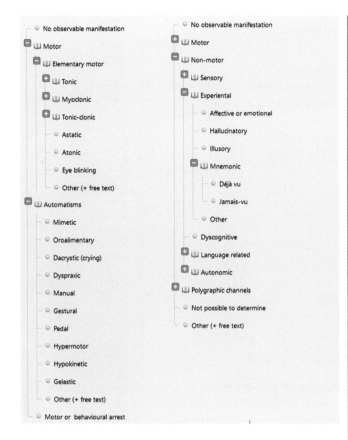

Figure 26.13. Terms for scoring ictal semiology.

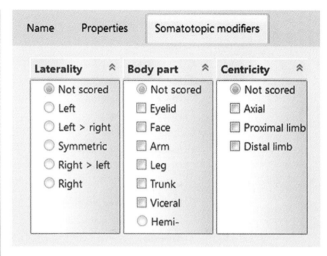

Figure 26.15. Scoring somatotopic modifiers.

pattern can be identified. If there is an observable ictal/postictal EEG pattern, its morphology is specified in the next step (Fig. 26.17). Then, the location is scored, using the same module already described for the interictal patterns. In the last step (properties), additional features (frequency and amplitude) are scored (Fig. 26.18). If several seizures are described under the same entry and there is some variation in the presence/absence of the various semiologic features or ictal EEG, the number of seizures in which the scored feature was present (event count) can be specified. Besides scoring the EEG and semiology that occurs during an episode, it the episode itself has to be classified and its timing and content must be scored. In the header of the episode entry, the reviewer can choose from the list shown in Figure 26.19.

After naming the episode, the timing and context box appears (Fig. 26.20). Clinically important features are scored here (e.g., consciousness, patient awareness of the seizure, time relationship between the appearance of EEG pattern and the semiology, time interval between them). The number of seizures scored under this entry is specified here (events per recording), as well as the state of consciousness from which the seizure starts (sleep/awake), the duration of the seizure and of the postictal phase, the presence of a prodrome, and tongue biting.

Factors influencing the occurrence of seizure are scored under modulators (facilitating and provoking factors). If medication was administered during the episode (e.g., AEDs during status epilepticus), its clinical effect and changes in the EEG are scored here (Fig. 26.21).

3.5. Rhythmic and Periodic Patterns in Critically Ill Patients

A special template for scoring rhythmic and periodic patterns in critically ill patients is available in SCORE. It was developed in accordance with the American Clinical Neurophysiology Society (ACNS) Critical Care EEG terminology, an official guideline of that society (the full description of the nomenclature, a self-guided training module, and clinical tools for this

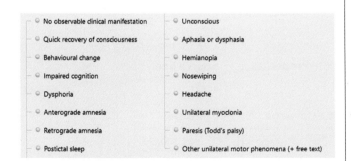

Figure 26.14. Terms for scoring postictal semiology.

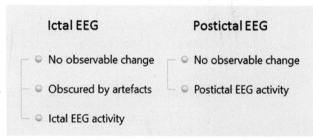

Figure 26.16. Scoring ictal and postictal EEG.

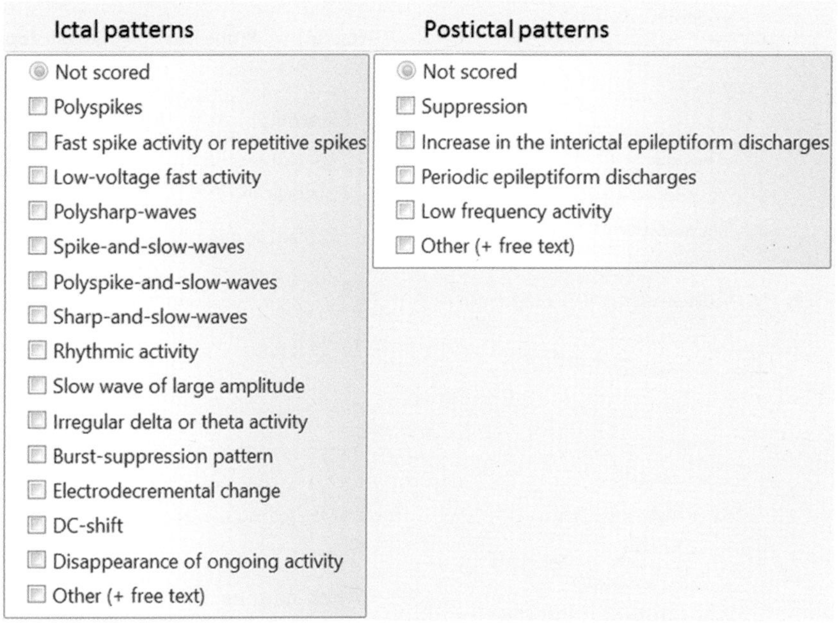

Figure 26.17. Ictal and postictal EEG patterns.

are available at http://www.acns.org/practice/guidelines)[11]. This terminology underwent numerous interrater reliability studies and revisions. This published version had very high interrater reliability for its main terms but more variable results for some of the many modifiers[12].

For each scored pattern, the user can attach a semiology scoring, provided the pattern is associated with a clinical manifestation (e.g., subtle myoclonus) (Fig. 26.22). In the first step, the user scores the name of the pattern to be described (at this stage it stands as "unclassified"). There are three possible choices: periodic discharges (PDs), rhythmic delta activity (RDA), or spike-and-wave, polyspike-and-wave or sharp-and-wave (SW). In the following step, the features related to the morphology of the pattern are scored. The features depend on the type of pattern. For PDs (Fig. 26.23) the user scores superimposed activity, sharpness, number of phases, triphasic morphology, absolute amplitude, relative amplitude (compared to baseline activity between discharges), and polarity. For RDA, the morphologic features are superimposed activity and amplitude (Fig. 26.24). For SWs the following can be scored: sharpness, number of phases, triphasic morphology, amplitude, and polarity (Fig. 26.25).

The location of the pattern is scored using the same module as for other EEG patterns. After scoring the location, the name of the pattern changes automatically, according to the type of location. If the location is scored as unilateral/focal, the name changes to "lateralized." If "bilateral" is selected, a new box appears, where the user has to score the synchrony. If "bilateral synchronous" is selected, the name changes to "generalized." If "bilateral independent" is selected, the name changes to "bilateral independent discharge." Time-related features contain prevalence, frequency (typical frequency and frequency range), duration, onset, and dynamics (Fig. 26.26).

The last features to be scored for the rhythmic and periodic patterns in critically ill patients are the modulators (Fig. 26.27). Here the user can score whether the pattern is spontaneous or stimulus-induced, and the type of stimulation can be specified. The clinical and EEG effects of medication administered or withdrawn during the recording are also scored here (see Fig. 26.27).

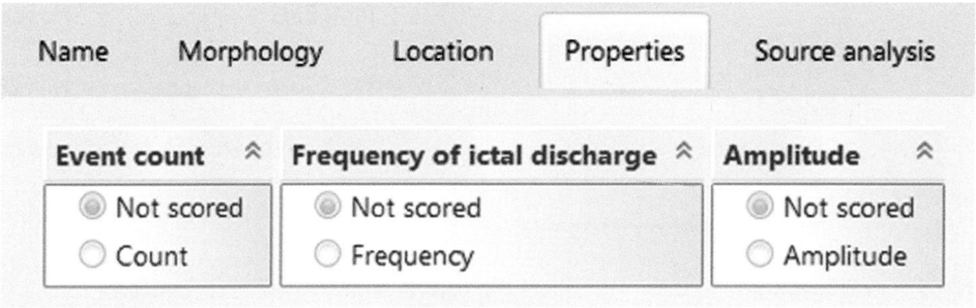

Figure 26.18. Properties of EEG ictal patterns.

Epileptic seizure
Focal onset
Generalized onset
Unknown onset
Subtle seizure
Psychogenic non-epileptic seizure (PNES)
Electroencephalographic seizure
Sleep-related events
Arousal (normal)
Benign sleep myoclonus
Confusional awakening
Periodic Limb Movement in Sleep (PLMS)
REM Sleep Behavioural Disorder (RBD)
Sleep-walking
Paediatric events
Hyperekplexia
Jactatio capitis nocturna
Pavor nocturnus
Stereotypical behaviour
Paroxysmal motor events
Other
Syncope
Cataplexy
Other (Specified in free text)
Not possible to determine

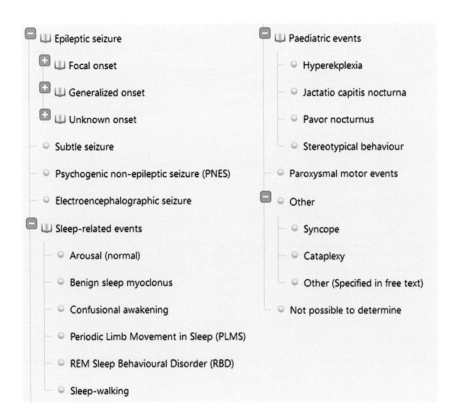

Figure 26.19. *List of episode names.*

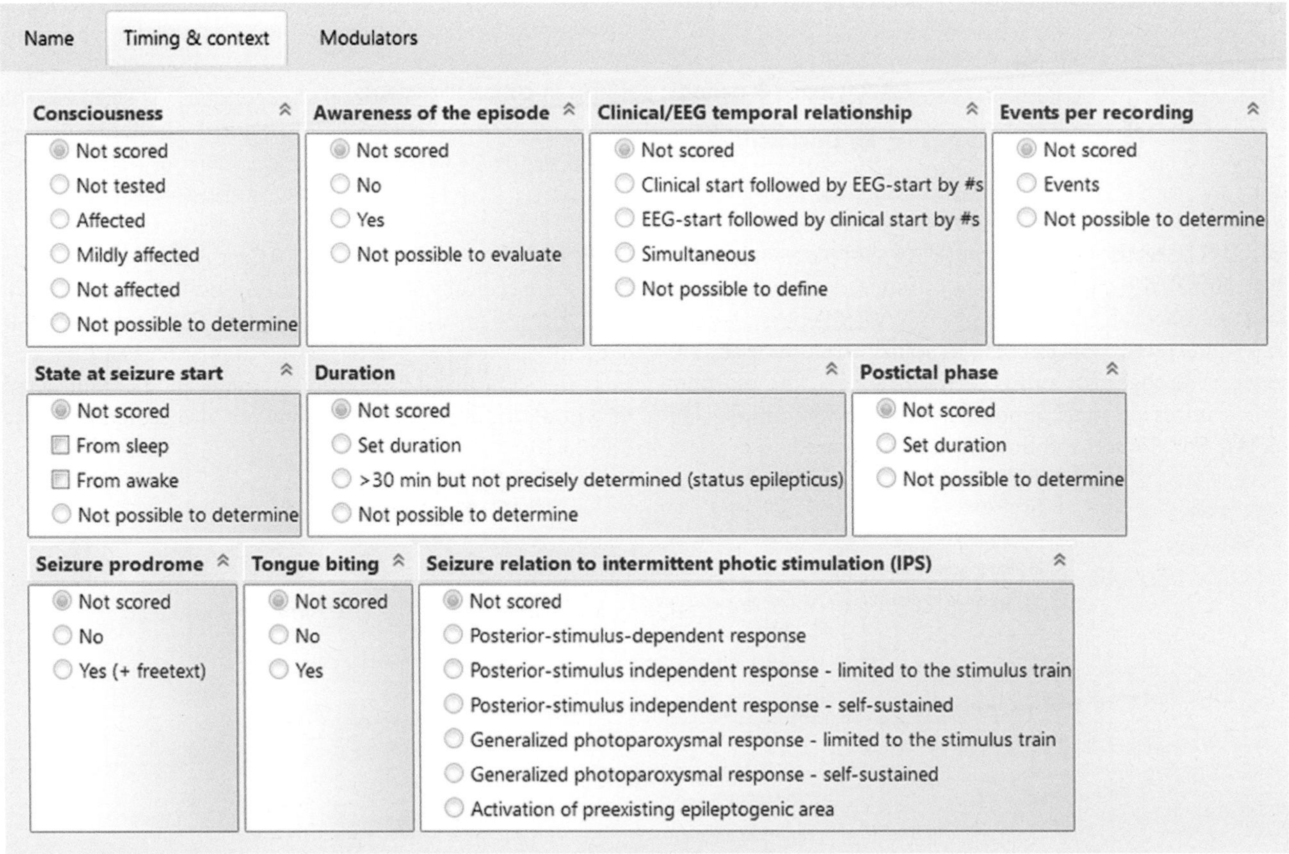

Name
Timing & context
Modulators
Consciousness
Not scored
Not tested
Affected
Mildly affected
Not affected
Not possible to determine
Awareness of the episode
Not scored
No
Yes
Not possible to evaluate
Clinical/EEG temporal relationship
Not scored
Clinical start followed by EEG-start by #s
EEG-start followed by clinical start by #s
Simultaneous
Not possible to define
Events per recording
Not scored
Events
Not possible to determine
State at seizure start
Not scored
From sleep
From awake
Not possible to determine
Duration
Not scored
Set duration
>30 min but not precisely determined (status epilepticus)
Not possible to determine
Postictal phase
Not scored
Set duration
Not possible to determine
Seizure prodrome
Not scored
No
Yes (+ freetext)
Tongue biting
Not scored
No
Yes
Seizure relation to intermittent photic stimulation (IPS)
Not scored
Posterior-stimulus-dependent response
Posterior-stimulus independent response - limited to the stimulus train
Posterior-stimulus independent response - self-sustained
Generalized photoparoxysmal response - limited to the stimulus train
Generalized photoparoxysmal response - self-sustained
Activation of preexisting epileptogenic area

Figure 26.20. *Scoring the timing and context of episodes.*

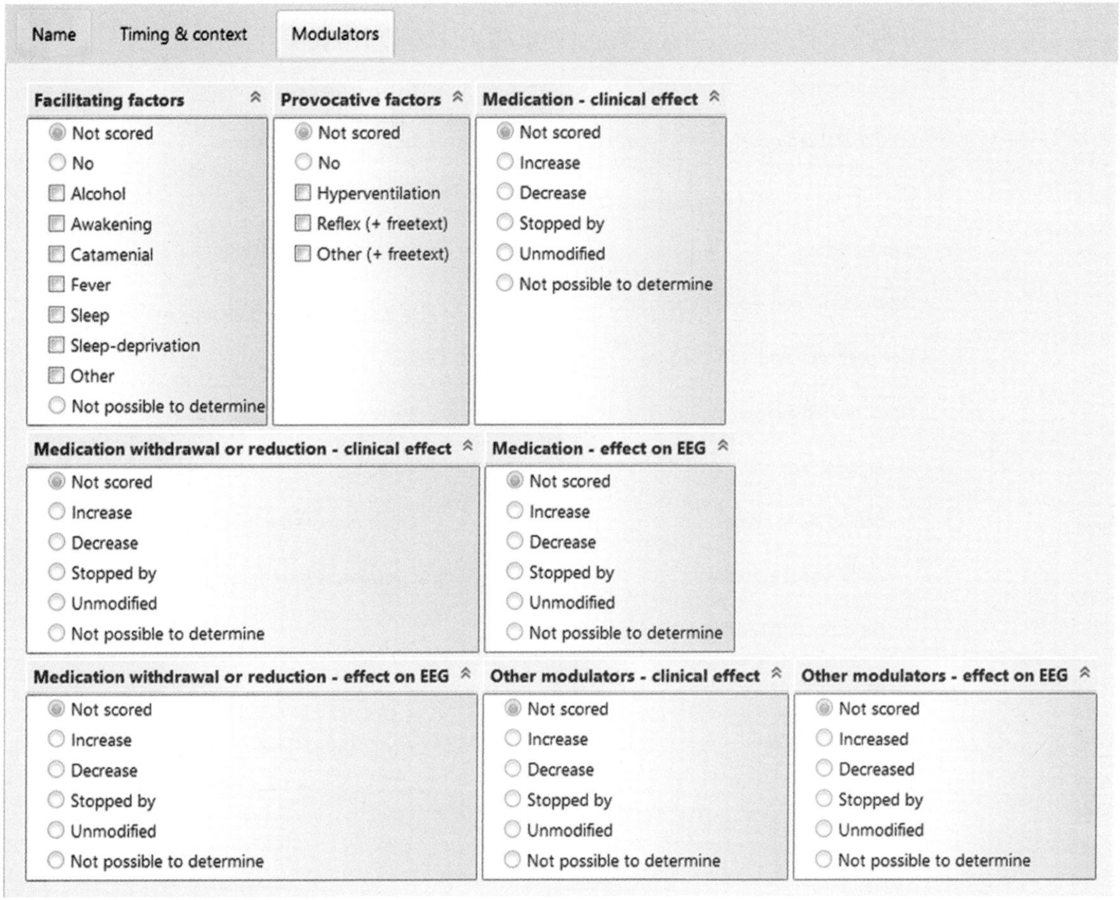

Figure 26.21. Scoring seizure modulators.

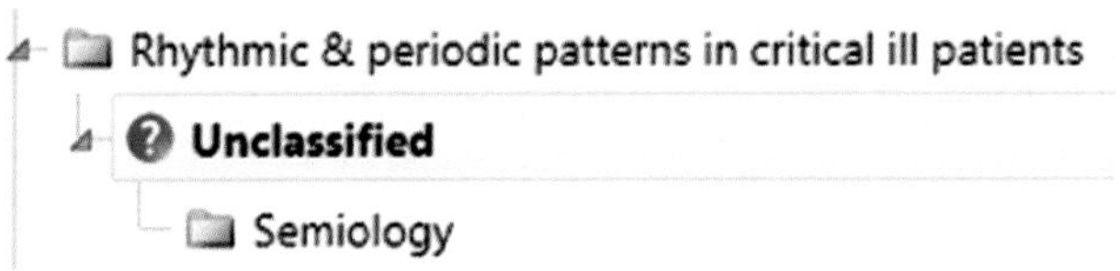

Figure 26.22. The folder for scoring the rhythmic and periodic patterns in critically ill patients, and the attached folder for scoring any semiologic finding, if time-locked to the pattern.

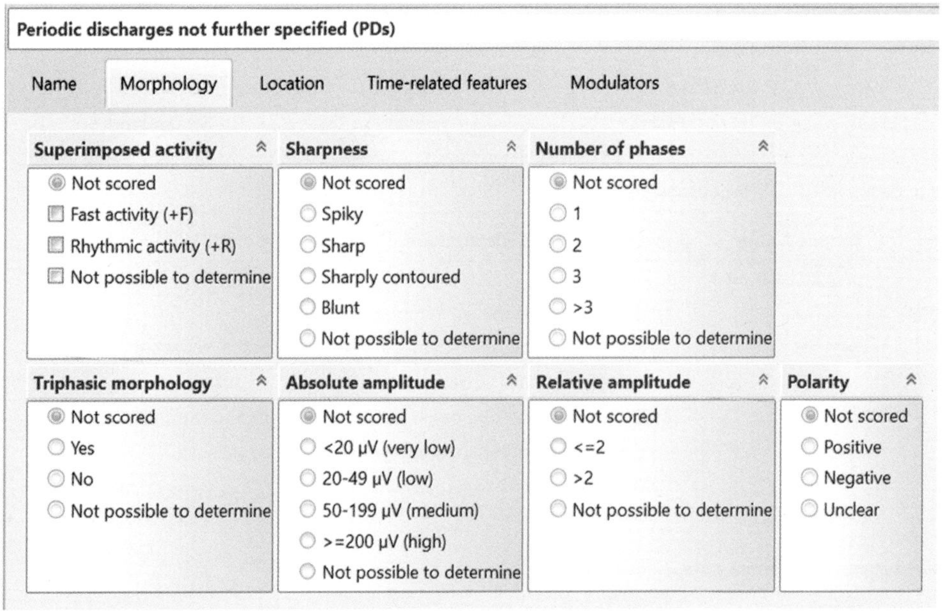

Figure 26.23. Features scored for periodic discharges.

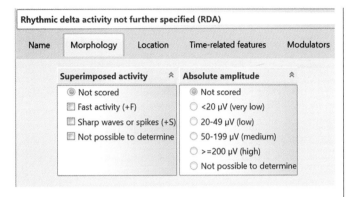

Figure 26.24. Features scored for rhythmic delta activity.

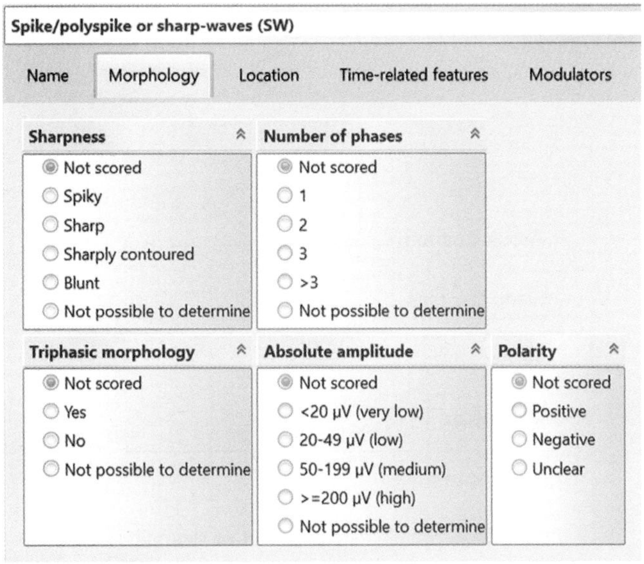

Figure 26.25. Features scored for spikes or sharp-waves.

3.6. Physiologic Patterns and Patterns of Uncertain Significance; Artifacts

When the EEG-er considers it important, the presence of physiologic patterns can be specified. First the name is selected, and then the location is specified using the SCORE location module (Fig. 26.28). Patterns of normal variants are scored in their own folder (Fig. 26.29). The procedure is the same as for physiologic patterns: first a name is chosen, and then the location is specified.

A separate folder contains a list of biological and nonbiological artifacts. Besides the name and location of the artifact, the user must score its significance (i.e., the impact on the quality and clinical utility of the recording) (Fig. 26.30).

3.7. Polygraphic Channels

Polygraphic channels provide valuable information, especially during long-term and neonatal recordings, but occasionally also during standard recordings. The modalities available for detailed scoring polygraphic channels are shown in Figure 26.31.

Electrocardiographic (ECG) channels should be included in all EEG recordings. The type of ECG finding is selected from the property list (Fig. 26.32). If any ECG abnormality is detected, its possible relationship to the clinical episode can be specified here. ECG changes can be either the cause of the clinical episode (e.g., syncope) or the consequence (e.g., ictal changes in heart rate). In addition, the value of the QT period can be saved here.

Surface electromyelographic (EMG) recordings provide valuable information on motor seizures. The type of EMG

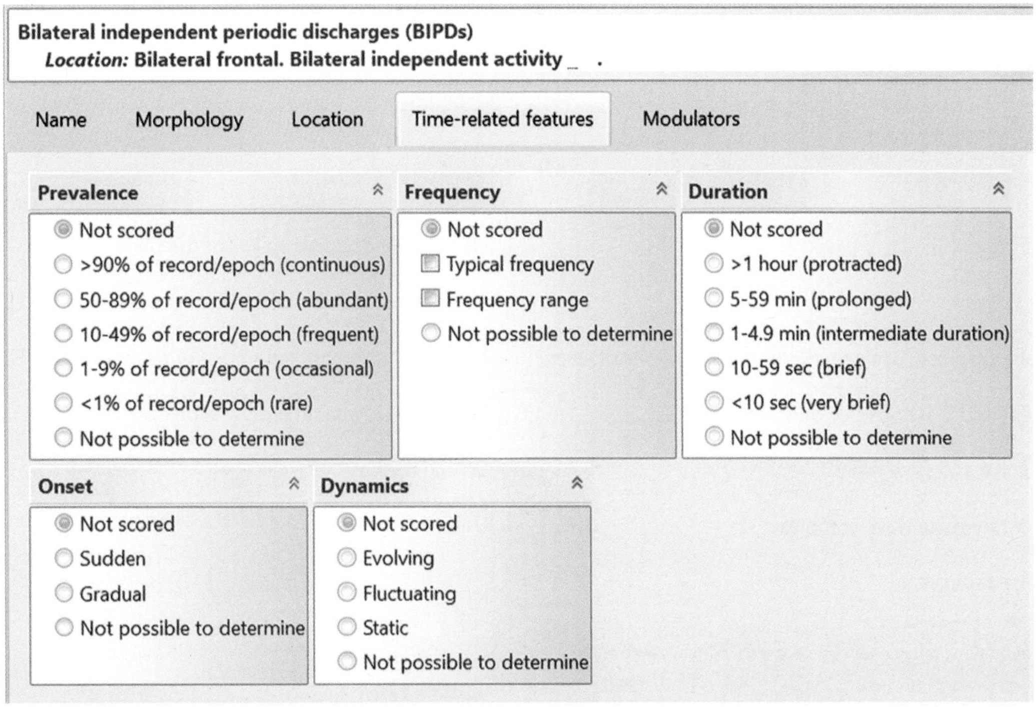

Figure 26.26. Time-related features of the rhythmic and periodic patterns.

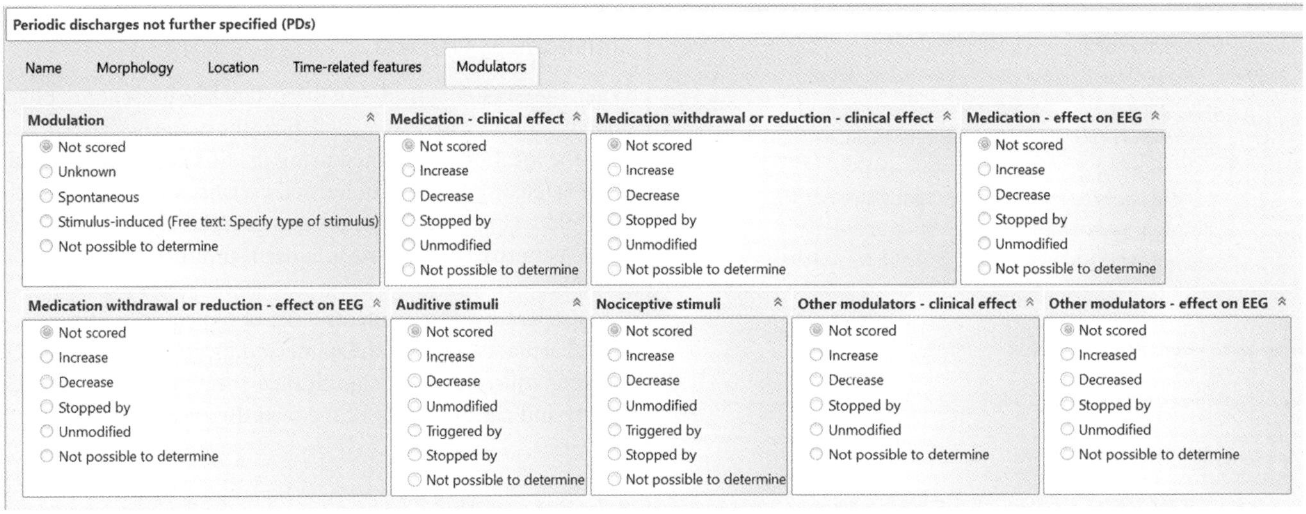

Figure 26.27. Scoring the effect of modulators on the rhythmic and periodic patterns.

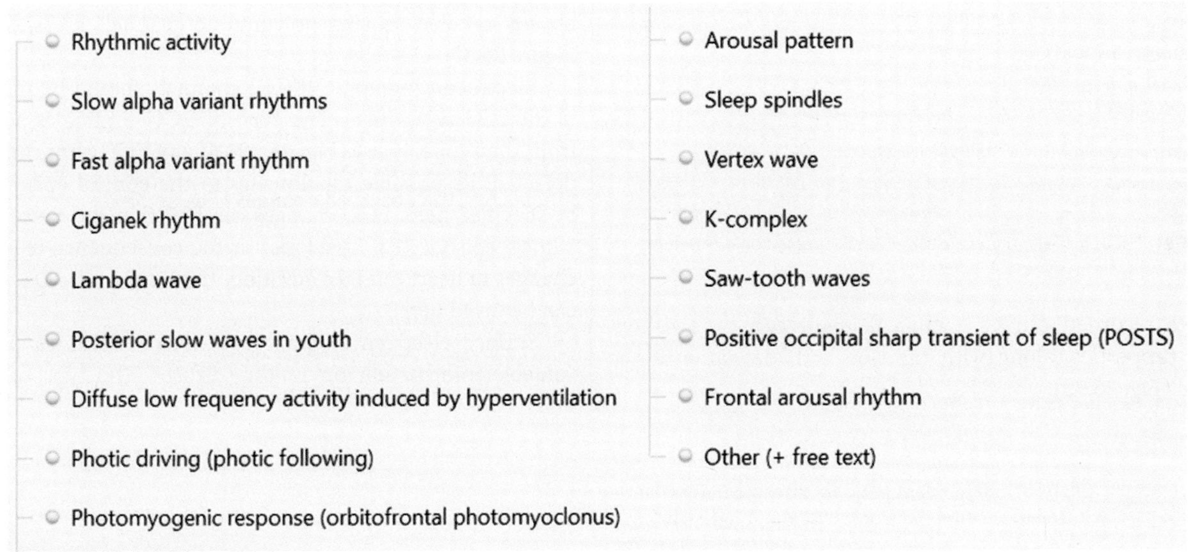

Figure 26.28. List of physiologic patterns.

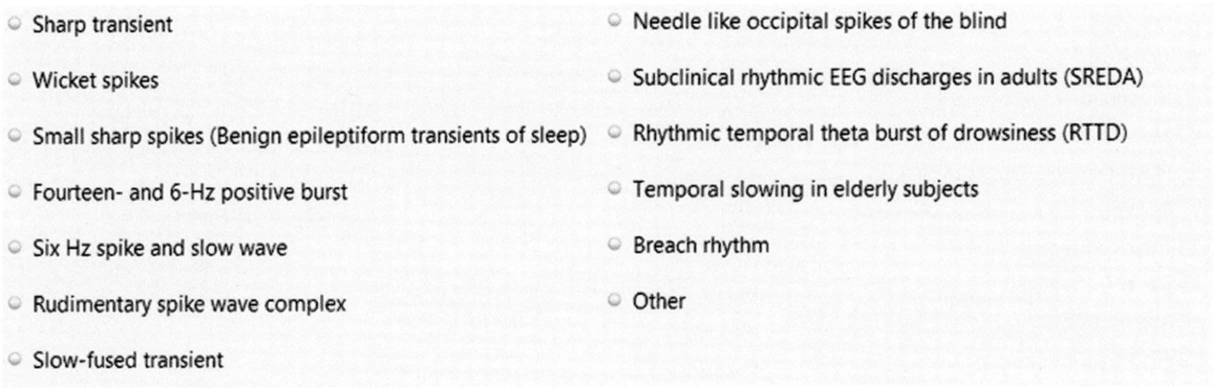

Figure 26.29. List of patterns of uncertain significance ("normal variants").

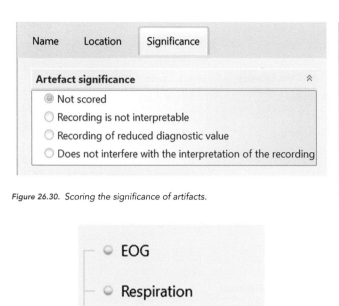

Figure 26.30. Scoring the significance of artifacts.

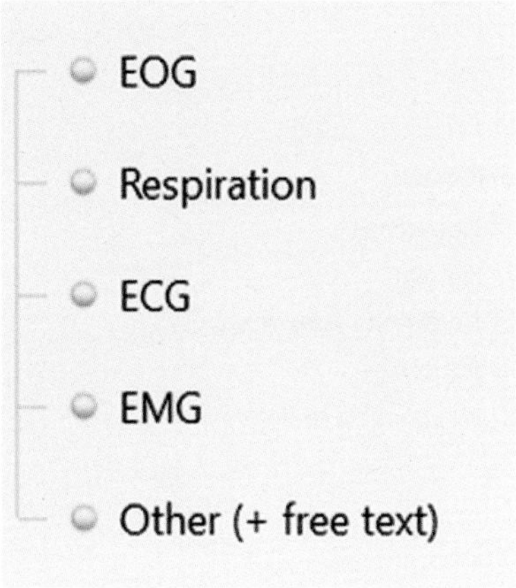

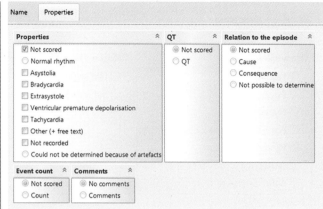

Figure 26.32. Scoring the electrocardiogram.

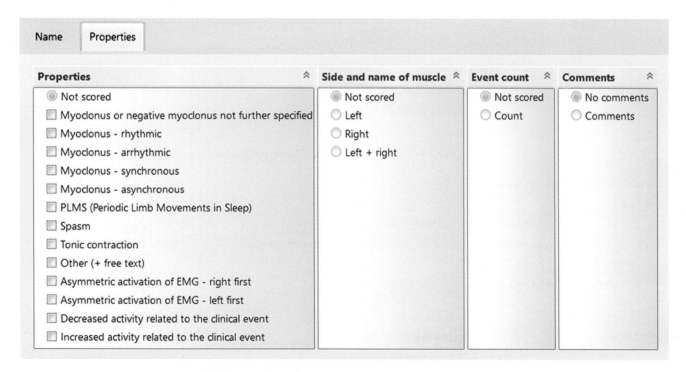

Figure 26.31. List of modalities that are scored under polygraphic channels.

changes recorded during a clinical event can be specified under properties, along with the side and the name of the muscle (Fig. 26.33).

The choices for respiration changes are listed in Figure 26.34. Similar to ECG changes, the possible relationship to the clinical episode is specified here.

3.8. Trend Analysis

If trend analysis was done, the results can be scored using a specific folder. For amplitude-integrated EEG, the user can score its characteristics, the sleep–wake cycling, and the significance of the observed changes (Fig. 26.35).

3.9. Diagnostic Significance

After extracting all clinically relevant EEG features and scoring them, they must be interpreted in their clinical context, which takes into account the additional clinical data provided

Figure 26.33. Scoring the surface electromyelogram.

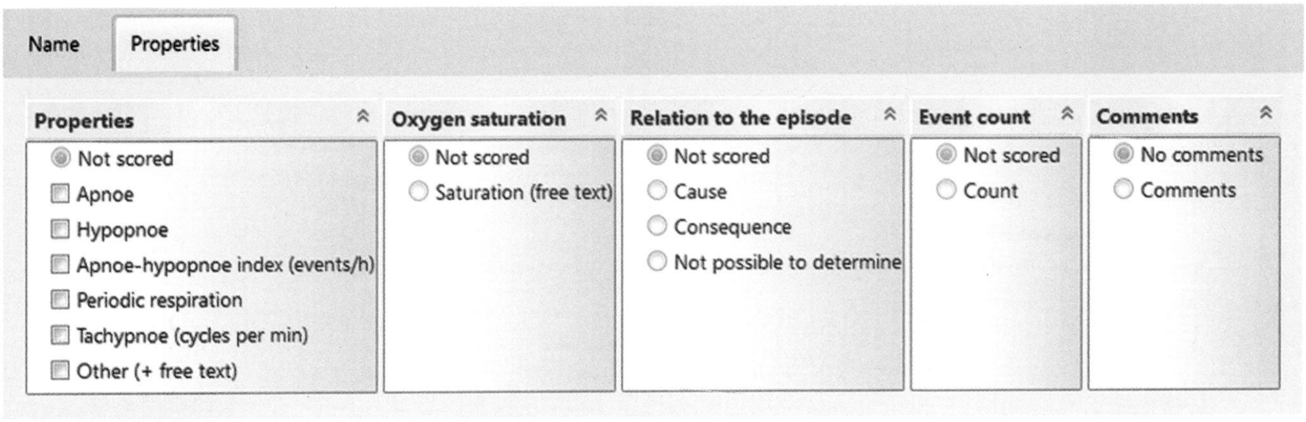

Name
Properties
Properties
Not scored
Apnoe
Hypopnoe
Apnoe-hypopnoe index (events/h)
Periodic respiration
Tachypnoe (cycles per min)
Other (+ free text)
Oxygen saturation
Not scored
Saturation (free text)
Relation to the episode
Not scored
Cause
Consequence
Not possible to determine
Event count
Not scored
Count
Comments
No comments
Comments

Figure 26.34. *Scoring respiration.*

Characteristics
Not scored
Continuous
Burst suppression
Low voltage
Seizure activity
Artefacts
Not possible to assess
Sleep-wake cycling
Not scored
Yes
No
Unspecified state changes
Unknown
Not possible to evaluate
Significance
Not scored
Normal
No definite abnormality
Abnormal
Not possible to determine

Figure 26.35. *Scoring the results of trend analysis/amplitude-integrated EEG.*

Normal
No definite abnormality
Abnormal recording
Epilepsy
Focal
Unifocal
Multifocal
Generalized
Combined generalized and focal epilepsy
Epilepsy of unknown type
Status epilepticus
Continuous spikes and waves during slow sleep (CSWS) or electrical status epilepticus in sleep (ESES)
Psychogenic non-epileptic seisure (PNES)
Other non-epileptic clinical episode
Focal central nervous system (CNS) dysfunction
Diffuse central nervous system (CNS) dysfunction
Coma
Brain death
EEG abnormality of uncertain clinical significance

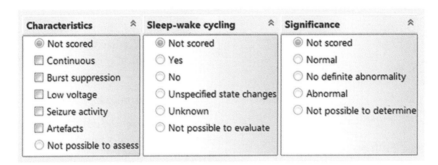

Figure 26.36. *Scoring diagnostic significance.*

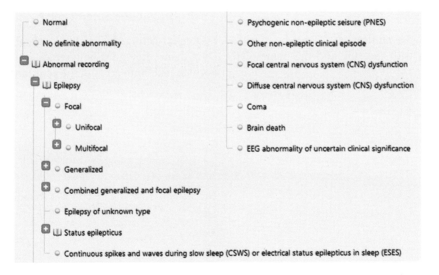

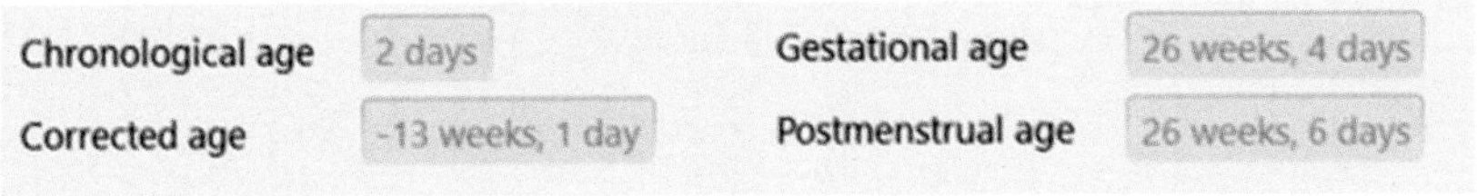

Chronological age
2 days
Corrected age
-13 weeks, 1 day
Gestational age
26 weeks, 4 days
Postmenstrual age
26 weeks, 6 days

Figure 26.37. *Corrected age and gestational age.*

Ongoing activity (1)
Unclassified
Graphoelement
Awake
Asleep
Alertness not possible to determine

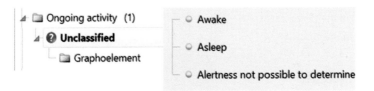

Figure 26.38. *Selecting alertness for a neonatal recording.*

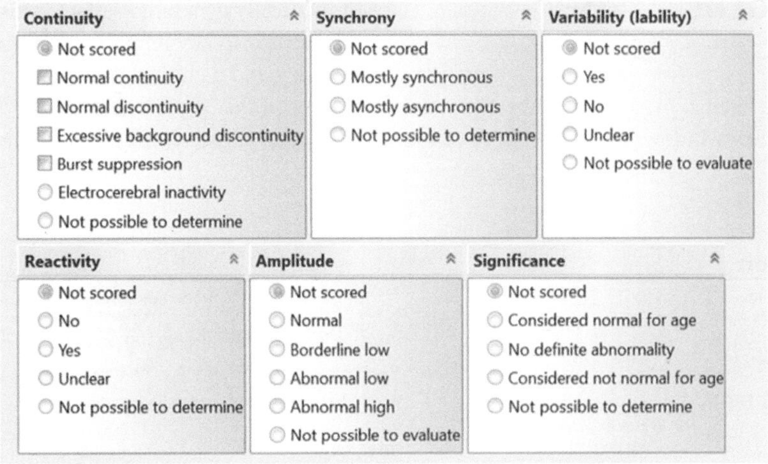

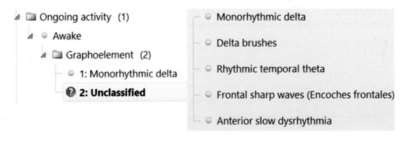

Figure 26.39. *Scoring ongoing activity for an awake neonatal recording.*

in the referral. Three main categories of clinical significance can be selected: normal, abnormal, and no definite abnormality. If a recording is scored as abnormal, the type is further specified (Fig. 26.36). If a previous recording exists in the database, the changes can be scored as no change, improved, or worsened.

3.10. The Neonatal Template in SCORE

Based on the date of birth and the date of recording, SCORE automatically opens a neonatal template. The folder for the background activity is replaced by a specific module for neonates, called "ongoing activity." Two additional neonatal folders are inserted: "transient patterns" and "rhythmic activity." For all patients <3 months of age, gestational age must be provided. Then, SCORE calculates chronological age, corrected age, and postmenstrual age at the time of the study (Fig. 26.37).

The steps of scoring the neonatal ongoing activity are the following: scoring alertness → behavioral state → properties → graphoelements. First, under "ongoing activity," the alertness has to be selected: awake or asleep (Fig. 26.38). Ongoing activity is scored separately, if both alertness types are present in the recording. In the next step, the features of the behavioral state(s) observed during the selected type of alertness are specified. For "awake," these are quiet, moving, upset, or crying. For "sleep," two aspects are scored under behavioral state: type of sleep (active, quiet, transitional, spontaneous, drug-induced) and sleep–wake cycling (yes, no, unspecified). Then, specific

features of the ongoing activity are scored, under "properties": continuity, synchrony, variability, reactivity, amplitude, and significance (Fig. 26.39).

For scoring continuity, for "asleep" an additional choice is presented (*tracé alternant*) for babies with a gestational age of >30 weeks. The graphoelements that constitute the ongoing activity of the selected type of alertness are scored in the subfolder belonging to the selected alertness. The user can add several graphoelements to the same alertness state (Fig. 26.40). Then, location and time-related features are scored for each graphoelement, similar to the adult module. Transient patterns (specific folder in the neonatal template) are scored by specifying first the morphology (negative sharp transients or positive sharp transients). Then location and time-related features are scored. The third folder specifically inserted for neonates is rhythmic activity. One can choose between rhythmic activity (delta, theta, alpha, beta) and brief rhythmic discharges. Location and time-related features are scored subsequently.

For preterm babies with a gestational age or corrected gestational age at the time of the study of <30 weeks, SCORE will automatically go into the preterm module. The structure of the template is the same as for babies >30 weeks, but its content is different for several features. Types of sleep are drug-induced and indeterminate. *Tracé alternant* is not presented as an option for scoring the continuity of sleep recordings for babies <30 weeks. The other folders, containing interictal and ictal features and rhythmic and periodic patterns, are available for neonates too.

Figure 26.40. *Scoring graphoelements of neonatal ongoing activity.*

4. PREVIEW AND GENERATION OF THE REPORT

After scoring all relevant items in a recording, the icon "Report" triggers the preview window, where the draft of the automatically generated report is displayed. Here the user can add free text to any item. In addition, the user can add a short summary and a clinical comment in the designated boxes. By clicking on the "sign" icon, the user who is logged in electronically signs it. The report is automatically generated, and it can

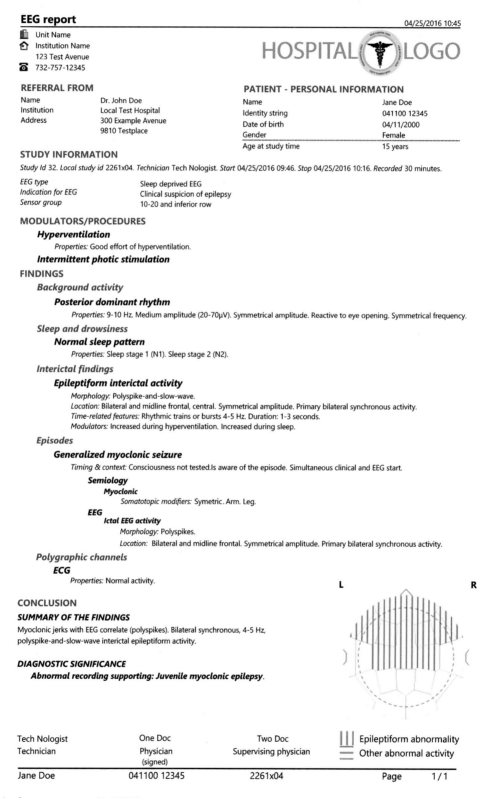

EEG report   04/25/2016 10:45

Unit Name
Institution Name
123 Test Avenue
☎ 732-757-12345

HOSPITAL LOGO

REFERRAL FROM

Name	Dr. John Doe
Institution	Local Test Hospital
Address	300 Example Avenue
	9810 Testplace

PATIENT - PERSONAL INFORMATION

Name	Jane Doe
Identity string	041100 12345
Date of birth	04/11/2000
Gender	Female
Age at study time	15 years

STUDY INFORMATION

Study Id 32. *Local study id* 2261x04. *Technician* Tech Nologist. *Start* 04/25/2016 09:46. *Stop* 04/25/2016 10:16. *Recorded* 30 minutes.

EEG type   Sleep deprived EEG
Indication for EEG   Clinical suspicion of epilepsy
Sensor group   10-20 and inferior row

MODULATORS/PROCEDURES

Hyperventilation
     Properties: Good effort of hyperventilation.
Intermittent photic stimulation

FINDINGS

Background activity
Posterior dominant rhythm
     Properties: 9-10 Hz. Medium amplitude (20-70µV). Symmetrical amplitude. Reactive to eye opening. Symmetrical frequency.

Sleep and drowsiness
Normal sleep pattern
     Properties: Sleep stage 1 (N1). Sleep stage 2 (N2).

Interictal findings
Epileptiform interictal activity
     Morphology: Polyspike-and-slow-wave.
     Location: Bilateral and midline frontal, central. Symmetrical amplitude. Primary bilateral synchronous activity.
     Time-related features: Rhythmic trains or bursts 4-5 Hz. Duration: 1-3 seconds.
     Modulators: Increased during hyperventilation. Increased during sleep.

Episodes
Generalized myoclonic seizure
     Timing & context: Consciousness not tested.Is aware of the episode. Simultaneous clinical and EEG start.
       Semiology
       Myoclonic
         Somatotopic modifiers: Symetric. Arm. Leg.
       EEG
         Ictal EEG activity
           Morphology: Polyspikes.
           Location: Bilateral and midline frontal. Symmetrical amplitude. Primary bilateral synchronous activity.

Polygraphic channels
ECG
     Properties: Normal activity.

CONCLUSION

SUMMARY OF THE FINDINGS
Myoclonic jerks with EEG correlate (polyspikes). Bilateral synchronous, 4-5 Hz, polyspike-and-slow-wave interictal epileptiform activity.

DIAGNOSTIC SIGNIFICANCE
Abnormal recording supporting: Juvenile myoclonic epilepsy.

L   R

Tech Nologist	One Doc	Two Doc	⦀ Epileptiform abnormality
Technician	Physician	Supervising physician	═ Other abnormal activity
	(signed)		
Jane Doe	041100 12345	2261x04	Page 1 / 1

Figure 26.41. Example of a report generated in SCORE.

be printed and/or saved in the electronic patient administration system. When the report is generated, all scored features are saved in the database (Fig. 26.41).

5. SEARCH FUNCTIONALITY

SCORE EEG provides a tool to search previous EEGs defined by specific criteria according to EEG findings and patient demographics. Simple individual searches can be combined to produce comprehensive searches to find the EEGs of interest.

REFERENCES

1. Noachtar S, Binnie C, Ebersole J, et al. A glossary of terms most commonly used by clinical electroencephalographers and proposal for the report for the EEG findings. Electroencephal Clin Neurophysiol 1999;Suppl 52:21–41.
2. Morgan TA, Helibrun ME, Kahn CE Jr. Reporting initiative of the Radiological Society of North America: progress and new directions. Radiology 2014;273:642–645.
3. Ellis DW, Srigley J. Does standardised structured reporting contribute to quality in diagnostic pathology? The importance of evidence-based datasets. Virchows Arch 2016;468:51–59.
4. Bretthauer M, Aabakken L, Dekker E, et al. Reporting systems in gastrointestinal endoscopy: Requirements and standards facilitating quality improvement: European Society of Gastrointestinal Endoscopy position statement. Endoscopy 2016;48:9291–294.
5. Aurlien H, Gjerde IO, Gilhus NE, et al. A new way of building a database of EEG findings. Clin Neurophysiol 1999;110:986–995.
6. Finnerup NB, Fuglsang-Frederiksen A, Røssel P, Jennum P. A computer-based information system for epilepsy and electroencephalography. Int J Med Inform 1999;55:127–134.
7. Aurlien H, Gjerde IO, Aarseth JH, et al. EEG background activity described by a large computerized database. Clin Neurophysiol 2004;115:665–673.
8. Aurlien H, Aarseth JH, Gjerde IO, et al. Focal epileptiform activity described by a large computerised EEG database. Clin Neurophysiol 2007;118:1369–1376.
9. Aurlien H, Gjerde IO, Eide GE, et al. Characteristics of generalised epileptiform activity. Clin Neurophysiol 2009;120:3–10.
10. Beniczky S, Aurlien H, Brøgger JC, et al. Standardized computer-based organized reporting of EEG: SCORE. Epilepsia 2013;54:1112–1124.
11. Hirsch LJ, LaRoche SM, Gaspard N, et al. American Clinical Neurophysiology Society's Standardized Critical Care EEG Terminology: 2012 version. J Clin Neurophysiol 2013;30:1–27.
12. Gaspard N, Hirsch LJ, LaRoche SM, Hahn CD, Westover MB; the Critical Care EEG Monitoring Research Consortium. Interrater agreement for Critical Care EEG Terminology. Epilepsia 2014;55:1366–1373.

27 | AUTOMATIC INTEGRATED EEG INTERPRETATION AND REPORTING

HIROSHI SHIBASAKI, MD AND MASATOSHI NAKAMURA†, MD

ABSTRACT: Automatic interpretation of electroencephalograms (EEG) is complicated due to fluctuation of background activity, paroxysmal activities, artifacts, and use of different electrode montages. Previous attempts at automatic EEG interpretation focused on a certain feature such as background activity and paroxysmal abnormalities. The authors' group has developed a computer-assisted, offline system for automatic comprehensive interpretation of EEG that takes into account all features of the adult waking EEG and provides the results in a written report. The system is not aimed at standardization of EEG interpretation, but its results can match the results of visual inspection by a limited number of qualified EEG-ers. Thus, this system can be adjusted in accordance with the strategy of visual inspection adopted by any EEG-er. Artifacts, spikes, and the vigilance level and attention level of subjects are automatically detected. This system can be used to supplement visual inspection and for training purposes.

KEYWORDS: electroencephalograph, EEG, automatic, interpretation, artifact, report, vigilance, attention, background activity

PRINCIPAL REFERENCES

1. Nakamura M, Nishida S, Neshige R, Shibasaki H. Quantitative analysis of 'organization' by feature extraction of the EEG power spectrum. Electroenceph Clin Neurophysiol 1985;60:84–89.
2. Marcuse LV, Schneider M, Mortati KA, Donnelly KM, Arnedo V, Grant AC. Quantitative analysis of the EEG, posterior-dominant rhythm in healthy adolescents. Clin Neurophysiol 2008;119:1778–1781.
3. Lodder SS, van Putten MJAM. Automated EEG analysis: characterizing the posterior dominant rhythm. J Neurosci Methods 2011;200:86–93.
4. Matsuoka S, Arakaki Y, Numaguchi K, Ueno S. The effect of dexamethasone on electroencephalograms in patients with brain tumors. With specific reference to topographic computer display of delta activity. J Neurosurg 1978;48:601–608.
5. Anderson NR, Doolittle LM. Automated analysis of EEG: opportunities and pitfalls. J Clin Neurophysiol 2010;27:453–457.
6. Nakamura M, Shibasaki H, Imajoh K, Nishida S, Neshige R, Ikeda A. Automatic EEG interpretation: a new computer-assisted system for the automatic integrative interpretation of awake background EEG. Electroenceph Clin Neurophysiol 1992;82:423–431.
7. Nakamura M, Sugi T, Ikeda A, Kakigi R, Shibasaki H. Clinical application of automatic integrative interpretation of awake background EEG: quantitative interpretation, report making, and detection of artifacts and reduced vigilance level. Electroenceph Clin Neurophysiol 1996;98:103–112.
8. Shibasaki H, Nakamura M, Sugi T, Nishida S, Nagamine T, Ikeda A. Automatic interpretation and writing report of the adult waking electroencephalogram. Clin Neurophysiol 2014;125:1081–1094.
9. Nishida S, Nakamura M, Shibasaki H. An EEG model expressed by the sinusoidal waves with the Markov process amplitude. [Abstract in English.] Iyodenshi To Seitai Kogaku 1986;24:8–14.
10. Bai O, Nakamura M, Ikeda A, Shibasaki H. Nonlinear Markov process amplitude EEG model for nonlinear coupling interaction of spontaneous EEG. IEEE Trans Biomed Eng 2000;47:1141–1146.
11. Noachtar S, Binnie C, Ebersole J, Mauguiere F, Sakamoto A, Westmoreland B. A glossary of terms most commonly used by clinical electroencephalographers and proposal for the report form for the EEG findings. In Deuschl G, Eisen A (Eds), Recommendations for the Practice of Clinical Neurophysiology: Guidelines of the International Federation of Clinical Neurophysiology, Electroenceph Clin Neurophysiol 1999;Suppl. 52:21–40.
12. Akaike H. A new look at the statistical model identification. IEEE Trans Automat Control 1974;AC-19:716–723.
13. Sugi T, Nakamura M, Ikeda A, Kakigi R, Shibasaki H. Automatic detection of artifacts for pre-processing of automatic EEG interpretation. [Abstract in English.] Iyodenshi To Seitai Kogaku 1995;33:203–213.
14. Sugi T, Nakamura M, Ikeda A, Shibasaki H. Adaptive EEG spike detection: determination of threshold values based on conditional probability. Front Med Biol Eng 2002;11:261–277.
15. Bai O, Nakamura M, Ikeda A, Shibasaki H. Automatic detection of open and closed eye states in the electroencephalographic (EEG) record for background EEG interpretation by the trigger method. Front Med Biol Eng 2000;10:1–15.
16. Nakamura M, Shibasaki H, Imajoh K, Ikeda A, Kakigi R. Automatic EEG report making for awake background EEG. [Abstract in English.] Jpn J Clin Neurophysiol 1993;21:47–56.
17. Beniczky S, Aurlien H, Brøgger JC, Fuglsang-Frederiksen A, Martins-da-Silva A, Trinka E, et al. Standardized computer-based organized reporting of EEG: SCORE. Epilepsia 2013;54:1112–1124.
18. Lodder SS, van Putten MJAM. Quantification of the adult EEG background pattern. Clin Neurophysiol 2013;124:228–237.

1. INTRODUCTION

Automatic interpretation of electroencephalograms (EEGs) has been faced with significant technical difficulties for the following reasons:

1. EEGs contain a large amount of spatial and temporal information.

2. Background activity on EEG recordings changes depending on the subject's vigilance level and attention level.

3. Paroxysmal activities must be distinguished from background activity.

4. EEG is often contaminated with a variety of artifacts.

5. Different kinds of electrode montage are used.

6. The criteria used for the interpretation are not necessarily the same among EEG-ers.

There have been a number of attempts to interpret EEGs automatically, but most of them have been focused on certain components, such as the posterior dominant rhythm (PDR) (1–3) and the scalp topography of slow waves (4). The integrated automatic interpretation of the entire EEG for practical purposes has not been achieved (5). The authors' group, a close collaboration between clinical EEG-ers and experts in systems engineering including Akio Ikeda, MD, PhD, Kyoto University Graduate School of Medicine, Kyoto, Japan; Takenao Sugi, PhD, Saga University Graduate School of Science and Engineering, Saga, Japan; Shigeto Nishida, PhD, Fukuoka Institute of Technology, Fukuoka, Japan and Takashi Nagamine, MD, PhD, Sapporo Medical University, Sapporo, Japan, has developed over a period of >30 years a computer-assisted system of systematic, comprehensive, integrated, and automatic interpretation and reporting of the adult waking EEG (6–8).

2. STEPS TAKEN TO DEVELOP THE AUTOMATIC SYSTEM OF EEG INTERPRETATION

We first extracted features of visual inspection based on the strategy adopted by the qualified EEG-ers in our group and expressed those features quantitatively (6) (Table 27.1). Based on those quantitative data, we prepared algorithms for calculating parameters of each frequency band (Table 27.2). All algorithms were constructed so that the results of automatic

analysis could match the results of visual inspection by the qualified EEG-ers as closely as possible (6).

The PDR is defined as a rhythmic activity, usually in the alpha frequency band in healthy adults, that is maximally located at the occipital or parietal region and is seen predominantly in time; it is the most important component of the waking background EEG (8). To determine whether PDR exists in a given EEG record, the following three criteria are taken into account:

1. The power of the dominant frequency band $(\bar{S}_d)$ at the occipital or parietal electrode, which is >10% of the total power $(\bar{S}_T)$ (Eq. 1 for the dominance in time)

2. The power at the occipital or parietal electrode $(\bar{S}_d)$, which is larger than the power at other electrodes $(\tilde{S}_d)$ (Eq. 2 for the dominance in space)

3. The amplitude of at least 10μV (Eq. 3 for the amplitude criteria). The amplitude information was estimated from the power spectrum based on our EEG model, which is expressed by the sinusoidal waves with the Markov process amplitude (9,10).

TABLE 27.1. Quantitative Scoring of the Adult Waking EEG Based on Visual Inspection by Qualified EEG-ers

ITEMS			NORMAL	ABNORMAL		
				MILD	MODERATE	MARKED
			SCORE 0	SCORE 1	SCORE 2	SCORE 3
Posterior dominant rhythm	Existence		Present			Absent
	Organization	Left or right	Good	Poorly organized	Disorganized	Markedly disorganized
		L–R difference	<0.3	0.3 ≤ <0.6	0.6 ≤ <1.0	1.0 ≤
	Frequency	Left or right (Hz)	9 ≤	8 < <9	6 < ≤8	
		L–R difference (Hz)	<0.5	0.5 ≤ < 1.0	1.0 ≤ < 2.0	2.0 ≤
	Amplitude	Left or right (μV)	<100	100 ≤ < 130	130 ≤	
		L–R difference (%)	<50	50 ≤ < 60	60 ≤ < 80	80 ≤
	Extension (electrode)		To C, MT	To F, AT	To Fp (low)	To Fp (high)
Beta	Amplitude	Left or right (μV)	≤50	50 < < 100	≤ 100	
		L–R difference (%)	<50	50 ≤ < 60	60 ≤ < 80	80 ≤
Theta	Duration (%)		0	< 5	5 ≤ < 50	50 ≤
	Electrodes		Active electrodes			
Delta	Duration (%)		0	-	<50	50 ≤
	Electrodes		Active electrodes			
Alpha	Duration (%)		<10	10 ≤ < 30	30 ≤ < 75	75 ≤
	Electrodes		Active electrodes			

Left or right: left or right, whichever better in organization, faster in frequency, or larger in amplitude; L–R difference: difference between left and right; Extension: C = central, MT = midtemporal, F = frontal, AT = anterior temporal, Fp = frontopolar; Alpha: nondominant alpha rhythm (alpha rhythm not attributed to the posterior dominant alpha rhythm).
Modified from reference 6 with permission.

TABLE 27.2. Equations Employed for Computer-Assisted Calculation of Parameters for Each Frequency Band of the Adult Waking EEG

ITEMS			EEG PARAMETERS
Posterior dominant rhythm	Existence		$\bar{S}_d / \bar{S}_T \geq 0.1, \ldots \bar{S}_d / \tilde{S}_d \geq 1.0, \ldots 10\sqrt{\bar{S}_d} \geq 10\mu V$
	Organization	Left or right	$y_d = 0.49 + 0.58\sigma_\alpha - 0.13S_\alpha + 4.82 \times 10^{-5}(S_\alpha)^2 - 0.41S_\alpha / S_T + 3.12S_\delta / S_T$
		L–R difference	$|y_d(X_2) - y_d(X_1)|$
	Frequency	Left or right (Hz)	f_d
		L–R difference (Hz)	$|f_d(X_2) - f_d(X_1)|$
	Amplitude	Left or right (μV)	$10\sqrt{\bar{S}_d} \geq 10\mu V$
		L–R difference (%)	$\left(\sqrt{\bar{S}_d(X_2)} - \sqrt{\bar{S}_d(X_1)}\right) / \max\left\{\sqrt{\bar{S}_d(X_1)}, \sqrt{\bar{S}_d(X_2)}\right\} \times 100$
	Extension		$10\sqrt{\bar{S}_{d'}}$
Beta	Amplitude	Left or Right (μV)	$6\sqrt{S_\beta} \geq 10\mu V$
		L–R difference (%)	$\left\{S_\beta(X_2) - S_\beta(X_1)\right\} / \max\left\{S_\beta(X_1), S_\beta(X_2)\right\} \times 100$
Theta	Duration (%)		$(S_\theta / S_T) \times 100 \quad$ if $6\sqrt{S_\theta} \geq 15\mu V$
	Location		Active electrodes
Delta	Duration (%)		$(S_\delta / S_T) \times 100 \quad$ if $6\sqrt{S_\delta} \geq 25\mu V$
	Location		Active electrodes
Alpha	Duration (%)		$(S_\alpha / S_T) \times 100 \quad$ if $6\sqrt{S_\alpha} \geq 15\mu V$
	Location		Active electrodes

S_d, S_β, S_θ, S_δ, S_α: power within the respective band where d is dominant rhythm and α is non-dominant α rhythm; S_d': power of the dominant rhythm at anterior electrodes; S_T: total power; σ_α: standard deviation of α rhythm; y_d: organization; f_d: peak frequency of dominant rhythm; X1: left, X2: right. Otherwise the same designation as for Table 27.1.
Modified from reference 6 with permission.
Reproduced from reference 8 with permission.

When all of these three criteria are fulfilled, PDR is judged to be present.

$$\bar{S}_d / \bar{S}_T \geq 0.1 \qquad \text{Eq. 1}$$

$$\bar{S}_d / \tilde{S}_d \geq 1.0 \qquad \text{Eq. 2}$$

$$10\sqrt{\bar{S}_d} \geq 10 \qquad \text{Eq. 3}$$

According to the glossary of terms proposed by the International Federation of Clinical Neurophysiology (IFCN) (11), the organization of PDR is defined as "the degree to which physiologic EEG rhythms conform to certain ideal characteristics displayed by a majority of subjects in the same age group, without personal or family history of neurologic and psychiatric diseases, or other illnesses that might be associated with dysfunction of the brain." In the present system of automatic EEG interpretation, the organization score of PDR (y_d) is calculated based on the Akaike Information Criteria (12) for determining the number of variables in an auto-regression model (Eq. 4).

A combination of the following four variables was judged to be the best selection out of all possible combinations:

1. Standard deviation of the alpha rhythm frequency (σ_α)

2. Integrated power of the alpha rhythm (S_α)

3. The ratio of the integrated power of alpha rhythm to the power of all frequency activities (S_α/S_T)

4. The ratio of the integrated power of delta rhythm to the power of all frequency activities (S_δ / S_T)

$$y_d = 0.49 + 0.58\sigma_\alpha - 0.13S_\alpha + 4.82 \times 10^{-5}(S_\alpha)^2 - 0.41S_\alpha / S_T + 3.12S_\delta / S_T$$
$$\text{Eq. 4}$$

Then a system of automatic detection of artifacts (13) and a system of automatic spike detection (14) were incorporated. Both systems were developed by our group. Furthermore, a system for evaluating the vigilance level of the subjects was developed so that we could select the appropriate segments for the final analysis (7,15). Finally, a comprehensive system of

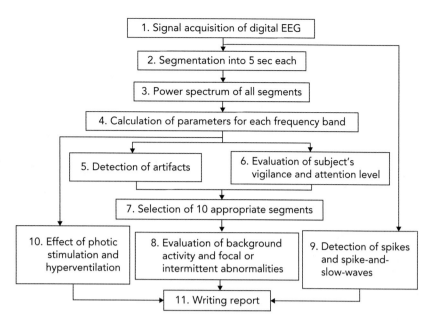

```
┌─────────────────────────────────┐
│ 1. Signal acquisition of digital EEG │
└─────────────────────────────────┘
┌─────────────────────────────┐
│ 2. Segmentation into 5 sec each │
└─────────────────────────────┘
┌─────────────────────────────┐
│ 3. Power spectrum of all segments │
└─────────────────────────────┘
┌──────────────────────────────────────┐
│ 4. Calculation of parameters for each frequency band │
└──────────────────────────────────────┘
┌──────────────────────┐   ┌──────────────────────┐
│ 5. Detection of artifacts │   │ 6. Evaluation of subject's │
│                          │   │ vigilance and attention level │
└──────────────────────┘   └──────────────────────┘
┌──────────────────────────────────┐
│ 7. Selection of 10 appropriate segments │
└──────────────────────────────────┘
┌─────────────────┐ ┌─────────────────┐ ┌─────────────────┐
│ 10. Effect of photic │ │ 8. Evaluation of background │ │ 9. Detection of spikes │
│ stimulation and │ │ activity and focal or │ │ and spike-and- │
│ hyperventilation │ │ intermittent abnormalities │ │ slow-waves │
└─────────────────┘ └─────────────────┘ └─────────────────┘
┌──────────────────┐
│ 11. Writing report │
└──────────────────┘
```

Figure 27.1. *Flowchart showing the steps of the present system of automatic interpretation of the adult waking EEG. Reproduced from reference 8 with permission.*

automatic interpretation was developed so that we could obtain the results in a written form. Thus, the present system has little to do with the standardization of EEG interpretation, but it is characterized by the fact that it can be adjusted in accordance with the strategy of visual inspection adopted by any individual EEG-er.

3. FLOW OF STEPS OF THE PRESENT AUTOMATIC EEG INTERPRETATION SYSTEM

The present system of automatic EEG interpretation is processed in the order of steps as illustrated in the flowchart in Figure 27.1. For this automatic interpretation, the EEG data acquired in a referential montage with respect to the ipsilateral earlobe electrode are primarily analyzed, and the standard bipolar montage is taken into account as necessary. In Step 2, the whole time series of digital EEG is split into consecutive 5-sec segments (the segment length of 5 sec was chosen to achieve the frequency resolution of 0.2 Hz). In Step 3, the power spectrum is obtained for all segments. In Step 4, by using the algorithm constructed as described in Table 27.2, parameters are calculated for each frequency band for all segments. In Step 5, artifacts such as blinks, lateral eye movements, and electromyographic and electrode artifacts are automatically detected (13) so that the segments containing any of those artifacts are automatically rejected from the final analysis.

In Step 6, the vigilance level and the attention level of the subject are evaluated. PDR may be decreased or even disappear completely in two physiologic conditions: a decrease in the subject's vigilance level and an increase in the subject's attention level. Differentiating these two physiologic states from pathologic conditions is one of the most important issues for automatic interpretation of background activity. It is especially important to avoid misinterpreting a highly attentive

condition of the subject as "lack of PDR." Blocking of the PDR by eye opening is a typical example of the highly attentive state. In the present system, these two conditions are differentiated by taking into account the amount of slow waves (7). Namely, slow waves are either absent or decreased during the highly attentive condition but are increased during decreased vigilance or in pathologic conditions.

After rejecting segments containing artifacts and segments judged to show either decreased vigilance or a highly attentive condition, 10 segments that are judged to be most appropriate for automatic interpretation are automatically selected and subjected to the final analysis (Step 7). All segments are arranged in the order of organization score of PDR, and the top 10 segments are subjected to the final analysis of background activity as well as to the detection of focal or intermittent abnormalities (Step 8).

In parallel with these steps, paroxysmal activities such as spikes and spike-and-slow-waves are automatically detected from the whole time series (Step 9). In the present system, the template waveform shown in Figure 27.2 is adopted for spike

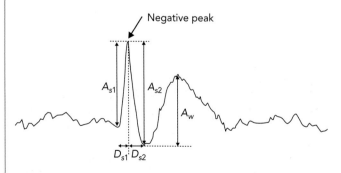

Figure 27.2. *Template waveform adopted for the automatic spike detection in the present system. Ds1 + Ds2: duration of spike, As1/Ds1, As2/Ds2: sharpness of spike, Aw: amplitude of slow wave, Aw/AT: prominence of slow wave from background activity, where AT is the mean amplitude of the whole background activities. Reproduced from reference 8 with permission.*

detection. We take into account the duration of spike ($Ds1 + Ds2$) and its sharpness ($As1/Ds1$, $As2/Ds2$), the amplitude of the slow wave immediately following the spike (Aw), and the prominence of the slow wave from background activity (Aw/AT) (14). The effects of intermittent photic stimulation and hyperventilation, if applicable, are analyzed from each corresponding segment in the frequency domain (Step 10).

Finally, a report of the interpretation is automatically obtained in a written form (Step 11). To make the written report, we prepared the terminology for each parameter of each frequency band and for the scalp distribution of abnormalities (Table 27.3) (16). To judge whether the whole EEG is normal or abnormal, and in order to score the degree of abnormality of the whole EEG, each parameter is weighted depending on the significance of each abnormality as judged by the qualified EEG-ers, and the scores are summed to calculate the degree of abnormalities of the whole EEG. Recently, the European group of EEG-ers led by Beniczky has developed a software program called Standardized Computer-Based Organized Reporting of EEG (SCORE) (17) (see Chapter 26).

An example of a written report prepared using the present system of automatic EEG interpretation is shown in Figure 27.3.

TABLE 27.3. Terminology Prepared for Automatic Report Writing of the Adult Waking EEG

NO.	ITEMS	SCORE	TERMINOLOGY	WEIGHT
Posterior dominant rhythm				
1	Existence	3	lack of dominant rhythm	10.0
2	Organization	3	markedly disorganized	7.0
		2	disorganized	4.5
		1	poorly organized	2.0
3	Asymmetry	3	marked asymmetry of dominant rhythm organization, poor on (L, R)	5.0
		2	asymmetry of dominant rhythm organization, poor on (L, R)	3.5
		1	slight asymmetry of dominant rhythm organization, poor on (L, R)	2.0
4	Frequency	3	markedly slow dominant rhythm (Hz)	8.0
		2	slow dominant rhythm (Hz)	5.0
		1	slow alpha rhythm	2.0
5	Asymmetry	3	marked asymmetry of dominant rhythm frequency, slower on (L, R)	5.0
		2	asymmetry of dominant rhythm frequency, slower on (L, R)	3.5
		1	slight asymmetry of dominant rhythm frequency, slower on (L, R)	2.0
6	Amplitude	2	excessively high amplitude dominant rhythm	3.0
		1	high amplitude dominant rhythm	2.0
7	Asymmetry	3	suppression of dominant rhythm on (L, R)	5.0
		2	depression of dominant rhythm on (L, R)	3.5
		1	mild depression of dominant rhythm on (L, R)	2.0
8	Extension	3	excessive anterior extension of alpha rhythm	2.0
		2	anterior extension of alpha rhythm	1.5
		1	mild anterior extension of alpha rhythm	1.0
Beta rhythm				
9	Amplitude	2	excessively high amplitude rhythmic fast activity	3.0
		1	high amplitude rhythmic fast activity	2.0

TABLE 27.3. Continued

NO.	ITEMS	SCORE	TERMINOLOGY	WEIGHT
10	Asymmetry	3	suppression of rhythmic fast activity on (L, R)	5.0
		2	depression of rhythmic fast activity on (L, R)	3.5
		1	mild depression of rhythmic fast activity on (L, R)	2.0
Theta rhythm				
11	Duration	3	continuous, rhythmic and/or irregular theta waves	8.0
		2	intermittent, rhythmic and/or irregular theta waves	5.0
		1	occasional theta waves	2.0
12	Electrodes			
Delta rhythm				
13	Duration	3	continuous, rhythmic and/or irregular delta waves	8.0
		2	intermittent, rhythmic and/or irregular delta waves	5.0
		1	occasional delta waves	2.0
14	Electrodes			
Non-dominant alpha rhythm				
15	Duration	3	continuous non-dominant alpha frequency	4.0
		2	intermittent non-dominant alpha frequency	3.0
		1	occasional non-dominant alpha frequency	2.0
16	Electrodes			

Reproduced from reference 8 with permission.

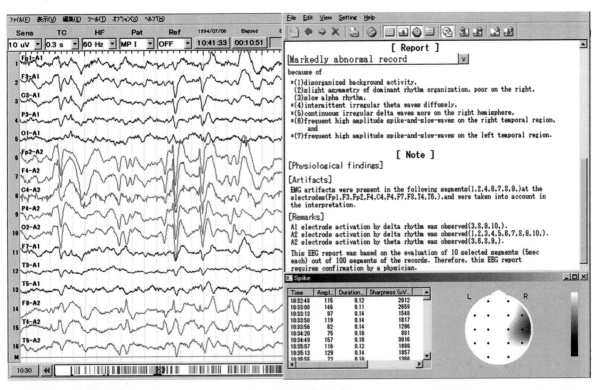

Figure 27.3. *A written report of automatic interpretation of an EEG in a 46-year-old man with temporal lobe epilepsy following acute encephalitis in childhood (right upper panel). A 5-sec segment of the recording is shown in the left panel. Distribution of the spike detected by the automatic analysis is shown in the right lower panel. The report of visual inspection of the same EEG, independently prepared by an EEG-er, reads, "Markedly abnormal waking record because of (1) lack of dominant rhythm, (2) continuous irregular delta and theta waves diffusely more on the right hemisphere, and (3) frequent high amplitude spike-and-waves on the right hemisphere, and occasionally on the left." Modified from reference 8 with permission.*

The automatic analysis in this patient reports a markedly abnormal record because of disorganized background activity, asymmetry of organization of PDR (which is poor on the right), slow alpha rhythm, intermittent irregular theta and delta waves, and frequent high-amplitude spike-and-slow-waves in the right and the left temporal regions. In the EEG trace shown in the left panel, which was recorded in a referential montage with respect to the ipsilateral ear electrode, the spike appears much larger over the right fronto-central leads than over the right temporal leads, but this is the result of activation of the right ear reference electrode (A2) by the spike, which is correctly detected by this automatic system. The report of visual inspection of the same record, obtained by a qualified EEG-er independently of the automatic analysis, is shown in the legends of Figure 27.3 for comparison. The distribution of spike thus detected is automatically illustrated, showing that this system can detect the ear reference activation by the spike and correctly identify the localization of the spike in the right temporal region.

4. DISCUSSION

This automatic program is operated offline. It starts from the beginning of the EEG recording unless otherwise specified, but it can be started at any time in the whole series. For an EEG record of ordinary length, the entire automatic analysis is completed within a few seconds, including the time for automatic report writing.

Some problems with the program remain, but they should be improved in the future. The present system selects 10 segments (overall 50 sec long) according to the organization score of PDR and subjects them to the final analysis. In ordinary EEG records of good quality, it is expected that analysis of a longer trace of EEG would produce more reasonable results from automatic analysis. However, if inappropriate segments, such as those containing artifacts or those recorded in a state of decreased vigilance or high attentiveness, are included in an attempt to increase the number of segments, the quality of automatic analysis may be lowered.

Our system of automatic analysis was not aimed at standardizing the EEG interpretation but was based on the criteria adopted by a limited number of qualified EEG-ers for visual inspection. Theoretically, in view of (1) the significant differences in the techniques of data acquisition among laboratories, (2) differences in the criteria of visual inspection even among qualified EEG-ers, and (3) possible differences in EEG features among different races and between genders of the subjects, standardization of EEG interpretation is expected to face significant difficulties. However, if an ideal standard were established, then the standard criteria could be incorporated into our system (18).

Application of the present system is limited to adult subjects, but it might be applied to children and the elderly population by adjusting the criteria for each age group. By the same token, it could also be modified for automatic interpretation of the sleep EEG.

REFERENCES

1. Nakamura M, Nishida S, Neshige R, Shibasaki H. Quantitative analysis of 'organization' by feature extraction of the EEG power spectrum. Electroenceph Clin Neurophysiol 1985;60:84–89.
2. Marcuse LV, Schneider M, Mortati KA, Donnelly KM, Arnedo V, Grant AC. Quantitative analysis of the EEG, posterior-dominant rhythm in healthy adolescents. Clin Neurophysiol 2008;119:1778–1781.
3. Lodder SS, van Putten MJAM. Automated EEG analysis: characterizing the posterior dominant rhythm. J Neurosci Methods 2011;200:86–93.
4. Matsuoka S, Arakaki Y, Numaguchi K, Ueno S. The effect of dexamethasone on electroencephalograms in patients with brain tumors. With specific reference to topographic computer display of delta activity. J Neurosurg 1978;48:601–608.
5. Anderson NR, Doolittle LM. Automated analysis of EEG: opportunities and pitfalls. J Clin Neurophysiol 2010;27:453–457.
6. Nakamura M, Shibasaki H, Imajoh K, Nishida S, Neshige R, Ikeda A. Automatic EEG interpretation: a new computer-assisted system for the automatic integrative interpretation of awake background EEG. Electroenceph Clin Neurophysiol 1992;82:423–431.
7. Nakamura M, Sugi T, Ikeda A, Kakigi R, Shibasaki H. Clinical application of automatic integrative interpretation of awake background EEG: quantitative interpretation, report making, and detection of artifacts and reduced vigilance level. Electroenceph Clin Neurophysiol 1996;98:103–112.
8. Shibasaki H, Nakamura M, Sugi T, Nishida S, Nagamine T, Ikeda A. Automatic interpretation and writing report of the adult waking electroencephalogram. Clin Neurophysiol 2014;125:1081–1094.
9. Nishida S, Nakamura M, Shibasaki H. An EEG model expressed by the sinusoidal waves with the Markov process amplitude. [Abstract in English.] Iyodenshi To Seitai Kogaku 1986;24:8–14.
10. Bai O, Nakamura M, Ikeda A, Shibasaki H. Nonlinear Markov process amplitude EEG model for nonlinear coupling interaction of spontaneous EEG. IEEE Trans Biomed Eng 2000;47:1141–1146.
11. Noachtar S, Binnie C, Ebersole J, Mauguiere F, Sakamoto A, Westmoreland B. A glossary of terms most commonly used by clinical electroencephalographers and proposal for the report form for the EEG findings. In Deuschl G, Eisen A (Eds), Recommendations for the Practice of Clinical Neurophysiology: Guidelines of the International Federation of Clinical Neurophysiology, Electroenceph Clin Neurophysiol 1999;Suppl. 52:21–40.
12. Akaike H. A new look at the statistical model identification. IEEE Trans Automat Control 1974;AC-19:716–723.
13. Sugi T, Nakamura M, Ikeda A, Kakigi R, Shibasaki H. Automatic detection of artifacts for pre-processing of automatic EEG interpretation. [Abstract in English.] Iyodenshi To Seitai Kogaku 1995;33:203–213.
14. Sugi T, Nakamura M, Ikeda A, Shibasaki H. Adaptive EEG spike detection: determination of threshold values based on conditional probability. Front Med Biol Eng 2002;11:261–277.
15. Bai O, Nakamura M, Ikeda A, Shibasaki H. Automatic detection of open and closed eye states in the electroencephalographic (EEG) record for background EEG interpretation by the trigger method. Front Med Biol Eng 2000;10:1–15.
16. Nakamura M, Shibasaki H, Imajoh K, Ikeda A, Kakigi R. Automatic EEG report making for awake background EEG. [Abstract in English.] Jpn J Clin Neurophysiol 1993;21:47–56.
17. Beniczky S, Aurlien H, Brøgger JC, Fuglsang-Frederiksen A, Martins-da-Silva A, Trinka E, et al. Standardized computer-based organized reporting of EEG: SCORE. Epilepsia 2013;54:1112–1124.
18. Lodder SS, van Putten MJAM. Quantification of the adult EEG background pattern. Clin Neurophysiol 2013;124:228–237.

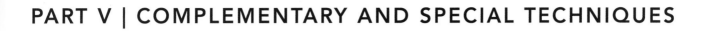

PART V | COMPLEMENTARY AND SPECIAL TECHNIQUES

28 | TRANSCRANIAL ELECTRICAL AND MAGNETIC STIMULATION

ALEXANDER ROTENBERG, MD, PHD, ALVARO PASCUAL-LEONE, MD, PHD, AND ALAN D. LEGATT, MD, PHD

ABSTRACT: Noninvasive magnetic and electrical stimulation of cerebral cortex is an evolving field. The most widely used variant, transcranial electrical stimulation (TES), is routinely used for intraoperative monitoring. Transcranial magnetic stimulation (TMS) and transcranial direct current stimulation (tDCS) are emerging as clinical and experimental tools. TMS has gained wide acceptance in extraoperative functional cortical mapping. TES and TMS rely on pulsatile stimulation with electrical current intensities sufficient to trigger action potentials within the stimulated cortical volume. tDCS, in contrast, is based on neuromodulatory effects of very-low-amplitude direct current conducted through the scalp. tDCS and TMS, particularly when applied in repetitive trains, can modulate cortical excitability for prolonged periods and thus are either in active clinical use or in advanced stages of clinical trials for common neurological and psychiatric disorders such as major depression and epilepsy. This chapter summarizes physiologic principles of transcranial stimulation and clinical applications of these techniques.

KEYWORDS: transcranial electrical stimulation, TES, transcranial magnetic stimulation, TMS, transcranial direct current stimulation, tDCS, intraoperative monitoring, mapping

PRINCIPAL REFERENCES

1. Legatt AD, Emerson RG, Epstein CM, et al. ACNS Guideline: transcranial electrical stimulation motor evoked potential monitoring. *Journal of Clinical Neurophysiology*. 2016;33(1):42–50.
2. Legatt AD. Ellen R. Grass Lecture: motor evoked potential monitoring. *American Journal of Electroneurodiagnostic Technology*. 2004;44(4):223–243.
3. Purpura DP, McMurtry JG. Intracellular activities and evoked potential changes during polarization of motor cortex. *Journal of Neurophysiology*. 1965;28(1):166–185.
4. Sun Y, Lipton JO, Boyle LM, et al. Direct current stimulation induces mGluR5-dependent neocortical plasticity. *Annals of Neurology*. 2016;80(2):233–2465.
5. Nitsche MA, Paulus W. Noninvasive brain stimulation protocols in the treatment of epilepsy: current state and perspectives. *Neurotherapeutics*. 2009;6(2):244–2505.
6. Kobayashi M, Pascual-Leone A. Transcranial magnetic stimulation in neurology. *Lancet Neurology*. 2003;2(3):145–156.
7. Picht T, Schmidt S, Brandt S, et al. Preoperative functional mapping for rolandic brain tumor surgery: comparison of navigated transcranial magnetic stimulation to direct cortical stimulation. *Neurosurgery*. 2011;69(3):581–589.
8. Picht T, Krieg SM, Sollmann N, et al. A comparison of language mapping by preoperative navigated transcranial magnetic stimulation and direct cortical stimulation during awake surgery. *Neurosurgery*. 2013;72(5):808–819.
9. Shafi MM, Vernet M, Klooster D, et al. Physiological consequences of abnormal connectivity in a developmental epilepsy. *Annals of Neurology*. 2015;77(3):487–503.
10. Rossi S, Hallett M, Rossini PM, Pascual-Leone A, Safety of TMS Consensus Group. Safety, ethical considerations, and application guidelines for the use of transcranial magnetic stimulation in clinical practice and research. *Clinical Neurophysiology*. 2009;120(12):2008–2039.

1. NONINVASIVE BRAIN STIMULATION

Noninvasive magnetic and electrical stimulation of cerebral cortex is an evolving field that includes a range of diagnostic and therapeutic protocols for conduction or induction of electrical current in the brain. Among clinical applications for these methods are electrical brain stimulation for intraoperative monitoring of the motor pathways, extraoperative assessment and mapping of motor and language cortical regions, and several techniques aimed at measuring or modifying cortical excitability. While the most mature and most widely tested techniques in this field are transcranial electrical stimulation (TES), transcranial direct current stimulation (tDCS), and transcranial magnetic stimulation (TMS), other protocols, such as transcranial alternating current stimulation, transcranial random noise stimulation, and low-field magnetic stimulation, are also in early testing phases. In this chapter, we focus on TES, tDCS, and TMS as examples of noninvasive brain stimulation techniques that are already in wide clinical and experimental use.

TES and TMS both rely on pulsatile stimulation with electrical current intensities sufficient to trigger action potentials within the stimulated cortical volume. In practical applications, TES, especially if delivered in brief trains of stimulus pulses, is most useful for intraoperative monitoring in an anesthetized patient [1], while single-pulse TMS is more useful for extraoperative diagnostic motor evoked potential (MEP) studies in awake subjects, as well as for research applications aimed at establishing and mapping causal brain–behavior relations in non-motor cortical areas. tDCS and TMS, particularly if delivered in repetitive trains (repetitive TMS [rTMS]), also share a capacity to modulate cortical excitability for prolonged periods and thus are either in active clinical use or in advanced stages of clinical trials for common neurological and psychiatric disorders such as major depression and other psychiatric disorders, post-stroke motor and language deficits, and epilepsy [2–4].

2. TES AND INSIGHTS FROM ELECTRICAL MOTOR CORTEX STIMULATION

Applied to the motor cortex, a single electrical stimulus can produce multiple volleys within the descending motor tracts that can be recorded with epidural electrodes placed over the spinal cord. Studies in experimental animals have elucidated the mechanisms underlying this [5] (Fig. 28.1). The first volley reflects direct stimulation of the pyramidal neuron axons that leave cerebral cortex and make up the corticobulbar and corticospinal tracts; this volley has been labeled the D-wave ("D" for "Direct"). Subsequent volleys, labeled I-waves ("I" for "Indirect"), derive from activation of the pyramidal neurons via excitatory synaptic input from other cortical neurons that were themselves activated, either directly or indirectly, by the externally applied stimulus. The delay from that stimulus to an I-wave reflects the time required for the intervening synaptic transmission(s), and thus is the sum of an integral number of cortical synaptic transmission delays. This accounts for the relatively consistent intervals between the D-wave and the first I-wave and between successive I-waves (e.g., see Fig. 28.1A).

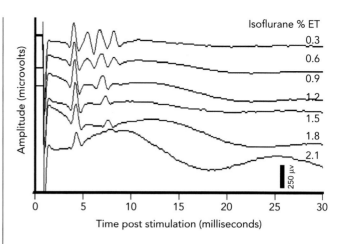

Figure 28.2. MEPs to single-pulse TES, recorded by an epidural electrode in the mid-thoracic region in a baboon anesthetized with ketamine and isoflurane, at varying isoflurane concentrations. The D-wave persists, but the I-waves are lost at the highest anesthetic dose. Reprinted from [7].

Since the production of I-waves depends on cortical synaptic transmission, factors that depress cortical synaptic function will reduce or eliminate the I-waves (see Fig. 28.1B). Most anesthetic agents depress cortical synaptic function, and will reduce or eliminate the I-waves [6–8] (Fig. 28.2).

In TES, stimulating current passes between an anode and a cathode that are at different locations on the scalp. With electrical stimulation of peripheral nerves, the action potential volleys are predominantly initiated under the cathode [9], whereas with TES the D-waves are predominantly initiated under the anode [5] (Fig. 28.3). Why is this? Outward transmembrane current depolarizes the neuronal membrane and is excitatory, whereas inward transmembrane current hyperpolarizes the neuronal membrane and is inhibitory. When stimulating peripheral nerve, the outward transmembrane current depolarizes the axonal membrane and initiates the action potential under the cathode (Fig. 28.4). When stimulating cerebral cortex, it is the action potentials that are propagating in the corticofugal motor tracts that generate the MEPs, and these action potentials are initiated at the axon hillocks of the cortical pyramidal neurons. Current flows under the scalp anode result in inward (inhibitory) transmembrane current in the superficial portion of the pyramidal neuron but outward (excitatory) current at the axon hillock [10] (Fig. 28.5), which produces the D-waves that can be recorded with epidural electrodes over the spinal cord. Current flows under the TES cathode are opposite in direction; they may excite the superficial portion of the pyramidal neuron as well as cortical interneurons, but the hyperpolarization at the axon hillock may block the initiation or propagation of action potentials along the motor tracts that would give rise to D-waves. Under surgical anesthesia, when I-waves are largely suppressed and the MEPs are predominantly generated by D-waves, the myogenic MEPs elicited by TES are predominantly recorded from muscles contralateral to the TES anode (Fig. 28.6).

While I-waves are mediated by cortical synaptic activity, D-waves can be elicited by stimulation of corticospinal tract axons within the white matter (see Fig. 28.1A, 28.1C). As the TES stimulus intensity is increased, intraparenchymal current

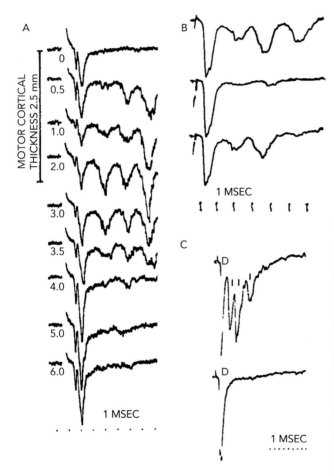

Figure 28.1. Data from animal experiments using direct electrical stimulation of cerebral cortex that illustrate the physiology of D-waves and I-waves. A: Stimulation within or near motor cortex elicits both D-waves and I-waves, here recorded from the ipsilateral medullary pyramid. When the stimulating electrode is advanced to the subcortical white matter so that the corticospinal tract axons but not the cortex itself are stimulated (lower traces), only D-waves are produced. B: Motor cortex stimulation initially produces both D-waves and I-waves (upper trace). Temporary depression of cortical function due to mechanical trauma eliminates the I-waves, but the D-waves persist (middle trace). Subsequently, the I-waves reappear as the cortex recovers (lower trace). C: Motor cortex stimulation produces a D-wave and multiple I-waves (upper trace), here recorded from the contralateral spinal cord. The cortex was then ablated. This eliminated the I-waves, but direct stimulation of the exposed subcortical white matter still produced D-waves (lower trace). Modified from [12].

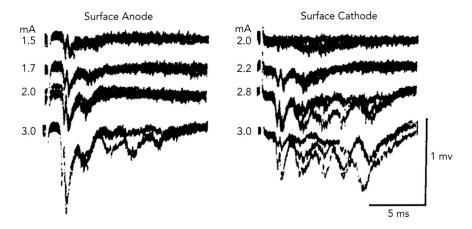

Surface Anode

mA
1.5
1.7
2.0
3.0

Surface Cathode

mA
2.0
2.2
2.8
3.0

1 mv

5 ms

Figure 28.3. Corticospinal tract responses (recorded from the contralateral spinal cord) to surface anodal and cathodal stimulation of motor cortex in a monkey, using a silver ball stimulating electrode resting on the pial surface. Note that anodal stimulation produces the largest D-waves, whereas I-waves are produced under both the anode and the cathode. Reprinted from Amassian et al. [12].

densities capable of stimulating these axons are produced farther and farther away from the surface of the head, and may be able to stimulate them as far caudally as the medulla [11]. During intraoperative monitoring of the brainstem and of the corticospinal tracts within the cerebrum, this could prevent recognition of surgery-related motor tract compromise if the motor tracts were stimulated caudal to that dysfunction.

Due to the relatively high impedance of the skull, high-intensity electrical stimuli (hundreds of volts, and currents of the order of magnitude of 100 mA) must be applied to the surface of the scalp in order to effectively stimulate brain tissue. These current levels powerfully stimulate pain fibers in the scalp. Thus, while TES has been performed on conscious subjects as part of a research protocol [12], it is not practical for use as a neurodiagnostic tool in awake patients. It is, however, the procedure of choice for eliciting MEPs for intraoperative monitoring [13].

In awake subjects TES (as well as TMS, see below) will produce a series of volleys, derived from D-waves and I-waves, in the corticospinal tract. The postsynaptic potentials that these produce will summate to bring the lower motor neurons to threshold, causing muscle contractions and allowing the recording of myogenic MEPs, also called M-waves. Under anesthesia, a single TES pulse will most likely produce a single

D-wave, which may not be sufficient to fire the anterior horn cells and produce reliable M-waves. Multiple stimuli will produce multiple D-waves; these will produce multiple excitatory postsynaptic potentials that will summate in the lower motor neurons, causing them to fire (Fig. 28.7) and producing muscle contractions (Fig. 28.8, right side). When stimulated repetitively, cerebral cortex may also produce I-waves [14], providing further excitatory drive to the anterior horn cells (see Fig. 28.8, left side). The development of stimulators capable of delivering brief trains of high-intensity electrical stimuli with short inter-stimulus intervals (ISIs) has permitted the recording of myogenic MEPs suitable for intraoperative monitoring in most patients.

The repetition rate of the pulses within the train has a marked influence on the size of the M-wave, as demonstrated by a paired-pulse experiment [14] (Fig. 28.9). If the ISI is too short, pulses after the first may not effectively stimulate the

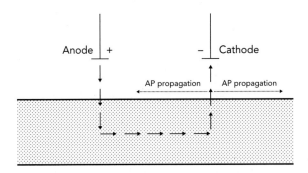

Anode | +   – | Cathode

AP propagation   AP propagation

Figure 28.4. Diagram of current flow during electrical stimulation of peripheral nerve. The action potential (AP) is initiated by outward transmembrane current under the cathode, and propagates in both directions. The membrane under the anode is hyperpolarized; this can cause "anodal block." Current flow is indicated as movement of positive charge. Reprinted from Legatt [1].

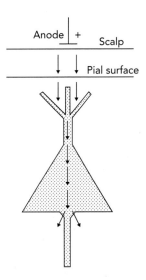

Anode | + Scalp

Pial surface

Figure 28.5. Diagram of current flow during electrical stimulation of cerebral cortex. Radially oriented currents under the anode produce inward trans membrane current in the apical dendrites of this cortical pyramidal neuron, and depolarizing outward transmembrane current in the axon hillock and proximal axon. Reprinted from Legatt [1].

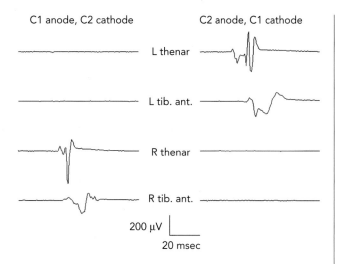

C1 anode, C2 cathode   C2 anode, C1 cathode

L thenar

L tib. ant.

R thenar

R tib. ant.

200 µV

20 msec

Figure 28.6. *Myogenic MEPs elicited by multi-pulse TES between electrodes at scalp positions C1 and C2 with both stimulus polarities, recorded bilaterally from thenar and tibialis anterior muscles during an occipitocervical fusion. TES elicited MEPs in the muscles contralateral to the anode. Reprinted from Legatt [1].*

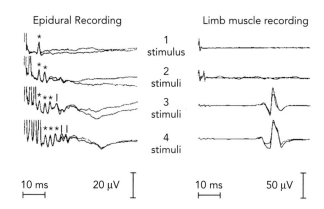

Epidural Recording   Limb muscle recording

1 stimulus

2 stimuli

3 stimuli

4 stimuli

10 ms   20 µV   10 ms   50 µV

Figure 28.8. *Epidural recordings of D-waves (marked with asterisks) and I waves (marked "I") (left) and recordings of M-waves from electrodes in limb muscles (right) following electrical stimulation of motor cortex with stimulus trains consisting of one, two, three, and four stimuli. D-waves are present in all cases, and I-waves appear following multi-pulse stimulation. The M-wave is only present when trains of at least three stimuli are used. Modified from Deletis and Kothbauer [14].*

corticospinal tract axons due to their refractory periods (note the falloff of both the M-waves and of the second D-waves, "D2," at the shortest ISIs). If the interval between the pulses is too long, the excitatory postsynaptic potentials within the alpha motor neurons will decay during the intervals between successive pulses, losing the benefit of the temporal summation (note the falloff of the M-waves at the longest ISIs as well). ISIs of 2 to 3 msec are typically used for intraoperative MEP monitoring. As needed, multiple stimulation trains can also be delivered to enhance the MEP size [15].

Even with high-intensity, short-ISI pulse train TES, only a small fraction of the motor neuron pool fires each time an MEP is recorded—and it is a different subset of the motor neuron pool each time, similar to the situation with F-waves to peripheral nerve stimulation. Thus, even though the stimulus is unchanged, successive M-wave recordings may differ markedly in amplitude and wave shape (Fig. 28.10), just as F-waves

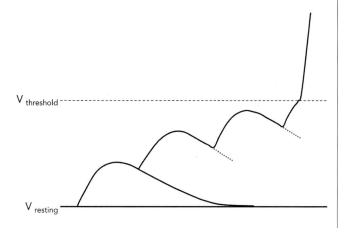

V threshold

V resting

Figure 28.7. *Cartoon showing summation of successive excitatory postsynaptic potentials (EPSPs) within an anterior horn cell; the curve represents the intracellular potential at the axon hillock. A single EPSP (shown in its entirety) would not make the lower motor neuron fire, but the summation of multiple EPSPs (in this example, four of them) is sufficient to bring the neuron to threshold and initiate an action potential.*

do. Because of this variability, signal averaging should not be applied to M-waves. However, these myogenic signals are usually sufficiently large that averaging is not necessary. D-waves can also be monitored using electrodes placed near the spinal cord; they are smaller than M-waves and more consistent in amplitude and wave shape (Fig. 28.11), so it is appropriate to use signal averaging (usually with a small number of sweeps per average) when recording D-waves.

The difficulty of activating the anterior horn cells under surgical anesthesia, even with repetitive train stimulation, makes myogenic MEPs highly susceptible to anesthetic effects, more sensitive than the sensory evoked potentials that are also used for intraoperative monitoring (Fig. 28.12). The choice of the anesthetic regimen is particularly critical when M-waves are being monitored. Halogenated inhalational agents prominently suppress them, and are best avoided. Intravenous anesthetics such as propofol and ketamine also affect MEPs, but to a lesser extent. Opioids have only minor effects on MEPs. Nitrous oxide produces marked changes in MEPs, but myogenic MEPs can be successfully recorded using a "nitrous-narcotic" technique. Total intravenous anesthesia using propofol and opioid infusions is an optimal anesthetic regimen for monitoring myogenic TES-MEPs. Complete neuromuscular blockade must obviously be avoided. If partial neuromuscular blockade is used, it should be maintained with a continuous infusion of muscle relaxant titrated to maintain a consistent degree of neuromuscular blockade, rather than with intermittent bolus doses, since the latter could cause misleading fluctuations in the degree of neuromuscular blockade and thus in the MEPs [7].

The electrical stimuli for TES are most often delivered using paired corkscrew electrodes inserted into the scalp, though alternative configurations such as a distributed or "ring" cathode covering a large region of the head have also been used. Electrode pairs Fz (anode)/Cz (cathode), C1/C2, and C3/C4 (Fig. 28.13) are most often used. The Fz/Cz electrode pair predominantly stimulates the corticospinal tracts to the legs, while C3/C4 preferentially stimulates the corticospinal tracts to the arms; stimulation between C1 and C2 may produce MEPs in both upper

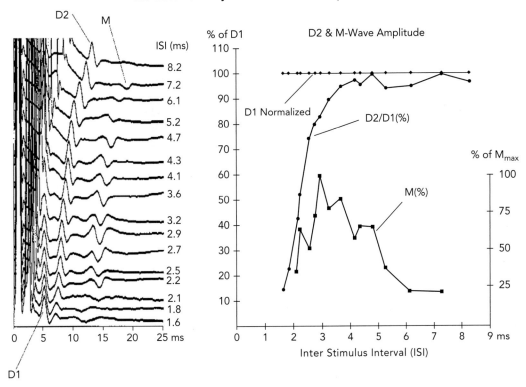

D2-Wave Recovery Time/MEP Muscle Amplitude

Figure 28.9. Left panel: *Epidural recordings of D-waves from the spinal cord following pairs of transcranial electrical stimuli with varying ISIs. The first D-wave ("D1") is obscured by the electrical stimulus artifact at the larger ISIs; the D-wave elicited by the second stimulus ("D2") is visible in all waveforms. An M-wave originating in paraspinal musculature ("M") is visible in some of the waveforms.* Right panel: *The amplitudes of the M-waves and the D2-waves (the latter expressed as a percentage of the amplitude of the D1 wave) are plotted as a function of the ISI. Modified from Deletis and Kothbauer [14].*

and lower extremities (see Figs. 28.6, 28.10). TES between electrodes Fz and Cz will stimulate the corticospinal tracts to the legs bilaterally. If M-waves are being monitored, this will permit assessment of the motor pathways to both legs simultaneously. However, if D-waves recorded from the spinal cord are being monitored, simultaneous bilateral stimulation may prevent recognition of unilateral corticospinal tract compromise. Use of laterally displaced electrode pairs permits selective stimulation of the hemisphere under the anode (see Fig. 28.6).

3. NEUROMODULATION AND SEIZURE SUPPRESSION BY TDCS

In contrast to high-voltage/high-current pulsatile stimulation in TES, neuronal activity in cerebral cortex may also be modulated by low-amplitude (typically 1–2 mA) transcranial direct current (DC) delivered by scalp electrodes. tDCS is based on decades-old observations that neuronal firing is modulated by low-amplitude electrical DC [16] that is, in contrast to TES, beneath the threshold necessary to trigger cortical action potentials. Specifically, when applied at the pial surface or at the scalp, anodal DC facilitates neuronal firing whereas cathodal DC inhibits neuronal firing. The mechanisms by which anodal tDCS facilitates neuronal firing likely relate to depolarization of the axon hillock cell membrane, which occurs when the dendrites of a neuron are oriented toward the anode in a constant electric field (see Fig. 28.5). The reverse may occur with cathodal

tDCS with the axon hillock becoming hyperpolarized, inhibiting neuronal firing. This mechanism is supported by in vitro studies in isolated brain slices where the direction of change in regional excitability, whether toward activation or depression, is dependent on the orientation of the axonal input into that area relative to the anodal or cathodal terminal of the DC field [17].

Notably, the change in cortical excitability outlasts the duration of a tDCS stimulus (typically 10–30 minutes), and enables tDCS applications as a neuromodulation tool in disorders where regional over-activation or under-activation of the cortex is part of the pathophysiology. The mechanisms by which tDCS produces lasting changes in cortical excitability are not fully understood, though preclinical data indicate involvement of both glutamatergic and GABAergic signaling [18,19].

The practical application of tDCS is simple: low-amplitude DC is administered via broad scalp electrodes (typically saline-saturated sponges) such that the cortical target is exposed to either anodal or cathodal DC beneath one of the electrodes, while one or more electrodes of the opposite polarity are positioned elsewhere on the head or on an extracephalic site such as the shoulder. In some indications, such in neuromodulation aimed to facilitate motor or expressive language recovery after stroke, paired anodal and cathodal tDCS administered to both sides of the head may be useful because, in patients with lateralized strokes, the facilitatory effect of anodal tDCS on the lesioned cortex and the inhibitory effect of cathodal tDCS over the homologous area in the unlesioned hemisphere may both be beneficial [20].

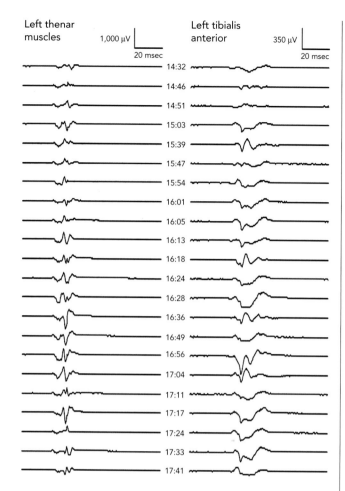

Left thenar muscles — 1,000 µV — 20 msec

Left tibialis anterior — 350 µV — 20 msec

14:32
14:46
14:51
15:03
15:39
15:47
15:54
16:01
16:05
16:13
16:18
16:24
16:28
16:36
16:49
16:56
17:04
17:11
17:17
17:24
17:33
17:41

Figure 28.10. *M-waves recorded from the left tibialis anterior and thenar muscles following multi-pulse TES with the anode over the right hemisphere (electrode position C2) over a 3-hour time period during an occipitocervical fusion. Note the large run-to-run variability of the MEP amplitudes and wave shapes. The numbers in the middle are the clock times of each run. Reprinted from Legatt [1].*

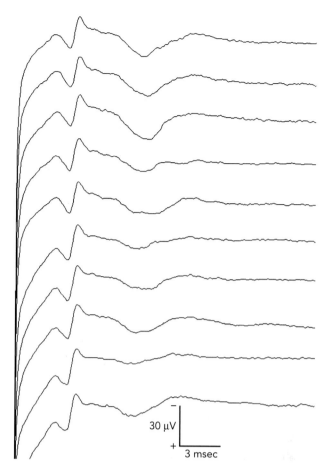

30 µV — 3 msec

Figure 28.11. *Consecutive D-wave recordings obtained over a half-hour time period during resection of an ependymoma of the cervical spinal cord in a 45-year-old man. The D-waves were recorded from an epidural electrode placed over the spinal cord caudal to the tumor. Each waveform is the average of the responses to eight single-pulse TES stimuli.*

In epilepsy, the capacity of cathodal tDCS to reduce cortical excitability has prompted research into its antiepileptic potential [21]. Clinical tDCS experience in epilepsy is limited, but published reports suggest a realistic role for tDCS in seizure suppression [22]. In one randomized controlled study of adults with intractable epilepsy (N = 19) referable to malformations of cortical development, interictal epileptiform discharges on EEG were reduced for up to 30 days followed one 20-minute application of 1 mA cathodal tDCS over the seizure focus [23]. In a pediatric controlled trial (N = 36), 1-mA cathodal tDCS for 20 minutes corresponded to a significant decrease in the EEG spike frequency for up to 48 hours after stimulation. Clinical seizure reduction in the active cohort of this cohort was small (~5%), but also statistically significantly different from control, and supports continued efforts to test whether multiple tDCS courses will result in a meaningful antiepileptic effect [24]. Another small (N = 12) crossover controlled trial identified an antiepileptic effect with active (2-mA cathodal tDCS for 30 minutes) stimulation over the seizure focus in a cohort of patients with temporal lobe epilepsy with hippocampal sclerosis [25].

As with other noninvasive brain stimulation protocols, the incomplete efficacy of human tDCS trials underscores the value of preclinical studies, the results of which can help to optimize future clinical tDCS study designs. Some preclinical studies underscore the antiepileptic potential of tDCS and demonstrate increased seizure thresholds in focal electroshock and amygdala seizure kindling models [26,27], as well as a neuroprotective effect in a rat pup pilocarpine-induced status epilepticus model [28]. In a more recent experiment, cathodal tDCS electrographic seizure suppression was seen within minutes of stimulation in a rat pentylenetetrazole status epilepticus model. Of translational relevance for plausible clinical tDCS application, cathodal tDCS in this experiment worked synergistically with lorazepam to suppress seizures [18]. These data underscore an important direction for translational neuromodulation research toward systematic testing of combination drug and device therapy in epilepsy [18,19].

4. TMS: TECHNICAL ASPECTS

During TMS, high-intensity current pulses are passed through a coil that is held in close proximity to the patient's head. The

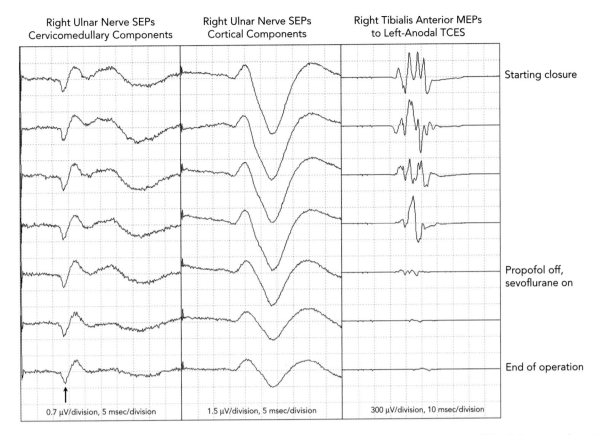

Right Ulnar Nerve SEPs
Cervicomedullary Components

Right Ulnar Nerve SEPs
Cortical Components

Right Tibialis Anterior MEPs
to Left-Anodal TCES

Starting closure

Propofol off,
sevoflurane on

End of operation

0.7 µV/division, 5 msec/division   1.5 µV/division, 5 msec/division   300 µV/division, 10 msec/division

Figure 28.12. Anesthetic effects on cervicomedullary somatosensory evoked potentials (SEPS) (left), cortical SEPs (center), and MEPs during surgery for revision of spinal instrumentation and fusion. Total intravenous anesthesia had been used during most of the operation, but during closing the propofol infusion was turned off and sevoflurane was turned on. The halogenated inhalational agent almost completely eliminated the MEPs; the cortical SEPs were attenuated but not eliminated, and the cervicomedullary SEPs were relatively unaffected. Reprinted from [100].

magnetic field produced by this coil passes through the skull without significant attenuation and induces rotatory currents within the patient's brain that flow in the opposite direction to the current in the stimulating coil [12] (Fig. 28.14). In essence,

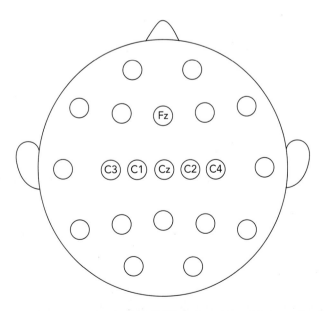

Figure 28.13. Cartoon showing the EEG electrode positions of the International 10-20 System along with additional electrode positions C1 and C2, which are midway between C3 or C4 (respectively) and Cz. The electrode positions that are most often used for TES are labeled.

this system functions as a transformer, with the brain parenchyma acting as the secondary coil. It is the current induced by the time-varying magnetic field within the brain that stimulates the neurons. Thus, TMS is a form of electrical brain stimulation, though the delivery of electromagnetic energy to the head is via a rapidly changing magnetic field pulse rather than by directly conducted currents. The advantage of TMS is that it does not activate scalp pain fibers as strongly as TES, and it is therefore useful for assessing central motor pathways in conscious subjects. TMS can also be applied to non-motor regions in the brain convexity. Depth penetration is limited, as the magnetic field strength decreases as a cube of the distance and is always maximal closer to the stimulation coil. Therefore, while relatively broad stimulation is possible with specialized H-coil TMS arrays [29], selective stimulation of deep brain structures is not possible.

Pyramidal tract axons are most effectively stimulated by radial currents, those flowing normal to the cortical surface (see Fig. 28.5). Depending on the position and orientation of the coil, the intraparenchymal currents induced by TMS may be largely tangential in orientation (see Fig. 28.14), preferentially stimulating horizontally coursing neurites within the cortical neuropil rather than the axon hillocks of pyramidal neurons (Fig. 28.15). Thus, when monitored by epidural spinal cord recordings, TMS often produces predominantly I-waves rather than D-waves [30,31] (Fig. 28.16). Since the I-waves are suppressed by surgical anesthesia (see Fig. 28.2), anesthesia

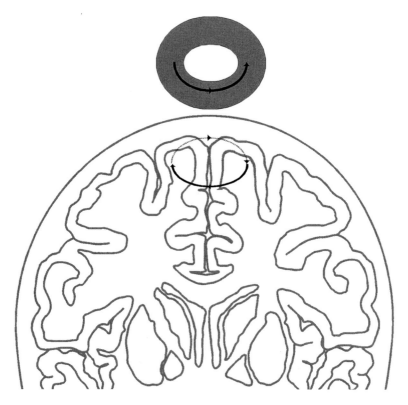

Figure 28.14. Diagram of TMS of the brain, showing the currents induced in the brain. Reprinted from [12].

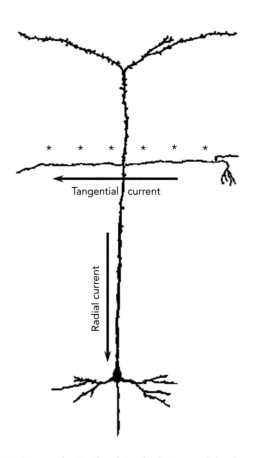

Tangential current

Radial current

Figure 28.15. Diagram showing the relationship between radial and tangential stimulating currents and cellular elements within cerebral cortex. Shown are the horizontally coursing process of a cortical interneuron, marked by the row of asterisks, and a cortical pyramidal neuron. Reprinted from [1].

may also markedly suppress the MEPs elicited by TMS. In addition, small changes in the position and orientation of the stimulating coil may produce dramatic changes in TMS-MEPs [32], and it is difficult to maintain the coil in the exact same position relative to the patient's head during operations lasting several hours. In addition, the magnetic field-pulse induced by TMS can affect other equipment in the operating room, necessitating appropriate placement and shielding of equipment. For these practical considerations, TES (see above), rather than TMS, is the procedure of choice for eliciting MEPs for intraoperative monitoring [13].

With a circular TMS coil, the intraparenchymal current density is relatively consistent within the torus of brain tissue underlying the coil (see Fig. 28.14). To obtain more focal stimulation of cerebral cortex, a figure-of-eight coil or other non-circular coil geometries may be used to obtain a focally higher current density within a more restricted volume [33–35] (Fig. 28.17). During diagnostic TMS-MEP studies, maintenance of a mild degree of tension in the muscle group(s) from which the MEPs are being recorded can augment the MEPs and decrease their onset latencies, or cause previously absent MEPs to appear [12,36]. This is most likely due to the voluntary contraction maintaining the spinal motor neurons in a partially depolarized state [36].

Single-pulse TMS can elicit an immediate MEP but does not induce changes in cortical excitability lasting more than a few milliseconds after the stimulus. rTMS, in contrast, induces changes in cortical excitability that outlast the stimulation [37]. Although the precise mechanisms by which rTMS alters cortical excitability are not completely understood, they resemble those of long-term-potentiation and long-term depression of

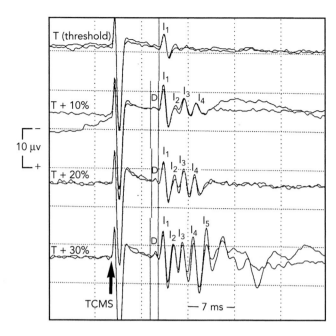

Figure 28.16. *Spinal cord potentials following brain TMS, recorded by an epidural electrode in a patient undergoing placement of a dorsal column stimulator for pain control. Note the multiple I-waves and the relatively insignificant D-wave. The stimulating coil was positioned for optimal activation of the left tibialis anterior muscle. Reprinted from [31].*

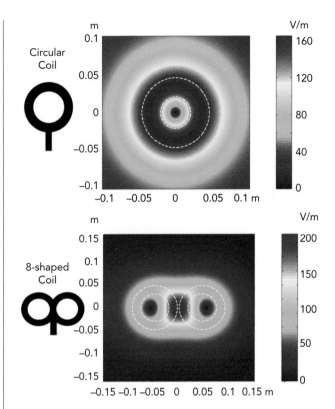

Figure 28.17. *Diagram of the voltage gradients produced in the brain by TMS using a circular coil (top) and a figure-of-eight coil (bottom). Note that the figure-of-eight coil produces more focal stimulation. Reprinted from [18].*

excitatory synaptic strength that can be induced by high (≥10 Hz) or low (≤1 Hz) repetitive electrical stimulation of the cortex or hippocampus [38–41]. It is this capacity to produce a durable and focal change in cortical excitability that appears to be the basis of the therapeutic effect of rTMS, which is supported by favorable clinical trials in several prevalent neuropsychiatric diseases states such as major depression, chronic pain, and epilepsy [3,42,43].

5. TMS AS A DIAGNOSTIC AND THERAPEUTIC TOOL

In clinical applications, TMS is unique among the neurostimulation methods in its realistic roles as both a therapeutic intervention and a diagnostic tool. As diagnostic procedures, single-pulse TMS and paired-pulse TMS may be used to noninvasively map cortical function and to measure regional cortical excitability [44,45], as underscored by U.S. Food and Drug Administration (FDA) clearance of one device for this indication. In therapeutic applications, the capacity of rTMS to induce a lasting change in cortical excitability has been tested in several disease states, including epilepsy [46–49]. The 2008 FDA clearance of a first device and protocol for treatment of some patients with medication-resistant major depression as well as subsequent clearance of several rTMS devices via the FDA 510k (equivalence to previously approved technology) mechanism indicates acceptance of rTMS in the clinical setting.

In most common protocols, TMS is coupled with surface electromyelography (TMS-EMG) such that the motor cortex is stimulated and the magnitude of the evoked muscle contraction in a contralateral limb (typically a hand muscle) can be quantified by skin electrodes and the recording of an MEP [43]. From the MEP, a number of measures can be derived to probe cortico-spinal excitability, and a number of them characterize cortical and intracortical excitation/inhibition balance. One is the threshold to muscle activation, or motor threshold (MT). The MT, obtained by single-pulse TMS, appears to reflect largely sodium channel–mediated membrane excitability in efferent pyramidal cells, and is increased by anticonvulsants, such as phenytoin and carbamazepine, that inhibit voltage-gated sodium channels. Additionally, paired-pulse TMS (Fig. 28.18) provides measures of γ-aminobutyric acid (GABA)-mediated cortico-cortical inhibition and glutamate-dependent cortico-cortical excitability. In the most common paired-pulse TMS protocols, a subthreshold conditioning stimulus is delivered before each succeeding TMS pulse [43,49]. Short ISIs (1–5 msec) lead to reduction of the MEP, and likely reflect $GABA_A$ receptor–mediated short-interval intracortical inhibition. Slightly longer ISIs (6–20 msec) augment the MEP, reflecting glutamate-mediated intracortical facilitation. Benzodiazepine ($GABA_A$ receptor agonist) anticonvulsants such as diazepam and lorazepam enhance short-interval intracortical inhibition and suppress intracortical facilitation [50]. Still longer ISIs (50–300 msec) paired-pulse TMS-EMG protocols can also measure $GABA_B$ receptor–mediated long-interval intracortical inhibition, which is enhanced by the $GABA_B$ receptor agonist baclofen [51,52]. The extent

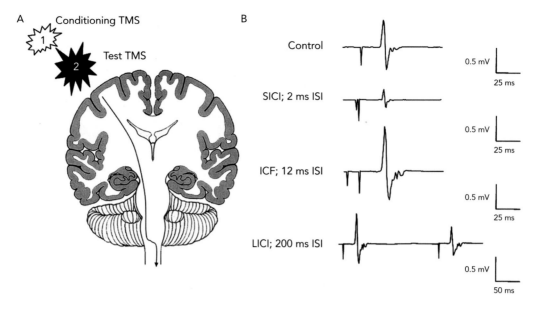

Figure 28.18. Paired-pulse TMS illustration. **A:** Schematic shows a paired-pulse protocol where two successive stimuli are delivered unilaterally to the motor cortex. **B:** Representative MEPs modulated in size as a function of the ISI are shown. Relative to the control stimulus, a short (2 ms) ISI results in short interval intracortical inhibition (SICI) of the test MEP, a slightly longer (12 ms) ISI leads to intracortical facilitation (ICF), and a still longer ISI (200 ms) produces long-interval intracortical inhibition (LICI) of the test MEP.

of cortical inhibition may also be measured by the cortical silent period, a transient EMG silence observed when TMS is delivered to the motor cortex during an active motor contraction. The cortical silent period too appears mediated by GABA receptors, although the contributions of GABA$_A$ and GABA$_B$ receptors to the cortical silent period are less defined than for paired-pulse measures [50,53,54].

These single-pulse TMS and paired-pulse TMS measures appear useful in detecting abnormalities in the excitation:inhibition (E:I) ratio in patients with epilepsy. Although findings vary between studies, published reports where parameters derived from TMS-EMG in patients with epilepsy were compared to values obtained from nonepileptic controls indicate that either primary or compensatory abnormalities in the cortical E:I ratio can be measured by TMS. In particular, pathologic suppression of intracortical inhibition as detected by paired-pulse stimulation appears to be a common finding in patients with epilepsy.

Detection of abnormalities in cortical inhibition by TMS-EMG data suggests its possible utility in epilepsy but also underscores a limitation, as global cortical excitability must be inferred from stimulation of the motor cortex. However, this anatomic limitation may be overcome by coupling TMS and EEG (TMS-EEG) such that TMS-evoked surface potentials can be recorded with scalp electrodes and used to estimate regional excitability of the areas of cerebral cortex other than motor cortex [55,56]. As a number of TMS-EMG experiments show motor cortex abnormalities in patients with extra-motor and generalized epilepsies, further studies will be required to test whether interrogating focal cortical excitability outside of the motor cortex by TMS-EEG is of any greater clinical value than checking TMS-EMG measures [57–60].

6. TMS IN PRESURGICAL FUNCTIONAL MAPPING

In presurgical motor cortex mapping, TMS, delivered by a figure-of-eight coil, is coupled with magnetic resonance imaging (MRI)-guided frameless stereotaxy to record the coil position over the stimulated cortex, while MEPs are recorded by skin surface electrodes from selected muscle groups (Fig. 28.19). The TMS operator, guided by the patient's brain MRI, thus tests whether stimulation of a specified brain region evokes an MEP from a specific muscle. These data are then registered to the patient's MRI to generate a precise motor map. TMS motor map spatial resolution approximates that which can be obtained by intraoperative cortical electrical stimulation and monitoring of the MEP [61]. In addition to motor mapping, TMS offers a unique tool for mapping the language cortex [62].

For language mapping, rTMS in short (~1 sec) 5- to 10-Hz trains is delivered repetitively to potential cortical language areas while a subject performs a linguistic task such as object naming, and the operator then identifies regions where stimulation interrupts the task performance. As with motor maps, the cortical region where stimulation produced a language error is documented and forms the basis of a functional language map [63,64]. Although language lateralization by rTMS-induced speech arrest shows a fairly high concordance with the results of intra-carotid amytal (Wada) testing in epilepsy patients [65–67], caution is warranted when administering rTMS for cortical mapping of linguistic functions. Early reports indicated relatively poor rTMS sensitivity for determination of language dominance, as some studies reported difficulties in obtaining speech arrest in more than one third of all tested patients [66,68]. Even when

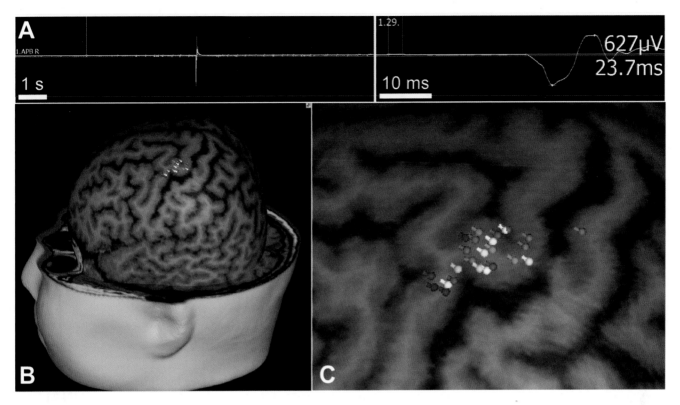

Figure 28.19. TMS motor map: a representative hand motor map in a child. A: Abductor pollicis brevis (APB) MEP obtained by motor cortex single-pulse TMS. B: Multiple MEPs are color-coded by amplitude, with white corresponding to maximum and gray corresponding to minimum, and projected onto the patient's brain MRI. C: Enlarged motor map shows APB localizing to the "hand knob" region of the precentral gyrus.

rTMS parameters are adjusted to reliably induce speech arrest, rTMS showed a relatively poor prognostic value for postoperative language deficits. Compared to the Wada test, the results of rTMS-induced speech arrest more often favor the right hemisphere and match less often the postoperative outcome with respect to language deficits [69]. This is most likely accounted for by the fact that speech arrest is obtained most easily over facial motor areas, where true aphasia is rarely observed [70]. Speech arrest might thus not represent an optimal marker for language lateralization. In future studies, rTMS protocols will have to be adapted in order to target aspects of language other than speech production, if online rTMS is to become a useful tool in presurgical evaluation of epileptic patients [69,71]. Of special interest in this respect is a study on the susceptibility of Wernicke's area to rTMS-induced language disruption (in a picture–word matching task) and the relationship to language lateralization in the same, healthy subjects as assessed through functional MRI [72,73].

7. SEIZURE SUPPRESSION BY RTMS

Encouraging open-label trials show a potential for seizure reduction by rTMS when applied over the epileptogenic region, or even when applied in a neutral scalp location, such as over the vertex. The positive response of some patients to stimulation outside of the epileptogenic zone, and in one series a favorable response of patients with primary generalized seizures to rTMS [3,21], raises the possibility that the antiepileptic mechanism of rTMS is not just local suppression of intracortical excitability but rather a network effect, where excitability is modulated at sites distal to the locus of stimulation [74–76].

In contrast to the open-label data, placebo-controlled rTMS trials have yielded inconsistent results. The first trial, in patients with temporal lobe epilepsy, did not reveal an antiepileptic benefit [49]. A second trial showed a significant reduction in seizures and improvement of the interictal electroencephalogram (EEG) in patients with intractable seizures attributable to cortical dysplasia [23]. The third, which investigated rTMS in a mixed group of patients with either focal or primary generalized seizures, found that rTMS was no better than placebo for seizure reduction but that active treatment significantly reduced epileptiform abnormalities in the interictal EEG [77]. However, the most recent large randomized, single-blinded controlled clinical trial (N = 60) reveals a substantial antiepileptic capacity. In subjects randomized to a 2-week high-intensity treatment group (90% resting motor threshold), 0.5-Hz rTMS over the epileptogenic focus showed an 80% reduction in mean seizure frequency along with decreased interictal EEG discharges as compared to the low-intensity (20% resting motor threshold) control group, with a mean seizure reduction of 2%. The antiepileptic effects were relatively long-lasting and maintained up to 2 months after treatment [78].

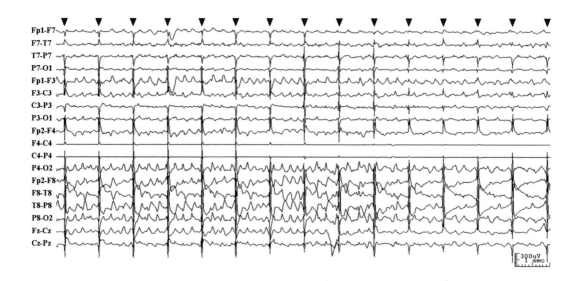

Figure 28.20. [101] (with author's permission from) Minimal rTMS artifact on EEG in a human patient. 15-second tracing shows a seizure terminating during rTMS (arrowhead). The C4 lead has been removed for rTMS coil placement. Note that 1-Hz rTMS artifact (vertical lines) does not obscure EEG. Similar recording enables accurate assessment of seizure duration as well as real-time monitoring for seizure exacerbation. Reprinted from [102].

In some clinical circumstances, such as treatment of ongoing seizures, TMS-EEG can be applied in the ictal state to identify real-time EEG changes induced by rTMS. Here, TMS-EEG may be of use to detect either improvement or exacerbation of seizures—both potentially valuable findings in the clinical setting. In patients with frontal lobe epilepsy and frequent interictal EEG spikes, TMS-EEG can demonstrate relative shortening of bursts of epileptiform activity [79]. In a small number of cases of epilepsia partialis continua, TMS-EEG has been used to detect seizure suppression as well as to exclude seizure exacerbation during rTMS [80]. Encouragingly, seizure exacerbation by rTMS was not seen, while seizure suppression was detected in some instances. A representative EEG obtained from a patient with epilepsia partialis continua undergoing 1-Hz rTMS is shown in Figure 28.20. In realistic applications, similar techniques for real-time EEG during therapeutic rTMS may be of use to monitor for epileptiform activity when rTMS is administered to treat nonepileptic symptoms such as mood disorder, motor dysfunction, or chronic pain in seizure-prone patients, such as those with recent stroke, neurodegenerative disease, or underlying epilepsy.

8. SAFETY CONCERNS

Among the safety concerns when stimulating the brain are physical damage to brain tissue, triggering of seizures or creation of an epileptic focus, and persistent changes in brain functions such as memory. Neuronal damage due to toxic electrochemical and electrolytic reactions at the electrode–tissue interface are a concern with direct electrical brain stimulation, but not with noninvasive brain stimulation protocols. On the other hand, TES and tDCS can induce similar skin reactions on the skin and lead to burns due to edge effects at the border of the electrodes.

Energy delivery to brain tissue and tissue heating are also negligible with all three techniques. The total charge and total charge density produced in brain tissue are less than those produced by direct cortical stimulation and by electroconvulsive therapy. Even in the relatively high-voltage TES protocols, the amount of current conducted to the cortex is orders of magnitude less than those values that have been found to be thresholds for tissue damage in animal experiments using 50-Hz stimulus trains sustained for several hours [81–83]. The major concern is with neuronal damage due to excitotoxicity. However, TES should not be performed with stimulating electrodes over a skull breach or a metal plate in the skull, lest unusually high current levels reach the brain.

Yet stimulation levels that do not produce histological damage in these animal studies can nonetheless produce seizures [84]. Seizures have occurred following both TES (Fig. 28.21) and TMS [85]. MacDonald [82] reported five seizures in a series of 15,000 patients having intraoperative MEP monitoring using TES, though it is not clear that the TES itself caused the seizures. In rTMS, seizure risk has been estimated in two patient populations: patients with major depression and patients with epilepsy. In patients with major depression, without epilepsy, the risk of seizure is less than 1 in 30,000 treatment sessions or less than 1 in 1,000 persons with a Neuronetis Neurostar device, and approximately 6 in 5,000 with the Brainsway Deep TMS device [86].

In patients with epilepsy, the crude per-subject risk of a seizure in patients with epilepsy during single- and paired-pulse TMS is estimated at 1.7% and 1.8%, respectively, and it has not been associated with a long-term adverse outcome [87]. Encouragingly, the risk of TMS-induced seizures is not appreciably higher in patients with epilepsy who receive rTMS.

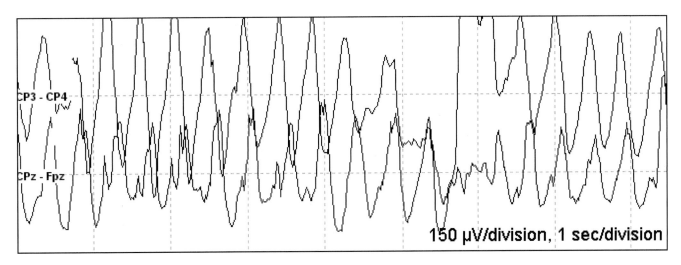

Figure 28.21. *EEG during an electroclinical seizure triggered by MEP monitoring; a repetitive spike-wave pattern is visible in the CPz-Fpz recording channel. The seizure occurred immediately following TES. A bolus dose of propofol was given, and the seizure stopped within 1 minute. The patient had no prior history of seizures. The anesthetic regimen was total intravenous anesthesia with propofol and remifentanil, and the surgery was for an arachnoid cyst that was compressing the brainstem. Reprinted from [100].*

Pereira et al. [87a], in a recent meta-analysis, estimated the per-subject risk at 2.9% (CI 1.3–4.4%), which includes the risk estimated previously by Bae et al. [88] of approximately 0.5% per 1,000 rTMS stimuli (0.41 ± 0.08% mean weighted by stimulus number). Further, seizures during low-frequency rTMS appear to be identical to the patients' habitual seizures [80], and thus the causal relationship between stimulation and the documented seizures could not be ascertained in all cases.

The safety of TMS has been the focus of a number of studies as well as several consensus conferences. Safety recommendations and precautions have been developed by panels of experts and endorsed by the International Federation of Clinical Neurophysiology. The most recent of these consensus conferences took place in 2008, and the conclusions are summarized by Rossi et al. [85]. These include specific discussion of applications of the various forms of TMS in the population with epilepsy who are, by definition, seizure-prone. In general, the side effects of TMS in patients with epilepsy are mild and short-lived. They include headache and scalp pain that result from direct activation of the pericranial scalp muscles. However, in some instances, seizures have been induced by rTMS in patients with epilepsy.

Beyond seizures, the side effects associated with TES, TMS, and tDCS are mild and short-lived. With TES, high current levels are delivered to the scalp, which may cause strong contractions of the temporalis muscle and forceful jaw closure. In MacDonald's study of 15,000 cases of intraoperative MEP monitoring using high-intensity pulse train TES [82], the most common adverse effect was mouth injury, with several tongue or lip lacerations and one case of mandibular fracture. The use of soft bite blocks can help to prevent these complications.

Transient headache is commonly reported following rTMS [85,89]. Higher stimulus intensities and frequencies worsen the headaches, but they typically respond to simple analgesics [90]. rTMS can also alter mood in non-depressed subjects [47]. However, rTMS has been reported to induce mania or a hypomanic state in some subjects [90].

The safety profile of tDCS is overall favorable. Skin irritation has been reported as a rare mild adverse event after tDCS [24,91]. However, a review of safety reports from trials of conventional tDCS settings (≤40 min, ≤4 mA, ≤7.2 Coulombs) did not identify any reports of a serious adverse event or an irreversible injury across >33,200 sessions and in 1,000 subjects with repeated tDCS sessions [92].

Additional safety concerns related to the high magnetic fields produced during TMS and rTMS, which are of the order of magnitude of 2 Tesla, are the possibility that metallic objects nearby will be moved. This could produce a dangerous projectile if an object of the proper shape (the worst would be a ring of approximately the same dimensions as the coil) were close to the coil. Forces on small objects, such as an aneurysm clips and titanium skull plates and screws, are miniscule and not of clinical concern [80,93,94]. Eddy currents in nearby conductors can produce heating during repetitive TMS; a scalp burn in a patient with a scalp electrode has been reported [95].

The high-intensity and rapidly varying magnetic field in TMS causes a transient deformation of the stimulating coil, producing an audible and at times loud click [96,97]. With rTMS, transient increases in the hearing threshold can occur [98]; if ear protection is not used, permanent hearing loss can even be possible under certain circumstances [98]. In animal studies, the hearing loss could be prevented with earphones that blocked external noise [99], suggesting that it is a noise-induced hearing loss rather than the result of direct effects of the pulsed magnetic field on the inner ear or the auditory pathways. Therefore, subjects receiving repetitive TMS, and personnel administering it, should wear earphones [85,98].

Implanted electronics such as cochlear prostheses and deep brain stimulators are considered contraindications to the performance of both TES and TMS. However, TMS is well tolerated in patients with extracranial stimulators such as a vagal nerve stimulator.

REFERENCES

1. Legatt AD, Emerson RG, Epstein CM, et al. ACNS Guideline: transcranial electrical stimulation motor evoked potential monitoring. *Journal of Clinical Neurophysiology.* 2016;33(1):42–50.
2. Padberg F, George MS. Repetitive transcranial magnetic stimulation of the prefrontal cortex in depression. *Experimental Neurology.* 2009;219(1):2–13.
3. Rotenberg A. Epilepsy. Chapter 39 in Lozano AM, Hallett M, eds. *Brain Stimulation* (Handbook of Clinical Neurology, Vol. 116). Amsterdam: Elsevier Inc.; 2013.
4. Kim DR, Pesiridou A, O'Reardon JP. Transcranial magnetic stimulation in the treatment of psychiatric disorders. *Current Psychiatry Reports.* 2009;11(6):447–452.
5. Amassian V, Stewart M, Quirk G, et al. VII Referenzen. *Neurosurgery.* 1987;20:74–93.
6. Hicks R, Burke D, Stephen J, Woodforth I, Crawford M. Corticospinal volleys evoked by electrical stimulation of human motor cortex after withdrawal of volatile anaesthetics. *Journal of Physiology.* 1992;456:393.
7. Sloan TB, Heyer EJ. Anesthesia for intraoperative neurophysiologic monitoring of the spinal cord. *Journal of Clinical Neurophysiology.* 2002;19(5):430–443.
8. Woodforth IJ, Hicks RG, Crawford MR, Stephen JP, Burke D. Depression of I waves in corticospinal volleys by sevoflurane, thiopental, and propofol. *Anesthesia & Analgesia.* 1999;89(5):1182–1187.
9. Brown W. Needle electromyographic abnormalities in neurogenic and muscle diseases. In Brown W. *The Physiological and Technical Basis of Electromyography.* Boston: Butterworth Publishers; 1984:317–338.
10. Legatt AD, Ellen R. Grass Lecture: motor evoked potential monitoring. *American Journal of Electroneurodiagnostic Technology.* 2004;44(4):223–243.
11. Rothwell J, Burke D, Hicks R, Stephen J, Woodforth I, Crawford M. Transcranial electrical stimulation of the motor cortex in man: further evidence for the site of activation. *Journal of Physiology.* 1994;481(Pt 1):243.
12. Amassian VE, Cracco RQ, Maccabee PJ. Basic mechanisms of magnetic coil excitation of nervous system in humans and monkeys and their applications. Paper presented at: Biomedical Engineering, Proceedings of a Special Symposium on Maturing Technologies and Emerging Horizons in 1988.
13. Legatt AD. Current practice of motor evoked potential monitoring: results of a survey. *Journal of Clinical Neurophysiology.* 2002;19(5):454–460.
14. Deletis V, Kothbauer K. Intraoperative neurophysiology of the corticospinal tract. In Stålberg E, Sharma HS, Olsson Y, eds. *Spinal Cord Monitoring.* Vienna: Springer; 1998:421–444.
15. Tsutsui S, Iwasaki H, Yamada H, et al. Augmentation of motor evoked potentials using multi-train transcranial electrical stimulation in intraoperative neurophysiologic monitoring during spinal surgery. *Journal of Clinical Monitoring and Computing.* 2015;29(1):35–39.
16. Purpura DP, McMurtry JG. Intracellular activities and evoked potential changes during polarization of motor cortex. *Journal of Neurophysiology.* 1965;28(1):166–185.
17. Kabakov AY, Muller PA, Pascual-Leone A, Jensen FE, Rotenberg A. Contribution of axonal orientation to pathway-dependent modulation of excitatory transmission by direct current stimulation in isolated rat hippocampus. *Journal of Neurophysiology.* 2012;107(7):1881–1889.
18. Dhamne SC, Ekstein D, Zhuo Z, et al. Acute seizure suppression by transcranial direct current stimulation in rats. *Annals of Clinical and Translational Neurology.* 2015;2(8):843–856.
19. Sun Y, Lipton JO, Boyle LM, et al. Direct current stimulation induces mGluR5-dependent neocortical plasticity. *Annals of Neurology.* 2016;80(2):233–2465.
20. Sparing R, Thimm M, Hesse M, Küst J, Karbe H, Fink G. Bidirectional alterations of interhemispheric parietal balance by non-invasive cortical stimulation. *Brain.* 2009;132(11):3011–3020.
21. Nitsche MA, Paulus W. Noninvasive brain stimulation protocols in the treatment of epilepsy: current state and perspectives. *Neurotherapeutics.* 2009;6(2):244–250.
22. San-juan D, Morales-Quezada L, Garduño AJO, et al. Transcranial direct current stimulation in epilepsy. *Brain Stimulation.* 2015;8(3):455–464.
23. Fregni F, Thome-Souza S, Nitsche MA, Freedman SD, Valente KD, Pascual-Leone A. A controlled clinical trial of cathodal DC polarization in patients with refractory epilepsy. *Epilepsia.* 2006;47(2):335–342.
24. Auvichayapat N, Rotenberg A, Gersner R, et al. Transcranial direct current stimulation for treatment of refractory childhood focal epilepsy. *Brain Stimulation.* 2013;6(4):696–700.
25. Tekturk P, Erdogan ET, Kurt A, et al. The effect of transcranial direct current stimulation on seizure frequency of patients with mesial temporal lobe epilepsy with hippocampal sclerosis. *Clinical Neurology and Neurosurgery.* 2016;149:27–32.
26. Kamida T, Kong S, Eshima N, Fujiki M. Cathodal transcranial direct current stimulation affects seizures and cognition in fully amygdala-kindled rats. *Neurological Research.* 2013;35(6):602–607.
27. Liebetanz D, Klinker F, Hering D, et al. Anticonvulsant effects of transcranial direct-current stimulation (tDCS) in the rat cortical ramp model of focal epilepsy. *Epilepsia.* 2006;47(11):1216–1224.
28. Kamida T, Kong S, Eshima N, Abe T, Fujiki M, Kobayashi H. Transcranial direct current stimulation decreases convulsions and spatial memory deficits following pilocarpine-induced status epilepticus in immature rats. *Behavioural Brain Research.* 2011;217(1):99–103.
29. Roth Y, Amir A, Levkovitz Y, Zangen A. Three-dimensional distribution of the electric field induced in the brain by transcranial magnetic stimulation using figure-8 and deep H-coils. *Journal of Clinical Neurophysiology.* 2007;24(1):31–38.
30. Burke D, Hicks RG. Surgical monitoring of motor pathways. *Journal of Clinical Neurophysiology.* 1998;15(3):194–205.
31. Houlden DA, Schwartz ML, Tator CH, Ashby P, MacKay WA. Spinal cord-evoked potentials and muscle responses evoked by transcranial magnetic stimulation in 10 awake human subjects. *Journal of Neuroscience.* 1999;19(5):1855–1862.
32. Gugino LD, Romero JR, Aglio L, et al. Transcranial magnetic stimulation coregistered with MRI: a comparison of a guided versus blind stimulation technique and its effect on evoked compound muscle action potentials. *Clinical Neurophysiology.* 2001;112(10):1781–1792.
33. Cadwell J. Principles of magnetoelectric stimulation. In: Chokroverty S, ed. *Magnetic Stimulation in Clinical Neurophysiology.* Boston, MA: Butterworth; 1990:13–32.
34. Maccabee P, Amassian V, Cracco R, Cracco J, Eberle L, Rudell A. Stimulation of the human nervous system using the magnetic coil. *Journal of Clinical Neurophysiology.* 1991;8(1):38–55.
35. Walsh V, Pascual-Leone A. *Transcranial Magnetic Stimulation: A Neurochromometrics of Mind.* Cambridge, MA: MIT Press; 2003.
36. Thompson PD, Rothwell JC, Day BL, et al. Mechanisms of electrical and magnetic stimulation of human motor cortex. In: Chokroverty S, ed. *Magnetic Stimulation in Clinical Neurophysiology.* Boston: Butterworths; 1990:121–143.
37. Pascual-Leone A, Bartres-Faz D, Keenan JP. Transcranial magnetic stimulation: studying the brain–behaviour relationship by induction of 'virtual lesions'. *Philosophical Transactions of the Royal Society B: Biological Sciences.* 1999;354(1387):1229–1238.
38. Bliss TV, Lømo T. Long-lasting potentiation of synaptic transmission in the dentate area of the anaesthetized rabbit following stimulation of the perforant path. *Journal of Physiology.* 1973;232(2):331–356.
39. Dudek SM, Bear MF. Homosynaptic long-term depression in area CA1 of hippocampus and effects of N-methyl-D-aspartate receptor blockade. *Proceedings of the National Academy of Sciences USA.* 1992;89(10):4363–4367.
40. Hallett M. Transcranial magnetic stimulation: a primer. *Neuron.* 2007;55(2):187–199.
41. Huang Y-Z, Edwards MJ, Rounis E, Bhatia KP, Rothwell JC. Theta burst stimulation of the human motor cortex. *Neuron.* 2005;45(2):201–206.
42. Fregni F, Pascual-Leone A. Technology insight: noninvasive brain stimulation in neurology—perspectives on the therapeutic potential of rTMS and tDCS. *Nature Clinical Practice Neurology.* 2007;3(7):383–393.
43. Kobayashi M, Pascual-Leone A. Transcranial magnetic stimulation in neurology. *Lancet Neurology.* 2003;2(3):145–156.
44. Krings T, Chiappa KH, Foltys H, Reinges MH, Cosgrove RG, Thron A. Introducing navigated transcranial magnetic stimulation as a refined brain mapping methodology. *Neurosurgical Review.* 2001;24(4–6):171–179.
45. Staudt M, Krägeloh-Mann I, Holthausen H, Gerloff C, Grodd W. Searching for motor functions in dysgenic cortex: a clinical transcranial magnetic stimulation and functional magnetic resonance imaging study. *Journal of Neurosurgery: Pediatrics.* 2004;101(2):69–77.
46. Boggio PS, Castro LO, Savagim EA, et al. Enhancement of non-dominant hand motor function by anodal transcranial direct current stimulation. *Neuroscience Letters.* 2006;404(1):232–236.
47. Pascual-Leone A, Catala MD, Pascual AP-L. Lateralized effect of rapid-rate transcranial magnetic stimulation of the prefrontal cortex on mood. *Neurology.* 1996;46(2):499–502.
48. Töpper R, Foltys H, Meister IG, Sparing R, Boroojerdi B. Repetitive transcranial magnetic stimulation of the parietal cortex transiently ameliorates phantom limb pain-like syndrome. *Clinical Neurophysiology.* 2003;114(8):1521–1530.

49. Theodore W, Hunter K, Chen R, et al. Transcranial magnetic stimulation for the treatment of seizures A controlled study. *Neurology*. 2002;59(4):560–562.

50. Ziemann U, Lönnecker S, Steinhoff B, Paulus W. Effects of antiepileptic drugs on motor cortex excitability in humans: a transcranial magnetic stimulation study. *Annals of Neurology*. 1996;40(3):367–378.

51. Sanger TD, Garg RR, Chen R. Interactions between two different inhibitory systems in the human motor cortex. *Journal of Physiology*. 2001;530(2):307–317.

52. Müller-Dahlhaus JFM, Liu Y, Ziemann U. Inhibitory circuits and the nature of their interactions in the human motor cortex—a pharmacological TMS study. *Journal of Physiology*. 2008;586(2):495–514.

53. Fedi M, Berkovic SF, Macdonell RA, Curatolo JM, Marini C, Reutens DC. Intracortical hyperexcitability in humans with a GABAA receptor mutation. *Cerebral Cortex*. 2008;18(3):664–669.

54. Roick H, Von Giesen H, Benecke R. On the origin of the postexcitatory inhibition seen after transcranial magnetic brain stimulation in awake human subjects. *Experimental Brain Research*. 1993;94(3):489–498.

55. Kähkönen S, Komssi S, Wilenius J, Ilmoniemi RJ. Prefrontal TMS produces smaller EEG responses than motor-cortex TMS: implications for rTMS treatment in depression. *Psychopharmacology*. 2005;181(1):16–20.

56. Lioumis P, Kičić D, Savolainen P, Mäkelä JP, Kähkönen S. Reproducibility of TMS—Evoked EEG responses. *Human Brain Mapping*. 2009;30(4):1387–1396.

57. Cincotta M, Borgheresi A, Guidi L, et al. Remote effects of cortical dysgenesis on the primary motor cortex: evidence from the silent period following transcranial magnetic stimulation. *Clinical Neurophysiology*. 2000;111(8):1340–1345.

58. Groppa S, Siebner HR, Kurth C, Stephani U, Siniatchkin M. Abnormal response of motor cortex to photic stimulation in idiopathic generalized epilepsy. *Epilepsia*. 2008;49(12):2022–2029.

59. Löscher WN, Dobesberger J, Szubski C, Trinka E. rTMS reveals premotor cortex dysfunction in frontal lobe epilepsy. *Epilepsia*. 2007;48(2):359–365.

60. Rotenberg A. Prospects for clinical applications of transcranial magnetic stimulation and real-time EEG in epilepsy. *Brain Topography*. 2010;22(4):257–266.

61. Picht T, Schmidt S, Brandt S, et al. Preoperative functional mapping for rolandic brain tumor surgery: comparison of navigated transcranial magnetic stimulation to direct cortical stimulation. *Neurosurgery*. 2011;69(3):581–589.

62. Picht T, Krieg SM, Sollmann N, et al. A comparison of language mapping by preoperative navigated transcranial magnetic stimulation and direct cortical stimulation during awake surgery. *Neurosurgery*. 2013;72(5):808–819.

63. Krieg SM, Tarapore PE, Picht T, et al. Optimal timing of pulse onset for language mapping with navigated repetitive transcranial magnetic stimulation. *Neuroimage*. 2014;100:219–236.

64. Picht T. Current and potential utility of transcranial magnetic stimulation in the diagnostics before brain tumor surgery. *CNS Oncology*. 2014;3:299–310.

65. Pascual-Leone A, Gates JR, Dhuna A. Induction of speech arrest and counting errors with rapid-rate transcranial magnetic stimulation. *Neurology*. 1991;41(5):697–702.

66. Jennum P, Friberg L, Fuglsang-Frederiksen A, Dam M. Speech localization using repetitive transcranial magnetic stimulation. *Neurology*. 1994;44(2):269–269.

67. Wassermann E, Blaxton T, Hoffman E, et al. Repetitive transcranial magnetic stimulation of the dominant hemisphere can disrupt visual naming in temporal lobe epilepsy patients. *Neuropsychologia*. 1999;37(5):537–544.

68. Michelucci R, Valzania F, Passarelli D, et al. Rapid-rate transcranial magnetic stimulation and hemispheric language dominance: Usefulness and safety in epilepsy. *Neurology*. 1994;44(9):1697–1697.

69. Epstein C, Woodard J, Stringer A, et al. Repetitive transcranial magnetic stimulation does not replicate the Wada test. *Neurology*. 2000;55(7):1025–1027.

70. Epstein CM, Woodard JL, Stringer A, Henry TR, Pennell PB, Litt B. Repetitive transcranial magnetic stimulation does not replicate the Wada test. *Neurology*. 1999;52(6):A469.

71. Epstein CM, Davey KR. Transcranial brain stimulation. Google Patents; 2000.

72. Knecht S, Flöel A, Dräger B, et al. Degree of language lateralization determines susceptibility to unilateral brain lesions. *Nature Neuroscience*. 2002;5(7):695–699.

73. Babajani-Feremi A, Narayana S, Rezaie R, et al. Language mapping using high gamma electrocorticography, fMRI, and TMS versus electrocortical stimulation. *Clinical Neurophysiology*. 2016;127(3):1822–1836.

74. Chang BS. TMS: a tailored method of stimulation for refractory focal epilepsy? *Epilepsy Currents*. 2013;13(4):162–163.

75. Shafi MM, Vernet M, Klooster D, et al. Physiological consequences of abnormal connectivity in a developmental epilepsy. *Annals of Neurology*. 2015;77(3):487–503.

76. Vernet M, Bashir S, Yoo W-K, Perez JM, Najib U, Pascual-Leone A. Insights on the neural basis of motor plasticity induced by theta burst stimulation from TMS–EEG. *European Journal of Neuroscience*. 2013;37(4):598–606.

77. Cantello R, Rossi S, Varrasi C, et al. Slow repetitive TMS for drug-resistant epilepsy: clinical and EEG findings of a placebo-controlled trial. *Epilepsia*. 2007;48(2):366–374.

78. Sun W, Mao W, Meng X, et al. Low-frequency repetitive transcranial magnetic stimulation for the treatment of refractory partial epilepsy: a controlled clinical study. *Epilepsia*. 2012;53(10):1782–1789.

79. Kimiskidis VK, Kugiumtzis D, Papagiannopoulos S, Vlaikidis N. Transcranial magnetic stimulation (TMS) modulates epileptiform discharges in patients with frontal lobe epilepsy: a preliminary EEG-TMS study. *International Journal of Neural Systems*. 2013;23(01):1250035.

80. Rotenberg A, Bae EH, Muller PA, et al. In-session seizures during low-frequency repetitive transcranial magnetic stimulation in patients with epilepsy. *Epilepsy & Behavior*. 2009;16(2):353–355.

81. Barker AT, Freeston IL, Jarratt JA, Jalinous JA. Magnetic stimulation of the human nervous system: an introduction and basic principles. In: Chokroverty S, ed. *Magnetic Stimulation in Clinical Neurophysiology*. Boston: Butterworths; 1990:55–72.

82. MacDonald DB. Safety of intraoperative transcranial electrical stimulation motor evoked potential monitoring. *Journal of Clinical Neurophysiology*. 2002;19(5):416–429.

83. Barker A. Magnetic stimulation of the human nervous system; an introduction and basic principles. In: Chokroverty S, ed. *Magnetic Stimulation in Clinical Neurophysiology*. Boston: Butterworths; 1990:55–72.

84. Agnew W, McCreery D. Considerations for safety in the use of extracranial stimulation for motor evoked potentials. *Neurosurgery*. 1987;20(1):143–147.

85. Rossi S, Hallett M, Rossini PM, Pascual-Leone A, Safety of TMS Consensus Group. Safety, ethical considerations, and application guidelines for the use of transcranial magnetic stimulation in clinical practice and research. *Clinical Neurophysiology*. 2009;120(12):2008–2039.

86. Perera T, George MS, Grammer G, Janicak PG, Pascual-Leone A, Wirecki TS. The Clinical TMS Society consensus review and treatment recommendations for TMS therapy for major depressive disorder. *Brain Stimulation*. 2016;9(3):336–346.

87. Schrader LM, Stern JM, Koski L, Nuwer MR, Engel J. Seizure incidence during single- and paired-pulse transcranial magnetic stimulation (TMS) in individuals with epilepsy. *Clinical Neurophysiology*. 2004;115(12):2728–2737.

87a. Pereira LS, Müller VT, da Mota Gomes M, Rotenberg A, Fregni F. Safety of repetitive transcranial magnetic stimulation in patients with epilepsy: a systematic review. *Epilepsy & Behavior*. 2016;57:167–176.

88. Bae EH, Schrader LM, Machii K, et al. Safety and tolerability of repetitive transcranial magnetic stimulation in patients with epilepsy: a review of the literature. *Epilepsy & Behavior*. 2007;10(4):521–528.

89. Machii K, Cohen D, Ramos-Estebanez C, Pascual-Leone A. Safety of rTMS to non-motor cortical areas in healthy participants and patients. *Clinical Neurophysiology*. 2006;117(2):455–471.

90. Loo CK, McFarquhar TF, Mitchell PB. A review of the safety of repetitive transcranial magnetic stimulation as a clinical treatment for depression. *International Journal of Neuropsychopharmacology*. 2008;11(1):131–147.

91. Rodriguez N, Opisso E, Pascual-Leone A, Soler MD. Skin lesions induced by transcranial direct current stimulation (tDCS). *Brain Stimulation*. 2014;7(5):765–767.

92. Bikson M, Grossman P, Thomas C, et al. Safety of transcranial direct current stimulation: evidence-based update 2016. *Brain Stimulation*. 2016;9(5):641–661.

93. Hsieh T-H, Dhamne SC, Chen J-JJ, et al. Minimal heating of aneurysm clips during repetitive transcranial magnetic stimulation. *Clinical Neurophysiology*. 2012;123(7):1471.

94. Rotenberg A, Harrington MG, Birnbaum DS, et al. Minimal heating of titanium skull plates during 1Hz repetitive transcranial magnetic stimulation. *Clinical Neurophysiology*. 2007;118(11):2536–2538.

95. Pascual-Leone A, Dhuna A, Roth B, Cohen L, Hallett M. Risk of burns during rapid-rate magnetic stimulation in presence of electrodes. *Lancet*. 1990;336(8724):1195–1196.

96. Dhamne SC, Kothare RS, Yu C, et al. A measure of acoustic noise generated from transcranial magnetic stimulation coils. *Brain Stimulation*. 2014;7(3):432–434.

97. Goetz SM, Lisanby SH, Murphy DL, Price RJ, O'Grady G, Peterchev AV. Impulse noise of transcranial magnetic stimulation: measurement, safety,

and auditory neuromodulation. *Brain Stimulation: Basic, Translational, and Clinical Research in Neuromodulation*. 2015;8(1):161–163.

98. Pascual-Leone A, Houser C, Reese K, et al. Safety of rapid-rate transcranial magnetic stimulation in normal volunteers. *Electroencephalography and Clinical Neurophysiology/Evoked Potentials Section*. 1993;89(2):120–130.

99. Counter SA, Borg E, Lofqvist L, Brismar T. Hearing loss from the acoustic artifact of the coil used in extracranial magnetic stimulation. *Neurology*. 1990;40(8):1159–1162.

100. Legatt A. *Intraoperative Neurophysiology: Interactive Case Studies*. New York: Demos Medical Publishing; 2015.

101. Rotenberg A, Pascual-Leone A. Safety of 1Hz repetitive transcranial magnetic stimulation (rTMS) in patients with titanium skull plates. *Clinical Neurophysiology*. 2009;120(7):1417.

102. Rotenberg A, Depositario-Cabacar D, Bae EH, Harini C, Pascual-Leone A, Takeoka M. Transient suppression of seizures by repetitive transcranial magnetic stimulation in a case of Rasmussen's encephalitis. *Epilepsy & Behavior*. 2008;13(1):260–262.

29 | INTRACRANIAL EEG MONITORING: DEPTH, SUBDURAL, FORAMEN OVALE, AND MICROARRAYS

MARGITTA SEECK, MD AND DONALD L. SCHOMER, MD

ABSTRACT: Intracranial electroencephalography (iEEG) is used to localize the focus of seizures and determine vital adjacent cortex before epilepsy surgery. The two most commonly used electrode types are subdural and depth electrodes. Foramen ovale electrodes are less often used. Combinations of electrode types are possible. The choice depends on the presumed focus site. Careful planning is needed before implantation, taking into account the results of noninvasive studies. While subdural recordings allow better mapping of functional cortex, depth electrodes can reach deep structures. There are no guidelines on how to read ictal intracranial EEG recordings, but a focal onset (<5 contacts) and a high-frequency onset herald a good prognosis. High-frequency oscillations have been described as a potential biomarker of the seizure onset zone. Intracranial recordings provide a focal but magnified view of the brain, which is also exemplified by the use of microelectrodes, which allow the recording of single-unit or multi-unit activity.

KEYWORDS: depth electrodes, subdural electrodes, intracranial, electroencephalography, EEG, epilepsy, seizure

PRINCIPAL REFERENCES

1. Talairach J, Bancaud J. Stereotaxic exploration and therapy in epilepsy. In: Vinken PJ, Bruyn G (Eds): The epilepsies. Handbook of Clinical Neurology, Vol 15. Amsterdam, North Holland, 1974, pp 758–782.
2. Mégevand P, Spinelli L, Genetti M, Brodbeck V, Momjian S, Schaller K, Michel CM, Vulliemoz S, Seeck M. Electric source imaging of interictal activity accurately localises the seizure onset zone. J Neurol Neurosurg Psychiatry. 2014;85:38–43.
3. Grouiller F, Delattre BM, Pittau F, et al. All-in-one interictal presurgical imaging in patients with epilepsy: single-session EEG/PET/(f)MRI. Eur J Nucl Med Mol Imaging. 2015 Jun;42(7):1133–1143.
4. Ebersole JS, Hawes-Ebersole S. Clinical application of dipole models in the localization of epileptiform activity. J Clin Neurophysiol. 2007; 24:120–129.
5. Knowlton RC, Elgavish RA, Limdi N, et al. Functional imaging: I. Relative predictive value of intracranial electroencephalography. Ann Neurol. 2008 Jul;64(1):25–34.
6. Hamer HM, Morris HH, Mascha EJ, et al. Complications of invasive video-EEG monitoring with subdural grid electrodes. Neurology. 2002;58:97–103.
7. Sperling MR, O'Connor MJ. Comparison of depth and subdural electrodes in recording temporal lobe seizures. Neurology. 1989;39:1497.
8. Palmini A, Gambardella A, Andermann F, et al. Intrinsic epileptogenicity of human dysplastic cortex as suggested by corticography and surgical results. Ann Neurol. 1995;37:476–487.
9. Worrell GA, Gardner AB, Stead SM, et al. High-frequency oscillations in human temporal lobe: simultaneous microwire and clinical macroelectrode recordings. Brain. 2008;131:928–937.

1. INTRODUCTION

In most Western societies, epilepsy affects around 0.7% of the population—that is, 2.1 million in the United States, 3.5 million in Europe, and 47 million worldwide. In ~20% to 30%, drug treatment cannot control seizures and the possibility of surgical treatment is considered. While the optimal profiles of surgical candidates continue to be defined, the precise localization of a focal onset remains a cornerstone of successful surgical treatment. In many patients, localization requires electroencephalographic (EEG) recording directly from the cortex. This is done either by perioperative corticography (i.e., directly from the brain in the operating room; see Chapter 30) or by means of electrodes that are chronically implanted for a few days to several weeks. The major goals of intracranial EEG recordings are to determine the seizure onset and to distinguish the focus from vital cortex (Box 29.1). There are no true evidence-based studies on the yield of chronic intracranial EEG monitoring (iEEG)—that is, studies assigning subjects randomly to "intracranial monitoring" or "no intracranial monitoring." Consequently, there are no guidelines on when and whom to implant, and each center has a different threshold based on local experience and resources.

Most patients who are candidates for iEEG fall into an intermediate category of operability: a focal onset is suspected or at least not completely ruled out on the basis of the results of noninvasive EEG exams, but evidence is too weak to schedule immediate resective surgery or it is considered too risky in terms of neurological complications (i.e., proximity of vital cortex). Statistically speaking, the need for iEEG represents an unfavorable predictor for postoperative success (1).

The definition of candidacy for iEEG has changed over recent decades, due in large part to more sophisticated brain imaging. Today, in most centers, a patient with a glioma in the anterior mesial temporal lobe or hippocampal sclerosis and consistent EEG findings would not be considered an iEEG candidate, even if he or she had few contralateral interictal spikes. In contrast, a patient with multiple lesions and discordant EEG findings, or with no magnetic resonance imaging (MRI) abnormality at all, would be considered an appropriate iEEG candidate. However, to the best of our knowledge, there are no published consensus guidelines regarding the utility of iEEG.

The need for invasive recordings has been discussed extensively for different clinical scenarios for patients with temporal lobe epilepsy. It has been proposed that the concordance of unilateral hippocampal atrophy and interictal EEG is sufficient to proceed to surgery—that is, even without (scalp) ictal recordings, which may sometimes misleadingly show bilateral or even contralateral epileptic discharges (2). However, some centers would envision not only ictal recordings but even intracranial iEEG in order to determine unambiguously EEG onset

(3). In any case, careful evaluation of each patient is mandatory, including functional imaging and neuropsychological data. Ictal scalp recordings help to better identify the patient's seizure semiology, verify the presumed ictal onset by analysis of the clinical picture, and help to estimate the burden of epilepsy, as well as following up on postoperative persistent seizures. Rare case reports of idiopathic seizures and psychogenic seizures, incorrectly diagnosed as focal seizures, underscore the need for ictal recordings (4). Apart from persistent epileptic seizures, postoperative new-onset nonepileptic (psychogenic) seizures have been described in 2% to 8%. These can be difficult to diagnose if the preoperative semiology is not known (5). Finally, medicolegal issues could be raised if a complication occurs and post hoc the ictal nature of the transient changes of behavior is not ascertained. Thus, the authors believe that ictal recordings should be obtained before surgery or implantation.

Despite improvements to our understanding about who benefits most from this otherwise costly and labor-intensive procedure, each center has its own strategies that depend on the experience of the epilepsy surgery team, the availability and quality of the noninvasive exams, and overall national healthcare systems that facilitate (or not) access to the highest-level epilepsy surgery centers and iEEG. Requirements for the equipment and staffing of such centers have been published (6). The diversity in presurgical epilepsy evaluation across nations or continents became evident in the recent survey conducted by the Pediatric Epilepsy Surgery subcommittee of the International League Against Epilepsy in Europe, the United States, and Australia (7). It appeared that, in the United States, children are more often evaluated with intracranial electrodes, even in the presence of an MRI lesion. There is also more access to functional imaging in the United States compared to Europe and Australia. On the other hand, more patients are treated with a vagal nerve stimulator, a palliative procedure, in the United States compared to Europe and Australia. While

other characteristics of the patient populations were not different (e.g., underlying pathology, affected lobe), the reasons for these differences are not entirely clear but are probably of multiple origins, which include different national "schools" with different algorithms of epilepsy care or different regulations from healthcare providers. However, while sophisticated epilepsy centers exist today in all Western countries, there are still countries where epilepsy surgery is not done or is only rarely available and iEEG is even more difficult to obtain (8).

In the past 30 years, the development of new noninvasive imaging techniques has been readily embraced in the presurgical epilepsy evaluation (9–14), starting with the entry of high-definition MRI and special imaging protocols for epilepsy patients (15). A recent prospective study on 190 surgical candidates underlined the powerful combination of high-density EEG and MRI; however, positron emission tomography (PET) and ictal single-photon emission computed tomography (SPECT) also made a significant contribution to successful localization of the focus (16). Indeed, the knowledge obtained from these techniques has helped to identify patient populations where iEEG is more likely to be diagnostic. For example, >10 years ago, invasive monitoring was considered in patients with hippocampal sclerosis but bilateral temporal spikes or seizures. However, the presence of an MRI abnormality is a good prognostic indicator for a seizure-free outcome postoperatively (17), and patients with bilateral spikes or even seizures may very well benefit from surgery on the sclerotic hippocampus (18,19), even without iEEG. However, truly bitemporal lobe epilepsy, as determined by iEEG and MRI, is associated with a lower success rate and only 50% of patients became seizure-free in a study on 11 patients (20). On the other hand, severe unilateral hippocampal atrophy, the so-called burned-out hippocampus, may present with aberrant, even contralateral, scalp ictal discharges. Those patients nevertheless benefit from surgery (21). In some of these patients, iEEG was used to verify ictal onset in the affected hippocampus, but care must be taken to correctly insert enough contacts in the severely atrophied hippocampus so as not to miss the true seizure onset.

More recently, it has become recognized that the presence of a localized or lateralized temporal hypometabolism equals the presence of an MRI lesion. Patients with both MRI lesional and non-lesional temporal lobe epilepsy have the same postoperative prognosis (i.e., a chance of seizure control of ~80%) if the temporal hypometabolism in the PET is obvious and unilateral (22–24). Thus, patients with non-lesional temporal lobe epilepsy may not need iEEG if they undergo good-quality PET imaging and its results are concordant with the remainder of the evaluation. Over the next few years, other investigative measures such as studies on other pathologies (e.g., dysplasia or tuberous sclerosis), identifying reliable noninvasive markers of the epileptogenic zone, may reduce further the overall number of patients who need iEEG (25–27) (see also Chapter 46).

2. HISTORY

Intracranial EEG focus evaluation has a relatively brief history, starting in Germany with Berger's discovery of the EEG published in 1929 (28). Otfrid Foerster used preoperative EEG during epilepsy surgery and became a pioneer in using EEG to determine the epileptogenic zone. Foerster worked with Wernicke, with whom he published a brain atlas—as an aside, he was the treating neurologist for Lenin when he suffered a stroke in 1922. The rising Nationalist government basically destroyed Germany's scientific culture for the next decades and many researchers left the country. Foerster was the mentor of Wilder Penfield, who himself became widely known for the corticography of the human neocortex. Thanks to his research on patients, the cortical representations of the motor cortex ("homunculus") became standard knowledge. Penfield was a neurosurgeon and founded the Montreal Neurological Institute. Herbert Jasper joined him as a neurologist and clinical neurophysiologist, and together they trained numerous neurosurgeons and neurologists in the field of epilepsy surgery. They probably represent the first example of a successful relationship between a neurologist and a neurosurgeon. This combination remains a prerequisite for any successful epilepsy surgery team (29).

Wires and a type of "strip" electrode, placed in the epidural space, were the first to be used in epilepsy patients by Jasper and Penfield. Later, subdural electrodes and other electrode types were developed and applied. Bancaud and Talairach, another successful team of neurologist and neurosurgeon, from Hôpital Sainte-Anne in Paris, introduced multi-contact depth electrodes penetrating directly into the cerebral tissue (30,31), allowing a systematic investigation of deep structures. This was a major step forward in epilepsy surgery investigations, since at that time MRI did not yet exist and the evaluation of surgical candidates relied more on neurophysiologic methods. Ten years later, Wyler developed and introduced another electrode type into the field: the subdural electrode, which can be placed onto the brain's surface without the risks of an intracerebral insertion (32). Initially, strips with four electrodes were described, evolving into more complex and larger arrangements.

While the number of inserted electrodes has steadily increased (or at least became technically possible), simultaneous recording of >100 electrodes was difficult for EEG systems, requiring the selection of recorded electrodes and even changes during the evaluation. Upgrading of established systems and innovative setups finally overcome this obstacle (33), and today EEG systems with up to 256 channels are on the market.

Today, depth and subdural electrodes are the most established electrode types. Most centers have a preference for one or the other electrode type, based on personal experience or the technical equipment in the neurosurgical clinic. Around the same time that subdural electrodes were introduced, foramen ovale electrodes (34) and epidural peg electrodes were described by the Zurich group of Wieser et al. and the Cleveland Clinic group of Lüders et al. (35), respectively. The use of the latter two types remains relatively limited; they are often used as an intermediate step in determining if and which larger set of intracranial electrode setups would be more effective or as a complementary electrode type if depth or subdural electrodes alone do not appear sufficient.

3. BASIC CONCEPTS

iEEG should be considered if it is thought that surgery can cure or at least significantly ameliorate the epilepsy disorder but pertinent localizing information is still missing from the noninvasive evaluation. This implies that every patient should undergo first a noninvasive evaluation to understand the size and nature of the problem. A clear clinical hypothesis is mandatory before implantation, because implanted electrodes record from only a limited cortical volume. While the exact volume is not known, there are estimates indicating that a cortical area of 10 to 20 cm^2 is necessary to generate a scalp spike (36). Detailed analysis of scalp discharges and the simultaneously recorded subdural EEG showed that only the early components of spikes and seizures arise from a limited volume, which is, however, still larger than 10 cm^2. With further propagation, the active brain areas attain 30 cm^2 or more (37). In this context, imaging methods that suggest point sources of the underlying spikes represent more of a simplification rather than the true estimate of the size of epileptogenic cortex (38). Two studies on simultaneous recordings of intracranial depth (39) and subdural electrodes (40) and scalp electrodes showed that in some patients, discharges recorded on the scalp correspond to the intracranial sources. However, in several cases, only averaging of the intracranial discharges could identify the corresponding scalp spike due to a low signal-to-noise ratio on a single trial level.

The surgical act and the fact that the electrodes remain in place for several days or weeks are associated with a significant risk of morbidity but a relatively small risk for mortality; therefore, careful elaboration of the goal of the investigation, sites of implantation, and documentation of the patient's information will be needed.

Several concepts need to be recognized and defined as well as possible before any epilepsy surgical procedure is proposed (41). The epileptogenic area (i.e., the area that needs to be resected and that will be sufficient to abolish further seizures) must be clearly identified. This zone is not to be confused with the following:

- The lesional zone: the area that appears morphologically altered but may be smaller than or even remote to the epileptogenic zone
- The irritative zone: the area of interictal spikes, which can be more widespread than the epileptogenic zone and can even include contralateral structures
- The symptomatic zone: the area whose activation produces the clinical symptoms, such as nausea or dystonic posturing
- The functional deficit zone: the area whose activation/deactivation leads to neurological or neuropsychological deficits (e.g., verbal memory impairment or Todd's paresis)

Overall, intracranial EEG data look different compared to scalp EEG data and appear to be more "epileptogenic" due to the lack of the filter qualities of the skull, although the same rhythms known from scalp EEG can be also retrieved in the iEEG. The determination of the ictal EEG pattern is usually at the center of the investigation, although careful analysis of interictal epileptogenic discharges is probably more important than previously appreciated.

There are few data on the overall yield of iEEG. A recent study, with access to modern imaging tools, described the results in 77 patients with mesial temporal (39%), lateral temporal (12%), and extratemporal (43%) epilepsy (42). In the remaining five patients (6%), seizures could not be captured and they remained unclassified. Localizing results were obtained in 74%, which corresponds to numbers from other studies (43,44) and to our experience. Thus, despite the invasive nature of the procedure and the physical and psychological investment by the patient, it is not always certain that iEEG will be followed by a resective procedure. In ~25% of patients, surgery cannot be proposed, and this possibility needs to be addressed and emphasized during preparatory talks with patients.

4. DETERMINATION OF PRECISE ELECTRODE PLACEMENT

Independent of the chosen electrode type, knowledge of the exact position of the electrodes with respect to the individual brain anatomy is of utmost importance for successful surgery in terms of complete focus removal while sparing eloquent cortex. Previously, only radiographs of the skull were possible, which provided only a gross idea of the electrode position (45,46). Three-dimensional reconstruction of CT and MRI with co-registration of X-rays will provide superior electrode localization results. Co-registration of CT, MRI before and after electrode placement, or digital photos taken intraoperatively with the patient's MRI (47–52) provides good results in terms of localizing electrode recording sites. While making electrode localization estimates for depth electrode contacts is somewhat easier, correct identification of individual subdural contacts is more challenging. Mean mismatch between real and virtual electrode placement was found between 2 and 4 mm but could be as large as 13 mm (53). The main problem is the nonlinear deformation of the brain surface due to fluid collection under the bone flap. In most studies, electrode positions are captured by a postoperative CT and merged with a preoperative MRI, which causes the electrodes to appear buried in the brain. However, electrodes farther away from the implantation site are less affected, which adds to the imprecision. Algorithms using intraoperative high-resolution photographs and reconstructions from the MRI appear to provide significantly more precise localization (i.e., ~1 mm), but this is a very tedious process (54). A recently proposed method, recursive grid partitioning, uses four grid electrodes obtained from intraoperative photographs, but the remaining electrodes are then interpolated (55). A mean error of 2 mm was noted, and most are within 4 mm, which compares favorably to most other methods. Alternatively, external or implantable fiducial markers were proposed (56), but they are less often used today.

Figure 29.1 summarizes the different co-registration algorithms. The exact localization of depth electrodes is simpler, given that there is less brain shift. Otherwise, similar algorithms to reconstruct the position of the electrodes are employed.

5. DEPTH ELECTRODES

5.1. Technical Aspects

Taking all patient studies together, depth electrodes are probably the most frequently used electrode type (Fig. 29.2), given that they were already in use in the 1960s and 1970s in the medical field. They are inserted through burr holes by stereotactic methods, using guidance from previously acquired brain imaging. Depth electrodes are built as wires containing evenly spaced electrode contacts of conductive material. The insertion is done by a gauge needles whose trajectory is determined by the site of the target(s) in the CT and/or MRI of the patient's brain. Sometimes additional arteriography or magnetic resonance angiography is required to identify crucial vessels and reduce the risk of hemorrhage. In many centers today, a stereotactic setup is used that includes the patient's MRI. More recently, frameless robot-guided insertion has been reported (57), and the future will show if the application of such sophisticated methods will decrease the risk of depth electrode placement and/or shorten the operative time significantly.

Electrode spacing is most often between 5 and 10 mm, but any configuration, distance, and number of electrodes can be chosen—that is, either at regular distances or only at sites that cover the gray matter. Most electrodes contain six to 15 electrodes. The electrodes themselves can be rigid or flexible, but most neurosurgeons prefer flexible electrodes. The use of flexible electrodes may lead to less precise electrode placement (due to involuntary deviation from the initial target), but they are associated with a lower risk of bleeding. Most companies that produce intracranial electrodes offer the choice between platinum-iridium and nickel-chrome alloys. Only the first combination is MR-compatible, but they are more expensive. The electrodes have multiple contacts (usually between eight and 12) and can be inserted orthogonally (i.e., perpendicular to the lateral surface or longitudinal-parasagittally). Oblique insertions into the frontal lobe toward the basal ganglia have also been employed. However, in all cases, there is only very limited sampling of the neocortical-lateral cortex, so additional subdural or scalp electrodes may be needed if the cortex needs larger coverage.

Given that this electrode type is the only one that goes into the brain parenchyma, the major advantage of depth electrode recordings is the opportunity to record from deep, buried cortex, such as hippocampus, amygdala, or mesial frontal structures. Furthermore, the simultaneous sampling of mesial and lateral cerebral structures, associated with an excellent EEG quality, is a favorable aspect of depth electrodes. They also permit bilateral and multilobar sampling, but there is limited spatial sampling in a given region—for instance, identification of language cortex and its extent is not possible with depth electrodes alone. Another significant advantage is the easy removal, which can be accomplished without anesthesia. They can even be removed at the bedside.

5.2. Risks

The major risk of using depth electrodes is intracranial or intracerebral hemorrhage, which occurs in 1% to 4% of cases (58). With modern imaging, the rate seems to be lower. In a

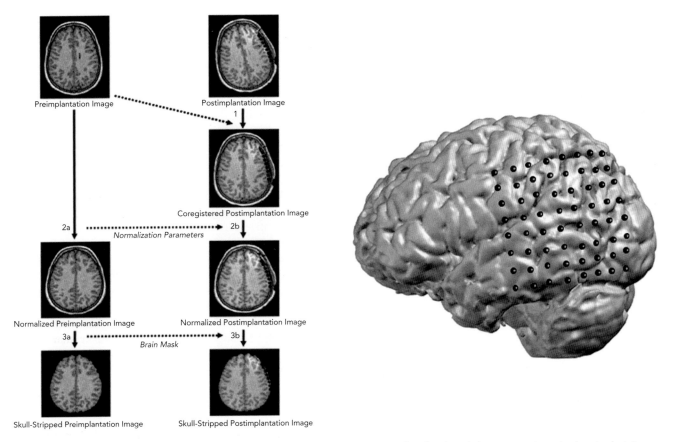

Figure 29.1. *Co-registration of intracranial electrodes and the patient's individual MRI. Proposition for a flowchart aiming to merge the patient's preimplantation MRI with the postimplantation MRI or postimplantation high-resolution CT. The preimplantation image is normalized and skull stripped, then merged with the postimplantation MRI, which underwent the same computation. In this example, particular care is taken to compensate for the brain shift due to compression by subdural grids. This is less of an issue in patients with depth electrodes. Courtesy of L. Spinelli, PhD.*

study of 50 patients with depth and subdural strip electrodes (59), no deaths, no infections, and no new neurological deficits were reported. Ross et al. (59) reviewed previously reported series of depth electrode patients; for the entire group of 1,656 patients, the relative risk was highest for intracranial

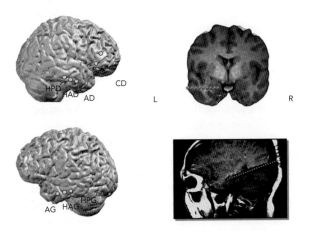

Figure 29.2. *Depth electrodes. Left: Co-registration of the orthogonally inserted electrodes and the patient's MRI. The insertion sites of depth electrodes in both hemispheres are marked in white. Upper right: Same patient as shown on left, showing his depth electrode inserted in the left amygdala. In this co-registration, each contact is identified separately (light gray balls). Lower right: Longitudinal insertion of depth electrodes (light gray).*

hemorrhage (1.1%) followed by infection (0.8%). In a recent review of 259 patients, the risk of symptomatic intracranial hemorrhage was 1.2% and the risk of permanent neurological deficit was 0.7% (60). The Montreal group reported the absence of major complications in a total of 6,415 electrode implantations (491 patients) between 1976 and 2006, representing a time span before and after introduction of MRI. Hematoma and infection were noted in 0.8% and 1.8%, respectively (61). Overall, in this study, complications were more frequent in the frontal lobe, perhaps due to the higher number of implanted electrodes. Mortality is basically zero in the series after 1990. Among the hemorrhages, few are life-threatening; in our experience the incidence should be <0.1%.

Patient counseling on the avoidance of antiplatelet drugs is recommended as well as the implementation of preoperative coagulation parameters. There is no agreement on the use of prophylactic antibiotic treatment in patients during depth electrode investigations. If contact between the intra- and extracranial milieu is minimized with sterile bandages and the patient is prevented from scratching under the bandage, the risk of infection is even less than 0.8%.

Even years after depth electrode investigations, discrete gliotic changes along the insertion channel are seen in MRI images, but, to date, there is no evidence that these changes become epileptogenic or are related to new neurological or cognitive deficits.

6. SUBDURAL ELECTRODES

6.1. Technical Aspects

These electrodes were introduced into the field of epilepsy surgery somewhat later than the depth electrodes and are used for epidural recordings. When Penfield recorded epidurally from the left parieto-temporal region in a patient with posttraumatic epilepsy in 1939 (62), he can probably be considered the first to have used this electrode type. Subdural or epidural electrodes consist of disc-shaped electrodes, embedded in transparent Silastic or Teflon material, arranged in rows or arrays of all shapes (Fig. 29.3). As with depth electrodes, they are made of platinum-iridium and nickel-chrome; MR imaging is possible only if they are made of platinum. The contacts are put freehand on the cortex, subdurally on the pia mater. If necessary, they can be reduced with sterile scissors or along perforated lines to create smaller arrays directly in the operating room. There are recent reports in which neuronavigation and stereotactic methods are used to improve the precision of placement, in particular for strips, or for merging imaging datasets that help to take all preoperative imaging information into consideration (63,64). Similar to depth electrodes, determination of electrode positions by MRI or CT imaging is an important issue because smaller or larger shifts may occur after the implantation, in particular with small arrays. The contacts are usually 5 to 10 mm apart, are 4 to 5 mm in diameter, and can be arranged as one line (strip) or in a larger array (e.g., 8×8 contacts, grids of 64 electrodes; see Fig. 29.3). Strip electrodes arranged in a single row can be inserted through burr holes. However, a large grid (e.g., an array of 4×4 or 8×8 electrodes) needs a full craniotomy. This is a more invasive procedure than the stereotactic procedure employed for the placement of depth electrodes.

There have been a number of technical developments in the past 10 years with respect to improvement of subdural electrodes, including smaller and thinner grid arrays, notches and holes allowing cerebrospinal fluid circulation, and better fitting to the curved brain (65). Wireless transmission reduces the number of intra–extracranial tunnels and therefore the risk of infection. Use of smaller contacts allows more contacts to be packed on a given surface, thus providing higher spatial sampling of the cortical surface and leading to more precise focus localization (66).

The main indication for subdural electrodes is the precise localization of a seizure focus within a suspicious area. When using grid arrays, two or three lobes can be covered with a single grid (e.g., frontal posterior, temporal, and parietal). This requires that noninvasive evaluation narrow the possible site of the focus to one or two lobes. Subdural electrodes also allow for preoperative corticography, with the aim of determining vital cortex (this procedure is described later in the chapter in the section on pediatric patients). By stimulation with short (2–5 sec) intermittent electrical currents, sensations or involuntary movements are produced that supposedly reflect the characteristics of the underlying cortex. Primary cortex can thus be reliably identified. However, higher-order cortical phenomena, like language, are not always easily identified, as shown by Seeck et al. (67). These electrodes do not necessarily require knowledge of stereotactic procedures and/or a neuronavigation device and thus can be performed in neurosurgical centers without experience in stereotactic methods. Subdural electrodes record from a larger cortical surface and capture incompletely signals from the sulci as well as from radial sources. It is a well-established finding that only one third of the brain is accessible from the surface, which means also that only one third is accessible in terms of recording. Thus, most brain tissue underneath a subdural grid will not be directly recorded, but may be involved only after propagation to these more superficial cortical regions has occurred.

6.2. Risks

The morbidity is low for strip electrodes. Risks include infections (~1%) and bleeding when bridge veins are damaged (68). Larger grid arrays are more likely to be associated with more significant complications. The infection rate is higher than with depth or strip electrodes alone and is reported to be ~8%. This risk can be diminished if the cables exit through a tunnel via a second incision a few centimeters away from the original incision. As for depth electrodes, no consensus exists as to whether prophylactic antibiotic therapy should be given, although this issue is more relevant with subdural electrodes. Based on personal experience, prophylactic antibiotic treatment in patients with large arrays of subdural electrodes is associated with a lower incidence of infectious problems (e.g., intravenous cefazolin 4 × 500 mg). Most patients with grids experience local edema of the underlying cortex, leading to headache and photo-phonophobia. This complication occurs less often with strips. Rigorous symptomatic treatment with pain relievers is helpful, as well as positioning of the head at a 30- to 450-degree elevation. Major or near-fatal increased intracranial pressure is extremely rare; if discovered, immediate surgical decompression may be needed. Consequently, a neurosurgeon on call nearby is a necessity.

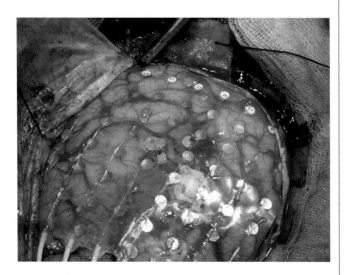

Figure 29.3. Intraoperative subdural grid placement. Each contact (platinum disk, 0.8 mm in diameter) is recorded through a wire, which is led out of the skull through a larger white cable (in the lower left of the image; in this grid, bundles of eight wires each).

In a recent study, delayed subdural hematoma was noted to be the most frequent complication (8%) (69). Hematoma occurred up to 3 days after implantation. This "fragile" period is probably somewhat longer and, as for most brain surgeries, spans up to 5 days. A recent study in a pediatric group noted problems after implantation in >20% of their patients, with predominance of hematoma, but this may be due to the fact that 43% of their patients had already undergone a prior epilepsy surgery procedure (70). Another pediatric series reported a lower complication rate, including hematoma (6%) (71).

Implantation of larger arrays of subdural electrodes remains a relatively delicate procedure, requiring unambiguous agreement about the indication, in particular in children. Patients with a history of high-dose radiotherapy and chemotherapy may develop significant persistent neurological deficits after subdural grid placement, not explained by brain swelling (72). iEEG in this patient group may be associated with more severe complications than in patients without this history.

Experience is also an important factor. The Cleveland Clinic group reported a 33% rate of minor and more serious complications in the beginning of their epilepsy program, but it dropped to 19% in more recent years. Overall, the use of more than 100 electrodes, longer recording sessions (i.e., >2 weeks), and more than one cable exit are related to an increase in complication rates (73,74). It is probably safe to say that a complication rate of between 10% and 20% can be expected, so close monitoring by specialized personnel and in a center with 24-hour access to a scanner and an intensive care unit will be needed. Regular neurological exams and monitoring for infectious diseases are mandatory (Box 29.2).

If bleeding complications are present, it is safer to remove the electrodes as soon as possible. If there are signs of local infections, and if enough seizures are recorded, removal of electrodes is recommended. An increase in the C-reactive protein (CRP) level, after attaining normal or near-normal values postoperatively, is a valuable marker. If no or too few seizures were recorded, introduction or reinforcement of the antibiotic treatment with prolongation of the recording period, perhaps with more rigorous drug and sleep withdrawal, should be considered. Since intracranial electrode implantation is a costly and intensive intervention in terms of manpower and, more importantly, the physical and psychological strain on the patient, reimplantation at another time is not easily done or recommended. General guidelines are difficult to establish since every center has its own resources and patients differ in their willingness to cope with unforeseen clinical situations.

Despite the higher complication rates with subdural electrodes, the rates of permanent neurological deficits do not seem to differ from those for depth electrodes and are ~1% to 2%. Removal can be done at the bedside, if strips are used. If grids are used, another craniotomy will be needed during which the surgical resection of the focus is carried out as well, if indicated.

7. FORAMEN OVALE ELECTRODES AND EPIDURAL ELECTRODES

Foramen ovale electrodes (FOEs), initially developed in 1985 by the Zurich group, are used somewhat less frequently in most centers. FOEs record epidurally and extracerebrally from the mesial temporal lobe structures. They contain four to six contacts and can be inserted under local anesthesia (Fig. 29.4). They are also easily removed at the bedside, similar to depth electrodes. Major complications are rare, but they are not "semi-invasive" as initially advocated. Subarachnoid hemorrhage and transient brainstem symptoms (e.g., trigeminal neuralgia) are observed. Complication rates of 1% to 9% are reported (i.e., similar to rates reported for depth or subdural electrodes), but complications are mostly transient. FOEs yield good recordings from the middle and posterior portion of the hippocampus; they are not as good at recording from its anterior aspect of the hippocampus and the amygdala and/or small subcompartments of the mesial temporal structures. The classical indication for FOEs is to lateralize (mesial) temporal lobe onset. They may be combined with subdural or scalp electrodes for more extensive sampling from lateral temporal or extratemporal structures, and consequently the indication may be extended to other indications.

Epidural peg electrodes share similar configuration aspects with subdural electrodes and are inserted through burr holes or twist drill holes. They can be placed bilaterally, similar to scalp electrodes, but cannot be used for cortical mapping. Electrical stimulation through epidural electrodes is painful because the dura is innervated and irritated by electrical current. Precise sublobar focus localization is not possible with epidural electrodes alone since their spatial sampling is not sufficient. However, they have a low morbidity (<0.5%), consisting mainly of discomfort when the electrodes are inserted through the temporalis muscle and some superficial wound infections. Their main indication is the verification of the absence of epileptogenic discharges and/or recording of selected sites where scalp electrodes would be too contaminated by muscle artifacts.

BOX 29.2. PROPOSED SURVEILLANCE ALGORITHM FOR PATIENTS ADMITTED FOR SUBDURAL INTRACRANIAL EEG MONITORING

- 24-hour supervision by nurses, technicians, and/or other persons (e.g., medical students or family members)
- Postimplantation 24-hour surveillance in the intensive care unit
- When admitted for EEG monitoring
  - C-reactive protein (CRP), blood: every day or every other day
  - Temperature: twice a day
  - Brief neurologic exam (pupils, responsiveness, motor functions) every 2–4 hours for the first 2 days, then every 4–6 hours for the next 3–4 days
- Optional: prophylactic antibiotic treatment (e.g., cefazolin) starting from the day of the implantation through the monitoring period
- Optional: dexamethasone during the first 3–4 days

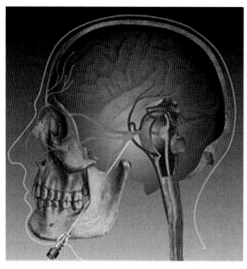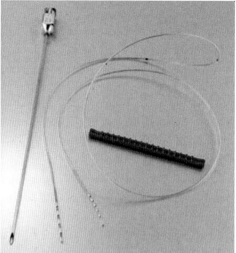

Figure 29.4. *Foramen ovale electrodes. Left: Insertion procedure through the base of the skull (i.e., through the foramen ovale). (Courtesy of CCND Winnipeg.) Right: Foramen ovale electrodes. (Courtesy of Dixi Electronics.)*

8. SURVEILLANCE

There are no consensus guidelines concerning the degree of medical and paramedical staff surveillance and concomitant treatment in patients admitted for EEG monitoring. However, a "semi-intensive" care unit with a lower nurse/patient ratio compared to normal care units appears the most appropriate setting. There are still many centers that cannot offer professional surveillance at night or on weekends, leading to seizure-related complications (e.g., autonomous electrode removal during the postictal confusional state).

The choice on whom to rely during the patient's monitoring session is influenced by budget and legal considerations. While we know relatively well the risk of iEEG complications such as bleeding or infection, there is disagreement across surgical epilepsy centers on who should watch the patient: parent/close family member, non-medical staff (e.g., out-of-work people recruited on through a placement agency), EEG technicians, or nurses. Patients whose recordings are made after drug withdrawal have a risk for more prolonged or more intense seizures (i.e., more often generalized tonic–clonic seizures) resulting in trauma and/or prolonged postictal confusion. Pulling out the electrodes is also encountered: in a review (61), 3 of 491 implanted patients (0.6%) pulled out their electrodes during a seizure or during the early postimplantation period. Cerebrospinal fluid leakage, bleeding, or infection may result

from such an act, particularly if larger subdural electrodes arrays are removed.

Family members or non-medical personnel may not be optimal for monitoring, since they are often unable to judge the clinical context or severity of a given situation. There are no studies on the guidelines for the size and composition of the surveillance staff necessary to minimize these complications and to reduce the recording time. For obvious reasons, professional surveillance by trained nurses and technicians, in collaboration with an experienced epileptologist or neurologist, is the optimal setting.

Legal aspects also need to be considered in order to be protected against "under-surveillance," and these differ markedly between countries. In some countries, like the United States, legal action against the hospital is more readily taken if complications are encountered; therefore, different solutions and their legal implications need to be more thoroughly studied.

Clinical observation of patients with iEEG should include close monitoring of the neurological status, cognitive function, and blood values indicating infections or bleeding. The "algorithm" proposed in Box 29.2 stems from our personal experiences. Close monitoring for the first 5 days is recommended by most neurosurgeons, due to an increased risk of intracranial bleeding during this period. From then on, daily neurological surveillance may be sufficient, aiming particularly at the detection of infectious complications.

Since the introduction of chronic iEEG, there is ongoing debate if, when, and for how long antibiotic therapy or corticosteroids should be administered. Informal review of the protocols from different centers shows that changes in such protocols have emerged. The most frequent pattern included the regular use of steroids during the initial period, but this pattern has been abandoned for most patients. In most centers, steroids and antibiotics are considered with subdural implants but very rarely with depth electrodes. The placement of large grids is almost always followed by focal cerebral edema of variable degree and clinical symptoms, but these usually improve

---

BOX 29.3. INTRACRANIAL ICTAL ONSET PATTERN

Low-voltage fast activity (LVFA; >13–20 Hz)

- Beta range (13–30 Hz)
- Gamma range (>30 Hz)

Rhythmic spiking (1–2 Hz)
Rhythmic sinusoidal pattern in alpha-theta range (~5–9 Hz)
Rhythmic spiking in the alpha-theta range
Semirhythmic slow waves (<5 Hz)
High-amplitude beta spike activity

---

spontaneously within 3 to 5 days postoperatively, with or without steroid use.

There are two studies on the use of dexamethasone in patients undergoing monitoring with subdural electrodes. The prophylactic use in children was thought to be efficacious for brain swelling, as determined by CT changes manifest by midline shift, decrease of ventricular size, and so forth, although it led to a slightly longer (~1 day) seizure-monitoring time (75). The benefit of steroids during a limited period of 3 days in adults seems to be less clear (76). In a randomized, placebo-controlled study of 30 patients, less pain and nausea were reported, but the effect was limited over time.

There is no study on the yield of antibiotics during iEEG. Most centers are more likely to consider administering a prolonged course of antibiotics with subdural recordings compared to depth electrodes. Other centers give a single dose or a short course of antibiotics during and shortly after the operation, while others use them also in patient with depth electrodes. To date there is no study supporting the view that antibiotic therapy offers better protection against nosocomial infections.

9. COMPARISON OF YIELD BETWEEN DIFFERENT ELECTRODE TYPES

Depth and subdural electrodes are the intracranial electrodes that are most frequently used, but each center has its own preferences and experiences that may influence the choice of one over the other. Depth electrodes yield better results when recording from deep temporal structures, in particular from the amygdala (77–79). Subdural electrodes are helpful in identifying a mesial temporal focus. However, if they are placed or moved too laterally, in particular lateral to the collateral sulcus, false localization and lateralization may occur due to propagation to orbitofrontal or contralateral temporal cortex before recruitment of the affected mesial temporal structure becomes visible (80).

Mesial extratemporal (i.e., interhemispheric) structures are explored well with both depth and subdural electrodes. Subdural electrodes are more easily placed given the larger cortical surface compared to mesial temporal structures. However, comparative studies do not exist.

In extratemporal lobe epilepsy, subdural electrodes seem to be slightly better than depth electrodes if convexity structures need to be recorded. Since they have the advantage of allowing cortical mapping, subdural electrodes may be preferred if focus localization includes mainly extratemporal cortex where there is a question of the involvement and/extent of eloquent cortex. The combination of depth and subdural electrodes is also more and more frequently used. However, comparative studies on the yield of combined depth and subdural electrodes compared to each electrode type alone are missing.

Comparisons between FOEs and other electrode types have been also performed. In seven patients with FOEs and depth electrodes, interictal and ictal discharges were picked up by FOEs if amygdala, hippocampus, and parahippocampal gyrus discharged simultaneously, but less reliably if only

a subcompartment of the mesial temporal structures was active (81).

Intracranial electrodes served also as the "gold standard" to determine the accuracy of scalp and sphenoidal electrodes. Compared to discharges recorded by FOEs, scalp electrodes over the anterior temporal lobe (1 cm anterior to T1/T2) recorded 95.6% of the discharges but midtemporal scalp electrodes recorded only 77.7% (T3/T4) (82). Rarely (3%) did the interictal discharges show up in the anterior temporal scalp electrode but not in the FOE. Discharges noted in sphenoidal electrodes arose mainly in mesial temporal cortex, but not exclusively: in the group of 21 patients studied, three also had spikes originating from the orbitofrontal and temporal neocortex (83).

10. INTERICTAL INTRACRANIAL EEG

All normal physiologic rhythms (e.g., alpha, theta during drowsiness, mu) that can be seen in scalp recordings appear also in intracranial EEG at the corresponding cortical sites (i.e., mu over sensory-motor cortex). However, due to the absence of scalp and skull, all EEG patterns look more "spiky." Scalp and skull filter out in particular high frequencies, including spikes, whereas slow frequencies pass. Thus, only a small fraction of intracranial spikes are visible in scalp EEG. If areas <6 cm^2 are active, no recognizable spike activity was found on the scalp. Discharges from areas between 6 and 10 cm^2 resulted in 10% in spikes, and in areas >10 cm^2, 90% were retrievable in scalp EEGs (36).

Intracranial EEG is thought to have the advantage of being devoid of muscle artifacts; however, this might not be entirely true, as indicated by a recent case report (84). In this 17-year-old boy, muscle artifacts appeared at infero-lateral temporal subdural electrodes, using another intracranial electrode as reference, while eating or during involuntary facial movement as part of the seizure semiology. Thus, muscle activity may be picked up by intracranial recordings, similar to any other interfering electrical activity, although its appearance may differ from muscle artifacts in scalp recordings.

If high frequencies remain in the EEG, everything appears "epileptogenic," which occasionally has led to incorrect EEG interpretation. This may be why most authorities in the field recommend relying mainly on the ictal data and less on the interictal EEG. Consequently, in intracranial recordings, interictal discharges appear more often multifocal and more frequently than in surface recordings.

To determine the relevance of the interictal iEEG spikes in a given location, several approaches are possible. The first is to determine the underlying area (see above): if the spikes are seen over an area of 10 cm^2 or more (as estimated by the number of simultaneously active electrodes), they are more likely to arise from the epileptogenic zone (see above). Second, doing a quantitative analysis of the relative frequency of spikes from different regions may help to determine their relevance. This could be done by visual analysis or through automatic or semi-automatic detection algorithms. The latter were used in a study of iEEG in 32 patients (24 with temporal lobe epilepsy,

8 with extratemporal lobe epilepsy), with mostly combined depth and subdural electrode recordings (85). Spikes with the highest frequency, the highest amplitude, and a shorter duration originated most often from the ictal onset zone (i.e., 2 cm from the site of seizure origin). Another study in 13 children, including also patients with cortical dysplasia, came to similar conclusions. In that study, subdural electrodes were implanted. Electrodes with the highest spike frequency and amplitude were closest to the area of seizure onset in most of the patients (86), and 11 of the 13 were seizure-free (Engel's class I) (87). The yield of careful interictal analysis was studied in patients with exclusively extratemporal lobe epilepsy, including cortical dysplasia. No quantification for different locations of interictal spikes was provided, but mapping of the extension of the interictal epileptogenic zone including depth and subdural electrodes was done. If the resection volume included the area of dominant interictal spikes, a good surgical outcome was significantly more likely (88).

The definition of iEEG spikes is mostly qualitative and adopted from scalp EEG. Criteria included a morphological pattern that (a) has a triangular waveform, with or without a following slow wave, (b) has a duration of <70 msec, and (c) stands out clearly from the background with its amplitude and steep component. Given the difficulties involved in determining unambiguously the presence or absence of spikes, spike-detection programs for scalp EEGs were developed and applied also for iEEG (89). Three of those algorithms were tested for iEEG from seven patients (six with temporal lobe epilepsy) and compared to analysis by visual inspection from two human reviewers. The agreement between the two EEG experts was relatively small, with <50% of all spikes identified by both reviewers, a number similar to scalp EEG. Compared to the human reviewers, the automatic algorithms were concordant in only 24% to 32%. However, despite the low agreement between the human experts and the computer, this affected the number of detected spikes but not the location: both reviewers and automatic systems identified the spikes in the same anatomical locations.

The intracranial interictal EEG correlates of dysplastic tissue have been investigated, since dysplasia and/or its extent are often invisible on the MRI. Rhythmic spike-wave complexes in a continuous or quasi-continuous fashion are most likely to be associated with cortical dysplasia (90,91). In fact, in patients with dysplasia, the analysis of "interictal" anomalies seemed to be more promising than that of ictal intracranial recordings (92). Other studies did not find any difference in the interictal spiking pattern between dysplastic and nondysplastic cortex (93). Continuous discharge patterns are also found with severely gliotic tissue (94), but the difference between dysplasia and severe gliosis should be obvious already from the patient's MRI.

In conclusion, disregard for interictal discharges in the EEG and concentration only on ictal recordings is an obsolete concept if only "true" interictal spikes are considered. Careful analysis of the location and frequency of interictal spikes in iEEG can significantly add to the detection of the epileptogenic zone. Recently, studies were presented that aimed at the brain "current source" reconstruction from intracranial recordings

(95), similar to algorithms for scalp EEG. Future studies will determine their feasibility and utility in a clinical environment (see also Chapter 45). If sophisticated analysis of interictal iEEG can provide sufficient data on the seizure onset area and resection leads to seizure freedom in most cases, recording time could be significantly shortened, resulting in lower morbidity and costs. Electric source localization of interictal *scalp* EEG corresponds most often to the intracranial ictal onset zone (2), and its resection leads to seizure freedom in the majority of patients (96,97).

11. ICTAL INTRACRANIAL EEG PATTERNS AND THEIR RELEVANCE TO OUTCOME

Despite promising results from interictal intracranial studies in terms of localization of the epileptogenic zone, ictal recording remains the chief goal of intracranial EEG. To date, there is no consensus of how many seizures are required to be confident enough to recommend surgery. Most centers try to obtain a minimum of five seizures or more if multifocal origin is suspected. The goal is to determine a principal seizure-onset focus. However, strict rules are probably not possible, given that intracranial recordings cannot be extended indefinitely due to medical concerns.

As a rule, the chances of seizure control are markedly better if the EEG onset precedes the clinical onset. The reasons are obvious: if the seizure is already ongoing clinically, even without focal EEG changes, there is a strong risk that the electrodes do not cover the zone of seizure generation, and any conclusion about the true area of epilepsy onset remains obscure. Furthermore, the chance of postoperative seizure control is higher if there is only one type of seizure semiology. This is true for ictal scalp recordings and also for ictal intracranial workups. However, since the noninvasive "phase 1" workup precedes the invasive "phase 2" workup, the information about how many different seizure types are involved is usually already provided.

A large body of studies looked into a possible relationship between the intracranial ictal EEG pattern, its location, and the surgical outcome. While most early studies included patients with temporal lobe epilepsy using depth electrode recordings, later observations were extended to subdural electrode recordings and/or extratemporal epilepsies.

Concerning iEEG, the impact of focal versus regional or diffuse onset has also been examined in several studies. A higher chance of postoperative seizure freedom is associated with onset in only few electrodes (98–100). Focal onset, defined as ictal activity in less than four or five electrode contacts, appears to be a sign of proximity of the recording contacts to the epileptogenic zone, so its resection is likely to result in seizure control or major seizure reduction (up to 85% of patients with fast frequency onset) (101). This relationship was less evident in another study of neocortical, mostly extratemporal, epilepsy (102), which reported no difference between focal and nonfocal onset.

Concerning the intracranial ictal EEG pattern, onset rhythms were classified either in terms of frequency bands or as certain morphological patterns. Since fast rhythms of cortical origin are filtered by skull and scalp, ictal onset, often characterized by low-amplitude rapid beta or gamma frequencies, was seen more easily in iEEG but most importantly earlier than on scalp EEG. In fact, fast EEG onset frequencies (in the beta or gamma range) are the most frequently reported EEG pattern at onset (103,104), significantly related to class I and II outcome (105,106). According to Lee et al. (100), extratemporal onset is faster and found in the gamma range (>30 Hz), whereas temporal lobe onset was seen in the beta range. These initial fast EEG patterns are also often associated with focal onset and, therefore, evocative of the proximity of the electrodes to the seizure-onset zone. Slower EEG onset frequencies (<5 Hz) probably indicate that there is already propagation from a focus elsewhere (107). During a slow iEEG pattern, the patient may show loss of responsiveness, automatisms, and other behavioral signs of already ongoing seizure activity. Consequently, a better surgical outcome is reported with focal, faster ictal EEG onset, although other evidence indicated that slow onset is not always a bad sign. If iEEG ictal slow onset contains poor prognosis, it was associated with developmental pathology, regional distribution, or an extratemporal location (only one in 16 became seizure-free) (100).

Other ictal iEEG patterns include a sinusoidal pattern, pre-ictal spiking, or high-amplitude beta spiking. A sinusoidal pattern were only seen with mature pathologic substrates. Its prognosis is unclear. It was thought to be a sign of propagation (106), although this was less clear in another report (100).

Next to low-voltage fast beta activity, periodic spiking before seizure onset was frequently observed. This represents another ictal onset pattern and was found to be related to seizures of hippocampal and amygdala onset (108–110). Ictal spiking at seizure onset is correlated with the presence of hippocampal sclerosis and/or neuronal decrease in the CA1 region of the hippocampus, which is in itself a favorable sign with respect to postoperative outcome. Consequently, ictal onset spiking is associated with a good prognosis in terms of seizure control. Finally, high-amplitude beta spike activity has been also described (111) in temporal lobe epilepsy, but it is rare and its prognosis is still unclear.

Although the intracranial ictal onset pattern was not predictive of the underlying pathology, low-voltage fast activity and rhythmic alpha-theta spike-wave were more common in developmental substrates (e.g., dysplasia) (100).

Another study subject is the variability of ictal onset. The rationale behind it is that variable onset patterns could indicate multiple seizure origins. In a study of 18 patients with temporal lobe epilepsy, more than one ictal EEG onset pattern was found in most patients (99). An earlier study found that the variability of the onset frequency is a characteristic of temporal lobe epilepsy and rarely found in extratemporal cases (104). However, in both studies, surgical outcome was not reported—in other words, it remains unknown whether the variability of the onset EEG pattern holds prognostic significance.

Apart from the onset iEEG pattern, the evolution of the seizure pattern and its prognostic significance have been addressed. The speed of propagation represents an important factor. Fast propagation (i.e., within one to a few seconds) to remote regions

is associated with a less favorable surgical result (112). This appears to be equally true for temporal and extratemporal lobe epilepsies. Interhemispheric propagation time in patients with temporal lobe epilepsy was analyzed, and a delay of only 0.5 to 5 sec was associated with a poor prognosis (113). It is assumed that rapid or even almost simultaneous EEG onset at two distant sites, such as both temporal lobes, points to a pacemaker elsewhere with rapid propagation to the two sites. Alternatively, rapid propagation could suggest diffuse damage to remote areas, each with significant epileptogenic properties of its own.

Propagation may occur through different EEG patterns. Two propagation patterns at distant sites were identified by Schiller et al. (114) in temporal and extratemporal lobe epilepsies: (1) rhythmic theta-delta activity correlating with the activity at the seizure onset site and (2) continuation of the seizure pattern of the seizure onset site. No significant correlation between the onset and propagation EEG patterns and the outcome was found. The visual analysis of iEEG during propagation is probably less relevant in the clinical context, and may even differ within a patient from one seizure to the other. It remains to be shown whether coherence-based measurements are more informative (i.e., if they help to identify nonfocal epilepsies) (115).

Finally, the end of the intracranial ictal EEG pattern ("offset") was studied to determine whether offset outside the generating structures is related to a worse outcome. Theoretically, it could indicate the presence of epileptogenic tissue in remote sites, ready to pick up seizure activity from elsewhere. However, there was no prognostic difference between patients with an ipsilateral and contralateral offset (116), but this finding is challenged by reports finding that patients with a contralateral offset have a poorer surgical outcome (117,118). However, just as for the onset, the offset pattern can vary within one patient, and more studies are probably needed to determine the prognostic relevance of the offset pattern.

While there have been many studies on the value of ictal iEEG, many questions remain as to the prognostic significance of a given EEG pattern. It appears that several variables influence the creation of an ictal iEEG pattern, such as the affected lobe, the underlying histopathology, the type of electrode and sites of contacts, the patient's age, and the speed of medication withdrawal. So many variables exist, in fact, that most studies are underpowered. Multicenter studies making use of modern three-dimensional localization of all contacts could help to better identify the significance of ictal iEEG patterns.

The various ictal EEG pattern are shown in Figures 29.7–29.21 and summarized in Box 29.3.

12. HIGH-FREQUENCY OSCILLATIONS

In recent years, research on the markers of epileptogenic tissue in the interictal EEG has been restarted, given that the new generation of recording systems with higher EEG sampling rates can capture very fast rhythms (30–500 Hz). Probably the first study on that subject was published by Fisher et al. (119); they found increased high-frequency activity (in this study >40 Hz) in the seizure onset zone. Many more studies followed, supporting the notion that high-frequency oscillations (HFOs) are more frequently co-localized with the seizure onset zone; however, the exact shape and frequency band of what is truly evocative of the epileptic focus still need to be defined (120). HFOs are believed to reflect inhibitory field potentials that facilitate information transfer by synchronizing neuronal activity over long distances. These recordings require a high sampling rate (i.e., 2,000–5,000 Hz) and a 500- to 1,000-Hz low-pass filter instead of the usual 200- to 250-Hz sampling rate and 70- to 100-Hz low-pass filter used for the routine iEEG. HFOs are recorded with the commercially available subdural or depth electrodes or with micro-wires that are inserted together with macro-electrodes (Figs. 29.5, 29.6).

HFOs are short bursts of high-frequency pattern that become visible if the EEG is sampled with a wide bandwidth up to 5,000 Hz. Bradin et al. (121) differentiated ripples (60–160 Hz) and fast ripples (250–500 Hz), and this nomenclature has been used in similar studies, although the lower and upper limits of the ripple frequencies are slightly different from study to study. Both ripple types increase during slow-wave sleep (122,123), which may explain the propensity of seizures to occur during periods of decreased vigilance or sleep. However, there is evidence that HFOs of ripple frequency are also found in the nonepileptogenic temporal lobe, whereas fast ripples are equally predominant in wakefulness and sleep; that is, they do not appear to be a physiologic event (see Chapter 33).

Across several studies and groups, it was claimed that fast ripples are more likely to pinpoint the ictal epileptogenic zone than HFOs of lower frequency (124,125), although not all studies reached the same conclusion (126). They may occur alone, or superposed on the spike. Overall, fast ripples appear to be a more localized event than HFOs of lower ripple frequency (127). They may also precede the seizure onset by up to several seconds to 20 minutes (128) but are not present in all patients. If HFOs indeed indicate the zone of seizure onset, longer EEG recordings requiring the capture of several seizures to confirm the presence of a unifocal ictal onset zone would become obsolete. However, the issue is far from resolved. Recordings from both macro- and microelectrodes showed that both types (fast ripples and ripples) can occur together—that is, the burst may start with ripples and evolve to fast ripples, or vice versa. Fast ripples were often recorded from a single microwire, indicating a very local event from a neuronal assembly. How and

when such a local and short discharge (20–50 ms) evolves to clinical seizures of several minutes remains to be elucidated.

Research on human HFOs is relatively recent. Most of the studies have been done in mesial temporal lobe structures, given that patients with temporal lobe epilepsy are more common in the surgical patient population and/or more frequently investigated with intracranial and micro-wire electrodes together. The existence of ripples or fast ripples in extratemporal lobe epilepsy is less well known up to now, but preliminary data suggest that they are also present in extratemporal areas. Thus, the most important question to be resolved concerns which type of HFO is truly pathologic and can potentially serve as a biomarker. Recent studies have found paroxysmal fast activity even in scalp recordings, mainly in pediatric patients in the beta and gamma frequency band (15–70 Hz) (129,130).

13. MICROELECTRODES

This type of electrode has been introduced recently and allows the recording of a few neurons, or even single neurons, in the form of extracellular signals. Microelectrodes are mainly used for research purposes and are "piggybacked" onto commercially available depth or subdural electrodes. Microelectrodes cover a bandwidth of 0.5 to 10 KHz recorded from electrodes of 5 kΩ impedance requiring special amplifiers (131). They are able to record action potentials (spiking). A review on the origin of extracellular fields and currents was published by Buzsaki et al. (132). Multiunit electrodes can be arranged in arrays, such as the "Utah array" (see Fig. 29.5), usually of 96 electrodes arranged in a rectangular form or as a "brush" at the tip of a depth electrode (usually six to 10 microelectrodes), which unfold in the mesial temporal or frontal structures after the depth (macro) electrode is placed. With new hybrid systems, both macro- and microelectrodes can be recorded simultaneously. Adequate amplifiers are now commercially available for use in human subjects, allowing the recording of up to 256 microwires.

Apart from cognitive studies (133,134), a number of studies in patients were conducted to better characterize the origin and propagation of ictal discharges. Shevon et al. coined the term "ictal penumbra." In five patients, microelectrode arrays

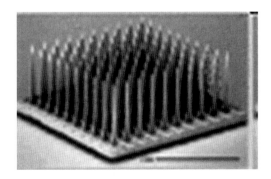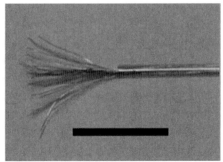

Figure 29.5. Microelectrode arrays. Left: So-called Utah microarray made of multiple silicon spikes 1.0 or 1.5 mm in length. A pressure applicator is used to insert the silicon array into the cortex across the pia. Right: Microelectrodes as a bundle at the end of a depth electrode. The scale bar represents 1 cm. From Turner DA, Patil PG, Nicolelis MAL. Conceptual and Technical Approaches to Human Neural Ensemble Recordings. Methods for Neural Ensemble Recordings, Frontiers in Neuroscience. CRC Press; 2008.)

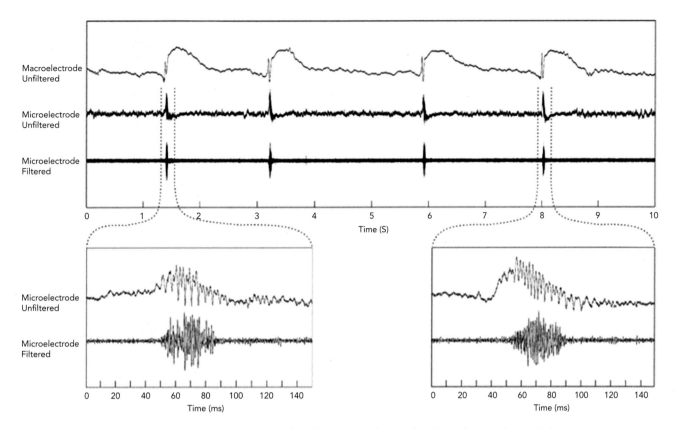

Figure 29.6. *High-frequency oscillations recorded from macroelectrodes and microelectrodes from the left mesial temporal cortex, harboring also the seizure onset zone. Note the coincidence of the spike in the macroelectrodes and ripples recorded in the microelectrodes. (From Worell et al., Brain, 2008.)*

of 96 electrodes were placed near, although not directly in, the seizure onset zone. Areas of high synchronous discharges were next to areas of unstructured firing, and only the areas with synchronous dischargers were recruited during a full seizure, whereas the latter appeared to serve as an inhibitory zone to prevent propagation (135). Somewhat in contrast to this finding, another study reported the lack of hypersynchronous activity at seizure onset; however, seizure termination occurs in a synchronous fashion (136). Interestingly, even neurons outside the seizure onset zone change their spike pattern during and before a seizure, indicating once more that seizures are a network phenomenon and not (only) a local dysfunction. However, synchrony may differ between electrophysiologically different seizure types. Neuronal synchrony appears to be present in particular in seizures with spike-wave onset, and during the spike phase corresponding to HFOs, but not in seizures with high-frequency (40–60 Hz) onset (137). In another study, recordings of "microseizures" with microelectrodes that were not detectable with macroelectrodes were reported, with an unclear relationship to the true seizure onset zone (138). They were also found in two nonepileptic patients (implantation for facial pain), albeit less dense. Further studies will elucidate the meaning of "microseizures." Macroelectrodes, although they provide highly interesting data, are particularly prone to be contaminated with electronic noise (139).

As mentioned above, careful analysis of interictal data may also lead to the identification of the seizure onset zone. In a recent study of 17 patients with temporal lobe epilepsy, the

relationship between high-frequency discharges and interictal spikes was revised. The authors showed that spikes preceded by gamma activity (30–100 Hz) and HFOs (100–600 Hz) were more likely to reflect the true seizure onset zone than interictal epileptiform discharges without gamma or HFO activity (140). Nine patients were operated on (eight seizure-free, one almost seizure-free), four of whom had gamma interictal epileptiform discharges. While microelectrodes offered an additional view of high-frequency activity, gamma activity had the highest specificity (and the lowest sensitivity) and the highest positive predictive value with respect to the identification of the seizure onset zone. Interestingly, the preceding gamma activity had already been recorded with macroelectrodes and could probably be seen also with the scalp EEG. Multicenter studies are mandatory to determine the true yield of microelectrode recordings of ictal or interictal events, given the high costs of microelectrodes.

14. SPECIAL CONSIDERATIONS IN PEDIATRIC PATIENTS

Invasive procedures are rare in infants younger than 3 years, but if they are indicated they should be done at specialized epilepsy surgery centers. Close collaboration with the (neuro) pediatricians is mandatory if the center is not already located in a pediatric department. In contrast to previous attitudes, children with epilepsy should be investigated as soon as pharmacoresistance is documented. To wait until the epilepsy

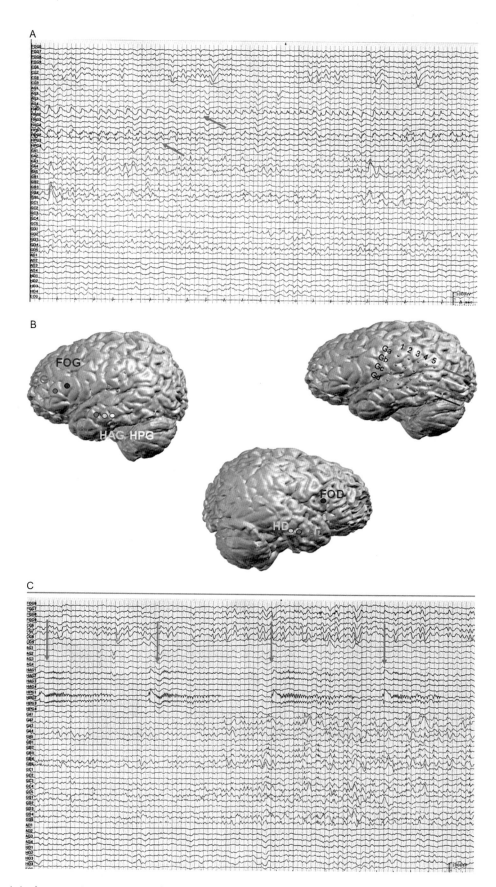

Figure 29.7. *A: Dissociation between seizure onset zone and symptomatic zone. Patient CA, 22-year-old male with left hippocampal sclerosis but nonlocalizing ictal scalp pattern. Continuous discharges in the left hippocampus (depth electrodes; HAG1, HPG1, HPG2) as interictal EEG (→) AD: right amygdala/ant temporal lobe; AG: amygdala/ant temporal lobe; HAG: left hippocampus/mid temporal lobe, HPG: left posterior hippocampis/mid temp lobe. G-contacts: subdural grid electrodes overlying the lateral temporo-parietal cortex. B: Position of depth electrodes in the left and right temporal and frontal cortex, and subdural grids over temporoparietal cortex. Co-registration of high-resolution CT (with the electrodes) and the patient's MRI. C: The interictal rhythm changes to rhythmic appearance of bursts of rapid 30- to 40-Hz pattern, appearing every 6 sec. D: The hippocampal bursts stop and are replaced by widespread 10-Hz rhythms in the lateral fronto-orbital cortex (FOG7) and lateral temporal subdural contacts (contacts GA, GB, GC, GD), coinciding with the onset of clinical symptoms that is, lip smacking, manual automatisms, loss of contact. E: The extrahippocampal discharges persist while the left hippocampus remains silent. This case represents an example of dissociation between areas of onset and the symptomatic propagation, which implicates rather lateral neocortical contacts.*

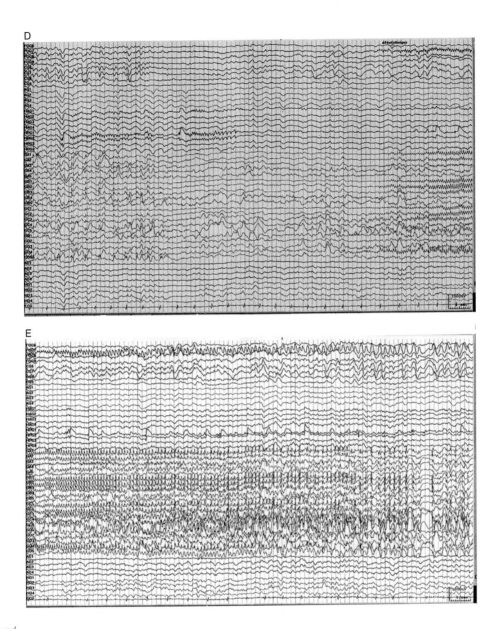

Figure 29.7. Continued

"grows" out is no longer appropriate unless the underlying syndrome is well determined and surgical treatment is clearly not indicated (e.g., Dravet's syndrome). Thorough workup helps to determine the underlying syndrome and potential usefulness of surgical therapy. Not all children with early-onset refractory epilepsy are surgical candidates, but if they are, any period of persistent seizures has deleterious effects on their development. If the indication for iEEG is given, the same implantation strategies, electrode types, and most importantly clinical reasoning regarding the goals apply as for adults.

Pediatric patients suffer more frequently from extratemporal lobe epilepsy. Consequently they are considered as candidates for intracranial monitoring if the exact focus localization is not yet evident from noninvasive monitoring. As in adults, additional electrocorticography may be necessary to identify eloquent cortex.

In older children, the corticography procedure is similar to that in adults (141). Trains of 50-Hz, alternating polarity square-wave pulses of fixed pulse duration (0.3 msec) are most often used, starting with low currents (e.g., 0.5 or 1 mA). The stimulation intensity is gradually augmented in 1-mA steps until a sensation or movement is elicited or the maximal value has been reached (up to a maximum of 10 to 15 mA, without any perceptible sensation or movement). However, in very young children, this approach is often ineffective, since motor responses are virtually unobtainable under 1 year of age, and are obtained only with difficulty until age 4 to 5 years (142). The Miami group described a different stimulation procedure in children younger than 5 years that results more often in motor movements: they propose a dual increment in the pulse duration and the stimulus intensity instead of only in stimulus intensity (143). The minimal current intensity (in mA) required to elicit a response at a very long pulse duration (in msec) is called the rheobase. The double of rheobase, called chronaxie, corresponds to the pulse duration required to elicit a response twice as intense as the rheobase. In nonmyelinated

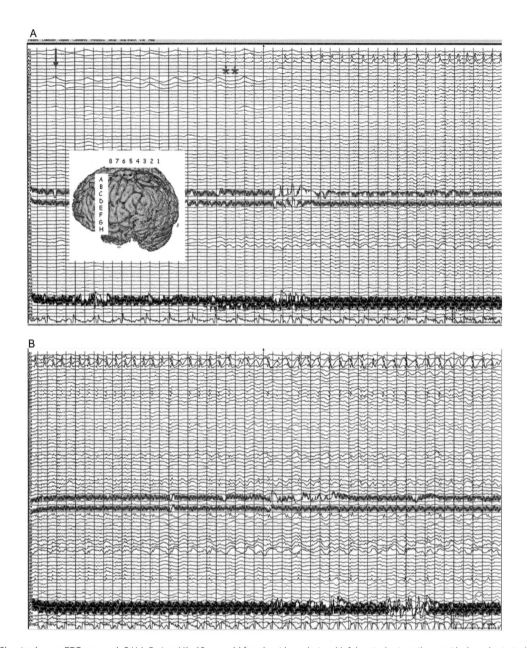

Figure 29.8. **A:** *Slow ictal onset EEG pattern (<5 Hz). Patient VA, 12-year-old female with nonlesional left hemispheric epilepsy with dysesthesia in the right foot. Slow onset (2-Hz waves) in the left superior parietal region (→), corresponding to the circled contacts. Five seconds later: rhythmic spikes in the adjacent region (**). IA and IP, anterior and posterior temporal subdural strips (not shown in the cartoon).* **B:** *Continuous rhythmic 5-Hz spiking in the contacts close to the sensory foot area, related to the patient's typical aura. However, persistent seizures postoperatively after a limited superior parietal resection suggest that the site of ictal onset does not coincide with the epileptogenic zone. Slow-onset rhythms (<5 Hz) are considered to be less likely associated to the true epileptogenic zone. This is true even when the slow onset pattern evolves to rhythmic discharges. Seizures continued after limited resection in the postcentral region.*

fibers the chronaxie is longer than that of myelinated fibers. In very young children, myelination is still incomplete; it gradually increases with age and is also site-dependent (i.e., myelination starts in the posterior cortices). Jayakar et al. (143) investigated the dual-increment approach in six patients between 1 and 10 years using pulse durations between 0.3 and 1 msec and increasing intensity starting at 1 mA up to 15 mA. With dual increment (i.e., alternating 1–2 mA and 0.1–0.2 msec increments), motor responses were obtained in three patients ages 1, 3, and 4.5 years and afterdischarges in 12 of the 14 electrodes, but there was no response with the adult paradigm. In three older children, ages 5.5, 7, and 10 years, the adult paradigm (i.e., with a fixed pulse duration of 0.3 msec)

and the dual-increment paradigm both elicited responses and afterdischarges in 16 of the 16 contacts.

An alternative approach in children (or adults) who cannot describe their feelings or collaborate with the examiner is the use of evoked potentials. In preoperative or perioperative monitoring, somatosensory or motor evoked potentials identified the localization of the central sulcus (144,145).

15. OUTLOOK

The indications for the use of intracranial electrodes in patient evaluation have undergone changes. Most patients with mesial

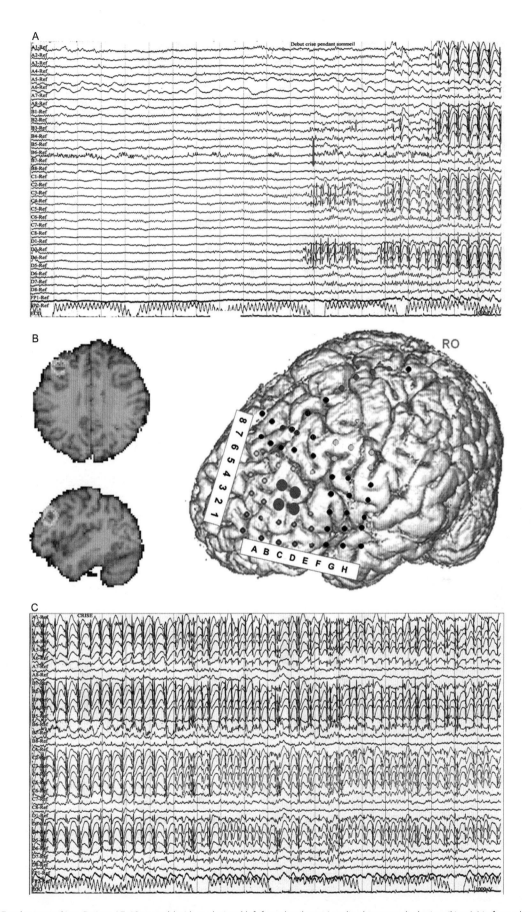

Figure 29.9. A: *Focal onset spiking. Patient AF, 18-year-old with nonlesional left frontal epilepsy. Localized onset as rhythmic spiking (→) in four selective subdural contacts (C3, C4, D3, D4) over the lateral anterior left frontal cortex. Within 5 seconds there is spread to other adjacent contacts. **B:** (Right) Localization of subdural electrodes co-registered with the patient's MRI. Contacts of seizure onset (see Fig. 29.8) are shown as large, dark gray circles. The iEEG localization of the ictal focus was concordant with the localization obtained by noninvasive electric source localization (left; see also Chapter 46). **C:** Persistent rhythmic spike-wave pattern continued. No clinical symptoms were seen or noted by the patient. A topectomy of the cortex underlying the four contacts resulted in marked improvement of the epilepsy disorder (i.e., one or two generalized tonic–clonic seizures per year if the patient forgot to take antiepileptic drugs). Focal onset (that is, onset in less than five contacts) is more likely related to a good outcome, as was the case here. Independently, ictal onset spiking has been described as another favorable sign in hippocampal seizures; it may also be truefor extratemporal lobe epilepsy.*

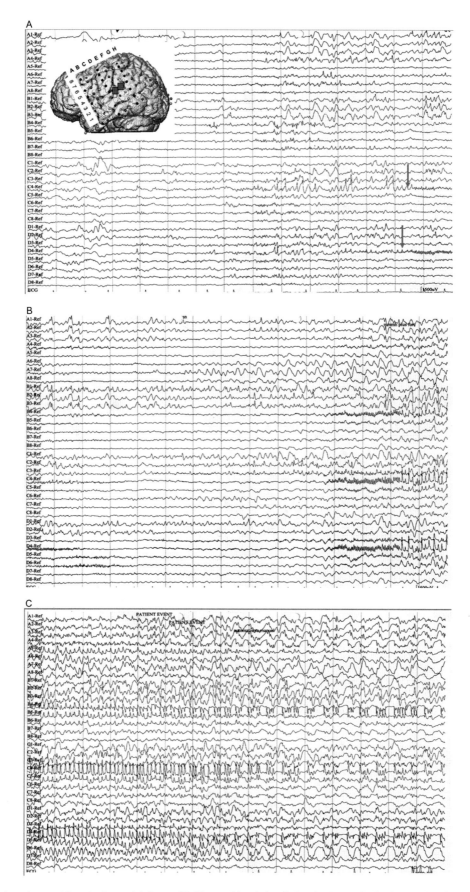

Figure 29.10. **A:** *Low-voltage beta activity at ictal onset (→). Patient CR, 20-year-old, right-handed, with transmantle dysplasia in the left posterior temporal cortex. Onset was characterized by rapid rhythms (>25 Hz) in two distinct contacts (D4 > C4). Left: Schema of electrodes co-registered to the patient's brain. Contacts corresponding to early ictal activity in black.* **B:** *Propagation to other contact over other temporal lateral cortex is noted. Discharges remain relatively well localized but become associated with clinical symptoms.* **C:** *Discharges continue, implicating the whole temporal lobe now, and to a lesser degree the frontal regions as well. The onset contacts remain the most active. Low-amplitude beta activity onset is considered a favorable sign in terms of seizure control. Indeed, resection of this area resulted in persistent seizure freedom (>5 years). Language comprehension was found to be localized in the contralateral hemisphere.*

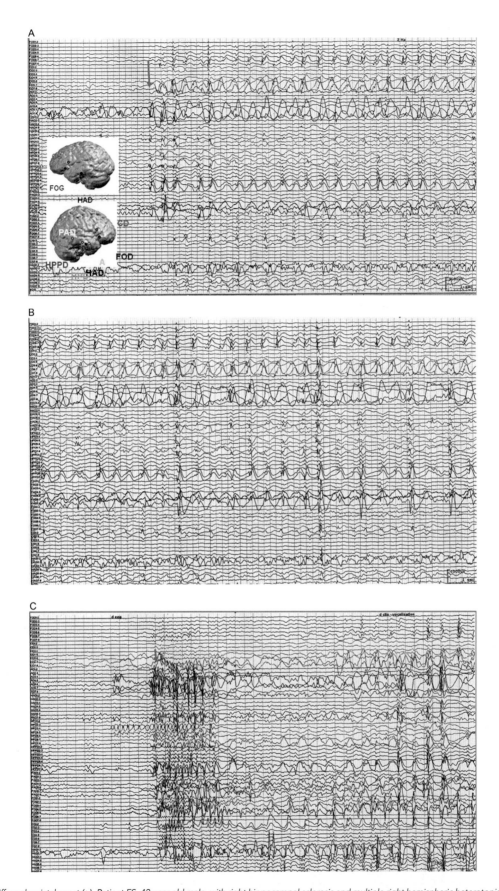

Figure 29.11. **A:** *Diffuse slow ictal onset (→). Patient FS, 42-year-old male, with right hippocampal sclerosis and multiple right hemispheric heterotopia. Poorly defined ictal onset: diffuse onset with 1- to 2-Hz sharp slow waves in right frontal (CD7-8), right lateral temporal (AD6-8), right parietal periventricular heterotopia (HPPD6-8). Left: Depth electrode position co-registered with the patient's brain.* **B:** *No further localization, but synchronous 1- to 2-Hz discharges of a network comprising fronto-orbital (FOD), right frontal lateral (CD), lateral temporal (AD), both right periventricular temporal (HPPTD), and parietal (PAD) heterotopia.* **C:** *Recording of another seizure, with simultaneous onset of the temporal lobe, heterotopias, and frontal structures, preceded by a brief hippocampal burst (HPD) of 6-Hz sharp waves. Resection of the hippocampus and partially the anterior heterotopia brought only partial seizure relief (decrease of 50%). Diffuse onset, even in the presence of structural lesions, is lesslikely related to good postoperative seizure control. Moreover, variable seizure-onset patterns were noted, another unfavorable prognostic factor.*

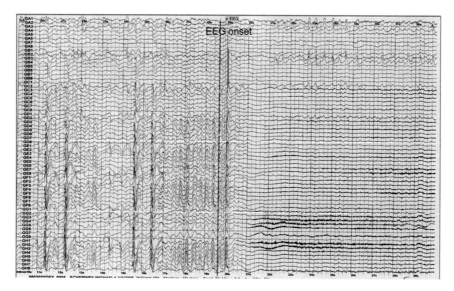

Figure 29.12. Gamma activity at onset. Patient MS, 15-year-old female with tuberous sclerosis. Largest tuber in the left posterior temporal lobe. Seizure onset presents as rapid gamma activity (>100 Hz; GG5-8; GH1-2). Interictally (before seizure onset) there are more widespread discharges over the left posterior cortex.

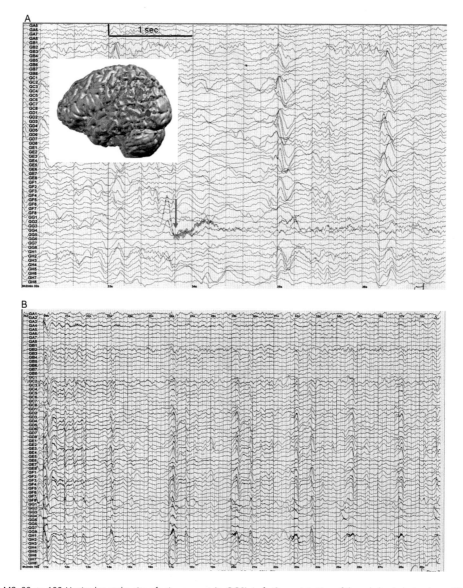

Figure 29.13. A: Patient MS: 80- to 100-Hz ripples at the site of seizure onset (→, GG3). Left: Co-registration of the subdural electrode positions with her brain. Site of ripple is indicated by dark gray circle. **B:** Patient MS: Diffuse semirhythmic sharp waves. Close analysis reveals the presence of rapid ripples riding on the discharges (max. GH2). Resection of the tissues underlying these ripples resulted in seizure freedom (follow-up 2 years) despite more diffuse spike and sharp wave discharges. Not only focal beta but also gamma activity at seizure onset is a good prognostic factor, despite the presence of multifocal lesions.

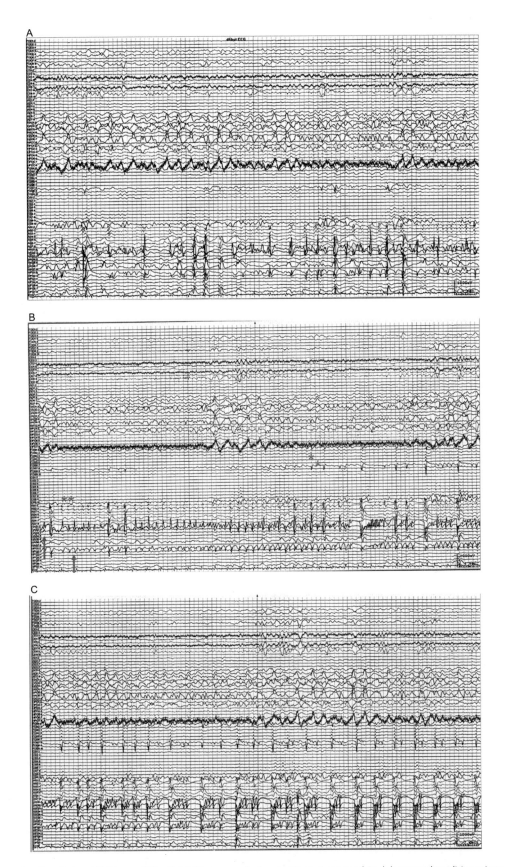

Figure 29.14. A: *Preictal spiking. Patient VT, 28 years old, with left hippocampal sclerosis. Monitoring was advised due to nonlateralizing seizure onset in ictal scalp EEGs. Depth electrodes were inserted orthogonally in both hemispheres. (Right: FOD, fronto-orbital; CD, frontal lateral cortex/anterior cingulate gyrus; AD, anterior temporal lobe/amygdala; HAD/HPD, anterior/posterior hippocampus. Left: FOG, CG, AG, HAG, HPG). Before the seizure, preictal spiking is noted in the sclerotic left hippocampus (HAG2-3, HPG2-3).* **B:** *Same patient. Unusual propagation pattern. Preictal spiking is replaced by rhythmic spiking in the left hippocampus (HAG2, HPG2, →). Recruitment occurs first in the lateral frontal cortex (FOG7-8, *). Small-amplitude discharges in the left amygdala become more rhythmic (AG1-2, 2-3, **). The smaller amplitude is explained by the closed electrical field of the amygdala as compared to the hippocampus.* **C:** *Recruitment in the lateral frontal cortex (FOG7-8) continues. Close analysis of the temporal pattern reveals that the discharges in the fronto-orbital cortex are 50 to 100 msec later than the large hippocampal spikes, indicating that the hippocampus drives the fronto-orbital discharges. There is no propagation to lateral temporal contacts (HAG7,8; HPG7,8), explaining retrospectively why the scalp EEG was unrevealing. The propagation pattern can show significant variability between patients and may even involve structures outside the lobe of onset, including the contralateral hemisphere.*

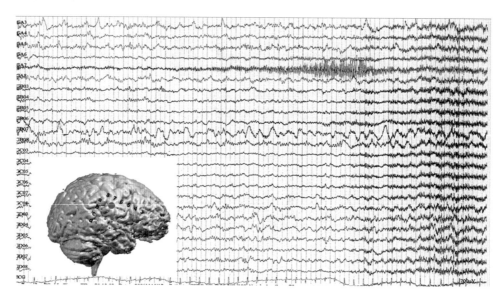

Figure 29.15. Low-amplitude gamma activity in extratemporal lobe epilepsy. Patient SC, 17 years old, with nonlesional right frontal epilepsy with daily nocturnal generalized tonic–clonic seizures (GTCS). Seizure onset is characterized by a very focal beta activity (GA7), which diffuses to other subdural contacts. Resection of the epileptogenic zone including the cortex underlying GA7 resulted in disappearance of GTCS (except once after sleep withdrawal), but persistence of short simple partial seizures (sensory–motor symptoms of the tongue). Focal low-amplitude rapid ictal onset activity is a favorable sign in extratemporal lobe epilepsy.

temporal epilepsy and hippocampal sclerosis do not need intracranial EEG monitoring if they have access to modern imaging techniques. Even patients with nonlesional epilepsy may not always need intracranial evaluation (146).

Despite advances in brain imaging, the rate of freedom from seizures is still lower in patients with extratemporal compared to temporal lobe epilepsy. The precision and yield of noninvasive imaging for patients with extratemporal lobe epilepsy remain under evaluation and will further improve. In the meantime, patients with conflicting results from noninvasive exams are still candidates for intracranial monitoring. Each intracranial evaluation needs a solid hypothesis as to where the seizures might have their origin. Intracranial EEG should not be a "fishing expedition," because even with EEG systems of 200 or more channels, not all possible brain regions can be covered; more importantly, the complication risk increases and may outweigh the benefit of the iEEG procedure. To obtain a valid hypothesis, co-registration and multimodal imaging may help to increase the yield of the invasive phase (147) (see also Chapter 46). Whole-head scalp EEG (or magnetoencephalographic) arrays of 200 or more electrodes/sensors, together with EEG source localization algorithms, were successfully employed in pediatric and adult patients with temporal and extratemporal lobe epilepsy for focus localization (148.149). Use of high-density intracranial recordings (200 or more electrodes) may overcome the difficulty involved in precisely locating the focus. Intracranial recordings pick up near-field activity and 1 cm farther away, the attenuation of the interictal epileptiform discharge might be already too high and impair its detection.

Intracranial EEG may be used for other purposes in addition to determining the seizure focus. A number of studies have tried to use intracranial EEG recordings to determine the neuropsychological functionality of distinct brain structures. For example, ongoing seizure activity was used as an "electrical Wada test" (150), the presence or absence of N400 components as well as HFOs was used as an indicator of (healthy) mnestic processes (151–154), or event-related gamma activity was used during naming to localize language cortex (155). In the past 5 years, the use of commercially available microelectrodes has opened a new view on the human brain, allowing the recording of single spikes from a few or single neurons. The future will tell us if microelectrodes need to be added to the macroelectrodes setup to determine unambiguously the seizure onset zone.

Intracranial monitoring imposes a certain burden on the patient and family, both on the psychological and physical level, and the indication must be carefully weighed against the possible benefit. In most centers and studies, the proportion of patients who cannot be offered surgery, despite intracranial monitoring, is around ~25% to 30%. Future studies will show if with the addition of sophisticated noninvasive brain imaging this percentage can be lowered, either because nonsurgical candidates can be more easily identified or because the seizure onset zone is already identified and iEEG is no more required.

ACKNOWLEDGMENTS

Supported by the Swiss National Science Foundation (grant No 146633 and 140332). M.S. is grateful to Karl Schaller for helpful comments on the neurosurgical aspects of intracranial EEG. Dr. Vitalo Chiosa and Dr. Laurent Spinelli provided invaluable help in the preparation of figures.

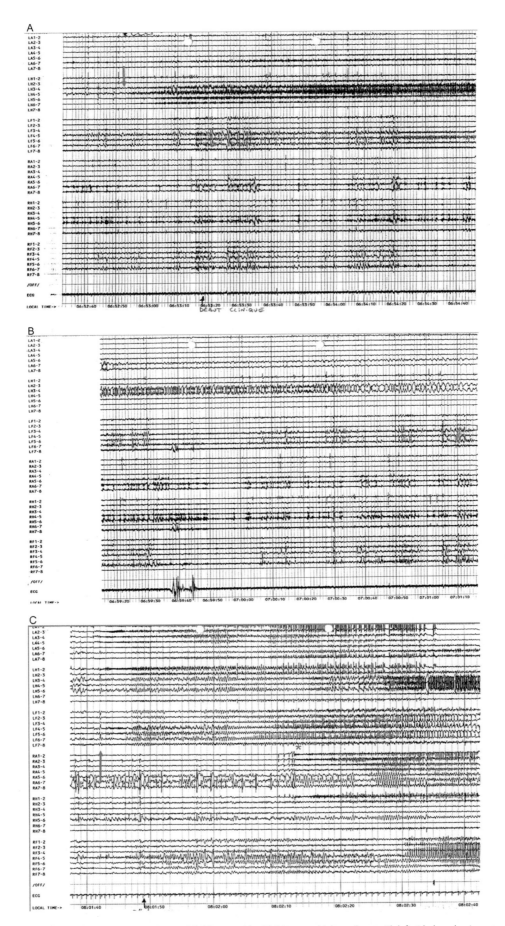

Figure 29.16. A: *Significance of different onset patterns. Patient BE, 43 years old, with bitemporal lobe epilepsy with left-sided predominance, which started after vaccination at the age of 7 years. MRI shows bilateral atrophy. Onset is characterized by beta activity in the left parahippocampal gyrus (LH4-5 and adjacent contacts, →). RF/LF, right/left fronto-orbital cortex; RA, toward right amygdala (LA, left amygdala); RH/LH, toward right/left hippocampus.* **B:** *Offset pattern of this seizure in the same contacts as the seizure onset (parahippocampal gyrus, LH3-4, LH4-5).* **C:** *Another seizure that also started with focal beta activity but is now in the left amygdala and hippocampus (LH1-2, LA2-3, LA1-2, →), leading to recruitment of right mesial temporal structures (RA1-2, RA2-3, RH-1-2, *). Variable onset patterns are less favorable signs. Indeed, selective resection of left mesial temporal structures did not lead to persistent seizurefreedom, although the incidence was reduced by ~70%.*

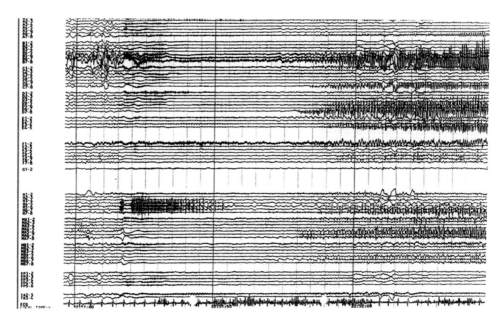

Figure 29.17. Diffuse EEG onset. Patient SG, 20-year-old male, with epilepsy onset at the age of 3. The scalp EEG showed almost continuous discharges over the left frontal lateral cortex. An 8×8 subdural grid was implanted over the left frontal and temporal cortex. Seizure onset was noted simultaneously over frontal and temporal regions (B5-6, 6-7, 7-8; H5-6, 6-7, 7-8). Limited resection of left frontal cortex due to the presence of language cortex (histopathology: severe cortical dysplasia) did not control seizures persistently.

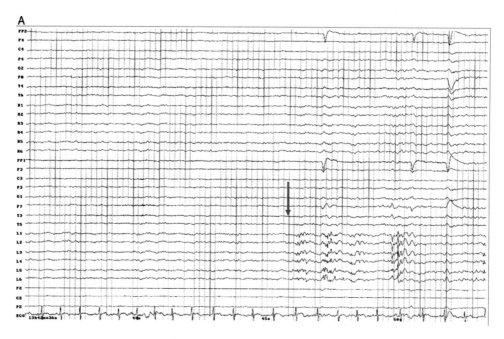

Figure 29.18. A: Ictal recording with FOEs. Patient ES: 21 years old, left-handed, known for seizures since the age of 9. Left hippocampal sclerosis. Scalp ictal EEG showed left, right, or bitemporal onset. Interictal spikes were found over left and right temporal lobes with variable predominance. FOEs were inserted bilaterally (left: L1-6; right: R1-6) and recorded together with scalp electrodes. Ictal recording with first changes in the left FOE. **B:** The seizure evolves, with few changes in the corresponding scalp electrodes. **C:** A low-amplitude beta activity starts (*). **D:** Beta activity persists, with still few changes in the scalp EEG and no clinical symptoms. Thus, FOEs can record focal hippocampal ictal activity with higher sensitivity than scalp EEG.

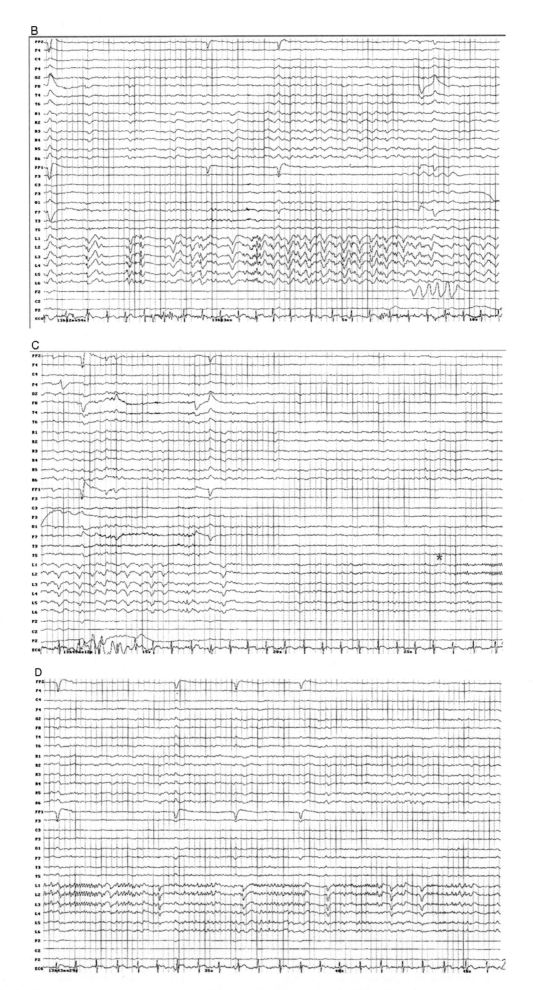

Figure 29.18. Continued

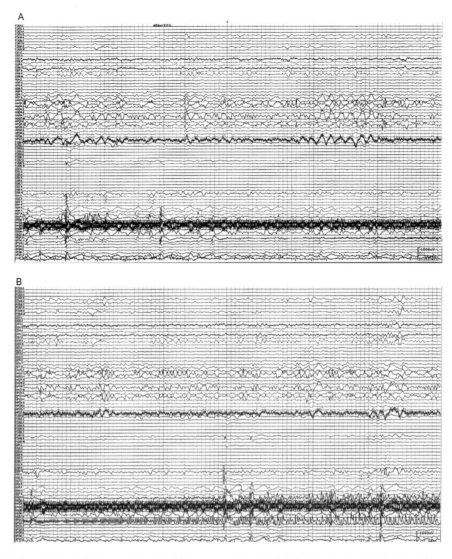

Figure 29.19. A: *Subclinical seizures. Patient VT, 28 years old, with left hippocampal sclerosis. Subclinical seizure in the left sclerotic hippocampus (>30-Hz beta activity) with very focal onset (in one contact, HPG2). No further recruitment is observed. Clinical symptoms are limited to deficient verbal memory. **B:** Subclinical seizure pattern gradually stops and discharges are of lower frequency. Multichannel iEEGs need to be carefully scrutinized because they may involve only one channel. If frequent, they usually indicate a high epileptogenicity of the recorded structure.*

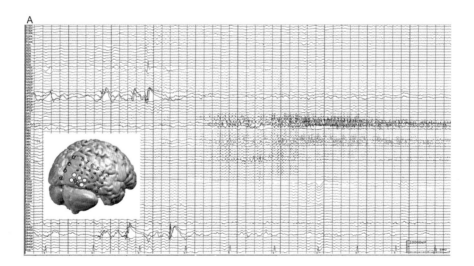

Figure 29.20. A: *Ictal beta activity, less focal. Patient RP, 24 years old, diagnosed with nonlesional right temporal epilepsy. Noninvasive workup found right anterior and posterior temporal discharges. After ESI localizing the focus to posterior temporal regions, careful review of the MRI showed focal polymicrogyria in the temporo-occipital junction. A subdural grid was placed there, as well as depth electrodes in the left and right temporal (right: AD, HAD, HPD; left: AG, HMG) and frontal regions (CD, FOD). **B:** Beta activity persists, becoming more rhythmic and organized. Around 10 sec after EEG onset in the temporo-occipital cortex, there is recruitment of the right hippocampus (→). **C:** Persistence of right-sided seizure activity, with left hippocampal recruitment (→). **D:** Posterior and bihippocampal discharges persist. This recruitment pattern may explain why the patient is amnesic of the entire event. Seizures came back 2 years after resection of the polymicrogyric cortex but subsided again after adaptation of drug treatment. Less focal (>5 Hz) EEG onset, together with a less organized rhythm at the beginning, may reflect a more widespread epileptogenic zone.*

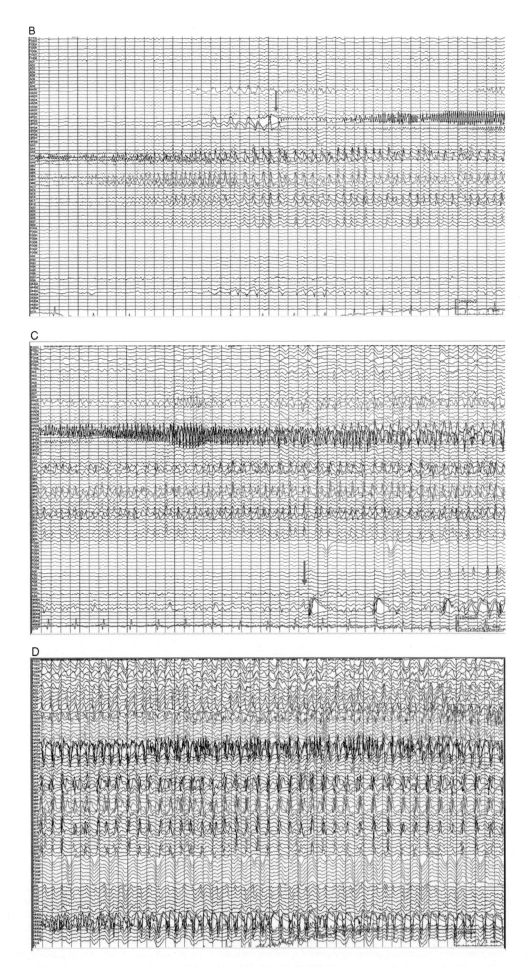

Figure 29.20. Continued

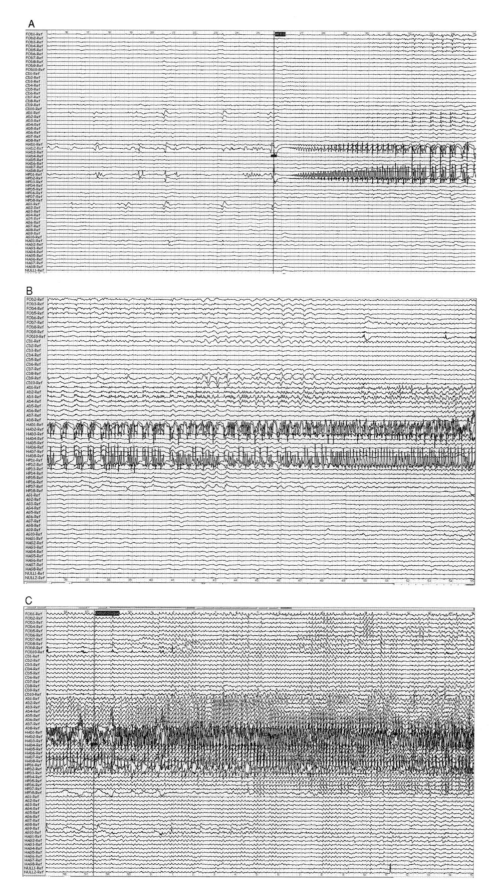

Figure 29.21. *A: Focal onset with late recruitment and contralateral offset. Patient SS, 37 years old, right-handed, with non-lesional right temporal lobe epilepsy. Depth electrodes were implanted in both temporal lobes and right frontal lobe. Onset is characterized by high-amplitude spiking, mixed with beta activity. Onset is restricted to four contacts in the right mesial temporal lobe (HAD1,2, HPD1,2; AG and HAG, left anterior and midtemporal lobe, respectively; FOD, fronto-orbital; CD, right frontal lateral).* ***B:*** *Focal discharges persist, with somewhat more recruitment of the right amygdala (AD1-3). Each page contains 20 sec of EEG.* ***C:*** *After 29 sec there is recruitment of lateral temporal and fronto-orbital contacts.* ***D:*** *Only very late (>40 sec) is there recruitment of the contralateral hippocampus (*).* ***E:*** *While the right-sided discharges subside, ictal spiking in the left hippocampus persists until the end of the seizure.* ***F:*** *The patient underwent a selective right antero-mesial temporal resection and has been seizure-free since (histopathology: cortical dysplasia). Focal onset (<5 contacts) and persistent focality are advantageous findings. However, offset in the contralateral hemisphere is obviously less predictive of postoperative outcome.*

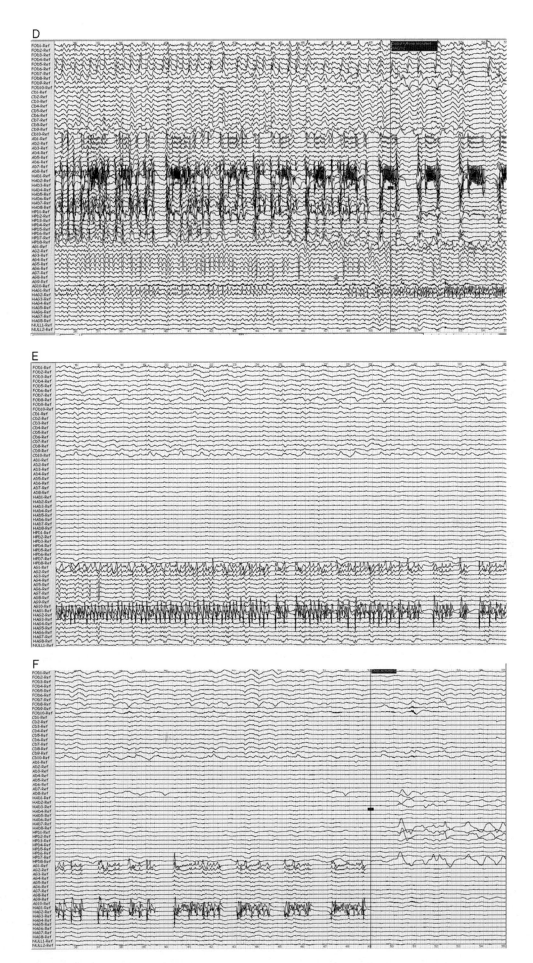

Figure 29.21. Continued

REFERENCES

1. Tonini C, Beghi E, Berg AT, et al. Predictors of epilepsy surgery outcome: a meta-analysis. Epilepsy Res. 2004;62:75–87.
2. Cendes F, Li LM, Watson C, et al. Is ictal recording mandatory in temporal lobe epilepsy? Arch Neurol. 2000;57:497–500.
3. Diehl B, Lüders HO. Temporal lobe epilepsy: when are invasive recordings are needed? Epilepsia. 2000;41(supp 3):S61–S74.
4. Hurst R, Chiota-McCollum N, Tatum W. Adult absence semiology misinterpreted as mesial temporal lobe epilepsy. Epileptic Disord. 2014;16:471–476.
5. Reuber M, Kral T, Kurthen M, Elger CE. New-onset psychogenic seizures after intracranial neurosurgery. Acta Neurochir (Wien). 2002;144:901–907.
6. Fourth level-epilepsy surgical center for epilepsy. Epilepsia. 1990;31(suppl 1):S7–S8.
7. Harvey S, Cross JH, Shinnar S, Mathern GW, and ILAE Pediatric Epilepsy Surgery Survey Taskforce. Defining the spectrum of internation practice in pediatric epilepsy surgery patients. Epilepsia. 2008;49:146–155.
8. Srikijvilaikul T, Locharernkul C, Deesudchit T, et al. The first invasive EEG monitoring for surgical treatment of epilepsy in Thailand. J Med Assoc Thai. 2006;89:527–532.
9. Seeck M, Lazeyras F, Michel CM, et al. Non-invasive epileptic focus localization using EEG-triggered functional MRI and electromagnetic tomography. Electroencephalogr Clin Neurophysiol. 1998;106:508–512.
10. O'Brien TJ, Miles K, Ware R, et al. The cost-effective use of 18F-FDG PET in the presurgical evaluation of medically refractory focal epilepsy. J Nucl Med. 2008;49:931–937.
11. O'Brien TJ, So EL, Mullan BP, et al. Subtraction ictal SPECT co-registered to MRI improves clinical usefulness of SPECT in localizing the surgical seizure focus. Neurology. 1998;50:445–454.
12. Laxer KD. Clinical applications of magnetic resonance spectroscopy. Epilepsia. 1997;38(Suppl 4):S13–17.
13. Knowlton RC, Elgavish RA, Limdi N, et al. Functional imaging: I. Relative predictive value of intracranial electroencephalography. Ann Neurol. 2008;64:25–34.
14. Duncan JS. The current status of neuroimaging for epilepsy. Curr Opin Neurol. 2009;22:179–184.
15. Briellmann RS, Pell GS, Wellard RM, et al. MR imaging of epilepsy: state of the art at 1.5 T and potential of 3 T. Epileptic Disord. 2003;5:3–20.
16. Lascano AM, Perneger T, Vulliemoz S, et al. Yield of non-invasive state-of-the-art imaging techniques in epilepsy surgery candidates. Clin Neurophysiol. 2016;127:150–155.
17. Sirven JI, Malamut BL, Liporace JD, et al. Outcome after temporal lobectomy in bilateral temporal lobe epilepsy. Ann Neurol. 1997;42:873–878.
18. Holmes MD, Dodrill CB, Ojemann GA, et al. Outcome following surgery in patients with bitemporal interictal epileptiform patterns. Neurology. 1997;48:1037–1040.
19. Hirsch LJ, Spencer SS, Spencer DD, et al. Temporal lobectomy in patients with bitemporal epilepsy defined by depth electroencephalography. Ann Neurol. 1991;30:347–356.
20. Boling W, Aghakhani Y, Andermann F, Sziklas V, Olivier A. Surgical treatment of independent bitemporal lobe epilepsy defined by invasive recordings. J Neurol Neurosurg Psychiatry. 2009;80:533–538.
21. Mintzer S, Cendes F, Soss J, et al. Unilateral hippocampal sclerosis with contralateral temporal scalp ictal onset. Epilepsia. 2004;45:792–802.
22. Carne RP, O'Brien TJ, Kilpatrick CJ, et al. MRI-negative PET-positive temporal lobe epilepsy: a distinct surgically remediable syndrome. Brain. 2004;127:2276–2285.
23. Gok B, Jallo G, Hayeri R, et al. The evaluation of FDG-PET imaging for epileptogenic focus localization in patients with MRI positive and MRI negative temporal lobe epilepsy. Neuroradiology. 2013; 55:541–550.
24. LoPinto-Khoury C, Sperling M, Skidmore C, et al. Surgical outcome in PET-positive, MRI negative patients with temporal lobe epilepsy. Epilepsia. 2012;53:342–348.
25. Michel CM, Lantz G, Spinelli L, et al. 128-channel EEG source imaging in epilepsy: clinical yield and localization precision. J Clin Neurophysiol. 2004;21:71–83.
26. Brodbeck V, Lascano A, Spinelli L, et al. Accuracy of electrical source imaging of epileptic spikes in patients with large brain lesions. J Clin Neurophysiol. 2009;120:679–685.
27. Grouiller F, Delattre BM, Pittau F, et al. All-in-one interictal presurgical imaging in patients with epilepsy: single-session EEG/PET/(f)MRI. Eur J Nucl Med Mol Imaging. 2015 Jun;42(7):1133–1143.
28. Berger H. Über das Elektrenkephalogramm des Menschen. Arch fur Psychiatr. 1929;87:527–570.
29. Penfield W, Jasper H. Epilepsy and the Functional Anatomy of the Human Brain. Boston: Little, Brown, 1954.
30. Talairach J, Bancaud J. Stereotaxic exploration and therapy in epilepsy. In: Vinken PJ, Bruyn G (Eds): The epilepsies. Handbook of Clinical Neurology, Vol 15. Amsterdam: North Holland, 1974:758–782.
31. Talairach J, Bancaud J. Stereotactic approach to epilepsy. Prog Neurol Surg, 1973;5:297–354,
32. Wyler AR, Ojemann GA, Lettich E, Ward AA. Subdural strip electrodes for localizing epileptogenic foci. J Neurosurg. 1984;60:1195–1200.
33. Ives JR, Mainwaring NR, Gruber LJ, et al. 128-channel cable-telemetry EEG recording system for long-term invasive monitoring. Electroencephalogr Clin Neurophysiol. 1991;79:69–72.
34. Siegfried J, Wieser HG, Stodieck SR. Foramen ovale electrodes: a new technique enabling presurgical evaluation of patients with mesiobasal temporal lobe seizures. Appl Neurophysiol. 1985;48(1–6):408–417.
35. Barnett GH, Burgess RC, Awad IA, et al. Epidural peg electrodes for the presurgical evaluation of intractable epilepsy. Neurosurgery. 1990;27:113–115.
36. Tao JX, Ray A, Hawes-Ebersole S, Ebersole JS. Intracranial EEG substrates of scalp EEG interictal spikes. Epilepsia. 2005;46:669–676.
37. Ray A, Tao JX, Hawes-Ebersole SM, Ebersole JS. Localizing value of scalp EEG spikes: a simultaneous scalp and intracranial study. Clin Neurophysiol. 2007;118:69–79.
38. Ebersole JS, Hawes-Ebersole S. Clinical application of dipole models in the localization of epileptiform activity. J Clin Neurophysiol. 2007;24:120–129.
39. Koessler L, Cecchin T, Colnat-Coulbois S, et al. Catching the invisible: mesial temporal source contribution to simultaneous EEG and SEEG recordings. Brain Topogr. 2015;28(1):5–20.
40. Ramantani G, Dümpelmann M, Koessler L, et al. Simultaneous subdural and scalp EEG correlates of frontal lobe epileptic sources. Epilepsia. 2014;55(2):278–288.
41. Rosenow F, Lüders H. Presurgical evaluation of epilepsy. Brain. 2001;124:1683–1700.
42. Knowlton RC, Elgavish RA, Limdi N, et al. Functional imaging: I. Relative predictive value of intracranial electroencephalography. Ann Neurol. 2008;64(1):25–34.
43. Wong CH, Birkett J, Byth K, et al. Risk factors for complications during intracranial electrode recording in presurgical evaluation of drug resistant partial epilepsy. Acta Neurochir. 2009;151:37–50.
44. Burneo JG, Steven DA, McLachlan RS, Parrent AG. Morbidity associated with the use of intracranial electrodes for epilepsy surgery. Can J Neurol Sci. 2006;33:223–227.
45. Cordova JE, Rowe RE, Furman MD, et al. A method for imaging of intracranial EEG electrodes using magnetic resonance imaging. Comput Biomed Res. 1994;27:337–341.
46. Winkler PA, Vollmar C, Krishnan KG, et al. Usefulness of 3-D reconstructed images of the human cerebral cortex for localization of subdural electrodes in epilepsy surgery. Epilepsy Res. 2000;41:169–178.
47. Silberbusch MA, Rothman MI, Bergey GK, et al. Subdural grid implantation for intracranial EEG recording: CT and MR appearance. AJNR Am J Neuroradiol. 1998;19:1089–1093.
48. Kovalev D, Spreer J, Honegger J, et al. Rapid and fully automated visualization of subdural electrodes in the presurgical evaluation of epilepsy patients. AJNR Am J Neuroradiol. 2005;26:1078–1083.
49. Sebastiano F, Di Gennaro G, Esposito V, et al. A rapid and reliable procedure to localize subdural electrodes in presurgical evaluation of patients with drug-resistant focal epilepsy. Clin Neurophysiol. 2006;117:341–347.
50. Mahvash M, König R, Wellmer J, et al. Coregistration of digital photography of the human cortex and cranial magnetic resonance imaging for visualization of subdural electrodes in epilepsy surgery. Neurosurgery. 2007;61:340–344.
51. Tao JX, Hawes-Ebersole S, Baldwin M, et al. The accuracy and reliability of 3D CT/MRI co-registration in planning epilepsy surgery. Clin Neurophysiol. 2009;120:748–753.
52. Seeck M, Spinelli L. Intracranial monitoring [Review]. Suppl Clin Neurophysiol. 2004;57:485–493.
53. Dykstra AR, Chan AM, Quinn BT, et al. Individualized localization and cortical surface-based registration of intracranial electrodes. Neuroimage. 2012;59(4):3563–3570.
54. Mahvash M, König R, Urbach H, et al. FLAIR-/T1-/T2-co-registration for image-guided diagnostic and resective epilepsy surgery. Neurosurgery. 2008;62(Suppl 2):482–488.
55. Pieters TA, Conner CR, Tandon N. Recursive grid partitioning on a cortical surface model: an optimized techniques for the localization of implanted subdural electrodes. J Neurosurg. 2013;118:1086–1097.

56. Maurer Jr CR, Fitzpatrick JM, Wang MY, et al. Registration of head volume images using implantable fiducial markers. IEEE Trans Med Imaging. 1997;16:447–562.
57. Spire WJ, Jobst BC, Thadani VM, et al. Robotic image-guided depth electrode implantation in the evaluation of medically intractable epilepsy. Neurosurg Focus. 2008;25:E19.
58. Van Buren JM. Complications of surgical procedures in the diagnosis and treatment of epilepsy. In: Engel J, ed. Surgical Treatment of the Epilepsies. New York: Raven Press, 1987:465–475.
59. Ross DA, Brunberg JA, Drury I, Henry TR. Intracerebral depth electrode monitoring in partial epilepsy: the morbidity and efficacy of placement using magnetic resonance image-guided stereotactic surgery. Neurosurgery. 1996;39:327–334.
60. Sansur CA, Frysinger RC, Pouratian N, et al. Incidence of symptomatic hemorrhage after sterotactic electrode placement. J Neurosurg. 2007;107:998–1003.
61. Tanriverdi T, Ajlan A, Poulin N, Olivier A. Morbidity in epilepsy surgery: an experience based on 2449 epilepsy surgery procedures from a single institution. J Neurosurg. 2009;110:1111–1123.
62. Almeida AN, Martinez V, Feindel W. The first case of invasive EEG monitoring for the treatment of epilepsy: historical significance and context. Epilepsia. 2005;46:1082–1085.
63. Erőss L, Bagó AG, Entz L, et al. Neuronavigation and fluoroscopy-assisted subdural strip electrode positioning: a simple method to increase intraoperative accuracy of strip localization in epilepsy surgery. J Neurosurg. 2009;110:327–331.
64. Chamoun RB, Nayar VV, Yoshor D. Neuronavigation applied to epilepsy monitoring with subdural electrodes. Neurosurg Focus. 2008;25:E21.
65. Salam MT, Gelinas S, Desgent S, et al. Subdural porous and notched mini-grid electrodes for wireless intracranial electroencephalographic recordings. J Multidisciplinary Healthcare. 2014;7:573–586.
66. Viventi J, Kim DH, Vigeland L, et al. Flexible, foldable, actively multiplexed, high-density electrode array for mapping brain activity in vivo. Nat Neurosci. 2011;14:1599–1605.
67. Seeck M, Pegna A, Ortigue S, et al. Speech arrest with stimulation may not reliably predict language deficit after epilepsy surgery. Neurology. 2006;66:592–594.
68. Wyler AR, Walker G. The morbidity of long-term seizure monitoring using subdural strip electrodes. J Neurosurg. 1991;74:734–737.
69. Lee WS, Lee JK, Lee SA, et al. Complications and results of subdural grid electrode implantation in epilepsy surgery. Surg Neurol. 2000;54:346–351.
70. Onal C, Otsubo H, Araki T, et al. Complications of invasive subdural grid monitoring in children with epilepsy. J Neurosurg. 2003;98:1017–1026.
71. Musleh W, Yassari R, Hecox K, et al. Low incidence of subdural grid-related complications in prolonged pediatric EEG monitoring. Pediatr Neurosurg. 2006;42:284–287.
72. Jobst BC, Williamson PD, Coughlin CT, et al. An unusual complication of intracranial electrodes. Epilepsia. 2000;41:898–902.
73. Hamer HM, Morris HH, Mascha EJ, et al. Complications of invasive video-EEG monitoring with subdural grid electrodes. Neurology. 2002;58:97–103.
74. Wiggins GC, Elisevich K, Smith BJ. Morbidity and infection in combined subdural grid and strip electrode investigation for intractable epilepsy. Epilepsy Res. 1999;37:73–80.
75. Araki T, Otsubo H, Makino Y, et al. Efficacy of dexamethasone on cerebral swelling and seizures during subdural grid EEG recording in children. Epilepsia. 2006;47:176–180.
76. Sahjpaul RL, Mahon J, Wiebe S. Dexamethasone for morbidity after subdural electrode insertion—a randomized controlled trial. Can J Neurol Sci. 2003;30:340–348.
77. Sperling MR, O'Connor MJ. Comparison of depth and subdural electrodes in recording temporal lobe seizures. Neurology. 1989;39:1497.
78. Spencer SS, Spencer DD, Williamson PD, Mattson R. Combined depth and subdural electrode investigation in uncontrolled epilepsy. Neurology. 1990;40:74–9.
79. Brekelmans GJF, Van Emde Boas W, Velis DN, et al. Comparison of combined versus subdural or intracerebral electrodes alone in presurgical focus localization. Epilepsia. 1998; 39:1290–1301.
80. Eisenschenk S, Gilmore RL, Cibula JE, Roper SN. Lateralization of temporal lobe foci: depth versus subdural electrodes. Clin Neurophysiol. 2001;112:836–844.
81. Wieser HG, Elger CE, Stodieck SR. The "foramen ovale electrode": a new recording method for the preoperative evaluation of patients suffering from mesio-basal temporal lobe epilepsy. Electroencephalogr Clin Neurophysiol. 1985;61:314–322.
82. Fernandez Torre JL, Alarcon G, Binnie CD, Polkey CE. Comparison of sphenoidal, foramen ovale and anterior temporal placements for detecting interictal epileptiform discharges in presurgical assessment for temporal lobe epilepsy. Clin Neurophysiol. 1999;110:895–904.
83. Marks DA, Katz A, Booke J, et al. Comparison and correlation of surface and sphenoidal electrodes with simultaneous intracranial recording: an interictal study. Electroencephalogr Clin Neurophysiol. 1992;82:23–29.
84. Otsubo H, Ochi A, Imai K, et al. High-frequency oscillations of ictal muscle activity and epileptogenic discharges on intracranial EEG in a temporal lobe epilepsy patient. Clin Neurophysiol. 2008;119:862–868.
85. Hufnagel A, Dümpelmann M, Zentner J, et al. Clinical relevance of quantified intracranial interictal spike activity in presurgical evaluation of epilepsy. Epilepsia. 2000;41:467–478.
86. Asano E, Muzik O, Shah A, et al. Quantitative interictal subdural EEG analyses in children with neocortical epilepsy. Epilepsia. 2003;44:425–434.
87. Engel J. Outcome with respect to epileptic seizures. In: Engel J Jr, ed. Surgical Treatment of the Epilepsies. New York: Raven Press, 1987:553–571.
88. Bautista RE, Cobbs MA, Spencer DD, Spencer SS. Prediction of surgical outcome by interictal epileptiform abnormalities during intracranial EEG monitoring in patients with extrahippocampal seizures. Epilepsia. 1999;40:880–890.
89. Dümpelmann M, Elger CE. Visual and automatic investigation of epileptiform spikes in intracranial EEG recordings. Epilepsia. 1999;40:275–285.
90. Palmini A, Gambardella A, Andermann F, et al. Intrinsic epileptogenicity of human dysplastic cortex as suggested by corticography and surgical results. Ann Neurol. 1995;37:476–487.
91. Gambardella A, Palmini A, Andermann F, et al. Usefulness of focal rhythmic discharges on scalp EEG of patients with focal cortical dysplasia and intractable epilepsy. Electroencephalogr Clin Neurophysiol. 1996;98:243–249.
92. Hirabayashi S, Binnie CD, Janota I, Polkey CE. Surgical treatment of epilepsy due to cortical dysplasia: clinical and EEG findings. J Neurol Neurosurg Psychiatry. 1993;56:765–770.
93. Turkdogan D, Duchowny M, Resnick T, Jayakar P. Subdural EEG patterns in children with Taylor-type cortical dysplasia: comparison with nondysplastic lesions. Clin Neurophysiol. 2005;22:37–42.
94. Guerreiro MM, Quesney LF, Salanova V, Snipes GJ. Continuous electrocorticogram epileptiform discharges due to brain gliosis. J Clin Neurophysiol. 2003;20:239–242.
95. Zhang Y, van Drongelen W, Kohrman M, He B. Three-dimensional brain current source reconstruction from intra-cranial ECoG recordings. Neuroimage. 2008;42:683–695.
96. Michel CM, Lantz G, Spinelli L, et al. 128-channel EEG source imaging in epilepsy: clinical yield and localization precision. J Clin Neurophysiol. 2004;21:71–83.
97. Sperli F, Spinelli L, Seeck M, et al. EEG source imaging in pediatric epilepsy surgery: a new perspective in presurgical workup. Epilepsia. 2006;47:981–990.
98. Jung WY, Pacia SV, Devinsky O. Neocortical temporal lobe epilepsy: intracranial EEG features and surgical outcome. J Clin Neurophysiol. 1999;16:419–425.
99. Wennberg R, Arruda F, Quesney LF, Olivier A. Preeminence of extrahippocampal structures in the generation of mesial temporal seizures: evidence from human depth electrode recordings. Epilepsia. 2002;43:716–726.
100. Lee SA, Spencer DD, Spencer SS. Intracranial EEG seizure-onset patterns in neocortical epilepsy. Epilepsia. 2000;41:297–307.
101. Wetjen N, Marsh WR, Myer FB, et al. Intracranial electroencephalography seizure onset patterns and surgical outcomes in non-lesional extratemporal epilepsy. J Neurosurg. 2009;110:1147–1152.
102. Kutsy RL, Farrell DF, Ojemann GA. Ictal patterns of neocortical seizures monitored with intracranial electrodes: correlation with surgical outcome. Epilepsia. 1999;40:257–266.
103. McGonigal A, Bartolomei F, Régis J, et al. Stereoelectroencephalography in presurgical assessment of MRI-negative epilepsy. Brain. 2007;130:3169–3183.
104. Spencer SS, Guimaraes P, Katz A, et al. Morphological patterns of seizures recorded intracranially. Epilepsia. 1992;33:537–545.
105. Fisher R, Weber W, Lesser R, et al. High-frequency EEG activity at the start of seizures. J Clin Neurophysiol. 1992;83:229–235.
106. Schiller Y, Cascino GD, Busacker NE, Sharbrough FW. Characterization and comparison of local onset and remote propagated electrographic seizures recorded with intracranial electrodes. Epilepsia. 1998;39:380–388.
107. Blumenfeld H, Rivera M, McNally KA, et al. Ictal neocortical slowing in temporal lobe epilepsy. Neurology. 2004;63:1015–1021.

108. Spencer SS, Kim J, Spencer DD. Ictal spikes: a marker of specific hippocampal cell loss. Electroencephalogr Clin Neurophysiol. 1992;83:104–111.

109. Townsend JB, Engel J Jr. Clinicopathological correlation of low voltage fast and high amplitude spike and wave mesial temporal stereoencephalographic ictal onsets. Epilepsia. 1991;32 (suppl 3):21.

110. Schuh LA, Henry TR, Ross DA, et al. Ictal spiking patterns recorded from temporal depth electrodes predict good outcome after anterior temporal lobectomy. Epilepsia. 2000;41:316–319.

111. Faught E, Kuzniecky RI, Hurst DC. Ictal EEG wave forms from epidural electrodes predictive of seizure control after temporal lobectomy. Electroencephalogr Clin Neurophysiol. 1992;83:229–235.

112. Adam C, Saint-Hilaire JM, Richer F. Temporal and spatial characteristics of intracerebral seizure propagation: predictive value in surgery for temporal lobe epilepsy. Epilepsia. 1994;35:1065–1072.

113. Lieb JP, Engel J Jr, Babb TL. Interhemispheric propagation time of human hippocampal seizures. I. Relationship to surgical outcome. Epilepsia. 1986;27:286–293.

114. Schiller Y, Cascino GD, Busacker NE, Sharborough FW. Characterization and comparison of local onset and remote propagated electrographic seizures recorded with intracranial electrodes. Epilepsia. 1998;39:380–388.

115. Zaveri HP, Pincus SM, Goncharova II, et al. Localization-related epilepsy exhibits significant connectivity away from the seizure-onset area. NeuroReport 2009;20:891–895.

116. Brekelmans GJF, Velis DN, van Veelen CWM, et al. Intracranial EEG seizure off-set termination patterns: relation to outcome of epilepsy surgery in temporal lobe epilepsy. Epilepsia. 1998;39:259–266.

117. Spencer SS, Spencer DD. Implication of seizure termination location in temporal lobe epilepsy. Epilepsia. 1996;37:455–458.

118. Verma A, Lewis D, VanLandingham KE, et al. Lateralized seizure termination: relationship to outcome following anterior temporal lobectomy. Epilepsy Res. 2001;47:9–15.

119. Fisher RS, Webber WR, Lesser RP, et al. High-frequency EEG activity at the start of seizures. J Clin Neurophysiol. 1992;9:441–448.

120. Engel J Jr, Bragin A, Staba R, Mody I. High-frequency oscillations: what is normal and what is not? Epilepsia. 2009;50:598–604.

121. Bragin A, Wilson CL, Staba RJ, et al. Interictal high-frequency oscillations (80–500 Hz) in the human epileptic brain: entorhinal cortex. Ann Neurol. 2002;52(4):407–415.

122. Staba RJ, Wilson CL, Bragin A, et al. High-frequency oscillations recorded in human medial temporal lobe during sleep. Ann Neurol. 2004;56:108–115.

123. Worrell GA, Parish L, Cranstoun SD, et al. High-frequency oscillations and seizure generation in neocortical epilepsy. Brain. 2004;127(Pt 7):1496–1506.

124. Urrestarazu E, Chander R, Dubeau F, Gotman J. Interictal high-frequency oscillations (100–500 Hz) in the intracerebral EEG of epileptic patients. Brain. 2007;130:2354–2366.

125. Worrell GA, Gardner AB, Stead SM, et al. High-frequency oscillations in human temporal lobe: simultaneous microwire and clinical macroelectrode recordings. Brain. 2008;131:928–937.

126. Jacobs J, Levan P, Chander R, et al. Interictal high-frequency oscillations (80–500 Hz) are an indicator of seizure onset areas independent of spikes in the human epileptic brain. Epilepsia. 2008;49(11):1893–1907.

127. Jirsch JD, Urrestarazu E, LeVan P, et al. High-frequency oscillations during human focal seizures. Brain. 2006;129:1593–1608.

128. Khosravani H, Mehrotra N, Rigby M, et al. Spatial localization and time-dependent changes of electrographic high frequency oscillations in human temporal lobe epilepsy. Epilepsia. 2009;50:605–616.

129. Yamazaki M, Chan D, Tovar-Spinoza Z, et al. Interictal epileptogenic fast oscillatons on neonatal and infantile EEGs in hemimegalencephaly. Epilepsy Res. 2009;83:198–206.

130. Wu JY, Koh S, Sankar R, Mathern GW. Paroxysmal fast activity: an interictal scalp EEG marker of epileptogenesis in children. Epilepsy Res. 2008;82:99–106.

131. Homer ML, Nurmikko AV, Donoghue JP, Hochberg LR. Implants and decoding for intracortical brain computer interfaces. Annu Rev Biomed Eng. 2013;15:383–405.

132. Buzsaki G, Anastassiou CA, Koch C. The origin of extracellular fields and currents: EEG, EcoG, LFP and spikes. Nature Rev Neurosci. 2012;13:407–420.

133. Mormann F, Kornblith S, Quiroga RQ, et al. Latency and selectivity of single neurons indicate hierarchical processing in the human medial temporal lobe. Neurosci. 2008;28(36):8865–8872.

134. Miller JF, Neufang M, Solway A, et al. Neural activity in human hippocampal formation reveals the spatial context of retrieved memories. Science. 2013;342:1111–1114.

135. Schevon CA, Weiss SA, McKhann G, et al. Evidence of an inhibitory restraint of seizure activity in humans. Nature Communications. 2012;3:1060.

136. Truccolo W, Donoghue JA, Hochberg LR, et al. Single-neuron dynamics in human focal epilepsy. Nature Neurosci. 2011;14:635–641.

137. Truccolo W, Ahmed OJ, Harrison MT, et al. Neuronal ensemble synchrony during human focal seizures. J Neurosci. 2014;34:9927–9944.

138. Stead M, Bower M, Brinkmann BH, et al. Microseizures and the spatio-temporal scales of human partial epilepsy. Brain. 2010;133:2789–2797.

139. Stacey WC, Kellis S, Greger B, et al. Potential for unreliable interpretation of EEG recorded withmicroelectrodes. Epilepsia. 2013;54:1391–1401.

140. Ren L, Kucewicz MT, Cimbalnik J, et al. Gamma oscillations precede interictal epileptiform spikes in the seizure onset zone. Neurology. 2015;84:602–608.

141. Lesser RP, Lüders H, Klem G, et al. Extraoperative cortical functional localization in patients with epilepsy. J Clin Neurophysiol. 1987;4:27–53.

142. Duchowny M, Jayakar P. Functional cortical mapping in children. In: Devinsky O, Beric A, Dogali M, eds. Electrical and Magnetic Stimulation of the Brain and Spinal Cord. New York: Raven Press, Ltd, 1993:149–154.

143. Jayakar P, Alvarez LA, Duchowny MS, Resnick TJ. A safe and effective paradigm to functionally map the cortex in childhood. J Clin Neurophysiol. 1992;9:288–293.

144. Allison T, McCarthy G, Luby M, et al. Localization of functional regions of human mesial cortex by somatosensory evoked potential recording and by cortical stimulation. Electroencephalogr Clin Neurophysiol. 1996;100:126–140.

145. Neuloh G, Schramm J. Motor evoked potential monitoring for the surgery of brain tumours and vascular malformations. Adv Tech Stand Neurosurg. 2004;29:171–228.

146. Carne RP, O'Brien TJ, Kilpatrick CJ, et al. MRI-negative PET-positive temporal lobe epilepsy: a distinct surgically remediable syndrome. Brain. 2004;127:2276–2285.

147. Kurian M, Spinelli L, Delavelle J, et al. Multimodality imaging for focus localization in pediatric pharmacoresistant epilepsy. Epileptic Disord. 2007;9:20–31.

148. Michel CM, Grave de Peralta R, Lantz G, et al. Spatiotemporal EEG analysis and distributed source estimation in presurgical epilepsy evaluation. J Clin Neurophysiol. 1999;16:239–266.

149. Lantz G, Grave de Peralta R, Spinelli L, et al. Epileptic source localization with high density EEG: how many electrodes are needed? Clin Neurophysiol. 2003;114:63–69.

150. Regard M, Cook ND, Wieser HG, Landis T. The dynamics of cerebral dominance during unilateral limbic seizures. Brain. 1994;117:91–104.

151. Seeck M, Mainwaring N, Cosgrove R, et al. Neurophysiologic correlates of implicit face memory in intracranial visual evoked potentials. Neurology. 1997;49:1312–1316.

152. Grunwald T, Lehnertz K, Heinze HJ, et al. Verbal novelty detection within the human hippocampus proper. Proc Natl Acad Sci U S A. 1998;95:3193–3197.

153. Axmacher N, Elger CE, Fell J. Ripples in the medial temporal lobe are relevant for human memory consolidation. Brain. 2008;131:1806–1817.

154. Vannucci M, Pezer N, Helmstaedter C, et al. Hippocampal response to visual objects is related to visual memory functioning. Neuroreport. 2008;19:965–968.

155. Sinai A, Bowers CW, Crainiceanu CM, et al. Eletrocorticographic high gamma activity versus electrical cortical stimulation mapping of naming. Brain. 2005;128:1556–1570.

30 | ELECTROCORTICOGRAPHY

MARC R. NUWER, MD, PHD AND STEPHAN SCHUELE, MD, MPH

ABSTRACT: Electrocorticography (ECoG) is the method of recording electroencephalographic signals directly from surgically exposed cerebral cortex. It detects intraoperatively the cortical regions with substantial epileptiform interictal discharges. Direct cortical stimulation during ECoG provides a method of identifying language, motor, and sensory regions during a craniotomy. Both techniques—the identification of cortex with epileptic activity and cortex with important eloquent functional activity—help determine limits for surgical cortical resection. These are used most commonly during epilepsy and tumor surgery. Anesthetic agents can adversely affect the recording, and ECoG restricts the types of anesthesia that can be used. The amount of spiking from diffuse or remote cortical regions on ECoG can predict the success of postoperative seizure control.

KEYWORDS: electrocorticography, ECoG, surgery, epilepsy, direct cortical stimulation, anesthesia, craniotomy

PRINCIPAL REFERENCES

1. Ritaccio, A., Brunner, P., Gunduz, A., et al. (2014). Proceedings of the Fifth International Workshop on Advances in Electrocorticography. *Epilepsy Behav, 41,* 183–192.
2. Fernández, I. S., & Loddenkemper, T. (2013). Electrocorticography for seizure foci mapping in epilepsy surgery. *J Clin Neurophysiol, 30,* 554–570.
3. Chui, J., Manninen, P., Valiante, T., & Venkatraghavan, L. (2013). The anesthetic considerations of intraoperative electrocorticography during epilepsy surgery. *Anesth Analg, 117,* 479–486.
4. Devinsky, O., Canevini, M. P., Sato, S., et al. (1992). Quantitative electrocorticography in patients undergoing temporal lobectomy. *J Epilepsy, 5,* 178–185.
5. Gallentine, W. B., & Mikati, M. A. (2009). Intraoperative electrocorticography and cortical stimulation in children. *J Clin Neurophysiol, 26,* 95–108.
6. Guenot, M., Isnard, J., Ryvlin, P., et al. (2001). Neurophysiological monitoring for epilepsy surgery: the Talairach SEEG method (StereoElectroEncephaloGraphy): indications, results, complications and therapeutic applications in a series of 100 consecutive cases. *Stereotact Funct Neurosurg, 77,* 29–32.
7. McGonigal, A., Bartolomei, F., Regis, J., et al. (2007). Stereo-electroencephalography in presurgical assessment of MRI-negative epilepsy. *Brain, 130,* 3169–3183.
8. Bancaud, J., Talairach, J., Bonis, A., & Schaub, C. (1965). *La stéréoélectro-encephalographie dans l'épilepsie: informations neurophysiopathologiques apportées par l'investigation fonctionelle stéréotaxique.* Paris: Masson & Cie.
9. Jasper, H. H. (1954). Electrocorticography. In: Penfield, W., & Jasper, H. H., eds. *Epilepsy and the Functional Anatomy of the Human Brain.* Boston: Little, Brown.
10. Nuwer, M. R., ed. (2008). *Intraoperative Monitoring of Neural Function.* Handbook of Clinical Neurophysiology: 8. Amsterdam: Elsevier.
11. Quesney, L. F., Binnie, C., & Chatrian, G. E., eds. (1998). *Electrocorticography.* Electroencephalogr Clin Neurophysiol Suppl: 48, Amsterdam: Elsevier.

1. INTRODUCTION

Electrocorticography (ECoG) is intraoperative electroencephalography (EEG) recorded directly from the exposed cerebral cortex. The technique is used for localizing epileptic discharges and regions of impaired cortex prior to resection. During direct electrical cortical stimulation mapping, ECoG is used to monitor for after-discharges to ensure that elicited responses are not due to the spread of electrical activity. The goal of ECoG is to separate regions suitable for resection from those that should be left intact. Extraoperative monitoring using invasive electrodes will be discussed in a separate chapter on Intracranial EEG Monitoring.

ECoG was the first application of intraoperative neurophysiology, a field that has since evolved to include many other techniques (1,2). Since the 1940s up to modern days, ECoG has been used to localize epileptogenic tissue prior to the neurosurgical treatment of partial epilepsy (3–7). The equipment for ECoG has evolved but the clinical goal remains relatively unchanged.

Around two decades after the introduction of invasive subdural recordings in the operating room, a group at St. Anne in Paris, France, developed a method called stereoencephalography (stereo EEG or SEEG) (8–10) to record from deep structures and buried cortex, areas that are not readily accessible by subdural or cortical methods of recording. In this way, ECoG can be obtained simultaneously from superficial and deep brain structures with the intent to understand the three-dimensional propagation of the epileptic activity rather than the two-dimensional map of cortical activity provided by subdural recordings. SEEG was introduced for recordings in the operating room as well but quickly evolved as a technique for extraoperative monitoring of the ictal onset zone. SEEG, in comparison to other methods of invasive EEG recording, is well tolerated by the majority of patients and overall complication rates of SEEG are reported to be on the order of 5% (11–14). This is similar to the complication rates of subdural strips (15) and is less than those of subdural grids (16). For intraoperative recordings, adding acute depth electrodes may appear to be "more invasive" than subdural recordings alone, but the complication rate is not higher and the depth electrodes can be accurately placed using a frameless stereotactic system (17,18).

2. ELECTRODES AND METHODS OF RECORDING DIRECTLY FROM CEREBRAL CORTEX

Intraoperative ECoG from the exposed cerebral cortex most often uses strip and grid electrodes. These electrodes are arrays of 3-mm metal discs embedded in a flexible silicon rubber matrix. Each disc is 1 cm apart measured center to center.

Discs are stainless steel or platinum alloy. Fine flexible wires connect to each disc. These wires course through the silicon rubber matrix and are gathered together to exit at one end of the strip or grid. Together they form a ribbon cable or braided wire connector cable leading to a multi-pin connector. A matched multi-pin connector with grounded heavier wiring transmits the signal to the EEG machine electrode junction box. Strips and grids come in many different sizes. Sizes used more often in surgery are 1×6 or 1×8 strips and 2×6 and 4×5 grids. For patients in whom these are left in place in the subdural space for days or weeks to catch epileptic seizures in an epilepsy monitoring unit, grid sizes up to 8×8 are available.

When used in surgery, ECoG grids and strips tend to curl up or pull slightly away from the cortex, especially in sulci. This results in a poor electrical connection to some contacts. To prevent corners from pulling up, the surgeon should place saline-wetted surgical cottonoid over each strip or grid to weigh it down. These strips and grids can be moved around to record from various regions of exposed cortex, or even under the dura or skull edges, to record from as many regions as needed (Fig. 30.1).

Acute multi-contact depth electrodes are used by some centers. This has been reported as very helpful for an acute exploration of deep limbic and neocortical structures during temporal lobectomy (see Fig. 30.1) (17,19). Intraoperative computed tomography has become a useful tool to confirm placement of subtemporal strips and grids, which can end up in unpredictable locations and confound the interpretation (20).

Montages are either bipolar among the adjacent contacts or referential to a distant site. A clip electrode on muscle or a disc scalp electrode can serve as a distant neutral reference. Some users prefer the mastoid site. Because the amplitude of ECoG is several-fold higher in amplitude than EEG picked up by electrodes on the muscle or scalp, referential recordings are often used without excessive channel contamination by an active reference.

Use of a low-frequency filter of 0.5 Hz and a high-frequency filter of 70 Hz ensures adequate recording of epileptiform discharges and background activity. The amplitude of EEG recorded directly from the cortex is several-fold higher than EEG recorded from the scalp. This allows for a relatively low sensitivity of 30 to 50 μV/mm to be used for ECoG recordings. A collection of 20 to 40 cortical electrodes is recommended, which often are composed of signals from more than one grid or strip. To record slow oscillations including DC shift, a low-pass filter with a time constant over 10 sec is necessary. For

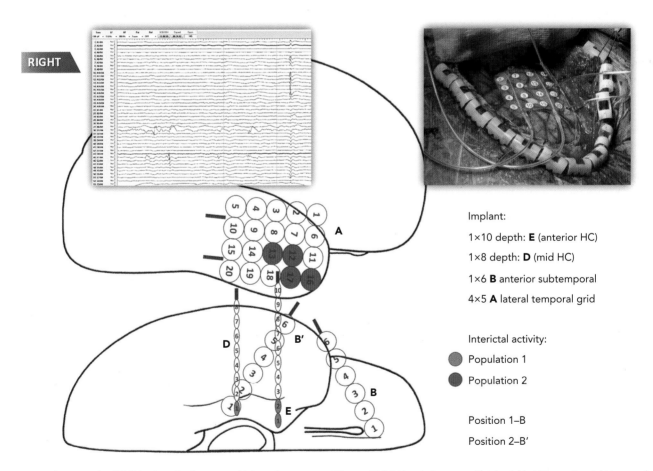

Figure 30.1. Intraoperative ECoG implantation for temporal lobe epilepsy surgery. 37-year-old right-handed woman with intractable MRI-negative right temporal lobe epilepsy confirmed by ictal SPECT and FDG-PET. Our standard temporal intraoperative implantation includes a lateral temporal grid, subtemporal strip(s), and one or two mesial depth electrodes as depicted. Frequent mesial spikes and sporadic lateral temporal spikes were noted. One spike subset (population 1) is seen in the top right portion of the EEG tracing, in channels corresponding to a maximum field at four electrodes in grid A. A second spike subset (population 2) is seen in the bottom left portion of the EEG tracing, in channels corresponding to a maximum field at three electrodes in grids D and E. The patient underwent anterior temporal resection, with pathology demonstrating focal cortical dysplasia type IIA.

high-frequency oscillations between 80 and 600 Hz, a high-pass filter at 500 to 700 Hz and a sampling rate of 2,000 Hz is required; this poses a variety of technical challenges (21).

3. DIRECT CORTICAL STIMULATION TECHNIQUE

Direct cortical stimulation is used to localize functional cortex. This technique requires special instrumentation and precautions. In general, equipment specifically designed for this purpose is used. Contact with the cortical surface usually is made using a bipolar stimulation wand or probe held against the cortex (e.g., the Ojemann Cortical Stimulator). The wand stimulation technique is more convenient during surgery where the cortex is directly exposed. The typical stimulating wand or probe is 30 cm long, with two round metal ball tips separated by a few millimeters. Such a wand can move among cortical locations quickly. This allows for testing many different locations in a short time but limits the ability to exactly mark a stimulation site, to reproduce a response, or to record EEG for after-discharges in the immediate vicinity of the stimulus (Fig. 30.2). Alternatively, the stimulation may be delivered directly through the grid or strip electrodes; the latter stimulation technique is used more often for subdural studies with indwelling electrodes in epilepsy monitoring units, but technical advancements may allow increasing use in the operating room. Stimuli through the handheld probe or grid are bipolar and biphasic. Bipolar means that electric current runs between the two adjacent active contacts; biphasic means that the current switches polarity halfway through each stimulus pulse. Biphasic stimulation is preferred in the ECoG setting so as not to leave a net electrical polarization at either metal–cortex contact. Polarization could allow metal ions to move onto the brain, which is undesirable, especially for iron ions, which would serve as a source of future cortical irritation. Polarization alters the electrical sensitivity of the underlying cortex to subsequent stimulus pulses. Monophasic stimulation equipment is unsuitable for direct cortical stimulation studies.

Typical direct cortical stimuli are 300- to 1,000-microsecond (0.3–1 msec) pulses delivered in trains of 50 pulses per second for several seconds. In adults, a 5- to 7-sec stimulation train is used for language testing, whereas shorter trains are used for motor testing. Stimulus pulses are delivered using currents up to 14 milliamperes (mA) for a stimulus duration of 300 msec and 2 to 4 mA for a 1-msec stimulus duration (Table 30.1 lists typical stimulation settings used in the operative room). This is sufficient to disrupt function at the cortex underlying the wand's location. Often one starts with a lower intensity, increasing gradually to higher intensities if no desired or adverse effects are seen at the lower intensities at each site. Either constant current or constant voltage stimulation may be used. A duration >8 sec should be avoided in adults but can be necessary for children, who have a longer chronaxis (22,23).

During direct cortical stimulation, ECoG should be recorded from nearby sites (see Fig. 30.2). This is carried out to check whether epileptic-like discharges occur with the stimulations. When epileptic-like discharges last longer than the stimulation, they are referred to as *after-discharges*. After-discharges appear as rhythmic repetitive high-voltage spikes or polyspike-wave complexes lasting seconds or occasionally minutes. Such prolonged after-discharges can be subclinical or associated with subtle clinical manifestations (24). When after-discharges occur, stimulation may have spread to other cortical regions; therefore, those stimulation trials cannot be used to localize cortical functions, since they reflect functional activation (or inactivation) of areas away from the wand's tip. After-discharges may herald epileptic seizures occurring with further stimulation at that site or intensity. This may prompt moving the stimulating wand to a different site or to reducing the stimulus intensity. Cortical stimulation can provoke epileptic seizures, and cold Ringer's lactate solution can readily be used to treat those seizures (25).

4. INTERPRETATION OF ECOG AND DIRECT CORTICAL STIMULATION

The goal of ECoG is to determine the location of epileptogenic or otherwise impaired cortex and its relation to eloquent cortex. The recording usually shows EEG features similar to those seen with scalp EEG. Fronto-central fast activity, low-amplitude generalized slowing, and fronto-polar triangular slow waves are seen during many types of anesthesia. Recordings above and below the sylvian fissure show more fast activity above and less below. ECoG background activity is more sharply contoured than typically seen on scalp EEG recordings; the EEG activity is similar to the scalp EEG over a skull breach. This sharply contoured background needs to be distinguished from epileptic activity during interpretation. Some ECoG epileptiform spikes may not be apparent on concurrent scalp-recorded EEG (26). Areas of impaired cortex may show relatively decreased fast activity or increased slow activity indicating focal dysfunction or a structural lesion (27). A knowledgeable and experienced physician neurophysiologist will be able to recognize these changes and thereby identify regions with impaired function or epileptogenic potential.

ECoG is used for selected patients during epilepsy surgery. Most often this is when the epileptogenic zone can be attributed to a particular lobe but needs to be further localized—for instance, some patients with suspected mesial temporal lobe epilepsy or patients with lesional neocortical epilepsy. ECoG is typically used to further define the resection limits in those patients (Fig. 30.3). In the rare situation of a patient with very frequent seizures during either scalp or invasive EEG monitoring, intraoperative ictal ECoG may be useful to demarcate the electrographic ictal onset zone more precisely. More commonly, the limited time in the operating room allows for only interictal ECoG to be obtained. Interictal spike discharges usually arise from the epileptogenic zone (i.e., the area that needs to be resected to make the patient seizure-free) but may also extend to cortex beyond it. Placement of invasive electrodes should be discussed ahead of time and the results of the presurgical evaluation, semiology, interictal and ictal surface findings, lesion if present, and nuclear imaging results need to be

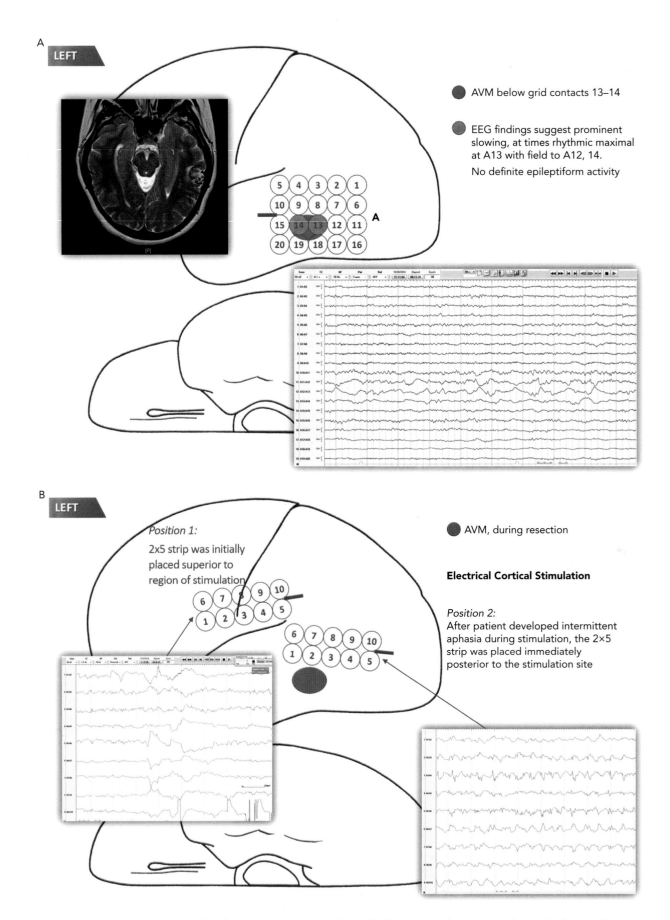

Figure 30.2. ECoG during lesionectomy (**A**) and for after-discharges (**B**). 36-year-old right-handed woman with new-onset epilepsy and left temporal arteriovenous malformation. Intraoperative ECoG to evaluate for epileptiform activity (**A**) was negative aside from irregular delta slowing. The lower half of the grid was used to monitor for after-discharges (**B**) and demonstrates the need to record close to the stimulation site.

TABLE 30.1. Stimulation Parameters: Comparison

	SUBDURAL	DEPTH/OJEMANN WAND
Polarity	Biphasic	Biphasic
Stimulated electrode	Monopolar or bipolar	Bipolar
Stimulus intensity	1–15 mA (Grass S88) 1–17.5 mA (Grass S12)	1–3 mA
Duration of stimulus	0.3 msec	1–3 msec
Frequency	50 Hz	50 Hz
Duration of train	5 sec	<5 sec

considered. Electrical or magnetic source imaging can provide a hypothesis for the source of the interictal activity, and image co-registration can be used to guide placement of invasive electrodes, including depth electrodes (Fig. 30.4). Areas of attenuation, slowing, and epileptiform activity are defined and discussed with the surgeon so that the resection can be tailored to the needs of the individual patient.

Epileptiform discharges observed at the resection margins may represent just "injury potentials" or "injury spikes,"

not the location of actual epileptic tissue. Epileptic spikes distant from the resection margin are more concerning, and in patients with frontal lobe epilepsy, epileptiform discharges three or more gyri away from the resection site indicate the likelihood of seizure recurrence.

5. ANESTHETIC CONSIDERATIONS AND PROTOCOLS FOR CORTICAL MAPPING

To avoid anesthetic effects, the anesthesia is lightened or minimized during ECoG. Many anesthetics can alter the presence of the epileptiform discharges sought in ECoG. The effects of the anesthetic on the ECoG are less important than the anesthetic's clearance time. Propofol (2,6 di-isopropyl phenol) clears adequately to allow good ECoG in most patients. Nitrous oxide and narcotics may be used during the ECoG to avoid pain or consciousness during the procedure, although these may affect the epileptiform discharges seen on the recording.

Direct cortical stimulation testing is interpreted by the presence of movement or sensation or the disruption of language. Neuromuscular blockade needs to be avoided. For motor testing, anesthesia cannot be deep. Observations of responses can be made visually, or electromyographic (EMG) electrodes can be placed in various muscles to record movements under

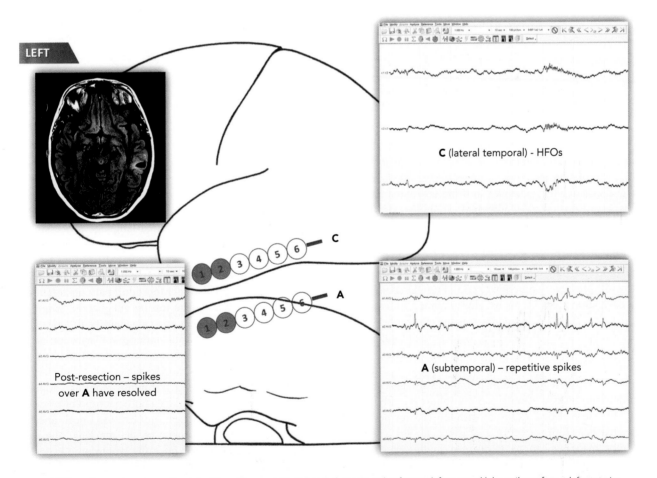

Figure 30.3. HFOs, spikes, and post-resection recordings. 29-year-old right-handed woman with refractory left temporal lobe epilepsy from a left posterior temporal cystic lesion. ECoG shows lateral temporal HFOs (and small spikes, not shown) as well as repetitive subtemporal spikes that subsided after resection. Pathology was consistent with a ganglioglioma.

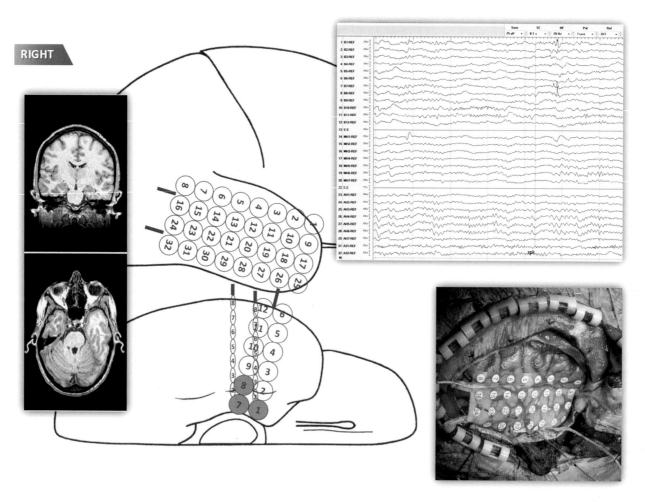

Figure 30.4. MEG DICOM co-registration for planning of ECoG placement. 39-year-old right-handed woman with intractable, MRI-negative right temporal lobe epilepsy with congruent FDG PET and MEG. Single dipole source model was exported to DICOM images and co-registered onto the stereotactic system. Intraoperative ECoG showed spikes in the basal temporal area indicated by the MEG. Patient underwent a standard anterior temporal resection. Pathology showed focal cortical dysplasia type IIA.

the surgical drapes to identify face, arm, and leg regions (28). Finding stimulation effects at some cortical areas shows that the anesthetic depth is adequate and the technique is working properly. Considerable individual variability exists in the location of eloquent cortex regions for language, motor, and sensory function (29–31). Anatomic locations need to be determined for each eloquent function for each individual patient. Stimulation mapping allows for best resection of pathologic tissue while preserving function (32,33). Functional neuroimaging navigation methods are usually combined with stimulation mapping; such a dual approach is the current best guide for the limits of a resection (34,35). Larger craniotomies allow mapping of eloquent cortex and maximum resection within functional boundaries. However, in glioma surgery it has also been advocated that negative mapping and the absence of a functional response to stimulation may allow a more limited craniotomy and cortical exposure with low risk for persisting language deficits (36).

Motor mapping can be performed in the anesthetized patient. In contrast, the patient is awake during surgery for sensory and language testing. The conscious patient is extubated while restrained on the table (37). The primary sensory

cortex can be mapped using such stimulation in the awake patient.

For language testing, a neuropsychologist or other trained language specialist administers language tasks for different aspects of auditory and visual language processing and short-term memory. The clinical neurophysiologist delivers the stimulations and observes for after-discharges while the surgeon holds the wand and the language specialist administers oral and visual testing. Most adult patients tolerate this awake craniotomy language testing adequately. Stimulation at a series of cortical locations can identify functional language areas. Regions without noticeable disruption at 12 to 14 mA (300-msec pulse width) are considered candidates for resection.

The asleep-awake-asleep technique requires cooperative patients (37). Initial anesthesia is often propofol or sodium thiopental with endotracheal intubation. Local anesthetic is infiltrated around the operative site margins. The patient is awakened and extubated once the craniotomy exposure is achieved. Consistent intraoperative language performance baseline is needed before stimulation testing. Without baseline consistency, any observed language disruption might be due to inconsistent performance rather than specific anatomic disruption due to stimulation. After mapping is completed, the patient is re-intubated and remains under general anesthesia for the remainder of the procedure.

Language mapping includes several types of tasks. *Visual object naming* involves the naming of objects presented as line drawings from the Boston Naming Test (38). Drawings are presented that the patient could name quickly in preoperative testing (29). Naming is a useful screening task for language during cortical stimulation mapping because naming deficits are frequently part of aphasia syndromes. Speech arrest or anomia may occur upon stimulating a cortical region important for language, although not all cortical language sites produce naming deficits (29,39). Different cortical sites may reveal stimulation deficits in *sentence reading* (39). Another easily accomplished stimulation language test is *word generation*, in which patients generate lists of words that begin with a certain letter or are of a certain category (e.g., animals). In *auditory responsive naming* the patient names objects: for instance, the answer for "tall pink bird" would be "flamingo." Auditory responsive naming and word-generation tasks activate frontal language areas (40). *Visual responsive naming* differs from auditory responsive naming because the question is written on a flash card.

The effect of stimulation mapping is well localized. Moving the stimulating electrodes 0.5 to 2 cm, even along the same gyrus, yields different functional effects (39,41). A site with consistent language function can be 2 cm from a site on the same gyrus without language disruption (29). Language function often is localized to small 1- to 2-cm^2 regions (39,42). Postoperative language deficits occur when resection margins are within 1.5 to 2.0 cm of language function sites. No permanent language deficits were reported if the surgical margins remain >2.0 cm from language sites (42,43).

6. GENERAL ANESTHESIA AND CORTICAL EEG ACTIVITY

Anesthetic drugs tend to either excite or depress the EEG and follow a pattern summarized by Winters (44). The activating or exciting anesthetic agents are *propofol* and *etomidate*. They inhibit brainstem arousal mechanisms through GABA$_A$ receptor mechanisms (45,46). Propofol also selectively suppresses persistent Na$^+$ currents and L-type high-voltage-activated Ca^{2+} conductance in cortical neurons (47). Together with opening of GABA$_A$ chloride channels, its action achieves depression of cortical activity during both anesthesia and status epilepticus. Resulting EEG patterns resemble slow-wave sleep, including vertex sharp waves and spindles. Propofol does not produce or affect EEG epileptiform activity in constant infusions (48–50), but it does reduce the number of epileptic high-frequency oscillations (HFOs) (51). Reducing the propofol infusion rate may decrease spikes in the epileptogenic zone (51). To record HFOs during surgery, the propofol infusion should be interrupted for some minutes to improve detection.

Propofol is a popular agent for use during direct cortical stimulation. Because of its rapid metabolism, propofol can induce unconsciousness during portions of the craniotomy while allowing awakening during awake language testing (52,53). Some evidence suggests that propofol-induced unconsciousness is associated with disruption of functional connectivity among cortical areas (54). Etomidate is another activating or exciting anesthetic agent. It enhances epileptic activity at low doses (0.1 mg/kg). It may produce seizures in patients with epilepsy (55).

The commonly used volatile inhalation anesthetic agents are sedating anesthetics. They include *halothane, desflurane, isoflurane*, and *sevoflurane*. They cause immobility through multiple molecular targets predominantly in the spinal cord, including GABA$_A$ receptors, glycine receptors, glutamate receptors, and two-pore-domain potassium channels (56). These agents cause rhythmic fronto-central alpha activity. This rhythmic fast activity can be abolished by nitrous oxide (57). Hyperventilation with high concentrations of these agents, except for desflurane, can produce epileptiform spikes or even electrographic nonconvulsive seizures. These agents can reduce or increase epileptiform discharges at standard anesthetic levels (58,59). They have little effect at low levels (60).

Barbiturates are similar to inhalational agents in producing activation and fast activity at low doses and a depressant effect leading to burst suppression at higher doses. These bursts may have very sharp components that could be misinterpreted as epileptiform. At low doses the short-acting barbiturate methohexital (0.5 mg/kg) does activate epileptic spike activity during ECoG, so it has been used deliberately to identify seizure foci (55,61–63). Methohexital also can produce seizures. *Benzodiazepines* produce frontal beta activity with a decrease in alpha activity at low doses. Some patients show epileptiform spike activity in that beta activity. Slowing of higher frequencies through inhibitory mechanisms may produce the barbiturate beta activity (64). Higher benzodiazepine doses produce generalized slowing. As an anticonvulsant, benzodiazepines are avoided if ECoG is planned for identification of seizure foci. *Nitrous oxide* produces a fronto-central fast activity when used by itself. When used with inhalational agents, it produces variable results. Nitrous oxide is a proconvulsant when combined with some agents. It may increase or suppress epileptic spike activity during ECoG depending on which other agents are used (65,66). *Droperidol* and *dexmedetomidine* are other adjunctive agents sometimes used during ECoG procedures. These seem compatible with ECoG. Narcotic drugs can increase epileptiform spiking, including spiking or seizures from sites outside the epileptogenic area (67–69). *Remifentanyl* may increase epileptiform discharges at higher doses but not with lower-dose continuous infusions (70,71).

Overall, light anesthesia enhances the ability to find epileptiform spiking during ECoG. Propofol is an example of an anesthetic agent that can be reduced quickly enough to achieve a light anesthesia. Varying the infusion rate may change how frequently spikes are seen (51). Methohexital or other drugs sometimes are used to enhance epileptiform abnormalities during ECoG (72).

7. APPLICATION IN EPILEPSY SURGERY

Spikes occur not only in the epileptogenic zone but also in other cortical areas. Even the most active spiking area may not coincide with the location of the lesion (6). The goal in ECoG is to localize the region to be resected without taking out areas unnecessarily. Interictal epileptic disturbances recorded at ECoG in patients with temporal lobe epilepsy often involve adjacent regions (24,73–85). Some reports suggest that interictal epileptic disturbance recorded intraoperatively should guide surgical resection (24,79,86–91). Others have emphasized that standardized lobectomy could be performed without ECoG control for patients with typical mesial temporal epilepsy (92–94). ECoG recording after a temporal resection is similarly controversial (95). Some authors believe that the persistence of spike activity after surgical excision is of little or no prognostic value (7,96–98). Other investigators advocate that persistent spike activity after surgical removal predicts an unsatisfactory outcome (19,86,99,100).

Recent reports showed that intraoperative ECoG activities can be analyzed with respect to more complex spike patterns, particularly in temporal lobe epilepsies (101); namely, in addition to focal spiking with or without propagation, focal slowing in the theta or delta range and ictal ECoG patterns were found. Furthermore, HFOs in the range of 250 to 600 Hz (fast ripples) have been identified in the ECoGs recorded from the hippocampus and parahippocampal areas of patients with temporal lobe epilepsy and may be used to identify brain epileptogenic areas (102). Rates and durations of HFOs were found to be significantly higher in the seizure onset zone than outside, and they occurred to a large extent independently of spikes (103). Propofol infusion rates may affect these HFOs and spikes, and do so differentially in the epileptogenic zone (51).

In extratemporal surgery, interictal epileptiform spiking is often widespread even when the patient has a circumscribed lesion (17,104–108). In neocortical temporal and extratemporal lobe epilepsy, ECoG mapping of the interictal epileptogenic area is useful to tailor the surgical resection (109). The distribution and the abundance of interictal spiking recorded via ECoG are prognostic indicators of postsurgical seizure control (108). A pre-excision epileptic abnormality recorded from less than two gyri and absence of post-excision epileptic activity distant to the resection border both strongly predicted a favorable outcome (see Fig. 30.3). Residual spiking limited to the resection border did not significantly correlate with the outcome. The presence of a circumscribed frontal lobe lesion was also significantly correlated with a favorable outcome. In frontal lobe epilepsy, post-excision residual spiking indicates a poor outcome in terms of seizure control (110).

ECoG is useful for localizing cortical dysplasia. The region of the lesion shows rhythmic electrographic seizure discharges corresponding to magnetic resonance imaging (MRI) evidence for cortical dysplasia. A good surgical outcome in these patients is proportional to the completeness of the lesion's surgical removal (111).

After-discharge locations during direct cortical stimulation do not correlate with impaired function or pathology, and often arise at normal cortex. Stimulation at certain anatomical sites (e.g., hippocampus) is more likely to elicit after-discharges (112–114). Electrical stimulation thresholds are often increased in damaged areas (115,116), so impaired regions tend not to have after-discharges (19,116).

REFERENCES

1. Foerster, O., & Altenburger, H. (1935). Elektrobiologische Vorgaenge an der menschlichen Hirnrinde. *J Neurol, 135*, 277–288.
2. Nuwer, M. R. (2008). *Intraoperative Monitoring of Neural Function. Handbook of Clinical Neurophysiology.* Amsterdam: Elsevier.
3. Jasper, H. H. (1949). Electrocorticogram in man. *Electroencephalogr Clin Neurophysiol Suppl*, 16–29.
4. Marshall, C., & Walker, A. E. (1949). Electrocorticography. *Bull Johns Hopkins Hosp, 85*, 344–359.
5. Meyers, R., Knott, J. R., Hayne, R. A., & Sweeney, D. B. (1950). The surgery of epilepsy; limitations of the concept of the cortico-electrographic "spike" as an index of the epileptogenic focus. *J Neurosurg, 7*, 337–346.
6. Penfield, W., & Jasper, H. H. (1954). Epilepsy and the functional anatomy of the human brain. *Science, 119*, 645–646.
7. Ajmone, M. C., & Baldwin, M. (1958). Electrocorticography. In: Baldwin, M., & Bailey, P., eds. *Temporal Lobe Epilepsy.* Springfield, IL: Charles C Thomas, pp. 368–395.
8. Bancaud, J., Talairach, J., Bonis, A., & Schaub, C. (1965). *La stéréoélectroencephalographie dans l'épilepsie: informations neurophysiopathologiques apportées par l'investigation fonctionelle stéréotaxique.* Paris: Masson & Cie.
9. Talairach, J., Bancaud, J., Szikla, G., et al. (1974). New approach to the neurosurgery of epilepsy. Stereotaxic methodology and therapeutic results. 1. Introduction and history. *Neurochirurgie, 20*, 1–240.
10. Chauvel, P., Buser, P., Badier, J. M., et al. (1987). The "epileptogenic zone" in humans: representation of intercritical events by spatio-temporal maps. *Rev Neurol, 143*, 443–550.
11. Guenot, M., Isnard, J., Ryvlin, P., et al. (2001). Neurophysiological monitoring for epilepsy surgery: the Talairach SEEG method (StereoElectroEncephaloGraphy): indications, results, complications and therapeutic applications in a series of 100 consecutive cases. *Stereotact Funct Neurosurg, 77*, 29–32.
12. Cossu, M., Cardinale, F., Castana, L., et al. (2005). Stereoelectroencephalography in the presurgical evaluation of focal epilepsy: a retrospective analysis of 215 procedures. *Neurosurgery, 57*, 706–718.
13. McGonigal, A., Bartolomei, F., Regis, J., et al. (2007). Stereoelectroencephalography in presurgical assessment of MRI-negative epilepsy. *Brain, 130*, 3169–3183.
14. Cardinale, F., Cossu, M., Castana, L., et al. (2013). Stereoelectroencephalography: surgical methodology, safety, and stereotactic application accuracy in 500 procedures. *Neurosurgery, 72*, 353–366.
15. Alarcon, G., Valentin, A., Watt, C., et al. (2006). Is it worth pursuing surgery for epilepsy in patients with normal neuroimaging? *J Neurol Neurosurg Psychiatry, 77*, 474–480.
16. Hamer, H. M., Morris, H. H., Mascha, E. J., et al. (2002). Complications of invasive video-EEG monitoring with subdural grid electrodes. *Neurology, 58*, 97–103.
17. Wennberg, R., Quesney, F., Olivier, A., & Dubeau, F. (1997). Mesial temporal versus lateral temporal interictal epileptiform activity: comparison of chronic and acute intracranial recordings. *Electroencephalogr Clin Neurophysiol, 102*, 486–494.
18. Mehta, A.D., Labar, D., Dean, A., et al. (2005). Frameless stereotactic placement of depth electrodes in epilepsy surgery. *J Neurosurg, 102*, 1040–1045.
19. Gloor, P. (1975). Contributions of electroencephalography and electrocorticography to the neurosurgical treatment of the epilepsies. *Adv Neurol, 8*, 59–105.
20. Lee, D. J., Zwienenberg-Lee, M., Seyal, M., & Shahlaie, K. (2015). Intraoperative computed tomography for intracranial electrode implantation surgery in medically refractory epilepsy. *J Neurosurg, 122*, 526–531.
21. Amiri, M., Lina, J. M., Pizzo, F., & Gotman, J. (2016). High-frequency oscillations and spikes: separating real HFOs from false oscillations. *Clin Neurophysiol, 127*, 187–196.
22. Jayakar, P., Alvarez, L. A., Duchowny, M. S., & Resnick, T. J. (1992). A safe and effective paradigm to functionally map the cortex in childhood. *J Clin Neurophysiol, 9*, 288–293.

23. Gallentine, W. B., & Mikati, M. A. (2009). Intraoperative electrocorticography and cortical stimulation in children. *J Clin Neurophysiol, 26,* 95–108.

24. Stefan, H., Quesney, L. F., Abou-Khalil, B., & Olivier, A. (1991). Electrocorticography in temporal lobe epilepsy surgery. *Acta Neurol Scand, 83,* 65–72.

25. Sartorius, C. J., & Berger, M. S. (1998). Rapid termination of intraoperative stimulation-evoked seizures with application of cold Ringer's lactate to the cortex. Technical note. *J Neurosurg, 88,* 349–351.

26. Tao, J. X., Ray, A., Hawes-Ebersole, S., & Ebersole, J. S. (2005). Intracranial EEG substrates of scalp EEG interictal spikes. *Epilepsia, 46,* 669–676.

27. Kim, A. J., Nangia, S., Berg, A. T., & Nordli, D. R. (2014). Interictal attenuation in pediatric electrocorticography can be reliably detected by EEG readers. *Epilepsy Res, 108,* 1367–1377.

28. Yingling, C. D., Ojemann, S., Dodson, B., et al. (1999). Identification of motor pathways during tumor surgery facilitated by multichannel electromyographic recording. *J Neurosurg, 91,* 922–927.

29. Ojemann, G., & Mateer, C. (1979). Human language cortex: localization of memory, syntax, and sequential motor-phoneme identification systems. *Science, 205,* 1401–1403.

30. Uematsu, S., Lesser, R., Fisher, R. S., et al. (1992). Motor and sensory cortex in humans: topography studied with chronic subdural stimulation. *Neurosurgery, 31,* 59, 71–72.

31. Tate, M. C., Herbet, G., Moritz-Gasser, S., et al. (2014). Probabilistic map of critical functional regions of the human cerebral cortex: Broca's area revisited. *Brain, 137,* 2773–2782.

32. Duffau, H., Capelle, L., Sichez, J., et al. (1999). Intra-operative direct electrical stimulations of the central nervous system: the Salpetriere experience with 60 patients. *Acta Neurochir, 141,* 1157–1167.

33. Duffau, H., Lopes, M., Arthuis, F., et al. (2005). Contribution of intraoperative electrical stimulations in surgery of low-grade gliomas: a comparative study between two series without (1985-96) and with (1996-2003) functional mapping in the same institution. *J Neurol Neurosurg Psychiatry, 76,* 845–851.

34. Duffau, H. (2000). Intraoperative direct subcortical stimulation for identification of the internal capsule, combined with an image-guided stereotactic system during surgery for basal ganglia lesions. *Surg Neurol, 53,* 250–254.

35. Kamada, K., Todo, T., Masutani, Y., et al. (2005). Combined use of tractography-integrated functional neuronavigation and direct fiber stimulation. *J Neurosurg, 102,* 664–672.

36. Sanai, N., Mirzadeh, Z., & Berger, M. S. (2008). Functional outcome after language mapping for glioma resection. *N Engl J Med, 358,* 18–27.

37. Huncke, K., Van de Wiele, B., Fried, I., & Rubinstein, E. H. (1998). The asleep-awake-asleep anesthetic technique for intraoperative language mapping. *Neurosurgery, 42,* 1312–1317.

38. Kaplan, E., Goodglass, H., & Weintraub, S. (1976). *Boston Naming Test.* Philadelphia: Lea & Febiger.

39. Ojemann, G. A. (1983). Brain organization for language from the perspective of electrical cortical mapping. *Behav Brain Sci, 2,* 230.

40. Bookheimer, S. Y., Zeffiro, T. A., Blaxton, T. A., et al. (1998). Regional cerebral blood flow during auditory responsive naming: evidence for cross-modality neural activation. *Neuroreport, 9,* 2409–2413.

41. Ojemann, G. A., & Whitaker, H. A. (1978). Language localization and variability. *Brain Lang, 6,* 239–260.

42. Ojemann, G. A. (1991). Cortical organization of language. *J Neurosci, 11,* 2281–2287.

43. Haglund, M. M., Berger, M. S., Shamseldin, M., et al. (1994). Cortical localization of temporal lobe language sites in patients with gliomas. *Neurosurgery, 34,* 567– 576.

44. Winters, W. D. (1976). Effects of drugs on the electrical activity of the brain: anesthetics. *Annu Rev Pharmacol Toxicol, 16,* 413–426.

45. Nelson, L. E., Guo, T. Z., Lu, J., et al. (2002). The sedative component of anesthesia is mediated by GABA(A) receptors in an endogenous sleep pathway. *Nat Neurosci, 5,* 979–984.

46. Rudolph, U., & Antkowiak, B. (2004). Molecular and neuronal substrates for general anaesthetics. *Nat Rev Neurosci, 5,* 709–720.

47. Martella, G., De-Persis, C., Bonsi, P., et al. (2005). Inhibition of persistent sodium current fraction and voltage-gated L-type calcium current by propofol in cortical neurons: implications for its antiepileptic activity. *Epilepsia, 46,* 624–635.

48. Ebrahim, Z. Y., Schubert, A., Van Ness, P., et al. (1994). The effect of propofol on the electroencephalogram of patients with epilepsy. *Anesth Analg, 78,* 275–279.

49. Samra, S. K., Sneyd, J. R., Ross, D. A., & Henry, T. R. (1995). Effects of propofol sedation on seizures and intracranially recorded epileptiform activity in patients with partial epilepsy. *Anesthesiology, 82,* 843–851.

50. Cheng, M. A., Tempelhoff, R., Silbergeld, D. L., et al. (1996). Large-dose propofol alone in adult epileptic patients: electrocorticographic results. *Anesth Analg, 83,* 169–174.

51. Zijlmans, M., Huiskamp, G. M., Cremer, O. L., et al. (2012). Epileptic high-frequency oscillations in intraoperative electrocorticography: the effect of propofol. *Epilepsia, 53,* 1799–1809.

52. Soriano, S. G., Eldredge, E. A., Wang, F. K., et al. (2000). The effect of propofol on intraoperative electrocorticography and cortical stimulation during awake craniotomies in children. *Paediatr Anaesth, 10,* 29–34.

53. Skucas, A. P., & Artru, A. A. (2006). Anesthetic complications of awake craniotomies for epilepsy surgery. *Anesth Analg, 102,* 882–887.

54. Lewis, L. D., Weiner, V. S., Mukamel, A. E., et al. (2012). Rapid fragmentation of neuronal networks at the onset of propofol-induced unconsciousness. *Proc Natl Acad Sci USA, 109,* E3377–3386.

55. Rampil, I. J. (1997). Electroencephalogram. In: Albin, M. A., ed. *Textbook of Neuroanesthesia with Neurosurgical and Neuroscience Perspective.* New York: McGraw-Hill, pp. 193–220.

56. Grasshoff, C., Rudolph, U., & Antkowiak, B. (2005). Molecular and systemic mechanisms of general anaesthesia: the "multi-site and multiple mechanisms" concept. *Curr Opin Anaesthesiol, 18,* 386–391.

57. Yli-Hankala, A. (1990). The effect of nitrous oxide on EEG spectral power during halothane and isoflurane anaesthesia. *Acta Anaesthesiol Scand, 34,* 579–584.

58. Endo, T., Sato, K., Shamoto, H., & Yoshimoto, T. (2002). Effects of sevoflurane on electrocorticography in patients with intractable temporal lobe epilepsy. *J Neurosurg Anesthesiol, 14,* 59–62.

59. Asano, E., Benedek, K., Shah, A., et al. (2004). Is intraoperative electrocorticography reliable in children with intractable neocortical epilepsy? *Epilepsia, 45,* 1091–1099.

60. Fiol, M. E., Boening, J. A., Cruz-Rodriguez, R., & Maxwell, R. (1993). Effect of isoflurane (Forane) on intraoperative electrocorticogram. *Epilepsia, 34,* 897–900.

61. Musella, L., Wilder, B. J., & Schmidt, R. P. (1971). Electroencephalographic activation with intravenous methohexital in psychomotor epilepsy. *Neurology, 21,* 594–602.

62. Ajmone, M. C., & O'Connor, M. (1973). Electrocorticography. In: Remond, A., ed. *Handbook of Electroencephalography and Clinical Neurophysiology.* Amsterdam: Elsevier, pp. 3–49.

63. Wennberg, R., Quesney, F., Olivier, A., & Dubeau, F. (1997) Induction of burst-suppression and activation of epileptiform activity after methohexital and selective amygdalo-hippocampectomy. *Electroencephalogr Clin Neurophysiol, 102,* 443–451.

64. Jensen, O., Goel, P., Kopell, N., et al. (2005). On the human sensorimotor-cortex beta rhythm: sources and modeling. *Neuroimage, 26,* 347–355.

65. Artru, A. A., Lettich, E., Colley, P. S., & Ojemann, G. A. (1990). Nitrous oxide: suppression of focal epileptiform activity during inhalation, and spreading of seizure activity following withdrawal. *J Neurosurg Anesthesiol, 2,* 189–193.

66. Hosain, S., Nagarajan, L., Fraser, R., et al. (1997). Effects of nitrous oxide on electrocorticography during epilepsy surgery. *Electroencephalogr Clin Neurophysiol, 102,* 340–342.

67. Tempelhoff, R., Modica, P. A., Bernardo, K. L., & Edwards, I. (1992). Fentanyl-induced electrocorticographic seizures in patients with complex partial epilepsy. *J Neurosurg, 77,* 201–208.

68. Cascino, G. D., So, E. L., Sharbrough, F. W., et al. (1993). Alfentanil-induced epileptiform activity in patients with partial epilepsy. *J Clin Neurophysiol, 10,* 520–525.

69. Manninen, P. H., Burke, S. J., Wennberg, R., et al. (1999). Intraoperative localization of an epileptogenic focus with alfentanil and fentanyl. *Anesth Analg, 88,* 1101–1106.

70. Wass, C. T., Grady, R. E., Fessler, A. J., et al. (2001). The effects of remifentanil on epileptiform discharges during intraoperative electrocorticography in patients undergoing epilepsy surgery. *Epilepsia, 42,* 1340–1344.

71. Herrick, I. A., Craen, R. A., Blume, W. T., et al. (2002). Sedative doses of remifentanil have minimal effect on ECoG spike activity during awake epilepsy surgery. *J Neurosurg Anesthesiol, 14,* 55–58.

72. Cascino, G. D. (1998). Pharmacological activation. *Electroencephalogr Clin Neurophysiol Suppl, 48,* 70–76.

73. Walker, A. E. (1967). Temporal lobectomy. *J Neurosurg, 26,* 642–649.

74. Walker, A. E. (1974). Surgery for epilepsy. In: Magnus, O., Lorentz de Haas, A.M., editors. *The Epilepsies (Handbook of Clinical Neurology).* Amsterdam: North Holland, pp. 739–757.

75. Engel, J. Jr., Driver, M. V., & Falconer, M. A. (1975). Electrophysiological correlates of pathology and surgical results in temporal lobe epilepsy. *Brain, 98,* 129–156.

76. Gastaut, H., Gastaut, J. L., Goncalves, E., et al. (1975). Relative frequency of different types of epilepsy: a study employing the classification of the International League Against Epilepsy. *Epilepsia, 16,* 457–461.

77. Niedermeyer, E. (1982). Electrocorticography. In: Niedermeyer, E., Lopes da Silva, F., eds. *Electroencephalography*. Munich: Urban & Schwarzenberg, pp. 537–541.
78. Rasmussen, T. B. (1983). Surgical treatment of complex partial seizures: results, lessons, and problems. *Epilepsia, 24,* S65–S76.
79. Graf, M., Niedermeyer, E., Schiemann, J., et al. (1984). Electrocorticography: information derived from intraoperative recordings during seizure surgery. *Clin Electroencephalogr, 15,* 83–91.
80. Niedermeyer, E. (1987). Electrocorticography. In: Niedermeyer, E., Lopes da Silva, F., eds. *Electroencephalography: Basic Principles, Clinical Applications and Related Fields*. Baltimore: Urban & Schwarzenberg, pp. 613–617.
81. Quesney, L. F., Abou-Khalil, B., Cole, A., & Olivier, A. (1988). Preoperative extracranial and intracranial EEG investigation in patients with temporal lobe epilepsy: trends, results and review of pathophysiologic mechanisms. *Acta Neurol Scand Suppl, 117,* 52–60.
82. Devinsky, O., Canevini, M. P., Sato, S., et al. (1992). Quantitative electrocorticography in patients undergoing temporal lobectomy. *J Epilepsy,* 178–185.
83. Cendes, F., Dubeau, F., Olivier, A., et al. (1993). Increased neocortical spiking and surgical outcome after selective amygdalo-hippocampectomy. *Epilepsy Res, 16,* 195–206.
84. Quesney, L. F., & Niedermeyer, E. (1993). Electrocorticography. In: Niedermeyer, E., & Lopes de Silva, F., eds. *Electroencephalography: Basic Principles, Clinical Applications and Related Fields*. Baltimore: Williams & Williams, pp. 695–699.
85. Tuunainen, A., Nousiainen, U., Mervaala, E., et al. (1994). Postoperative EEG and electrocorticography: relation to clinical outcome in patients with temporal lobe surgery. *Epilepsia, 35,* 1165–1173.
86. Bengzon, A. R., Rasmussen, T., Gloor, P., et al. (1968). Prognostic factors in the surgical treatment of temporal lobe epileptics. *Neurology, 18,* 717–731.
87. Ajmone, M. C. (1980). Depth electrography and electrocorticography. In: Aminoff, M. J., ed. *Electrodiagnosis in Clinical Neurology*. Churchill Livingstone, pp. 167–196.
88. Ojemann, G. A. (1980). Basic mechanisms implicated in surgical treatments of epilepsy. In: Lockard, J. S., Ward, A. A., eds. *Window to Brain Mechanisms*. New York: Raven Press, pp. 261–277.
89. Fiol, M. E., Gates, J. R., Torres, F., & Maxwell, R. E. (1991). The prognostic value of residual spikes in the postexcision electrocorticogram after temporal lobectomy. *Neurology, 41,* 512–516.
90. Primrose, D. C., & Ojemann, G. A. (1992). Outcome of resective surgery for temporal lobe epilepsy. In: Luders, H., ed. *Epilepsy Surgery*. New York: Raven Press, pp. 601–611.
91. Jennum, P., Dhuna, A., Davies, K., et al. (1993). Outcome of resective surgery for intractable partial epilepsy guided by subdural electrode arrays. *Acta Neurol Scand, 87,* 434–437.
92. Engel, J. Jr. (1987). Approaches to the localization of the epileptogenic lesion. In: Engel, J., Jr., ed. *Surgical Treatment of the Epilepsies*. New York: Raven Press, pp. 75–100.
93. Spencer, D. D., & Inserni, J. (1992). Temporal lobectomy. In: Luders, H. O., ed. *Epilepsy Surgery*. New York: Raven Press, pp. 533–545.
94. Doyle, W. K., & Spencer, D. D. (1997). Anterior temporal resection. In: Engel, J., Jr., & Pedley, T., eds. *Epilepsy: A Comprehensive Textbook*. Vol. 2. Philadelphia: Lippincott-Raven Publishers, pp. 1807–1817.
95. Schwartz, T. H., Bazil, C. W., Forgione, M., et al. (2000). Do reactive postresection "injury" spikes exist? *Epilepsia, 41,* 1463–1468.
96. Gibbs, F. A., Amador, L., & Rich, C. (1958). Electroencephalographic findings and therapeutic results in surgical treatment of psychomotor epilepsy. In: Baldwin, M., & Bailey, P., eds. *Temporal Lobe Epilepsies*. Springfield, IL: Charles C Thomas, pp. 358–367.
97. Walker, A. E., Lichtenstein, S., & Marshall, C. (1960). A critical analysis of electrocorticography in temporal lobe epilepsy. *Arch Neurol,* 172–182.
98. Chatrian, G. E., & Quesney, L. F. (1997). Intraoperative electrocorticography. In: Engel, J., Jr., & Pedley, T. A., eds. *Epilepsy: A Comprehensive Textbook*. Philadelphia: Lippincott-Raven Publishers, pp. 1749–1765.
99. Jasper, H. H., Arfel-Capdeville, G., & Rasmussen, T. (1961). Evaluation of EEG and cortical electrographic studies for prognosis of seizures following surgical excision of epileptogenic lesions. *Epilepsia, 2,* 130–137.
100. McBride, M. C., Binnie, C. D., Janota, I., & Polkey, C. E. (1991). Predictive value of intraoperative electrocorticograms in resective epilepsy surgery. *Ann Neurol, 30,* 526–532.
101. Stefan, H., Hopfengartner, R., Kreiselmeyer, G., et al. (2008). Interictal triple ECoG characteristics of temporal lobe epilepsies: an intraoperative ECoG analysis correlated with surgical outcome. *Clin Neurophysiol, 119,* 642–652.
102. Engel, J. Jr., Bragin, A., Staba, R., & Mody, I. (2009). High-frequency oscillations: what is normal and what is not? *Epilepsia, 50,* 598–604.
103. Jacobs, J., LeVan, P., Chander, R., et al. (2008). Interictal high-frequency oscillations (80–500 Hz) are an indicator of seizure onset areas independent of spikes in the human epileptic brain. *Epilepsia, 49,* 1893–1907.
104. Quesney, L. F., Constain, M., Fish, D. R., & Rasmussen, T. (1990). Frontal lobe epilepsy—field of recent emphasis. *Am J EEG Technol, 30,* 177–193.
105. Quesney, L. F., Constain, M., Rasmussen, T., et al. (1992). How large are frontal lobe epileptogenic zones? EEG, ECoG, and SEEG evidence. *Adv Neurol, 57,* 311–323.
106. Salanova, V., Andermann, F., Olivier, A., et al. (1992). Occipital lobe epilepsy: electroclinical manifestations, electrocorticography, cortical stimulation and outcome in 42 patients treated between 1930 and 1991. Surgery of occipital lobe epilepsy. *Brain, 115,* 1655–1680.
107. Salanova, V., Andermann, F., Rasmussen, T., et al. (1995). Parietal lobe epilepsy. Clinical manifestations and outcome in 82 patients treated surgically between 1929 and 1988. *Brain, 118,* 607–627.
108. Wennberg, R. A., Quesney, L. F., & Villemure, J. G. (1997). Epileptiform and non-epileptiform paroxysmal activity from isolated cortex after functional hemispherectomy. *Electroencephalogr Clin Neurophysiol, 102,* 437–442.
109. Quesney, L. F., Wennberg, R., Olivier, A., & Rasmussen, T. (1998). ECoG findings in extratemporal epilepsy: the MNI experience. *Electroencephalogr Clin Neurophysiol Suppl, 48,* 44–57.
110. Wennberg, R., Quesney, F., Olivier, A., & Rasmussen, T. (1998). Electrocorticography and outcome in frontal lobe epilepsy. *Electroencephalogr Clin Neurophysiol, 106,* 357–368.
111. Palmini, A., Gambardella, A., Andermann, F., et al. (1995). Intrinsic epileptogenicity of human dysplastic cortex as suggested by corticography and surgical results. *Ann Neurol, 37,* 476–487.
112. Walker, A. E. (1949). Electrocorticography in epilepsy. A surgeon's appraisal. *Electroencephalogr Clin Neurophysiol, 2,* 30–37.
113. Jasper, H. H. (1954). Electrocorticography. In: Penfield, W., & Jasper, H. H., eds. *Epilepsy and the Functional Anatomy of the Human Brain*. Boston: Little, Brown, pp. 692–738.
114. Ajmone, M. C. (1972). Focal electrical stimulation. In: Purpura, D. P., Penry, J. K., & Tower, D. B., eds. *Experimental Models of Epilepsy: A Manual for the Laboratory Worker*. New York: Raven Press, pp. 147–172.
115. Cherlow, D. G., Dymond, A. M., Crandall, P. H., et al. (1977). Evoked response and after-discharge thresholds to electrical stimulation in temporal lobe epileptics. *Arch Neurol, 34,* 527–531.
116. Bernier, G. P., Richer, F., Giard, N., et al. (1990). Electrical stimulation of the human brain in epilepsy. *Epilepsia, 31,* 513–520.

31 | PRINCIPLES AND TECHNIQUES FOR LONG-TERM EEG RECORDING (EPILEPSY MONITORING UNIT, INTENSIVE CARE UNIT, AMBULATORY)

MARC R. NUWER, MD, PHD, RONALD G. EMERSON, MD, AND CECIL D. HAHN, MD, MPH

ABSTRACT: Long-term monitoring is a set of methods for recording electroencephalographic (EEG) signals over a period of 24 hours or longer. Patient video recording is often synchronized to the EEG. Interpretation aids help physicians to identify events, which include automated spike and seizure detection and various trending displays of frequency EEG content. These techniques are used in epilepsy monitoring units for presurgical evaluations and differential diagnosis of seizures versus nonepileptic events. They are used in intensive care units to identify nonconvulsive seizures, to measure the effectiveness of therapy, to assess depth and prognosis in coma, and other applications. The patient can be monitored at home with ambulatory monitoring equipment. Specialized training is needed for competent interpretation of long-term monitoring EEGs. Problems include false-positive events flagged by automated spike and seizure detection software, and muscle and movement artifact contamination during seizures.

KEYWORDS: EEG, electroencephalogram, long-term monitoring, critical care, ambulatory, epilepsy, seizure

PRINCIPAL REFERENCES

1. Herman, S. T., Abend, N. S., Bleck, T. P., et al. Consensus statement on continuous EEG in critically ill adults and children, part I: indications; part II: personnel, technical specifications, and clinical practice. *J Clin Neurophysiol*, 2015;32(2):87–108.
2. Hirsch, L. J., LaRoche, S. M., Gaspard, N., et al. American Clinical Neurophysiology Society's Standardized Critical Care EEG Terminology: 2012 version. *J Clin Neurophysiol*, 2013;30(1):1–27.
3. Tsuchida, T. N., Wusthoff, C. J., Shellhaas, R. A., et al. American Clinical Neurophysiology Society standardized EEG terminology and categorization for the description of continuous EEG monitoring in neonates: report of the American Clinical Neurophysiology Society critical care monitoring committee. *J Clin Neurophysiol*, 2013;30(2):161–173.
4. Abend, N. S., Arndt, D. H., Carpenter, J. L., et al. Electrographic seizures in pediatric ICU patients: cohort study of risk factors and mortality. *Neurology*, 2013;81(4):383–391.
5. Vespa, P., Tubi, M., Claassen, J., et al. Metabolic crisis occurs with seizures and periodic discharges after brain trauma. *Ann Neurol*, 2016;879(4):579–590.
6. Arndt, D. H., Lerner, J. T., Matsumoto, J. H., et al. Subclinical early posttraumatic seizures detected by continuous EEG monitoring in a consecutive pediatric cohort. *Epilepsia*, 2013;54(10):1780–1788.
7. Sivaraju, A., Gilmore, E. J., Wira, C. R., et al. Prognostication of postcardiac arrest coma: early clinical and electroencephalographic predictors of outcome. *Intensive Care Med*, 2015;41(7):1264–1272.
8. Husain, A., and Sinha, A. R. (Eds.). *Critical Care EEG Monitoring*. New York: Springer Clinical Medicine, 2016.
9. Tatum, W. (Ed.). *Fundamentals of Ambulatory EEG*. New York: Demos, 2017.
10. Sirven, J., and Stern, J. (Eds.). *Atlas of Video-EEG Monitoring*. New York: McGraw-Hill, 2011.

1. INTRODUCTION

Most standard electroencephalographic (EEG) recordings last 20 to 40 minutes, with some extended to a few hours. EEG recorded over many hours, days, or weeks is considered *long-term monitoring* (LTM). This chapter reviews their applications, recording, and analysis techniques. Most LTM is provided for identification and characterization of episodic disorders. Video recording of the patient, synchronized with the EEG, is an integral part of some LTM.

Long-term EEG telemetry techniques date to a 1960s-era U.S. National Aeronautics and Space Administration (NASA) program to record EEG on astronauts during space exploration. This NASA radio telemetry technology allowed the recorded subject to move around distant from the recording base station, in our case the patients on an inpatient epilepsy monitoring unit (EMU) (1). The application became more widely applied in the early 1980s (2). The technology has considerably improved since then, but fundamental aspects have not really changed. LTM application expanded in the 1980s (3) to the intensive care unit (ICU), a role that has become more popular since 2000.

The recording of behavior at first was limited to film and subsequently to time-lapse video at a few frames per second. Development of VCRs in the 1980s allowed much simpler, higher-quality images. EEG recording and storage initially was limited 12 hours of recording of 14 channels on a high-capacity, industrial-quality tape. Those tapes were changed twice daily to allow continuous monitoring over days. By 1990 the sampling rates, tape recording durations, and channel capacity had all expanded. Today the LTM storage requirements are easy to meet, except with large numbers of channels (100 or more) at very high sampling rates (2,000 Hz).

2. LONG-TERM MONITORING FOR EPILEPSY

2.1. Indications

The International League Against Epilepsy published guidelines for the use of LTM in epilepsy (4). To diagnose epilepsy and identify the type of epilepsy, a description is needed of the behavioral and cognitive manifestations of seizures. This is obtained most often by history from patients and relatives. In many cases, however, the history is incomplete or even erroneous: patients are often not aware of their seizures or parts of their symptoms, and relatives too frequently are poor observers. To make a correct diagnosis, it is important to know the behavioral correlates of EEG manifestations. For example, behavioral arrest occasionally occurs with generalized epilepsy, and a secondarily generalized spike and wave with a localization-related epilepsy. We can summarize the indications for LTM as follows (4):

- The diagnosis of epilepsy needs to be made or ruled out because the events cannot be unambiguously classified based on the historical information. Some patients have epileptic and nonepileptic seizures.

- The diagnosis of epilepsy has been made but the type of seizure or syndrome is unclear.

- Epilepsy is medically intractable and surgery is considered. This requires a full characterization of the electroclinical manifestations of seizures, at first with scalp EEG, and possibly with subsequent intracranial electrodes in case scalp LTM does not provide sufficient information.

- Seizures need to be quantified to assess response to medical treatment, as may be the case for brief but frequent seizures.

LTM allows recording throughout the sleep–wake cycle. Some patients have predominantly or exclusively seizures during sleep, others predominantly upon awakening. Interictal activity in focal epilepsy is activated by non-rapid eye movement (REM) sleep and in some patients is present only during that stage.

2.2. Equipment and Personnel

The basic components of an LTM system are the electrodes, amplifier, camera, and transmission and recording system.

2.2.1. Electrodes

Electrode attachment is particularly important for obtaining high-quality LTM EEG over days while the patient moves during daily activities (e.g., eating and walking) and especially during seizures themselves. Electrode problems are the most common cause of poor-quality recordings. Scalp electrodes must make good contact for long periods, even if technicians are not available to regel them daily or over weekends. Collodion or other durable electrode–scalp adhesive is recommended. Wrapping a bandage or placing elastic netting over the patient's head minimizes artifacts caused by wire movements, a common problem during seizures. The wrap serves also to limit the patient's access to electrodes during head scratching. Bundling wires together provides greater rigidity than individual wires and also reduces movement artifact.

If a patient undergoing LTM requires a magnetic resonance imaging (MRI) scan, the electrodes must be removed and then replaced after the study. This can require a considerable time. Electrodes that can be kept in place during MRI studies have been developed recently. They include MR-compatible material for the electrodes and the wires and an MR-compatible connector system. Such electrodes include gold, silver–silver chloride, subdermal silver wire, and conductive plastic electrodes (5,6). Some of these electrodes are also compatible with computed tomography (CT), greatly facilitating EEG monitoring of patients in the ICU (6).

Electrodes recording from regions lower than the standard 10–20 electrodes can help characterize some temporal and inferior frontal discharges. The 10% system, or 10–10 system, of the expanded 10–20 International Electrode Nomenclature system (Nuwer 10% system, Jasper 10–20 system) describes a process for naming electrode sites that can be extended onto the face or behind the ear. These superficial cheek electrodes have become more popular than placement of implanted sphenoidal electrodes.

Recordings are most often referential so that they later can be reconstructed to any referential or bipolar montage (1). A good-quality reference is therefore important. The electrocardiogram (EKG) must be included in the montage since cardiac changes can be an important component of seizures or seizure-like events. We will not discuss here the various types of intracerebral electrodes, as this subject is addressed elsewhere in this volume (see Chapter 29 on Intracranial EEG Monitoring).

2.2.2. EEG Amplification and Transmission

The patient can carry a sufficiently small amplifier, usually in a chest pouch, on a belt, or under the head wraps. An amplifier signal can be transmitted with much less artifact contamination. Characteristics should be those of a standard EEG amplifier. These are typically a low filter at 0.3 Hz, a high filter at least 60 to 70 Hz, and sampling at 200 or 250 Hz. Higher frequencies in intracerebral EEG (7–9) and low frequencies in newborns (10) may also be of interest. To capture those well, amplifier characteristics would include lower frequencies (low filter at 0.1 Hz) and higher frequencies (high filter at 600 Hz and sampling at 2,000 Hz). Digital techniques can filter unwanted low or high frequencies during review, and down-sample for faster review speeds if desired. Recording with a high sampling rate otherwise has the disadvantage of increasing memory requirements and slowing down display reviews. Twelve-bit digitizing is common and often sufficient, whereas 16-bit digitizing is more than sufficient for intracerebral EEG's dynamic range (Chapters 32 and 33 deal with infra-slow and high-frequency EEG activities).

The patient-worn amplifier, cable system, or wireless telemetry transmitter should be not only light and comfortable, but also robust enough to withstand the stress of falls and convulsions. Cable or wireless telemetry is used to transmit the EEG signal. Cable may provide power to the amplifier. Wireless transmission gives freedom of movement but requires the patient to carry the battery power. This increases weight and risks battery depletion.

2.2.3. Video Recording

Digital video cameras are most commonly used. Whereas a color camera is used during the day, black-and-white recording with an infrared illuminator provides excellent image quality even in darkness. Recording in darkness increases patient nighttime comfort. The digital video signal is synchronized with the EEG recording. Because the EEG and camera have separate timing clocks, maintaining signal synchronization is important.

2.2.4. Display, Network, and Archive

EEG and video signals are transmitted to monitoring and recording computers and servers. This is accomplished either by dedicated cable or through a standard digital network. The digital transmission network may be a devoted local area network or the hospital's main backbone digital network.

Modern digital technology can now store many days of EEG recording, even when it is sampled at high rates on many channels with video recording. Large monitors display 15 to 20 seconds of EEG on the screen, and multiple adjacent screens allow simultaneous display of video and electronic medical record. EEG display gain, time scale, montage, and filters easily can be changed (1). By recording EEG referentially, alternate montages can be reconstructed as bipolar, other referential, average reference, and so forth (1). Network facilities allow remote EEG review from any station that can access the record, even from an offsite virtual private network (VPN) Internet connection (3).

Archiving data is challenging because of its size, especially the video size. Permanent storage on durable media, such as DVDs, is difficult because of the number that would be produced. Furthermore, technical issues present problematic planned obsolescence of media in future years. No hard medium is expected to be readable in a decade or two without eventual data copying onto another future hard medium. Soft storage has instead become common, in which long-term records are kept on an archive server. These servers can be maintained and routinely backed up. This is similar to the solution developed by radiology for imaging. Video is the source of most data for video-EEG, so archiving is less burdensome if the video can be trimmed by selecting only those clips most relevant for archiving. At the same time, the EEG can be trimmed by selecting the most relevant portion. Data for archives must be selected by a person familiar with patient's video-EEG presentation, seizure type, and EEG interpretation to ensure that relevant information is retained. As an example, a week-long EMU's video-EEG recording might be condensed to EEG alone for the first 24 hours plus video-EEG for the 10 to 15 minutes of each of the half-dozen seizure events. That consumes only 1% of storage capacity compared to saving the entire week's video-EEG.

2.2.5. Personnel and Certification

Trained observers need to be near the patients to provide close clinical observation during seizures as well as to ensure patient safety. Identifying convulsions is easier, whereas identifying subtle partial seizures and auras is more difficult in a long-term monitoring setting. Several tactics are used. To identify seizures, patients are constantly observed by trained staff using a video link. Patients and family press an alarm button to self-report any auras or seizures. Automatic seizure detection software flags suspicious EEG events. A relative or companion in the patient's room can alert staff to seizures or reported auras. Each event is logged for video-EEG review and each triggers a nurse responding to the bedside for an evaluation and safety check.

Experienced EEG technologists are vital in LTM to obtain the best-quality recording. They not only secure electrodes well in proper locations but also provide preliminary data review to mark record segments for physician interpretation. Full record review directly by the physician often is considered too time-consuming, which is why the technologist is used to provide this allied health staff preliminary review step. After physician review, selecting segments to be retained for archiving is a task that can be delegated to the well-trained technologist.

In some locations, technologists can obtain specific certification for EEG as practiced in the LTM setting. For example, the American Board of Registration of Electroencephalographic and Evoked Potential Technologists (ABRET) grants a Certification in Long Term Monitoring (CLTM). This is available to EEG technologists who have advanced training and experience, and who take and pass an examination to demonstrate their competence in LTM. The certification allows physicians and hospitals to identify technologists who have this demonstrated competence in LTM (11).

LTM services can demonstrate their adherence to the standards and principles of high-quality LTM also through ABRET accreditation. LTM Laboratory Board Accreditation is available typically for EMUs or critical care monitoring units. This ABRET LTM Lab accreditation flags a hospital service as meeting a high degree of quality and service. This can be useful for patients who choose which hospital to use for their admission, and for insurance carriers who choose to which hospitals to direct their patients for services (12). In these days of growing attention to healthcare economics and the public need for quality assurance processes, these CLTM and LTM Lab accreditation processes are ways in which the EEG LTM field contributes to what the public wants from the healthcare community.

2.3. Duration of Monitoring and Drug Withdrawal

The duration of EMU admission depends on its purpose. In general, it is best to try to be generous with the duration of monitoring because unexpected events are commonly discovered. Patients may have more than one seizure type, and capturing each is needed before a surgical decision can be made. Patients may report that they have only one seizure type, but may not be aware of a second type. Some patients are unaware of nocturnal, unwitnessed, or subtle types. A sample of only two to four seizures may be too few to use for major clinical decisions such as surgery. The historical description reported by the patient or family is often incomplete or erroneous, and it may require the recording of several seizures to fully document a seizure disorder that is different from what was expected. In the context of presurgical evaluation, it has been estimated that five seizures with the same region of onset and no contradictory information provide a reasonable sample to decide that the onset is indeed in that region (13).

Antiepileptic medications frequently are reduced or discontinued during LTM to induce more frequent seizures. In presurgical evaluation, the question of whether seizures occurring after medication withdrawal are similar to habitual seizures has been raised. Symptomatology and the EEG pattern at onset are similar after medication withdrawal (14–17). There is no evidence that seizures spread more rapidly from one hemisphere to the other after drug withdrawal. Seizures do more often secondarily generalize after drug reduction (18,19), so the EMU staff should be prepared for generalized seizures.

It is sometimes claimed that reducing antiepileptic medication causes increased spiking activity. However, careful studies of the timing of drug withdrawal, seizure occurrence, and changes in spiking (20,21) showed no increased spiking following drug withdrawal. Spiking does increase following seizures. When drugs are reduced, seizures occur and spiking increases as a result of increased seizures. Spiking may even *decrease* as a result of drug withdrawal in the absence of seizures (22).

2.4. Considerations for Children or Infants

LTM can be performed at all ages, including newborns (23). In newborns and young infants, a subset of the standard 10–20 electrodes is used. Since seizures can be very focal, the montage does need to be reasonably complete. The frontopolar electrodes often are moved somewhat more posteriorly. Collodion should be avoided in young children, because of their very delicate skin. Young patients often have seizures much more frequently than adults, so LTM can be shorter (e.g., 1–2 days).

In children, a full syndromic definition often requires that different seizure patterns be recorded, as well as the interictal activity (4). A parent in the room during monitoring helps to identify the events being investigated. (Specific aspects of recordings of seizures in neonates, infants, and children are presented in Chapter 18.)

2.5. Seizure and Spike Detection

2.5.1. SEIZURES IN LTM

Since seizure detection is performed from analyzing the EEG, only seizures that have a clear manifestation in the EEG can be detected. Some subtle seizures occur in deep or distant structures and EEG electrodes are not well positioned to detect them. EEG generally will detect seizures that cause a lapse of consciousness, but scalp EEG alone may miss many auras or focal motor seizures without a lapse of consciousness. Depth electrodes placed in deep structures, typically the hippocampus and nearby locations, detect auras even when they have no scalp correlate, or at a moment when those seizures have yet to spread to the scalp.

Figures 31.1 and 31.2 show examples of seizures recorded from the scalp, and Figure 31.3 shows a seizure recorded from intracerebral electrodes. In Figures 31.1 and 31.3, the specific moment of onset is not easily identified. In Figure 31.2, the onset is clear, consisting of a few seconds of rhythmic discharge followed by irregular slow waves.

Seizure patterns are quite different in the newborn EEG than in older children and adults: the discharges are often much slower and sometimes very focal (limited to one electrode). For these reasons, methods specific to the newborn have been

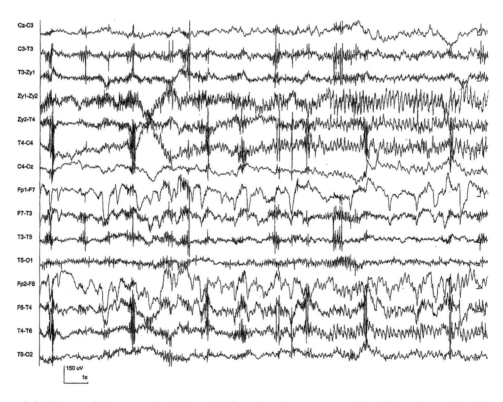

Figure 31.1. *Scalp-recorded right temporal seizure occurring in the context of muscle and eye movement artifacts. This early part of the seizure consists of a discharge in the theta range of frequencies, commonly seen in temporal lobe seizures. From (24).*

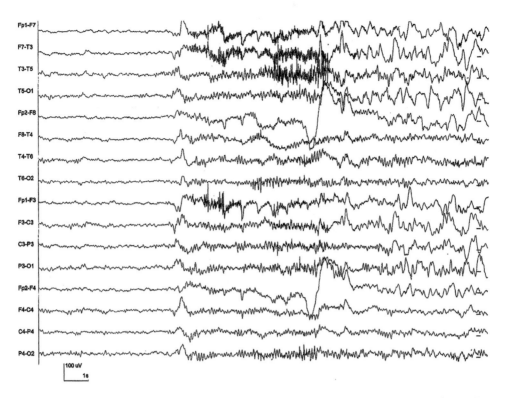

Figure 31.2. Scalp-recorded seizure with a generalized and abrupt onset. A few seconds of rhythmic theta-frequency activity are followed by irregular slow waves in the delta range. From (24).

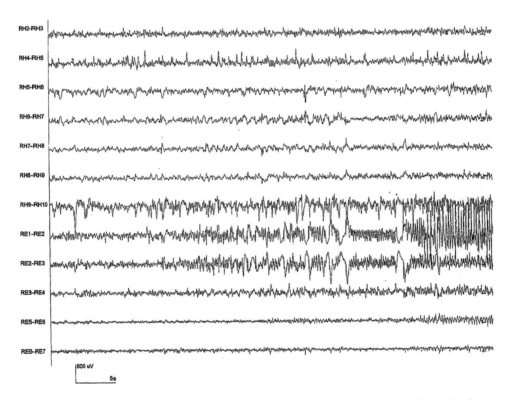

Figure 31.3. Seizure recorded from intracerebral electrodes placed on the temporal lobe. The RH contacts are along an orthogonal multicontact depth electrode having its deepest contacts (lower numbers) in the hippocampus and most superficial contacts in the second temporal convolution. The RE electrodes are epidural electrodes placed along the first temporal convolution. The seizure onset consists of mixed-frequency activity, followed by a more rhythmic discharge. Note compressed time scale. For the purpose of clarity, this EEG illustrates only a fraction of the electrodes implanted in this patient's brain. From (24).

developed, with the particular aim of detecting the very slow discharges often present during newborn seizures (25–27).

2.5.2. Automatic Seizure Detection

During LTM, patients are usually asked to press a button when they feel a seizure coming. If patients could always feel their seizure coming, there would be no need for automatic seizure detection. Often, though, patients are not aware of their seizures, and observers are not always present or able to recognize a seizure. Furthermore, some seizures have very minimal clinical signs—sometimes no visible signs at all. Finding seizures is long and tedious and may miss short seizures. Automatic seizure detection can be helpful in this context, since it provides a means for marking the EEG sections that are likely to include seizure patterns. For this purpose, the detection can take place at any time during the seizure (not necessarily early) because the EEG will be reviewed a posteriori.

Seizures in an EEG are "paroxysmal, rhythmic, and evolving," and adapting that to a software algorithm is difficult. The detection method may characterize each 2-sec epoch by its frequency, rhythmicity, and amplitude, and compare these measurements to background (28,29). Empirical rules across epochs and channels are used to reach a detection decision. The background criterion repeatedly is updated because EEG is nonstationary—that is, the background content changes over time due to factors such as the patient's states of drowsiness. A variety of these methods follow a similar empirical approach (30,31).

An extension of the above concept is to incorporate a particular patient's seizure characteristics into the context. In this case, the method is aimed at detecting seizures in that particular patient, and only seizures that look like the sample seizures (which have been incorporated in the context) are detected. The method can then be labeled "patient-specific"—or more correctly, "seizure-specific," since a patient can have several types of seizure. Better detection performance can thus be obtained if it is acceptable to detect only a specific seizure pattern in a given patient (32–35).

The false-detection rate, the most common measure of failure, is in the range of one per hour for scalp recordings. Contributing factors are scalp artifacts from electromyography, movement, chewing, and eye blinks. False detections from intracerebral recordings are fewer because they contain fewer such artifacts and seizure patterns are often more prominent in intracerebral EEG (30).

Artificial neural networks (ANNs) require no a priori algorithm for seizure detection (36–38). Using a large number of training examples of seizures and non-seizure data, a network gradually learns to differentiate seizure examples from non-seizure EEG examples. Features of amplitude, rhythmicity, and dominant frequency are specified in advance as relevant, but it is not necessary to explicitly describe seizure patterns. The ANN automatically determines which combinations of features are characteristic of seizures by adapting its internal structure to reflect the training data. The performance of ANN methods depends on an appropriate set of features and on exposure to a sufficiently large training set containing a variety of seizure patterns.

2.5.3. Automatic Spike Detection

Many patients with epilepsy have interictal EEG abnormalities such as spikes, polyspikes, sharp waves, and bursts of spike and wave. These paroxysmal events may occur unpredictably and sometimes rarely. They play an important role in defining some epileptic syndromes and they contribute to localizing the seizure onset zone. They themselves can subtly or more overtly disturb brain function (39,40).

Automated spike detection is far from perfect for two reasons: (a) individual spikes can represent a poorly defined pattern, leading to low inter-rater agreement (41), and (b) spike detection involves a complex analysis of temporal and spatial features as well as context, an analysis that is not easily reproduced in an algorithm.

Routine EEG interpretation does not use automatic spike detection because expert readers find the spikes visually. Unfortunately, non-experts may incorrectly interpret artifacts or normal variants as epileptiform transients (42). This can result in incorrect patient care. A reliable automatic detection method might become useful for the non-expert in the future, but at present automatic spike detection is useful to screen the extensive recordings made during LTM (43). Automatic detection is most difficult in this setting because the recording includes multiple confounding transients such as eye blinks, movement, chewing, and muscle artifacts, electrode artifacts, and normal sleep transients.

3. CRITICAL CARE EEG MONITORING

When it is used in the critical care unit, LTM often is referred to as continuous electroencephalography (cEEG). The current generation of cEEG technology was applied first in the 1980s (3) and gradually spread in the 1990s. In recent years its use has rapidly increased such that it is becoming standard practice at many academic centers in North America (44,45). Recent guidelines proposed indications for the use of cEEG in critically ill neonates, (46) children, and adults, (47) and have defined minimum technical standards and terminology for cEEG interpretation (48–50).

3.1. Classification of Seizures During Critical Illness

The clinical neurological examination of the critically ill patient is often challenging. Encephalopathy or altered mental status is common, the cause of which is often unclear and multifactorial. In this challenging clinical setting, cEEG monitoring can provide valuable insights into cortical function, in particular the occurrence of seizures, the majority of which are known to be subtle or entirely subclinical.

Seizures in the critical care unit are classified according to their clinical and electrographic characteristics. *Electrographic seizures* are defined by characteristic EEG features: a rhythmic electrographic pattern lasting ≥10 sec (or shorter if associated with clinical change) with a clear onset and offset, and evolution in frequency, amplitude, or morphology (Box 31.1) (51). When electrographic seizures are accompanied by clinical signs such as motor, sensory, or autonomic changes,

The term "ictal-interictal continuum" has been coined to describe this dilemma (51). Terminology for the consistent description of rhythmic and periodic EEG patterns occurring during critical care EEG recordings has been developed to facilitate standardized multicenter research and clinical care (48). The Critical Care EEG Monitoring Research Consortium has developed an open-access database using this terminology for standardized critical care EEG reporting that is freely available (53).

3.2. Indications for Critical Care EEG Monitoring

A recent evidence-based consensus statement from the American Clinical Neurophysiology Society (ACNS) has outlined *recommended* and *suggested* indications for cEEG monitoring in critically ill children and adults (Box 31.2) (47,50). According to surveys of current practice, (45,54) the most common indications for critical care cEEG monitoring in North American centers are to screen for subclinical or subtle seizures among patients with altered mental status, to diagnose clinical events suspected to represent epileptic seizures, and to guide titration of antiepileptic therapy in patients with recurrent seizures or status epilepticus. Most centers perform cEEG monitoring for at least 24 hours, based on evidence that 1 hour of monitoring may identify only 50% to 60% of patients destined to develop seizures whereas 24 hours is likely to identify >80% (55–57). Recent ACNS guidelines for cEEG monitoring in neonates recommend at least 24 hours of cEEG monitoring for the detection of seizures in certain high-risk groups (e.g., hypoxic-ischemic encephalopathy, encephalitis, stroke) to clarify whether clinical paroxysmal events represent epileptic seizures, and to monitor the evolution of the EEG background activity to assist with prognostication (Box 31.3) (46).

3.3. Prevalence and Risk Factors for Seizures in Critical Care Units

Seizures are remarkably common among critically ill adults, children, and neonates. Numerous studies have now reported the prevalence of seizures among cohorts of ICU patients who underwent cEEG monitoring at the request of a treating physician, often according to institutional guidelines. However, it has become clear that there is substantial inter-institutional variability in the indications for cEEG monitoring, the timing of cEEG initiation, the duration of monitoring, and the case mix of patients in the ICU (45). Therefore, it is not surprising that the reported prevalence of seizures also varies between institutions. Prospective and retrospective observational studies of broad groups of critically ill patients undergoing clinically indicated cEEG monitoring identified electrographic seizures in between 30% and 46% of children and between 8% and 37% of adults (44,55,56,58–68).

An important recurring theme from these publications is that the majority of seizures identified by cEEG in critically ill adults and children either are subclinical or are accompanied by only very subtle clinical signs, and would likely go undetected without cEEG monitoring. For example, studies have demonstrated that at least 70% of encephalopathic children who experience electrographic seizures will experience some subclinical

they are termed *electroclinical seizures*. Often, however, these clinical manifestations are very subtle, such that seizures go unrecognized by bedside caregivers and are appreciated only during review of the cEEG with time-locked video. When electrographic seizures occur without any clinical signs, they are termed *subclinical, nonconvulsive*, or *EEG-only seizures*. As discussed further below, subclinical seizures constitute the majority of ICU seizures, and frequently occur in the setting of an acute brain injury such as encephalitis, trauma, or hypoxic-ischemic injury, or following convulsive seizures. Therefore, cEEG monitoring is required to accurately quantify the burden of subclinical and subtle seizures among critically ill patients.

When reviewing critical care EEG, distinguishing between recurrent *interictal* epileptiform discharges and *ictal* discharges can be challenging. Electrographic patterns frequently wax and wane, or evolve from patterns that are clearly ictal to those that are clearly interictal and vice versa. Various periodic and rhythmic EEG patterns are frequently encountered (e.g., generalized and lateralized periodic discharges, rhythmic delta activity). These phenomena often present challenges to clinicians who must decide which EEG patterns are potentially harmful and warrant more or less aggressive treatment (52). Most experts would treat unequivocal nonconvulsive seizures and equivocal EEG patterns when they have a clear clinical correlate. There is less consensus on the treatment of equivocal patterns without clinical correlate.

seizures, and 29% to 83% of these children will experience *exclusively* subclinical seizures (56,62,63,66–70). Furthermore, in several studies *all* children found to have electrographic status epilepticus experienced some subclinical seizures, and at least 30% experienced *exclusively* subclinical seizures (62,68,69). Similar observations have been made in critically ill adults.

In the neonatal ICU, the best data on seizure prevalence comes from the most common group undergoing cEEG monitoring: neonates with encephalopathy due to presumed perinatal hypoxia-ischemia. Among this population, electrographic seizures were detected in 34% to 48% and status epilepticus in 10% of patients (57,71).

Among broad ICU populations undergoing cEEG monitoring, the risk factors for seizures in critically ill adults and children are remarkably similar. Clinical factors associated with seizures on cEEG have included younger age (<18 years in adult cohorts, <3 years in pediatric cohorts), coma at the start of cEEG monitoring, a past medical history of epilepsy, and the occurrence of convulsive seizures prior to monitoring. EEG factors associated with seizures on cEEG have included the presence of interictal epileptiform discharges, periodic discharges, and abnormal initial background activity (e.g., burst suppression) (55,56). In fact, in an adult cohort, the absence of epileptiform discharges during the first 30 minutes of a cEEG recording was associated with a marked reduction in seizure risk from 22% to 3%, indicating that early EEG features may permit risk stratification (72).

cEEG monitoring has also been applied to specific subpopulations, which has identified several other patient groups at high risk for electrographic seizures. In adults, electrographic seizures were identified following convulsive status epilepticus in 48%

(73), following traumatic brain injury in 22% (74), following intracranial hemorrhage in 18% (75), and following subarachnoid hemorrhage in 8% (76). Even adults admitted to a medical ICU without evidence of acute neurological injury were found to be at risk, with 10% experiencing electrographic seizures, of which two thirds were entirely subclinical. Among these patients, sepsis was the only independent risk factor for seizures (77).

Among children, seizures have been detected in 63% with suspected encephalitis (78), 47% of those suffering a hypoxic brain injury following cardiac arrest (79), 11% to 20% of infants undergoing cardiac surgery (80,81), and 21% of children undergoing treatment with extracorporeal membrane oxygenation (82). In addition, electrographic seizures have been observed in 43% to 57% of children following traumatic brain injury, particularly following abusive brain trauma and when a concomitant hemorrhage is identified (83–85). Furthermore, seizures are frequently identified following childhood stroke and often represent the presenting symptom (62,86–88). Electrographic seizures are especially common following hemorrhagic stroke but also frequently occur after arterial or venous ischemic infarction (87,89).

Among neonates, the only reliable predictor of seizures following hypoxic-ischemic encephalopathy is an abnormal initial EEG background (excessively discontinuous, depressed, and undifferentiated, burst suppression, or extremely low voltage). In contrast, clinical factors such as the Apgar score and evidence of acidosis were not helpful in identifying neonates who developed seizures (57).

3.4. Impact of Seizures on Outcomes

One of the main motivations for cEEG monitoring in critically ill patients is the concern that electrographic seizures, especially when prolonged or repetitive, may be independently contributing to brain injury and worsening outcome. Thus, early detection and treatment of electrographic seizures represents an attractive neuroprotective strategy. Although a definitive causal link between seizures, secondary brain injury, and worse outcome remains to be proven, there is a growing body of evidence supporting this hypothesis.

In critically ill adults, a longer duration of nonconvulsive seizures and a delay to their diagnosis have been independently associated with mortality (90). The occurrence of seizures and periodic discharges in adults with traumatic brain injury has been associated with a state of "metabolic crisis," evidenced by an elevated lactate/pyruvate ratio and elevated glutamate levels on cerebral microdialysis (91,92). Nonconvulsive seizures in critically ill patients are known to increase glucose metabolism and raise intracranial pressure (93). These mechanisms most likely underlie the observation that nonconvulsive seizures after intracerebral hemorrhage are associated with increased cerebral edema and midline shift, and a greater risk of mortality (94). Furthermore, nonconvulsive seizures after traumatic brain injury have been associated with ipsilateral hippocampal atrophy, suggesting that these seizures may cause permanent neuropathologic changes (95).

In critically ill children, electrographic seizures have also been independently associated with worse short-term and long-term outcome in several different cohorts (65,68,96–100).

A recent cohort study of critically ill children demonstrated that increasing electrographic seizure burden was independently associated with neurological decline, even after controlling for diagnosis and illness severity (68). A maximum seizure burden of >12 minutes in a given hour was associated with a greater probability and magnitude of neurological decline. Electrographic status epilepticus has been associated with short-term neurological decline and mortality (97), as well as unfavourable long-term global health outcome, lower health-related quality-of-life scores, and an increased risk of subsequently diagnosed epilepsy (99). Among infants with congenital heart disease, the occurrence of clinical and electrographic seizures in the postoperative period has also been associated with worse long-term outcomes (101,102).

In critically ill neonates, after controlling for the severity of brain injury, clinical seizures have been independently associated with elevated lactate/choline ratio by magnetic resonance spectroscopy (103). Electrographic neonatal seizures have been associated with microcephaly, severe cerebral palsy, failure to thrive, and mortality(104). However, in another study of neonates with hypoxic-ischemic encephalopathy who underwent therapeutic hypothermia, the evolution of EEG background activity over time was more predictive of MRI brain injury than seizures (71).

Despite mounting evidence for an association between increasing seizure burden and worse neurological outcome, it remains to be proven that more timely identification and treatment of seizures can actually lower seizure burden and improve outcomes (68,98). It remains possible that seizures are only a symptom of primary brain injury and not a contributor to secondary brain injury. The reported associations between seizure burden and outcome in many studies may simply be due to incomplete adjustment for the severity of the underlying brain injury, despite the authors' best efforts. A randomized controlled trial would eliminate these confounders, but such a trial faces numerous methodological and ethical challenges. Despite the current level of evidence, recent consensus guidelines have chosen to recommend cEEG monitoring to detect and manage status epilepticus in critically ill patients, and to recommend that both clinical *and* electrographic seizure activity be controlled as quickly as possible (105). Finally, it is important to consider that the potential for electrographic seizures to cause harm likely depends on both the seizure burden and the type and severity of the underlying brain injury (106).

3.5. cEEG Monitoring for Prognostication

Certain cEEG features have been associated with better and worse prognosis in comatose or deeply encephalopathic patients. Favorable prognostic features include the presence of an organized posterior dominant rhythm, sleep spindles, reactivity, and variability. Unfavorable prognostic features include an attenuated, suppressed, or burst-suppression EEG background, or invariant polymorphic slow background activity without evidence of reactivity or variability (107,108).

Reactivity is defined as a change in EEG background activity that is temporally correlated to auditory, visual, or tactile stimulation. Reactivity should be evaluated and reported on a daily basis during cEEG monitoring. *Variability* is defined as a spontaneous change in EEG background activity, which may only become apparent over minutes to hours—for example, cycling through various sleep stages. Quantitative EEG (qEEG) techniques can be very helpful to appreciate these slowly evolving EEG changes. Early recovery of sleep–wake cycling visualized by amplitude-integrated EEG is a particularly favorable prognostic sign in neonates following hypoxic-ischemic encephalopathy (109,101). Techniques for automated assessment of sleep–wake cycling are under development (111,112).

The prognostic value of cEEG in post-anoxic coma has been particularly extensively studied (113). Reports have consistently shown that in comatose patients undergoing therapeutic hypothermia following cardiac arrest, an unreactive, discontinuous, or suppression-burst, or low-voltage (20μV) background, or the presence of electrographic seizures, is strongly associated with unfavorable outcome (114–118). A unique EEG pattern of "burst suppression with identical bursts" has been described among comatose adults with diffuse cerebral ischemia, which was invariably associated with poor outcome (119). In newborns with hypoxic-ischemic encephalopathy, electrographic seizures and persistently abnormal EEG background activity over time have been associated with poor outcome (71,104,110).

3.6. cEEG Monitoring for Cerebral Ischemia

The rationale for using cEEG to monitor for cerebral ischemia is based on the fact that EEG generators located in cortical layers 3 and 5 are particularly sensitive to hypoxia and ischemia (120–123). Notably, EEG changes already begin to manifest when cerebral blood flow (CBF) drops to 25 mL/100 g/min, whereas ischemic injury typically requires CBF to drop below 12 to 18 mL/100 g/min (124–126). Therefore, in the setting of a slowly progressive decline in CBF, recognition of early EEG changes could provide a "window of opportunity" for therapeutic intervention before irreversible ischemic injury takes place.

As CBF declines, the EEG background activity first demonstrates a loss of fast activity, followed by polymorphic delta activity and eventually diffuse attenuation (127). Upon CBF restoration, EEG activity may improve before recovery of the clinical exam (121).

cEEG monitoring may be used to screen for acute ischemic stroke; however, confirmation with MRI or CT is required since EEG changes such as focal slowing or attenuation are not specific for stroke. The amount of EEG slowing does correlate with perfusion-weighted MRI lesion volume (128) and with clinical control of hypertension and hypotension (129). An acute EEG index has been shown to reflect the therapeutic effects of tissue plasminogen activator (tPA) (128,130). In the setting of severe focal ischemia the EEG may demonstrate a characteristic pattern termed regional attenuation without delta (RAWOD) (131).

3.7. cEEG Monitoring for Vasospasm After Subarachnoid Hemorrhage

Subarachnoid hemorrhage causes EEG slowing (132), disrupts the posterior dominant rhythm (133), and may also cause focal or lateralized slowing. Among 116 consecutive subarachnoid hemorrhage patients with ICU EEG monitoring in one study (134), 16% showed periodic epileptiform discharges, 6% non-convulsive seizures, and 4% nonconvulsive status epilepticus. The EEG was nonreactive to external stimuli in 14% and showed no state changes in 14%, and stage II sleep transients were absent in 85%. Other EEG findings included frontal intermittent rhythmic delta activity (FIRDA; 8%) and stimulus-induced rhythmic, periodic, or ictal discharges (SIRPIDs; 8%) (134,135).

Delayed cerebral ischemia due to vasospasm is a major complication of SAH. Angiographic vasospasm is detected in 50% to 70% of subarachnoid hemorrhage patients (136), whereas delayed cerebral ischemia is seen in 19% to 46% of patients (137–143). Vasospasm may develop slowly over hours to days, creating an opportunity for early detection by cEEG monitoring and intervention before irreversible ischemic injury occurs. However, because vasospasm-related EEG changes occur so slowly, they can be difficult to recognize on conventional EEG review. Several qEEG techniques have been shown to herald the onset of vasospasm: total power trends (144), relative alpha variability (145), and post-stimulation alpha/delta ratio (55). EEG in one study was 100% sensitive for angiographically defined vasospasm (145). Focal ischemia from vasospasm may produce bilateral EEG changes (55,145).

3.8. Technical Considerations

Many of the techniques now used for critical care EEG monitoring have been adopted from other EEG applications. Continuous EEG recording was adopted from the EMU, with the later addition of time-locked video. The practice of frequent surveillance to observe for complications, deterioration, or improvement was adopted from intraoperative monitoring. Visualization techniques for prolonged recordings such as time compression were adopted from polysomnography.

Critical care EEG monitoring was initially performed using two- or four-channel compressed spectral array (CSA) monitors (146,147), which were difficult to understand and use. In the early 1990s, a new generation of ICU EEG monitoring equipment introduced innovations that went beyond CSA (148), including recording from full-head EEG channel coverage, more intuitive quantitative trending displays, remote review access from outside the unit, and digital storage of the raw EEG, which permitted confirmation of suspicious activity identified by qEEG. The ability to display both the qEEG trends and the raw EEG tracings continuously at the bedside of critically ill patients permitted ICU nurses and physicians to participate in basic EEG interpretation. Automated seizure detection algorithms, initially developed for use in the EMU, began to be applied in the critical care setting.

On qEEG frequency trending, seizures may appear as events that begin with faster frequencies, then slow and dissipate (Fig. 31.4).

Simple automated flags for surges in total power, amplitude integrated EEG, or amount of fast activity also can alert for possible seizures. While the simple systems may have a modest loss of sensitivity and specificity, they can perform reasonably well under more ideal circumstances especially to detect higher amplitude, more widespread seizure discharges (Fig. 31.5).

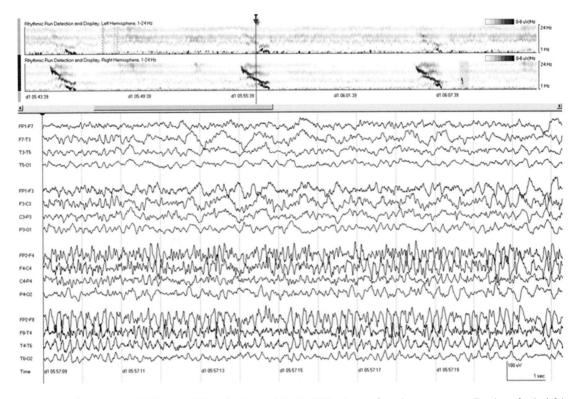

Figure 31.4. Seizures occur three times in this 30-minute ICU monitoring trend display. EEG review confirms these are seizures. Trends are for the left hemisphere (top trend) and right hemisphere (bottom trend). Trends measure frequencies from 1 to 24 Hz. Dark color represents intense activity at that frequency at that moment of time. Seizures begin at faster frequencies and then slow, as can be seen clearly on the trends. The cursor marks the time of the 13-sec routine EEG displayed below. The use of trend shows the laterality and recurrence of the seizures, and allows the interpreting physician the opportunity to get a quick overview of long stretches of the record. Illustration courtesy of Suzette LaRoche.

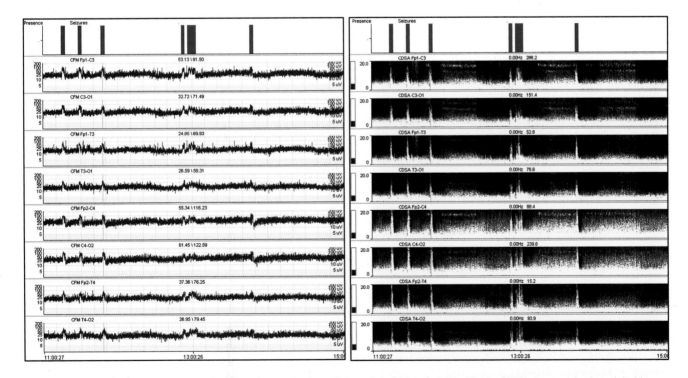

Figure 31.5. qEEG trending displays provide an overview of seizure burden. qEEG trending displays depicting 4 hours of EEG using an eight-channel double-distance longitudinal bipolar montage. Electrographic seizures identified by conventional EEG review are indicated by the blue bars in the top channel. **A:** On the amplitude-integrated EEG display, seizures are associated with a rise in both the upper and lower margin of the amplitude-integrated EEG tracing. **B:** On the color spectrogram display, seizures are associated with bright "flame-shaped" bands of color, indicating higher-power EEG activity across a wider range of frequencies.

Successful critical care EEG monitoring requires a dedicated interdisciplinary team comprising EEG technologists, neurophysiologists, ICU nurses, and ICU physicians. Support from the hospital's information technology department is essential to ensure reliable remote access to continuous EEG recordings from within the hospital's network, and secure remote access from outside the hospital, usually over a VPN connection. Because cEEG recordings provide time-sensitive information on the health of critically ill patients, an information technology infrastructure that can provide >99% uptime is essential.

Critical care EEG recordings must be interpreted by individuals with formal training and certification in clinical neurophysiology. However, at many centers EEG technologists also play an important role in the continuous or periodic surveillance of ongoing cEEG recordings. It is important to establish institutional standards for cEEG review and reporting, and to ensure that ICU caregivers and a patient's family members are aware of these standards so that they have realistic expectations. According to a survey of institutional practice in North America, cEEG recordings are most commonly reviewed twice daily, with more frequent review guided by clinical need (45). In addition to routine review, neurophysiologists should be prepared to review the cEEG at the request of ICU caregivers when they are concerned about a suspicious clinical behavior or EEG pattern. Excellent communication between the clinical neurophysiology team and the neurology and critical care teams is essential to ensure that significant changes in the cEEG can be acted upon in a timely manner.

Conventional full-montage EEG is the best technique for identifying electrographic seizures and distinguishing seizures from the many forms of EEG artifact that may occur in the ICU setting. Inclusion of time-locked digital video is essential to identify the subtle clinical manifestations of seizures, to confirm whether a given clinical behavior represents an electrographic seizure, and to determine sources of physiologic and nonphysiologic artifact. The use of fewer recording electrodes limits the extent of cortex being monitored and reduces the ability to detect seizures and distinguish seizures from artifacts. Therefore, reduced EEG montages should be used with caution. In adults, certain reduced montages may permit reasonably accurate seizure detection (e.g., a seven-electrode montage) (149), while others do not (e.g., a hairline montage) (150,151). In neonatal ICUs, one- or two-channel "cerebral function monitors" based on amplitude-integrated EEG are in widespread use, particularly in Europe. Although amplitude-integrated EEG-based monitors can provide an accurate indication of the EEG background, their sensitivity and specificity for seizure detection are relatively low (152–154).

Electrode application should be performed by registered EEG technologists according to the International 10–20 System. Electrodes should be fixed with paste or collodion adhesive. Skin integrity underneath electrodes should be checked daily and electrodes repositioned as needed. Skin ulceration most commonly occurs beneath occipital electrodes due to pressure from the weight of the head, and beneath frontopolar electrodes due to pressure from head bandages that are wrapped too tightly. The use of conductive plastic electrodes that cause only minimal artifact on CT and MRI can reduce the need to remove and replace electrodes for neuroimaging (155–157). Both disposable and reusable EEG electrode systems are available, and some are prewired to a quick connector that can be easily disconnected and reconnected by bedside nurses without the need for assistance from an EEG technologist.

At many institutions qualified EEG technologists are often unavailable after normal working hours. Creative strategies can be applied to enable after-hours electrode application. For instance, ICU nurses can be taught to apply a limited array of EEG electrodes or an electrode cap until an EEG technologist becomes available to apply a conventional electrode montage. When applied by trained critical care physicians or nurse practitioners, electrode caps can achieve EEG recordings with acceptable electrode impedances and signal quality, at considerable time saving (158).

qEEG trending displays that time compress and simplify the EEG display can both facilitate EEG interpretation by clinical neurophysiologists, and enable bedside caregivers to more easily screen for seizures (159–162). qEEG displays provide an overview of the temporal evolution in seizure burden and can highlight slowly evolving changes in the EEG background indicative of impending ischemia that would be difficult to appreciate on a conventional EEG display. Amplitude-integrated EEG, power spectrograms, and rhythmicity spectrograms are generally best suited to highlighting electrographic seizures. The alpha/delta ratio, alpha variability, and asymmetry indexes are best suited to ischemia monitoring. Importantly, reliance on qEEG displays alone is not recommended because seizures can be missed (particularly seizures of short duration or low amplitude), and various kinds of artifacts can easily be mistaken for seizures, resulting in false positives. Therefore, any suspicious patterns identified by qEEG should be verified by review of the underlying raw EEG. However, when used judiciously, qEEG displays can result in significant time saving, with minimal reduction in sensitivity for seizures and other significant electrographic patterns (159,162). Finally, although much effort has been devoted to developing automated seizure detection algorithms (163,164), until now the sensitivity of these algorithms has been too low or their false-detection rates too high to replace clinical EEG interpretation.

4. AMBULATORY MONITORING

Ambulatory EEG is the recording of EEG typically lasting 24 to 72 hours using portable devices carried home by patients. Recently, chronic recording has appeared using implanted devices. These fill a useful niche between routine laboratory-based EEGs and inpatient video-EEG LTM. Ambulatory EEG provides the ability to extend the duration of EEG surveillance from the 30 minutes typical of a routine EEG to several days. In the past, ambulatory EEG devices offered limited fidelity and flexibility, and could record relatively few channels. Those limitations no longer apply, and current ambulatory EEG systems can produce recordings equivalent in quality to recordings obtained using standard laboratory systems.

4.1. Clinical Utility of Ambulatory EEG

The ability to record EEG over extended periods of time increases the likelihood of capturing interictal discharges and seizures. This information is often critical for accurate diagnosis and clinical management. In one study, the yield of ambulatory EEG monitoring for providing evidence to support the diagnosis of epilepsy was 2.5 times that of a standard EEG, and 83% that of inpatient video-EEG monitoring (165). Importantly, the chances of capturing *seizures* is far greater on ambulatory EEG than standard EEG; in a study comparing sleep-deprived and ambulatory EEGs in patients with normal or nondiagnostic standard EEGs, a sleep-deprived EEG captured no seizures while seizures were recorded in 15% of patients on ambulatory EEG, including in several patients who were unaware of them (166). Underreporting of seizures is well recognized, in part because amnesia for the ictus is common; in one study, patients were unaware of 63% of all seizures occurring in an inpatient EMU (167).

While the ability to record EEG as the patient goes about normal activity is an advantage, daytime recordings often contain substantially more movement- and muscle-related artifacts than recordings made in an EEG laboratory. Nighttime recordings are more likely to be artifact-free, and indeed the ability to obtain prolonged sleep recording is an attractive feature of ambulatory EEG. Mathematical techniques for removal of electromyographic and eye-movement artifact from EEG, which has recently been incorporated into commercially available EEG reading software, may serve to increase the utility of daytime ambulatory EEG recordings (168,169). Perhaps the greatest limitation of ambulatory EEG is that it is not possible for a technician to monitor recording quality and electrode integrity, and to adjust electrodes if necessary. Failure of electrode contacts, and also occasionally of ambulatory equipment itself, can compromise the quality of ambulatory EEG recordings.

Although ambulatory EEG can provide days of continuous EEG monitoring, it is generally not a substitute for inpatient video-EEG, because simultaneous time-locked video provides substantial diagnostic information not provided by EEG alone. Most commercial ambulatory EEG systems are not designed to record time-locked video along with EEG. Although some systems do support video, the requirement that the patient remains "on camera" defeats one advantage of ambulatory EEG, the ability to record EEG as the patient goes about routine activities. Further, inpatient video-EEG monitoring allows trained personnel to observe, to interact with, and to test patients during seizures or seizure-like episodes, acquiring important information regarding semiology that is not captured by unsupervised video recording. The inpatient setting makes it possible to safely withdraw medication to increase the likelihood of recording seizures, and, of course, the inpatient setting is uniquely suited to invasive EEG recording (170).

These limitations notwithstanding, one group has reported the successful use of outpatient monitoring as part of the presurgical evaluation of a group of patients with temporal lobe epilepsy (171). Further, seizure frequency is often reported to *decrease* upon hospitalization (172,173), perhaps related to medication compliance or environment stressors (171). Some have suggested a role for ambulatory EEG in conjunction with inpatient video-EEG monitoring, either prior to or following hospitalization (174).

4.2. Indications for Ambulatory EEG

Given these considerations, the principal indications for ambulatory EEG monitoring are as follows (175):

1. Diagnosis: In patients with suspected epilepsy, ambulatory EEG may help to establish the diagnosis of epilepsy by recording interictal epileptiform discharges (IEDs) and seizures, and may help to distinguish epilepsy from "nonepileptic seizures" and other behavior disorders, syncope, cardiac arrhythmias, and disturbances of sleep.

2. Classification: The electrographic patterns and scalp distributions of IEDs and seizures, their temporal patterns of occurrence including relationship to precipitating events and stimuli, as well as the EEG background activity, may provide useful information for refining the seizure type and the epilepsy diagnosis.

3. Quantification: Ambulatory EEG may provide important information regarding the frequency of IEDs and seizures, as well as documentation of response to medication. This may be particularly important in patients with frequent seizures, of which they may not be aware.

4.3. Ambulatory EEG Equipment

Since the early days of galvanometers and photographic recording devices, clinical neurophysiology has progressed in lock-step with available technology. The first commercial devices recorded four channels of EEG (or three EEG channels plus a time code) using four-channel analog eighth-inch cassette tape recorders designed for general industrial applications (176). A standard tape cassette could store 24 hours of EEG. EEG signals were amplified using specially designed small single-channel preamplifiers that were affixed, along with electrodes, to the scalp with collodion. A video display reader station permitted rapid visual review, as fast as 1 hour of EEG per minute.

In the early 1980s, eight-channel ambulatory EEG systems became commercially available. A "block analog" technique was used to store eight channels of EEG plus timing data on four-channel analog cassette tape; three channels of EEG were digitized, combined, and reconverted back to analog form, and written to a single analog tape channel. Subsequently, a nine-channel analog device was introduced that used standard quarter-inch recording tape. An important advantage of these devices was that eight-channel EEG proved easier to interpret than three- or four-channel EEG; with eight channels, montages could be constructed that more closely resembled traditional montages. While sensitivity for identification of epileptiform abnormalities was similar for three and eight channels, review of eight-channel data afforded a lower false-positive rate (177). Additionally, these newer devices offered greater flexibility for adjustment of filters and gain, printouts of selectable segments, and ability to easily locate the EEG recorded at specific times during the study. Importantly, they provided that the ability to convert one or several EEG channels to audio, allowing seizures to be identified by listening to high-speed playback (175).

Attachment of eight on-head preamplifiers to the scalp with collodion proved cumbersome and time-consuming. Further, although in principle on-head amplification can reduce artifact related to electrode lead length and movement, it became apparent that on-head amplification could not reduce artifact from some important sources, including the electromyogram and eye movement. Further, fixing a standard EEG lead wire to the scalp with collodion next to an electrode cup effectively mitigates electrode artifacts produced by movement at the interface of the electrode cup and the scalp (175). Accordingly, with the introduction of eight-channel ambulatory EEG devices, there was a move to off-head amplification and standard EEG electrodes. Despite this move to off-head amplification, on-head amplification may be superior under conditions of vigorous movement (e.g., during a convulsive seizure). Direct bipolar recordings can provide signal quality superior to that produced by referential recordings reformatted into bipolar montages (175,178).

Later in the 1980s, 16-channel digital ambulatory EEG devices were introduced, still using tape as the storage medium. Initially, the tradeoff for 16 channels was limited storage capabilities; instead of retaining the complete recording, intermittent samples (e.g., 15 sec every 10 minutes), as well as a longer period of time before and after manual activation of a push button by the patient, were stored. Subsequently hybrid "computer-assisted" ambulatory EEG systems combined a 16-channel waist-worn device with a portable computer, connected by a wire tether that processed EEG in real time using automated spike and seizure detection software (179,180). Data available for clinical review consisted of intermittent samples, manually recognized events, and automatic detections, in much the same manner as the inpatient video-monitoring systems in use at the time.

Current ambulatory EEG devices represent an important departure from past designs. Present-day digital technology makes possible portable EEG devices that are not much larger than a cellphone and are able to record EEG with fidelity and number of channels equal to standard laboratory EEG machines. Indeed, the designs of ambulatory EEG systems and standard EEG systems have largely merged. In a typical EEG machine, amplification and analog-to-digital conversion are performed in the "head box"; the computer performs control, data storage, and display functions. An ambulatory EEG system simply adds battery power and solid-state memory to the head box. Since some head boxes, particularly those intended for use in inpatient monitoring units, often contain memory and rechargeable batteries, permitting the patient to disconnect from the wired system for several hours, real differences between ambulatory EEG systems and other EEG systems relate to packaging, quantity of storage, battery life, and marketing.

The typical modern ambulatory EEG recorder provides for 21 or more referential channels of EEG that can be reformatted in the same manner as standard laboratory EEG. It samples EEG with 16-bit resolution at typically 200 or 256 Hz per channel. It also has several channels for inputs such as pulse oximetry and other polysomnographic devices, electromyography, and electrocardiography. It connects to a desktop computer using USB or Ethernet for startup, and for download and review of data. It weighs just over 1 lb, is powered by several AA or rechargeable batteries, and has 2 to 4 GB of flash memory capable of storing two to four days of continuous data. Ambulatory EEG systems are also available that support time-synchronized video. While no currently available ambulatory EEG system provides for real-time upload of data over mobile broadband, implementation of this feature would not be technically challenging.

Real-time processing of EEG for spike and seizure detection was important to the design of earlier computer-assisted ambulatory EEG systems that had insufficient storage capacity to retain entire 16-channel day-long EEG recordings, and instead stored only samples and automatic detections. Storage capacity is no longer a limiting factor, and present-day systems retain all EEG recorded. When the study is complete, data are easily transferred to a desktop computer for review, and if desired, processed by automatic spike and seizure detection software (181,182). As with inpatient EMU recordings, the physician has the option of exhaustively reviewing the entire recording, or relying on periodic samples, "push button events," and automated detections.

4.4. Future Directions in Ambulatory Monitoring

Ambulatory EEG has the potential to provide accurate information about seizure frequency that, in some patients, may be difficult to obtain otherwise (183). Underreporting of seizures by patients is well recognized (167), in part because reporting requires the patient to remember events that commonly produce amnesia. When seizures go undetected and under-reported, medical management may be compromised because the efficacy of treatment can be difficult to ascertain. The apparent relationship between seizure frequency and the risk of sudden unexplained death in patients with epilepsy underscores the importance of accurate measurement (184).

Proof of concept for chronic ambulatory EEG is provided by Neuropace® Inc.'s responsive neurostimulation (RNS) device (185–187) and by NeuroVista®, Inc.'s investigational seizure prediction device (183). The Neuropace device is implanted within the skull and connects to subdural or depth electrodes. Designed to detect and then abort seizures using electrical stimulation (188), the device contains memory sufficient to store about 30 minutes of four-channel EEG corresponding to seizure detections, allowing it to function as a chronic ambulatory EEG recorder. The NeuroVista system consists of a telemetry unit implanted in the chest, connecting to a pair of eight subdural electrodes and communicating wirelessly to an external handheld "personal advisory device" (PAD). The telemetry unit transmits EEG continuously to the PAD, which implements a real-time seizure prediction algorithm and also stores the EEG, allowing it also to function as an ambulatory EEG recording device. Using the system, Cook et al. observed a marked disparity between reported seizures and electrographically detected seizures in 15 patients over many months (183) (see also discussion in Chapter 22).

Newly developed power harvesting techniques may provide a solution to the problems of power consumption and battery size and life that have, until now, plagued implantable devices (189,190). In contrast to standard near-field inductive coupling, which is commonly used to recharge consumer devices and which requires that the power source and powered device be in direct proximity, power can be transmitted using radiofrequency (RF) energy over greater distances. A cardiac pacing application using a miniature focused midfield power transfer device capable of providing milliwatt power to deep tissues was recently demonstrated (191). Although not specifically designed for implanted medical devices, commercial systems are available that are capable of safely providing milliwatt-range power over even greater distances (192).

It is easy to envision a device that records full-fidelity EEG through implanted subgaleal or epidural peg electrodes that would provide high-quality, stable EEG signals, relatively immune from artifacts. At night, as the patient sleeps, the device would recharge while data automatically download to a computer that runs seizure detection software, logging the results or transmitting them, along with raw data if desired, back to the physician. Rather than wired connections between multiple passive electrodes and implanted electronics, a wireless local network could provide communication between active electrodes (193) and the ambulatory EEG electronics, implanted perhaps in the skull, or the chest or abdominal wall. The network could use the Medical Implant Communication Service band, 402 to 405 KHz, recently established by the Federal Communications Commission for radio transmission to implanted medical devices (194). This concept is readily extended to include continuous recording of other physiological signals, such as the electrocardiogram, respiration, and blood oxygen saturation. The relatively liberal power budget afforded by RF power transfer might permit the functionality of implanted ambulatory EEG systems to include not only data storage but also real-time seizure detection and, if effective methodologies emerge, seizure prediction and warning (183,195).

REFERENCES

1. Nuwer, M. R., Sutherling, W. W., Babb, T. L., & Engel, J. J. Monitoring at the University of California, Los Angeles. *Electroenceph Clin Neurophysiol*, 1985;37S:385–402.
2. Gotman, J. Seizure recognition and analysis. In: J. Gotman, J. R. Ives, & P. Gloor (Eds.). *Long-Term Monitoring in Epilepsy*. Amsterdam: Elsevier; 1985:133–145.
3. Nuwer, M. R. EEG and evoked potentials: monitoring cerebral function in the neurosurgical ICU. *Neurosurg Clin North Am*, 1994;5:647–659.
4. Velis, D., Plouin, P., Gotman, J., et al. ILAE DMC Subcommittee on Neurophysiology. Recommendations regarding the requirements and applications for long-term recordings in epilepsy. *Epilepsia*, 2007;48(2):379–384.
5. Mirsattari, S. M., Tapsell, L. M., Ives, J. R., et al. MR imaging-compatible electroencephalography electrode system for an epilepsy monitoring unit. *Am J Neuroradiol*, 2008;29(9):1649–1651.
6. Mirsattari, S. M., Davies-Schinkel, C., Young, G. B., et al. Usefulness of a 1.5 T MRI-compatible EEG electrode system for routine use in the intensive care unit of a tertiary care hospital. *Epilepsy Res*, 2009;84(1):28–32.
7. Jirsch, J. D., Urrestarazu, E., LeVan, P., et al. High-frequency oscillations during human focal seizures. *Brain*, 2006;129:1593–1608.
8. Urrestarazu, E., Chander, R., Dubeau, F., et al. Interictal high-frequency oscillations (100–500 Hz) in the intracerebral EEG of epileptic patients. *Brain*, 2007;130:2354–2366.
9. Jacobs, J., LeVan, P., Chander, R., et al. Interictal high-frequency oscillations (80–500 Hz) are an indicator of seizure onset areas independent of spikes in the human epileptic brain. *Epilepsia*, 2008;49:1893–1907.
10. Vanhatalo, S., Voipio, J., Kaila, K. Full-band EEG (fbEEG): a new standard for clinical electroencephalography. *Clin EEG Neurosci*, 2005;36(4):311–317.
11. ABRET; CLTM Exam Eligibility Requirements (2015). Available from: http://abret.org/candidates/credentials/cltm/
12. ABRET; LTM Lab Accreditation (2015). Available from: http://abret.org/lab/ltm/introduction/
13. Blum, D. Prevalence of bilateral partial seizure foci and implications for electroencephalographic telemetry monitoring and epilepsy surgery. *Electroencephalogr Clin Neurophysiol*, 1994;91(5):329–336.
14. Marciani, M. G., & Gotman, J. Effects of drug withdrawal on location of seizure onset. *Epilepsia*, 1986;27(4):423–431.
15. So, N., & Gotman, J. Quantitative EEG analysis of carbamazepine effects on amygdaloid kindled seizures in cats. *Electroencephalogr Clin Neurophysiol*, 1990;76(1):63–72.
16. Zhou, D., Wang, Y., Hopp, P., et al. Influence on ictal seizure semiology of rapid withdrawal of carbamazepine and valproate in monotherapy. *Epilepsia*, 2002;43(4):386–393.
17. Theodore, W. H., Porter, R. J., Albert, P., et al. The secondarily generalized tonic–clonic seizure: a videotape analysis. *Neurology*, 1994;44(8):1403–1407.
18. Spencer, S. S., Spencer, D. D., Williamson, P. D., et al. Ictal effects of anticonvulsant medication withdrawal in epileptic patients. *Epilepsia*, 1981;22(3):297–307.
19. Marciani, M. G., Gotman, J., Andermann, F., et al. Patterns of seizure activation after withdrawal of antiepileptic medication. *Neurology*, 1985;35(11):1537–1543.
20. Gotman, J., & Marciani, M. G. Electroencephalographic spiking activity, drug levels, and seizure occurrence in epileptic patients. *Ann Neurol*, 1985;17(6):597–603.
21. Gotman, J., & Koffler, D. J. Interictal spiking increases after seizures but does not after decrease in medication. *Electroencephalogr Clin Neurophysiol*, 1989;72(1):7–15.
22. Spencer, S. S., Goncharova, I. I., Duckrow, R. B., et al. Interictal spikes on intracranial recording: behavior, physiology, and implications. *Epilepsia*, 2008;49(11):1881–1892.
23. Mizrahi, E. M. Pediatric electroencephalographic video monitoring. *J Clin Neurophysiol*, 1999;16(2):100–110.
24. Gotman, J., Nuwer, M. R., & Emerson, R. Principles and techniques for long-term EEG recording (EMU, ICU, ambulatory). In: D. L. Schomer & F. Lopes da Silva (Eds.). *Niedermeyer's Electrocephalography: Basic Principles, Clinical Applications, and Related Fields*. Philadelphia: Lippincott Williams & Wilkins, 2011:725–740.
25. Gotman, J., Flanagan, D., Rosenblatt, B., et al. Evaluation of an automatic seizure detection method for the newborn EEG. *Electroencephalogr Clin Neurophysiol*, 1997;103(3):363–369.
26. Celka, P., & Colditz, P. A computer-aided detection of EEG seizures in infants: a singular-spectrum approach and performance comparison. *IEEE Trans Biomed Eng*, 2002;49(5):455–462.
27. Aarabi, A., Wallois, F., & Grebe, R. Automated neonatal seizure detection: a multistage classification system through feature selection based on relevance and redundancy analysis. *Clin Neurophysiol*, 2006;117(2):328–340.
28. Gotman, J. Interhemispheric relations during bilateral spike-and-wave activity. *Epilepsia*, 1981;22(4):453–466.
29. Gotman, J. Automatic seizure detection: improvements and evaluation. *Electroencephalogr Clin Neurophysiol*, 1990;76(4):317–324.
30. Grewal, S., & Gotman, J. An automatic warning system for epileptic seizures recorded on intracerebral EEGs. *Clin Neurophysiol*, 2005;116(10):2460–2472.
31. Saab, M. E., & Gotman, J. A system to detect the onset of epileptic seizures in scalp EEG. *Clin Neurophysiol*, 2005;116(2):427–442.
32. Qu, H., & Gotman, J. A seizure warning system for long-term epilepsy monitoring. *Neurology*, 1995;45(12):2250–2254.
33. Qu, H., & Gotman, J. A patient-specific algorithm for the detection of seizure onset in long-term EEG monitoring: possible use as a warning device. *IEEE Trans Biomed Eng*, 1997;44(2):115–122.
34. Shoeb, A., Edwards, H., Connolly, J., et al. Patient-specific seizure onset detection. *Epilepsy Behav*, 2004;5(4):483–498.
35. Wilson, S. B. A neural network method for automatic and incremental learning applied to patient-dependent seizure detection. *Clin Neurophysiol*, 2005;116(8):1785–1795.
36. Gabor, A. J., Leach, R. R., & Dowla, F. U. Automated seizure detection using a self-organising neural network. *Electroencephalogr Clin Neurophysiol*, 1996;99:257–266.
37. Webber, W. R. S., Lesser, R. P., Richardson, R. T., et al. An approach to seizure detection using an artificial neural network. *Electroencephalogr Clin Neurophysiol*, 1996;98:250–272.
38. Wilson, S. B., Scheuer, M. L., Emerson, R. G., et al. Seizure detection: evaluation of the Reveal algorithm. *Clin Neurophysiol*, 2004;115(10):2280–2291.

39. Aarts, J. H., Binnie, C. D., Smit, A. M., et al. Selective cognitive impairment during focal and generalized epileptiform EEG activity. *Brain*, 1994;107(pt 1):293–308.

40. Shewmon, D. A., & Erwin, R. J. Transient impairment of visual perception induced by single interictal occipital spikes. *J Clin Exp Neuropsychol*, 1989;11(5):675–691.

41. Wilson, S. B., Harner, R. N., Duffy, F. H., et al. Spike detection. I. Correlation and reliability of human experts. *Electroencephalogr Clin Neurophysiol*, 1996;98(3):186–198.

42. Benbadis, S. R., & Lin, K. Errors in EEG interpretation and misdiagnosis of epilepsy. Which EEG patterns are overread? *Eur Neurol*, 2008;59:267–271.

43. Halford, J. J. Computerized epileptiform transient detection in the scalp electroencephalogram: obstacles to progress and the example of computerized ECG interpretation. *Clin Neurophysiol*, 2009;120(11):1909–1915.

44. Sanchez, S. M., Arndt, D. H., Carpenter, J. L., et al. Electroencephalography monitoring in critically ill children: current practice and implications for future study design. *Epilepsia*, 2013;54(8):1419–1427.

45. Gavvala, J., Abend, N., LaRoche, S., et al. Continuous EEG monitoring: a survey of neurophysiologists and neurointensivists. *Epilepsia*, 2014;55(11):1864–1871.

46. Shellhaas, R. A., Chang, T., Tsuchida, T., et al. The American Clinical Neurophysiology Society's Guideline on Continuous Electroencephalography Monitoring in Neonates. *J Clin Neurophysiol*, 2011;28(6):611–617.

47. Herman, S. T., Abend, N. S., Bleck, T. P., et al. Consensus statement on continuous EEG in critically ill adults and children, part I: indications. *J Clin Neurophysiol*, 2015;32(2):87–95.

48. Hirsch, L. J., LaRoche, S. M., Gaspard, N., et al. American Clinical Neurophysiology Society's Standardized Critical Care EEG Terminology: 2012 version. *J Clin Neurophysiol*, 2013;30(1):1–27.

49. Tsuchida, T. N., Wusthoff, C. J., Shellhaas, R. A., et al. American Clinical Neurophysiology Society standardized EEG terminology and categorization for the description of continuous EEG monitoring in neonates: report of the American Clinical Neurophysiology Society critical care monitoring committee. *J Clin Neurophysiol*, 2013;30(2):161–173.

50. Herman, S. T., Abend, N. S., Bleck, T. P., et al. Consensus statement on continuous EEG in critically ill adults and children, part II: personnel, technical specifications, and clinical practice. *J Clin Neurophysiol*, 2015;32(2):96–108.

51. Chong, D. J., & Hirsch, L. J. Which EEG patterns warrant treatment in the critically ill? Reviewing the evidence for treatment of periodic epileptiform discharges and related patterns. *J Clin Neurophysiol*, 2005;22(2):79–91.

52. Claassen, J. How I treat patients with EEG patterns on the ictal-interictal continuum in the neuro ICU. *Neurocrit Care*, 2009;11(3):437–444.

53. Lee, J. W., LaRoche, S., Choi, H., et al. Development and Feasibility Testing of a Critical Care EEG Monitoring Database for Standardized Clinical Reporting and Multicenter Collaborative Research. *J Clin Neurophysiol*, 2016;33(2):133–140.

54. Sanchez, S. M., Carpenter, J., Chapman, K. E., et al. Pediatric ICU EEG monitoring: current resources and practice in the United States and Canada. *J Clin Neurophysiol*, 2013;30(2):156–160.

55. Claassen, J., Mayer, S. A., Kowalski, R. G., Emerson R. G., & Hirsch, L. J. Detection of electrographic seizures with continuous EEG monitoring in critically ill patients. *Neurology*, 2004;62(10):1743–1748.

56. McCoy, B., Sharma, R., Ochi, A., et al. Predictors of nonconvulsive seizures among critically ill children. *Epilepsia*, 2011;52(11):1973–1978.

57. Glass, H. C., Wusthoff, C. J., Shellhaas, R. A., et al. Risk factors for EEG seizures in neonates treated with hypothermia: a multicenter cohort study. *Neurology*, 2014;82(14):1239–1244.

58. Privitera, M., Hoffman, M., Moore J. L., & Jester, D. EEG detection of nontonic-clonic status epilepticus in patients with altered consciousness. *Epilepsy Res*, 1994;18(2):155–166.

59. Towne, A. R., Waterhouse, E. J., Boggs, J. G., et al. Prevalence of nonconvulsive status epilepticus in comatose patients. *Neurology*, 2000;54(2):340–345.

60. Pandian, J. D., Cascino, G. D., So, E. L., et al. Digital video-electroencephalographic monitoring in the neurological-neurosurgical intensive care unit: clinical features and outcome. *Arch Neurol*, 2004;61(7):1090–1094.

61. Jette, N., Claassen, J., Emerson, R. G., & Hirsch, L. J. Frequency and predictors of nonconvulsive seizures during continuous electroencephalographic monitoring in critically ill children. *Arch Neurol*, 2006;63(12):1750–1755.

62. Abend, N. S., Gutierrez-Colina, A. M., Topjian, A. A., et al. Nonconvulsive seizures are common in critically ill children. *Neurology*, 2011;76(12):1071–1077.

63. Williams, K., Jarrar R., & Buchhalter, J. Continuous video-EEG monitoring in pediatric intensive care units. *Epilepsia*, 2011;52(6):1130–1136.

64. Greiner, H. M., Holland, K., Leach, J. L., et al. Nonconvulsive status epilepticus: the encephalopathic pediatric patient. *Pediatrics*, 2012;129(3):e748–755.

65. Kirkham, F. J., Wade, A. M., McElduff, F., et al. Seizures in 204 comatose children: incidence and outcome. *Intensive Care Med*, 2012;38(5):853–862.

66. Schreiber, J. M., Zelleke, T., Gaillard, W. D., et al. Continuous video EEG for patients with acute encephalopathy in a pediatric intensive care unit. *Neurocrit Care*, 2012;17(1):31–38.

67. Abend, N. S., Arndt, D. H., Carpenter, J. L., et al. Electrographic seizures in pediatric ICU patients: cohort study of risk factors and mortality. *Neurology*, 2013;81(4):383–391.

68. Payne, E. T., Zhao, X. Y., Frndova, H., et al. Seizure burden is independently associated with short term outcome in critically ill children. *Brain*, 2014;137(5):1429–1438.

69. Jette, N., Claassen, J., Emerson R. G., & Hirsch, L. J. Frequency and predictors of nonconvulsive seizures during continuous electroencephalographic monitoring in critically ill children. *Arch Neurol*, 2006;63(12):1750–1755.

70. Shahwan, A., Bailey, C., Shekerdemian, L., & Harvey, A. S. The prevalence of seizures in comatose children in the pediatric intensive care unit: a prospective video-EEG study. *Epilepsia*, 2010;51(7):1198–1204.

71. Nash, K. B., Bonifacio, S. L., Glass, H. C., et al. Video-EEG monitoring in newborns with hypoxic-ischemic encephalopathy treated with hypothermia. *Neurology*, 2011;76(6):556–562.

72. Shafi, M. M., Westover, M. B., Cole, A. J., et al. Absence of early epileptiform abnormalities predicts lack of seizures on continuous EEG. *Neurology*, 2012;79(17):1796–1801.

73. DeLorenzo, R. J., Waterhouse, E. J., Towne, A. R., et al. Persistent nonconvulsive status epilepticus after the control of convulsive status epilepticus. *Epilepsia*, 1998;39(8):833–840.

74. Vespa, P. M., Nuwer, M. R., Nenov, V., et al. Increased incidence and impact of nonconvulsive and convulsive seizures after traumatic brain injury as detected by continuous electroencephalographic monitoring. *J Neurosurg*, 1999;91(5):750–760.

75. Claassen, J., Jette, N., Chum, F., et al. Electrographic seizures and periodic discharges after intracerebral hemorrhage. *Neurology*, 2007;69(13):1356–1365.

76. Claassen, J., Perotte, A., Albers, D., et al. Nonconvulsive seizures after subarachnoid hemorrhage: Multimodal detection and outcomes. *Ann Neurol*, 2013;74(1):53–64.

77. Oddo, M., Carrera, E., Claassen, J., et al. Continuous electroencephalography in the medical intensive care unit. *Crit Care Med*, 2009;37(6):2051–2056.

78. Gold, J. J., Crawford, J. R., Glaser, C., et al. The role of continuous electroencephalography in childhood encephalitis. *Pediatr Neurol*, 2014;50(4):318–323.

79. Abend, N. S., Topjian, A., Ichord, R., et al. Electroencephalographic monitoring during hypothermia after pediatric cardiac arrest. *Neurology*, 2009;72(22):1931–1940.

80. Helmers, S. L., Wypij, D., Constantinou, J. E., et al. Perioperative electroencephalographic seizures in infants undergoing repair of complex congenital cardiac defects. *Electroencephalogr Clin Neurophysiol*, 1997;102(1):27–36.

81. Clancy, R. R., Sharif, U., Ichord, R., et al. Electrographic neonatal seizures after infant heart surgery. *Epilepsia*, 2005;46(1):84–90.

82. Piantino, J. A., Wainwright, M. S., Grimason, M., et al. Nonconvulsive seizures are common in children treated with extracorporeal cardiac life support. *Pediatr Crit Care Med*, 2013;14(6):601–609.

83. Arndt, D. H., Lerner, J. T., Matsumoto, J. H., et al. Subclinical early posttraumatic seizures detected by continuous EEG monitoring in a consecutive pediatric cohort. *Epilepsia*, 2013;54(10):1780–1788.

84. Gallentine, W. B. Utility of continuous EEG in children with acute traumatic brain injury. *J Clin Neurophysiol*, 2013;30(2):126–133.

85. Hasbani, D. M., Topjian, A. A., Friess, S. H., et al. Nonconvulsive electrographic seizures are common in children with abusive head trauma. *Pediatr Crit Care Med*, 2013;14(7):709–715.

86. Singh, R. K., Zecavati, N., Singh, J., et al. Seizures in acute childhood stroke. *J Pediatr*, 2012;160(2):291–296.

87. Beslow, L. A., Abend, N. S., Gindville, M. C., et al. Pediatric intracerebral hemorrhage: acute symptomatic seizures and epilepsy. *JAMA Neurol*, 2013;70(4):448–454.

88. Fox, C. K., Glass, H. C., Sidney, S., et al. Acute seizures predict epilepsy after childhood stroke. *Ann Neurol*, 2013;74(2):249–256.

89. Abend, N. S., Beslow, L. A., Smith, S. E., et al. Seizures as a presenting symptom of acute arterial ischemic stroke in childhood. *J Pediatr*, 2011;159(3):479–483.

90. Young, G. B., Jordan, K. G., & Doig, G. S. An assessment of nonconvulsive seizures in the intensive care unit using continuous EEG monitoring: an investigation of variables associated with mortality. *Neurology*, 1996;47(1):83–89.

91. Vespa, P., Prins, M., Ronne-Engstrom, E., et al. Increase in extracellular glutamate caused by reduced cerebral perfusion pressure and seizures after human traumatic brain injury: a microdialysis study. *J Neurosurg,* 1998;89(6):971–982.

92. Vespa, P., Tubi, M., Claassen, J., et al. Metabolic crisis occurs with seizures and periodic discharges after brain trauma. *Ann Neurol.* 2016;79(4):579–590.

93. Vespa, P. M., Miller, C., McArthur, D., et al. Nonconvulsive electrographic seizures after traumatic brain injury result in a delayed, prolonged increase in intracranial pressure and metabolic crisis. *Crit Care Med,* 2007;35(12):2830–2836.

94. Vespa, P. M., O'Phelan, K., Shah, M., et al. Acute seizures after intracerebral hemorrhage: a factor in progressive midline shift and outcome. *Neurology,* 2003;60:1441–1446.

95. Vespa, P. M., McArthur, D. L., Xu, Y., et al. Nonconvulsive seizures after traumatic brain injury are associated with hippocampal atrophy. *Neurology,* 2010;75(9):792–798.

96. Lambrechtsen, F. A., & Buchhalter, J. R. Aborted and refractory status epilepticus in children: a comparative analysis. *Epilepsia,* 2008;49(4):615–625.

97. Topjian, A. A., Gutierrez-Colina, A. M., Sanchez, S. M., et al. Electrographic status epilepticus is associated with mortality and worse short-term outcome in critically ill children. *Crit Care Med,* 2013;41(1):215–223.

98. Holmes, G. L. To know or not to know: does EEG monitoring in the paediatric intensive care unit add anything besides cost? *Brain,* 2014;137(5):1276–1277.

99. Wagenman, K. L., Blake, T. P., Sanchez, S. M., et al. Electrographic status epilepticus and long-term outcome in critically ill children. *Neurology,* 2014;82(5):396–404.

100. Abend, N. S., Wagenman, K. L., Blake, T. P., et al. Electrographic status epilepticus and neurobehavioral outcomes in critically ill children. *Epilepsy Behav,* 2015;49:238–244.

101. Bellinger, D. C., Wypij, D., Rivkin, M. J., et al. Adolescents with d-transposition of the great arteries corrected with the arterial switch procedure: neuropsychological assessment and structural brain imaging. *Circulation,* 2011;124(12):1361–1369.

102. Gaynor, J. W., Jarvik, G. P., Gerdes, M., et al. Postoperative electroencephalographic seizures are associated with deficits in executive function and social behaviors at 4 years of age following cardiac surgery in infancy. *J Thorac Cardiovasc Surg,* 2013;146(1):132–137.

103. Miller, S. P., Weiss, J., Barnwell, A., et al. Seizure-associated brain injury in term newborns with perinatal asphyxia. *Neurology,* 2002;58(4):542–548.

104. McBride, M. C., Laroia N., & Guillet, R. Electrographic seizures in neonates correlate with poor neurodevelopmental outcome. *Neurology,* 2000;55(4):506–513.

105. Brophy, G. M., Bell, R., Claassen, J., et al. Guidelines for the evaluation and management of status epilepticus. *Neurocrit Care,* 2012;17(1):3–23.

106. Hahn, C. D., & Jette, N. Neurocritical care: Seizures after acute brain injury—more than meets the eye. *Nat Rev Neurol,* 2013;9(12):662–664.

107. Bergamasco, B., Bergamini, L., & Doriguzzi, T. Clinical value of the sleep electroencephalographic patterns in post-traumatic coma. *Acta Neurol Scand,* 1968a;44(4):495–511.

108. Bergamasco, B., Bergamini, L., Doriguzzi, T., & Fabiani, D. EEG sleep patterns as a prognostic criterion in post-traumatic coma. *Electroencephalogr Clin Neurophysiol,* 1968;24(4):374–377.

109. Osredkar, D., Toet, M. C., van Rooij, L. G., et al. Sleep-wake cycling on amplitude-integrated electroencephalography in term newborns with hypoxic-ischemic encephalopathy. *Pediatrics,* 2005;115(2):327–332.

110. Murray, D. M., Boylan, G. B., Ryan, C. A., & Connolly, S. Early EEG findings in hypoxic-ischemic encephalopathy predict outcomes at 2 years. *Pediatrics,* 2009;124(3):e459–467.

111. Scher, M. S. Automated EEG-sleep analyses and neonatal neurointensive care. *Sleep Med,* 2004;5(6):533–540.

112. Stevenson, N. J., Palmu, K., Wikstrom, S., et al. Measuring brain activity cycling (BAC) in long term EEG monitoring of preterm babies. *Physiol Meas,* 2014;35(7):1493–1508.

113. Juan, E., Kaplan, P. W., Oddo, M., & Rossetti, A. O. EEG as an indicator of cerebral functioning in postanoxic coma. *J Clin Neurophysiol,* 2015;32(6):465–471.

114. Rossetti, A. O., Urbano, L. A., Delodder, F., et al. Prognostic value of continuous EEG monitoring during therapeutic hypothermia after cardiac arrest. *Crit Care,* 2010;14(5):R173.

115. Thenayan, E. A., Savard, M., Sharpe, M. D., et al. Electroencephalogram for prognosis after cardiac arrest. *J Crit Care,* 2010;25(2):300–304.

116. Kessler, S. K., Topjian, A. A., Gutierrez-Colina, A. M., et al. Short-term outcome prediction by electroencephalographic features in children treated with therapeutic hypothermia after cardiac arrest. *Neurocrit Care,* 2011;14(1):37–43.

117. Sadaka, F., Doerr, D., Hindia, J., et al. Continuous electroencephalogram in comatose postcardiac arrest syndrome patients treated with therapeutic hypothermia: outcome prediction study. *J Intensive Care Med,* 2015;30(5):292–296.

118. Sivaraju, A., Gilmore, E. J., Wira, C. R., et al. Prognostication of postcardiac arrest coma: early clinical and electroencephalographic predictors of outcome. *Intensive Care Med,* 2015;41(7):1264–1272.

119. Hofmeijer, J., Tjepkema-Cloostermans, M. C., & van Putten, M. J. Burst-suppression with identical bursts: a distinct EEG pattern with poor outcome in postanoxic coma. *Clin Neurophysiol,* 2014;125(5):947–954.

120. Courville, C. B. Etiology and pathogenesis of laminar cortical necrosis; its significance in evaluation of uniform cortical atrophies of early life. *AMA Arch Neurol Psychiatry,* 1958;79(1):7–30.

121. Jordan, K. G. Continuous EEG monitoring in the neuroscience intensive care unit and emergency department. *J Clin Neurophysiol,* 1999;16(1):14–39.

122. Ebersole, J. S., & Pedley, T. M. Cortical generators and EEG voltage fields. In: *Current Practice of Clinical Electroencephalography.* New York: Lippincott, Williams & Wilkins, 2003:12–31.

123. Jordan, K. G. Emergency EEG and continuous EEG monitoring in acute ischemic stroke. *J Clin Neurophysiol,* 2004;21(5):341–352.

124. Astrup, J., Siesjo, B. K., & Symon, L. Thresholds in cerebral ischemia—the ischemic penumbra. *Stroke,* 1981;12(6):723–725.

125. Sundt, T. M. Jr., Sharbrough, F. W., Piepgras, D. G., et al. Correlation of cerebral blood flow and electroencephalographic changes during carotid endarterectomy: with results of surgery and hemodynamics of cerebral ischemia. *Mayo Clin Proc,* 1981;56(9):533–543.

126. Baron, J. C. Perfusion thresholds in human cerebral ischemia: historical perspective and therapeutic implications. *Cerebrovasc Dis,* 2001;11:2–8.

127. Nuwer, M. R., Jordan, S. E., & Ahn, S. S. Evaluation of stroke using EEG frequency analysis and topographic mapping. *Neurology,* 1987;37(7):1153–1159.

128. Finnigan, S. P., Rose, S. E., Walsh, M., et al. Correlation of quantitative EEG in acute ischemic stroke with 30-day NIHSS score: comparison with diffusion and perfusion MRI. *Stroke,* 2004;35(4):899–903.

129. Suzuki, A., Yoshioka, K., & Yasui, N. Clinical application of EEG topography in cerebral ischemia: detection of functional reversibility and hemodynamics. *Brain Topogr,* 1990;3(1):167–174.

130. van Putten, M. J., & Tavy, D. L. Continuous quantitative EEG monitoring in hemispheric stroke patients using the brain symmetry index. *Stroke,* 2004;35(11):2489–2492.

131. Schneider, A. L., & Jordan, K. G. Regional attenuation without delta (RAWOD): a distinctive EEG pattern that can aid in the diagnosis and management of severe acute ischemic stroke. *Am J Electroneurodiagnostic Technol,* 2005;45(2):102–117.

132. Daly, D. D., & Markand, O. N. Focal brain lesions. In D. D. Daly & T. M. Pedley (Eds.). *Current Practice of Clinical Electroencephalography.* New York: Raven Press, Ltd., 1990:335–370.

133. Niedermeyer, E. Cerebrovascular disorders and EEG. In E. Niedermeyer & F. H. Lopes da Silva (Eds.). *Electroencephalography.* Baltimore: Urban & Schwarzenberg Inc., 2005:339–362.

134. Claassen, J., Hirsch, L. J., Frontera, J. A., et al. Prognostic significance of continuous EEG monitoring in patients with poor-grade subarachnoid hemorrhage. *Neurocrit Care,* 2006;4(2):103–112.

135. Hirsch, L. J., Claassen, J., Mayer S. A., & Emerson, R. G. Stimulus-induced rhythmic, periodic, or ictal discharges (SIRPIDs): a common EEG phenomenon in the critically ill. *Epilepsia,* 2004;45(2):109–123.

136. Weir, B., Grace, M., Hansen, J., & Rothberg, C. Time course of vasospasm in man. *J Neurosurg,* 1978;48(2):173–178.

137. Hijdra, A., van Gijn, J., Nagelkerke, N. J., et al. Prediction of delayed cerebral ischemia, rebleeding, and outcome after aneurysmal subarachnoid hemorrhage. *Stroke,* 1988;19(10):1250–1256.

138. Murayama, Y., Malisch, T., Guglielmi, G., et al. Incidence of cerebral vasospasm after endovascular treatment of acutely ruptured aneurysms: report on 69 cases. *J Neurosurg,* 1997;87(6):830–835.

139. Charpentier, C., Audibert, G., Guillemin, F., et al. Multivariate analysis of predictors of cerebral vasospasm occurrence after aneurysmal subarachnoid hemorrhage. *Stroke,* 1999;30(7):1402–1408.

140. Hop, J. W., Rinkel, G. J., Algra, A., & van Gijn, J. Initial loss of consciousness and risk of delayed cerebral ischemia after aneurysmal subarachnoid hemorrhage. *Stroke,* 1999;30(11):2268–2271.

141. Qureshi, A. I., Sung, G. Y., Razumovsky, A. Y., et al. Early identification of patients at risk for symptomatic vasospasm after aneurysmal subarachnoid hemorrhage. *Crit Care Med,* 2000;28(4):984–990.

142. Claassen, J., Bernardini, G. L., Kreiter, K., et al. Effect of cisternal and ventricular blood on risk of delayed cerebral ischemia after subarachnoid hemorrhage: the Fisher scale revisited. *Stroke*, 2001;32(9):2012–2020.

143. Schmidt, J. M., Wartenberg, K. E., Fernandez, A., et al. Frequency and clinical impact of asymptomatic cerebral infarction due to vasospasm after subarachnoid hemorrhage. *J Neurosurg*, 2008;109(6):1052–1059.

144. Labar, D. R., Fisch, B. J., Pedley, T. A., et al. Quantitative EEG monitoring for patients with subarachnoid hemorrhage. *Electroencephalogr Clin Neurophysiol*, 1991;78(5):325–332.

145. Vespa, P. M., Nuwer, M. R., Juhasz, C., et al. Early detection of vasospasm after acute subarachnoid hemorrhage using continuous EEG ICU monitoring. *Electroencephalogr Clin Neurophysiol*, 1997;103(6):607–615.

146. Bickford, R. G., Fleming, N., & Billinger, T. Compression of EEG data. *Trans Am Neurol Assoc*, 1971;96:118–122.

147. Karnaze, D. S., Marshall, L. F., & Bickford, R. G. EEG monitoring of clinical coma: the compressed spectral array. *Neurology*, 1982;32(3):289–292.

148. Nuwer, M. R. EEG and evoked potentials: Monitoring cerebral function in the neurosurgical ICU. *Neurosurg Clin North Am*, 1994;5:647–659.

149. Karakis, I., Montouris, G. D., Otis, J. A., et al. A quick and reliable EEG montage for the detection of seizures in the critical care setting. *J Clin Neurophysiol*, 2010;27(2):100–105.

150. Kolls, B. J., & Husain, A. M. Assessment of hairline EEG as a screening tool for nonconvulsive status epilepticus. *Epilepsia*, 2007;48(5):959–965.

151. Tanner, A. E., Sarkela, M. O., Virtanen, J., et al. Application of subhairline EEG montage in intensive care unit: comparison with full montage. *J Clin Neurophysiol*, 2014;31(3):181–186.

152. Shellhaas, R. A., Soaita, A. I., & Clancy, R. R. Sensitivity of amplitude-integrated electroencephalography for neonatal seizure detection. *Pediatrics*, 2007;120(4):770–777.

153. Shah, D. K., Mackay, M. T., Lavery, S., et al. Accuracy of bedside electroencephalographic monitoring in comparison with simultaneous continuous conventional electroencephalography for seizure detection in term infants. *Pediatrics*, 2008;121(6):1146–1154.

154. Shah, D. K., & Mathur, A. Amplitude-integrated EEG and the newborn infant. *Curr Pediatr Rev*, 2014;10(1):11–15.

155. Mirsattari, S. M., Davies-Schinkel, C., Young, G. B., et al. Usefulness of a 1.5 T MRI-compatible EEG electrode system for routine use in the intensive care unit of a tertiary care hospital. *Epilepsy Res*, 2009;84(1):28–32.

156. Vulliemoz, S., Perrig, S., Pellise, D., et al. Imaging compatible electrodes for continuous electroencephalogram monitoring in the intensive care unit. *J Clin Neurophysiol*, 2009;26(4):236–243.

157. Schultz, T. L. Technical tips: MRI compatible EEG electrodes: advantages, disadvantages, and financial feasibility in a clinical setting. *Neurodiagn J*, 2012;52(1):69–81.

158. Kolls, B. J., Olson, D. M., Gallentine, W. B., et al. Electroencephalography leads placed by nontechnologists using a template system produce signals equal in quality to technologist-applied, collodion disk leads. *J Clin Neurophysiol*, 2012;29(1):42–49.

159. Stewart, C. P., Otsubo, H., Ochi, A., et al. Seizure identification in the ICU using quantitative EEG displays. *Neurology*, 2010;75(17):1501–1508.

160. Akman, C. I., Micic, V., Thompson, A., & Riviello, J. J. Jr. Seizure detection using digital trend analysis: Factors affecting utility. *Epilepsy Res*, 2011;93(1):66–72.

161. Pensirikul, A. D., Beslow, L. A., Kessler, S. S., et al. Density spectral array for seizure identification in critically ill children. *J Clin Neurophysiol*, 2013;30(4):371–375.

162. Moura, L. M., Shafi, M. M., Ng, M., et al. Spectrogram screening of adult EEGs is sensitive and efficient. *Neurology*, 2014;83(1):56–64.

163. Sackellares, J. C., Shiau, D. S., Halford, J. J., et al. Quantitative EEG analysis for automated detection of nonconvulsive seizures in intensive care units. *Epilepsy Behav*, 2011;22(1):S69–73.

164. Sierra-Marcos, A., Scheuer M. L., & Rossetti, A. O. Seizure detection with automated EEG analysis: A validation study focusing on periodic patterns. *Clin Neurophysiol*. 2015;126(3):456–462.

165. Bridgers, S. L., & Ebersole, J. Ambulatory cassette EEG in clinical practice: experience with 500 patients. *Neurology*, 1985;35(12):1167–1168.

166. Liporace, J., Tatum, W. O., Morris, G. L., French, J. Clinical utility of sleep-deprived versus computer-assisted ambulatory 16-channel EEG in epilepsy patients: a multi-center study. *Epilepsy Res*, 1998;32:357–362.

167. Blum, D. E., Eskola, J., Bortz, J. J., & Fisher, R. S. Patient awareness of seizures. *Neurology*, 1966;47:260–264.

168. De Clercq, W., Vergult, A., Vanrumste, B., et al. Canonical correlation analysis applied to remove muscle artifacts from the electroencephalogram. *IEEE Trans Biomed Eng*, 2006;53:2583–2587.

169. Wilson, S. Personal communication, Persyst, Inc., 2015.

170. Velis, D., Plouin, P., Gotman, J., & Lopes da Silva, L. Recommendations regarding the requirements and applications for long-term recordings in epilepsy. *Epilepsia*, 2007;48(2):379–384.

171. Chang, B. S., Ives, J. R., Schomer, D. L., & Drislane, F. W. Outpatient EEG monitoring in the presurgical evaluation of patients with refractory temporal lobe epilepsy. *J Clin Neurophysiol*, 2002;19(2):152–156.

172. Nuwer, M. R., Engel, J. Jr., Sutherling, W. W., & Babb, T. L. Monitoring at the University of California, Los Angeles. *Electroencephalogr Clin Neurophysiol*, 1985;37:S385–402.

173. Riley, T., Porter, R. J., White, B. G., & Penry, J. K. The hospital experience and seizure control. *Neurology*, 1981;31:912–915.

174. Schomer, D. L. Ambulatory EEG telemetry: how good is it? *J Clin Neurophysiol*, 2006;23(4):294–305.

175. Ebersole, J. Ambulatory cassette EEG. *J Clin Neurophysiol*, 1985;2(4):397–418.

176. Ives, J. R., & Woods, J. 4-channel 24 hour cassette recorded for long-term EEG monitoring of ambulatory patients. *Electroencephalogr Clin Neurophysiol*, 1975;39:88–92.

177. Ebersole, J. S., & Bridgers, S. L. Direct comparison of 3- and 8-channel ambulatory cassette EEG with intensive inpatient monitoring. *Neurology*, 1985;35:846–854.

178. Schomer, D. L., Ives, J. R., & Schachter, S. C. The role of ambulatory EEG in the evaluation of patients for epilepsy surgery. *J Clin Neurophysiol*, 1999;16(2):116–129.

179. Gotman, J. Automatic recognition of epileptic seizures in the EEG. *Electroencephalogr Clin Neurophysiol*, 1982;54:530–540.

180. Morris, G. L., Jalezowska, J., Leroy, R., & North, R. The results of computer-assisted ambulatory 16-channel EEG. *Electroencephalogr Clin Neurophysiol*, 1994;91:229–231.

181. Saab, M. E., & Gotman, J. A system to detect the onset of epileptic seizures in scalp EEG. *Clin Neurophysiol*, 2005;116:427–442.

182. Wilson, S. B., Scheuer, M. L., Emerson, R. G., & Gabor, A. J. Seizure detection: evaluation of the Reveal algorithm. *Clin Neurophysiol*, 2004;115:2280–2291.

183. Cook, M., O'Brien, T., Berkovic, F., et al. Prediction of seizure likelihood with a long-term, implanted seizure advisory system in patients with drug-resistant epilepsy: a first-in-man study. *Lancet Neurol*, 2013;12:563–571.

184. Tomson, T., Nashef, L., & Ryvlin, P. Sudden unexpected death in epilepsy: current knowledge and future directions. *Lancet Neurol*, 2008;7(11):1021–1031.

185. Spanaki, M., Smith, B., Burdette, D., et al. Chronic measurement of increased epileptiform activity during menses using the responsive neurostimulator system (RNS) in a menses with catamenial seizures 2005 [1/22/2009]. Available from: http://www.neuropace.com/resources/publications/0512.html#8

186. Vossler, D. G., & Tcheng, T. Ambulatory intracranial ictal electroencephalogram patterns recorded chronically using the first implanted, self-contained ECOG recording and analysis instruments 2005 [1/22/2009]. Available from: http://www.neuropace.com/resources/publications/0512.html#9

187. Morrell, M. Responsive cortical stimulation for treatment of medically intractable partial epilepsy. *Neurology*, 2011;77:1295–1304.

188. Fischell, R. E., & Rischell, D. R. InventorsIntegrated system for EEG monitoring and electrical stimulation with a multiplicity of electrodes. U.S. Patent No. 6,320,049 B1 patent 6,320,049 B1., 2001.

189. Sauer, C., Stanacevic, M., Cauwenberghs, G., & Thakor, N. Power harvesting and telemetry in CMOS for implanted devices. *IEEE Trans Circuits Systems I: Regular Papers*, 2005;52(10):2605–2613.

190. Pan, C., Li, Z., Guo, W., Zhu, J., & Want, Z. Fiber-based hybrid nanogenerators for/as self-powered systems in biological liquid. *Agnew Chem*, 2011;123:11388–11392.

191. Ho, J., Yeh, A., Neofytou, E., et al. Wireless power transfer to deep-tissue microimplants. *Proc Nat Acad Sci USA*, 2014;111:7974–7979.

192. Powercast. Available from: http://powercastco.com/lifetime_power_app.html

193. Bhutani, A., McGarvey, Z., Frye, J., et al. Remote monitoring of EEG signals through wireless sensor networks 2008. Available from: edge.rit.edu/content/P08050/public/PDF%20Documentation/P08050_TechPaper.pdf

194. Yuce, M. R., Ng, W. P. S., Myo, N. L., et al. Wireless body sensor network using medical implant band. *J Med Sys*, 2007;31:467–474.

195. Mormann, F., Andrzejak, R. G., Elger, C. E., & Lehnertz, K. Seizure prediction: the long and winding road. *Brain*, 2007;130(2):v314–333.

32 | INFRASLOW EEG ACTIVITY

SAMPSA VANHATALO, MD AND J. MATIAS PALVA, PHD

ABSTRACT: Infraslow electroencephalographic (EEG) activity refers to frequencies below the conventional clinical EEG range that starts at about 0.5 Hz. Evidence suggests that salient EEG signals in the infraslow range are essential parts of many physiological and pathological conditions. In addition, brain is known to exhibit multitude of infraslow processes, which may be observed directly as fluctuations in the EEG signal amplitude, as infraslow fluctuations or intermittency in other neurophysiological signals, or as fluctuations in behavioural performance. Both physiological and pathological EEG activity may range from 0.01 Hz to several hundred Hz. In the clinical context, infraslow activity is commonly observed in the neonatal EEG, during and prior to epileptic seizures, and during sleep and arousals. Laboratory studies have demonstrated the presence of spontaneous infraslow EEG fluctuations or very slow event-related potentials in awake and sleeping subjects. Infraslow activity may not only arise in cortical and subcortical networks but is also likely to involve non-neuronal generators such as glial networks. The full, physiologically relevant range of brain mechanisms can be readily recorded with wide dynamic range direct-current (DC)-coupled amplifiers or full-band EEG (FbEEG). Due to the different underlying mechanisms, a single FbEEG recording can even be perceived as a multimodal recording where distinct brain modalities can be studied simultaneously by performing data analysis for different frequency ranges. FbEEG is likely to become the standard approach for a wide range of applications in both basic science and in the clinic.

KEYWORDS: electroencephalogram, EEG, infraslow, full-band EEG, direct current, sleep, epilepsy, neonatal EEG, FbEEG

PRINCIPAL REFERENCES

1. Vanhatalo S, Voipio J, Kaila K. Full-band EEG (FbEEG): An emerging standard in electroencephalography. *Clin Neurophysiol.* 2005;116:1–8.
2. Monto S, Palva S, Voipio J, Palva JM. Very slow EEG fluctuations predict the dynamics of stimulus detection and oscillation amplitudes in humans. *J Neurosci.* 2008;28:8268–8272.
3. Hiltunen T, Elseoud AA, Lepola P, et al. Infra-slow EEG fluctuations are correlated with resting-state network dynamics in fMRI. *J Neurosci.* 2014;34:356–362.
4. Palva JM, Palva S. Infra-slow fluctuations in electrophysiological recordings, blood-oxygenation-level-dependent signals, and psychophysical time series. *Neuroimage.* 2012;62:2201–2211.
5. Thompson S, Krishnan B, Gonzalez-Martinez J, et al. Ictal infraslow activity in stereoelectroencephalography: Beyond the "DC shift." *Clin Neurophysiol.* 2016;127:117–128.
6. van Putten MJ, Tjepkema-Cloostermans MC, Hofmeijer J. Infraslow EEG activity modulates cortical excitability in postanoxic encephalopathy. *J Neurophysiol.* 2015;113:3256–3267.
7. Thompson GJ, Pan WJ, Magnuson ME, Jaeger D, Keilholz SD. Quasi-periodic patterns (QPP): Large-scale dynamics in resting state fMRI that correlate with local infraslow electrical activity. *Neuroimage.* 2014;84:1018–1031.

1. INTRODUCTION

The prevailing standards for electroencephalography (EEG) were defined over half a century ago, and they aimed to allow adequate recording of the most salient EEG features. It was realized very early that faithful recording of brain-born slow events is challenging, because amplifiers were easily saturated by technical artifacts, such as electrode drifts, and even by high-amplitude cortical activities. This issue was solved by building EEG amplifiers with an inbuilt high-pass filter at the expense of eliminating all very-low-frequency components, whether physiological or artifactual. Such amplifiers have a poor low-frequency response. They attenuate and distort slow signals in ways that are not comparable between amplifier types, and often not even disclosed by the manufacturers. Therefore, clinicians have neglected the slowest EEG signals.

This standard practice is in sharp contrast with the growing literature showing that EEG signals range from infraslow (<0.1 Hz; this chapter) to ultrafast (up to several hundreds of Hz; next chapter) frequencies, which are collectively referred to as *full-band EEG* (FbEEG)[1].

For historical reasons, the terminology related to infraslow EEG phenomena and their recording methods has been confusing. Older literature uses the term *direct-current EEG* (DC-EEG) to emphasize that the signal was recorded with a by-then-uncommon DC-coupled amplifier. However, the term *DC-EEG* has become obsolete because many current EEG devices are built using DC-coupled amplifier circuits. These modern amplifiers are indeed able to record simultaneously the full physiological range from infraslow to ultrafast frequencies.

The term *DC* refers to, by definition, a 0-Hz response, which is not physiologically relevant in the EEG context as it only means the constant "standing potential" between two electrodes. It has hence become more common to use the term *infraslow*, which refers to periodic (oscillations), aperiodic (fluctuations), and unimodal (shifts) EEG events with a nominal frequency at the very low end of the conventional delta range. Notably, there is an overlap in the frequency response between the very-well-characterized slow oscillations (see Chapter 2) and some of the events described here using the concept of infraslow activity, which collectively refers to a wide range of brain mechanisms.

This chapter will review the current evidence of the presence of infraslow processes in the brain, their underlying mechanisms, their relationships to brain function and its disorders, and some clinical applications.

2. DEFINING INFRASLOW ACTIVITY: OSCILLATIONS, FLUCTUATIONS, AND EVENTS

Infraslow brain activity can be measured and perceived in different ways. It can be seen as spontaneous infraslow fluctuations (ISFs) in the EEG signal or more indirectly in infraslow modulations of several features of EEG activity, such as in infraslow-amplitude modulations of fast oscillations or modulations of the occurrence of fast events. Infraslow brain activity also includes discrete infraslow events, such as baseline shifts during epileptic seizures.

In the context of infraslow signals, it is important to acknowledge the distinction between discrete events and continuous oscillations or fluctuations[2], where "continuous" activity may be fluctuating but cannot be unequivocally split into periods of activity and no activity. Sometimes this distinction is more technical than physiological, because the underlying brain processes, such as preterm EEG events or sleep arousals, are distinct events even though they give rise to an apparently continuous aperiodic infraslow fluctuation in the EEG signal.

Whether the continuous infraslow activity as a phenomenon would correspond to transient quasi-periodic oscillations[3] or fluctuations[4] or rather to arrhythmic 1/f-like noise[5] has been a matter of debate[6], and it will be discussed further below. For the purpose of both the analysis design and interpretation of findings, it is important to recognize that activities in any EEG frequency range, including the infraslow, are phenomenologically heterogeneous and likely to arise through several distinct mechanisms and hence lack a direct one-to-one correspondence with specific physiological processes.

3. INFRASLOW PHENOMENA CHARACTERIZE BEHAVIORAL AND ALL SCALES OF ELECTROPHYSIOLOGICAL BRAIN ACTIVITY

ISFs are a salient feature in behavioral measurements of psychophysical and cognitive performance[4–8]. Behavioral ISFs were originally discovered through the observation that consecutive trials in psychophysical experiments have a greater probability of producing similar behavioral outcomes, such as successes or failures, than expected by chance[7,9]. More recent studies have revealed ISFs in a wide range of continuous-performance tasks where the subject performs a constant-difficulty task for up to tens of minutes. The ISFs in psychophysical performance (e.g., in hit rates or reaction times) exhibit autocorrelations over several minutes, specifically in a scale-free and fractal-like fashion[4,8]. Fluctuations in psychophysical performance are thus governed by scaling laws where a variable k is a nonlinear function $\mathbf{f}$ of another variable raised to the power a so that $\mathbf{f}(k) \approx k^{-a}$. Taking the log of both sides of this expression yields a straight line with slope $-a$. Scaling laws are observed in many branches of science and imply that the underlying system exhibits *scale-free* behavior or "fractal dynamics" (see Chapter 44). These systems often also exhibit *long-range temporal correlations* with an autocorrelation function $\mathbf{C}(k) \approx k^{-a}$ that decays slowly as function of time lag. In the frequency domain the corresponding spectral power $\mathbf{S}(f)$ can be expressed as $\mathbf{S}(f) \approx f^{-a}$, where f is the frequency. For $a = 1$, $\mathbf{S}(f)$ has the commonplace 1/f scaling.

The electrophysiological correlates of ISFs in psychophysical performance would conceivably be spontaneous neuronal processes with comparable scale-free ISFs. Indeed, recent studies have demonstrated that such ISFs are abundant in the dynamics of fast neuronal activities as well as in FbEEG signals per se.

ISFs in the amplitude envelope of alpha-frequency-band (8–14 Hz) oscillations[10] were among the first observations of this kind in the human EEG. Later studies using both EEG and magnetoencephalography (MEG)[11,12], as well as invasive electrocorticography[13,14], have shown that the amplitude fluctuations of human cortical oscillations in theta-frequency (4–8 Hz), alpha-frequency, and beta-frequency (14–30 Hz) bands exhibit long-range temporal correlations in time scales from tens to hundreds of seconds and thus display scale-free, fractal-like dynamics as observed in psychophysics (Fig. 32.1). Infraslow amplitude fluctuations in the EEG are not specific to human; they have been reported in a wide phylogenetic range of species from monkeys to rats, rabbits, and cats[6]. Moreover, cortical recordings from both monkeys[15] and humans[14] show that, in addition to the amplitudes, inter-areal coherence of a wide spectrum of oscillations have ISFs and power-law frequency scaling.

At the cellular level, in vivo single-unit recordings of neuronal firing rates have shown ISFs or infraslow oscillations (ISOs) in monkeys[16] as well as in rat thalamus[17] and basal ganglia[18]. Further insight into the mechanistic basis of ISFs/ISOs has recently been obtained in vitro with observations that neuronal firing rates of rat thalamocortical neurons exhibit ISOs through an ATP-dependent mechanism (see below)[19].

To our knowledge, the first "FbEEG" recordings of infraslow scalp potentials with DC-stable electrodes and amplifiers were carried out by Aladjalova[20]. Recordings of spontaneous infraslow potentials in rabbit[20] and cat cortex[21] in vivo provided the first evidence for ISFs and ISOs in EEG signals per se[22]. Since Aladjalova, spontaneous infraslow potential fluctuations have been observed in rats (e.g., in hippocampus[23], in primary auditory and visual cortex, as well as in several thalamic and brainstem nuclei[24] in both awake and anaesthetized animals). Notably, some forms of anesthesia eliminate ISFs[18,22]. In human scalp FbEEG, spontaneous ISFs are characteristic to preterm neonates[25] as well as to sleeping[3,26], awake[27], and task-engaged adults[4] (Figs. 32.2 and 32.3, for review, see[6]).

Taken together, electrophysiological data across a wide range of species, brain structures, and spatial scales show that ISFs are salient both in direct electric potential fluctuations and in firing rate and oscillation amplitude dynamics.

4. TECHNICAL ASPECTS

The technical requirements for a successful study vary between different forms of infraslow brain activity. The main factor is the frequency of signal amplitude fluctuations. When the infraslow process is studied from a signal derivative, such as fluctuation of power in a defined frequency band[11,28,29], it can be successfully studied using conventional EEG recording methods. However, a faithful recording of infraslow changes in signal amplitude requires special technical considerations. An ideal, uncompromised recording of infraslow changes in the EEG signal requires a DC-coupled amplifier and a DC-stable electrode–skin interface (for more technical details, see[1,30]).

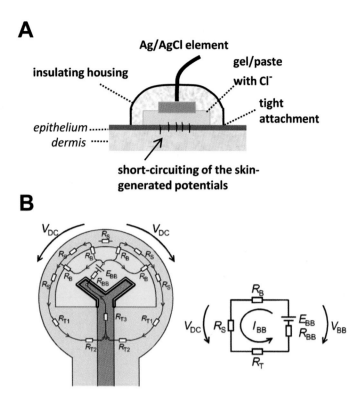

A

Ag/AgCl element

insulating housing

gel/paste
with Cl⁻

tight
attachment

epithelium

dermis

short-circuiting of the skin-
generated potentials

B

Figure 32.1. **A:** *Electrode–skin interface of a DC-stable recording requires removing and/or avoiding sources of potential fluctuations. The electrode–gel interface needs to be nonpolarizing; this is typically achieved by using an Ag/AgCl electrode and chloride-containing gel. Skin-born potentials need short-circuiting at the epithelium. The electrode element needs an insulated housing, such as plastic, and a firm mechanical attachment to the skin to avoid movement, as well as drying of the gel.* **B:** *A model of the non-neuronal mechanism underlying infraslow signals via volume currents generated by the blood–brain barrier potential. The schematic drawing (left) shows compartments of a human head: brain (yellow), blood–brain barrier (thick black), blood vessel (pink), and the other tissues (light green). EBB is the electromotive force of the voltage source across the blood–brain barrier that has internal resistance RBB. This voltage source generates a volume current that flows through the distributed resistance of brain (RB) and other cranial tissue (RS) until it returns back into blood vessel outside of the blood–brain barrier. RT1 is the tissue resistance below the cranium, RT2 refers to resistance into blood vessel, and RT3 refers to resistance within blood vessel. An equivalent but simplified technical drawing of the circuitry is shown on the right. (IBB denotes the current driven in the circuit by EBB.) Adapted with permission from* [33].

As in any neurophysiological recordings, it is sometimes necessary to make compromises in recording setup due to, for instance, clinical recording conditions, lack of a DC-coupled amplifier or DC-coupled intracranial electrodes, or inability to fully short-circuit the transepithelial skin potentials[31]. It is then imperative that the results are interpreted in keeping with the degree of uncertainty imposed on the signal. For instance, any compromise in terms of the electrode material or in preparation of the electrode–skin interface will always affect the reliability of infraslow waveforms, including signal amplitudes, due to introduction of several poorly controllable sources of technical (e.g., baseline drifts) and biological (e.g., skin potential) noise. The significance of technical compromise depends on the EEG phenomena of interest as well as on the type of analysis carried out for the signal. For instance, source localization is unpredictably distorted in non-ideal recordings, because it depends on the global combination of signal amplitudes at each time point. It is mostly not possible to recover or estimate the original signal if it was distorted during the recording; hence, it is strongly advisable to obtain undistorted recordings in the first place.

A faithful detection of infraslow amplitude change requires a DC-stable electrode–skin interface (see Fig. 32.1), which is achieved by combining (1) a non-polarizable (in practice Ag/AgCl) electrode, (2) chloride-containing gel[32], (3) a good mechanical fixation to minimize artifacts caused by gel leakage (or drying), and (4) elimination of skin-born signals seen during electrode movements or galvanic skin reactions. Skin-born signals are best avoided by short-circuiting the transepithelial potential, which can be done by scratching through the epithelium[33] or by using minimally invasive techniques[31,34]. An unstable electrode–skin interface makes it challenging if not impossible to fully distinguish genuine brain-born infraslow signals from non-cerebral artifacts[1]. However, a suboptimal electrode–skin interface may still give reasonably good recordings in calm and/or sleeping subjects when the EEG events of interests are phasic with relatively short duration.

The principles of choosing the recording reference and montages for recording infraslow activities are the same as for any EEG studies. Notably, the spatial extent of infraslow activity is often significantly larger than the extent of conventional EEG activity. This implies that the typical clinically used bipolar derivations computed from nearby electrodes may not appropriately disclose the actual infraslow activity that spans multiple electrodes. The same care needs to be taken when using grand average or Laplacian montages. It is hence advisable to select the montage only after first studying the spatial extent

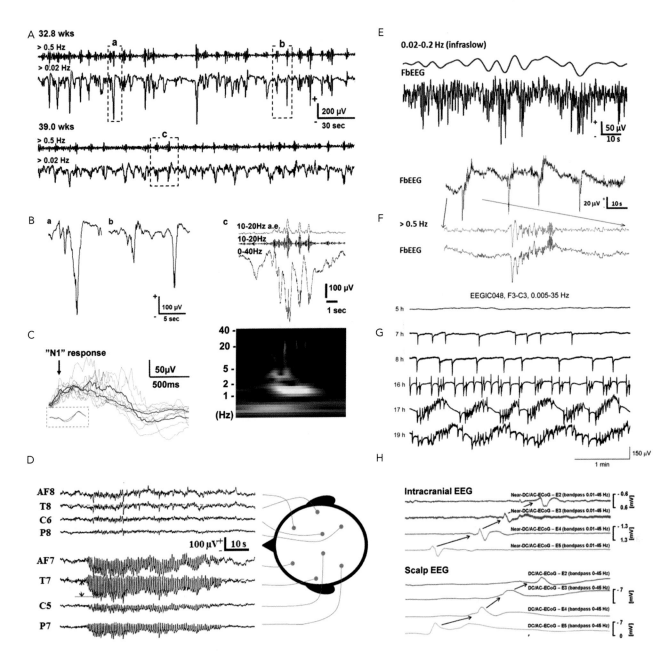

Figure 32.2. Examples of infraslow EEG activity recorded in clinical research. **A:** Four-minute-long FbEEG recordings of a preterm (above) and a full-term (below) infant, showing comparison between conventionally filtered signal (high-pass 0.5 Hz) and the signal where only slow trend is removed using high-pass filter at 0.02 Hz. Note the large-amplitude, slow spontaneous activity transients (SATs) that dominate the EEG signal. **B:** Examples of SATs shown in A (insets a, b, c) depict the details of the SAT events, while the band-specific filtering and the time–frequency representation of inset c depicts how the SATs consist of grouped multiband activity. **C:** Infraslow cortical response to tactile stimulation of a preterm infant. The early sensory responses consist of a long-duration, high-amplitude, multiband event, which has a somewhat variable waveform, making it escape capture by conventional averaging. For comparison, the inset below depicts a conventional somatosensory response with the typically measured N1 wave. **D:** Infraslow ictal (DC) shift during a subclinical temporal lobe epileptic seizure. Note the maximum of shift at the site of maximal seizure activity, as well as ISF of the amplitude during the seizure. **E:** ISO in a 2-minute FbEEG epoch during sleep. The trace above shows the infraslow component (0.02–0.2 Hz) to visualize the phase-amplitude relationship with higher frequencies. **F:** DC shifts seen at the vertex during transient arousals during sleep. One arousal is depicted on an expanded scale for an unfiltered (FbEEG) as well as a conventionally filtered trace. **G:** Evolution of infraslow activity associated with burst-suppression patterns during recovery from coma. Note the phase-amplitude coupling between the phase of infraslow and the amplitude of conventional EEG frequencies. **H:** Spreading depolarization after head trauma. Comparison of intracranial and scalp EEG signals shows a similar spatial evolution between electrodes. Adapted with permission from [3,42,60,111,112].

of the infraslow activity of interest. Recordings of very-long-duration shifts, in time scales from tens of minutes to hours, in DC potentials of brain-born EEG signals are inherently inaccurate because of the uncontrollable instabilities that may arise from potential gradients across other tissues, or changes at different components of the electrode–skin interface.

5. INFRASLOW EEG AND CLINICAL APPLICATIONS

5.1. Neonatal EEG

The abundance of slow activity is a well-known feature of EEG activity in the preterm human EEG[35] (see also Chapters 7 and 18).

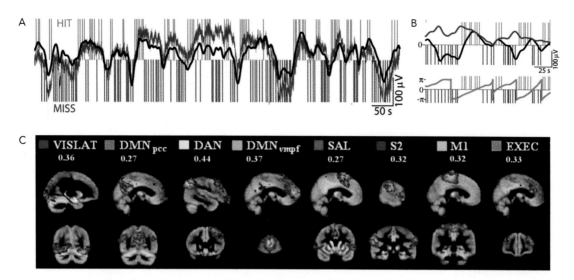

Figure 32.3. **A:** *Data from a representative subject shows that 0.01- to 0.1-Hz ISFs in human scalp FbEEG (black line) are large in comparison with the broadband EEG (gray line), observable during task execution, and locked to task performance. In this task, the subject performed a threshold-stimulus detection task where weak constant-intensity somatosensory stimuli intermittently became detected (blue ticks) or remained unperceived (red ticks). **B:** The phase (green line), but not the magnitude (black line) or amplitude (gray line), of ISFs is correlated with behavioral performance. **C:** In concurrent FbEEG and fMRI recordings, independent components of FbEEG scalp potentials are correlated with fMRI-voxel-BOLD signals (green regions) with neuroanatomical patterns matching those of fMRI resting-state networks (orange-yellow regions). Adapted with permission from[4,72].*

After the introduction of clinically compatible FbEEG recordings, it was shown that most of the spectral power in the neonatal EEG is at infraslow range, well below the conventional EEG frequency bands[25,36]. Comparison of recordings from infants at different conceptional ages shows that the dominance of infraslow activity declines rapidly from the early preterm period toward the early infantile period[25]. This early decline in infraslow activity is physiologically different from the later developmental change in frequency distribution[37]. Most importantly, the early ISFs arise from the developmentally unique brain events that are considered to play a crucial role as an endogenous guidance of neuronal growth, survival, and networking prior to onset of external sensory input[38].

These developmental events, also known as spontaneous activity transients, delta brushes, or bursts[39], have a characteristic duration of several seconds, and they give rise to FbEEG spectral power of <0.1 Hz. More recent studies have shown that such infraslow events can be readily triggered by delivering tactical, auditory, or photic stimulations to the preterm baby[40–42]. These early responses are now known to arise from a complex interplay between cortical plate and the transiently present subcortical layer, subplate[43], which opens a unique opportunity for bedside testing of subcortical brain function in preterm infants[44].

Taken together, while FbEEG recordings unravel a fully novel type of cortical activity in the low-frequency range, they also call for a revised, physiologically sound interpretation of the perinatal EEG[45], and open the potential for direct translational bridging between human and experimental studies.

5.2. Sleep and Infraslow EEG Activity

Recording of FbEEG during non–rapid-eye-movement sleep discloses prominent ISOs with amplitudes up to tens of microvolts over a wide range of frequencies (from ~0.02 to 0.2 Hz)[3,46]. The sleep-related ISOs are likely to reflect a more pervasive physiological brain process, because the phase of ISO is robustly correlated with higher-frequency EEG oscillations, sleep events, and even the occurrence of interictal epileptiform activity[3]. ISOs may reflect slow spontaneous fluctuation in cortical excitability under both physiological and pathophysiological conditions, an idea that fits well with results obtained in in vivo experiments on humans[47], rats[23], and monkeys[15].

In addition to the direct ISFs in scalp EEG potential, it has been shown that transient arousals during sleep are coupled with a high-amplitude vertex-positive DC shift that might last several tens of seconds. Moreover, overnight recordings have reported DC shifts with polarity and magnitude consistent with sleep stage as well[26,48]. Another type of infraslow activity is represented in the cyclic occurrence of cortical arousal patterns that usually repeat with a periodicity of 20 to 60 seconds during sleep. These are phenomenologically referred to as cyclic alternating patterns, and they have been intensively studied in different populations[47]. It is conceivable that cyclic alternating patterns reflect the higher-frequency component of the infraslow brain activity during sleep.

5.3. Epileptic Seizures and Infraslow EEG Activity

An abundant experimental literature has shown that the fast ictal spiking discharge is usually associated with a slow change in the EEG baseline, referred to as an ictal DC shift[49–51]. The pioneering work in the 1960s showed that ictal DC shifts can be recorded from the scalp during generalized seizures[52], and they were studied extensively in experimental animal models by Speckmann et al.[53] However, due to technical difficulties their routine recording did not become more general until the 1990s[49,54,55]. Both scalp-recorded and intracranial studies suggest that the ictal DC shifts may provide an independent marker of the ictal onset zone[50,51,56,57]. It is possible that ictal DC shifts may become clinically useful as an independent modality in the presurgical epilepsy evaluation[51,54,58]. The invasive studies are challenged by the fact that intracranial electrodes are not DC-coupled[32], which will lead to some distortion of infraslow signals, and this needs to be taken into account during the analysis. A similar situation holds for the attempts to analyze infraslow activity from the scalp EEG that was initially recorded with AC-coupled amplifiers[59]; all results from such recordings are inherently confounded by the inbuilt filtering property of the amplifier, precluding, for instance, a reliable source localization of the kind that can be informative in genuine DC-coupled recordings[50].

5.4. Other Brain Disorders

Several other disorders of brain function are also shown to exhibit robust infraslow activity. For instance, post-anoxic coma is associated with an infraslow activity that modulates cortical excitability[60]. Recent studies have also demonstrated that prominent infraslow shifts can be recorded both on the scalp and in the intracranial electrodes during acute brain trauma[61,62]. The attention-deficit disorders are characterized by abnormalities in behavioral ISFs[63]. This suggests that ISFs play a fundamental mechanistic role in healthy and diseased brain processing, and suggests that further research on ISFs may also have translational value in shedding light on disorder mechanisms and future therapeutic targets.

5.5. ISFs/ISOs in Functional Magnetic Resonance Imaging and Their Relationship with FbEEG ISFs

Investigations of spontaneous brain activity in functional magnetic resonance imaging (fMRI) recordings have revealed a slow waxing and waning of the spontaneous blood-oxygenation-level-dependent (BOLD) signal[29,64,65] (see also Chapter 46). These BOLD ISFs are correlated between bilateral homologous regions as well as among specific stable constellations of brain regions, of which the so-called default mode network was among the first to be recognized. An extensive body of later fMRI studies has shown similar correlations in several distributed brain networks in the resting state[66,67]. These correlations have a scale-free, power-law-governed spatiotemporal architecture[68]. Infraslow network dynamics characterize neuronal activity also during cognitive tasks, and thus these "resting-state networks" have also been termed "intrinsic connectivity networks"[69,70] or "brain systems"[71].

Several lines of indirect evidence suggest that ISFs in FbEEG signals and in fMRI reflect the same underlying intrinsic neuronal dynamics (reviewed in[6]). Direct evidence for the correlation of FbEEG and BOLD ISFs was recently obtained with combined FbEEG and fMRI recordings[72] (see Fig. 32.3C). In this study, the authors used independent components analysis to segregate both the 32-channel FbEEG and the fMRI data to independent components. First, an fMRI voxel-level analysis showed that in significant numbers of voxels, the BOLD time series was correlated with the FbEEG independent components time series. The anatomical patterns of these FbEEG-correlated voxels were matched with the patterns of specific fMRI independent components (i.e., with the classical fMRI resting-state networks). This finding thus shows both that FbEEG signals at the scalp are directly correlated with BOLD signals and that separable FbEEG signals are likely to originate from distinct BOLD resting-state networks. Taken together, these data strongly support the notion that spontaneous infraslow electrophysiological rhythms and intrinsic BOLD signal fluctuations have significant overlap in their underlying physiological phenomena.

6. GENERATORS OF INFRASLOW EEG SIGNALS

Recent work has shown that infraslow changes in the EEG signals may arise from multiple different intracranial sources that include both neuronal (neurons and glial cells) and non-neuronal mechanisms (other cellular structures; see Chapter 2, Fig. 2.1)[33]. In addition to these genuinely brain-born signals, some extracranial sources, such as tongue movements[73] or changes in voltage gradients across other tissues, might cause slow shifts in the EEG signal.

The slow DC shifts during many long-latency cortical responses (see below) have been traditionally explained by a tonic depolarization of apical dendrites[74]. This idea is supported by direct invasive recordings that show intracortical potential gradient compatible with the excitation of the apical dendrite layer. The glial networks have also been implicated in the generation of some slow activity by generating ionic gradients in a manner that can be detected at epicortical electrodes (see Chapter 2)[75].

The non-neuronal source of infraslow amplitude change is most obvious after hyperventilation, which induces a pH-dependent, millivolt-scale DC shift in human[33], and there is an absence of intracortical potential gradient in a comparable animal model[75]. Moreover, other physical maneuvers may also generate DC shifts that correlate with hemodynamic changes as measured using near-infrared spectroscopy[76]. These seemingly enigmatic observations can be fully explained by changes of electric potential across the blood–brain barrier[73].

Acknowledging the multitude of generators, and the presence of the blood–brain barrier as an EEG generator, has a number of implications. In particular, this can readily explain at least part of the ictal DC shifts during epileptic seizures, and the correlations between infraslow activities in the EEG and fMRI or near-infrared spectroscopy signals[46]. In addition, slow signals related to extracranial sources, especially the uncontrolled tongue movements or changes in respiration, need to be considered in cognitive paradigms that measure infraslow EEG activity.

The above-described relationship of ISFs in FbEEG signals and in BOLD/near-infrared spectroscopy signals adds another dimension to their intimate relationship. First, maneuvers and pharmacological modulations affecting regional cerebral blood flow are associated with shifts in FbEEG potential[33,76–78]; conversely, event-related slow cortical potentials are correlated with BOLD signals[79]. Second, several studies using DC-EEG, DC-MEG, fMRI, and near-infrared spectroscopy[80,81] reveal direct and regionally specific associations between task-performance-evoked slow shifts in scalp electric potentials and magnetic fields with concurrent BOLD signals in fMRI and near-infrared spectroscopy. However, here it is necessary to note that the exact mechanistic relationship of these task-evoked potential shifts with the spontaneous EEG and BOLD ISFs remains unknown.

7. ARE ISFS GENERATED BY EMERGENT SLOW FLUCTUATIONS OF FAST NEURONAL ACTIVITIES?

Theoretically ISFs in the fbEEG scalp potentials, oscillation amplitude envelopes, and BOLD signals could arise from the emergent slow dynamics of fast (>1 Hz) activities without any underlying slow cellular-level mechanisms[82,83]. Emergence of ISFs in the dynamics of fast activities would be predicted by, for instance, the framework of brains operating near a critical state[11,84,85] (see, however, discussion in Chapter 46). In critical-state systems, spatially and temporally local interactions give rise to long-range spatiotemporal correlations of power-law form like those observed in ISFs, as has been observed with neuronal network models exhibiting critical dynamics[83]. Similar emergence of ISFs has also been observed in other kinds of large-scale models composed of exclusively fast neuronal mechanisms and realistic structural connectivity[4,11,82,86,87,88].

A counterpoint to this notion is provided by findings that in rodent brain slices in vitro, periodic adenosine-triphosphate release that is associated with astrocytic calcium oscillations hyperpolarizes thalamocortical neurons in the lateral geniculate nucleus and drives the generation of infraslow membrane potential oscillations in these neurons. These fluctuations underlie the amplitude fluctuations of thalamic alpha oscillations[19,89], which suggests that infraslow membrane potential oscillations could drive the amplitude modulations of fast cortical and subcortical activities. As crucial and direct evidence for a similar mechanism in vivo, Du et al.[90] showed that low-frequency calcium oscillations are correlated with BOLD ISFs/ISOs in rat somatosensory cortex. Comparable infraslow astrocytic-calcium oscillations are prominent also in visual cortex, hippocampus[91], and thalamus[92,93]. It appears likely that emergent scale-free ISFs arising in the dynamics of fast neuronal activities cooperate with and are modulated by slow-time-scale-specific cellular-level mechanisms.

8. IS INFRASLOW ACTIVITY ARRHYTHMIC NOISE OR QUASI-PERIODIC OSCILLATIONS?

ISFs have been argued to be an exclusively arrhythmic, $1/f$-noise-like phenomenon[5,94]. This view is seemingly supported by the $1/f$-like power spectrum that FbEEG and BOLD signals have. The notion of arrhythmicity would also be plausible if ISFs were generated exclusively through the emergent dynamics of fast neuronal activities. However, both the presence of cellular-level ISF/ISO generating mechanisms and other lines of evidence appear to be incompatible with the arrhythmic $1/f$ noise hypothesis and suggest that ISFs could phenomenologically be composed of quasi-periodic oscillations[6,95]. Here quasi-periodicity indicates a pattern of recurrence without a fixed period, which is phenomenologically common to systems that mechanistically exhibit a potential for (periodic) oscillations but lack an external drive. Evidence for this alternative includes findings that the thalamocortical ISFs may arise through time-scale-specific cellular-level mechanisms that are in vitro known to produce oscillatory or at least quasi-periodic activity[19,89]. In line with these data, low-frequency calcium oscillations are correlated with BOLD oscillations in rat cortex[90]. In addition, electrical stimulation of thalamic and brainstem nuclei leads to different modulations of <0.01-Hz, 0.01- to 0.1-Hz, and 0.1- to 1-Hz band activities in the auditory cortex and suggests a mechanistic double dissociation among these bands[24,96]. Furthermore, quantitative analyses of periodicity as well as visual inspection suggest that at the cellular level, a large fraction of infraslow activities are oscillatory[18–20,22,89,97,98]. Also, scalp EEG ISFs may exhibit significant periodicity and even power-spectral peaks in some conditions[3,99,100]. Likewise, in fMRI data, correlations among ISFs in different brain regions are phase-dependent, involve band-limited infraslow interactions[101,102], and emerge transiently in narrow-frequency bands[103,101,102]. Finally, as key evidence for such transient periodicity being functionally significant, the phase of electrophysiological ISFs, rather than their magnitude or potential level, predicts stimulus detection probability[4], reaction times[104], occurrence of fast neuronal transients[3], and the amplitude dynamics of fast neuronal oscillations[3,14]. Several lines of findings thus converge to suggest that ISFs and infraslow inter-areal interactions are at least transiently periodic rather than exclusively arrhythmic.

9. INFRASLOW EVENT-RELATED POTENTIALS

Most of the past literature on low-frequency EEG has focused on slow potentials that are seen during various kinds of cognitive tasks and states, such as contingent stimulation (contingent negative variation), motor movements (Bereitschaftspotential), and the orienting paradigm[105,106]. More recent work on the development of brain–computer interfaces has shown that subjects may even learn to deliberately induce slow scalp-recorded potentials[107,108]. These slow potentials have a duration of up to several seconds, although their amplitude is typically only a few microvolts. Their recording needs particular care in order to reliably distinguish the genuine brain-born components from a non-neuronal contamination elicited by changes in respiration patterns or tongue movements (see above).

In addition to the slow EEG responses recorded during cognitive tasks, there is evidence that very-long-latency components (up to ~2,500 msec) of evoked potentials might provide clinically useful information in brain monitoring. For instance, long-latency auditory evoked potentials correlate with the depth of anesthesia or coma[109,110]; however, the full clinical exploitation of this potential has remained untapped so far. Moreover, developmentally unique infraslow responses can be recorded from preterm infants after somatosensory, visual, and auditory stimulations[40-42]. The network mechanism of these responses is supposed to involve both the developmentally transient subplate structure and the intracortical circuitry implicated in evoked responses later in life[40,43].

10. CONCLUDING POINTS

- Infraslow EEG activity is an integral part of brain function.

- Undistorted recordings of infraslow potential fluctuations can be achieved with a DC-stable skin interface and a DC amplifier.

- Brain activity in the infraslow range can be observed as fluctuations in the EEG potential or as infraslow periodicity in EEG features.

- Infraslow EEG potentials are correlated with spontaneous BOLD signal fluctuations.

- Infraslow activity can be phase-amplitude-coupled to faster EEG oscillations.

- Cerebral ISFs are strongly correlated with fluctuations in task performance.

- ISFs are likely to reflect fluctuations in cortical excitability.

REFERENCES

1. Vanhatalo S, Voipio J, Kaila K. Full-band EEG (FbEEG): An emerging standard in electroencephalography. *Clin Neurophysiol.* 2005;116(1):1–8.
2. Bullock TH, Mcclune MC, Enright JT. Are the electroencephalograms mainly rhythmic? Assessment of periodicity in wide-band time series. *Neuroscience.* 2003;121(1):233–252.
3. Vanhatalo S, Palva JM, Holmes MD, Miller JW, Voipio J, Kaila K. Infraslow oscillations modulate excitability and interictal epileptic activity in the human cortex during sleep. *Proc Natl Acad Sci USA.* 2004;101(14):5053–5057.
4. Monto S, Palva S, Voipio J, Palva JM. Very slow EEG fluctuations predict the dynamics of stimulus detection and oscillation amplitudes in humans. *J Neurosci.* 2008;28(33):8268–8272.
5. He BJ. Scale-free brain activity: Past, present, and future. *Trends Cogn Sci.* 2014;18(9):480–487.
6. Palva JM, Palva S. Infra-slow fluctuations in electrophysiological recordings, blood-oxygenation-level-dependent signals, and psychophysical time series. *Neuroimage.* 2012 ;62(4):2201–2211.
7. Verplanck WS, Collier GH, Cotton JW. Nonindependence of successive responses in measurements of the visual threshold. *J Exp Psychol.* 1952;44(4):273–282.
8. Gilden DL, Wilson SG. On the nature of streaks in signal detection. *Cognit Psychol.* 1995;28(1):17–64.
9. Wertheimer M. An investigation of the randomness of threshold measurements. *J Exp Psychol.* 1953;45(5):294–303.
10. Pfurtscheller G. Ultralangsame schwankungen innerhalb der rhythmischen aktivität im alpha-band und deren mögliche ursachen. *Pflügers Archiv Eur J Physiol.* 1976;367(1):55–66.
11. Linkenkaer-Hansen K, Nikouline VV, Palva JM, Ilmoniemi RJ. Long-range temporal correlations and scaling behavior in human brain oscillations. *J Neurosci.* 2001;21(4):1370–1377.
12. Linkenkaer-Hansen K, Monto S, Rytsala H, Suominen K, Isometsa E, Kahkonen S. Breakdown of long-range temporal correlations in theta oscillations in patients with major depressive disorder. *J Neurosci.* 2005;25(44):10131–10137.
13. Monto S, Vanhatalo S, Holmes MD, Palva JM. Epileptogenic neocortical networks are revealed by abnormal temporal dynamics in seizure-free subdural EEG. *Cerebral Cortex.* 2007;17(6):1386–1393.
14. Ko AL, Darvas F, Poliakov A, Ojemann J, Sorensen LB. Quasi-periodic fluctuations in default mode network electrophysiology. *J Neurosci.* 2011;31(32):11728–11732.
15. Leopold DA, Murayama Y, Logothetis NK. Very slow activity fluctuations in monkey visual cortex: Implications for functional brain imaging. *Cereb Cortex.* 2003;13(4):422–433.
16. Werner G, Mountcastle VB. The variability of central neural activity in a sensory system, and its implications for the central reflection of sensory events. *J Neurophysiol.* 1963;26:958–977.
17. Albrecht D, Gabriel S. Very slow oscillations of activity in geniculate neurones of urethane-anaesthetized rats. *Neuroreport.* 1994;5(15):1909–1912.
18. Ruskin DN, Bergstrom DA, Kaneoke Y, Patel BN, Twery MJ, Walters JR. Multisecond oscillations in firing rate in the basal ganglia: Robust modulation by dopamine receptor activation and anesthesia. *J Neurophysiol.* 1999;81(5):2046–2055.
19. Hughes SW, Lorincz ML, Parri HR, Crunelli V. Infraslow (<0.1 Hz) oscillations in thalamic relay nuclei basic mechanisms and significance in health and disease states. *Prog Brain Res.* 2011;193:145–162.
20. Aladjalova NA. Infra-slow rhythmic oscillations of the steady potential of the cerebral cortex. *Nature.* 1957;179(4567):957–959.
21. Norton S, Jewett RE. Frequencies of slow potential oscillations in the cortex of cats. *Electroencephalogr Clin Neurophysiol.* 1965;19(4):377–386.
22. Aladjalova NA. Infraslow potential oscillations in the cerebral cortex. In: Aladjalova NA, ed. *Progress in Brain Research, Vol. 7: Slow Electrical Processes in the Brain.* Elsevier Publishing Company; 1964:39–58.
23. Penttonen M, Nurminen N, Miettinen R, et al. Ultra-slow oscillation (0.025 Hz) triggers hippocampal afterdischarges in wistar rats. *Neuroscience.* 1999;94(3):735–743.
24. Filippov IV, Williams WC, Krebs AA, Pugachev KS. Dynamics of infraslow potentials in the primary auditory cortex: Component analysis and contribution of specific thalamic-cortical and non-specific brainstem-cortical influences. *Brain Res.* 2008;1219(0):66–77.
25. Vanhatalo S, Palva JM, Andersson S, Rivera C, Voipio J, Kaila K. Slow endogenous activity transients and developmental expression of K+-Cl- cotransporter 2 in the immature human cortex. *Eur J Neurosci.* 2005;22(11):2799–2804.
26. Marshall L, Molle M, Fehm HL, Born J. Scalp recorded direct current brain potentials during human sleep. *Eur J Neurosci.* 1998;10(3):1167–1178.
27. Trimmel M, Mikowitsch A, Groll-Knapp E, Haider M. Occurrence of infraslow potential oscillations in relation to task, ability to concentrate and intelligence. *Int J Psychophysiol.* 1990;9(2):167–170.
28. Goncalves SI, de Munck JC, Pouwels PJ, et al. Correlating the alpha rhythm to BOLD using simultaneous EEG/fMRI: Inter-subject variability. *Neuroimage.* 2006;30(1):203–213.
29. Mantini D, Perrucci MG, Del Gratta C, Romani GL, Corbetta M. Electrophysiological signatures of resting state networks in the human brain. *Proc Natl Acad Sci USA.* 2007;104(32):13170–13175.
30. Vanhatalo S, Voipio J, Kaila K. Full-band EEG (fbEEG): A new standard for clinical electroencephalography. *Clin EEG Neurosci.* 2005;36(4):311–317.
31. Stjerna S, Alatalo P, Maki J, Vanhatalo S. Evaluation of an easy, standardized and clinically practical method (SurePrep) for the preparation of electrode-skin contact in neurophysiological recordings. *Physiol Meas.* 2010;31(7):889–901.
32. Tallgren P, Vanhatalo S, Kaila K, Voipio J. Evaluation of commercially available electrodes and gels for recording of slow EEG potentials. *Clin Neurophysiol.* 2005;116(4):799–806.
33. Voipio J, Tallgren P, Heinonen E, Vanhatalo S, Kaila K. Millivolt-scale DC shifts in the human scalp EEG: Evidence for a nonneuronal generator. *J Neurophysiol.* 2003;89(4):2208–2214.
34. Sinisalo L, Maki J, Stjerna S, Vanhatalo S. SurePrep, an easy alternative for skin preparation in neonatal EEG monitoring. *Acta Paediatr.* 2012;101(8):e378–381.
35. Andre M, Lamblin MD, d'Allest AM, et al. Electroencephalography in premature and full-term infants. developmental features and glossary. *Neurophysiol Clin.* 2010;40(2):59–124.
36. Vanhatalo S, Tallgren P, Andersson S, Sainio K, Voipio J, Kaila K. DC-EEG discloses prominent, very slow activity patterns during sleep in preterm infants. *Clin Neurophysiol.* 2002;113(11):1822–1825.
37. Fransson P, Metsaranta M, Blennow M, Aden U, Lagercrantz H, Vanhatalo S. Early development of spatial patterns of power-law frequency scaling in FMRI resting-state and EEG data in the newborn brain. *Cereb Cortex.* 2013;23(3):638–646.

38. Hanganu-Opatz IL. Between molecules and experience: Role of early patterns of coordinated activity for the development of cortical maps and sensory abilities. *Brain Res Rev.* 2010;64(1):160–176.

39. Vanhatalo S, Kaila K. Spontaneous and evoked activity in the early human brain. In: Lagercrantz H, Hanson MA, Ment LR, Peebles DM, eds. *The Newborn Brain: Neuroscience & Clinical Applications.* 2nd ed. Cambridge University Press; 2010:229–243.

40. Colonnese MT, Kaminska A, Minlebaev M, et al. A conserved switch in sensory processing prepares developing neocortex for vision. *Neuron.* 2010;67(3):480–498.

41. Chipaux M, Colonnese MT, Mauguen A, et al. Auditory stimuli mimicking ambient sounds drive temporal "delta-brushes" in premature infants. *PLoS One.* 2013;8(11):e79028.

42. Vanhatalo S, Jousmaki V, Andersson S, Metsaranta M. An easy and practical method for routine, bedside testing of somatosensory systems in extremely low birth weight infants. *Pediatr Res.* 2009;66(6):710–713.

43. Vanhatalo S, Lauronen L. Neonatal SEP—back to bedside with basic science. *Semin Fetal Neonatal Med.* 2006;11(6):464–470.

44. Stjerna S, Voipio J, Metsaranta M, Kaila K, Vanhatalo S. Preterm EEG: A multimodal neurophysiological protocol. *J Vis Exp.* 2012;(60):3774.

45. Vanhatalo S, Kaila K. Development of neonatal EEG activity: From phenomenology to physiology. *Semin Fetal Neonatal Med.* 2006;11(6):471–478.

46. Picchioni D, Horovitz SG, Fukunaga M, et al. Infraslow EEG oscillations organize large-scale cortical-subcortical interactions during sleep: A combined EEG/fMRI study. *Brain Res.* 2011;1374:63–72.

47. Parrino L, Halasz P, Tassinari CA, Terzano MG. CAP, epilepsy and motor events during sleep: The unifying role of arousal. *Sleep Med Rev.* 2006;10(4):267–285.

48. Marshall L, Molle M, Born J. Spindle and slow wave rhythms at slow wave sleep transitions are linked to strong shifts in the cortical direct current potential. *Neuroscience.* 2003;121(4):1047–1053.

49. Vanhatalo S, Holmes MD, Tallgren P, Voipio J, Kaila K, Miller JW. Very slow EEG responses lateralize temporal lobe seizures: An evaluation of non-invasive DC-EEG. *Neurology.* 2003;60(7):1098–1104.

50. Miller JW, Kim W, Holmes MD, Vanhatalo S. Ictal localization by source analysis of infraslow activity in DC-coupled scalp EEG recordings. *Neuroimage.* 2007;35(2):583–597.

51. Thompson SA, Krishnan B, Gonzalez-Martinez J, et al. Ictal infraslow activity in stereoelectroencephalography: Beyond the "DC shift." *Clin Neurophysiol.* 2016;127(1):117–128.

52. Chatrian GE, Somasundaram M, Tassinari CA. DC changes recorded transcranially during "typical" three per second spike and wave discharges in man. *Epilepsia.* 1968;9(3):185–209.

53. Caspers H, Speckmann EJ, Lehmenkuhler A. DC potentials of the cerebral cortex. seizure activity and changes in gas pressures. *Rev Physiol Biochem Pharmacol.* 1987;106:127–178.

54. Kanazawa K, Matsumoto R, Imamura H, et al. Intracranially recorded ictal direct current shifts may precede high frequency oscillations in human epilepsy. *Clin Neurophysiol.* 2015;126(1):47–59.

55. Ikeda A, Taki W, Kunieda T, et al. Focal ictal direct current shifts in human epilepsy as studied by subdural and scalp recording. *Brain.* 1999;122 (Pt 5):827–838.

56. Ikeda A, Taki W, Kunieda T, et al. Focal ictal direct current shifts in human epilepsy as studied by subdural and scalp recording. *Brain.* 1999;122 (Pt 5):827–838.

57. Wu S, Kunhi Veedu HP, Lhatoo SD, Koubeissi MZ, Miller JP, Luders HO. Role of ictal baseline shifts and ictal high-frequency oscillations in stereo-electroencephalography analysis of mesial temporal lobe seizures. *Epilepsia.* 2014;55(5):690–698.

58. Wu S, Kunhi Veedu HP, Lhatoo SD, Koubeissi MZ, Miller JP, Luders HO. Role of ictal baseline shifts and ictal high-frequency oscillations in stereo-electroencephalography analysis of mesial temporal lobe seizures. *Epilepsia.* 2014;55(5):690–698.

59. Constantino T, Rodin E. Peri-ictal and interictal, intracranial infraslow activity. *J Clin Neurophysiol.* 2012;29(4):298–308.

60. van Putten MJ, Tjepkema-Cloostermans MC, Hofmeijer J. Infraslow EEG activity modulates cortical excitability in postanoxic encephalopathy. *J Neurophysiol.* 2015;113(9):3256–3267.

61. Hartings JA, Wilson JA, Hinzman JM, et al. Spreading depression in continuous electroencephalography of brain trauma. *Ann Neurol.* 2014;76(5):681–694.

62. Gongolo A, Spreafico G, Buttazzoni L, Giraldi E, Ravasini R, Pinzani A. Duplex-sonography in the preoperative evaluation of the small saphenous vein. *Radiol Med.* 1990;80(3):234–238.

63. Adamo N, Di Martino A, Esu L, et al. Increased response-time variability across different cognitive tasks in children with ADHD. *J Atten Disord.* 2014;18(5):434–446.

64. Cooper R, Crow HJ, Walter WG, Winter AL. Regional control of cerebral vascular reactivity and oxygen supply in man. *Brain Res.* 1966;3(2):174–191.

65. Biswal B, Yetkin FZ, Haughton VM, Hyde JS. Functional connectivity in the motor cortex of resting human brain using echo-planar MRI. *Magn Reson Med.* 1995;34(4):537–541.

66. Gusnard DA, Raichle ME. Searching for a baseline: Functional imaging and the resting human brain. *Nat Rev Neurosci.* 2001;2(10):685–694.

67. Fox MD, Raichle ME. Spontaneous fluctuations in brain activity observed with functional magnetic resonance imaging. *Nat Rev Neurosci.* 2007;8(9):700–711.

68. Expert P, Lambiotte R, Chialvo DR, et al. Self-similar correlation function in brain resting-state functional magnetic resonance imaging. *J R Soc Interface.* 2011;8(57):472–479.

69. Greicius MD, Krasnow B, Reiss AL, Menon V. Functional connectivity in the resting brain: A network analysis of the default mode hypothesis. *Proc Natl Acad Sci USA.* 2003;100(1):253–258.

70. Lowe MJ, Dzemidzic M, Lurito JT, Mathews VP, Phillips MD. Correlations in low-frequency BOLD fluctuations reflect cortico-cortical connections. *Neuroimage.* 2000;12(5):582–587.

71. Power JD, Cohen AL, Nelson SM, et al. Functional network organization of the human brain. *Neuron.* 2011;72(4):665–678.

72. Hiltunen T, Elseoud AA, Lepola P, et al. Infra-slow EEG fluctuations are correlated with resting-state network dynamics in fMRI. *J Neurosci.* 2014;34:356–362.

73. Vanhatalo S, Voipio J, Dewaraja A, Holmes MD, Miller JW. Topography and elimination of slow EEG responses related to tongue movements. *Neuroimage.* 2003;20(2):1419–1423.

74. Caspers H, Speckmann EJ, Lehmenkuhler A. Electrogenesis of cortical DC potentials. *Prog Brain Res.* 1980;54:3–15.

75. Nita DA, Vanhatalo S, Lafortune FD, Voipio J, Kaila K, Amzica F. Nonneuronal origin of CO_2-related DC EEG shifts: An in vivo study in the cat. *J Neurophysiol.* 2004;92(2):1011–1022.

76. Vanhatalo S, Tallgren P, Becker C, et al. Scalp-recorded slow EEG responses generated in response to hemodynamic changes in the human brain. *Clin Neurophysiol.* 2003;114(9):1744–1754.

77. Tschirgi RD, Taylor JL. Slowly changing bioelectric potentials associated with the blood-brain barrier. *Am J Physiol—Legacy Content.* 1958;195(1):7–22.

78. Besson JM, Woody CD, Aleonard P, Thompson HK, Albe-Fessard D, Marshall WH. Correlations of brain D-C shifts with changes in cerebral blood flow. *Am J Physiol.* 1970;218(1):284–291.

79. Khader P, Schicke T, Roder B, Rosler F. On the relationship between slow cortical potentials and BOLD signal changes in humans. *Int J Psychophysiol.* 2008;67(3):252–261.

80. Leistner S, Sander T, Burghoff M, Curio G, Trahms L, Mackert B-. Combined MEG and EEG methodology for non-invasive recording of infraslow activity in the human cortex. *Clin Neurophysiol.* 2007;118(12):2774–2780.

81. Leistner S, Sander TH, Wuebbeler G, et al. Magnetoencephalography discriminates modality-specific infraslow signals less than 0.1 Hz. *Neuroreport.* 2010;21(3):196–200.

82. Deco G, Jirsa VK. Ongoing cortical activity at rest: Criticality, multistability, and ghost attractors. *J Neurosci.* 2012;32(10):3366–3375.

83. Poil SS, Hardstone R, Mansvelder HD, Linkenkaer-Hansen K. Critical-state dynamics of avalanches and oscillations jointly emerge from balanced Excitation/Inhibition in neuronal networks. *J Neurosci.* 2012;32:9817–9823.

84. Hahn G, Petermann T, Havenith MN, et al. Neuronal avalanches in spontaneous activity in vivo. *J Neurophysiol.* 2010.

85. Klaus A, Yu S, Plenz D. Statistical analyses support power law distributions found in neuronal avalanches. *PLoS One.* 2011;6(5):e19779.

86. Honey CJ, Kotter R, Breakspear M, Sporns O. Network structure of cerebral cortex shapes functional connectivity on multiple time scales. *Proc Natl Acad Sci USA.* 2007;104(24):10240–10245.

87. Deco G, Jirsa VK, McIntosh AR. Emerging concepts for the dynamical organization of resting-state activity in the brain. *Nat Rev Neurosci.* 2011;12(1):43–56.

88. Nikulin VV, Linkenkaer-Hansen K, Nolte G, et al. A novel mechanism for evoked responses in the human brain. *Eur J Neurosci.* 2007;25(10):3146–3154.

89. Lorincz ML, Geall F, Bao Y, Crunelli V, Hughes SW. ATP-dependent infra-slow (<0.1 Hz) oscillations in thalamic networks. *PLoS One.* 2009;4(2):e4447.

90. Du C, Volkow ND, Koretsky AP, Pan Y. Low-frequency calcium oscillations accompany deoxyhemoglobin oscillations in rat somatosensory cortex. *Proc Natl Acad Sci USA.* 2014;111(43):E4677–4686.

91. Pasti L, Volterra A, Pozzan T, Carmignoto G. Intracellular calcium oscillations in astrocytes: A highly plastic, bidirectional form of communication between neurons and astrocytes in situ. *J Neurosci.* 1997;17(20):7817–7830.

92. Parri HR, Gould TM, Crunelli V. Spontaneous astrocytic Ca^{2+} oscillations in situ drive NMDAR-mediated neuronal excitation. *Nat Neurosci.* 2001;4(8):803–812.

93. Parri HR, Crunelli V. Pacemaker calcium oscillations in thalamic astrocytes in situ. *Neuroreport.* 2001;12(18):3897–3900.

94. He BJ, Zempel JM, Snyder AZ, Raichle ME. The temporal structures and functional significance of scale-free brain activity. *Neuron.* 2010;66(3):353–369.

95. Thompson GJ, Pan WJ, Magnuson ME, Jaeger D, Keilholz SD. Quasi-periodic patterns (QPP): Large-scale dynamics in resting state fMRI that correlate with local infraslow electrical activity. *Neuroimage.* 2014;84:1018–1031.

96. Filippov IV, Williams WC, Krebs AA, Pugachev KS. Sound-induced changes of infraslow brain potential fluctuations in the medial geniculate nucleus and primary auditory cortex in anaesthetized rats. *Brain Res.* 2007;1133(0):78–86.

97. Allers KA, Ruskin DN, Bergstrom DA, et al. Multisecond periodicities in basal ganglia firing rates correlate with theta bursts in transcortical and hippocampal EEG. *J Neurophysiol.* 2002;87(2):1118–1122.

98. Ruskin DN, Bergstrom DA, Tierney PL, Walters JR. Correlated multisecond oscillations in firing rate in the basal ganglia: Modulation by dopamine and the subthalamic nucleus. *Neuroscience.* 2003;117(2):427–438.

99. Marshall L, Molle M, Fehm HL, Born J. Changes in direct current (DC) potentials and infra-slow EEG oscillations at the onset of the luteinizing hormone (LH) pulse. *Eur J Neurosci.* 2000;12(11):3935–3943.

100. Demanuele C, James CJ, Sonuga-Barke EJ. Distinguishing low frequency oscillations within the 1/f spectral behaviour of electromagnetic brain signals. *Behav Brain Funct.* 2007;3:62.

101. Baria AT, Baliki MN, Parrish T, Apkarian AV. Anatomical and functional assemblies of brain BOLD oscillations. *J Neurosci.* 2011;31(21):7910–7919.

102. Zuo X, Di Martino A, Kelly C, et al. The oscillating brain: Complex and reliable. *Neuroimage.* 2010;49(2):1432–1445.

103. Chang C, Glover GH. Time-frequency dynamics of resting-state brain connectivity measured with fMRI. *Neuroimage.* 2010;50(1):81–98.

104. Helps SK, Broyd SJ, James CJ, Karl A, Sonuga-Barke EJS. The attenuation of very low frequency brain oscillations in transitions from a rest state to active attention. *J Psychophysiol.* 2010;23(4):191–198.

105. Kononowicz TW, Sander T, van Rijn H. Neuroelectromagnetic signatures of the reproduction of supra-second durations. *Neuropsychologia.* 2015;75:201–213.

106. Cui RQ, Huter D, Egkher A, Lang W, Lindinger G, Deecke L. High resolution DC-EEG mapping of the bereitschaftspotential preceding simple or complex bimanual sequential finger movement. *Exp Brain Res.* 2000;134(1):49–57.

107. Mayer K, Wyckoff SN, Strehl U. One size fits all? Slow cortical potentials neurofeedback: A review. *J Atten Disord.* 2013;17(5):393–409

108. Yilmaz O, Birbaumer N, Ramos-Murguialday A. Movement related slow cortical potentials in severely paralyzed chronic stroke patients. *Front Hum Neurosci.* 2015;8:1033.

109. Koenig MA, Kaplan PW. Clinical applications for EPs in the ICU. *J Clin Neurophysiol.* 2015;32(6):472–480.

110. Haenggi M, Ypparila H, Takala J, et al. Measuring depth of sedation with auditory evoked potentials during controlled infusion of propofol and remifentanil in healthy volunteers. *Anesth Analg.* 2004;99(6):1728–1736.

111. Tolonen M, Palva JM, Andersson S, Vanhatalo S. Development of the spontaneous activity transients and ongoing cortical activity in human preterm babies. *Neuroscience.* 2007;145(3):997–1006.

112. Drenckhahn C, Winkler MK, Major S, et al. Correlates of spreading depolarization in human scalp electroencephalography. *Brain.* 2012;135(Pt 3):853–868.

33 | HIGH-FREQUENCY EEG ACTIVITY

JEAN GOTMAN, PHD AND NATHAN E. CRONE, MD

ABSTRACT: Activities with frequencies between 60 and 80 Hz and approximately 500 Hz are labeled here as high-frequency activities. They were largely ignored until the beginning of the millennium, but their importance is now well recognized. They can be divided into activities occurring in the healthy brain in relation to sensory, motor, and cognitive or memory activity and activities occurring in the epileptic brain in the form of brief events (high-frequency oscillations), which appear to be an important marker of the brain regions that are able to generate seizures of focal origin. In humans, most of the work related to these activities has been done in intracerebral electrodes, where they are relatively frequent and easy to identify. They have been recorded in scalp electroencephalograms in some circumstances, however. This chapter reviews the recording methods, the circumstances in which they occur, their mechanism of generation, and their clinical significance.

KEYWORDS: high frequency, electroencephalogram, epilepsy, seizure, oscillations

PRINCIPAL REFERENCES

1. Lachaux JP, Axmacher N, Mormann F, Halgren E, Crone NE. High-frequency neural activity and human cognition: past, present and possible future of intracranial EEG research. *Progress Neurobiol.* 2012;98(3):279–301.
2. Crone NE, Korzeniewska A, Franaszczuk PJ. Cortical gamma responses: searching high and low. *Int J Psychophysiol.* 2011;79(1):9–15.
3. Pfurtscheller G, Lopes da Silva FH. Event-related EEG/MEG synchronization and desynchronization: basic principles. *Clin Neurophysiol.* 1999;110(11):1842–1857.
4. Bragin A, Engel J, Jr., Wilson CL, Fried I, Mathern GW. Hippocampal and entorhinal cortex high-frequency oscillations (100–500 Hz) in human epileptic brain and in kainic acid–treated rats with chronic seizures. *Epilepsia.* 1999;40(2):127–137.
5. Urrestarazu E, Chander R, Dubeau F, Gotman J. Interictal high-frequency oscillations (100–500 Hz) in the intracerebral EEG of epileptic patients. *Brain.* 2007;130(Pt 9):2354–2366.
6. Kobayashi K, Watanabe Y, Inoue T, Oka M, Yoshinaga H, Ohtsuka Y. Scalp-recorded high-frequency oscillations in childhood sleep-induced electrical status epilepticus. *Epilepsia.* 2010;51(10):2190–2194.
7. Jacobs J, Staba R, Asano E, et al. High-frequency oscillations (HFOs) in clinical epilepsy. *Prog Neurobiol.* 2012;98(3):302–315.
8. Matsumoto A, Brinkmann BH, Matthew Stead S, et al. Pathological and physiological high-frequency oscillations in focal human epilepsy. *J Neurophysiol.* 2013;110(8):1958–1964.
9. van 't Klooster MA, van Klink NE, Leijten FS, et al. Residual fast ripples in the intraoperative corticogram predict epilepsy surgery outcome. *Neurology.* 2015;85(2):120–128.

1. INTRODUCTION

The electroencephalogram (EEG) is traditionally recorded and clinically interpreted with a low-pass filter set at 60 or 70 Hz. The most common EEG activities are divided into the delta, theta, alpha and beta bands, the latter term usually used for activity extending up to ~30 Hz. There has been much interest recently in the gamma band, a term commonly used for activity faster than beta (>30 Hz). Because of considerable variability in the frequency bounds of gamma band activity reported across different studies, it may be premature, or even altogether inappropriate, to select a specific frequency range to define it. Nevertheless, there is a practical need for consistent terminology in order to facilitate communication in both scientific discourse and translation to clinical practice. Based on accumulating evidence from studies of both physiological and pathological responses in gamma frequencies (see below), it may be useful to arbitrarily, but provisionally, define the gamma band as 30 to 70 Hz. It has recently been discovered that frequencies higher than 70 Hz can also be recorded and can have both physiological and pathological significance. A variety of terms have been used to describe physiological EEG activity above 70 Hz, such as high-gamma[1,2] and the chi-band[3]. In the context of epilepsy, pathological patterns at high frequencies have also been described, for example ripples between 100 and 200 Hz (sometimes between 80 and 160, sometimes between 100 and 250), and fast ripples between 160, 200, or 250 Hz and 500 or 600 Hz. These events have other properties besides their frequency, and in general we think that frequency bands should be defined independently from specific EEG phenomena at a time when much exploration is taking place. Rather than using a name, we will therefore refer to bands by their boundaries (e.g., the 100- to 250-Hz band). A special issue of *Progress in Neurobiology* devoted to high-frequency activity was published following the workshop held in Montreal in 2011[4].

At the other end of the frequency spectrum, it has been shown that low frequencies below the traditional filter at ~0.5 Hz have meaningful information, particularly in newborns and infants. Direct-current (DC) shifts have been studied for a long time, particularly in the context of epileptic seizures. Equipment to record DC shifts is, however, complex, and recent studies have used alternating-current (AC) amplifiers with a very low high-pass filter (as low as 0.01 Hz) as a surrogate for DC equipment, opening the door to the evaluation of very slow EEG changes. The development in high and low frequencies (see also Chapter 32) has given rise to the concept of *full-band EEG*, which may more correctly be called *wide-band EEG* since there always remain unexplored frequencies below and above the currently explored limits.

2. THE SKULL, THE GENERATOR VOLUME, AND THE ELECTRODES

2.1. The Generator Volume and the Effect of the Skull

It is often said and sometimes written that "the skull filters out high frequencies." This would imply that high frequencies, for instance above 60 Hz, would be more attenuated by the skull than lower frequencies, making it essentially impossible to record high frequencies except with intracranial electrodes or with magnetoencephalography (MEG), which is not sensitive to skull conductivity. In fact, the skull does not attenuate any frequency until ~10,000 Hz; this has been clearly demonstrated in the excellent study by Oostendorp et al.[5] The confusion may have arisen from the fact that there seems to be an inverse relationship between the frequency of an EEG rhythm and the volume of brain that generates it. For instance, very large regions can generate synchronous delta activity, and smaller regions can generate synchronous higher frequencies. Following this scheme, very high frequencies would be generated in a very small volume and would be unlikely to be "seen" from the scalp, simply because of the small angle under which they would be seen[6]. In addition to this issue of geometry, the skull attenuates the electrical field because of its resistivity, and a signal that is already small becomes even smaller and at some point may be lost in the noise. For these reasons (distance from generator to sensor and small amplitude of signal), it may be just as difficult to record high frequencies with MEG as it is with scalp EEG.

Spontaneous activity up to 200 Hz and evoked activity up to 600 Hz have, however, been recorded from the scalp. This is puzzling, since it is often said that it takes a generator of 6 to 10 cm^2 of cortex for its activity to be seen on the scalp[7,8] and generators of high-frequency activity are thought to be at most a few square millimeters, possibly less than one square millimeter[9]. A recent simulation study[10] may shed light on this question. It emphasizes two points: (i) generators of *the same cortical surface* can result in scalp signals differing in amplitude by as much as a factor of 10 as a result of the location and orientation of the generator (on a gyrus, sulcus, in between), of the skull thickness and composition in the region of the generator (highly variable between head regions), and on the thickness of the cerebrospinal fluid layer; and (ii) the detectability of a signal on the scalp is essentially a function of the signal-to-noise ratio *in the frequency band of interest*. When evaluating spikes (as in the study by Tao et al.[8]), the noise is composed of the standard EEG in the theta, alpha, and beta bands, with typical amplitude of 30 to 50 μV; when evaluating bursts of activity at 130 Hz, the "noise" is the spontaneous EEG around 130 Hz and this is very low (Fig. 33.1), making it possible to detect 130-Hz ripples having only a few μV and possibly generated by a few square millimeters[11,12].

2.2. Electrode Size in Relation to Generator Size

In the context of a small generator volume, the size of recording electrodes becomes a potentially important factor, although the question of electrode size has rarely been

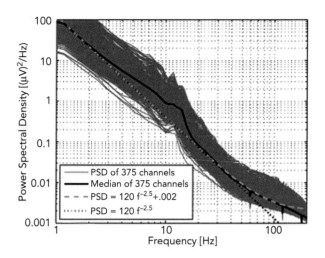

Figure 33.1. Power spectral density (PSD) of 375 scalp EEG channels during non-REM sleep (gray), median (black full line), and approximations: background brain activity (dotted black line), and background brain activity plus electronic noise (dashed gray line). This illustrates that HFOs may be detected on the scalp because the background activity in their frequency range is of very low amplitude. From von Ellenrieder N, Beltrachini L, Perucca P, Gotman J. Size of cortical generators of epileptic interictal events and visibility on scalp EEG. Neuroimage. 2014;94:47–54; Fig. 4.

addressed in the field of intracranial EEG (iEEG). If a generator is on the order of a few hundred microns, two issues can be raised. The first is that of spatial sampling: if such small generators are scattered and present in a small number of locations, the likelihood that an electrode would be in their vicinity is low. This is one extreme of the general problem of poor spatial sampling of intracranial investigations. The second one is that an electrode larger than the field generator and in contact with it could significantly alter that field; an electrode much larger than the generator field could attenuate it, possibly to the point of making it undetectable. It is very difficult to know the size of a generator unless one performs a systematic exploration with microelectrodes[9]. It is therefore not easy to determine the optimal electrode size. Electrodes have usually been designed to allow electrical stimulation without an excessive current density[13,14]; for this purpose a relatively large contact surface is important, but this requirement may be in conflict with that of optimizing the recording of high-frequency activity. In one set of studies in rats and in humans, it was shown that macroelectrodes with highly variable electrode sizes (0.02–0.09 mm^2 in rats and 0.2–0.8 mm^2 in humans) recorded almost the same high-frequency activity[15,16]. On the other hand, comparing more extreme sizes of subdural electrodes (typically 5 mm^2) and microelectrodes (typically 0.001 mm^2), it was found that microelectrodes were more sensitive in the recording of high-frequency activity[17].

Another issue influences what can be recorded on the scalp, or generally at some distance from brain generators. Whereas a single generator, as typically observed with microelectrodes, probably contributes little to what is recorded at a distant electrode, it may be that many neighboring generators are active at the same time; even if they are not all synchronized, their activities at the same frequency will partially sum up and contribute to the appearance of a larger generator (see also a discussion of underlying biophysical factors in Chapter 2). This has been observed at the larger scale of combined scalp–intracerebral studies of sleep spindles[18] and in earlier experimental studies of the alpha rhythm[19].

It may be useful to discuss terminology issues. In the animal experimentation domain, the notion of "local field potential" is often used. For instance, filtering an extracellular microelectrode recording such that only activity below 100 Hz, or below 500 Hz, remains (i.e., removing action potentials) is said to produce the local field potential (LFP). This extracellular potential fluctuation is not easily differentiated from the EEG, as recorded locally with a small electrode. Although the term "EEG" is most often associated with relatively large electrodes, there is nothing in the definition of the EEG that implies electrode size. It is rather defined as potential fluctuations within a certain frequency range. From our point of view, there is no formal difference between LFP and EEG, but the terms tend to be used in different contexts.

We will first discuss the high frequencies that are recorded in the context of normal function. These have been documented in experimental animals as well as in humans in response to specific sensory, motor, or cognitive activities. In humans, some of these high frequencies can be recorded from the scalp, but most were investigated in patients with intracerebral electrodes in the context of evaluation for surgical treatment of medically refractory epilepsy. We will then discuss the high-frequency activities that have been related to focal epilepsy, here again investigated in experimental animals and in patients with intracerebral electrodes.

3. HIGH-FREQUENCY ACTIVITY AND NORMAL CORTICAL FUNCTION

3.1. Experimental Background and Theoretical Significance

The importance of high-frequency EEG activity to normal brain physiology has been the subject of many investigations over the past several decades in both animals and humans and is still hotly debated. Some of the earliest studies using EEG recognized that cortical activation was associated with the disappearance of low-frequency activity (alpha) and the appearance of fast activity, though the extent of this fast activity was difficult to ascertain given the technical limitations of existing equipment[20]. Subsequent microelectrode recordings in rabbit olfactory cortex showed that different odors elicited different spatial patterns in the amplitude of sniff-triggered gamma oscillations (38–80 Hz), suggesting a mechanistic role in stimulus discrimination[21]. A decade later, local field recordings in cat visual cortex found that oscillatory neuronal firing in a frequency range of 40 to 60 Hz can become synchronized during visual stimulation between spatially separate columns[22], between striate, parastriate, and extrastriate visual cortex[23,24], and even between areas 17 of the two hemispheres[24], and that this synchronization depends on global stimulus properties. In these studies bursts of single-unit activity were commonly synchronized with gamma oscillations in the LFP, suggesting that LFP oscillations facilitated and/or were facilitated by the

synchronization of neuronal firing among functionally related neurons.

Synchronization of neural firing has been hypothesized to form the basis for temporal coding by which temporary assemblies of neurons represent higher-order, or global, stimulus properties[25]. This hypothesis is not widely accepted as it may be viewed as complementary or contrary to traditional models of neural coding based on firing rates alone[26], but it has been recognized as a potential solution to the binding problem in sensory segmentation and invariant object recognition[27]. More recent theories have proposed that subthreshold gamma oscillations, driven by synchronous inhibitory neuron firing, produce temporal windows for cortical–cortical communication, whereby coherently oscillating ensembles of neurons interact more effectively because their communication windows are open at the same time[28]. Another theory proposes that rhythmic gamma oscillations from inhibitory interneuron firing interact with excitatory inputs to pyramidal cells such that more excited cells fire earlier in the gamma cycle. This re-coding of the amplitude of excitatory drive into phase values relative to the gamma cycle would provide a more efficient coding mechanism by enabling the readout of amplitude information within a single gamma cycle without requiring the temporal integration of firing rates[29].

3.2. 40-Hz Gamma In Human EEG

Inspired by experiments in animals and theories relating gamma oscillations to neural coding[30], many investigators have attempted to correlate band-limited gamma oscillations in human EEG with cognitive and perceptual operations in cortex. Early attempts to relate band-limited gamma oscillations to human cortical function were designed to demonstrate task-specific lateralization of 40-Hz activity in scalp-recorded EEG during long blocks of task performance. These studies did show lateralization of 40 Hz to the left hemisphere during verbal tasks[31] and to the contralateral central scalp region during both simple and complex choice reaction time tasks[32,33]. Like block designs in functional magnetic resonance imaging (fMRI) experiments, however, block designs in EEG experiments are susceptible to variance in brain state measures due to experimentally irrelevant behavioral fluctuations. Furthermore, this block-design approach does not exploit the fine temporal scale at which gamma activity can change during task performance. For these reasons, event-related designs have been used much more extensively when studying gamma responses.

3.3. Phase-Locked Gamma Responses

Using event-related analyses of MEG, Pantev et al. observed band-limited gamma responses to tone bursts at 35 to 40 Hz[34]. This was consistent with previous reports of 40-Hz clicks driving large steady-state evoked responses in auditory cortex[35]. Notably, these gamma-band responses were obtained by filtering event-related potentials (ERPs), in turn produced by averaging raw signal from many individual trials in the time domain. This procedure reveals phase-locked *evoked*

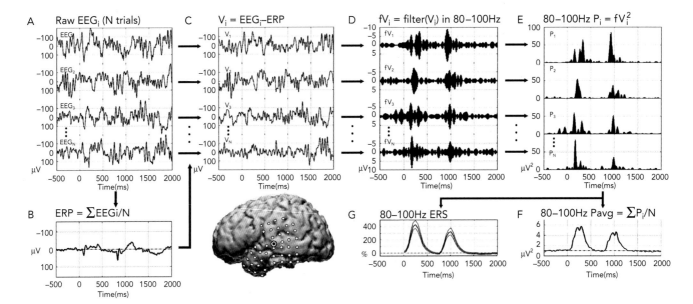

Figure 33.2. *Signal analysis of phase-locked and non–phase-locked responses using bandpass filtering. Schematic of signal analyses for one channel of intracranial EEG recorded over dominant (left) superior temporal gyrus (filled circle on brain) during an auditory speech discrimination task. To minimize the contribution of phase-locked responses to subsequent analyses of non–phase-locked responses, the ERP may be subtracted from the raw EEG signal in each individual trial (depicted in steps A, B, and C; for alternative approaches, see Kalcher et al.[44] and Trautner et al.[83]). In this approach, the raw signal (A) is averaged across N trials to obtain the ERP (B), and the ERP is then subtracted from each individual trial (C) prior to bandpass filtering (D, 80–100 Hz in this illustration). Bandpass filtered signals from each individual trial are then squared to obtain power values (E). These band-specific power estimates, which are all positive, may then be averaged across trials to obtain the power average (F), or submitted to statistical analyses to calculate the percentage change in post-stimulus power from pre-stimulus baseline power (G). Event-related power increases (F, G) are also known as induced responses and are dominated by non–phase-locked response components. Note the variability in the latency and magnitude of these responses across individual trials (E). From Crone NE, Boatman D, Gordon B, Hao L. Induced electrocorticographic gamma activity during auditory perception. Clin Neurophysiol. 2001;112:565–582; Fig. 1.*

gamma-band responses, consisting of gamma components in the ERP. It is important to distinguish these evoked gamma-band responses from *induced* gamma band activity that is time-locked but not phase-locked (Fig. 33.2; see the section below on non–phase-locked gamma responses)[36].

Phase-locked gamma responses have been investigated in a variety of experimental contexts. In many cases narrow-bandpass filters have been used to focus on ERP components in and around 40 Hz. This practice is potentially susceptible to artifacts from filtering ERP impulses containing a wide range of frequencies. Nevertheless, evoked gamma-band responses have been observed in both animals and humans during cortical activation in a variety of functional-anatomical domains[37,38], and in humans this class of responses has been used to explore mind–brain relationships[39,40].

In addition to ERP components in the gamma band, ERP components have also been observed in even higher frequencies, such as ultrafast frequencies (400–1,000 Hz), in both animals and humans. For example, both scalp and intracranial EEG recordings have shown that somatosensory evoked potentials from electrical stimulation of the median nerve contain a brief (10–15 msec) burst of ~600-Hz spike-like wavelets, called sigma bursts[41,42]. Sigma bursts temporally overlap the thalamic P15 component and the N20 primary cortical response and, based on converging evidence from animals and humans, are thought to represent both far-field and near-field potentials generated by highly synchronized population spikes in cuneothalamic and thalamocortical relay cells and a variety of cortical neurons.

3.4. Non–Phase-Locked Gamma Responses

Averaging electrophysiological (e.g., EEG, MEG, LFP) responses in the time domain extracts phase-locked signal components as ERPs and discards non–phase-locked components as noise. In contrast, averaging these responses in the frequency domain focuses on event-related changes in the spectral energy of responses that may have both phase-locked and non–phase-locked components[43]. The latter approach is still temporally linked to an event across multiple trials, but the result is not limited to phase-locked components, as in ERPs. Different methods have been used to recognize and minimize the contribution of phase-locked components (ERPs) to analyses of non–phase-locked electrophysiological responses[44,45]. However, the distinction between phase-locked responses (ERPs) and non–phase-locked increases in signal energy (often termed "induced" responses) could depend more on the methods by which they are extracted than on fundamental differences between their generators.

Averaging in the time domain necessarily yields phase-locked responses. However, significant variability (jitter) in the latency (or phase) of ERPs can distort their appearance in time-averaged responses. High-frequency components of electrophysiological responses are more susceptible to latency jitter, and there is usually more jitter of these responses (and their corresponding cognitive processes) at longer latencies. This may explain why ERPs with high-frequency components (e.g., the sigma bursts described above) are usually confined to early latencies. On the other hand, ERPs at longer latencies (e.g.,

P300) usually consist of low-frequency components that are more resistant to jitter[46,47]. Because averaging in the frequency domain does not require phase locking, it may be better suited to investigate cortical processing at longer and/or more variable latencies and to investigate high-frequency electrophysiological responses at longer latencies. It may therefore be useful to conceive of electrophysiological responses as having different combinations of frequencies, latencies, and phase-locking. Nevertheless, the distinction between phase-locked and non–phase-locked responses is often still a practical one to make (this issue is also discussed in Chapter 36 referring to methods of blind-source separation). Furthermore, many studies suggest that these different classes of EEG responses may have distinct functional response properties[48].

One of the first event-related analyses of non–phase-locked gamma activity (i.e., on a temporal scale commensurate with task performance) was made by Pfurtscheller et al.[49], who demonstrated a lateralized increase in 40-Hz activity during self-paced finger movements in three subjects. One of these subjects was later shown to have a somatotopic pattern of this activity during movements of the tongue, finger, and toes[50]. Similar non–phase-locked gamma activity has also been observed in a variety of experimental contexts, such as during the perception of illusory triangles[51].

3.5. Intracranial EEG and "High-Gamma" Activity

Throughout the history of epilepsy surgery, iEEG, including recordings from subdural electrodes (electrocorticography; ECoG) and depth electrodes (stereo-EEG), has been used to localize the seizure onset zone when scalp EEG has not been sufficiently precise. Because of the greater proximity between sensors and sources, as well as the inverse relationship between the frequency of EEG activity and the size of neural populations generating it (see above), iEEG generally records high-frequency electrocortical activity with greater signal quality than scalp EEG. Consequently, iEEG has allowed the discovery and investigation of event-related, non–phase-locked responses in gamma frequencies higher than those previously studied noninvasively in humans. In one of the earliest of these studies[1], non–phase-locked responses were observed in multiple frequency bands ranging from 75 to 100 Hz during a visually cued motor task. These responses were observed in somatotopically defined regions of sensorimotor cortex contralateral to the cued movement and corresponded well to electrocortical stimulation maps of motor function[1]. The spatial patterns of these responses were more discrete and somatotopically specific than those of power changes in mu (alpha) and beta bands, and their temporal patterns were also more discrete, occurring in brief bursts limited to the onset of movement, with latencies that co-varied with the latencies of movement onset. Because these spatial and temporal response characteristics appeared distinct from those of responses in lower frequencies, particularly those at 40 Hz, the frequency range above 70 Hz was provisionally termed "high-gamma." Subsequent studies have found that the lower and upper frequency boundaries of high-gamma responses have been quite variable, but they have most commonly ranged from ~60 Hz to ~200 Hz, with the majority of event-related energy changes occurring between 80 and 150 Hz[52,53].

Studies in both humans and animals have shown that non–phase-locked responses in the traditional 40-Hz gamma band are more variable and less sensitive to functional activation of cortex than responses in high-gamma frequencies[45,54]. This may be due to variability in the frequency range of event-related power suppression. If this power suppression extends into low-gamma frequencies, it may mask power augmentation in this frequency range. This is a potential pitfall for analyses of responses with narrow-bandpass filters at low-gamma frequencies (e.g., at 40 Hz). Although the lower boundary of broadband gamma power increases may extend down into 40-Hz frequencies, the most consistent responses occur above 60 Hz. Moreover, the functional response properties of high-gamma activity are distinct (typically more discrete spatially and temporally) from both phase-locked responses (ERPs) and non–phase-locked responses in other frequency bands[2,55,56].

High-gamma responses have been demonstrated not only in motor cortex[1,57] but also in many other functional–anatomical domains, including frontal eye fields[58], auditory cortex[45,59,60], visual cortex[61,62], and language cortex[63,64]. The functional–anatomical ubiquity of these responses has thus suggested that they may serve as a general electrophysiological index of cortical neurophysiological mechanisms important for neural representation and computation.

3.6. Mechanisms Generating Broadband "High-Gamma" Responses

The neurophysiological mechanisms responsible for "high-gamma" responses were first hypothesized within the context of experiments showing neural synchronization at 40 Hz, as well as theories of temporal coding derived from these observations[2,65]. A common feature of temporal coding theories is that they require rhythmic oscillations of membrane potentials and/or action potentials at band-limited gamma frequencies. However, high-gamma responses consistently have a broadband spectral profile; in other words, power is increased over a range of frequencies, most often including 80 to 150 Hz[52,53].

To be reconciled with gamma oscillations and related theories of temporal coding, high-gamma power changes were hypothesized to arise from the summation of multiple, spatially overlapping neuronal assemblies, each oscillating at different frequencies[1,65]. Given a sufficient number of assemblies oscillating at overlapping, broadly tuned, or changing frequencies, a broadband response might be observed. To date there has been no direct experimental support for this hypothesis. One iEEG study, however, has demonstrated that high-gamma spectral responses during speech production are not strictly broadband, but emphasize different frequencies at different recording sites[66]. Within the aforementioned framework of summated oscillators, this observation could potentially arise from variability in the size of assemblies tuned to different frequencies within large-scale cortical language networks, resulting in some oscillation frequencies dominating others.

In a recent computational modeling study, a cortical network model receiving thalamic input generated high-gamma

LFP responses in a range of frequencies from 60 to 200 Hz, with spectral signatures comparable to those observed in LFP recordings from monkey somatosensory cortex during vibrotactile stimulation[67,68]. High-gamma oscillations were dependent on an excited population of inhibitory fast-spiking interneurons firing at high-gamma frequencies and pacing excitatory regular-spiking pyramidal cells, which fired at lower rates but in phase with the population rhythm. In the model, high-gamma responses to constant levels of thalamocortical input were observed in narrower bands than what is typically observed experimentally, with center frequencies that increased logarithmically with increasing inputs. If thalamocortical inputs were to vary across the total neuronal population recorded with iEEG, and/or if these inputs were to change over time, it could generate a broadband response in high-gamma frequencies.

An alternative explanation for the broadband spectral profile of high-gamma responses is that they are the time-frequency representations of transient responses with a broad range of frequency components. Intertrial jitter in the latency of these transients presumably renders them invisible when averaged across trials in the time domain. Microelectrode recordings from macaque secondary somatosensory (SII) cortex during tactile stimulation have observed broadband high-gamma responses with spectral profiles identical to those recorded in human iEEG[67,69]. Detailed time-frequency analyses of these responses using matching pursuits revealed that they are temporally tightly linked to neuronal spikes, though their precise generating mechanisms could not be determined[69]. In addition, LFP power in the high-gamma range was strongly correlated, both in its temporal profile and in its trial-by-trial variation, with the firing rate of the recorded neural population[69].

Whether the underlying signals giving rise to broadband gamma responses are oscillations or transients, activity in such a high frequency range is much more likely to be recorded at the mesoscale of subdural ECoG if there is some degree of synchronization across a population of neural generators. In a recent simulation of intracranial EEG responses using different firing patterns in the underlying cortical population, both an increase in firing rate and an increase in neuronal synchrony resulted in broadband high-gamma power increases[69]. These responses were, however, much more sensitive to increases in neuronal synchrony than to increases in firing rate. Thus, broadband gamma responses may index neuronal synchronization to some extent even if the underlying firing pattern is not a band-limited oscillation. Synchronization, as mentioned above, could be used as a temporal code that complements rate coding and could also play a role in attention[70,71]. However, at this time there is greater experimental support and consensus for high-gamma responses arising from an increase in the overall firing rate of the neural population being recorded. Regardless of the relative contribution of firing rates versus synchronization, there is ample evidence that high-gamma responses index the functional activation of cortical neurons that is useful for applications in cognitive neuroscience, functional brain mapping, and brain–machine interfaces.

3.7. Applications to Cognitive Neuroscience

Because high-gamma responses measure overall population firing rates with outstanding spatial and temporal resolution, they have been increasingly used in studies probing higher cortical functions in humans. For example, several human iEEG studies have found an augmentation of broadband high-gamma activity in association with selective attention in a variety of sensory modalities[53,63,72–77].

Because of the frequency with which iEEG electrodes are implanted over the temporal lobe, high-gamma responses have been used extensively to investigate the cortical mechanisms of auditory function[78–83]. The earliest of these studies demonstrated high-gamma responses during tone and speech discrimination[45], concentrated over posterior superior temporal gyrus, with greater magnitude in dominant superior temporal gyrus during discrimination of speech stimuli than during discrimination of tone stimuli. More recently, high-gamma responses recorded while patients listened to natural continuous speech were used to map acoustic-phonetic representations in the dominant superior temporal gyrus for the entire English phonetic inventory[84]. At single electrodes in high-density iEEG arrays with 5-mm spacing, Mesgarani et al.[84] found response selectivity to distinct phonetic features, which were based on tuning for spectral-temporal acoustic cues.

Another cortical region commonly recorded with iEEG is the ventral temporal lobe, and here many investigators have used high-gamma responses to probe higher-order visual representations using a variety of tasks[61,62,85,86]. Likewise, high-gamma responses have been used to probe cortical function in the frontal lobe, including attention, goal maintenance, response inhibition, and working memory[76,87–89].

Because of the risk of language impairments from epilepsy surgery, iEEG recordings are more common in the dominant hemisphere, and high-gamma responses have been used here to probe not only various cortical areas that make up language cortex[64,90–93] but also how these sites interact with each other during speech production and related language tasks[94,95]. For example, a recent study examined the timing of activation in Broca's area and its interactions with other language cortices during spoken-word production[96]. Because of the effects of lesions in Broca's area, it is commonly understood to be important for speech production, but its precise role in this task is not fully understood. Surprisingly, iEEG high-gamma responses peak in Broca's area well before the onset of articulation (Fig. 33.3) and are essentially absent during articulation (Fig. 33.4A). Using a measure of the magnitude, timing, and direction of high-gamma propagation between iEEG recording sites, this study also found that during auditory word repetition, Broca's area acts as a network hub (see Fig. 33.4B) that mediates a temporal cascade of reciprocal feed-forward and feedback interactions between sensory representations of words in temporal cortex and their corresponding articulatory gestures in motor cortex.

3.8. Applications to Functional Mapping

Although neurosurgeons are increasingly using fMRI to map cortical function prior to brain tumor resections[97], clinicians

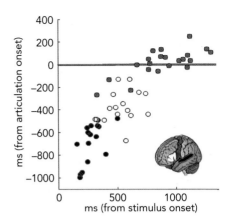

Figure 33.3. Peak latencies of high-gamma responses locked to stimulus onset (x axis) and locked to response (articulation) onset (y axis) are plotted for electrodes in three anatomical regions of interest: superior temporal gyrus (black), Broca's area (white), and motor cortex (gray). Activity in both dimensions temporally propagates from superior temporal gyrus to Broca's area and culminates in the precentral gyrus. Note that activation in Broca's area peaks at least 100 msec before speech onset. Reproduced with permission from Flinker A, Korzeniewska A, Shestyuk AY, et al. Redefining the role of Broca's area in speech. Proc Nat Acad Sci USA. 2015;112(9):2871–2875; Fig. 2B.

still turn to electrocortical stimulation mapping (ESM), which temporarily simulates the effects of a lesion prior to permanent resection[98,99]. When the seizure onset zone has been mapped with iEEG, this allows a direct comparison between normal and pathological cortical function. However, ESM can trigger after-discharges and clinical seizures[100–102] or pain[103], which can limit mapping, and it is time-consuming, particularly as the number and density of iEEG electrodes increase[104]. Furthermore, the effects of stimulation on local or distant brain networks are not well controlled or understood, often manifesting as all-or-none behavioral effects, and cannot account for functional reserve or reorganization following permanent lesions. These limitations have motivated the investigation of passive iEEG recordings for mapping cortical function. Intracranial EEG recordings cannot trigger seizures or pain and can assess function at all recording sites simultaneously, yielding a complete map of graded task-related neural activation. Until recently, it was not clear which of the many potential iEEG signal components would be most useful for this purpose, but the consensus at this point is that high-gamma responses are particularly useful for this purpose. Since they index task-related increases in population firing rates, demonstrated in single-unit activity recorded by microelectrodes[69,105,106], it is not surprising that they are highly correlated with blood-oxygen-level–dependent (BOLD) responses in fMRI[107–110]. Unlike fMRI, the temporal resolution of iEEG high-gamma maps is on the order of tens of milliseconds, sufficient to track the dynamics of brain activation associated with human behavior. In spite of these advantages, ESM is still considered by many to be the clinical gold standard, and thus the accuracy of iEEG has typically been assessed through comparisons with ESM.

3.8.1. Motor Cortex

In an iEEG study of 22 subjects, Miller et al. compared the topographic patterns of power suppression in low frequencies (8–32 Hz) with power augmentation in high-gamma frequencies (76–100 Hz) during a variety of motor tasks[57]. As in a previous study[1], high-gamma responses had a more focused spatial distribution than did power suppression in low frequencies. In addition, these responses had a somatotopic organization corresponding to the movement of different body parts and corresponded well to the results of ESM. In a subsequent study by Brunner et al.[111], the utility of iEEG for motor mapping was demonstrated using the SIGFRIED system[112] implemented within the BCI2000 framework[113]. This system uses a block design to measure differences in high-gamma signal between rest and active periods to produce a map of cortical activation at the patient's bedside. In a next-neighbor comparison with ESM, Brunner et al. found no false negatives, and only 0.46% and 1.1% false positives for hand and tongue maps, respectively[111]. Subsequent studies using a variety of methods have shown that high-gamma responses localize motor cortex with high sensitivity and specificity relative to ESM[114–116].

3.8.2. Language Cortex

Intracranial EEG high-gamma responses have also been used to map language cortex in neurosurgical patients[64,90,91,115,117–123]. For a variety of reasons, mapping language cortex is more challenging than mapping motor cortex. First, the functional anatomy of language is not as discretely organized as that of motor function and involves multiple cortical areas, including Broca's, Wernicke's, and surrounding association cortices that are distributed over large-scale cortical networks. This distributed organization, particularly for semantic knowledge[124], presents challenges for using iEEG or ESM maps to predict postoperative impairments, because discrete lesions may have little or no effect on task proficiency if sufficient functional reserve exists in other areas. Second, language task performance employs different brain areas at different times, and it may be necessary to measure the timing of activation at a given site, relative to other sites, to appreciate its function and contribution to a given task. A recent study illustrated this using a bedside procedure for online spatial-temporal functional mapping using iEEG high-gamma responses (Fig. 33.5)[125]. Last, language cortex can be activated with a variety of experimental tasks. Because different tasks probe different combinations of sites within cortical networks supporting language function, a battery of complementary tasks is usually needed to completely map areas where lesions could impair language. For iEEG mapping these tasks must be adapted either for a block design, as in SIGFRIED and fMRI, or for an event-related design, which allows analysis of the timing of activation along with its location.

To date, there is no widely accepted battery for testing language with either ESM or iEEG. The task most commonly used for functional mapping with ESM, largely because it is one of the tasks most likely to be impaired by lesions in language cortex, is visual object (confrontation) naming[126]. Most studies of iEEG mapping have tested its accuracy relative to ESM using this task alone or in combination with other tasks.

In general, studies that have compared iEEG mapping with ESM using tasks that are closely related have found that

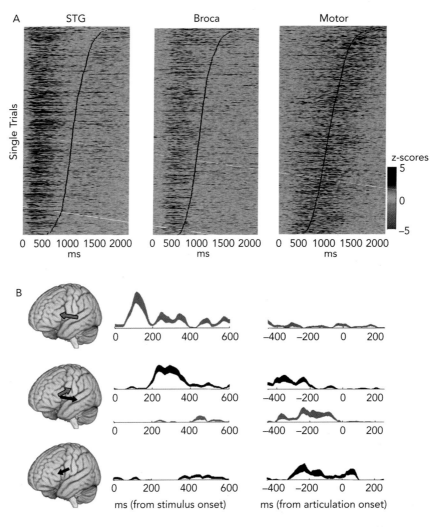

Figure 33.4. **A:** *Vertically stacked single trials are shown for seven patients performing auditory word repetition. Single-trial high-gamma responses (z-scores within each trial compared with a baseline distribution) are sorted by spoken response latency (black curve). Neural activity proceeds in a temporal cascade from superior temporal gyrus (STG) to Broca's area and culminates in motor cortex. STG is activated strongly during speech perception and to a lesser degree during feedback from spoken responses. Activation of Broca's area overlaps activation of STG and motor cortex.* **B:** *Significant Granger causal influences in high-gamma frequencies summarized by region of interest from five patients. Causal influences are shown from STG to Broca (top row, gray arrow and traces), Broca to STG (middle, black), Broca to motor cortex (middle, gray), and motor cortex to Broca (bottom, black). The shaded area in each trace represents the standard error of the mean. Reproduced with permission from Flinker A, Korzeniewska A, Shestyuk AY, et al. Redefining the role of Broca's area in speech. Proc Nat Acad Sci USA. 2015;112:2871–2875; Fig. 3.*

its specificity and sensitivity, relative to ESM, are highly variable but often less than ideal[115,117,119,121,127]. In one study of visual object naming in 13 subjects, for example, iEEG high-gamma mapping had a specificity of 84% and a sensitivity of 43%[121]. Another study found a specificity and sensitivity of 78% and 71%, respectively[117], while yet another found a specificity and sensitivity of 85% and 20%, respectively[119]. In a more recent study using bedside spatial-temporal functional mapping, the specificity and sensitivity of iEEG relative to ESM were 69.9% and 83.5%[125]. The variability of results across these studies could be due to a number of factors, including the effect of different thresholds for high-gamma responses on sensitivity and specificity calculations[121], a problem shared with fMRI. Indeed, comparisons between fMRI and ESM have also yielded variable results[128–131]. Comparisons across multiple language tasks generally increase sensitivity but reduce specificity, and comparisons for individual tasks generally yield good specificity at the expense of sensitivity. Similarly, a recurrent finding in iEEG mapping studies is a poor sensitivity relative to ESM. One possible explanation for this is that stimulation may sometimes interfere with task performance through distant effects on functional critical sites with tight functional connectivity with the stimulation site[101]. Alternatively, it is possible that the neuronal populations affected by ESM are critical to function but are too small to generate high-gamma responses. A study of intracranial gamma responses suggested an optimal electrode spacing of <5 mm to avoid missing discrete populations generating gamma activity[132].

In spite of these concerns, a few recent reports have suggested that in some instances iEEG can be more predictive of postoperative language impairments than ESM.[79,80,91] Undoubtedly, more work will be required to correlate surgical outcomes with the location of resected and preserved sites identified by ESM and iEEG.

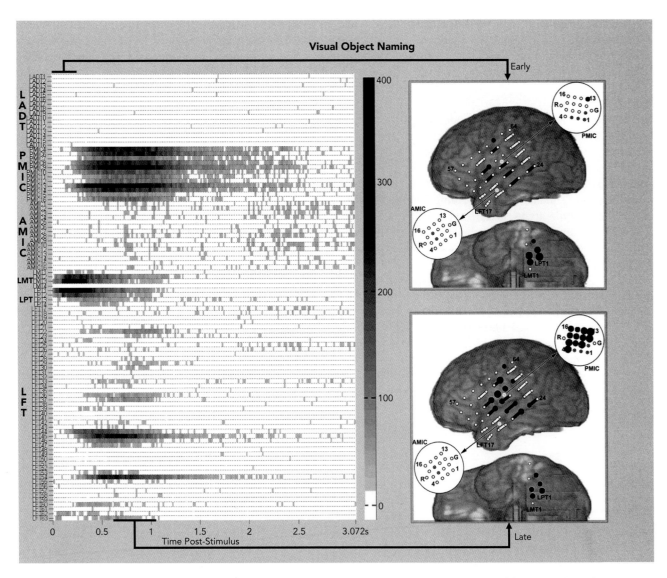

Figure 33.5. Spatial-temporal functional mapping (STFM) of visual object naming in one patient also reported by Wang et al.[125] STFM results are shown as a raster of high-gamma (HG = 70–110 Hz) responses on the left and as brain maps of HG responses (black disks, magnitude represented by size) on the right. Each raster plot displays the spatial-temporal distribution of significant increases in HG energy relative to pre-cue baseline in 16-ms windows (percentage change represented by gray scale, x axis = time in seconds). Each row corresponds to a different electrode as displayed on the right brain maps. All times are relative to cue onset (t = 0 sec). To highlight the spatial pattern of cortical activation at early (visual/auditory perception) and late (response production) stages, HG responses are integrated across early and late temporal windows (horizontal black bars at top and bottom margins of raster) and shown in separate brain maps (early stage in the top brain and late stage in the bottom brain). Microelectrode arrays (labeled AMIC and PMIC for anterior and posterior microarrays, respectively) are enlarged for better visualization of HG responses. "R" and "G" indicate reference and ground electrodes, respectively. Macroelectrode grids and strips are labeled LFT (left frontal-temporal), LMT (left middle temporal), and LPT (left posterior temporal). Contacts at extremes of grids, strips, and microarrays are numbered. Early and late stages can be modified by the user offline, based on the spatial-temporal evolution observed in the raster, to visualize the spatial distribution of activation during different observed task stages. In this illustration, the early sections were chosen manually and post hoc to map perceptual processing stages and the late sections were chosen to map response production. Electrocortical stimulation mapping (ESM) maps are also shown as bars between pairs of electrodes. Black bars: ESM interfered with visual object naming or affected tongue/mouth motor and/or somatosensory function; white bars: ESM had no effect on these functions. From Wang Y, Fifer MS, Flinker A, et al. Spatial-temporal functional mapping of language at the bedside with electrocorticography. Neurology. 2016;86(13):1181–1189, Fig. 1.

3.9. Applications to Brain–Computer Interfaces

While searching for components of LFPs in monkey motor cortex that could be used to drive prosthetics, investigators found that if the signal was filtered between 80 and 250 Hz and then rectified and smoothed, it was reliably correlated with the monkey's movements[133]. However, this observation in 1972 was not followed by additional experiments, and its significance was not appreciated until high-gamma responses were independently discovered 20 years later during cognitive neuroscience and functional mapping research. Since then, spectral perturbations in high-gamma frequencies have proven useful in research on human brain–computer and brain–machine interfaces based on iEEG recordings[134–136]. High-gamma responses are particularly useful in this context because they are sufficiently robust to be detected in single trials, without any averaging across trials. This allows increases in population firing rates to be detected in real time with extraordinary spatial and temporal resolution, which is also useful for real-time functional mapping (see above). Although low-frequency signal components (<4 Hz) can also be used to achieve similar decoding performance in brain–computer interface applications[137,138], these components come from smoothing iEEG signals over large temporal windows, limiting their utility in real-time decoding applications.

Although the most impressive control of robotic prosthetics to restore upper-limb function have come from brain–machine interfaces based on penetrating microelectrode arrays that are capable of simultaneously recording from >100 single units, microelectrode arrays suffer from attrition of reliable single units over time and do not sample from a wide enough area of cortex to take advantage of native cortical representations for limb movements. High-gamma responses have been used in iEEG-based brain–machine interfaces providing continuous online control of reaching and/or grasping movements by a robotic prosthetic upper limb[139–142]. For example, a recent iEEG study mapped cortical sites activated during reaching and grasping movements and used these sites to independently and continuously control reaching and grasping movements in a modular prosthetic limb[140]. Likewise, iEEG maps of cortical sites activated during individuated finger movements were recently used to identify the best sites for online control of individual fingers on the modular prosthetic limb

(Fig. 33.6)[143]. A similar strategy of mapping cortical representations and then exploiting them for a brain–computer interface may also be useful in efforts to develop speech prostheses for patients with severe impairments of articulation. A recent study using high-gamma responses recorded from high-density iEEG arrays showed a population-level representation of phonetic features in ventral precentral and postcentral gyri[144]. In another study, single-trial neural decoding of vowel acoustic features was achieved using high-gamma responses[145]. (See also Chapter 47, where several specific aspects of EEG-based brain–computer interface applications are described.)

4. HIGH-FREQUENCY ACTIVITY IN EPILEPSY

Ripple activity, in the range of 100 to 200 Hz, had been recorded in the LFPs of hippocampus in normal experimental animals and, like the gamma responses discussed above, were considered to be normal physiological activity. It was then found that the hippocampal formation of experimental animal models of epilepsy presented a ripple type of activity, but at an even higher frequency[146,147]. These were termed *fast ripples*. Ripples and fast ripples were also found in the mesial temporal structures of epileptic patients in whom microelectrodes were inserted[146]. This discovery started an extensive series of

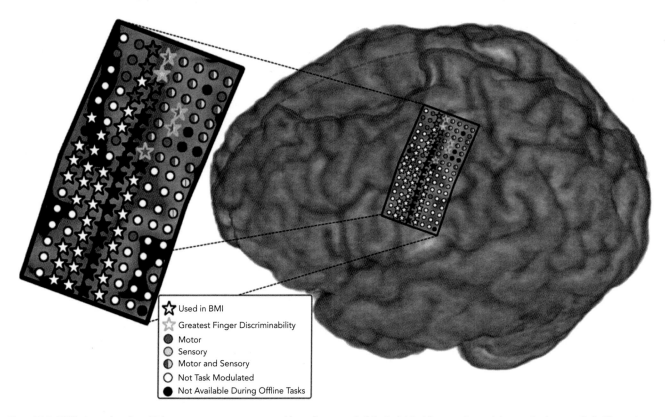

Figure 33.6. *iEEG electrodes where high-gamma responses were used for online control of the individual fingers of a modular prosthetic upper limb. Electrodes labeled by black stars were selected for online brain–machine interface (BMI) control. Sulci are accentuated in the inset for improved visibility, with the central sulcus highlighted in gray. Post hoc analysis showed the electrodes with gray stars contributed the most to decoding accuracy on the training set. Electrodes with white semicircles showed significant activation during vibrotactile stimulation, and electrodes with gray semicircles were active during the motor task. The electrodes that were not available for the offline analysis are filled black. On the brain, the interhemispheric fissure is outlined in gray, with a dotted line indicating the medial margin of the previously resected superior frontal gyrus. Reproduced with permission from Hotson G, McMullen DP, Fifer MS, et al. Individual finger control of a modular prosthetic limb using high-density electrocorticography in a human subject. J Neural Eng. 2016;13:026017; Fig. 2.*

investigations in experimental animals and in humans using microelectrodes. It was then found that low-amplitude activity in the same frequency range (100–500 Hz) could also be recorded from clinical EEG macroelectrodes[148]. This was followed by a series of studies with clinical EEG recordings. We will review separately the microelectrode and the macroelectrode studies and then discuss the issues in interpreting their similarities and differences. Relatively recent reviews can be found in Zijlmans et al.[149] and Jacobs et al.[150]

4.1. High-Frequency Activity from Microelectrodes

Microelectrodes are normally used to record the activity of one or a small number of cells (we discuss here extracellular recordings) in the form of action potentials. This requires a small electrode tip (usually 40 microns in diameter or smaller) and a sampling rate sufficient to identify action potentials (typically 20 kHz). Equipment required for such recordings is common in the experimental laboratory but is not normally used when investigating epileptic patients. Standard EEG equipment cannot record properly from microelectrodes because of their high impedance compared to EEG electrodes and because it cannot deal with such high sampling rates. Microelectrode investigations in humans therefore require a complex setup where the EEG is recorded with a standard clinical EEG system at the same time that microelectrode activity is recorded with a parallel system dedicated to this task.

In addition to providing action potentials, microelectrodes also record the field potential, or the local EEG. This can be revealed by filtering out action potentials (removing frequencies above ~600 Hz). Figure 33.7 shows how the different components of a microelectrode recording are obtained. The

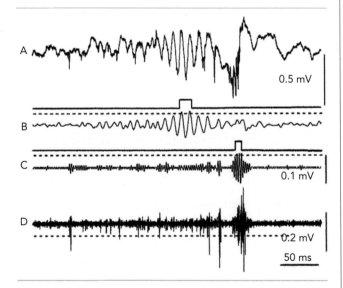

Figure 33.7. Example of bandpass filter settings used to detect specific activities recorded from microelectrodes. A: Unfiltered EEG. B: Ripple frequency (80–160 Hz). C: Fast ripple frequency (250–500 Hz). D: Unit activity (600 Hz–5 kHz). Marker pulses shown in B and C indicate trigger points used for waveform averaging. From Bragin A, Wilson CL, Staba RJ, Reddick M, Fried I, Engel J, Jr. Interictal high-frequency oscillations (80–500 Hz) in the human epileptic brain: entorhinal cortex. Ann Neurol. 2002;52:407–415; Fig. 2.

knowledge of when action potentials fire is of course important in interpreting the high frequencies of the LFP.

As indicated above, Bragin et al.[146] recorded ripples in the frequency range of 80 to 200 Hz and fast ripples between 200 and 500 Hz in the hippocampal region of rats in whom chronic epilepsy was induced with intrahippocampal injection of kainic acid, and in human hippocampal regions of epileptic patients investigated with intracerebral electrodes, through which microelectrodes were inserted. They noted that fast ripples were not present in the recordings from kindled animals. The same group then demonstrated that ripples were the more frequent pattern in the least abnormal temporal lobe (in patients with electrodes implanted on both sides because of possible bitemporal epilepsy) whereas fast ripples were more frequent on the more abnormal side[151]. They also showed[9] that fast ripple are generated over a smaller volume than ripples in patients; in animals the fast-ripple generator appeared to be <1 mm³. In rats, it was found that the regions generating fast ripples were stable over time (days and weeks) and that the broader the region in which fast ripples were found, the more frequent were the seizures, implying that the fast ripples represented the epileptogenic region and seizures were more frequent if the epileptogenic region was larger. Fast ripples appeared to be generated in multiple discrete clusters of hyperexcitable neurons.

Engel et al.[152] concluded that fast ripples may be a more efficient marker of epileptogenic tissue than synchronized cellular activity because the field potential of fast ripples can be recorded more easily than cellular activity, given the small fraction of neurons that participate in the synchronous activity of epileptic discharges.

In a different experimental context (ketamine-induced anesthesia in the cat), Grenier et al.[153] argued that fast oscillations result from a vicious cycle in which bursts of population spikes generate a field potential that itself facilitates neuronal firing.

Recent work has elucidated in part the mechanisms of generation of ripples and fast ripples. Ripples are thought to reflect abnormal network activity during epileptogenesis since they only occur in animals that develop seizures and can predict seizure occurrence[154,155]. Ripples are also seen during seizures, especially during low-voltage fast-onset seizures[155,156]. Low-voltage fast-onset seizures and ripples are thought to originate from GABAergic interneurons[157–159]. The optogenetic activation of parvalbumin-positive interneurons in the 4-aminopyridine model induces low-voltage fast-onset seizures associated to ripples[160], providing evidence for this hypothesis.

Fast ripples are also observed during epileptogenesis in various models of temporal lobe epilepsy, such as in the kainic acid model[147,154], the pilocarpine model[155], and the non-lesional tetanus toxin model[161]. Interestingly, when analyzing high-frequency oscillations (HFOs) over time, Jones et al.[162] found that fast ripples are prolonged in duration and display complex spectral characteristics at the transition to the chronic stage. It was also shown that regions generating fast ripples express few genes associated to presynaptic and postsynaptic functions. This could induce dysfunctional synaptic transmission and the generation of fast ripples in epileptic regions[163]. Neuronal loss would thus not be required for the generation of such fast oscillations, as previously proposed[161].

Fast ripples also occur during seizures. They are preferentially associated to hypersynchronous-onset seizures, whether spontaneous[154,155] or acutely induced with picrotoxin, a GABA$_A$ receptor antagonist[156]. The mechanisms underlying fast ripples are still unclear, but it is thought that they reflect the in-phase[164,165] or out-of-phase[166,167] firing of clusters of principal cells. Ephaptic transmission was suggested as a mechanism that could trigger highly synchronized principal cell firing[168]. In vitro, it was shown that the optogenetic activation of principal cells in the 4-aminopyridine model produces hypersynchronous-onset seizures associated to fast ripples[160], supporting the hypothesis that fast ripples and these seizures are generated by principal cell activity.

In humans, it was observed that ripples and fast ripples were more frequent in non-rapid eye movement (REM) sleep than during wakefulness and REM sleep. In addition, REM sleep suppressed ripples but not fast ripples, compared to wakefulness[169]. In patients with temporal lobe epilepsy, Staba et al.[170] found that the ratio of fast ripples to ripples increased with increased hippocampal atrophy, thus establishing a direct link between the generation of fast ripples and the pathology underlying mesial temporal lobe epilepsy. In an attempt to try to link directly the generation of HFOs (including ripples and fast ripples) and the generation of seizures, Bragin et al.[154] studied the evolution of HFOs after kianic acid injection, a model in which status epilepticus is generated, followed by a latent period and then spontaneous recurrent seizures. They found that if no HFOs developed, no seizure developed. They also found that the earlier HFOs appeared following the status, the earlier seizures developed, indicating that HFOs appear to reflect epileptogenicity in this model. In a subsequent study of the same model, they attempted to link seizure onset and HFOs, but found that seizures started with an EEG wave before the first ictal HFO was observed, concluding that HFOs do not seem to be the immediate trigger of seizure discharges[171].

4.2. High-Frequency Activity from Macroelectrodes

4.2.1. Filtering the EEG to See High-Frequency Activity

High-frequency activity is most often of much lower amplitude than low-frequency activity (see Fig. 33.1). To see it better, a high-pass filter is most often used, largely eliminating the components of the traditional EEG. Depending on what is to be observed, a filter cutoff frequency can be at 40, 100, or 200 Hz, for instance. This is a very effective way of enhancing the detectability of the low-amplitude high frequencies, and most of the work on HFOs in epilepsy uses this approach. It has one drawback, however, when the original EEG includes sharp transients such as artifacts or epileptic spikes or polyspikes. Such sharp transients are in fact broadband signals, including low- and high-frequency components. When the low-frequency components are removed, the high-frequency components remain and can be indistinguishable from high-frequency activity that is not part of a wide-band transient. This problem can be exacerbated by the type of filter used. This

is discussed extensively by Bénar et al.[172]; some methods have been developed to deal with this issue[173]. The same situation can occur when filtering physiological fast transients: it was, for instance, demonstrated in one type of experiment that what was originally thought to be scalp gamma activity of neuronal origin was actually the result of filtering rapid eye saccades[174].

4.2.2. Automatic Detection of HFOs

How to detect HFOs is a challenging issue due to lack of a formal and global definition of HFOs. The detection can be done by visual inspection in which clear oscillations standing out of the background in high-frequency filtered signal represent HFOs. The screen time resolution has to be high and only a few channels can be evaluated simultaneously[175]. Visual marking is therefore time-consuming, tedious, and inconsistent. It is also subjective and biased by the reviewer's experience. To overcome these limitations, automatic detectors have been implemented. They can analyze long periods of data in a short time with consistency and can facilitate HFO studies. The main idea of most HFO detectors is to compare the signal energy in a specific frequency band with the energy threshold derived from the background. Different types of energy functions have been proposed, including root mean square, line length, Hilbert transform, and short time energy[151,176]. In some studies, a dynamically adjusted threshold is used instead of a constant threshold by estimating the background in short segments[177]. HFOs have also been detected by frequency and time-frequency analysis of EEG signal, and by neural networks or feature-based classification methods[178,179]. A technical issue in HFO detection is that spikes, artifacts, and sharp activities can disturb the detection process by generating false oscillations in the filtered signal[172]. There are methods to solve this problem[173].

HFOs have also been described in the scalp EEG (see below) and it is particularly delicate to detect them because of the possible confound created by short muscle twitches. A first attempt at scalp HFO detection is presented by von Ellenrieder et al.[180].

4.2.3. EEG Activity Between 40 and 120 Hz in Epilepsy

Activity in the range of 80 to 120 Hz was reported in subdural recordings at the time of electro-decremental seizure onset, and this activity appeared limited to the region of seizure onset[181]. The same year, Allen et al.[182] reported that frequencies around 100 Hz might be useful in localizing the seizure onset in frontal lobe epilepsy. It took quite a few years until significant studies evaluated further the importance of activity faster than the beta band in epileptic patients.

There have been several studies relating activity in the 40- to 150-Hz band and different types of epileptic syndromes. Worrell et al.[183] found that bursts of interictal activity in the 60- to 100-Hz range were often found in the intracerebral EEG of patients with neocortical epilepsy, were indicative of the seizure onset region, and became more frequent as seizures were approaching. Studying the scalp EEG of a large group of children, Wu et al.[184] found that interictal paroxysmal beta and gamma activity was an accurate indicator of epilepsy and

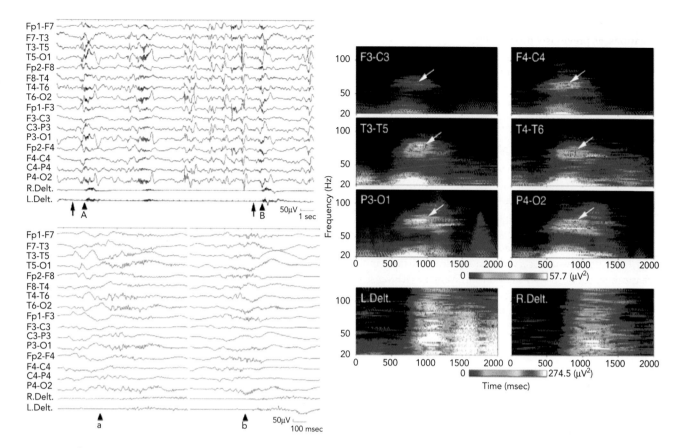

Figure 33.8. Left: Ictal EEG of spasms in series in patient with symptomatic West syndrome. Top: A conventional trace. Bottom: A temporally expanded trace. The time points of A and B (arrowheads) in the conventional trace correspond to those of a and b (arrowheads) in the expanded trace. Rhythmic gamma activity at ~60 Hz is dominant over the posterior head area and is associated with each spasm in the expanded trace. The power spectra in the right part of the figure correspond to the 2-sec ictal EEG segments, with each segment beginning from each arrow in the conventional trace. L and RDelt., left and right deltoid muscle. Right: Time evolution of spasm-associated gamma activity in averaged power. Spectral peaks of the ictal gamma activity are indicated by arrows at ~60 or 70 Hz in the EEG. Activity from the deltoid muscles has much broader and noisier spectra than does gamma activity. The peaks of gamma activity on the scalp precede those of muscle activity by about 200 msec. From Kobayashi K, Oka M, Akiyama T, et al. Very fast rhythmic activity on scalp EEG associated with epileptic spasms. Epilepsia. 2004;45:488–496; Figs. 1 and 2.

of the seizure onset region, particularly in children younger than 3 years. In young children with hemimegalencephaly, Yamazaki et al.[185] frequently saw activity around 40 to 50 Hz. Kobayashi et al.[186] showed that gamma activity (50–100 Hz) was present at the time of infantile spasms in the vast majority of spasms. The power spectrum of this activity showed a clear peak, thus differentiating it from muscle activity with energy in the same frequency range (Fig. 33.8). Akiyama et al.[187] also showed activity between 60 and 150 Hz at the onset of spasms, and suggested that high-frequency activity triggers the spasm.

Moving into frequencies above 120 Hz, but in relation to infantile spasms, Ramachandranair et al.[188] demonstrated activity between 150 to 250 Hz at spasm onset, localized to frontal or rolandic areas in intracranial recordings.

4.2.4. EEG Activity Higher than 80 Hz (Ripples and Fast Ripples)

Given the size of the presumed generators of HFOs, it would seem unlikely that such activity can be recorded from the standard macroelectrodes used in the presurgical evaluation of some patients with intractable epilepsy. Electrodes used for subdural recordings are usually disks of 4 to 5 mm² with an exposed diameter of 2.3 mm, and depth electrodes used for intracerebral implantation are made of cylinders of approximately the same surface area. This size is approximately 4,000 times larger than a microelectrode. The group at the Montreal Neurological Institute has used electrodes made in house with a surface contact of 0.8 mm², smaller than commercial electrodes. Sampling the EEG at 2,000 Hz after 500-Hz low-pass filtering, they demonstrated that HFOs in the range of 100 to 500 Hz could be recorded with these macroelectrodes and had a strong relationship with the seizure-generating region. Subsequent studies demonstrated that HFOs could also be recorded with standard electrodes.

The first study demonstrated HFOs during epileptic seizures[148]. High-frequency activity, in the form of either brief oscillations or prolonged discharges, was found most often in the electrodes in which the seizure had started and rarely in regions to which the seizure had propagated (Fig. 33.9). It was also found that patients for whom it was felt that the seizure onset had been missed (e.g., if clinical signs preceded the first EEG change) did not have high-frequency activity at seizure onset. It was then demonstrated that interictal HFOs were also relatively frequent in the ripple frequency band (i.e., not just in the fast ripple frequency band)[189]. These HFOs occurred in three situations (Fig. 33.10): (i) riding on top of traditional

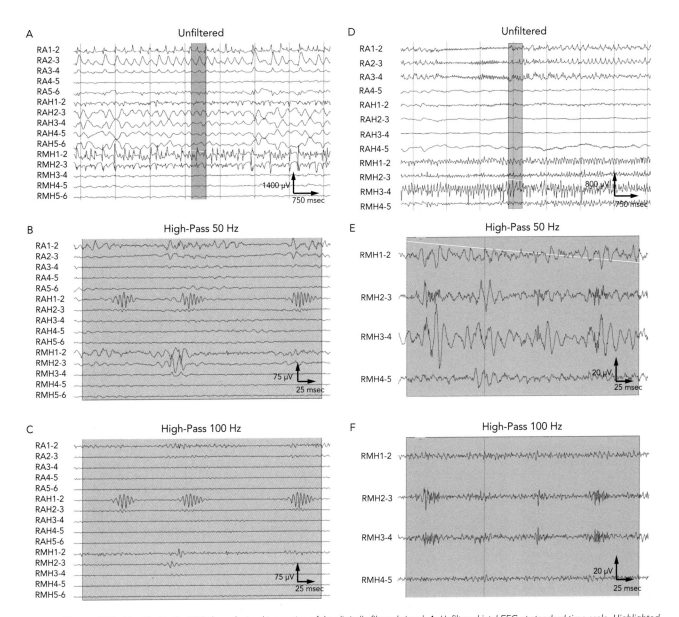

Figure 33.9. Discrete HFOs identified in the EEG through visual inspection of the digitally filtered signal. *A:* Unfiltered ictal EEG at standard time scale. Highlighted sample for further visual analysis in *B* and *C*. Ictal EEG is shown at an expanded time scale and increased vertical gain with high-pass filtering at 50 Hz and 100 Hz in *B* and *C*. A brief 160- to 210-Hz segmental oscillation is well visualized in the RAH1-2 channel at both filter settings. *D:* Unfiltered ictal EEG at standard time scale. A highlighted sample is shown at increased vertical and horizontal gain in *E* and *F* with filtering. A discrete 285- to 375-Hz segmental oscillation is clearly visualized in RMH2-3 and to a lesser extent RMH3-4 at both filter settings. From Jirsch JD, Urrestarazu E, LeVan P, Olivier A, Dubeau F, Gotman J. High-frequency oscillations during human focal seizures. Brain. 2006;129:1593–1608; Fig. 3.

EEG spikes (as was most often the case for fast ripples recorded with microelectrodes); (ii) totally independently of spikes; and (iii) at the same time as a spike but not visible on the spike. As we discussed above in the section on filtering, in such a situation it is difficult to exclude the possible contribution of the filter itself. In both above studies, HFOs were found in neocortical regions as well as in mesial temporal lobe structures. In one recent study, Kobayashi et al.[190], recording with a 3,000-Hz filter, demonstrated activity up to 900 Hz from subdural electrodes at seizure onset, in the form of short oscillations superimposed on spikes.

It is known that the zone of interictal spiking and the seizure onset zone are related to each other, but the relationship is not always tight. By examining the spatial relationship between the seizure onset zone, the region in which interictal spiking took place, and the region in which HFOs were found, it could be determined that HFOs had a tighter correspondence with the seizure onset zone than did interictal spikes (Fig. 33.11)[175,191,192]. HFOs therefore appeared to be a better candidate for a biomarker of ictogenesis than spikes. These results were largely confirmed for mesial and polar structures of the temporal lobe in the study by Crépon et al.[176] In a study that was not directly related to HFOs as discrete entities but rather to activity in the ripple and fast ripple frequency bands as calculated by spectral analysis, Urrestarazu et al.[193] showed that high-frequency activity was suppressed during the slow wave following spikes, compared to the background. The suppression was most pronounced in the region closest to the maximum of the spike

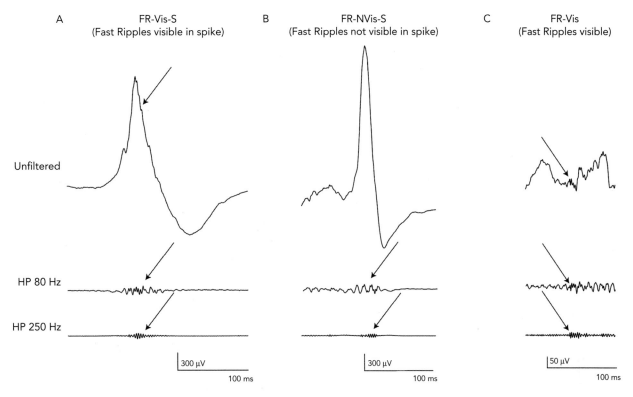

Figure 33.10. *Different types of HFOs, with and without spikes. **A:** Fast ripple visible in spike. **B:** Fast ripple not visible in spike. **C:** Fast ripple visible, independently of a spike. Top: nonfiltered EEG; middle: EEG filtered with high-pass filter of 80 Hz; bottom: EEG filtered with high-pass filter of 250 Hz. From Urrestarazu E, Chander R, Dubeau F, Gotman J. Interictal high-frequency oscillations (100–500 Hz) in the intracerebral EEG of epileptic patients. Brain. 2007;130:2354–2366; Fig. 2.*

and was most prominent in the hippocampus compared to the amygdala or neocortical region. This suppression was interpreted as reflecting the strength of the inhibition that follows a spike. A statistical approach to the demonstration of this phenomenon and of other high-frequency changes was presented by Kobayashi et al.[194]

The importance of HFOs was further underlined when it was found that, in patients with lesions, HFOs were more closely coupled with the region of seizure onset than with the lesion, which is sometimes but not always the source of seizures[195]. It was also found, however, that HFO rates vary widely according to the type of pathology[196]: for instance, they are much more frequent in hippocampal sclerosis and focal cortical dysplasia than in atrophic lesions, even if the latter is just as epileptogenic.

4.2.5. FLUCTUATIONS OF HFOS OVER TIME

The above studies were performed by measuring HFO rates during non-REM sleep, since it was shown that, as in microelectrode recordings, HFOs are most frequent during non-REM sleep but their relative distribution across brain regions is not state-dependent[197]. Looking closely within slow-wave sleep, it was found that HFOs (and spikes) were activated by large-amplitude slow waves compared to periods of lower-amplitude slow waves or periods without slow waves (but within slow-wave sleep), emphasizing the modulating role of thalamocortical circuits[18]. Examining also the different phases of REM sleep, it was observed that spikes and HFOs are more suppressed in the phasic (with rapid eye movements) than

in the tonic (no eye movements) part of REM sleep[198]. It was found, however, that REM sleep generates HFOs that are spatially more specific than slow-wave sleep to the epileptogenic zone[199]. It was also found that the different brain regions do not all fluctuate in the same way with wakefulness and sleep[200]. Coupling between HFOs and slow waves was also studied in a different context, that of infantile spasms[201]. It is also interesting to note that high-frequency activity elicited by single-pulse stimulation appears to localize to the same regions as spontaneous HFOs[202].

If there is a good spatial correspondence between the region of seizure onset and HFOs, one can naturally wonder if there is also a temporal coupling. The most natural question is whether HFOs become more frequent as a seizure approaches. Khorsravani et al.[203] found that HFOs often increased in the few seconds immediately preceding a seizure. In a study that examined fluctuations in HFO rate and energy in the 15-, 5-, and 1-minute intervals preceding seizure occurrence, Jacobs et al.[204] did not find any systematic change. These two studies appear to indicate that if there is a change in HFOs prior to seizures, it is only immediately prior to their occurrence and thus it may be difficult to distinguish them from the seizure onset itself. The question of the use of high-frequency activity in seizure prediction is reviewed in greater detail in Chapter 23. When studying high-frequency activity during seizures with clinical electrodes and with microelectrodes, Weiss et al.[205] demonstrated that some regions are invaded by high-frequency activity and represent the core of the seizure discharge with intense neuronal firing; others are not, and they

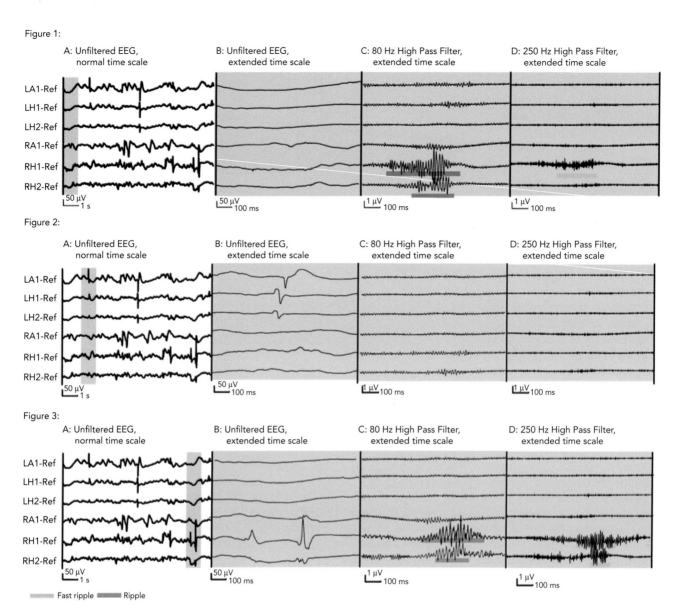

Figure 33.11. HFOs are most prominent in the seizure onset region. This patient presented with interictal and ictal signs of bitemporal epilepsy on scalp EEG. He was implanted bitemporally aiming at the amygdala (LA, RA) and hippocampus (LH, RH). The MRI revealed a malrotation of the right hippocampus. All seizures originated from the right mesial temporal structures, where the highest rates of HFOs were found. The figure shows three sections selected from the same few seconds of EEG. In each panel the original EEG is on the left and the thin section marked in gray is expanded at the right, after filtering and changing the gain as indicated. The unfiltered EEG shows frequent spikes in both mesial TL structures. **Top panel (Figure 1):** Co-occurrence of ripples and fast ripples outside spikes in channel RH1. Additionally a ripple is seen in channel RH2. **Middle panel (Figure 2):** The selection includes two spikes over LA1 and LH1. Both spikes lay outside the seizure onset zone and in the healthier mesial TL. The expanded sections show no HFOs during this time period. **Bottom panel (Figure 3):** The gray selection shows two spikes simultaneously at RH1 and RH2 in the seizure onset zone. No oscillation is visible in the spike at RH1 in the extended unfiltered EEG, while the spike in RH2 shows a very short and small oscillation. The filtered EEG segments clearly reveal a ripple and fast ripple oscillation during these spikes. Spikes looking similar in the unfiltered EEG might differ in whether they carry HFOs. From Jacobs J, LeVan P, Chander R, Hall J, Dubeau F, Gotman J. Interictal high-frequency oscillations (80–500 Hz) are an indicator of seizure onset areas independent of spikes in the human epileptic brain. Epilepsia. 2008;49:1893–1907; Figs. 1, 2, and 3.

represent a sort of penumbra in which neuronal firing is much less intense.

Looking at HFO fluctuations at the time scale of days in relation to seizure occurrence and to changing antiepileptic medication, Zijlmans et al.[206] demonstrated that medication reduction results directly in an increase in the rate of HFO occurrence. Seizures, on the other hand, when they occurred in the context of stable medication use, did not cause any change in HFO occurrence rates. This is in contrast to interictal spikes[207–209], for which medication reduction does not result directly in an increased occurrence rate; seizures, however, are followed by increased spiking (this explains the increase in spiking often seen after medication withdrawal, as seizures occur more often in this context and mediate the increase in spiking). Comparing HFOs and spikes, one therefore can conclude that HFOs behave more like seizures than spikes do in the context of changing medication levels. A similar effect on spikes and HFOs was induced by the anesthetic agent propofol[210]. HFOs may therefore be a better marker of disease activity than spikes.

4.2.6. HFOs and Surgery for Epilepsy

Given these results, the question naturally arises regarding the possible use of HFOs in the surgical evaluation of epileptic patients. In a first small study, Ochi et al.[211] noted some correlation between the removal of regions generating HFOs and a successful surgery outcome. In a larger patient group and a study evaluating systematically the correlation between regions generating HFOs, spikes, and the seizure onset, Jacobs et al.[212] showed that the outcome of surgery was more closely related to whether the HFO-generating region was removed than to whether spike- or seizure-generating regions were removed. Similar findings were obtained in a study based on ECoG in children[127], and several publications have since confirmed these findings, some using interictal HFOs and some using-high frequency activity at seizure onset[213-219]. A recent study performed during acute ECoG in adults indicates that leaving unresected regions generating fast ripples carries a poor prognosis with respect to seizure freedom[220]. These multiple studies strongly suggest that regions generating HFOs are *potential* seizure-generating regions.

When looking for HFOs in intracerebral EEG, recorded by depth or subdural recordings, an important word of caution is necessary: artifacts from contracting scalp muscles can appear surprisingly like HFOs[221]. Just as EEG activity is transmitted through the skull and can be recorded on the scalp, activity generated outside the skull is measurable in intracerebral recordings. This has been shown for eye blinks[222]. Similarly, Electromyelographic (EMG) activity from scalp muscles is transmitted through the skull and can be recorded on subdural electrodes and on the most superficial contacts of depth electrodes. Because of skull attenuation and because of the small surface of synchronized activity in muscles, EMG recorded with intracerebral EEG electrodes is of small amplitude, just like HFOs. This is a particular concern during seizures, when scalp muscles can have strong contractions. One way to become aware of this possibility and to observe the intracerebral distribution of EMG activity is to ask patients to contract their jaws and observe in intracranial contacts the changes directly related to the contractions.

A recent set of reports indicate that activity between 1,000 and 2,500 Hz can also be recorded in subdural recordings and that this activity is indicative of the epileptogenic zone[223]. It is difficult to imagine how such activity can be generated by neurons, and this finding remains intriguing.

4.2.7. Activity Above 80 Hz in the Scalp EEG and MEG

Given the presumed size of HFO generators, it was surprising to record HFOs with the large clinical subdural and intracerebral electrodes. It is even more surprising to see that oscillations in the 100- to 200-Hz range can be recorded from the scalp. This was first reported by Kobayashi et al. in a group of children with electrical status epilepticus during slow-wave sleep[224]. It has since been reported in other pediatric conditions[225,226] and also in adult patients with focal epilepsy, primarily in the seizure onset zone[11]. In patients with focal epilepsy, ripples appear almost exclusively around the time of EEG spikes and are largely absent in patients with rare spikes or no

spikes[227]. Interestingly, the ripples tend to appear just before spikes or at the time of their rising phase[228] and are absent during the slow wave following the spike, confirming earlier results in intracerebral EEG[193]. Kobayashi et al.[229] found that scalp ripples (40–150 Hz) were very common during periods of hypsarrhythmia in patients with West syndrome, and that their occurrence rate decreased in the course of adrenocorticotropic hormone (ACTH) treatment. Great caution must be exercised when identifying scalp ripple activity, as brief bursts of EMG activity can easily be misinterpreted as activity originating from the brain (Fig. 33.12). This issue is discussed in detail in[11].

It remains difficult to understand why the ripples recorded in intracranial EEG, with low amplitude and a small generator, can be recorded on the scalp. Combined subdural and scalp recordings were obtained in epileptic patients in an attempt to clarify this question[12]. The study concluded that there was no direct correspondence between ripples recorded on subdural EEG and on the scalp, and that both recording modalities are probably spatially undersampled, making the evaluation of their correspondence difficult. This study may have been complicated by the presence of the grid, which acts as an isolator[230]. As was discussed in the introduction of this chapter it is possible that small generators are visible on the scalp because they are at frequencies (~100–150 Hz) at which the amplitude of spontaneous brain signals is very low[10].

Distinct ripples have also been recorded with MEG. In one study they were not apparent in raw signal traces but became apparent with a spatial filter targeted at the regions likely to generate spikes[231]. In another study, they were detected automatically and subjected to frequency-dependent source localization[232].

4.2.8. Physiological and Pathological HFOs

An important issue that has not yet been fully resolved in intracerebral EEG studies is the differentiation between normal HFOs related to cognitive activity and pathological HFOs related to epilepsy, which may occur in overlapping frequency ranges. As discussed above, oscillations occur as a result of sensory, motor, cognitive, and memory activity in the normal brain. Even during sleep, a time when most of the studies of interictal HFOs are performed in epileptic patients, several studies have shown that high-frequency activity is present in channels that never present any spike or seizure activity and are therefore in presumably quite normal brain regions, even if they belong to epileptic patients[233-235]. These studies also show that in terms of amplitude, duration, and frequency, there are statistical differences but a large overlap between pathological and physiological ripples. In the study by Frauscher et al.[18] on the activation of HFOs and spikes by the large-amplitude slow waves of slow-wave sleep, it was also found that the ripples in normal channels were activated at a different phase of the slow wave than the ripples in channels of the seizure onset zone. It may therefore be possible to separate channels with predominantly pathological ripples from channels with predominantly normal ripples by their pattern of activation by slow waves[236]. In this approach, one does not try to separate individual ripples; rather, one tries to separate EEG channels.

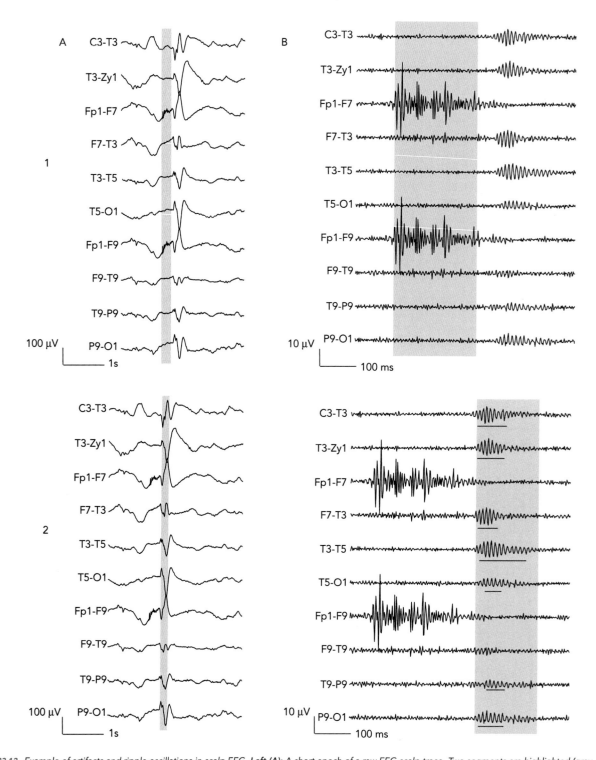

Figure 33.12. Example of artifacts and ripple oscillations in scalp EEG. **Left (A):** A short epoch of a raw EEG scalp trace. Two segments are highlighted (gray area): in part 1(above) focusing on an EMG burst, and in part 2 (below) on an immediately following sharp wave co-occurring with ripples. The two gray sections in A are expanded in time and amplitude in B (note different calibrations in A and B). Ripple oscillations are underlined. The waveform morphology of nonartifactual fast oscillations is more rhythmic and regular in amplitude and frequency than artefactual oscillations[11]. From Andrade-Valença LP, Dubeau F, Mari F, Zelmann R, Gotman J. Interictal scalp fast oscillations as a marker of the seizure onset zone. Neurology. 2011;77:524–531; Fig. 1.

There are also considerable variations according to brain regions in the distribution of physiological HFOs. Alkawadri et al.[235] found that they were most frequent in the perirolandic, occipital, and basal temporal regions. In the process of investigating HFOs, Melani et al.[227] found that some patients display continuous or semi-continuous activity in the ripple band; this activity was largely confined to the occipital lobe and mesial temporal structures and was not related to epileptogenicity. The study did not evaluate the central region, and these results may thus be compatible with the findings of Alkawadri et al.[235]

4.3. Discussion

In a review, Engel et al.[237] discussed the origin and possible meaning of normal and pathological microelectrode-recorded HFOs in the context of mesial temporal lobe epilepsy. They concluded that ripples appear to reflect synchronized inhibitory postsynaptic potentials and that fast ripples probably reflect bursts of population spikes. It was possible to demonstrate in human recordings that interneurons and pyramidal cells fire in sequence, thus supporting the generation of ripples by inhibitory activity[238]. Engel et al.[237] also concluded that not all ripples represent normal phenomena since, for instance, ripples are not normally seen in the dentate gyrus but appear there prior to seizures in kainic acid–treated rats[154]. Abnormal ripples could be generated by slow bursts of population spikes. It is also possible that not all fast ripples represent abnormal phenomena. These hypotheses are compatible with the results found by Avoli and colleagues[155–157], who have studied HFOs mainly in the pilocarpine model of temporal lobe epilepsy. They concluded that epileptic ripples mainly reflect GABAergic interneuronal activation, whereas fast ripples reflect the activity of principal glutamatergic cells. Ripples and fast ripples may also reflect different seizure-generating mechanisms[160] (see also computational models of the generation of ripples and fast ripples in Chapter 3).

From the studies of HFOs recorded with intracranial EEG macroelectrodes, one can conclude that HFOs are an important marker of the epileptogenic region not only in mesial temporal structures, where they are particularly abundant, but also in neocortical regions. Although fast ripples were sometimes more specific than ripples, the distinction that was possible with microelectrodes has not fully carried over with macroelectrodes. There is clearly a relationship between the events recorded with microelectrodes and those recorded with macroelectrodes, but the nature of this relationship is uncertain. From microelectrode recordings, it would seem that the field of HFOs should be too small to be clearly visible with macroelectrodes, and a fortiori from scalp EEG. Microelectrode recordings are made with a local reference, however, and they may therefore be blind to broader field changes that take place at the same time as the very local event that they are best suited to detect. The properties of these broader events may not be identical to those of the very local events. We also do not have a clear understanding of how multiple small generators with activity at similar frequencies add up at a distance. There is a need for a systematic study of the distribution of these HFO fields and of the electrode sizes most appropriate for recording the most discriminating events. Whereas microelectrodes record activity that is easier to interpret scientifically because it relates directly to the basic building block of the nervous system (i.e., the neuron), macroelectrodes record potentials that are more difficult to interpret in terms of the activity of individual cells. However, activity recorded with macroelectrodes may be more significant from the clinical point of view because it represents what happens to neuronal populations on a larger scale.

There is a frequent overlap between the spike-generating region and the seizure-generating region, justifying the interest in spikes. The relationship is, however, uncertain, and it is not clear how information about spikes should be integrated in the definition of the epileptogenic region. The investigations of HFOs recorded with macroelectrodes suggest that they are more tightly coupled to seizures than are spikes, in both time and in space. They may therefore be of greater clinical utility. Several studies suggest that HFOs may be a better spatial indicator of epileptogenicity than the region of seizure onset itself. A clinical trial is currently under way to try to answer this question[239].

It is common now that clinical EEG systems allow recordings of activity up to 500 or 600 Hz, but these systems are not equipped for microelectrode recordings, requiring very-high-input impedance amplifiers. If it is shown conclusively that microelectrode recordings provide useful clinical information that cannot be obtained from EEG electrodes, it may be necessary for future clinical equipment to allow microelectrode recordings in addition to the EEG.

We started this chapter with a mention of *wide-band EEG*, encompassing very high and very low frequencies. Studies have shown that at the onset of seizures, it is common that very slow fluctuations are combined with HFOs[240,241]. In some cases, the slow fluctuations appear to precede the first HFOs.

REFERENCES

1. Crone NE, Miglioretti DL, Gordon B, Lesser RP. Functional mapping of human sensorimotor cortex with electrocorticographic spectral analysis. II. Event-related synchronization in the gamma band. *Brain*. 1998;121(Pt 12):2301–2315.
2. Crone NE, Sinai A, Korzeniewska A. High-frequency gamma oscillations and human brain mapping with electrocorticography. *Prog Brain Res*. 2006;159:275–295.
3. Miller KJ, Shenoy P, den Nijs M, Sorensen LB, Rao RN, Ojemann JG. Beyond the gamma band: the role of high-frequency features in movement classification. *IEEE Trans Biomed Eng*. 2008;55(5):1634–1637.
4. High-frequency oscillations in cognition and epilepsy. *Progress Neurobiol*. 2012;98(3):239–318.
5. Oostendorp TF, Delbeke J, Stegeman DF. The conductivity of the human skull: results of in vivo and in vitro measurements. *IEEE Trans Biomed Eng*. 2000;47(11):1487–1492.
6. Gloor P. Neuronal generators and the problem of localization in electroencephalography: application of volume conductor theory to electroencephalography. *J Clin Neurophysiol*. 1985;2(4):327–354.
7. Cooper R, Winter AL, Crow HJ, Walter WG. Comparison of subcortical cortical and scalp activity using chronically indwelling electrodes in man. *Electroencephalogr Clin Neurophysiol*. 1965;18(3):217.
8. Tao JX, Baldwin M, Hawes-Ebersole S, Ebersole JS. Cortical substrates of scalp EEG epileptiform discharges. *J Clin Neurophysiol*. 2007;24(2):96–100.
9. Bragin A, Mody I, Wilson CL, Engel J, Jr. Local generation of fast ripples in epileptic brain. *J Neurosci*. 2002;22(5):2012–2021.
10. von Ellenrieder N, Beltrachini L, Perucca P, Gotman J. Size of cortical generators of epileptic interictal events and visibility on scalp EEG. *Neuroimage*. 2014;94:47–54.
11. Andrade-Valenca LP, Dubeau F, Mari F, Zelmann R, Gotman J. Interictal scalp fast oscillations as a marker of the seizure onset zone. *Neurology*. 2011;77(6):524–531.
12. Zelmann R, Lina JM, Schulze-Bonhage A, Gotman J, Jacobs J. Scalp EEG is not a blur: it can see high frequency oscillations although their generators are small. *Brain Topography*. 2014;27(5):683–704.
13. McCreery DB, Agnew WF, Yuen TG, Bullara L. Charge density and charge per phase as cofactors in neural injury induced by electrical stimulation. *IEEE Trans Biomed Eng*. 1990;37(10):996–1001.
14. Wei XF, Grill WM. Current density distributions, field distributions and impedance analysis of segmented deep brain stimulation electrodes. *J Neural Eng*. 2005;2(4):139–147.

15. Chatillon CE, Zelmann R, Bortel A, Avoli M, Gotman J. Contact size does not affect high frequency oscillation detection in intracerebral EEG recordings in a rat epilepsy model. *Clin Neurophysiol*. 2011;122(9):1701–1705.

16. Chatillon CE, Zelmann R, Hall JA, Olivier A, Dubeau F, Gotman J. Influence of contact size on the detection of HFOs in human intracerebral EEG recordings. *Clin Neurophysiol*. 2013;124(8):1541–1546.

17. Blanco JA, Stead M, Krieger A, et al. Data mining neocortical high-frequency oscillations in epilepsy and controls. *Brain*. 2011;134:2948–2959.

18. Frauscher B, von Ellenrieder N, Ferrari-Marinho T, Avoli M, Dubeau F, Gotman J. Facilitation of epileptic activity during sleep is mediated by high amplitude slow waves. *Brain*. 2015;138:1629–1641.

19. da Silva FH, van Lierop TH, Schrijer CF, van Leeuwen WS. Organization of thalamic and cortical alpha rhythms: spectra and coherences. *Electroencephalogr Clin Neurophysiol*. 1973;35(6):627–639.

20. Adrian ED, Matthews BHC. The Berger rhythm: potential changes from the occipital lobes in man. *Brain*. 1934;57:355–385.

21. Freeman WJ. Spatial properties of an EEG event in the olfactory bulb and cortex. *Electroencephalogr Clin Neurophysiol*. 1978;44:586–605.

22. Gray CM, König P, Engel AK, Singer W. Oscillatory responses in cat visual cortex exhibit inter-columnar synchronization which reflects global stimulus properties. *Nature*. 1989;338:334–337.

23. Eckhorn R, Bauer R, Jordan W, et al. Coherent oscillations: a mechanism of feature linking in the visual cortex? Multiple electrode and correlation analyses in the cat. *Biol Cybernetics*. 1988;60:121–130.

24. Engel AK, Konig P, Kreiter AK, Singer W. Interhemispheric synchronization of oscillatory neuronal responses in cat visual cortex. *Science*. 1991;252:1177–1179.

25. Singer W, Gray CM. Visual feature integration and the temporal correlation hypothesis. *Annu Rev Neurosci*. 1995;18:555–586.

26. Gray CM. The temporal correlation hypothesis of visual feature integration: still alive and well. *Neuron*. 1999;24(1):31–47, 111–125.

27. Von der Malsburg C. Binding in models of perception and brain function. *Curr Opin Neurobiol*. 1995;5:520–526.

28. Fries P. A mechanism for cognitive dynamics: neuronal communication through neuronal coherence. *Trends Cogn Sci*. 2005;9(10):474–480.

29. Fries P, Nikolic D, Singer W. The gamma cycle. *Trends Neurosci*. 2007;30(7):309–316.

30. Bressler SL. The gamma wave: a cortical information carrier? [news]. *Trends Neurosci*. 1990;13:161–162.

31. Spydell JD, Ford MR, Sheer DE. Task dependent cerebral lateralization of the 40 Hertz EEG rhythm. *Psychophysiology*. 1979;16:347–350.

32. Sheer DE, Grandstaff NW, Benignus VA. Behavior and 40-c.-sec. electrical activity in the brain. *Psychol Rep*. 1966;19:1333–1334.

33. DeFrance J, Sheer DE. Focused arousal, 40-Hz EEG, and motor programming. In: Giannitrapani D, Murri L, eds. *The EEG of Mental Activities*. New York: Karger; 1988:153–168.

34. Pantev C, Makeig S, Hoke M, Galambos R, Hampson S, Gallen C. Human auditory evoked gamma-band magnetic fields. *Proc Nat Acad Sci USA*. 1991;88:8996–9000.

35. Galambos R, Makeig S, Talmachoff PJ. A 40-Hz auditory potential recorded from the human scalp. *Proc Nat Acad Sci USA*. 1981;78:2643–2647.

36. Pantev C. Evoked and induced gamma-band activity of the human cortex. *Brain Topography*. 1995;7(4):321–330.

37. Barth DS, MacDonald KD. Thalamic modulation of high-frequency oscillating potentials in auditory cortex. *Nature*. 1996;383(6595):78–81.

38. Basar-Eroglu C, Struber D, Schurmann M, Stadler M, Basar E. Gamma-band responses in the brain: a short review of psychophysiological correlates and functional significance. *Int J Psychophysiol*. 1996;24(1-2):101–112.

39. Sheer DE. Focused arousal and the cognitive 40-Hz event-related potentials: differential diagnosis of Alzheimer's disease. *Prog Clin Biol Res*. 1989;317:79–94.

40. Tiitinen H, Sinkkonen J, Reinikainen K, Alho K, Lavikainen J, Naatanen R. Selective attention enhances the auditory 40-Hz transient response in humans. *Nature*. 1993;364(6432):59–60.

41. Curio G. Linking 600-Hz "spikelike" EEG/MEG wavelets ("sigma-bursts") to cellular substrates: concepts and caveats. *J Clin Neurophysiol*. 2000;17(4):377–396.

42. Curio G. Ultrafast EEG activities. In: Niedermeyer E, Lopes da Silva F, eds. *Electroencephalography: Basic Principles, Clinical Applications, and Related Fields*. Fifth ed. Philadelphia: Lippincott, Williams, & Wilkins; 2005:495–504.

43. Pfurtscheller G, Lopes da Silva FH. Event-related EEG/MEG synchronization and desynchronization: basic principles. *Clin Neurophysiol*. 1999;110(11):1842–1857.

44. Kalcher J, Pfurtscheller G. Discrimination between phase-locked and non-phase-locked event-related EEG activity. *Electroencephalogr Clin Neurophysiol*. 1995;94:381–384.

45. Crone NE, Boatman D, Gordon B, Hao L. Induced electrocorticographic gamma activity during auditory perception. *Clin Neurophysiol*. 2001;112(4):565–582.

46. Spencer KM, Polich J. Poststimulus EEG spectral analysis and P300: attention, task, and probability. *Psychophysiology*. 1999;36(2):220–232.

47. Demiralp T, Ademoglu A, Comerchero M, Polich J. Wavelet analysis of P3a and P3b. *Brain Topography*. 2001;13(4):251–267.

48. Herrmann CS, Knight RT. Mechanisms of human attention: event-related potentials and oscillations. *Neurosci Biobehav Rev*. 2001;25(6):465–476.

49. Pfurtscheller G, Neuper C, Kalcher J. 40-Hz oscillations during motor behavior in man. *Neurosci Lett*. 1993;164:179–182.

50. Pfurtscheller G, Flotzinger D, Neuper C. Differentiation between finger, toe and tongue movement in man based on 40 Hz EEG. *Electroencephalogr Clin Neurophysiol*. 1994;90:456–460.

51. Tallon-Baudry C, Bertrand O, Delpuech C, Pernier J. Stimulus specificity of phase-locked and non-phase-locked 40 Hz visual responses in human. *J Neurosci*. 1996;16(13):4240–4249.

52. Ray S, Jouny CC, Crone NE, Boatman D, Thakor NV, Franaszczuk PJ. Human ECoG analysis during speech perception using matching pursuit: a comparison between stochastic and dyadic dictionaries. *IEEE Trans Biomed Eng*. 2003;50(12):1371–1373.

53. Ray S, Niebur E, Hsiao SS, Sinai A, Crone NE. High-frequency gamma activity (80–150Hz) is increased in human cortex during selective attention. *Clin Neurophysiol*. 2008;119(1):116–133.

54. Steinschneider M, Fishman YI, Arezzo JC. Spectrotemporal analysis of evoked and induced electroencephalographic responses in primary auditory cortex (A1) of the awake monkey. *Cereb Cortex*. 2008;18:610–625.

55. Crone NE, Korzeniewska A, Franaszczuk PJ. Cortical gamma responses: searching high and low. *Int J Psychophysiol*. 2011;79(1):9–15.

56. Lachaux JP, Axmacher N, Mormann F, Halgren E, Crone NE. High-frequency neural activity and human cognition: past, present and possible future of intracranial EEG research. *Progr Neurobiol*. 2012;98(3):279–301.

57. Miller KJ, Leuthardt EC, Schalk G, et al. Spectral changes in cortical surface potentials during motor movement. *J Neurosci*. 2007;27(9):2424–2432.

58. Lachaux JP, Hoffinann D, Minotti L, Berthoz A, Kahane P. Intracerebral dynamics of saccade generation in the human frontal eye field and supplementary eye field. *Neuroimage*. 2006;30(4):1302–1312.

59. Chang EF, Rieger JW, Johnson K, Berger MS, Barbaro NM, Knight RT. Categorical speech representation in human superior temporal gyrus. *Nat Neurosci*. 2010;13(11):1428–1432.

60. Eliades SJ, Crone NE, Anderson WS, Ramadoss D, Lenz FA, Boatman-Reich D. Adaptation of high-gamma responses in human auditory association cortex. *J Neurophysiol*. 2014;112(9):2147–2163.

61. Tanji K, Suzuki K, Delorme A, Shamoto H, Nakasato N. High-frequency gamma-band activity in the basal temporal cortex during picture-naming and lexical-decision tasks. *J Neurosci*. 2005;25(13):3287–3293.

62. Lachaux JP, George N, Tallon-Baudry C, et al. The many faces of the gamma band response to complex visual stimuli. *Neuroimage*. 2005;25(2):491–501.

63. Jung J, Mainy N, Kahane P, et al. The neural bases of attentive reading. *Hum Brain Mapp*. 2008;29(10):1193–1206.

64. Crone NE, Hao L, Hart J, Jr., et al. Electrocorticographic gamma activity during word production in spoken and sign language. *Neurology*. 2001;57(11):2045–2053.

65. Crone NE, Hao L. The functional significance of event-related spectral changes (ERD/ERS) from the perspective of electrocorticography. In: Reisin RC, Nuwer MR, Hallett M, Medina C, eds. *Advances in Clinical Neurophysiology (Supp to Clin Neurophysiol)*. Vol 54. Amsterdam: Elsevier Science; 2002:435–442.

66. Gaona CM, Sharma M, Freudenburg ZV, et al. Nonuniform high-gamma (60–500 Hz) power changes dissociate cognitive task and anatomy in human cortex. *J Neurosci*. 2011;31(6):2091–2100.

67. Ray S, Hsiao SS, Crone NE, Franaszczuk PJ, Niebur E. Effect of stimulus intensity on the spike-local field potential relationship in the secondary somatosensory cortex. *J Neurosci*. 2008;28(29):7334–7343.

68. Suffczynski P, Crone NE, Franaszczuk PJ. Afferent inputs to cortical fast-spiking interneurons organize pyramidal cell network oscillations at high-gamma frequencies (60–200 Hz). *J Neurophysiol*. 2014;112(11):3001–3011.

69. Ray S, Crone NE, Niebur E, Franaszczuk PJ, Hsiao SS. Neural correlates of high-gamma oscillations (60–200 Hz) in macaque local field potentials and their potential implications in electrocorticography. *J Neurosci*. 2008;28(45):11526–11536.

70. Fries P, Reynolds JH, Rorie AE, Desimone R. Modulation of oscillatory neuronal synchronization by selective visual attention. *Science*. 2001;291(5508):1560–1563.

71. Steinmetz PN, Roy A, Fitzgerald PJ, Hsiao SS, Johnson KO, Niebur E. Attention modulates synchronized neuronal firing in primate somatosensory cortex. *Nature*. 2000;404(6774):187–190.

72. Brovelli A, Lachaux JP, Kahane P, Boussaoud D. High gamma frequency oscillatory activity dissociates attention from intention in the human premotor cortex. *Neuroimage*. 2005;28(1):154–164.

73. Jensen O, Kaiser J, Lachaux JP. Human gamma-frequency oscillations associated with attention and memory. *Trends Neurosci*. 2007;30(7):317–324.

74. Vidal JR, Chaumon M, O'Regan JK, Tallon-Baudry C. Visual grouping and the focusing of attention induce gamma-band oscillations at different frequencies in human magnetoencephalogram signals. *J Cogn Neurosci*. 2006;18(11):1850–1862.

75. Mesgarani N, Chang EF. Selective cortical representation of attended speaker in multi-talker speech perception. *Nature*. 2012;485(7397):233–236.

76. Martin A, Wang L, Saalmann Y, et al. Modulation of intracranial field potential responses in the human large-scale attention network during a spatial attention task. *J Vis*. 2015;15(12):1055.

77. Tallon-Baudry C, Bertrand O, Henaff MA, Isnard J, Fischer C. Attention modulates gamma-band oscillations differently in the human lateral occipital cortex and fusiform gyrus. *Cereb Cortex*. 2005;15(5):654–662.

78. Potes C, Gunduz A, Brunner P, Schalk G. Dynamics of electrocorticographic (ECoG) activity in human temporal and frontal cortical areas during music listening. *Neuroimage*. 2012;61(4):841–848.

79. Cervenka MC, Corines J, Boatman-Reich DF, et al. Electrocorticographic functional mapping identifies human cortex critical for auditory and visual naming. *Neuroimage*. 2013;69:267–276.

80. Cervenka MC, Boatman-Reich DF, Ward J, Franaszczuk PJ, Crone NE. Language mapping in multilingual patients: electrocorticography and cortical stimulation during naming. *Frontiers Hum Neurosci*. 2011;5:13.

81. Edwards E, Soltani M, Deouell LY, Berger MS, Knight RT. High gamma activity in response to deviant auditory stimuli recorded directly from human cortex. *J Neurophysiol*. 2005;94(6):4269–4280.

82. Nourski KV, Howard MA. Chapter 13—Invasive recordings in the human auditory cortex. In: Aminoff MJ, Boller F, Dick FS, eds. *Handbook of Clinical Neurology*. Vol 129: Elsevier; 2015:225–244.

83. Trautner P, Rosburg T, Dietl T, et al. Sensory gating of auditory evoked and induced gamma band activity in intracranial recordings. *Neuroimage*. 2006;32(2):790–798.

84. Mesgarani N, Cheung C, Johnson K, Chang EF. Phonetic feature encoding in human superior temporal gyrus. *Science*. 2014;343(6174):1006–1010.

85. Engell AD, McCarthy G. Repetition suppression of face-selective evoked and induced EEG recorded from human cortex. *Hum Brain Mapp*. 2014;35(8):4155–4162.

86. Rangarajan V, Hermes D, Foster BL, et al. Electrical stimulation of the left and right human fusiform gyrus causes different effects in conscious face perception. *J Neurosci*. 2014;34(38):12828–12836.

87. Iijima M, Mase R, Osawa M, Shimizu S, Uchiyama S. Event-related synchronization and desynchronization of high-frequency electroencephalographic activity during a visual go/no-go paradigm. *Neuropsychobiology*. 2015;71(1):17–24.

88. Voytek B, Kayser AS, Badre D, et al. Oscillatory dynamics coordinating human frontal networks in support of goal maintenance. *Nat Neurosci*. 2015;18(9):1318–1324.

89. Noy N, Bickel S, Zion-Golumbic E, et al. Intracranial recordings reveal transient response dynamics during information maintenance in human cerebral cortex. *Hum Brain Mapp*. 2015;36(10):3988–4003.

90. Brown EC, Rothermel R, Nishida M, et al. In vivo animation of auditory-language-induced gamma-oscillations in children with intractable focal epilepsy. *Neuroimage*. 2008;41(3):1120–1131.

91. Kojima K, Brown EC, Rothermel R, et al. Multimodality language mapping in patients with left-hemispheric language dominance on Wada test. *Clin Neurophysiol*. 2012;123(10):1917–1924.

92. Edwards E, Nagarajan SS, Dalal SS, et al. Spatiotemporal imaging of cortical activation during verb generation and picture naming. *Neuroimage*. 2010;50(1):291–301.

93. Wu HC, Nagasawa T, Brown EC, et al. γ-oscillations modulated by picture naming and word reading: intracranial recording in epileptic patients. *Clin Neurophysiol*. 2011;122(10):1929–1942.

94. Kingyon J, Behroozmand R, Kelley R, et al. High-gamma band frontotemporal coherence as a measure of functional connectivity in speech motor control. *Neuroscience*. 2015;305:15–25.

95. Korzeniewska A, Franaszczuk PJ, Crainiceanu CM, Kus R, Crone NE. Dynamics of large-scale cortical interactions at high gamma frequencies during word production: event related causality (ERC) analysis of human electrocorticography (ECoG). *Neuroimage*. 2011;56(4):2218–2237.

96. Flinker A, Korzeniewska A, Shestyuk AY, et al. Redefining the role of Broca's area in speech. *Proc Nat Acad Sci USA*. 2015;112(9):2871–2875.

97. Bailey PD, Zacà D, Basha MM, et al. Presurgical fMRI and DTI for the prediction of perioperative motor and language deficits in primary or metastatic brain lesions. *J Neuroimag*. 2015;25(5):776–784.

98. Ojemann G, Ojemann J, Lettich E, Berger M. Cortical language localization in left, dominant hemisphere. An electrical stimulation mapping investigation in 117 patients. *J Neurosurg*. 1989;71(3):316–326.

99. Lesser R, Gordon B, Uematsu S. Electrical stimulation and language. *J Clin Neurophysiol*. 1994;11:191–204.

100. Blume WT, Jones DC, Pathak P. Properties of after-discharges from cortical electrical stimulation in focal epilepsies. *Clin Neurophysiol*. 2004;115(4):982–989.

101. Hamberger MJ. Cortical language mapping in epilepsy: a critical review. *Neuropsychol Rev*. 2007;17(4):477–489.

102. Lesser RP, Lüders H, Klem G, Dinner DS, Morris HH, Hahn J. Cortical after-discharge and functional response thresholds: results of extraoperative testing. *Epilepsia*. 1984;25:615–621.

103. Lesser RP, Luders H, Klem G, Dinner DS, Morris HH, Hahn J. Ipsilateral trigeminal sensory responses to cortical stimulation by subdural electrodes. *Neurology*. 1985;35:1760–1763.

104. Viventi J, Kim DH, Vigeland L, et al. Flexible, foldable, actively multiplexed, high-density electrode array for mapping brain activity in vivo. *Nat Neurosci*. 2011;14(12):1599–1605.

105. Manning JR, Jacobs J, Fried I, Kahana MJ. Broadband shifts in local field potential power spectra are correlated with single-neuron spiking in humans. *J Neurosci*. 2009;29(43):13613–13620.

106. Ray S, Maunsell JH. Different origins of gamma rhythm and high-gamma activity in macaque visual cortex. *PLoS Biol*. 2011;9(4):e1000610.

107. Genetti M, Tyrand R, Grouiller F, et al. Comparison of high gamma electrocorticography and fMRI with electrocortical stimulation for localization of somatosensory and language cortex. *Clin Neurophysiol*. 2015;126(1):121–130.

108. Khursheed F, Tandon N, Tertel K, Pieters TA, Disano MA, Ellmore TM. Frequency-specific electrocorticographic correlates of working memory delay period fMRI activity. *Neuroimage*. 2011;56(3):1773–1782.

109. Siero JCW, Hermes D, Hoogduin H, Luijten PR, Ramsey NF, Petridou N. BOLD matches neuronal activity at the mm scale: A combined 7 T fMRI and ECoG study in human sensorimotor cortex. *Neuroimage*. 2014;101:177–184.

110. Lachaux JP, Fonlupt P, Kahane P, et al. Relationship between task-related gamma oscillations and BOLD signal: new insights from combined fMRI and intracranial EEG. *Hum Brain Mapp*. 2007;28(12):1368–1375.

111. Brunner P, Ritaccio AL, Lynch TM, et al. A practical procedure for real-time functional mapping of eloquent cortex using electrocorticographic signals in humans. *Epilepsy Behav*. 2009;15(3):278–286.

112. Schalk G, Leuthardt EC, Brunner P, Ojemann JG, Gerhardt LA, Wolpaw JR. Real-time detection of event-related brain activity. *Neuroimage*. 2008;43(2):245–249.

113. Schalk G, McFarland DJ, Hinterberger T, Birbaumer N, Wolpaw JR. BCI2000: a general-purpose brain-computer interface (BCI) system. *IEEE Trans Biomed Eng*. 2004;51(6):1034–1043.

114. Ogawa H, Kamada K, Kapeller C, Hiroshima S, Prueckl R, Guger C. Rapid and minimum invasive functional brain mapping by real-time visualization of high gamma activity during awake craniotomy. *World Neurosurg*. 2014;82(5):912.e911–910.

115. Ruescher J, Iljina O, Altenmüller D-M, Aertsen A, Schulze-Bonhage A, Ball T. Somatotopic mapping of natural upper- and lower-extremity movements and speech production with high gamma electrocorticography. *Neuroimage*. 2013;81:164–177.

116. Vansteensel MJ, Bleichner MG, Dintzner LT, et al. Task-free electrocorticography frequency mapping of the motor cortex. *Clin Neurophysiol*. 2013;124(6):1169–1174.

117. Cheung C, Chang EF. Real-time, time-frequency mapping of event-related cortical activation. *J Neural Eng*. 2012;9(4):046018.

118. Arya R, Wilson JA, Vannest J, et al. Electrocorticographic language mapping in children by high-gamma synchronization during spontaneous conversation: comparison with conventional electrical cortical stimulation. *Epilepsy Res*. 2015;110:78–87.

119. Bauer PR, Vansteensel MJ, Bleichner MG, et al. Mismatch between electrocortical stimulation and electrocorticography frequency mapping of language. *Brain Stimul*. 2013;6(4):524–531.

120. Miller KJ, Abel TJ, Hebb AO, Ojemann JG. Rapid online language mapping with electrocorticography. *J Neurosurg Pediatr*. 2011;7(5):482–490.

121. Sinai A, Bowers CW, Crainiceanu CM, et al. Electrocorticographic high gamma activity versus electrical cortical stimulation mapping of naming. *Brain*. 2005;128(Pt 7):1556–1570.

122. Crone NE, Hart J, Jr., Boatman D, Lesser RP, Gordon B. Regional cortical activation during language and related tasks identified by direct cortical electrical recording. *Brain Language*. 1994;47(3):466–468.

123. Wu M, Wisneski K, Schalk G, et al. Electrocorticographic frequency alteration mapping for extraoperative localization of speech cortex. *Neurosurgery*. 2010;66(2):E407–409.

124. Binder JR, Desai RH, Graves WW, Conant LL. Where is the semantic system? A critical review and meta-analysis of 120 functional neuroimaging studies. *Cerebral Cortex.* 2009;19(12):2767–2796.

125. Wang Y, Fifer MS, Flinker A, et al. Spatial-temporal functional mapping of language at the bedside with electrocorticography. *Neurology.* 2016;86(13):1181–1189.

126. Hamberger MJ, Williams AC, Schevon CA. Extraoperative neurostimulation mapping: Results from an international survey of epilepsy surgery programs. *Epilepsia.* 2014;55(6):933–939.

127. Wu JY, Sankar R, Lerner JT, Matsumoto JH, Vinters HV, Mathern GW. Removing interictal fast ripples on electrocorticography linked with seizure freedom in children. *Neurology.* 2010;75(19):1686–1694.

128. FitzGerald DB, Cosgrove GR, Ronner S, et al. Location of language in the cortex: a comparison between functional MR imaging and electrocortical stimulation. *Am J Neuroradiol.* 1997;18(8):1529–1539.

129. Pouratian N, Bookheimer SY, Rex DE, Martin NA, Toga AW. Utility of preoperative functional magnetic resonance imaging for identifying language cortices in patients with vascular malformations. *J Neurosurg.* 2002;97(1):21–32.

130. Roux FE, Boulanouar K, Lotterie JA, Mejdoubi M, LeSage JP, Berry I. Language functional magnetic resonance imaging in preoperative assessment of language areas: correlation with direct cortical stimulation. *Neurosurgery.* 2003;52(6):1335–1345.

131. Rutten GJ, Ramsey NF, van Rijen PC, Noordmans HJ, van Veelen CW. Development of a functional magnetic resonance imaging protocol for intraoperative localization of critical temporoparietal language areas. *Ann Neurol.* 2002;51(3):350–360.

132. Menon V, Freeman WJ, Cutillo BA, et al. Spatio-temporal correlations in human gamma band electrocorticograms. *Electroencephalogr Clin Neurophysiol.* 1996;98:89–102.

133. Brindley GS, Craggs MD. The electrical activity in the motor cortex that accompanies voluntary movement. *J Physiol.* 1972;223(1):28P–29P.

134. Leuthardt EC, Schalk G, J.R. W, Ojemann JG, Moran DW. A brain-computer interface using electrocorticographic signals in humans. *J Neural Eng.* 2004;1:63–71.

135. Kubanek J, Miller KJ, Ojemann JG, Wolpaw JR, Schalk G. Decoding flexion of individual fingers using electrocorticographic signals in humans. *J Neural Eng.* 2009;6(6):66001.

136. Anderson NR, Blakely T, Schalk G, Leuthardt EC, Moran DW. Electrocorticographic (ECoG) correlates of human arm movements. *Exp Brain Res.* 2012;223(1):1–10.

137. Acharya S, Fifer MS, Benz HL, Crone NE, Thakor NV. Electrocorticographic amplitude predicts finger positions during slow grasping motions of the hand. *J Neural Eng.* 2010;7(4):046002.

138. Schalk G, Kubanek J, Miller KJ, et al. Decoding two-dimensional movement trajectories using electrocorticographic signals in humans. *J Neural Eng.* 2007;4(3):264–275.

139. Chestek CA, Gilja V, Blabe CH, et al. Hand posture classification using electrocorticography signals in the gamma band over human sensorimotor brain areas. *J Neural Eng.* 2013;10(2):026002.

140. Fifer M, Hotson G, Wester B, et al. Simultaneous neural control of simple reaching and grasping with the modular prosthetic limb using intracranial EEG. *IEEE Trans Neural Systems Rehab Eng.* 2014;22(3):695–705.

141. Yanagisawa T, Hirata M, Saitoh Y, et al. Electrocorticographic control of a prosthetic arm in paralyzed patients. *Ann Neurol.* 2012;71(3):353–361.

142. Wang W, Collinger JL, Degenhart AD, et al. An electrocorticographic brain interface in an individual with tetraplegia. *PLoS One.* 2013;8(2):e55344.

143. Hotson G, McMullen DP, Fifer MS, et al. Individual finger control of a modular prosthetic limb using high-density electrocorticography in a human subject. *J Neural Eng.* 2016;13(2):026017.

144. Bouchard KE, Mesgarani N, Johnson K, Chang EF. Functional organization of human sensorimotor cortex for speech articulation. *Nature.* 2013;495(7441):327–332.

145. Bouchard KE, Chang EF. Neural decoding of spoken vowels from human sensory-motor cortex with high-density electrocorticography. *Conference proceedings of the Annual International Conference of the IEEE Engineering in Medicine and Biology Society.* 2014;2014:6782–6785.

146. Bragin A, Engel J, Jr., Wilson CL, Fried I, Mathern GW. Hippocampal and entorhinal cortex high-frequency oscillations (100–500 Hz) in human epileptic brain and in kainic acid–treated rats with chronic seizures. *Epilepsia.* 1999;40(2):127–137.

147. Bragin A, Engel J, Jr., Wilson CL, Fried I, Buzsaki G. High-frequency oscillations in human brain. *Hippocampus.* 1999;9(2):137–142.

148. Jirsch JD, Urrestarazu E, LeVan P, Olivier A, Dubeau F, Gotman J. High-frequency oscillations during human focal seizures. *Brain.* 2006;129(Pt 6):1593–1608.

149. Zijlmans M, Jiruska P, Zelmann R, Leijten FSS, Jefferys JGR, Gotman J. High-frequency oscillations as a new biomarker in epilepsy. *Ann Neurol.* 2012;71(2):169–178.

150. Jacobs J, Staba R, Asano E, et al. High-frequency oscillations (HFOs) in clinical epilepsy. *Prog Neurobiol.* 2012;98(3):302–315.

151. Staba JR, Wilson CL, Bragin A, Fried I, Engel J. Quantitative analysis of high-frequency oscillations (80–500 Hz) recorded in human epileptic hippocampus and entorhinal cortex. *J Neurophysiol.* 2002;88(4):1743–1752.

152. Engel J, Jr., Wilson C, Bragin A. Advances in understanding the process of epileptogenesis based on patient material: what can the patient tell us? *Epilepsia.* 2003;44(Suppl 12):60–71.

153. Grenier F, Timofeev I, Steriade M. Neocortical very fast oscillations (ripples, 80–200 Hz) during seizures: intracellular correlates. *J Neurophysiol.* 2003;89(2):841–852.

154. Bragin A, Wilson CL, Almajano J, Mody I, Engel J, Jr. High-frequency oscillations after status epilepticus: epileptogenesis and seizure genesis. *Epilepsia.* 2004;45(9):1017–1023.

155. Levesque M, Bortel A, Gotman J, Avoli M. High-frequency (80–500 Hz) oscillations and epileptogenesis in temporal lobe epilepsy. *Neurobiol Dis.* 2011;42(3):231–241.

156. Salami P, Levesque M, Gotman J, Avoli M. Distinct EEG seizure patterns reflect different seizure generation mechanisms. *J Neurophysiol.* 2015;113(7):2840–2844.

157. Avoli M, de Curtis M. GABAergic synchronization in the limbic system and its role in the generation of epileptiform activity. *Prog Neurobiol.* 2011;95(2):104–132.

158. Ylinen A, Bragin A, Nadasdy Z, et al. Sharp wave-associated high-frequency oscillation (200 Hz) in the intact hippocampus: network and intracellular mechanisms. *J Neurosci.* 1995;15(1 Pt 1):30–46.

159. Klausberger T, Marton LF, Baude A, Roberts JD, Magill PJ, Somogyi P. Spike timing of dendrite-targeting bistratified cells during hippocampal network oscillations in vivo. *Nat Neurosci.* 2004;7(1):41–47.

160. Shiri Z, Manseau F, Levesque M, Williams S, Avoli M. Activation of specific neuronal networks leads to different seizure onset types. *Ann Neurol.* 2016;79(3):354–365.

161. Jiruska P, Finnerty GT, Powell AD, Lofti N, Cmejla R, Jefferys JG. Epileptic high-frequency network activity in a model of non-lesional temporal lobe epilepsy. *Brain.* 2010;133(Pt 5):1380–1390.

162. Jones RT, Barth AM, Ormiston LD, Mody I. Evolution of temporal and spectral dynamics of pathologic high-frequency oscillations (pHFOs) during epileptogenesis. *Epilepsia.* 2015;56(12):1879–1889.

163. Winden KD, Bragin A, Engel J, Geschwind DH. Molecular alterations in areas generating fast ripples in an animal model of temporal lobe epilepsy. *Neurobiol Dis.* 2015;78:35–44.

164. Bragin A, Benassi SK, Kheiri F, Engel J, Jr. Further evidence that pathologic high-frequency oscillations are bursts of population spikes derived from recordings of identified cells in dentate gyrus. *Epilepsia.* 2011;52(1):45–52.

165. Dzhala VI, Staley KJ. Mechanisms of fast ripples in the hippocampus. *J Neurosci.* 2004;24(40):8896–8906.

166. Ibarz JM, Foffani G, Cid E, Inostroza M, Menendez de la Prida L. Emergent dynamics of fast ripples in the epileptic hippocampus. *J Neurosci.* 2010;30(48):16249–16261.

167. Simeone TA, Simeone KA, Samson KK, Kim do Y, Rho JM. Loss of the Kv1.1 potassium channel promotes pathologic sharp waves and high frequency oscillations in in vitro hippocampal slices. *Neurobiol Dis.* 2013;54:68–81.

168. Jiruska P, Csicsvari J, Powell AD, et al. High-frequency network activity, global increase in neuronal activity, and synchrony expansion precede epileptic seizures in vitro. *J Neurosci.* 2010;30(16):5690–5701.

169. Staba RJ, Wilson CL, Bragin A, Jhung D, Fried I, Engel J, Jr. High-frequency oscillations recorded in human medial temporal lobe during sleep. *Ann Neurol.* 2004;56(1):108–115.

170. Staba RJ, Frighetto L, Behnke EJ, et al. Increased fast ripple to ripple ratios correlate with reduced hippocampal volumes and neuron loss in temporal lobe epilepsy patients. *Epilepsia.* 2007;48(11):2130–2138.

171. Bragin A, Wilson CL, Fields T, Fried I, Engel J, Jr. Analysis of seizure onset on the basis of wideband EEG recordings. *Epilepsia.* 2005;46(Suppl 5):59–63.

172. Benar CG, Chauviere L, Bartolomei F, Wendling F. Pitfalls of high-pass filtering for detecting epileptic oscillations: a technical note on "false" ripples. *Clin Neurophysiol.* 2010;121(3):301–310.

173. Amiri M, Lina JM, Pizzo F, Gotman J. High frequency oscillations and spikes: separating real HFOs from false oscillations. *Clin Neurophysiol.* 2016;127(1):187–196.

174. Yuval-Greenberg S, Tomer O, Keren AS, Nelken I, Deouell LY. Transient induced gamma-band response in EEG as a manifestation of miniature saccades. *Neuron.* 2008;58(3):429–441.

175. Jacobs J, LeVan P, Chander R, Hall J, Dubeau F, Gotman J. Interictal high-frequency oscillations (80–500 Hz) are an indicator of seizure onset areas independent of spikes in the human epileptic brain. *Epilepsia*. 2008;49(11):1893–1907.
176. Crepon B, Navarro V, Hasboun D, et al. Mapping interictal oscillations greater than 200 Hz recorded with intracranial macroelectrodes in human epilepsy. *Brain*. 2010;133(Pt 1):33–45.
177. Zelmann R, Mari F, Jacobs J, Zijlmans M, Dubeau F, Gotman J. A comparison between detectors of high frequency oscillations. *Clin Neurophysiol*. 2012;123(1):106–116.
178. Dumpelmann M, Jacobs J, Kerber K, Schulze-Bonhage A. Automatic 80–250Hz "ripple" high frequency oscillation detection in invasive subdural grid and strip recordings in epilepsy by a radial basis function neural network. *Clin Neurophysiol*. 2012;123(9):1721–1731.
179. Burnos S, Hilfiker P, Surucu O, et al. Human intracranial high frequency oscillations (HFOs) detected by automatic time-frequency analysis. *PloS One*. 2014;9(4).
180. von Ellenrieder N, Andrade-Valenca LP, Dubeau F, Gotman J. Automatic detection of fast oscillations (40–200 Hz) in scalp EEG recordings. *Clin Neurophysiol*. 2012;123(4):670–680.
181. Fisher RS, Webber WR, Lesser RP, Arroyo S, Uematsu S. High-frequency EEG activity at the start of seizures. *J Clin Neurophysiol*. 1992;9(3):441–448.
182. Allen PJ, Fish DR, Smith SJ. Very high-frequency rhythmic activity during SEEG suppression in frontal lobe epilepsy. *Electroencephalogr Clin Neurophysiol*. 1992;82(2):155–159.
183. Worrell GA, Parish L, Cranstoun SD, Jonas R, Baltuch G, Litt B. High-frequency oscillations and seizure generation in neocortical epilepsy. *Brain*. 2004;127(Pt 7):1496–1506.
184. Wu JY, Koh S, Sankar R, Mathern GW. Paroxysmal fast activity: an interictal scalp EEG marker of epileptogenesis in children. *Epilepsy Res*. 2008;82(1):99–106.
185. Yamazaki M, Chan D, Tovar-Spinoza Z, et al. Interictal epileptogenic fast oscillations on neonatal and infantile EEGs in hemimegalencephaly. *Epilepsy Res*. 2009;83(2-3):198–206.
186. Kobayashi K, Oka M, Akiyama T, et al. Very fast rhythmic activity on scalp EEG associated with epileptic spasms. *Epilepsia*. 2004;45(5):488–496.
187. Akiyama T, Otsubo H, Ochi A, et al. Focal cortical high-frequency oscillations trigger epileptic spasms: confirmation by digital video subdural EEG. *Clin Neurophysiol*. 2005;116(12):2819–2825.
188. Ramachandrannair R, Ochi A, Imai K, et al. Epileptic spasms in older pediatric patients: MEG and ictal high-frequency oscillations suggest focal-onset seizures in a subset of epileptic spasms. *Epilepsy Res*. 2008;78(2-3):216–224.
189. Urrestarazu E, Chander R, Dubeau F, Gotman J. Interictal high-frequency oscillations (100–500 Hz) in the intracerebral EEG of epileptic patients. *Brain*. 2007;130(Pt 9):2354–2366.
190. Kobayashi K, Agari T, Oka M, et al. Detection of seizure-associated high-frequency oscillations above 500Hz. *Epilepsy Res*. 2010;88(2-3):139–144.
191. Guggisberg AG, Kirsch HE, Mantle MM, Barbaro NM, Nagarajan SS. Fast oscillations associated with interictal spikes localize the epileptogenic zone in patients with partial epilepsy. *Neuroimage*. 2008;39(2):661–668.
192. Brazdil M, Halamek J, Jurak P, et al. Interictal high-frequency oscillations indicate seizure onset zone in patients with focal cortical dysplasia. *Epilepsy Res*. 2010;90(1-2):28–32.
193. Urrestarazu E, Jirsch JD, LeVan P, et al. High-frequency intracerebral EEG activity (100–500 Hz) following interictal spikes. *Epilepsia*. 2006;47(9):1465–1476.
194. Kobayashi K, Jacobs J, Gotman J. Detection of changes of high-frequency activity by statistical time-frequency analysis in epileptic spikes. *Clin Neurophysiol*. 2009;120(6):1070–1077.
195. Jacobs J, LeVan P, Chatillon CE, Olivier A, Dubeau F, Gotman J. High-frequency oscillations in intracranial EEGs mark epileptogenicity rather than lesion type. *Brain*. 2009;132:1022–1037.
196. Ferrari-Marinho T, Perucca P, Mok K, et al. Pathologic substrates of focal epilepsy influence the generation of high-frequency oscillations. *Epilepsia*. 2015;56(4):592–598.
197. Bagshaw AP, Jacobs J, LeVan P, Dubeau F, Gotman J. Effect of sleep stage on interictal high-frequency oscillations recorded from depth macroelectrodes in patients with focal epilepsy. *Epilepsia*. 2009;50(4):617–628.
198. Frauscher B, von Ellenrieder N, Dubeau F, Gotman J. EEG desynchronization during phasic REM sleep suppresses interictal epileptic activity in humans. *Epilepsia*. 2016;57(6):879–888.
199. Sakuraba R, Iwasaki M, Okumura E, et al. High-frequency oscillations are less frequent but more specific to epileptogenicity during rapid eye movement sleep. *Clin Neurophysiol*. 2016;127(1):179–186.
200. Dumpelmann M, Jacobs J, Schulze-Bonhage A. Temporal and spatial characteristics of high-frequency oscillations as a new biomarker in epilepsy. *Epilepsia*. 2015;56(2):197–206.
201. Nariai H, Matsuzaki N, Juhasz C, et al. Ictal high-frequency oscillations at 80–200 Hz coupled with delta phase in epileptic spasms. *Epilepsia*. 2011;52(10):E130–E134.
202. van 't Klooster MA, Zijlmans M, Leijten FS, Ferrier CH, van Putten MJ, Huiskamp GJ. Time-frequency analysis of single pulse electrical stimulation to assist delineation of epileptogenic cortex. *Brain*. 2011;134(Pt 10):2855–2866.
203. Khosravani H, Mehrotra N, Rigby M, et al. Spatial localization and time-dependent changes of electrographic high frequency oscillations in human temporal lobe epilepsy. *Epilepsia*. 2009;50(4):605–616.
204. Jacobs J, Zelmann R, Jirsch J, et al. High-frequency oscillations (80–500 Hz) in the preictal period in patients with focal seizures. *Epilepsia*. 2009;50(7):1780–1792.
205. Weiss SA, Banks GP, McKhann GM, Jr., et al. Ictal high-frequency oscillations distinguish two types of seizure territories in humans. *Brain*. 2013;136(Pt 12):3796–3808.
206. Zijlmans M, Jacobs J, Zelmann R, Dubeau F, Gotman J. High-frequency oscillations mirror disease activity in patients with epilepsy. *Neurology*. 2009;72(11):979–986.
207. Gotman J, Marciani MG. Electroencephalographic spiking activity, drug levels, and seizure occurrence in epileptic patients. *Ann Neurol*. 1985;17(6):597–603.
208. Gotman J, Koffler DJ. Interictal spiking increases after seizures but does not after decrease in medication. *Electroencephalogr Clin Neurophysiol*. 1989;72(1):7–15.
209. Spencer SS, Goncharova, II, Duckrow RB, Novotny EJ, Zaveri HP. Interictal spikes on intracranial recording: behavior, physiology, and implications. *Epilepsia*. 2008;49(11):1881–1892.
210. Zijlmans M, Huiskamp GM, Cremer OL, Ferrier CH, van Huffelen AC, Leijten FS. Epileptic high-frequency oscillations in intraoperative electrocorticography: the effect of propofol. *Epilepsia*. 2012;53(10):1799–1809.
211. Ochi A, Otsubo H, Donner EJ, et al. Dynamic changes of ictal high-frequency oscillations in neocortical epilepsy: using multiple band frequency analysis. *Epilepsia*. 2007;48(2):286–296.
212. Jacobs J, Zijlmans M, Zelmann R, et al. High-frequency electroencephalographic oscillations correlate with outcome of epilepsy surgery. *Ann Neurol*. 2010;67(2):209–220.
213. Modur PN, Zhang S, Vitaz TW. Ictal high-frequency oscillations in neocortical epilepsy: implications for seizure localization and surgical resection. *Epilepsia*. 2011;52(10):1792–1801.
214. Akiyama T, McCoy B, Go CY, et al. Focal resection of fast ripples on extraoperative intracranial EEG improves seizure outcome in pediatric epilepsy. *Epilepsia*. 2011;52(10):1802–1811.
215. Fujiwara H, Greiner HM, Lee KH, et al. Resection of ictal high-frequency oscillations leads to favorable surgical outcome in pediatric epilepsy. *Epilepsia*. 2012;53(9):1607–1617.
216. Kerber K, Dumpelmann M, Schelter B, et al. Differentiation of specific ripple patterns helps to identify epileptogenic areas for surgical procedures. *Clin Neurophysiol*. 2014;125(7):1339–1345.
217. Cho JR, Koo DL, Joo EY, et al. Resection of individually identified high-rate high-frequency oscillations region is associated with favorable outcome in neocortical epilepsy. *Epilepsia*. 2014;55(11):1872–1883.
218. Okanishi T, Akiyama T, Tanaka SI, et al. Interictal high-frequency oscillations correlating with seizure outcome in patients with widespread epileptic networks in tuberous sclerosis complex. *Epilepsia*. 2014;55(10):1602–1610.
219. Leung H, Zhu CX, Chan DT, et al. Ictal high-frequency oscillations and hyperexcitability in refractory epilepsy. *Clin Neurophysiol*. 2015;126(11):2049–2057.
220. van 't Klooster MA, van Klink NE, Leijten FS, et al. Residual fast ripples in the intraoperative corticogram predict epilepsy surgery outcome. *Neurology*. 2015;85(2):120–128.
221. Otsubo H, Ochi A, Imai K, et al. High-frequency oscillations of ictal muscle activity and epileptogenic discharges on intracranial EEG in a temporal lobe epilepsy patient. *Clin Neurophysiol*. 2008;119(4):862–868.
222. Ball T, Kern M, Mutschler I, Aertsen A, Schulze-Bonhage A. Signal quality of simultaneously recorded invasive and non-invasive EEG. *Neuroimage*. 2009;46(3):708–716.
223. Usui N, Terada K, Baba K, et al. Significance of very-highFrequency oscillations (over 1,000Hz) in epilepsy. *Ann Neurol*. 2015;78(2):295–302.
224. Kobayashi K, Watanabe Y, Inoue T, Oka M, Yoshinaga H, Ohtsuka Y. Scalp-recorded high-frequency oscillations in childhood sleep-induced electrical status epilepticus. *Epilepsia*. 2010;51(10):2190–2194.

225. Kobayashi K, Yoshinaga H, Toda Y, Inoue T, Oka M, Ohtsuka Y. High-frequency oscillations in idiopathic partial epilepsy of childhood. *Epilepsia.* 2011;52(10):1812–1819.

226. Iwatani Y, Kagitani-Shimono K, Tominaga K, et al. Ictal high-frequency oscillations on scalp EEG recordings in symptomatic West syndrome. *Epilepsy Res.* 2012;102(1-2):60–70.

227. Melani F, Zelmann R, Dubeau F, Gotman J. Occurrence of scalp-fast oscillations among patients with different spiking rate and their role as epileptogenicity marker. *Epilepsy Res.* 2013;106(3):345–356.

228. van Klink N, Frauscher B, Zijlmans M, Gotman J. Relationships between interictal epileptic spikes and ripples in surface EEG. *Clin Neurophysiol.* 2016;127(1):143–149.

229. Kobayashi K, Akiyama T, Oka M, Endoh F, Yoshinaga H. A storm of fast (40–150Hz) oscillations during hypsarrhythmia in West syndrome. *Ann Neurol.* 2015;77(1):58–67.

230. von Ellenrieder N, Beltrachini L, Muravchik CH, Gotman J. Extent of cortical generators visible on the scalp: effect of a subdural grid. *Neuroimage.* 2014;101:787–795.

231. van Klink N, Hillebrand A, Zijlmans M. Identification of epileptic high-frequency oscillations in the time domain by using MEG beamformer-based virtual sensors. *Clin Neurophysiol.* 2016;127(1):197–208.

232. von Ellenrieder N, Pellegrino G, Hedrich T, et al. Detection and magnetic source imaging of fast oscillations (40–160 Hz) recorded with magnetoencephalography in focal epilepsy patients. *Brain Topogr.* 2016;29(2):218–231.

233. Matsumoto A, Brinkmann BH, Matthew Stead S, et al. Pathological and physiological high-frequency oscillations in focal human epilepsy. *J Neurophysiol.* 2013;110(8):1958–1964.

234. Wang S, Wang IZ, Bulacio JC, et al. Ripple classification helps to localize the seizure-onset zone in neocortical epilepsy. *Epilepsia.* 2013;54(2):370–376.

235. Alkawadri R, Gaspard N, Goncharova II, et al. The spatial and signal characteristics of physiologic high frequency oscillations. *Epilepsia.* 2014;55(12):1986–1995.

236. von Ellenrieder N, Frauscher B, Dubeau F, Gotman J. Interaction with sleep slow waves improves discrimination of physiologic and pathologic high frequency oscillations (80–500 Hz). *Epilepsia.* 2016;57(6):869–878.

237. Engel J, Jr., Bragin A, Staba R, Mody I. High-frequency oscillations: what is normal and what is not? *Epilepsia.* 2009;50(4):598–604.

238. Le Van Quyen M, Bragin A, Staba R, Crepon B, Wilson CL, Engel J, Jr. Cell type-specific firing during ripple oscillations in the hippocampal formation of humans. *J Neurosci.* 2008;28(24):6104–6110.

239. van 't Klooster MA, Leijten FS, Huiskamp G, et al. High frequency oscillations in the intra-operative ECoG to guide epilepsy surgery ("The HFO Trial"): study protocol for a randomized controlled trial. *Trials.* 2015;16(1):422.

240. Wu SS, Veedu HPK, Lhatoo SD, Koubeissi MZ, Miller JP, Luders HO. Role of ictal baseline shifts and ictal high-frequency oscillations in stereo-electroencephalography analysis of mesial temporal lobe seizures. *Epilepsia.* 2014;55(5):690–698.

241. Kanazawa K, Matsumoto R, Imamura H, et al. Intracranially recorded ictal direct current shifts may precede high frequency oscillations in human epilepsy. *Clin Neurophysiol.* 2015;126(1):47–59.

242. Bragin A, Wilson CL, Staba RJ, Reddick M, Fried I, Engel J, Jr. Interictal high-frequency oscillations (80–500 Hz) in the human epileptic brain: entorhinal cortex. *Ann Neurol.* 2002;52(4):407–415.

34 | INTRAOPERATIVE MONITORING OF CENTRAL NEUROPHYSIOLOGY

ALAN D. LEGATT, MD, PHD, MARC R. NUWER, MD, PHD, AND RONALD G. EMERSON, MD

ABSTRACT: This chapter covers neurophysiological intraoperative monitoring (NIOM). It describes the relevant neurophysiological signals, their anatomical sources, the techniques used to record them, the manner in which they are assessed, and possible causes of intraoperative signal changes. Techniques used include electroencephalography (EEG), electromyography, and auditory, somatosensory, and motor evoked potentials. Some of these techniques can be used to localize and identify areas of cerebral cortex or the corticospinal tract. Recording of the electromyogram generated by reflex activity can be used to evaluate central nervous system function in some circumstances. EEG can be used to assess depth of anesthesia. Signals can be affected by anesthesia, and the chapter discusses various anesthetic agents, their effects on signals, and considerations for anesthetic management during NIOM. Personnel performing NIOM must be knowledgeable about the anatomy and physiology underlying the signals, the technology used to record them, and the factors (including anesthesia) that can affect them.

KEYWORDS: EEG, electroencephalography, electromyography, anesthesia, evoked potentials, intraoperative monitoring, NIOM, BAEPs, MEPs, SSEPs

PRINCIPAL REFERENCES

1. Deletis V, Shils J, eds. *Neurophysiology in Neurosurgery: A Modern Intraoperative Approach*. New York: Academic Press, 2002.
2. Galloway GM, Nuwer MR, Lopez JR, Zamel KM. *Intraoperative Neurophysiologic Monitoring*. Cambridge: Cambridge University Press. 2010.
3. Husain A, ed. *A Practical Approach to Neurophysiologic Intraoperative Monitoring*. 2nd ed. New York: Demos Medical, 2014.
4. Legatt AD. *Intraoperative Neurophysiology: Interactive Case Studies*. New York: Demos Medical Publishing, 2015.
5. Loftus CM, Biller J, Baron EM, eds. *Intraoperative Neuromonitoring*. New York: McGraw Hill, 2014.
6. Møller AR. *Intraoperative Neurophysiological Monitoring*. 3rd ed. New York: Springer, 2011.
7. Nuwer MR, ed. *Intraoperative Monitoring of Neural Function. Handbook of Clinical Neurophysiology*, Vol. 8. Amsterdam: Elsevier, 2008.
8. Simon MV, ed. *Intraoperative Neurophysiology: A Comprehensive Guide to Monitoring and Mapping*. New York: Demos Medical, 2010.
9. Zouridakis G, Papanicolaou AC. *A Concise Guide to Intraoperative Monitoring*. Boca Raton, FL: CRC Press, 2001.

1. INTRODUCTION

A variety of clinical neurophysiological techniques can be used to assess central nervous system (CNS) function during surgery in which portions of the CNS are at risk. The signals most often recorded for neurophysiological intraoperative monitoring (NIOM) are several types of evoked potentials (EPs) and the electroencephalogram (EEG). Sensory EPs are the electrical signals produced by the nervous system in response to a sensory stimulus, whereas the EEG is the ongoing electrical activity of the brain independent of sensory stimulation.

Auditory, visual, and somatosensory EPs are used as extra-operative diagnostic tests to noninvasively assess the sensory pathways within the central and peripheral nervous systems, and also to identify dysfunction of sensory organs—the eyes and the ears. Somatosensory evoked potentials (SSEPs) and auditory evoked potentials (AEPs) have also found wide utility in NIOM to detect neural compromise during surgery, when the patient is anesthetized and a conventional neurological examination cannot be performed. The anesthetic sensitivity of visual EPs limits their utility for NIOM.

The central motor tracts can also be monitored by stimulating them rostrally and recording either from muscles or from the neural motor pathways caudal to the part of the nervous system that is at risk. By analogy to SSEPs, the signals that are recorded are typically called motor evoked potentials (MEPs). The brain can be stimulated either electrically or magnetically in order to elicit MEPs. MEP recordings for extraoperative diagnostic testing are elicited by transcranial magnetic brain stimulation, because electrical stimulation would be too painful in an awake subject. But MEPs to magnetic stimulation are difficult to record consistently in anesthetized patients during surgery; intraoperative MEP monitoring is therefore typically performed using transcranial electrical stimulation (TES).

Several other neurophysiological techniques are useful for intraoperative assessment of the CNS. Direct electrical brain stimulation can be used to locate anatomical structures, including eloquent cortex, and also for monitoring of the central motor pathways in some surgical situations. Recordings of reflex activity to peripheral nerve or nerve root stimulation can be used to assess the CNS substrates of these reflexes. Continuous recording of the electromyogram (EMG), while usually done to detect mechanical stimulation or irritation of peripheral nerves, may also detect surgery-related stimulation of motor pathways within the CNS.

All of the electrophysiologic measures used for NIOM can be affected by the anesthetic regimen, including anesthetic drugs and neuromuscular blocking agents. Different anesthetic agents act via different mechanisms, and anesthetic agents affect different NIOM signals in different ways.

Personnel performing NIOM must be knowledgeable about the anatomy and physiology underlying the signals being recorded, the technology used to record them, and factors (including anesthesia) that can affect them. The practice of NIOM is subject to both governmental and hospital regulations and policies.

2. EVOKED POTENTIALS

The EP modalities commonly used for NIOM are described in this chapter. For the sensory EPs, the description includes the anatomical generators of the components that are useful for NIOM. Recording techniques, assessment of the NIOM data, causes of adverse EP changes, and typical intraoperative applications are described.

2.1. Factors Common to Multiple EP Modalities

2.1.1. RECORDING TECHNIQUES
Sensory EPs are in general too small to be seen in the raw data following a single stimulus. Signal averaging is therefore employed—multiple stimuli are delivered and the data epochs or sweeps recorded following the individual stimuli are averaged together, after rejecting those that contain large artifacts. Signal averaging (Fig. 34.1) improves the signal-to-noise ratio

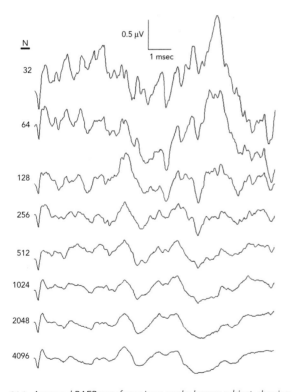

Figure 34.1. Averaged BAEP waveforms in an awake human subject, showing the improvement in the signal-to-noise ratio as the number of epochs in the average is increased. The BAEPs were elicited by right ear stimulation with rarefaction clicks delivered a rate of 11.3/sec; the number of epochs included in the average is shown to the left of each waveform. Amplifier bandpass 150–3,000 Hz, vertex (Cz) to right mastoid recording. In this and subsequent BAEP figures, Cz positivity is plotted as an upward deflection. Reprinted from Legatt AD. Intraoperative evoked potential monitoring. In: Schomer DL, Lopes da Silva FH, eds. Niedermeyer's Textbook of Electroencephalography: Basic Principles, Clinical Applications, and Related Fields. 6th ed. Philadelphia: Lippincott Williams & Wilkins, 2011:767–786, Fig. 38.1.

of the averaged EP waveforms by a factor equal to the square root of the number of sweeps included in the average[1]. If the EP data are noisy and/or the EP amplitudes are small, the number of sweeps per average may have to be increased. Conversely, if the signal-to-noise ratio of the raw data is favorable, the number of sweeps per average can be decreased, allowing averages to be acquired more frequently and thus facilitating more rapid notification to the surgeons should adverse EP changes occur.

Evoked potentials should be recorded to unilateral stimulation, so that the presence of a normal EP to stimulation of one side will not prevent recognition of an abnormal or absent EP to stimulation of the other side, as might occur if simultaneous bilateral stimulation were employed. Modern EP recording systems permit interleaving of sensory stimuli (e.g., auditory stimuli are delivered alternately to the left and to the right ears). The data sweeps are then sorted (after artifact rejection) into separate left- and right-sided averages. Thus, even though left- and right-sided averages are acquired concurrently, simultaneous bilateral stimulation is never actually delivered.

2.1.2. ASSESSMENT OF EP DATA DURING NIOM
Sensory EP amplitudes vary substantially across different subjects whereas component latencies are much more consistent. Therefore, interpretation of extraoperative EP studies performed for diagnostic purposes is predominantly based on latencies[2,3]. However, EP component amplitudes on repeated recordings in the same subject are usually quite consistent if the recording techniques and anesthesia are not altered. Moreover, if parts of the nervous system are compromised, amplitude changes may occur earlier than, or in the absence of, latency changes. Therefore, both the amplitudes and latencies should be assessed during intraoperative monitoring of SSEPs and AEPs.

For extraoperative sensory EP studies performed for diagnostic purposes, the patient's EP waveforms are compared to those recorded in a control population of normal subjects. For this comparison to be valid, the techniques used and the state of the subjects must be identical in the patient's study and in the control studies. During NIOM, the anesthetic regimen, the body temperature, the delivered stimulus intensity, and other factors will differ from patient to patient. Therefore, during NIOM each patient serves as his or her own control; EPs recorded during the time when parts of the nervous system are at risk are compared to those recorded earlier during the same operation[4]. If the anesthetic regimen or other factors that will affect the EP data are changed, the baseline amplitude and latency values should be reassessed.

2.1.3. CAUSES OF ADVERSE EP CHANGES
Changes in the signals recorded during NIOM can be classified into three categories: "true-positive" changes, which reflect compromise of the structures that the monitoring is intended to safeguard (e.g., Figs. 34.2, 34.3), changes produced by other physiological mechanisms such as anesthetic effects (e.g., Fig. 34.4) or hypothermia, and changes due to technical problems (e.g., Fig. 34.5) rather than to actual changes in neuronal function[5]. True-positive changes can reflect tissue damage due to direct mechanical or thermal injury. They can also reflect ischemia caused by compromise of the blood supply

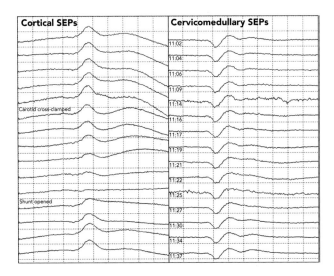

Figure 34.2. Consecutive SSEP runs recorded to left median nerve stimulation during a right carotid endarterectomy in a 78-year-old man. There was a delayed attenuation of the cortical SSEPs (left) following carotid cross-clamping. The surgeons were notified and placed a shunt; the SSEPs then returned to baseline. The patient was unchanged neurologically after the surgery. The simultaneously recorded cervicomedullary SSEPs (right) did not change, demonstrating that the left median nerve was still being stimulated and that afferent somatosensory activity was still reaching the level of the medulla. Vertical calibration: 3 μV/division. Horizontal calibration: 5 msec/division. In this and subsequent SSEP figures, negativity at input 1 is plotted as an upward deflection. Reprinted from Legatt AD. Intraoperative evoked potential monitoring. In: Schomer DL, Lopes da Silva FH, editors. Niedermeyer's Textbook of Electroencephalography: Basic Principles, Clinical Applications, and Related Fields. 6th ed. Philadelphia: Lippincott Williams & Wilkins, 2011:767–786, Fig. 38.2.

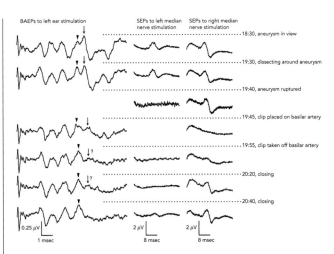

Figure 34.3. BAEP and SSEP changes due to brainstem ischemia and infarction during surgery for a basilar artery aneurysm in a 50-year-old woman. Cortical SSEPs to stimulation of both median nerves and BAEPs to left ear stimulation are shown. The aneurysm ruptured during an attempt to place a clip on it and the cortical SSEP to left median nerve stimulation disappeared. A clip was placed on the basilar artery to control the bleeding and the cortical SSEP to right median nerve then disappeared as well. A BAEP run was not obtained between the aneurysm rupture and clipping of the basilar artery, but following the clipping BAEP wave V (arrow) became delayed and attenuated, while BAEP wave IV (triangle) persisted. The cortical SSEP to right median nerve stimulation reappeared and returned to baseline; the cortical SSEP to left median nerve stimulation recovered only partially The patient suffered multiple brainstem infarcts. In the SSEP waveforms, cortical negativity is shown as an upward deflection. The first 8 msec of each SSEP waveform was cropped off to remove the large stimulus artifacts. Reprinted with permission from Legatt AD. Mechanisms of intraoperative brainstem auditory evoked potential changes. J Clin Neurophysiol. 2002;19(5):396–408; Fig. 4.

to the neural tissue (see Figs. 34.2, 34.3), by vasospasm, by generalized hypotension, or by a combination of these acting synergistically.

EPs can be lost due to technical problems such as equipment malfunction, dislodged electrodes or stimulators (see Fig. 34.5), disconnected or broken wires, and operator error (the use of incorrect protocols or settings). A variety of artifacts can obscure the EPs (Fig. 34.6). The artifact from the cavitational ultrasonic suction aspiration (CUSA) device (see Fig. 34.6C) deserves special mention, as it may manifest as a low-voltage, high-frequency artifact that obscures the EP but does not trigger automatic artifact rejection[4]. Monopolar cautery use can saturate the EP recording system's input amplifiers, preventing recording of valid EP data for some time after the cautery is stopped.

Anesthesia (see Fig. 34.4), systemic hypothermia, and hypotension can produce EP changes that do in fact reflect changes in neural function, but are different from the neural dysfunction due to surgical manipulations that the NIOM is specifically intended to detect. Irrigation of the surgical field with cold fluids can produce localized tissue hypothermia, causing reversible EP changes that resemble those that would be caused by surgical compromise of the neural tissue there (Fig. 34.7).

2.2. AEPs

The earliest electrical signals recorded following a transient auditory stimulus are generated within the cochlea, and are recorded as part of the electrocochleogram. The subsequent neurally generated signals have been divided into latency classes—short-latency AEPs (latencies<10 msec), long-latency AEPs (latencies>50 msec), and middle-latency AEPs (intermediate latencies). The long-latency AEPs are generated within cerebral cortex, including cortical association areas, and are profoundly affected by the degree to which the subject is attending to the auditory stimulus and extracting information from it. The long-latency AEPs are suppressed by surgical anesthesia, and thus are not useful for NIOM. Middle-latency AEPs are also generated within cerebral cortex, including primary auditory cortex and surrounding areas[6]. They are also markedly affected by surgical anesthesia, which limits their utility for NIOM to detect surgery-related focal neurological dysfunction. However, this anesthetic sensitivity has led to attempts to use middle-latency AEPs as an indicator of the depth of anesthesia[7].

The short-latency AEPs are the most useful AEPs for neurological and otological diagnosis because they are relatively easy to record and their waveforms and latencies are highly consistent across normal subjects[8]. They are also useful for NIOM because surgical anesthesia produces only minor changes in them[5,9,10]; some of the intraoperative changes that are observed in them may be due more to changes in body temperature than to anesthetic effects[11–13]. Although the earliest components are generated, at least in part, in the eighth

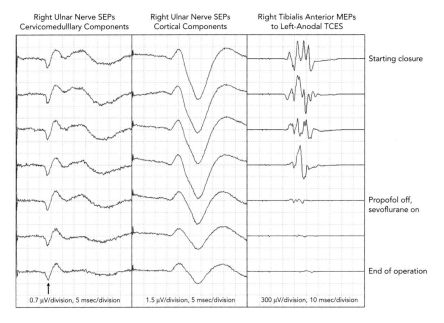

Right Ulnar Nerve SEPs
Cervicomedulllary Components

Right Ulnar Nerve SEPs
Cortical Components

Right Tibialis Anterior MEPs
to Left-Anodal TCES

Starting closure

Propofol off,
sevoflurane on

End of operation

0.7 µV/division, 5 msec/division   1.5 µV/division, 5 msec/division   300 µV/division, 10 msec/division

Figure 34.4. Anesthetic effects on cervicomedullary SSEPS (left), cortical SSEPs (center), and MEPs during surgery for revision of spinal instrumentation and fusion in a patient with a T11 compression fracture and progressive kyphosis following failure of a previous spinal fusion. TIVA had been used during most of the operation, but during closing the propofol infusion was turned off to allow propofol in body fat stores to return to the bloodstream and be metabolized, and sevoflurane was turned on to keep the patient anesthetized. The halogenated inhalational agent almost completely eliminated the MEPs. The cortical SSEPs were attenuated but not eliminated, and the cervicomedullary SSEPs were relatively unaffected. Reprinted with permission from Legatt AD. Intraoperative Neurophysiology: Interactive Case Studies. New York: Demos Medical Publishing, 2015; case 14, p. 11.

nerve, most of the components are generated in the parts of the brainstem auditory pathways; these short-latency AEPs are most commonly referred to as brainstem auditory evoked potentials (BAEPs).

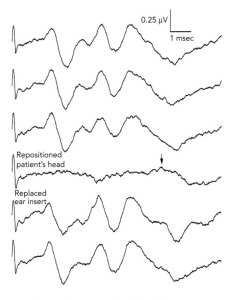

0.25 µV

1 msec

Repositioned
patient's head

Replaced
ear insert

Figure 34.5. Loss of BAEPs due to a technical problem in a patient undergoing surgery for a left-sided vestibular schwannoma. Consecutive BAEP recordings (Cz-A1 recording) to right ear stimulation are shown, with the earliest waveform at the top. During positioning of the patient's head, these BAEPs disappeared. Investigation revealed that the tube carrying the acoustic stimulus had been pulled out of the patient's ear. The tube was replaced and the BAEPs reappeared. The arrow indicates a possible delayed BAEP peak when the tube was dislodged, reflecting acoustic stimulus reaching the ear at a reduced intensity. Reprinted with permission from Legatt AD. Mechanisms of intraoperative brainstem auditory evoked potential changes. J Clin Neurophysiol. 2002;19(5):396–408, Fig. 1.

2.2.1. BAEP COMPONENTS, GENERATORS, AND RECORDING ELECTRODE LOCATIONS

BAEP components are typically recorded between the vertex (position "Cz" of the International 10-20 System) and both earlobes or both mastoids (labeled "Ai" or "Mi" for the ipsilateral ear and mastoid, respectively, and "Ac" or "Mc" for the ear and mastoid contralateral to the stimulated ear); recording the two channels provides a measure of redundancy in case one of the ear/mastoid electrodes becomes unusable during surgery and may also help in the identification of wave V (see next paragraph). Positive BAEP peaks are most often displayed as upward deflections (the opposite polarity convention from SSEPs and from EEG and EMG, in which negativity is displayed as an upward deflection), and the positive peaks in the Cz-Ai recording channel are typically labeled with Roman numerals according to the convention of Jewett and Williston[14] (Fig. 34.8). Most of the BAEP components are recorded from the scalp as far-field potentials, which means that small displacements of the recording electrodes do not significantly alter the BAEP waveform. Thus, if a CPz electrode is being placed to record lower-limb SSEPs, it can be used in place of the Cz electrode to record BAEPs, with minimal effect on the waveforms obtained. Wave I, however, is recorded as a near-field potential on the surface of the head in the vicinity of the stimulated ear.

Waves I, III, and V are the most consistent BAEP peaks, and those upon which interpretation of both extraoperative BAEP studies and intraoperative BAEP monitoring is based. Wave I is recorded as a negativity by the ipsilateral ear/mastoid electrode and is largely absent in the Cz-Ac recording (see Fig. 34.8). Wave III is typically seen in both channels, though it is smaller in Cz-Ac than in the Cz-Ai recording. Waves IV and

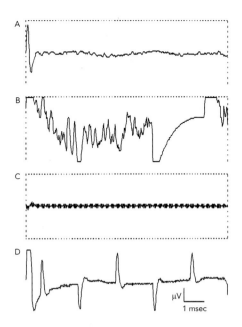

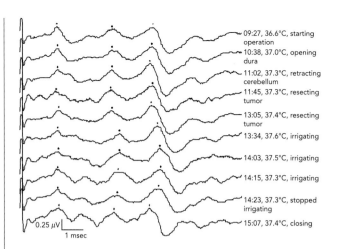

Figure 34.7. BAEPs to right ear stimulation recorded during surgery for a right cerebellopontine angle meningioma. The BAEPs were stable during cerebellar retraction and tumor resection. After the tumor had been removed, copious irrigation of the surgical field with cold fluids produced a transient prolongation of the I–III interpeak interval, reflecting slowed neural conduction within the eighth nerve resulting from local cooling. The peak latencies of waves I, III, and V are marked by the small diamonds, and the clock times, esophageal temperatures, and surgical procedures corresponding to each of the BAEP waveforms are noted at the right. Modified with permission from Legatt AD. Mechanisms of intraoperative brainstem auditory evoked potential changes. J Clin Neurophysiol. 2002;19(5):396–408, Fig. 3.

Figure 34.6. Single (unaveraged) data epochs recorded during intraoperative BAEP monitoring. A: An electrical stimulus artifact is present at the beginning of the epoch. The BAEP, which is <1 μV in amplitude, is not visible in this single epoch of raw data. B: Bipolar cautery produces a large artifact that triggers automatic artifact rejection. C: The cavitational ultrasonic surgical aspirator (CUSA) device produces a very high-frequency but low-voltage artifact that completely obliterates the neurophysiological data but does not trigger automatic artifact rejection. D: The light source of the operating microscope produces a repetitive, sharply contoured artifact that recurs at a harmonic of the line frequency but is composed of higher frequencies that would not be removed by a line-frequency notch filter. In A, B, and C, the horizontal dotted lines show the input window of the analog-to-digital converter and the threshold for automatic artifact rejection. In D, the amplifier gain was reduced to show the light source artifacts in their entirety. Voltage calibration bar: 10 μV in A, B, and C, 40 μV in D. Reprinted with permission from Legatt AD. Mechanisms of intraoperative brainstem auditory evoked potential changes. J Clin Neurophysiol. 2002;19(5):396–408, Fig. 2.

wave I. Because wave I arises from the most distal portion of the auditory nerve, it may persist after the nerve is sectioned at a more proximal location, such as during surgery for eighth nerve tumors[20, 21] (Fig. 34.10).

Subsequent BAEP components are the composites of contributions of multiple generators. The complexity of the generators of human BAEPs derives in part from the anatomy of the brainstem auditory pathways, with ascending fibers both synapsing in and bypassing various relay nuclei[22–24]. It also reflects

V are seen in both channels at similar amplitudes and typically overlap, forming a IV–V complex with variable morphology[15] (Fig. 34.9). In the Cz-Ac channel, the latency of wave IV is typically a little shorter than that in the Cz-Ai channel, and that of wave V is typically a little longer (see Fig. 34.8). The increased separation of waves IV and V in the Cz-Ac channel may make wave V easier to identify in that channel. However, if wave V in the Cz-Ac channel is followed during the surgery, the baseline latency and amplitude values should also have been obtained in the Cz-Ac channel.

Wave I originates in the first volley of action potentials in the auditory nerve as it begins in the most distal portion of the nerve[16]. It represents the same electrical phenomenon as the N1 component of the eighth nerve compound action potential in the electrocochleogram[17], and at the skin surface it appears as a negativity in a circumscribed area around the stimulated ear[18,19]. The negativity picked up by the Ai electrode gives rise to the upgoing (positive) peak in the Cz-Ai recording. Since wave I is recorded as a near-field potential around the stimulated ear, repositioning of the Ai/Mi recording electrode can substantially alter it, and alternate electrode positions can be used to obtain a clearer wave I. An electrode within the external auditory canal may pick up an even larger

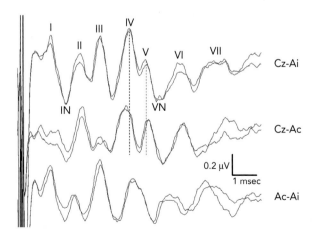

Fig. 34.8. BAEPs recorded simultaneously from three different recording electrode linkages following monaural stimulation in a normal subject. The vertical dashed lines indicate the peak latencies of waves IV and V in the Cz-Ai waveforms; these peaks are more widely separated in the Cz-Ac waveforms. Reprinted from Legatt AD. Brainstem auditory evoked potentials: Methodology, interpretation, and clinical application. In: Aminoff MJ, ed. Aminoff's Electrodiagnosis in Clinical Neurology. 6th ed. New York: Churchill Livingstone; 2012:519–552, Fig. 24-6.

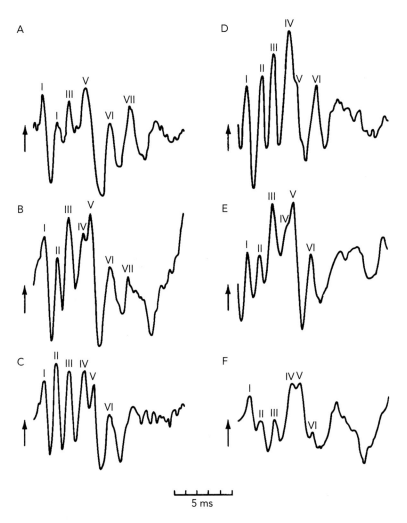

Figure 34.9. Various IV–V complex morphologies in Cz-Ai waveforms recorded in normal subjects. *Reprinted from Chiappa K, Gladstone KJ, Young RR. Brain stem auditory evoked responses. Studies of waveform variations in 50 normal human subjects. Arch Neurol. 1979;36(2):81–87, Fig. 2. Copyright © 1979 American Medical Association. All rights reserved.*

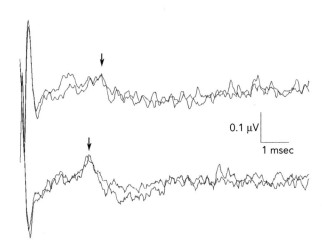

Figure 34.10. Intraoperative BAEPs to left ear stimulation recorded during surgery for left vestibular schwannomas in two different patients, showing persistence of wave I (arrows) after transection of the intracranial eighth nerve. The nerves were intentionally sacrificed to permit total resection of the tumors. *Reprinted with permission from Legatt AD. Mechanisms of intraoperative brainstem auditory evoked potential changes. J Clin Neurophysiol. 2002;19(5):396–408, Fig. 6.*

the presence of at least two bursts of activity in the auditory nerve (corresponding to the N1 and N2 components of the eighth nerve compound action potentials in the electrocochleogram), which can drive the more rostral pathways. Because of both of these factors, several different structures within the infratentorial auditory pathways may be active simultaneously, and thus contribute to the same BAEP component[16]. Wave II originates, in part, in the first auditory nerve volley (the N1 component of the eighth nerve compound action potential, which gave rise to wave I when it began in the distal eighth nerve) that has propagated to the proximal end of the auditory nerve and to the cochlear nucleus. However, this occurs simultaneously with the onset of the second auditory nerve volley (the N2 component of the eighth nerve compound action potential) in the distal nerve[17]. The latter contributes to the scalp-recorded BAEP in the same manner as the N1 component did when it was at the same location. This can cause persistence of a wave II in cases where the proximal eighth nerve has been destroyed[8].

Wave III predominantly originates in the caudal pontine tegmentum, including the region of the superior olivary complex[8]. Since ascending projections from the cochlear nucleus are bilateral, wave III may receive contributions from

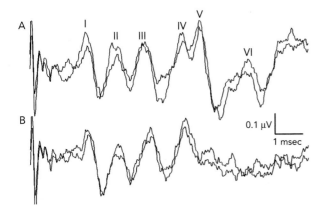

Figure 34.11. *Intraoperative BAEPs to left ear stimulation recorded during the surgery of Figure 34.2. A: Clear waves I through VI were present in these BAEPs, recorded just before the aneurysm ruptured. B: BAEPs recorded after the aneurysm had been clipped and the basilar artery had been reopened show a loss of waves V and VI; waves I through IV were unaffected. Modified from Legatt AD, Arezzo JC, Vaughan HG, Jr. The anatomic and physiologic bases of brain stem auditory evoked potentials. Neurol Clin. 1988;6(4):681–704, Fig. 9.*

brainstem auditory structures both ipsilateral and contralateral to the stimulated ear. In patients with asymmetrical lesions of the brainstem, wave III abnormalities are usually most pronounced following stimulation of the ear ipsilateral to the lesion[25–27], though occasionally they are more pronounced following contralateral stimulation[28].

The anatomical generators of waves IV and V are most likely in close anatomical proximity, since they are usually either both affected or both unaffected by brainstem lesions[28–30]. They may, however, be differentially affected[16,28,31], including by intraoperative brainstem damage (Fig. 34.11). Wave IV appears to reflect activity predominantly in ascending auditory fibers within the dorsal and rostral pons, just caudal to the inferior colliculus, while wave V predominantly reflects activity at the level of the inferior colliculus, perhaps including activity in the rostral portion of the lateral lemniscus as it terminates in the inferior colliculus[8]. As is the case with wave III, wave V abnormalities due to unilateral brainstem lesions are usually most pronounced following stimulation of the ear ipsilateral to the lesion[25–27,32,33], though there are exceptions[34,35].

Waves VI and VII are absent in some normal subjects. While they may in part reflect activity in more rostral structures such as the medial geniculate nucleus, they also receive contributions from activity in the inferior colliculus[8]; the latter generator may cause persistence of these waves in patients with auditory pathway damage rostral to the inferior colliculus. Therefore, BAEPs cannot be used to assess or monitor the auditory pathways rostral to the mesencephalon.

2.2.2. BAEP Recording Techniques

Acoustic clicks, produced by delivering trains of 100-μsec-duration electrical square pulses to the acoustic transducer, are most often used to elicit BAEPs for NIOM; brief tone pips can also be used. Since the responses to rarefaction and compression clicks may differ[36,37], extraoperative diagnostic BAEP studies typically employ a single click polarity. Stimulation with alternating click polarities and averaging the responses to rarefaction and compression clicks together is useful to cancel a large stimulus artifact and/or the cochlear microphonic, and is often employed during intraoperative BAEP monitoring.

Since headphones would be impractical for NIOM, the acoustic stimuli are typically delivered using ear inserts, incorporating foam cylinders that can be compressed and then gradually expand to achieve a tight fit with the ear canal. The foam can be covered with a thin layer of metal foil, to serve as a near-field electrode for recording of wave I from the external auditory canal. The ear insert can be held in place with bone wax or cotton padding, and secured with nonporous tape or an adhesive waterproof dressing pad[4,38]. This is to prevent fluids from entering the ear canal, where they might interfere with transmission of sound to the inner ear. The ear insert is connected to the acoustic transducer using a segment of plastic tubing. Care should be taken to ensure that this tubing remains in place during positioning of the patient and is not kinked. The time required for the acoustic signal to propagate through the tubing typically prolongs the latencies of all BAEP components by approximately 0.9 to 1.0 msec compared to those recorded using headphones. This causes no problems in the evaluation of the BAEPs, since each patient serves as his or her own control and the acoustic propagation delay is constant. Moreover, the delay helps to prevent obscuration of wave I by the electrical stimulus artifact, because (1) it prolongs the latency of wave I, helping to separate it in time from the electrical stimulus artifact (which remains simultaneous with the activation of the acoustic transducer), and (2) it permits increasing the distance between the acoustic transducer and the recording electrodes, reducing the amplitude of the electrical stimulus artifact.

The stimulus intensity delivered during intraoperative BAEP monitoring cannot be precisely controlled, due to variability in the positioning of the ear insert, but this does not cause a problem since each patient serves as his or her own control. The intensity setting chosen should be loud enough to produce a clear BAEP but not loud enough to cause ear damage. A stimulus rate of approximately 10 per second is typical, but a rate of exactly 10 Hz or another submultiple of the power line frequency should be avoided; if such a submultiple were chosen, signal averaging would not eliminate line-frequency artifact that is present in the data. Contralateral white noise masking, such as is typically used to during extraoperative diagnostic BAEP studies to prevent acoustic crosstalk, cannot be used during NIOM if left and right ear stimuli are interleaved. This is not a problem because acoustic crosstalk is much smaller with ear-insert transducers than with headphones[39]. Also, the major reason for white noise masking is to prevent acoustic crosstalk from producing a BAEP when a deaf ear is stimulated during a diagnostic BAEP study; absence of white noise masking will not prevent recognition of new auditory pathway compromise when a functioning ear is stimulated.

Typical filter settings for BAEP recordings are 100 to 150 Hz for the low-frequency (high-pass) filter and 2,500 to 3,000 Hz for the high-frequency (low-pass) filter. Line-frequency (e.g., 60 Hz) "notch" filters can be used for BAEP recordings but are of limited utility, since 60-Hz interference would have already been attenuated by the high-pass filter; a 60-Hz notch

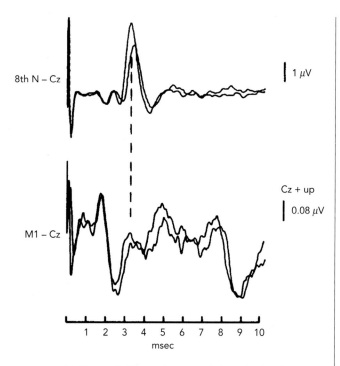

Figure 34.12. *BAEPs recorded from a platinum pad electrode placed on the intracranial eighth nerve (top) compared to surface-recorded BAEPs (bottom) during surgery in a 52-year-old woman with a left-sided intracanalicular acoustic neuroma. Note the voltage calibrations; the near-field response is considerably larger. The patient had transient BAEP changes during the resection, but BAEPs were at baseline at its end, and postoperative hearing was normal. Courtesy of Dr. Timothy A. Pedley.*

filter would not eliminate artifact that is a harmonic of 60 Hz. The analog gain depends on the input window of the analog-to-digital converter; a value of approximately 100,000 is typical.

While an averaging epoch duration of 10 msec is often used for extraoperative diagnostic BAEP recordings in adults, a longer epoch duration, typically 15 msec, should be used during intraoperative BAEP monitoring because component latencies can be prolonged by preexisting pathology, hypothermia, or intraoperative compromise of the auditory system. The choice of the number of sweeps per average will depend on the signal-to-noise ratio of the raw data. A value of 1,000 to 2,000 sweeps per average is typical.

If the risk is to the eighth nerve (e.g., during surgery for an intracanalicular eighth nerve tumor) and the surgical exposure permits placement of a recording electrode on the proximal eighth nerve, a near-field eighth nerve compound action potential that is typically much larger than the far-field BAEP can be recorded[4,40] (Fig. 34.12). This permits averaging using fewer sweeps, facilitating more frequent assessment and more rapid notification to the surgeons should adverse changes occur. Near-field recordings do not assess the auditory pathways rostral to the eighth nerve recording electrode; BAEPs would have to be recorded from the scalp at intervals to do that.

2.2.3. Assessment of BAEP Data
The peak latencies of waves I, III, and V are measured, and the amplitude of each of these components is measured with respect to the trough that follows it. The central transmission time, the interval between the peaks of waves I and V, can also

be calculated. Typical alarm criteria are a 50% drop in component amplitudes and a 1-msec increase in component latencies or in the central transmission time.

Loss or delay of wave V with preservation of waves I and III (see Fig. 34.11) reflects compromise of the auditory pathways within the brainstem, between the lower pons and the mesencephalon. If the BAEP changes are unilateral or asymmetrical, the predominant pathology is most often, though not always, ipsilateral to the ear whose stimulation gives the most abnormal BAEPs.

Loss or delay of waves III and V with preservation of wave I (see Fig. 34.10) reflects compromise of the eighth nerve (though not of its most distal part, within the modiolus) or of the lower pons. If the BAEP changes are unilateral or asymmetrical, the predominant pathology is again most often ipsilateral to the ear whose stimulation gives the most abnormal BAEPs.

Loss or delay of wave I and subsequent waves (Fig. 34.13), if not due to technical problems, reflects cochlear dysfunction. This may include cochlear ischemia or infarction due to compromise of the blood supply to the cochlea.

2.2.4. Causes of Adverse BAEP Changes
As previously noted, true-positive BAEP changes may reflect direct mechanical or thermal tissue injury as well as ischemia/

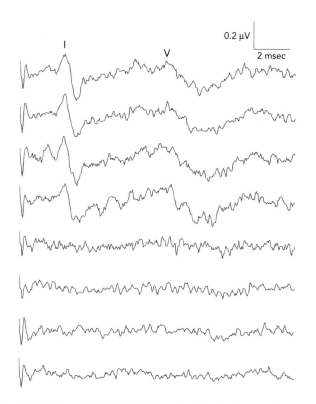

Figure 34.13. *Consecutive BAEPs to left ear stimulation (earliest waveform at the top) recorded in a patient undergoing surgery for a left acoustic neuroma. A clear wave I and a poorly formed wave V were initially present and were stable during the initial dissection, but all BAEP components disappeared simultaneously during dissection within the internal auditory canal and remained absent through the end of the operation. This was most likely due to interruption of the blood supply to the cochlea via the internal auditory artery. Reprinted with permission from Legatt AD. Mechanisms of intraoperative brainstem auditory evoked potential changes. J Clin Neurophysiol. 2002;19(5):396–408, Fig. 7.*

infarction. Two situations specifically pertaining to BAEPs deserve special mention: internal auditory artery compromise and eighth nerve stretch.

The cochlea receives its blood supply from the intracranial circulation via the internal auditory artery. This vessel, which is usually a branch of the anterior inferior cerebellar artery, passes through the internal auditory canal alongside the eighth nerve[41]. Damage to this artery will cause cochlea ischemia or infarction, affecting wave I and all subsequent BAEP components. Internal auditory artery compromise probably accounts for most of the cases where all BAEP components, including wave I, are suddenly lost (see Fig. 34.13), during surgery for cerebellopontine angle tumors[42].

When the cerebellum is retracted to gain access to the cerebellopontine angle (e.g., for a cerebellopontine angle tumor or during microvascular decompression surgery), this also moves the brainstem away from the internal auditory meatus and stretches the eighth nerve, which can cause hearing loss. BAEP monitoring can be used to detect excessive eighth nerve stretch (Fig. 34.14) and to notify the surgeons that the retraction needs to be reduced or readjusted. Uncorrected excessive traction on the eighth nerve can lead to avulsion of the distal nerve from the cochlea[43], causing hearing loss.

Drilling of bone produces high noise levels in both ears via bone conduction, and can alter the BAEPs due to acoustic masking[44], simulating cochlear dysfunction. This would represent a change due to physiological factors; it is not a "true-positive" change reflecting compromise of the auditory system. It is best to pause BAEP recording during drilling.

2.2.5. Typical Intraoperative Applications of BAEPs

BAEPs can be used for NIOM of the ears, the eighth nerves, and the infratentorial auditory pathways up through the level of the mesencephalon. They are not useful for monitoring the

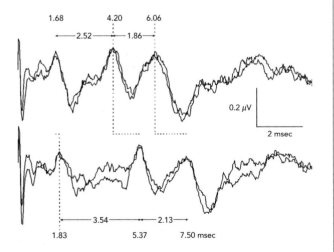

Figure 34.14. *Intraoperative BAEPs to right ear stimulation recorded during surgery for a right acoustic neuroma, showing two runs recorded prior to (top) and after (bottom) retraction of the cerebellum. The most prominent change in the BAEPs was an increase in the I–III interpeak interval of >1 msec, reflecting stretching of the eighth nerve. The smaller change in the III–V interpeak interval may reflect effects of the retraction on the brainstem. Reprinted with permission from Legatt AD. Mechanisms of intraoperative brainstem auditory evoked potential changes. J Clin Neurophysiol. 2002;19(5):396–408, Fig. 5.*

thalamus (medial geniculate) or the auditory pathways within the cerebrum. They are most often used to monitor surgery for eighth nerve tumors such as vestibular schwannomas (formerly called acoustic neuromas) and for tumors or vascular abnormalities within the posterior fossa, both extra-axial and within the brainstem. BAEPs are also useful to detect excessive eighth nerve stretch, which can lead to hearing loss, from cerebellar retraction during surgery in the cerebellopontine angle, such as microvascular decompression procedures[45].

2.3. SSEPs

While SSEPs can be elicited by mechanical stimulation, for NIOM and for extraoperative diagnostic studies SSEPs are elicited by electrical stimulation of mixed peripheral nerves, most often the median and ulnar nerves in the upper extremities and the peroneal and posterior tibial nerves in the lower extremities[46] (Fig. 34.15). Components generated in the peripheral nerves, the spinal cord, the brainstem, and cerebral cortex can be identified. SSEP components are typically named by their scalp polarity and their average latency in unanesthetized normal subjects; for example, N20 is a negativity with a typical latency of 20 msec.

Upper-extremity SSEPs are most often elicited by stimulation of the median or ulnar nerves just proximal to the wrist. Median nerve SSEPs are most often used for extraoperative diagnostic SSEP studies, because of the common occurrence of a degree of ulnar neuropathy at the elbow; carpal tunnel syndrome will not affect them because the stimulation site is proximal to the wrist. Sensory fibers of the median nerve gain access to the spinal cord through the C6 and C7 spinal roots[47]. If the spinal cord pathways were compromised at a level below C6, the afferent activity traversing the C6 nerve root could generate SSEPs and mask the presence of more caudal spinal cord dysfunction. Thus, median nerve SSEPs by themselves are not adequate for monitoring the spinal cord below the C6 level. Similarly, ulnar nerve SSEPs are not adequate for monitoring the spinal cord below the C8 level, because sensory fibers of the ulnar nerve gain access to the spinal cord through the C8 and T1 nerve roots[47].

In the lower extremity, the common peroneal nerve is typically stimulated at the level of the knee, behind the head of the fibula. The posterior tibial nerve is stimulated at the ankle, behind the medial malleolus; this permits recording of the peripheral nerve compound action potential behind the knee, which can help in the determination of the cause of a change in the more rostrally recorded SSEPs. Other advantages of posterior tibial nerve SSEPs as compared to peroneal nerve SSEPs are that (1) posterior tibial nerve SSEPs are typically larger[48], (2) stimulating electrodes at the ankle are usually easier to reach and replace than those at the knee should they become dislodged during surgery, when the patient is draped, and (3) if the patient is not pharmacologically paralyzed, posterior tibial nerve stimulation causes less patient movement than does peroneal nerve stimulation. If posterior tibial nerve SSEPs cannot be used due to peripheral neuropathy, the anatomy at the ankle, or a distal amputation, then peroneal nerve SSEPs offer another way to monitor the afferent somatosensory pathways from the legs.

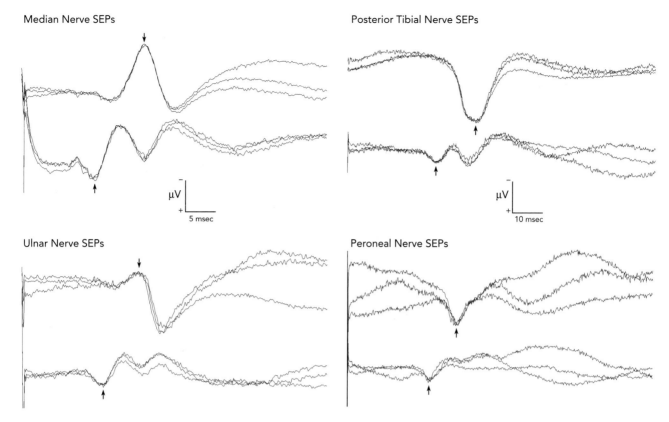

Median Nerve SEPs

Posterior Tibial Nerve SEPs

μV
5 msec

μV
10 msec

Ulnar Nerve SEPs

Peroneal Nerve SEPs

Figure 34.15. *Examples of the four most common SSEPs used for NIOM, recorded in four different patients. Data from three consecutive runs are superimposed. The arrows indicate the primary cortical SSEPs (upper waveforms in each pair) and the cervicomedullary SSEP components (lower waveforms in each pair). Vertical calibration bar = 1 μV for the cortical SSEPs to peroneal nerve stimulation, 2 μV for the cortical SSEPs to median nerve and to posterior tibial nerve stimulation, and 1.5 μV for all of the other waveforms.* Reprinted from Legatt AD. Intraoperative evoked potential monitoring. In: Schomer DL, Lopes da Silva FH, eds. Niedermeyer's Textbook of Electroencephalography: Basic Principles, Clinical Applications, and Related Fields. 6th ed. Philadelphia: Lippincott Williams & Wilkins; 2011:767–786, Fig. 38.16.

Similar to auditory EPs, a complex series of SSEPs with latencies ranging from a few msec to hundreds of msec can be recorded following a single peripheral nerve shock. The shorter-latency SSEP components, generated in the peripheral nerves, in the spinal cord, and at the level of the cervicomedullary junction, are relatively insensitive to anesthetic effects. The primary cortical SSEP components—N20 to stimulation of the median or ulnar nerve at the wrist, P37 to stimulation of the posterior tibial nerve at the ankle, and P27 to stimulation of the peroneal nerve at the knee—are affected more by anesthesia (see Fig. 34.4), but can be recorded and used for NIOM if the anesthesia is not excessive. Longer-latency SSEP components are even more attenuated by anesthesia, and may be completely suppressed, which limits their utility for NIOM. Thus, SSEPs can be used to monitor the central somatosensory pathways only up through the level of primary somatosensory cortex.

2.3.1. SSEP COMPONENTS, GENERATORS, AND RECORDING ELECTRODE LOCATIONS

For extraoperative diagnostic studies of upper-limb SSEPs, the signal generated by the afferent peripheral nerve volley as it traverses the brachial plexus is typically recorded by an electrode at Erb's point as the N9 component. This can also be done during NIOM, but in some cases Erb's point is too close to the surgical field, or the positioning of the patient may preclude

secure placement of an electrode there. The afferent peripheral volley can also be recorded by an electrode near the nerve at, or just proximal to, the elbow; use of a reference electrode on the lateral or medial aspect of the limb, at the same level, maximizes in-phase cancellation of the electrocardiogram[4]. Axillary electrodes are another alternative to Erb's point electrodes[49]. The peripheral nerve volley to posterior tibial nerve stimulation is recorded from a midline electrode behind the knee, referred to either the lateral or medial aspect of that knee or to the midline electrode on the other knee.

Components originating in the gray matter of the spinal cord at the level of root entry, N13 following median nerve stimulation and N22 following posterior tibial nerve stimulation, are used during clinical SSEP studies[2] but are of limited utility during NIOM. They are often small and difficult to record, their recording sites may be too close to the surgical field, and they are generated caudal to the CNS structures that the NIOM is intended to safeguard.

Activity in the afferent somatosensory pathways at the level of the dorsal column nucleus/cervicomedullary junction is typically recorded as a far-field potential, P14 for upper limb stimulation and P31 for posterior tibial nerve stimulation (see Fig. 34.15), with the positivity of the equivalent dipole field directed upwards and anteriorly and the negativity directed downwards and posteriorly. These cervicomedullary far-field potentials are best recorded between an electrode in the area

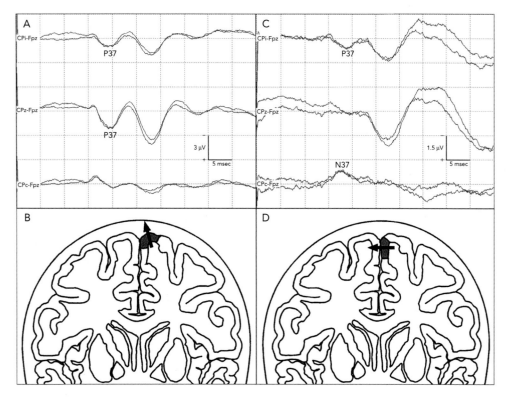

Figure 34.16. *Extraoperative recordings of cortical SSEPs to posterior tibial nerve stimulation during diagnostic SSEP testing in two different patients, and P37 generator locations (gray shading) and equivalent dipole orientations (arrows) that would explain them. A P37 component that is largest in the midline (**A**) is explained by an almost vertically oriented P37 dipole (**B**). A P37 component that is "paradoxical," largest over the hemisphere ipsilateral to the stimulated nerve and inverted over the contralateral hemisphere (**C**), is explained by a generator in the mesial wall of the hemisphere that produces a horizontally oriented P37 dipole (**D**). Note that an electrode at CPz would not pick up a P37 component that is suitable for NIOM in the example shown in **C**. The larger peak that follows P37 has a wider distribution; suppression by anesthesia makes it not useful for NIOM. Reprinted from Legatt AD. Intraoperative evoked potential monitoring. In: Schomer DL, Lopes da Silva FH, eds. Niedermeyer's Textbook of Electroencephalography: Basic Principles, Clinical Applications, and Related Fields. 6th ed. Philadelphia: Lippincott Williams & Wilkins, 2011:767–786, Fig. 38.17.*

where the dipole field is positive and one in which the dipole field is negative. In extraoperative diagnostic SSEP studies, these components are typically recorded between the dorsal scalp and a noncephalic electrode[2]. During NIOM, recording electrode pairs with such large inter-electrode distances tend to pick up more noise. A forehead-to-inion recording linkage can also pick up the SSEP components generated at the level of the cervicomedullary junction; if the inion is within the surgical field, a forehead-to-earlobe recording linkage can also be used[50].

The primary cortical SSEP to upper limb stimulation, N20, is recorded from the scalp over the parietal region contralateral to the stimulated arm, for example at positions CP3 and CP4 of the International 10-10 System[51] for right arm and left arm stimulation, respectively. The reference can be either the electrode over the other parietal region (CPi, ipsilateral to the stimulus) or an electrode on the forehead. Recordings to a forehead reference may also contain the N18 component, which is generated in the rostral brainstem (upper pons or lower mesencephalon), caudal to the thalamus[52]. If SSEPs are being used to monitor the cerebrum, a CPc-Cpi recording linkage can be used to cancel the N18 component, which has a symmetrical distribution over the top of the head[53], to ensure that the SSEPs being monitored are entirely of cerebral origin. However, if the spinal cord is being monitored, the use of a forehead reference

may give a somewhat larger SSEP waveform, and is acceptable because N18 and N20 would both be affected by spinal cord dysfunction.

The scalp topographies of the primary cortical SSEPs to lower-limb stimulation—P37 following posterior tibial nerve stimulation at the ankle and P27 following peroneal nerve stimulation at the knee—vary from one subject to another because of anatomical variability in the location and orientation of the foot area of primary somatosensory cortex[54]. These components are typically largest in the midline or over the parietal area ipsilateral to the stimulated limb—a so-called paradoxical localization (Fig. 34.16). Preoperative SSEPs studies can be performed to determine the optimal location for recording electrodes for NIOM of lower-limb SSEPs in each individual patient, or electrodes can be placed at multiple recording positions (e.g., CP3, CPz, and CP4) to permit adequate recording of the cortical SSEPs in all patients no matter what the scalp topographies of their cortical SSEPs are.

The primary cortical SSEP to median or ulnar nerve stimulation (N20) is generated in the posterior bank of the central sulcus (Fig. 34.17) and thus inverts in polarity across the central sulcus in recordings from the cortical surface[55–57]. This inversion can be used to identify the central sulcus during resective surgery[58–60]. For this application, the SSEPs are typically recorded from metal disk electrodes embedded in a sheet

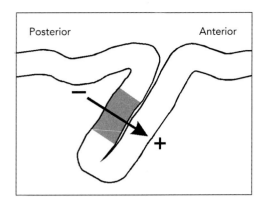

Figure 34.17. Diagram showing generation of the N20/P20 component of the median nerve SSEP in primary somatosensory cortex located in the posterior bank of the central sulcus (shaded area). The arrow represents the equivalent voltage dipole produced by activation of this area of cortex. Reprinted with permission from Legatt AD, Kader A. Topography of the initial cortical component of the median nerve somatosensory evoked potential: relationship to central sulcus anatomy. J Clin Neurophysiol. 2000;17(3):321–325, Fig. 1.

of Silastic that is placed on the exposed cortical surface after the dura is opened. Electrode strips containing several electrodes arranged in a linear array can be used, but use of an electrode grid containing a rectangular grid of electrodes may make identification of the central sulcus easier and faster[61]. SSEPs recorded from the cortical surface may also be used to monitor for compromise of cortical somatosensory tracts during resection of cerebral lesions or during surgery for aneurysms or vascular malformations when the craniotomy opening permits placement of cortical surface electrodes.

2.3.2. SSEP Recording Techniques

SSEPs are elicited using a pair of stimulating electrodes over each tested peripheral nerve, with the cathode proximal to prevent the possibility of anodal block of the afferent signal. Either surface electrodes or subdermal needle stimulating electrodes can be used. The spacing between the surface electrodes, or between the skin entry points of needle electrodes, should be ~3 cm. If subdermal needles are used, they should be directed away from each other; otherwise, the tips could be too close to each other and the stimulating current could travel between them without effectively stimulating the underlying nerve. If surface cup electrodes with electrode gel are used, care should be taken to ensure that the gel does not leak out and form a salt bridge between the paired stimulating electrodes, since this would shunt the stimulus current between them. Were this to happen, the nerve would not be stimulated but the stimulating equipment would not indicate an open-circuit condition[4].

During extraoperative SSEP studies, the stimulus intensity is typically adjusted to just above the threshold level necessary to obtain a consistent muscle twitch, so as not to cause undue patient discomfort. During NIOM, higher stimulus intensities are used, to give a safety margin should the efficacy of peripheral nerve stimulation decrease during the surgery due to technical factors, such as the development of edema that would increase the distance between the nerve and the stimulating electrodes.

Peripheral nerve stimulation is typically accomplished using trains of 200-μsec-duration constant-current stimulus

pulses. Stimulus rates of 2 to 8 per second have been used for SSEP monitoring, but rates that are exact submultiples of the line frequency (e.g., 5 or 6 Hz in North America) should be avoided; if such a submultiple were chosen, signal averaging would not eliminate line-frequency artifact that is present in the data. Typical filter settings are 5 to 30 Hz for the low-frequency (high-pass) filter and 1,000 to 3,000 Hz for the high-frequency (low-pass) filter. Line-frequency (e.g., 60 Hz) "notch" filters should not be used for SSEP recordings because they can cause a "ringing" oscillatory artifact[62].

The epoch or sweep duration used for averaging should be at least twice the latency of the longest EP component that is of interest. A typical epoch duration for recording of upper-limb SSEPs is 50 msec; epoch durations in the 80- to 100-msec range are appropriate for recording of lower-limb SSEPs. The choice of the number of sweeps per average will depend on the signal-to-noise ratio of the raw data, and may range from 200 to 1,000. SSEPs recorded from the cortical surface are typically much larger than those recorded from the scalp, and the number of sweeps per average can be smaller.

In some patients with spinal cord lesions, the volleys along the afferent pathways may be sufficiently desynchronized that the cortical and cervicomedullary SSEP components are not identifiable. In such patients, recording electrodes placed directly on the spinal cord rostral to the lesion may pick up signals that are sufficiently reproducible to be used for NIOM[4].

2.3.3. Assessment of SSEP Data

The peak latencies of the peripheral nerve potentials (if applicable), the cervicomedullary far-field potentials, and the primary cortical SSEPs are measured, and the amplitude of each of these components is measured with respect to the following peak of the opposite polarity. Depending on the configuration of the SSEP and the degree to which the SSEP waveform is contaminated by lower-frequency noise, it may also be useful to measure the amplitude of the SSEP peak with respect to the preceding peak of the opposite polarity or with respect to the baseline level of the waveform preceding the SSEP. Typical alarm criteria are a 50% drop in component amplitudes and a 10% increase in component latencies.

If the rostrally recorded SSEPs are lost, recording of the peripheral nerve compound action potential permits immediate categorization of the cause of the SSEP change. If the peripheral nerve compound action potential also disappears, the cause of the SSEP change is most likely due to either technical factors leading to inadequate stimulation of the peripheral nerve or mechanical or ischemic compromise of the peripheral nerve in the limb. If the peripheral nerve compound action potential persists but the rostral SSEPs disappear, the cause is most likely compromise of the afferent somatosensory pathways due to surgical manipulations, and the surgeons should be notified accordingly.

If the region of the neuraxis that is at risk is caudal to the cervicomedullary junction (e.g., the spinal cord), then both the primary cortical SSEPs and the cervicomedullary far-field SSEP components are generated rostral to the region that is at risk, and either may serve to monitor the condition of the spinal cord. If, however, the part of the nervous system that is at risk during the surgery is above the cervicomedullary junction, then the subcortical far-field potentials can be used to verify that the peripheral nerves are being adequately stimulated and that the afferent activity has reached the level of the cervicomedullary junction, but the cortical potentials must be examined to assess the region of the brain or brainstem that is at risk during the operation (see Fig. 34.2).

2.3.4. Causes of Adverse SSEP Changes

As with all NIOM, true-positive SSEP changes may reflect direct mechanical or thermal tissue injury as well as ischemia/infarction of the tissue due to compromise of its blood supply (see Figs. 34.2, 34.3). Since cortical SSEPs are affected by surgical anesthesia much more than are cervicomedullary SSEPs (see Fig. 34.4), increases in the anesthetic regimen can cause SSEP changes that resemble the effects of surgery-related compromise of the intracranial somatosensory pathways (compare Fig. 34.2 and Fig. 34.4, left and center).

During aortic surgery with retrograde bypass via the femoral artery, anterograde blood flow in the femoral artery is blocked, and the peripheral nerve in that leg may become ischemic. This may lead to disappearance of all SSEP components, including the peripheral nerve components, to stimulation of that leg following the placement of the femoral artery catheter. The absence of the peripheral nerve volley would preclude NIOM of the central somatosensory pathways from that leg.

Compression of the peripheral nerve in a limb or limb ischemia due to positioning of the limb may also lead to attenuation or disappearance of the SSEPs to stimulation of a nerve in that limb. Recording of the peripheral nerve SSEP in that limb may help to recognize that situation. If peripheral nerve SSEPs are not being recorded, investigations to determine the cause of an adverse change in the rostral SSEPs should include assessment of the stimulated limb.

If the constant-current SSEP stimulator is unable to deliver the preset current level, most contemporary NIOM equipment will indicate a high-impedance or open-circuit stimulus condition, which can help to identify technical problems with stimulation such as broken wires or dislodged electrodes. If, however, the paired stimulating electrodes are short-circuited together, as by a salt bridge, then the nerve will not be stimulated effectively and the SSEPs will deteriorate, but the equipment will not indicate the error condition.

As previously mentioned, an increase in the anesthetic concentration can cause attenuation and latency prolongation of the cortical SSEPs that resembles SSEP changes caused by somatosensory pathway compromise. If the region of the neuraxis at risk is caudal to the cervicomedullary junction and cervicomedullary far-field SSEPs adequate for NIOM are obtained, they can be used to determine whether the changes in the cortical SSEPs are due to anesthesia or to surgical manipulations.

2.3.5. Typical Intraoperative Applications of SSEPs

SSEPs can be used to monitor the condition of the central somatosensory pathways during surgery on the brain, brainstem, or spinal cord that places those structures at risk or during orthopedic surgery that poses a risk to the spinal cord (Fig. 34.18). Neural structures are at risk of ischemic injury during vascular surgery on the aorta or on the carotid arteries, and during surgery for aneurysms or arteriovenous malformations of vessels that supply the brain and spinal cord.

During surgery on the thoracic and lumbar spine, the brachial plexus or nerves in the arms may be stretched due to the

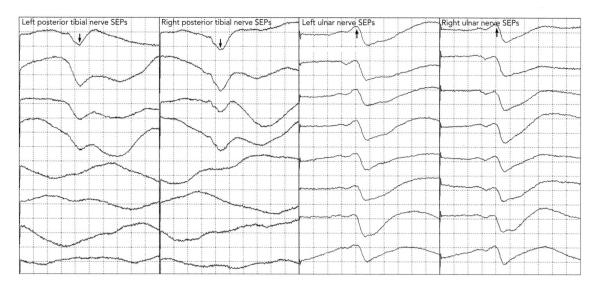

Figure 34.18. Consecutive SSEP runs recorded during spinal instrumentation and fusion surgery for congenital kyphoscoliosis with multiple hemivertebrae in a 15-year-old boy; only the cortical SSEPs are shown. The lower-limb SSEPs and MEPs disappeared bilaterally during placement of pedicle screws; upper-limb SSEPs and MEPs remained present. The surgeons were notified and the most recently placed screws were removed. A wakeup test was performed and the patient had left leg weakness. The patient was reanesthetized and the remaining hardware was removed. Postoperatively the patient had motor and sensory deficits in the left leg, with subsequent improvement. Shown here are the cortical SSEPs from the last four runs recorded before the adverse changes (top) and the first four runs recorded after them (bottom). The arrows indicate the primary cortical SSEP components (P37 for posterior tibial nerve stimulation and N20 for ulnar nerve stimulation). Calibrations: 10 msec/division and 1.5 µV/division for posterior tibial nerve SSEPs, 5 msec/division and 2 µV/division for ulnar nerve SSEPs. Reprinted from Legatt AD. Intraoperative evoked potential monitoring. In: Schomer DL, Lopes da Silva FH, eds. Niedermeyer's Textbook of Electroencephalography: Basic Principles, Clinical Applications, and Related Fields. 6th ed. Philadelphia: Lippincott Williams & Wilkins, 2011:767–786, Fig. 38.19.

positioning of the patient's arms. Monitoring of upper-limb SSEPs can be used to detect nerve stretch during surgery[63,64], permitting intraoperative correction of the arm positioning to reduce postoperative morbidity.

Afferent somatosensory activity is carried rostrally, within the spinal cord, in both the dorsal columns and the spinotha-lamic tracts. However, due to the slower conduction velocities and temporal dispersion within the spinothalamic tracts, the activity in them does not contribute significantly to the earliest SSEP components generated in the brain. The rostral SSEPs used for NIOM are mediated almost entirely by the dorsal columns[54,65] and therefore directly assess only that portion of the spinal cord that is supplied by the posterior spinal arteries. Since intraoperative spinal cord damage during spinal surgery may be on a vascular basis[66], SSEP monitoring may fail to detect ischemic spinal cord compromise that involves the anterior spinal artery territory but spares the dorsal columns; SSEPs may also remain unchanged following mechanical trauma limited to the anterior spinal cord. Therefore, SSEP monitoring may fail to detect damage that is limited to the motor tracts in the anterolateral funiculus of the spinal cord[67-69]. Fortunately such "false-negative" SSEP studies are rare; surgical situations that compromise the anterior spinal cord usually compromise the posterior spinal cord as well. MEP monitoring was developed to directly monitor the central motor pathways.

Even if MEPs are employed during surgery on the spinal cord, SSEPs should still be monitored. Because of the anatomical separation between the somatosensory and motor pathways and their different blood supplies, the somatosensory pathways can be damaged without effects on the motor pathways[70,71], and SSEPs may show changes in the absence of MEP changes during NIOM[72].

2.4. MEPs

MEP monitoring is used to directly assess the motor pathways within the brain and spinal cord during surgery. If the dura is opened and motor cortex is accessible, MEPs can be elicited by direct cortical stimulation, but most often the brain is stimulated through the intact skull using transcranial electrical stimulation (TES). As discussed in Chapter 43, transcranial magnetic stimulation is of limited use in anesthetized patients.

Stimulation of the spinal cord rostral to the region that is at risk coupled with recording of responses from peripheral nerves in the legs has been proposed as another way of monitoring the spinal cord motor tracts[73], but the responses obtained in this way predominantly reflect retrograde conduction within somatosensory fibers in the dorsal columns[74]. Therefore, like SSEPs, they may fail to detect intraoperative damage to the corticospinal tracts[75]. Responses recorded from muscles may be mediated both by descending motor tracts and by retrograde conduction in somatosensory tracts with reflex connections to the alpha motor neurons[76-78]; thus, they also do not convey the desired specificity. The only way to be sure that the signals being monitored are mediated solely by the motor tracts within the spinal cord is to stimulate rostral to the somatosensory synapses in the dorsal column nuclei[79].

2.4.1. MEP COMPONENTS, GENERATORS, AND RECORDING ELECTRODES

MEPs to TES can be recorded from the spinal cord or from muscles. Myogenic MEPs ("M-waves"), recorded from muscles (Fig. 34.19, left), are more sensitive to anesthetic effects than are the other EPs commonly used for NIOM (see Fig. 34.4) due to anesthetic effects at the anterior horn cell synapse, and total

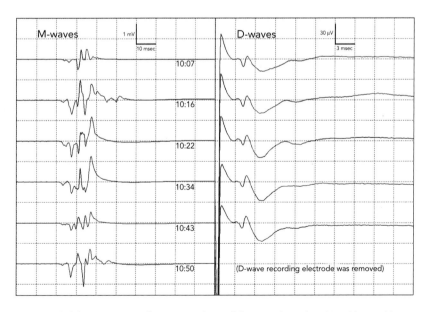

Figure 34.19. M-waves and D-waves recorded during resection of a recurrent glioma of the cervical spinal cord in a 22-year-old woman. Left: Consecutive recordings of M-waves in right hand muscles to multiple-pulse TES with the anode on the left. Right: D-waves recorded from an epidural electrode placed over the spinal cord caudal to the tumor to single-pulse TES with the anode on the left. D-waves were recorded more frequently than M-waves; the D-wave runs included in this figure are those that were recorded closest in time to the M-waves that are shown. M-waves are single sweeps; D-waves are averages of the responses to 25 stimuli. Tumor resection was completed at 10:34. Reprinted from Legatt AD. Intraoperative evoked potential monitoring. In: Schomer DL, Lopes da Silva FH, eds. Niedermeyer's Textbook of Electroencephalography: Basic Principles, Clinical Applications, and Related Fields. 6th ed. Philadelphia: Lippincott Williams & Wilkins, 2011:767–786, Fig. 38.20.

intravenous anesthesia (TIVA; e.g., a combination of propofol and narcotic infusions) with avoidance of any inhalational agents may be required to record MEPs in some patients. M-waves will also be attenuated or eliminated by neuromuscular blockade (NMB). They may be recordable under partial NMB, but that NMB should be maintained by a continuous infusion of paralytic drug rather than by intermittent bolus doses[80].

MEPs recorded from the spinal cord ("D-waves") (see Fig. 34.19, right) are generated by propagating action potentials within corticospinal tract axons. They are relatively insensitive to anesthetic effects, since there are no intervening synapses between the site of corticospinal tract stimulation in the brain and the spinal cord recording site. They are also more consistent from run to run, and can be recorded in some patients in whom M-waves are not identifiable due to preexisting pathology or anesthetic effects. However, invasive electrodes must be placed close to the spinal cord to record them, and they may miss unilateral deficits if the motor tracts in the brain are stimulated bilaterally[81]. Also, M-waves can be used to monitor the lower spinal cord where D-waves are not usable, may show adverse changes earlier than D-waves when the motor tracts are compromised, and may be monitorable in some patients in whom preexisting spinal cord pathology has desynchronized the descending corticospinal tract volley so that there are no identifiable D-waves[82]. The relative advantages and disadvantages of M-waves and D-waves are described in greater detail in Legatt et al.[83]

2.4.2. MEP RECORDING TECHNIQUES

M-waves can be recorded from surface or needle electrodes placed in or over the muscles of interest, and reflect the compound motor action potentials elicited within the muscles. D-waves can be recorded using an epidural recording electrode placed percutaneously via a Tuohy needle, or by multiple contacts within a tubular electrode array that is placed within the surgical field close to the spinal cord. Sutures can be used to hold the cable leading to the electrode array in place to minimize the chances of the electrodes being dislodged during the surgery.

A high-intensity electrical stimulator is typically used to stimulate the corticospinal tract within the brain, through the intact skull. Both constant-current and constant-voltage stimulators can be used. To record M-waves to TES, a high-intensity multi-pulse stimulator is used to produce multiple closely spaced descending volleys in the corticospinal tract, so that temporal summation of the excitatory postsynaptic potentials that they produce can fire the anterior horn cells (see Chapter 43). Typical train parameters[72] are 3 to 7 stimulus pulses per train and inter-pulse intervals of 2 to 4 msec within the train. Wide-open filters (e.g., 5 to 3,000 Hz) permit recording of both lower- and higher-frequency components of the MEP waveform.

Only a small percentage of the alpha motor neuron pool is activated with each TES stimulus, and the subset of alpha motor neurons that are activated varies from run to run. Therefore, M-waves typically vary substantially in wave shape from trial to trial (see Fig. 34.19, left), and signal averaging should not be employed—nor is it required, since the single-trial myogenic

MEPs are typically quite large, often hundreds of microvolts in amplitude.

D-waves are much smaller, and signal averaging of a small number of sweeps (e.g., 5 to 25) is useful to obtain a clearer and more consistent waveform. Since there is no intervening synapse, TES with single pulses, rather than pulse train stimulation, is used. This makes it less likely that the stimulation will cause undesirable patient movement.

When TES is used to elicit M-waves, as the stimulus intensity is increased intraparenchymal current densities capable of stimulating corticospinal tract axons are produced farther and farther away from the surface of the head, and may be able to stimulate the motor pathways as far caudally as the medulla[84]. During intraoperative monitoring of the brainstem and of the corticospinal tracts within the cerebrum and of cerebral cortex, this could prevent recognition of surgery-related motor tract compromise if the motor tracts were stimulated caudal to that dysfunction. Therefore, when monitoring these surgeries, the TES stimulus intensity should be kept relatively low, for instance to a level that produces MEPs in one limb but not in multiple limbs. For example, during clipping of a middle cerebral artery aneurysm, the TES stimulus can be titrated to elicit MEPs in the contralateral arm but not in the leg, and during clipping of an anterior cerebral artery aneurysm, the TES stimulus can be titrated to elicit MEPs in the leg but not in the arm (see Legatt[85], case 36). This stimulates the motor pathways near their origins, before the motor fibers for the arm and for the leg converge in the internal capsule.

D-waves can be elicited by stimulation of subcortical white matter[86]; therefore, M-waves to multi-pulse stimulation can also be elicited by stimulation of subcortical white matter. During resection of intracerebral lesions, pulse train stimulation within the surgical cavity can be used to estimate the distance from the stimulating electrode tip to the corticospinal tract. The threshold for eliciting an MEP is measured; the distance in mm is approximately equal to the threshold in mm[87,88].

2.4.3. ASSESSMENT OF MEP DATA

D-waves are highly consistent from run to run (see Fig. 34.19, right) and are evaluated by criteria similar to those used for sensory EPs; for example, a 50% decrease in amplitude or a 10% increase in latency would constitute a significant change.

M-waves typically show substantial run-to-run variability (see Fig. 34.19, left), and uniform use of a 50% amplitude criterion would lead to an unacceptably high level of false alarms. In many centers, the alarm criterion is complete disappearance of the MEP, although a higher percentage amplitude criterion (e.g., a 75% or a 90% drop in amplitude) may also be used[83]. When evaluating M-waves, the anesthetic regimen should be taken into account. Increases in the anesthetic doses, especially the addition of an inhalational agent to an intravenous regimen, may cause substantial amplitude attenuation or eliminate the MEPs (see Fig. 34.4). In addition, during surgeries lasting several hours, MEP amplitudes tend to decrease and thresholds to elicit MEPs tend to rise, a phenomenon known as "anesthetic fade"[89,90]. This may require reassessment of the MEP baseline.

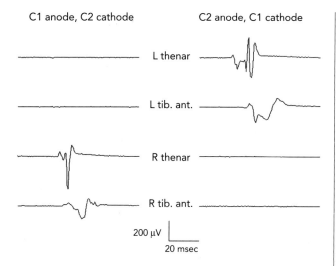

C1 anode, C2 cathode   C2 anode, C1 cathode

L thenar

L tib. ant.

R thenar

R tib. ant.

200 µV

20 msec

Figure 34.20. *Myogenic MEPs to TES between electrodes at scalp positions C1 and C2 with both TES stimulus polarities, recorded bilaterally from thenar and tibialis anterior muscles during an occipitocervical fusion. Reprinted with permission from Legatt AD, et al. ACNS guideline: Transcranial electrical stimulation motor evoked potential monitoring. J Clin Neurophysiol. 2016;33(1):42–50, Fig. 3.*

Since TES preferentially stimulates the corticospinal tract under the anode (see Chapter 43), it predominantly elicits M-waves in muscles contralateral to the anode (Fig. 34.20). M-waves may also be present in muscles contralateral to the TES cathode, but these cathodal stimulation–elicited MEPs may disappear due to anesthetic-related changes in cortical excitability, in the absence of corticospinal tract compromise. Therefore, adverse changes in cathodal stimulation–elicited MEPs should not be interpreted as definite evidence of spinal cord compromise. Instead, MEPs elicited by anodal stimulation should be used to more accurately assess the motor pathways

to the limb(s) in which the cathodal stimulation–elicited MEPs had deteriorated[91].

2.4.4. CAUSES OF ADVERSE MEP CHANGES

The causes of adverse MEP changes are similar to those described for SSEPs, including direct mechanical or thermal tissue injury and ischemia/infarction of neural or muscle tissue due to compromise of its blood supply. Apparently significant MEP attenuations due to changes in the anesthetic regimen are even more common for M-wave monitoring than for SSEP monitoring. If the spinal cord below the neck is at risk (as in scoliosis or aortic surgery), then MEPs recorded from upper-limb muscles can be used as controls to identify anesthetic effects on MEPs in lower-limb muscles.

2.4.5. TYPICAL INTRAOPERATIVE APPLICATIONS OF MEPs

MEPs are used to monitor the condition of the corticospinal tracts during surgery on the brain, brainstem, or spinal cord that places those structures at risk; during orthopedic surgery that poses a risk to the spinal cord (Fig. 34.21); or during surgery on the aorta or on other blood vessels that supply the brain and spinal cord. They can also be used to assess the function of cranial nerves or spinal nerve roots by recording the MEPs in the muscles that they innervate following stimulation of the corticospinal and corticobulbar tracts within the brain.

As noted above, the somatosensory pathways may be damaged without MEP changes, so SSEP monitoring should also be employed when MEPs are used to monitor the spinal cord. Also, monitoring both SSEPs and MEPs provides a measure of redundancy for monitoring the integrity of the spinal cord; two independent monitoring techniques are employed, each capable of detecting most cases of spinal cord compromise in case the other technique cannot provide effective NIOM due to

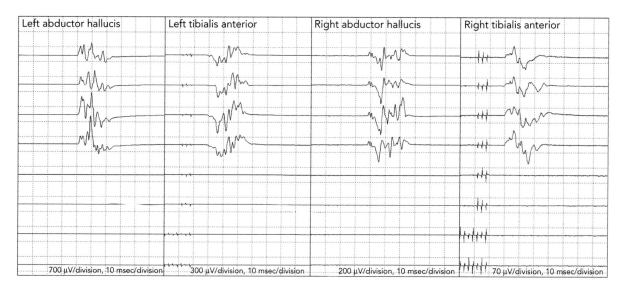

Left abductor hallucis	Left tibialis anterior	Right abductor hallucis	Right tibialis anterior
700 µV/division, 10 msec/division	300 µV/division, 10 msec/division	200 µV/division, 10 msec/division	70 µV/division, 10 msec/division

Figure 34.21. *Consecutive MEP runs recorded during the same operation as the data shown in Figure 34.18. Shown here are the last four MEP runs recorded from the abductor hallucis and tibialis anterior muscles to contralateral anodal TES before the adverse changes (top) and the first four runs recorded after them (bottom). The MEPs recorded from the hand muscles did not change. Reprinted from Legatt AD. Intraoperative evoked potential monitoring. In: Schomer DL, Lopes da Silva FH, eds. Niedermeyer's Textbook of Electroencephalography: Basic Principles, Clinical Applications, and Related Fields. 6th ed. Philadelphia: Lippincott Williams & Wilkins, 2011:767–786, Fig. 38.21.*

preexisting neurological compromise, anesthetic effects, NMB, excessively noisy data, or other technical problems[92].

3. EEG

The EEG is the ongoing electrical activity of the brain, as recorded from the surface of the head. Electrocorticography—recording of the EEG directly from the surface of the brain during surgery—is covered in Chapter 28. During surgery, scalp-recorded EEG is used to monitor the cerebral hemispheres to determine if there is adequate perfusion and oxygenation and to identify any new focal impairment or epileptic seizures. EEG monitoring is most often used during carotid endarterectomy, intracranial aneurysm clipping, and certain other craniotomies, but may also be used during surgery on the heart or aorta. It may also be used during other types of surgeries where MEP monitoring is employed (e.g., spinal surgery) to detect seizures triggered by TES.

3.1. EEG Recording Techniques

EEG is recorded from the scalp in the operating room using techniques similar to those used for extraoperative EEG recordings. Electrodes should be secured well at the usual International 10-20 System placements[93] because loose electrodes are not conveniently regelled during surgery. Sometimes midline electrodes are not used and only the 16 electrodes of the parasagittal and temporal chains are used for surgical monitoring. Filter settings of 0.3 to 70 Hz allow for adequate recording of slow and fast activities, both of which are important during monitoring. The page speed, formerly known as paper speed, may be changed to compress the record, so that the EEG over a greater amount of time is displayed at once, which is advantageous for monitoring for changes over time. Onset of slow activity may be more noticeable at 5 to 10 mm/sec than at a standard page speed (30 mm/sec). Modern digital viewing screens allow simultaneous monitoring of a patient's baseline data alongside the current moment's recording. Such visual comparisons are of great assistance for identifying by eye any relative changes in fast or slow activity.

As for most NIOM, adequate grounding is needed to avoid excessive line frequency (50 or 60 Hz) noise. The operating room EEG machine generally uses an isoground rather than a true ground. A true ground may be employed for the surgeon's electrocautery device. A second true ground would risk electrical burns in case of a ground or equipment malfunction. The EEG user should check that the EEG machine's ground is optically isolated or otherwise protected from a double-ground situation. Older-generation equipment, which uses a true ground, is not appropriate for use in the operating room.

3.2. EEG Alarm Criteria

Interpretation of EEG changes during NIOM is based on the patient's own baseline. Each patient has a somewhat different EEG under anesthesia, or at least there is considerable variability among the general population. The first degree of adverse change with cerebral ischemia is a decrease in background fast activity; this meets an alarm criterion when the fast activity decreases by >50%. The second degree of adverse change is increased slow activity; this meets an alarm criterion when the slow activity increases by >50%. Sometimes decreased fast activity and increased slow activity occur concurrently. The third degree of change is decreased amplitude of the EEG activity; this meets an alarm criterion when the overall EEG amplitude decreases by >50%. In the worst extent the EEG disappears entirely (i.e., it becomes isoelectric). Changes may be seen unilaterally or bilaterally. Ischemia from unilateral surgery may be seen over both hemispheres on EEG, because the circle of Willis can share ischemia between the hemispheres. As such, physicians who assess only for asymmetry can miss significant ischemia that affects both hemispheres.

At the end of inhalational anesthesia, the anesthesiologist may initiate hyperventilation to eliminate the gas. As in the outpatient setting, hyperventilation is accompanied by generalized EEG slowing. The monitoring team should not confuse the onset of this slowing for a clinical alarm circumstance.

At times, the anesthesiologist will administer a bolus of centrally active medication, such as a bolus of propofol. Such a sudden medication administration often provokes a change in the EEG frequency content, sometimes mimicking an adverse change. Good communication with the anesthesia team will help prevent confusion.

3.3. Quantitative Trending of EEG

Computer EEG analysis can now be used to produce frequency analysis and automated trending of the amount of EEG in fast- and slow-frequency bands. These automated trend displays can be helpful in supplementing the traditional visual analysis. Visual reading of paper EEG, or its electronic version displayed on a video screen, is hampered by the fact that changes over long periods of time may be missed because they have been so gradual. By using a supplemental frequency analysis trend, one can observe the gradual changes in EEG over arbitrarily short or long time spans, including watching the changes over the entire course of the operative procedure. Such quantitative EEG analysis has been shown to be more sensitive than routine EEG for detecting changes occurring with ischemia[94-96]. The rate of shunting may increase to as high as 40% when predicated upon the subtle degrees of EEG change detected by quantitative techniques.

3.4. Typical Intraoperative Applications of EEG

3.4.1. Carotid Endarterectomy

Carotid artery clamping, such as is performed during carotid endarterectomy, can produce significant cerebral ischemia if there is insufficient collateral vascular supply. EEG monitoring is used to determine which patients have substantial cerebral ischemia due to clamping. When EEG detects ischemia, a vascular shunt is considered to restore adequate cerebral perfusion (Fig. 34.22). When an EEG shows no ischemia upon clamping, the patient may be spared a shunt. Vascular shunts are associated with a 1% to 3% risk of iatrogenic problems, so shunts

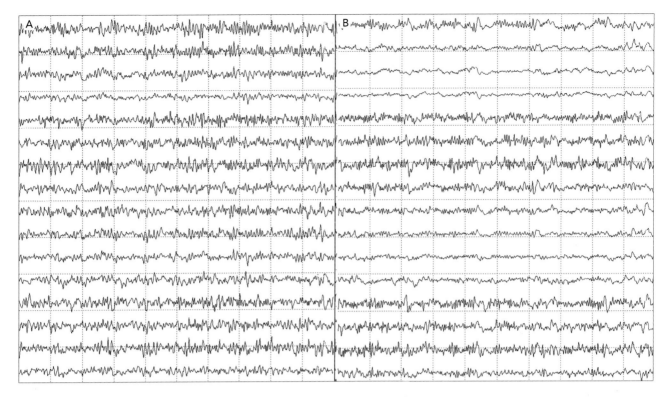

Figure 34.22. EEG changes with carotid clamping. Bipolar chains, parasagittal above temporal, 1 sec/div. **A:** Before clamping, symmetric fast activity. **B:** Within seconds of clamping, unilateral loss of fast activity.

are best avoided unless they are truly needed. Shunt problems may arise from arterial wall damage or from emboli. Selective shunting is a common surgical tactic, with the choice based on the EEG findings at the time of clamping. Other responses, such as increasing the systemic arterial blood pressure, can also be made when the EEG detects ischemia.

Redekop and Ferguson[97] studied 293 patients undergoing carotid endarterectomy in an extension of a previously reported study[98]. EEG was monitored without using shunts. Major EEG changes occurred in 11/77 patients (14%) with significant contralateral carotid stenosis or occlusion. Major EEG changes occurred in 11/216 patients (5%) without significant contralateral carotid stenosis or occlusion. Among their patients, the risk of immediate postoperative deficit was significantly higher among the patients who had major EEG changes (4/22, 18%) compared with those who had no such major EEG changes (5/271, 2%). This showed that major EEG changes are infrequent but identify patients with a significantly higher risk of intraoperative stroke. On this basis, they recommended selective vascular shunting of patients with EEG change.

Sundt et al.[99] and later McKay et al.[100] established relationships among EEG changes, cerebral blood flow, and carotid artery stump pressure. Cerebral blood flow and EEG changes correlated well. A normal EEG requires a cerebral blood flow of at least 18 mL/100 g/min; below that, the degree of the EEG change reflects the severity of reduced blood flow. Regional cerebral blood flow also corresponds to stump pressure in the cross-clamped carotid artery. However, the stump pressures do not reflect stenosis above the circle of Willis and clinically only are measured on a single test occasion upon clamping. Overall the EEG is more readily related to cerebral function than is

stump pressure, and therefore it is a more reliable test for cerebral ischemia. EEG also can be monitored throughout the procedure, whereas stump pressure is only tested once. EEG reliably measures cerebral function during clamping, allowing the surgeon to understand whether the hemispheres are tolerating the procedure. SSEPs can also be used to monitor for cerebral ischemia during carotid cross-clamping[101].

3.4.2. CARDIOTHORACIC SURGERY

The EEG is monitored continuously during some types of cardiothoracic surgery[102]. The brain may become relatively ischemic during extracorporeal perfusion. EEG can identify ischemia, prompting an increase in pump pressure. During surgery in which hypothermic cardioplegia is used, EEG may be used to gauge when hypothermia is sufficiently deep. At temperatures well below 25°C, the EEG may become isoelectric. This is typically below 18°C, but may vary from patient to patient[103]. A principal goal of hypothermia is to prevent ischemia brain damage during deliberate cardiac standstill. Monitoring EEG can identify the isoelectric point when sufficient hypothermia is attained and then ensure that it is maintained.

3.4.3. CRANIOTOMIES

During clipping of intracranial aneurysms and resection of tumors, and in certain other settings, EEG monitoring is advantageous. EEG assesses cerebral perfusion, and for intracranial procedures it also evaluates for seizures. EEG recording techniques for craniotomy necessarily eliminate some recording sites from where the bone flap will be removed. Monitoring is accomplished from remaining electrode sites. Sometimes sterile metal strip electrodes embedded in silicone plastic are placed along the edge of the craniotomy, epidurally or subdurally, and tucked out of the way of the surgical team. These either can be left in place, weighted down by wet cottonoid, tucked under dura, or otherwise held in a secure position. Significant decreases in fast activity or increases in slow activity are considered typical of ischemia. When this accompanies placement of a vascular clip, the presence of ischemia signals in an EEG suggests that the clip is occluding significant vessels serving cortex.

3.4.4. EEG DURING MEP MONITORING

EEG can be monitored for safety when MEPs are used during surgery. Many such cases are spinal surgery. A few channels are used for EEG monitoring to identify whether the patient experiences any seizures or brief after-discharges upon MEP stimulation. The same electrodes used to record SSEPs can be used for EEG recording, and additional recording channels can be used as well. Surgical MEP is rarely associated with seizures: MacDonald[104] noted five seizures reported among 15,000 surgeries. The association is so infrequent that some of the seizures that have occurred may not be the result of MEP itself but rather coincidental spontaneous seizures. Nevertheless, caution is commonly warranted. A seizure temporally and causally related to TES has been reported, however[85] (Fig. 34.23). Among patients with epilepsy, TES does not appear frequently to provoke seizures. Seizures may be rare because the stimuli were very brief and the patients generally did not have conditions predisposing to seizures.

When performed with an abundance of caution to identify seizures or brief seizure-like after-discharges, EEG monitoring might forewarn that a patient is not tolerating MEP stimulation. More likely, the patient may suffer spontaneous seizures that may be nonconvulsive. Noting that can be clinically helpful in patients who are not under NMB so that treatment can be started before the problem progresses to a convulsive seizure.

3.4.5. EEG MEASUREMENT OF DEPTH OF ANESTHESIA

The effects of various anesthetic agents on the EEG are described in the section on anesthesia and NIOM below. The characteristic sequence of EEG patterns corresponding to increasing

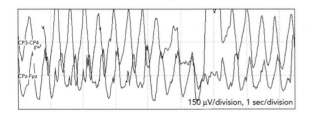

Figure 34.23. *EEG during an electroclinical seizure triggered by MEP monitoring; a repetitive spike-wave pattern is visible in the CPz-Fpz recording channel. The seizure occurred immediately following TES. A bolus dose of propofol was given, and the seizure stopped within 1 minute. The patient had no prior history of seizures. The anesthetic regimen was TIVA with propofol and remifentanil, and the surgery was for an arachnoid cyst that was compressing the brainstem. Reprinted with permission from Legatt AD. Intraoperative Neurophysiology: Interactive Case Studies. New York: Demos Medical Publishing, 2015, case 23, p. 5.*

doses of anesthetic agents, especially the GABAergic agents, potentially provides a way of assessing the effect of anesthetic agents on the brain, measuring the depth of anesthesia more directly than by monitoring reflexes, movement, and cardiovascular parameters.

Depth of anesthesia has been tracked using indices computed from the EEG and displayed on brain monitoring devices[105,106]. The goal for routine use of these automated devices has been to avoid awareness under general anesthesia. The devices are better used for patients who are not at the extremes of age and whose nervous systems have no preexisting neurological impairment. Because these indices do not relate directly to the neurophysiology of how a specific anesthetic exerts its effects in the brain, they cannot give an accurate picture of the brain's responses to the drugs[107]. They often assume that slower is deeper, yet not all agents produce similar EEG changes that can be captured in a linear manner among all patients. Artifacts can influence automated readings, and anesthesiologists have been encouraged to understand how to assess the raw EEG so as to avoid readings based on artifact[108]. Automated devices have achieved a common use in guiding some anesthesiologists in judging depth of anesthesia.

Commercial devices are available that encode the EEG patterns into single numerical scales putatively reflecting the depth of anesthesia. The best-known is the BIS™ (Covidien, Mansfield, MA), which records EEG from four forehead electrodes and produces the "bispectral index" (BIS), a unit-less number between 0 and 100, where 0 and 100 correspond respectively to absence of brain activity and to wakefulness. BIS values between 40 and 60 are said to indicate a level of general anesthesia appropriate for surgery[109]. The BIS™ algorithm remains proprietary but apparently derives from a combination of the 95% spectral edge frequency (SEF95, the frequency below which 95% of the EEG power is located), the ratio of spectral power in the 30- to 47-Hz to 11- to 20-Hz bands, the ratio of bispectral power (related to both signal amplitude and phase coupling in 40- to 47-Hz to 0.5- to 47-Hz bands), and the burst suppression ratio[110]. Other manufacturers offer variations on the BIS™ theme, also using algorithms based on power spectral parameters and measures of synchrony.

At present, the utility of EEG-based anesthesia monitors remains controversial. The BIS™ is, by far, the most studied. Three large trials are of particular note. One large randomized controlled study, conducted in >2,400 patients at risk for awareness under anesthesia, demonstrated an 82% reduction in the incidence of postoperative awareness in patients monitored using the BIS™ (B-Aware Trial[111]). A second similar randomized controlled study and third larger multicenter study both failed to confirm this finding (B-Unaware Trial[112] and BAG-RECALL Trial[113]). A possibly important difference between these studies is that in the B-Aware Trial >40% of patients received TIVA, whereas in the B-Unaware and BAG-RECALL trials all patients received potent inhalational agents[112].

Apart from the concerns that apply in general when signal processing is used to extract salient information from the EEG (e.g., contamination by EMG, electrical interference, and electrode-related artifact), along with potential confounds such as the effects of hypoxia, ischemia, or preexisting cerebral pathology, an important limitation to the use of BIS™ and similar devices as depth-of-anesthesia monitors is the assumption that a single EEG-derived numerical value would similarly reflect the effects of all anesthetic agents. Initial validation studies showed good correlations between both the probabilities of consciousness and recall and the BIS for the largely GABAergic agents (e.g., propofol, midazolam, isoflurane)[114]. However, non-GABAergic drugs whose EEG effects differ substantially from these agents not surprisingly deviate from this pattern; nitrous oxide and ketamine produce high BIS values when patient is, in fact, unconscious, and dexmedetomidine produces misleadingly low BIS values when the patient is not adequately anesthetized[107]. Further, even among volatile agents, equivalent median alveolar concentration (MAC) concentrations of different drugs have been shown to produce substantially different BIS values; in one study, at both 0.5 and 1 MAC, BIS values for halothane and isoflurane differed by over 10 units[115]. Moreover, wide inter-individual differences in the BIS value at loss of consciousness have been observed both with GABAergic (propofol and isoflurane) and non-GABAergic (dexmedetomidine) agents[116].

Recently, attention has focused on application of more sophisticated analyses of EEG dynamics to characterize and measure the effects of anesthetics on the brain. Although not widely utilized in currently practice, many current EEG-based anesthesia monitoring systems provide power spectrographic displays similar to those now commonly used to supplement continuous EEG monitoring in the intensive care unit, along with displays of the raw EEG. Characteristic power spectral and coherence patterns have been identified for many agents. It is possible that measures based on these and similar parameters will provide the basis for more effective approaches to intraoperative assessment of the effects of anesthetic drugs on the brain, including the monitoring of the depth of anesthesia, than can be provided by a single, highly data-reduced, number (Fig. 34.24) [107,117–119].

4. EMG

Recordings of spontaneous EMG activity and of EMG activity triggered by electrical stimulation within the surgical field are most often used to detect mechanical stimulation, irritation, or injury of peripheral nerve tissue and to locate and identify peripheral nerves (including cranial nerves) when their location is not apparent from visual inspection of the surgical field. However, recording of spontaneous and triggered EMG activity may also be used to assess CNS structures.

4.1. Spontaneous EMG Activity

Mechanical or thermal stimulation or injury of peripheral nerve fibers can cause them to fire. When motor fibers fire (and the patient is not pharmacologically paralyzed), the muscle fibers they innervate will as well, producing EMG discharges in a variety of patterns[120] with both diagnostic and prognostic implications. Such monitoring has found wide utility during surgery in which peripheral nerves, nerve roots, and cranial nerves are at risk.

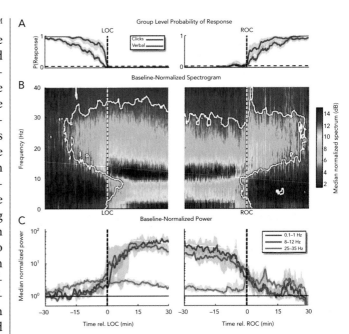

Figure 34.24. Loss (LOC) and subsequent regaining of consciousness (ROC) coincide with appearance and disappearance of prominent alpha and very-low-frequency EEG activity as the propofol target effect-site concentration is gradually raised from 0 to 5 µg/mL, and then decreased back to zero. A: Group probability of LOC and ROC to clicks and verbal stimulation. B: Group EEG spectrogram. The white outline surrounds regions where power significantly exceeds baseline. C: Power in low-frequency, alpha and gamma bands over time. It is proposed that structured alpha frequency oscillation may interfere with communication in thalamocortical circuits, and that disrupted intracortical communication may be reflected in widespread 0.1- to 1-Hz activity, both effects leading the loss of consciousness. Modified from Purdon PL, et al. Electroencephalogram signatures of loss and recovery of consciousness from propofol. Proc Natl Acad Sci USA. 2013;110(12):E1142–1151, Fig. 2.

Mechanical stimulation of fibers within spinal cord motor tracts can cause them to fire as well, especially in cases of impacts with high kinetic energies[121]. If the activity in spinal cord motor tracts is sufficient to fire the lower motor neurons in more caudal levels of the spinal cord, this will produce EMG bursts. These bursts have been labeled suprasegmentally generated EMG discharges and have predictive value for adverse MEP changes[121]. Monitoring of spontaneous EMG activity generated in segmental levels caudal to where the spinal cord is at risk may therefore help to detect spinal cord compromise.

4.2. Triggered EMG Activity

Stimulation of peripheral nerves and nerve roots can cause muscle contraction via reflex mechanisms within the spinal cord. The corresponding EMG activity can be recorded to quantitate reflex activity during surgery. This modality has been most useful during selective posterior rhizotomy surgery.

4.3. Selective Posterior Rhizotomy

Selective posterior rhizotomy is a neurosurgical procedure used to treat spastic cerebral palsy. Cutting selected posterior spinal sensory rootlets reduces spasticity by decreasing excessive feedback to spinal motor neurons. Neuromonitoring signs of a relatively higher degree of spasticity select rootlets for transection. Peacock, working with Nuwer in 1986, popularized the procedure[122,123], and several technical variations have evolved[124]. Surgical testing techniques are described in greater detail in Staudt et al.[125] Clinical outcome assessments using objective measures of muscle tone, range of motion, functional skills, and gait analysis[125–127] showed improved abilities that were retained over years.

4.3.1. STIMULATION

Each sensory root is separated surgically into four to 12 individual rootlets. Their higher threshold for muscle activity identifies sensory roots, which usually require more than 10-fold greater intensity to elicit a muscle response compared to a motor root. Constant-voltage stimulation is delivered to individual rootlets in the cauda equina from L2 to S2. Constant-voltage technique is used because of the unequal size of rootlets.

Individual 0.1-msec square-wave electrical pulse stimuli are delivered through a pair of blunt-tipped nerve hook electrodes, over which the surgeon holds the rootlet. Delivery of individual stimuli is applied at increasing voltages until a motor threshold is found. Trains of electrical pulses then are delivered at 50/sec for 1 sec to test each rootlet around its motor threshold.

4.3.2. RECORDING

Continuous EMG is recorded bilaterally from adductors longus, vastus lateralis, hamstrings, tibialis anterior, and gastrocnemius muscles, as well as from the anal sphincter. Display speed is set at 30 to 60 mm/sec to visualize responses to several successive 1-sec stimulus trains.

Stimulus artifact must be differentiated from EMG activity. Stimulus artifact with trains is a series of equally spaced, equal-amplitude lines proportional to stimulus intensity, often greatest at the sphincter and proximal recording channels.

Background muscle artifact is a common problem. The reflex activity sought is seen only with light anesthesia in these patients with chronic spasticity. Deeper anesthesia abolishes the reflex responses, a problem that has caused some controversy in this field. When excess background EMG interferes with recording, slight deepening of anesthesia can help. Pausing the procedure for many minutes also may allow background muscle activity to resolve.

4.3.3. TRAIN RESPONSES

Several different EMG amplitude patterns are commonly encountered after delivery of a 1-sec train of 50/sec stimuli (Fig. 34.25): (1) decremental: the response gradually decreases; (2) squared: the response remains unchanged; (3) decremental–squared: there is a brief higher EMG response followed by an unchanged response; (4) incremental: increasing response; (5) multiphasic: there is a fluctuating response, sometimes with brief inhibitory pauses; (6) clonic: there are six to 12 bursts of EMG; (7) irregular: there are uneven responses without interludes of absent activity; (8) sustained: EMG activity continues beyond the 1-sec stimulus; (9) spread: there are EMG responses in muscle groups inconsistent with the level tested.

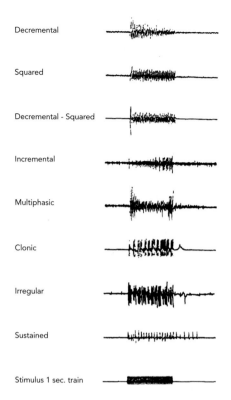

Figure 34.25. Examples of EMG patterns commonly encountered during the rhizotomy procedure. Rootlets associated with multiphasic and clonic patterns are cut. The bottom tracing shows the timing of the stimulus train. Reprinted with permission from Staudt LA, Nuwer MR, Peacock WJ. Intraoperative monitoring during selective posterior rhizotomy: technique and patient outcome. Electroencephalogr Clin Neurophysiol. 1995;97(6):296–309, Fig. 1.

4.3.4. CRITERIA FOR DIVISION OF ROOTLETS

Abnormal responses to the stimulus train are clonic, multiphasic, incremental, and spread of responses, analogous to abnormal physical examination findings with a reflex hammer. An accessory criterion is reflexes that are hyperactive compared to others (i.e., with a substantially lower threshold to evoke a response). The abnormal findings are believed to represent failure of temporal and spatial inhibition associated with spasticity. Typically the worst one third of the rootlets are cut. S1 and S2 rootlets are spared if the sphincter responds, or if testing shows substantial pudendal afferent activity coursing through a root[128]. Further details are given in Staudt et al.[125]

5. ANESTHESIA AND NIOM

Anesthetic agents profoundly affect most of the signals recorded for NIOM. Many anesthetics depress SSEPs and MEPs (see Fig. 34.4). Providing anesthesia compatible with NIOM imposes requirements and constraints on the anesthesiologist that do not apply to unmonitored surgeries. Optimal patient management therefore requires understanding of relevant effects of anesthetic drugs by the monitoring team as well as an understanding of NIOM by the anesthesiologist; cooperation and communication are essential.

Contrary to the popular notion, anesthesia is not simply sleep, nor is it a nonspecific scrambling of brain function.

Rather, anesthesia can be thought of as consisting of four discrete components: unconsciousness, amnesia, analgesia, and immobility. Some anesthetic agents provide all four; others are more specific. The anesthesiologist must select an agent, or combination of agents, that provides all four components while still permitting monitoring of neurophysiological signals.

The effectiveness of anesthetic agents is assessed in terms of their ability to affect specific measurable endpoints (e.g., suppression of movement and blunting of autonomic responses to surgical stimuli). Other endpoints, in particular awareness and memory formation, are more difficult to measure, contributing to the possibility of failure to provide adequate unconsciousness and amnesia.

The incidence of accidental awareness during general anesthesia (AAGA) has been reported to be one in 19,000 cases based upon spontaneous patient reporting[129], but it was an order of magnitude greater when patients were queried specifically about it[113,130,131]. In one study[129], 41% of patients reporting AAGA suffered long-term psychological harm, including symptoms resembling posttraumatic stress disorder. In this study, risk factors for AAGA included TIVA and NMB; also, the risk of AAGA was elevated for cardiothoracic surgery, during which (as with neurophysiologically monitored cases) low doses of anesthetic agents may intentionally be used. These findings underscore the challenge of providing anesthesia during NIOM, and the importance for effective cooperation and communication between neurophysiologist and anesthesiologist.

5.1. Anesthetic Agents

5.1.1. INHALATIONAL AGENTS

5.1.1.1. HALOGENATED INHALATIONAL AGENTS
The halogenated inhalational agents, also commonly referred to as "potent agents" or "volatile agents," are halogenated ethers and are probably the most commonly used general anesthetics. The term "potent agent" derives from the fact that halogenated inhalational agents are effective at relatively low concentrations. The term "volatile agent" refers to their common property of being liquids at room temperature that are easily volatilized for administration. They are "complete" anesthetics, providing unconsciousness, amnesia, analgesia, and immobility through their actions at a host of receptors, including gamma-aminobutyric acid type A (GABA-A), N-methyl-D-aspartate (NMDA), nicotinic acetylcholine (nACh) and glycine receptors, and K^+ channels.

The potency of the inhalational anesthetics is most commonly measured by the MAC of the gas, expressed in terms of percentage at 1 atmosphere of pressure that is required to achieve the desired endpoint in 50% of subjects. The acronym MAC originally referred to the "minimum alveolar concentration" required in an individual subject. Its meaning has changed, but the acronym is still often erroneously defined as abbreviating the "minimum" rather than the "median" alveolar concentration. In practice, end-expiratory concentration serves as a surrogate for alveolar concentration. The most common endpoint is abolition of movement to surgical stimulation, and "MAC" is often used synonymously with

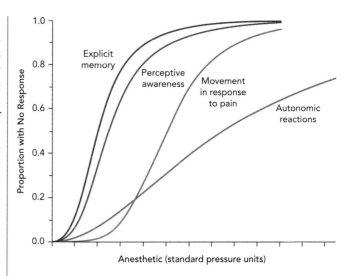

Figure 34.26. The general relationship between the concentration of inhalational agents and each of the four anesthetic actions. Awareness and recall are lost at lower concentrations than are movement to pain and autonomic responses. The intersection of a horizontal line drawn at 0.5 on the vertical axis with each of the four curves corresponds to the MAC for the corresponding action. Inter-individual variability in potency is reflected by the shape of the curve for each response. Modified from Campagna JA, Miller KW, Forman SA. Mechanisms of actions of inhaled anesthetics. N Engl J Med. 2003;348(21):2110–2124, Fig. 2.

"MAC-immobility." Importantly, concentrations required to abolish explicit memory and perceptive awareness are lower than those required to prevent movement to surgical pain and to blunt autonomic responses (Fig. 34.26).

The inhalational agents differ in both potency and speed of action (Table 34.1). MAC-immobility is 1.2% for isoflurane and 6% for desflurane, making desflurane approximately five times less potent than isoflurane. The inhalational agents also differ in their solubility in blood, brain, fat, and other tissues. Solubility is inversely related to the speed at which partial pressures equilibrate between compartments, and to rapidity of onset and offset of anesthetic effects of the gas (Fig. 34.27).

The halogenated inhalational agents do not significantly affect the brainstem-generated (subcortical) SSEP signals but produce dose-related attenuation of the cortical components of SSEPs[80] (see Fig. 34.4). This effect can be nonlinear, with small changes in concentration producing large changes in the cortical SSEPs. In some patients, the cortical SSEPs may be relatively unaffected at one dose, generally <0.5 MAC, but be prominently attenuated at a minimally greater dose[132].

The halogenated inhalational agents suppress myogenic MEPs and spinal cord recorded I-waves (I-waves are additional corticospinal tract volleys following the D-wave that are produced by cortical synaptic activity); D-waves are unaffected at clinically relevant concentrations. The suppression of myogenic MEPs is the combined result of attenuation of cortically generated I-waves plus suppression of synaptic transmission in the anterior horn of the spinal cord and possibly also at the myoneural junction[80,133] (Fig. 34.28). The various halogenated inhalational agents similarly affect MEPs and SSEPs on a MAC-equivalent basis; the less soluble agents may, however, appear to be more potent, probably because of their more rapid

TABLE 34.1. MAC Values and Partition Coefficients for Various Anesthetic Gases

AGENT	MAC (VOL %)	PARTITION COEFFICIENTS @ 37°C		
		BLOOD:GAS	BRAIN:BLOOD	FAT:BLOOD
Nitrous oxide	105	0.47	1.1	2.3
Desflurane	6	0.45	1.3	27
Sevoflurane	2	0.65	1.7	48
Isoflurane	1.2	1.4	2.6	45
Halothane	0.75	2.3	2.9	51

Adapted from Patel PM, Patel HH, Roth DM. General anesthetics and therapeutic gases. In: Brunton LL, Chabner BA, Knollmann BC, eds. *Goodman & Gilman's The Pharmacological Basis of Therapeutics.* 12th ed. New York: McGraw-Hill, 2011, Table 19.1.

onset and offset coupled with nonlinear dose–amplitude relationships[80,133,134]. Short-latency brainstem AEPs are well preserved in the presence of halogenated inhalational agents but do demonstrate small increases in both I–III and III–V interpeak latencies with increasing concentration[135].

5.1.1.2. Nitrous Oxide
Nitrous oxide is an effective analgesic and also contributes to unconsciousness, immobility, and amnesia. At atmospheric pressure, however, it has a MAC of 104%, and so it is a not an effective general anesthetic when used as the sole agent. Its mechanism of action is not fully understood, but it is thought to work primarily through NMDA and kappa opioid receptors, along with additional actions at GABA-A, glycine, nACh, central alpha-2 adrenergic receptors, and 2-pore-domain K⁺

channels[136,137]. Nitrous oxide is highly insoluble and, accordingly, has rapid onset and offset of action.

Like the halogenated inhalational agents, nitrous oxide attenuates MEPs and the cortical components of SSEPs without significantly affecting brainstem components. On a MAC-equivalent basis, nitrous oxide appears to have a greater depressant effect than the volatile agents on MEPs and cortical SSEPs; when used along with halogenated inhalational agents, their depressant effects appear to be synergistic—that is, greater than the sum of the expected depressant effects of each agent alone[80,138–140].

5.1.2. Intravenous Agents
5.1.2.1. Propofol
Propofol is a potent sedative and amnestic agent, with only minor analgesic and immobilizing properties. It acts primarily at GABA-A receptors, inducing an inward chloride current that hyperpolarizes the postsynaptic neurons, thus leading to inhibition[141], with small effects on glycine and nACh receptors[142]. It is often used in combination with other agents (e.g., opioids, ketamine, or dexmedetomidine) to provide analgesia. Propofol is metabolized rapidly, but it is fat-soluble and redistributes quickly into fatty tissues, including the brain. The pharmacokinetics of propofol are complex, and at a constant infusion rate, the propofol plasma concentration increases over time. The effect is pronounced at higher infusion rates (Fig. 34.29). In contrast to the inhalational agents for which end-expiratory partial pressure is monitored, plasma concentrations of intravenous agents, including propofol, are not routinely measured. To maintain an approximately constant blood level, the propofol infusion rate is generally decreased over time, particularly when used at higher doses and for longer

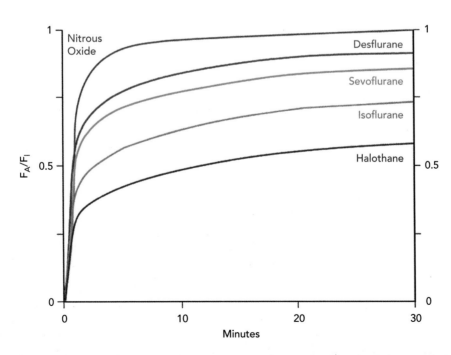

Figure 34.27. *Equilibration of end-tidal alveolar partial pressure (F_A) and inspired partial pressure (F_I) of anesthetic gases over time. The least soluble gases (see Table 34.1) equilibrate most rapidly. Reprinted from Eger EI, II. Inhaled anesthetics: uptake and distribution. In: Miller RD, Eriksson LI, Fleisher LA, Wiener-Kronish JP, Young WL, eds. Miller's Anesthesia. 7th ed. Philadelphia: Churchill Livingstone, 2010:540.*

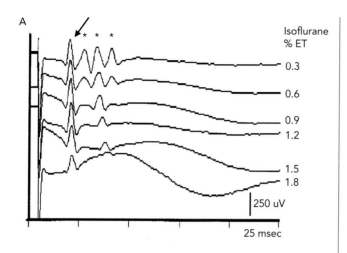

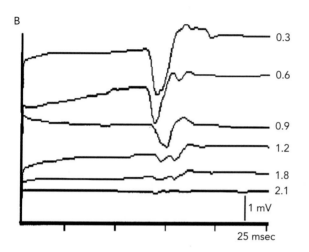

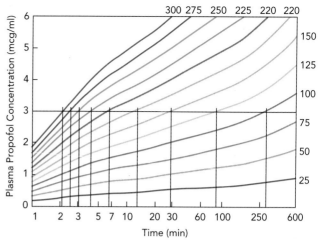

Figure 34.29. Plasma propofol concentrations versus infusion duration at various infusion rates. Each curve represents the plasma propofol concentration versus infusion duration for an infusion at the rate specified along the right and upper borders, in µg/mL/min. The horizontal line shows the infusion rate changes needed to maintain a constant propofol plasma concentration of 3 µg/mL. The plots represent calculations based on the pharmacokinetic model of Schnider et al.[204] Reprinted with permission from Barash PG, et al. Clinical Anesthesia. 7th ed. New York: Wolters Kluwer, 2013, Fig. 7-14.

Figure 34.28. Increasing the concentration of isoflurane attenuates I-waves (asterisks in A) and muscle MEP (B). D-waves (arrow in A) are relatively unaffected. Epidural (A) and hypothenar muscle (B) recordings in a baboon anesthetized with ketamine and isoflurane, following stimulation with a single-pulse transcranial electrical stimulus. Modified with permission from Sloan T, Heyer EJ. Anesthesia for intraoperative neurophysiologic monitoring of the spinal cord. J Clin Neurophysiol. 2002;19(5):430–443, Figs. 4 and 5 combined.

cases. Special infusion pumps are available that automatically adjust the infusion rate to achieve target plasma or "effect-site" concentration based on pharmacodynamics models[143].

An important consequence of accumulation in fatty tissue is that the elimination half-time of propofol increases with the duration of infusion. The term "context-sensitive half-time" refers to the elimination half-time in context of the infusion duration. Propofol has a context-sensitive half-time of about 10 minutes following a 3-hour infusion, but of about 40 minutes following an 8-hour infusion[144]. This can result in slow emergence from anesthesia after long procedures, and can present problems should a wakeup test be required.

Propofol produces only minimal attenuation of cortical SSEPs when used alone[145,146]. In the presence of other agents (e.g., nitrous oxide), however, propofol may exert a synergistic depressant effect[147]. Minimal increase in BAEP interpeak latencies have been reported with high propofol doses in children[148].

Propofol attenuates MEPs in a dose-related manner. The effect, however, is mitigated by optimal stimulus train

paradigms, including the use of dual train facilitation. When used along with an opioid infusion, MEPs can generally be monitored throughout the range of clinically relevant plasma concentrations, up to 6 to 8 µg/mL corresponding to deep anesthesia[146,149–151]. When combined with other agents, however, depressant effects may be synergistic[152]. At propofol concentrations sufficient to produce a burst-suppression EEG pattern[153], MEPs may be abolished.

TIVA using propofol, along with an opioid, is considered by many to be an optimal anesthetic regimen when MEPs will be monitored. However, this is tempered by concerns related to delayed emergence as well as the propofol infusion syndrome (PRIS). PRIS is a potentially fatal but reversible condition characterized by acute refractory bradycardia and lactic acidosis, thought to be related to inhibition of the mitochondrial respiratory chain or impairment of mitochondrial fatty acid metabolism. It is most often seen in children exposed to high doses of propofol for prolonged periods of time, particularly in association with acute head injury and elevated corticosteroid and catecholamine levels. It has been reported, however, to occur with brief (several hours), high-dose (e.g., 150 µg/kg/min) exposure[154].

5.1.2.2. Etomidate

Etomidate is also a GABA-A agonist with potent sedative and amnestic properties; it has no analgesic properties. Etomidate enhances cortical SSEPs and also augments MEPs by increasing the number of I-waves. It also produces myoclonus on induction, and can produce seizures in patients with epilepsy. Although both are GABA-A agonists, propofol and etomidate bind to different sites on the GABA-A receptor and differentially alter inhibitory postsynaptic current kinetics[155], potentially accounting for etomidate's unique properties in producing increased cortical excitability at low doses.

Etomidate also produces adrenal suppression; there is no consensus on the need for corticosteroid supplementation[156].

5.1.2.3. BENZODIAZEPINES

The benzodiazepines, including diazepam and midazolam, are GABA-A agonists; they are often used as supplemental agents because of their amnestic properties, and may also be used to reduce the hallucinatory effects of ketamine. They produce mild attenuation of cortical SSEP signals[80], but when used with multi-pulse train stimulation, they have minimal effects on MEPs[157].

5.1.2.4. OPIOIDS

Opioid drugs, including fentanyl, sufentanil, alfentanil, and remifentanil, are excellent analgesics, exerting their effect though μ-opioid receptors. They do not reliably effect unconsciousness or produce amnesia. Opioids do not affect sub-cortical SSEP signals but at high doses can produce modest attenuation of cortical SSEP signals. This effect can be particularly pronounced following bolus administration[158,159]. Opioids do not affect spinal cord D-waves and I-waves but can depress MEPs recorded from muscle at high doses, probably at the level of spinal motor neurons or interneuronal circuits[159]. Fentanyl, sufentanil, and alfentanil will abolish MEPs at high concentrations, roughly twice that required to abolish movement to noxious stimulation[160,161]. Remifentanil, in contrast, has a much wider dosing window, with MEPs being maintained at up to 20 times the concentration required to prevent movement to surgical stimulation[157]. Remifentanil has a very short clinical half-life (~3–10 minutes) even after prolonged infusion; alfentanil, sufentanil, and particularly fentanyl exhibit prominent prolongation of their context-sensitive half-lives for infusion durations of several hours[162]. Remifentanil, particularly in high doses, has been associated with acute opioid tolerance[163]; to facilitate postoperative pain management, it is commonly administered along with longer-acting opioids.

5.1.2.5. KETAMINE

Ketamine is an effective analgesic. It binds to a specific site within the channel of the NMDA glutamate receptor and also acts on opioid receptors. Additionally, it contributes to amnesia and unconsciousness through minor effects on GABA-A and nACh receptors[164]. Ketamine increases the amplitude of the cortical SSEPs[165]. It has minimal effects on muscle-recorded MEPs and has no effect on D-waves or I-waves[160,166,167]. Ketamine may, however, facilitate MEP recording by decreasing the requirements for other agents. Ketamine can increase intracranial pressure and produce hallucinations; postoperative hallucinations can be largely avoided by the concomitant use of a sedative such as benzodiazepine or propofol.

5.1.2.6. DEXMEDETOMIDINE

Dexmedetomidine is an effective analgesic and sedative agent. It is a selective alpha-adrenergic agonist that acts presynaptically to inhibit norepinephrine release[168]. Side effects of hypotension and bradycardia, along with its lack of amnestic effects, preclude its standalone use. It is generally used along with other agents, including propofol and the halogenated agents. Dexmedetomidine does not significantly affect cortical SSEPs.

When used with propofol, it appears to have minimal effect on MEPs at low doses but attenuates MEPs at higher doses (0.6–0.8 ng/mL target plasma concentration)[152].

5.1.2.7. LIDOCAINE

Intravenous lidocaine can be used as an adjunctive agent to general anesthesia, providing analgesia as well as contributing to unconsciousness[169]. Its antinociceptive effects extend into the postoperative period and have been shown to decrease postoperative opioid usage[170,171]. Lidocaine is thought to act through blockade of sodium channels, as well as modulation of the effects of other agents on GABA-A receptors, and antagonism of NMDA and G-protein-coupled receptors[169,170,172]. While boluses and higher doses of lidocaine produce modest attenuation of cortical SSEP components, the standard antiarrhythmic dose of 1.5 mg/kg/hr was found to have no effect on SSEP amplitudes or MEP amplitudes or stimulation voltages, while reducing propofol and sufentanil requirements[169].

5.1.3. NEUROMUSCULAR BLOCKING AGENTS

Neuromuscular blocking agents (NMBAs) are commonly given at the time of intubation, as well as during surgery to facilitate both ventilation and certain surgical procedures.

Succinylcholine binds to postsynaptic ACh receptors, causing initial depolarization accompanied by visible muscle fasciculations. This is followed by flaccid paralysis, typically lasting 10 to 12 minutes after administration. Its short duration of action makes succinylcholine attractive from the NIOM perspective because it permits rapid acquisition of MEP baselines after intubation but before positioning. Some anesthesiologists prefer to avoid its use because of adverse side effects, including increased intragastric, intraocular, and intracranial pressure, hyperkalemia, and the potential to trigger malignant hyperthermia. Further, in patients with plasma butyrylcholinesterase deficiency (incidence ~1 in 2,000), its duration of action is prolonged to several hours; there is no reversal agent. Vecuronium, rocuronium, and cis-atracurium are commonly used nondepolarizing NMBAs. These bind reversibly to ACh receptors, producing NMB blockade by competing with ACh. Their durations of action are longer than that of succinylcholine, typically about 30 minutes for vecuronium and rocuronium and 45 minutes for cis-atracurium following a typical intubating dose[173]. Recovery time, however, varies considerably between patients; in one study, 10% of patients had residual blockade (train-of-four ratio <0.7, see below) after 2 hours[174].

The effects of nondepolarizing NMBAs can be reversed by anticholinesterase medication, such as neostigmine, that blocks the degradation of ACh, resulting in higher concentrations in the synaptic cleft to compete with receptor-bound NMBA. Reversal with neostigmine is usually incomplete, and to be effective requires sufficient prior metabolism of the NMBA; it is ineffective in patients with "deep" blockade (i.e., zero twitches on train-of-four testing)[175, p. 205]. Sugammadex is a new NMBA reversal agent that works by an entirely different mechanism. It is a ring of eight sugar molecules with a central cavity proportioned to encapsulate the rocuronium molecule. It is also effective for reversing vecuronium but is ineffective against cis-atracurium and similar agents[176].

NMB can be assessed by measuring muscle response to supramaximal peripheral nerve stimulation (T1). T1 amplitude (assessed mechanically or by EMG measurement) will begin to diminish at about 70% post-junctional ACh receptor blockage. Between 80% and 85% receptor blockade, T1 amplitude will be ~20% of baseline, and it will become zero at ~95% receptor blockade. The reduction in T1 amplitude compared to baseline is often referred to as the "percent blockade." For clinical purposes, it is more convenient to use the "train of four" test, which takes advantage of a presynaptic action of the non-depolarizing NMBAs that incrementally reduces the amount of ACh released to successive stimulation. The train-of-four test entails four supramaximal stimuli delivered at 2 Hz. The number of observable twitches is counted; if four twitches are elicited, the ratio of the amplitude of the forth twitch (T4) to that of the first can be calculated (TOF ratio). Below ~75% to 80% receptor blockade, four twitches will be elicited; between 80% and 85% receptor blockade, two twitches are elicited; twitches are absent at >95% receptor blockade[173]. The major practical advantage of train-of-four testing is that no T1 amplitude baseline is required; however, it is probably a less reliable index of NMB than T1 amplitude measurement[177].

The sensitivity of different muscle groups to NMBA action is not uniform; for example, diaphragmatic and laryngeal muscles are less sensitive than limb muscles. Beyond that, differences in NMBA effect are observed between limb muscles. In one study, the abductor hallucis, in the foot, was generally found to be more resistant to nondepolarizing NMBAs and to have faster recovery than the first dorsal interosseous, in the hand; in a small fraction of patients, however, the reverse relationship was observed[178]. Accordingly, when NMB is measured to assess the effect of NMBAs on EMG or MEPs, it is best measured in the muscle of interest.

NMBAs have no effect on SSEPs signals per se, but that they can substantially improve SSEP monitoring by eliminating muscle artifact. NMBAs interfere with NIOM tests that depend on the integrity of neuromuscular transmission (i.e., myogenic MEPs, and triggered and free-run EMG). Although most commonly avoided, successfully monitoring of MEPs is possible in the presence of partial NMB, with T1 amplitude suppression of no more than 80%, or at least two twitches on train-of-four testing[156,173]. Partial NMB may, however, increase trial-to-trial variability[179] and confound interpretation of MEPs based on amplitude or waveform complexity criteria, rather than the simpler "presence or absence" criteria. If MEP monitoring is conducted with partial NMB, constant blockade must be maintained using a continuous infusion, ideally controlled using a closed-loop system; bolus administration of NMBAs must be avoided. Triggered EMG testing for assessment of the pedicle screw stimulation threshold has similarly been employed successfully with partial NMB, where T1 amplitude reduction was <80%; the effect of partial NMB on the sensitivity of pedicle screw testing in the presence of chronically compressed roots, however, is not known. Similarly, insufficient data exist concerning the use of NMBAs along with free-run EMG monitoring, but it reasonable that its sensitivity for detection of mechanical nerve injury would be reduced in a dose-related manner.

5.2. Anesthetic Effects on the EEG

Anesthetic effects on the EEG were noted beginning with early observations of effects of ether and pentobarbital[180]. Most anesthetics produce widespread synchronous rhythmic fast activity at induction, maximal in the frontal and central regions, mixed with varying degrees of generalized slow activity. The frontocentral fast activity is greater above the sylvian fissure and is better seen in the parasagittal chain than in the temporal chain. Some inhalational anesthetic agents produce frontopolar sharply contoured slow waves, known as frontal triangular waves. Specific EEG patterns differ among anesthetic agents[181].

Anesthetic agents that are largely or partially GABA-A agonists (e.g., the halogenated inhalational agents, propofol, etomidate, and the barbiturates and benzodiazepines) produce EEG changes that follow a generally similar dose-related pattern. At low doses, there are prominent alpha or lower beta-range frequency frontally maximal oscillations that, with increasing dosage, become more widely distributed. These can be abolished by nitrous oxide[182]. At deeper levels of anesthesia, delta and theta become more prominent; this is followed by the development of a burst-suppression pattern (Fig. 34.30). Finally, continuous EEG suppression is seen. Although the volatile agents and propofol have generally similar effects on the EEG, power spectral and coherence analysis reveal differences; sevoflurane, for example, produces both increases in beta and theta band power as well as an increase in theta band coherence not seen with propofol[117]. Etomidate and sevoflurane have pro-convulsant properties, enhancing epileptiform activity and potentially producing seizures. In high concentrations, sevoflurane can produce seizures in patients without a history of epilepsy[181].

Barbiturates are similar to halogenated inhalational agents in producing activation and beta activity at low doses and a depressant effect leading to burst suppression at higher doses. In the latter, the bursts may have very sharp components that could be misinterpreted as epileptiform activity. Slowing of higher frequencies through inhibitory mechanisms may produce the barbiturate beta activity seen at low doses[183].

Benzodiazepines produce frontal beta activity with a decrease in alpha activity at low doses. Some patients show epileptiform spike activity within that beta activity. Higher benzodiazepine doses produce generalized slowing, but not burst suppression.

The effects on the EEG of the non-GABAergic anesthetics differ from those of the GABAergic agents. The effects of nitrous oxide are "context sensitive." Used alone, nitrous oxide produces high-frequency (>30 Hz) frontal activity. When used along with a volatile agent, nitrous oxide produces rhythmic delta oscillations in a previously continuous EEG, but causes a burst-suppression pattern to become more continuous[107,184]. Ketamine produces prominent beta and low gamma activity along with theta and at high doses produces polymorphic delta, also admixed with beta[107,185]. Dexmedetomidine produces a pattern resembling stage 2 sleep, with spindle-like activity superimposed on slow waves, at low doses[186], and slow-wave sleep at higher doses.

Opioids produce dose-related increases in theta and then delta activity, but not burst suppression or attenuation of the

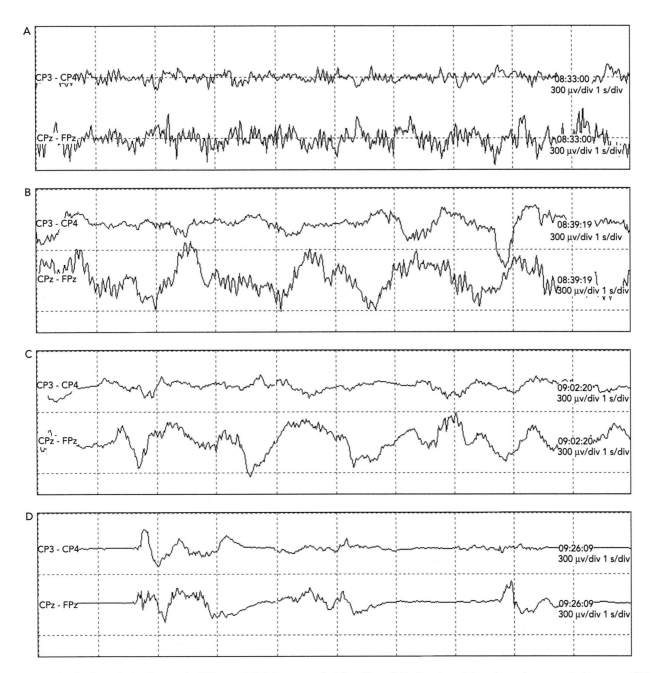

Figure 34.30. Depth-of-anesthesia effects on the EEG, recorded during surgery for idiopathic scoliosis. Two channels in each panel, upper cortical transverse (CP3-CP4) and lower cortical anterior-posterior (CPz-Fpz). **A:** After induction (with infusions of propofol at 100 mcg/kg/min and sufentanil at 20 mcg/hr), fast activity is seen. **B:** As the level of anesthesia grows deeper, increased slow activity is added. **C:** Even deeper (the propofol infusion was increased to 300 mcg/kg/min a few minutes before), fast activity is greatly attenuated. **D:** Deeper still (the propofol is still at 300 mcg/kg/min and the sufentanil has been increased to 40 mcg/hr), suppressions are encountered.

EEG[187]. They can increase epileptiform spiking[188] and also have pro-convulsant properties[189]. Remifentanil may increase epileptiform discharges at higher doses but not with lower-dose continuous infusions[190,191].

5.3. Anesthetic Considerations During NIOM

5.3.1. Baselines and Stable Anesthesia

Since most anesthetics affect MEPs and cortical SSEP signals, it is desirable that stable anesthesia be maintained during NIOM. As discussed earlier, anesthetic effects can be nonlinear, with a small increase of, for example, the concentration of a potent inhalational agent causing a large decrease in the amplitude of cortical SSEPs or complete loss of MEPs. High doses of inhalational agents, especially high doses of multiple agents, are undesirable. Large changes in the anesthetic regimen are as problematic as high anesthetic doses, however. It is particularly important to avoid large changes in the anesthetic regimen (i.e., a sudden increase in the concentration of an inhalational anesthetic or a bolus dose of an intravenous anesthetic), especially around the time of critical surgical maneuvers such as positioning of the head and neck in a patient with cervical spinal stenosis or instability, clamping of important blood vessels, or distraction during spinal deformity surgery[4].

Stable anesthesia is, of course, not always possible, and it is important that changes in the anesthetic regimen be communicated to the monitoring team to avoid unnecessary confusion and possible errors.

Cortical SSEPs are affected by surgical anesthesia, and increases in the anesthesia can cause cortical SSEP amplitude changes resembling those due to surgical compromise of neural structures (compare Fig. 34.2 and Fig. 34.4, left and center). If the anesthetic regimen is changed, the baselines for MEPs and cortical SSEPs may have to be reassessed. Even with "stable anesthesia," the effects of anesthetic agents on SSEPs and MEPs can change with time. Over the course of lengthy procedures (e.g., > 6 hours), cortical SSEP amplitudes often gradually diminish, and MEPs stimulation thresholds increase. This effect, known as "anesthetic fade," is seen both with lipid-soluble and lipid-insoluble agents, and is often more pronounced in myelopathic patients. The cause is not known, but it may relate to longer times required for penetration of brain or spinal cord than to reach equilibration in blood, or to anesthetic effects, such as prolongation of refractory periods, that may have slow time courses[89,192]. For intravenous agents such as propofol, for which the blood concentration is not measured but is known to increase with time at constant infusion rates, anesthetic fade, in some cases, may simply reflect increased unrecognized increases in blood concentration. For these reasons as well, baselines must be readjusted over time. Importantly, the effects of anesthetic fade on SSEPs and MEPs can mimic, and must be distinguished from, those of systemic factors that are common with some lengthy procedures, in particular blood loss and hypervolemia.

5.3.2. ANESTHETIC PROTOCOLS FOR NIOM

Selection of anesthesia for monitored cases is ultimately determined by specific patient requirements, the requirements of monitoring, and the preferences of the anesthesiologist. In most cases, there is no single "correct" protocol; flexibility and good communication are keys to successful monitoring.

BAEPs are largely resistant to anesthetic effects, and selection of anesthetic agents generally has no significant effect on BAEP monitoring. However, a change from 0% to 1% isoflurane was reported to produce a modest (up to 0.4 msec) increase in the wave I to V interpeak latency[135]; conceivably, a large change in the concentration of a volatile anesthetic could confound interpretation of BAEP monitoring based on latency criteria.

For SSEP monitoring, the availability of cortical and brainstem signals often provides for considerable flexibility during NIOM of the spinal cord. While cortical SSEPs are attenuated by many anesthetics, particularly the inhalational agents, the concentrations at which these agents interfere with monitoring vary considerably between individuals (Fig. 34.31). When brainstem signals cannot be monitored, it is often necessary to adjust anesthetics to allow for adequate monitoring of cortical signals; in these cases, the considerations regarding stability of anesthesia, discussed above, apply. For patients in whom robust brainstem SSEPs are recorded, substantial attenuation of cortical SSEPs by anesthetic agents may not pose a problem for monitoring and adjustment of anesthetics may not be necessary. Occasionally, when EMG artifact obscures otherwise high-quality brainstem signals, increasing the concentration of a potent inhalational agent may facilitate monitoring by reducing muscle artifact while leaving the brainstem SSEPs unaffected.

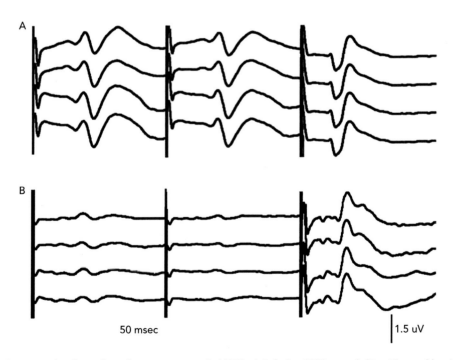

Figure 34.31. *Individual differences in the effects of anesthetic agents on cortical SSEPs. A: Left ulnar SSEPs recorded in a 17-year-old patient receiving propofol 50 μg/kg/hr, nitrous oxide 50%, and isoflurane 0.73%. Easily monitored cortical (CP4-CP3, CP4-Cz) as well as brainstem (CP3-SC5, denoting an electrode placed over the fifth cervical vertebra) SSEPs are recorded. B: Left ulnar SSEPs recorded in a 42-year-old receiving propofol 30 μg/kg/hr, nitrous oxide 56%, and isoflurane 0.74%. Easily monitored brainstem SSEPs are recorded, but cortical signals are attenuated and cannot be monitored.*

MEP monitoring imposes considerable restrictions on anesthetic selection. Muscle MEPs are commonly more sensitive than cortical SSEPs to anesthetic effects (see Fig. 34.4). Further, for motor monitoring there is most often no equivalent to the redundancy afforded by anesthetic-resistant brainstem SSEPs. Although D-waves are substantially unaffected by anesthetic agents, they are not routinely monitored in most situations, and when D-waves are monitored during intramedullary spinal cord surgery, they are usually monitored along with muscle MEPs[193]. TIVA using propofol in combination with remifentanil or another opioid is often recommended as the ideal anesthetic regimen for MEP monitoring[193–195]. As discussed above, this combination permits MEP monitoring even at high propofol blood levels, and high doses of remifentanil will leave MEPs unaffected. Other intravenous agents may be added to reduce propofol requirements. Ketamine can be added without affecting MEPs; dexmedetomidine may be added, but it may attenuate MEPs in a dose-related manner[152,196]. Many anesthesiologists prefer to use balanced anesthesia, for example a reduced dose of propofol in combination with a low dose of volatile agent, rather than TIVA for a variety of reasons, including concerns regarding delayed emergence and opioid tolerance. Satisfactory MEP monitoring is most often possible with either approach, although adjustment of anesthetic doses is more commonly required with balanced anesthesia, likely due to inter-patient differences, as well as nonlinear and synergistic depressant effects. A recent retrospective study comparing 156 patients routinely treated during spine surgery with either TIVA (propofol, average dose 115 µg/kg/min plus opioid) or balanced anesthesia (0.5 MAC of desflurane along with propofol, average dose 49 µg/kg/min, or opioids as needed) at the anesthesiologist's discretion found that, although MEPs occasionally (3/61 patients) could not be obtained in the presence of desflurane, in the remaining patients, there were no significant differences in MEP or cortical SSEP amplitudes or trial-to-trial variability between the two groups[132]. It should be noted that this study examined MEPs from only the abductor pollicis brevis and tibialis anterior muscles, which are commonly used to monitor spinal cord integrity because they are relatively easily elicited. It is likely that more stringent anesthetic requirements will apply if MEPs are used to assess possible nerve root injury because of differences in the stimulation thresholds and stability of individual muscle responses, as well the requirement for stricter interpretive criteria[197].

6. STAFFING FOR NIOM

Many political jurisdictions' standard public policy restricts care of patients to licensed personnel who provide services within a regulatory scope of practice. These practice requirements provide public safety by restricting privileges to individuals with proper skills, knowledge, and abilities based on their training and experience. These regulations generally license individuals to provide advanced care, which gives the government authorities tools to discipline, restrict, or remove from practice individuals who fail to meet standards. Those standards pertain to topics such as competence, ethics, and continuing education.

Operating room neuromonitoring requires three types of personnel skills: (1) someone in the operating room to apply electrodes and run equipment, (2) a professional with advanced knowledge of neurophysiological monitoring, and (3) a licensed physician with knowledge of clinical neurophysiology and patient care[198,199]. In this way, best neuromonitoring tactics and techniques are applied for the patient's clinical circumstances. In many settings, a physician highly skilled in neuromonitoring serves both the second and third roles. In some settings, an advanced non-physician serves both the first and second roles. In some cases, a three-tier model may be employed. Occasionally, one person simultaneously fills all three roles.

Government healthcare regulations generally restrict rendering a diagnosis to a licensed physician. Diagnosis is the rendering of a professional opinion about the presence, absence, type, location, or severity of an illness, injury, or other pathology. The interpretation of medical tests involves rendering a diagnosis, so it is generally restricted to licensed physicians. Interpretation of a diagnostic test or monitoring is the rendering of a professional opinion about the presence, absence, type, location, or severity of an illness, injury, or other pathology based upon the findings of a test or monitoring. Certain other licensed professionals usually also are allowed to render diagnoses and diagnostic interpretations, either based on a limited practice license (e.g., dentists for the mouth, podiatrist for the feet, psychologists for mental health) or under the structured supervision of a physician (e.g., nurse practitioners, physician's assistants). For this reason, NIOM is the practice of medicine.

Technologists and other non-physicians provide services under the rules of a hospital and within the government regulation. They neither render diagnoses nor diagnostic interpretations, nor do they offer medical recommendations about treatment plans. That is the role of the physician involved in the monitoring case. During surgical procedures the technologist works as part of a monitoring team under the supervision of a physician neurophysiologist who is responsible for interpreting the data and making recommendations for actions.

In general, the operating surgeon lacks the suitable knowledge, training, and experience to ensure high-quality monitoring services. The surgeon also is busy during the case and so is unable to keep close watch on the peak identification, artifacts, technical problems, and the meaning of the changes when they occur.

Each hospital's medical staff office provides privileging, credentialing, and proctoring processes to ensure that each physician meets appropriate standards. These determine whether an individual has licensure, insurance, and lack of professional disciplinary actions or criminal convictions to practice in that institution. They also evaluate an individual's training and board certifications for the specific fields of practice and particular techniques proposed. Proctoring involves checking on actual performance during an initial period.

Certification is conducted by national organizations generally known as examining boards. Boards develop written and oral examinations in a specialty or subspecialty, and administer them to qualified individuals. Qualifications for board examinations usually include an extended period of relevant formal supervised training. The validity of board organizations is based in part on their community acceptance and the reputation of their sponsoring organizations. The validity also depends on the skills, knowledge, abilities, training, and experience required of candidates.

Physicians involved in intraoperative monitoring should be well trained about EEG, EMG, and evoked potentials, as well as in the ethics, professionalism, regulations, and other topics relevant to the field.

Technologists and other non-physicians are trained and privileged to provide the technical portion of monitoring[200,201]. They provide immediate feedback about findings, such as latencies, amplitudes, and changes to those readings. The technologist defers to the physician about the meaning of and responses to changes, which are diagnostic opinions restricted to the practice of medicine. Hospital neurodiagnostic departments should evaluate technologists for their skills, knowledge, abilities, training, and experience for intraoperative monitoring. Each technologist should be matched with individual intraoperative procedures for which he or she is qualified. Technologists gain further privileges through learning and proctoring until each is judged competent for a further skill set.

A technologist can monitor without physician or supervisor backup in the room when a physician is monitoring continuously online[202]. A physician clinical neurophysiologist is always involved directly in procedures either in the room or online.

Modern healthcare strives to avoid errors[203]. Communications errors are the most common types of errors in intraoperative monitoring. The surgeon needs to be kept appropriately aware of the state of the at-risk nervous system structure being monitored. The surgeon should also understand the role of monitoring and the possible occurrence of neurological injury despite monitoring. The monitoring team should obtain quality tracings, or else let the surgeon know if problems have been encountered. Likewise, when significant changes occur, clear communication should be made and documented.

Monitoring teams should be aware of professional and public policy as it pertains to NIOM. Some policies regulate background issues such as procedural coding. Many others are in place to ensure patient safety and quality of services. The latter include policies on supervision, staffing, privileging, credentialing, and certifying clinical neurophysiologists and monitoring technologists. These are ways that the profession passes judgment on an individual's skills, knowledge, abilities, and training relevant to monitoring. Good practice also includes good record documentation, clear communications with the surgeon, and professional conduct of the monitoring team.

REFERENCES

1. Epstein CM, Boor DR. Principles of signal analysis and averaging. *Neurol Clin.* 1988;6(4):649–656.
2. American Clinical Neurophysiology Society. Guideline 9C: Guidelines on short-latency auditory evoked potentials. *J Clin Neurophysiol.* 2006;23(2):157–167.
3. American Clinical Neurophysiology Society. Guideline 9D: Guidelines on short-latency somatosensory evoked potentials. *J Clin Neurophysiol.* 2006;23(2):168–179.
4. Legatt AD. Intraoperative neurophysiologic monitoring. In: Frost EAM, ed. *Clinical Anesthesia in Neurosurgery.* 2nd ed. Boston, MA: Butterworth-Heinemann, 1991:63–127.
5. Legatt AD. Mechanisms of intraoperative brainstem auditory evoked potential changes. *J Clin Neurophysiol.* 2002;19(5):396–408.
6. Yvert B, Crouzeix A, Bertrand O, Seither-Preisler A, Pantev C. Multiple supratemporal sources of magnetic and electric auditory evoked middle latency components in humans. *Cerebral Cortex.* 2001;11(5):411–423.
7. Schneider G, Hollweck R, Ningler M, Stockmanns G, Kochs EF. Detection of consciousness by electroencephalogram and auditory evoked potentials. *Anesthesiology.* 2005;103(5):934–943.
8. Legatt AD. Brainstem auditory evoked potentials: Methodology, interpretation, and clinical application. In: Aminoff MJ, ed. *Aminoff's Electrodiagnosis in Clinical Neurology.* 6th ed. New York: Churchill Livingstone, 2012:519–552.
9. Banoub M, Tetzlaff JE, Schubert A. Pharmacologic and physiologic influences affecting sensory evoked potentials: implications for perioperative monitoring. *Anesthesiology.* 2003;99(3):716–737.
10. Stockard JJ, Pope-Stockard JE, Sharbrough FW. Brainstem auditory evoked potentials in neurology: Methodology, interpretation, and clinical application. In: Aminoff MJ, ed. *Electrodiagnosis in Clinical Neurology.* 3rd ed. New York: Churchill Livingstone, 1992:503–536.
11. Litscher G. Continuous brainstem auditory evoked potential monitoring during nocturnal sleep. *Int J Neurosci.* 1995;82(1-2):135–142.
12. Markand ON, Lee BI, Warren C, Stoelting RK, King RD, Brown JW, et al. Effects of hypothermia on brainstem auditory evoked potentials in humans. *Ann Neurol.* 1987;22(4):507–513.
13. Rodriguez RA, Edmonds HL, Jr., Auden SM, Austin EH, III. Auditory brainstem evoked responses and temperature monitoring during pediatric cardiopulmonary bypass. *Can J Anaesth.* 1999;46(9):832–839.
14. Jewett DL, Williston JS. Auditory-evoked far fields averaged from the scalp of humans. *Brain.* 1971;94(4):681–696.
15. Chiappa K, Gladstone KJ, Young RR. Brain stem auditory evoked responses. Studies of waveform variations in 50 normal human subjects. *Arch Neurol.* 1979;36(2):81–87.
16. Legatt AD, Arezzo JC, Vaughan HG, Jr. The anatomic and physiologic bases of brain stem auditory evoked potentials. *Neurol Clin.* 1988;6(4):681–704.
17. Gersdorff MCH. Simultaneous recordings of human auditory potentials: transtympanic electrocochleography (ECoG) and brainstem-evoked responses (BER). *Arch Otorhinolaryngol.* 1982;234(1):15–20.
18. Hughes JR, Fino JJ. A review of generators of the brainstem auditory evoked potential: contribution of an experimental study. *J Clin Neurophysiol.* 1985;2(4):355–381.
19. Grandori F. Field analysis of auditory evoked brainstem potentials. *Hearing Res.* 1986;21(1):51–58.
20. Raudzens PA, Shetter AG. Intraoperative monitoring of brain-stem auditory evoked potentials. *J Neurosurg.* 1982;57(3):341–348.
21. Legatt AD, Pedley TA, Emerson RG, Stein BM, Abramson M, Dowling K, et al. Electrophysiological monitoring of seventh and eighth nerve function during surgery for acoustic neuromas. *Electroencephalogr Clin Neurophysiol.* 1986;64(2):30P.
22. Strominger NL. The origins, course and distribution of the dorsal and intermediate acoustic striae in the rhesus monkey. *J Comp Neurol.* 1973;147(2):209–234.
23. Strominger NL, Nelson LR, Dougherty WJ. Second-order auditory pathways in the chimpanzee. *J Comp Neurol.* 1977;172(2):349–366.
24. Strominger NL, Strominger AI. Ascending brain stem projections of the anteroventral cochlear nucleus in the rhesus monkey. *J Comp Neurol.* 1971;143(2):217–242.
25. Brown RH, Jr., Chiappa KH, Brooks E. Brain stem auditory evoked responses in 22 patients with intrinsic brain stem lesions: implications for clinical interpretations. *Electroencephalogr Clin Neurophysiol.* 1981;51(2):38P.
26. Faught E, Oh SJ. Brainstem auditory evoked responses in brainstem infarction. *Stroke.* 1985;16(4):701–705.
27. Oh SJ, Kuba T, Soyer A, Choi IS, Bonikowski FP, Vitek J. Lateralization of brainstem lesions by brainstem auditory evoked potentials. *Neurology.* 1981;31(1):14–18.
28. Stockard JJ, Rossiter VS. Clinical and pathologic correlates of brain stem auditory response abnormalities. *Neurology.* 1977;27(4):316–325.
29. Starr A, Hamilton AE. Correlation between confirmed sites of neurological lesions and abnormalities of far-field auditory brainstem responses. *Electroencephalogr Clin Neurophysiol.* 1976;41(6):595–608.

30. Stockard JJ, Stockard JE, Sharbrough FW. Detection and localization of occult lesions with brainstem auditory responses. *Mayo Clin Proc.* 1977;52(12):761–769.

31. Hirsch BE, Durrant JD, Yetiser S, Kamerer DB, Martin WH. Localizing retrocochlear hearing loss. *Am J Otol.* 1996;17(4):537–546.

32. York DH. Correlation between a unilateral midbrain-pontine lesion and abnormalities of brain-stem auditory evoked potential. *Electroencephalogr Clin Neurophysiol.* 1986;65(4):282–288.

33. Scaioli V, Savoiardo M, Bussone G, Rezzonico M. Brain-stem auditory evoked potentials (BAEPs) and magnetic resonance imaging (MRI) in a case of facial myokymia. *Electroencephalogr Clin Neurophysiol.* 1988;71(2):153–156.

34. Zanette G, Carteri A, Cusumano S. Reappearance of brain-stem auditory evoked potentials after surgical treatment of a brain-stem hemorrhage: contributions to the question of wave generation. *Electroencephalogr Clin Neurophysiol.* 1990;77(2):140–144.

35. Fischer C, Bognar L, Turjman F, Lapras C. Auditory evoked potentials in a patient with a unilateral lesion of the inferior colliculus and medial geniculate body. *Electroencephalogr Clin Neurophysiol.* 1995;96(3):261–267.

36. Emerson RG, Brooks EB, Parker SW, Chiappa KH. Effects of click polarity on brainstem auditory evoked potentials in normal subjects and patients: unexpected sensitivity of wave V. *Ann NY Acad Sci.* 1982;388:710–721.

37. Schwartz DM, Morris MD, Spydell JD, Brink CT, Grim MA, Schwartz JA. Influence of click polarity on the brain-stem auditory evoked response (BAER) revisited. *Electroencephalogr Clin Neurophysiol.* 1990;77(6):445–457.

38. Little JR, Lesser RP, Lueders H, Furlan AJ. Brain stem auditory evoked potentials in posterior circulation surgery. *Neurosurgery.* 1983;12(5):496–502.

39. Roeser RJ, Clark JL. Clinical masking. In: Roeser RJ, Valente M, Hosford-Dunn H, eds. *Audiology: Diagnosis.* New York: Thieme, 2000:253–279.

40. Møller AR, Jannetta PJ. Monitoring auditory functions during cranial nerve microvascular decompression operations by direct recording from the eighth nerve. *J Neurosurg.* 1983;59(3):493–499.

41. Kim HN, Kim YH, Park IY, Kim GR, Chung IH. Variability of the surgical anatomy of the neurovascular complex of the cerebellopontine angle. *Ann Otol Rhinol Laryngol.* 1990;99(4 Pt 1):288–296.

42. Nadol JB, Jr., Levine R, Ojemann RG, Martuza RL, Montgomery WW, de Sandoval PK. Preservation of hearing in surgical removal of acoustic neuromas of the internal auditory canal and cerebellar pontine angle. *Laryngoscope.* 1987;97(11):1287–1294.

43. Sekiya T, Møller AR. Avulsion rupture of the internal auditory artery during operations in the cerebellopontine angle: a study in monkeys. *Neurosurgery.* 1987;21(5):631–637.

44. Levine RA, Ronner SF, Ojemann RG. Auditory evoked potential and other neurophysiologic monitoring techniques during tumor surgery in the cerebellopontine angle. In: Loftus CM, Traynelis VC, eds. *Intraoperative Monitoring Techniques in Neurosurgery.* New York: McGraw-Hill, 1994:175–191.

45. Radtke RA, Erwin CW, Wilkins RH. Intraoperative brainstem auditory evoked potentials: significant decrease in postoperative morbidity. *Neurology.* 1989;39(2 Pt 1):187–191.

46. Nuwer MR, Packwood JW. Somatosensory evoked potential monitoring with scalp and cervical recording. In: Nuwer MR, ed. *Intraoperative Monitoring of Neural Function Handbook of Clinical Neurophysiology, Volume 8.* Amsterdam: Elsevier, 2008:180–189.

47. Kimura J, ed. *Electrodiagnosis in Diseases of Nerve and Muscle: Principles and Practice.* 3rd ed. Oxford: Oxford University Press, 2001.

48. Pelosi L, Cracco JB, Cracco RQ, Hassan NF. Comparison of scalp distribution of short latency somatosensory evoked potentials (SSEPs) to stimulation of different nerves in the lower extremity. *Electroencephalogr Clin Neurophysiol.* 1988;71(6):422–428.

49. Draughn LR, Swanson TH. Axillary somatosensory evoked potential response: an alternate peripheral recording site. *J Clin Neurophysiol.* 1998;15(1):64–68.

50. Fried SJ, Legatt AD. The utility of a forehead-to-inion derivation in recording the subcortical far-field potential (P14) during median nerve somatosensory-evoked potential testing. *Clin EEG Neurosci.* 2012;43(2):121–126.

51. American Clinical Neurophysiology Society. Guideline 5: Guidelines for standard electrode position nomenclature. *J Clin Neurophysiol.* 1996;23(2):107–110.

52. Philips M, Kotapka M, Patterson T, Bigelow DC, Zager E, Flamm ES, et al. Brainstem origins of the N18 component of the somatosensory evoked response. *Skull Base Surg.* 1998;8(3):133–140.

53. Desmedt JE, Cheron G. Non-cephalic reference recording of early somatosensory potentials to finger stimulation in adult or aging normal man: differentiation of widespread N18 and contralateral N20 from pre-rolandic P22 and N30 components. *Electroencephalogr Clin Neurophysiol.* 1981;52(6):553–570.

54. Emerson RG. Anatomic and physiologic bases of posterior tibial nerve somatosensory evoked potentials. *Neurol Clin.* 1988;6(4):735–749.

55. Allison T, Goff WR, Williamson PD, VanGilder JC. On the neural origin of early components of the human somatosensory evoked potential. In: Desmedt JE, ed. *Clinical Uses of Cerebral, Brainstem and Spinal Somatosensory Evoked Potentials: Progress in Clinical Neurophysiology, Vol. 7.* Basel: S. Karger, 1980:51–68.

56. Broughton R, Rasmussen T, Branch C. Scalp and direct cortical recordings of somatosensory evoked potentials in man (circa 1967). *Can J Psychol.* 1981;35(2):136–158.

57. Lueders H, Lesser RP, Hahn J, Dinner DS, Klem G. Cortical somatosensory evoked potentials in response to hand stimulation. *J Neurosurg.* 1983;58(6):885–894.

58. Gregorie EM, Goldring S. Localization of function in the excision of lesions from the sensorimotor region. *J Neurosurg.* 1984;61(6):1047–1054.

59. King RB, Schell G. Cortical localization and monitoring during cerebral operations. *J Neurosurg.* 1987;67(2):210–219.

60. Wood CC, Spencer DD, Allison T, McCarthy G, Williamson PD, Goff WR. Localization of human sensorimotor cortex during surgery by cortical surface recording of somatosensory evoked potentials. *J Neurosurg.* 1988;68(1):99–111.

61. Legatt AD, Kader A. Topography of the initial cortical component of the median nerve somatosensory evoked potential: relationship to central sulcus anatomy. *J Clin Neurophysiol.* 2000;17(3):321–325.

62. Yamada T. The anatomic and physiologic bases of median nerve somatosensory evoked potentials. *Neurol Clin.* 1988;6(4):705–733.

63. O'Brien MF, Lenke LG, Bridwell KH, Padberg A, Stokes M. Evoked potential monitoring of the upper extremities during thoracic and lumbar spinal deformity surgery:a prospective study. *J Spinal Disord.* 1994;7(4):277–284.

64. Chung I, Glow JA, Dimopoulos V, Walid MS, Smisson HF, Johnston KW, et al. Upper-limb somatosensory evoked potential monitoring in lumbosacral spine surgery: a prognostic marker for position-related ulnar nerve injury. *Spine J.* 2009;9(4):287–295.

65. Cusick JF, Myklebust JB, Larson SJ, Sances A, Jr. Spinal cord evaluation by cortical evoked responses. *Arch Neurol.* 1979;36(3):140–143.

66. Machida M, Weinstein SL, Yamada T, Kimura J, Toriyama S. Dissociation of muscle action potentials and spinal somatosensory evoked potentials after ischemic damage of spinal cord. *Spine.* 1988;13(10):1119–1124.

67. Ben-David B, Haller G, Taylor P. Anterior spinal fusion complicated by paraplegia: a case report of a false-negative somatosensory-evoked potential. *Spine.* 1987;12(6):536–539.

68. Zornow MH, Grafe MR, Tybor C, Swenson MR. Preservation of evoked potentials in a case of anterior spinal artery syndrome. *Electroencephalogr Clin Neurophysiol.* 1990;77(2):137–139.

69. Jones SJ, Buonamassa S, Crockard HA. Two cases of quadriparesis following anterior cervical discectomy, with normal perioperative somatosensory evoked potentials. *J Neurol Neurosurg Psychiatry.* 2003;74(2):273–276.

70. Ben-David B, Taylor PD, Haller GS. Posterior spinal fusion complicated by posterior column injury. A case report of a false-negative wake-up test. *Spine.* 1987;12(6):540–543.

71. Chatrian G-E, Berger MS, Wirch AL. Discrepancy between intraoperative SSEPs and postoperative function. *J Neurosurg.* 1988;69(3):450–454.

72. Legatt AD. Current practice of motor evoked potential monitoring: results of a survey. *J Clin Neurophysiol.* 2002;19(5):454–460.

73. Owen JH, Laschinger J, Bridwell K, Shimon S, Nielsen C, Dunlap J, et al. Sensitivity and specificity of somatosensory and neurogenic-motor evoked potentials in animals and humans. *Spine.* 1988;13(10):1111–1118.

74. Toleikis JR, Skelly JP, Carlvin AO, Burkus JK. Spinally elicited peripheral nerve responses are sensory rather than motor. *Clin Neurophysiol.* 2000;111(4):736–742.

75. Minahan RE, Sepkuty JP, Lesser RP, Sponseller PD, Kostuik JP. Anterior spinal cord injury with preserved neurogenic "motor" evoked potentials. *Clin Neurophysiol.* 2001;112(8):1442–1450.

76. Machida M, Weinstein SL, Yamada T, Kimura J, Itagaki T, Usui T. Monitoring of motor action potentials after stimulation of the spinal cord. *J Bone Joint Surg.* 1988;70(6):911–918.

77. Mochida K, Shinomiya K, Komori H, Furuya K. A new method of multisegment motor pathway monitoring using muscle potentials after train spinal stimulation. *Spine.* 1995;20(20):2240–2246.

78. Su CF, Haghighi SS, Oro JJ, Gaines RW. "Backfiring" in spinal cord monitoring. High thoracic spinal cord stimulation evokes sciatic response by antidromic sensory pathway conduction, not motor tract conduction. *Spine.* 1992;17(5):504–508.

79. Legatt AD, Ellen R. Ellen R. Grass Lecture: Motor evoked potential monitoring. *Am J Electroneurodiagn Technol.* 2004;44(4):223–243.

80. Sloan T, Heyer EJ. Anesthesia for intraoperative neurophysiologic monitoring of the spinal cord. *J Clin Neurophysiol.* 2002;19(5):430–443.

81. Burke D, Hicks RG. Surgical monitoring of motor pathways. *J Clin Neurophysiol.* 1998;15(3):194–205.

82. Deletis V, Kothbauer K. Intraoperative neurophysiology of the corticospinal tract. In: Stålberg E, Sharma HS, Olsson Y, eds. *Spinal Cord Monitoring.* Wein: Springer, 1998:421–444.

83. Legatt AD, Emerson RG, Epstein CM, MacDonald DB, Deletis V, Bravo RJ, et al. ACNS guideline: transcranial electrical stimulation motor evoked potential monitoring. *J Clin Neurophysiol.* 2016;33(1):42–50.

84. Rothwell J, Burke D, Hicks R, Stephen J, Woodforth I, Crawford M. Transcranial electrical stimulation of the motor cortex in man: further evidence for the site of activation. *J Physiol.* 1994;481(Pt 1):243–250.

85. Legatt AD. *Intraoperative Neurophysiology: Interactive Case Studies.* New York: Demos Medical Publishing, 2015.

86. Amassian VE, Stewart M, Quirk GJ, Rosenthal JL. Physiological basis of motor effects of a transient stimulus to cerebral cortex. *Neurosurgery.* 1987;20(1):74–93.

87. Kamada K, Todo T, Ota T, Ino K, Masutani Y, Aoki S, et al. The motor-evoked potential threshold evaluated by tractography and electrical stimulation. *J Neurosurg.* 2009;111(4):785–795.

88. Nossek E, Korn A, Shahar T, Kanner AA, Yaffe H, Marcovici D, et al. Intraoperative mapping and monitoring of the corticospinal tracts with neurophysiological assessment and 3-dimensional ultrasonography-based navigation. *J Neurosurg.* 2011;114(3):738–746.

89. Lyon R, Feiner J, Lieberman JA. Progressive suppression of motor evoked potentials during general anesthesia: the phenomenon of "anesthetic fade." *J Neurosurg Anesthesiol.* 2005;17(1):13–19.

90. MacDonald DB, Al Zayed Z, Khoudeir I, Stigsby B. Monitoring scoliosis surgery with combined multiple pulse transcranial electric motor and cortical somatosensory-evoked potentials from the lower and upper extremities. *Spine.* 2003;28(2):194–203.

91. Legatt AD. MEPs elicited by cathodal stimulation during transcranial electrical stimulation-MEP monitoring. *Neurology.* 2006;66(Suppl. 2):A68.

92. Nagle KJ, Emerson RG, Adams DC, Heyer EJ, Roye DP, Schwab FJ, et al. Intraoperative monitoring of motor evoked potentials: a review of 116 cases. *Neurology.* 1996;47(4):999–1004.

93. Silverman D. The rationale and history of the 10–20 system of the International Federation. *Am J EEG Technol.* 1973;3(1):17–22.

94. Chiappa KH, Burke SR, Young RR. Results of electroencephalographic monitoring during 367 carotid endarterectomies. Use of a dedicated minicomputer. *Stroke.* 1979;10(4):381–388.

95. Ahn SS, Jordan SE, Nuwer MR. Computerized EEG topographic brain mapping. In: Moore WS, ed. *Surgery for Cerebrovascular Disease.* New York: Churchill Livingstone, 1987:275–280.

96. Ahn SS, Jordon SE, Nuwer MR, Marcus DR, Moore WS. Computed electroencephalographic topographic brain mapping: a new and accurate monitor of cerebral circulation and function for patients having carotid endarterectomy. *J Vasc Surg.* 1988;8(3):247–254.

97. Redekop G, Ferguson G. Correlation of contralateral stenosis and intraoperative electroencephalogram change with risk of stroke during carotid endarterectomy. *Neurosurgery.* 1992;30(2):191–194.

98. Blume WT, Ferguson GG, McNeill DK. Significance of EEG changes at carotid endarterectomy. *Stroke.* 1986;17(5):891–897.

99. Sundt TM, Sharbrough FW, Anderson RE, Michenfelder JD. Cerebral blood flow measurements and electroencephalograms during carotid endarterectomy. *J Neurosurg.* 1974;41(3):310–320.

100. McKay RD, Sundt TM, Jr., Michenfelder JD, Gronert GA, Messick JM, Sharbrough FW, et al. Internal carotid artery stump pressure and cerebral blood flow during carotid endarterectomy: modification by halothane, enflurane, and Innovar. *Anesthesiology.* 1976;45(4):390–399.

101. Haupt WF, Horsch S. Evoked potential monitoring in carotid surgery: a review of 994 cases. *Neurology.* 1992;42(4):835–838.

102. Mizrahi EM, Patel VM, Crawford ES, Coselli JS, Hess KR. Hypothermic-induced electrocerebral silence, prolonged circulatory arrest, and cerebral protection during cardiovascular surgery. *Electroencephalogr Clin Neurophysiol.* 1989;72(1):81–85.

103. James ML, Andersen ND, Swaminathan M, Phillips-Bute B, Hanna JM, Smigla GR, et al. Predictors of electrocerebral inactivity with deep hypothermia. *J Thorac Cardiovasc Surg.* 2014;147(3):1002–1007.

104. MacDonald DB. Safety of intraoperative transcranial electrical stimulation motor evoked potential monitoring. *J Clin Neurophysiol.* 2002;19(5):416–429.

105. Rampil IJ. A primer for EEG signal processing in anesthesia. *Anesthesiology.* 1998;89(4):980–1002.

106. Schneider G, Gelb AW, Schmeller B, Tschakert R, Kochs E. Detection of awareness in surgical patients with EEG-based indices—bispectral index and patient state index. *Br J Anaesth.* 2003;91(3):329–335.

107. Purdon PL, Sampson A, Pavone KJ, Brown EN. Clinical electroencephalography for anesthesiologists: Part I: Background and basic signatures. *Anesthesiology.* 2015;123(4):937–960.

108. Bennett C, Voss LJ, Barnard JP, Sleigh JW. Practical use of the raw electroencephalogram waveform during general anesthesia: the art and science. *Anesth Analg.* 2009;109(2):539–550.

109. Kelly S. Monitoring consciousness using the bispectral index (BIS) during anesthesia. Available from:http://solutionscontent.covidien.com/uploads/0/871-10PM6809v1_updated-1441832714.pdf

110. Morimoto Y, Hagihira S, Koizumi Y, Ishida K, Matsumoto M, Sakabe T. The relationship between bispectral index and electroencephalographic parameters during isoflurane anesthesia. *Anesth Analg.* 2004;98(5):1336–1340.

111. Myles PS, Leslie K, McNeil J, Forbes A, Chan MT. Bispectral index monitoring to prevent awareness during anaesthesia: the B-Aware randomised controlled trial. *Lancet.* 2004;363(9423):1757–1763.

112. Avidan MS, Zhang L, Burnside BA, Finkel KJ, Searleman AC, Selvidge JA, et al. Anesthesia awareness and the bispectral index. *N Engl J Med.* 2008;358(11):1097–1108.

113. Avidan M, Jacobson E, Glick D, Burnside B, Zhang L, Villafranca A, et al. Prevention of intraoperative awareness in a high-risk surgical population. *N Engl J Med.* 2011;365(7):591–600.

114. Glass PS, Bloom M, Kearse L, Rosow C, Sebel P, Manberg P. Bispectral analysis measures sedation and memory effects of propofol, midazolam, isoflurane, and alfentanil in healthy volunteers. *Anesthesiology.* 1997;86(4):836–847.

115. Bharti N, Devrajan J. Comparison of bispectral index values produced by isoflurane and halothane at equal end-tidal MAC concentrations. *Indian J Anaesth.* 2007;51(5):401–404.

116. Kaskinoro K, Maksimow A, Langsjo J, Aantaa R, Jaaskelainen S, Kaisti K, et al. Wide inter-individual variability of bispectral index and spectral entropy at loss of consciousness during increasing concentrations of dexmedetomidine, propofol, and sevoflurane. *Br J Anaesth.* 2011;107(4):573–580.

117. Akeju O, Westover MB, Pavone KJ, Sampson AL, Hartnack KE, Brown EN, et al. Effects of sevoflurane and propofol on frontal electroencephalogram power and coherence. *Anesthesiology.* 2014;121(5):990–998.

118. Purdon PL, Pierce ET, Mukamel EA, Prerau MJ, Walsh JL, Wong KF, et al. Electroencephalogram signatures of loss and recovery of consciousness from propofol. *Proc Natl Acad Sci USA.* 2013;110(12):E1142–E1151.

119. Akeju O, Pavone KJ, Westover MB, Vazquez R, Prerau MJ, Harrell PG, et al. A comparison of propofol- and dexmedetomidine-induced electroencephalogram dynamics using spectral and coherence analysis. *Anesthesiology.* 2014;121(5):978–989.

120. Romstöck J, Strauss C, Fahlbusch R. Continuous electromyography monitoring of motor cranial nerves during cerebellopontine angle surgery. *J Neurosurg.* 2000;93(4):586–593.

121. Skinner SA, Transfeldt EE, Mehbod AA, Mullan JC, Perra JH. Electromyography detects mechanically-induced suprasegmental spinal motor tract injury: review of decompression at spinal cord level. *Clin Neurophysiol.* 2009;120(4):754–764.

122. Fasano VA, Broggi G, Barolat-Romana G, Sguazzi A. Surgical treatment of spasticity in cerebral palsy. *Childs Brain.* 1978;4(5):289–305.

123. Peacock WJ, Arens LJ, Berman B. Cerebral palsy spasticity. Selective posterior rhizotomy. *Pediat Neurosci.* 1987;13(2):61–66.

124. Galloway G. Selective dorsal rhizotomies: technique and protocol for monitoring. In: Galloway G, Nuwer MR, Lopez J, Zamel K, eds. *Intraoperative Neurophysiological Monitoring.* Cambridge, UK: Cambridge University Press, 2010:196–206.

125. Staudt LA, Nuwer MR, Peacock WJ. Intraoperative monitoring during selective posterior rhizotomy: technique and patient outcome. *Electroencephalogr Clin Neurophysiol.* 1995;97(6):296–309.

126. Peacock WJ, Staudt LA. Functional outcomes following selective posterior rhizotomy in children with cerebral palsy. *J Neurosurg.* 1991;74(3):380–385.

127. Mittal S, Farmer JP, Al-Atassi B, Montpetit K, Gervais N, Poulin C, et al. Functional performance following selective posterior rhizotomy: long-term results determined using a validated evaluative measure. *J Neurosurg.* 2002;97(3):510–518.

128. Huang JC, Deletis V, Vodusek DB, Abbott R. Preservation of pudendal afferents in sacral rhizotomies. *Neurosurgery.* 1997;41(2):411–415.

129. Pandit J, Cook T. Accidental awareness during general anaesthesia in the United Kingdom and Ireland 2014 [Available from: http://www.nationalauditprojects.org.uk/NAP5report]; accessed 2/14/2016.

130. Sandin R, Enlund G, Samuelsson P, Lennmarken C. Awareness during anaesthesia: a prospective case study. *Lancet*. 2000;355(9205):707–711.

131. Davidson A, Huang G, Czarnecki C, Gibson M, Stewart S, Jamsen K, et al. Awareness during anesthesia in children: a prospective cohort study. *Anesth Analg*. 2005;100(3):653–661.

132. Sloan TB, Toleikis JR, Toleikis SC, Koht A. Intraoperative neurophysiological monitoring during spine surgery with total intravenous anesthesia or balanced anesthesia with 3% desflurane. *J Clin Monit Comput*. 2015;29(1):77–85.

133. Sekimoto K, Nishikawa K, Ishizeki J, Kubo K, Saito S, Goto F. The effects of volatile anesthetics on intraoperative monitoring of myogenic motor-evoked potentials to transcranial electrical stimulation and on partial neuromuscular blockade during propofol/fentanyl/nitrous oxide anesthesia in humans. *J Neurosurg Anesthesiol*. 2006;18(2):106–111.

134. Peterson DO, Drummond JC, Todd MM. Effects of halothane, enflurane, isoflurane, and nitrous oxide on somatosensory evoked potentials in humans. *Anesthesiology*. 1986;65(1):35–40.

135. Manninen PH, Lam AM, Nicolas JF. The effects of isoflurane and isoflurane-nitrous oxide anesthesia on brainstem auditory evoked potentials in humans. *Anesth Analg*. 1985;64(1):43–47.

136. Ohara A, Mashimo T, Zhang P, Inagaki Y, Shibuta S, Yoshiya I. A comparative study of the antinociceptive action of xenon and nitrous oxide in rats. *Anesth Analg*. 1997;85(4):931–936.

137. Fukagawa H, Koyama T, Fukuda K. kappa-Opioid receptor mediates the antinociceptive effect of nitrous oxide in mice. *Br J Anaesth*. 2014;113(6):1032–1038.

138. Thornton C, Creagh-Barry P, Jordan C, Luff NP, Doré CJ, Henley M, et al. Somatosensory and auditory evoked responses recorded simultaneously: differential effects of nitrous oxide and isoflurane. *Br J Anaesth*. 1992;68(5):508–514.

139. Kunisawa T, Nagata O, Nomura M, Iwasaki H, Ozaki M. A comparison of the absolute amplitude of motor evoked potentials among groups of patients with various concentrations of nitrous oxide. *J Anesth*. 2004;18(3):181–184.

140. Sloan T, Sloan H, Rogers J. Nitrous oxide and isoflurane are synergistic with respect to amplitude and latency effects on sensory evoked potentials. *J Clin Monit Comput*. 2010;24(2):113–123.

141. Devor M, Zalkind V. Reversible analgesia, atonia, and loss of consciousness on bilateral intracerebral microinjection of pentobarbital. *Pain*. 2001;94(1):101–112.

142. Veselis RA, Reinsel RA, Feshchenko VA, Wronski M. The comparative amnestic effects of midazolam, propofol, thiopental, and fentanyl at equisedative concentrations. *Anesthesiology*. 1997;87(4):749–764.

143. Absalom AR, Mani V, De Smet T, Struys MM. Pharmacokinetic models for propofol: defining and illuminating the devil in the detail. *Br J Anaesth*. 2009;103(1):26–37.

144. Patel PM, Patel HH, Roth DM. General anesthetics and therapeutic gases. In: Brunton LL, Chabner BA, Knollmann BC, eds. *Goodman & Gilman's The Pharmacological Basis of Therapeutics*. 12th ed. New York: McGraw-Hill, 2011.

145. Boisseau N, Madany M, Staccini P, Armando G, Martin F, Grimaud D, et al. Comparison of the effects of sevoflurane and propofol on cortical somatosensory evoked potentials. *Br J Anaesth*. 2002;88(6):785–789.

146. Chen Z. The effects of isoflurane and propofol on intraoperative neurophysiological monitoring during spinal surgery. *J Clin Monit Comput*. 2004;18(4):303–308.

147. Maurette P, Simeon F, Castagnera L, Esposito J, Macouillard G, Heraut LA. Propofol anaesthesia alters somatosensory evoked cortical potentials. *Anaesthesia*. 1988;43(Suppl):44–45.

148. Purdie JA, Cullen PM. Brainstem auditory evoked response during propofol anaesthesia in children. *Anaesthesia*. 1993;48(3):192–195.

149. Nathan N, Tabaraud F, Lacroix F, Moulies D, Viviand X, Lansade A, et al. Influence of propofol concentrations on multipulse transcranial motor evoked potentials. *Br J Anaesth*. 2003;91(4):493–497.

150. Scheufler KM, Reinacher PC, Blumrich W, Zentner J, Priebe HJ. The modifying effects of stimulation pattern and propofol plasma concentration on motor-evoked potentials. *Anesth Analg*. 2005;100(2):440–447.

151. Journée HL, Polak HE, De Kleuver M. Conditioning stimulation techniques for enhancement of transcranially elicited evoked motor responses. *Neurophysiol Clin*. 2007;37(6):423–430.

152. Mahmoud M, Sadhasivam S, Salisbury S, Nick TG, Schnell B, Sestokas AK, et al. Susceptibility of transcranial electric motor-evoked potentials to varying targeted blood levels of dexmedetomidine during spine surgery. *Anesthesiology*. 2010;112(6):1364–1373.

153. van Hemelrijck J, Tempelhoff R, White PF, Jellish WS. EEG-assisted titration of propofol infusion during neuroanesthesia: effect of nitrous oxide. *J Neurosurg Anesthesiol*. 1992;4(1):11–20.

154. Liolios A, Guerit JM, Scholtes JL, Raftopoulos C, Hantson P. Propofol infusion syndrome associated with short-term large-dose infusion during surgical anesthesia in an adult. *Anesth Analg*. 2005;100(6):1804–1806.

155. Drexler B, Jurd R, Rudolph U, Antkowiak B. Distinct actions of etomidate and propofol at beta3-containing gamma-aminobutyric acid type A receptors. *Neuropharmacology*. 2009;57(4):446–455.

156. Sloan T. Anesthesia and intraoperative neurophysiological monitoring in children. *Childs Nerv Syst*. 2010;26(2):227–235.

157. Scheufler KM, Zentner J. Total intravenous anesthesia for intraoperative monitoring of the motor pathways: an integral view combining clinical and experimental data. *J Neurosurg*. 2002;96(3):571–579.

158. Pathak KS, Brown RH, Cascorbi HF, Nash CL, Jr. Effects of fentanyl and morphine on intraoperative somatosensory cortical-evoked potentials. *Anesth Analg*. 1984;63(9):833–837.

159. Kalkman CJ, Leyssius AT, Bovill JG. Influence of high-dose opioid anesthesia on posterior tibial nerve somatosensory cortical evoked potentials: effects of fentanyl, sufentanil, and alfentanil. *J Cardiothorac Anesth*. 1988;2(6):758–764.

160. Scheufler KM, Thees C, Nadstawek J, Zentner J. S(+)-ketamine attenuates myogenic motor-evoked potentials at or distal to the spinal alpha-motoneuron. *Anesth Analg*. 2003;96(1):238–244.

161. Thees C, Scheufler KM, Nadstawek J, Pechstein U, Hanisch M, Juntke R, et al. Influence of fentanyl, alfentanil, and sufentanil on motor evoked potentials. *J Neurosurg Anesthesiol*. 1999;11(2):112–118.

162. Egan TD, Lemmens HJ, Fiset P, Hermann DJ, Muir KT, Stanski DR, et al. The pharmacokinetics of the new short-acting opioid remifentanil (GI87084B) in healthy adult male volunteers. *Anesthesiology*. 1993;79(5):881–892.

163. Guignard B, Bossard AE, Coste C, Sessler DI, Lebrault C, Alfonsi P, et al. Acute opioid tolerance: intraoperative remifentanil increases postoperative pain and morphine requirement. *Anesthesiology*. 2000;93(2):409–417.

164. Kohrs R, Durieux ME. Ketamine: teaching an old drug new tricks. *Anesth Analg*. 1998;87(5):1186–1193.

165. Schubert A, Licina MG, Lineberry PJ. The effect of ketamine on human somatosensory evoked potentials and its modification by nitrous oxide. *Anesthesiology*. 1990;72(1):33–39.

166. Inoue S, Kawaguchi M, Kakimoto M, Sakamoto T, Kitaguchi K, Furuya H, et al. Amplitudes and intrapatient variability of myogenic motor evoked potentials to transcranial electrical stimulation during ketamine/N2O- and propofol/N2O-based anesthesia. *J Neurosurg Anesthesiol*. 2002;14(3):213–217.

167. Zaarour C, Engelhardt T, Strantzas S, Pehora C, Lewis S, Crawford MW. Effect of low-dose ketamine on voltage requirement for transcranial electrical motor evoked potentials in children. *Spine*. 2007;32(22):E627–E630.

168. Gertler R, Brown HC, Mitchell DH, Silvius EN. Dexmedetomidine: a novel sedative-analgesic agent. *Bayl Univ Med Cent Proc*. 2001;14(1):13–21.

169. Sloan TB, Mongan P, Lyda C, Koht A. Lidocaine infusion adjunct to total intravenous anesthesia reduces the total dose of propofol during intraoperative neurophysiological monitoring. *J Clin Monit Comput*. 2014;28(2):139–147.

170. Lauwick S, Kim DJ, Michelagnoli G, Mistraletti G, Feldman L, Fried G, et al. Intraoperative infusion of lidocaine reduces postoperative fentanyl requirements in patients undergoing laparoscopic cholecystectomy. *Can J Anaesth*. 2008;55(11):754–760.

171. Kaba A, Laurent SR, Detroz BJ, Sessler DI, Durieux ME, Lamy ML, et al. Intravenous lidocaine infusion facilitates acute rehabilitation after laparoscopic colectomy. *Anesthesiology*. 2007;106(1):11–18.

172. Gottschalk A, McKay AM, Malik ZM, Forbes M, Durieux ME, Groves DS. Systemic lidocaine decreases the Bispectral Index in the presence of midazolam, but not its absence. *J Clin Anesth*. 2012;24(2):121–125.

173. Sloan TB. Muscle relaxant use during intraoperative neurophysiologic monitoring. *J Clin Monit Comput*. 2013;27(1):35–46.

174. Debaene B, Plaud B, Dilly MP, Donati F. Residual paralysis in the PACU after a single intubating dose of nondepolarizing muscle relaxant with an intermediate duration of action. *Anesthesiology*. 2003;98(5):1042–1048.

175. Barash PG, Cullen BF, Stoelting RK, Cahalan MK, Stock MC, Ortega R, et al. *Clinical Anesthesia Fundamentals*. New York: Wolters Kluwer, 2015.

176. Fink H, Hollmann MW. Myths and facts in neuromuscular pharmacology. New developments in reversing neuromuscular blockade. *Minerva Anestesiol*. 2012;78(4):473–482.

177. Minahan RE, Riley LH, Lukaczyk T, Cohen DB, Kostuik JP. The effect of neuromuscular blockade on pedicle screw stimulation thresholds. *Spine*. 2000;25(19):2526–2530.

178. Gavrancic B, Lolis A, Beric A. Train-of-four test in intraoperative neurophysiologic monitoring: differences between hand and foot train-of-four. *J Clin Neurophysiol*. 2014;31(6):575–579.

179. van Dongen EP, ter Beek HT, Schepens MA, Morshuis WJ, Langemeijer HJ, de Boer A, et al. Within-patient variability of myogenic motor-evoked potentials to multipulse transcranial electrical stimulation during two levels of partial neuromuscular blockade in aortic surgery. *Anesth Analg.* 1999;88(1):22–27.

180. Gibbs FA, Gibbs EL, Lennox WG. Effects on the electro-encephalogram of certain drugs which influence nervous activity. *Arch Intern Med.* 1937;60(1):154–166.

181. Jäntti V, Sloan TB. EEG and anesthetic effects. In: Nuwer MR, ed. *Intraoperative Monitoring of Neural Function Handbook of Clinical Neurophysiology, Volume 8.* Amsterdam: Elsevier, 2008:77–93.

182. Yli-Hankala A. The effect of nitrous oxide on EEG spectral power during halothane and isoflurane anaesthesia. *Acta Anaesthesiol Scand.* 1990;34(7):579–584.

183. Jensen O, Goel P, Kopell N, Pohja M, Hari R, Ermentrout B. On the human sensorimotor-cortex beta rhythm: sources and modeling. *Neuroimage.* 2005;26(2):347–355.

184. Porkkala T, Jantti V, Kaukinen S, Hakkinen V. Nitrous oxide has different effects on the EEG and somatosensory evoked potentials during isoflurane anaesthesia in patients. *Acta Anaesthesiol Scand.* 1997;41(4):497–501.

185. Hirota K. Special cases: ketamine, nitrous oxide and xenon. *Best Pract Res Clin Anaesthesiol.* 2006;20(1):69–79.

186. Huupponen E, Maksimow A, Lapinlampi P, Sarkela M, Saastamoinen A, Snapir A, et al. Electroencephalogram spindle activity during dexmedetomidine sedation and physiological sleep. *Acta Anaesthesiol Scand.* 2008;52(2):289–294.

187. Scott JC, Cooke JE, Stanski DR. Electroencephalographic quantitation of opioid effect: comparative pharmacodynamics of fentanyl and sufentanil. *Anesthesiology.* 1991;74(1):34–42.

188. Cascino GD, So EL, Sharbrough FW, Strelow D, Lagerlund TD, Milde LN, et al. Alfentanil-induced epileptiform activity in patients with partial epilepsy. *J Clin Neurophysiol.* 1993;10(4):520–525.

189. McGuire G, El-Beheiry H, Manninen P, Lozano A, Wennberg R. Activation of electrocorticographic activity with remifentanil and alfentanil during neurosurgical excision of epileptogenic focus. *Br J Anaesth.* 2003;91(5):651–655.

190. Wass CT, Grady RE, Fessler AJ, Cascino GD, Lozada L, Bechtle PS, et al. The effects of remifentanil on epileptiform discharges during intraoperative electrocorticography in patients undergoing epilepsy surgery. *Epilepsia.* 2001;42(10):1340–1344.

191. Herrick IA, Craen RA, Blume WT, Novick T, Gelb AW. Sedative doses of remifentanil have minimal effect on ECoG spike activity during awake epilepsy surgery. *J Neurosurg Anesthesiol.* 2002;14(1):55–58.

192. Kalkman CJ, ten Brink SA, Been HD, Bovill JG. Variability of somatosensory cortical evoked potentials during spinal surgery. Effects of anesthetic technique and high-pass digital filtering. *Spine.* 1991;16(8):924–929.

193. Sala F, Palandri G, Basso E, Lanteri P, Deletis V, Faccioli F, et al. Motor evoked potential monitoring improves outcome after surgery for intramedullary spinal cord tumors: a historical control study. *Neurosurgery.* 2006;58(6):1129–1143.

194. Sutter M, Eggspuehler A, Muller A, Dvorak J. Multimodal intraoperative monitoring: an overview and proposal of methodology based on 1,017 cases. *Eur Spine J.* 2007;16(Suppl 2):S153–S161.

195. Macdonald DB. Intraoperative motor evoked potential monitoring: overview and update. *J Clin Monit Comput.* 2006;20(5):347–377.

196. Mahmoud M, Sadhasivam S, Sestokas AK, Samuels P, McAuliffe J. Loss of transcranial electric motor evoked potentials during pediatric spine surgery with dexmedetomidine. *Anesthesiology.* 2007;106(2):393–396.

197. Macdonald DB, Stigsby B, Al Homoud I, Abalkhail T, Mokeem A. Utility of motor evoked potentials for intraoperative nerve root monitoring. *J Clin Neurophysiol.* 2012;29(2):118–125.

198. Nuwer MR. Regulatory and medical-legal aspects of intraoperative monitoring. *J Clin Neurophysiol.* 2002;19(5):387–395.

199. Nuwer MR. Regulatory issues in intraoperative monitoring. In: Loftus CM, Biller J, Baron EM, eds. *Intraoperative Neuromonitoring.* New York: McGraw-Hill, 2014:1–7.

200. Beacham AG. Kathleen Mears Lecture: Intraoperative neurophysiological monitoring—a contemporary perspective. *Am J Electroneurodiagn Technol.* 2001;41(2):99–115.

201. Mullikin E. IONM education. *Am J Electroneurodiagn Technol.* 2001;41(4):339–341.

202. Nuwer MR, Cohen BH, Shepard KM. Practice patterns for intraoperative neurophysiologic monitoring. *Neurology.* 2013;80(12):1156–1160.

203. Kohn LT, Corrigan JM, Donaldson MS. *To Err is Human: Building a Safer Health Care System.* Washington, D.C.: National Academies Press, 2000.

204. Schnider TW, Minto CF, Gambus PL, Andresen C, Goodale DB, Shafer SL, et al. The influence of method of administration and covariates on the pharmacokinetics of propofol in adult volunteers. *Anesthesiology.* 1998;88(5):1170–1182.

35 | MAGNETOENCEPHALOGRAPHY: METHODS AND CLINICAL ASPECTS

RIITTA HARI, MD, PHD

ABSTRACT: This chapter introduces magnetoencephalography (MEG), a tool to study brain dynamics in basic and clinical neuroscience. MEG picks up brain signals with millisecond resolution, as does electroencephalography, but without distortion by skull and scalp. The chapter describes current instrumentation based on superconducting quantum interference devices (SQUIDs). It delineates basic characteristics of measured signals: (1) brain rhythms and their reactivity during sensory processing and various tasks and (2) evoked responses elicited by sensory stimuli, and the dependence of these responses on various stimulus characteristics. Signals are described from healthy and diseased brains. The chapter presents studies of the brain basis of cognition and social interaction studied in dual-MEG setups and describes how MEG applications can be broadened by innovative setups, including frequency tagging. Progress in the field is predicted regarding sensor technology, data analysis, and multimodal brain imaging, all of which could strengthen MEG's role in the study of brain dynamics.

KEYWORDS: brain, magnetoencephalography, MEG, electroencephalography, SQUID, rhythm, evoked response, sensor, imaging

PRINCIPAL REFERENCES

1. Hämäläinen M, Hari R, Ilmoniemi R, Knuutila J, Lounasmaa OV. Magnetoencephalography—theory, instrumentation, and applications to noninvasive studies of signal processing in the human brain. *Rev Mod Phys.* 1993;65:413–497.
2. Hari R, Salmelin R. Human cortical oscillations: a view through the skull. *Trends Neurosci.* 1997;20:44–49.
3. Hari R, Parkkonen L, Nangini C. The brain in time: Insights from neuromagnetic recordings. *Ann NY Acad Sci.* 2010;1191:89–109.
4. Hari R, Salmelin R. Magnetoencephalography: From SQUIDs to neuroscience. *Neuroimage.* 2012;61:386–396.
5. Hari R, Parkkonen L. The brain timewise: How timing shapes and supports brain function. *Phil Trans Royal Soc B.* 2015;370:20140170.
6. Hansen P, Kringelbach M, Salmelin R, eds. *MEG: An Introduction to Methods.* New York: Oxford University Press, 2010.
7. Supek S, Aine CJ, eds. *Magnetoencephalography: From Signals to Dynamic Cortical Networks.* Berlin/Heidelberg: Springer, 2014.
8. Hari R, Puce A. *MEG-EEG Primer.* New York: Oxford University Press, 2017.

1. INTRODUCTION

Recording of weak magnetic fields outside the head by means of magnetoencephalography (MEG) emerged in the late 1960s, 40 years after the invention of the human electroencephalography (EEG). The first instrument was an induction coil magnetometer with two million turns of wire, used to detect the magnetic alpha rhythm by means of signal averaging, with the electric alpha activity as the time reference.[1] The MEG method became more practical with the introduction of SQUID (Superconducting QUantum Interference Device) magnetometers in the early 1970s, and since then it has been possible to record both spontaneous and evoked magnetic signals of the human brain without any electric reference. Sensor arrays with whole-scalp coverage are commercially available, and signal-analysis methods have progressed quickly. At present, over 200 laboratories worldwide utilize MEG for exploration of normal and abnormal functions of the human brain, and MEG results continue to influence interpretation of the EEG recordings.

A PubMed search in December 2015 with search words "((magnetoencephalograph*) OR (meg AND brain) OR (meg AND cortex))" resulted in over 8,150 hits, which means that this chapter can cover only about 2.5% of the available literature. Therefore the reader is advised to consult review papers and textbooks whenever more information is desirable. This chapter* reviews the basic principles of MEG briefly, focusing on the basic concepts, and with most examples from our own laboratory at Aalto University (former Helsinki University of Technology), Finland; consequently, the figures present recordings with planar gradiometers used in our laboratory since 1989. Spontaneous and evoked activity, both in normal subjects and in some neurological patients, are discussed to the extent that will be of immediate interest to a clinical neurophysiologist.

The main advantages of MEG are its good spatial resolution in locating cortical events and its selectivity to activity of the fissural cortex. The sites of active brain areas can be located with respect to external landmarks on the head, brain structures, or functional brain regions (identified by means of, for instance, sources of evoked responses). Several review articles and books are available for consulting MEG findings related to basic brain research and relevant methodology.[2-16]

Although the main advantage of MEG is its ability to obtain time-sensitive information about brain function, it is also important to obtain information about the sites of neural generators of various signals. The EEG research has

---

* Compared with the previous version of this chapter (Hari R. Magnetoencephalography: Methods and applications. In Schomer DL, Lopes da Silva FH, eds, *Niedermeyer's Electroencephalography: Basic Principles, Clinical Applications, and Related Fields.* 6th ed. Philadelphia: Lippincott Williams & Wilkins, 2011:865–900), the main changes include deletion of detailed literature regarding MEG abnormalities in various brain disorders (encephalitis, migraine, infantile neuronal ceroid lipofuscinosis, multiple sclerosis, and the effects of electroconvulsive therapy in depressive patients). Similarly, the description of various evoked responses and brain rhythms has been reduced to give space for some newer developments.

traditionally focused on temporal waveforms, and an entire branch of electrophenomenology has arisen around EEG "graphoelements" that have been correlated with different tasks and stimulation parameters, clinical states, and even personality factors. It is clear that a better understanding of the generators underlying the EEG signals would permit a more precise and physiological interpretation of abnormalities. Here MEG has advanced the field both at the conceptual and practical level.

2. COMPARISON OF EEG AND MEG

MEG is closely related to EEG. In spite of the different sensitivities of EEG and MEG to currents of different orientations and locations, the primary currents causing the signals are the same. Similarities between the MEG and EEG time courses are therefore to be expected. The advantage of MEG over EEG in source identification results mainly from the transparency of the skull and other extracerebral tissues to the magnetic field, in contrast to the substantial distortion and smearing of the electric potentials. The MEG recording is also reference-free, whereas the EEG maps depend on the location of the reference electrode. As a result it is often more straightforward to make reasonable first guesses of the source locations by visual inspection of the MEG data. Reference-free EEG presentations that facilitate the interpretation of the potential distributions can be obtained by calculating "surface Laplacians."[17] However, even then one has to proceed to neural sources for proper interpretation, and problems arise in the presence of several simultaneous sources. Moreover, the Laplacians cannot be calculated for the outermost electrodes, which reduces the brain areas that can be characterized.

Figure 35.1 shows a current dipole in a spherical volume conductor consisting of four layers of different conductivities that simulate the brain, the cerebrospinal fluid, the skull, and the scalp. The resulting distributions of electric potential and

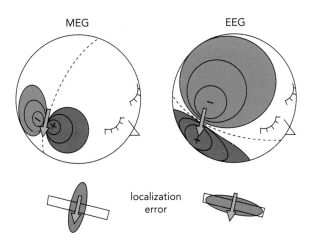

Figure 35.1. MEG and EEG patterns over a concentric four-layer sphere when a tangential current dipole (arrow) is active in the auditory cortex in the lower lip of the sylvian fissure. The red areas indicate the magnetic flux out of the head (MEG) and positive scalp potential (EEG). The lower part of the figure illustrates schematically, with shadowed ellipsoids, the inaccuracy region of the dipole location when determined "backwards" from the measured signals.

magnetic field are "dipolar"—that is, they both display two extrema of opposite polarities but are rotated by 90 degrees with respect to each other. The isocontour lines are relatively tighter in the magnetic than in the electric pattern because concentric electric inhomogeneities smear only the electric potential, while the magnetic pattern is not influenced. Consequently, in an ideal sphere, a single superficial tangential dipole can be found one-third more accurately on the basis of magnetic than electric recordings. For interpretation of MEG signals recorded from the real brain, it is sufficient to use a realistically shaped model consisting of the brain only, while accurate EEG calculations require a full multicompartmental model with known conductivities and shapes for the brain, skull, cerebrospinal fluid, and scalp.

MEG's selectivity to tangential currents in the presence of several simultaneous sources is an important advantage in practical work, as is illustrated, for example, by the early differentiation between multiple cortical areas activated by somatosensory stimuli.[18–20]

It is often more straightforward to interpret MEG than EEG data as they have a smaller number of potential sources. However, since both electric and magnetic signals are generated by the same primary currents that flow in the brain, one should pay attention to both MEG and EEG results when drawing conclusions on brain function from either type of recordings. For example, a dipolar potential distribution could be explained equally well with two radial current dipoles or with one tangential dipole. However, the existence of a clear magnetic pattern, rotated 90 degrees with respect to the electric one, would imply that the latter explanation should be favored, as happens in the case of early cortical somatosensory responses.[21] The minimum requirement for sound data interpretation is that the conclusions based on EEG and MEG do not contradict.

Some current sources (very deep and radial) are more easily picked up by EEG than MEG, although reliable MEG counterparts of auditory brainstem responses have been detected after averaging of a large number of single responses.[22] The contribution of deep activity to the MEG signals can be probed by means of forward modeling, inserting sources to interesting brain structures (e.g., thalamus or hippocampus) and then calculating the best fit of these sources, as a function of time, to the measured signals.[23]

For maximum information, the MEG and EEG techniques should be combined, and the simultaneously recorded data should be interpreted with methods that take advantage of the complementarity of the records. In practice, all cerebral currents that give rise to MEG signals are expected to generate EEG signals as well, although, in theory, current loops are electrically silent but magnetically visible. However, so far ideal current loops have not been observed in the brain, and the occasional appearance of epileptic spikes only in MEG, but not in EEG, is likely due to different contributions of background noise to the two recordings. Recent animal recordings have shown that "monopolar" charges—resembling the "closed fields" of Lorente de No (see Chapter 4)—can considerably contribute to intracortical laminar EEG recordings. Such charge configurations would not be associated with systematically directed currents and thus would be invisible in MEG. For further considerations of these neuronal mechanisms, see Chapter 2.

3. MEG INSTRUMENTATION

The magnetic fields generated by cerebral currents are only about a hundredth part of the field produced by the heart, and only a tiny part of the steady magnetic field of the earth (Table 35.1). To avoid contamination by external magnetic artifacts due to moving vehicles, power lines, radio transmission, and so forth, it is common to carry out the recordings within a magnetically shielded room, usually made of several layers of aluminum and mu-metal. Cheaper lightweight magnetically shielded rooms, especially designed for clinical environments, comprise just a single shell of interleaved mu-metal and aluminum layers added by active shielding; they provide sufficient attenuation of external magnetic disturbances for recording of both spontaneous and evoked MEG

TABLE 35.1. Orders of Magnitude of Magnetic Fields

Magnetic resonance imaging	3 000 000 000 000 000 (= 3 T)
Steady magnetic field of the earth	100 000 000 000
Magnetocardiogram	100 000
Cerebral alpha rhythm	1 000
Cerebral evoked response	100
Sensitivity of magnetometers	3
Noise within a shielded room	1

Data in femtotesla, fT = 10^{-15} T. Note that the sensitivity of the present-day magnetometers is < 5 fT/$\sqrt{Hz}$.

signals.[24] Biomagnetic measurements have been performed also without magnetic shielding using sensors with special configurations (higher-order gradiometers). In general, however, it is better to prevent than to compensate for artifacts

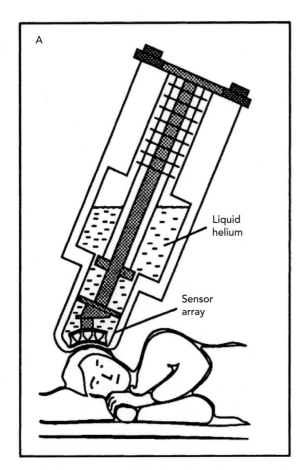

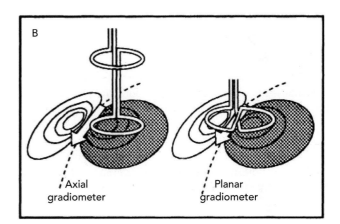

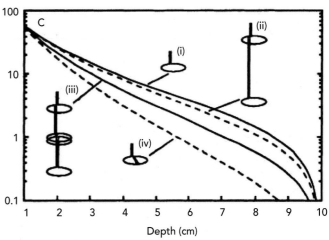

Figure 35.2. **A:** MEG recording before the advent of whole-scalp-covering neuromagnetometers. The subject is lying in a magnetically shielded room with his head supported by a vacuum cast. The dewar containing the SQUID sensors is brought as close to the head as possible, without direct contact, and the magnetic field (or its gradient) is picked up outside the head at several locations simultaneously. **B:** Two flux-transformer configurations. The first-order axial gradiometer (left) measures essentially the radial magnetic-field component B_r and detects the maximum signals at both sides of the dipole. The planar gradiometer (right) measures the tangential derivative $\partial B_r/\partial x$ or $\partial B_r/\partial y$; the maximum signal is detected just above the dipole. **C:** Dependence of signal strength (in arbitrary units) on the depth of a current dipole when measured by (i) a magnetometer, (ii) a first-order axial gradiometer, (iii) a second-order axial gradiometer, and (iv) a planar figure-of-eight gradiometer. The computations have been made in a sphere 10 cm in diameter. The calculations are based on Hari R, Joutsiniemi S-L and Sarvas J. Spatial resolution of neuromagnetic recordings: Theoretical calculations in a spherical model. Electroenceph Clin Neurophysiol. 1988; 71:64–72.

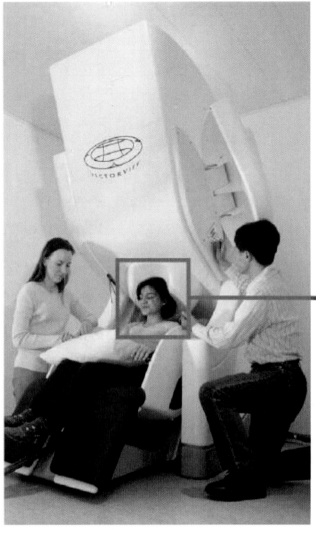
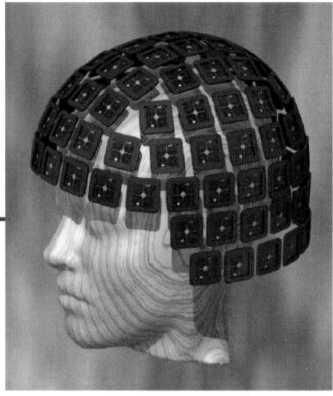

Figure 35.3. A 306-SQUID whole-scalp-covering neuromagnetometer (Vectorview™, Neuromag Ltd., Finland; currently Elekta Neuromag™, Elekta Oy, Helsinki, Finland) in our laboratory. Each of the 102 three-channel sensor elements comprises two orthogonal planar gradiometers and one magnetometer; the helmet-shaped arrangement of the elements is shown on the right covering a surface rendering of a real subject. Courtesy of Mika Seppä, Aalto University, Finland.

and to record the original signals in as undistorted a form as possible.

Figure 35.2A gives a schematic illustration of a now old-fashioned arrangement during the MEG recording. The subject lies in a magnetically shielded room and the neuromagnetometer, containing SQUID sensors immersed in liquid helium (at −269°C), is positioned close to the head. To replace the evaporating helium, the dewar container has to be refilled regularly, in the present systems typically once a week, but cryocooler-based helium-circulation devices have already been developed. Figure 35.3 shows an example of the modern-day MEG setup where the subject can be either sitting or lying during the measurement.

The cerebral magnetic field is coupled into the SQUID sensors through superconducting flux transformers. The transformer configuration is important for the device's sensitivity to different source current configurations and to artifacts. A magnetometer, containing a single pickup loop in

the flux transformer, is most sensitive to signals but also to artifacts (see Fig. 35.2C). A more elaborate axial first-order gradiometer contains a compensation coil, wound in the direction opposite to the pickup coil (see Fig. 35.2B,C); this configuration decreases the influence of distant disturbances that link the same magnetic flux into both coils. Therefore, the output of the axial first-order gradiometer is essentially determined by the signal of the nearby neuronal source itself. Furthermore, since the distance between the pickup and compensation coils of a first-order axial gradiometer is several centimeters, the measured signal approximates the amplitude of the radial field component B_r rather than its axial derivative. In higher-order gradiometers the sensitivity is reduced to the distant artifacts but also, to some extent, to the nearby brain currents.

The contour plots in Figure 35.2B illustrate the pattern of B_r, the magnetic field radial to the surface, generated by a tangential current dipole in a sphere. The signal strengths measured with an axial gradiometer form a spatial pattern similar to the field itself, with extrema of opposite polarities at the two sides of the dipole. In contrast, the planar gradiometer yields the maximum signal when centered just over the dipole at the location of the steepest field gradient. The planar gradiometer is able to detect the location of the source even at the edge of the sensor array, and the essential information from the field pattern can thus be obtained from a rather small measurement area. On the other hand, information about the depth of the source is more accurate with axial than planar sensors since the gradient decreases relatively more rapidly as a function of source depth than does the field itself (see Fig. 35.2C). However, whole-scalp sensor coverage largely counterbalances the latter drawback. Although the patterns measured by both axial and planar gradiometers are easily interpreted, in practice it is often useful that the maximum signal detected by the planar gradiometers already provides a good first guess of the approximate source location. Methods are available to present data measured with different coil configurations in a standard format. On the basis of axial gradiometers, some users compute virtual planar gradiometers from nearby sensors; these work well as indicators of the most likely source areas, but the resulting signals have $\sqrt{2}$ times more noise than the original signals.

To determine the current distribution within the brain, the magnetic field must be sampled at several locations, preferably simultaneously. With the first single-channel magnetometers it took several hours or even days to complete a field map, and changes in the subject's attentive state and vigilance from one measurement point to the other were thus unavoidable. With the present-day helmet-shaped neuromagnetometers that cover the whole scalp (see Fig. 35.3), the whole field pattern can be measured with a single shot. This progress of instruments has made MEG recordings feasible for comprehensive studies of integrative brain functions in healthy adults and children as well as in different patient groups. Importantly, the intrinsic noise of the present-day SQUIDs is no longer a problem, and the main "noise" arises from the brain itself.

The optimal spacing of the sensors is determined by the spatial frequency of the signal distribution and, therefore, only marginal benefit can be obtained by reducing the sensor spacing below the distance between the source and the sensor. As this distance is > 3 cm in the current multichannel devices, about 150 sensors would suffice to cover the whole cortex. Therefore, the modern instruments with > 300 sensors provide dense enough spatial sampling for MEG recordings. However, the situation will change with the development of sensor technology that allow the sensors to be put closer to the skull (see the section "Future Perspectives" at the end of the chapter).

The diameter of the sensor coil ("pickup coil") is a matter of compromise: the larger the coil, the more sensitive it is, but also the more it averages spatially the magnetic field, thereby leading to loss of information. Taking into account the distance of the sensors from the source, pickup coils with diameters ~2 cm are reasonably sensitive and do not lose significant information.

An essential part of the measurement system is the head-position indicator, which gives the exact measurement sites and the orientations of the sensors with respect to the head. This information can be obtained, for example, by placing three or four small coils on known sites on the scalp. The field pattern produced by currents led through the coils is then measured with the multichannel magnetometer. The head-position indicator devices allow the position of the magnetometer to be determined with respect to external landmarks on the head with 2- to 3-mm accuracy. The coordinate system in which the source locations are expressed is typically fixed on the basis of the nasion, the inion, and the preauricular points so that it can be easily transported to Talairach space or other anatomical atlases commonly used in functional magnetic resonance imaging (fMRI). The important landmarks on the head and the shape of the skull can be determined with a three-dimensional (3D) digitizer, or the shape of the whole head can be quickly scanned with a portable 3D scanner.

Currently (as of December 2016) ~200 whole-scalp neuromagnetometers are in use worldwide in clinical and research settings. The available devices vary in the number of channels, in the pickup coil configuration (e.g., first-, second-, or third-order axial gradiometer, planar gradiometer, or magnetometer), as well as in the area covered by the sensor array. Still, the different devices provide comparable information about the brain's neurodynamics.

4. SOURCE IMAGING

Since the aim of MEG studies is to obtain information about well-specified brain functions, the field pattern should be interpreted in terms of cerebral currents. Yet, due to the non-uniqueness of the inverse problem—namely, because several current distributions can, in principle, produce identical magnetic field patterns outside the head—the interpretation usually requires the use of both source and volume-conductor models. Thus the situation is more complicated than in fMRI or in positron emission tomography (PET) where the inverse problem can be solved uniquely. However, meaningful source models of MEG patterns can be constrained by the brain's known anatomy and physiology.

4.1. Current Dipole

The most commonly used source model in MEG studies is a current dipole within a sphere. In an ideal sphere, only primary currents tangential to the surface produce magnetic fields outside the volume. Therefore a current dipole can be characterized by means of five parameters: three for its 3D location, one for its orientation (only the plane parallel to the local surface of the sphere is relevant for MEG), and one for its strength.

As will be explained below, the tangential currents picked up with MEG likely arise in the parallel apical dendrites of the fissural cortex because the main direction of the dendritic tree is perpendicular to the cortical surface. In reality, signals may also be detected from the convexial cortex where the currents are considerably closer to the detector than are the currents within the wall of a fissure. Deviation of the convexial source by only 10 to 20 degrees from the radial orientation is enough to give a signal as large as that produced by a tangential dipole of the same size but 2 cm deeper in the fissural cortex. It therefore seems likely that under realistic conditions nearly radial sources can contribute significantly to the MEG signals. This notion is supported by simulations that took into account the real geometry of the cerebral cortex.[25]

In dipole modeling, the location of the "equivalent current dipole" (ECD) is found by a least-squares fit to the data, typically at the time of a clearly dipolar field pattern. In progressing toward a multidipole model, one may extract the field patterns produced by the already identified sources to facilitate further analysis. However, if the first source was wrong, so are all the further sources. Multidipole models with time-varying source strengths are useful in interpreting the resulting complex field patterns, but one should examine the time courses of all sources at the same time to rule out possible interactions of oppositely directed nearby dipoles.

The success of dipole models in MEG interpretation derives, in part, from the difficulty in discerning the details of the brain activation pattern from the typical measurement distance of at least 3 cm from the source (Fig. 35.4). Consequently, a single current dipole provides a feasible accurate description of a local active cortical area of < 2 to 3 cm in diameter, whatever the local current configuration is.

The adequacy of the source model can be evaluated by calculating the goodness-of-fit (g) value,[6,26] which is the squared correlation coefficient between the measured signals and those predicted by the model. The g-value, however, depends on several factors, such as the number and distribution of the measurement locations. A low g-value means that either the brain source significantly deviates from the model or that the signal-to-noise ratio is poor, or both. It is often useful to examine the residual field (i.e., the difference between the measured field and the field predicted by the model) and to compare the measured and predicted waveforms. If the residual field shows systematic features that cannot be explained by noise, a different source configuration has to be considered.

The inaccuracy of MEG source localization is smallest in the direction transverse to dipole orientation (cf. Fig. 35.1) and largest (about double) in the direction of depth. The locating accuracy depends drastically on the signal-to-noise ratio, which is improved by signal averaging for evoked responses but cannot be affected much—except by filtering—for spontaneous activity. For comparison, note that the best localization accuracy for EEG is in the direction along the dipole (see Fig. 35.1), again emphasizing the complementarity of MEG and EEG recordings. Since the ECDs mainly reflect synchronous activation of the cortical pyramidal cells and thus are perpendicular to the cortical surface, MEG

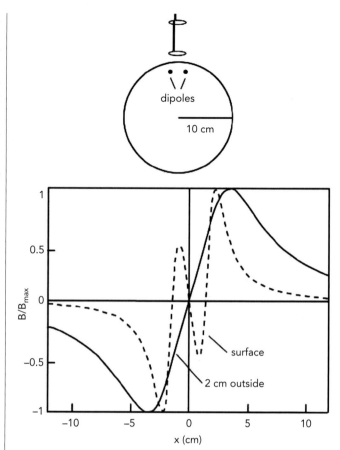

Figure 35.4. *The dependence of the radial component of the magnetic field on the distance between the source and the detector. Two current dipoles are situated in a homogeneous sphere (radius 10 cm), 1 cm beneath the surface, 3 cm from each other, and symmetrically with respect to the origin. The field was calculated on an arc perpendicular to the orientation of the dipoles (x-axis). The pattern is complex on the surface, whereas 2 cm outside the sphere the higher spatial frequencies have faded away and the dipolar term dominates. The amplitudes have been normalized according to the maximum value; the field would be about seven times stronger on the surface than 2 cm above it. Adapted from Hari R. Interpretation of cerebral magnetic fields elicited by somatosensory stimuli. In: Basar E, ed. Springer Series of Brain Dynamics. Berlin/Heidelberg: Springer-Verlag, 1988:305–310.*

indicates more easily than does EEG changes in the focus of activation along the cortex, for example along the finger representation area of the primary somatosensory cortex during stimulation of different fingers. On the other hand, EEG may be more accurate in indicating which wall of a fissure was activated, since here the distinction must be made along the direction of the dipole.

When a single current dipole is used to model an extended cortical area consisting of a layer of dipoles, the estimates of dipole depth and, consequently, of dipole strengths may be erroneous (Fig. 35.5). Better source models are thus needed for extended areas and other distributed sources (see below). When multiple brain regions are simultaneously active, the relative contribution of each area to the measured signal depends on its site, strength, and synchrony.

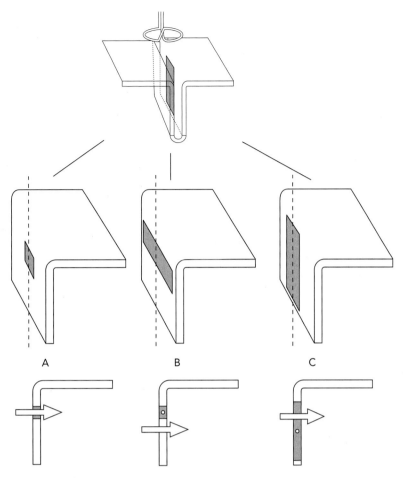

Figure 35.5. *Schematic illustration of ECD locations when the source is (A) a layer < 2 cm in diameter, (B) a layer with angular extension, and (C) a layer extended along the radius of the sphere. The activity is assumed to occur in the wall of a cortical fissure. Adapted from Hari R. On brain's magnetic responses to sensory stimuli. J Clin Neurophysiol. 1991;8:157–169.*

4.2. Neural Currents Underlying the Current Dipole

To understand the basic cellular events underlying the ECD, it is reasonable to divide the currents associated with postsynaptic potentials (PSPs)—the main contributors to local field potentials (LFPs)—to transmembrane currents at the active synaptic area, intracellular currents within the neuron, and extracellular "volume" currents. Transmembrane currents are the driving force ("battery") for both intra- and extracellular current flow. ECD calculated from the measured MEG signals reflects the direction of the net intracellular current flow. A single PSP at the end of one dendrite produces an "elementary" dipole moment—which strongly depends on the cell size—of the order of $Q = I \times \lambda$ ($\approx 10^{-14}$ nA $\times$ m for a single synapse), where I is the intracellular current driven by the synapse and λ is the length constant of the cell membrane. The strength of the observed dipole moment can be strongly affected, in addition to sodium and potassium currents, by the simultaneous calcium currents. See Chapters 2 and 4 for more details of the biophysics of these processes.

Since it is not known how many PSPs occur synchronously in each pyramidal cell and how much cancellation takes place within the cortex due to oppositely directed currents in different cortical layers, it is not possible to derive accurate estimates for the source area of a typical evoked response on the basis of cell/synapse density and the size of the elementary dipole. Interestingly, however, many animal species across a wide phylogenetic scale (turtle, guinea pig, and swine) show an apparent invariance in the maximum current dipole moment density of 1 to 2 nAm per squaremillimeter.[27,28] Considerably smaller dipole moment densities have been estimated on the basis of available information on intracortical current densities and values of cortical λ.[4] However, intracortical current densities also depend on the degree of neuronal synchrony, and thus on the specimen studied. Importantly, λ may vary according to background activity. Since λ is proportional to the square root of the fiber diameter, the dipole moments weigh the larger neurons. Many other factors besides synchrony, size, shape, and location of cortical neurons may affect the net dipole moment. For example, glial cells change the return paths of volume currents, and giant synapses in pyramidal cells might dominate the local current flow; the quantitative contributions of both of these effects are still unknown.

Several important electrical events likely remain beyond the reach of both MEG and EEG measurements. For example, intracortical short-distance interactions are—when viewed from the top of the cortex—radially symmetrical, and thus only their net effect along the apical dendrites of the pyramidal cells can give rise to a detectable MEG signal (see also Chapters 2 and 4).

4.3. Minimum-Norm Estimates

An example of a different approach to the neuromagnetic inverse problem is the minimum-norm estimate (MNE) presentation of the source currents.[29] MNE gives the most probable current distribution, in the sense of the minimum norm, giving rise to the recorded magnetic field. Calculation of MNE does not require specific assumptions about the source configuration (one dipole, multiple dipoles, quadrupoles, etc.), which is an advantage when the basis for such explicit models is missing. On the other hand, the unconstrained MNE solution favors superficial currents and does not give a reliable estimate of the source depth. Therefore MNE solutions have been weighted with constraints based on the known brain anatomy and physiology, especially source depth.[30] Minimum-current estimates,[31] a subclass of MNE solutions that give more local solutions, have been applied for visualization and analysis of single-subject and group-level MEG data.

The distributed MNE-based source activations often look "more physiological" than the point-like current dipoles, and therefore current dipoles have been considered less appropriate than the distributed models to describe the complex brain activity. However, a word of caution has its place here because the appearance of the result depends strongly on the method used: the MNE approach will give a distributed solution and the dipole approach a local solution (dipole), whatever the real current distribution is, as demonstrated in Figure 35.6.[32] In general, both dipole and MCE solutions give rather similar results, although the temporal accuracy may be better with dipole modeling and the group data may be easier to visualize with MCE. According to our experience, even well-informed users tend to report more false positives with MCE than with current-dipole modeling. For a detailed discussion of distributed sources in EEG modeling, see Chapter 45.

4.4. Combination of MEG with MRI/fMRI/PET Data

All source estimates can be improved by constraints based on the known anatomy of the brain, derived from MRI data, and forcing the dipoles/currents to the cortex. In preoperative evaluation, reconstruction of the 3D outer surface of the brain from MRI scans may help the surgeon to recognize the landscape after opening the skull when the brain tissue retracts and the relationship between the brain and the landmarks on the skull changes. Adding surface vessels to the reconstruction further facilitates the orientation during surgery (see Fig. 35.21).[33]

Compared with PET and fMRI, the advantage of MEG is its good temporal resolution that allows monitoring of

ORIGINAL SOURCES

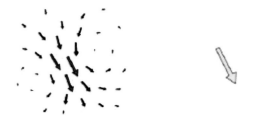

FIELD PATTERNS

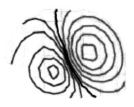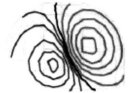

CURRENT-DIPOLE MODEL

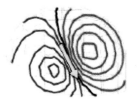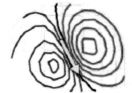

MINIMUM-NORM ESTIMATES

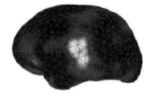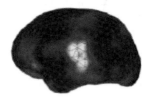

Figure 35.6. Minimum current estimate and dipole model give similar results for local sources. The picture illustrates the actual sources (distributed on left, local current dipole on right), the resulting magnetic field patterns, and the results of both current-dipole modeling and minimum-norm estimates.

cortical dynamics on millisecond scale. In combined use of multiple methods, active brain regions have been first determined with PET/fMRI and then used as source constraints in the inverse solution of the MEG data to reveal the corresponding temporal behavior. However, not all changes in the synchronization of a neuronal population, reflected in the MEG/EEG signals, induce significant changes in the mean neuronal firing rates or the blood flow and metabolism, and vice versa. Therefore MEG and fMRI results may significantly differ,[34,35] and the MEG/EEG and fMRI/PET methods remain complementary in studies of human brain function. Importantly, different MEG/EEG frequency bands can correlate either negatively (as in 10-Hz "alpha" range)[36] or positively (as in the > 40-Hz "gamma" range)[37] with the strength of the fMRI signal. Moreover, fMRI may weigh activity transferred by the dense and slow fibers whereas MEG and EEG mainly rely on activations transmitted by the fastest-conducting axons.[16]

5. VOLUME-CONDUCTOR MODELS

The sphere model works well in most areas of the head when the radius of the sphere is fitted to the local radius of curvature of the measurement area.[38] However, realistic head models that take more computing time may be needed for modeling of the temporobasal and frontobasal brain areas. Fortunately, it is sufficient for MEG to model the intracranial space since only a relatively small proportion of the currents flow in the poorly conducting skull. In contrast, proper modeling of the EEG signals necessitates a multicompartmental model consisting of three or four concentric layers with resistivities that are typically unknown.

Some nonspherical electric inhomogeneities may also affect MEG distributions. For example, the falx cerebri may change volume current paths and lead to slight mislocalizations of current dipoles in the mesial wall of the hemisphere. An intact human skull also contains holes, the largest ones in the base of the skull and in the orbits, in principle providing low-resistance current paths. However, from the absence of electro-oculographic artifacts in intracranial recordings from the frontal lobe[39] one can predict that the normal skull holes do not considerably affect MEG distributions.

6. PRACTICAL ISSUES

The practical benefits of multichannel MEG recordings include the short preparation time and the exact knowledge of the relative locations of the sensors, required for accurate source analysis. Since the subject's head has to be immobile during MEG recordings, problems are encountered in studies of uncooperative subjects who either cannot keep still during the recording or who are not willing or able to perform the tasks. Moreover, recordings cannot be performed during major motor seizures. However, continuous monitoring of the head position will considerably help studies of restless subjects.

Figure 35.7 illustrates some common MEG artifacts. Eye blinks and movements cause large artifacts[40] that can be easily recognized and rejected if simultaneous electro-oculogram recordings are available. Muscular artifacts may occur spontaneously but also time-locked to strong stimuli. Magnetic lung contamination or magnetic material in clothing can cause respiration-related slow shifts. Cardiac MEG contamination can include magnetocardiographic signals,[41] picked up at distance, and ballistocardiographic fluctuations, caused by the movement of magnetized material at the rhythm of the cardiac cycle. For recognition of both artifacts, a simultaneously recorded electrocardiogram (ECG) is most useful: the magnetocardiographic artifact coincides with the ECG signals, being similar in both timing and shape (although the shapes of both signals depend on the measurement locations), whereas the main peak of the magnetic ballistocardiogram is broader and lags the ECG-QRS complex by hundreds of milliseconds.

All magnetic materials must be avoided in the clothing of the subject. Although intraoral metallic devices for orthodontics or magnetized material used in staples, and sutures during brain surgery may contaminate the MEG measurement, efficient methods are currently available to remove the artifacts in the postprocessing phase,[42,43] so that it is possible to clean the MEG data even from artifacts elicited by a deep brain stimulator (Fig. 35.8).[44] Such efficient postprocessing methods have considerably widened the clinical applicability of the MEG recordings.

Special attention must also be paid to the proper design of stimulators. High-quality sounds can be produced with electroacoustic transformers placed outside the shielded room and connected through plastic tubes to the subject; the system may need sophisticated equalizing to guarantee flat frequency transfer. Excessive artifacts from electric somatosensory stimuli can be avoided by twisting the stimulator wires tightly together. Multichannel devices with balloon diaphragms driven by compressed air[45] provide a nice and artifact-free method for tactile

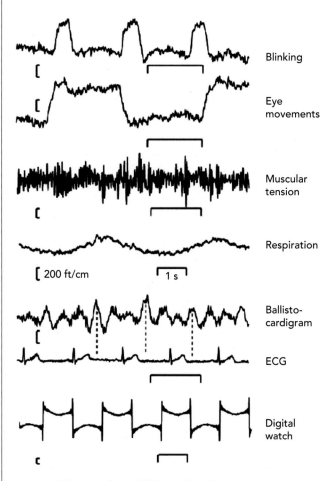

Figure 35.7. *Different artifacts in MEG recordings of spontaneous brain activity over the temporal area; the measurements were made with a planar gradiometer. Eye blinking and vertical eye movements produce signals of about equal size; for horizontal eye movements the signals are similar in waveform but have different spatial distributions. Muscular tension was produced by biting the teeth together. Respiration artifacts were due to a metallic piece over the subject's chest. The magnetic ballistocardiogram was due to movement of magnetized metal on the bed, on which the subject was lying on his left side. Note the timing differences between the maximum signals in the ECG and the ballistocardiogram. The lowest artifact was due to a digital watch, worn by the child subject's parent, 70 cm from the measuring device.*

Raw data

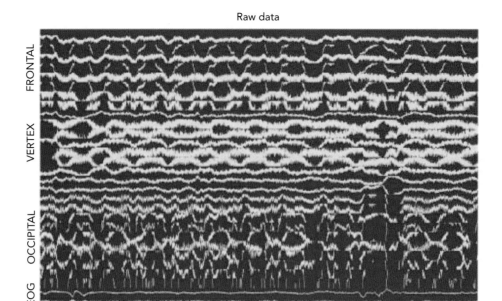

After tSSS-cleaning

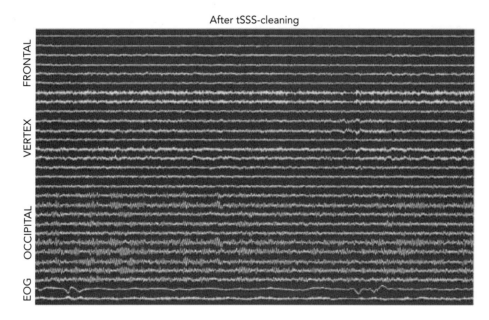

Figure 35.8. The effect of tSSS (temporal spectral space separation) artifact suppression on spontaneous MEG of a person with a deep brain stimulator. Above: Before tSSS. Below: After tSSS, when even the normal posterior alpha activity can be seen. Courtesy of Jyrki Mäkelä, Helsinki University Central Hospital, Finland.

stimulation. A handheld bundle of optical fibers, half emitting red light and the other half detecting the reflected light from the skin, can be used to evoke reliable somatosensory responses to taps to any part of the skin (Fig. 35.9).[46] MEG-compatible devices that produce passive finger, hand, or foot movements can be used to study cortical effects of proprioceptive afference.[47]

Noxious laser heat stimuli for pain studies can be brought to the shielded room via optical cables. Visual stimuli can be transmitted through mirrors, a data projector, or a bundle of optic fibers, or the subject can view a monitor through a hole in the wall. EEG can be measured simultaneously with MEG using nonmagnetic electrodes and wires without causing problems to the MEG recordings. Eye tracking can be performed during the MEG recordings with an infrared camera.[48]

Figure 35.10 draws attention to dangers of filtering. A high-pass filter setting that is too high will cause well-known distortions in the signal waveforms but—what may be less obvious—also transfer the dipolar field patterns, with opposite polarities, to latencies distant from the real signal and thereby lead to erroneous interpretations of the timing and site of brain activation. Such distorted timing would be especially harmful in studies addressing, say, the earliest input to the sensory projection cortex.[49]

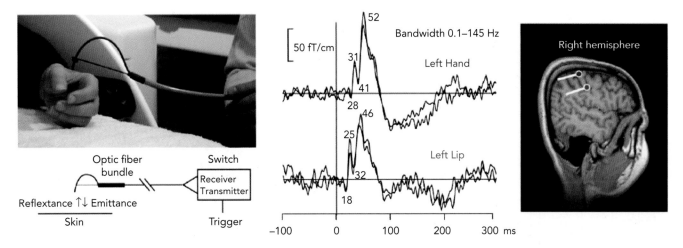

Figure 35.9. Tactile stimulator made of a bundle of optical fibers and the somatosensory responses obtained by stimulating the left hand and the left lip. Adapted from Jousmäki V, Nishitani N, Hari R. Brush stimulator for functional brain imaging. Clin Neurophysiol. 2007;118: 2620–2624.

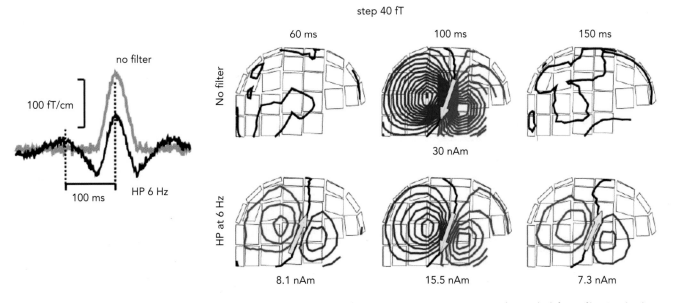

Figure 35.10. Dangers of filtering, illustrated with simulated data. A current dipole with a monophasic activation curve (gray line on the left, "no filter") and with 30-nAm dipole moment was inserted to a site corresponding to the right auditory cortex. The field patterns above show a dipolar field pattern at peak activation at 100 ms. After high-pass filtering at 6 Hz the waveform changes (black curve on the left, "HP 6 Hz") and ghost sources appear at 60 and 150 ms.

7. ANALYSIS OF SPONTANEOUS ACTIVITY

Very useful information about spontaneous MEG activity can be obtained by calculating frequency spectra of the signals (Fig. 35.11) and by mapping the abundance of different frequencies at various sensor sites. The sources can then be identified in either time or frequency domain. In multichannel recordings, cross-spectra between channels suggest which signals arise from the same source, and time lags may tell about the sequence of activation.

One may quantify the level of different brain rhythms by examining the temporal behavior of selected frequency bands in time–frequency representations, or more simply—if the frequencies of interest are approximately known—using the temporal spectral evolution (TSE) method[50] by focusing on the temporal behavior of one frequency band at a time. For TSE, the brain signals are first bandpass filtered, then rectified (taking absolute values of the signals), and thereafter averaged with respect to the triggering event. In these analyses, all signals that are time-locked but not necessarily phase-locked to the event will be detected. TSE (as well as amplitude but not power spectrum) preserves the original units, and the signal levels can thus be directly compared with the sizes of evoked responses.

Sometimes one may be interested in just the signal waveform and the temporal changes of the field patterns. This type of analysis, which resembles the classical use of EEG recordings, can be helpful in screening candidates for epilepsy surgery: clear changes of the field pattern from one irritative phenomenon to the next discourage the assumption of a single local onset of the discharge, although they do not rule out a deeper common trigger.

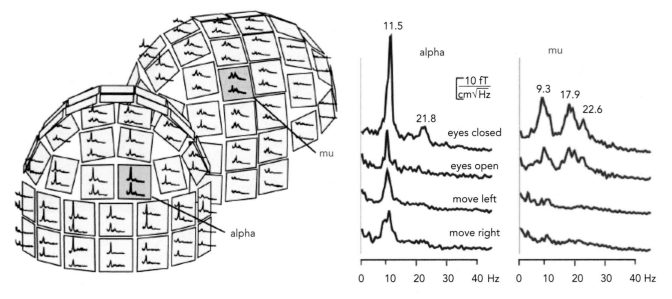

Figure 35.11. *Amplitude spectra from a 1-min period of spontaneous activity when the subject was resting with the eyes closed. Two orthogonal derivatives of the radial magnetic field were measured at each location, along the longitude and latitude, with a helmet-shaped 122-channel planar gradiometer (left). The panels on the right show reactivity of the alpha and mu rhythms to opening of the eyes and to movements of the left and right hand. Adapted from Hari R, Salmelin R. Human cortical oscillations: a view through the skull. Trends Neurosci. 1997;20:44–49.*

Due to noise problems and the use of single-channel instruments, the first studies of epileptic MEG activity employed averaging, with the simultaneously recorded EEG signal as a trigger.[51] The drawback of such a procedure is that the choice of the trigger channel largely determines the observed activity, and the method works only if easily discernible spikes or sharp waves are present in the EEG. With multichannel low-noise MEG instruments, averaging is typically necessary only for the detection of *prespikes*, which might be accurate indicators of the onset area of the paroxysmal activity. With template matching, spikes can be automatically classified and the source locations determined separately for each class.

8. SPONTANEOUS ACTIVITY OF AWAKE NORMAL SUBJECTS

8.1. Alpha Rhythm from Parieto-Occipital Areas

The typical parieto-occipital alpha rhythm, with a peak frequency around 10 Hz, is damped by opening the eyes (see the middle panel in Fig. 35.11). In the first study of the human magnetic alpha rhythm,[1] a phase reversal was observed between signals measured from the right and left hemispheres and the generator currents were therefore suggested to be parallel to the longitudinal fissure.

The sources of the alpha rhythm cluster around the calcarine and parieto-occipital sulcus (POS), the latter being the most dominant source of the MEG alpha rhythm. Importantly, one local source typically lives for only a few hundred milliseconds,[52] meaning that several sources likely contribute to a single alpha spindle. As its EEG counterpart, the parieto-occipital MEG alpha[7] is suppressed during visual stimuli, visual imagery, and various attention-demanding tasks, and its level has been related to memory load.[53]

8.2. Mu Rhythm from Sensorimotor Areas

The EEG mu rhythm has a magnetic counterpart that consists of two main frequency components, one around 10 Hz and the other around 20 Hz (see the right panel in Fig. 35.11). These two frequencies are usually not exact harmonics: they can show independent temporal behaviors both spontaneously[54] and in relation to voluntary movements.[55] Moreover, the source locations cluster on average 5 mm more anterior for the 20-Hz than the 10-Hz rhythm.[50] These findings suggest the existence of separate precentral (20 Hz) and postcentral (10 Hz) rhythms (Fig. 35.12), although they do not by any means rule out the possibility that a part of the ~20-Hz sensorimotor activity would represent the first harmonic of the ~10-Hz rolandic rhythm. Although these two frequency components of the sensorimotor MEG/EEG rhythms are in the literature often called beta and mu,[56] it is good to remember that the mu rhythm, in its original sense,[57] has an arch-like shape and thus has to include more than one frequency component. Thus—to avoid confusion—the whole movement-reactive rolandic rhythm, with both 10- and 20-Hz components, is the proper mu rhythm.

The magnetic mu rhythm starts to dampen already 1 to 2 s before a voluntary movement. In association with unilateral movements, the suppression is bilateral, although contralaterally dominant;[58] for a detailed description of the suppression and enhancement phenomena ("desynchronization" and "synchronization") of cortical rhythms, see Chapter 40. In addition to movements, the magnetic mu rhythm is modified by electric stimulation of peripheral nerves, with a more clear increase, "rebound," of the 20-Hz than the 10-Hz component around 400 ms after the stimulus.[50] The poststimulus rebound is abolished when the subject moves the fingers of the same hand. Interestingly, a similar, but weaker, suppression is seen when the subject just imagines making the movements, indicating

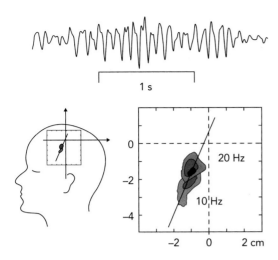

Figure 35.12. *Above: A 5-s trace of magnetic mu rhythm from the rolandic region. Below: Isodensity clusters of sources of 10- and 20-Hz oscillations over the rolandic region of one subject, based on thousands of ECD locations. The black oval over the upper (red) cluster shows the area activated by median nerve stimulation at the wrist, and the line shows the estimated course of the rolandic fissure. Adapted from Salmelin R, Hari R. Spatiotemporal characteristics of rhythmic neuromagnetic activity related to thumb movement. Neuroscience. 1994;60:537–550.*

involvement of the primary motor cortex in motor imagery.[59] Suppression of the rebound, as a sign of motor-cortex activation, also occurs when the subject just views another person making certain movements (Fig. 35.13).[60]

The 20-Hz rebounds do—whereas the 10-Hz rebounds do not—follow the moved body part in a somatotopical manner: they appear at lateral rolandic areas after mouth movements, more medially after finger movements, and close to midline after foot movements.[61]

8.3. Oscillatory Cortex–Muscle Coupling

The human rolandic MEG activity has a close temporal relationship to rhythmic motor-unit activity in skeletal muscles.[62–64] During isometric contraction of different muscles, the muscular and cortical signals are coherent at frequencies varying between 15 and 33 Hz in individual subjects.[63] The sites of maximum coherence in the motor cortex show

gross somatotopical organization, with activations during foot-muscle contraction closer to the head midline than during hand-muscle contractions (Fig. 35.14). The MEG signals lead the EMG signals in time, with increasing time lags with increasing brain–muscle distance. Such data suggest that the 20-Hz rolandic rhythm reflects, at the population level, the common central drive to spinal motoneurons.[65,66] Cortex–muscle coherence can be demonstrated also with EEG recordings.[67]

Although the early MEG recordings implied the M1 cortex as the main source of the cortex–muscle coherence, intracranial recordings have shown sources also in pre-supplementary motor area (pre-SMA) and SMA proper.[68] Still, the MEG–EMG coherence predominantly reflects M1 activity as MEG is poorly sensitive to SMA activity.

The functional role of the cortex–muscle coherence is still unclear but the coherence level seems to be related to the stability of the isometric contraction. Studies with different gripping tasks have led to the proposal that the cortical oscillations have a role in recalibrating the control system after a change in the cortex–muscle relationship.[69,70] At strong contractions, the frequency of the coherence jumps from 20 Hz to 40 Hz ("Piper rhythm") for reasons that are still unknown.[71] Similarly it is still unknown why the Piper-rhythm coherence is significantly slower in lower-limb than upper-limb muscles,[71] whereas the 20-Hz coherence occurs at approximately the same frequency for upper and lower limbs.

The normal 15- to 30-Hz cortex–muscle coherence is abolished in patients with Parkinson's disease who are withdrawn from medication from the preceding evening, and it is restored with the patients' normal levodopa treatment.[72] This finding is in line with the suggestion that abolishment of the normal 15- to 30-Hz synchronized oscillatory activity leads to bradykinesia.[73]

Gross et al.[74] demonstrated, using the dynamic imaging of coherent sources (DICS) method to characterize synchronously firing neural networks in different parts of the brain, that 6- to 9-Hz velocity changes, known to occur during slow finger movements, are directly correlated to oscillatory activity of the primary motor cortex. Moreover, the coherence patterns suggested that the pulsatile velocity changes were sustained by a cerebellar drive through thalamus and premotor cortex.

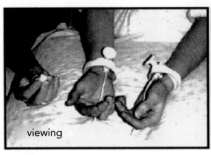
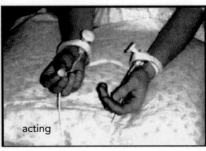
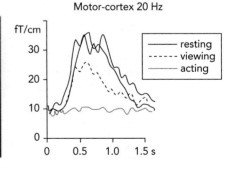

Figure 35.13. *Level of the 20-Hz rolandic activity after stimulation of the contralateral median nerve when the subject either rested (two solid lines), viewed another person manipulating a small object with the right-hand fingers (dashed line; "viewing" image), or manipulated the same object herself (dotted line; "acting" image). The sources of these 20-Hz signals were in the precentral primary motor cortex. Adapted from Hari R, Forss N, Avikainen S, et al. Activation of human primary motor cortex during action observation: A neuromagnetic study. Proc Natl Acad Sci USA. 1998;95:15061–15065.*

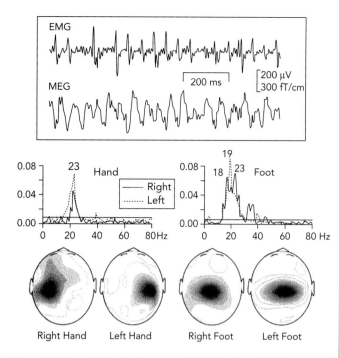

Figure 35.14. Top: Surface electromyogram (EMG) from isometrically contracted left hallucis brevis muscle and simultaneously recorded MEG over the parietal midline (3–100 Hz). Middle: Coherence spectra between MEG and EMG during isometric contraction of small hand and foot muscles (left- and right-sided contractions superimposed). Below: Spatial distributions of the strongest peaks of the coherence spectra. Adapted from Salenius S, Portin K, Kajola M., Salmelin R, Hari R. Cortical control of human motoneuron firing during isometric contraction. J Neurophysiol. 1997;77:3401–3405.

8.4. Tau Rhythm from Auditory Cortex

MEG τ-rhythm (τ, tau, according to *temporal lobe*) refers to 8- to 10-Hz oscillatory activity best seen in planar-gradiometer recordings just over the auditory cortex.[54] The rhythm is occasionally reduced by sounds, such as bursts of noise, but it is not dampened by opening the eyes—a feature clearly distinct from the occipital alpha. The sources of single tau oscillations cluster to the supratemporal auditory cortex close to the generation site of strongest auditory evoked fields, with right-hemisphere dominance (Fig. 35.15).[75]

On the basis of the observed current orientations, the corresponding electric τ-rhythm should be seen mostly in the frontocentral midline where the tau sources, with dipole moments of 40 nAm, would lead to potentials of about 10 to 20 μV. In fact, such an EEG rhythm may appear during drowsiness: decreased vigilance is often considered to be associated with a "spread" of occipital EEG alpha toward more anterior regions, with simultaneously slightly decreasing frequency.[76] A real spread of the alpha would be in clear contrast to the fixed, although distributed, generators of alpha activity, and a more plausible explanation is that the anterior "alpha" in fact reflects "tau" generated in the supratemporal auditory cortex.

The combined MEG and EEG data[77] would agree with such a hypothesis. During the awake state (the first panel of Fig. 35.16) the occipital EEG displays rhythmic 10- to 11-Hz alpha activity, and the simultaneous MEG in the

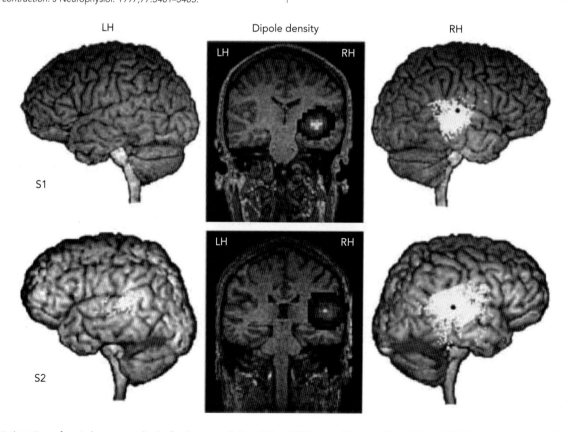

Figure 35.15. Locations of equivalent current dipoles for the tau oscillations (6.5- to 9.5-Hz range) in two subjects (S1 and S2). The sources (clusters of white dots) are projected to the surface of the brain and shown on the subject's own MRI. The black dot indicates the source of the auditory N100m response. In the coronal sections in the middle, the dipole distributions are presented as contour plots, with highest dipole densities in white and lowest in black. Adapted from Lehtelä L, Salmelin R, Hari R. Evidence for reactive magnetic 10-Hz rhythm in the human auditory cortex. Neurosci Lett 1997;222:111–114.

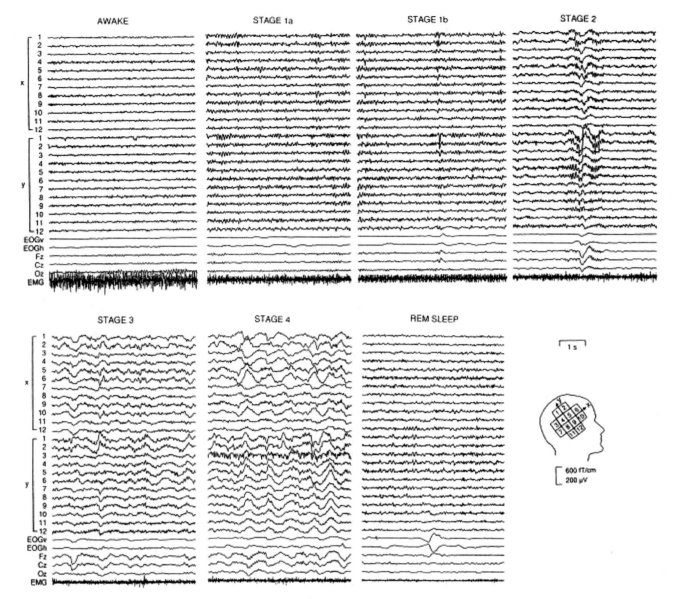

Figure 35.16. *Different vigilance stages in one subject. The recording locations (24-channel planar gradiometer used in early 1990s) are indicated on the schematic head; the x-gradients at 12 locations are plotted above and the y-gradients below. In the electric channels EOGv and EOGh refer to vertical and horizontal oculograms, respectively. The electric amplitude scale refers to all other electric recordings except the EMG, for which only relative amplitudes are of importance. Note the increase of rhythmic MEG activity during Stage 1a, compared with the awake stage. A typical V-wave occurs during Stage 1b. During Stage 2, light sleep, K-complexes occur both in MEG and EEG. In deep sleep, Stages 3 and 4, slow activity is seen in the whole measurement area. Note the eye movements and the decreased EMG activity during the REM stage. Adapted from Lu ST, Kajola M, Joutsiniemi SL, et al. Generator sites of spontaneous MEG activity during sleep. Electroenceph Clin Neurophysiol. 1992;82:182–196.*

temporal region is of low amplitude, with little rhythmic activity. However, when the occipital electric alpha becomes discontinuous during light drowsiness (Stage 1a) and seems to spread more anteriorly with slightly slower frequency, rhythmic activity of the same frequency appears in the MEG sensors over the temporal lobe.

Therefore, the apparent spread of the EEG "alpha" during drowsiness might reflect changed relative contributions from the occipital alpha and from the temporal-lobe tau generators rather than, say, traveling waves. Epidural recordings[78] show that also the temporal-lobe 6- to 11-Hz activity arising from the convexial cortex is strikingly resilient to decreased vigilance. Further studies are needed to confirm this relationship of tau and vigilance, as well as the recently suggested relationship of tau and speech perception.[79]

8.5. Other Brain Rhythms

It is possible that all cortical areas have their characteristic brain rhythms, many of which react to specific stimuli. Single median nerve stimuli have been shown to elicit in the second somatosensory cortex 7- to 9-Hz MEG oscillations, with enhanced amplitudes during stimulation at the rhythm's dominant frequency.[80]

Theta-range MEG activity has been scarcely studied. Sasaki et al.[81] observed 5- to 7-Hz MEG signals from the frontal cortex during mental calculation and intensive thinking. Tesche[23] estimated the temporal waveforms of sources (computationally) inserted to the hippocampus and found in some subjects ~5-Hz rhythmic activity during mental calculation.

Since the 1980s, much attention has been paid to the 40-Hz frequency band, often supposed to have a role in perceptual binding. Both stimulus-related activity and later "induced" 40-Hz activity have been reported in EEG recordings, less prominently so in MEG.[82] MEG frequencies (from 30 to 150 Hz) have been used to demonstrate dissociation between visual awareness and spatial attention.[83]

Theta- and gamma-range rhythms and their coupling have been suggested to form representational codes of multiple items for both sensory and memory processes.[84] Moreover, network analysis has implied frequency-specific oscillatory interactions between different nodes of the brain's resting-state network.[85]

8.6. A Note on Nomenclature

The existence of several local cortical rhythms explains in part the confusion in the literature concerning the effects of various tasks on the overlapping frequency bands of spontaneous EEG and MEG. The classical alpha rhythm refers to the parieto-occipital "Berger rhythm" that is dampened by opening of the eyes. However, many authors call any signals falling in the 8- to 13-Hz frequency range "alpha," independently of the brain area where they are generated. To avoid confusion, it would be necessary to characterize each rhythm both by its site of origin and by its frequency range, such as "parieto-occipital 10-Hz rhythm" or "rolandic 20-Hz rhythm." A comment was made above about the arch-like shape of the rolandic mu rhythm and the need for at least two underlying oscillators.

8.7. Spontaneous Activity During Sleep

Figure 35.16 illustrates multichannel MEG recording of sleep, with clearly distinct stages of vigilance.[77] The activity during the awake stage and the appearance of τ rhythm during Stage 1a were discussed above. During deep drowsiness and light sleep (Stages 1b and 2), vertex waves of 150- to 250-ms duration appeared in the frontocentral EEG leads and on several MEG channels, but the electric and magnetic V-waves did not always coincide.

MEG spindles of 11 to 15 Hz in frequency and 0.3 to 2 s in duration appeared during Stage 2. The spindles were occasionally superimposed on high-amplitude transients, thereby resembling the typical K-complexes seen in the EEG. A typical MEG K-complex lasted 0.8 to 1.2 s. Often the successive MEG V-waves and K-complexes differed in waveform and spatial distribution, implying that the K-complexes are not stereotypical responses of the cortex to external or internal stimuli but rather reflect a diffuse and variable reaction involving large cortical areas. Despite the spatial variability of the MEG K-complexes, the corresponding EEG patterns always had the maximum amplitudes around the vertex, dismissing the clear variability of the widespread generator areas demonstrated in intracranial recordings as well.[86]

The sources of the spindles also seemed complex so that a single local source did not explain the whole spindle. Such complexity of spindle generation, with a multitude of sources and frequencies, has been earlier observed in human depth-electrode and scalp-topography studies.[87,88]

During slow-wave sleep (Stages 3 and 4 in Fig. 35.16), 0.5- to 2-Hz polymorphic MEG activity was widely spread over the measurement area. During the REM stage, defined on the basis of rapid eye movements and decreased submental muscular tone, MEG activity was lower in amplitude and faster in frequency than during the other sleep stages. Sharp magnetic transients, resembling the V-waves, were frequently seen.

9. MEG IN EPILEPSY

The earliest clinical MEG recordings were used to locate both single and multiple brain areas giving rise to epileptic discharges.[89,90] Differentiation between ictal and interictal spikes is as difficult in MEG as it is in EEG. Since MEG recordings can only infrequently be performed during major motor seizures, the relevance of the interictal MEG focus has been questioned. Sometimes the activity just preceding the seizure, assumed to have the best localizing value, can be detected. One possibility to reveal the significance of the observed focus is to tailor an EEG electrode array on the basis of the interictal MEG distribution, by calculating the forward potential solution from the identified sources, and then to monitor the ictal activity during telemetric EEG recordings to ascertain whether the interictal focus is responsible for triggering the seizure.

In preoperative evaluation of epileptic patients it is important to know whether the epileptic discharges are focal, whether there are multiple foci, and whether these foci show any systematic time lags. One should also find how close the foci are to functionally irretrievable brain regions, such as the sensorimotor and speech areas, and whether the source configuration is stable over time. MEG seems especially suitable for identifying epileptic foci in the convexial neocortex. Moreover, MEG results have been used to guide placement of intracranial electrodes and to suggest reevaluation of structural MRI data.[91]

Figure 35.17 shows spikes, field patterns, and dipole moments from an early 122-channel MEG recording of a 18-year-old female who suffered from complex partial epilepsy.[92] Her nighttime seizures lasted for 20 to 30 seconds and included awakening and bilateral increase of muscular tone, as well as tonic jerks in left extremities. During the daytime she had epochs of paresthesia and loosening of the grip in the left hand. The abundant spikes, recorded with a 122-channel whole-scalp magnetometer, were adequately

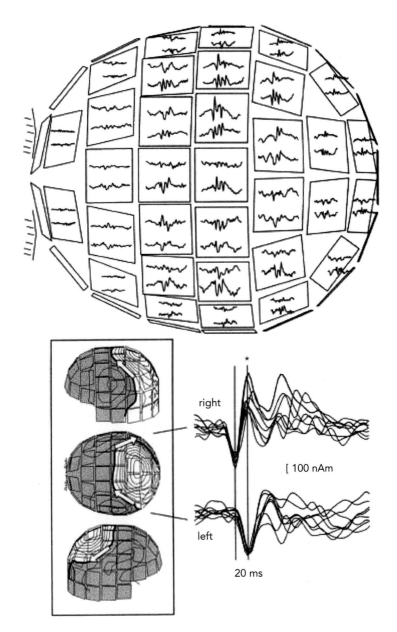

Figure 35.17. MEG recording of an epileptic patient. Top: Spatial distribution of one multispike displayed on the 122-channel sensor array viewed from top. Bottom left: Field pattern during the spike (asterisk above the curves); the sensor array is viewed from left, top, and right. The shadowed areas indicate magnetic flux emerging from the head; the isocontours are separated by 400 fT/cm. The arrows indicate the sites and orientations of the two ECDs of different directions required to account for the field pattern. Bottom right: Dipole moments as a function of time in both hemispheres. Each trace corresponds to one unaveraged spike, whose distribution was explained by the two-dipole model. Adapted from Hari R, Ahonen A, Forss N, et al. Parietal epileptic mirror focus detected with a whole-head neuromagnetometer. Neuroreport 1993;5:45–48.

modeled with two current dipoles, one in each posterior parietal cortex. The peak activity occurred consistently 20 ms later in the left than the right hemisphere, suggesting callosal conduction of the signals from right to left. Such time lags are useful in differentiating the primary and the secondary (mirror) foci.

In patients with Landau–Kleffner syndrome, MEG has displayed stereotypic 3 c/s spike-and-wave complexes in the auditory cortex.[93,94] It is obvious that such continuous epileptic discharges prevent the proper analysis of sounds, including speech, and thereby can explain the clinical symptoms in children with Landau–Kleffner syndrome.

10. ABNORMAL SPONTANEOUS ACTIVITY IN BRAIN DISEASE

In general, the MEG abnormalities found in various brain disorders resemble EEG abnormalities in time domain but often give spatially more accurate information about the affected brain area.

Ischemic hemispheric lesions are associated with considerable slowing of both MEG and EEG activity. Recent studies have suggested that the reactivity of the brain rhythms, especially in the rolandic cortex, to finger movements or median-nerve stimuli could serve as an index of recovery from stroke.[95]

One important advantage of electrophysiological methods in stroke recovery is that they are not affected by the damaged neurovascular coupling that can impair the interpretation of fMRI signals obtained from stroke patients.

In patients with Parkinson's disease, strong MEG–muscle coherence has been observed at the frequency of the 3- to 6-Hz resting tremor in several cortical and subcortical areas.[96] According to current knowledge,[97] however, such coherence likely reflects proprioceptive afference to the cortex, time-locked to the frequency of the tremor. In addition to the frequency of the parkinsonian tremor, the coherence also occurs, even more strongly, at its double,[98] again in line with proprioceptive drive that will be received separately during flexion and extension movements. Tremors occurring in both parkinsonism and in hepatic encephalopathy seem to involve widely spread cortical circuits.[99]

More abnormalities of spontaneous MEG activity were briefly discussed in the previous version of this chapter.[100]

11. AUDITORY EVOKED FIELDS

The first demonstrations of the generation of the main auditory-evoked field in the superior surface of the temporal lobe,[101,102] deduced from the measured field patterns, provided considerable insight into the origin of the coinciding electric evoked potentials, which had been previously believed to be "nonspecific" due to their maximum amplitude at the vertex.[4] Consequently, various long-latency EEG and MEG responses are today widely used as tools to study functions of the supratemporal auditory cortex.

11.1. Transient Responses

Figure 35.18 shows examples of middle-latency and long-latency auditory evoked magnetic fields, obtained using different stimulus repetition rates, different filter settings, different analysis periods, and different number of averaged responses. After the earliest cortical auditory responses peaking at 19 to 20 ms, or even at 11 ms,[103] the interindividually variable but otherwise reliable middle-latency responses peak around 30 ms and are followed by longer-latency responses around 50, 100, and 200 ms (P50m, N100m, and P200m, respectively), and a sustained field is seen during long sounds.[102,104] All these responses have cortical origin and their generation sites differ slightly, indicating contribution from several cytoarchitectonic areas in the supratemporal auditory cortex. The clear dependence of the auditory N100m response on the interstimulus interval (ISI), with saturation at ISIs of 4 to 8 s,[104,105] has been related to the duration ("lifetime") of sensory memory.[13,106,107]

The reactivity of the auditory cortex to physical changes in the stimuli in an otherwise monotonous sequence has been

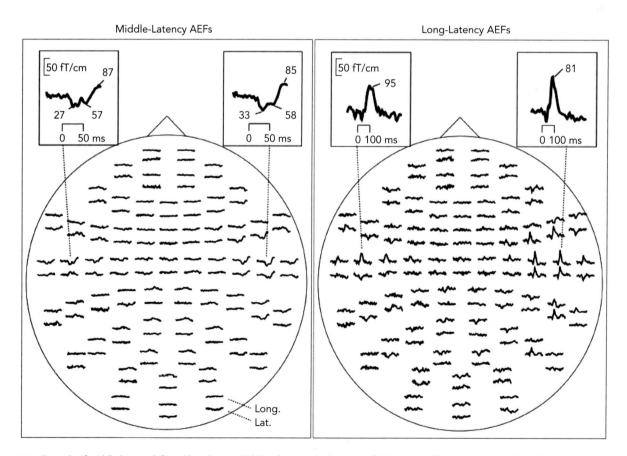

Figure 35.18. Example of middle-latency (left) and long-latency (right) auditory evoked magnetic fields recorded from one subject with a 122-channel device. Adapted from McEvoy L, Mäkelä JP, Hämäläinen M et al. Effect of interaural time differences on middle-latency and late auditory evoked magnetic fields. Hear Res. 1994;78:249–257.

studied and reviewed extensively.[4,108–110] Infrequent deviations in a monotonous sound sequence evoke "mismatch fields" (MMFs) in the close vicinity of the generation site of the auditory N100m, often with right-hemisphere dominance. MMF can in the predictive-coding framework[111] be considered as an outcome of a violation of expectations. As MMF is related to automatic sound processing, it has been widely used in testing of auditory cortical functions, including the duration of echoic memory.[112] MMFs are very sensitive indicators of different sensory and brain disorders at the group level but lack specificity; thus, their clinical usefulness at the single-subject level remains to be shown. On the other hand, only few measures can serve as clinical standalone applications, and it is always good to base clinical decisions on several measures.

11.2. Steady-State Responses

Sounds repeated at frequencies of >10 Hz elicit steady-state responses (SSRs) with nearly sinusoidal waveforms. SSRs are powerful tools to explore the reactivity of sensory projection cortices because a good signal-to-noise ratio can be obtained within a short time due to of the high stimulus repetition rate. In fact, tonotopic organization of the human auditory cortex was first shown by steady-state recordings.[113] The amplitude of the auditory SSR reaches its maximum at repetition rates around 40 Hz. This so-called 40-Hz response[114] has a cortical origin.[115] [To avoid confusion, it is important to emphasize that the notion of "cortical origin" refers to the major contributor to the *measured* signal but it does not, by any means, deny the possibility of a subcortical trigger, or simultaneous activity in some subcortical areas. In other words, saying that a measured MEG/EEG signal has a cortical origin does not take any position regarding simultaneous activity in other parts of the brain. It only tells that in many cases the adequate explanation of the signal patterns by cortical sources indicates negligible contribution from subcortical areas to the *measured* MEG/EEG signals.]

The amplitude enhancement of the SSR around 40 Hz has been adequately explained by summation of subsequent single responses, each with a 40-Hz content, thereby suggesting linearity of the responses at stimulation rates from 10 to 40 Hz.[116,117] In other words, the amplitude enhancement can occur without "resonance" (increase of responses to single stimuli) at stimulation rates of 40 Hz. However, its appearance does imply that the original responses contain frequencies of ~40 Hz.

During normal binaural hearing, sounds from each ear reach the auditory cortices of both hemispheres. Therefore the binaural cortical responses, even when recorded from one hemisphere only, are unknown mixtures of inputs from both ears. One solution to this problem is to mark ("frequency tag") the inputs from both ears.[118] Continuous tones, presented either monaurally (to the left or right ear) or binaurally, can be amplitude modulated with different frequencies in the two ears, and the MEG signals of each hemisphere can then be analyzed either in time or frequency domain. Such analysis demonstrates significantly stronger suppression of the ipsilateral than contralateral input during binaural hearing, and the effect is robust despite interaural intensity differences.[119]

Frequency tagging of auditory input has been used to unravel the brain basis of the curious dichotic octave illusion[120] and to study attentional modulation of auditory-cortex activation.[121]

12. SOMATOSENSORY EVOKED FIELDS

12.1. Responses from SI

The earliest cortical somatosensory evoked field (SEF) to median nerve stimulation peaks at ~20 ms. It is the magnetic counterpart of the electric N20 and thus often called N20m (or M20). The field pattern of N20m can be explained by a local source in the posterior wall of the central sulcus, in cytoarchitectonic area 3b, with intracellular current flow pointing from back to front. When the recording band is opened and up to 20,000 single responses are averaged, brief bursts of about 600-Hz oscillations can be seen superimposed on N20m.[122] These high-frequency responses will be discussed in detail in Chapters 33 and 39.

Since MEG mainly picks signals from tangential currents, the signals arising from the SI hand area tend to reflect activity of fissural (rather than convexial) cortex. Instead, in the SI foot area all cortical areas produce currents tangential to the skull, and thus their changed relative contributions as a function of time should be seen as rotation of the field patterns. Evoked fields to lower-limb stimulation in fact support such rotations as signs of successive activation of several cytoarchitectonic areas, as is illustrated below.

Figure 35.19 shows one subject's responses to left tibial nerve stimuli, with largest signals at the top of the head.[123] The field patterns rotate as a function of time, as predicted above. A two-dipole model, with one dipole in area 3b and the other in area 5, both in the mesial wall of the hemisphere, explained the data during the first 100 ms, with a consistent 3-ms time difference in their initial peak latencies. Other source models were rejected on the basis of their inconsistencies with experimental data and/or anatomical information. A slightly different two-source model for tibial nerve SEFs has been suggested on the basis of beamformer analysis.[124]

SEFs from the SI cortex are typically strictly contralateral, although some long-latency MEG responses from the ipsilateral SI have been reported. However, transfer of stimulus- or movement-related vibrations to the other hand (e.g., by means of a table on which both hands are resting during a finger-pressing task) has been demonstrated as one prominent contributor to 60-ms ipsilateral responses.[125]

During development, SEF latencies, polarities, and relative amplitudes of successive deflections change (Fig. 35.20),[126] likely reflecting differences in myelination (conduction velocity), connectivity, and the effects of transmitter substances.

Careful quantification of source strengths may be very useful in some applications. For example, Elbert et al.,[127] determining source strengths for tactile finger stimulation at SI cortex, found increased cortical representations for the left hands of string players, indicative of practice-related cortical reorganization.

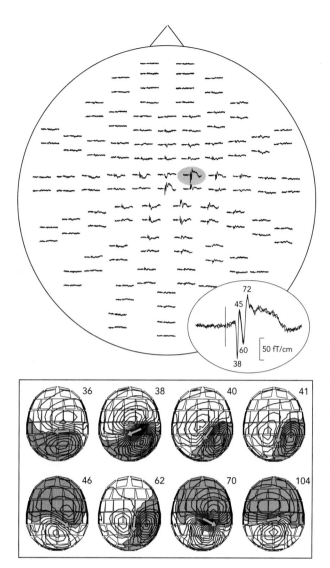

Figure 35.19. Top: *Responses of one subject to electric stimulation of the left tibial nerve at the ankle. The traces are averages of 800 single responses. The insert shows two enlarged sets of 400 responses from successive experiments superimposed, indicating excellent replicability of the responses. The passband is 0.03 to 275 Hz. Bottom: Magnetic field patterns and equivalent current dipoles of the same subject as a function of time (indicated in milliseconds). The isocontours are separated by 20 fT. Adapted from Hari R, Nagamine T, Nishitani N, et al. Time-varying activation of different cytoarchitectonic areas of the human SI cortex after tibial nerve stimulation. Neuroimage 1996;4:111–118.*

The generation sites of SEFs can in the preoperative evaluation of the sensorimotor strip be complemented by cortex–muscle coherence recordings (Fig. 35.21) to pinpoint both the postcentral cortex (by means of SEFs) and the primary motor cortex anterior to the central sulcus. Visualization of the somatosensory and motor landmarks on a brain rendering (right), with veins superimposed, further helps the neurosurgeon to navigate during the operation.[33]

12.2. Responses from SII and Other Nonprimary Cortical Areas

MEG recordings were the first to demonstrate noninvasively that peripheral stimuli activate bilaterally the upper lip of the Sylvian fissure—that is, the region of the second somatosensory

area, SII.[19,128–130] Although the SI/SII differentiation was possible already using small MEG sensor arrays, only the whole-scalp recordings have given detailed information about the whole cortical somatosensory network, with spatially and temporally distinct activations also in the posterior parietal cortex, in the mesial cortex, and in the frontal lobes.[20] Tactile stimulation activates essentially the same brain regions as does electric stimulation, but with slightly different latencies and relative amplitudes. The interstimulus dependence of the main SII response, peaking at ~100 ms,[19] resembles that of the auditory 100-ms response on the other side of the sylvian fissure.[105]

12.3. Abnormal SEFs in Patients

In addition to differentiation of various source areas, recordings of SEFs in patients with various lesions[131] and analysis of, say, phase-locking between areas[132] have brought new information about the cortical somatosensory network, also regarding the debate on parallel versus serial processing in different somatosensory cortical areas.

Figure 35.22 gives a striking example of abnormal SEFs in a patient with Unverricht–Lundborg-type progressive myoclonus epilepsy (PME).[133] "Giant" SEFs are seen in the contralateral SI as a sign of hyperreactivity. The ipsilateral SI also reacts to the stimuli which is in contrast to the healthy control subject; the latency delay of ~20 ms suggests callosal transfer to the ipsilateral side. In spite of the enhanced SI responses, no clear SII responses are seen in the patient. Findings like this encourage the clinical neurophysiologist to assess functions of the whole cortical somatosensory network beyond the primary somatosensory cortex, as such dysfunctions may have direct consequences to the prognosis and rehabilitation of the patient.

12.4. Proprioception

Proprioception is crucial for proper motor control and omnipresent during movements, but no reliable clinical neurophysiological tools have been available to assess proprioceptive afference to the cortex. Recent results suggest that corticokinematic coherence (CKC)—computed between cortical MEG activity and the acceleration of a moving limb—could provide such a new clinical tool. Figure 35.23 shows that CKC is of the same strength to active and passive finger movements, which implies that it is mainly driven by proprioceptive afference.[97] CKC is robust against simultaneous magnetic artifacts and thus in principle well suited for clinical environments.[134]

One may produce well-controlled passive movements for CKC purposes with a MEG-compatible stimulator.[47] If movements are produced only transiently, at intervals from 1 to 8 s, prominent transient responses peak at 80 to 90 ms in the contralateral rolandic cortex; for clinical purposes, an interstimulus interval of 2 to 3 s would produce the best signal-to-noise ration within a given time slot.[135]

12.5. Noxious Stimulation

Painful electric stimulation of the tooth pulp, carbon dioxide stimulation of the nasal mucosa, and electric or laser

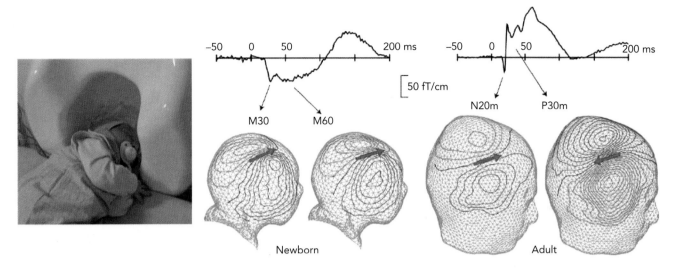

Figure 35.20. Somatosensory evoked fields and field patterns to median nerve stimulation in a newborn (left) and an adult (right). The signals are from one planar gradiometer channel over the right somatosensory cortex. The photograph on the left (courtesy of Elina Pihko) illustrates how signals can be recorded with an adult-shape neuromagnetometer from the small bably brain one hemisphere at the time. Adapted from Lauronen L, Nevalainen P, Wikström H, et al. Immaturity of somatosensory cortical processing in human newborns. Neuroimage. 2006;33:195–203.

stimulation of the skin all elicit MEG responses around SII and/or the frontal operculum.[136–142]

With laser heat it is possible to stimulate rather selectively Aδ- and C-fibers by applying different stimulus intensities to stimulus areas of different sizes,[139,142,143] but this opportunity has not yet been adopted to clinical pain research. Figure 35.24 shows that the evoked responses from the contralateral SII cortex peak to Aδ-fiber stimuli at ~160 ms and to C-fiber stimuli at ~800 ms, in agreement with the conduction velocities of these two fiber types.[142] C-fibers can be selectively activated also with intra-epidermal electric

stimuli, with MEG responses peaking over 1,300 ms after foot stimulation.[144]

Reactivity of the 20-Hz motor-cortex rhythm to laser-heat pain suggests that these noxious stimuli automatically activate the primary motor cortex, which might be related to mechanisms of pathological muscle contraction in tension pain.[145,146]

In patients with chronic complex regional pain syndrome (CRPS), the motor cortex was activated abnormally strongly to innocuous tactile stimuli, suggesting decreased inhibition; accordingly, the somatosensory responses were stronger to stimulation of the painful than the healthy

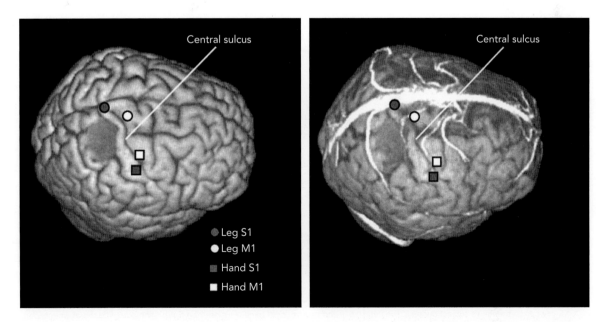

Figure 35.21. Preoperative functional localization in a patient with a parietal-lobe tumor. The postcentral somatosensory cortex (S1) has been identified by measuring SEFs to median-nerve (hand) and tibial-nerve (leg) stimulation. In addition, cortex–muscle coherence for hand and foot small muscles has been used to identify the precentral primary motor cortex (M1). On the right, veins are superimposed on the surface rendering. Courtesy of CliniMEG, Brain Research Unit, Aalto University, Finland.

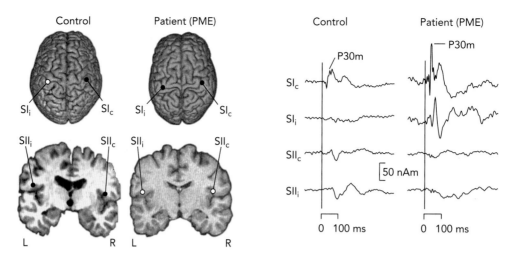

Figure 35.22. Source locations (left) and source waveforms as a function of time (right) to electric stimulation of the left median nerve in a healthy control subject and in a patient with Unverricht–Lundborg-type progressive myoclonus epilepsy. The black circles indicate source locations and the white circles indicate possible source locations that did not show any activation; c and i refer to contralateral and ipsilateral hemispheres. Adapted from Forss N, Silén T, Karjalainen T. Lack of activation of human secondary somatosensory cortex in Unverricht-Lundborg type of progressive myoclonus epilepsy. Ann Neurol. 2001;49:90–97.

side.[147] MEG recordings have demonstrated in one CRPS patient that the pain-related abnormalities of somatosensory processing progress with time from one hemisphere to another,[148] in agreement with the spread of the patient's symptoms.

13. VISUAL EVOKED FIELDS

Visual evoked fields (VEFs) were reported for the first time in 1975.[149,150] The retinotopic organization is clearly seen in the occipitally generated MEG responses, with different spatial distributions to left and right, to upper and lower, and to central and peripheral visual fields.[151,152] Outside the occipital cortex the response patterns are quite complex, and VEFs have not yet found their way to clinical toolboxes.

Figure 35.25 shows that responses to half-field pattern and luminance stimuli differ in their spatial distributions. For both stimuli, the first responses are generated in the occipital cortex but a later response occurs, especially for luminance stimuli, in the region of the POS, with no dependence on the visual field stimulated.[153] The very same POS area, a likely human

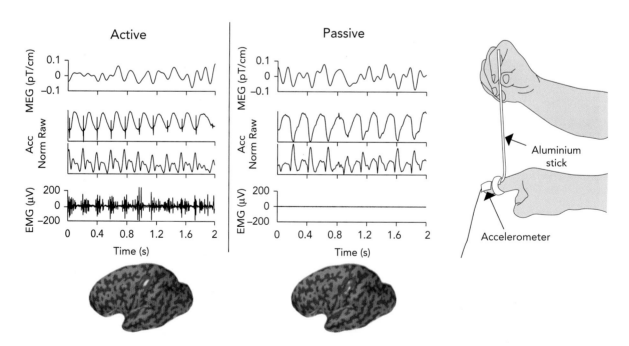

Figure 35.23. CKC of one representative subject during active (left panel) and passive (right panel and insert on right) right index-finger movements during 2 s. Traces from top to bottom: Single-trial MEG recorded with a planar gradiometer over the left rolandic cortex (filtered from 1 to 10 Hz), raw accelerometer signals, norm of 3D accelerometer signals, and surface EMG from flexor carpi radialis. The brain renderings below show the locations of the maximum coherence, with the strength coded in color. Adapted from Piitulainen H, Bourguignon M, De Tiège X, et al. Corticokinematic coherence during active and passive finger movements. Neuroscience 2013;238:361–370.

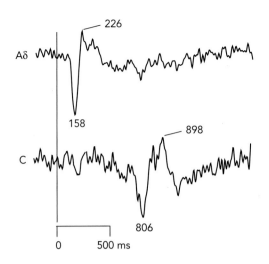

Figure 35.24. *Averaged responses (N = 100) of a single subject from right SII region to selective A-delta- (upper trace; weak pricking pain) and C-fiber (lower trace; weak burning pain) thulium-laser stimuli presented to the dorsum of the left hand once every 4.5 to 5.5 s. Modified from Forss N, Raij TT, Seppä M, et al. Common cortical network for first and second pain. Pain. 2005;24:132–142.*

homologue of the monkey V6/V6A region, is activated about 230 ms after voluntary eye blinks,[154] as well as after voluntary saccades (Fig. 35.26).[155] The POS activation after the subject's own blinks has been suggested to be related to the maintenance of visual continuity despite the interruption of visual input during lid closure.[154]

The human homologue of the monkey MT/V5 cortex, a brain area selective to visual motion, has also been identified by MEG recordings.[156–158] Interestingly, the activation order of human visual cortices, especially between V1/V2 and MT/V5, can deviate from the simple serial activation pattern.[156,159,160] The experimental results agree with monkey recordings[161] and with the importance of interareal feed-forward and feedback connections in the hierarchically connected network.

14. RESPONSES TO MORE COMPLEX VISUAL STIMULI

Some percepts change so unexpectedly that it is not possible to time-lock the analysis of MEG signals to the event. Figure 35.27 shows how frequency tagging can help to follow cortical activation changes related to the spontaneous switching of percepts of the ambiguous Rubin's vase stimulus.[162] Dynamic noise was superimposed to the picture and updated at 12 Hz in the vase region and at 15 Hz in the face region. The subjects were not able to tell the difference between the update frequencies, but their occipital MEG signals displayed distinct, very prominent frequency peaks at both 12 and 15 Hz.

On the basis of the changes in the relative strengths of the 12-Hz and 15-Hz frequencies during the percepts it was possible to conclude that the activation of the early visual cortices co-varied with the percept, most likely because of top-down influences. Eye tracking ruled out the possibility that the changes in the MEG signals could have been related to gaze deviations.[162]

In agreement with both clinical and other imaging data, MEG responses to pictures of faces, socially very relevant

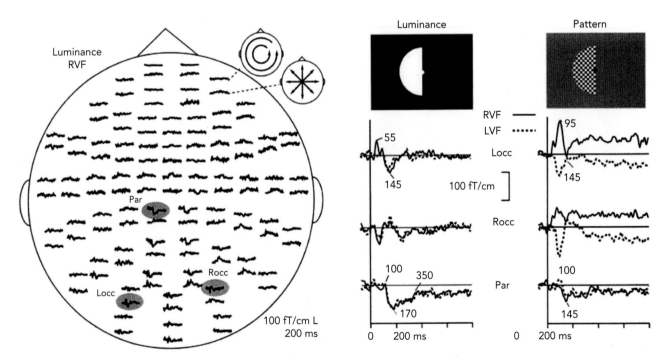

Figure 35.25. *Responses of a single subject to left and right hemifield (LVF, RVF) luminance and pattern stimuli (radius 8 deg) from the parietal region (Par) and from left and right occipital areas (Locc, Rocc). Note the predominance of the parietal response to luminance stimuli and the very clear LVF versus RVF difference in the occipital channels for pattern, but not for luminance, stimuli. Adapted from Portin K, Salenius S, Salmelin R, et al. Activation of the human occipital and parietal cortex by pattern and luminance stimuli: Neuromagnetic measurements. Cereb Cortex. 1998;18:253–260.*

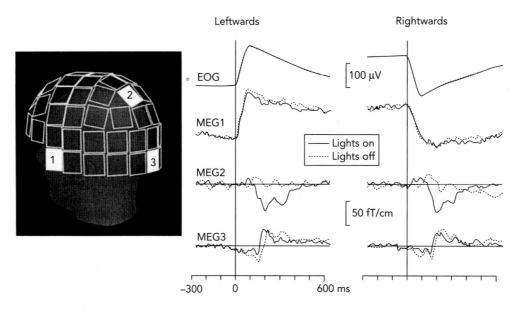

Figure 35.26. MEG signals from three locations (shown on the schematic head) during a visually guided saccade task. The signals were averaged with respect to the onset of horizontal saccades (leftwards or rightwards); the horizontal electro-oculogram (EOG) used as the trigger is depicted above. Signals recorded during darkness and with lights on are illustrated with dashed and solid lines, respectively. Adapted from Jousmäki V, Hämäläinen M, Hari R. Magnetic source imaging during a visually guided task. Neuroreport. 1996;7:2961–2964.

stimuli, indicate activation of extrastriate visual areas, predominantly in the right posterior fusiform gyrus 140 to 170 ms after the stimulus onset,[34] with a systematic amplitude dependence on the degree of "faceness" of the stimulus.[163] Observed eye blinks activate the viewer's visual cortex even during a conversation when the blinks are embedded within a rich audiovisual stimulus flow and the viewer does not consciously pay attention to them.[164] This finding agrees with the suggestion that eye blinks have functions beyond moisturizing the eyeball, possibly indicating "punctuations of thought," which makes them socially relevant to the other person.

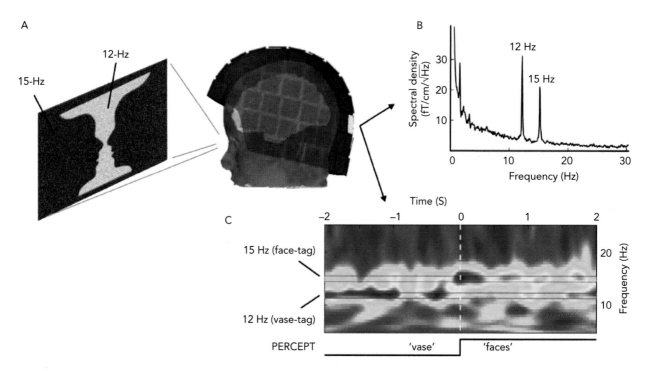

Figure 35.27. An example of frequency tagging. **A:** The Rubin's vase/faces figure used as the stimulus. The vase and faces areas are superimposed with dynamical noise that is updated at 12 Hz in the vase area and at 15 Hz in the face areas (insert on the right). **B:** Frequency spectrum from one occipital MEG channel, based on 10-min recording. **C:** Cortical current estimate as a function of time for one subject computed with respect to the change in cortical tag-related activity during the change of percept. Adapted from Parkkonen L, Andersson J, Hämäläinen M, et al. Early visual areas reflect the percept of an ambiguous scene. Proc Nat Acad Sci USA. 2008;105:20500–20504.

The next step in the complexity of visual stimuli is to let the subject view real live actions of another person, and we will discuss such progress below after the brief visit to language and speech.

15. LANGUAGE AND SPEECH

MEG's excellent temporal resolution is of high value in studies of language perception and production (speech). In the first MEG study of picture naming,[165] the cortical activation sequence progressed in both hemispheres from the posterior brain areas toward more anterior regions. Signs of considerable parallel processing were evident and both hemispheres were activated by the task. Since then, MEG has been increasingly applied in studies of reading and naming, both in healthy subjects and in, for example, aphasic patients, stuttering subjects, and dyslexic individuals.[166] Other interesting approaches include the analysis of long-range connectivity[167] and the study of language development.[168]

MEG (as well as EEG) also allows sophisticated analyses of the temporal windows of speech perception,[169] cortical tracking of the hierarchical linguistic structures of speech,[170] and the decoding of the heard segments of continuous speech.[171] Future studies will certainly apply increasingly naturalistic setups and include studies of dialogues to assess the real essence of speech as a tool of interpersonal communication.

In clinical settings, studies of speech and language are most relevant for presurgical planning to identify the essential language cortices and to eventually even replace invasive examinations with noninvasive methods.[172]

16. TIME-SENSITIVE IMAGING OF SOCIAL INTERACTION

MEG recordings have since the late 1990s been used to study brain activation to live actions of other humans.[60] These rather complex studies are motivated by the omnipresence of social interaction that shapes human brains and minds throughout lifetime.

The first MEG study of action observation[60] was inspired by the discovery of motor mirror neurons in the monkey frontal cortex, in area F5.[173] MEG recordings have since then indicated in humans a sequence of activation from the visual cortex to the superior temporal sulcus, then to the inferior parietal cortex, next to the inferior frontal cortex, and finally to the primary motor cortex within 250 to 400 ms of seeing another person's live motor acts or still faces.[174,175] Using median-nerve stimuli to probe the function of the somatosensory network while the subjects were viewing another person's finger manipulations demonstrated that the primary and secondary somatosensory cortices of the viewer also react to the observed hand actions.[176]

Reactivity of the motor-cortex 20-Hz MEG rhythm has demonstrated that the primary motor cortex is activated before and during observed actions (that the viewer already more or less knows because they have occurred previously), and that

it is stabilized afterwards, very much like what happens during the person's own actions.[55] The human mirroring systems have been suggested to play an important role both in action imitation and in understanding the action goals, thereby likely having relevance in social interaction.[177] However, the exact functional roles of the mirroring systems are currently under strong debate. MEG studies of action observation have been recently reviewed.[178]

Despite the extensive results of human mirroring systems and the increasing complexity of the stimuli one can use in brain imaging, one can criticize the applied setups to represent "spectator science," in which one is studying passive subjects who only spectate the stimuli instead of actively participating in the events.[179,180] We have therefore tried to advance toward "two-person neuroscience" (2PN) to study the brain basis of social interaction.[181] Specifically, we have developed a dual-MEG setting where one can record MEG activity simultaneously from two interacting subjects. One experimental goal would be to differentiate interactive from reactive states of human social interaction as the previous ones cannot be studied in the traditional one-person settings where the interaction is not present.[180] The 2PN setups seem particularly important for rapid interactions, such as conversation, where turn-takings take place with a mean latency of 200 ms and thus cannot be just responses to the end of the other person's turn. Turn-taking is evident in prelinguistic children (as protoconversation), is universal across languages, and is present in many primates, either in vocal or gestural communication.[182] Turn-taking can thus be considered a very basic form of interaction that could be studied in the dual-MEG setups.

In our first dual-MEG setup, the subjects had telephone-like audio connection between two MEG labs 5 km apart in the Helsinki area.[183] An updated version[184] includes a video connection via the Internet to allow the same setup to be copied to any geographical location; the obtained end-to-end delay of about 130 ms allows smooth and natural interaction. Another dual-MEG setup has been established in Japan, where a mother and her child, lying on their backs in side-by-side MEG scanners, can be studied at the same time; mirrors allow them to see each other's facial expressions.[185]

Compared with the earlier EEG hyperscanning studies,[186] MEG has the advantage that source locations of the signals of interest (brain rhythms and their modulations or evoked responses) can be estimated in a rather straightforward and accurate manner.

Figure 35.28 shows recent dual-MEG recordings where the subjects were online interacting with each other like during a normal telephone conversation.[183] In another study, with an audiovisual connection, the subjects were imitating each other's finger movements.[187] Both these feasibility studies confirmed that good-quality MEG data can be collected from both partners during social interaction. Tiny differences in beta-range modulation in the early visual cortices of the subjects in the imitation study depended on the subject's role as a follower or leader in a joint hand-action task and probably reflected different strategies needed in the two roles to integrate kinematics-related visual information.[187] Much work is still needed to develop suitable analysis methods for the 2PN recordings to

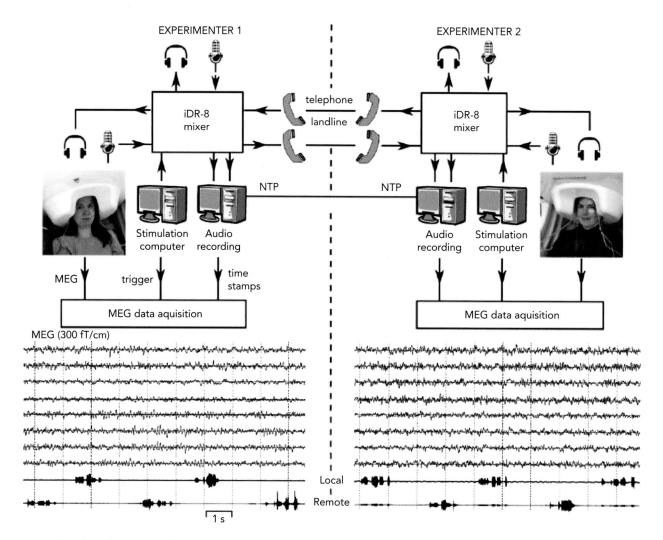

Figure 35.28. Experimental setup in a dual-MEG study. The subjects were located in laboratories 5 km apart; in this particular setup the subjects were only hearing each other via an audiolink. The bottom panels show a few MEG channels from both sites, accurately time-locked to each other, and the sound channels from the two sites (local and remote) with respect to each subject Modified from Baess P, Zhdanov A, Mandel A, Parkkonen L, Hirvenkari L, Mäkelä JP, Jousmäki V, Hari R. MEG dual scanning: A procedure to study interacting humans. Front Human Neurosci. 2012;6: Article 83.

catch the details of intersubject synchrony, alignment, and turn-taking within different time windows. Novel innovative experimental setups are also needed. Some ideas about the future 2PN MEG studies have been recently proposed.[179]

17. FUTURE PERSPECTIVES

MEG has established a firm position as a tool of basic neuroscience in unraveling brain dynamics in perception, cognition, action, and interaction. Clinical applications are still few but are slowly increasing with the installation of whole-scalp neuromagnetometers in hospital environments. Co-registration of functional information from MEG with structural information from MRI is currently routine, and the results are frequently compared with other imaging methods, especially fMRI. Commercial multichannel MEG instruments allow convenient recordings of adult brains. MEG has a clear potential also in developmental neuroscience,[188] and for that purpose a few specific devices for infants have been recently developed.

With the whole-scalp neuromagnetometers, and with improved head-position monitoring tools and sophisticated artifact-suppression methods, MEG can be applied in a variety of behavioral conditions. The noise levels of the current low-T_c SQUIDs are so low that the "noise" coming from the brain far exceeds the instrument noise. However, some benefits might be still obtained from even lower-noise SQUIDs at higher (say, > 60 Hz) frequencies, as was discussed recently.[16]

To improve the spatial resolution of MEG, the sensors should be put closer to the skull, even directly on the scalp, where the distance to the closest sources in cortex would still be ~1.5 to 2 cm. With low-T_c SQUIDs such close placing is not possible because of the space needed for liquid helium (4 K = –269°C), but high-T_c SQUIDS operated at liquid nitrogen temperature (77 K = –196°C) could be taken closer to the skull. MEG signals have been recorded with high-T_c SQUIDs,[189] although with a sensitivity of an order of magnitude worse than with the low-T_c SQUIDs.

Other new sensor options include optically pumped atomic magnetometers[190,191] and magnetoresistive sensors[192] that both could be placed close to the scalp. These sensors are currently under active development.

The neuromagnetism community is at present focusing on development of new signal-analysis approaches that employ methods of machine learning and predictive coding.[49,193,194] It is likely that MEG signals contain much more information than we can at present extract, and they thus appear as ideal tools to decode subtle brain states.[195]

Other sophisticated analysis methods have been used to analyze data collected during naturalistic stimulation, for example while the subjects are viewing a movie[196] or listening to natural connected speech.[170,171]

Further progress is expected with respect to innovative combination of several existing methods with new instruments, for example for recording both MEG and MRI at the same time with an ultralow-field MEG–MRI hybrid device.[197]

It is encouraging for MEG/EEG users to realize that the brain imaging community is now increasingly emphasizing the importance of temporal information to complement the detailed structural information obtained by human brain imaging. We can thus expect the electrophysiological methods, both MEG and EEG, to have a prosperous future.

ACKNOWLEDGMENTS

The studies reported here have been supported by the Academy of Finland, the Sigrid Jusélius Foundation (Finland), the European Research Council (Advanced Grant #232946), Louis Jeantet Foundation (award; Switzerland), and the multidisciplinary research project aivoAALTO of the Aalto University. The skill, support, and enthusiasm of the research-team members have been decisive for collecting the MEG data presented in this chapter.

REFERENCES

1. Cohen D. Magnetoencephalography: Evidence of magnetic fields produced by alpha-rhythm currents. *Science.* 1968;161:784–786.
2. Hari R, Lounasmaa OV. Recording and interpretation of cerebral magnetic fields. *Science.* 1989;244:432–436.
3. Grandori F, Hoke M, Romani G-L, eds. *Auditory Evoked Magnetic Fields and Potentials. Advances in Audiology, Vol. 6.* Basel: Karger, 1990.
4. Hari R. The neuromagnetic method in the study of the human auditory cortex. In: Grandori F, Hoke M, Romani G, eds. *Auditory Evoked Magnetic Fields and Potentials. Advances in Audiology, Vol. 6.* 1st ed. Basel: Karger, 1990:222–282.
5. Sato S, ed. *Magnetoencephalography. Advances in Neurology, Vol. 54.* New York: Raven Press, 1990.
6. Hämäläinen M, Hari R, Ilmoniemi RJ, Knuutila J, Lounasmaa OV. Magnetoencephalography—theory, instrumentation, and applications to noninvasive studies of the working human brain. *Rev Mod Phys.* 1993;65:413–497.
7. Hari R, Salmelin R. Human cortical oscillations: a neuromagnetic view through the skull. *Trends Neurosci.* 1997;20:44–49.
8. Hari R, Forss N. Magnetoencephalography in the study of human somatosensory cortical processing. *Proc Royal Soc Lond B.* 1999;354:1145–1154.
9. Forss N, Nakasato N, Ebersole J, Nagamine T, Salmelin R. Clinical use of magnetoencephalography. *Clin Neurophysiol.* 2000;Suppl. 53:287–297.
10. Baillet S, Mosher J, Leahy R. Electromagnetic brain mapping. *IEEE Signal Processing Magazine.* 2001; 18:14–30.
11. Del Gratta C, Pizzella V, Tecchio F, Romani GL. Magnetoencephalography—a noninvasive brain imaging method with 1 ms time resolution. *Reports on Progress in Physics.* 2001;64:1759–1814.
12. Hansen PC, Kringelbach ML, Salmelin R, eds. *MEG. An Introduction to Methods.* New York: Oxford University Press, 2010.
13. Hari R, Parkkonen L, Nangini C. The brain in time: insights from neuromagnetic recordings. *Ann New York Acad Sci.* 2010;1191:89–109.
14. Supek S, Aine C, eds. *Magnetoencephalography. From Signals to Dynamic Cortical Networks.* Berlin/Heidelberg: Springer-Verlag, 2014.
15. Pizzella V, Marzetti L, Della Penna S, de Pasquale F, Zappasodi F, Romani GL. Magnetoencephalography in the study of brain dynamics. *Funct Neurol.* 2014;29:197–203.
16. Hari R, Parkkonen L. The brain timewise: how timing shapes and supports brain function. *Philos Trans R Soc Lond B Biol Sci.* 2015;370:20140170.
17. Nunez PL. Estimation of large scale neocortical source activity with EEG surface Laplacians. *Brain Topogr.* 1989;2:141–154.
18. Hari R, Reinikainen K, Kaukoranta E, et al. Somatosensory evoked cerebral magnetic fields from SI and SII in man. *Electroenceph Clin Neurophysiol.* 1984;57:254–263.
19. Hari R, Karhu J, Hämäläinen M, et al. Functional organization of the human first and second somatosensory cortices: A neuromagnetic study. *Eur J Neurosci.* 1993;5:724–734.
20. Mauguière F, Merlet I, Forss N, et al. Activation of a distributed somatosensory cortical network in the human brain. A dipole modelling study of magnetic fields evoked by median nerve stimulation. Part I: Location and activation timing of SEF sources. *Electroenceph Clin Neurophysiol.* 1997;104:281–289.
21. Hari R. On brain's magnetic responses to sensory stimuli. *J Clin Neurophysiol.* 1991;8:157–169.
22. Parkkonen L, Fujiki N, Mäkelä JP. Sources of auditory brainstem responses revisited: contribution by magnetoencephalography. *Hum Brain Mapp.* 2009;30:1772–1782.
23. Tesche CD. Non-invasive detection of ongoing neuronal population activity in normal human hippocampus. *Brain Res.* 1997;749:53–60.
24. Taulu S, Simola J, Nenonen J, Parkkonen L. Novel noise reduction methods. In: Supek S, Aine C, eds. *Magnetoencephalography. From Signals to Dynamic Cortical Networks.* Berlin/Heidelberg: Springer-Verlag, 2014.
25. Hillebrand A, Barnes GR. A quantitative assessment of the sensitivity of whole-head MEG to activity in the adult human cortex. *Neuroimage.* 2002;16:638–650.
26. Kaukoranta E, Hämäläinen M, Sarvas J, Hari R. Mixed and sensory nerve stimulations activate different cytoarchitectonic areas in the human primary somatosensory cortex SI. *Exp Brain Res.* 1986;63:60–66.
27. Okada YC, Papuashvili N, Xu C. What can we learn from MEG studies of the somatosensory system of the swine? *Electroencephalogr Clin Neurophysiol Suppl.* 1996;47:35–46.
28. Murakami S, Okada Y. Invariance in current dipole moment density across brain structures and species: physiological constraint for neuroimaging. *Neuroimage.* 2015;111:49–58.
29. Hämäläinen M, Ilmoniemi R. Interpreting magnetic fields of the brain: minimum norm estimates. *Med Biol Engineer Comp.* 1994;32:35–42.
30. Ribary U, Ioannides A, Singh K, et al. Magnetic field tomography of coherent thalamocortical 40-Hz oscillation in humans. *Proc Natl Acad Sci USA.* 1991;88:11037–11041.
31. Uutela K, Hämäläinen M, Somersalo E. Visualization of magnetoencephalographic data using minimum current estimates. *Neuroimage.* 1999;10:173–180.
32. Hämäläinen M, Hari R. Magnetoencephalographic characterization of dynamic brain activation: Basic principles, and methods of data collection and source analysis. In: Toga A, Mazziotta J, eds. *Brain Mapping, The Methods.* 2nd ed. Amsterdam: Academic Press, 2002:227–253.
33. Mäkelä J, Kirveskari E, Seppä M, et al. Three-dimensional integration of brain anatomy and function to facilitate intraoperative navigation around the sensorimotor strip. *Hum Brain Mapp.* 2001;12:181–192.
34. Furey ML, Tanskanen T, Beauchamp MS, et al. Dissociation of face-selective cortical responses by attention. *Proc Natl Acad Sci USA.* 2006;103:1065–1070.
35. Liljeström M, Hulten A, Parkkonen L, Salmelin R. Comparing MEG and fMRI views to naming actions and objects. *Hum Brain Mapp.* 2009;30:1845–1856.
36. Laufs H, Krakow K, Sterzer P, et al. Electroencephalographic signatures of attentional and cognitive default modes in spontaneous brain activity fluctuations at rest. *Proc Natl Acad Sci USA.* 2003;100:11053–11058.
37. Lachaux JP, Fonlupt P, Kahane P, et al. Relationship between task-related gamma oscillations and BOLD signal: new insights from combined fMRI and intracranial EEG. *Hum Brain Mapp.* 2007;28:1368–1375.

38. Hari R, Ilmoniemi RJ. Cerebral magnetic fields. *CRC Crit Rev Biomed Engineer.* 1986;14:93–126.
39. Cooper R, Winter A, Crow H, Grey Walter W. Comparison of subcortical, cortical and scalp activity using chronically indwelling electrodes in man. *Electroenceph Clin Neurophysiol.* 1965;18:217–228.
40. Antervo A, Hari R, Katila T, Ryhänen T, Seppänen M. Magnetic fields produced by eye blinking. *Electroenceph Clin Neurophysiol.* 1985;61:247–254.
41. Jousmäki V, Hari R. Cardiac artifacts in magnetoencephalogram. *J Clin Neurophysiol.* 1996;13:172–176.
42. Taulu S, Simola J, Kajola M. Applications of the signal space separation method. *IEEE Trans Sign Proc* 2005;53:3359–3372.
43. Taulu S, Hari R. Removal of magnetoencephalographic artifacts with temporal signal-space separation: demonstration with single-trial auditory-evoked responses. *Hum Brain Mapp.* 2009;30:1524–1534.
44. Mäkelä JP, Taulu S, Pohjola J, Ahonen A, Pekkonen E. Effects of subthalamic nucleus stimulation on spontaneous sensorimotor MEG activity in a Parkinsonian patient. In: Cheyne D, Ross B, Stroink G, Weinberg H, eds. *New Frontiers in Biomagnetism. Proceedings of the 15th International Conference on Biomagnetism, 2006. International Congress Series.* Vol 13002007:345–348.
45. Mertens M, Lütkenhöner B. Efficient neuromagnetic determination of landmarks in the somatosensory cortex. *Clin Neurophysiol.* 2000;111:1478–1487.
46. Jousmäki V, Nishitani N, Hari R. Brush stimulator for functional brain imaging. *Clin Neurophysiol.* 2007;118:2620–2624.
47. Piitulainen H, Bourguignon M, Hari R, Jousmäki V. MEG-compatible pneumatic stimulator to elicit passive finger and toe movements. *Neuroimage.* 2015;112:310–317.
48. Hirvenkari L, Jousmäki V, Lamminmäki S, Saarinen VM, Sams ME, Hari R. Gaze-direction-based MEG averaging during audiovisual speech perception. *Front Hum Neurosci.* 2010;4:17.
49. Ramkumar P, Jas M, Pannasch S, Hari R, Parkkonen L. Feature-specific information processing precedes concerted activation in human visual cortex. *J Neurosci.* 2013;33:7691–7699.
50. Salmelin R, Hari R. Spatiotemporal characteristics of sensorimotor neuromagnetic rhythms related to thumb movement. *Neurosci.* 1994;60:537–550.
51. Barth DS, Sutherling W, Beatty J. Fast and slow magnetic phenomena in focal epileptic seizures. *Science.* 1984;226:855–857.
52. Salmelin R, Hari R. Characterization of spontaneous MEG rhythms in healthy adults. *Electroenceph Clin Neurophysiol.* 1994;91:237–248.
53. Tuladhar AM, ter Huurne N, Schoffelen JM, Maris E, Oostenveld R, Jensen O. Parieto-occipital sources account for the increase in alpha activity with working memory load. *Hum Brain Mapp.* 2007;28:785–792.
54. Tiihonen J, Kajola M, Hari R. Magnetic mu rhythm in man. *Neuroscience.* 1989;32:793–800.
55. Caetano G, Jousmäki V, Hari R. Actor's and observer's primary motor cortices stabilize similarly after seen or heard motor actions. *Proc Natl Acad Sci USA.* 2007;104:9058–9062.
56. Cheyne DO. MEG studies of sensorimotor rhythms: a review. *Exp Neurol.* 2013;245:27–39.
57. Gastaut H. Etude électrocorticographique de la réactivité des rythmes rolandiques. *Rev Neurologique.* 1952;87:176–182.
58. Salenius S, Schnitzler A, Salmelin R, Jousmäki V, Hari R. Modulation of human cortical rolandic rhythms during natural sensorimotor tasks. *Neuroimage.* 1997;5:221–228.
59. Schnitzler A, Salenius S, Salmelin R, Jousmäki V, Hari R. Involvement of primary motor cortex in motor imagery: a neuromagnetic study. *Neuroimage.* 1997;6:201–208.
60. Hari R, Forss N, Avikainen S, Kirveskari E, Salenius S, Rizzolatti G. Activation of human primary motor cortex during action observation: A neuromagnetic study. *Proc Natl Acad Sci USA.* 1998;95:15061–15065.
61. Salmelin R, Hämäläinen M, Kajola M, Hari R. Functional segregation of movement-related rhythmic activity in the human brain. *Neuroimage.* 1995;2:237–243.
62. Conway BA, Halliday DM, Farmer SF, et al. Synchronization between motor cortex and spinal motoneuronal pool during the performance of a maintained motor task in man. *J Physiol.* 1995;489 917–924.
63. Salenius S, Portin K, Kajola M, Salmelin R, Hari R. Cortical control of human motoneuron firing during isometric contraction. *J Neurophysiol.* 1997;77:3401–3405.
64. Salenius S, Salmelin R, Neuper C, Pfurtscheller G, Hari R. Human cortical 40-Hz rhythm is closely related to EMG rhythmicity. *Neurosci Lett.* 1996;21:75–78.
65. Hari R, Salenius S. Rhythmical corticomotor communication. *Neuroreport.* 1999;10:R1–R10.

66. Salenius S, Hari R. Synchronous cortical oscillatory activity during motor action. *Curr Opin Neurobiol.* 2003;13:678–684.
67. Mima T, Hallett M. Corticomuscular coherence: a review. *J Clin Neurophysiol.* 1999;16:501–511.
68. Ohara S, Mima T, Baba K, et al. Increased synchronization of cortical oscillatory activities between human supplementary motor and primary sensorimotor areas during voluntary movements. *J Neurosci.* 2001;21:9377–9386.
69. Kilner JM, Baker SN, Salenius S, Hari R, Lemon RN. Human cortical muscle coherence is directly related to specific motor parameters. *J Neurosci.* 2000;20:8838–8845.
70. Kilner JM, Salenius S, Baker SN, Jackson A, Hari R, Lemon RN. Task-dependent modulations of cortical oscillatory activity in human subjects during a bimanual precision grip task. *Neuroimage.* 2003;18:67–73.
71. Brown P, Salenius S, Rothwell JC, Hari R. The cortical correlate of the Piper rhythm in man. *J Neurophysiol.* 1998;80:2911–2917.
72. Salenius S, Avikainen S, Kaakkola S, Hari R, Brown P. Defective cortical drive to muscle in Parkinson's disease and its improvement with levodopa. *Brain.* 2002;125:491–500.
73. Brown P, Marsden J, Defebvre L, et al. Intermuscular coherence in Parkinson's disease: relationship to bradykinesia. *Neuroreport.* 2001;12:2577–2581.
74. Gross J, Timmermann L, Kujala J, et al. The neural basis of intermittent motor control in humans. *Proc Natl Acad Sci USA.* 2002;99:2299–2302.
75. Lehtelä L, Salmelin R, Hari R. Evidence for reactive magnetic 10-Hz rhythm in the human auditory cortex. *Neurosci Lett.* 1997;222:111–114.
76. Santamaria J, Chiappa K. The EEG of drowsiness in normal adults. *J Clin Neurophysiol.* 1987;4:327–382.
77. Lu S-T, Kajola M, Joutsiniemi S-L, Knuutila J, Hari R. Generator sites of spontaneous MEG activity during sleep. *Electroenceph Clin Neurophysiol.* 1992;82:182–196.
78. Niedermeyer E. The 'third rhythm': further observations. *Clin Electroencephalogr.* 1991;22:83–96.
79. Weisz N, Hartmann T, Müller N, Lorenz I, Obleser J. Alpha rhythms in audition: cognitive and clinical perspectives. *Front Psychol.* 2011;2:73.
80. Narici L, Forss N, Jousmäki V, Peresson M, Hari R. Evidence for a 7- to 9-Hz 'sigma' rhythm in the human SII cortex. *Neuroimage* 2001;13:662–668.
81. Sasaki K, Tsujimoto T, Nambu A, Matsuzaki R, Kyuhou S. Dynamic activities of the frontal association cortex in calculating and thinking. *Neurosci Res.* 1994;19:229–233.
82. Tallon-Baudry C, Bertrand O, Wienbruch C, Ross B, Pantev C. Combined EEG and MEG recordings of visual 40 Hz responses to illusory triangles in human. *Neuroreport.* 1997;8:1103–1107.
83. Wyart V, Tallon-Baudry C. How ongoing fluctuations in human visual cortex predict perceptual awareness: baseline shift versus decision bias. *J Neurosci.* 2009;29:8715–8725.
84. Lisman JE, Jensen O. The theta-gamma neural code. *Neuron.* 2013;77:1002–1016.
85. Marzetti L, Della Penna S, Snyder AZ, et al. Frequency specific interactions of MEG resting state activity within and across brain networks as revealed by the multivariate interaction measure. *Neuroimage.* 2013;79:172–183.
86. Cash SS, Halgren E, Dehghani N, et al. The human K-complex represents an isolated cortical down-state. *Science.* 2009;324:1084–1087.
87. Niedermeyer E. Depth electroencephalography. In: Niedermeyer E, Lopes da Silva F, eds. *Electroencephalography. Basic Principles, Clinical Applications and Related Fields.* Baltimore/Munich: Urban & Schwarzenberg, 1982:519–536.
88. Scheuler W, Kubicki S, Scholz G, Marquardt J. Two different activities in the sleep spindle frequency band—discrimination based on the topographical distribution of spectral power and coherence. In: Horne J, ed. *Sleep '90.* Bochum: Pontenagel Press, 1990:13–16.
89. Barth D, Sutherling W, Engel JJ, Beatty J. Neuromagnetic localization of epileptiform spike activity in the human brain. *Science.* 1982;218:891–894.
90. Modena I, Ricci GB, Barbanera S, Leoni R, Romani GL, Carelli P. Biomagnetic measurements of spontaneous brain activity in epileptic patients. *Electroenceph Clin Neurophysiol.* 1982;54:622–628.
91. Bagic A. Look back to leap forward: The emerging new role of magnetoencephalography (MEG) in nonlesional epilepsy. *Clin Neurophysiol.* 2015.
92. Hari R, Ahonen A, Forss N, et al. Parietal epileptic mirror focus detected with a whole-head neuromagnetometer. *Neuroreport.* 1993;5:45–48.
93. Paetau R, Kajola M, Korkman M, Hämäläinen M, Granström M, Hari R. Landau-Kleffner syndrome: epileptic activity in the auditory cortex. *Neuroreport.* 1991;2:201–204.
94. Paetau R. Magnetoencephalography in Landau-Kleffner syndrome. *Epilepsia.* 2009;50(Suppl. 7):51–54.
95. Laaksonen K, Helle L, Parkkonen L, et al. Alterations in spontaneous brain oscillations during stroke recovery. *PLoS One.* 2013;8:e61146.

96. Volkmann J, Joliot M, Mogilner A, et al. Central motor loop oscillations in parkinsonian resting tremor revealed by magnetoencephalography. *Neurology.* 1996;46:1359–1370.
97. Piitulainen H, Bourguignon M, De Tiege X, Hari R, Jousmäki V. Corticokinematic coherence during active and passive finger movements. *Neuroscience.* 2013;238:361–370.
98. Timmermann L, Gross J, Dirks M, Volkmann J, Freund HJ, Schnitzler A. The cerebral oscillatory network of parkinsonian resting tremor. *Brain.* 2003;126:199–212.
99. Butz M, Timmermann L, Gross J, et al. Cortical activation associated with asterixis in manifest hepatic encephalopathy. *Acta Neurol Scand.* 2014;130:260–267.
100. Hari R. Magnetoencephalography: Methods and applications. In: Schomer DL, Lopes da Silva FH, eds. *Niedermeyer's Electroencephalography: Basic Principles, Clinical Applications, and Related Fields.* 6th ed. Philadelphia: Lippincott Williams & Wilkins, 2011:865–900.
101. Elberling C, Bak C, Kofoed B, Lebech J, Saermark K. Magnetic auditory responses from the human brain. A preliminary report. *Scand Audiol.* 1980;9:185–190.
102. Hari R, Aittoniemi K, Järvinen ML, Katila T, Varpula T. Auditory evoked transient and sustained magnetic fields of the human brain. Localization of neural generators. *Exp Brain Res.* 1980;40:237–240.
103. Kuriki S, Nogai T, Hirata Y. Cortical sources of middle latency responses of auditory evoked magnetic field. *Hear Res.* 1995;92:47–51.
104. Hari R, Pelizzone M, Mäkelä JP, Hällström J, Leinonen L, Lounasmaa OV. Neuromagnetic responses of the human auditory cortex to on- and offsets of noise bursts. *Audiology.* 1987;25:31–43.
105. Hari R, Kaila K, Katila T, Tuomisto T, Varpula T. Interstimulus-interval dependence of the auditory vertex response and its magnetic counterpart: Implications for their neural generation. *Electroenceph Clin Neurophysiol.* 1982;54:561–569.
106. Lu Z-L, Williamson S, Kaufman L. Behavioral lifetime of human auditory sensory memory predicted by physiological measures. *Science.* 1992;258:1668–1670.
107. Mäkelä JP, Ahonen A, Hämäläinen M, et al. Functional differences between auditory cortices of the two hemispheres revealed by whole-head neuromagnetic recordings. *Hum Brain Mapp.* 1993;1:48–56.
108. Näätänen R, Picton T. The N1 wave of the human electric and magnetic response to sound: a review and analysis of the component structure. *Psychophysiology.* 1987;24:375–425.
109. Alho K. Cerebral generators of mismatch negativity (MMN) and its magnetic counterpart (MMNm) elicited by sound changes. *Ear Hear.* 1995;16:38–51.
110. Näätänen R. Mismatch negativity: clinical research and possible applications. *Int J Psychophysiol.* 2003;48:179–188.
111. Auksztulewicz R, Friston K. Attentional enhancement of auditory mismatch responses: a DCM/MEG study. *Cereb Cortex.* 2015;25:4273–4383.
112. Sams M, Hari R, Rif J, Knuutila J. The human auditory sensory memory trace persists about 10 s: neuromagnetic evidence. *J Cogn Neurosci.* 1993;5:363–370.
113. Romani GL, Williamson SJ, Kaufman L. Tonotopic organization of the human auditory cortex. *Science.* 1982;216:1339–1340.
114. Galambos R, Makeig S, Talmachoff PJ. A 40-Hz auditory potential recorded from the human scalp. *Proc NY Acad Sci.* 1981;78:2643–2647.
115. Mäkelä J, Hari R. Evidence for cortical origin of the 40-Hz auditory evoked response in man. *Electroenceph Clin Neurophysiol.* 1987;66:539–546.
116. Hari R, Hämäläinen M, Joutsiniemi SL. Neuromagnetic steady-state responses to auditory stimuli. *J Acoust Soc Am.* 1989;86:1033–1039.
117. Gutschalk A, Mase R, Roth R, et al. Deconvolution of 40 Hz steady-state fields reveals two overlapping source activities of the human auditory cortex. *Clin Neurophysiol.* 1999;110:856–868.
118. Fujiki N, Jousmäki V, Hari R. Neuromagnetic responses to frequency-tagged sounds: A new method to follow inputs from each ear to the human auditory cortex during binaural hearing. *J Neurosci.* 2002;22:RC205(201–204).
119. Kaneko K-I, Fujiki N, Hari R. Binaural interaction in the human auditory cortex revealed by neuromagnetic frequency tagging: no effect of stimulus intensity. *Hear Res.* 2003;183:1–6.
120. Lamminmäki S, Mandel A, Parkkonen L, Hari R. Binaural interaction and the octave illusion. *J Acoust Soc Am.* 2012;132:1747–1753.
121. Ahveninen J, Hämäläinen M, Jääskeläinen IP, et al. Attention-driven auditory cortex short-term plasticity helps segregate relevant sounds from noise. *Proc Natl Acad Sci USA.* 2011;108:4182–4187.
122. Curio G, Mackert BM, Burghoff M, Koetitz R, Abraham-Fuchs K, Harer W. Localization of evoked neuromagnetic 600 Hz activity in the cerebral somatosensory system. *Electroencephalogr Clin Neurophysiol.* 1994;91:483–487.
123. Hari R, Nagamine T, Nishitani N, et al. Time-varying activation of different cytoarchitectonic areas of the human SI cortex after tibial nerve stimulation. *Neuroimage.* 1996;4:111–118.
124. Hashimoto I, Sakuma K, Kimura T, Iguchi Y, Sekihara K. Serial activation of distinct cytoarchitectonic areas of the human S1 cortex after posterior tibial nerve stimulation. *Neuroreport.* 2001;12:1857–1862.
125. Hari R, Imada T. Ipsilateral movement-evoked fields reconsidered. *Neuroimage.* 1999;10:582–588.
126. Lauronen L, Nevalainen P, Wikström H, Parkkonen L, Okada Y, Pihko E. Immaturity of somatosensory cortical processing in human newborns. *Neuroimage.* 2006;33:195–203.
127. Elbert T, Pantev C, Wienbruch C, Rockstroh B, Taub E. Increased cortical representation of the fingers of the left hand in string players. *Science.* 1995;270:305–307.
128. Hari R, Hämäläinen M, Kaukoranta E, Reinikainen K, Teszner D. Neuromagnetic responses from the second somatosensory cortex in man. *Acta Neurol Scand.* 1983;68:207–212.
129. Hari R, Hämäläinen H, Tiihonen J, Kekoni J, Sams M, Hämäläinen M. Separate finger representations at the human second somatosensory cortex. *Neuroscience.* 1990;37:245–249.
130. Kaukoranta E, Hari R, Hämäläinen M, Huttunen J. Cerebral magnetic fields evoked by peroneal nerve stimulation. *Somatosens Res.* 1986;3:309–321.
131. Forss N, Hietanen M, Salonen O, Hari R. Modified activation of somatosensory cortical network in patients with right-hemisphere stroke. *Brain.* 1999;122:1889–1899.
132. Simoes C, Jensen O, Parkkonen L, Hari R. Phase locking between human primary and secondary somatosensory cortices. *Proc Natl Acad Sci USA.* 2003;100:2691–2694.
133. Forss N, Silén T, Karjalainen T. Lack of activation of human secondary somatosensory cortex in Unverricht-Lundborg type of progressive myoclonus epilepsy. *Ann Neurol.* 2001;49:90–97.
134. Bourguignon M, Whitmarsh S, Piitulainen H, Hari R, Jousmäki V, Lundqvist D. Reliable recording and analysis of MEG-based corticokinematic coherence in the presence of strong magnetic artifacts. *Clin Neurophysiol.* 2016;127:1460–1469.
135. Smeds E, Piitulainen H, Bourguignon M, Jousmäki V, Hari R. Cortical recovery rates of proprioceptive responses to passive finger movements. 2016, submitted.
136. Hari R, Kaukoranta E, Reinikainen K, Huopaniemi T, Mauno J. Neuromagnetic localization of cortical activity evoked by painful dental stimulation in man. *Neurosci Lett.* 1983;42:77–82.
137. Huttunen J, Kobal G, Kaukoranta E, Hari R. Cortical responses to painful CO_2 stimulation of the nasal mucosa. *Electroenceph Clin Neurophysiol.* 1986;64:347–349.
138. Kakigi R, Koyama S, Hoshiyama M, Kitamura Y, Shomojo M, Watanabe S. Pain-related magnetic fields following painful CO_2 laser stimulation in man. *Neurosci Lett.* 1995;192:45–48.
139. Kakigi R, Tran TD, Qiu Y, et al. Cerebral responses following stimulation of unmyelinated C-fibers in humans: electro- and magneto-encephalographic study. *Neurosci Res.* 2003;45:255–275.
140. Ploner M, Freund HJ, Schnitzler A. Pain affect without pain sensation in a patient with a postcentral lesion. *Pain.* 1999;81:211–214.
141. Kanda M, Nagamine T, Ikeda A, et al. Primary somatosensory cortex is actively involved in pain processing in human. *Brain Res.* 2000;853:282–289.
142. Forss N, Raij TT, Seppä M, Hari R. Common cortical network for first and second pain. *Neuroimage.* 2005;24:132–142.
143. Bragard D, Chen AC, Plaghki L. Direct isolation of ultra-late (C-fibre) evoked brain potentials by CO_2 laser stimulation of tiny cutaneous surface areas in man. *Neurosci Lett.* 1996;209:81–84.
144. Motogi J, Kodaira M, Muragaki Y, Inui K, Kakigi R. Cortical responses to C-fiber stimulation by intra-epidermal electrical stimulation: an MEG study. *Neurosci Lett.* 2014;570:69–74.
145. Hari R, Forss N, Raij T. Neuromagnetic exploration of the connection between pain and the motor cortex. In: Kalso E, Estlander A-M, Klockars M, eds. *Psyche, Soma and Pain. Acta Gyllenbergiana IV.* Helsinki: The Signe and Ane Gyllenberg Foundation, 2003:145–153.
146. Raij TT, Forss N, Stancak A, Hari R. Modulation of motor-cortex oscillatory activity by painful A-delta- and C-fiber stimuli. *Neuroimage.* 2004;23:569–573.
147. Juottonen K, Gockel M, Silén T, Hurri H, Hari R, Forss N. Altered central sensorimotor processing in patients with complex regional pain syndrome. *Pain.* 2002;98:315–323.

148. Forss N, Kirveskari E, Gockel M. Mirror-like spread of chronic pain. *Neurology*. 2005;65:748–750.
149. Brenner D, Williamson SJ, Kaufman L. Visually evoked magnetic fields of the human brain. *Science*. 1975;190:480–481.
150. Teyler TJ, Cuffin BN, Cohen D. The visual magnetoencephalogram. *Life Sci*. 1975;17:683–692.
151. Ahlfors S, Ilmoniemi R, Hämäläinen M. Estimates of visually evoked cortical currents. *Electroenceph Clin Neurophysiol*. 1992;82:225–236.
152. Aine C, Supek S, George J, et al. Retinotopic organization of human visual cortex: Departures from the classical model. *Cereb Cortex*. 1996;6:354–361.
153. Portin K, Salenius S, Salmelin R, Hari R. Activation of the human occipital and parietal cortex by pattern and luminance stimuli: neuromagnetic measurements. *Cereb Cortex*. 1998;8:253–260.
154. Hari R, Salmelin R, Tissari S, Kajola M, Virsu V. Visual stability during eyeblinks. *Nature*. 1994;367:121–122.
155. Jousmäki V, Hämäläinen M, Hari R. Magnetic source imaging during a visually guided task. *Neuroreport*. 1996;7:2961–2964.
156. ffytche DH, Guy CN, Zeki S. The parallel visual motion inputs into areas V1 and V5 of human cerebral cortex. *Brain*. 1995;118:1375–1394.
157. Anderson SJ, Holliday IE, Singh KD, Harding GF. Localization and functional analysis of human cortical area V5 using magneto-encephalography. *Proc Biol Sci*. 1996;263:423–431.
158. Uusitalo M, Jousmäki V, Hari R. Activation trace lifetime of human cortical responses evoked by apparent visual motion. *Neurosci Lett*. 1997;224:45–48.
159. Vanni S, Tanskanen T, Seppä M, Uutela K, Hari R. Coinciding early activation of the human primary visual cortex and anteromedial cuneus. *Proc Natl Acad Sci USA*. 2001;98:2776–2780.
160. Prieto EA, Barnikol UB, Soler EP, et al. Timing of V1/V2 and V5+ activations during coherent motion of dots: an MEG study. *Neuroimage*. 2007;37:1384–1395.
161. Schmolesky MT, Wang Y, Hanes DP, et al. Signal timing across the macaque visual system. *J Neurophysiol*. 1998;79:3272–3278.
162. Parkkonen L, Andersson J, Hämäläinen M, Hari R. Early visual brain areas reflect the percept of an ambiguous scene. *Proc Natl Acad Sci USA*. 2008;105:20500–20504.
163. Halgren E, Raij T, Marinkovic K, Jousmäki V, Hari R. Cognitive response profile of the human fusiform face area as determined by MEG. *Cereb Cortex*. 2000;10:69–81.
164. Mandel A, Helokunnas S, Pihko E, Hari R. Brain responds to another person's eye blinks in a natural setting—the more empathetic the viewer the stronger the responses. *Eur J Neurosci*. 2015;42:2508–2514.
165. Salmelin R, Hari R, Lounasmaa OV, Sams M. Dynamics of brain activation during picture naming. *Nature*. 1994;368:463–465.
166. Salmelin R. MEG and reading: from perception to linguistic analysis In: Hansen PC, Kringelbach ML, Salmelin RM, eds. *An Introduction to Methods*. New York: Oxford University Press, 2010:346–372.
167. Salmelin R, Kujala J. Neural representation of language: activation versus long-range connectivity. *Trends Cogn Sci*. 2006;10:519–525.
168. Kuhl PK. Early language learning and the social brain. *Cold Spring Harb Symp Quant Biol*. 2014;79:211–220.
169. Giraud AL, Poeppel D. Cortical oscillations and speech processing: emerging computational principles and operations. *Nat Neurosci*. 2012;15:511–517.
170. Ding N, Melloni L, Zhang H, Tian X, Poeppel D. Cortical tracking of hierarchical linguistic structures in connected speech. *Nat Neurosci*. 2016;19:158–164.
171. Koskinen M, Viinikanoja J, Kurimo M, Klami A, Kaski S, Hari R. Identifying fragments of natural speech from the listener's MEG signals. *Hum Brain Mapp*. 2013;34:1477–1489.
172. Papanicolaou AC, Rezaie R, Narayana S, et al. Is it time to replace the Wada test and put awake craniotomy to sleep? *Epilepsia*. 2014;55:629–632.
173. Rizzolatti G, Fadiga L, Gallese V, Fogassi L. Premotor cortex and recognition of motor actions. *Cogn Brain Res*. 1996;3:131–141.
174. Nishitani N, Hari R. Temporal dynamics of cortical representation for action. *Proc Natl Acad Sci USA*. 2000;97:913–918.
175. Nishitani N, Hari R. Viewing lip forms: cortical dynamics. *Neuron*. 2002;36:1211–1220.
176. Avikainen S, Forss N, Hari R. Modulated activation of the human SI and SII cortices during observation of hand actions. *Neuroimage*. 2002;15:640–646.
177. Rizzolatti G, Sinigaglia C. The functional role of the parieto-frontal mirror circuit: interpretations and misinterpretations. *Nat Rev Neurosci*. 2010;11:264–274.
178. Hari R. Magnetoencephalography studies of action observation. In: Ferrari PF, Rizzolatti G, eds. *New Frontiers in Mirror Neurons Research*. New York: Oxford University Press, 2015:58–70.
179. Hari R, Henriksson L, Malinen S, Parkkonen L. Centrality of social interaction in human brain function. *Neuron*. 2015;88:181–193.
180. Hari R, Sams M, Nummenmaa L. Attending and neglecting people: Bridging neuroscience, psychology and sociology. *Phil Trans Royal Soc B*. 2016;371:1693.
181. Hari R, Kujala MV. Brain basis of human social interaction: from concepts to brain imaging. *Physiol Rev*. 2009;89:453–479.
182. Levinson SC. Turn-taking in human communication—Origins and implications for language processing. *Trends Cogn Sci*. 2016;20:6–14.
183. Baess P, Zhdanov A, Mandel A, et al. MEG dual scanning: a procedure to study real-time auditory interaction between two persons. *Front Hum Neurosci*. 2012;6:83.
184. Zhdanov A, Nurminen J, Baess P, et al. An Internet-based real-time audiovisual link for dual MEG recordings. *PLoS One*. 2015;10:e0128485.
185. Hirata M, Ikeda T, Kikuchi M, et al. Hyperscanning MEG for understanding mother–child cerebral interactions. *Front Hum Neurosci*. 2014;8:118.
186. Babiloni F, Astolfi L. Social neuroscience and hyperscanning techniques: past, present and future. *Neurosci Biobehav Rev*. 2014;44:76–93.
187. Zhou G, Bourguignon M, Parkkonen L, Hari R. Neural signatures of hand kinematics in leaders vs. followers: A dual-MEG study. *Neuroimage*. 2016;125:731–738.
188. Nevalainen P, Lauronen L, Pihko E. Development of human somatosensory cortical functions—What have we learned from magnetoencephalography. *Front Hum Neurosci*. 2014;8:158.
189. Öisjöen F, Schneiderman JF, Figueras GA, et al. High-T_c superconducting quantum interference device recordings of spontaneous brain activity: Towards high-T_c magnetoencephalography. *App Phys Lett*. 2012;100:132601–132604.
190. Kominis IK, Kornack TW, Allred JC, Romalis MV. A subfemtotesla multichannel atomic magnetometer. *Nature*. 2003;422:596–569.
191. Sander TH, Preusser J, Mhaskar R, Kitching J, Trahms L, Knappe S. Magnetoencephalography with a chip-scale atomic magnetometer. *Biomed Opt Express*. 2012;3:981–990.
192. Pannetier M, Fermon C, Le Goff G, Simola J, Kerr E. Femtotesla magnetic field measurement with magnetoresistive sensors. *Science*. 2004;304:1648–1650.
193. Kauppi JP, Parkkonen L, Hari R, Hyvärinen A. Decoding magnetoencephalographic rhythmic activity using spectrospatial information. *Neuroimage*. 2013;83:921–936.
194. Cichy RM, Ramirez FM, Pantazis D. Can visual information encoded in cortical columns be decoded from magnetoencephalography data in humans? *Neuroimage*. 2015;121:193–204.
195. Stokes MG, Wolff MJ, Spaak E. Decoding rich spatial information with high temporal resolution. *Trends Cogn Sci*. 2015;19:636–638.
196. Lankinen K, Saari J, Hari R, Koskinen M. Intersubject consistency of cortical MEG signals during movie viewing. *Neuroimage*. 2014;92:217–224.
197. Vesanen PT, Nieminen JO, Zevenhoven KC, et al. Hybrid ultra-low-field MRI and magnetoencephalography system based on a commercial whole-head neuromagnetometer. *Magn Res Med*. 2013;69:1795–1804.

36 | POLYSOMNOGRAPHY: TECHNICAL AND CLINICAL ASPECTS

SUDHANSU CHOKROVERTY, MD AND ROBERTO VETRUGNO, MD

ABSTRACT: This chapter covers the technical and clinical aspects of poly-somnography (PSG). Section 1 includes a brief review of the historical mile-stones, functional neuroanatomy of sleep, physiological changes (emphasizing those pertinent to overnight PSG interpretation) and clinical relevance as well as homeostatic and circadian factors, and functions of sleep. Section 2 deals with laboratory procedures, including PSG recording and scoring techniques, indications for PSG, video-PSG, ambulatory and computerized PSG, artifacts during PSG recording, and pitfalls of PSG. Section 3 includes clinical consid-erations, briefly describing the clinical presentation, diagnosis, and treatment but mainly focusing on PSG findings in common sleep disorders as well as sleep-related movement disorders, neurological disorders, and sleep-related epilepsies. Section 4 addresses related laboratory procedures for the assess-ment of sleep, including the multiple sleep latency test, the maintenance-of-wakefulness test, and actigraphy.

KEYWORDS: polysomnography, PSG, sleep, sleep disorders, epilepsy, actigraphy

PRINCIPAL REFERENCES

1. Rechtschaffen K, Kales A. *A Manual of Standardized Terminology, Techniques and Scoring System for Sleep Stages of Human Subjects.* Washington DC: US Government Printing Office, 1968.
2. Saper CB, Scammell TE, Lu J. Hypothalamic regulation of sleep and circa-dian rhythms. *Nature.* 2005;437:1257–1263.
3. McCarley RW. Neurobiology of REM and NREM sleep. *Sleep Med.* 2007;8:302–330.
4. Lu J, Sherman D, Devor M, et al. A putative flip-flop switch for control of REM sleep. *Nature.* 2006;441:589.
5. Luppi PH, Clement O, Sapin E, et al. The neuronal network responsible for paradoxical sleep and its dysfunctions causing narcolepsy and rapid eye movement (REM) behavior disorder. *Sleep Med Rev.* 2011;15:153–163.
6. Luppi P-H, Clement O, Fort P. Paradoxical (REM) sleep genesis by the brainstem is under hypothalamic control. *Curr Opin Neurobiol.* 2013; 23:786–792.
7. Chen MC, Yu H, Huang Z-L, Lu J. Rapid eye movement sleep behavior disorder. *Curr Opin Neurobiol.* 2013; 23: 793–798.
8. Chokroverty S. Physiological changes in sleep. In: Chokroverty S, ed. *Sleep Disorders Medicine: Basic Science, Technical Considerations and Clinical Aspects.* 4th ed. New York: Springer 2017.
9. Scammell TE. Narcolepsy. *N Engl J Med.* 2015; 373:2654–2662.
10. American Academy of Sleep Medicine. *International Classification of Sleep Disorders.* 3rd ed. Darien, IL: American Academy of Sleep Medicine, 2014.

Polysomnography (PSG) is the single most important labora-tory technique for assessment of sleep and its disorders. PSG consists of recordings of multiple physiological characteris-tics during sleep, whereas polygraphy indicates the record-ing of similar characteristics at any time during the day. An understanding of the importance of the laboratory evaluation of sleep and its disorders has been evolving slowly, but in the last century great advances have been made in this direction.

The discoveries of the human electroencephalogram (EEG) by Berger (1) in 1929 and rapid eye movements (REMs) during sleep by Aserinsky and Kleitman (2) in 1953 are the real driv-ing forces behind this understanding. In 1974, Holland et al. (3), during a presentation at the 14th annual meeting of the Association of the Psychophysiological Study of Sleep (aka the American Sleep Disorders Association and now the American Academy of Sleep Medicine [AASM]), coined the term PSG.

This chapter is divided into four sections: (1) histori-cal milestones and basic science; (2) laboratory techniques, addressing mainly PSG and video-PSG recordings and their indications; (3) clinical considerations focusing on PSG find-ings; and (4) related laboratory procedures.

1. HISTORICAL MILESTONES AND FUNCTIONAL NEUROANATOMY AND PHYSIOLOGY OF SLEEP

In 1875, Richard Caton (4), an English neurophysiologist, first recorded electrical activities from rabbit and monkey brains. It was, however, Hans Berger (1), an Austrian psychiatrist, who in 1924 first obtained electrical activities from the surface of a 17-year-old young man with a skull defect and published his findings in 1929. Although sleep was known since antiquity, brain activities in sleep could not have been recorded before the discovery of EEG. It was in 1937 that Loomis et al. clas-sified sleep into five stages (A–E) based on the EEG activities during the deepening stages of sleep (5). It is notable to note that Kohlschutter (6,7), a 19th-century German physiolo-gist, thought that sleep was deepest in the first few hours and became lighter as time went on. This is reminiscent of mod-ern concept of stage N3 (deep sleep) predominating in the first third of the night. He also described the varying arousal thresh-olds throughout the night. The REMs of sleep were not known in those days. In 1953, Aserinsky and Kleitman (2) obtained characteristic REMs during sleep using surface electrodes over the eyelids. Over a 4-year period, Loomis et al. (5) published 12 papers, describing the oscillating nature of EEG along with five distinct stages of sleep as well as arousals manifested by increased body movements and respiratory effort. In 1957, Dement and Kleitman (8) described sleep evolving through non-rapid eye movement (NREM) and REM sleep states in a cyclic manner throughout the night. All the components of REM sleep, however, were not described until Jouvet and

Michel (9) in 1959 observed clearly decreased muscle tone during REM sleep in cats. In 1961, Berger (10) recorded markedly decreased muscle tone from extrinsic laryngeal muscles during human REM sleep.

To standardize the scoring of different stages of sleep, an ad hoc committee led by Rechtschaffen and Kales (11) in 1968 produced the now-famous sleep scoring technical manual (*The R–K Scoring Technique*). This remained the "gold standard" until the AASM published the *AASM Manual for the Scoring of Sleep and Associated Events* (12), which modified the R and K technique and extended the scoring rules. The R and K sleep scoring manual (11) was devised only for normal sleeping adults, but later an infant sleep scoring manual was developed. The R and K sleep scoring technique is based on three physiological characteristics: EEG, electro-oculography (EOG), and electromyography (EMG). PSG, however, includes more than just sleep staging: other physiological characteristics such as respiration, limb muscle activity, blood oxygen saturation, electrocardiogram (ECG), body position, snoring, and other special recordings have been incorporated, which are described later in this chapter.

Since the discovery of REM sleep, dreaming was thought to be associated with REM sleep during 80% of the time. In 1868 Griesinger (13) suggested that dreaming was associated with eye movements, and in 1895, Freud (14) indicated that dreaming was associated with relaxation of the major muscles of the body. Amazingly, centuries ago (ca. 1000 BC), the *Upanishads* (15), the ancient Indian scriptures of Hinduism, sought to divide human existence into four states: the waking, the dreaming, the deep dreamless sleep, and the superconscious ("the very self"). This is reminiscent of the modern classification of three states of existence.

1.1. Functional Neuroanatomy of Sleep

The control of sleep is quite complex. Whereas for the most part during the whole sleep period we are in an unconscious state, changes occur that are physiologically quite distinct. During slow-wave sleep, the cortical neurons fire in relative synchrony; slow-wave sleep is so named after the polygraphic pattern of this brain activity. During REM sleep, the eyes show phasic, rapid conjugate movements, whereas at the same time skeletal muscle tone is at its lowest levels. Brain activity during REM sleep is rapid and desynchronous, almost like waking, which is why it is also referred to as "paradoxical sleep."

1.2. Anatomical Substrates for Wakefulness

There are two major branches to the ascending arousal or reticular activating system (ARAS) (16), which determine the states of wakefulness. One is an ascending pathway from pedunculopontine (PPT) and laterodorsal tegmental (LDT) nuclei to the reticular nucleus and thalamic relay nuclei in the thalamus. These thalamic relay neurons transmit signals to the cortex. Pedunculopontine and laterodorsal tegmental neurons fire most rapidly during REM and wakefulness, and are at their most inactive state during NREM.

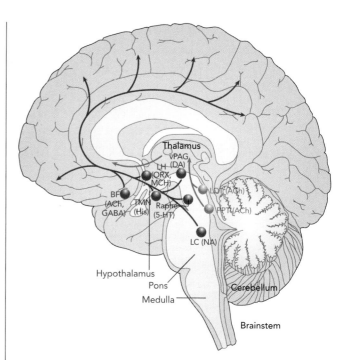

Figure 36.1. *The ascending arousal system. Two major pathways are shown. One, shown in yellow, provides upper brainstem input to the thalamic-relay nuclei and to the reticular nucleus of the thalamus coming from the pedunculopontine and laterodorsal tegmental (PPT/LDT) nuclei. This is an acetylcholine (ACh)-producing neuronal group. The second major group of neurons, shown in red, come from the noradrenergic (NA) locus coeruleus (LC), serotoninergic (5-HT) dorsal and median raphe nuclei, dopaminergic (DA) periaqueductal gray matter (vPAG), and histaminergic (His) tuberomamillary neurons (TMN). Additional cortical input merges from the basal forebrain (BF) neurons containing GABA or ACh, and by lateral hypothalamic (LH) peptidergic neurons that contain melanin-concentrating hormone (MCH) or orexin (hypocretin) (ORX). Reproduced from Saper CB, Scammell TE, Lu J. Hypothalamic regulation of sleep and circadian rhythms. Nature. 2005;437:1257–1263, with permission.*

The second branch of the ARAS comes from locus coeruleus (LC), dorsal and median raphe nuclei, periaqueductal gray matter, and tuberomammillary neurons. Cortical input goes through lateral hypothalamic neurons and basal forebrain neurons. The neuron groups in the two branches of the ARAS are shown in Figure 36.1 along with their respective neurotransmitters. The hypocretin (orexin) peptidergic system (17, 18) located in the lateral hypothalamic and perifornical regions, with its widespread ascending and descending projections, is thought to play an important role in the control of arousal and wakefulness (Fig. 36.2). A reduction of activities of the hypocretin projections to the LC, midline raphe, mesopontine, and posterior hypothalamic and tuberomedullary regions will cause sleepiness.

1.3. REM-Generating Neurons

The existence of REM sleep-generating neurons in the pons has been proved by transection experiments in cats through different regions of the midbrain, pons, and medulla (19) (Fig. 36.3). A transection of the pontomesencephalic (see Fig. 36.3A) and pontomedullary (see Fig. 36.3B) junctions produced an isolated pons that shows all the signs of REM sleep.

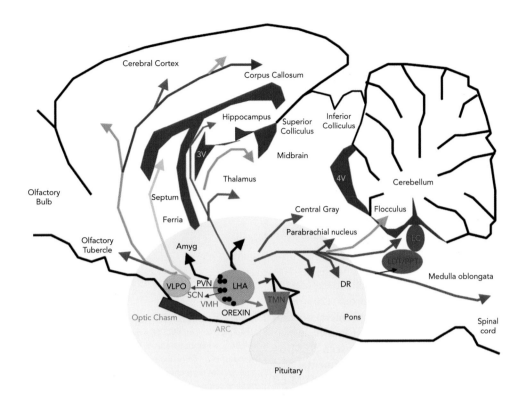

Figure 36.2. Widespread ascending and descending hypocretin (orexin) projections throughout the central nervous systems (CNS) shown schematically.

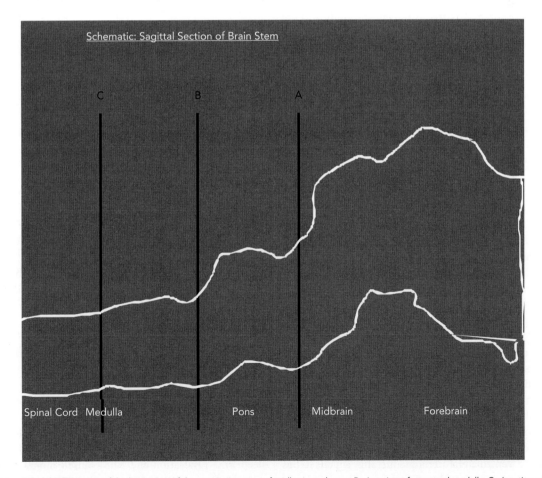

Figure 36.3. Schematic sagittal section of the brainstem of the cat. *A, Junction of midbrain and pons. B, Junction of pons and medulla. C, Junction of medulla and spinal cord. Reproduced from Chokroverty S. Sleep Disorders Medicine: Basic Science, Technical Considerations and Clinical Aspects. 3rd ed. Philadelphia: Saunders/Elsevier; 2009, with permission.*

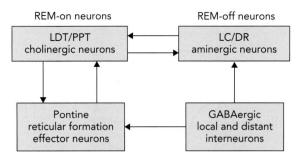

Figure 36.4. Schematic diagram of McCarley-Hobson model of REM sleep mechanism. GABA, γ-aminobutyric acid; LC/DR, locus coeruleus/dorsal raphe; LDT/PPT, laterodorsal tegmental/pedunculopontine tegmental nuclei. Modified from McCarley RW. Neurobiology of REM and NREM sleep. Sleep Med. 2007;8:302.

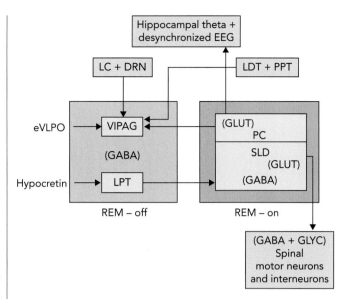

Figure 36.5. Lu-Saper "flip-flop" model shown schematically to explain REM sleep mechanism. eVLPO, extended region of ventrolateral preoptic nucleus; GABA, γ-aminobutyric acid; GLUT, glutamatergic neurons; GLYC, glycinergic neurons; LC + DRN, locus coeruleus + dorsal raphe nuclei; LDT + PPT, laterodorsal tegmental + pedunculopontine tegmental nuclei; LPT, lateral pontine tegmentum; PC, precoeruleus; SLD, sublaterodorsal nucleus; VlPAG, ventrolateral periaqueductal gray. Reproduced from Chokroverty S, ed. Sleep Disorders Medicine: Basic Science, Technical Considerations and Clinical Aspects. 3rd ed. Philadelphia: Elsevier/Saunders, 2009.

There are mainly three animal models available to explain the mechanism of REM sleep. McCarley–Hobson's (20) reciprocal interaction model based on reciprocal interactions of REM-on and REM-off neurons is the earliest known model. A reciprocal interaction in the brainstem between REM-on neurons (the cholinergic pedunculopontine tegmental and LDT nuclei in the pontomesencephalic region) and REM-off neurons (the aminergic LC and dorsal raphe [DR] nuclei) is responsible for REM generation and maintenance (Fig. 36.4). The role of gamma-aminobutyric acid (GABA) in REM sleep generation has been emphasized in the latest modification of the reciprocal interaction model by McCarley (20). Lu et al. (21) described a "flip-flop" switch interaction model in rats (Fig. 36.5) between GABAergic REM-off neurons in the deep mesencephalon, ventral periaqueductal gray, and lateral pontine tegmentum, and GABAergic REM-on neurons in the sublaterodorsal (SLD) nucleus (equivalent to perilocus coeruleus alpha in the cat) and the dorsal extension of the SLD named precoeruleus to explain REM sleep mechanism. Ascending glutamatergic projections from precoeruleus neurons to the medial septum are responsible for the hippocampal EEG theta rhythm during REM sleep. Muscle atonia during REM sleep is related to descending glutamatergic projections from the ventral SLD directly to the spinal interneurons inhibiting spinal ventral horn cells by both glycinergic and GABAergic mechanisms. Cholinergic and aminergic neurons play a modulatory role in this model and are not part of the "flip-flop" switch.

The third model proposed by Luppi's group (22) is a refinement of the "flip-flop" switch model of Lu-Saper (21) [Figs. 36.6 and 36.6A]. In this model neurons active during REM sleep are identified in a small area in the dorsolateral pontine tegmentum called the SLD nucleus in rats (corresponding to the dorsal subceruleus nucleus in humans or peri-LC alpha region in cats). At the onset of REM sleep there is an activation of REM-on glutamatergic neurons from the SLD. During NREM sleep and wakefulness, these neurons in the SLD would be inhibited by tonic GABAergic input from GABAergic REM-off neurons located in the deep mesencephalic and pontine reticular nuclei, and ventrolateral periaqueductal gray (vlPAG) as well as by monoaminergic REM-off and lateral hypothalamic hypocretinergic neurons. Ascending dorsal SLD REM-on glutamatergic neurons can cause cortical activation through projections to thalamocortical neurons along with REM-on cholinergic and glutamatergic neurons from the LDT/PPT mesencephalic and pontine reticular nuclei, and basal forebrain regions. Descending ventral REM-on glutamatergic SLD neurons would cause muscle atonia through excitatory both direct and indirect projections via ventromedial medulla (VMM) to glycinergic and GABAergic premotor neurons in the magnocellularis and parvocellularis reticular nuclei in the medulla, causing hyperpolarization of the motor neurons of the spinal cord and brainstem. In the Luppi model, therefore, the glutamatergic neurons play a crucial role in REM generation. GABAergic neurons are responsible for inactivation of monoaminergic neurons during REM sleep, and cholinergic neurons do not play a crucial role in activating REM executive neurons in this model.

The essential similarities and differences between these two contemporary models (Lu-Saper and Luppi) can be summarized as follows. SLD in pons plays a critical role for REM generation in both models. In the Luppi model glutamatergic SLD neurons play a crucial role, proven by immunohistochemical study showing that 85% of c-fos-labeled SLD neurons during recovery hypersomnia after REM sleep deprivations in rats express the vesicular 2 glutamate (VGlut 2) transporter, a specific marker for glutamatergic neurons. In contrast, the Lu-Saper model postulates that GABAergic neurons in both REM-off and REM-on (SLD) regions play a critical role in activating dorsal and ventral glutamatergic pathways in the SLD for REM sleep EEG generation and REM muscle atonia. Both of these models recognize the importance of the glutamatergic system for REM muscle atonia and EEG desynchronization. The Luppi model initially suggested both a direct projection from

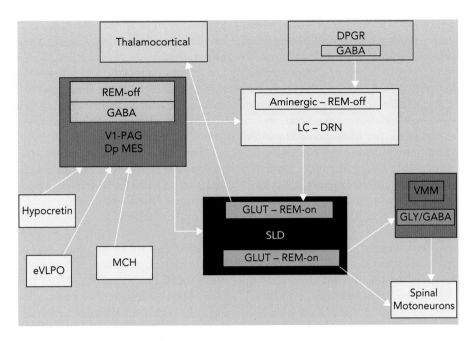

Figure 36.6. Luppi model schematically shown to explain mechanism of REM sleep generation. DPGR = dorsal paragigantocellular reticular nucleus; Dp-MES = deep mesencephalic; eVLPO = extended ventrolateral preoptic region; GABA = γ-aminobutyric acid; GLUT = glutamatergic; GLY = glycinergic neurons; LC-DRN = locus coeruleus–dorsal raphe nuclei; MCH =melanin concentrating hormone; VlPAG = ventrolateral periaqueductal gray; VMM ventromedial medulla.

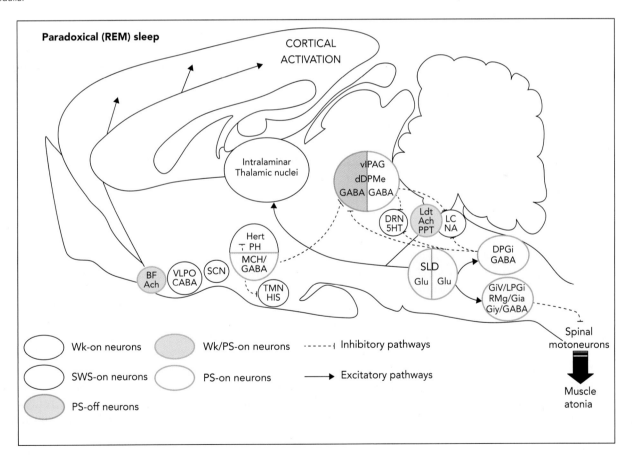

Figure 36.6A. Neuronal network responsible for REM sleep. PS = paradoxical (REM) sleep; BF = basal forebrain; Ach = acetylcholine; VLPO = ventrolateral preoptic nucleus; GABA = gamma aminobutyric acid; SCN = suprachiasmatic nucleus; Hcrt = hypocretinergic neurons; PH = posterior hypothalamus; MCH = melanin concentrating hormone-containing neurons; TMN = tuberomammillary nucleus; HIS = histamine; vlPAG = ventrolateral periaqueductal gray; dDPMe = deep mesencephalic reticular nucleus; DRN = dorsal raphe nucleus; 5HT = 5-hydroxtryptamine; Ldt = laterodorsal tegmental nucleus; PPT = pedunculopontine tegmental nucleus; LC = locus coeruleus; NA = noradrenaline; SLD = sublaterodorsal nucleus; Glu = glutamic acid; DPGi = dorsal paragigantocellular reticular nucleus; Giv = ventral gigantocellular nucleus; LPGi = lateral paragigantocellular reticular nucleus; Rmg = nucleus raphe magnus; Gia = alpha gigantocellular reticular nucleus; Gly = glycine. Reproduced with permission from reference 22a in the text.

SLD and an indirect projection to spinal cord via relay in the VMM. The latest report from this group (22a, 22b) suggested that muscle atonia during REM sleep is mediated mainly by an indirect projection to the VMM and to a minor extent by a direct projection to spinal cord. Saper's group (21) initially suggested a direct projection from SLD to spinal cord without a relay in the VMM. However, the latest report (22c) from this group suggested that REM atonia is mainly due to a direct projection from SLD to spinal cord, but may also be mediated by the VMM, which also sends glutamatergic projections to inhibitory spinal interneurons to inhibit spinal motor neurons. Thus these two models (Lu-Saper and Luppi) seem to be merging in finding a common ground to explain REM atonia.

The latest hypothesis from Luppi's group (22a) for REM sleep generation highlights the important role played by the lateral hypothalamus. This postulates that melanin concentrating hormone (MCH)/GABAergic neurons (REM-on) in the lateral hypothalamus constitute a master generator of REM sleep by a direct projection to the vlPAG region and deep mesencephalic reticular nucleus (inhibiting these REM-off GABAergic neurons) controlling REM sleep onset and maintenance.

1.4. Anatomical Substrates for NREM Sleep

NREM sleep-generating neurons are located primarily in the ventrolateral preoptic area (VLPO) and the median preoptic nucleus (MnPn) of the hypothalamus, the basal forebrain area, as well as the solitary nucleus region and the parafacial zone (PZ) of the medulla. The reticular nucleus of the thalamus is thought to be responsible for sleep spindle generation. Both passive and active mechanisms play a role in the generation of sleep. The contemporary theory (23) for the mechanism of NREM sleep suggests a reciprocal interaction between two antagonistic neurons in the VLPO and MnPn region of the anterior hypothalamus and wake-promoting neurons in the tuberomammillary nuclei of the posterior hypothalamus and the hypocretinergic neurons in the lateral hypothalamus, as well as the LC, DR nuclei, basal forebrain, and mesopontine tegmentum. The extended VLPO input to LC and DR is thought to be involved in regulating REM sleep. Reciprocal interaction between sleep-promoting neurons in the region of the solitary nucleus and Pz, and the wake-promoting neurons within the ARAS of the brainstem independent of the reciprocal interaction of the neurons of the forebrain, also plays a minor role in the generation of NREM sleep. It has been suggested that adenosine, a neuromodulator, may act as a physiological sleep factor modulating the somnogenic effects of prolonged wakefulness (24).

1.5. Physiological Changes During Sleep

A vast number of physiological changes take place during sleep in humans, affecting almost every system in the body (Table 36.1) (25). It is important to have a basic knowledge about these changes during sleep and how they affect various sleep disorders. These changes may be documented in PSG. A case in point is obstructive sleep apnea (OSA), which causes dramatic changes in the respiratory control of the upper airway muscles during sleep, directing our attention to a very important pathophysiological mechanism and the therapeutic intervention for this disorder. These physiological changes are most commonly noted in the respiratory, cardiovascular, gastrointestinal, and endocrine systems. Respiration is controlled by the automatic or metabolic and behavioral systems complemented by the third system known as the arousal system or the system for wakefulness stimulus. These respiratory systems receive inputs from various peripheral and central neural structures to maintain acid–base regulation and respiratory homeostasis. The location of the respiratory neurons makes them easily vulnerable to a variety of neurological disorders, particularly those involving the brainstem. Some conditions may affect control of breathing only during sleep, causing undesirable, often catastrophic, results such as cardiorespiratory failure or even sudden death. The two control systems (metabolic and voluntary) are active during wakefulness, but during NREM sleep, the voluntary system is inactive and respiration is entirely dependent upon the metabolic controller. The behavioral mechanism is probably responsible for controlling breathing, at least in part during REM sleep. Tidal volume and alveolar ventilation decrease during sleep. Arterial oxygen tension is slightly decreased and arterial carbon dioxide tension is increased during both NREM and REM sleep. Hypoxic ventilatory response is impaired in NREM sleep in adult men but not in women. Hypoxic ventilatory response during REM sleep is significantly decreased in both sexes. Hypercapnic ventilatory response is also decreased during NREM and further decreased during REM sleep. Thus, ventilation is unstable during sleep and a few periods of apneas may occur particularly at sleep onset and during REM sleep in normal individuals. Respiratory homeostasis is thus relatively unprotected during sleep, making those individuals with intrinsic respiratory disease, such as chronic obstructive pulmonary disease (COPD) or bronchial asthma, highly vulnerable to respiratory failure during sleep.

As a result of increased parasympathetic and decreased sympathetic activity during sleep, heart rate, blood pressure, cardiac output, and peripheral vascular resistance decrease during NREM sleep and decrease still further during REM sleep. In REM sleep, however, there is an intermittent activation of the sympathetic nervous system, accounting for rapid fluctuations in blood pressure and heart rate. Cardiac output falls progressively during sleep, with the greatest decrement occurring during the last sleep cycle, particularly during the last REM sleep cycle early in the morning. This may explain why normal individuals and patients with cardiopulmonary disease are most likely to die during the early morning hours. Cerebral blood flow and cerebral metabolic rates for glucose and oxygen decrease during NREM sleep but increase to that of the waking values during REM sleep. Because of these hemodynamic and sympathetic changes in REM sleep during the last third of the sleep cycle in the early hours of the morning, there could be increased platelet aggregability, plaque rupture, and coronary arterial spasms, possibly triggering thrombotic events causing myocardial infarction, ventricular arrhythmias, or even sudden cardiac death. These circadian variations in

TABLE 36.1. Physiological Changes During Wakefulness, NREM Sleep, and REM Sleep

PHYSIOLOGY	WAKEFULNESS	NREM SLEEP	REM SLEEP
Parasympathetic activity	++	+++	++++
Sympathetic activity	++	+	Decreases or variable (++)
Heart rate	Normal sinus rhythm	Bradycardia	Bradytachyarrhythmia
Blood pressure	Normal	Decreases	Variable
Cardiac output	Normal	Decreases	Decreases further
Peripheral vascular resistance	Normal	Normal or decreases slightly	Decreases further
Respiratory rate	Normal	Decreases	Variable; apneas may occur
Alveolar ventilation	Normal	Decreases	Decreases further
Upper airway muscle tone	++	+	Decreases or absent
Upper airway resistance	++	+++	++++
Hypoxic and hypercapnic ventilatory responses	Normal	Decreases	Decreases further
Cerebral blood flow[a]	++	+	+++
Thermoregulation	++	+	–
Gastric acid secretion	Normal	Variable	Variable
Gastric motility	Normal	Decreases	Decreases
Swallowing	Normal	Decreases	Decreases
Salivary flow	Normal	Decreases	Decreases
Migrating motor complex (a special type of intestinal motor activity)	Normal	Slow velocity	Slow velocity
Penile or clitoral tumescence	Normal	Normal	Markedly increased

[a]There is, in general, a global decrease in cerebral blood flow with regional variation during NREM sleep, but this is not homogeneous. It may not decrease in some areas and may even show phasic increase in certain areas.
NREM, non-rapid eye movement; REM, rapid eye movement; +, mild; ++, moderate; +++, marked; ++++, very marked; —, absent.
Reproduced from Chokroverty S. *Sleep Disorders Medicine: Basic Science, Technical Considerations, and Clinical Aspects*, 3rd ed. Philadelphia: Elsevier/ Saunders, 2009.

cardiovascular and cerebrovascular events, with the highest rates of events occurring during the early morning hours, have been documented by meta-analysis of epidemiological studies.

There are profound changes in endocrine secretions during sleep. There is a pulsatile increase of growth hormone during NREM sleep in the first third of the normal sleep period. Prolactin secretion also rises 30 to 90 minutes after sleep onset. Cortisol secretion is inhibited by sleep, whereas thyroid-stimulating hormone levels reach a peak in the evening and then decrease throughout the night. Testosterone levels in men increase during sleep, rising from low levels at 8 p.m. to peak levels at 8 a.m., but there is no clear relationship noted between levels of gonadotrophic hormones and the sleep–wake cycle in children or adults. Melatonin, the hormone of darkness released by the pineal gland, reaches its highest secretion level between 3 and 5 a.m. and then decreases to low levels during the day. Thermoregulation is maintained during NREM sleep, but it is nonexistent in REM sleep: body temperature begins to

fall at sleep onset and reaches its lowest point during the third sleep cycle.

1.6. Homeostatic and Circadian Factors and Functions of Sleep

The normal sleep–wake rhythm is controlled by both the circadian and homeostatic systems. The circadian system is entrained by the normal light–dark cycle, and the hormone controlling the circadian timing of physiological systems is the pineal hormone, melatonin. Bright light suppresses melatonin, and it is released during the dark phase. Human circadian rhythm has a cycle close to 24 hours (24.2). The paired suprachiasmatic nuclei (SCNs) of the hypothalamus above the optic chiasm serve as the master biological clock. SCN receives afferent information from the retinohypothalamic tract sending signals to multiple synaptic pathways, including other parts of the hypothalamus and the pineal gland, where melatonin is released. Remarkable progress has been made, including identification of many genes and their protein products within the circadian clock in both fruit flies (*Drosophila*) and mammals (26). Dysfunction of the circadian rhythm results in several important sleep disorders, including delayed sleep phase syndrome and advanced sleep phase syndrome.

During wakefulness, it is thought that a buildup of some sleep factor, or process "S," occurs and is burned off or dissipated at night through sleep (27). In the morning after waking, cognitive and physiological functioning takes a while to get to a full waking state due to an inertia from the sleep system (28). The wake system takes a while to fully prime and synchronize all components for optimal output. This mechanistic framework has explanatory utility and does a reasonable job of providing a framework for much of the physiological and cognitive data. Notably, the concept of homeostasis is exemplified by the finding of recovery sleep following a period of sleep deprivation that is intensified with respect to slow-wave activity. This suggests that physiological systems need slow-wave sleep and therefore attempt to catch up for what was lost by intensifying and lengthening the sleep bout as well (29).

The function of sleep remains the greatest biological mystery of all times. Sleep is essential, and sleep deprivation leads to impaired attention and decreased performance in addition to sleepiness. Sleep is thought to have restorative, conservative, adaptive, thermoregulatory, and consolidative functions, as well as maintenance of synaptic and neuronal network integrity. Recent scientific data have strengthened the theory that memory reinforcement and consolidation take place during sleep. The recent discovery of lymphatic system (29a) in the central nervous system of mice (named glymphatic system because of its dependence on glial cells performing a lymphatic-like cleansing of the brain interstitial fluid in the perivascular space) directs our attention to the increased clearance of brain metabolic waste products during sleep: there is 60% more expansion of this interstitial space in sleep than in wakefulness.

1.7. Sleep Architecture

The term "sleep architecture" refers to the pattern of sleep stages that cycle through the night in what is known as the REM–NREM cycle. During development, there are changes that occur in the general pattern of sleep stages, but the adult shows a pattern of stages N1, N2, and N3 followed by REM sleep (Stage R), and the periodicity of this REM–NREM cycle throughout the night is generally 90 to 120 minutes in duration. The first REM period of the night is very often brief and may even be missed in young healthy sleepers. The first third of sleep is dominated by slow-wave sleep (Stage N3), and the last third is dominated by Stage R.

In the newborn, the sleep–wake cycle is approximately 50% dominated by REM sleep, and the sleep pattern involves frequent napping through the day. As the infant matures, there is a consolidation of sleep into the night period. During infancy, the mother's melatonin rhythm is conveyed to the infant through breast milk, helping to consolidate the sleep period into the nocturnal dark phase. The last sleep to be given up during the day period is generally the afternoon nap.

2. TECHNICAL ASPECTS

2.1. Polysomnographic Techniques

In 2007, the AASM (12) published a new manual for the scoring of sleep and associated events, almost 40 years after the first consensus on the technical standards for the field was published by Rechtschaffen and Kales in 1968 (11). The AASM has a website (http://www.aasmnet.org/) with links to resources for sleep medicine clinicians, scientists, technical personnel, and laboratory managers, and to several position papers.

2.2. Technical Personnel

The hiring of motivated and competent technologists is a critical step in the operations of a sleep laboratory. A feeling of trust between the patient and technologist is very important for sleeping in an unusual environment because electrodes and other sensors attached to the body can put the patient in a somewhat uneasy state. Coupled with the fact that patients are in the laboratory for reasons of disturbed sleep and/or wakefulness, and that continuous positive pressure may be tested, even on their first night in the laboratory, it is very important that they have a trusting professional interaction with the technologist.

In addition to professionalism, maturity, and an excellent bedside manner, the technologist needs to be able to function well at night, and, as much as possible, maintain a consistent shift. Frequent rotations from night to day lead to stress and result in unnecessary sleep loss and misalignment of biological rhythms. This can in turn lead to impaired performance and mood dysregulation.

Sleep technologists frequently have full EEG technician training or training as a respiratory therapist. In addition, they require well-supervised training in specialized polygraphic recording methods and in visual sleep staging, including identification and classification of arousals, leg movements, and respiratory disturbance. Technologists are responsible for maintaining equipment and for identifying and fixing technical problems at night during a recording if they should arise. Although most recordings are now performed using commercially available digital systems, the technologists still need to quickly and correctly identify problems and swap out parts as necessary. Therefore, they must make sure that adequate supplies and backup equipment are available. The American Association of Sleep Technologists has developed standards of training, practice, and certification for registration of technologists in North America (http://www.aastweb.org/).

2.3. Setting: Equipment and Recording Room

A report for the technologist that includes the patient's presenting symptoms and reason for the referral needs to be provided. The technologist should also have access to a list of medications and other information pertinent to the care of the patient through the night in the laboratory. It is most common for patients to be studied outside of a hospital setting, but even within the hospital setting, the technologist should have explicit instructions for when and whom to call with respect to critical levels of oximetry, abnormal ECG, or other medical needs of the patient. As in any hospital ward setting, for safety reasons it is not desirable for a technologist to work alone, without any backup personnel immediately available.

The equipment and technologist are usually housed in a room separate from that of the sleeping subject. Rather than an institutional-like bedroom, it is preferable for the patient to have an environment that is as home-like as possible, with a comfortable mattress, a closet, and a night stand. The sleeping room should be quiet and sound attenuated so that noises from outside the sleep laboratory and the technologist's area do not disturb the sleeping patient. An intercom system for contact with the patient is essential. Toilet facilities should preferably be attached to the bedroom and a shower should also be readily available.

Patients are generally asked to report to the laboratory facility one to three hours before their normal bedtimes. They are shown to their room and given a brief tour of the facility, as appropriate. The technician asks them to change into their bedclothes and then begins to attach the electrodes and recording devices. The technologist turns the lights out after he or she conducts a test of the equipment and performs biological calibrations. These calibrations enable the technologist to demonstrate to the individual who will review the recording the patient's normal waking eye movement pattern, and pattern of gritting teeth, breathing deeply, coughing, and pointing and flexing the toes and feet. All of these need to be documented by the technologist at the outset of the recording. When lights are turned off for the night, the technologist must document the time in the recording.

2.4. The Electrode Setup

2.4.1. EEG

Sleep EEG has always been based on the standard International 10–20 System derivations originally defined by Jasper in 1958 (30). According to the most recent AASM scoring guidelines (12), the recommended EEG derivations for sleep include scalp EEG derivations (from the frontal, central, and occipital regions) linked to the left mastoid (M1) or right mastoid (M2). Recommendations for sleep stage discrimination are F4–M1, C4–M1, and O2–M1, with backup electrodes placed at F3, C3, O1, and M2 to allow for re-referencing to F3–M2, C3–M2, and O1–M2 if problems develop over the course of the recording with the right hemisphere selections (Fig. 36.7). An alternative montage for stage scoring is F_z–C_z, C_z–O_z, and C4–M1 with backup electrodes FP_z, C3, O1, and M2. The EEG is the most important physiological information for the determination of sleep stages. Of course, for studies where epileptic discharge during sleep is under investigation, additional electrodes would be included depending on the brain regions of interest.

2.4.2. EOG

For routine EOG, the AASM scoring manual (12) recommends referential recordings from each outer canthus (1 cm below the left outer canthus [LOC] and 1 cm above the right outer canthus) to the ipsilateral mastoid (Fig. 36.8). These derivations show horizontal out-of-phase potentials very well,

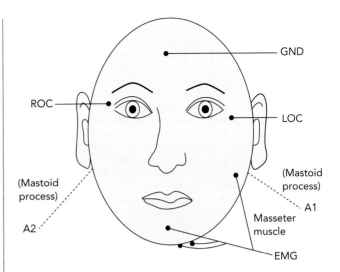

Figure 36.7. Schematic diagram to show electrode placement for electrooculography (EOG) (in right outer canthus [ROC] and left outer canthus [LOC]) and electromyography (EMG) (muscle activity from mentalis and submental muscles [mylohyoid and anterior belly of digastric]) as well as masseter muscle (for patient with bruxism). GND = ground electrode. Reproduced from Chokroverty S, ed. Sleep Disorders Medicine: Basic Science, Technical Considerations and Clinical Aspects. 3rd ed. Philadelphia: Elsevier/Saunders, 2009.

which are used to identify REMs associated with REM sleep. EOG electrodes should be attached with soft tape made for use on skin, and they should never be attached with collodion-soaked gauze because of the potential for corneal damage and also because collodion becomes inflexible when dry, so not only itchy and uncomfortable but prone to lifting and coming off during sleep. A micropore surgical tape maintains good contact for >48 hours of continuous recording and can be easily trimmed to needed dimensions. Tape width is usually twice the diameter of the electrode and about 5 to 8 cm along the wire. A length of tape added at right angles over the end of the first tape helps anchor the latter. A high-frequency filter of 35 Hz is used to reduce EMG artifact on the tracing. The low-frequency filter is generally selected at 0.3 to 0.5 sec (time constant) and permits recording of both the slow rolling eye movements of drowsiness and the REMs of REM sleep.

2.4.3. EMG

EMG is recorded with surface electrodes placed on the skin, secured with flexible sticky tape. It is recommended that three electrodes be attached, one electrode positioned midline just above the inferior rim of the mandible and two other electrodes each 2 cm below the inferior edge of the mandible, to the right and left. In this arrangement, EMG activity is recorded from mentalis, mylohyoid, and anterior belly of digastric muscles (see Fig. 36.8). The technologist can in this way select the bipolar combination of electrodes giving the best tonic EMG. Pairs of electrodes have also been used on the jaw edge or over the masseter muscles to record axial muscle tone (31,32). There is a great deal of variability in the resting chin tone EMG level that is related to adipose tissue and age, so it is important for the technologist to adjust the EMG amplification such that the background level during drowsiness shows some baseline

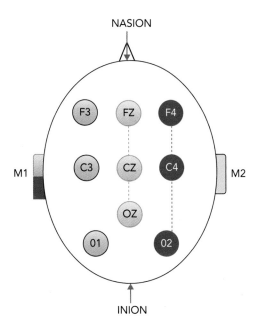

NASION

INION

Figure 36.8. AASM recommendation for EEG derivation during PSG recording (see text). International electrode placement.

elevation so that the transition into sleep and particularly REM can be easily discerned.

In addition to submental EMG, muscle activity is routinely recorded from the legs to document leg muscle activation. These extra-long electrodes are placed on the anterior tibialis muscles and again fixed with soft flexible skin tape such as micropore. They need to be well fixed with tape so that they do not come off with normal leg movements during sleep.

Patients with a history of abnormal movement or behavior in sleep may require a more extended EMG montage (known as "multiple muscle montage") (32a), which includes extra channels recording from additional cranially innervated and upperlimb muscles as well as axial and other lowerlimb muscles. This is of particular interest in patients with suspected REM behavior disorder (RBD), in whom REM without atonia may be missed if not enough muscles are sampled.

2.4.4. ECG

A single lead that is modified from lead II used in clinical cardiology is used to monitor the heartbeat during sleep, with an electrode placed on the right subclavicle area and left torso over the lower ribcage beneath the heart. Standard EEG electrodes may be used, but ECG electrode applications are preferable in that they are more resistant to artifact. Heart rate, extrasystoles, and other arrhythmias can be monitored using this lead, but due to differences in sampling rate and amplifier characteristics, this tracing is not suitable for detecting PQRST complex abnormalities.

2.5. Respiratory Monitoring

The measurement of respiration during sleep is critical to the diagnosis of sleep disorders and includes chest and abdominal excursion, most often using inductance plethysmography or sometimes strain gauges, and also a means of assessing nasal

airflow. Syndrome definitions and measurement techniques are described for sleep-disordered breathing in the AASM taskforce report (33), and more recent guidelines for the classification and scoring of respiratory events were published in the *AASM Manual for the Scoring of Sleep and Associated Events* in 2007 (12).

Careful monitoring of both upper airway airflow and thoracoabdominal movement in the respiratory tracings is used to categorize central, mixed, and obstructive sleep apnea, which is further discussed below. In addition, the monitoring and quantification of blood oxygen levels are necessary and accomplished using pulse oximetry. Endoesophageal (intrathoracic) pressure recording is also sometimes used in the detection of partial obstructions or upper airway resistance that can exist without actual apneas or hypopneas. The nasal pressure transducer (NPT) is recommended for the measurement of subtle reductions in airflow and can also be used to identify absent airflow, characteristic of apnea.

2.5.1. CAPNOGRAPHY

Capnography refers to the monitoring of the concentration of carbon dioxide (CO_2) in the respiratory gases and is measured in the breath at the end of complete expiration (end-tidal). A CO_2 analyzer is sometimes used to document CO_2 retention in sleep-related respiratory disorders, especially COPD and hypoventilation syndromes.

2.5.2. END-TIDAL CO_2

End-tidal CO_2 refers to the measurement of the CO_2 in the air exhaled from the lungs, and the normal range is 4% to 6% (equivalent to 35–45 mmHg).

2.5.3. PNEUMOTACHOGRAPHY

This technique is rarely used in diagnostic testing because it involves the placement of an airtight mask on the face and uses a pressure transducer system to measure flow rate, tidal volume, and other respiratory variables. This method is adopted frequently in the sleep testing laboratory during continuous positive airway pressure (CPAP) titration in order to monitor the adequacy of pressure and flow (see "Nasal Flow Using Nasal Airway Pressure" above).

2.6. Respiratory Effort

2.6.1. PIEZOELECTRIC STRAIN GAUGES

Thoracoabdominal movement is frequently monitored with piezoelectric crystal sensors incorporated into bands that are fitted around the torso at the level of the chest and abdomen. Generally these sensors can be plugged directly into the headbox and connected to the AC amplifier. Respiratory excursion is monitored and the traces are used to detect reductions in breathing effort, but it does not produce a measured signal, rather only a relative one.

2.6.2. INDUCTANCE PLETHYSMOGRAPHY

Inductive plethysmography uses wire coils placed around the chest and abdomen, sometimes woven into a vest, to monitor separate movements and then add them together, mimicking total spirometric volume. In contrast to the piezoelectric belts, this measuring technique is not only adjusted for visual characteristics of the wave but also calibrated before the sleep period begins. It produces a measured output for chest movement, abdominal movement, and total volume. This system has an advantage in being able to clearly distinguish paradoxical breathing associated with obstruction in contrast with central cessation of breathing that is reflected in a loss of signal in all three tracings.

2.7. Intercostal EMG

Long electrode leads are sometimes applied to record intercostal muscles to aid in detecting effort during breathing, and the placement is sensitive to muscle activity during coughing. The intercostal EMG recorded from the seventh to ninth intercostal space with the active electrode on the anterior axillary line and the reference electrode on the mid-axillary line may also include some diaphragmatic muscle activity in addition to the intercostal activity.

2.8. Snoring Monitor

In addition to the NPT method mentioned earlier in this chapter, both piezo sensors (encased in a rubber disk attached to the throat and plugged into the headbox) and microphones are used to monitor snoring. Snoring is associated with reduced upper airway diameter, and bursts of loud guttural inspiratory snorting are signs of OSA.

2.9. Indirect Measurement of Blood Gases

2.9.1. TRANSCUTANEOUS MEASUREMENT
Transcutaneous (T_cCO_2) measurement is the measurement of CO_2 gas tension of tissue underlying a specialized electrode that is usually placed on the chest or forearm. The electrode method uses a Stow–Severinghaus glass/ceramic electrochemical sensor, with a small heater unit to facilitate blood flow. Transcutaneous monitoring of CO_2 tension is more reliable than transcutaneous measurement of O_2 because CO_2 diffuses better through the skin.

2.9.2. FINGER OXIMETRY FOR OXYGEN SATURATION
Standard polygraphic diagnostic recording must include monitoring of an index of blood oxygen saturation or the percentage of available circulating hemoglobin that is saturated with oxygen (SaO_2). Probes are easily attached to the finger with a specially designed clip or with tape. Measurement is achieved with an optical device that uses a DC channel involving computation of absorption of certain wavelengths of light.

2.10. Body Position

Body position is useful information to have when interpreting a pattern of respiratory disturbance and can be obtained visually through infrared camera monitoring and/or with the aid of a position sensor. Such sensors can be attached to respiratory bands with accurate output of information including prone, supine, right side, and left side. Table 36.2 lists appropriate filter settings and sensitivity for recording various physiological characteristics in the PSG.

2.11. Sleep Staging Criteria

In 1968, the publication of the R and K sleep scoring atlas (11) represented the consensus agreement between sleep researchers of the time to the scoring of sleep stages. Remarkably, this document remains the dominant force in sleep scoring and analysis. With the recent publication of the *AASM Manual for the Scoring of Sleep and Associated Events*, the standardization of sleep and event scoring has reached a new level of consensus (12). The scoring of sleep in this recent document varies only slightly from that published in 1968 (11); however, this document addresses scoring rules for other physiological characteristics and rules for scoring in children.

The nomenclature of sleep stages has changed with the recent AASM scoring manual. NREM Stage 1 is now called Stage N1, and NREM Stage 2 is now Stage N2. What had previously been NREM Stages 3 and 4 (or slow-wave sleep) is now unified into a single Stage N3. Stage REM is now Stage R.

A sleep study is scored in 30-second epochs with each stage labeled as Stage W (or wakefulness), Stage N1, Stage N2, Stage N3, or Stage R. If two or more stages coexist in an epoch, the epoch is labeled as the stage that represents the greatest portion of the epoch.

1. Stage W represents the waking state, ranging from full alertness through early drowsiness. Stage W is scored when >50% of the epoch demonstrates alpha frequency activity over the occipital region (Fig. 36.9). Stage W is

TABLE 36.2 Filter Settings for PSG Recordings

CHARACTERISTICS	HIGH-FREQUENCY FILTER (HZ)	TIME CONSTANT (SECOND)	LOW-FREQUENCY FILTER (HZ)	SENSITIVITY
Electroencephalogram	70 or 35	0.4	0.3	5–7 µV/mm
Electro-oculogram	70 or 35	0.4	0.3	5–7 µV/mm
Electromyogram	90	0.04	5.0	2–3 µV/mm
Electrocardiogram	15	0.12	1.0	1 mv/cm to start; adjust
Airflow and effort	15	1	0.1	5–7 µV/mm; adjust

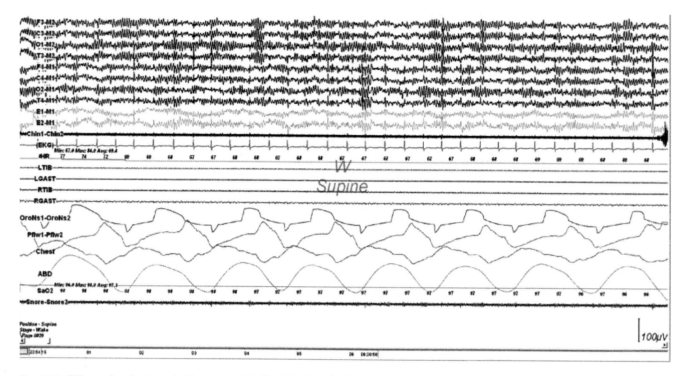

Figure 36.9. *PSG recording showing wakefulness in an adult. Top eight channels of EEG show posterior dominant 10-Hz alpha rhythm intermixed with a small amount of low-amplitude beta rhythms (international nomenclature). M2, right mastoid; M1, left mastoid. Waking eye movements are seen in the EOG of the left (E1) and right (E2) eyes, referred to the left mastoid. Chin1 (left) and Chin2 (right) submental EMG shows tonic muscle activity. EKG = electrocardiogram; HR= heart rate per minute. LTIB (left tibialis), LGAST (left gastrocnemius), RTIB (right tibialis), and RGAST (right gastrocnemius), EMG shows very little tonic activity. OroNs1-OroNs2 = oronasal airflow; Pflw1-Pflw2 = nasal pressure transducer recording airflow; Chest and ABD = respiratory effort (chest and abdomen); SaO2 = oxygen saturation by finger oximetry; Snore = snoring. Reproduced from Chokroverty S, ed. Sleep Disorders Medicine: Basic Science, Technical Considerations and Clinical Aspects. 3rd ed. Philadelphia: Elsevier/Saunders, 2009.*

scored in the absence of alpha activity (which occurs in 10–20% of individuals) if eye blinks, reading eye movements, or irregular conjugate REMs (waking eye movements) are identified with accompanying normal or elevated chin muscle tone. The chin EMG during Stage W is variable but is usually higher than that seen during sleep stages.

2. Stage N1 represents late drowsiness and light sleep. It is scored when >50% of an epoch shows alpha attenuation and is replaced by low-amplitude, mixed-frequency EEG activity (Fig. 36.10). K-complexes and sleep spindles are absent by definition. If an individual does not generate alpha activity, Stage N1 is scored when >50% of the epoch demonstrates theta range slowing (4–7 Hz), vertex sharp waves, or slow eye movements. In individuals who do generate alpha activity, slow eye movements are frequently seen before the disappearance of alpha activity, so individuals who do not generate alpha activity may have Stage N1 scored slightly earlier than those who do generate alpha activity. During Stage N1, chin EMG is variable but usually lower than that seen in Stage W.

3. Stage N2 represents the predominant sleep stage during an overnight recording and is scored when there is the appearance of a K-complex or sleep spindle (Fig. 36.11). In sleep medicine, a K-complex is defined as a biphasic

negative sharp wave maximum at the vertex or frontal regions that lasts ≥ 0.5 sec. Sleep spindles are 11- to 16-Hz sinusoidal activity lasting at least 0.5 sec, seen maximally in the central head region. Less than 20% of an epoch of Stage N2 can have slow wave activity (0.5–2 Hz, ≥75 μV in amplitude). Stage N2 is scored from the first epoch of Stage N2 until a clear epoch of Stage W or another stage of sleep is identified. Although eye movements are usually absent in Stage N2, slow eye movements can sometimes be seen. Chin or axial EMG is variable but usually lower than in Stage W.

4. Stage N3, which encompasses both former Stages 3 and 4 of the R and K criteria (11), is the deepest stage of sleep and is associated with increasing slow wave activity. Stage N3 is scored when 20% or greater of an epoch has slow wave activity (Fig. 36.12). For the purposes of sleep scoring, slow wave activity is defined as activity of 0.5 to 2 Hz that is at least 75 μV in amplitude when measured over the frontal or central regions. Sleep spindles may persist into Stage N3, but eye movements are usually absent. Axial EMG is usually lower than stage N2 and may approach that seen in stage R.

5. Stage R (formerly Stage REM) requires three components for it to be scored: low-amplitude mixed-frequency EEG, low chin EMG, and REMs (Fig. 36.13). Phasic EMG activity may occur, but tonic EMG activity must be at a

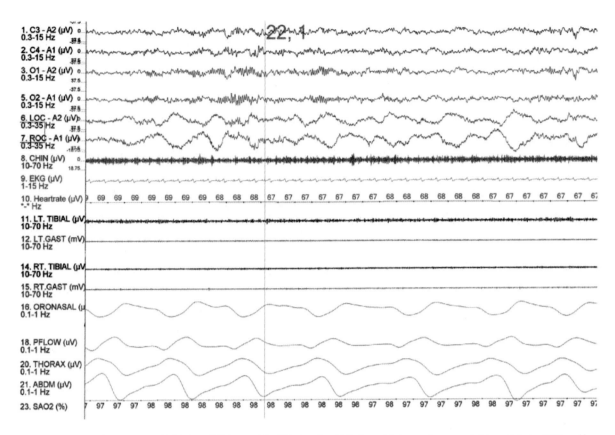

Figure 36.10. PSG recording shows stage 1 NREM sleep (N1) in an adult. EEGs (top four EEG channels) show a decrease of alpha activity to <50% and low-amplitude beta and theta activities. EOG (LOC, left; ROC, right) show slow rolling eye movements. A1, left ear; A2, right ear; Thorax, respiratory effort (chest). Rest of the montage is same as in Figure 36.9. Reproduced from Chokroverty S, ed. Sleep Disorders Medicine: Basic Science, Technical Considerations and Clinical Aspects. 3rd ed. Philadelphia: Elsevier/Saunders, 2009.

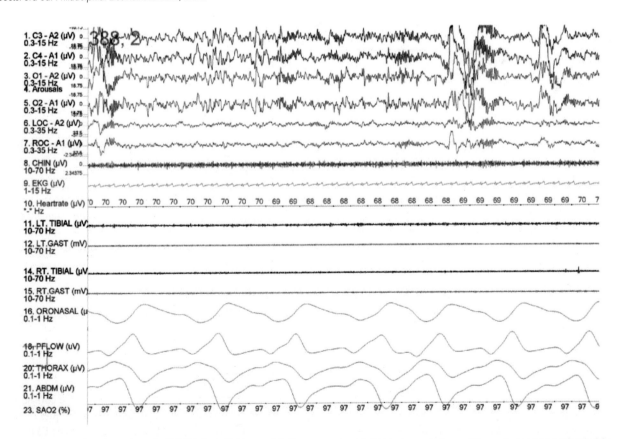

Figure 36.11. PSG recording shows Stage 2 of NREM sleep (N2) in an adult. Note approximately 14-Hz sleep spindles and K-complexes intermixed with delta waves (0.5–2 Hz) and up to 75 µV in amplitude occupying <20% of the epoch. See Figure 36.10 for description of rest of the montage. Reproduced from Chokroverty S, ed. Sleep Disorders Medicine: Basic Science, Technical Considerations and Clinical Aspects. 3rd ed. Philadelphia: Elsevier/Saunders, 2009.

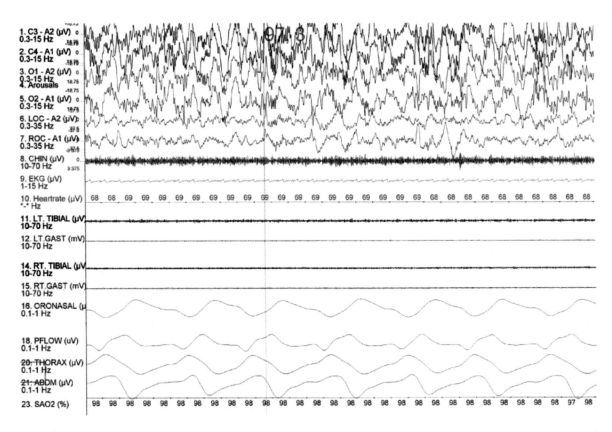

Figure 36.12. *PSG recording shows Stage 4 (N3) NREM sleep in an adult. Delta waves occupy 20% or more of the epoch in the traditional R–K scoring technique. See Figures 36.9 and 36.10 for description of rest of the montage. Reproduced from Chokroverty S, ed.* Sleep Disorders Medicine: Basic Science, Technical Considerations and Clinical Aspects. *3rd ed. Philadelphia: Elsevier/Saunders, 2009.*

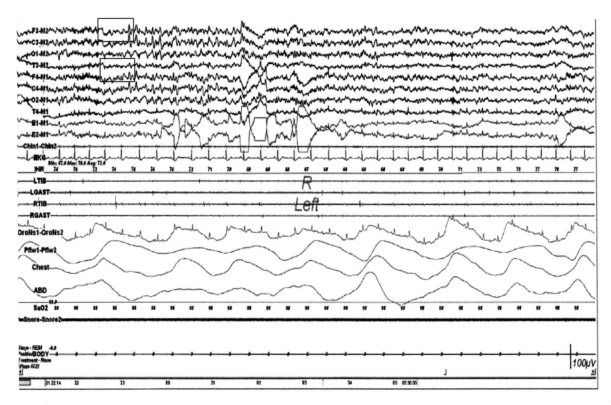

Figure 36.13. *PSG recording shows REM sleep in an adult. EEG (top eight channels) shows mixed-frequency theta, low-amplitude beta, and a small amount of alpha activity. Note the characteristic sawtooth waves (seen prominently in channels 1, 2, 5, and 6 from the top) of REM sleep preceding bursts of REMs (boxes) in the EOGs (E1-M1; E2–M2). Chin EMG shows marked hypotonia, whereas TIB and GAST EMG channels show very low-amplitude phasic myoclonic bursts. See Figure 36.10 for description of the montage. Reproduced from Chokroverty S, ed.* Sleep Disorders Medicine: Basic Science, Technical Considerations and Clinical Aspects. *3rd ed. Philadelphia: Elsevier/Saunders, 2009.*

level that is lower than that occurring at any other time during the study. Sleep spindles and K-complexes are absent. Series of 2- to 5-Hz vertex negative "sawtooth" waves occur, particularly just before phasic REM activity.

Movement time (or Stage M as described by Rechtschaffen and Kales (11)) is no longer scored. During major body movements that obscure >50% of an epoch, the epoch is scored as Stage W if alpha activity is present at any time in the epoch. If no alpha activity is identified, but an epoch of Stage W precedes or follows the epoch with a major body movement, then the epoch is scored as Stage W. If neither of these requirements can be met, the movement is scored the same as the epoch that follows it.

2.12. Hypnograms

Normal sleep has a clearly defined architecture that occurs each night. Hypnograms are a graphic display of the ultradian cycle within a night's sleep (34). Sleep stage is depicted in the vertical axis with the hours of sleep on the horizontal axis (Fig. 36.14). Sleep onset begins with a transition to Stage N1 sleep followed quickly by Stage N2. Stage N3 (formerly NREM Stage 3 and 4 or slow-wave sleep) comes next and is particularly sustained in this first sleep cycle in children and young adults. Sleep then briefly lightens to Stage N2 and transitions into Stage R for the first time, usually about 60 to 90 minutes after sleep onset. This completes the first sleep cycle, a pattern that repeats itself three to five times during the typical night's sleep. With each ensuing 90-minute sleep cycle, there is a decreasing amount of Stage N3 sleep and an increasing amount of Stage R sleep.

Predictable changes are noted in sleep architecture with aging and are illustrated by the histograms in Figure 36.14. Beginning in middle age, Stage 3 sleep lessens and more wakefulness after sleep onset is noted. The number of arousals and awakening continues to increase with aging, becoming particularly notable in the elderly (35,36).

2.13. Arousal Scoring

The original R–K scoring guidelines (11) focused primarily on the scoring of the stages of sleep (as discussed above). According to these criteria, the appearance of 15 sec or more of waking background (which resulted in the epoch being labeled as wake) would be labeled an awakening. The R–K manual made reference to movement arousals, but no other mention of brief EEG frequency changes was made. There was little standardization to the scoring of arousals before the publication of the position paper by the American Sleep Disorder Association (ASDA; now known as American Academy of Sleep Medicine) taskforce in 1992 (37). This consensus paper carefully defined rules for scoring an arousal. In the recent AASM scoring manual (12), these rules were distilled to a single rule: an arousal should be scored during Stages N1, N2, N3, or R if there is an abrupt shift of EEG frequency including alpha, theta, and/or frequencies of >16 Hz (but not spindles) that lasts at least 3 sec, with a minimum of 10 sec of stable sleep preceding the change. To be scored as an arousal during REM, there must be a concurrent increase in submental EMG lasting at least 1 sec (Figs. 36.15 and 36.16).

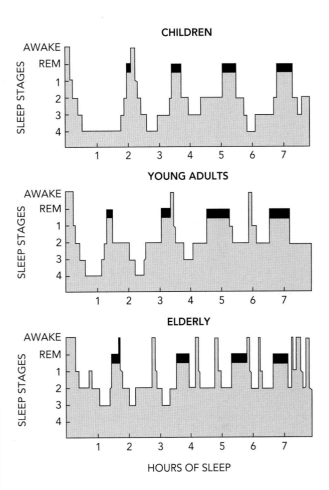

Figure 36.14. *Histograms representing normal sleep cycles for age. REM sleep represented by darkened area. Note that NREM Stages 3 and 4 would now be combined into Stage N3. Horizontal axis is 8 hours of PSG recording. From Kales A, Kales J. Recent findings in the diagnosis and treatment of disturbed sleep. N Engl J Med. 1974;487–499, with permission.*

The use of the 3-sec duration of EEG change is not based on any judgment of physiological impact; rather, it is an arbitrary value chosen by the taskforce partly due to increased inter-observer reproducibility of arousal scoring (as compared to shorter-duration events). The requirement for an accompanying EMG change in Stage R is due to the routine appearance of faster EEG frequencies during normal sustained Stage R sleep.

2.13.1. Periodic Limb Movements in Sleep Scoring
Periodic limb movements in sleep (PLMS) (also called periodic leg movements of sleep) are repetitive, stereotyped movements of the legs characterized by tonic extension of the great toe (with occasional superimposed clonic activity) variably accompanied by ankle dorsiflexion and knee flexion (38). These periodic movements can rarely preferentially involve the arm, and thus the use of the term PLMS. These periodic movements may sometimes be associated with an accompanying EEG arousal. PLMS are commonly seen on PSGs, particularly in the setting of disrupted sleep or in the elderly. The clinical significance of PLMS is often unclear, but they may sometimes contribute to insomnia or daytime sleepiness. In 1980, Coleman et al. (38) made a major contribution in understanding PLMS,

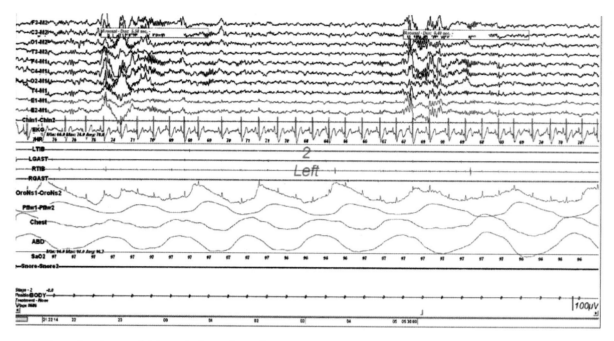

Figure 36.15. PSG recording shows two brief periods of arousals out of Stage N2 sleep in the left- and right-hand segments of the recording, lasting for 5.58 and 6.40 sec and separated by >10 sec of sleep. Note delta waves followed by approximately 10-Hz alpha activities during brief arousals.

and various rules of scoring the movements have been proposed, including that from the ASDA taskforce in 1993 (39), the World Association of Sleep Medicine and the International Restless Legs Syndrome Study Group in 2006 (40). From here on we will focus on the recent guidelines given in the AASM scoring manual, which are essentially similar to the criteria of the World Association of Sleep Medicine and the International Restless Legs Syndrome Study Group (40).

During PSG, the reviewer counts how many events occurred and notes whether an EEG arousal was associated with them (Fig. 36.17). A significant leg movement is defined as an increase in EMG lasting 0.5 to 10 seconds. The EMG increase

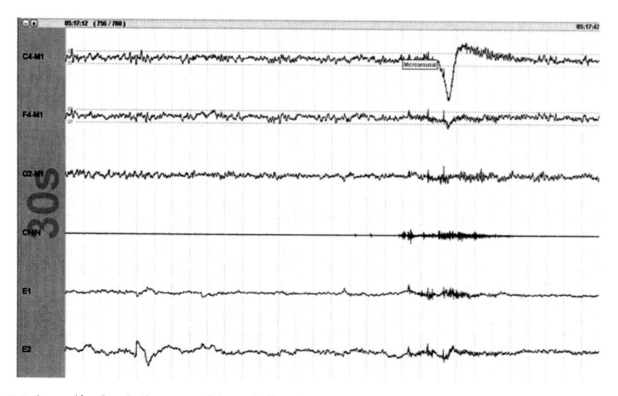

Figure 36.16. An arousal from Stage R with appearance of >3 seconds of faster frequencies accompanied by the appearance of EMG in the axial (chin) EMG channel (30-sec epoch).

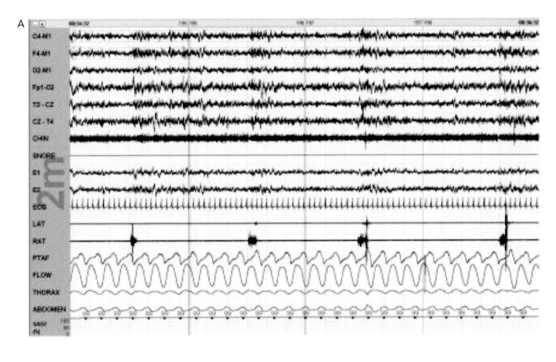

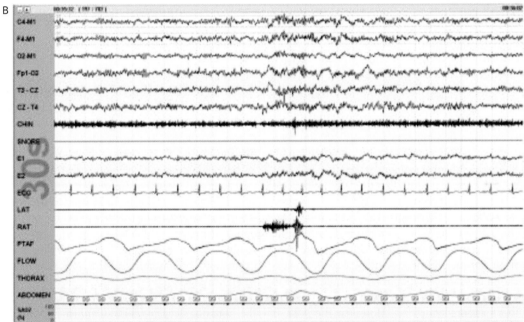

*Figure 36.17. **A:** An illustration of periodic limb movements of sleep. This is a 2-minute epoch with the appearance of EMG activity in the right anterior tibialis (RAT) channel occurring approximately every 30 sec. The patient is in NREM sleep (which is not able to be confidently determined in this 2-minute epoch). **B:** A 30-sec epoch taken from the time period illustrated in **A**. Note the appearance of faster frequencies on the EEG demonstrating an arousal associated with this periodic movement.*

has to be at least 8 μV above the resting EMG. The leg movement is labeled as part of a series of one of the four consecutive leg movement events occurring with an interval between 5 and 90 sec. If each leg movement event is separated by <5 sec, the movements are considered a single leg movement. Arousals are scored as associated with the leg movement if there is an interval of <0.5 sec between the end of one event and the onset of the other, regardless of which is first. Limb movements should not be scored if they occur within 0.5 sec of the onset or end of an apnea or hypopnea (these are respiratory-related leg

movements, the scoring of which is somewhat controversial and is undergoing modification [40a]).

Similar periodic leg movements can be seen in wakefulness, particularly in patients with restless legs syndrome (RLS). RLS is a neurological movement disorder where patients get an urge to move the legs, usually but not always associated with an uncomfortable sensation in their legs; it is worse at night, worse while at rest, and relieved with movement. RLS is a clinical diagnosis made in the clinic based primarily on the history and does not require PSG evaluation. PLMS is a diagnosis made on the PSG as most patients do not have daytime symptoms and observer history is not usually helpful. Most patients with RLS will also have PLMS, but PLMS most commonly occur in the absence of RLS symptoms. Periodic limb movements in wakefulness are not part of the recently published AASM scoring guidelines (12), but several investigators have suggested the utility of periodic limb movements in wakefulness in assessing patients with RLS. The scoring criteria are exactly the same as those outlined above for the scoring of PLMS. These investigators have also proposed a suggested immobilization test (SIT) with associated quantification of periodic limb movements in wakefulness as a diagnostic test for patients with RLS (41).

2.13.2. Scoring of Respiratory Events

With the advent of the recognition of apneic events during sleep (42), the cessation of identified airflow for 10 sec has been the standard definition of an apneic event. With subsequent recognition of the significance of partial airflow interruption (hypopneas), no consistent standard definition was accepted and technical and scoring standards varied widely. The recent AASM scoring manual defines technical recording requirements as well as scoring rules (12), which may lead to an improvement in the standardization of quantifying respiratory abnormalities during sleep.

The sensor used to score apnea is the oronasal thermal sensor (thermistor or thermocouple) that has long been used to qualitatively assess airflow during PSG recording. The sensor for detection of a hypopnea is the NPT. The NPT is much more sensitive to a decrease in airflow and is appropriate to use for the identification of a hypopnea. Frequently during a study a clear decrease in airflow is identified in the NPT, with no evidence of change in the thermal sensor. Previously, it was common to recognize cyclical arousals associated with loud snoring and oxygen desaturation that could not be scored using the less sensitive thermal sensors. This led to the recognition of the upper airway resistance syndrome, in which the patient had a clinical syndrome consistent with OSA but without scorable apneic events. With the use of NPT and the associated identification of scorable hypopneas, it is much rarer to have a clinical suspicion of unrecognized respiratory events contributing to a patient's symptoms. However, the NPT is frequently overly sensitive in that it demonstrates no airflow (an apnea) while the thermal sensor continues to demonstrate obvious airflow. As such, the NPT is not to be used for determination of apneic events, which are to be scored using the thermal sensor recording.

An apnea is scored using the thermal sensor when there is a >90% decrease in identified airflow lasting at least 10 sec. The apnea is classified based on the accompanying inspiratory effort identified using the inductive plethysmography belts from the chest and abdomen. An apnea is labeled as *obstructive* if there is continued or increased respiratory effort throughout the entire period of absent airflow (Fig. 36.18B). The apnea is classified as *central* if the event has no associated inspiratory effort throughout the entire apneic period (see Fig. 36.18A). The event is scored as a *mixed* apnea if there is initially an absence of inspiratory effort followed by resumption of inspiratory effort

in the later portion of the event (Fig. 36.18C). The duration of the absent respiratory effort needed to score a mixed apnea is not defined, but usually would be at least one complete breath cycle (4–6 sec). There is no requirement for any accompanying oxygen desaturation or EEG arousal to score an apnea.

Two separate rules for scoring hypopneas were presented in the AASM scoring manual (12). The "recommended" rule is that used by Medicare and was chosen in an attempt to be in concert with Medicare definitions and decision regarding coverage of CPAP and other therapies. However, the "alternative" set of rules for scoring hypopneas is actually more widely used and captures a larger number of hypopneas, particularly in individuals with healthy lungs where oxygen desaturations occur much less frequently. The "recommended" rule requires that (1) NPT signal decreases by >50% for at least 10 sec and (2) there is an accompanying oxygen desaturation of 4% or more. The "alternative" rule requires that (1) NPT signal decreases by >30% for at least 10 sec and (2) there is an accompanying oxygen desaturation of 3% or more, or the event is accompanied by an EEG arousal within 3 sec of the event.

Either scoring method is acceptable, but the rules used should be clearly defined in the PSG report. Most labs do not attempt to classify hypopneic events as obstructive or central due to the inaccuracy of assessing respiratory effort in the absence of more invasive monitoring techniques such as esophageal manometry.

An optional scoring rule outlines the scoring of respiratory effort–related arousals. This may be particularly helpful in identifying potential clinically significant respiratory events if only the "recommended" rule for hypopnea identification is used. A respiratory effort–related arousal is scored if there is a sequence of events lasting at least 10 seconds characterized by increasing respiratory effort or flattening of the nasal pressure waveform leading to an arousal from sleep when the sequence of breaths does not meet criteria for an apnea or hypopnea. Flattening of NPT waveform is thought to identify increased airway pressure reflecting partial airway occlusion. The flattening of the NPT waveform is illustrated in Figure 36.19.

The number of scored respiratory events is then divided by the hours of sleep to yield an apnea–hypopnea index (AHI), which represents the number of respiratory events per hour of sleep. This value is most commonly used to categorize the severity of respiratory abnormality. The consensus statement from the AASM classifies apnea severity as per the following criteria:

AHI <5: normal

AHI >5 but <15: mild apnea

AHI >15 but <30: moderate apnea

AHI >30: severe apnea (33).

Many observers suggest this categorization of apnea severity may be too severe, particularly given the lack of normative data. Several large studies have demonstrated that 20% of

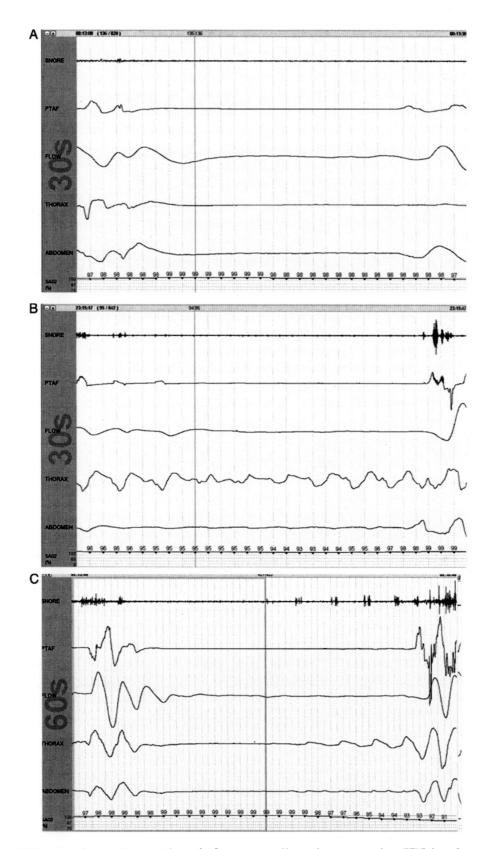

Figure 36.18. A: *Limited PSG montage demonstrating no evidence of airflow as measured by nasal pressure transducer (PTAF channel), oronasal thermocouple (flow channel) accompanied by the absence of ventilatory effort in the thorax, and abdominal channels (measured by respiratory inductive plethysmography belts). This is an example of a central apnea lasting ~16 sec. B: Limited PSG montage demonstrating no evidence of airflow as measured by nasal pressure transducer (PTAF channel), oronasal thermocouple (flow channel) accompanied by the evidence of continued ventilatory effort in the thorax channel (measured by respiratory inductive plethysmography belts). This is an example of an obstructive apnea lasting ~18 sec. Note the appearance of snore artifact (in snore and PTAF channel) with resumption of airflow. C: Limited PSG montage demonstrating an apneic event lasting ~40 sec (in this 60-sec epoch). No evidence of airflow is noted by the nasal pressure transducer (PTAF channel) or the oronasal thermocouple (flow channel) throughout the event identifying it as an apnea. During the first half of the apneic period, there is no evidence of ventilatory effort, but then increasing evidence of effort in the thorax channel is seen leading up to the termination of the apneic event. This is an illustration of a mixed apnea, having central features at onset but then demonstrating obstructive features as the event progresses.*

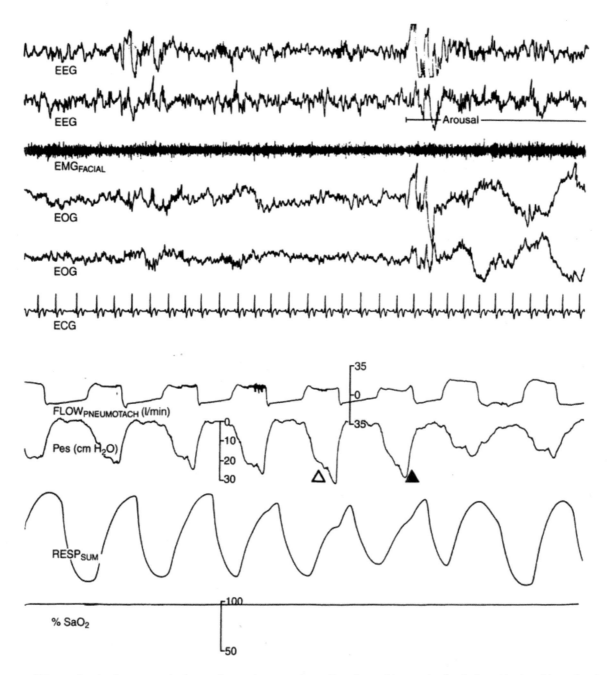

Figure 36.19. *PSG recording showing an example of upper airway resistance syndrome. Note that peak increase in effort (indicated by the solid arrowhead) is associated with a small drop in peak flow and tidal volume, triggering a transient EEG arousal. ECG = electrocardiogram; EMGFACIAL = facial muscle electromyogram; EOG = electro-oculogram (right and left); FLOWPNEUMOTACH = pneumotachometer to quantify airflow; Pes = esophageal manometry to record esophageal pressure; RESPSUM = respiratory effort; SaO2 = saturation with oxygen. Reproduced from Chokroverty S, ed. Sleep Disorders Medicine: Basic Science, Technical Considerations and Clinical Aspects. 3rd ed. Philadelphia: Elsevier/Saunders, 2009.*

non-obese healthy middle-aged adults have an AHI >5, and ~6% have an AHI >15. The AHI is also recognized to increase with age, even in individuals with no sleep complaint (43–45).

2.13.3. Scoring of Cardiac Events

Before the AASM scoring manual (12), there had been no attempt to define or standardize the documentation or scoring of cardiac events during a PSG. The AASM scoring manual defined the use of a modified ECG lead II (recording electrodes placed on torso at approximately the second rib to the

right of the sternum and the sixth rib near the apex of the heart on the left chest). The following ECG scoring rules for adults were defined:

1. Score sinus tachycardia for sustained sinus heart rate >90 beats per minute (bpm).

2. Score sinus bradycardia for sustained sinus heart rate <40 bpm.

3. Score asystole for cardiac pauses >3 sec.

4. Score wide complex tachycardia for a rhythm of at least three consecutive beats at a rate >100 bpm and a QRS duration of >120 msec.

5. Score narrow complex tachycardia for a rhythm of at least three consecutive beats at a rate >100 bpm and a QRS duration of <120 msec.

6. Score atrial fibrillation if there is an "irregularly irregular" ventricular rhythm associated with replacement of consistent P-waves with variable rapid oscillations.

7. Other significant arrhythmias (such as heart block) should be reported if the quality of the single lead is sufficient for accurate identification.

2.13.4. SCORING OF CYCLIC ALTERNATING PATTERN

The cyclic alternating pattern (CAP) was first described by Terzano et al. in 1985 (46). CAP has been proposed as a tool for the comprehensive analysis of sleep microstructure in both normal and pathologic conditions. Traditional sleep scoring using the R–K criteria (11) has been the gold standard for looking at sleep macrostructure. CAP presents another way of looking at NREM sleep within those sleep stages. NREM sleep has been recognized to have high-amplitude EEG bursts such as K-complexes or delta bursts. These are often seen as an arousal response to external stimuli but also occur when sleep disturbance was not evident. An alternative view to this arousal process is that these phenomena are associated with sleep instability (due to an internal or external challenge to the sleep process) and that this type of slow-wave activity marks the brain's attempt to preserve or sustain the sleep state. If sleep becomes too unstable, the preservation attempt fails and the high-amplitude activity is accompanied by a more complete EEG arousal. It is proposed that the addition of a periodicity dimension to the concept of sleep stability and arousal will provide a valuable perspective on sleep and its relationship to underlying physiological and pathophysiological mechanisms.

CAP represents a slow oscillation of EEG activity that manifests in the appearance of EEG arousal patterns with a periodicity of 20 to 40 sec. It is represented by three characteristics:

1. The recurring high-amplitude EEG activity (Phase A of the period)

2. The intervening background EEG activity (Phase B of the period)

3. The period or cycle that is the sum of Phases A and B

A CAP sequence is composed of repetitive CAP cycles, with each cycle composed of a Phase A and a Phase B. Each phase of the CAP is 2 to 60 sec in duration. If there is no CAP activity for >60 sec, then that portion of NREM sleep is scored as a non-CAP. Figure 36.20 illustrates an example of the CAP in Stage 2 sleep. Figure 36.21 illustrates a brief period of CAP surrounded by non-CAP sleep on either side. Phase A can take on three patterns:

1. A1 is primarily slow (<4 Hz) delta activity with a small degree of autonomic activation.

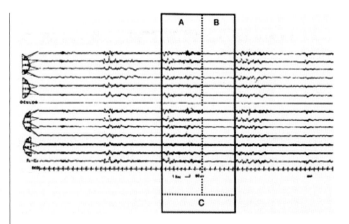

Figure 36.20. An example of CAP in Stage N2. The box outlines a CAP cycle (C) composed of Phase A and following Phase B. Bipolar EEG channels 1 to 6 from top to bottom: Fp2–F4, F4–C4, C4–P4, P4–O2, F8–T4, and T4–T6; channels 8 to 14 from top to bottom: Fp1–F3, F3–C3, C3–P3, F7–T3, T3–T5, P3-01, P3–O2, F2-C2. EOG (channel 7 from top) and ECG (bottom channel). From Terzano MG, et al. Atlas, rules, and recording techniques for the scoring of cyclic alternating pattern (CAP) in human sleep. Sleep Med. 2001;2:537–553, with permission.

2. A3 demonstrates an increase in fast rhythms with strong autonomic activation (an EEG arousal as per ASDA rules) (37).

3. A2 represents a middle ground between the A1 and A3 subtypes (Fig. 36.22).

A summary paper outlining the rules for scoring CAP and including an atlas to illustrate those rules was published by Terzano et al. in 2001 (47).

In several studies, CAP Phase A is identified as the "gate" or "amplifier" that allows pathologic events such as PLMS, bruxism, sleepwalking, and sleep-disordered breathing to occur. The majority of nocturnal partial seizures presenting during NREM sleep also occur predominantly in CAP in association with Phase A (in particular in association with K-complexes and delta bursts) (48). At this point, the clinical significance of CAP remains unclear, but further research is warranted.

2.14. Indications for PSG

The indications for PSG have been summarized by the published practice parameters of the AASM (49,50). The dominant indication for PSG is for the evaluation of sleep-related breathing disorders. The increasing awareness of sleep apnea and its possible impact on long-term cardiovascular health has led to a marked increase in evaluation of sleep-disordered breathing. While the obese individual who presents with snoring, witnessed apneas, and excessive daytime sleepiness (EDS) represents the obvious candidate for PSG evaluation, there are many others who likely need PSG evaluation. Symptoms of concern for possible sleep apnea include daytime sleepiness, loud snoring, witnessed apneas, and unrefreshing sleep. Additional medical conditions that warrant exploring a possible role of OSA include intractable hypertension, new-onset atrial fibrillation (particularly with onset in sleep), intractable congestive heart failure, and stroke.

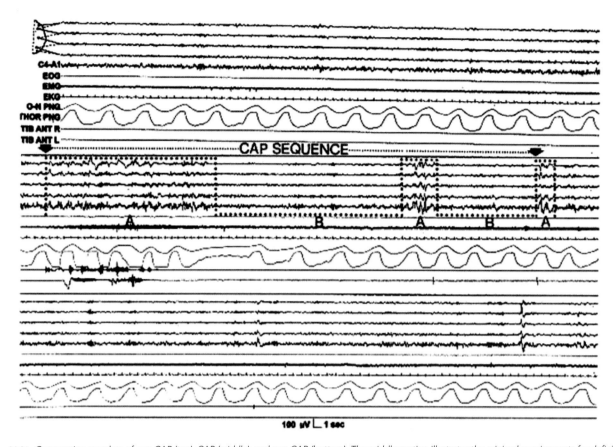

Figure 36.21. *Consecutive stretches of non-CAP (top), CAP (middle), and non-CAP (bottom). The middle section illustrates the minimal requirements for definition of a CAP sequence (at least three Phase A's in succession). The CAP sequence occurs between two black arrows and the transition between phases is delineated by the dotted line. EEG derivation is Fp2–F4, F4–C4, C4–P4, P4–O2, and C4–A1. From Terzano MG, et al. Atlas, rules, and recording techniques for the scoring of cyclic alternating pattern (CAP) in human sleep. Sleep Med. 2001;2:537–553, with permission.*

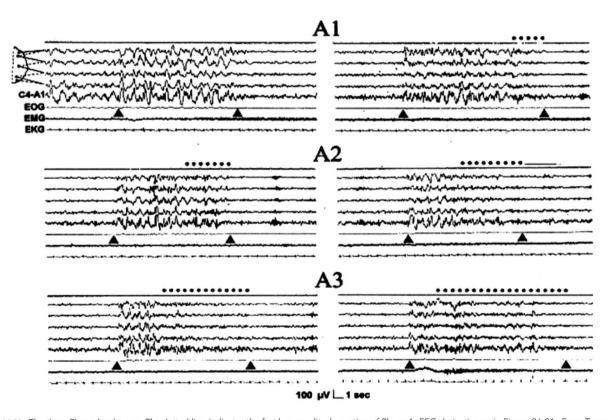

Figure 36.22. *The three Phase A subtypes. The dotted line indicates the fast low-amplitude portion of Phase A. EEG derivation as in Figure 36.21. From Terzano MG, et al. Atlas, rules, and recording techniques for the scoring of cyclic alternating pattern (CAP) in human sleep. Sleep Med. 2001;2:537–553, with permission.*

Once the diagnosis of sleep apnea has been documented, patients usually return for a repeat study for CPAP titration. The goal is to document the minimum CPAP pressure that eliminates apnea, hypopneas, and arousals, with particular attention to Stage R and supine sleep. It is recommended that patients undergoing upper airway surgery to treat snoring or apnea have a study prior to surgery to document apnea severity and ensure the appropriate choice of therapy and perioperative management. Similarly, after upper airway surgery or oral appliance to treat apnea, a follow-up PSG is warranted to document the residual degree of sleep apnea and to determine whether additional therapeutic efforts are warranted. If the patient has lost or gained substantial weight (e.g., 10% of body weight since the last study), a repeat PSG is indicated to reassess the clinical situation.

In addition to the evaluation of sleep-disordered breathing, PSGs are also used to evaluate other causes of EDS, sleep disruption, and unusual nocturnal behavior. In an individual with EDS where sleep apnea is not a concern, a PSG can be done to evaluate possible PLMS as a contributor to the patient's complaint. PSG is routinely done the night before a multiple sleep latency test (MSLT, discussed later in this chapter) to document adequate sleep quantity and quality to allow interpretation of the multiple nap study.

In patients with RLS, PSG is not routinely done, as this is a clinical diagnosis and the restrained environment of the sleep lab can be very uncomfortable for the symptomatic patient with RLS. PSG may be appropriate if a patient with RLS does not respond to therapy or has other potential sleep pathology. Similarly, PSG is not routinely indicated in patients presenting with insomnia. Both behavioral and pharmacological therapies are pursued before considering PSG evaluation in a patient with insomnia, to exclude sleep apnea comorbid with insomnia.

Most PSG recordings are today done with video accompanying the polygraph recording. Video recording is essential if the goal is to evaluate unusual nocturnal behavior. The diagnosis of a parasomnia can usually be made on a clinical basis and a video-PSG is not required in many patients. However, if there are unusual features or a concern about coexistent sleep problems, PSG may be warranted. If the differential diagnosis includes nocturnal seizures, additional EEG channels covering both the temporal and parasagittal regions bilaterally are often helpful in more confidently differentiating parasomnias from epileptic seizures (32a).

2.15. Home Sleep Apnea Testing (Ambulatory PSG Recording)

Home sleep apnea testing (HSAT), also known as portable or ambulatory recording of sleep in the evaluation of sleep disorders, has been rarely utilized in the past due to the limitations of the technique and the lack of third-party reimbursement (51). With the recent Centers for Medicare and Medicaid Services (CMS) approval for coverage and the push to control healthcare costs, the role of ambulatory or HSAT is being reevaluated (52). As outlined earlier in this chapter, in-lab PSG is the gold standard for the evaluation of sleep disorders and is classified as a type 1 study. A full but unattended PSG (seven or more channels, including the recording of EEG) is classified as a type 2 study. The focus on the HSAT has been with the use of type 3 studies, which have four to seven channels and focus on the evaluation of respiratory parameters; however, they do not record EEG and therefore there is no evaluation of sleep stages or arousals. A type 4 study is a one- or two-channel overnight recording, with at least one of them being oximetry (53).

In the typical HSAT, the patient presents to the lab during the day and is educated regarding use of the equipment and placement of electrodes and recording devices. After preparing for bed, the patient places the recording sensors and pushes a button indicating that he or she is retiring for the night. The button is pressed again upon awakening in the morning and a total recording time is obtained, which is supplemented by a brief sleep log from the patient outlining any sustained periods of wakefulness or other important information. Usual recorded parameters include nasal/oral airflow, respiratory effort, oxygen saturation, body position, snoring, and heart rate. The studies are scored by automated scoring systems, but the data should be reviewed and edited by a technologist or a sleep specialist to ensure that artifactual information is discarded and that the results represent a reasonable interpretation of the data. From this recording, an estimate of an AHI and oxygen desaturation index is obtained.

The guidelines from the AASM for unattended sleep studies outline minimal technical expectations for portable monitoring (53). They should at a minimum record airflow, respiratory effort, and blood oxygenation and should use the same sensors used in the laboratory studies. Accurate data collection is paramount to successful use of the techniques, so the devices should not be used by technologists or physicians who are inexperienced in sleep disorders and their evaluation. The devices must also allow review of the raw data so that manual scoring and/or adjustment of the automated scoring algorithms can be made.

Recently there has been a trend toward increasing referrals and a push by the third-party insurance payers for HSAT disregarding the AASM guidelines (53) for HSAT including patients with high pretest probability of having moderate to severe OSA resulting in false-negative studies. Thus in many patients, OSA remains undiagnosed, with potentially serious consequences. A case in point is a study published in 2014 (54) showing that 90% of symptomatic patients with negative HSAT results had OSA (43% moderate and 21% severe) in an in-lab PSG study. The reason could be any of the following factors (55): an inability of HSAT to detect arousal-associated OSA, use of total recording time rather than total sleep time in calculating respiratory event index, and recording in a particular patient population who may not have the highest pretest probability of having moderate or severe OSA. As Collop (56) mentioned in an editorial, the definition of "high pretest probability" has not been clarified, thus creating such confusion. The clinical history is key in assessing a patient's appropriateness for HSAT (56). Also, HSAT should never be used to exclude OSA in asymptomatic individuals.

Since the introduction of HSAT, there have been improvements in its technology, including the method of applying the sensors. In a recent review, Bruyneel and Ninane (57) analyzed five acceptable randomized controlled trials comparing unattended HSAT to in-lab PSG studies in symptomatic patients with a high index of suspicion for OSA. The authors concluded that HSAT is reliable for diagnosis of OSA. The use of HSAT, however, still remains hotly debated. In the following paragraphs we summarize its advantages, disadvantages, and contraindications.

The advantages of HSAT include the following (55,57):

1. Relatively inexpensive

2. Comfortable for the patients having the study in their home environment

3. More readily available than in-lab PSG

4. Feasible for those with relative immobility and difficulty traveling to the sleep laboratory

5. Better quality of sleep

6. An important tool if used in the right population and interpreted properly.

The disadvantages of HSAT are many, as listed below (55,57):

1. Potential loss of data (3–18%) (58), which means less cost savings

2. Most HSATs do not have EEG leads and hence cannot detect arousals and sleep staging including REM sleep, and thus cannot assess the severity of OSA as OSA tends to be worse in REM sleep.

3. Many HSATs do not have position sensors and therefore cannot assess the severity of OSA which becomes worse in the supine position.

4. Technical problems due to loss of sensor signal cannot be corrected in the absence of a technologist.

5. Inability to perform CPAP titration and inability to perform split-night study

6. Cannot distinguish central from obstructive sleep apnea and identify hypopnea

7. Unreliability of automatic scoring performed in HSAT compared with manual scoring performed in general in-lab PSG recording

8. HSAT tends to overestimate the severity of sleep apnea in patients with mild or moderate OSA but tends to underestimate the severity for severe OSA based on determination of the respiratory event index due to inability to determine the exact sleep monitoring time

9. Inability to have video documentation for parasomnias, nocturnal seizures, and complex nocturnal behavior

10. Inability to diagnose hypoventilation in absence of a CO_2 sensor

11. Difficult to perform MSLT next day for central hypersomnolence disorders

12. Inability to detect other sleep disorders.

AASM guidelines list the following contraindications for HSAT (53):

1. Significant comorbid conditions (e.g., moderate or severe COPD, heart failure, neuromuscular disorders)

2. Patients suspected to have sleep disorders other than OSA (e.g., narcolepsy, central sleep apnea, REM behavior disorder, circadian rhythm sleep disorder)

3. Screening for asymptomatic population

4. Patients suspected to have nocturnal seizures, nocturnal cardiac arrhythmias, and hypoventilation (e.g., opiate use, neuromuscular disorders)

5. Pediatric population (<18 years)

6. Patients on supplemental O_2 or those with low baseline O_2 saturation.

Figures 36.23 and 36.24 are examples from an HSAT recording showing a sleep histogram and a graphic representation.

2.16. Computerized PSG and Computer-Assisted Scoring

Visual sleep scoring has been the standard for analyzing sleep from the very beginning, and subsequent standardizations of sleep scoring has emphasized that (11,12) any attempt to utilize computerized sleep scoring in clinical sleep studies has been modeled on the visual sleep analysis. Although it is extremely useful for quantifying easily identified events (e.g., oxygen desaturations), its inability to adjust to hostile "pathologic states" such as frequent apneas, disrupted sleep, and movement artifacts has limited its clinical application. Although many of the commercially available PSG equipment do come with computerized analysis of sleep stage, the clinical standard remains visual scoring by a trained technologist or, at least, the review and scoring of the computerized sleep staging by a technologist. Similarly, computerized identification of respiratory or movement events also requires review and editing by a technologist.

As part of the efforts to create the new scoring manual, there was a critical evidence-based look at computerized analysis of PSG. The individuals in charge of this section suggested that "computer scoring and quantitative analysis are still in the formative stage of development" and have not been proved to be useful in clinical practice (59).

The real strength of computerized analysis of sleep is in its ability to look at sleep as a continuum rather than the arbitrary definitions provided for identifying Stages N1, N2, N3, and R sleep. Similarly, the microstructure of sleep is likely lost in the 30-secepoch. Research is still needed to determine whether this technology will contribute to new methods for understanding sleep and its disorders (60).

2.17. Pitfalls of PSG

One of the biggest pitfalls of PSG is the recognition of respiratory events that may be clinically significant but may not be

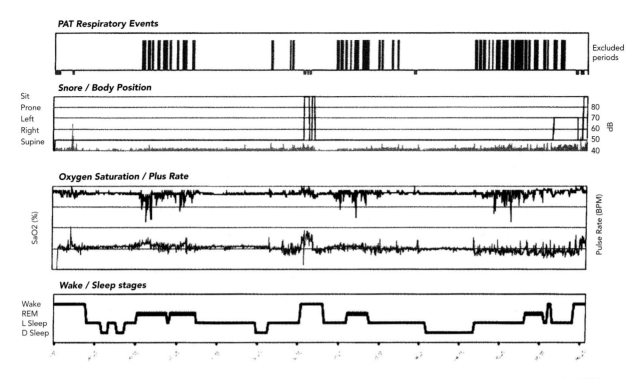

Figure 36.23. *Sleep histogram taken from HSAT recording using principle of peripheral arterial tonometry (PAT) to record respiratory event index (REI) from a 390year-old obese (BMI 31) man with a high pretest probability of moderate OSA based on symptoms of snoring, EDS, and witnessed apneas. Histogram shows, from top to bottom, PAT/respiratory events; snore/body position; oxygen saturation (SaO2)/pulse rate; sleep stages (L sleep: Light sleep; D sleep: Deep sleep; REM: rapid eye movement sleep) and wake state estimated indirectly.*

consistently recognized by the sensors used for the recording. The clearest example of this is the upper airway resistance syndrome (61,62), in which patients experience repetitive increases in upper airway resistance that result in brief arousals with associated EDS. Not all of these individuals snore, and the repetitive arousals can sometimes be attributed to other causes such as PLMS. The gold standard of documenting this disorder is the use of esophageal manometry to document large negative intrathoracic pressure swings that correlate with the EEG arousals. Esophageal manometry is not commonly used in the sleep lab due to its effect on sleep and patient comfort.

In the past several years, the consistent use of NPTs to monitor airflow and airway pressure has markedly increased our sensitivity to this phenomenon, with many of these events now being recognized as hypopneas due to the superior identification of airflow resistance by NPT (63–65). However, the sleep physician needs to be sensitive to the possibility of the underrecognition of respiratory events in the sleep laboratory.

2.18. Artifacts During PSG Recording

PSG recordings frequently contain extraneous electrical activities that do not originate from the brain, eyes, heart, or other regions of interest and that interfere with the biological signals of interest (66). These include physiological, environmental, and instrumental artifacts.

2.18.1. PHYSIOLOGICAL ARTIFACTS

It is important to recognize physiological artifacts resulting from movements of the head, eyes, and other body parts (Figs. 36.25, 36.26, 36.27), rhythmic leg movements causing tremor-like artifacts (Fig. 36.28), movements originating from muscles causing myogenic artifacts (Fig. 36.29), and movements of the heart giving rise to ECG artifacts (Fig. 36.30), which may interfere with recordings from the regions of interest and may sometimes be mistaken for slow waves in the EEG. Sweating, by causing excessive baseline swaying, produces very slow oscillations lasting for 1 to 3 sec, mainly during non-REM sleep, as a result of action potentials generated by the salt content of the sweat glands (Fig. 36.31).

2.18.2. ENVIRONMENTAL ARTIFACTS

The most important environmental artifact is the 60-Hz artifact (Fig. 36.32) resulting from electromagnetic radiation from AC current in power lines (in many other countries the mains frequency is 50 Hz). Most often this results from high impedance of the electrodes. The impedance should be kept at <5 K.

2.18.3. INSTRUMENTAL ARTIFACTS

These artifacts result from faulty electrodes (Fig. 36.33), resembling transient sharp or slow waves limited to one electrode, wires, switches, and the PSG machine itself due to random fluctuations of charges causing instrumental noise artifacts.

3. CLINICAL CONSIDERATIONS

3.1. Narcolepsy and Other Hypersomnias

Narcolepsy is a disorder of EDS that is usually accompanied by other "auxiliary" symptoms such as cataplexy, hypnagogic

Sleep Study Report

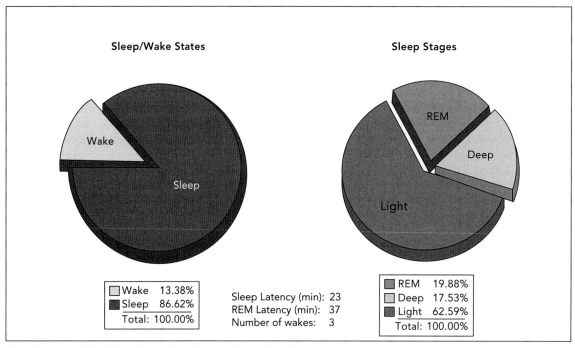

Sleep/Wake States

Wake

Sleep

Wake	13.38%
Sleep	86.62%
Total:	**100.00%**

Sleep Latency (min): 23
REM Latency (min): 37
Number of wakes: 3

Sleep Stages

REM

Deep

Light

REM	19.88%
Deep	17.53%
Light	62.59%
Total:	**100.00%**

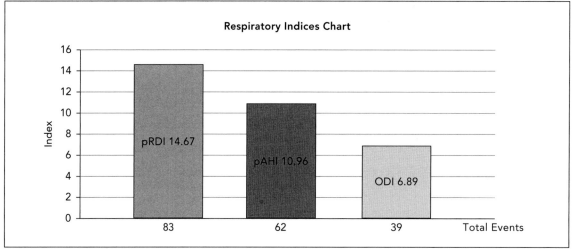

Respiratory Indices Chart

pRDI 14.67

pAHI 10.96

ODI 6.89

Index

83   62   39   Total Events

Figure 36.24. Graphic representation from the same patient's (Fig. 36.23) HSAT recording showing sleep–wake states; sleep stages; respiratory disturbance index (RDI); apnea–hypopnea index (AHI); and oxygen desaturation index (ODI). The data are consistent with mild OSA.

hallucinations, and sleep paralysis. Additional features commonly include disrupted nighttime sleep and excessive motor activity in sleep. A more complete review of the clinical features of narcolepsy can be found in the literature (67,68). Nevertheless, the *International Classification of Sleep Disorders—3rd Edition* (ICSD-3) (69) distinguishes between Type 1 narcolepsy (characterized by EDS, sleep fragmentation, and cataplexy with cerebrospinal fluid hypocretin deficiency) and Type 2 narcolepsy (with absence of cataplectic features and normal cerebrospinal fluid hypocretin levels) (69).

During the initial diagnostic evaluation of a patient with possible narcolepsy, a PSG is usually done in tandem with an MSLT. Excessive and pathologic motor activity during sleep (i.e., PLMS and RBD) and sleep-disordered breathing are

common in individuals with narcolepsy. Nevertheless, sleep-disordered breathing and PLMS seem to be rarely severe, suggesting an overall limited effect on clinical manifestations (70). Even more remarkable is the high incidence of RBD in narcolepsy. In a group of narcolepsy patients off medication, 60% provided a history of RBD and 40% demonstrated RBD during PSG (71). Another 14% had evidence of REM sleep without atonia. Studies have expanded on the observations of PSG in narcolepsy patients (71,72). The nighttime sleep of narcoleptics is characterized by increased awakenings, decreased Stage N1, decreased Stage N3, and shortened REM latency. Abnormal sleep transitions during a nocturnal polysomnography can be identified in narcolepsy (73). Moreover, nocturnal sleep onset Stage REM period (SOREMP; a REM sleep latency

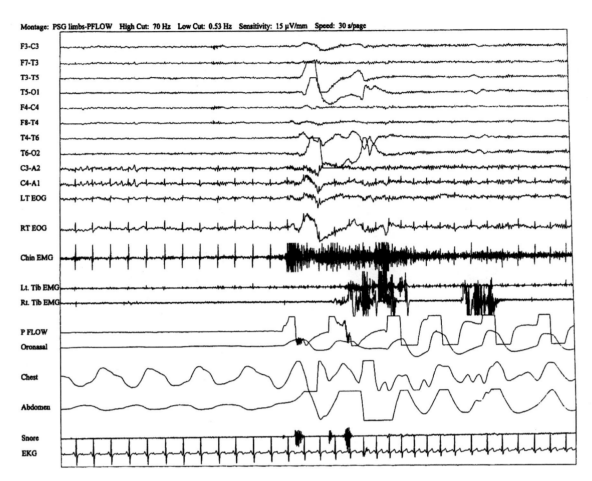

Montage: PSG limbs-PFLOW   High Cut: 70 Hz   Low Cut: 0.53 Hz   Sensitivity: 15 µV/mm   Speed: 30 s/page

Figure 36.25. A 30-sec excerpt from overnight PSG recording shows body movement artifact following an obstructive apnea as demonstrated by variable, high-voltage, asymmetrical and asynchronous slow activity on EEG channels and increased EMG activity on chin and tibialis anterior electrode channels. Top 10 channels, EEG; LT and RT EOG, left and right electro-oculograms; chin EMG, electromyography of chin muscles; Lt. and Rt. Tib EMG, left and right tibialis anterior electromyography; P Flow, peak flow; oronasal thermistor; chest and abdomen effort channels; snore monitor; EKG, electrocardiography. *Reproduced from Chokroverty S, Thomas R, Bhatt M, eds. Atlas of Sleep Medicine. Philadelphia: Elsevier; 2005, with permission.*

<15 minutes during a nocturnal polysomnographic study) has been found to be highly specific (~99%) for narcolepsy (74,75) and was added back as a diagnostic criterion in the ICSD-3. The PSG is also used to document adequate sleep duration (usually >6 hours) and sleep quality to allow confident interpretation of the MSLT performed the following day. The focus of the MSLT is to document the pathologic hypersomnolence (as a shortened sleep latency) and to evaluate any abnormal REM sleep pressure through the identification of SOREMP in the brief nap trials.

Idiopathic hypersomnia is another disorder of EDS that also presents in adolescence or young adulthood. Generally, idiopathic hypersomnia categorizes individuals who have prominent EDS but lack the classic features of narcolepsy or evidence of another disorder known to cause such sleepiness. Moreover, the sleepiness of idiopathic hypersomnia is usually less severe than that seen in narcolepsy, but it has a more pervasive all-day character that is not impacted by daytime naps. Nighttime sleep in idiopathic hypersomnia is usually described as long and uninterrupted (76). An early study of nighttime sleep in narcolepsy and idiopathic hypersomnia confirmed most of these clinical impressions (77). Patients with idiopathic hypersomnia usually show shortened initial

sleep latency, normal or increased total sleep time, and normal sleep architecture, in contrast to narcoleptic patients, who exhibit significant sleep fragmentation. Mean sleep latency at MSLT is typically <8 minutes in idiopathic hypersomnia, but SOREMPs are not typically seen as in narcolepsy (Fig. 36.34 and Fig. 36.35). In addition, the coexistence of sleep-disordered breathing and PLMS was less frequently noted in idiopathic hypersomnia. Episodic hypersomnias are also described and include Kleine–Levin syndrome (KLS) and menstrual-associated hypersomnia.

KLS is a rare recurrent encephalopathy primarily affecting teenagers, characterized by relapsing-remitting episodes of hypersomnia along with cognitive, psychiatric, and behavioral disturbances. During episodes, patients suddenly present with hypersomnia (with sleep lasting 15–21 hours/day), cognitive impairment (major apathy, confusion, slowness, amnesia), and a specific feeling of derealization (dreamy state, altered perception). Less frequently, they may also experience hyperphagia (66%), hypersexuality (53%, principally men), depressed mood (53%, principally women), anxiety, hallucinations, and acute brief psychosis (33%). The first episode of hypersomnia is often triggered by an infection, with relapses occurring every 1 to 12 months for a median of 14 years. Disease duration can

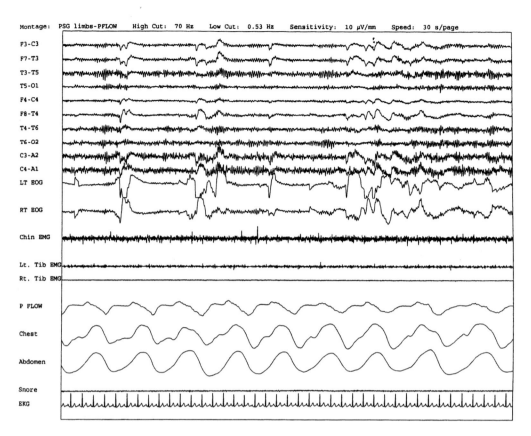

Figure 36.26. A 30-sec epoch from overnight PSG showing repetitive blink artifact best noted in the EOG channels and on the frontal and anterior temporal EEG electrode recordings. This can be misinterpreted as abnormal cerebral activity. Top 10 channels: EEGs; LT and RT EOG, left and right electro-oculograms; chin EMG, electromyography of chin muscles; Lt. and Rt. Tib EMG, left and right tibialis anterior electromyography; P. Flow, peak flow; chest and abdomen effort channels; snore monitor; EKG, electrocardiography. Reproduced from Chokroverty S, Thomas R, Bhatt M, eds. Atlas of Sleep Medicine. Philadelphia: Elsevier; 2005, with permission.

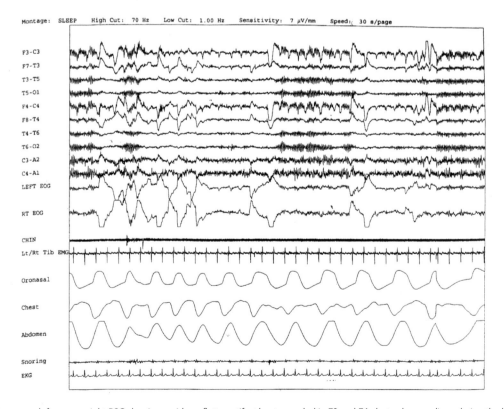

Figure 36.27. A 20-sec epoch from overnight PSG showing rapid eye flutter artifact best recorded in F3 and F4 electrode recordings during the latter half of the epoch. A blink artifact is noted in the initial part of the recording and is best seen on the EOG channels. Well-formed alpha rhythm is noted in the background on all EEG channels when eyes are closed. Reproduced from Chokroverty S, Thomas R, Bhatt M, eds. Atlas of Sleep Medicine. Philadelphia: Elsevier; 2005, with permission.

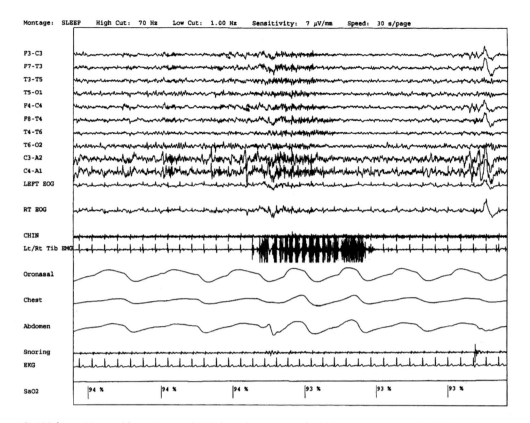

Figure 36.28. Overnight PSG from a 50-year-old man. Nocturnal PSG shows the presence of mild sleep apnea with an AHI of 12.3. A 30-sec excerpt from nocturnal PSG shows bursts of rhythmic foot and leg movements on the left/right tibialis anterior muscle recording channel during Stage 2 of NREM sleep. The movement is not associated with respiratory events, oxygen desaturation, or arousal from sleep. Top 10 channels: EEGs; LEFT and RT EOG, left and right electro-oculograms; chin EMG, electromyography of chin muscles; Lt/Rt Tib EMG, left/right tibialis anterior EMG; oronasal thermistor; chest and abdomen effort channels; snore monitor; EKG, electrocardiography; SaO2, oxygen saturation by finger oximetry. Reproduced from Chokroverty S, Thomas R, Bhatt M, eds. Atlas of Sleep Medicine. Philadelphia: Elsevier; 2005, with permission.

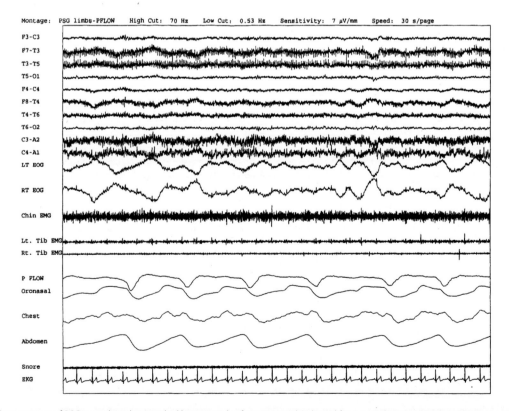

Figure 36.29. A 30-sec excerpt of PSG recording shows spike-like potentials of varying amplitude and frequency denoting muscle activity not only on the chin EMG channel but also in all EEG channels, particularly prominent in T3, T4, A2, and A1 electrode derivations. Top 10 channels: EEGs; LT and RT EOG, left and right electro-oculograms; chin EMG, electromyography of chin muscles; Lt. and Rt. Tib EMG, left and right tibialis anterior electromyography; P Flow, peak flow; oronasal thermistor; chest and abdomen effort channels; snore monitor; EKG, electrocardiography. Reproduced from Chokroverty S, Thomas R, Bhatt M, eds. Atlas of Sleep Medicine. Philadelphia: Elsevier; 2005, with permission.

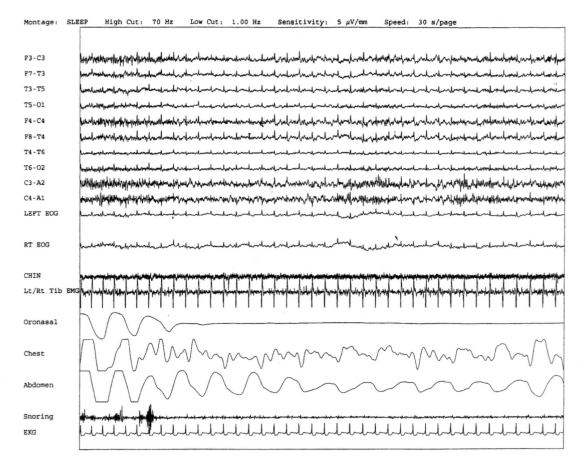

Figure 36.30. *A 30-sec excerpt from an overnight PSG selected to show ECG artifact, which is characterized by its morphology, rhythm, and synchrony with ECG recording. It is seen throughout the epoch on EEG, EOG, and tibialis EMG channels. Incidentally, an obstructive apnea is seen in the airflow and effort channels. Top 10 channels: EEGs; LEFT and RT EOG, left and right electro-oculograms; CHIN, electromyography of chin; Lt/Rt Tib EMG, left and right tibialis anterior electromyography; oronasal thermistor; chest and abdomen effort channels; snore monitor; EKG, electrocardiography. Reproduced from Chokroverty S, Thomas R, Bhatt M, eds. Atlas of Sleep Medicine. Philadelphia: Elsevier; 2005, with permission.*

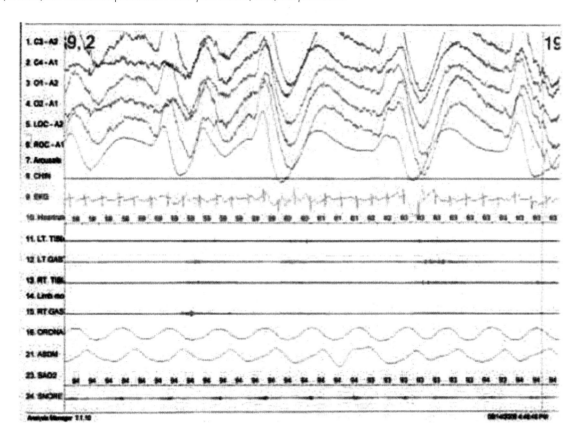

Figure 36.31. *Sweat artifact at 30 sec. Reproduced from Siddiqui F, Osuna E, Walters AS, et al. Sweat artifact and respiratory artifact occurring simultaneously in polysomnogram. Sleep Med. 2006;7(2):197–199, with permission.*

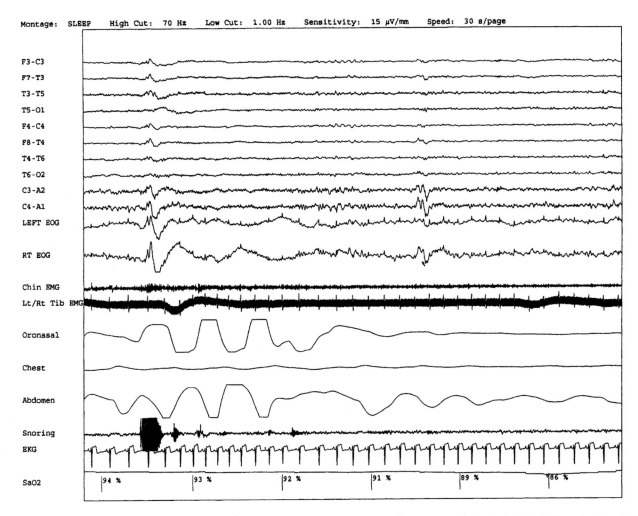

Montage: SLEEP   High Cut: 70 Hz   Low Cut: 1.00 Hz   Sensitivity: 15 µV/mm   Speed: 30 s/page

F3-C3
F7-T3
T3-T5
T5-O1
F4-C4
F8-T4
T4-T6
T6-O2
C3-A2
C4-A1
LEFT EOG
RT EOG
Chin EMG
Lt/Rt Tib EMG
Oronasal
Chest
Abdomen
Snoring
EKG
SaO2 |94 % |93 % |92 % |91 % |89 % |86 %

Figure 36.32. A 30-sec excerpt from an overnight PSG recording shows a uniform monorhythmic artifact at 60 Hz on left/right tibialis EMG channel, which is further superimposed by an ECG artifact. The 60-Hz artifact is due to electrical interference from power lines and equipment occurring at a frequency of 60 Hz in North America (but at 50 Hz in many other countries). Maximum interference is seen in the presence of poor electrode contact. Incidentally, an obstructive apnea is noted in the airflow and respiratory effort channels. Top 10 channels: EEGs; LEFT and RT EOG, left and right electro-oculograms; chin EMG, electromyography of chin muscles; Lt/Rt Tib EMG, left and right tibialis anterior electromyography; oronasal thermistor; chest and abdomen effort channels; snore monitor; EKG, electrocardiography; SaO2, oxygen saturation. *Reproduced from Chokroverty S, Thomas R, Bhatt M, eds.* Atlas of Sleep Medicine. *Philadelphia: Elsevier; 2005, with permission.*

be much longer with childhood or adult onset than in patients with adolescent onset. Between episodes, patients generally have normal sleep patterns, cognition, mood, and eating habits (78,79). The pathogenesis of KLS is unknown, with hypotheses centering on neurotransmitter imbalance or autoimmune mechanisms. There is no consensus on accompanying PSG findings in KLS, likely related to variability in the timing of the studies with reference to the hypersomnolent period. Up to 30% of patients have completely normal EEG findings during episodes. In 70% of cases, nonspecific diffuse slowing of background activity is seen, including the alpha frequency, which is notably higher between episodes (80). Low-frequency high-amplitude waves (delta or theta) also occur, in isolation or in sequence, mainly in the bilateral temporal or temporofrontal areas when patients are awake, which parallels the findings on single photon emission computed tomography (SPECT) (78).

The findings in PSG sleep studies are often difficult to interpret and are affected by whether sleep is monitored for one night or during a 24-hour period, at the beginning or at the end of an episode, and during the first or a later episode. In 18 patients monitored for 24 hours during episodes, the total sleep duration recorded by PSG was ~11 to 12 hours per patient (81). In another study of 14 patients, nighttime sleep lasted 9 to 10 hours, compared with 6 to 7 hours between episodes (82). In 17 Taiwanese children, the proportion of slow-wave sleep at night was decreased during the first half of episodes and that of REM sleep was decreased during the second half of episodes (83).

MSLT is difficult to do in patients with KLS during episodes, but it might show a narcolepsy-like pattern (SOREMPs) and be abnormal during and between episodes (83). Overall, sleep studies have shown that even if sleep is extended for up to 12 hours during episodes, between 3 and 9 hours per day are spent in a state with eyes closed that seems closer to a state of withdrawal and apathy than to sleep.

Episodes of hypersomnia have been rarely reported just before or during menstruation (84–86). Episodes in these cases may be associated with compulsive eating, sexual disinhibition, and depressive mood, last 3 to 15 days, and occur fewer

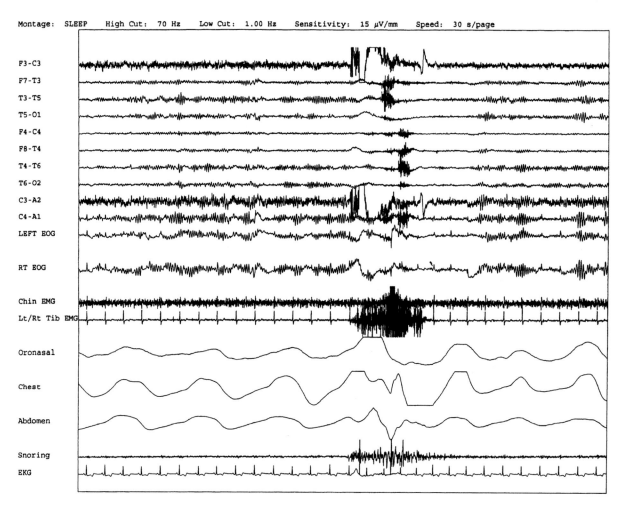

Figure 36.33. A 30-sec excerpt from an overnight PSG recording shows the presence of a C3 electrode pop artifact. Near the middle of the epoch, it is accentuated by a movement artifact simultaneously recorded on the chin EMG, left and right tibialis anterior EMG, and snoring channel. Top 10 channels: EEGs; LEFT and RT EOG, left and right electro-oculograms; chin EMG, electromyography of chin muscles; Lt/Rt Tib EMG, left and right tibialis anterior electromyography; oronasal thermistor; chest and abdomen effort channels; snore monitor; EKG, electrocardiography. *Reproduced from Chokroverty S, Thomas R, Bhatt M, eds. Atlas of Sleep Medicine. Philadelphia: Elsevier; 2005, with permission.*

than three times per year on average. Decreased frequency of episodes has been reported in response to treatment with estrogen-containing contraceptive pills in some cases (87).

3.2. Parasomnias

Parasomnias are defined as unpleasant or undesirable behavioral or experiential phenomena that occur predominantly or exclusively during the sleep period. The parasomnias are conveniently classified according to the sleep state of origin as NREM sleep parasomnias, REM sleep parasomnias, or miscellaneous (i.e., those not related to the sleep state).

NREM parasomnias refer to disorders of arousal that occur on a broad spectrum ranging from confusional arousal, through sleepwalking, to sleep terrors. Disorders of arousal typically arise from slow-wave sleep (N3), and therefore usually occur in the first third of the night, and they are common in childhood. During *confusional arousal* the individual whimpers, moans, moves about slowly, may speak in short phrases, and resists consoling or attention from others. These events may last up to 30 minutes. *Sleep terrors* tend to be briefer but

are associated with screams and autonomic activation (sweating, tachycardia, flushed face). A universal feature is inconsolability, and amnesia for the activity is typical. *Sleepwalking* events are similar to confusional arousal in terms of time of the night, duration, and character of the behavior, but the individual moves about the house. Sleepwalking may be either calm or agitated, with varying degrees of complexity and duration. In disorders of arousal at the start of an event, the PSG recording usually shows sudden arousals from slow-wave sleep, without anticipatory tachycardia, sometimes accompanied by bursts of high-amplitude rhythmic delta or theta activity (Fig. 36.36).

RBD is the most common and best-studied REM sleep parasomnia. In patients with RBD, somatic muscle atonia, one of the defining features of REM sleep, is absent, permitting the acting out of dream mentation, often with violent or injurious results (Fig. 36.37; ◑ Video 36.1: RBD). It usually comes to medical attention when the aggressive dream enactment has resulted in injury to the patient or bed partner (88,89). Two striking demographic characteristics of RBD are that it predominantly affects males (~90%) and usually begins after the age of 50 years. RBD in humans occurs in both an acute

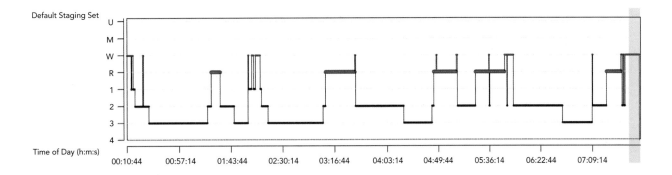

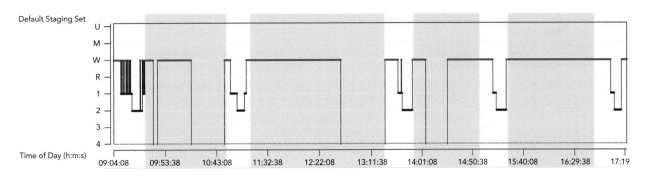

Figure 36.34. Idiopathic hypersomnia sleep histogram and MSLT. Upper panel: *Nocturnal sleep histogram of a patient with idiopathic hypersomnia showing shortened initial sleep latency, with quite normal total sleep time and normal sleep architecture.* Lower panel: *MSLT histogram of the same patient with idiopathic hypersomnia showing mean sleep latency <8 minutes but without SOREMPS.*

and chronic form. The acute form is often due to undesirable side effects of prescribed medications, most commonly antidepressant medications, particularly selective serotonin reuptake inhibitors (SSRIs). The chronic form of RBD is usually either idiopathic or most commonly associated with neurological disorders. One of the most interesting implications of chronic RBD is its growing association as a prodromal manifestation with neurodegenerative disorders, particularly

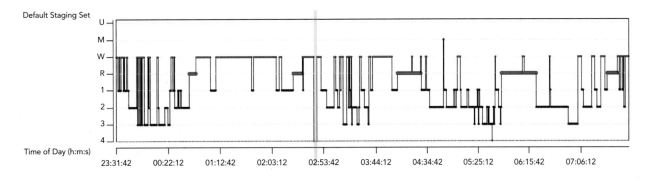

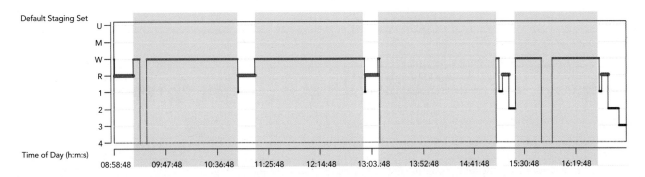

Figure 36.35. Narcolepsy sleep histogram and MSLT. Upper panel: *Nocturnal sleep histogram of a patient with narcolepsy showing significant sleep fragmentation.* Lower panel: *MSLT histogram of the same patient with narcolepsy showing mean sleep latency <2 minutes with five SOREMPS.*

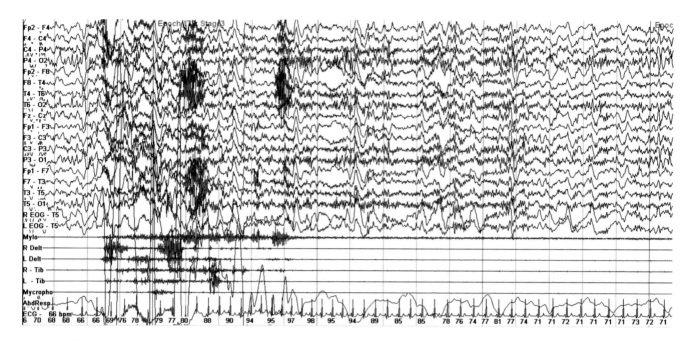

Figure 36.36. *PSG example of disorder of arousal. Note the precipitous arousal from slow-wave sleep (NREM Stage N3 sleep) without anticipatory tachycardia, with the EEG showing persistent slowing even though the patient was talking and appeared to be awake (half-awake/half-aroused).*

the synucleinopathies (Parkinson's disease, multiple system atrophy, or dementia with Lewy body disease). RBD may be the first manifestation of these conditions and may precede any other manifestation of the underlying neurodegenerative process by >10 years (90,91). RBD is also seen more frequently in other neurological disorders with brainstem dysfunction, including multiple sclerosis (92) and narcolepsy (93).

The behavioral events of RBD occur during REM sleep and tend to be more frequent in the early morning. Frequency is variable, so a single-night PSG recording will often not record any of the dream-enacted behaviors. Greater attention has been

paid to objectively evaluating the degree of muscle atonia present in REM sleep as a way to identify patients with an increased risk of dream enactment (94). The *AASM Scoring Manual* defined criteria for scoring pathologic muscle activity during REM sleep (12). Sustained muscle activity (tonic activity) in REM sleep is defined as an epoch of REM in which at least 50% of the epoch duration has a chin EMG amplitude greater than the minimum amplitude in NREM sleep. Excessive transient muscle activity (phasic activity) in REM sleep is defined as when at least five of the 10 "3-sec mini-epochs" (in a 30-sec epoch) have bursts of transient muscle activity. In RBD, the

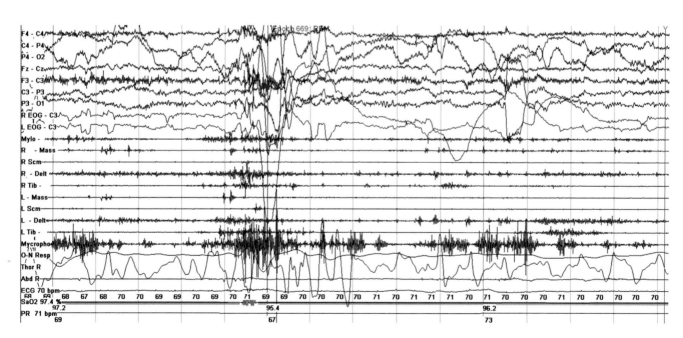

Figure 36.37. *PSG correlates of RBD. Note REM sleep features with activated EEG, rapid eye movements, and quite constant ECG rate about 70 beats (despite vigorous limb movements); prominent phasic and tonic submental EMG activity; and prominent recurrent EMG activity in the other muscle recording channels.*

excessive transient muscle activity bursts are 0.1 to 5.0 sec in duration and at least four times the amplitude of background EMG activity. The PSG characteristics of RBD can include either or both the tonic and phasic EMG observations. REM sleep without atonia can occur without accompanying clinical behaviors; as such, RBD remains a clinical diagnosis that can be complemented by the abnormal observations of muscle activity during REM sleep as defined by the AASM guidelines (12). SSRIs and selective norepinephrine reuptake inhibitors (SNRIs) commonly provoke REM sleep without atonia, with or without associated clinical RBD episodes. Most investigations have also reported an increased incidence of PLMS in individuals with RBD. Other abnormalities are not usually described on PSG.

3.3. Sleep-Related Epilepsies

The interface between sleep and epilepsy is vast and compelling, because sleep affects seizures and seizures affect sleep. The myriad of sleep and epileptic phenomena may perfectly counterfeit one another. An extensive overview of sleep and epilepsy is beyond the scope of this chapter, and epilepsy is extensively discussed elsewhere. However, sleep-related epilepsies will be briefly discussed here, with a focus on their differentiation from other sleep disorders, namely disorders of arousal and RBD. We will also briefly review the role of PSG in the evaluation of a patient with epilepsy.

An EEG recording during sleep is more sensitive to the identification of interictal epileptiform abnormality than an EEG recording only during wakefulness. Given the difficulties in recording a sleep EEG during the daytime (usually requiring sleep deprivation or sedation), the use of an all-night sleep recording to identify interictal epileptiform activity may be useful (95,96). PSG recordings may be used to assist in the diagnosis of unusual nocturnal behavior. In most settings prolonged video-EEG recording is used as the primary diagnostic tool if the primary diagnostic concern is seizures. Overnight PSG may be used to evaluate potential epileptic seizures, particularly if prolonged video-EEG monitoring is unavailable. PSG does more confidently identify sleep stage (and any accompanying sleep abnormality, such as sleep apnea) than video-EEG recordings. However, the limited EEG montage used on routine PSG represents a significant disadvantage. An extended EEG montage or continuous video-EEG recording with extended sleep parameters is required for neurophysiological investigation of patients with nocturnal spells. This recording should include greater EEG coverage of the frontal and temporal head region and must be reviewed at the 20-sec/page display, as opposed to the typical 30-sec/page display, to better discriminate epileptiform activity from other background activity (95,96).

Nocturnal frontal lobe epilepsy (NFLE) is a remarkable disorder in which the seizures manifest by bizarre motor behavior that occurs almost exclusively during sleep. On the basis of the different intensity, duration, and features of the motor patterns, the NFLE epileptic seizures have been classified into three groups:

1. Paroxysmal arousals: brief (<20 sec) episodes in which patients suddenly open their eyes, raise their heads, or sit up in bed with a bizarre posture of the limbs, staring around with a frightened or surprised expression, and sometimes screaming; they then return to sleep (⦿ Video 36.2: NFLE Paroxysmal Arousal).

2. Nocturnal paroxysmal dystonia: episodes are longer (20 seconds to 2 minutes) and include more complex behaviors characterized by wide-ranging, often violent, and sometimes ballistic movements, with dystonic posturing of the head, trunk, and limbs, such as head rotation, torsion of the trunk, and choreoathetoid movements of the arms and legs, with vocalization (Fig. 36.38).

3. Episodic nocturnal wandering: episodes last up to 1 to 3 minutes and the characteristic feature is stereotypic paroxysmal ambulation during sleep, often with agitation and accompanied by screaming and bizarre, dystonic movements (97,98).

NFLE should always be suspected in the presence of paroxysmal nocturnal motor events characterized by a high frequency of same-night or inter-night recurrence, persistence beyond puberty into adulthood, quasi-extrapyramidal features, agitated behavior, and remarkable stereotypy of the attacks. Although EEG recordings during the attacks can fail to disclose ictal epileptic activity, the stereotyped movements and behaviors mark again the epileptic nature of the nocturnal events. The absence of scalp EEG ictal epileptic activity during the NFLE seizure attacks in some patients can be explained by the seizure focus being located in deep brain regions (98). Parasomnias need to be carefully considered in the differential diagnosis of NFLE (99). Disorders of arousals rarely occur more than once per night, very rarely occur nightly, almost never occur nightly for months or years, and are not stereotyped, and the usual EEG pattern seen during the episode is a diffuse hypersynchronous slowing in the theta or delta range. During RBD, the EEG is that of REM sleep. In both cases, superimposed EMG and movement artifact complicates the interpretation.

Disorders of arousals are common in childhood, usually decreasing in frequency with increasing age. The seizures of NFLE can begin at any age, occur more frequently (often many times per night), are briefer (several seconds up to a minute), and have a stereotyped pattern. Several reviews in the literature attempt to review how clinical information may help in differentiating the character of these nocturnal events (100,101).

3.4. Sleep Apnea-Hypopnea Syndrome

Sleep-related breathing disorders include several conditions broadly divided into two types: upper airway obstructive sleep apnea syndrome (OSAS) and central sleep apnea syndrome (CSAS). OSAS is the most common sleep-related breathing disorder and the most common indication for referral of patients to sleep laboratories for PSG. Two groups of neurologists, Gastaut and Tassinari from France (42) and Jung and Kuhlo from Germany (102), in 1965 independently discovered

the site of obstruction in the upper airway. In CSAS the problem lies in an imbalance of CNS respiratory control.

3.4.1. UPPER AIRWAY OBSTRUCTIVE SLEEP APNEA SYNDROME

OSAS is characterized by recurrent pharyngeal collapses during sleep. The pathophysiology of OSAS is multifactorial and includes a reduction in upper airway dimensions that can result from both anatomical and functional alterations (obesity or maxillofacial changes), and increased pharyngeal collapsibility owing to reduced neuromuscular compensation and lack of pharyngeal protective reflex during sleep (103–105). The decreased upper airway size and increased resistance might result in snoring by vibration of the soft palate, the uvula,

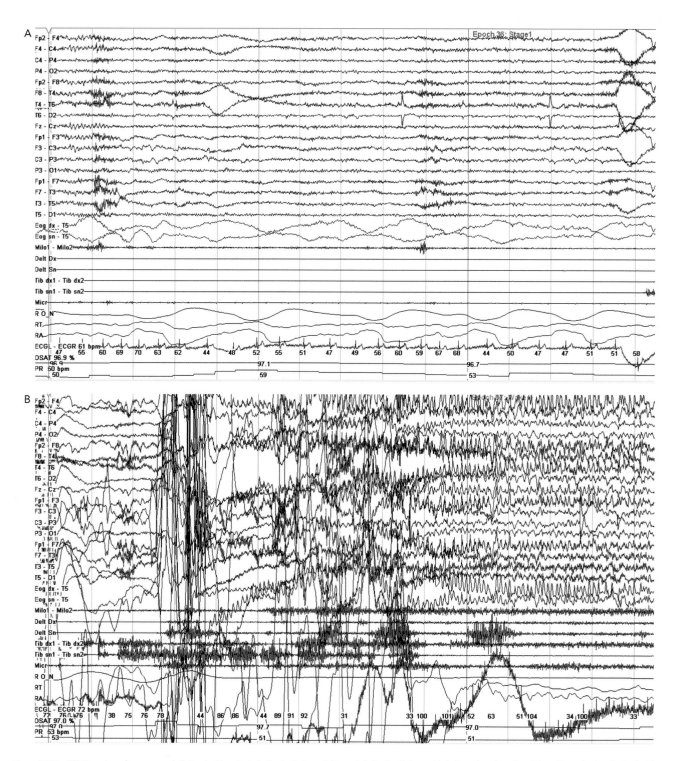

Figure 36.38. NFLE nocturnal paroxysmal dystonia. Transient rhythmic theta activity mainly in the right and left frontal regions is evident (*A*, at the beginning). After ~30 sec (*B* and *C*), a spell with the features of nocturnal paroxysmal dystonia is registered with the patient turning the head toward the left side and displaying a bizarre motor behavior characterized by asymmetric bilateral dystonic posture and choreoathetoid movements, with generalized paroxysmal rhythmic activity on the EEG.

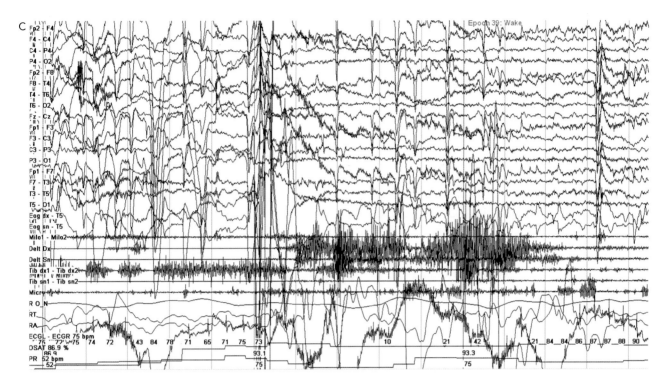

Figure 36.38. *Continued*

and/or the lateral walls of the pharynx (106). The upper airway collapse can be complete, leading to an obstructive apnea, defined as a reduction of air flow of >90% associated with persistent respiratory movement. Partial closure corresponds to hypopnea, defined as a reduction in ventilation of >30% from baseline and oxygen desaturation of >3% from baseline or microarousal (12,69). Owing to their short duration (3–15 sec), microarousals are not perceived by the patients but still cause sleep fragmentation. In particular, obstructive apnea and hypopnea cause intermittent hypoxia, which has a large role in the pathophysiology of OSAS (107) and in its major consequences, including EDS, cardiovascular comorbidities, and increased risk of death from any cause, at least in severe OSAS (107,108). OSAS is now considered a major public health issue, affecting 5% to 15% of the general population, increasing linearly with age up to at least 60 to 65 years (43,109,110).

The diagnosis of OSAS can be made during a sleep study. A diagnosis is made if there are more than five predominantly obstructive respiratory events (obstructive and mixed apneas, hypopneas, or respiratory effort-related arousals) per hour of sleep (see Fig. 36.18B and 36.18C) in a patient with at least one of the following symptoms or clinical signs: EDS, nonrestorative sleep, fatigue or insomnia, waking up with choking, breath holding or gasping, witnessed habitual snoring and/or breathing interruptions, and hypertension, mood disorder, cognitive dysfunction, coronary artery disease, stroke, congestive heart failure, atrial fibrillation, or type 2 diabetes mellitus. OSAS severity depends on the severity of daytime sleepiness, the AHI and/or oxygen desaturation index (ODI) range based on overnight monitoring (mild, AHI 5–15; moderate, AHI 15–30; severe, AHI > 30). Of note, sleep apnea events discovered in a sleep recording in individuals without any symptoms do *not* constitute OSAS except when the AHI exceeds 15 (69,111).

The sleep study is the most important investigative tool in the process of making the diagnosis of OSAS. Full PSG, respiratory polygraphy, and overnight oximetry are the three major types of sleep studies for OSAS. Full PSG is regarded as the diagnostic gold standard and usually includes assessment of oximetry, snoring, body and leg movements, oronasal airflow, excursion of chest and abdomen, as well as an ECG, EEG, EOG, and EMG to identify sleep stages. Respiratory polygraphy usually includes all these assessments but without an EEG, EOG, and EMG. The equipment for respiratory polygraphy and oximetry is suitable for HSAT, which allows the patients to sleep in their own environment and potentially reflects normal ambient conditions better than a sleep laboratory. By contrast, full PSG generally requires a sleep laboratory and a trained technician to set up and supervise the sleep study during the entire night and, accordingly, is resource-intensive (Fig. 36.39; ⬤ Video 36.3: OSAS). However, there are some limitations in the interpretation of results obtained from HSAT, such as a higher rate of technically unsatisfactory studies compared with full PSG, the limitation of not knowing whether the patient was awake or asleep, and the fact that other diagnoses, such as PLMS, might be missed (described above). Nonetheless, limited sleep studies, such as respiratory polygraphy, have become the routine investigation in cases where OSAS is suspected. Although oximetry alone can identify OSAS in most patients with a high clinical likelihood, false-positive oximetry results occur in patients with Cheyne-Stokes breathing and when there is a low baseline oximetry saturation, as in patients with COPD. False-negative results can occur in non-obese patients and those with primarily hypopneas, as in milder cases of OSAS.

Management of OSAS should be tailored to the severity of the condition. Severe OSAS always requires treatment,

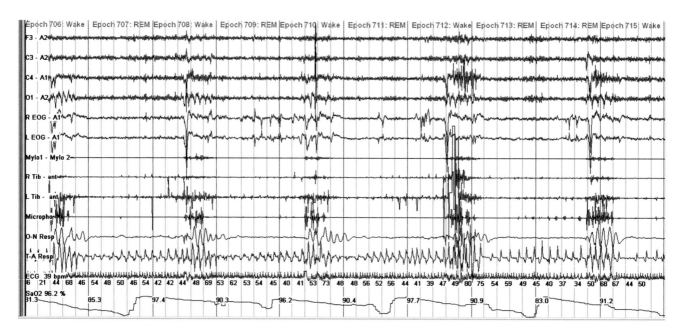

Figure 36.39. *PSG in a patient with OSAS. Each OSA episode is associated with a cessation of flow, a progressive increase in respiratory effort, and a reduction in oxygen saturation, which is delayed. Note the persistence of the thoracic and abdominal movements, which correspond to persistent respiratory effort despite the closure of the pharynx and subsequent cessation of flow. Each OSA episode is also associated with an arousal visible on the ECG, EMG, and EOG.*

and CPAP is the first-line option to prevent collapse of the pharynx (Fig. 36.40). Mild to moderate OSAS should be also treated with CPAP or oral appliances such as a mandibular advancement device, the latter with video-PSG documentation of the efficacy and maintenance of efficacy over time. Upper airway surgery can be considered when the patient has craniofacial abnormalities. Regardless, weight loss is mandatory when overweight or obesity is present. CPAP works as a pneumatic splint to keep the airways open. The optimal CPAP pressure must first be determined by an overnight PSG study (see Fig. 36.40) and the patient can then purchase a home unit for use during the night's sleep. Adherence to CPAP is a crucial issue. Moreover, CPAP has limitations, and combination therapies (CPAP plus weight loss or CPAP plus specific antihypertensive treatments) may be required to reverse the chronic consequences of OSAS (i.e., EDS and cardiovascular and metabolic outcomes) (112,113).

3.4.2. Central Sleep Apnea Syndrome

The term "central sleep apnea" encompasses a heterogeneous group of sleep-related breathing disorders in which respiratory effort is diminished or absent in an intermittent or cyclical fashion during sleep. In most cases, central sleep apnea is caused by an underlying medical condition, recent ascent to high altitude, or narcotic use. Primary central sleep apnea is a rare condition, the etiology of which is not entirely understood. During PSG, a central apneic event is conventionally defined as cessation of airflow for 10 sec or longer without an identifiable respiratory effort (🔘 Video 36.4: Central Sleep Apnea). In general, treatment of central sleep apnea is often more difficult than treatment of obstructive sleep apnea, and treatment varies according to the specific syndrome. The ICSD-3 (69) describes several different entities grouped under central sleep apnea with varying signs, symptoms, and clinical and PSG features.

Those that affect adults include primary central sleep apnea, Cheyne-Stokes breathing/central sleep apnea (CSB-CSA) pattern, high-altitude periodic breathing, central sleep apnea due to medical conditions other than Cheyne-Stokes, and central sleep apnea due to drugs or substances. The primary central sleep apnea of infancy primarily affects premature newborns and is excluded from this discussion.

CSB-CSA is characterized by a classic crescendo/decrescendo pattern (Fig. 36.41) that typically occurs with a periodicity of 45-sec or greater cycles with at least five central apneas per hour of sleep accompanied by arousals and derangement of sleep structure. The arousals occur at the peak of the hyperpnea phase. Patients usually have predisposing factors such as heart failure, stroke, or renal failure, as well as a lower resting $PaCO_2$ than normal.

Two types of pathophysiological phenomena can cause CSAS: (1) ventilatory instability or (2) depression of the brainstem respiratory centers or chemoreceptors. Ventilatory instability is the mechanism behind CSB-CSA, high-altitude periodic breathing, and probably primary central sleep apnea (104). Central sleep apnea-hypoventilation syndromes such as those associated with narcotic use or brainstem lesions are due to disturbances of the central respiratory pattern center or peripheral chemoreceptors (or both) that may become more evident during sleep because of the suppression of wakefulness or behavior drive. Predominant central apnea is uncommon and is seen in <10% of patients presenting for PSG. In the general population, the prevalence of central sleep apnea is <1% (44,114). CSB-CSA has been reported in 25% to 40% of patients with heart failure and in 10% of patients who have had a stroke. Primary central sleep apnea mostly affects middle-aged or elderly individuals. CSB-CSA increases in prevalence among individuals older than 60 years (115). The most common reported symptoms in CSAS are insomnia, daytime sleepiness, and fatigue. In general, the degree of daytime hypersomnolence is less than that observed with obstructive sleep apnea, and insomnia is more prominent. Notably, the presence of insomnia may actually put these patients at increased risk of central apneas because a greater number of sleep–wake transitions provide more opportunities for an unstable breathing pattern (116).

3.5. Circadian Rhythm Sleep Disorders

Circadian rhythm disorders are disruptions in a person's circadian rhythm—a name given to the "internal body clock" (i.e., the suprachiasmatic nucleus) that regulates the ~24-hour cycle of biological processes in animals and plants. The word "circadian" comes from Latin words that literally mean "around the day." The key feature of circadian rhythm disorders is a continuous or occasional disruption of sleep patterns. The disruption

results from either a malfunction in the internal body clock or a mismatch between the internal body clock and the external environment regarding the timing and duration of sleep. As a result of the circadian mismatch, individuals with these disorders usually complain of insomnia at certain times and excessive sleepiness at other times of the day, resulting in work, school, or social impairment (117).

3.5.1. Jet Lag Sleep Disorder
Jet lag results from a conflict between the pattern of sleep and wakefulness between the internal biological clock and that of a new time zone. Individuals find it hard to adjust and function optimally in the new time zone. Eastward travel is more difficult than westward travel because it is easier to delay sleep than to advance sleep. This desynchronization causes sleepiness, tiredness, and general malaise, impairment of judgment and concentration, and sometimes disorientation. Sleep problems

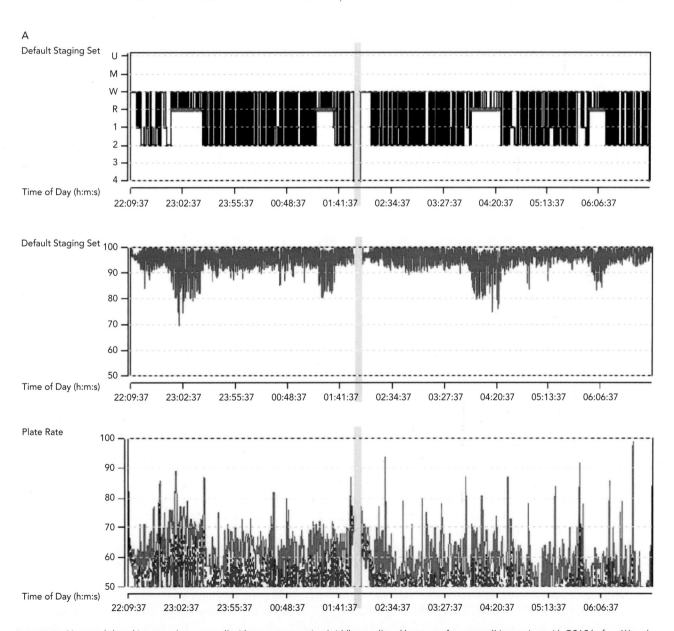

Figure 36.40. *Nocturnal sleep histogram* (upper panel) *with oxygen saturation* (middle panel) *and heart rate* (lower panel) *in a patient with OSAS before (A) and after (B) CPAP treatment.*

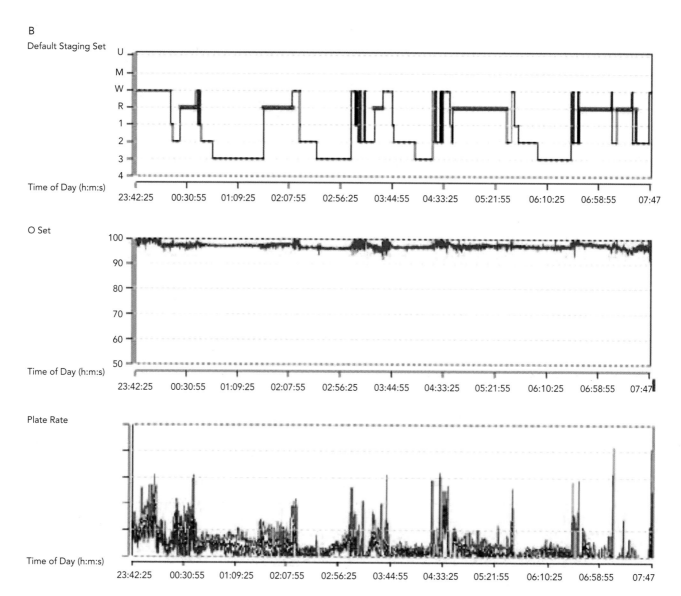

B

Default Staging Set

Time of Day (h:m:s)

O Set

Time of Day (h:m:s)

Plate Rate

Time of Day (h:m:s)

Figure 36.40. Continued

include difficulty maintaining sleep, frequent arousals, and daytime sleepiness. These symptoms may also be associated with gastrointestinal problems and the body's other rhythms, including those that control endocrine secretions, and body temperature. The symptoms may last for several days, depending on the direction of travel and the number of time zones traversed. It takes ~1.5 hours per day to readjust the internal body clock when traveling east as compared with 1 hour per day when traveling west. Symptoms also depend on age: older individuals take a longer time to readjust than younger ones.

3.5.2. Shift Work Sleep Disorder

Shift work disorder affects up to 5 million people in the United States who work irregular shifts, particularly night shifts. When work schedules conflict with the body's natural circadian rhythm, some individuals have difficulty adjusting to the change. Shift work sleep disorder is identified by a constant or recurrent pattern of sleep interruption that results in insomnia or excessive sleepiness, increasing chances of being involved in traffic accidents and making errors on the job.

3.5.3. Delayed Sleep Phase Disorder

Delayed sleep phase disorder is a circadian rhythm disorder most common in adolescents and young adults whose "night owl" tendencies delay sleep onset, often until 2 a.m. or later. If allowed to sleep in late (often as late as 3 p.m.), sleep deprivation does not occur. However, earlier wakeup times can lead to daytime sleepiness and impaired work and school performance. These individuals are often perceived as lazy, unmotivated, or poor performers who are chronically tardy for morning obligations. People with delayed sleep phase syndrome are often most alert, productive, and creative late at night.

3.5.4. Advanced Sleep Phase State

Advanced sleep phase state is usually seen in the elderly. This disorder is identified by regular early evening bedtimes (6 to 9 p.m.) and early morning awakenings (2 to 5 a.m.). People with advanced sleep phase syndrome are "morning larks" and typically complain of early morning awakening or insomnia as well as sleepiness in the late afternoon or early evening.

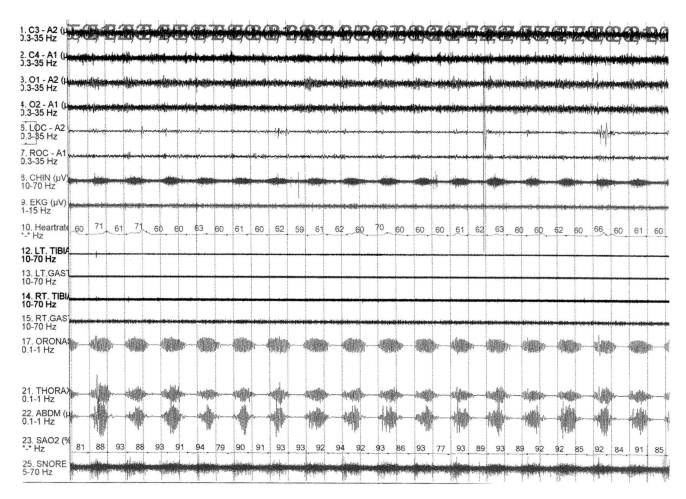

Figure 36.41. *Snapshot from overnight PSG study in a 69-year-old woman with heart failure showing crescendo/decrescendo pattern of breathing with central sleep apnea (Cheyne-Stokes breathing) seen in the respiratory channels (oronasal thermistor, thoracic [thorax], and abdominal [ABDM] effort channels), seen also in recording from chin (CHIN) muscle and snore (SNORE) channel. Top four channels: EEG (international nomenclature); EOG: left outer canthus (LOC) and right outer canthus (ROC) eyes referred to right (A2) and left (A1) mastoid, respectively; EKG: electrocardiogram; LT and RT TIB; left and right tibialis anterior muscles (EMG); LT and RT GAST: left and right Gastrocnemius muscle (EMG); SaO2; Oxygen saturation by finger oximetry.*

Familial advanced sleep phase state has been ascribed to mutation in the hPer 2 gene.

3.5.5. Free-Running Circadian Rhythm Disorder

This circadian rhythm sleep disorder (non-entrained type or non-24-hour sleep–wake syndrome) is characterized by a patient's inability to maintain a regular bedtime and wake time, and sleep onset occurs at irregular hours. In each 24-hour sleep–wake cycle the patient displays increasing delay of sleep onset by ~1 hour, causing an eventual progression of sleep onset to the daytime hours into the evening. This disorder is most often seen in blind people.

3.5.6. Irregular Sleep–Wake Circadian Rhythm Disorder

This circadian rhythm sleep disorder is characterized by lack of a clearly defined circadian rhythm of sleep and wake. Patients are seen to be napping throughout the 24-hour period, but total sleep time is normal. This condition may be seen in patients with degenerative neurological disorders such as dementia and children with mental retardation.

Actigraphy recordings are very useful in diagnosing this condition or any of the circadian rhythm sleep disorders (discussed later in Section 4).

3.6. Sleep-Related Movement Disorders

Sleep-related movement disorders are diagnosed when complaints of insomnia, daytime sleepiness and fatigue, or nonrestorative sleep are due to movements that occur during sleep or near the onset of sleep. These movements may be typically simple and stereotyped (i.e., short limb twitches), monophasic (i.e., sleep-related leg cramps), periodic (i.e., PLMS), and rhythmic (i.e., rhythmic movement disorders). Restless legs syndrome (RLS) is included here because of its close association with PLMS.

3.6.1. Restless Legs Syndrome

RLS is a heterogeneous, distressing, sensorimotor neurological movement disorder whose cardinal clinical features include an urge to move the legs, usually (but not always) with an uncomfortable sensation in the extremities described as crawling, muscle ache, or tension, that is partially or totally relieved by motor activity. It is worse at night. RLS may be idiopathic, or primary, when symptoms are not related to any other medical condition, or secondary to other medical or neurological disorders, or even drug use. Although the pathophysiology of RLS is not fully understood, evidence exists for both iron/transferrin and dopaminergic abnormalities being factors in its etiology. As iron is a major cofactor in dopaminergic neurotransmission, iron deficits may produce dopaminergic changes that exacerbate RLS symptoms. Although it occurs in 2% to 15% of the general population (118,119), RLS is often underrecognized and misdiagnosed, which may lead to significant physical and emotional disability. A female preponderance has been described in several studies (120–122). The mean age of patients with RLS falls within middle age (age 40 to 60); however, onset can occur from infancy to old age. RLS in children should be differentiated from or may be associated with attention-deficit/hyperactive disorder (ADHD) and growing pains (123,124). Although symptoms may arise before 30 years of age, most individuals do not seek medical attention until they reach their mid-30s, and many are not appropriately diagnosed until their 50s. Typically, RLS is gradually progressive over time, and the remission rate is generally low.

Familial aggregation has been widely shown since Ekbom's description of the condition (125). The high familial aggregation of RLS suggests a genetic component. Through genome-wide association studies (GWAS) analysis, an association with variants in gene *MEIS1, BTBD9,* and *MAP2K5/LBXCOR1* on chromosomes 2p, 6p, and 15q was identified in RLS (126,127). These findings were confirmed in several studies (128,129). Another GWAS identified two additional RLS susceptibility loci within an intergenic region on chromosome 2p14 and 16q12.1 (130). Opportunities now exist to study the functionality of the RLS risk susceptibility loci and the potential molecular pathways involved. Some illustrative examples include the study reporting that the *MEIS1* risk variant influences iron metabolism (131) and *BTBD9* regulates brain dopamine levels and controls iron homeostasis through the iron regulatory protein-2 (132), adding to the growing body of evidence that dopaminergic neurotransmission and iron dysregulation might contribute to the pathogenesis of RLS.

Essential criteria for diagnosis of RLS include (1) an urge to move the legs, usually accompanied by an uncomfortable sensations in the legs, (2) beginning or worsening during periods of rest or inactivity such as lying or sitting, (3) partly or totally relieved by movements such as walking, bending, stretching, and so forth, at least for as long as the activity continues, (4) worse in the evening or at night than during the day, or only occurring in the evening or night, and (5) these symptoms are not solely explained by another medical or behavioral condition (RLS mimic). A positive family history, a positive response to dopaminergic treatment, and the presence of periodic limb movements while awake (PLMA) and/or during sleep (PLMS) are supportive criteria for the diagnosis of RLS, whereas an age of onset-related progression of the disease, and a normal neurological examination, at least in the idiopathic form, constitute associated features of the disease (69,133).

The main merit of the new diagnostic criteria for RLS is that they specify that frequent confounders of RLS or RLS mimics (133a) must be specifically excluded before making a positive RLS diagnosis (69,133). Mimics may account for up to 16% of individuals diagnosed with RLS in a primary RLS population (134) and possibly even more in comorbid conditions in which symptoms similar to RLS occur as part of the primary disease (i.e., polyneuropathy or Parkinson's disease) (135).

Several types of excessive motor activity have been reported in RLS, such as hypnic fragmentary myoclonus, pacing, fidgeting, repetitive kicking, tossing and turning in bed, slapping the legs on the mattress, cycling movements of the lower limbs, repetitive foot tapping, rubbing the feet together, and inability to remain seated. Rhythmic movement disorder (i.e., body rocking), marching in place (136,137), pelvic rhythmic movements (138), alternating leg muscles activation, and propriospinal myoclonus (139) have also been described associated with RLS. However, the most common motor phenomenon seen in patients with RLS is the presence of unilateral or bilateral recurring movements of the lower limbs (PLMW or PLMS). About 80% of patients with RLS have PLMS (140), and in severely affected patients the arms may also be involved.

There are only limited PSG studies to characterize sleep in RLS patients. The typical PSG findings in an RLS patient are prolonged sleep onset latency, increased wake after sleep onset, increased PLMS, evidence of sleep-related breathing disorders in some patients, and a transient rise of blood pressure and heart rate associated with PLMS and arousal (141–143).

There is no diagnostic laboratory test for RLS. However, in the "suggested immobilization test" (SIT), RLS patients are asked to lie still and not to move while EMG activity is recorded from the tibialis anterior muscles. Depending on the severity of the syndrome, patients start to complain about sensory symptoms, and PLMWs occurring over a period of 1 hour are collected. SIT can be used to quantify the RLS, to study its circadian variability, and to monitor treatment (41). A modified SIT is also available (144).

Levodopa and dopamine agonists are the main treatment for RLS. Although their efficacy has been well documented over the short term, long-term dopaminergic treatment is often complicated by augmentation, loss of efficacy, and other side effects. Recent large randomized controlled trials provide new evidence for the efficacy of high-potency opioids and alpha2-delta ligands (145).

3.6.2. PERIODIC LIMB MOVEMENT IN SLEEP AND PERIODIC LIMB MOVEMENT DISORDER

Periodic limb movements (PLMs) are characterized by stereotyped, repetitive, nonepileptic movements of the limbs, more frequently in legs. They occur during wakefulness preceding sleep onset (PLMA) and during sleep (PLMS). The first polygraphically documented cases occurred in RLS (146). In fact, most of what we know about PLMs derives from studies of patients with RLS. In their simplest form, PLMs consist of withdrawal-like dorsiflexion of the big and other toes and of the ankle, resembling the spinal flexor reflex, occurring more frequently at the beginning of the night and exponentially declining across sleep cycles according to circadian influence(s)

(Fig. 36.42; ⏺ Video 36.5: PLMS). However, although the leg muscles are the most frequently affected, followed by the upper-limb muscles (sometimes involved) and by the axial muscles (rarely involved), the movements are less stereotyped than previously believed, with individual variations of the movement patterns (147,148). What's more, the EMG activity during PLMS may assume different forms. They include a tonic activity lasting several hundreds of milliseconds possibly followed by myoclonic activity, an initial myoclonic jerk followed by tonic activity, or several myoclonic jerks in clusters sometimes followed by tonic activity. Sometimes PLMs may be seen to occur only in one leg or on one side of the body or to alternate between the two sides.

From a polysomnographic point of view, PLMs are scored only if they occur in series of at least four consecutive movements each lasting 0.5 to 10 sec and separated by intervals of 5 to 90 sec (69). The number of PLMs per hour of total sleep time is assessed by the periodic limb movement index (PLMI), with a pathological cutoff of >15 per hour in adults and more than 5 per hour in children. An increased PLMI may be associated with poor sleep, including reduced sleep efficiency, increased wakefulness after sleep onset, more time spent in Stages 1 and 2 of non-REM sleep, and less time spent in Stage N3 and REM sleep. However, asymptomatic PLMS can occur, and the clinical significance of excessive PLMs remains controversial. There is a growing body of evidence that PLMs may simply be a PSG phenomenon and may not have any specific clinical significance, except their presence in the majority of patients with RLS (149).

The standard method to detect PLMs is a polysomnography recording. However, there have been efforts to detect PLMs by means of actigraphy, which is more convenient for both patient and investigator, since it permits multiple-night recordings in an outpatient setting. Actigraphy offers a convenient and economical alternative to PSG in the study of large populations to increase our understanding of the epidemiology and clinical significance of the PLMs (150). However, actigraphy alone should not be used for diagnostic decisions. Periodic limb movement disorder (PLMD) is defined as a PLMI of 15 or greater that is associated with otherwise unexplained sleep–wake complaints. It requires PSG confirmation along with the exclusion of other causes of sleep disturbances (69).

3.6.3. SLEEP-RELATED RHYTHMIC MOVEMENT DISORDER

Sleep-related rhythmic movement disorder (SRMD) is characterized by repetitive, stereotyped, and rhythmic motor activity involving large muscle groups occurring near sleep onset or during drowsiness or sleep. The movements or behaviors result in at least one referable complaint: interference with normal sleep, significant impairment of daytime function, and self-inflicted bodily injury or risk of injury without use of protective measures (69,151). Also known as "jactatio capitis nocturna" or "headbanging" or "headrolling," the term SRMD is preferred as different body areas may be involved in the movement activity. The head is typically rolled from side to side, or may be forcibly banged into the pillow and mattress. The whole body or parts of it, such as hands, arms, or legs, may also be rolled ("body or leg rolling") and rocked repetitively ("bodyrocking"). These stereotypic movements may last a few or several minutes, repeating at a frequency of 0.5 to 2 per second.

Rhythmic feet movement, formerly hypnagogic foot tremor (0.5–3 Hz), occurring during pre-sleep wakefulness and light sleep may be considered a new kind of RMD arising in adults, in some cases associated with insomnia, sleep apnea, PLMs, and RLS (69). Brief activation of the tibialis anterior in one leg alternating with similar activation in the other leg, so-called alternating leg muscles activity, has been described. Such activations, similar to rhythmic feet movements while falling asleep, occur

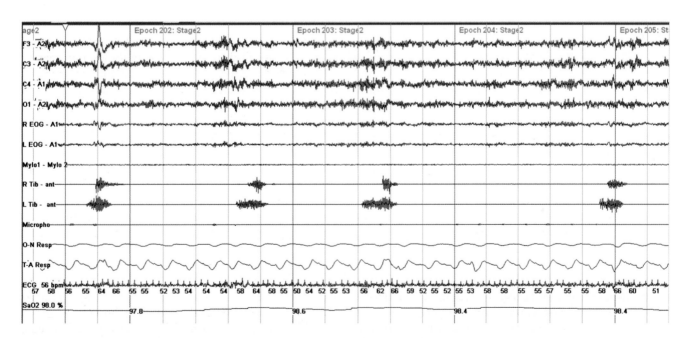

Figure 36.42. PSG recordings in a patient with primary RLS-PLMS during Stage 2 of NREM sleep showing the periodic (every 15–20 sec) repetition of EMG bursts over the tibialis anterior muscles, typical of PLMS. Note the clear-cut transient rhythmic heart rate acceleration and EEG arousals associated with PLMS.

at a frequency of 0.5 to 3 Hz, each lasting up to 0.5 sec, with sequences of several to 20 sec and recurring particularly during arousal. Alternating leg muscles activity has been described in patients with sleep apnea, those taking antidepressant medication, and those with PLMs and RLS (139,152). SRMD is commonly noted in otherwise normal children, but it has also been reported in mentally retarded and autistic patients. More than 60% of 9-month-old infants experience SRMD to some degree. By age 4, only 18% of children persist in having bedtime rhythmic movements. Moreover, SRMD may persist during wakefulness and into adulthood, particularly in autistic or mentally retarded individuals, not rarely associated with other "stereotypies" (i.e., the rhythmic habit pattern).

For particularly violent forms of SRMD, use of protective measures is appropriate. Clonazepam (1 mg nightly), oxazepam (10–20 mg nightly), citalopram, imipramine, and behavioral therapies have been reported to produce significant improvement in some cases (151).

3.6.4. Nocturnal Leg Cramps
Nocturnal leg cramps are sudden, involuntary, painful contractions of the calf muscles that occur during the night or at rest, not explained by another sleep disorder, medical or neurological disorder, medication use, or substance use disorder. They may last a few seconds to several minutes. The prevalence ranges from 37% to 95%, depending on the population studied (153,154). The cramps can occur in otherwise healthy individuals but are also common in patients with a variety of diseases such as chronic polyneuropathies/myopathies, radiculopathy, metabolic or electrolyte disorders, and neuromyotonia. Several drugs are known to cause nocturnal leg cramps: beta sympathomimetics, beta-receptor blockers with partial agonism, cholinergic/acetylcholinesterase blockers, statins, calcium antagonists, clofibric acid derivatives, and diuretics. The origin of and mechanisms responsible for muscle cramps are poorly understood (154,155). Polysomnographic recordings show increased EMG activity in the affected leg and associated awakening (156).

3.6.5. Sleep-Related Bruxism (Nocturnal Tooth Grinding)
Sleep-related bruxism is defined as involuntary and repetitive movements of the jaw muscles during sleep that cause grinding and/or clenching of the teeth. Sleep-related bruxism has a prevalence of 8% in the general population. Consequences of sleep-related bruxism include temporomandibular joint pain, chronic headache, disrupted sleep of the patient and bed partner, and dental wear. The diagnosis is based on a history of tooth grinding and clenching and is confirmed by the PSG recording of the EMG activity of jaw muscles during sleep (Fig. 36.43; 🎥 Video 36.6: Sleep Bruxism). According to motor activity type, sleep bruxism may be classified as "tonic" (with muscular contraction sustained for >2 sec), "phasic" (with brief, repeated contraction of the masticatory musculature with three or more consecutive bursts of EMG activity that last 0.25–2 sec apiece), and "combined" (with alternating appearance of tonic and phasic episodes) (157). Jaw muscle contraction may be extremely brief and sudden, lasting for <0.25 sec, with tooth tapping and/or tongue biting as in nocturnal faciomandibular myoclonus

(158). As a familial form of this activity has been recorded (158), and sleep-related epilepsy is a possible concomitant finding (159), a full EEG montage is recommended.

3.6.6. Sleep-Related Eating Disorder
Sleep-related eating disorder is defined as dysfunctional eating after a partial or complete arousal from sleep with consumption of food or inedible or toxic substances. Patients are often not aware of their eating behavior until the next morning upon seeing a mess in the kitchen or on their bedclothes. Some patients, however, may be aware of their nocturnal eating behavior and report recurrent awakenings with the inability to return to sleep without eating or drinking. The condition can be idiopathic or can be comorbid with other sleep disorders (e.g., sleep walking, RLS, PLMS, OSAS, narcolepsy, irregular sleep–wake circadian rhythm sleep disorder) and with use of medications such as zolpidem, triazolam, and other psychotropic agents. Patients who report for clinical attention often have a chronic course, with multiple eating episodes per night and a variety of daytime consequences of this behavior, including weight gain, daytime fatigue, and mood disorders. The most common PSG findings are multiple arousals with or without eating, arising predominantly from Stage N3 sleep but also from other stages of NREM sleep and occasionally from REM sleep. Currently, treatment is directed toward the underlying sleep disorder, when present, or otherwise involve the empirical use of a serotonergic antidepressant or topiramate (69,160,161).

3.6.7. Catathrenia
Catathrenia is a rare idiopathic condition characterized by high-pitched, monotonous, irregular groans that occur during prolonged expiration in sleep (162). The hallmark of catathrenia is that sleep inspiration is followed by protracted expiration during which a sound is produced, repetitively recurring during NREM and especially REM sleep. From a PSG point of view, episodes of catathrenia are characterized by a sudden switch from eupneic breathing to bradypneic breathing with prolonged expiratory phase and without significant alteration of gas exchange (i.e., normal and unchanged oxygen saturation) (Fig. 36.44; 🎥 Video 36.7). During this protracted expiration, continuous or fragmented sounds are produced. In contrast to central apnea (163), where the apneic pause is associated with oxygen desaturation and is preceded by an exhalation, the breath preceding the catathrenia is a large inhalation. Catathrenia should be clearly differentiated from other respiratory disturbances with or without noise during sleep. The course of catathrenia appears to be chronic. The available follow-up data are still incomplete, but they seem to exclude substantial clinical progression or complications (69,162,164,165).

3.6.8. Propriospinal Myoclonus at Sleep Onset
This is discussed below.

3.7. Neuromuscular Disorders

Several types of chronic neuromuscular diseases adversely affect respiration during sleep, with consequent insidiously

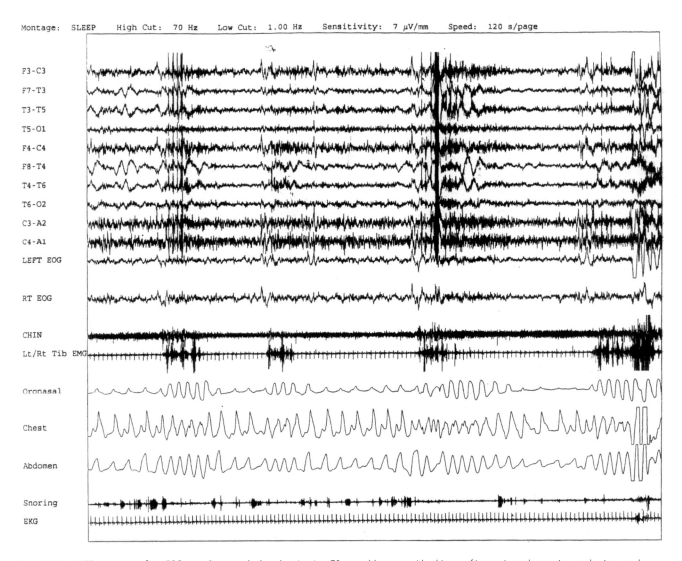

Figure 36.43. A 120-sec excerpt from PSG recording reveals sleep bruxism in a 70-year-old woman with a history of insomnia, early morning awakenings, and EDS. Overnight PSG revealed the presence of mild to moderate OSA with an AHI of 21.5. Episodes of bruxism are recorded repeatedly as part of the arousal response following respiratory events accompanied by tooth grinding on simultaneous audio and video recording. Respiratory-related limb movements are recorded on tibialis anterior channel in association with the arousal response. PSG sleep bruxism is characterized by a series of teeth grinding associated with rhythmic EMG artifacts with a frequency of ~0.5–1.0 Hz in Stage 1 NREM sleep. Top 10 channels: EEGs; LEFT and RT EOG, left and right electrooculograms; CHIN, EMG of chin; Lt/Rt Tib EMG, left/right tibialis anterior EMG; oronasal thermistor; chest and abdomen effort channels; snore monitor EKG, electrocardiography. Reproduced from Chokroverty S, Thomas R, Bhatt M, eds. Atlas of Sleep Medicine. Philadelphia: Elsevier; 2005, with permission.

developing chronic respiratory failure. Sleep-disordered breathing is indeed the leading cause of mortality in patients with chronic neuromuscular diseases; therefore, early detection and treatment are very important to improve outcome and save lives (166,167).

The most common sleep-disordered breathing in neuromuscular disorders is sleep-related, especially REM-related, hypoventilation. Both central and upper airway obstructive apneas also occur. Nocturnal hypoventilation giving rise to hypoxemia and hypercapnia during sleep in the initial stage of neuromuscular disorders causes chronic respiratory failure. In later stages of the illness, abnormal blood gasses may persist even during the daytime. Nocturnal hypoventilation and chronic respiratory failure, however, in neuromuscular disorders may present insidiously and may initially remain asymptomatic. To make the diagnosis, a high index of clinical suspicion is needed. Historical clues include the presence of EDS, daytime fatigue, morning headache, restless and disturbed nocturnal sleep, and unexplained leg edema. Patients with neuromuscular disorders manifesting these symptoms should undergo investigation to uncover nocturnal hypoventilation to prevent the serious consequences of chronic respiratory failure such as pulmonary hypertension and congestive cardiac failure (167).

Neuromuscular disorders causing chronic respiratory failure include primary muscle disease, neuromuscular junctional disorders, motor neuron diseases, acute and chronic inflammatory demyelinating polyneuropathies, hereditary sensorymotor neuropathy, and phrenic neuropathy (167a). The characteristic PSG findings in neuromuscular disorders consist of central, mixed, and upper airway obstructive apneas and hypopneas associated with oxygen desaturation. Sleep hypoventilation consists of non-apneic oxygen desaturation that is worse during REM sleep (166,167).

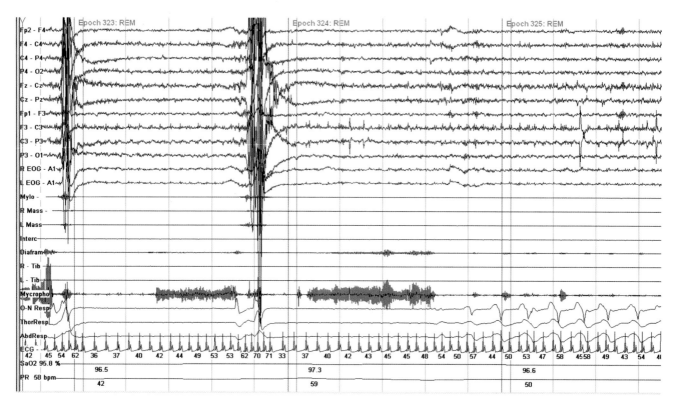

Figure 36.44. PSG recordings of catathrenia. Eupneic breathing switches to catathrenic breathing during REM sleep. Note the dramatic slowing down of breathing rate during catathrenia, with the cycle length now mainly occupied by the expiratory phase. Groaning sounds are shown on the microphone trace. Inspiration is associated with increased submental and intercostal/diaphragm EMG activity, speeding of EEG frequency, and waxing of heart rate. After inspiration and during groaning intercostal/diaphragm EMG activity is absent, and heart rate wanes during the expiratory phase. Oxygen saturation remains normal throughout.

3.8. Neurodegenerative Disorders

Neurodegenerative diseases are often divided into two categories: the synucleinopathies and the tauopathies. These names derive from the abnormalities in underlying molecular mechanisms. In the tauopathies (including Alzheimer's disease, progressive supranuclear palsy, Pick disease, and corticobasal degeneration), abnormal structure or phosphorylation of microtubule-associated proteins leads to both intra- and extracellular protein deposition. The synucleinopathies (Parkinson's disease, diffuse Lewy body dementia, multiple system atrophy, striatonigral degeneration, and olivo-ponto-cerebellar atrophy) result from abnormalities of the protein alpha-synuclein, which accumulates abnormally in neurons and glia, as well as extracellularly. Abnormalities in the related proteins ubiquitin and parkin are also important in the synucleinopathies.

Sleep disorders are relatively common in neurodegenerative diseases. They include insomnia, hypersomnia, parasomnias, respiratory dysrhythmias (nocturnal stridor; central, obstructive, or mixed apneic events; as well as cluster breathing, Cheyne-Stokes respiration, and other abnormalities in the rate, rhythm, and amplitude of respiration), disturbed sleep–wake cycles with the "sundowning" phenomenon, and excessive nocturnal motor activity (167,168). RBD, in particular, is a parasomnia frequently seen in patients with Parkinson's disease and other synucleinopathies and can sometimes predate the motor and cognitive symptoms of the condition by several years or longer. It is the first time that a sleep disorder can be

used as a biomarker to predict a neurodegenerative disorder (169,170). For patients with neurodegenerative diseases, and dementia in particular, sleep disturbances may have a dramatic impact on function and quality of life.

In patients with Alzheimer's disease, sleep abnormalities may appear early in the disease process and may be a prominent feature. In dementia in general, reported abnormalities have included low sleep efficiency, high percentage of Stage N1 sleep relative to other stages, decrease in slow-wave sleep, and increased frequency of arousals and awakenings (171). Early in the disease course, circadian sleep–wake cycles are disturbed, and there is an increase in nighttime wakefulness, which worsens with disease progression (172). Later in the disease, REM sleep time is decreased, and there is increased REM sleep latency, which, along with abnormalities of the circadian rhythm, may result in EDS (171,172). Sundowning and other disturbances of the sleep–wake cycle are common in Alzheimer's disease and may be influenced and exacerbated by a number of factors, including a foreign environment, medications, and infection (173). Other abnormalities on PSG of patients with Alzheimer's disease are sleep apnea and PLMS.

Parkinson's disease has been among the most studied of the neurodegenerative disorders with respect to sleep disorders. Complaints of insomnia, parasomnias, daytime sleepiness and fatigue, and sleep onset and maintenance difficulties are common (168,174). Sleep studies in Parkinson's patients have revealed reduction of total sleep time, frequent awakenings, decreased slow-wave sleep, decreased sleep spindles and K-complexes in Stage 2, and intrusions of REM sleep into NREM with altered sleep structure (175,176). Sleep apnea and RLS/PLMS are also common in Parkinson's disease (168,177). The prevalence of RBD is increased in Parkinson's disease, as is REM sleep without atonia (178). Circadian rhythms and sleep cycles are also affected in Parkinson's disease (179,180). Regarding hypersomnia, medication side effects (particularly of dopamine agonists and L-dopa) can result in increased daytime sleepiness, though large population studies have also demonstrated increased daytime sleepiness in Parkinson's disease patients irrespective of medications (175). Central hypersomnia has also been described in patients with Parkinson's disease, including a narcolepsy phenotype with low hypocretin levels measured in the cerebrospinal fluid (181).

In patients with *diffuse Lewy body dementia*, PSG findings include decreased total sleep time, frequent awakenings, and absence of muscle atonia in REM sleep with RBD, which may be a preclinical sign of the disease (90,168). Because of sleep fragmentation and repeated awakenings, the patient may have EDS, as reflected in an abnormal MSLT (182).

Patients with *progressive supranuclear palsy* have a high prevalence of comorbid sleep disorders. Initially, the most common problems are insomnia and delayed sleep onset. Decreased REM sleep and spindle formation have also been reported. As the disease progresses, sleep latency shortens and insomnia becomes more severe due to associated increased sleep fragmentation (183). PSG findings include increased sleep fragmentation, reduced sleep time, variable latency to REM sleep, reduction or absence of REM sleep, and a general reduction in sleep spindles and K-complexes (184). Other problems associated with progressive supranuclear palsy, such as immobility and dysphagia, contribute to interrupted sleep patterns. RBD and sleep-related respiratory disturbances have also been described in these patients (185,186).

Patients with *Huntington's disease* show decreased sleep efficiency, an increase in Stage N1 with increased arousals and awakenings, and reduced slow-wave sleep. Sleep-disordered breathing, PLMS, REM sleep disturbances, and an increased density of sleep spindles have also been reported (187–190). The involuntary movements decrease progressively from wake to Stage N1 and N2 to REM sleep. The dyskinetic movements in sleep are of shorter duration, are of lower amplitude, and are more fragmented as compared to wakefulness.

Patients with *torsion dystonia* suffer from a markedly reduced quality of life. This might, at least in part, be mediated by non-motor symptoms, including sleep disturbances (191). PSG findings in torsion dystonia show frequent awakenings, reduced sleep efficiency, and increased sleep latency. High-amplitude sleep spindles have been described in some cases, but this has been an inconsistent finding in other studies. Segawa et al. recorded movement counts in PSG studies in patients with hereditary progressive dystonia (192) and reported a decrease in gross body movements in Stage N1, an increase in Stage N2, and a decrease in REM sleep.

In patients with *olivo-ponto-cerebellar atrophy*, PSG studies have been reported to show increased awakenings, reduced slow-wave sleep, and reduced or absent REM sleep. In several cases, REM sleep without muscle atonia, accompanied by features of RBD, has been described (193). Central, obstructive, and mixed apneas have been reported by several authors.

Sleep-disordered breathing of various types can occur in *multiple system atrophy* (MSA). Obstructive and/or central sleep apnea can be observed. Nocturnal stridor is one of the most serious sleep disorders associated with MSA (194–196). Nocturnal stridor is potentially fatal, with several case reports of MSA patients dying during sleep (197,198). RBD is frequently observed: early series reported a clinical prevalence of RBD in up to 69% of MSA patients (199). REM sleep without atonia is even more prevalent and was found in 90% of PSGs performed in this population. Excessive daytime sleepiness has been reported in 28% of Caucasian MSA patients (200) and 24% of Japanese MSA patients (201). PLMs are reported in MSA patients (202); they may have a decrease in the cortical and autonomic arousal responses to PLMs (203) and a loss of the normal nocturnal dip in blood pressure (204).

3.9. Insomnia, Including Fatal Familial Insomnia

Dissatisfaction with sleep owing to difficulty falling asleep or staying asleep or to waking up too early is present in roughly one third of adults on a weekly basis (205). For most, such sleep difficulties are transient or of minor importance. However, prolonged sleeplessness is often associated with substantial distress, impairment in daytime functioning, or both. In such cases, a diagnosis of insomnia disorder is appropriate. Reductions in perceived health (206) and quality of life (207), increases in workplace injuries and absenteeism (208), and even fatal injuries (209) are all associated with chronic insomnia. Insomnia symptoms may also be an independent risk factor for suicide attempts and deaths from suicide, independent of depression (210). Neuropsychological testing reveals deficits in complex cognitive processes, including working memory and attention switching, which are not simply related to impaired alertness (211).

Older diagnostic systems attempted to distinguish "primary" from "secondary" insomnia on the basis of the inferred original cause of the sleeplessness. However, because causal relationships between different medical and psychiatric disorders and insomnia are often bidirectional, such conclusions are unreliable. In addition, owing to the poor reliability of insomnia subtyping (212) based on phenotype or pathophysiology, the fifth edition of the *Diagnostic and Statistical Manual of Mental Disorders* (213) takes a purely descriptive approach that is based on the frequency and duration of symptoms, allowing a diagnosis of insomnia disorder to be made independent of, and in addition to, any coexisting psychiatric or medical disorders. The clinician should monitor whether treatment of such coexisting disorders normalizes sleep; if it does not, the insomnia disorder should be treated independently.

Fatal familial insomnia (FFI) is a rare autosomal dominant human prion disease characterized clinically by a disordered sleep–wake cycle, dysautonomia, and motor signs, and pathologically by predominant thalamic degeneration (214). Data indicate that the neurodegenerative process associated with FFI begins in the thalamus 13 to 21 months before the clinical presentation of the disease (215). Severe thalamic neuronal loss and gliosis are characteristically seen in postmortem studies of FFI, usually without concomitant spongiform change, except in very advanced stages of the disease. The most seriously affected thalamic nuclei are the anteroventral and mediodorsal nuclei and the pulvinar (216). Atrophy of the inferior olive with neuronal loss and gliosis is also commonly observed.

FFI was first described in 1986 in an Italian family (214). Although rare, sporadic cases are also described. Genetically, FFI is linked to a GAC-to-AAC point mutation at codon 178 of the prion protein gene (PRNP) that leads to a substitution of asparagine for aspartic acid (D178N) (216). In FFI the D178N mutation is always associated with methionine at the polymorphic position 129 of the mutant allele. More than 30 pathogenic mutations of the PRNP have been reported to date worldwide (217).

Usually, the onset of FFI is between ages 32 and 62 (mean 51 years) (218). Disease onset is earlier and duration is shorter in those who are homozygous for methionine at codon 129. It is a rapidly fatal disease in which patients characteristically develop progressive insomnia with loss of the normal circadian pattern, along with dysautonomia and endocrine disturbances. Progressive sleep disruption with loss of the normal circadian sleep–activity pattern may manifest as a dream-like confusional state during waking hours. Inattention, impaired concentration and memory, confusion, and hallucinations are frequent, but overt dementia is rare (219). Methionine-homozygous patients are more likely to have hallucinations and myoclonus as prominent disease features, while methionine-heterozygous patients are more likely to develop early problems with ataxia, bulbar signs, and nystagmus. Catatonia and psychotic symptoms may belong to the clinical phenotype of early stage FFI. Dysautonomia is characterized by hyperhidrosis, hyperthermia, tachycardia, and hypertension. Endocrine disturbances include decreased ACTH secretion, increases in cortisol secretion, and loss of the normal diurnal variations in levels of growth hormone, melatonin, and prolactin. Sleep studies demonstrate a dramatic reduction in total sleep time and disruption of the normal sleep architecture.

3.10. Uncommon and Atypical PSG Patterns

In certain normal individuals, particularly following sleep deprivation, withdrawal of medications, and alteration of sleep habits, certain atypical and uncommon sleep patterns may be observed in the PSG (220). Similar patterns, however, have also been described in a variety of sleep disorders. Some of these patterns include alpha–delta or alpha-NREM sleep, REM-spindle sleep, REM intrusion into NREM sleep, REM sleep without atonia in conditions other than RBD, abnormal REM–NREM cycling, rhythmic leg movements, bruxism with arousals after termination of apnea, alternating leg muscle activation, propriospinal myoclonus at sleep onset, ataxic (Biot's) breathing in patients taking opiates for pain management, effect of body and head position on respiratory pattern, antiarrhythmic effects of sleep, and phasic tongue movements in REM sleep.

3.10.1. ALPHA–DELTA SLEEP
An EEG pattern of alpha intrusion into NREM sleep was first noted in 1973 in patients with psychiatric disorders (221). The EEG appearance was that of intrusion of prominent alpha activity (frequency of 8–13 cycles per second) on delta waves (frequency of 0.5–2.0 per second with amplitude >75 microvolts). A similar pattern, termed *alpha–delta sleep* (Fig. 36.45), has been found to be related to a complaint of nonrestorative sleep in patients with musculoskeletal pain or fibrositis and nondepressed patients with chronic fatigue. Other disorders in which alpha–delta sleep, nonrestorative sleep, and pain or fatigue symptoms are evident include rheumatoid arthritis and systemic lupus erythematosus. Alpha–delta sleep is also reported in patients with psychophysiological insomnia and other primary sleep disorders (e.g., PLMD, circadian rhythm sleep disorders, sleep apnea, and narcolepsy) (222).

3.10.2. REM-SPINDLE SLEEP
On many occasions bursts of sleep spindles are noted during REM sleep, giving rise to a pattern called REM-spindle sleep pattern (Fig. 36.46). This is noted in many normal individuals, particularly in the beginning of the first REM period. Similar REM-sleep spindle pattern is noted also in many patients with hypersomnia and narcolepsy-cataplexy syndrome.

3.10.3. REM SLEEP WITHOUT MUSCLE ATONIA
REM sleep without muscle atonia (RSWA) is characterized by increased phasic or tonic muscle activity seen on the EMG channels of PSG. RSWA is a requisite diagnostic feature of RBD (see Fig. 36.37) but may also be seen in patients without clinical symptoms or signs of dream enactment as an incidental finding in neurologically normal individuals, especially in patients receiving tricyclic antidepressants, monoamine oxidase inhibitors, selective serotonin reuptake inhibitors, and phenothiazines. RSWA may be observed also in patients with Parkinson's disease or narcolepsy in absence of the typical behavioral manifestation of RBD. Longitudinal studies must investigate whether patients with isolated RSWA are at an increased risk of developing fully expressed RBD and/or neurodegenerative disease (223).

3.10.4. MIXTURE OF REM BURSTS IN NREM SLEEP
Occasionally REM-like bursts are noted during NREM sleep in normal persons. Such a pattern, however, is seen particularly in patients with narcolepsy and patients with depression who have been treated with REM suppressant medications. This pattern may also be seen in Parkinson's disease.

3.10.5. ABNORMAL REM–NREM CYCLING
REM–NREM sleep goes through a normal cycling of four or five cycles throughout the night. The initial cycle is of brief duration and the longest period of REM is noted toward the end of the night, when it may last up to 1 hour. Such cycling may be disrupted in patients with narcolepsy-cataplexy and patients with narcolepsy who have been taking REM-suppressant medications. Such abnormal cycling may also be seen in patients with head injury and Parkinson's disease. In addition, some normal individuals may display abnormal REM–NREM cycling.

A case of alpha–delta sleep

Montage: SLEEP   High Cut: 70 Hz   Low Cut: 1.00 Hz   Sensitivity: 7 µV/mm   Speed: 10 s/page

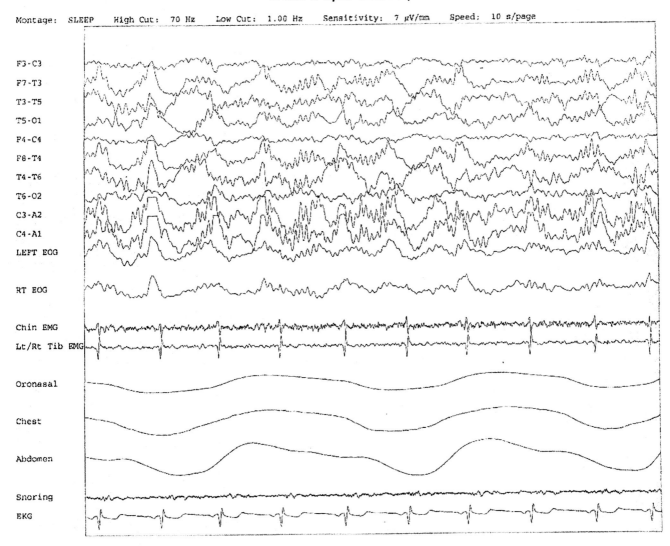

Figure 36.45. A ten-sec excerpt from a nocturnal PSG showing alpha–delta sleep in a 30-year-old man with history of snoring for many years. He denied any history of joint or muscle aches and pains. The alpha frequency is intermixed with and superimposed on underlying delta activity. Alpha–delta sleep denotes a nonspecific sleep architectural change noted in many patients with complaints of muscle aches and fibromyalgia. It is also seen in other conditions and many normal individuals. Top 10 channels: EEGs; LEFT EOG and RT EOG, left and right electro-oculograms; chin EMG, EMG of chin; Lt/Rt Tib EMG, left/right tibialis anterior EMG; oronasal thermistor; chest and abdomen effort channels; snore monitor; EKG, electrocardiography. Reproduced from Chokroverty S, Thomas R, Bhatt M, eds. Atlas of Sleep Medicine. Philadelphia: Elsevier; 2005, with permission.

3.10.6. RHYTHMIC LIMB AND BODY MOVEMENTS ON AROUSAL AFTER TERMINATION OF APNEIC-HYPOPNEIC EVENTS

Rhythmic movement disorder is an abnormal sleep-related movement disorder characterized by rhythmic oscillations of the head, trunk, or limbs during the wake–sleep transition. As an unusual manifestation this also has been noted in patients with OSAS on arousals after termination of apneic-hypopneic events (224,225) (Fig. 36.47).

3.10.7. RHYTHMIC LEG MOVEMENTS

Rhythmic leg movements in wakefulness, NREM sleep, and REM sleep are sometimes noted as unusual PSG findings in normal individuals (Fig. 36.48) as well as in patients with sleep pathologies (225).

3.10.8. SLEEP BRUXISM (TOOTH GRINDING)

As an unusual manifestation, bruxism may rarely be noted on arousal after termination of apneic events in patients with OSAS (66,225) (see Fig. 36.43).

3.10.9. ALTERNATING LEG MUSCLE ACTIVATION

Alternating leg muscle activation is an unusual PSG observation characterized by alternating leg muscle activation preceding or following an arousal or awakening (Fig. 36.49). Such activations, similar to rhythmic feet movements while falling asleep (i.e., hypnagogic foot tremor), occur at a frequency of 1 to 1.5 Hz (range 0.5–3 Hz), each lasting up to 0.5 sec, with sequences of several to 20 sec showing at least four discrete and alternating muscle activations (12) and recurring in all sleep stages but particularly during arousal (227). Alternating

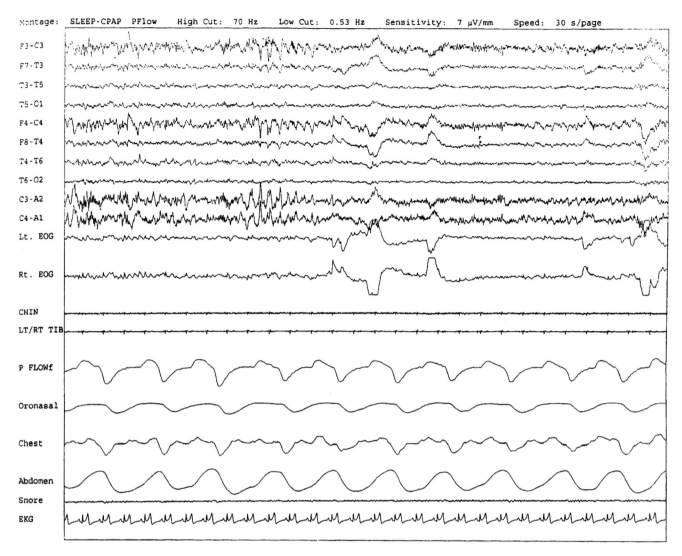

Figure 36.46. *A 67-year-old man with difficulty sleeping, loud snoring, and EDS for 5 years. Medical history is significant for high blood pressure and coronary artery disease. Nocturnal PSG showed the presence of moderate sleep apnea with an AHI of 29.5. A 30-sec excerpt from nocturnal PSG showing the presence of frequent sleep spindles throughout the epoch of REM sleep. Prominent sawtooth waves of REM sleep in C3- and C4-derived EEG channels, prominent phasic eye movements of REM sleep on EOG channels, and decreased chin muscle tone characteristic of REM atonia are seen. Reproduced from Chokroverty S, Thomas R, Bhatt M, eds. Atlas of Sleep Medicine. Philadelphia: Elsevier; 2005, with permission.*

leg muscle activation has been described in patients with sleep apnea, PLMS, and RLS (139) and those taking antidepressant medication (227).

3.10.10. PROPRIOSPINAL MYOCLONUS IN PRE-DORMITUM

Propriospinal myoclonus is a syndrome of spontaneous or, in rare instances stimulus-sensitive, axial myoclonic jerks that originate at a spinal segmental level and spread up and down the spinal cord via supposedly propriospinal pathways. A typical feature in some cases is its occurrence and intensification when patients sit or lie flat and in which the triggering factor is the reduction in vigilance level at the transition from alert to relaxed wakefulness (i.e., the pre-dormitum) (228–230) (Figs. 36.50, 36.51, 36.52; ⬤ Video 36.8: Propriospinal Myoclonus). The etiology remains undetermined, but at the wake–sleep transition it may prevent the patient from falling asleep, causing sleep-onset insomnia. As a sleep-related movement disorder, propriospinal

myoclonus has also been found in patients with a long history of RLS (139). In these cases, it arises during relaxed wakefulness but gives way with the appearance of spindles and K-complexes on the EEG to typical PLMS with characteristic EMG activity limited to the leg muscles (Fig. 36.53).

3.10.11. ATAXIC OR BIOT'S BREATHING IN PATIENTS TAKING OPIATES

Ataxic breathing is a type of periodic breathing with central apnea without a crescendo/decrescendo pattern resulting from an unstable or destabilized central controller for breathing (medullary respiratory neurons). This is well known to occur in medullary pathology (231) but has recently been observed in patients taking large doses of opiates for pain management (232,233). Biot's breathing is a type of ataxic breathing with two or three normal breaths interspersed with periodically recurring central apnea (Fig. 36.54).

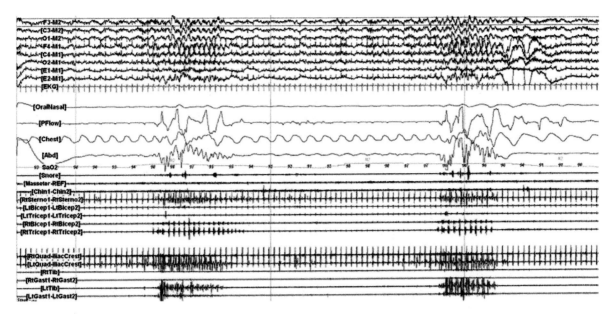

Figure 36.47. A 90-sec excerpt from overnight PSG during Stage 2 (N2) of NREM sleep in a 51-year-old man with upper airway OSA, RLS, and rhythmic movement disorder showing two episodes of rhythmic EMG bursts (~0.75 Hz) beginning in the right biceps (RtBiceps) and right triceps (RtTriceps) and spreading to other muscles. These bursts were noted following termination of the apneic events and were accompanied by arousals and resumption of normal breathing as well as rhythmic body and head-rolling movements. Top six channels (international nomenclature): EEGs; E1–M1, left electro-oculogram; E2–M1, right electro-oculogram; EKG, electrocardiogram; OralNasal, oronasal thermistor (air flow); PFlow, nasal pressure recording for airflow; Chest, thoracic breathing effort; Abd, abdominal breathing effort; SaO2, oxygen saturation by finger oximetry; Snore, snoring recording; Masseter, right masseter EMG; Chin: submental EMG; RtSterno: right sternocleidomastoideus EMG; LtBiceps, left biceps EMG; LtTriceps, left triceps EMG; RtBiceps, right biceps EMG; RtTriceps, right triceps EMG; RtQuad, right quadriceps (biceps femoris) EMG; LtQuad, left quadriceps EMG; RtTib, right tibialis EMG; RtGast, right gastrocnemius EMG; LtTib, left tibialis EMG; LtGast, left gastrocnemius EMG. Reproduced from Gharagozlou P, Seyffert M, Santos R, et al. Rhythmic movement disorder associated with respiratory arousals and improved by CPAP titration in a patient with restless legs syndrome and sleep apnea. Sleep Med. 2009;10(4):501–503, with permission.

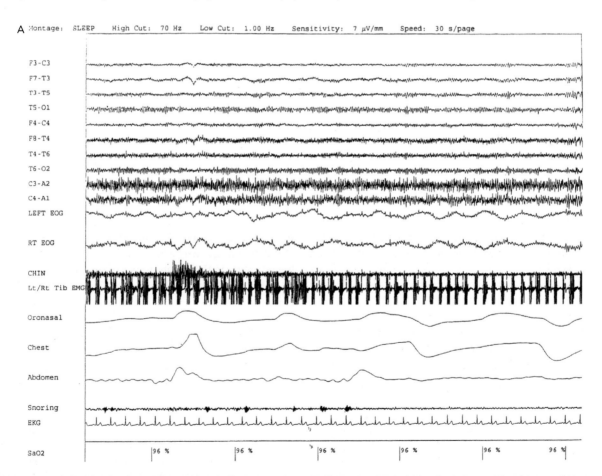

Figure 36.48. A: A 50-year-old man with history of loud snoring, choking in sleep, and intermittent leg jerking at night. Nocturnal PSG shows the presence of mild sleep apnea with an AHI of 12.3. This 30-sec excerpt from nocturnal PSG shows bursts of rhythmic foot and leg movements on the left/right tibialis anterior muscle recording channel during wakefulness. The movement was not associated with respiratory events, oxygen desaturation, or arousal from sleep. EEG, Top 10 channels: EEGs; LEFT and RT EOG, left and right electro-oculograms; CHIN, EMG of chin; Lt/Rt Tib EMG, left/right tibialis anterior EMG; oronasal thermistor; chest and abdomen effort channels; snore monitor; EKG, electrocardiography; SaO2, oxygen saturation by finger oximetry.

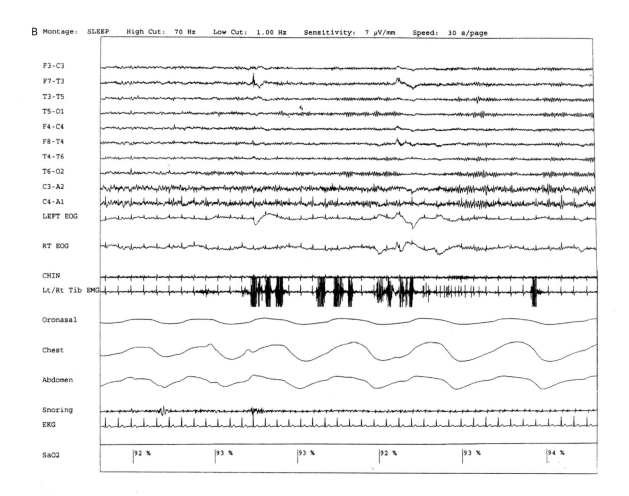

Montage: SLEEP   High Cut: 70 Hz   Low Cut: 1.00 Hz   Sensitivity: 7 µV/mm   Speed: 30 s/page

*Figure 36-48. **B:** Same patient as in Figs 36-48 A. This 30-second excerpt from nocturnal polysomnography shows bursts of rhythmic foot and leg movements on the left/right tibialis anterior muscle recording channel during REM sleep. The movement is not associated with respiratory events, oxygen desaturation, or arousal from sleep. PSG montage: same as in Figure 36-48A.*

3.10.12. Effect of Body and Head Position on Breathing Events in Sleep

Cheyne-Stokes breathing, commonly seen in patients with heart failure or stroke, generally gets worse or sometimes may be seen only in the supine position due to destabilization of central respiratory controllers resulting from stimulation of irritant lung receptors related to pulmonary congestion in the supine position. This may improve when the patient is in the lateral position (Fig. 36.55). In some patients Cheyne-Stokes breathing may not be seen in the supine position but appears when the patient turns the head to the left or the right, still staying in the supine position (Fig. 36.56).

3.10.13. Antiarrhythmic Effect of Sleep on Ventricular Ectopy

The effect of sleep on ventricular ectopic beats has been inconsistent, but in many patients, sleep, especially NREM sleep, may show an improvement (Fig. 36.57).

3.10.14. Rhythmic Tongue Movements in Phasic REM Sleep

Rhythmic tongue movements may be seen as another phasic manifestation of REM sleep in normal individuals as well as in pathological conditions (Fig. 36.58).

4. RELATED LABORATORY PROCEDURES FOR DIAGNOSIS OF SLEEP DISORDERS

PSG and video-PSG recordings remain the most important laboratory tests for the diagnosis of sleep disorders. Three other technical procedures, however, have found an important place in the assessment of sleep disorders: the MSLT, the maintenance-of-wakefulness test (MWT), and actigraphy. Two other procedures (234,235) also have some place in the assessment of sleep disorders (peripheral arterial tonometry and pulse transit time), but these will not be described in this chapter.

4.1. MSLT

The most common indication for MSLT is EDS. The initial step in the assessment of a patient with EDS is a detailed sleep history covering not only sleep at night but also daytime function as well as a history and physical examination. The first step prior to ordering the laboratory tests is an assessment of EDS. Certain clinical clues may suggest EDS (236): falling asleep in inappropriate places and inappropriate circumstances, such as while sitting and relaxing on a couch, watching television, reading, watching movies, sitting in classes or conferences,

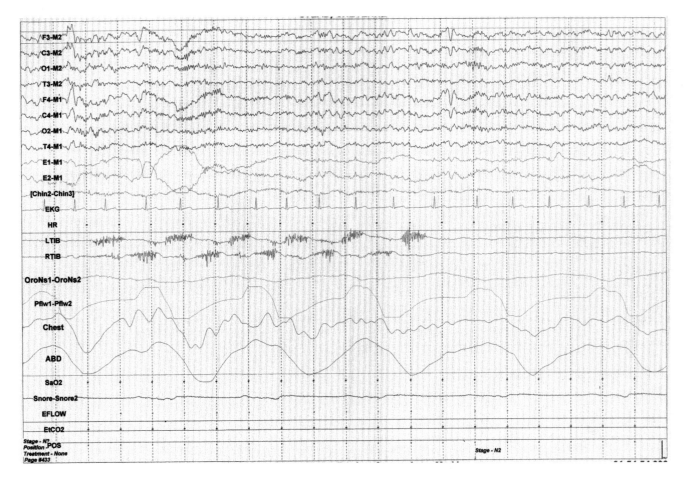

Figure 36.49. *A 20-sec except of PSG showing alternating leg muscle activation (ALMA) in the left and right tibialis anterior muscles (LTIB and RTIB) at a rate of ~1.5 Hz in an adult man during Stage N2 sleep. Top 8 channels: EEGs; E1–M1 and E2–M1, left and right electro-oculograms; Chin 2–Chin 3, chin muscle EMG; EKG, electrocardiogram; HR, heat rate; OroNs1–OroNs2 and Pflw1-Pflw2, respiratory airflow; Chest and ABD, respiratory Effort; SaO2, oxygen saturation by finger oximetry; EtCO2, expiratory carbon dioxide.*

listening to a lecture, and in very severe cases even talking on the telephone and giving the history to the physician; dozing off while driving; a poor attention span and difficulty coping with work and schoolwork; driving accidents or accidents at work; frequent naps during the day; and nonrefreshing sleep and feeling sleepy and tired upon waking up first thing in the morning.

For assessment of persistent sleepiness, the Epworth Sleepiness Scale (ESS) (237) is often used to assess the patient's general level of sleepiness. This is a subjective propensity to sleepiness assessed by the patient under eight situations on a scale of 0 to 3, with 3 indicating that the chances of dozing off are at the highest. The maximum score is 24; a score of 10 or above suggests the presence of EDS. The test has been weakly correlated with the MSLT score. However, the ESS and MSLT test different types of sleepiness: MSLT tests the propensity to sleepiness objectively and ESS tests the general feeling of sleepiness or subjective propensity to sleepiness.

The Stanford Sleepiness Scale (SSS) is a 7-point scale to measure subjective sleepiness at the time of testing, but it does not measure persistent sleepiness. There is a somewhat similar scale called the Karolinska Sleepiness Scale (238), which

is used mostly in Europe; it is a 9-point scale but again does not measure persistent sleepiness. In the visual analog scale, another method used to assess alertness and well-being, subjects indicate their feelings of alertness at an arbitrary point on a 0- to 100-mm scale, with 100 being the maximum sleepiness and 0 being the most alert.

4.1.1. Technique of MSLT

The MSLT has been standardized and includes several general and specific procedures (239,240). The general procedures before the actual recording include keeping a sleep diary for one to two weeks before the test in which the patient records information about bedtime, time of rising, napping, and any drug use. The patient should discontinue drugs with central nervous system activity before the test. The test is preceded by an overnight PSG study and is scheduled about 2 to 3 hours after the conclusion of the PSG study. The actual test consists of four to five nap opportunities at 2-hour intervals, and each recording session lasts for a maximum of 20 minutes. Between sessions, test subjects must remain awake. The subject must not smoke for 30 minutes before lights are turned out. Physiological calibrations (e.g., grit teeth, blink your eyes, look up, look down, look to the right, look to the left, open

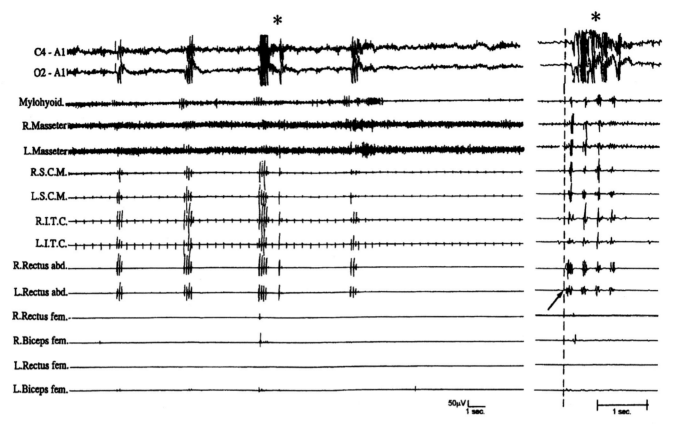

Figure 36.50. Propriospinal myoclonus at the wake–sleep transition. A 40-year-old man presented with a 4-year history of axial jerks during relaxed wakefulness impeding falling asleep. PSG recording shows repetitive myoclonic axial jerks. The EMG activity originates in the left rectus abdominis muscle, thereafter propagating to rostral (sternocleidomastoid, masseter, mylohyoid) and caudal (biceps femoris) muscles. The left panel shows jerks at low speed; the right panel shows one of the jerks at a high speed. R, right; L, left; Mylohyoid, mylohyoideus; S.C.M., sternocleidomastoideus; I.T.C., intercostalis; Rectus abd, abdominis; Rectus fem., rectus femoris; Biceps fem, biceps femoris. Reproduced from Chokroverty S, Thomas R, Bhatt M, eds. Atlas of Sleep Medicine. Philadelphia: Elsevier; 2005, with permission.

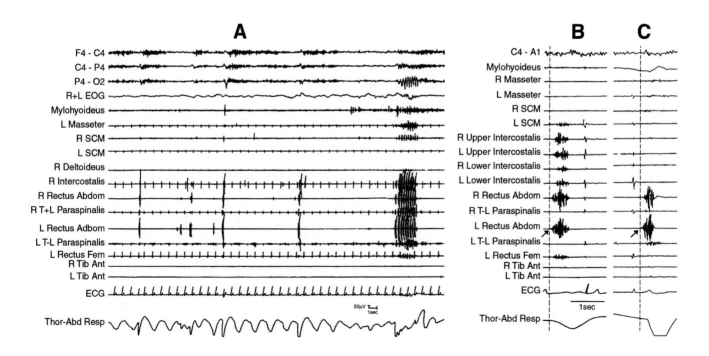

Figure 36.51. PSG recordings of propriospinal myoclonus recurring either isolated or in clusters (A). At higher paper speed, it is evident that jerks always start in the left rectus abdominis muscle with (B) or without (C) spreading to more rostral and caudal muscles. Arrows show onset of activity.

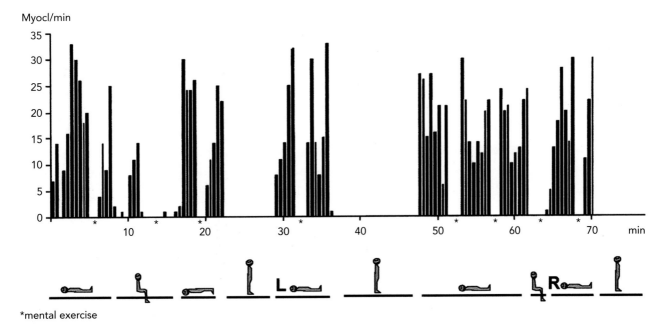

*mental exercise

Figure 36.52. *Picture highlighting the close relationship between propriospinal myoclonus and the level of vigilance as portrayed from the direct observation of a patient. Propriospinal myoclonus appears when the patient is seated or lying down, and the triggering factor is the reduction in vigilance level at the transition from alert to relaxed wakefulness. Mental exercise (*) re-establishes alert wakefulness and suppresses the jerks independent from the posture of the patient.*

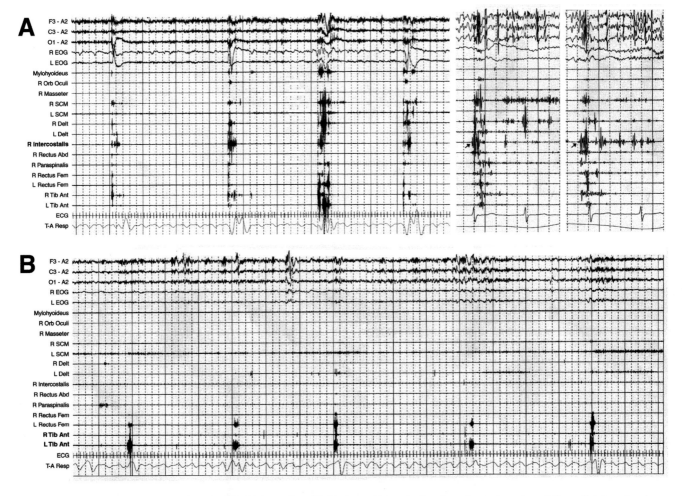

Figure 36.53. *Propriospinal myoclonus and PLMS in RLS. PSG recordings (**A**) showing multiple episodes of propriospinal myoclonus (left panel) during relaxed wakefulness with muscle activity starting in the intercostalis muscle (arrow in right panels: arrows) and spreading to the rostral and caudal muscles. The axial jerks disappear with sleep onset (**B**), at which time they are replaced by typical PLMS, with EMG activity now restricted mainly to the tibialis anterior muscles.*

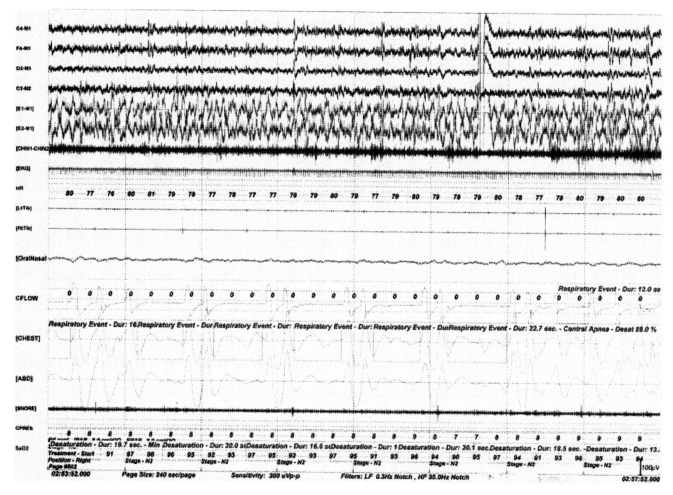

Figure 36.54. A 240-sec excerpt of PSG during Stage N2 sleep showing periodic breathing (ataxic or Biot's breathing, with two or three normal breaths interspersed with periodically recurring central apneas) in a 68-year-old woman on large doses of OxyContin (opiate) for pain management. Her abnormal breathing improved somewhat on bilevel positive upper airway pressurization, but this could not eliminate the events most of the time. Top four channels, EEGs; E1–M1 and E2–M1, left and right EOGs; CHIN1–CHIN2, chin EMG; EKG, electrocardiogram; HR, heart rate; LtTib and RtTib, left and right tibialis anterior EMG (); CFLOW, air flow during positive pressure titration; CHEST and ABD, respiratory effort; CPRES; positive pressure in centimeter; SaO2, oxygen saturation.

your eyes, close your eyes) are then performed and the patient is instructed to relax and fall asleep, and the lights are turned out. The test must be conducted in a quiet, dark room. The recordings may include three to six channels of EEG, submental EMG, and EOG recordings.

The measurements include average sleep onset latency and the presence of sleep-onset REMs (SOREMs), defined as the occurrence of REM sleep within the first 15 minutes of sleep onset. Sleep onset is defined as the time from lights out to the first epoch of any stage of sleep, including Stage N1 sleep. The first epoch of >15 seconds of sleep in a 30-sec epoch is considered sleep onset. If no sleep occurs, the test is concluded 20 minutes after lights out. Fifteen minutes after the first 30-sec epoch in any stage of sleep, the test is terminated. If the finding is indefinite, it is better to continue the test than to end it prematurely. Mean sleep latency is calculated as the average of the latencies to sleep onset for each of the four or five naps. A sleep latency of <8 minutes is consistent with pathological sleepiness. A mean sleep latency of 8 to 10 minutes is consistent with mild sleepiness, and a mean sleep latency of 10 to 15 minutes is considered normal.

A repeat MSLT is indicated if the patient is strongly suspected to have narcolepsy but did not show the characteristic findings of pathological sleepiness with sleep onset latency of <8 minutes and the presence of two or more SOREMs during four or five tests, as may be seen in certain percentage of narcolepsy patients after the first MSLT. If the preceding overnight PSG had shown a SOREM, that can substitute for one daytime SOREM (69). MSLT may not be diagnostic in the initial test, and the yield increases after the second test. The other situation for repeating MSLT is when the finding is ambiguous and the sleep onset or REM sleep cannot be adequately interpreted. Finally, if the MSLT guidelines have not been followed, the test results may be technically invalid.

4.1.2. INDICATIONS FOR MSLT

The AASM developed indications and practice parameters for clinical use of the MSLT (240). The single most important indication for performing MSLT is for the evaluation of patients with suspected narcolepsy. The MSLT may also be useful in the evaluation of patients with suspected idiopathic hypersomnia; in this condition the patient develops

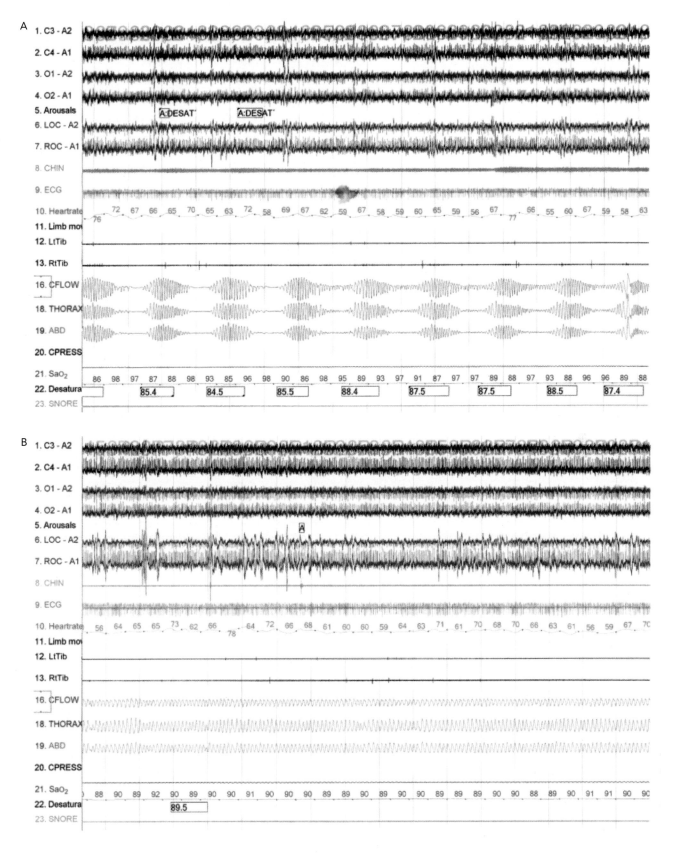

Figure 36.55. The effect of position on Cheyne-Stokes respiration. Epochs of 480 sec from the bilevel titration of a 68-year-old man with a history of myocardial infarction and congestive heart failure. His spouse reported irregular breathing and witnessed apneas in sleep, and he had EDS. He also had hypertension and asthma. A previously performed PSG showed severe central sleep apnea (AHI = 48/hr) with a mean arterial oxygen saturation (SaO$_2$) of 84% and an O$_2$ saturation nadir of 74%. *A:* Note the presence of Cheyne-Stokes respirations in Stage N2 sleep with the patient in the supine position The patient is on a pressure of 12/9 cm. *B:* Improvement of Cheyne-Stokes respirations when the patient assumes the lateral position. He remains in Stage N2 sleep at the same bilevel pressure. Top four channels, electroencephalograms (international nomenclature); LOC-A2, ROC-A1, electro-oculogram; CHIN, chin electromyogram (EMG); LtTib, RtTib, right and left lower limb EMGs; CFLOW, CPAP airflow channel; THORAX, ABD, thoracic and abdominal respiratory belts; Sao2, arterial oxygen saturation by finger pulse oximetry. Also included are channels for ECG, heart rate, and snoring. Reproduced from: Chokroverty S, Thomas RJ, eds. Atlas of Sleep Medicine. 2nd ed. Philadelphia: Elsevier, 2014.

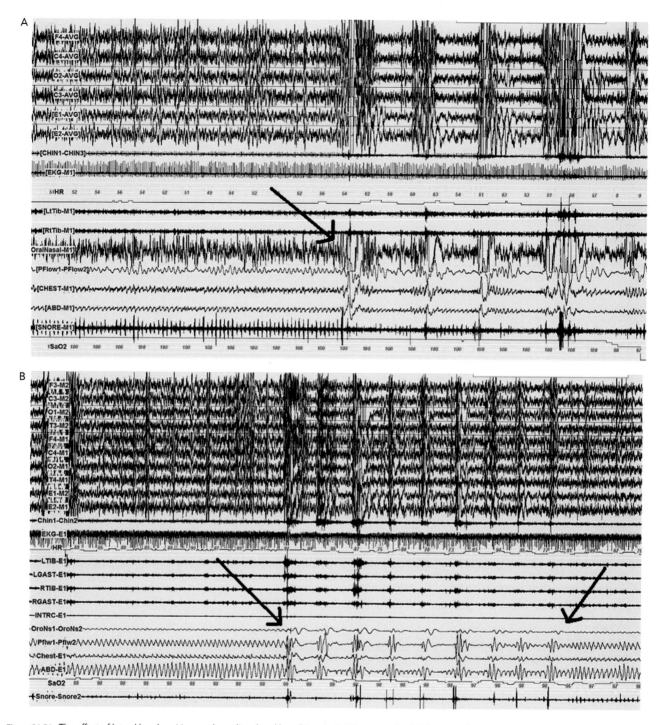

*Figure 36.56. The effect of lateral head position on sleep-disordered breathing. **A:** A 480-sec epoch of PSG tracing from Stage N2 sleep in a 63-year-old man showing supine body position with head initially turned to the left and then to the right (arrow marks point of head position change). Note the immediate appearance of respiratory events with the head turned to the right. **B:** A 480-second excerpt from Stage N2 sleep in a 6-year-old boy showing supine body position with head initially supine and then turned to the left (first arrow marks the point of this change). Respiratory events improved after 2 to 3 minutes in the same position (second arrow). Although OSA worsening with the supine body position is well known, recent reports have also confirmed that sleep-disordered breathing worsens with the head supine. However, worsening of sleep-disordered breathing with the head turned laterally to one side or the other and the body remaining supine, as illustrated in this example, is unusual. Top four channels in A and eight channels in B, Electroencephalography (international 10-20 electrode nomenclature); E1-M1 and E2-M1, left and right electro-oculogram; CHIN1-CHIN2, chin electromyography; ECG, electrocardiogram; HR, heart rate; LtTib and RtTib, left and right tibialis anterior electromyogram (EMG); LGAST and RGAST, left and right gastrocnemius EMG; OroNs and PFLOW, respiratory air flow; Chest and ABD, respiratory effort; Sao2, arterial oxygen saturation by finger oximetry; snore channel. Reproduced with permission from Riar S, Bhat S, Kabak B, Gupta D, Smith I, Chokroverty S. The effect of lateral head position on sleep disordered breathing: a case series. Sleep Med. 2013;14(2):220–221.*

pathological sleepiness or sleep onset of <8 minutes with one or no SOREMs during four or five nap tests. The MSLT is not routinely indicated in the initial evaluation and diagnosis of OSAS nor for the monitoring of the treatment effects after CPAP therapy. The MSLT is also not routinely indicated for patients complaining of EDS due to medical or neurological

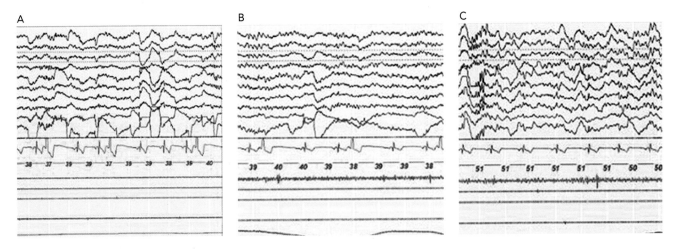

Figure 36.57. Snapshots from overnight PSG in a 24-year-old man with idiopathic cardiomyopathy presenting with dizziness and palpitations. The PSG showed predominantly central sleep apnea (apnea index of 17.4/hr), unrelated to frequent ventricular trigeminy present in wakefulness (A) and REM sleep (B) but absent in non-REM sleep (C). This is an example of the antiarrhythmic effect of sleep on ventricular ectopy. Top eight channels, Electroencephalogram (international nomenclature); E1-M1 and E2-M1, electro-oculograms of left (E1) and right (E2) eyes referred to left mastoid (M1); Chin1-Chin2, mentalis muscle electromyogram (EMG); ECG, electrocardiogram; HR, heart rate; LtTib and RtTib, left and right tibialis anterior muscle EMG; LGAST and RGAST, left and right gastrocnemius muscle EMG; OroNs1-OroNs2 and PFLOW1-PFLOW2, air flow by thermistor and nasal pressure transducer; Chest and ABD, effort channels; SaO2, arterial oxygen saturation by finger oximetry. Reproduced from: Chokroverty S, Thomas RJ, eds. Atlas of Sleep Medicine. 2nd ed. Philadelphia: Elsevier, 2014.

disorders except narcolepsy, insomnia, or circadian rhythm sleep disorders.

4.1.3. RELIABILITY, VALIDITY, AND LIMITATIONS OF MSLT

The sensitive and specificity of the MSLT in detecting sleepiness have not been clearly determined (241). Its test–retest reliability, however, has been documented in both normal subjects and patients with narcolepsy. In subjects with sleepiness caused by circadian rhythm sleep disorders, sleep deprivation, and ingestion of alcohol, pathologic sleepiness has been validated by the MSLT. There is, however, poor correlation between the MSLT and ESS. The patient's psychological and behavioral state also interferes with the MSLT results. The MSLT objectively measures tendency to sleep rather than the likelihood of falling asleep. If the patient suffers from severe anxiety or psychological disturbances causing behavioral stimulation, the MSLT may not show sleepiness even in a patient complaining of EDS.

4.2. The Maintenance-of-Wakefulness Test

The MWT, a variant of the MSLT, measures a patient's ability to stay awake (242,243). The MWT is performed similar to MSLT at 2-hour intervals in a quiet dark room beginning about 1.5 to 3 hours after waking up. Four or five such tests are performed, each lasting for 40 minutes. A PSG and sleep logs are not required before the MWT. The patient should be seated in bed with the back and head supported by a bed rest, ensuring that the neck is comfortable. The patient should not smoke at least 30 minutes prior to each test and should not have caffeinated beverages on the day of the test. The conventional recording montage for the MWT is similar to that used for the MSLT. At the start of the test, after lights out, the patient is instructed to sit still and remain awake for as long as possible. The patient is not allowed to use extraordinary measures to stay awake. Unequivocal sleep is defined as three consecutive epochs of N1 sleep or one epoch of any other stage of sleep. Trials are ended after 40 minutes if no sleep occurs and also after sleep onset as defined above.

The MWT 40-minute protocol may be indicated in assessment of an individual's ability to remain awake when the inability to remain awake constitutes a public or personal safety issue (240). The MWT is also indicated in patients with excessive sleepiness to assess response to treatment (e.g., response to stimulants in narcolepsy and idiopathic hypersomnia and response to CPAP titration in obstructive sleep apnea patients). The MWT is less useful and less sensitive than the MSLT as a diagnostic test for narcolepsy. However, the MSLT and the MWT do have separate functions. The MSLT unmasks physiological sleepiness, which depends on both the circadian and homeostatic factors. In contrast, the MWT reflects the individual's capability to resist sleep and is influenced by physiological sleepiness. The validity, reliability, and specificity of MWT need to be studied using large samples and different populations of sleep disorders.

No universally accepted normative data for the MWT are available. Using standard deviation criteria, the lower limit of normative data for sleep onset latency (mean minus 2 standard deviations) has been defined by Mittler et al. (244) as 19.4 minutes. In contrast, the AASM practice parameters (240) advocate the use of a percentile cutoff score. Accordingly, a mean sleep latency of <8 minutes on the 40-minute protocol is considered abnormal, and values greater than this but <40 minutes are of uncertain significance.

There is little evidence linking mean sleep latency on the MWT with the risk of accidents in real-world circumstances; therefore, the sleep clinician should not rely exclusively on mean sleep latency for determining the risk of accidents but should take into consideration the patient's clinical history, physical findings, and compliance with treatment. An important study by Philip et al. (245) correlated subjective and

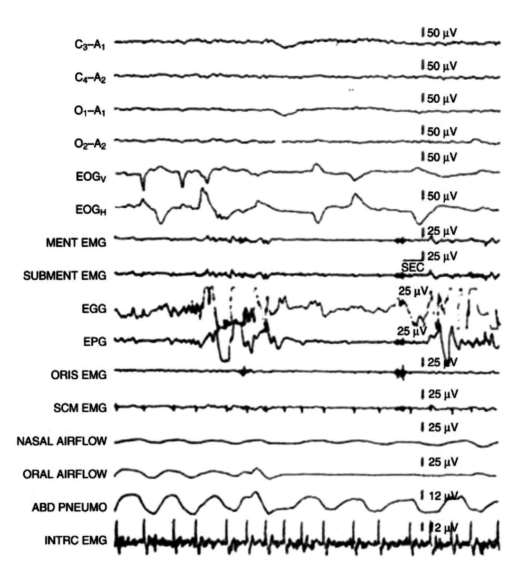

Figure 36.58. Rhythmic tongue movements in REM sleep. PSG recording of REM sleep in a healthy 31-year-old man. Rapid eye movements (seen in the EOG channels) are noted to occur concomitant with complex tongue movements (recorded in the electroglossogram (EGG) and electropharyngogram (EPG) channels). Complex tongue movements in REM may occur at the same time as or independent of rapid eye movements. Top four channels (C3-A1, C4-A2, O1-A1, O2-A2), Electroencephalogram; EOGV, vertical electro-oculogram, EOGH, horizontal electro-oculogram. The next six channels represent electromyography from mentalis (MENT), mylohyoid and anterior belly of digastric (SUBMENT), orbicularis oris (ORIS), sternocleidomastoideus (SCM), electroglossogram (EGG), electropharyngogram (EPG) and intercostal muscle (INTRC),. Nasal and oral airflow and an abdominal effort belt are also included. Reproduced with permission from Chokroverty S. Phasic tongue movements in human rapid eye-movement sleep. Neurology. 1980;30(6):665–668.

objective measures of sleepiness and driving performance in patients with EDS. The study included 38 untreated sleep apnea patients and 14 healthy controls. Based on the number of inappropriate line-crossings during a 90-minute real-life driving session, they determined the MWT sleep onset score as follows: very sleepy, 0 to 19 minutes; sleepy, 20 to 33 minutes; and alert, 34 to 40 minutes.

4.3. Actigraphy

Colburn et al. (246) first documented the use of accelerometers to record body movements. Tyron in 1991 gave a comprehensive account of activity monitoring in psychology and medicine (247). Actigraphy is defined as the technique of recording and quantifying movements. Monitoring of body movements and other activities can be performed continuously for days, weeks, or even months by using an actigraph, also known as an actometer or actimeter (248,249). This can be worn on the wrist or on the ankle to record arm, leg, and body movements. Actigraphy uses piezoelectric sensors, which generate electric currents in direct proportion to the amount of acceleration. The activity usually covers a frequency range of 0.5 to 15 Hz, which is generally the dominant range for human movements. The mechanical movements are converted into electrical signals, which are then sampled every 10th second over a predetermined time or epoch (generally 1 minute). These samples are stored in the memory of the actigraph and then retrieved and analyzed in a computer. The principle of analysis is based on the fact that increased movements (as indicated by black bars in the actigraphy) are seen during wakefulness in contrast to markedly

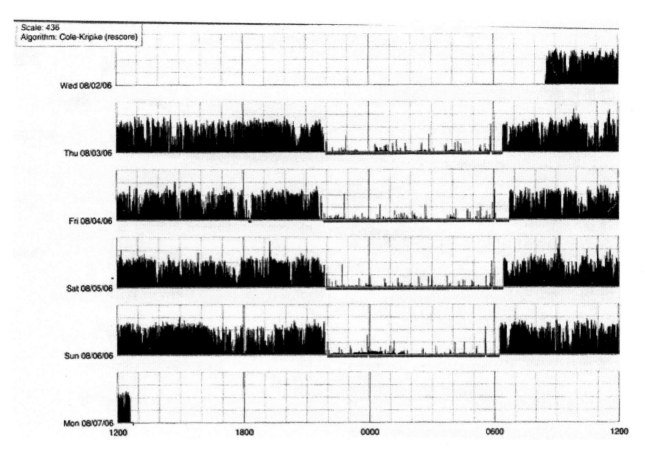

Figure 36.59. *Normal sleep–wake schedule. This shows a wrist actigraph recording from a healthy 60-year-old man with a regular sleep–wake schedule. The subject goes to bed around 10 p.m. and wakes up at 6 a.m. Physiological body shifts and movements are indicated by a few black bars in the white (sleep period) areas. The waking period is indicated by black bars reflecting activities.*

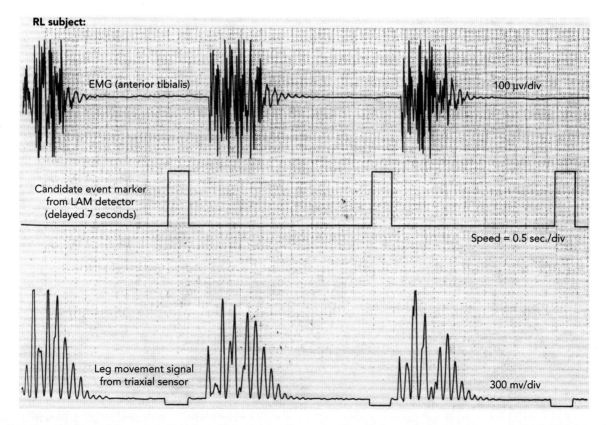

Figure 36.60. *Example of the real-time output of a high-precision activity monitor worn on the ankle (bottom line) compared to anterior tibialis EMG activity (top line). The middle line shows the real-time automatic detection of a significant leg movement made by the activity meter. The decision rules for the real-time leg movement detector create a 7-sec delay in the detection.* Reproduced from Chokroverty S. Sleep Disorders Medicine: Basic Science, Technical Considerations and Clinical Aspects. *3rd ed. Philadelphia: Saunders/Elsevier; 2009, with permission.*

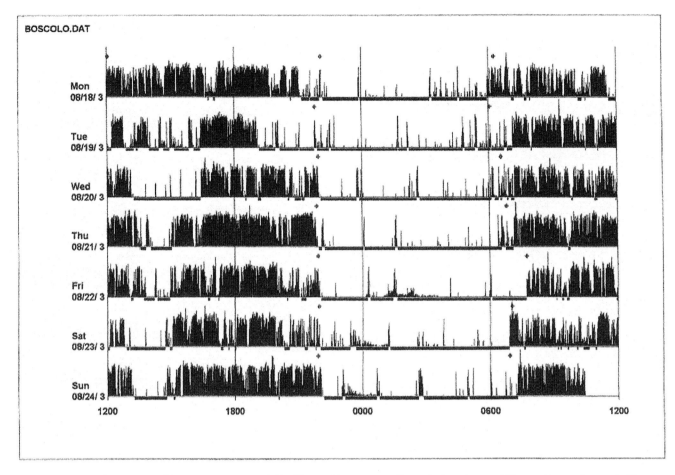

Figure 36.61. *Actigraphy in insomnia (sleep state misperception). This 59-year-old man reported insomnia since the age of 12 years. He was diagnosed with DSM IV Axis personality disorder (dependent personality) and panic attacks in the past, treated with benzodiazepines (clordemetildiazepam 3 mg, flurazepam 30 mg) and zolpidem 10 mg. He denies any symptoms of RLS, EDS, or daytime sleep attacks. Subjective sleep duration is 3 to 4 hours per night. In the past he tried numerous drugs for sleep amelioration but no clear and stable subjective improvement was noted. An actigraphic monitoring (during drug reduction: clordemetildiazepam 2 mg, flurazepam 15 mg, and no zolpidem) shows a clear misperception of sleep duration and quality. The recording shows normal nocturnal motor activity and sleep efficiency and duration. Note sleep period during the afternoon. He complained of sleeping not more than 3 hours each night. Reproduced from Chokroverty S, Thomas R, Bhatt M, eds.* Atlas of Sleep Medicine. *Philadelphia: Elsevier; 2005, with permission.*

decreased movements or no movements (as indicated by the white bars interrupting the black bars during sleep), although normal physiological body and limb movements and postural shifts during sleep will cause interruptions (small black bars) of the white background (Fig. 36.59).

Several actigraph models are in the development stage to carefully regulate the sampling frequencies, durations, filters, sensitivities, and dynamic range in order to detect and quantify PLMs, but no generally accepted standardized technique of quantifying and identifying PLMs as distinct from other movements (e.g., those resulting from parasomnia, nocturnal seizures, and other disordered movements) is currently available. The role of actigraphy in detecting, quantifying, and differentiating abnormal motor activities remains controversial, but there is immense potential for such applications with the development of sophisticated models and techniques. Sophisticated systems for counting movements have been developed and validated (250,251). This system therefore may be useful for therapeutic monitoring and for its diagnostic ability in patients with PLMS and RLS (252,253). One of the available monitors (PAM-RL, Respironics, Pittsburgh,

PA), using a fine-grained analysis with 40-Hz sampling and storage at 10 Hz, provides a description closely matching the EMG recordings for these movements. The data provide an excellent agreement with the EMG recordings of the legs (Fig. 36.60) and with the nocturnal PSG for number of leg movements (254).

Studies have been conducted using actigraphy and PSG recordings simultaneously to validate the ability of the actigraph to distinguish sleep from wakefulness. Assessment of sleep/wakefulness for a prolonged period of time (days to weeks) has been the main indication of actigraphy. Total sleep time and sleep onset time, however, have shown variable results with discrepancy from PSG results. Computer algorithms are available for automatic sleep–wake scoring, but visual inspection of the raw data is necessary. The reliability and validity of the data are available only for a specific actigraph model; no universally validated data are available. Actigraphs can differentiate sleep from wakefulness but cannot differentiate REM from NREM sleep and cannot identify different NREM sleep stages. Actigraphs and sleep logs are complementary.

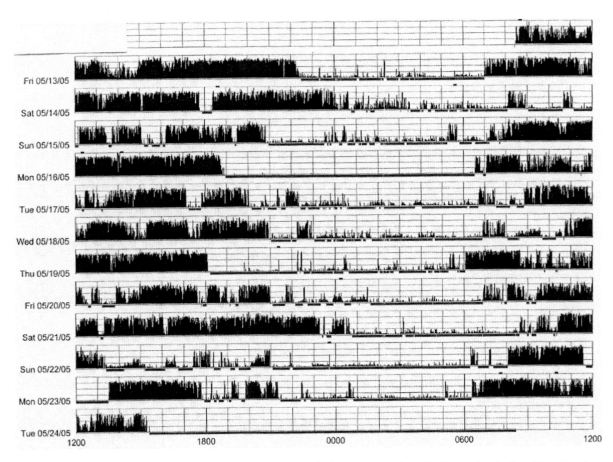

Figure 36.62. *This wrist actigraphic recording is taken from a 50-year-old woman with chronic insomnia due to inadequate sleep hygiene. The actigraph worn for 11 days shows highly irregular bedtime and wakeup time. The waking period is indicated by black bars and the sleep period by gray bars. Note excessive body movements (indicated by black bars) during sleep period and brief periods of sleepiness (white areas) during wakefulness (black bars). Note the subject did not wear the actigraph on Monday, 5/16/05, from 7 p.m. to 6:30 a.m. (fourth from the top showing a continuous, thick, black line).*

4.3.1. RECOMMENDATIONS FOR ACTIGRAPHY

The AASM standards of practice committee suggests the following recommendations for actigraphy (249):

- Actigraphy may be a useful adjunct to history and physical examination and sleep logs in patients with insomnia, including sleep state misperception and inadequate sleep hygiene (Figs. 36.61 and 36.62), circadian rhythm sleep disorders (255) (Figs. 36.63 and 36.64), and EDS.

- Actigraphy may be a useful adjunct to detect the rest time and activity patterns during modified HSAT.

- Actigraphy may be useful in assessing EDS in situations where MSLT is not practical.

- Actigraphy is useful to detect rest time and activity patterns over days and weeks when a sleep log or other methods cannot provide such data.

- Actigraphy may be useful for monitoring circadian rhythm disturbances in special populations (e.g., the elderly and nursing home patients); newborns, infants, children, and adolescents; hypertensive individuals (to monitor circadian patterns of blood pressure and circadian therapeutic effectiveness of medications); depressed or schizophrenic patients; and individuals during space flight.

- Actigraphy may be useful to measure outcomes in clinical trials.

- Actigraphs are not indicated for the diagnosis, assessment, or severity of any sleep disorder, including insomnia and OSAS.

4.3.2. ADVANTAGES OF ACTIGRAPH OVER PSG

Advantages include the following:

Easy accessibility

Inexpensive recording over extended periods (e.g., days, weeks, or even months)

Recording of 24-hour activities at all sites (home, work, or lab)

Useful in uncooperative and demented patients when a laboratory PSG study is not possible

Ability to conduct longitudinal studies to monitor disease progression, remission, and therapeutic responses

Ability to overcome the problem of nighttime variability noted in many sleep disorders and some nocturnal movement disorders

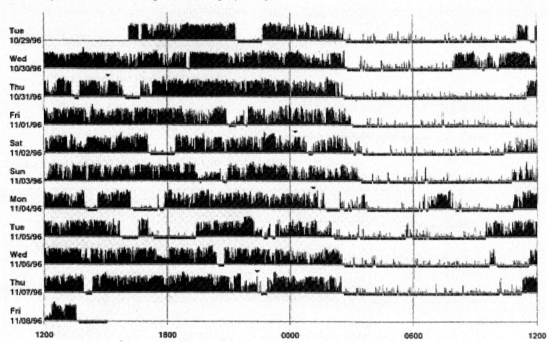

File: 11896DO.DAT   Epoch: 60   Scale: 377   Algorithm: Cole-Kripke (rescore)

Tue 10/29/96
Wed 10/30/96
Thu 10/31/96
Fri 11/01/96
Sat 11/02/96
Sun 11/03/96
Mon 11/04/96
Tue 11/05/96
Wed 11/06/96
Thu 11/07/96
Fri 11/08/96

1200   1800   0000   0600   1200

Figure 36.63. *Primary delayed sleep phase syndrome. This wrist actigraphic recording is taken from a 29-year-old man with a lifelong history of delayed sleep onset and delayed wakeup time. The actigram shows his typical sleep period from 3 to 4 a.m. to 9 a.m. to noon (white areas). If he has to wake up early in the morning, he feels exhausted and sleepy all day. He feels fine if he is allowed to follow his own schedule. Melatonin at night did not help him. Morning bright light therapy was suggested but the patient declined. Reproduced from Chokroverty S, Thomas R, Bhatt M, eds. Atlas of Sleep Medicine. Philadelphia: Elsevier; 2005, with permission.*

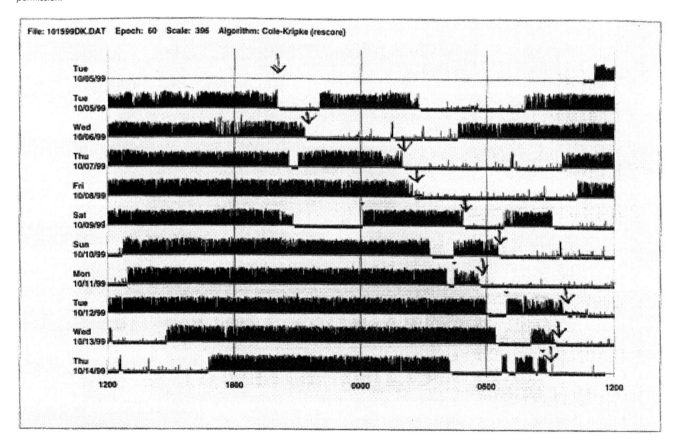

File: 161599DK.DAT   Epoch: 60   Scale: 395   Algorithm: Cole-Kripke (rescore)

Tue 10/05/99
Tue 10/05/99
Wed 10/06/99
Thu 10/07/99
Fri 10/08/99
Sat 10/09/99
Sun 10/10/99
Mon 10/11/99
Tue 10/12/99
Wed 10/13/99
Thu 10/14/99

1200   1800   0000   0600   1200

Figure 36.64. *Sleep–wake schedule disorder in a patient with acquired immunodeficiency syndrome (AIDS). This wrist actigram is taken from a 46-year-old man with AIDS. The patient presented with sleep difficulty due to inability to fall asleep and wake at desired bedtime and wakeup time. This 10-day recording shows disorganization of the sleep–wake schedule. There is a suggestion of non–24-hour (hypernychthemeral) syndrome with progressive delay of sleep onset (arrows) from day 1 to day 6, and again delayed sleep onset (arrows) from day 7 to day 10. Reproduced from Chokroverty S, Thomas R, Bhatt M, eds. Atlas of Sleep Medicine. Philadelphia: Elsevier; 2005, with permission.*

BOX 36.1. PSG MONTAGE FREQUENTLY USED IN OUR LABORATORY

Channel Number	Name
1	F3-M2
2	C3-M2
3	T3-M2
4	01-M2
5	F4-M1
6	C4-MI
7	T4-M1
8	02-M1
9	Left electro-oculogram (E1-M1)
10	Right electro-oculogram (E2-M1)
11	Chin EMG
12	ECG
13	Heart rate
14	Left gastrocnemius EMG
15	Left tibialis anterior EMG
16	Right gastrocnemius EMG
17	Right tibialis anterior EMG
18	Intercostal EMG
19	Oronasal thermistor*
20	Nasal pressure transducer*
21	Chest
22	Abdomen
23	Snoring
24	Arterial oxygen saturation

ECG, electrocardiogram; EMG, electromyogram.

Channels 1 to 8 record electroencephalographic activity from bilateral cerebral hemispheres in a referential chain; electrode designation per the International 10-20 System of electrode placement. M1 and M2, left and right mastoid, respectively. Channels 19 and 20 record airflow ("flow channels"). Channels 21 and 22 record respiratory effort ("effort channels").

*In a continuous positive airway pressure (CPAP) titration study, flow channels are replaced by a CPAP signal (C-flow signal).

BOX 36.2. EXTENDED EEG ("SEIZURE") MONTAGE USED DURING OVERNIGHT PSG RECORDING IN PATIENTS SUSPECTED TO HAVE NOCTURNAL SEIZURES

Channel Number	Name
1	F4-M1
2	C4-M1
3	02-M1
4	C3-M2
5	Fp1-F7
6	F7-T3
7	T3-T5
8	T5-01
9	Fp2-F8
10	F8-T4
11	T4-T6
12	T6-02
13	Fp1-F3
14	F3-C3
15	C3-P3
16	P3-01
17	Fp2-F4
18	F4-C4
19	C4-P4
20	P4-02
21	Left electro-oculogram (El-M1)
22	Right electro-oculogram (E2-M1)
23	Chin EMG
24	Right masseter EMG
25	Left biceps EMG
26	Right biceps EMG
27	Left tibialis anterior EMG
28	Right tibialis anterior EMG
29	Intercostal EMG
30	Oronasal thermistor*
31	Nasal pressure transducer*

(continued)

BOX 36.2. CONTINUED

32	Chest
33	Abdomen
34	Snoring
35	Arterial oxygen saturation
36	ECG
37	Heart rate

ECG, electrocardiogram; EMG, electromyogram.

Channels 1 to 20 record electroencephalographic activity from bilateral cerebral hemispheres with referential and bipolar montages, including both temporal and parasagittal chains; electrode designation per the International 10-20 System of electrode placement. Channels 30 and 31 record airflow ("flow channels"). Channels 32 and 33 record respiratory effort ("effort channels").

*In a continuous positive airway pressure (CPAP) titration study, flow channels are replaced by a CPAP signal (C-flow signal).

Ability to discriminate real movements from clinically insignificant EMG potentials

Usefulness in sleep state misperception

Ability to document delayed or advanced sleep-phase syndrome or non-24-hour circadian rhythm disorders (although sleep logs may suggest such diagnosis)

Finally, actigraphs are small, lightweight, easily maintained, and inexpensive in contrast to the bulky, labor-intensive, expensive, and inconvenient PSG recordings.

4.3.2. DISADVANTAGES AND LIMITATIONS OF ACTIGRAPH RECORDINGS

These include the following:

Inability to diagnose sleep apnea and to clarify the etiology of insomnia

Overestimation of sleep (some insomniacs may lie down in bed for prolonged periods without moving)

Inability to identify subjects who are feigning sleep problems

Inability to discriminate movements such as PLMs from other body movements

Inability to provide any information about other physiological characteristics (e.g., EEG, EOG, respiration)

Records are nonspecific because the actometer records all kinds of movements

Lack of standardization of placement of the actigraph may also be seen as a pitfall. Most commonly the actigraph is placed on the nondominant side. Activity is somewhat different between the two sides, with more activities being recorded from dominant than from nondominant limbs. The overall agreement, however, for sleep period between the two sites is not frequently different when compared with the PSG data.

In conclusion, the actigraph is an inexpensive, useful method for longitudinal assessment of sleep–wake pattern, can differentiate normal sleep patterns from those of disturbed sleep due to insomnia and sleep-disordered breathing, and can differentiate normal sleep from sleep–wake schedule disturbances by recording over long periods and longitudinal monitoring.

REFERENCES

1. Berger H. Uber Das elektroencephalogramm Des Menschen. *Arch Psychiatr Nervenkr.* 1929;87:527–570.
2. Aserinsky E, Kleitman N. Regularly occurring periods of eye motility and concomitant phenomenon during sleep. *Science.* 1953;119:273.
3. Holland JV, Dement WC, Raynal DM. Polysomnography: a response for a need for improved communication. Paper presented at the 14th annual meeting of the Association of the Psychophysiological Study of Sleep, Association of the Psychophysiological Study of Sleep, Jackson Hole, WY, 1974:121.
4. Caton R. The electric currents of the brain. *BMJ.* 1975;2:278.
5. Loomis AL, Harvey EN, Hobart GA. Cerebral states during sleep, as studied by human brain potentials. *J Exp Physiol.* 1937;21:127.
6. Kohlschutter E. Messeungen Dar Festigkei Des Schlafes. *Zeitschrift Fur Rationelle Medicin.* 1863;17(3):209–253.
7. Basner M. Arousal threshold determination in 1862: Kohlschutter's measurements on the firmness of sleep. *Sleep Med.* 2010;11:417–422.
8. Dement WC, Kleitman N. Cyclic variations of EEG during sleep and their relation to eye movements, body motility and dreaming. *Electroencephalogr Clin Neurophysiol.* 1957;9:673.
9. Jouvet M, Michel F. Correlations electromyographiques du sommeil chez le chat decortique et nesencephalique chroniue. *Comp Rend Soc Biol (Paris).* 1959;153:422–425.
10. Berger RJ. Tonus of extrinsic laryngeal muscles during sleep and dreaming. *Science.* 1961;134:840.
11. Rechtschaffen K, Kales A. *A Manual of Standardized Terminology, Techniques and Scoring System for Sleep Stages of Human Subjects.* Washington DC: US Government Printing Office, 1968.
12. American Academy of Sleep Medicine. *The AASM Manual 2007 for the Scoring of Sleep and Associated Events: Rules, Terminology and Technical Specifications.* Westchester, IL: American Academy of Sleep Medicine, 2007.
13. Griesinger W. Berliner medizinischpsychologische Gesclleschaft. *Arch Psychiatr Nervenkr.* 1868;1:200–204.
14. Freud S. Project for a scientific psychology. In: Bonaparte M, Freud A, Kris, E eds. *The Origins of Psychoanalysis: Letters to Wilhelm Fliess, Drafts and Notes, 1895 to 1902.* New York: Basic Books, 1954:400.
15. Wolpert S. *A New History of India.* New York: Oxford University Press, 1982:48.
16. Jones B. Neurology of NREM sleep. In: Montagna P, Chokroverty S, eds. *Sleep Disorders, Handbook of Clinical Neurology.* Amsterdam: Elsevier, 2011.
17. Saper CB, Scammell TE, Lu J. Hypothalamic regulation of sleep and circadian rhythms. *Nature.* 2005;437:1257–1263.
18. Peyron C, Tighe DK, Van den Pol AN, et al. Neurons containing hypocretin (orexin) project to multiple neuronal systems. *J Neurosci.* 1998;18:9996.
19. Siegel JM. Mechanisms of sleep control. *J Clin Neurophysiol.* 1990;7:49.
20. McCarley RW. Neurobiology of REM and NREM sleep. *Sleep Med.* 2007;8:302–330.
21. Lu J, Sherman D, Devor M, et al. A putative flip-flop switch for control of REM sleep. *Nature.* 2006;441:589.
22. Luppi PH, Clement O, Sapin E, et al. The neuronal network responsible for paradoxical sleep and its dysfunctions causing narcolepsy and rapid eye movement (REM) behavior disorder. *Sleep Med Rev.* 2011;15:153–163.
22a. Luppi P-H, Clement O, Fort P. Paradoxical (REM) sleep genesis by the brainstem is under hypothalamic control. *Curr Opin Neurobiol.* 2013;23:786–792.
22b. Luppi P-H, Clement O, Garcia SV, et al. New aspects in the pathophysiology of rapid eye movement sleep behavior disorders: the potential role of glutamate, gamma-aminobutyric acid and glycine. *Sleep Med,* 2013;14:714–718,

22c. Chen MC, Yu H, Huang Z-L, Lu J. Rapid eye movement sleep behavior disorder. *Curr Opin Neurobiol.* 2013;23:793–798.

23. Saper CB, Chou T, Scammell TE. The sleep switch: hypothalamic control of sleep and wakefulness. *Trends Neurosci.* 2001;24:726.

24. Porkka-Hieskanen T, Strecker RE, Thakkar M, et al. Adenosine: a mediator of the sleep-inducing effects of prolonged wakefulness. *Science.* 1997;276:1265.

25. Chokroverty S. Physiological changes in sleep. In: Chokroverty S, ed. *Sleep Disorders Medicine: Basic Science, Technical Considerations and Clinical Aspects.* 4th ed. New York: Springer Science, 2017: 153–194.

26. Moore RY. Circadian timing and sleep-wake regulation. In: Chokroverty S, ed. *Sleep Disorders Medicine: Basic Science, Technical Considerations and Clinical Aspects.* 3rd ed. Philadelphia: Elsevier, 2009:105–111.

27. Daan S, Beersma DGM, Borbely AA. The timing of human sleep: A recovery process gated by a circadian pacemaker. *Am J Physiol.* 1984;246:R161–R178.

28. Dinges DF, Broughton RJ. *Sleep and Alertness: Chronobiological, Behavioral and Medical Aspects of Napping.* New York: Raven Press, 1989.

29. Dijk DJ, Czeisler CA. Contribution of the circadian pacemaker and the sleep homeostat to sleep propensity, sleep structure, electroencephalographic slow waves and sleep spindle activity in humans. *J Neurosci.* 1995;15:3525–3538.

29a. Nedergaard M. Neuroscience garbage struck of the brain. Science 2014; 340: 1529-1530.

30. Jasper HH. The ten-twenty electrode system of the International Federation. *Electroencephalogr Clin Neurophysiol.* 1958;10:371.

31. Mouret J, Delorme F, Jouvet M. Activité des muscles de la face au cours du sommeil paradoxal chez l'homme. *Compt Rend Soc Biol Paris.* 1965;159:391–394.

32. Bliwise D, Coleman R, Bergmann B, et al. Facial muscle tonus during REM and NREM sleep. *Psychophysiology.* 1974;11:497–508.

32a. Bhat S, Chokroverty S. Electroencephalography, Electromyography, and Electro-oculography: General Principles and Basic Technology. In Chokroverty S, ed. Sleep Disorders Medicine: Basic Science, Technical Considerations and clinical aspects, 4th ed. New York: Springer Science, 2017;295–330.

33. AASM Task Force. Sleep-related breathing disorders in adults: recommendations for syndrome definition and measurement techniques in clinical research. *Sleep.* 1999;22(5):667–689.

34. Kales A, Kales J. Recent findings in the diagnosis and treatment of disturbed sleep. *N Engl J Med.* 1974;209:487–499.

35. Williams RI, Karacan I, Hursch CJ. *EEG of Human Sleep: Clinical Applications.* New York: Wiley, 1974.

36. Bonnet MH, Arand DL. EEG arousal norms by age. *J Clin Sleep Med.* 2007;3(3):271–274.

37. Bonnet M, Carley D, Carskadon M, et al. EEG arousals: scoring rules and examples: a preliminary report of the Sleep Disorders Atlas Task Force of the ASDA. *Sleep.* 1992;15:173–184.

38. Coleman RM, Pollak C, Weitzman ED. Periodic movements in sleep (nocturnal myoclonus): relation to sleep-wake disorders. *Ann Neurol.* 1980;8:416–421.

39. Bonnet M, Carley D, Carskadon M, et al. Recording and scoring leg movements. *Sleep.* 1993;16:748–759.

40. Zucconi M, Ferri R, Allen R, et al. The official World Association of Sleep Medicine standards for recording and scoring PLMS and PLMW developed in collaboration with a task force from the International RLS Study Group. *Sleep Med.* 2006;7:175–183.

40a. Ferri R, Fulda S, Allen RP, et al. World Association of Sleep Medicine (WASM) 2016 Standards for recording and scoring leg movements in polysomnograms developed by a joint task force from the International and the European Restless Legs Syndrome study groups (IRLSSG and EURLSSG). *Sleep Med* 2016;26:86–95.

41. Montplaisir J, Boucher S, Lesperance P, et al. Immobilization tests and periodic leg movements in sleep for the diagnosis of restless legs syndrome. *Mov Disord.* 1998;13(2):324–329.

42. Gastaut H, Tassinari C, Duron B. Etude polygraphique des manifestations épisodiques (hypniques et respiratoires) du syndrome de Pickwick. *Rev Neurol.* 1965;112:568–579.

43. Young T, Palta M, Dempsey J, et al. The occurrence of sleep disordered breathing among middle-ages adults. *N Engl J Med.* 1993;328:1230–1235.

44. Bixler EO, Vgontas AN, Ten Have T, et al. Effects of age on sleep apnea in men: prevalence and severity. *Am J Resp Cricial Care Med.* 1998;157:144–148.

45. Pavlova MK, Duffy JF, Shea SA. PSG respiratory abnormalities in asymptomatic individuals. *Sleep.* 2008;31:241–248.

46. Terzano MG, Mancia D, Salati MR, et al. The cyclic alternating pattern as a physiologic component of normal NREM sleep. *Sleep.* 1985;8:137–145.

47. Terzano MG, Parrino L, Sherieri A, et al. Atlas, rules, and recording techniques for the scoring of cyclic alternating pattern (CAP) in human sleep. *Sleep Med.* 2001;2:537–553.

48. Parrino L, Halasz P, Tassinari CA, et al. CAP, epilepsy, and motor events during sleep: the unifying role of arousal. *Sleep Med Rev.* 2006;10:267–285.

49. Indications for PSG Task Force. Practice parameters for the indications for PSG and related procedures. *Sleep.* 1997;20:406–422.

50. Kushida CA, Littner MR, Morgenthaler T, et al. Practice parameters for the indications for PSG and related procedures: an update for 2005. *Sleep.* 2005;28:499–521.

51. Chesson AL Jr, Berry RB, Pack A. Practice parameters for the use of portable monitoring devices in the investigation of suspected obstructive sleep apnea in adults. *Sleep.* 2003;26:907.

52. Department of Health and Human Services, Center for Medicare and Medicaid Services. Decision Memo for Continuous Positive Airway Pressure (CPAP) Therapy for Obstructive Sleep Apnea (OSA). CAG#0093R. March 13, 2008. Available at: http://www.cms.hhs.gov/mcd/viewdecisionmemo.asp?from2=viewdecisionmemo.asp&id=204&. Accessed August 7, 2010.

53. Collop NA, Anderson WM, Boehlecke B, et al. Clinical guidelines for the use of unattended portable monitors in the diagnosis of obstructive sleep apnea in adult patients. Portable Monitoring Task Force of the American Academy of Sleep Medicine. *J Clin Sleep Med.* 2007;3:737–747.

54. Nerfeldt P, Aoki F, Friberg D. Polygraphy vs. polysomnography: missing OSAS in symptomatic snorers; a reminder for clinicians. *Sleep Breath.* 2014;18(2):297–303.

55. Kapoor M, Greenough G. Home sleep tests for obstructive sleep apnea (OSA). *J Am Board Fam Med.* 2015;28(4):504–509.

56. Collop N. Home sleep testing: appropriate screening is the key. *Sleep.* 2012;35:1445–1446.

57. Bruyneel M, Ninane V. Unattended home-based polysomnography for sleep-disordered breathing: current concepts and perspectives. *Sleep Med Rev.* 2014;18(4):341–347.

58. Shah P, Gurubhagavatula I. Portable monitoring: practical aspects and case examples. *Sleep Med Clin.* 2011;186(3):355–366.

59. Penzel T, Hirshkowitz M, Harsh J, et al. Digital analysis and technical specifications. *J Clin Sleep Med.* 2007;3(2):109–120.

60. Schulz H. Rethinking sleep analysis: comment on the *AASM Manual for Scoring Sleep and Associated Events. J Clin Sleep Med.* 2008;4:99–103.

61. Guilleminault C, Stoohs R, Clerk A, et al. A cause of daytime sleepiness: the upper airway resistance syndrome. *Chest.* 1993;104: 781–787.

62. Exar E, Collop N. The upper airway resistance syndrome. *Chest.* 1999;115:1127–1139.

63. Norman RG, Ahmed MM, Walsleben JA, et al. Detection of respiratory events during NPSG: nasal cannula/pressure sensor versus thermistor. *Sleep.* 1997;20:1175–1184.

64. Epstein MD, Chicoine SA, Hanumara RC. Detection of UARS using a nasal cannula/pressure transducer. *Chest.* 2000;117:1073–1077.

65. Budhiraja R, Goodwin JL, Parthasarathy S, et al. Comparisons of NPT and thermistor for detection of respiratory events during PSG in children. *Sleep.* 2005;28(9):1117–1121.

66. Chokroverty S, Bhatt S. Polysomnographic recording technique. In: Chokroverty S, Thomas RJ, eds. *Atlas of Sleep Medicine.* 2nd ed. Philadelphia: Elsevier/Saunders, 2014:1–25

67. Scammell TE. Narcolepsy. *N Engl J Med.* 2015;373:2654–2662.

68. Nishino S. Clinical and neurobiological aspects of narcolepsy. *Sleep Med.* 2007;8:373–399.

69. American Academy of Sleep Medicine. *International Classification of Sleep Disorders.* 3rd ed. Darien, IL: American Academy of Sleep Medicine, 2014.

70. Pizza F, Tartarotti S, Poryazova R, Baumann CR, Bassetti CL. Sleep-disordered breathing and periodic limb movements in narcolepsy with cataplexy: a systematic analysis of 35 consecutive patients. *Eur Neurol.* 2013;70:22–26.

71. Mattarozzi K, Bellucci C, Campi C, et al. Clinical, behavioral and PSG correlates of cataplexy in patients with narcolepsy/cataplexy. *Sleep Med.* 2008;9:425–433.

72. Harsh J, Peszka J, Hartwig G, et al. Night-time sleep and EDS in narcolepsy. *J Sleep Res.* 2000;9:309–316.

73. Christensen J, Carrillo O, Leary E, et al. Sleep stage transitions during polysomnographic recordings as diagnostic features of type 1 narcolepsy. *Sleep Med.* 2015;16:1558–1566.

74. Andlauer O, Moore H, Jouhier L, et al. Nocturnal rapid eye movement sleep latency for identifying patients with narcolepsy/hypocretin deficiency. *JAMA Neurol.* 2013;70:891–902.

75. Reiter J, Katz E, Scammel T, et al. Usefulness of a nocturnal SOREMP for diagnosing narcolepsy with cataplexy in a pediatric population. *Sleep.* 2015;38:859–865.

76. Frenette E, Kushida CA. Primary hypersomnia of central origin. *Semin Neurol.* 2009;29:354–367.

77. Baker TL, Guilleminault C, Nino-Murcia G, Dement W. Comparative PSG study of narcolepsy and idiopathic CNS hypersomnia. *Sleep.* 1986;9:232–242.

78. Arnulf I, Rico TJ, Mignot E. Diagnosis, disease course, and management of patients with Kleine-Levin syndrome. *Lancet Neurol.* 2012;11:918–928.

79. Lavault S, Golmard JL, Groos E, Brion A, Dauvilliers Y, Lecendreux M, Franco P, Arnulf I. Kleine-Levin syndrome in 120 patients: differential diagnosis and long episodes. *Ann Neurol.* 2015;77:529–540.

80. Papacostas SS, Hadjivasilis V. The Kleine-Levin syndrome. Report of a case and review of the literature. *Eur Psychiatry.* 2000;15:231–235.

81. Dauvilliers Y, Mayer G, Lecendreux M, et al. Kleine-Levin syndrome: an autoimmune hypothesis based on clinical and genetic analyses. *Neurology.* 2002;59:1739–1745.

82. Gadoth N, Kesler A, Vainstein G, Peled R, Lavie P. Clinical and polysomnographic characteristics of 34 patients with Kleine-Levin syndrome. J Sleep Res. 2001;10:337–341.

83. Huang YS, Lin YH, Guilleminault C. PSG in Kleine–Levine syndrome. *Neurology.* 2008;70(10):795–801.

84. Kleine W. Periodische Schlafsucht. *Mschr Psychiat Neurol.* 1925;57:285–320.

85. Billiard M, Guilleminault C, Dement WC. A menstruation-linked periodic hypersomnia. Kleine-Levin syndrome or new clinical entity? *Neurology.* 1975;25:436–443.

86. Billiard M, Jaussent I, Dauvilliers Y, Besset A. Recurrent hypersomnia: a review of 339 cases. *Sleep Med Rev.* 2011;15:247–257.

87. Sachs C, Persson HE, Hagenfeldt K. Menstruation-related periodic hypersomnia: a case study with successful treatment. *Neurology.* 1982;32:1376–1379.

88. Schenck CH, Bundie SR, Ettinger MG, et al. Chronic behavioral disorders of human REM sleep. A new category of parasomnia. *Sleep.* 1986;9:293–308.

89. Schenck C, Mahowald M. REM sleep behavior disorder: clinical developmental, and neuroscience perspectives 16 years after formal identification. *Sleep.* 2002;25:120–138.

90. Boeve B, Silber M, Parisi J, et al. Synucleinopathy pathology and REM sleep behavior disorder plus dementia or parkinsonism. *Neurology.* 2003;61:40–45.

91. Claassen DO, Joseph KA, Ahlskog JE, Silber MH, Tippman-Peikert M, Boeve BF. REM sleep behavior disorder preceding other aspects of synucleinopathies by up to half a century. *Neurology.* 2010;75:494–499.

92. Brass SD, Duquette P, Proulx-Therrien J, Auerbach S. Sleep disorders in patients with multiple sclerosis. *Sleep Med Rev.* 2010;14:121–129.

93. Nightingale S, Orgill JC, Ebrahim IO, de Lacy SF, Agrawal S, Williams AJ. The association between narcolepsy and REM behavior disorder (RBD). *Sleep Med.* 2005;6:253–258.

94. Lapierre O, Montplaisir J. PSG features of REM sleep behavior disorder: development of a scoring method. *Neurology.* 1992;42:1371–1374.

95. Foldvary N, Caruso AC, Maschaa E, et al. Identifying montages that best detect EEG seizure activity during polysomnography. *Sleep.* 2000;23:221–229.

96. Foldvary-Schaefer N, DeOcamp J, Mascha E, et al. Accuracy of seizure detection using abbreviated EEG during polysomnography. *J Clin Neurophysiol.* 2006;23:68–71.

97. Montagna P. Nocturnal paroxysmal dystonia and nocturnal wandering. *Neurology.* 1992;42(7 Suppl 6):61–67.

98. Provini F, Plazzi G, Tinuper P et al. Nocturnal frontal lobe epilepsy: A clinical and polygraphic overview of 100 consecutive cases. *Brain.* 1999;122:1017–1031.

99. Boursoulian LJ, Schenck CH, Mahowald MW, Lagrange AH. Differentiating parasomnias from nocturnal seizures. *J Clin Sleep Med.* 2012;8:108–112.

100. Tinuper P, Provini F, Bisulli F, Vignatelli L, Plazzi G, Vetrugno R, Montagna P, Lugaresi E. Movement disorders in sleep: guidelines for differentiating epileptic from non-epileptic motor phenomena arising from sleep. *Sleep Med Rev.* 2007;11:255–267.

101. Derry CP, Harvey AS, Walker MC, Duncan JS, Berkovic SF. NREM arousal parasomnias and their distinction from nocturnal frontal lobe epilepsy: a video-EEG analysis. *Sleep.* 2009;32:1637–1644.

102. Jung R, Kuhlo W. Neurophysiological studies of abnormal night sleep and the Pickwickian syndrome. *Prog Brain Res.* 1965;18:140.

103. Mayer P, Pépin JL, Bettega G, Veale D, Ferretti G, Deschaux C, Lévy P. Relationship between body mass index, age and upper airway measurements in snorers and sleep apnoea patients. *Eur Respir J.* 1996;9:1801–1809.

104. White DP. Pathogenesis of obstructive and central sleep apnea. *Am J Respir Crit Care Med.* 2005;172:1363–1370.

105. Horner RL. Contribution of passive mechanical loads and active compensation to upper airway collapsibility during sleep. *J Appl Physiol.* 2007;102:510–512.

106. Malhotra A, White DP. Obstructive sleep apnoea. *Lancet.* 2002;360:237–245.

107. Levy P, Pepin JL, Arnaud C, et al. Intermittent hypoxia and sleep-disordered breathing: current concepts and perspectives. *Eur Respir.* 2008;32:1082–1095.

108. Yaggi HK, Concato J, Kernan WN, et al. Obstructive sleep apnea as a risk factor for stroke and death. *N Engl J Med.* 2005;353: 2024–2041.

109. Peppard PE, Young T, Barnet JH, et al. Increased prevalence of sleep-disordered breathing in adults. *Am J Epidemiol.* 2013;177:1006–1014.

110. Young T, Peppard PE, Gottlieb DJ. Epidemiology of obstructive sleep apnea: a population health perspective. *Am J Respir Crit Care Med.* 2002;165:1217–1239.

111. Sateia MJ. International classification of sleep disorders—third edition: highlights and modifications. *Chest.* 2014;146:1387–1394.

112. Chirinos JA, Gurubhagavatula I, Teff K, et al. CPAP, weight loss, or both for obstructive sleep apnea. *N Engl J Med.* 2014;370:2265–2275.

113. Thomasouli M, Brady EM, Davies MJ, Hall AP, Khunti K, Morris DH, Gray LJ. The impact of diet and lifestyle management strategies for obstructive sleep apnoea in adults: a systematic review and meta-analysis of randomised controlled trials. *Sleep Breath.* 2013;17:925–935.

114. Bixler EO, Vgontzas AN, Ten Have T, Tyson K, Kales A. Effects of age on sleep apnea in men: I. Prevalence and severity. *Am J Respir Crit Care Med.* 1998;157:144–148.

115. Johansson P, Alehagen U, Svanborg E, Dahlstrom U, Brostrom A. Sleep disordered breathing in an elderly community-living population: relationship to cardiac function, insomnia symptoms and daytime sleepiness. *Sleep Med.* 2009;10:1005–1011.

116. Eckert DJ, Jordan AS, Merchia P, Malhotra A. Central sleep apnea: Pathophysiology and treatment. *Chest.* 2007;131:595–607.

117. Bjorvatn B, Pallesen S. A practical approach to circadian rhythm sleep disorders. *Sleep Med Rev.* 2009;13:47–60.

118. Allen RP, Picchietti D, Hening WA, et al. Restless legs syndrome: diagnostic criteria, special considerations, and epidemiology. A report from the restless legs syndrome diagnosis and epidemiology workshop at the National Institute of Health. *Sleep Med.* 2003;4:101–119.

119. Phillips B, Young T, Finn L, Asher K, Hening WA, Purvis C. Epidemiology of restless legs symptoms in adults. *Arch Intern Med.* 2000;160:2137–2141.

120. Rothdach AJ, Trenkwalder C, Haberstock J, Keil U, Berger K. Prevalence and risk factors for RLS in an elderly population: the MEMO study. Memory and morbidity in Augsburg Elderly. *Neurology.* 2000;54:1064–1068.

121. Berger K, Luedemann J, Trenkwalder C, John U, Kessler C. Sex and the risk of restless legs syndrome in the general population. *Arch Intern Med.* 2004;164:196–202.

122. Allen RP, Walters AS, Montplaisir J, Hening W, Myers A, Bell TJ, Ferini-Strambi L. Restless legs syndrome prevalence and impact. REST general population study. *Arch Intern Med.* 2005;165:1286–1292.

123. Chervin RD, Archbold KH, Dillon JE, Pituch KJ, Panahi P, Dahl RE, Guilleminault C. Association between symptoms of inattention, hyperactivity, restless legs, and periodic limb movements. *Sleep.* 2002;25:213–218.

124. Rajaram SS, Walters AS, England SJ, Mehta D, Nizam F. Some children with growing pains may actually have restless legs syndrome. *Sleep.* 2004;27:767–773.

125. Ekbom KA. Restless legs: a clinical study. *Acta Med Scand.* 1945;158(Suppl):1–122.

126. Winkelmann J, Schormair B, Lichtner P, et al. Genome-wide association study of restless legs syndrome identifies common variants in three genomic regions. *Nat Genet.* 2007;39:1000–1006.

127. Stefansson H, Rye DB, Hicks A, et al. A genetic risk factor for periodic limb movements in sleep. *N Engl J Med.* 2007;357:639–647.

128. Yang Q, Li LL, Chen Q, et al. Association studies of variants in MEIS1, BTBD9, and MAP2K5/SKOR1 with restless legs syndrome in a US population. *Sleep Med.* 2011;12:800–804.

129. Kemlink D, Polo O, Frauscher B, et al. Replication of restless legs syndrome loci in three European populations. *J Med Genet.* 2009;46:315–318.

130. Winkelmann J, Czamara D, Schormair B, et al. Genome-wide association study identifies novel restless legs syndrome susceptibility loci on 2p14 and 16q12.1. *PLoS Genet.* 2011;7:e1002171.

131. Catoire H, Dion PA, Xiong L, et al. Restless legs syndrome-associated MEIS1 risk variant influences iron homeostasis. *Ann Neurol.* 2011;70:170–175.

132. Freeman A, Pranski E, Miller RD, et al. Sleep fragmentation and motor restlessness in a Drosophila model of restless legs syndrome. *Curr Biol.* 2012;22:1142–1148.

133. Allen RP, Picchietti DL, Garcia-Borreguero D, et al. Restless legs syndrome/Willis-Ekbom disease diagnostic criteria: updated International Restless Legs Syndrome Study Group (IRLSSG) consensus criteria—history, rationale, description, and significance. *Sleep Med.* 2014;15:860–873

133a. Chokroverty S. Differential diagnoses of restless legs syndrome/Willis-Ekbom disease: mimics and comorbidities. *Sleep Med Clin.* 2015;10:249–262.

134. Hening WA, Allen RP, Washburn M, Lesage S, Earley CJ. Validation of the Hopkins telephone diagnostic interview for restless legs syndrome. *Sleep Med.* 2008;9:283–289.

135. Muntean M-L, Sixel-Doring F, Trenkwalder C. Serum ferritin levels in Parkinson's disease patients with and without restless legs syndrome. *Mov Disord Clin Prac.* 2015;2:249–252.

136. Morgan LK. Restless limbs: a commonly overlooked symptom controlled by Valium. *Med J Aust.* 1967;2:589–594.

137. Walters AS. Frequent occurrence of myoclonus while awake and at rest, body rocking and marching in place in a subpopulation of patients with restless legs syndrome. *Acta Neurol Scand.* 1988;77: 418–421.

138. Lombardi C, Provini F, Vetrugno R, Plazzi G, Lugaresi E, Montagna P. Pelvic movements as rhythmic manifestation associated with restless legs syndrome. *Mov Disord.* 2003;18:110–113.

139. Vetrugno R, Provini F, Plazzi G, Cortelli P, Montagna P. Propriospinal myoclonus: a motor phenomenon found in restless legs syndrome different from periodic limb movements during sleep. *Mov Disord.* 2005;20:1323–1329.

140. Montplaisir J, Boucher S, Poirier G, Lavigne G, Lapierre O, Lesperance P. Clinical, polysomnographic, and genetic characteristics of restless legs syndrome: a study of 133 patients diagnosed with new standard criteria. *Mov Disord.* 1997;12:61–65.

141. Hornyak M, Feig B, Voderholzer U, et al. Polysomnography findings in patients with restless legs syndrome and in healthy controls: a comparative observational study. *Sleep.* 2007;30:861–865.

142. Saletu B, Anderer P, Saletu M, et al. EEG mapping, psychometric, and polysomnographic studies in Restless Legs Syndrome (RLS) and periodic limb movement disorder (PLMD) patients as compared with normal controls. *Sleep Med.* 2002;3(suppl):S35–42.

143. Winkelman JW, Redline S, Baldwin CM, et al. Polysomnographic and health-related quality of life correlates of restless legs syndrome in the Sleep Heart Health Study. *Sleep.* 2009;32:772–778.

144. Hening WA, Walters AS, Wagner M, et al. Circadian rhythm of motor restlessness and sensory symptoms in the idiopathic restless legs syndrome. *Sleep.* 1999;22:901–912.

145. Hogl B, Comella C. Therapeutic advances in restless legs syndrome (RLS). *Mov Disord.* 2015;30:1574–1579.

146. Lugaresi E, Cirignotta F, Coccagna G,Montagna P. Nocturnal myoclonus and restless legs syndrome. *Adv Neurol.* 1986;43:295–307.

147. Provini F, Vetrugno R, Meletti S, Plazzi G, Solieri L, Lugaresi E, Coccagna G, Montagna P. Motor pattern of periodic limb movements during sleep. *Neurology.* 2001;57:300–304.

148. Vetrugno R, D'Angelo R, Montagna P. Periodic limb movements in sleep and periodic limb movement disorder. *Neurol Sci.* 2007;28(Suppl 1):S9–14.

149. Mahowald M. Hope for the PLMS quagmire. *Sleep Med.* 2002;3:463–464.

150. King MA, Jaffre MO, Morrish E, Shneerson JM, Smith IE. The validation of a new actigraphy system for measurement of periodic leg movements in sleep. *Sleep Med.* 2005;6:507–513.

151. Vetrugno R, Montagna P. Sleep-to-wake transition movement disorders. *Sleep Med.* 2011;12(Suppl 2):S11–16.

152. Chokroverty S, Bhat S, Thomas R. Uncommon, atypical, and often unrecognized PSG patterns. In: Chokroverty S, Thomas R, eds. *Atlas of Sleep Medicine.* 2nd ed. Philadelphia: Elsevier/Saunders, 2014:184.

153. Miller TM, Layzer RB. Muscle cramps. *Muscle Nerve.* 2005;32:431–442.

154. Katzberg HD. Neurogenic muscle cramps. *J Neurol.* 2015;262:1814–1821.

155. Minetto MA, Holobar A, Botter A, Ravenni R, Farina D. Mechanisms of cramp contractions: peripheral or central generation? *J Physiol.* 2011;589:5759–5773.

156. Saskin P, Whelton C, Moldofsky H, et al. Sleep and nocturnal leg cramps. *Sleep.* 1988;11:307–308.

157. Carra MC, Huynh N, Fleury B, Lavigne G. Overview on sleep bruxism for sleep medicine clinicians. *Sleep Med Clin.* 2015;10:375–384.

158. Vetrugno R, Provini F, Plazzi G, et al. Familial nocturnal faciomandibular myoclonus mimicking sleep bruxism. *Neurology.* 2002;58:644–647.

159. Meletti S, Cantalupo G, Volpi L, et al. Rhythmic teeth grinding induced by temporal lobe seizures. *Neurology.* 2004;62:2306–2309.

160. Vetrugno R, Manconi M, Ferini-Strambi L, et al. Nocturnal eating: a sleep-related eating disorder or night eating syndrome?. A videopolysomnographic study. *Sleep.* 2006;29:949–954.

161. Winkelmann JW, Johnson EA, Richards LM. Sleep-related eating disorder. *Handb Clin Neurol.* 2011;98:577–585.

162. Vetrugno R, Provini F, Plazzi G. Catathrenia (nocturnal groaning): a new type of parasomnia. *Neurology.* 2001;56:681–683.

163. Siddiqui F, Walters AS, Chokroverty S. Catathrenia: A rare parasomnia which may mimic central sleep apnea on polysomnogram. *Sleep Med.* 2008;9:460–461.

164. Vetrugno R, Lugaresi E, Plazi G, et al. Catathrenia (nocturnal groaning): an abnormal respiratory pattern during sleep. *Eur J Neurol.* 2007;14:1236–1243.

165. Vetrugno R, Lugaresi E, Ferini-Strambi L, Montagna P. Catathrenia (nocturnal groaning): what is it? *Sleep.* 2008;31:308–309.

166. Chokroverty S. Sleep and breathing in neuromuscular disorders. *Hanb Clin Neurol.* 2011;99:1087–1108.

167. Bhat S, Gupta D, Chokroverty S. Sleep disorders in neuromuscular disease. *Neurol Clin.* 2012;30:1359–1387.

167a. Martin TJ, Sanders MH. Chronic alveolar hypoventilation: a review for the clinician. *Sleep.* 1995;18:617–634.

168. Chokroverty S. Sleep and neurodegenerative diseases. *Semin Neurol.* 2009;29:446–467.

169. Schenck CH, Bundlie SR, Mahowald MW. Delayed emergence of a parkinsonian disorder in 38% of 29 older men initially diagnosed with idiopathic rapid eye movement sleep behavior disorder. *Neurology.* 1996;46:388–393.

170. Iranzo A, Fernandez-Arcos A, Tolosa E, et al. Neurodegenerative disorder risk in idiopathic REM sleep behavior disorder: a study of 174 patients. *PLos One.* 2014;9:e89741.

171. Bliwise DL. Sleep in normal aging and dementia. *Sleep.* 1993;16:40–81.

172. Liguori C, Romigi A, Nuccetelli M, et al. Orexinergic system dysregulation, sleep impairment, and cognitive decline in Alzheimer disease. *JAMA Neurol.* 2014;71:1498–1505.

173. Hoyt BD. Sleep in patients with neurologic and psychiatric disorders. *Prim Care.* 2005;32:535–548.

174. Ylikoski A, Martikainen K, Partinen M. Parasomnias and isolated sleep symptoms in Parkinson's disease: a questionnaire study on 661 patients. *J Neurol Sci.* 2014;346:204–208.

175. Thorpy MJ, Adler CH. Parkinson's disease and sleep. *Neurol Clin.* 2005;23:1187–1208.

176. Yong MH, Fook-Chong S, Pavanni R, et al. Case control polysomnographic studies of sleep disorders in Parkinson's disease. *PLoS One.* 2011;6:e22511.

177. Moccia M, Erro R, Picillo M, Santangelo G, et al. A four-year longitudinal study on restless legs syndrome in Parkinson disease. *Sleep.* 2016;39:405–412.

178. Sixel-Doring F, Trautmann E, Mollenhauer B, Trenkwalder C. Associated factors for REM sleep behavior disorder in Parkinson disease. *Neurology.* 2011;77:1048–1054.

179. Breen DP, Vuono R, Nawarathna U, et al. Sleep and circadian rhythm regulation in early Parkinson disease. *JAMA Neurol.* 2014;71: 589–595.

180. Videnovic A, Noble C, Reid KJ, et al. Circadian melatonin rhythm and excessive daytime sleepiness in Parkinson disease. *JAMA Neurol.* 2014;71:463–469.

181. Wienecke M, Werth E, Poryazova R, et al. Progressive dopamine and hypocretin deficiencies in Parkinson's disease: is there an impact on sleep and wakefulness? *J Sleep Res.* 2012;21:710–717.

182. Ferman TJ, Smith GE, Dickson DW, et al. Abnormal daytime sleepiness in dementia with Lewy bodies compared to Alzheimer's disease using the Multiple Sleep Latency Test. *Alzheimers Res Ther.* 2014;16:76.

183. Aldrich MS, Foster NL, White RF, Bluemhein L, Prokopowicz G. Sleep abnormalities in progressive supranuclear palsy. *Ann Neurol.* 1989;25:577–581.

184. Petit D, Gagnon JF, Fantini ML, Ferini-Strambi L, Montplaisir J. Sleep and quantitative EEG in neurodegenerative disorders. *J Psychosom Res.* 2004;56:487–496.

185. Arnulf I, Merino-Andreu M, Bloch F, et al. REM sleep behavior disorder and REM sleep without atonia in patients with progressive supranuclear palsy. *Sleep.* 2005;28:349–354.

186. Sixel-Doring F, Schweitzer M, Mollenhauer B, Trenkwalder C. Polysomnographic findings, video-based sleep analysis and sleep perception in progressive supranuclear palsy. *Sleep Med.* 2009;10:407–415.

187. Wiegand M, Möller AA, Lauer CJ, Stolz S, Schreiber W, Dose M, Krieg JC. Nocturnal sleep in Huntington's disease. *J Neurol.* 1991;238:203–208.

188. Arnulf I, Nielsen J, Lohmann E, et al. Rapid eye movement sleep disturbances in Huntington disease. *Arch Neurol*. 2008;65: 482–488.

189. Goodman A, Barker RA. How vital is sleep in Huntington's disease? *J Neurol*. 2010;257:882–897.

190. Piano C, Losurdo A, Della Marca G, Solito M, Calandra-Buonaura G, Provini F, Bentivoglio AR, Cortelli P. Polysomnographic findings and clinical correlates in Huntington disease: a cross-sectional cohort study. *Sleep*. 2015;38:1489–1495.

191. Hertenstein E, Tang NK, Bernstein CJ, Nissen C, Underwood MR, Sandhu HK. Sleep in patients with primary dystonia: A systematic review on the state of research and perspectives. *Sleep Med Rev*. 2015;26:95–107.

192. Segawa M, Hysaka A, Miwakawa F, et al. Hereditary progressive dystonia with marked diurnal fluctuation. *Adv Neurol*. 1976;14:215–233.

193. Salva MA, Gulleminault C. Olivopontocerebellar degeneration, abnormal sleep and REM sleep without atonia. *Neurology*. 1986;36:576–577.

194. Silber MH, Levine S. Stridor and death in multiple system atrophy. *Mov Disord*. 2000;15:699–704.

195. Vetrugno R, Provini F, Cortelli P, et al. Sleep disorders in multiple system atrophy: a correlative video-polysomnographic study. *Sleep Med*. 2004;5:21–30.

196. Vetrugno R, Liguori P, Cortelli P, et al. Sleep-related stridor due to dystonic vocal cord motion and neurogenic tachypnea/tachycardia in multiple system atrophy. *Mov Disord*. 2007;22:673–678.

197. Munschauer FE, Loh L, Bannister R, Newsom-Davis J. Abnormal respiration and sudden death during sleep in multiple system atrophy with autonomic failure. *Neurology*. 1990;40:677–679.

198. Shimohata T, Ozawa T, Nakayama H, Tomita M, Shinoda H, Nishizawa M. Frequency of nocturnal sudden death in patients with multiple system atrophy. *J Neurol*. 2008;255:1483–1485.

199. Plazzi G, Corsini R, Provini F, et al. REM sleep behavior disorders in multiple system atrophy. *Neurology*. 1997;48:1094–1097.

200. Moreno-Lopez C, Santamaria J, Salamero M, et al. Excessive daytime sleepiness in multiple system atrophy (SLEEMSA study). *Arch Neurol*. 2011;68:223–230.

201. Shimohata T, Nakayama H, Tomita M, Ozawa T, Nishizawa M. Daytime sleepiness in Japanese patients with multiple system atrophy: prevalence and determinants. *BMC Neurol*. 2012;12:130.

202. Wetter TC, Collado-Seidel V, Pollmacher T, Yassouridis A, Trenkwalder C. Sleep and periodic leg movement patterns in drug-free patients with Parkinson's disease and multiple system atrophy. *Sleep*. 2000;23:361–377.

203. Vetrugno R, D'Angelo R, Cortelli P, Plazzi G, Vignatelli L, Montagna P. Impaired cortical and autonomic arousal during sleep in multiple system atrophy. *Clin Neurophysiol*. 2007;118:2512–2518.

204. Schmidt C, Berg D, Prieur S, et al. Loss of nocturnal blood pressure fall in various extrapyramidal syndromes. *Mov Disord*. 2009;24:2136–2142.

205. Ohayon MM. Epidemiology of insomnia: what we know and what we still need to learn. *Sleep Med Rev*. 2002;6:97–111.

206. Roth T, Coulouvrat C, Hajak G, et al. Prevalence and perceived health associated with insomnia based on DSM-IV-TR; International Statistical Classification of Diseases and Related Health Problems, tenth revision; and Research Diagnostic Criteria/International Classification of Sleep Disorders, second edition criteria: results from the America Insomnia Survey. *Biol Psychiatry*. 2011;69:592–600.

207. Kyle SD, Morgan K, Espie CA. Insomnia and health-related quality of life. *Sleep Med Rev*. 2010;14:69–82.

208. Shahly V, Berglund PA, Coulouvrat C, et al. The associations of insomnia with costly workplace accidents and errors: results from the America Insomnia Survey. *Arch Gen Psychiatry*. 2012;69:1054–1063.

209. Laugsand LE, Strand LB, Vatten LJ, Janszky I, Bjørngaard JH. Insomnia symptoms and risk for unintentional fatal injuries: the HUNT Study. *Sleep*. 2014;37:1777–1786.

210. Ribeiro JD, Pease JL, Gutierrez PM, et al. Sleep problems outperform depression and hopelessness as cross-sectional and longitudinal predictors of suicidal ideation and behavior in young adults in the military. *J Affect Disord*. 2012;136:743–750.

211. Shekleton JA, Flynn-Evans EE, Miller B, et al. Neurobehavioral performance impairment in insomnia: relationships with self-reported sleep and daytime functioning. *Sleep*. 2014;37:107–116.

212. Edinger JD, Wyatt JK, Stepanski EJ, et al. Testing the reliability and validity of DSM-IV-TR and ICSD-2 insomnia diagnoses: results of a multi-trait-multimethod analysis. *Arch Gen Psychiatry*. 2011;68:992–1002.

213. American Psychiatric Association. *Diagnostic and Statistical Manual of Mental Disorders*. 5th ed. Arlington, VA: American Psychiatric Publishing, 2013.

214. Lugaresi E, Medori R, Montagna P, Baruzzi A, Cortelli P, Lugaresi A, Tinuper P, Zucconi M, Gambetti P. Fatal familial insomnia and dysautonomia with selective degeneration of thalamic nuclei. *N Engl J Med*. 1986;315:997–1003.

215. Cortelli P, Perani D, Montagna P, et al. Pre-symptomatic diagnosis in fatal familial insomnia: serial neurophysiological and 18FDG-PET studies. *Brain*. 2006;129:668–675.

216. Hauw JJ, Hausser-Hauw C, De Girolami U, Hasboun D, Seilhean D. Neuropathology of sleep disorders: a review. *J Neuropathol Exp Neurol*. 2011;70:243–252.

216a. Goldfarb L, Petersen R, Tabaton M, et al. Fatal familial insomnia and familial Creutzfeldt-Jakob disease: disease phenotype determined by a DNA polymorphism. *Science*. 1992;258:806–808.

217. Krasnianski A, Bartl M, Sanchez Juan PJ, et al. Fatal familial insomnia: Clinical features and early identification. *Ann Neurol*. 2008;63:658–661.

218. Montagna P, Gambetti P, Cortelli P, Lugaresi E. Familial and sporadic fatal insomnia. *Lancet Neurol*. 2003;2:167–176.

219. Gambetti P, Petersen R, Monari L, et al. Fatal familial insomnia and the widening spectrum of prion diseases. *Br Med Bull*. 1993;49:980–994.

220. Broughton RJ, Mullington JM. Polysomnography; principles and applications in sleep and arousal disorders. In: Niedermeyer E, Lopes Da Silva F, eds. *Electroencephalography*. 5th ed. Philadelphia: Lippincott, Williams & Wilkins, 2005:899–936.

221. Hauri P, Hawkins DR. Alpha-delta sleep. *Electroencephalog Clin Nuerophysiol*. 1973;34:233–237.

222. Pivik RT, Harman KA. Reconceptualization of EEG alpha activity during sleep: all alpha activity is not equal. *J Sleep Res*. 1995;4:131–137.

223. Sasai-Sakuma T, Frauscher B, Mitterling T, et al. Quantitative assessment of isolated rapid eye movement (REM) sleep without atonia without clinical REM sleep behavior disorder: clinical and research implications. *Sleep Med*. 2014;15:1009–1015.

224. Gharagozlou P, Seyffert M, Santos R, Chokroverty S. Rhythmic movement disorder associated with respiratory arousals and improved by CPAP titration in a patient with restless legs syndrome and sleep apnea. *Sleep Med*. 2009;10:501–503.

225. Chokroverty S, Thomas RJ, Bhatt M. *Atlas of Sleep Medicine*. Philadelphia: Butterworth/Heinemann, 2005.

226. Chervin RD, Consens FB, Kutluay E. Alternating leg muscles activation during sleep and arousals: a new sleep-related motor phenomenon? *Mov Disord*. 2003;18:551–559.

227. Cosentino FL, Lero I, Tripodi M, Ferri R. The neurophysiology of the alternating leg muscle activation (ALMA) during sleep: study of one patient before and after treatment with pramipexole. *Sleep Med*. 2006;7:63.71.

228. Montagna P, Provini F, Plazzi G, et al. Propriospinal myoclonus upon relaxation and drowsiness: a cause of severe insomnia. *Mov Disord*. 1997;12:66–72.

229. Critchley M. The pre-dormitum. *Rev Neurol (Paris)*. 1955;93:101–106.

230. Vetrugno R, Provini F, Meletti S, et al. Propriospinal myoclonus at the sleep-wake transition: a new type of parasomnia. *Sleep*. 2001;24:835–843.

231. Fabbri M, Vetrugno R, Provini F, Bosi M, Santucci M. Breathing instability in Joubert syndrome. *Mov Disord*. 2012;27:64.

232. Alattar MA, Scharf SM. Opioid-associated central sleep apnea: a case series. *Sleep Breath*. 2009;13:201–206.

233. Farney RJ, Walker JM, Boyle KM, et al. Adaptive servoventilation (ASV) in patients with sleep disordered breathing associated with chronic opioid medication for non-malignant pain. *J Clin Sleep Med*. 2008;4: 311–319.

234. Pepin JL, Dale D, Argod J, Levy P. Recommendations for practical use of pulse transit time as a tool for respiratory effort measurements and microarousal recognition. In: Chokroverty S, Thomas R, Bhatt M, eds. *Atlas of Sleep Medicine*. Philadelphia: Elsevier/Butterworth-Heinemann, 2005:262–271.

235. Pittman SD, Thomas RJ. Peripheral arterial tonometry. In: Chokroverty S, Thomas R, Bhatt M, eds. *Atlas of Sleep Medicine*. Philadelphia: Elsevier/Butterworth-Heinemann, 2005:285–288.

236. Chokroverty S. Sleep disorders. In: Bradley W, Daroff R, Fenichel G, Jankovic J (eds), Neurology in Clinical Practice, Butterworth-Hinemann/ElSevier: Philadelphia, 2008.

237. Johns MW. A new method for measuring daytime sleepiness: The Epworth Sleepiness Scale. *Sleep*. 1991;14:540–545.

238. Ackersted T, Gilberg M. Subjective and objective sleepiness in the active individual. *Int J Neuroscience*. 1990;52:29–37.

239. Carskadon MA, Dement WC, Mitler M, et al. Guidelines for the multiple sleep latency test (MSLT): a standard measure of sleepiness. *Sleep*. 1986;9:519–524.

240. Littner MR, Kushaida C, Wise M, et al. Practice parameters for clinical use of the multiple sleep latency test and the maintenance of wakefulness test. *Sleep.* 2005;28:113–121.

241. Cherbin R. Assessment of sleepiness. In: Chokroverty S, Hening WA, Walters AS, eds. *Sleep and Movement Disorders.* Boston: Butterworth/Heinemann, 2002.

242. Doghramji K, Mitler M, Sangal RB, et al. A normative study of the maintenance of wakefulness test (MWT). *Electroencephalogr Clin: Neurophysiol.* 1997;103:554–562.

243. Doghramji K. The maintenance of wakefulness test. In: Chokroverty S, ed. *Sleep Disorders Medicine: Basic Science, Technical Considerations and Clinical Aspects.* Philadelphia: Saunders/Elsevier, 2009:224–228.

244. Mitler MM, Miller JC, Lipsitz JJ, et al. The sleep of long-haul truck drivers. *N Engl J Med* 1997;337:755–761.

245. Philip P, Sagaspe P, Taillard G, et al. Maintenance of wakefulness test, obstructive sleep apnea syndrome, and driving risk. *Ann Neurol.* 2008;64:410–416.

246. Colburn TR, Smith BM, Guarini JJ, et al. An ambulatory activity monitor with solid state memory. *ISA Transaction.* 1976;15:114–154.

247. Tyron WW. *Activity Measurement in Psychology and Medicine.* New York: Plenum Press, 1991.

248. Sadeh A, Hauri PJ, Kripke DF, Lavie P. The role of actigraphy in the evaluation of sleep disorders. *Sleep.* 1995;18:288–302.

249. Littner M, Kushida CA, Anderson WM, et al. Practice parameters for the role of actigraphy in the study of sleep and circadian rhythms: An update for 2002. *Sleep.* 2003;26:337–341.

250. Sforza E, Johannes M, Claudio B. The PAM-RL ambulatory device for detection of periodic leg movements: a validation study. *Sleep Med.* 2005;6:407–413.

251. Kemlink D, Pretal M, Sonka K, Nevsimalova S. A comparison of polysomnographic and actigraphic evaluation of periodic limb movements in sleep. *Neurol Res.* 2008;30:234–238.

252. Allen RP. Improving RLS diagnosis and severity assessment: Polysomnography, actigraphy and sleep log. *Sleep Med.* 2007;8:S13.

253. Kohnen R, Allen RP, Benes H, et al. Assessment of restless legs syndrome: methodological approaches for use in practice and clinical trials. *Mov Disord.* 2007;22:S485–494.

254. Allen RP. Activity monitoring to diagnose and evaluate motor abnormalities of sleep. In: Henning W, Chokroverty S, eds. Topics in Movement Disorders in Sleep, course syllabus: ASDA annual meeting, San Francisco, Rochester, MN, American Sleep Disorders Association, 1997.

255. Morganthaler TI, Lee-Chiung T, Friedman AG, et al. Practice parameters for the clinical evaluation of circadian rhythm sleep disorders; an American Academy of Sleep Medicine report. *Sleep.* 2007;30:1445–1459.

37 | THE NEUROPHYSIOLOGICAL BASIS OF MYOCLONUS

PHILIP D. THOMPSON, MD, HIROSHI SHIBASAKI, MD, AND MARK HALLETT, MD

ABSTRACT: There are several types of myoclonus, with a variety of classification schemes, and the clinician must determine what type of myoclonus a patient has and what type of neurophysiological assessment can facilitate diagnosis. The electromyographic (EMG) correlate of the myoclonus should be examined, including the response to sensory stimuli (C-reflex). The electroencephalographic (EEG) correlate of the myoclonus should then be examined, possibly including back-averaging from the myoclonus or looking at corticomuscular (EEG–EMG) coherence. The somatosensory evoked response (SEP) should be obtained. Such studies will help determine the myoclonus origin, most commonly cortical or brainstem. One form of cortical myoclonus has the clinical appearance of a tremor (cortical tremor). Brainstem myoclonus includes exaggerated startle (hyperekplexia). Other forms of myoclonus include spinal myoclonus and functional myoclonus, which have their own distinct physiological signature. Several causes of myoclonus are reviewed, including rare types such as Creutzfeldt-Jakob disease and subacute sclerosing panencephalitis.

KEYWORDS: myoclonus, EMG, electromyography, EEG, electroencephalography, back-averaging, C-reflex, somatosensory evoked response, SEP

PRINCIPAL REFERENCES

1. Fahn S, Marsden CD, Van Woert MH. Definition and classification of myoclonus. Adv Neurol 1986; 43: 1–5.
2. Shibasaki H. Hallett M. Electrophysiological studies of myoclonus. Muscle Nerve 2005; 31: 157–174.

1. DEFINITION AND CLASSIFICATION OF MYOCLONUS

Myoclonus refers to involuntary, brief shock-like movements caused by a sudden sharp involuntary muscular jerk or a quick muscle contraction and is derived from Greek for muscle (*myo-*) turmoil (*klonus*) (1,2). Sudden sharp or shock-like movements may be caused by brief muscle contraction (positive myoclonus, a muscle jerk) or a pause in muscle contraction, giving rise to a lapse in limb posture (negative myoclonus or asterixis) (Fig. 37.1). Myoclonus may be classified according to the clinical characteristics (distribution, pattern of occurrence, stimulus sensitivity), the neurophysiology, or the underlying disease or cause (Box 37.1). Diagnosis and classification of myoclonus can be made by careful clinical observation, but neurophysiological examination helps confirm these and the mechanisms generating myoclonus. In general, the term myoclonus implies a central nervous system origin. The neurophysiological mechanisms and evidence of anatomical site of origin are best established for cortical, brainstem, and spinal myoclonus. It is speculated that myoclonus may be generated within the thalamus or basal ganglia (so-called subcortical myoclonus), where there is no evidence of abnormal cortical excitability, though it is likely that the sensorimotor cortex mediates the myoclonic activity, as in the case of thalamic asterixis (3) and possibly myoclonus in dystonic syndromes. There are occasional references in the literature to peripheral myoclonus. This condition is rare, and available evidence suggests it is due to ectopic generation of impulses in a peripheral nerve, akin to hemifacial spasm.

2. ELECTROMYOGRAPHIC CORRELATES OF MYOCLONUS

The neurophysiological examination of myoclonus begins with recording an electromyograph (EMG) of the responsible muscle activity, whether spontaneous, on action, or after relevant stimuli in stimulus-sensitive reflex myoclonus. The EMG burst duration of myoclonic muscle activity is typically short (<50 msec) in cortical myoclonus (Fig. 37.2) and brainstem reticular reflex myoclonus. Longer burst durations, up to 120 msec or so, are seen in brainstem startle myoclonus and some cases of spinal myoclonus. Burst durations >200 msec are typical of propriospinal myoclonus and voluntary activity. A wide range of burst durations is recorded in myoclonus dystonia, in addition to very long bursts of dystonic muscle activity. Recording the activity of agonist and antagonist muscle pairs will demonstrate whether there is co-contraction, as in cortical myoclonus, or alternating activity, as in voluntary muscle jerks. The pattern and distribution of myoclonic activity in cranial and limb muscles will reveal the order of muscle recruitment, and the intervals between the onset of myoclonus in different muscle groups can be measured accurately to distinguish between myoclonus of cortical origin (rostral–caudal spread) and brainstem origin (spread up and down brainstem). Asterixis and cortical reflex negative myoclonus are associated with an isolated EMG silent period or a silent period interrupted by a brief EMG burst (3,4,5).

3. ELECTROENCEPHALOGRAPHIC CORRELATES OF MYOCLONUS AND "JERK-LOCKED" BACK AVERAGING

The routine electroencephalogram (EEG) may be abnormal in cortical myoclonus associated with focal cortical lesions, the progressive myoclonus epilepsies (see Fig. 37.2) and other causes listed in Box 37.2. Cortical myoclonus is usually associated with spikes or polyspikes on EEG, but it is often difficult to study

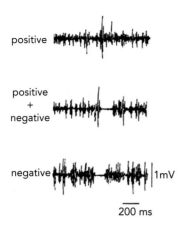

Figure 37.1. Surface EMG correlates of cortical myoclonus during sustained voluntary contraction in a patient with progressive myoclonus epilepsy. The illustration demonstrates a positive myoclonic jerk (upper trace), a positive myoclonic jerk followed by a period of EMG silence (negative myoclonus or asterixis) (middle trace), and negative myoclonus alone (lower trace). Reproduced with permission from reference 2.

precisely the spatial and temporal relationship between the EEG spike and myoclonus on routine EEG. The temporal relationship of the ongoing EEG activity to each myoclonic EMG burst is examined using the technique of "back-averaging" or "jerk-locked" back averaging (2). This is particularly useful when the EEG does not appear to show any discharges temporally related to myoclonus. The cortical correlate or myoclonus-related

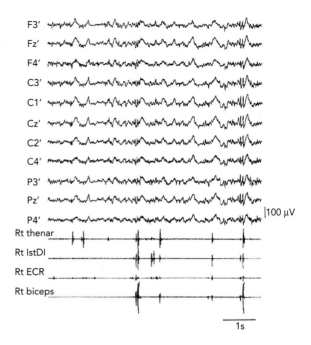

Figure 37.2. EEG–EMG polygraphic recordings in a patient with progressive myoclonus epilepsy illustrating positive myoclonus in the hands at rest. Note that most myoclonic jerks are associated with a spike-wave complex in the EEG. EEG recorded in reference to ipsilateral earlobe electrode. ECR = extensor carpi radialis, 1st DI = first dorsal interosseous muscle, Rt = right. Reproduced with permission from reference 2.

BOX 37.1. CLASSIFICATIONS OF MYOCLONUS

Myoclonus can be classified according to the clinical characteristics, the pathophysiology, or the anatomical site of origin.

Clinical Characteristics
Type of muscle involvement: positive, negative
Distribution: focal, segmental, generalized
Occurrence: spontaneous, action, stimulus-sensitive
Rhythmicity: regular, irregular

Pathophysiology
Epileptic
    Fragments of epilepsy (e.g., focal epilepsy)
    Juvenile myoclonic epilepsy
    Progressive myoclonus epilepsy
Non-epileptic
    Physiological: hypnic jerks, hiccough
    Dystonic myoclonus, DYT11
    Functional myoclonus

Site of Origin
Cortical myoclonus
    Focal: epilepsia partialis continua
    Multifocal or generalized
Brainstem myoclonus
    Hyperekplexia
    Reticular reflex myoclonus
Spinal myoclonus
    Spinal segmental myoclonus
    Propriospinal myoclonus

BOX 37.2. CAUSES OF CORTICAL MYOCLONUS ACCORDING TO SYNDROMIC PRESENTATION

Metabolic, toxic encephalopathies (asterixis)
Viral encephalitis
Focal central nervous system lesions
Post-anoxic myoclonus
Celiac disease
Creutzfeldt–Jakob disease (in advanced stage)
Neurodegeneration and myoclonus with or without dementia
    Alzheimer's disease
    Corticobasal syndrome
    Multiple system atrophy (olivo-ponto-cerebellar atrophy)
    Rett syndrome
Progressive myoclonus epilepsy/ataxia
    Myoclonus epilepsy with ragged red fibers (MERRF)
    Spinocerebellar degenerations
    Dentatorubropallidoluysian atrophy (DRPLA)
    Baltic myoclonus (Unverricht-Lundborg)
    Juvenile myoclonic epilepsy
    Lafora body disease
    Sialidosis
    Neuronal ceroid lipofuscinosis
    GM2 gangliosidosis
    Non-infantile Gaucher's disease
    Angelman syndrome
Familial cortical myoclonic tremor
Benign adult familial myoclonus epilepsy (BAFME)
The cause of progressive myoclonus epilepsy or ataxia (depending on whether epilepsy or ataxia is more prominent) remains unknown in many cases (and in some of these, new genetic abnormalities are being identified).

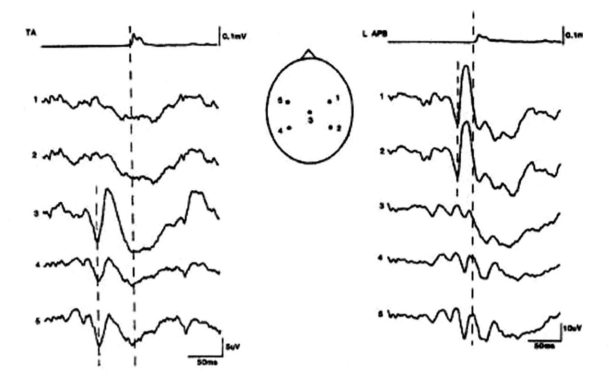

Figure 37.3. Jerk-locked back-averaging of myoclonus-related cortical discharges in a patient with celiac disease and cortical reflex and action myoclonus. Left panel shows back-averaged EEG preceding myoclonus in left tibialis anterior (n = 44). A positive wave was recorded 40 msec before the onset of myoclonus. The waveform was maximal over the vertex corresponding to the leg area of the sensorimotor cortex. Right panel shows back-averaged EEG preceding myoclonus in left abductor pollicis brevis (n = 128). A positive wave was recorded over the lateral aspect of the contralateral hemisphere, corresponding to the hand area of the sensorimotor cortex, preceding the myoclonus by 24 msec. Electrodes 2 and 4 were placed over the hand areas of the somatosensory cortex. Electrodes 1 through 5 were referred to linked mastoid electrodes. Reproduced with permission and modified from reference 6.

cortical potential recorded on back-averaging EEG is a biphasic positive/negative discharge over the corresponding cortical representation of the muscle used to trigger the collection of EEG waveforms (Fig. 37.3). Identifying a cortical potential preceding each myoclonic jerk provides definitive proof of a cortical origin for myoclonus. Spike discharges or spike-and-wave complexes on EEG may also be associated with asterixis in cortical negative myoclonus (Fig. 37.4) (5). The technique of "silent-period locked back-averaging" can be used to confirm a cortical origin for asterixis using an accelerometer to trigger the collection of EEG waveforms (3,4).

4. MEASUREMENT OF STIMULUS-SENSITIVE REFLEX MYOCLONUS

In cortical reflex myoclonus, the reflex response is referred to as a C-reflex (8) (Fig. 37.5). Typically the C-reflex is elicited by stimulating a mixed or cutaneous peripheral nerve. C-reflexes often appear at stimulus intensities that are below the threshold for a peripheral M-wave, indicating activation of large-diameter sensory afferents. Muscle stretch and tendon taps may also elicit a reflex response. Recording a C-reflex following sensory stimulation is useful when severe cortical action myoclonus makes it difficult to decide whether there is stimulus sensitivity on clinical examination. Measurement of the stimulus-induced response latency confirms the reflex nature of the response and distinguishes it from a voluntary reaction. The distribution of reflex activity provides important clues to the likely origin of the myoclonus. Peripheral sensory stimulation that evokes distally predominant myoclonus is usually cortical in origin. Auditory or facial stimulation that evokes bilateral proximal upper-body myoclonus is typical of brainstem myoclonus.

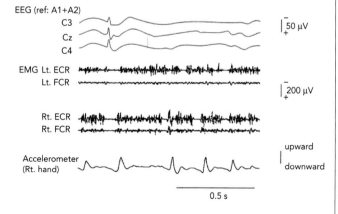

Figure 37.4. EEG–EMG polygraphic records in a patient with Lennox–Gastaut syndrome manifesting negative myoclonus in both hands. Note that negative myoclonus documented by accelerometer from the right (Rt) hand is associated with a silent period in the EMG and that the negative myoclonus with the longest silent period in the record is associated with a clear spike and wave discharge on EEG. A1 = left earlobe; A2 = right earlobe; ECR = extensor carpi radialis muscle; FCR = flexor carpi radialis muscle; Lt = left; Rt = right. Reproduced with permission from reference 2.

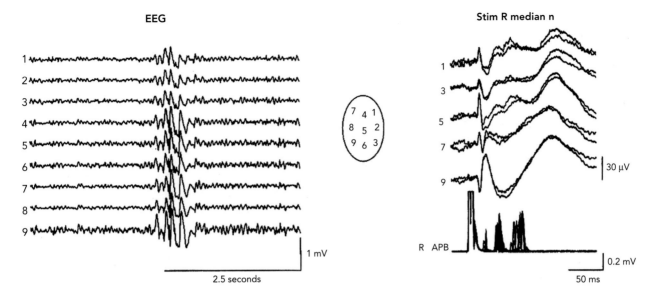

EEG   Stim R median n

Figure 37.5. EEG, cortical SEP, and C-reflexes in a patient with myoclonus epilepsy and ragged red fibers associated with the mitochondrial DNA point mutation at position 8344 and infrequent action and stimulus-sensitive myoclonus. The EEG (left panel) illustrates spontaneous generalized spike-and-wave discharges. The cortical SEP (right panel) following right median nerve stimulation shows an enlarged P1-N2 component of the SEP (two averages of 384 stimuli are superimposed; linked earlobe reference). Below the SEP are 10 superimposed single trials of abductor pollicis brevis (APB) rectified EMG after median nerve stimulation at the wrist. The stimulus artifact and M-wave are followed by an F-response (latency 27 msec) and two C-reflexes with latencies of 48 msec and 80 msec after the median nerve stimulus. Reproduced with permission from reference 7.

5. CORTICAL MYOCLONUS

Cortical myoclonus (9–11) can present as spontaneous, action-induced, or stimulus-sensitive reflex myoclonus, which may be focal or multifocal. Spontaneous myoclonus is typical of epilepsia partialis continua (11). The EMG consists of short-duration hypersynchronous bursts (<50 msec in duration) in agonist and antagonist muscle pairs synchronously. Cortical myoclonus is often most conspicuous in distal muscles, though any group of muscles may be affected. When multiple muscles are affected, spread from one muscle group to another occurs in a rostrocaudal manner at intervals compatible with central conduction in the corticospinal tract (Fig. 37.6). Stimulus sensitivity to light touch, muscle stretch, or mixed and cutaneous nerve stimulation elicits reflex myoclonus (C-reflex) at latencies between 50 and 60 msec in intrinsic hand muscles and ~80 to 90 msec in foot muscles. These intervals are consistent with a long reflex loop comprising afferent conduction in fast-conducting large-diameter afferents to sensorimotor cortex and efferent conduction in the corticospinal tract (9–11).

5.1. Cortical Somatosensory Evoked Potentials

Pathologic enlargement of the amplitude of the P25-N33 (P1-N2) component of the somatosensory evoked potential (SEP; an amplitude >10 µV is generally accepted as a "giant" SEP) is characteristic of cortical reflex myoclonus (10–14). In contrast, the initial N20 (N1) component is normal. The topography of the "giant" SEP is comparable to the normal SEP, and the "giant" SEP is considered an enlargement of the normal or physiological cortical sensory potential (Fig. 37.7) (13). The enlarged P25-N33 components of the SEP reflect abnormal

excitability of the primary sensorimotor cortex (15). In cortical myoclonus, the P25 component is commonly generated in the precentral gyrus, while other components of the SEP are generated in the postcentral gyrus (16).

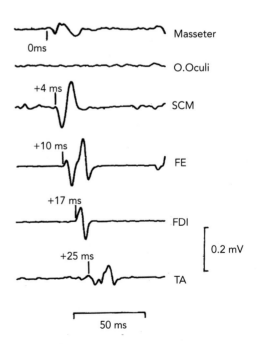

Figure 37.6. Rostral-caudal recruitment of activity in different muscles during a single generalized action myoclonic jerk. Latencies are recorded in each muscle after the masseter, and the intervals approximate conduction time down the corticospinal tract. Note the short duration of the EMG bursts (~25 msec). O = Oculi orbicularis oculi; SCM = sternocleidomastoid; FE = forearm extensors; FDI = first dorsal interosseous; TA = tibialis anterior. Reproduced with the kind permission of Professor J. C. Rothwell.

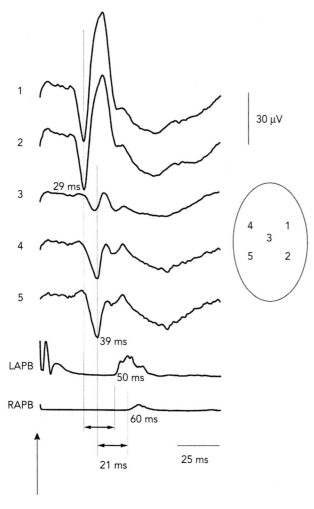

30 μV

29 ms

39 ms

50 ms

60 ms

21 ms

25 ms

Stimulate L Median nerve

Figure 37.7. Cortical SEP following stimulation of the left median nerve at the wrist in a patient with action and stimulus-sensitive myoclonus and ataxia. An enlarged SEP is recorded over the right sensorimotor cortex with a P1 latency of 29 msec. Left median nerve stimulation elicited an M-wave in left abductor pollicis brevis (APB) followed by a C-reflex at a latency of 50 msec. The right sensorimotor cortex SEP is followed by another SEP over the left sensorimotor cortex with an interval between the positive peaks in electrodes 2 and 5 of 10 msec, consistent with interhemispheric spread of the SEP. The latency of the left cortical positive peak was 39 msec, and it in turn was followed by a C-reflex in the right APB with a latency of 60 msec. The interval between the positive SEP peak and C-reflex was 21 msec on both sides, consistent with conduction in the corticospinal tract. Scalp electrodes referred to linked mastoids. Record is average of 256 trials.

5.2. Myoclonus-Related Cortical Discharge

The myoclonus-related cortical potential recorded on back-averaging is a positive/negative biphasic discharge recorded over the corresponding cortical representation of the muscle used to trigger the collection of back-averaged EEG. Accordingly, the scalp topography of the discharge corresponds to the somatotopy of the motor cortex (10,13). The positive peak of the cortical potential precedes each myoclonic jerk by an interval of the order of 20 msec for intrinsic hand muscles and 40 msec for intrinsic foot muscles, compatible with conduction from the cortex to periphery in large-diameter

fast-conducting fibers of the corticospinal tract (see Fig. 37.3). Since the P25 peak of the cortical SEP and the back-averaged myoclonus-related cortical discharge exhibit comparable waveforms and share similar scalp topography and temporal relationship to the myoclonic jerk (Fig. 37.8) it has been proposed that these share similar mechanisms (12). Both the giant SEP and myoclonus-related cortical discharge are also followed by a period of cortical hyperexcitability (17). Refining the spatial location of the myoclonus-related cortical discharge using magnetoencephalography (MEG) suggests that the P25 peak and the positive peak of the myoclonus-related cortical potential share closely spaced sources in the precentral gyrus (Fig. 37.9) (16). Studies of negative myoclonus using back-averaging can show a similar cortical abnormality (4,5). Presumably the discharge in the sensorimotor cortex produces net inhibition in this circumstance rather than excitation.

5.3. Corticomuscular (EEG–EMG) Coherence

The frequency of repetitive bursts of cortical myoclonus is often ~50 Hz, corresponding to an interburst interval of 20 msec. Studies correlating the frequency of EEG spikes and EMG discharges in cortical reflex and action myoclonus reveal coherence at a range of high frequencies and jitter in C-reflex latencies of 5 msec or so and 3 to 6 msec in the intervals between positive spike and muscle discharge (18). This might be explained by variation in spinal motoneuron excitability at the time of arrival of the descending discharges. The investigators of this phenomenon suggested the alternative explanation of a higher-frequency periodicity superimposed on the 50-Hz oscillations in the sensorimotor cortex (18). High-frequency corticomuscular coherence may indicate a cortical origin for myoclonus in cases where back-averaging has failed to identify a cortical discharge preceding myoclonus and SEPs are not enlarged (19).

5.4. Intrahemispheric and Interhemispheric Spread of Cortical Myoclonus

In many examples of cortical myoclonus, movement of one limb or peripheral sensory stimulation is followed by bilateral limb jerking, creating the clinical impression of multifocal or synchronous generalized myoclonus. Detailed EEG–EMG recordings indicate that the myoclonic activity can spread rapidly from the limb initially affected to other body parts, indicating that the apparently generalized myoclonus was not actually synchronous (20). Recording EMG from multiple muscles revealed intrahemispheric spread of myoclonus to other ipsilateral muscles, for example from the hand to the shoulder and leg, consistent with the cortical discharges spreading throughout the cortical motor territory in one hemisphere (20). Recording EEG spikes preceding myoclonus revealed interhemispheric spread of spikes from one hemisphere to the other accompanied by bilateral myoclonic EMG with an interval of 10 msec between bursts in contralateral homologous muscles (Fig. 37.10). A focal (unilateral) stimulus or movement can therefore recruit widespread ipsilateral myoclonus through intrahemispheric spread and contralateral myoclonus through transcallosal interhemispheric spread.

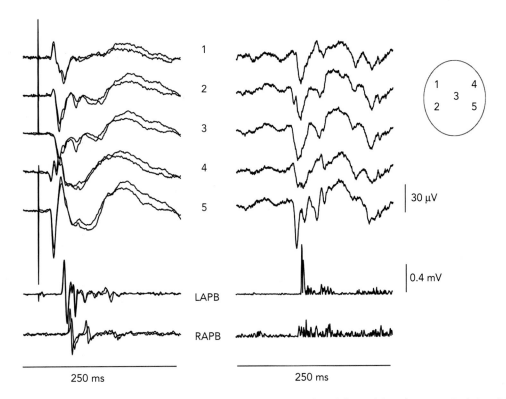

Figure 37.8. *Cortical SEP and back-averaged EEG in a patient with sialidosis. Left panel: Cortical SEP following left median nerve stimulation elicits a giant SEP with the enlarged P1-N2 component located over the right sensorimotor cortex (electrode 5). A C-reflex is also illustrated in the left abductor pollicis brevis (LAPB) EMG trace below (and, after interhemispheric spread to the left hemisphere, a C-reflex occurred in the right APB). Right panel: Back-averaging EEG triggered by myoclonic jerks in the left APB revealed a positive/negative wave over the right sensorimotor cortex (electrode 5). The enlarged positive peak of the SEP and the positive peak of the myoclonus-related cortical discharge share a similar topography over the right sensorimotor cortex.*

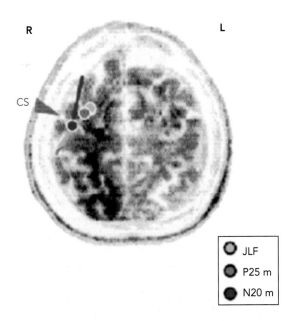

Figure 37.9. *Source localization of dipoles estimated from MEG of cortical magnetic fields associated with myoclonic jerks (JLF = jerk-locked field), SEP N20, and generators of the giant SEP (P25) in relation to the central sulcus (CS). The N20 is located in the postcentral region. The P25 is very close to the JLF of the spike preceding myoclonus. See reference 16 for further details.*

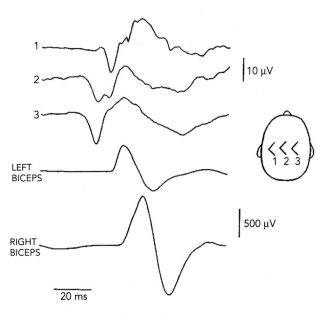

Figure 37.10. *Interhemispheric spread of cortical action myoclonus-related discharges revealed by back-averaged EEG preceding bilateral action myoclonus induced by voluntary movement of the left arm. EMG activity in muscles of the left upper limb was followed by myoclonus in the right upper limb (average of 33 myoclonic jerks). EEG was recorded from a bipolar montage with a frontal reference electrode. The cortical correlate of the left upper-limb myoclonus was recorded over the right sensorimotor cortex and followed by a later cortical correlate over the left sensorimotor cortex preceding the right upper-limb myoclonus. Reproduced with permission from reference 20.*

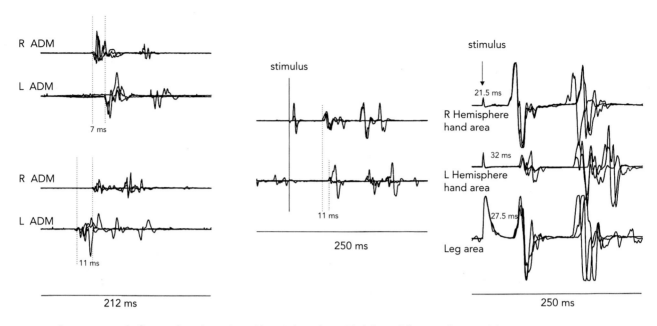

SPONTANEOUS JERKS   STIMULATE R MEDIAN N (wrist)   CORTEX STIMULATION

Figure 37.11. *Spontaneous and reflex myoclonus in a patient with cortical myoclonus. The left panel illustrates the intervals between spontaneous myoclonus of the right (R) and left (L) abductor digiti minimi (ADM). The intervals are reproducible from right to left and vice versa, reflecting interhemispheric spread of myoclonic activity. The middle panel illustrates the intervals for stimulus-induced interhemispheric spread of myoclonic activity between the two sides (R and L ADM). The right panel illustrates the responses in left ADM following focal (figure-of-8 coil) magnetic stimulation of different areas of the brain. The response evoked by right hemisphere stimulation (upper traces) occurs at a normal latency (and is followed by reflex myoclonus). The middle traces illustrate the response from stimulation of the left (i.e., ipsilateral) hemisphere and reveal a later response, 10.5 msec longer than that from left hemisphere stimulation, approximating the interhemispheric delay for spontaneous and stimulus-induced myoclonus. Stimulation over the leg area (lower traces) also elicits a response that is 6 msec longer than for stimulation of the hand area, consistent with the delay for intrahemispheric conduction. The right panel is reproduced from reference 21 with permission.*

The enlarged cortical SEP also may show a similar transcallosal interhemispheric spread from one sensorimotor cortex to the other (12) with the appearance of an ipsilateral cortical P25 following the contralateral SEP by 10 msec or so (see Fig. 37.6). In reflex myoclonus, the latency difference between homologous muscles on each side of the body is ~10 to 15 msec, accounting for the time taken to spread from one hemisphere to the other. In action myoclonus the interval for transcallosal interhemispheric spread is even shorter (~7 msec) (20). Estimated times for intracortical spread following a somatotopic pattern from hand to leg was ~10 msec (20). Intracortical and transcallosal interhemispheric spread after magnetic cortical stimulation has been demonstrated in cortical myoclonus with comparable intervals (Fig. 37.11) (21).

5.5. Mechanism of the Long Loop Transcortical Reflex and C-Reflex

It has been postulated that the physiological basis for cortical reflex myoclonus is enhancement of a component of long loop transcortical stretch reflexes (9,10). Peripheral sensory stimulation can elicit reflex responses in hand muscles of normal subjects during background contraction in two or three periods, the first around 35 to 45 msec, the second 50 to 60 msec, and a third 65 to 80 msec after stimulation (22–24). These latencies are consistent with a transcortical loop influencing the excitability of the sensorimotor cortex. These observations have some bearing on the pathophysiology of

cortical myoclonus. In cortical reflex myoclonus with giant SEPs, the C-reflex latency occurs between 50 and 60 msec after stimulation.

It should be noted that not all cases of cortical myoclonus exhibit all of these features (11,12). In some cases of cortical myoclonus, stimulus sensitivity with reflex myoclonus is not evident but there may be enlarged cortical SEPs. Conversely, stimulus sensitivity may occur with normal SEPs. Similarly, the presence of an enlarged cortical SEP does not imply that time-locked EEG potential will be recorded on back-averaging (and vice versa). There are a number of possible explanations for these apparent inconsistencies, including whether there is hyperexcitability of afferent or efferent sensorimotor cortex mechanisms (12). Drugs such as benzodiazepines reduce stimulus sensitivity and the occurrence of action, reflex, and spontaneous myoclonus but may or may not influence the size of the cortical SEP (11,12,14). In other cases it is suggested that the cortical dipoles responsible for the abnormal cortical discharge project unfavorably for surface EEG recordings. It is also likely there are further, as yet undefined, mechanisms for the generation of cortical myoclonus.

5.6. Causes of Cortical Myoclonus

The most common conditions identified in patients with cortical myoclonus are diseases of the cerebellum (11), particularly those affecting the cerebellar efferent neurons from the dentate nucleus. All exhibit typical cortical reflex and action myoclonus, giant SEPs, C-reflexes, and cortical correlates preceding myoclonus. These conditions (see Box 37.2) may present with a clinical picture of progressive myoclonus epilepsy or progressive myoclonus ataxia when seizures are less frequent and cognitive decline is less pronounced (24). The reason for the difference in these clinical manifestations is not clear. Similarly, the reason for the association of cortical myoclonus with certain patterns of cerebellar degeneration has been speculated to be that the cerebellar degeneration leads to withdrawal of tonic inhibition of the primary sensorimotor cortex and resultant heightened excitability (11,25).

5.7. Cortical Tremor

Repetitive high-frequency myoclonic jerks of the fingers resemble tremor. Tremor-like postural and action myoclonus occurs in autosomal dominant families with benign adult familial myoclonus epilepsy or familial cortical myoclonic tremor with epilepsy and is referred to as "cortical tremor" (26–28). The myoclonus has been shown to be of cortical origin and has the electrophysiological characteristics of cortical myoclonus (27). Tremor-like myoclonus of cortical origin is also seen in corticobasal syndrome, in which case myoclonus is unilateral or asymmetric (29–31).

5.8. Myoclonus in Corticobasal Syndrome

A different physiological mechanism may account for action and reflex myoclonus in corticobasal syndrome (29–33). Myoclonus is present in 50% of cases, is most conspicuous in distal muscles, and is often superimposed on dystonic postures in an apraxic limb. Action and reflex myoclonus is produced by short-duration (25–50 msec) muscle discharges, simultaneously activating antagonist muscle pairs, in bursts of discharges with interburst intervals of 60 to 80 msec. Reflex myoclonus elicited by cutaneous stimuli appears at intensities near or below sensory perceptual threshold even in patients with cortical sensory loss. Spike discharges are not present in the EEG and myoclonus-related cortical discharges are not recorded on back-averaged EEG in most cases, though cortical activity preceding myoclonus may be detected on back-averaged MEG (31). The latency of reflex myoclonus (C-reflex) in hand muscles after stimulation of the median nerve at the wrist is ~40 msec, in contrast to 50 to 60 msec in classical cortical reflex myoclonus. Estimates of the cortical delay for generation of myoclonus in "typical" cortical reflex myoclonus (6.9 ± 3.7 msec) are significantly longer than for corticobasal degeneration (1.4 ± 0.8 msec). The parietal N20-P25-N35 SEP components are poorly formed, with a broad-notched positive wave rather than the normal "W"- shaped waveform (29). Borderline enlargement of the P25-N30 component of the SEP is occasionally found, but giant SEPs do not occur. The prefrontal P22-N30 components are relatively preserved. Based on the latency difference it is suggested that reflex myoclonus in corticobasal degeneration is generated by the first period of transcortical excitability occurring 40 msec after peripheral nerve stimulation, possibly in response to a direct sensory relay

from ventrolateral thalamic nuclei to an abnormally excitable motor cortex (29).

5.9. Photic Cortical Reflex Myoclonus

Photic cortical reflex myoclonus with generalized muscle jerks following flash stimulation has been recorded in Lafora disease, Creutzfeldt–Jakob disease (CJD), myoclonus epilepsy with ragged red fibers, and multiple system atrophy (34,35). Action myoclonus and somatosensory reflex myoclonus were also present in some of these cases. Flash stimulation induced widespread cerebral cortical responses with an occipital potential followed 5 to 10 msec later by a frontal wave and then a myoclonic jerk (34,35). The latency of the frontal wave to the myoclonus was comparable to the interval between the giant SEP and myoclonus (29). Myoclonic responses in limb muscles exhibited inter-muscle intervals consistent with corticospinal conduction.

5.10. Combined Forms of Myoclonus

Post-anoxic myoclonus and possibly other myoclonic syndromes may exhibit more than one physiological mechanism. For example, combinations of cortical action and reflex myoclonus and brainstem myoclonus are described in post-anoxic encephalopathy (36).

5.11. Minipolymyoclonus

The term "minipolymyoclonus" has been used to describe the small-amplitude myoclonic movements of the fingers and hands in progressive epileptic encephalopathies. The action jerks were preceded by a frontally predominant negative cerebral potential of long duration and variable timing in relation to the jerks (37). This form of minipolymyoclonus was thought to be a fragment of primary generalized epilepsy (38). Note also this term has been used to describe low-amplitude trembling and twitching of the outstretched fingers produced by voluntary recruitment of enlarged motor units following denervation and reinnervation, also referred to as "contraction pseudotremor."

5.12. Myoclonus in Alzheimer's Disease

Spontaneous and action myoclonus in Alzheimer disease (including that associated with Down syndrome) may have the characteristics of cortical myoclonus (39,40). Stimulus sensitivity was variable, C-reflex latencies ranged from 40 to 75 msec, and the P1-N2 component of the cortical SEP was enlarged in some cases. Contralateral negative cortical potentials preceded the myoclonus in most cases with latencies from negative potential to myoclonus of 25 to 40 msec (39).

5.13. Myoclonus in Dystonia

Jerky movements are common in many dystonic syndromes and when prominent may even overshadow the abnormal postures of dystonia. This is particularly evident in myoclonus dystonia

(DYT11) and some cases of cervical dystonia. Myoclonus occurs only on action and is not stimulus-sensitive. Apart from clinical recognition of the signs of underlying dystonia, the EMG features of myoclonus in dystonia provide further important clues to the diagnosis. These include long-duration bursts of EMG activity (100–500 msec), intermixed with the longer bursts of dystonic spasm, often occurring rhythmically for short periods of time and alternating patterns of agonist–antagonist muscle activity such as described in DYT11. The myoclonus in dystonia, in addition to the above features, is not associated with enlarged cortical SEPs or EEG abnormalities. The site of origin of this form of myoclonus is not known. The characteristics and association with dystonia have led to the term "subcortical myoclonus," although the efferent pathway is most likely the corticospinal tract. It is probably simpler to view such movements as one of the wide spectrum of movements seen in dystonia.

6. PERIODIC MYOCLONUS IN CJD AND SUBACUTE SCLEROSING PANENCEPHALITIS

Approximately 50% of patients with CJD exhibit myoclonus at some stage, and the characteristics of myoclonus may vary (40). Myoclonus is usually not stimulus-sensitive and occurs continuously and quasi-periodically at rest with time intervals ranging from 600 msec to 1.5 sec (40) (Fig. 37.12). The duration of each myoclonic EMG discharge is usually longer than that of cortical myoclonus, but it can be as short as in cortical myoclonus. Myoclonus in CJD is commonly accompanied by a periodic synchronous discharge (PSD) on EEG, but either periodic myoclonus or PSD may appear independently. The relationship between the myoclonus and PSD also varies. In this disease, therefore, there is no causative relationship between the cortical activity recorded on EEG and the peripheral motor phenomena (40). Patients with CJD may also show typical cortical reflex myoclonus in advanced stages of the disease, when PSDs tend to disappear and the background EEG activity becomes very low in amplitude. In this case, myoclonus is often elicited not only by somatosensory stimuli but also by photic stimulation (34).

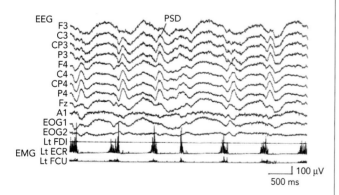

Figure 37.12. EEG–EMG polygraph of a patient with CJD, showing the PSDs on EEG and the EMG discharges associated with periodic myoclonus of the left hand. There is no constant relationship between PSDs and myoclonus.

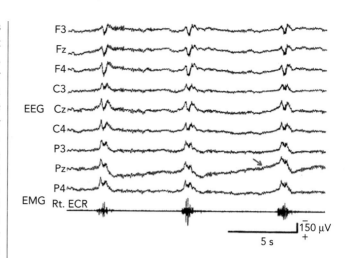

Figure 37.13. EEG–EMG polygraph of a patient with SSPE, showing PSDs and EMG discharges associated with periodic dystonic myoclonus of the right hand. There is a fixed relationship between PSDs and the periodic involuntary movements. Reproduced from reference 41 with permission.

In subacute sclerosing panencephalitis (SSPE), periodic myoclonus repeats at an interval of 4 to 13 sec and the frequency is often quite constant at each stage of the disease. Each movement is much longer in duration than cortical myoclonus, and thus it might be called periodic dystonic myoclonus. It is commonly seen in extremities but may also be evident in the eyes. Unlike CJD, PSDs in SSPE are constant in waveform and duration and are constantly associated with the involuntary movements, suggesting cortical participation in their generation (Fig. 37.13) (41).

7. MYOCLONUS OF BRAINSTEM ORIGIN

This form of myoclonus is identified by the presence of generalized or bilaterally synchronous upper-body myoclonus producing flexion of the trunk with flexion or extension of the head and neck, abduction (or adduction) of the shoulders, and flexion of the elbows. It is usually stimulus-induced (sound, fright, novel visual stimuli, taps to the mantle region) but can appear spontaneously or in response to an unexpected but otherwise innocuous stimulus. The generalized and bilaterally synchronous nature of this response suggests that it is conducted from brainstem reticular nuclei in the reticulospinal tracts (42,43).

One major distinguishing feature of brainstem myoclonus is the pattern of muscle recruitment after appropriate stimulation (Fig. 37.14). The initial response is recorded in the sternocleidomastoid or trapezius muscle followed a few milliseconds later by muscle recruitment proceeding in a rostral direction upward from the brainstem to the facial muscles (VIIth nerve) and masseter (Vth nerve) and caudally from the low brainstem to the limb and axial muscles innervated by spinal cord segments (42–44).

Two types of brainstem myoclonus have been defined, according to the efferent conduction velocity down the spinal cord, calculated from the intervals between muscle recruitment. In reticular reflex myoclonus (42) the efferent conduction velocity was rapid, approximating that of the corticospinal

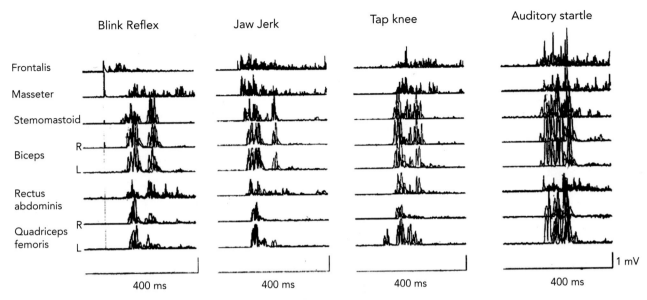

Figure 37.14. Surface EMG recordings from various muscles in response to four different stimuli in a patient with brainstem myoclonus and central nervous system sarcoidosis (Case 6 in reference 43). The responses to each stimulus consist of bilateral synchronous bursts of EMG activity beginning in the sternomastoid muscle and then spreading up the brainstem and down the spinal cord. Several single trials are superimposed. Note that the R1 and R2 components of the blink reflex (elicited by stimulation of the supraorbital nerve) occur in frontalis and tendon reflexes precede the myoclonic response in the masseter following the jaw jerk and the quadriceps following the knee jerk.

pathways. There were spontaneous and stimulus-sensitive generalized jerks, with stimulus sensitivity being greatest for taps to distal limbs, although sound and touch to the mantle area also were effective. This type of myoclonus is thought to be mediated by the nucleus reticularis gigantocellularis.

The second type of brainstem myoclonus, hyperekplexia, represents an exaggeration of the startle response where the efferent conduction velocity is slow (~30 m/sec, or half the conduction velocity of the corticospinal tract) (43,44). In this type the clinical appearance of the jerks is similar to reticular reflex myoclonus, but spontaneous jerks are rare and stimulus sensitivity is greatest for stimuli applied to the mantle region (taps to the nose, forehead, and upper chest) and sound. These electrophysiological characteristics of this response are identical to the normal startle response. The major difference is that the normal startle response to a loud noise habituates rapidly with repeated presentation of stimuli, whereas the pathological response does not. The startle response is mediated by the nucleus reticularis pontis caudalis, and the slowly conducting efferent pathway in hyperekplexia is thought to be part of the reticulospinal system.

A further feature of interest in hyperekplexia is the occurrence of prolonged generalized tonic spasms during which the patient is unable to move and may fall "like a tree trunk," without normal protective responses, often sustaining injuries to the face (45). Consciousness is preserved throughout. These may be precipitated by fright or an unexpected somaesthetic, visual, or auditory stimulus. The pathophysiology of these episodes is not known. They bear some resemblance to startle epilepsy, although there are several clinical differences between patients reported with startle epilepsy and those with hyperekplexia. In children with startle epilepsy, other neurological signs, such as hemiplegia, are common. In contrast, in hereditary hyperekplexia excessive stiffness in early infancy, particularly when the baby is handled, umbilical hernias, and delayed acquisition of walking skills with frequent falls (presumably as the result of tonic spasms) are common. Nevertheless, in some reported cases of hyperekplexia, the EEG has been abnormal (although it often is difficult to distinguish movement artifact associated with a massive generalized myoclonic jerk of the upper body from an abnormal cortical EEG discharge). Furthermore, in hereditary hyperekplexia (but not in other causes of brainstem myoclonus), cortical SEPs may be enlarged, as in cortical myoclonus (46). No EEG potentials have been proven to be time-locked to the reflex or spontaneous jerks in hyperekplexia. Hereditary hyperekplexia is caused by abnormalities of glycine transmission, usually due to mutations in the glycine receptor genes or, rarely, inflammatory immune-mediated brainstem disease (47). Other causes of brainstem myoclonus are listed in Box 37.3.

BOX 37.3. CAUSES OF BRAINSTEM MYOCLONUS

Pathologic exaggeration of the normal startle reflex
    Hereditary hyperekplexia
Symptomatic
    Static perinatal encephalopathy
    Post-anoxic encephalopathy
    Posttraumatic encephalopathy
    Brainstem encephalitis
    Sarcoidosis
    Viral encephalomyelitis
    Encephalomyelitis with rigidity and myoclonus (glycine receptor antibodies)
    Paraneoplastic encephalomyelitis (anti-Ri antibodies)
    Multiple sclerosis
    Brainstem hemorrhage, infarction
Reticular reflex myoclonus
    Post-anoxic encephalopathy

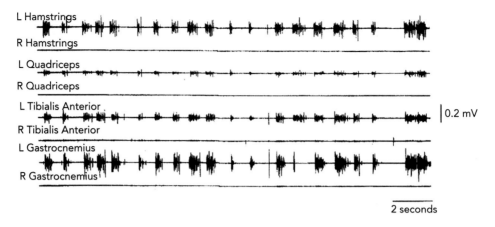

Figure 37.15. *Spinal myoclonus in spina bifida. Surface EMG recordings from right (R) and left (L) lower-limb muscles in a 5-year-old girl with a flaccid paraplegia, areflexia, and complete anesthesia below T12 due to a thoracolumbar meningomyelocele. Semirhythmic movements of the legs persisted throughout the day and night during sleep and were caused by bursts of muscle activity (duration 100–500 msec) in the left gastrocnemius, tibialis anterior, and hamstrings, with lesser activity in the left quadriceps. Reproduced with permission from reference 49.*

8. MYOCLONUS OF SPINAL CORD ORIGIN

Spinal myoclonus is a rare movement disorder. The concept of segmental myoclonus of spinal origin is based on the observation that isolated spinal cord preparations in animals are capable of developing rhythmic myoclonus. Spinal segmental myoclonus in humans has been defined as spontaneous rhythmic jerking of muscles innervated by one or a few contiguous spinal segments, which continues during sleep, at a rate of 30 to 130 per minute. The arms, legs, or trunk may be involved, and stimulus sensitivity is uncommon. The duration of the individual myoclonic EMG bursts is long and often variable. It is presumed that rhythmic firing of spinal neurons, including the anterior horn cells, generates this form of myoclonus, although the underlying mechanism is not known. The capacity of the isolated human spinal cord to generate rhythmic myoclonus has been illustrated in complete cervical cord transection (48) and spinal dysraphism (49), where continuous slow semirhythmic leg movements are caused by long-duration EMG bursts (500 msec to 1sec) (Fig. 37.15). The postulated mechanism was release of spinal locomotor generators.

A second type of spinal myoclonus, characterized by myoclonic flexion or extension movements of the trunk involving axial muscles innervated by multiple segments of the spinal cord, was designated "propriospinal myoclonus" on the grounds that it may be mediated by the slowly conducting propriospinal systems that link different segments of the spinal cord (50). The first burst of muscle activity in each truncal jerk appeared in the rectus abdominis muscles, followed by recruitment of rostral and caudal muscles innervated by other spinal segments at a presumed rate of conduction in the spinal cord of ~5 m/sec (50). Stimulus sensitivity was variable, the movements tended to become more severe when supine, and the movements persisted in sleep. Subsequently several studies have demonstrated that these patterns of truncal muscle activity can be mimicked voluntarily, and in many cases a premovement potential (Bereitschaftspotential) has been recorded along with other clinical features indicating a functional origin (51).

9. FUNCTIONAL MYOCLONUS

Functional (psychogenic) myoclonus is a common form of myoclonus seen in the clinic and should not be overlooked. The EMG patterns are similar to voluntary movements, and the myoclonus is typically preceded by a normal Bereitschaftspotential. The latency of reflex myoclonus is similar to voluntary reaction times and is highly variable (52). Distractibility and suggestibility are features common to other functional movement disorders.

REFERENCES

1. Fahn S, Marsden CD, Van Woert MH. Definition and classification of myoclonus. Adv Neurol 1986; 43: 1–5.
2. Shibasaki H. Hallett M. Electrophysiological studies of myoclonus. Muscle Nerve 2005; 31: 157–174.
3. Inoue M, Kojima Y, Mima T et al Pathophysiology of unilateral asterixis due to a thalamic lesion. Clin Neurophysiol 2012; 123: 1858–1864.
4. Ugawa Y, Shimpo T, Mannen T. Physiological analysis of asterixis: silent period locked averaging. J Neurol Neurosurg Psychiatry 1989; 52: 89–92.
5. Shibasaki H, Ikeda A, Nagamine T et al. Cortical reflex negative myoclonus. Brain 1994; 117: 477–486.
6. Lu CS, Thompson PD, Quinn NP, Parkes JD, Marsden CD. Ramsay Hunt syndrome and coeliac disease: A new association? Mov Disord 1986; 1: 209–219.
7. Thompson PD, Hammans SR, Harding AE. Cortical reflex myoclonus in patients with the mitochondrial DNA transfer RNA Lys(8344) (MERRF) mutation. J Neurol 1994; 241: 335–340.
8. Sutton GG, Mayer RF. Focal reflex myoclonus. J Neurol Neurosurg Psychiatry 1974; 37: 207–217.
9. Hallett M, Chadwick D, Marsden CD. Cortical reflex myoclonus. Neurology 1979; 29: 1107–1125.
10. Shibasaki H, Yamashita Y, Kuroiwa Y. Electroencephalographic studies of myoclonus. Myoclonus-related cortical spikes and high amplitude somatosensory evoked potentials. Brain 1978; 101: 447–460.
11. Obeso JA, Rothwell JC, Marsden CD. The spectrum of cortical myoclonus. From focal reflex jerks to spontaneous motor epilepsy. Brain 1985; 108: 193–224.
12. Shibasaki H, Yamashita Y, Neshige R, Tobimatsu S, Fukui R. Pathogenesis of giant somatosensory evoked potentials in progressive myoclonic epilepsy. Brain 1985; 108: 225–240.
13. Shibasaki H, Kakigi R, Ikeda A. Scalp topography of giant SEP and premyoclonus spike in cortical reflex myoclonus. Electroencephalogr Clin Neurophysiol 1991; 81: 31–37.
14. Rothwell JC, Obeso JA, Marsden CD. On the significance of giant somatosensory evoked potentials in cortical myoclonus. J Neurol Neurosurg Psychiatry 1984; 47:33–42.

15. Mima T, Nagamine T, Nishitani N, Mikuni N, Ikeda A, Fukuyama H, et al. Cortical myoclonus sensorimotor hyperexcitability. Neurology 1998; 50: 933–942.
16. Mima T, Nagamine T, Ikeda A, Yazawa S, Kimura J, Shibasaki H. Pathogenesis of cortical myoclonus studied by magnetoencephalography. Ann Neurol 1998; 43: 598–607.
17. Shibasaki H, Neshige R, Hashiba Y. Cortical excitability after myoclonus: jerk-locked somatosensory evoked potentials. Neurology 1985; 35: 36–41.
18. Brown P, Marsden CD. Rhythmic cortical and muscle discharge in cortical myoclonus. Brain 1996; 119: 1307–1316.
19. Brown P, Farmer SF, Halliday DM, Marsden J, Rosenberg JR. Coherent cortical and muscle discharge in cortical myoclonus. Brain 1999;122: 461–472.
20. Brown P, Day BL, Rothwell JC, Thompson PD, Marsden CD. Intrahemispheric and interhemispheric spread of cerebral cortical myoclonic activity and its relevance to epilepsy. Brain 1991; 114: 2333–2351.
21. Thompson PD, Rothwell JC, Brown P, Day BL, Asselman P. Transcallosal and intracortical spread of activity following cortical stimulation in a patient with generalized cortical myoclonus. J Physiol (Lond) 1993: 459; 64P.
22. Chauvel P, Louvel J, Lamarche M. Transcortical reflexes and focal motor epilepsy. Electroencephalogr Clin Neurophysiol 1978: 45; 309–318.
23. Deuschl G, Schenck E, Lucking CH, Ebner A. Cortical reflex myoclonus and its relation to normal long-latency reflexes. In: Benecke R, Conrad B, Marsden CD, eds. Motor Disturbances I. London: Academic Press, 1987:305–319.
24. Marseille Consensus Group. Classification of progressive myoclonus epilepsies and related disorders. Ann Neurol 1990; 28:113–116.
25. Tjissen MAJ, Thom M, Wilkins P et al Cortical myoclonus and cerebellar pathology. Neurology 2000; 54: 1350–1356.
26. Ikeda A, Kakigi R, Funai N, Neshige R, Kuroda Y, Shibasaki H. Cortical tremor: a variant of cortical reflex myoclonus. Neurology 1990; 40: 1561–1565.
27. Terada K, Ikeda A, Mima T, Kimura M, Nagahama Y, Kamioka Y, et al. Familial cortical myoclonic tremor as a unique form of cortical reflex myoclonus. Mov Disord 1997; 12: 370–377.
28. van Rootselaar AF, Aronica E, Steur EHNJ et al Familial cortical tremor with epilepsy and cerebellar pathological findings. Mov Disord 2004; 19: 213–217.
29. Thompson PD, Day BL, Rothwell JC, Brown P, Britton TC, Marsden CD. The myoclonus in corticobasal degeneration. Evidence for two forms of cortical reflex myoclonus. Brain 1994; 117: 1197–1207.
30. Carella F, Ciano C, Panzica F, Scaioli V. Myoclonus in corticobasal degeneration. Mov Disord 1997; 12: 598–603.
31. Lu CS, Ikeda A, Terada K, Mima T, Nagamine T, Fukuyama H, et al. Electrophysiological studies of early stage corticobasal degeneration. Mov Disord 1998; 13: 140–146.
32. Brunt ER, Van Weerden TW, Pruim J, Lakke JWF. Unique myoclonic pattern in corticobasal degeneration. Mov Disord 1995; 10: 132–142.
33. Chen R, Ashby P, Lang AE. Stimulus sensitive myoclonus in akinetic rigid syndromes. Brain 1992; 115: 1875–1888.
34. Shibasaki H, Neshige R. Photic cortical reflex myoclonus. Ann Neurol 1987; 22: 252–287.
35. Artieda J, Obeso JA. The pathophysiology and pharmacology of photic cortical reflex myoclonus. Ann Neurol 1993; 34: 175–184.
36. Brown P, Thompson PD, Rothwell JC, Day BL, Marsden CD. A case of post-anoxic encephalopathy with cortical action and brainstem reflex myoclonus. Mov Disord 1991; 6: 139–144.
37. Wilkins DE, Hallett M, Erba G. Primary generalized epileptic myoclonus: a frequent manifestation of minipolymyoclonus of central origin. J Neurol Neurosurg Psychiatry 1985; 48: 506–516.
38. Wilkins DE, Hallett M, Berardelli A, Walshe T, Alvarez N. Physiologic analysis of the myoclonus of Alzheimer's disease. Neurology 1984; 34: 898–903.
39. Ugawa Y, Kohara N, Hirasawa H, Kuzuhara S, Iwata M, Mannen T. Myoclonus in Alzheimer's disease. J Neurol 1987; 235: 90–94.
40. Shibasaki H, Motomura S, Yamashita Y, Shii H, Kuroiwa Y. Periodic synchronous discharge and myoclonus in Creutzfeldt-Jakob disease: diagnostic application of jerk-locked averaging method. Ann Neurol 1981; 9: 150–156.
41. Oga T, Ikeda A, Nagamine T, Sumi E, Matsumoto R, Akiguchi I, et al. Implication of sensorimotor integration in the generation of periodic dystonic myoclonus in subacute sclerosing panencephalitis (SSPE). Mov Disord 2000; 15: 1173–1183.
42. Hallett M, Chadwick D, Adam J, Marsden CD. Reticular reflex myoclonus: a physiological type of human post-hypoxic myoclonus. J Neurol Neurosurg Psychiatry 1977; 40: 253–264.
43. Brown P, Rothwell JC, Thompson PD, Britton TC, Day BL, Marsden CD. The hyperekplexias and their relationship to the normal startle reflex. Brain 1991; 114: 1903–1928.
44. Matsumoto J, Fuhr P, Nigro M, Hallett M. Physiological abnormalities in hereditary hyperekplexia. Ann Neurol 1992; 32: 41–50.
45. Suhren O, Bruyn GW, Tuynman JA. Hyperexplexia: a hereditary startle pattern. J Neurol Sci 1966; 3: 577–605.
46. Markand ON, Garg BP, Weaver DD. Familial startle disease (hyperekplexia). Arch Neurol 1984; 41: 71–74.
47. Rees MI, Lewis TM, Vafa F, et al Compound heterozygosity and nonsense mutations in the alpha (1) subunit of the inhibitory glycine receptor in hyperekplexia. Hum Genet 2001; 109: 267–270.
48. Bussel B, Roby-Brami A, Azouvi P, Biraben A, Yakovleff A, Held JP. Myoclonus in a patient with spinal cord transection. Possible involvement of the spinal stepping generator. Brain 1988; 111: 1235–1245.
49. Warren JE, Vidailhet M, Kneebone CS, Quinn NP, Thompson PD. Myoclonus in spinal dysraphism. Mov Disord 2003; 18: 961–964.
50. Brown P, Thompson PD, Rothwell JC, Day BL, Marsden CD. Axial myoclonus of propriospinal origin. Brain 1991; 114: 197–214.
51. Erro R, Bhatia KP, Edwards MJ, Farmer SF, Cordivari C. Clinical diagnosis of propriospinal myoclonus is unreliable. An electrophysiological study. Mov Disord 2013; 28: 1868–1873.
52. Brown P, Thompson PD. Electrophysiological aids to the diagnosis of psychogenic jerks, spasms and tremor. Mov Disord 2001; 16: 595–599.

38 | RECORDING TECHNIQUES RELATED TO DEEP BRAIN STIMULATION FOR MOVEMENT DISORDERS AND RESPONSIVE STIMULATION FOR EPILEPSY

JAY L. SHILS, PHD, DABNM, FASNM, FACNS, SEPEHR SANI, MD,

RYAN KOCHANSKI, MD, MENA KEROLUS, MD, AND JEFFREY E. ARLE, MD, PHD

ABSTRACT: Neuromodulation therapies are now common treatments for a variety of medically refractory disorders, including movement disorders and epilepsy. While surgical techniques for each disorder vary, electricity is used by both for relieving symptoms. During stereotactic placement of the stimulating electrode, either deep brain stimulation electrodes or cortical strip electrodes, intraoperative neurophysiology is used to localize the target structure. This physiology includes single-unit recordings, neurostimulation evoked response evaluation, and intracranial electroencephalography (EEG) to ensure the electrode leads are in the optimal location. Because the functional target for the responsive neurostimulator is more easily visualized on preoperative magnetic resonance imaging, intraoperative physiology is used more as a confirmatory tool, in contrast to the more functional localization-based use during electrode placement for movement disorders. This chapter discusses surgical placement of the electrodes for each procedure and the physiological guidance methodology used to place the leads in the optimal location.

KEYWORDS: movement disorders, epilepsy, neuromodulation, single-unit recording, deep brain stimulation, electroencephalography, EEG

PRINCIPAL REFERENCES

1. Sterio, D., Beric, A., Dogali, M., Fazzini, E., Alfaro, G., and Devinsky, O. (1994). Neurophysiological properties of pallidal neurons in Parkinson's disease. Ann. Neurol., 35, 586–591.
2. Vitek, J.L., Zhang, J., Evatt, M., Mewes, K., DeLong, M.R., Hashimoto, T., Triche, S., and Bakay, R.A. (1998). GPi pallidotomy for dystonia: Clinical outcome and neuronal activity. In Advances in Neurology (S. Fahn, C.D. Marsden, and M. DeLong, eds.), vol. 78, pp. 211–219. Philadelphia: Lippincott-Raven.
3. Hutchison, W.D., Allan, R.J., Opitz, H., Levey, R., Dostrovsky, J.O., Lang, A.E., and Lozano, A.M. (1998). Neurophysiological identification of the subthalamic nucleus in surgery for Parkinson's disease. Ann. Neurol., 44, 622–628.
4. Bakay, R.A.E., Vitek, J.L., and DeLong, M.R. (1992). Thalamotomy for tremor. In Neurosurgical Operative Atlas (S.S. Rengachary and R.N. Wilkins, eds.), vol. 2, pp. 299–312. Baltimore: Williams and Wilkins.
5. Alexander, G.E., Crutcher, M.D., and DeLong, M.R. (1990). Basal ganglia-thalamocortical circuits: Parallel substrates for motor, oculomotor, prefrontal and limbic functions. Prog. Brain Res., 85, 119–146.
6. Lenz, F.A., Tasker, R.R., Kwan, H.C., Schnider, S., Kwong, R., Murayama, Y., Dostrovsky, J.O., and Murphy, J.T. (1988). Single unit analysis of the human ventral thalamic nuclear group: Correlation of thalamic "tremor cells" with the 3–6 Hz component of parkinsonian tremor. J. Neurosci., 8, 754–764.
7. Morrell, M.J., RNS System in Epilepsy Study Group. (2011). Responsive cortical stimulation for the treatment of medically intractable partial epilepsy. Neurology, 77(13), 1295–304.

While deep brain stimulation (DBS) has become more refined over the past 40 years, responsive intracranial neural stimulation (RNS) (e.g., the NeuroPace device to treat refractory epilepsy) has only recently been introduced. Both involve placement of electrodes into or on the surface of brain tissue to modulate neuron activity within some therapeutic change. Both rely on recordings to determine targeting for electrode placement, but newer developments in DBS have incorporated recordings to inform stimulation parameters, while RNS largely relies on recordings to trigger stimulation.

Targeting between DBS and RNS, however is different in two regards. First, precision in DBS is paramount, with accuracy requirements on the order of 1 mm, whereas RNS typically requires ~2 to 3 mm precision (e.g., depth electrodes within the hippocampus) and sometimes even less. Second, DBS now uses a few common targets reliably for certain disorders; in fact, practitioners are particularly adamant about demanding the precision in targeting each time. In contrast, RNS is so customized to each patient and the location of seizure foci or circuitry nexuses that there is little consistency from case to case thus far.

1. DEEP BRAIN STIMULATION

1.1. Background

The full array of intraoperative neurophysiology techniques may be used during the performance of so-called functional neurosurgical procedures. During DBS interventions, stimulating electrodes are stereotactically placed within deep brain structures to treat movement disorders such as Parkinson's disease (PD), essential tremor, dystonia, epilepsy, affective disorders, and chronic neuropathic pain. The deep location of these structures precludes direct surgical approaches. Instead, surgeons rely on a combination of image-guided stereotactic techniques and intraoperative neurophysiology to place the stimulating electrodes both accurately and safely. Unlike tumors, which are relatively large and easily identified on computed tomography (CT) or magnetic resonance imaging (MRI), functional neurosurgical targets typically are small and poorly visualized with current imaging modalities. Moreover, these targets are not only anatomical but physiological; thus, image-based targeting may incompletely identify the desired location. Consequently, intraoperative recording and stimulation techniques have been developed to aid target localization.

These techniques complement anatomical targeting by providing real-time electrophysiological data concerning the probe position and the surgical target. The surgeon and physiologist use these data to fine-tune the anatomical targeting before placing the permanent electrode. Intraoperative neurophysiology does not simply monitor surgical activity; it guides it.

1.2. History and Theory

1.2.1. Surgery for Movement Disorders

The first successful basal ganglia surgery is credited to Meyers [2–4], who reported improvement in a patient with postencephalitic parkinsonism in 1939. Despite the high mortality rates (10–12%) that plagued these "open" procedures [2–5], Meyers demonstrated the potential benefits of basal ganglia surgery. Meyers' work also provided the first accounts of human basal ganglia physiology, describing the frequency, phase, and amplitude of neuronal signals from the striatum, pallidum, corpus callosum, internal capsule, subcallosal bundle, and dorsal thalamus in patients with and without movement disorders [3,4,6]. Meyers realized the potential value of the accumulated data, which he ultimately employed to help localize specific deep brain structures during his procedures. As for sterotactic approaches, Zernov in 1889, is credited with the first stereotactic frame which mapped the surface of the brain in 2D space. Robert Clarke, in 1908 is credited with the first 3D stereotactic frame [7]. It was not until 1947, after the introduction of ventriculography, that Spiegel and Wycis performed the first human stereotactic surgeries, for psychiatric illness [8] and Huntington's chorea [9]. The following years saw a number of human stereotactic atlases published with standard landmarks from which stereotactic coordinates could be determined.

It is interesting to note that some effective targets were discovered by accident. While performing a pedunculotomy, Cooper accidently ligated the anterior choroidal artery of a PD patient, and the patient woke with his tremor reduced and less rigidity [10]. Cooper used this finding to create lesions in the globus pallidus stereotactically, reporting favorable results and reduced surgical mortality rates (~3%) as compared to open procedures [11–14].

1.2.2. Neurophysiology and Movement Disorder Surgery

Most early electrophysiological studies of the human thalamus and basal ganglia were performed with macroelectrodes yielding local field potential (LFP) data [19–23]. Over time the electrodes, amplifiers, and recording techniques have allowed for single-unit recording to become a common technique in the operating room. Of note is the work of Albe-Fessard, who refined microelectrode techniques for experimental purposes

and paved the way for their intraoperative use [24,25]. She believed that microelectrode recording (MER) would "provide a powerful tool in improving stereotactic localization and that it would furthermore reduce the risk due to anatomical variability" [25].

The history of electrical brain stimulation can be dated to the 1870s, when Fritsch and Hitzig elicited limb movement in dogs by stimulating the frontal cortex and then defined the limits of the motor area electrophysiologically [26]. In 1950, Spiegel et al. described the use of stimulation during surgery at the H fields of Forel to both "test the position of the electrode and to avoid proximity to the corticospinal pathways ventrally, the sensory thalamic-relay nuclei dorsally, and the third nucleus posteriorly" [18]. At this juncture DBS has supplanted the prior technique of neuroablation [18, 26, 33-115].

1.3. Modern Movement Disorder Surgery

There is no single "best" surgical method for performing movement disorder surgery. Stereotactic surgeons modify historical approaches to target localization to suit their personal preferences, to include modern technology, and to take advantage of their institution's strengths. Currently accepted techniques involve both frame-based and frameless stereotactic anatomical localization methodologies supported by intraoperative physiological confirmation of proper targeting. No matter the approach, it is still generally accepted that some form of intraoperative physiological confirmation is needed. This chapter will describe the technique of intraoperative single-unit recordings followed by macroelectrode stimulation testing.

1.4. Initial Anatomical Targeting

To perform these procedures, brain locations are defined in the three-dimensional (3D) space of an applied coordinated system so the surgeon can both accurately and repeatedly access structures that cannot be directly visualized. This is known as the stereotactic technique. Today, most anatomical stereotactic targeting is still performed using either a frame application and MRI exam or a prior MRI fused to a post-frame-application CT scan. From the scans, with the frame space coordinates, the surgeon can choose the initial target coordinates for the electrodes.

1.5. Microelectrode Techniques

Microelectrodes provide the most detailed picture of the neural elements encountered during movement disorder surgery [20,34,38,53,71,73,74,102,111,154–159,167–169]. Microelectrode tips have diameters of 1 to 40 μm and impedances of ~1 MΩ. By recording individual neuronal activity (Fig. 38.1), microelectrodes provide real-time information

Figure 38.1. An example of a single-unit recording. Used with permission from reference 170.

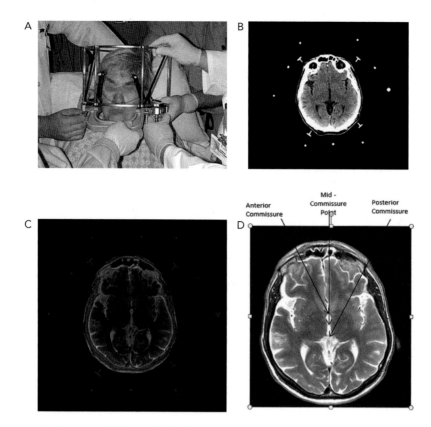

Figure 38.2. *An example of stereotactic placement and planning. A: The CRW frame with CT localizer placed on a patient. B: CT scan with the frame localizer bars. C: CT/MRI image fusion. D: MRI with anterior, posterior, and mid-commissure points.*

concerning the electrophysiological characteristics of a single neural unit and indirectly about the nucleus within which the cell is located. One drawback to the technique is that interpreting single-cell recordings is a skill that is mastered only with experience and patience. Yet our history has shown that, once mastered, MER can be performed both quickly and efficiently and yields invaluable data concerning electrode position. For example, Alterman et al. demonstrated that in 12% of 132 consecutive pallidotomies, final lesion placement, as guided by MER, was >4 mm removed from the site that was originally selected by the surgeon based on stereotactic MRI measurements [68]. This distance is considered significant because it is equivalent to the diameter of the typical pallidotomy lesion and the effective direct effects of the DBS electrode [166].

1.6. General Sterotactic Technique

Prior to surgery, an axial fast-spin-echo inversion recovery MRI sequence of the brain is performed. On the morning of surgery a stereotactic headframe (e.g. Integra CRW, Burlington, MA, USA) is applied in the holding area (Fig. 38.2A). Care is taken to center the head within the frame and to align the base of the frame with the zygoma, which approximates the orientation of the anterior commissure–posterior commissure (AC-PC) line. In this way, axial images obtained perpendicular to the axis of the frame will run parallel to the AC-PC plane. The patient is then transferred to radiology, where a stereotactic CT is performed. This CT (see Fig. 38.2B), which contains the fiducial markers to determine the 3D coordinates of any point in the patient's brain,

is then digitally fused (see Fig. 38.2C) with the prior MRI (see Fig. 38.2D). This fusion method is used because the MRI has inherent image distortions with the frame that are not found in CT scanners and could potentially cause inaccuracies in the coordinate determination. Obtaining the CT on the day of surgery is much more expeditious as well. The MRI is necessary, though, as certain structures are much more visible on the MRI (e.g., AC and PC). The target coordinates are then determined. The surgical target coordinates are based on a relationship to the AC, the PC, and/or the middle point between the AC and PC locations (see Fig. 38.2D). The localizations employed for the most commonly targeted sites are given in Table 38.1.

The patient is brought to the operating room and is positioned lounge-chair-like on the operating table. The target coordinates are set on the frame, bringing the presumptive

TABLE 38.1. Initial Target Coordinates

TARGET	MEDIAL LATERAL COORDINATE	ANTERIOR-POSTERIOR COORDINATE	VENTRAL-DORSAL COORDINATE
GPi	20 mm from midline	3 mm anterior to MCP	6 mm ventral to AC-PC
VIM	15 mm from midline	20% of the AC-PC length anterior to PC	2 mm dorsal to AC-PC
STN	11.5 mm from midline	3 mm posterior to MCP	6 mm ventral to AC-PC

target to the center of the operating arc. The scalp is incised in a curved fashion, exposing the area for a 14-mm burr hole ~11.5 cm posterior to the nasion (14–15 cm for a VIM target) and in the mid-pupillary line laterally. The dura mater is opened within the burr hole fully, taking care not to damage brain or surface veins. The included plastic ring (part of the electrode securing system) is inserted into the burr hole and a small pial opening is made where the cannulas are to be inserted. The base of the microdrive is mounted onto the operating arc. For the particular system in use at our facility, the microelectrode is back-loaded into the microdrive and zeroed to the guide tube that is set to be 15 mm from the target when inserted into the brain. For safe insertion, the electrode is withdrawn into the cannula (~5 mm). An insertion cannula is carefully advanced through the frontal lobe and then the drive system with the microelectrode is inserted. The guide tube containing the recording electrode is inserted into the insertion cannula and the microdrive apparatus is mounted to the X-Y adjustment stage. At this point, the guide tube, at the end of which the electrode tip position is zeroed, is flush with the end of the insertion cannula. Thus, recording begins 15 mm anterosuperior to the presumptive target.

The electrode is driven 1.0 mm into the brain and the impedance of the electrode–tissue system is measured. In our experience, impedances of 500 to 800 MΩ (theoretically, higher impedance values better isolate single units, practically, the impedance measured is a function of the microelectrode, the input impedance of the amplifier, and the operating room environment) provide the best single-unit recordings at our facility. If the electrode impedance is higher than this, the electrode is 'conditioned'. Conditioning, by passing an electrical current though the electrode, burns off any oxide that may have formed, lowering the impedance. If the electrode impedance starts below 650 KΩ, the electrode is replaced. Even with conditioning of the electrode and stimulation testing, these starting impedances allow for sufficient current passage without degradation of the recording electrode surface. If there is a large impedance drop following electrode conditioning, the electrode is deemed unacceptable and is replaced.

We correct any noise problems at this time and then proceed to data acquisition. Excess noise usually stems from poorly grounded equipment or bad cables. The systems in use today are much less susceptible to noise than in the past, but that does not preclude large noise sources such as intraoperative MRI units, even in shielded rooms, from causing significant problems. At the conclusion of each recording trajectory, the collected data are mapped onto scaled sagittal sections derived from the Schaltenbrand-Wahren stereotactic atlas [164]. Mapping is used to determine the most probable location and orientation in the brain employing a "best fit" model (see Data Organization section). When the data suggest that our targeting is correct, we proceed with electrode implantation and test stimulation.

1.7. GPi Procedures

Posteroventral GPi DBS procedures are reported to improve tremor, rigidity, and levodopa-induced dyskinesias, with reduced psychological complications as compared to STN DBS, in patients with medically refractory, moderately advanced PD. Profound improvements have also been reported in patients with DYT1- associated primary dystonia in whom GPi stimulation was performed. Successful pallidal interventions require targeting of the sensorimotor region of the GPi, which lies posterior and ventral in the nucleus. When recording in this region, three key nuclear structures must be recognized: the striatum, the external globus pallidus (GPe), and the GPi (Fig. 38.3). Our typical trajectory passes at a 60- to 70-degree angle above the horizontal of the AC-PC line, and at a medial-lateral angle of 90 degrees (i.e., true vertical). By employing this purely parasagittal trajectory, we can more readily fit the

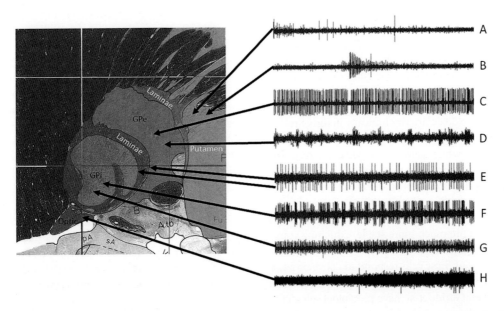

Figure 38.3. Sagittal slice through the GPi region and a graphical representation of the single units encountered in each structure. Modified and used with permission from reference 170.

operative recording data to the parasagittal sections provided in human stereotactic atlases.

The first cells encountered during recording are in the corpus striatum (caudate and putamen in Fig. 38.3). They exhibit characteristic low-amplitude action potentials, which sound like corn popping (*A* in Fig. 38.3, 🔊 GPi audio 38.1). Cellular activity in this area is extremely sparse, and the background is quiet. The electrode may also traverse some quiet regions that represent small fingerlike projections of the internal capsule into the striatum. Another cell that is encountered traversing all regions is called an *X-cell* and represents a dying cell that was injured by the microelectrode. It is important to differentiate bursters (see below) from X-cells (*B* in Fig. 38.3B, 🔊 GPi audio 38.2). Either the detection of a border cell or an increase in background activity marks entry into the GPe, the next structure to be encountered. Though rare in this region, border cells greatly facilitate localization of the boundaries within the globus pallidus.

Two major cell types are found within the GPe: *pausers* (*C* in Fig. 38.3, 🔊 GPi audio 38.3) and *bursters* (*D* in Fig. 38.3, 🔊 GPi audio 38.4). Pauser cells fire arrhythmically at a frequency of 30 to 80 Hz. They exhibit moderate- to high-amplitude discharges and lower amplitude than the border cells. They are distinguishable by their staccato-type, asynchronous pauses. An extremely small number of pauser cells (5%) may demonstrate somatotopically organized kinesthetic responses in PD, but more may be found in the dystonic patient. Burster cells are distinguished by short bursts of high-frequency discharges, achieving rates as high as 500 Hz. Amplitudes vary but are usually less than the amplitudes of the pauser cells. X-cells exhibit high-frequency discharges (near 500 Hz) with a time-related decrease in amplitude, representing death of the cell.

We may encounter anywhere from 4 to 8 mm of GPe during one recording tract. Border cells are again encountered at the inferior border of GPe and are more plentiful in this region. Border cells (*E* in Fig. 38.3, 🔊 GPi audio 38.5) exhibit very low frequencies (2–20 Hz) that are highly periodic, with high-amplitude spikes and moderate to long firing times. A quiet laminar area (see Fig. 38.3) is encountered upon exit from the GPe, marked by a steep drop-off in background activity. Border cells are again encountered upon entry into the GPi, and again, two classes of neurons predominate within the nucleus: tremor-related cells and high-frequency cells. Tremor cells (*F* in Fig. 38.3, 🔊 GPi audio 38.6) fire rhythmically in direct relation to the patient's tremor. Single-unit recordings show a frequency modulation pattern, while semi-microelectrode recordings show a frequency and amplitude modulation pattern. The firing rate of these cells is between 80 and 200 Hz.

High-frequency cells (*G* in Fig. 38.3G, 🔊 GPi audio 38.7) are characterized by firing rates that are similar to the tremor cells (80–100 Hz) but are much more stable, exhibiting consistent amplitude but asynchronous firing rates and no real repetitive patterning. Many of these cells respond to active or passive range of motion of a specific joint or extremity. When recording movement responses, Guridi et al. have physiologically defined a somatotopic organization of the kinesthetic cells in the GPi, with the face and arm region located ventrolaterally and the leg

dorsomedially [69]. Taha et al. found a slightly different arrangement, with the leg sandwiched centrally between the arm in both the rostral and caudal areas [74]. Vitek et al. have found the leg to be medial and dorsal with respect to the arm, and the face more ventral [16]. The GPi is subdivided into external and internal segments, labeled GPie (external GPi) and GPii (internal GPi), respectively. Both regions exhibit similar cellular recording patterns, but GPie may exhibit less cellularity than GPii. Total GPi recordings normally span from 5 to 12 mm. A steep drop-off in background activity denotes exit from the GPi inferiorly.

Three important white matter structures border the GPi and may be encountered during recording. The ansa lenticularis (AL), which emerges from the base of the GPi, carries motor-related efferents from the GPi to the ventrolateral thalamus, merging with its sister pathway, the lenticular fasciculus at the H field of Forel. The AL is an electrically quiet region, although rare cells of relatively low amplitudes and firing frequencies can be recorded. It has been proposed that lesioning within the AL generates the best results from posteroventral pallidotomy. The optic tract (OT) lies directly inferior to the AL (see Fig. 38.3, 🔊 GPi audio 38.8), accounting for the high rate of visual field complications reported in the early modern pallidotomy literature [17,60]. With quality recordings, it is possible to hear the microelectrode tip enter the OT, the sound of which is reminiscent of a waterfall. Upon hearing this background change, one may confirm entry into the OT by turning off the ambient lights and shining a flashlight in the patient's eyes. This will increase the recorded signal if the electrode is within the OT. Finally, one may encounter the internal capsule (IC). Background recordings within the IC are similar to those of the OT. Movement of the mouth or contralateral hemibody will generate a swooshing sound that is correlated to the movement. Obviously, one wishes to avoid the posterior internal capsule when placing the DBS lead, since a hemiparesis or hemiplegia may result.

Macroelectrode stimulation is performed prior to securing the DBS lead to ensure that the electrode is a safe distance from the internal IC and the OT and as a secondary check of the MER. We conduct test stimulation using the DBS lead itself using a bipolar stimulation montage at 130 Hz and 60 uSec for PD and 210 uSec for dystonia. Stimulation of contralateral muscular contractions at <2.5 V suggests that the DBS electrode is too close to the internal capsule and should be adjusted laterally. Induction of phosphenes at <2.0 V suggests that the electrode is too close to the OT and should be withdrawn slightly. Test stimulation should be performed at all DBS lead contacts to ensure that all leads are a safe distance from the IC and the OT. Decreasing voltage trends in the induction of muscular contractions and/or phosphenes should be monitored.

In addition to PD, GPi has been a target of choice for dystonia, Tourette syndrome, and status dystonicus. Recording GPi for other disorders demonstrates how the electrophysiology of one target structure varies with the disorder. Figure 38.4 shows GPi recordings from four different disorders. For PD the patterning is as described above with asynchronous high-frequency bursts with very short interspike intervals (ISI), intermingled with areas of larger ISI periods. Dystonia, on

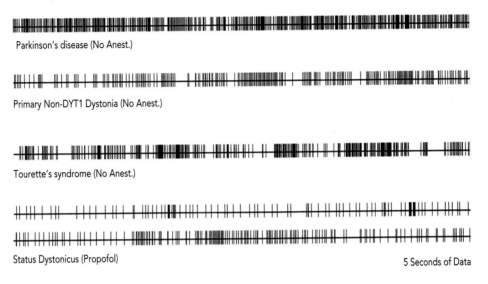

Parkinson's disease (No Anest.)

Primary Non-DYT1 Dystonia (No Anest.)

Tourette's syndrome (No Anest.)

Status Dystonicus (Propofol)   5 Seconds of Data

Figure 38.4. Raster plots of single-unit recordings from the GPi in various diseases.

the other hand, does not show areas of high-frequency (short ISI) bursts, and there are some areas with a very long pause between firings. Tourette syndrome shows a mix between both the PD and dystonia patterns, with areas of high-frequency bursts and areas of large ISI patterns. We have not performed a GPi recording on a patient with status dystonicus without anesthesia, so the patterning is probably affected by the propofol, but the firing rate is much lower with large ISIs.

1.8. VIM Procedures

Chronic high-frequency electrical stimulation within the ventral intermediate nucleus of the thalamus (VIM; Fig. 38.5) suppresses parkinsonian and essential tremor without adversely affecting voluntary motor activity to a significant degree. Thalamic interventions are extremely gratifying to perform because of the immediacy of the results and the well-defined physiology of the motor and sensory thalamic nuclei [41].

When targeting VIM, our standard angles of approach are 60 to 70 degrees relative to the AC-PC line and 5 to 10 degrees

lateral of the true vertical. Pure parasagittal trajectories cannot be employed as they are in GPi procedures due to the medial location of the target and a desire to avoid the ipsilateral lateral ventricle. Transit through the ventricle may increase the risk of hemorrhage and typically leads to more rapid loss of cerebrospinal fluid (CSF), with resulting brain shift and loss of targeting accuracy.

Recording begins in the dorsal thalamus, where cells characterized by low amplitudes and sparse firing patterns are encountered. Bursts of activity and small-amplitude single spikes (*A* in Fig. 38.5, ◐ Thal audio 38.1) are typical findings in this region. Upon exiting the dorsal thalamus, the electrode enters the VL nucleus, which is composed of nucleus ventralis oralis anterior (VOA), ventralis oralis posterior, and VIM. The dorsal third of the VL nucleus is sparsely populated such that cellular recordings in this area are similar to those of the dorsal thalamus. As the electrode passes ventrally within the VL complex, cellular density increases and cells with firing rates of 40 to 50 Hz (*B* in Fig. 38.5, ◐ Thal audio 38.2) are encountered. Kinesthetic cells with discrete somatotopic representation are routinely

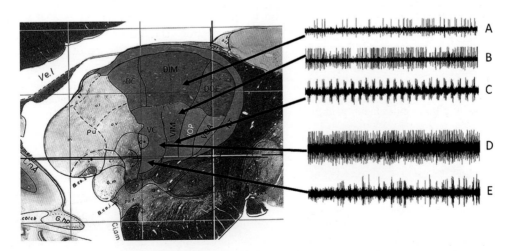

Figure 38.5. Sagittal slice through the VIM region and a graphical representation of the single units encountered in each structure. Modified and used with permission from reference 170.

encountered. This organization permits an assessment of the mediolateral position of the electrode. The homunculus of the ventrocaudal (Vc) and VIM nuclei are virtually identical: representation of the contralateral face and mouth lies 9 to 11 mm lateral of midline, the arm is represented lateral to this at 13 to 15 mm lateral of midline, and the leg is more lateral still, adjacent to the internal capsule. Thus, if one encounters a cell that responds to passive movement of the ankle, one knows that one has targeted too laterally to treat an upper-extremity tremor and should adjust the mediolateral position accordingly.

In addition to kinesthetic neurons, one will routinely encounter "tremor" cells (C in Fig. 38.5, 🔊 Thal audio 38.3) within the VIM of tremor patients. These cells exhibit a rhythmic firing pattern that can be synchronized to electromyographic recordings of the patient's tremor [37]. Lenz et al. demonstrated that these cells are concentrated within VIM, 2 to 4 mm above the AC-PC plane, a site that is empirically known to yield consistent tremor control [162]. The recording electrode may exit VIM inferiorly, passing into the zona incerta (ZI) with a resulting decrease in background signal, or it will enter Vc, the primary sensory relay nucleus of the thalamus. Entry into Vc is marked by a change in the background signal. Cells in this region are densely packed, exhibit high amplitudes, and respond to sensory phenomena (e.g., light touch) with a discrete somatotopic organization, which mirrors that of VIM (D in Fig. 38.5, 🔊 Thal audio 38.4). A typical cell, which responds to lightly brushing the patient's finger, is indicated by E in Figure 38.5 (🔊 Thal audio 38.5). Note the increase in firing rate as a light bristle paintbrush is dabbed against the finger (it has a "whoosh"-like sound quality). The bars represent the times that the brush is being dabbed against the finger. If Vc is encountered early in the recording trajectory, the electrode may be targeted posteriorly and should be adjusted anteriorly.

The nucleus ventrocaudalis parvocellularis (VCpc) rests inferiorly to Vc. Recordings within this nucleus are similar to those of Vc; however, stimulation in this location may yield painful or temperature-related sensations. Single-unit recordings in this area will respond to both painful and temperature-related stimuli applied within the cell's receptive field.

When performing VIM DBS, we use the lead itself to perform test stimulation. In such cases bipolar stimulation is performed so that a reference pad is unnecessary. In our experience, a properly positioned DBS lead results in tremor arrest at 3 V (pulse width 60 μsec, frequency 180 Hz). Transient paresthesias are common with a properly positioned electrode; however, persistent paresthesias, which are induced at low voltages, indicate that the electrode is positioned posteriorly, near or within Vc. Failure to suppress tremor or induce paresthesias, even at 5 V, suggests that the electrode is positioned anteriorly within VOA. Muscular contractions (typically of the contralateral face and/or hand) suggest that the lead is positioned too laterally and stimulation is affecting the internal capsule. It has been our experience that microelectrode stimulation may not suppress tremor at sites where macroelectrode stimulation is effective.

1.9. STN Procedures

Subthalamic DBS improves all of the cardinal features of PD, dampens the severity of "on–off" fluctuations, alleviates freezing spells, and dramatically reduces medication requirements. The STN is approached at an angle of 70 degrees relative to the AC-PC line and 10 to 15 degrees lateral of the true vertical. Microelectrode recording begins in the anterior thalamus and passes sequentially through the ZI, Forel's field H2, the STN, and the substantia nigra pars reticulata (SNr) (Fig. 38.6).

In the thalamus, one encounters cells that fire with low amplitude and frequency. Two patterns of activity may be identified: (1) bursts of activity (A in Fig. 38.6, 🔊 STN audio 38.1) and (2) irregular, low-frequency (1–30 Hz) activity (B in Fig. 38.6, 🔊 STN audio 38.2). The density of cellular

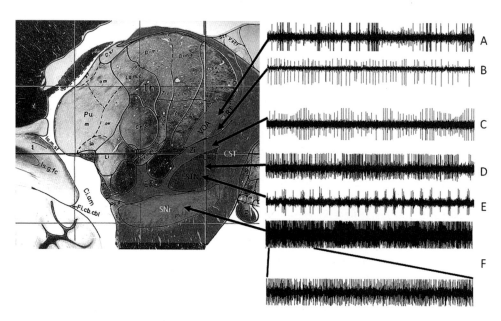

Figure 38.6. Sagittal slice through the STN region and a graphical representation of the single units encountered in each structure. Modified and used with permission from reference 170.

activity varies in this region. For example, we have observed that VOA is more cellular than the reticular thalamus. The border between the thalamus and ZI may be very distinct, but not in all cases. Developmentally, the ZI is a continuation of the reticular nucleus of the thalamus, and the transition from one to the other may not be clear. The ZI can be differentiated electrophysiologically from the thalamus in two ways. First, cellular firing rates slow and become a little more asynchronous, and the amplitudes decrease in intensity (*C* in Fig. 38.6, ◀) STN audio 38.3). These changes are subtle and can be missed by inexperienced observers. The second indication of transition from thalamus to ZI is a change in the background recordings. Whereas the background of the thalamus proper is somewhat active, the ZI background is much quieter. Typically, the recording electrode will exit the thalamus 6 to 10 mm anterosuperior to our presumptive target and will pass through 2.5 to 4.0 mm of ZI before entering H2. If >4 mm of relative "quiet" is encountered, a trajectory that is anterior or posterior to the STN should be suspected.

A decrease in background activity demarcates entry into Forel's field H2, which lies immediately superior to the STN, 10 to 12 mm lateral of midline. Sparse cellular activity is detected over a span of 1 to 2 mm. Background activity increases as the recording electrode enters STN. Additionally, dense cellular activity is now encountered. Two patterns of cellular activity are observed within STN: (1) tremor activity (*D* in Fig. 38.6, ◀) STN audio 38.4) similar to that encountered in VIM or GPi and (2) single-cell activity (*E* in Fig. 38.6, ◀) STN audio 38.5) with frequencies that vary from ~25 to 45 Hz. Cells in the dorsal segments of the STN exhibit slower firing rates than those of the ventral STN. Kinesthetic-related activity (see ◉ Video 38.1 and 38.2 for a responsive cell and a voluntary cell) is often observed, but a clear somatotopy is not evident. Upon exiting the STN, the microelectrode may pass through a thin quiet zone or will pass directly into the SNr. Entry into the SNr is demarcated by significant increases both in background neural activity and in cellular firing rates (*F* in Fig. 38.6, ◀) STN audio 38.6), which are usually >60 Hz. Up to 7 mm of SNr may be encountered, depending on the anteroposterior position of the trajectory.

We require 4 to 6 mm of STN, preferably with evidence of kinesthetic activity, for implantation of the DBS lead. This large span of STN recording ensures that the electrodes are implanted solidly within the nucleus and not near a border. The primary goal of test stimulation at the STN is to check for stimulation-induced adverse events because, aside from tremor arrest and some modest reductions in rigidity, positive STN stimulation effects may not be observed for hours or days.

Test stimulation is performed in bipolar configuration. Parameters are 60 μsec, 180 Hz, 0 to 4 V. We do not stimulate higher than 4.0 V for fear of inducing hemiballism. Moreover, we have yet to employ amplitudes greater than 4 V to achieve clinical benefit at this target. Transient paresthesias are frequently encountered with the onset of stimulation. Persistent paresthesias indicate stimulation of the medial lemniscal pathway, which lies posterolateral to the nucleus. Stimulation-induced contractions of the contralateral hemibody and/or face indicate anterolateral

misplacement of the lead. Finally, abnormal eye movements may be encountered if the lead is positioned too medially or deep to the nucleus.

The first test stimulation is performed using contacts 0+, 1- up to a voltage of 4.0 V. If no significant adverse effects are encountered with this focal test, we proceed to test stimulation employing each of the four contacts (i.e., 0, 1, 2, 3 up to a voltage of 4.0 V). This test covers the full contact space of the electrodes and focuses on identifying stimulation-induced adverse events in the ventral aspect of the stimulation field. This is the area where most adverse events have occurred in our experience. The final stimulation is performed using contacts 0+, 1-, 2-, 3- up to a voltage of 4.0 V. This examines the dorsal aspect of the stimulation field.

1.10. Data Organization

The data from each microrecording tract are plotted on scaled graph paper (1.0 cm = 1.0 mm) [17,163]. The borders of each encountered structure are marked, and the span of each region is represented by a different color for easy differentiation. To account for our angle of approach accurately, a line that is parallel to the intercommissural line is also drawn. The plotted tract is then traced onto a transparent plastic sheet. The transparency is placed on scaled maps (10:1) derived from the Schaltenbrand-Wahren human stereotactic atlas [164] (see ◉ Video 38.3 for an example of this procedure) to determine to which map the trajectory best fits. The accuracy of the fit depends upon the number of trajectories, upon the number of structures encountered along each trajectory, and finally upon how well the patient's anatomy fits the atlas, which is derived from a single human specimen. It can be difficult to find one place to which a single tract fits best, especially when performing pallidal or thalamic interventions. When mapping the STN, the many structures encountered along a single trajectory make fitting it to the atlas a little more straightforward. Knowing the spatial relationship between each tract, we can better fit all of the data to the atlas with each subsequent trajectory although most cases ire only 1-2 passes per side [186].

2. RESPONSIVE NEURAL STIMULATION

2.1. Background

In 2013, the U.S. Food and Drug Administration approved the Neuropace responsive neurostimulator (RNS)' system for treatment of refractory epilepsy with no more than two epileptic sources in patients with frequent and/or disabling seizures who are resistant to two or more antiepileptic drugs [171,172]. It is an additional option for those patients who have either failed to respond to or are not candidates for resective surgery. The system involves a battery-powered, closed-loop neurostimulator connected to two permanent leads or subdural grids, providing a system for detection and treatment of a seizure focus. The efficacy of the RNS system has been reported in double-blind, randomized control trials, with reports of 37.9% reduction in seizures compared to the 17.3% reduction in the sham group in long-term follow-up studies [171,173–175].

This system provides unique electrocorticographical recording and stimulation techniques to treat medically refractory epilepsy.

2.2. Anatomical Targeting

Unlike intraoperative lead implantation for movement disorders like PD, dystonia, or essential tremor, the final anatomical target for lead placement varies in each patient. Furthermore, physiological target confirmation using MER is at present not used to optimize lead placement. For these reasons, extensive efforts must be made to localize the seizure focus prior to surgery.

Commonly used modalities that provide insight into seizure focus location and guide RNS placement include MRI, CT, video-encephalography (vEEG) monitoring, and subtraction ictal SPECT co-registered to MRI (SISCOM). Each of these imaging modalities or a combination thereof can play an integral role in seizure focus identification and preoperative surgical implantation of the RNS system.

MRI is vital in detecting epileptogenic structural lesions and is a Level B classification for evaluation of a first unprovoked seizure [176]. At our institution, an MRI "epilepsy protocol" is employed that uses thin slices in the coronal plane to detail the anatomy and identify any pathology within the temporal lobes. From the surgical planning standpoint, MRI is imperative prior to RNS placement as it also serves as the foundation for stereotactic electrode placement if needed. At our institution, the MRI is merged preoperatively with a thin-cut CT scan after stereotactic headframe placement. Coordinates are then calculated and chosen based on the desired target.

Prolonged vEEG monitoring also plays an essential role in the presurgical evaluation and seizure focus localization. Optimally, a recording should capture several of the patient's typical seizures. The video recording in conjunction with scalp EEG can allow improved seizure localization. Postictal deficits can also be characterized in the inpatient setting, allowing for improved localization and lateralization [177]. Patients are monitored from several days to several weeks, and the adequacy of vEEG is mainly dependent on how quickly the patient experiences seizures after tapering of antiepileptic drugs. The total number of seizures required for localization varies and depends on a particular patient's distinct seizure types and their ability to be lateralized and localized upon review. Patients with unilateral interictal spikes and a single seizure type may require two or three seizures, whereas patients with multifocal discharges and multiple distinct seizure types may require two or three seizures of each type. Techniques to provoke seizure activity during inpatient monitoring include sleep deprivation, exercise, photic stimulation, and hyperventilation. Ictal EEG can provide valuable lateralizing and localizing information in temporal lobe epilepsy, but results can be inconsistent with extratemporal seizure foci [178]. The earliest ictal rhythms associated with a seizure identify the ictal onset zone, although in some patients the ictal onset appears to be essentially bilateral and lateralization is not possible, and thus invasive intracranial monitoring may be necessary. Ictal single-photon emission computed tomography (SPECT) is a nuclear medicine study where the patient is injected with a radioactive tracer during a seizure. Ideally, imaging must be obtained right after the radiotracer is injected, within seconds of seizure onset, and focal hyperperfusion in the seizure focus is typically demonstrated. Greater chances of positive surgical outcomes have been shown to occur when the findings on ictal EEG and ictal SPECT are concordant in cases of both temporal and extratemporal epilepsy with or without structural lesions [179]. Ictal SPECT can also be co-registered with MRI with computerized subtraction of interictal findings from ictal findings (SISCOM). SISCOM is commonly used to determine the utility of temporal depth electrode placement prior to RNS surgery. It has been shown to be helpful in patients who have focal epilepsy but normal MRI findings, and in patients with extensive focal cortical dysplasia [180,181]. Reliable ictal SPECCT is difficult to obtain in many centers, however.

For mesial temporal lobe epilepsy, there is no clear consensus on the ideal depth electrode location. A trajectory through the long axis of the hippocampus proper is advocated by some, several electrodes placed into the hippocampus orthogonally by others, while others prefer a hippocampal-sparing path along the parahippocampal white matter, although it has been reported that depth electrode placement for recording ictal onsets during resective epilepsy surgery only requires the contacts to touch rather than to reside within the intended structure [182]. However, in regards to depth electrode placement for RNS, no direct comparison studies have been done. The issue is complicated further in patients who have undergone prior amygdalohippocampectomy but have continued epileptiform discharges on the ipsilateral side.

Anatomical relationships of the mesial temporal structures and the long occipito-temporal trajectory necessitate accurate lead placement during surgery. Although the laterotemporal approach been shown to be a more accurate method of placing intracranial recording electrodes than an occipitotemporal approach, no significant differences in the efficacy of ictal monitoring, complications, or clinical outcome were reported [182,183].

2.3. Surgical Procedure

Patients are deemed appropriate for RNS placement following a multidisciplinary review by epileptologists, neurosurgeons, and neuropsychologists after completion of mandatory investigative studies, which at our institution include MRI, SISCOM, video-EEG, and neuropsychiatric and Wada testing. Contrast-enhanced T1- and T2-weighted 1-mm-thick MRI slices along with SISCOM sequence images are obtained prior to surgery and imported to the image guidance software workstation (Fig. 38.7). At our institution, the same stereotactic frame and software that are used during movement disorder surgery are also implemented during RNS implantation, with several modifications. There are multiple frame based and frameless methods for RNS implantation. Two will be described here. One method uses the Leksell Model G Stereotactic Frame (Elekta, Stockholm, Sweden) which is applied to the patient's head with the frame's posterior bars adjusted and secured in a more caudal location (compared to DBS procedures for

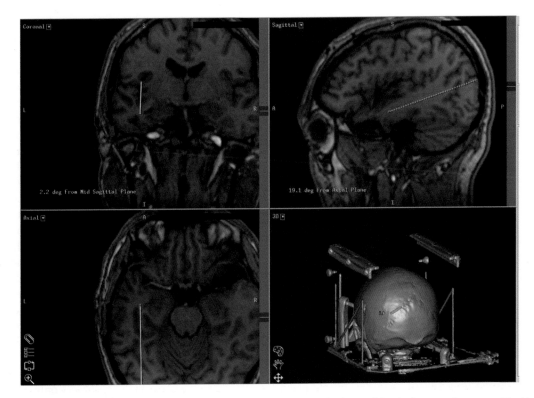

Figure 38.7. MRI-guided targeting using the Framelink software. Note that the trajectory of the lead is parallel and adjacent to the course of the hippocampus from the head to the point of reflection around the ambient cistern. Also note that the trajectory avoids crossing sulci, vascular structures, or the occipital horn of the lateral ventricle.

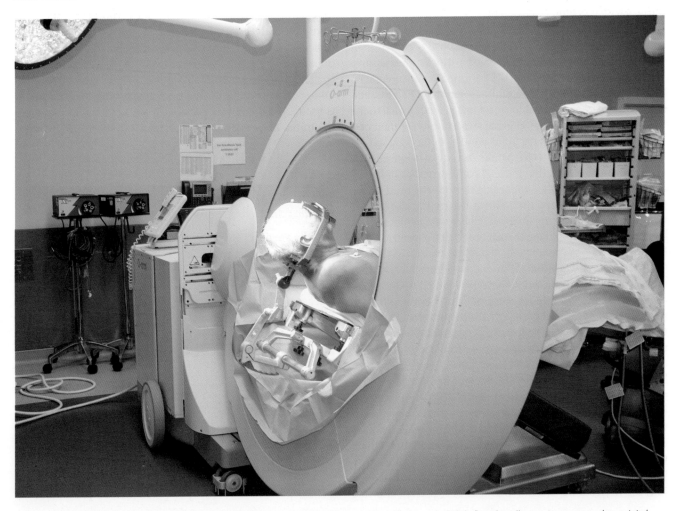

Figure 38.8. The patient is positioned on the operating table supine in the "recline" position with the neck slightly flexed to allow easier access to the occipital entry points. The frame is then secured to the table. Note the "parked" position of the intraoperative CT.

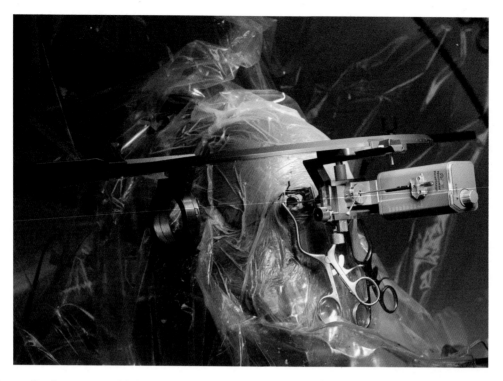

Figure 38.9. *Leksell arc and headstage are assembled and burr hole(s) placed. A sterile guide tube is inserted and the lead is subsequently assembled and advanced to the target.*

movement disorders) on the skull for ease of operative access at the occipital depth-electrode entry point, while taking care to maintain the parallel orientation of the frame to the AC-PC line in the axial plane. A high-resolution CT study is then obtained and computationally merged with the preoperative MRI studies. Direct targeting is performed with stereotactic image guidance software. Anatomical locations of AC, PC, and midline markers are defined to create images orthogonal to the AC-PC plane and midsagittal plane. Trajectories are then created, with an occipital entry point parallel to the long axis of the hippocampus within the parahippocampal white matter. Care is taken to ensure that the lead path is parallel and adjacent to the course of the hippocampus from the head to the point of reflection around the ambient cistern. It is also important that the planned trajectory avoids crossing sulci, vascular structures, or the occipital horn of the lateral ventricle (see Fig. 38.7).

The patient is positioned on the operating table supine in the "recline" position with the neck slightly flexed to allow easier access to the occipital entry points. The frame is then secured to the table (Fig. 38.8). After appropriate draping, the Leksell arc and headstage are assembled and burr hole(s) placed. A sterile guide tube is inserted to a depth of 45 mm above the target. The lead is then subsequently assembled and advanced to the target (Fig. 38.9). Intraoperative CT is subsequently used to verify final depth-electrode placement (Fig. 38.10). Once the surgeon is satisfied with the target accuracy, the guide tube and the Leksell arc are removed. Another method uses a frameless approach using the Brainlab (Munich, Germany) navigation system and their VarioGuide arm. A MRI is acquired the morning before surgery and entered into the navigational system. The head is registered allowing

the VarioGuide arm adjusted to target any point in the stereotactic field. At this time, subdural strips may also be placed. The next stage of the operation involves performing a custom-sized craniectomy. The responsive neurostimulator is subsequently implanted and connected to the leads (Fig. 38.11). This can be challenging when a craniotomy has already been performed on one or both sides for the prior intracranial monitoring. It is useful, but not always possible, if RNS can be considered in the initial planning stages of evaluation, before any intracranial surgery is performed.

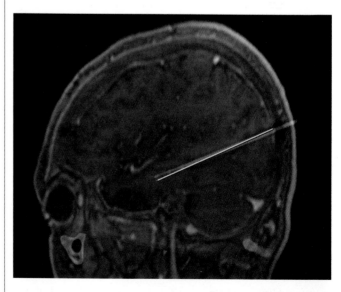

Figure 38.10. *Sagittal orthogonal MRI with merged intraoperative CT (iCT) study demonstrating the depth-electrode position in relation to planned trajectory (yellow line).*

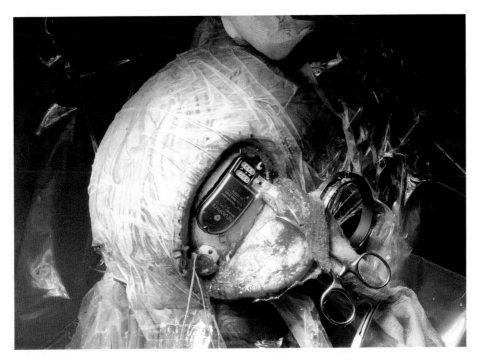

Figure 38.11. Right Neuropace generator placement at the prior planned craniectomy site. The depth leads have been connected and placed under the skin flap.

2.4. Intraoperative Electrophysiological Data

As previously mentioned, there exists no protocol for the use of real-time electrocorticography (ECoG) in guiding final strip or depth-electrode placement during RNS implantation. At present, unlike MER for movement disorders, intraoperative ECoG is not used to guide and/or optimize final electrode placement. After placement of subdural strip(s) and/or depth electrode(s), real-time intraoperative ECoG signals are useful for evaluating impedance and signal strength, allowing amplifier gain settings to be adjusted if necessary. Responses in ECoG can also be assessed while the stimulation settings are being programmed, which would allow for any immediate adjustments in stimulation parameters should an unfavorable acute response occur [172].

Figure 38.12 shows intraoperative ECoG signals for bilateral occipito-temporal depth electrodes implanted in three different patients. These recordings provide real-time ECoG over four different channels, which can each be programmed with up to five customized stimulations [172]. Figure 38.13 shows a burst-suppression pattern from general anesthesia during surgery. Although active spiking activity may be seen on the intraoperative ECoG recording, it is not necessary. Methohexital can also be used to induce epileptiform activity intraoperatively.

It is at the neurologist's discretion to choose which events trigger ECoG storage, and the stimulator is programmed to store ECoG recordings when those particular events occur. The three recommended ECoG triggers that are programmed at implantation are (1) magnet swipe performed by the patient when he or she feels a clinical seizure has or may have occurred and (2) saturation (high-amplitude ECoG) and (3) long episode (sustained changes in the ECoG), both of which could indicate an electrographic seizure [172].

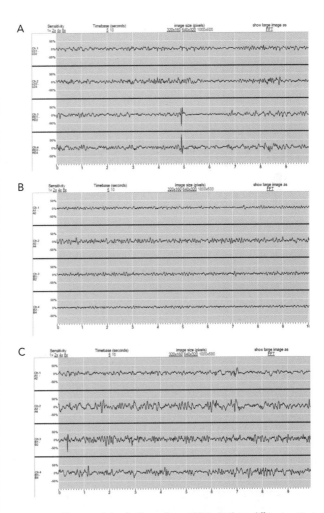

Figure 38.12. Bitemporal depth-electrode recordings in three different patients demonstrating variable levels of spontaneous ECoG activity. Typical ECoG recording (A); suppressed (B) and hyperactive (C) spontaneous ECoG activity.

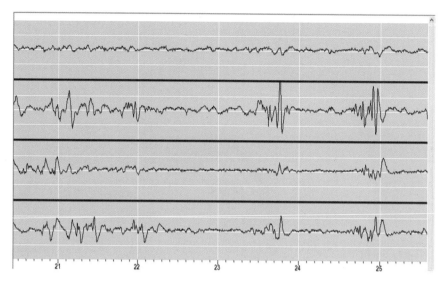

Figure 38.13. Burst-suppression pattern during general anesthesia.

When a specified ECoG signal is detected, therapeutic stimulation is then delivered. If the pattern is no longer detected, the remaining therapies in the sequence are not delivered.

Typical initial responsive therapy settings are a frequency of 200 Hz, pulse width of 160 μsec, and burst duration of 100 msec. Current is initially programmed at a low amplitude (e.g., 1.0 mA) and titrated upward as tolerated to a maximum of 12 mA [172]. Final skin closure is completed once impedances and ECoG recordings are deemed satisfactory [184]. The RNS Neuropace device allows for the connection of either two depth electrodes or two subdural strips or a combination thereof. Occasionally, more than two depth electrodes or subdural strips are implanted, with the unused leads left disconnected in the event that the desired areas of ECoG recording and/or stimulation change over time. In those cases, the preexisting skin incision is reopened and the desired strips or electrodes are then connected to the stimulator and the prior leads disconnected.

While the utility of intraoperative ECoG for RNS placement has yet to be fully realized, longer-term ECoG monitoring or chronic unlimited recording electrocorticography (CURE) by the RNS can occasionally provide seizure focus localization to guide resective surgery even for patients who do not receive a therapeutic benefit from the neurostimulator [185].

3. CONCLUSION

The neurophysiological techniques used in the operating room require trained and skilled personnel, not only to acquire but also to interpret the data. If everything goes perfectly, the data are relatively easy to interpret, but when the signals are not textbook cases, this interpretation needs to be done by very experienced personnel. No software-based interpretation scheme is likely going to replace the skilled human interpreter when recordings are difficult. The operating room is a very harsh electrically environment. As we learn about each area of interest, these procedures can take place more expeditiously and effectively.

REFERENCES

1. Horsley, V. (1909). The function of the so-called motor area of the brain. Br. Med. J., 2, 125–132.
2. Meyers, R. (1940). Surgical procedure for postencephalitic tremor, with notes on the physiology of the premotor fibers. Arch. Neurol. Psychiatry, 44, 455–459.
3. Meyers, R. (1942). Surgical interruption of the pallidofugal fibers: Its effect on the syndrome of paralysis agitans and technical considerations in its application. N.Y. State J. Med., 42, 317–325.
4. Meyers, R. (1968). The surgery of the hyperkinetic disorders. In The Handbook of Clinical Neurology (P.J. Vinken, and G. Bruyn, eds.), vol. 6, pp. 844–878. Amsterdam: North Holland Publishers.
5. Meyers, R. (1941). The modification of alternating tremors, rigidity and festination by surgery of the basal ganglia. Res. Pub. Assoc. Nerv. Ment. Dis., 21, 602–665.
6. Meyers, R. (1941). Cortical extinction in convulsions. J. Neurophysiol., 4, 250–256.
7. Fotlstad, H., Hariz, M., and Ljunggren, B. (1991). History of Clarke's stereotactic instrument. Stereot. Funct. Neurosurg., 57, 130–140.
8. Spiegel, E.A., Wycis, H.T., and Marks, M. (1947). Stereotactic apparatus for operations on the human brain. Science, 106, 349–350.
9. Spiegel, E.A. (1996). Development of stereoencephalatomy for extrapyramidal disease. J. Neurol., 24, 433–439.
10. Cooper, I.S. (1953). Ligation of the anterior choroidal artery for involuntary movements of parkinsonism. Psychiatry, 27, 317–319.
11. Cooper, I.S., and Bravo, G.O. (1958). Anterior choroidal artery occlusion, chemopallidectomy and chemothalarnectomy in parkinsonism: A consecutive series of 700 operations. In Pathogenesis and Treatment of Parkinsonism (W.S. Fields, ed.), pp. 325–352. Springfield, IL: Thomas.
12. Cooper, I.S. (1958). Chemopallidectomy. J. Neurosurg., 15, 244–250.
13. Narabayashi, H., and Okuxna, T. (1953). Procaine-oil blocking of the globus pallidus for the treatment of rigidity and tremor of parkinsonism. Proc. Jpn. Acad., 29, 134–137.
14. Guiot, G., and Brion, S. (1953). Traitement des mouvements anormaux par la coagulation pallidale. Rev. Neurol., 89, 578–580.
15. Laitinen, L.V., Bergenheim, A.T., and Hariz, M.I. (1992). Leksell's posteroventral pallidotomy in the treatment of Parkinson's disease. J. Neurosurg., 76, 53–61.
16. Yoshida, S., Nambu, A., and Jinnai, K. (1993). The distribution of the globus pallidus neurons with input from various cortical areas in the monkeys. Brain Res., 611(1),
17. Vitek, J.L., Bakay, R.A.E., Hashimoto, T., Kaneoke, Y., Mewes, K., Yu Zhang, J., Rye, D., Starr, P., Baron, M., Turner, R., and DeLong, M.R. (1998). Microelectrode-guided pallidotomy: Technical approach and its application in medically intractable Parkinson's disease. J. Neurosurg., 88, 1027–1043.
18. Spiegel, E.A., Wycis, H.T., Szekely, E.G., Adams, J., Flanaga, M., and Baird, W. (1963). Campotomy in various extrapyramidal disorders. J. Neurosurg., 20, 871–884.

19. Hughes, J.R. (1996). The electroencephalogram in parkinsonism. J. Neurosurg., 24, 369–376.
20. Tasker, R.R., Organ, L.W., and Hawrylyshyn, P.A. (1982). The Thalamus and Midbrain of Man. A Physiological Atlas Using Electrical Stimulation. Springfield, IL: Thomas.
21. Nakajima, H., Fukamachi, A., Isobe, I., Miyazaki, M., Shibazaki, T., and Ohye, C. (1978). Estimation of neural noise. Appl. Neurophysiol., 41, 193–201.
22. Bertrand, C., Poirier, L., Martinez, N., and Gauthier, C. (1958). Pneumotaxic localization, recording, stimulation, and section of basal brain structures in dyskinesia. Neurology, 8, 783–786.
23. Bertrand, G., Jasper, H., and Wong, A. (1967). Microelectrode study of the human thalamus: Functional organization in the ventro-basal complex. Confin. Neurol., 29, 81–86.
24. Albe-Fessard, D., Arfel, G., Guiot, G., Derome, P., Hertzog, E., Vourc'h, G., Brown, H., Aleonard, P., De La Herran, J., and Trigo, J.C. (1966). Electophysiological studies of some deep cerebral structures in man. J. Neurosci., 3, 37–51.
25. Albe-Fessard, D. (1973). Electrophysiological methods for the identification of thalamic nuclei. Z. Neurol., 205, 15–28.
26. Penfield, W., and Rasmussen, T. (1957). The Cerebral Cortex of Man: A Clinical Study of Localization and Function. New York: Macmillan.
27. Organ, L.W., Tasker, R.R., and Moody, N.F. (1967). The impedance profile of the human brain as a localization technique in stereoencephalotomy. Confin. Neurol., 29, 192–196.
28. Laitinen, L.V., and Johansson, G.G. (1967). Locating human cerebral structures by the impedance method. Confin. Neurol., 29, 197–201.
29. Albe-Fessard, D., Tasker, R., Yamashiro, K., Chodakiewitz, J., and Dostrovsky, J. (1986). Comparison in man of short latency averaged evoked potentials in thalamic hand and scalp zones of representation. Electroencephalogr. Clin. Neurophysiol., 65, 405–415.
30. Hassler, R., Riechert, T., Mundinger, F., Umbach, W., and Ganglberger, J.A. (1960). Physiologic observations in stereotaxic operations in extrapyramidal motor disturbances. Brain, 83, 337–350.
31. Narabayashi, H., and Ohye, C. (1974). Nucleus ventralis intermedius of human thalamus. Trans. Am. Neurol. Assoc., 99, 232–233.
32. Fukamachi, A., Ohye, C., and Narabayashi, H. (1973). Delineation of the thalamic nuclei with a microelectrode in stereotaxic surgery for parkinsonism and cerebral palsy. J. Neurosurg., 39, 214–225.
33. Yokoyama, T., Imamura, Y., Sugiyama, K., Nishizawa, S., Yokota, N., Ohta, S., and Uemura, K. (1999). Prefrontal dysfunction following unilateral posteroventral pallidotomy in Parkinson's disease. J. Neurosurg., 90, 1005–1010.
34. Bakay, R.A., DeLong, M.R., and Vitek, J.L. (1992). Posteroventral pallidotomy for Parkinson's disease. J. Neurosurg., 77, 487–488.
35. Lenz, F.A., Tasker, R.R., Kwan, H.C., Schider, S., Kwong, R., Dostrovsky, J.O., and Murphy, J.T. (1987). Selection of the optimal site for the relief of parkinsonian tremor on the basis of spectral analysis of neuronal firing patterns. Appl. Neurophysiol., 50, 338–343.
36. Lenz, F.A., Dostrovsky, J.O., Tasker, R.R., Yamashiro, K., Kwan, H.C., and Murphy, J.T. (1988). Single-unit analysis of the human ventral thalamic nuclear group: Somatosensory responses. J. Neurophysiol., 59, 299–316.
37. Lenz, F.A., Tasker, R.R., Kwan, H.C., Schneider, S., Kwong, R., Murayama, Y., Dostrovsky, J.O., and Murphy, J.T. (1988). Single unit analysis of the human ventral thalamic nuclear group: Correlation of thalamic tremor cells with the 3–6 Hz component of parkinsonian tremor. J. Neurosci., 8, 754–764.
38. Lenz, F.A., Kwan, H.C., Dostrovsky, J.O., Tasker, R.R., Murphy, J.T., and Lenz, Y.E. (1990). Single unit analysis of the human ventral thalamic nuclear group. Brain, 113, 1795–1821.
39. Levy, A. (1967). Stereotaxic brain operations in Parkinson's syndrome and related motor disturbances. Comparison of lesions in the pallidum and the thalamus with those in the internal capsule. Confin. Neurol., 29(Suppl.), 5–68.
40. Lenz, F.A., Dostrovsky, J.O., Kwan, H.C., Tasker, R.R., Yamashiro, K., and Murphy, J.T. (1988). Methods for microstimulation and recording of single neurons and evoked potentials in the human central nervous system. J. Neurosurg., 68, 630–634.
41. Tasker, R.R., and Kiss, Z.H.T. (1995). The role of the thalamus in functional neurosurgery. Neurosurg. Clin. North Am., 6, 73–99.
42. Dostrovsky, J.O., Davis, K.D., Lee, L., Sher, G.D., and Tasker, R.R. (1993). Electrical stimulation- induced effects in the human thalamus. In Electrical and Magnetic Stimulation of the Brain and Spinal Cord (O. Devinsky, A. Beric, and M. Dogali, eds.). New York: Raven Press.
43. Yoshida, M. (1989). Electrophysiological characteristics of human subcortical structures by frequency spectral analysis of neural noise (field potential) obtained during stereotactic surgery. Stereotac. Funct. Neurosurg., 52, 157–163.
44. Narabayashi, H., Yokochi, F., and Nakajima, Y. (1984). Levodopa-induced dyskinesia and thalamotomy. J. Neurol. Neurosurg. Psychiatry, 47, 831–839.
45. Sano, K., Mayanagi, Y., Sekino, H., Ogahiwa, M., and Ishijima, B. (1970). Results of stimulation and destruction of the posterior hypothalamus in man. J. Neurosurg., 33, 687–707.
46. Lang, A.E. (1998). Surgical treatment of dystonia. In Dystonia 3: Advances in Neurology (S. Fahn, C.D. Marsden, and M. DeLong, eds.), vol. 78, pp. 185–198. Philadelphia: Lippincott-Raven.
47. Vitek, J.L. (1998). Surgery for dystonia. Neurosurg. Clin. North Am., 9, 345–366.
48. Sterio, D., Beric, A., Dogali, M., Fazzini, E., Alfaro, G., and Devinsky, O. (1994). Neurophysiological properties of pallidal neurons in Parkinson's disease. Ann. Neurol., 35, 586–591.
49. Gillingham, F.J., Watson, W.S., Donaldson, A.A., and Naughton, J.A. (1960). The surgical treatment of Parkinsonism. Br. Med. J., 2, 1395–1402.
50. Baron, M.S., Vitek, J.L., Bakay, R.A., Green, J., Kaneoke, Y., Hashimoto, T., Turner, R.S., Woodard, J.L., Cole, S.A., McDonald, W.M., and DeLong, M.R. (1996). Treatment of advanced Parkinson's disease by posterior GPi pallidotomy: 1-year results of a pilot study. Ann. Neurol., 40, 355–366.
51. Sutton, J.P., Couldwell, W., Lew, M.F., Mallory, L., Grafton, S., DeGiorgio, C., Welsh, M., Apuzzo, M.L.J., Ahmadi, J., and Waters, C.H. (1995). Ventroposterior medial pallidotomy in patients with advanced Parkinson's disease. Neurosurgery, 36, 1112–1117.
52. Lang, A.E., Lozano, A.M., Montgomery, E., Duff, J., Tasker, R., and Hutchinson, W. (1997). Posteroventral medial pallidotomy in advanced Parkinson's disease. N. Engl. J. Med., 337, 1036–1042.
53. Dogali, M., Fazzini, E., Kolodny, E., Eidelberg, D., Sterio, D., Devinsky, O., and Beric, A. (1995). Stereotactic ventral pallidotomy for Parkinson's disease. Neurology, 45, 753–761.
54. Iacono, R.P., Shima, F., Lonser, R.R., Kuniyoshi, S., Maeda, G., and Yamada, S. (1995). The results, indications, and physiology of posteroventral pallidotomy for patients with Parkinson's disease. Neurosurgery, 36, 1118–1127.
55. Iacono, R.P., Lonser, R.R., Oh, A., and Yamada, S. (1995). New pathophysiology of Parkinson's disease revealed by posteroventral pallidotomy. Neurol. Res., 17, 178–180.
56. Iacono, R.P., Kuniyoshi, S.M., and Schoonenberg, T. (1998). Experience with stereotactics for dystonia: Case examples. In Dystonia 3: Advances in Neurology (S. Fahn, C.D. Marsden, and M. DeLong, eds.), vol. 78, pp. 221–226. Philadelphia: Lippincott-Raven.
57. Kondziolka, D., Bonaroti, E., Baser, S., Brandt, F., Kim, Y.S., and Lundsford, L.D. (1999). Outcomes after stereotactically guided pallidotomy for advanced Parkinson's disease. J. Neurosurg., 90, 197–202.
58. Lozano, A.M., Lang, A.E., Galvez-Jimenez, N., Miyasaki, J., Duff, J., Hutchinson, W.D., and Dostrovsky, J.O. (1995). Effect of GPi pallidotomy on motor function in Parkinson's disease. Lancet, 346, 1383–1387.
59. Laitinen, L.V., and Hariz, M.I. (1990). Pallidal surgery abolishes all Parkinsonian symptoms. Move. Disord, 5, 82.
60. Laitinen, L.V., Bergenheim, A.T., and Hariz, M.I. (1992). Ventroposterolateral pallidotomy can abolish all parkinsonian symptoms. Stereotact. Funct. Neurosurg., 58, 14–21.
61. Laitinen, L.V. (1994). Ventroposterolateral pallidotomy. Stereotact. Funct. Neurosurg., 62, 41–52.
62. Laitinen, L.V. (1995). Pallidotomy for Parkinson's disease. Neurosurg. Clin. North Am., 6, 105–112.
63. Krauss, J.K., Jankovic, J., Lai, E.C., Rettig, G.M., and Grossman, R.G. (1997). Posterioventral medial pallidotomy in levodopa-unresponsive Parkinsonism. Arch. Neurol., 54, 1026–1029.
64. Fazzini, E., Dogali, M., Sterio, D., Eidelberg, D., and Beric, A. (1997). Stereotactic pallidotomy for Parkinson's disease. Neurology, 48, 1273–1277.
65. Krack, P., Pollak, P., Limousin, P., Hoffmann, D., Benazzouz, A., Le Bas, J.F., Koudsie, A., and Benabid, A.L. (1998). Opposite motor effects of pallidal stimulation in Parkinson's disease. Ann. Neurol., 43, 180–192.
66. Honey, C.R., Phil, D., Stoessl, A.J., Tsui, J.C.K., Schulzer, M., and Calne, D.B. (1999). Unilateral pallidotomy for reduction of parkinsonian pain. J. Neurosurg., 91, 198–201.
67. Ghika, J., Ghika-Schmid, F., Fankhauser, H., Assal, G., Vingerhoets, F., Albanese, A., Bogousslavsky, J., and Favre, J. (1999). Bilateral contemporaneous posteroventral pallidotomy for the treatment of Parkinson's disease: Neuropsychological and neurologic side effects. J. Neurosurg., 91, 313–321.
68. Alterman, R.L., Sterio, D., Beric, A., and Kelly, P.J. (1999). Microelectrode recording during posterioventral pallidotomy: Impact on target selection and complications. Neurosurgery, 44, 315–323.
69. Guridi, J., Gorospe, A., Ramos, E., Linazasoro, G., Rodriguez, M.C., and Obeso, J.A. (1999). Stereotactic targeting of the globus pallidus internus

in Parkinson's disease: Imaging versus electrophysiological mapping. Neurosurgery, 45, 278–289.

70. Hassler, R., Mundinger, F., and Riechert, T. (1965). Correlations between clinical and autopic findings in stereotaxic operations of parkinsonism. Confin. Neurol., 25, 282–290.

71. Dogali, M., Beric, A., Sterio, D., Eidelberg, D., Fazzini, E., Takikawa, S., Samelson, D.R., Devinsky, O., and Kolodny, E.H. (1994). Anatomic and physiologic considerations for Parkinson's disease. Stereotact. Funct. Neurosurg., 62, 53–60.

72. Justesen, C.R., Penn, R.D., Kroin, J.S., and Egel, R.T. (1999). Stereotactic pallidotomy in a child with Hallervorden-Spatz disease. J. Neurosurg., 90, 551–554.

73. Taha, J.M., Favre, J., Baumann, T.K., and Burchiel, K.J. (1996). Functional anatomy of the pallidal base in Parkinson's disease. Neurosurgery, 39, 1164–1168.

74. Taha, J.M., Favre, J., Baumann, T.K., and Burchiel, K.J. (1996). Characteristics and somatotopic organization of kinesthetic cells in the globus pallidus of patients with Parkinson's disease. J. Neurosurg., 85, 1005–1012.

75. Taha, J.M., Favre, J., Baumann, T.K., and Burchiel, K.J. (1997). Tremor control after pallidotomy in patient with Parkinson's disease: Correlation with microrecording findings. J. Neurosurg., 86, 642–647.

76. Beric, A., Sterio, D., Dogali, M., Alterman, R., and Kelly, P. (1996). Electrical stimulation of the globus pallidus preceding stereotactic posteroventral pallidotomy. Stereotact. Funct. Neurosurg., 66, 161–169.

77. Limousin, P., Greene, J., Pollak, P., Rothwell, J., Benabid, A.L., and Frackowiak, R. (1997). Changes in cerebral activity pattern due to subthalamic nucleus or internal pallidum stimulation in Parkinson's disease. Ann. Neurol., 42, 283–291.

78. Svennilson, E., Torvik, A., Lowe, R., and Leksell, L. (1960). Treatment of parkinsonism bystereotactic thermolesions in the pallidal region: A clinical evaluation of 81 cases. Acta Psychiatr. Neurol. Scand., 35, 358–377.

79. Kelly, P.J. (1995). Pallidotomy in Parkinson's disease. Neurosurgery, 36, 1154–1157.

80. Young, M.S., Triggs, W.J., Bowers, D., Greer, M., and Friedman, W.A. (1997). Stereotactic pallidotomy lengthens the transcranial magnetic cortical stimulation silent period in Parkinson's disease. Neurology, 49, 1278–1283.

81. Kazumata, K., Antonini, A., Dhawan, V., Moeller, J.R., Alterman, R.L., Kelly, P., Sterio, D., Fazzini, E., Beric, A., and Eidelberg, D. (1997). Preoperative indicators of clinical outcome following stereotaxic pallidotomy. Neurology, 49, 1083–1090.

82. Vitek, J.L., Zhang, J., Evatt, M., Mewes, K., DeLong, M.R., Hashimoto, T., Triche, S., and Bakay, R.A. (1998). GPi pallidotomy for dystonia: Clinical outcome and neuronal activity. In Advances in Neurology (S. Fahn, C.D. Marsden, and M. DeLong, eds.), vol. 78, pp. 211–219. Philadelphia: Lippincott-Raven.

83. Lozano, A.M., Kumar, R., Gross, R.E., Giladi, N., Hutchison, W.D., Dostrovsky, J.O., and Lang, A.E. (1997). Globus pallidus internus pallidotomy for generalized dystonia. Move. Disord., 12, 865–870.

84. Lin, J.-J., Lin, S.-Z., Lin, G.-Y., Chang, D.-C., and Lee, C.-C. (1998). Application of bilateral sequential pallidotomy to treat a patient with generalized dystonia. Eur. Neurol., 40, 108–110.

85. Lin, J.-J., Lin, S.-Z., and Chang, D.-C. (1999). Pallidotomy and generalized dystonia. Move. Disord., 14, 1057–1059.

86. Lin, J.-J., Lin, G.-Y., Shih, C., Lin, S.-Z., Change, D.-C., and Lee, C.-C. (1999). Benefit of bilateral pallidotomy in the treatment of generalized dystonia. J. Neurosurg., 90, 974–976.

87. Alvarez, L., Macias, R., Guridi, J., Lopez, G., Alvarez, E., Maragoto, C., Teijeiro, J., Torres, A., Pavon, N., Rodriguez-Oroz, M.C., Ochoa, L., Hetherington, H., Juncos, J., DeLong, M.R., and Obeso, J.A. (2001). Dorsal subthalamotomy for Parkinson's disease. Move. Disord., 16, 72–78.

88. Andy, O.J., Jurko, M.F., and Sias, F.R. (1963). Subthalomotomy in treatment of parkinsonian tremor. Presented at meeting of Harvey Cushing Society, Philadelphia, PA.

89. Benabid, A.L., Pollak, P., Gao, D., Hoffmann, D., Limousin, P., Gay, E., Payen, I., and Benazzouz, A., (1996). Chronic electrical stimulation of the ventralis intermedius nucleus of the thalamus as a treatment of movement disorders. J. Neurosurg., 84, 203–214.

90. Koller, W., Pahwa, R., Busenbark, K., Hubble, J., Wilkinson, S., Lang, A., Tuite, P., Sime, E., Lazano, A., Hauser, R., Malapira, T., Smith, D., Tarsy, D., Miyawaki, E., Norregaard, T., Kormos, T., and Olanow, C.W. (1997). High-frequency unilateral thalamic stimulation in the treatment of essential and parkinsonian tremor. Ann. Neurol., 42, 292–299.

91. Hubble, J.P., Busenbark, K.L., Wilkinson, S., Pahwa, R., Paulson, G.W., Lyons, K., and Koller, W.C. (1997). Effects of thalamic deep brain stimulation based on tremor type and diagnosis. Move. Disord., 12, 337–341.

92. Hubble, J.P., Busenbark, K.L., Wilkinson, S., Penn, R.D., Lyons, K., and Koller, W.C. (1996). Deep brain stimulation for essential tremor. Neurology, 46, 1150–1153.

93. Geny, C., Nguyen, J.P., Pollin, B., Feve, A., Ricolfi, F., Cesaro, P., and Degos, J.D. (1996). Improvement of severe postural cerebellar tremor in multiple sclerosis by chronic thalamic stimulation. Move. Disord., 11, 489–494.

94. Whittle, I.R., Hooper, J., and Pentland, B. (1998). Thalamic deep-brain stimulation for movement disorders due to multiple sclerosis. Lancet, 351, 109–110.

95. Krack, P., Limousin, P., Benabid, A.L., and Pollak, P. (1997). Chronic simulation of subthalamic nucleus improves levodopa-induced dyskinesias in Parkinson's disease. Lancet, 350, 1676.

96. Krack, P., Pollak, P., Limousin, P., Benazzouz, A., and Benabid, A.L. (1997). Stimulation of subthalamic nucleus alleviates tremor in Parkinson's disease. Lancet, 350, 1675–1676.

97. Krack, P., Hamel, W., Mehdorn, H.M., and Deuschl, G. (1999). Surgical treatment of Parkinson's disease. Curr. Opin. Neurol., 12, 417–425.

98. Limousin, P., Krack, P., Pollak, P., Benazzouz, A., Ardouin, C., Hoffmann, D., and Benabid, A.L. (1998). Electrical stimulation of the subthalamic nucleus in advanced Parkinson's disease. N. Engl. J. Med., 339, 1105–1111.

99. Houeto, J.L., Damier, P., Bejjani, P.B., Staedler, P.B., Bonnet, A.M., Arnulf, I., Pidoux, B., Dormont, D., Cornu, P., and Agid, Y. (2000). Subthalamic stimulation in Parkinson disease: A multidisciplinary approach. Arch. Neurol., 57, 461–465.

100. Molinuevo, J.L., Valldeoriola, F., Tolosa, E., Rumia, J., Valls-Sole, J., Roldan, H., and Ferrer, E. (2000). Levodopa withdrawal after bilateral subthalamic nucleus stimulation in advanced Parkinson disease. Arch. Neurol., 57, 983–988.

101. Pinter, M.M., Alesch, F., Murg, M., Seiwald, M., Helscher, R.J., and Binder, H. (1999). Deep brain stimulation of the subthalamic nucleus for control of extrapyramidal features in advanced idiopathic Parkinson's disease: One-year follow-up. J. Neur. Trans., 106, 693–709.

102. Hutchison, W.D., Allan, R.J., Opitz, H., Levey, R., Dostrovsky, J.O., Lang, A.E., and Lozano, A.M. (1998). Neurophysiological identification of the subthalamic nucleus in surgery for Parkinson's disease. Ann. Neurol., 44, 622–628.

103. Gross, C., Rougier, A., Guehl, D., Boraud, T., Julien, J., and Bioulac, B. (1997). High-frequency stimulation of the globus pallidus internalis in Parkinson's disease: A study of seven cases. J. Neurosurg., 87, 491–498.

104. Bejjani, B., Damier, P., Arnuff, I., Bonnet, A.M., Vidailhet, M., Dormont, D., Pidoux, B., Cornu, P., Marsault, C., and Agid, Y. (1997). Pallidal stimulation for Parkinson's disease. Two targets? Neurology, 49, 1564–1569.

105. Tronnier, V.M., Fogel, W., Kronenbuerger, M., and Steinvorth, A. (1997). Pallidal stimulation: An alternative to pallidotomy? J. Neurosurg., 87, 700–705. 106.

106. Kumar, R., Dagher, A., Hutchison, W.D., Lang, A.E., and Lozano, A.M. (1999). Globus pallidus deep brain stimulation for generalized dystonia: Clinical and PET investigation. Neurology, 53, 871–874.

107. Lang, A.E. (2000). Surgery for Parkinson disease: A critical evaluation of the state of the art. Arch. Neurol., 57, 1118–1125.

108. Burchiel, K.J., Anderson, V.C., Favre, J., and Hammerstad, J.P. (1999). Comparison of pallidal and subthalamic nucleus deep brain stimulation for advanced Parkinson's disease: Results of a randomized, blinded pilot study. Neurosurgery, 45, 1375–1384.

109. Vayssiere, N., Hemm, S., Zanca, M., Picot, M.C., Bonafe, A., Cif, L., Frerebeau, P., and Coubes, P. (2000). Magnetic resonance imaging stereotactic target localization for deep brain stimulation in dystonic children. J. Neurosurg., 93, 784–790.

110. Coubes, P., Roubertie, A., Vayssiere, N., Hemm, S., and Echenne, B. (2000). Treatment of DYT1-generalized dystonia by stimulation of the internal globus pallidus. Lancet, 355, 2220–2221.

111. Bakay, R.A.E., Vitek, J.L., and DeLong, M.R. (1992). Thalamotomy for tremor. In Neurosurgical Operative Atlas (S.S. Rengachary, and R.N. Wilkins, eds.), vol. 2, pp. 299–312. Baltimore: Williams and Wilkins.

112. Limousin, P., Pollak, P., Benazzouz, A., Hoffmann, D., Le Bas, J.F., Broussolle, E., Perret, J.E., and Benabid, A.L. (1995). Effect on parkinsonian signs and symptoms of bilateral subthalamic nucleus stimulation. Lancet, 345, 91–95.

113. Limousin, P., Pollak, P., Hoffmann, D., Benazzouz, A., Perret, J.E., and Benabid, A.L. (1996). Abnormal involuntary movements induced by subthalamic nucleus stimulation in parkinsonian patients. Move. Disord., 11, 231–235.

114. Forster, A., Eljamel, M.S., Varma, T.R., Tulley, M., and Latimer, M. (1999). Audit of neurophysiological recording during movement disorder surgery. Stereotact. Funct. Neurosurg., 72, 154–156.

115. Bejjani, B.P., Dormont, D., Pidoux, B., Yelnik, J., Damier, P., Arnulf, I., Bonnet, A.M., Marsault, C., Agid, Y., Philippon, J., and Cornu, P. (2000). Bilateral subthalamic stimulation for Parkinson's disease by using three-dimensional stereotactic magnetic resonance imaging and electrophysiologic guidance. J. Neurosurg., 92, 615–625.

116. Tagliati, M., and Alterman, R.L. (2001). Guidelines for patient selection for ablative and deep brain stimulation surgery. Semin. Neurosurg., 12, 161–168.

117. Kretschmann, H.J., and Weinrich, W. (1999). Neurofunctional Systems (CD-ROM). New York: Thieme.

118. Miller, W.C., and DeLong, M.R. (1967). Altered tonic activity of neurons in the globus pallidus and subthalamic nucleus in the primate MPTP model of parkinsonism. In The Basal Ganglia II (M.B. Carpenter, and A. Jayarman, eds.), pp. 415–427. New York: Plenum.

119. Filion, M., and Tremblay, L. (1991). Abnormal spontaneous activity of globus pallidus neurons in monkeys with MPTP-induced parkinsonism. Brain Res., 547, 142–151.

120. DeLong, M.R. (1990). Primate models of movement disorders of basal ganglia origin. Trends Neurosci. Special Issue: Basal Ganglia Research, 13, 281–285.

121. DeLong, M.R., Crutcher, M.D., and Georgopoulos, A.P. (1985). Primate globus pallidus and subthalamic nucleus: Functional organization. J. Neurophysiol., 53, 530–543.

122. Alexander, G.E., and Crutcher, M.D. (1990). Functional architecture of basal ganglia circuits: Neural substrates of parallel processing. Trends Neurosci., 13, 266–271.

123. Alexander, G.E., Crutcher, M.D., and DeLong, M.R. (1990). Basal ganglia-thalamocortical circuits: Parallel substrates for motor, oculomotor, prefrontal and limbic functions. Prog. Brain Res., 85, 119–146.

124. Mink, J.W. (1996). The basal ganglia: Focused selection and inhibition of competing motor programs. Prog. Neurobiol., 50, 381–425.

125. DeLong, M.R., and Wichmann, T. (1993). Basal ganglia-thalamocortical circuits in Parkinsonian signs. Clin. Neurosci., 1, 18–26.

126. Kandel, E.R., Schwartz, J.H., and Jessell, T.M. (1991). Principles of neural science. Norwalk, CT: Appleton & Lange.

127. Obeso, J.A., Linazasoro, G., Gorospe, A., et al. (1997). Complication associated with chronic levodopa therapy in Parkinson's disease. In Beyond the Decade of the Brain (C.W. Olanow, and J.A. Obeso, eds.), vol. 2, pp. 11–31. Kent, UK:Wells Medical Limited.

128. Nutt, J.G. (1990). Leva-dopa–induced dyskinesia: Review, observations, and speculations. Neurology, 40, 340–345.

129. Crossman, A.R., Sambrook, M.A., and Jackson, A. (1984). Experimental hemichorea/hemiballismus in the monkey. Studies on the intracerebral site of action in a drug-induced dyskinesia. Brain, 107, 579–596.

130. Pal, P.K., and Samii, A., Kishore, A., et al. (2000). Long-term outcome of unilateral pallidotomy: Follow-up of 15 patients for 3 years. J. Neurol, Neurosurg. Psychiatry, 69, 337–344.

131. Arle, J.E., and Alterman, R.L., (1999). Surgical options in Parkinson's disease. Med. Clin. North Am., 83, 483–498.

132. Siegfried, J., and Lippitz, B. (1994). Bilateral chronic electrostimulation of ventroposterolateral pallidum: A new therapeutic approach for alleviating all parkinsonian symptoms. Neurosurgery, 35, 1126–1130.

133. Ambrose, J. (1974). Computerized x-ray scanning of the brain. J. Neurosurg., 40, 679–695.

134. Lunsford, L.D., Latchaw, R.E., and Vries, J. (1983). Stereotaxic implantation of deep brain electrodes using computed tomography. Neurosurgery, 13, 280–286.

135. Lunsford, L.D., and Martinez, A.J. (1984). Stereotactic exploration of the brain in the era of computed tomography. Surg. Neurol., 22, 222–230.

136. Leskell, L., Herner, T., and Leskell, D. (1985). Visualisation of stereotactic radiolesions by nuclear magnetic resonance. J. Neurol. Neurosurg. Psychiatry., 48,19–20.

137. Lunsford, L.D., Martinez, A.J., and Latchaw, R.E. (1986). Stereotaxic surgery with a magnetic resonance and computed tomography-compatible system. J. Neurosurg., 64, 872–878.

138. Kondziolka, D., Dempsey, P.K., Lunsford, L.D., Kestle, J.R., Dolan, E.J., Kanal, E., Tasker, R.R. (1992). A comparison between magnitude resonance imaging and computed tomography for stereotactic coordinate determination. Neurosurgery, 30, 402–407.

139. Alterman, R.L., Reiter, G.T., Shils, J., Skolnick, B., Arle, J.E., Lesutis, M., Simuni, T., Colcher, A., Stern, M., and Hurtig, H. (1999). Targeting for thalamic deep brain stimulation implantation without computer guidance: Assessment of targeting accuracy. Stereotact. Funct. Neurosurg., 72, 150–153.

140. Taren, J.A., Ross, D.A., and Gebarski, S.S. (1993). Stereotactic localization using fast spin-echo imaging in functional disorders. Acta Neurochir., 58 (suppl), 59–60.

141. Starr, P.A., Vitek, J.L., DeLong, M., and Bakay, R.A.E. (1999). Magnetic resonance imaging based stereotactic localization of the globus pallidus and subthalamic nucleus. Neurosurgery, 44, 303–314.

142. Reich, C.A., Hudgins, P.A., Sheppard, S.K., Starr, P.A., and Bakay, R.A.E. (2000). A high-resolution fast spin-echo inversion-recovery for preoperative localization of the internal globus pallidus. Am. J. Neuroradiol., 21, 928–931.

143. Zonenshayn, M., Rezai, A.R., Mogilner, A.Y., Beric, A., Sterio, D., and Kelly, P.J. (2000). Comparison of anatomic and neurophysiologic methods for subthalamic nucleus targeting. Neurosurgery, 47, 282–294.

144. Sumanaweera, T.S., Adler, J.R., Napel, S., and Glover, G.H. (1994). Characterization of spatial distortion in magnetic resonance imaging and its implications for stereotactic surgery. Neurosurgery, 35, 696–704.

145. Gerdes, J.S., Hitchon, P.W., Neerangun, W., and Torner, J.C. (1994). Computed tomography versus magnetic resonance imaging in stereotactic localization. Stereotact. Funct. Neurosurg., 63, 124–129.

146. Walton, L., Hampshire, A., Forster, D.M.C., and Kemeny, A.A. (1995). Stereotactic localization using magnetic resonance imaging. Stereotact. Funct. Neurosurg., 64 (suppl 1), 155–163.

147. Walton, L., Hampshire, A., Forster, D.M.C., and Kemeny, A.A. (1996). A phantom study to assess the accuracy of stereotactic localization, using T1-weighted magnetic resonance imaging with the Leksell stereotactic system. Neurosurgery, 38, 170–178.

148. Alterman, R.L., Shils, J.L, Tagliati, M., and Rogers, J. (2000), Relative accuracy of inversion recovery and T2-weighted MRI for targeting the subthalamic nucleus. Presented at the XIVth European Society for Stereotactic and Functional Neurosurgery, London, UK.

149. Shils, J.L., and Alterman, R.L. (2000). Comparative accuracy of stereotactic coordinates derived from various MRI acquisition techniques. Presented at the XIVth European Society for Stereotactic and Functional Neurosurgery, London, U.K.

150. Holtzheimer, P.E., Roberts, D.W., and Darcey, T.M. (1999). Magnetic resonance imaging versus computer tomography for target localization in functional stereotactic neurosurgery. Neurosurgery, 45, 290–298.

151. Axer, H., Stegelmeyer, J., and von Keyserlingk, D.G. (1999). Comparison of tissue impedance measurements with nerve fiber architecture in human telencephalon: Value in identification of intact subcortical structures. J. Neurosurg., 90, 902–909.

152. Organ, W.L., Tasker, R.R., and Moody, N.F. (1967). The impedance profile of the human brain as a localization technique in stereoecephalotomy. Confin. Neurol., 29, 192–196.

153. Yoshida, M., Yanagisawa, N., Shimazu, H., Givre, A., and Narabayashi, H. (1964). Physiological identification of the thalamic nucleus. Arch. Neurol., 11, 435–443.

154. Guridi, J., and Lozano, A.M. (1997). A brief history of pallidotomy. Neurosurgery, 41, 1169–1180.

155. Ohye, C., and Narabayashi, H. (1979). Physiological study of presumed ventralis intermedius neurons in the human thalamus. J. Neurosurg., 50, 290–297.

156. Hardy, J. (1966). Electrophysiological localization and identification. J. Neurosurg., 24, 410–414.

157. Lozano, A., Hutchison, W., Kiss, Z., Tasker, R., Davis, K., and Dostrovsky, J. (1996). Methods for microelectrode-guided posteroventral pallidotomy. J. Neurosurg., 84, 194–202.

158. Hirai, T., Miyazaki, M., Nakajima, H., Shibazaki, T., and Ohye, C. (1983). The correlation between tremor characteristics and the predicted volume of effective lesions in stereotaxic nucleus ventralis intermedius thalamotomy. Brain, 106, 1001–1018.

159. Gillingham, F.J. (1966). Depth recording and stimulation. J. Neurosurg., 24, 382–387.

160. Geddes, L.A. (1972). Electrodes and the Measurement of Bioelectric Events. New York: Wiley-Interscience.

161. Shils, J.L., Patterson, T., and Stecker, M.M. (2000). Electrical properties of metal microelectrodes. Am. J. Electrodiag. Technol., 40, 71–82.

162. Lenz, F.A., Tasker, R.R., Kwan, H.C., Schnider, S., Kwong, R., Murayama, Y., Dostrovsky, J.O., and Murphy, J.T. (1988). Single unit analysis of the human ventral thalamic nuclear group: Correlation of thalamic "tremor cells" with the 3–6 Hz component of parkinsonian tremor. J. Neurosci., 8, 754–764.

163. Starr, P.A., Vitek, J.L., and Bakay, R.A.E. (1998). Deep brain stimulation for movement disorders. Neurosurg. Clin. North Am., 9, 381–402.

164. Schaltenbrand, G., and Wahren, W. (1977). Atlas for Stereotaxy of the Human Brain. New York: Thieme.

165. Alterman, R.L., and Kelly, P.J. (1998). Pallidotomy technique and results. Neurosurg. Clin. North Am., 9, 337–343.

166. Arle, J.E., Mei, L.Z., and Shils, J.L. (2008). Modeling parkinsonian circuitry and the DBS electrode. I. Biophysical background and software. Stereo. Funct. Neurosurg., 86(1), 1–15.

167. Zaidel, A., Spivak, A., Shpigelman, L., et al. (2009). Delimiting subterritories of the human subthalamic nucleus by means of microelectrode recordings and a Hidden Markov Model. Move. Disord., 24(12), 1785–1793.

168. Coste, J., Ouchchane, L., Sarry, L., et al. (2009). New electrophysiological mapping combined with MRI in parkinsonian's subthalamic region. Eur. J. Neurosci., 29(8), 1627–1633.

169. Wong, S., Baltuch, G.H., Jaggi, J.L., et al. (2009). Functional localization and visualization of the subthalamic nucleus from microelectrode recordings acquired during DBS surgery with unsupervised machine learning. J. Neural Engin., 6(2), 026006.

170. Shils, J.L., Tagliati, M., and Alterman, R.L. (2002). Neurophysiological monitoring during neurosurgery for movement disorders. In Neurophysiology in Neurosurgery: A Modern Intraoperative Approach (V. Deletis and J.L. Shils), eds.). New York: Academic Press.

171. Morrell, M.J., RNS System in Epilepsy Study Group. (2011). Responsive cortical stimulation for the treatment of medically intractable partial epilepsy. Neurology, 77(13), 1295–304.

172. Sun, F.T., and Morrell, M.J. (2014).The RNS System: responsive cortical stimulation for the treatment of refractory partial epilepsy. Expert Rev Med Devices, 11(6), 563–572.

173. Bergey, G.K., Morrell, M.J., Mizrahi, E.M., et al. (2015). Long-term treatment with responsive brain stimulation in adults with refractory partial seizures. Neurology, 84(8), 810–817.

174. Lee, B., Zubair, M.N., Marquez, Y.D., et al. (2015). A single-center experience with the NeuroPace RNS System: a review of techniques and potential problems. World Neurosurg., 84(3), 719–726.

175. Parrent, A., and Almeida, C.S. (2006). Deep brain stimulation and cortical stimulation in the treatment of epilepsy. Adv. Neurol., 97, 563–572.

176. Krumholz, A., Wiebe, S., Gronseth, G., et al. (2007). Practice parameter: evaluating an apparent unprovoked first seizure in adults (an evidence-based review): report of the Quality Standards Subcommittee of the American Academy of Neurology and the American Epilepsy Society. Neurology, 69(21), 1996–2007.

177. French, J.A., and Delanty, N.M.D., eds. (2008). Therapeutic Strategies in Epilepsy. 1st edn. Oxford, UK/Ashland, OH: Clinical Pub. Serv.

178. Siegel, A.M. (2004). Presurgical evaluation and surgical treatment of medically refractory epilepsy. Neurosurg. Rev., 27(1), 1–21.

179. Thadani, V.M., Siegel, A., Lewis, P., et al. (2004). Validation of ictal single photon emission computed tomography with depth encephalography and epilepsy surgery. Neurosurg. Rev., 27(1), 27–33.

180. O'Brien, T.J., So, E.L., Mullan, B.P., et al. (2000). Subtraction perictal SPECT is predictive of extratemporal epilepsy surgery outcome. Neurology, 55(11), 1668–1677.

181. O'Brien, T.J., So, E.L., Cascino, G.D., et al. (2004). Subtraction SPECT coregistered to MRI in focal malformations of cortical development: localization of the epileptogenic zone in epilepsy surgery candidates. Epilepsia, 45(4), 367–376.

182. Mehta, A.D., Labar, D., Dean, A., et al. (2005). Frameless stereotactic placement of depth electrodes in epilepsy surgery. J Neurosurg., 102(6), 1040–1045.

183. Van Gompel, J.J., Meyer, F.B., Marsh, W.R., Lee, K.H., and Worrell, G.A. (2010). Stereotactic electroencephalography with temporal grid and mesial temporal depth electrode coverage: does technique of depth electrode placement affect outcome? J. Neurosurg., 113(1), 32–38.

184. Canavero, S. (2015). Textbook of Cortical Brain Stimulation. Berlin/Munich/Boston: Walter de Gruyter GmbH & Co KG.

185. DiLorenzo, D.J., Mangubat, E.Z., Rossi, M.A., and Byrne, R.W. (2014). Chronic unlimited recording electrocorticography-guided resective epilepsy surgery: technology-enabled enhanced fidelity in seizure focus localization with improved surgical efficacy. J. Neurosurg., 120(6), 1402–1414.

186. Arle, J.E., Zani, J, and Shils, JL. (2011). Intraoperative decisionmaking with MER for STN DBS in PD and the potential relationship to patient selsction. The open neurosurgery journal. 4(Suppl 1-M3), 36–41.

PART VI | EVOKED POTENTIALS AND EVENT-RELATED EEG PHENOMENA

39 | EVENT-RELATED POTENTIALS: GENERAL ASPECTS OF METHODOLOGY AND QUANTIFICATION

MARCO CONGEDO, PHD AND FERNANDO H. LOPES DA SILVA, MD, PHD

ABSTRACT: Event-related potentials (ERPs) can be elicited by a variety of stimuli and events in diverse conditions. This chapter covers the methodology of analyzing and quantifying ERPs in general. Basic models (additive, phase modulation and resetting, potential asymmetry) that account for the generation of ERPs are discussed. The principles and requirements of ensemble time averaging are presented, along with several univariate and multivariate methods that have been proposed to improve the averaging procedure: wavelet decomposition and denoising, spatial, temporal and spatio-temporal filtering. We emphasize basic concepts of principal component analysis, common spatial pattern, and blind source separation, including independent component analysis. We cover practical questions related to the averaging procedure: overlapping ERPs, correcting inter-sweep latency and amplitude variability, alternative averaging methods (e.g., median), and estimation of ERP onset. Some specific aspects of ERP analysis in the frequency domain are surveyed, along with topographic analysis, statistical testing, and classification methods.

KEYWORDS: event-related potentials, ERPs, wavelets, denoising, spatio-temporal filtering, principal component analysis, common spatial pattern, blind source separation, independent component analysis, statistical testing

PRINCIPAL REFERENCES

1. Holmes, A. P., Blair, R. C., Watson, J. D. G., Ford, I. Nonparametric analysis of statistic images from functional mapping experiments. *J. Cerebr. Blood Flow Metabol.*, 1996, 16(1), 7–22.
2. Jung, T.P., Makeig, S., McKeown, M.J., et al. Imaging brain dynamics using independent component analysis. *Proc. IEEE*, 2001, 89(7), 1107–1122.
3. Koles, Z.J., Soong, A. EEG source localization: Implementing the spatio-temporal decomposition approach. *Electroencephalogr. Clin. Neurophysiol.*, 1998, 107, 343–352.
4. Makeig, S., Jung, T.P., Bell, A.J., et al. Blind separation of auditory event-related brain responses into independent components. *Proc. Natl. Acad. Sci. USA*, 1997, 94(20), 10979–10984.
5. Quiroga R.Q., Garcia H. Single-trial event-related potentials with wavelet denoising. *Clin. Neurophysiol.*, 2003, 114(2), 376–390.
6. Shah, A.S., Bressler. S.L., Knuth, K.H., et al. Neural dynamics and the fundamental mechanisms of event-related brain potentials. *Cerebral Cortex*, 2004, 14, 476–483.
7. Blankertz, B., Lemm, S., Treder, M., et al. Single-trial analysis and classification of ERP components—a tutorial. *Neuroimage*, 2011, 56, 814–825.
8. Oostenveld, R., Fries, P., Maris, E., Schoffelen, J.M. FieldTrip: open source software for advanced analysis of MEG, EEG, and invasive electrophysiological data. *Comput. Intell. Neurosci.*, 2011, 156869.
9. Luck, S.J. *An Introduction to the Event-Related Potential Technique.* 2nd ed. Boston: MIT Press, 2014.
10. Regan, D. *Human Brain Electrophysiology: Evoked Potentials and Evoked Magnetic Fields in Science and Medicine.* New York: Elsevier, 1989.

1. INTRODUCTION

Electroencephalography (EEG) as a general method for investigating human brain function includes ways of determining the reactions of the brain to a variety of discrete events. Some of these reactions may be associated with clear-cut changes in the EEG; others, however, consist of changes that are difficult to visualize. Interest in the detection, quantification, and physiological analysis of those slight EEG changes that are related to particular events has steadily grown in recent decades. These EEG changes may be treated globally under the common term *event-related potentials* (ERPs); a subset of the ERPs is constituted by the classic sensory (e.g., visual, auditory, somatosensory) evoked potentials (EPs).

Generally there are three main areas of human research where ERPs play an important role:

1. *Clinical studies* that aim at identifying pathophysiological processes for diagnostic purposes and monitoring of brain and/or spinal cord functions

2. *Neurocognitive and psychophysiological studies* with the aim of disclosing neural mechanisms underlying, or associated with, cognitive and psychological phenomena

3. *Brain–computer interfaces* (BCI), where the classification of ERPs is used to convey messages directly from the brain to the external world without any muscle activity.

Methods of analysis of ERPs must fit the research question of interest appropriately. Thus, clinical applications need well-standardized ERPs, as much as possible in quantitative terms so that deviations from normal may be readily detectable. Neurocognitive applications imply paying special attention to single-trial ERPs with the emphasis on their time-varying properties that may be analyzed along the same time scale as cognitive processes evolve. BCI studies require the application of robust methods of ERP detection so that relevant brain signals may be used to operate external devices with a high level of reliability.

This chapter focuses on some general aspects of the methodology of analyzing ERPs, taking into consideration the different requirements alluded to above. Detailed descriptions of specific aspects of ERPs to stimuli of different modalities are presented in separate chapters of this book (visual modality in Chapter 41, auditory in Chapter 42, and somatosensory in Chapter 43), as well as general aspects of *event-related (de) synchronization* in Chapter 40. Specialized aspects of ERPs of children and infants are referred in Chapter 7 and the use of ERPs in the operating room is covered in Chapter 34. Frequency and time-frequency analysis methods that can be applied to the study of ERPs are presented in Chapter 44. There is a long list of important texts dedicated to the field of ERPs since the authoritative specialized textbook [1]. A recent comprehensive introduction to the ERP technique is provided in [2]. Time-frequency analysis methods are extensively and clearly treated in [3].

This field has benefited from theoretical advances in signal analysis and the development of techniques in various research areas, since the questions raised by the need to identify signals as ERPs of small amplitude in a varying EEG of much larger amplitude (this applies equally to event-related fields recorded by magnetoencephalography [MEG]) are similar to those encountered in many different areas of physics and engineering. Although several sophisticated methods have been introduced in the field of ERPs, in the setting of the clinical routine, simple averaging is still the dominant methodology used.

2. BASIC MODELS OF ERPS

For decades ERPs have been conceived as stereotyped fluctuations with approximately fixed polarity, shape, latency, amplitude, and spatial distribution. According to this view, ERPs are considered independent of the ongoing EEG; in other words, ERPs, time- and phase-locked with respect to a given event, would be simply added to the ongoing EEG. This concept constitutes the so-called *additive* generative model. Nonetheless, several observations show that the ongoing synchrony within a neuronal population, manifest in spontaneous EEG oscillations, changes as neurons are recruited by a sensory stimulus that elicits also an attention reaction.

The possibility that evoked responses may be caused by a process of *phase resetting* was put forward based on seminal findings [4–6] showing in the auditory system that stimuli at low intensity, near hearing threshold, evoke responses that can be discriminated better based on ensemble phase spectral measures than amplitude measures. These findings indicate that the ERP may consist, at least partially, of an enhanced alignment of phase components of the spontaneous neuronal activity. In line with these seminal observations, several authors [7–9] have proposed considering ERPs as time/frequency modulations of the activity of local neuronal populations. From a theoretical point of view, we noted [10] that it is not probable that two independent neuronal populations, one generating exclusively ongoing activity and another one responsible only for the evoked response, would coexist side by side as distinct and independent entities in a given brain area. It is more likely that the same neuronal elements contribute to the generation of both types of activity. This same idea was formulated in [11], where it was noted that EEG ongoing activity and EPs are generated by overlapping neuronal elements. According to this model, event-related responses may engage a group of neurons by way of two basic mechanisms: either by enhancing (or decreasing) synchrony of ongoing neuronal firing and/or by synchronizing the activity of specific neuronal populations. These two mechanisms are not mutually exclusive. Thus, several combinations of neural processes may take place in the generation of evoked responses: narrow-band

power decreases and increases (event-related spectral perturbations) as well as phase-locking and/or phase-resetting of ongoing EEG frequency components.

Furthermore, since the ongoing EEG activity is commonly nonsymmetric around zero, slow components may contribute to averaged responses, according to the *potential asymmetry* model in [12] and [13]. An editorial analyzing these and other fundamental aspects of the generation of evoked responses [14] stressed the need for a mathematical framework enabling the comparison of different models of ERP generation. We may add that a better understanding of the biophysics underpinning the generation of ERPs is a prerequisite for advancing our knowledge in this field. The methods described in this chapter are mainly based on the additive model. This may be considered a basic working hypothesis that may yield meaningful results even if the data do not precisely conform to this model, as decades of practice have confirmed.

3. TIME AVERAGING OF ERPS

3.1. Ensemble Averaging

According to the additive model, ERP analysis in the time domain is based on two assumptions: (i) the electrical response evoked by the brain is time- and phase-locked to the event and (ii) the ongoing activity is a stationary "noise." In this way, the observed ERP can be decomposed in a signal term (assumed fixed across sweeps, although amplitude and latency inter-sweep variability should be taken into account, as discussed further below) and a "noise" term, which actually includes all recordable activity besides the ERPs (e.g., instrumental noise, environmental artifacts, biological artifacts, induced EEG, and ongoing EEG) and is highly variable from sweep to sweep. The former constitutes the generally called *evoked response,* or in classic EEG literature "evoked potential." ERP detection becomes, accordingly, a matter of improving the signal-to-noise ratio (SNR).

Let us consider a real case where it is of interest to study EPs related to sensory stimuli. The presentation of the stimuli is repeated a number of times. Each repetition is named a *sweep* (or trial). The aim is to estimate the corresponding *event-related responses*. Throughout this chapter we will make use of the following notation and nomenclature: there is a set of K sweeps, which we will index by $k \in \{1,..,K\}$. EEG signals are recorded from N electrodes (also referred to as sensors or derivations) at a succession of equally spaced discrete time samples. T is the number of sampled time points in a sweep. A sweep starts at a given time related to the presentation of a stimulus. The kth observed sweep for a given class of ERP signals is held in matrix $X_k \in \mathbb{R}^{N \times T}$, where $\in \mathbb{R}^{N \times T}$ indicates that the matrix contains N rows and T columns of real numbers (the electric potential). The *additive* generative model for the observed sweep of a given class can then be written

$$X_k = \sigma_k Q(\tau_k) + N_k \tag{39.1}$$

where $Q \in \mathbb{R}^{N \times T}$ is a matrix representing the evoked responses for the class under analysis, σ_k are (optional) positive scaling factors accounting for inter-sweep variations in the amplitude of Q, τ_k are (optional) time-shifts, in samples units, accounting for inter-sweep variations in the latency of Q, and $N_k \in \mathbb{R}^{N \times T}$ are matrices representing the noise term added to the kth sweep. According to this model, the evoked responses in Q may be continuously *modulated in amplitude and latency* across sweeps. The single-sweep SNR is the ratio between the variance of $\sigma_k Q(\tau_k)$ and the variance of N_k. Since the amplitude of ERP responses on the average is in the order of a few μV, whereas the background EEG is in the order of several tens of μV, the SNR of single sweeps is very low. Therefore averaging, smoothing, and/or filtering is warranted to improve the SNR.

The weighted and aligned *arithmetic ensemble average* of the K sweeps is given by

$$\bar{X} = \frac{\sum_k \left(\hat{\sigma}_k X_k \left(\hat{\tau}_k \right) \right)}{\sum_k \left(\hat{\sigma}_k \right)}, \tag{39.2}$$

where the hat symbol ($\hat{\ }$) on σ_k and τ_k indicates that these quantities are unknown and therefore must be estimated. Of course, with all weights equal to one and time-shifts equal to zero, ensemble average estimation (Eq. 39.2) reduces to the usual *arithmetic mean*. Using equal weights, the above estimator is unbiased if the noise term is zero-mean, uncorrelated to the signal, spatially and temporally uncorrelated and stationary. It is actually optimal if the noise is also Gaussian [15]. However these conditions are never matched in practice. For instance, EEG data are highly spatially and temporally correlated and typically contain outliers and artifacts, and thus are non-stationary. As a rule of thumb, the SNR of the arithmetic ensemble average improves proportionally to the *square root of the number of sweeps*. In practice, it is well known that the arithmetic mean is an acceptable ensemble average estimator, provided that sweeps with low SNR are removed and that enough sweeps are available.

In the following we consider several methods that have been proposed to improve the arithmetic average estimator. We will first review briefly univariate methods, and thereafter describe in some detail multivariate methods. Nowadays ERP recordings most often involve several channels, and it is not uncommon to see studies using tens or hundreds of channels. The spatial diversity of the signal recorded at many derivations can be specifically exploited by spatial filtering to improve the ensemble average and single-sweep estimation; thus, in practice, univariate methods are slowly being replaced by multivariate methods.

3.2. Univariate Methods

The goal being suppressing noise while preserving the ERP components, early attempts addressed the *univariate* problem (i.e., at each available sensor separately) by using Wiener filtering [16,17]. To overcome deviations from signal stationarity, the researchers in [18,19] introduced an adaptive time-varying Wiener filter capable of optimizing the estimation of both low-frequency components of relatively long duration and high-frequency components of short duration. In the same vein several approaches, borrowed from the field of

signal processing, were proposed in the course of time: autoregressive models [20], autoregressive moving average models [21], Kalman filters [22], and wavelets denoising [23–29]. In the next section we consider the latter since it has interesting potentiality in neurocognitive studies, in particular.

Wavelet transforms yield a time-frequency decomposition of non-stationary signals [30], as described further in Chapter 44, where the reader may find the basic concepts of the methodology of wavelet decomposition. In [31] the authors noted that wavelet analysis provides reliable measures for the detection of ERPs, more robust than conventional filtering techniques, and summarize a number of applications of this methodology in the field of ERPs. Specifically regarding ERPs it is important to emphasize that these signals are non-stationary and present different frequency components with different durations distributed along the time signal. Typically the earlier components of ERPs have relatively high frequencies and short duration, while the later components have lower frequencies and extend over longer durations. These features make ERPs particularly suitable for an analysis using wavelet decomposition. The seminal papers [23,24,32] paved the way for the application of ERP wavelet decomposition.

The process of automatic denoising is, however, not simple. Several algorithms have been proposed with this purpose. Recently the researchers in [33] introduced an algorithm for the automatic selection of wavelet coefficients (the so-called NZT algorithm) based on the inter- and intra-scale correlation of neighboring wavelet coefficients. An example of this application is shown in Figure 39.1, illustrating the potential of this methodology to extract single-trial evoked potentials with an enhanced SNR. Such methods are being actively explored particularly in neurocognitive studies of perception, learning, and memory [34]. The possibility of reliably recording single-trial EPs is particularly relevant, for example, in studies where it is of interest to study trial-to-trial variability in relation to perceptual performance, or to follow changes in latency of a given component associated with a memory task, for instance. In this way it is possible to reliably extract single-trial EPs from a session consisting of many stimuli presentations, while the subject is performing a cognitive task.

3.3. Multivariate Methods

Several multivariate methods have been developed with the aim of improving the estimation of ERP ensemble averages by means of spatial, temporal, or spatio-temporal filtering. Spatial filtering is more common; according to the macroscopic model of EEG generation, the brain current sources of EEG/MEG signals contribute linearly to the scalp electric/magnetic fields (see Chapter 4). The aim of a *spatial filter* is to find an optimal linear combination of the data across sensors to enhance the SNR. The aim of a *temporal filter* is to find an optimal linear combination of data across samples. One can design a spatial filter, a temporal filter, or a spatio-temporal filter. The mathematical description of the three kinds of filters is presented in Box 39.1. In this context we introduce briefly three methods that have similar objectives: principal component analysis (PCA), the common spatial pattern (CSP), and blind

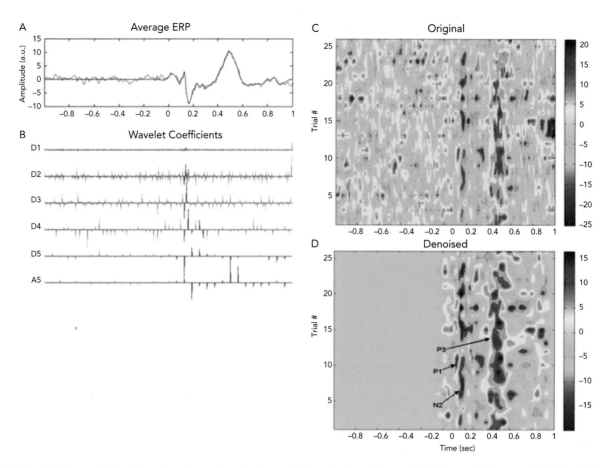

Figure 39.1. Result of the application of the automatic denoising algorithm applied to a visual evoked potential (VEP) recorded from an occipital site. A: The original VEP is in black and the denoised version of it in red. B: Wavelet decomposition showing the wavelet coefficients chosen automatically for denoising by the NZT algorithm. C: Contour plot of the amplitude of the original single-trial VEPs of successive trials as a function of time (stimulus presentation at moment 0). D: Same as (c) but for the denoised single-trial VEPs. The amplitude scale in color is indicated by the bar on the right. Note that the components (N2, P1, and P3) of the single-trial VEPs are much more evident in the denoised traces shown in (d). Adapted with permission from Ahmadi, M., Quian Quiroga, R. Automatic denoising of single-trial evoked potentials. Neuroimage, 2015, 66, 672–680.

source separation (BSS). The performance of these methods for removing eye artifacts is illustrated in Figures 39.2 and 39.3 using an example of a visual oddball paradigm eliciting a P300 for infrequent stimuli.

3.3.1. PRINCIPAL COMPONENT ANALYSIS

PCA was the first filter of this kind to be applied to ERP data [35,36] and has been often employed since then [37–40]. A long-lasting debate has concerned the choice of spatial versus temporal PCA [10,41]. This debate, however, could be resolved by performing a spatio-temporal PCA, which combines the advantages of both. The PCA seeks uncorrelated components maximizing the variance of the ensemble average estimation; the first component explains the maximum of the variance, while the remaining components explain the maximum of the remaining variance, assuming that it is uncorrelated to all the previous. Hence, the variance explained by the N-P discarded components (P is the subspace dimension; see Box 39.1) explains the variance of the "noise" that has been filtered out by the PCA. The spatial and/or temporal filter matrix B and D are found by singular value decomposition as the left and right singular vectors of the ensemble average given by (Eq. 39.2). An example of spatial PCA applied to a P300 data set is shown in Figure 39.2.

3.3.2. THE COMMON SPATIAL AND TEMPORAL PATTERN

The authors of [42,43] first adapted to EEG en extension of PCA proposed in [44]. The objective is to obtain a spatial filter separating EEG signals from distinct classes, with possible diagnostic value in the clinical domain or, more in general, distinguishing EEG signals obtained in different conditions [45]. Specifically, the aim is to find spatial filters maximizing the ratio of the variance of the EEG obtained in two conditions. Since the resulting spatial components are common to EEG signals obtained in two different conditions, the approach is named common spatial pattern (CSP). In contrast to the PCA, the CSP does not require orthogonality of the components. The ERP components resulting from a spatial filter are given by the first expression of (Eq. 39.3) in Box 39.1. A CSP adapted for time- and phase-locked activity such as ERPs was proposed in [46]; the two conditions in this case are defined as the evoked activity and the evoked activity plus the noise, respectively, the noise being defined in Section 3.1. Since the spatial filter maximizes the variance (energy) of the evoked activity with respect to the total EEG variance, it effectively seeks the optimal linear combinations of EEG derivations enhancing the SNR of the evoked activity. As for the PCA, the first P components are usually retained, with P smaller than N (see Box 39.1). A later

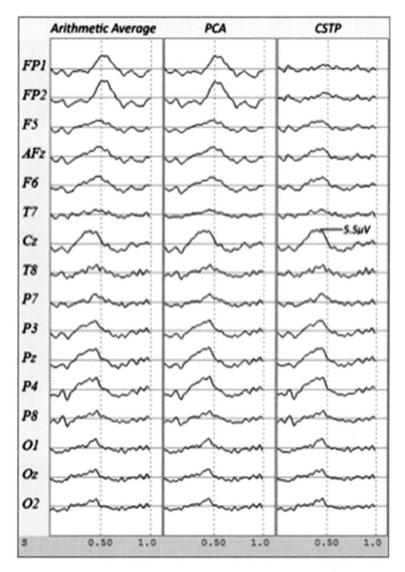

Figure 39.2. *Comparison of the arithmetic ensemble average estimations (EA) with the ensemble average estimation obtained by a PCA (with P = 4; see Box 39.1) and a CSTP (with P = 12). Data are from one subject performing a visual oddball ERP paradigm. The averages are computed on 80 1-sec sweeps following the infrequent stimulus (stimulus onset = time 0). All plots have the same horizontal and vertical scales. All available sweeps have been used and no artifact rejection has been performed on the recording. Note that only the CSTP method filters out the eye-related artifact peaking at about 500 msec, better visible at derivations FP1 and FP2.*

extension of this method accounted for inter-sweep latency variability as well [47]. Reference [48] extended the idea to the spatio-temporal setting, yielding the common spatio-temporal pattern (CSTP), in which components for ERPs are given by the third expression of (Eq. 39.3) in Box 39.1, A closed-form solution for the CSTP accounting for inter-sweep latency and amplitude variability has been provided in [49]. The reader can find comprehensive reviews on spatial filters and linear analysis of EEG in [50] and a tutorial on single-trial analysis and classification of ERP components in [51]. An example of CSTP applied to a P300 dataset is shown in Figure 39.2.

3.3.3. BLIND SOURCE SEPARATION

Blind source separation is introduced and described in Chapter 44, and for more details the reader is referred to that chapter. Here we briefly consider the specificities of its application as applied to ERP data. In Chapter 44 the two main families of BSS methods are considered: the methods based on *high-order statistics* (HOS), better known as independent component analysis (ICA), and those based on *second-order statistics* (SOS).

ICA (HOS-based BSS) has been applied to a collection of ERP ensemble averages (e.g., [52,53]) or to unaveraged single sweeps (e.g., [54]). In the former case the ICA decomposition focuses on evoked ERP components only, since time- but not phase-locked components have been drastically attenuated by the averaging process. The latter approach is more general, since it allows the decomposition at the same time of evoked components, induced components, background EEG, and artifact. It faces, however, the problem of the low SNR of evoked and induced ERP components in unaveraged data [52]; therefore, in practice, it requires a large and clean ERP recording set [55].

SOS-based BSS in the context of ERPs has been introduced in [56]. In that work evoked components, induced components, as well as background EEG and artifacts were modeled

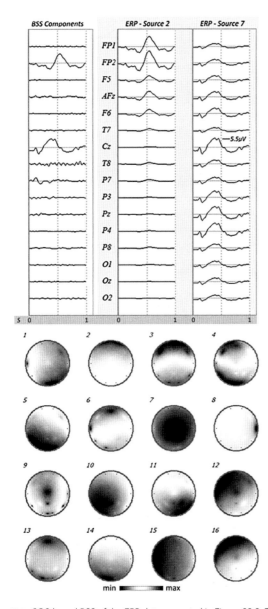

BSS Components		ERP - Source 2	ERP - Source 7
	FP1		
	FP2		
	F5		
	AFz		
	F6		
	T7		
	Cz		—5.5µV
	T8		
	P7		
	P3		
	Pz		
	P4		
	P8		
	O1		
	Oz		
	O2		

S 0   1   0   1 0   1

min ■▬▬■ max

Figure 39.3. SOS-based BSS of the ERP data presented in Figure 39.2. The left plot of the top figure shows the 16 temporal components separated by BSS. The associated spatial patterns are shown in the bottom figure in the form of monochromatic topographic maps (the numbers on top of each map indicate the corresponding temporal BSS component shown above). The sign of the potential is arbitrary in BSS analysis; thus, in these maps positive and negative potentials are plotted with the same color. The scale of the components is also arbitrary; thus, each map is scaled to its own (arbitrary) maximum. The plots in the top figures entitled "ERP—source 2" and "ERP—source 7" show the ensemble average of Figure 39.2 obtained retaining only the second and seventh BSS component; that is, they show the ERP ensemble average produced by these two components once all the others have been filtered out. Note that component 2 focuses on the eye-related artifact responsible for the peak visible in the ensemble average at ~500 msec at derivations FP1 and FP2 (see Fig. 39.2), separating this feature from the P300 component, which has a maximal amplitude at the vertex, which is clearly identified by component 7.

by means of spatial covariance matrices. Computing these covariance matrices separately for an "error" class and a "correct" class of ERPs in an error-related potential experiment, the author was able to separate the source responsible for an evoked negativity component and the source responsible for an induced event-related synchronization, even though the

two phenomena peaked at the same time (500 msec post-stimulus) and had very similar spatial distribution. An example of BSS based on second-order statistics applied to the same dataset used in Figure 39.2 is shown in Figure 39.3.

4. SPECIAL CONSIDERATIONS

4.1. Overlapping ERPs

Special care in ERP time-domain analysis must be undertaken when we record overlapping ERPs, since in this case estimation (Eq. 39.2) is biased [57,58]. ERPs are non-overlapping if the minimum inter-stimulus interval (ISI) is longer than the length of the latest recordable ERP component. There is today increasing interest in paradigms eliciting overlapping ERPs, such as some oddball paradigms and rapid image triage [48], which are heavily employed in BCI for increasing the transfer rate [59] and in the study of eye-fixation potentials, where the "stimulus onset" is the time of an eye fixation and saccades follow each other rapidly [60]. The strongest distortion is observed when the ISI is fixed; less severe is the distortion when the ISI is drawn at random from an exponential distribution [57]. Remedies for overlapping ERPs have been proposed by a few authors. The method in [58] takes into consideration only the case of a maximum of three overlapping ERPs, and thus it is not general. The multivariate regression method proposed in [46] and an improved version formulated in [47] consider any occurrence and any form of overlapping (i.e., overlapping of any number of ERPs of the same as well as of different classes, in any combination). A further extension of the multivariate regression method, accounting for amplitude weights and latency time-shifts in the resulting ensemble average estimation, has been considered in [49]. Reference [61] discusses a univariate regression method and other weighting procedures that can be used to refine the study of the ERPs in relation to some properties of a stimulus. Note that the regression method is very general in that it reduces to the usual averaging when no overlapping is present [49].

4.2. Latency and Amplitude Variability

In Section 3.2.1 we emphasized the use of methods with the aim of obtaining reliable estimates of single-trial ERPs, particularly in the case of neurocognitive studies, where it is relevant to relate dynamic changes of the amplitude of a peak or its latency of a single-trial ERP to the performance of a subject in tasks, where the neural correlates of attention, perception, or memory are the targets of the investigation. Another face of the same coin, however, consists in improving the estimation of an average ERP in the presence of latency jitter or amplitude variations. According to this perspective one assumes that inter-sweep latency variability should be eliminated.

The multivariate ensemble average estimation introduced in (Eq. 39.2) accounts for both latency and amplitude variability by means of the τ (latency) and σ (amplitude) variables therein introduced. Indeed, the usual approach in ERP studies requires the estimation of a time-shift (in sample units) and a (non-negative) weight for each sweep. An appropriate estimation of the time-shifts aims at aligning the ERP peaks. An appropriate estimation of weights dampens the contribution of sweeps contaminated by artifacts and strong spontaneous background activity. Using optimization techniques to estimate either variable, an improvement of the ensemble average SNR is expected. Of course, estimating both time shifts and weights is preferable.

In this context several approaches have been proposed to optimize the estimation of ERPs, starting from Woody's adaptive matched filter method [62], where the cross-correlation between each sweep and a template is computed to estimate the time by which each sweep should be shifted in order to obtain the maximal cross-correlation with the template. The method was extended in [63], allowing compensation not only for latency, but also for amplitude variability. Several modifications of this basic approach have been proposed (47,49,64).

4.3. Refining the ERP Averaging Procedure

In addition to the methods presented above, a number of other statistical techniques can be used for refining the averaging procedure applied to ERPs. Instead of computing the

average, according to (Eq. 39.2), it has been proposed to use the median, trimmed mean or trimmed L-mean [65,66]. The simplest method of this family is to use the median—that is, the middle observation in the case of an odd number of observations or the average of the two middle observations in the case of an even number of observations. In the computation of the "trimmed mean" a predefined percentage of extreme values are given weight zero (i.e., are discarded), while the remaining observations keep equal weights; the trimmed L-mean applies higher weights for the observations near the median. Examples of these different computational methods are given in [65]. Extensive testing has shown that the median leads to noisy ensemble average estimates with spurious high-frequency components [15,65]. Smoothing the ERP sweeps by low-pass filtering (e.g., by a moving average filter) can yield useful results in this context [67].

4.4. Estimating the Onset of an ERP

The researcher using ERPs is often confronted with the question of how to estimate the onset of an ERP. A useful method, the standard deviation (SD) method, based on the t-test, consists in setting a threshold at 3 SDs from the mean of the pre-stimulus baseline signal, as exemplified in Figure 39.4. Reference [69] proposed an alternative method called the

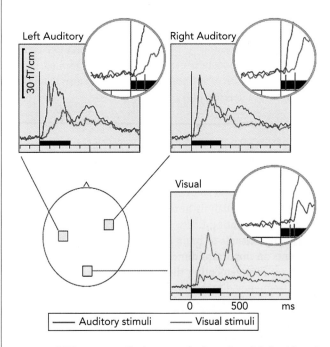

Figure 39.4. MEG source-specific time course for the auditory (A1, Heschl's gyri) cortex (light blue background) and visual (V1, calcarine fissure) cortex (yellow background) to stimuli of both modalities (auditory in dark blue and visual in red). The circular insets show the onset of each response, indicated by the vertical lines (red for visual and dark blue for auditory). Both sensory-specific and cross-sensory ERPs are shown. Note that the onset latencies of the sensory-specific stimulation are shorter than those of the cross-sensory activation, particularly in the case of the auditory modality. Time scales –200 to 1,000 msec post-stimulus, stimulus duration 300 msec (black bar). Adapted with permission from Raij, T., Ahveninen, J., Lin, F.H., Witzel, T., Jääskeläinen, I.P., Letham, B, et al. Onset timing of cross-sensory activations and multisensory interactions in auditory and visual sensory cortices. Eur J Neurosci., 2010;31(10), 1772-82, Fig. 1.

median rule. It makes use of boxplot rules for outlier detection using a threshold that is set based on the interquartile range. The onset latency is the first post-stimulus point above this threshold. Simulations studies demonstrated that the SD method is more sensitive to outliers than the median rule method. The latter does not make assumptions with respect to the distribution of the data and can be applied to single-sweep ERPs. In cases where the baseline is of good quality, like those presented in Figure 39.4, the differences between the two methods are small.

5. FREQUENCY AND TIME-FREQUENCY DOMAIN ANALYSIS

Analysis in frequency and time-frequency domains of EEG signals in general terms is described in detail in Chapter 44, to which the reader is referred. Although in ERP studies representations in the time domain are much more common, a large body of studies have used frequency domain analysis of ERPs, particularly elicited by steady-state visual evoked potentials (SSVEPs), since the pioneering work of the Amsterdam's school of van der Tweel [70] and in [1]. This early work has yielded significant contributions to a better understanding of the physiology of the visual system, as reviewed in [71]. Reference [72] pointed out the relevance of SSVEPs in new applications in BCI systems. Besides SSVEP studies, also steady-state amplitude- or frequency-modulated sound stimuli are used to investigate functional properties of the auditory system; the corresponding steady-state auditory evoked potentials (SSAEPs) can be analyzed using frequency analysis [73,74] and applied in the objective evaluation of auditory thresholds, and also to analyze suprathreshold hearing [75].

6. TOPOGRAPHY AND SOURCE LOCALIZATION

Scalp topography and source localization of ERPs are the basic tools to perform analysis in the *spatial domain* of the electrical activity generating ERPs. This is fundamental for linking experimental results to brain anatomy and physiology. It also represents an important dimension for studying ERP dynamics per se, complementing the information provided in time and/or frequency dimensions [76]. The spatial pattern of ERP scalp potential or of an ERP source component provides useful information to recognize and categorize ERP features, as well as to identify artifacts and background EEG. Current research typically uses several tens and even hundreds of electrodes covering the whole scalp surface. An increasing number of high-density EEG studies involve realistic head models for increasing the precision of source localization methods (for the biophysical aspects see Chapter 4, and for source imaging techniques see Chapter 45). Advanced spatial analysis with high spatial resolution has therefore become common practice in ERP research. A comprehensive tutorial of topographic ERP analyses can be found in [77]. In contrast to continuous EEG, ERP studies allow the generation of topographical and source localization maps for each time sample. This is due to the SNR gain engendered by averaging across sweeps. The SNR of spatial analysis increases with the number of averaged sweeps. One can further increase the SNR by using multivariate filtering methods, as discussed above. An example is given by the application of BSS to ERPs, yielding a number of time series with associated spatial patterns that are fixed for the whole duration of the sweeps (see Fig. 39.3).

7. STATISTICAL TESTING

ERP studies involve both *space* (scalp location) and *time* dimensions (latency and duration of the ERP components). Frequency and time-frequency-domain variables may also be added depending on the objective of the study. Typical hypotheses to be tested in ERP studies concern differences in central location (mean) between and within subjects (t-tests), the generalization of these tests to multiple experimental factors extending to more than two levels, including their interaction (ANOVA), and the correlation between ERP variables and subject characteristics or behavioral variables such as response time, age of the participants, complexity of the cognitive task, and so forth (linear and non-linear regression, ANCOVA). These questions entail statistical analysis of ERPs, which may be rather complex and cumbersome. This chapter cannot deal with these statistical questions in depth; nonetheless, it is useful to call attention to a number of specific questions that appear frequently in the field of ERP studies. In these studies it is common to have datasets constituted by ERPs recorded at, say, 32 scalp derivations and 128 sampling points, while the objective may be to test the null hypothesis that the mean ERP amplitude does not differ substantially in two experimental conditions (e.g., in a treatment vs. a control group), for each time point and each derivation. Such an experiment requires testing $128 \times 32 = 4{,}096$ hypotheses. This yields the well-known *multiple-comparisons problem* [78], which is very common in ERP studies: whereas a statistical test guarantees that the probability to reject a null hypothesis when it is actually true is inferior to a desired probability (the α level of the test), this is no longer guaranteed when multiple hypotheses are tested at once.

Two families of procedures have been applied in ERP studies to deal with the multiple comparison problem: those controlling the *family-wise error rate* (FWER) and those controlling the *false-discovery rate* (FDR). The FWER is the probability of making one or more false rejections among all tested hypotheses. The term "family" represents the collection of hypotheses that are being considered for joint testing [79]; this is what is meant by FWER. The popular Bonferroni procedure [80] belongs to this family. It consists in adjusting the alpha level to α/M, where M is the number of hypotheses being tested. All Bonferroni-like procedures fail to take into consideration explicitly the correlation structure of the hypotheses and thus are unduly conservative, the more so the higher the number of hypotheses to be tested.

An important general class of test procedures controlling the FWER while preserving power is known as *permutation tests* based on maximal statistics, tracing back to the seminal work of Ronald Fisher [81]. Permutation tests based on maximal statistics are able to account adaptively for any correlation structure of hypotheses, regardless of their form and degree. Also, they do not need a distributional model for the observed variables (e.g., Gaussianity), as required by t-tests, ANOVA, and so forth. Given these characteristics, permutation tests are ideal options for testing hypotheses in ERP studies and have received much attention in the neuroimaging community (for a review see [82] and for excellent treatises see [83,84]).

Another family of testing procedures controls the FDR, which is the expected proportion of falsely rejected hypotheses [85]. Indicating by R the number of rejected hypotheses and by F the number of those that have been falsely rejected, simply stated the FDR controls the expectation of the ratio F/R. This is a less stringent criterion than the FWER, since, as the number of discoveries increases, we allow proportionally more errors [85,86]. The FDR procedure and its version for dependent hypotheses have been the subject of several improvements (e.g., [87]).

A very efficient approach in ERP analysis is the suprathreshold cluster permutation test included in the EEG toolbox "Fieldtrip" in [88], as described in [89]. The reader can find in these references, as well as in the original and pioneering work of [90], useful tips to realize this kind of testing; in ERP data we may assume that the effect of interest is concentrated simultaneously along some specific dimensions. For example, in testing the mean amplitude difference of a P300 ERP, one expects the effect to be concentrated along time and space—the former at ~300 to 500 msec and the latter at midline central and adjacent parietal locations. This leads to a typical correlation structure of hypotheses in ERP data; under the basic null hypothesis the effect would instead be scattered all over both the whole time and spatial dimensions. The concentration of the effect along relevant dimensions is the rationale of the suprathreshold cluster size test. An example in the time-space ERP domain is shown in Figure 39.5.

Figure 39.6 illustrates the performance of this method compared to two others: the classic (uncorrected) t-test and the t-test adjusted by Bonferroni correction. The three methods were applied to MEG ERPs recorded from the temporal cortex in one subject, in a linguistic experiment separately for congruent and incongruent sentence endings (see also Chapter 48 and Fig. 48.9). It can be seen that the classic t-test yields too many rejections of the null hypothesis (i.e., of false discoveries), the Bonferroni-corrected test yields a very conservative result, and the permutation test yields a result that is consistent for eight different test statistics.

8. CLASSIFICATION OF SINGLE SWEEPS

The goal of a classification method is to automatically estimate the class to which a single sweep belongs. The task is challenging because of the very low amplitude of ERPs compared to the background EEG. Large EEG artifacts, the non-stationary nature of EEG, and inter-sweep variability exacerbate the difficulty of the task. Although single-sweep classification has been investigated for a long time [91], it has recently received

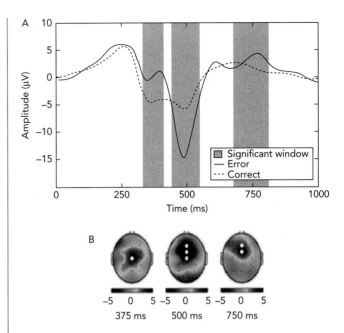

Figure 39.5. A: *Grand ensemble average error-related potentials (19 subjects) for "Correct" and "Error" trials at different electrodes, the location of which is schematically indicated in the circular heads below (B) for three time samples. The suprathreshold cluster size permutation test applied in time and spatial dimension, with α = 0.05, yields three time windows, indicated in A by the gray areas, where there were significant differences between the two sets of ERPs, corresponding to the "Correct" and "Error" trials. The three significant differences between the two sets of ERPs were the following: a significant positivity for Error trials was found at time window 320–400 msec at electrode Cz (p < .01); a significant negativity for Error trials at time window 450–550 msec at clustered electrodes Fz, FCz, Cz (p < .01); and a significant positivity for Error trials at time 650–775 msec at clustered electrodes Fz, FCz (p = .025). Significant clustered derivations are represented by white disks in B. Adapted, with permission, from Congedo, M. EEG Source Analysis.* HDR thesis *presented at Doctoral School EDISCE, University of Grenoble Alpes, 2013.*

a strong impetus thanks to development of ERP-based BCI ([59]). In fact, a popular family of such interfaces is based on the recognition of the P300 ERP. The most famous example is the P300 Speller [92,93], a system allowing the user to spell text without moving but just by focusing attention on symbols (e.g., letters) that are flashed on a virtual keyboard.

Classification methods typically involve the following steps:

1. Describing each ERP sweep by a *set of features*: in the simplest case, the amplitude values of time samples and derivations concatenated so as to form a vector

2. Using a *training set*—that is, a number of labeled sweeps for all classes—to find a *discriminant function* that can partition the space occupied by all objects so that unique patterns corresponding to different classes can be identified (e.g., pathologic vs. healthy subjects)

3. Determining the class to which a new object (i.e., an unlabeled single-sweep ERP) belongs; this is accomplished by computing a discriminant score for the object to be classified. Thus, each sweep is classified in the class corresponding to the subspace within which the discriminant score falls.

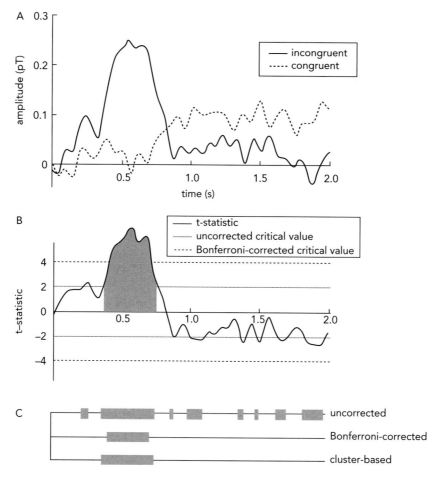

Figure 39.6. Statistical testing of MEG evoked responses obtained in an experiment where subjects heard sentences where the last word was either semantically congruent or incongruent. The response of interest is the ERP elicited by the last word in the two conditions. The aim was to test the differences between the latter. **A:** Evoked responses of one single subject at one sensor are shown separately for congruent (dotted line) and incongruent (solid line) sentence endings. **B:** The time series of sample-specific t-values. **C:** The significant samples shown separately for each of three statistical procedures: sample-specific t-tests at the uncorrected 0.05 level (two-sided); sample-specific t-tests at the Bonferroni-corrected level of 0.05/600 = 0.00008 (two-sided); and a nonparametric test based on clustering of adjacent time samples (cluster mass test). Note that the major result is an ERP that is most prominent in the interval 400–800 msec. The t-test procedure yields a large (8 clusters) number of samples where the uncorrected 0.05 level is crossed. In contrast, lowering the α level according to the Bonferroni procedure produces a very conservative estimate. The nonparametric test, based on the permutation distribution of the maximum of the cluster-level statistics, results in a more robust estimate (see methodological details in [88]). Adapted with permission from Figure 1 of Oostenveld, R., Fries, P., Maris, E., Schoffelen, J.M. FieldTrip: open source software for advanced analysis of MEG, EEG, and invasive electrophysiological data. Comput. Intell. Neurosci., 2011, 156869.

The fundamental criterion for choosing a classification method is the achieved *accuracy* for the data at hand. However, other criteria may be relevant. In most applications training of the classifier (step 2 above) starts with a calibration session carried out just before the actual session.

Classification methods are characterized by the set of features and the discriminant function they employ. The approaches emphasizing the definition of the set of features attempt to increase the SNR of single sweeps by using multivariate filtering, as discussed previously in this chapter, and are specifically designed to increase the separation of the classes in a reduced feature space where the filter projects the data [46,48]. Without entering into technical details of the methodologies involved in this process, we may refer the reader to the useful tutorial dealing with the single-trial analysis and classification of ERPs in [51].

Recently, it has been recommended to start regarding the preprocessing feature extraction and discrimination not as isolated processes, but jointly, as a whole [94,95]. An approach that features at the same time good accuracy, good generalization, and good adaptation capabilities in the case of ERP data has been recently borrowed from the field of Riemannian geometry [56,96,97].

REFERENCES

1. Regan, D. *Human Brain Electrophysiology: Evoked Potentials and Evoked Magnetic Fields in Science and Medicine.* New York: Elsevier, 1989.
2. Luck, S.J. *An Introduction to the Event-Related Potential Technique.* 2nd ed. Boston: MIT Press, 2014.
3. Cohen, M.X. *Analyzing Neural Time Series Data. Theory and Practice.* Boston: MIT Press, 2014.
4. Sayers, B.M., Beagley, H.A. Objective evaluation of auditory evoked EEG responses. *Nature,* 1974, 251(5476), 608–609.
5. Sayers, B.M., Beagley, H.A., Henshall, W.R. The mechanism of auditory evoked EEG responses. *Nature,* 1974, 247(5441), 481–483.
6. McClelland, R.J., Sayers, B.M. Towards fully objective evoked responses audiometry. *Br. J. Audiol.,* 1983, 17, 263–270.
7. Basar, E. *EEG-Brain Dynamics: Relation Between EEG and Brain Evoked Potentials.* Amsterdam: Elsevier, 1980.

8. Makeig, S., Westerfield, M., Jung, T.P., et al. Dynamic brain sources of visual evoked responses. *Science*, 2002, 295(5555), 690–694.
9. Penny, W.D., Kiebel, S.J., Kilner, J.M., et al. Event-related brain dynamics. *Trends Neurosci.*, 2002, 25(8), 387–389.
10. Lopes da Silva, F.H. Event-related neural activities: what about phase? *Prog. Brain Res.*, 2006, 159, 3–17.
11. Shah, A.S., Bressler. S.L., Knuth, K.H., et al. Neural dynamics and the fundamental mechanisms of event-related brain potentials. *Cerebr. Cortex*, 2004, 14, 476–483.
12. Mazaheri, A., Jensen, O. Rhythmic pulsing: linking ongoing brain activity with evoked responses. *Front. Hum. Neurosci.*, 2010, 4, 177.
13. Nikulin, V.V., Linkenkaer-Hansen, K., Nolte, G., Curio, G. Non-zero mean and asymmetry of neuronal oscillations have different implications for evoked responses. *Clin. Neurophysiol.*, 2010, 121, 186–193.
14. de Munck, J.C., Bijma, F. How are evoked responses generated? The need for a unified mathematical framework. *Clin. Neurophysiol.*, 2010, 121, 127–129.
15. Lęski, J.M. Robust weighted averaging, *IEEE Trans. Biomed. Eng.*, 2002, 49(8), 796–804.
16. Doyle, D.J. Some comments on the use of Wiener-filtering for the estimation of evoked potentials. *Electroencephalogr. Clin. Neurophysiol.*, 1975, 38, 533–534.
17. Albrecht, V., Lánský, P., Indra, M., Radil-Weiss, T. Wiener filtration versus averaging of evoked responses. *Biol. Cybern.*, 1977, 27(3), 147–154.
18. De Weerd, J.P. A posteriori time-varying filtering of averaged evoked potentials. I. Introduction and conceptual basis. *Biol. Cybern.*, 1981, 41(3), 211–222.
19. De Weerd, J.P., Kap, J.I. A posteriori time-varying filtering of averaged evoked potentials. II. Mathematical and computational aspects. *Biol. Cybern*, 1981, 41(3), 223–234.
20. Cerutti, S., Basselli, G., Pavesi, G. Single sweep analysis of visual evoked potentials through a model of parametric identification. *Biol. Cybern.*, 1987, 56(2–3), 111–120.
21. Heinze, H.J., Kunkel, H. ARMA-filtering of evoked potentials. *Meth. Inform. Med.*, 1984, 23(1), 29–26.
22. Tarvainen, M.P., Hiltunen, J.K., Ranta-aho, P.O., Karjalainen, P.A. Estimation of nonstationary EEG with Kalman smoother approach: an application to event-related synchronization (ERS). *IEEE Trans. Biomed. Eng.*, 2004, 51(3), 516–524.
23. Bartnik, A., Blinowska, K.J., Durka, P.J. Single evoked potential reconstruction by means of wavelet transform. *Biol. Cybern.*, 1992, 67, 175–181.
24. Bertrand, O., Bohorquez, J., Pernie, J. Time frequency digital filtering based on an invertible wavelet transform: An application to evoked potentials. *IEEE Trans. Biomed. Eng.*, 1994, 41(1), 77–88.
25. Schiff, S.J., Aldroubi, A., Unser, M., Sato, S. Fast wavelet transformation of EEG. *Electroenceph. Clin. Neurophysiol.*, 1994, 91, 442–455.
26. Demiralp, T., Ademoglu, A. Decomposition of event-related brain potentials into multiple functional components using wavelet transform. *Clin. Electroenceph.*, 2001, 32(3), 122–138.
27. Effern, A., Lehnertz, K., Schreiber, T., et al. Nonlinear denoising of transient signals with application to event-related potentials, *Physica D: Nonlinear Phenomena*, 2000, 140 (3-4), 257–266.
28. Quian Quiroga, R. Obtaining single stimulus evoked potential with wavelet denoising. *Physica*, 2000, 145, 278–292.
29. Quian Quiroga, R., Garcia, H. Single-trial event-related potentials with wavelet denoising. *Clin. Neurophysiol.*, 2003, 114(2), 376–390.
30. Mallat, S.G. A theory for multiresolution signal decomposition: the wavelet representation. *IEEE Trans. Patterns Analysis Machine Intell.*, 1989, 11(7), 674–693.
31. Aniyan, A.K., Sajeeth, N, Desjardins, J.A., Segalowitz, S.J. A wavelet-based algorithm for the identification of oscillatory event-related potential components. *J. Neurosci. Meth.*, 2014, 233, 63–72.
32. Tallon-Baudry, C., Bertrand, O., Delpuech, C., Pernier, J. Stimulus specificity of phase-locked and non-phase -locked 40 Hz visual responses in human. *J. Neurosci.*, 1996, 16, 4240–4249.
33. Ahmadi, M., Quian Quiroga, R. Automatic denoising of single-trial evoked potentials. *Neuroimage*, 2015, 66, 672–680.
34. Rey, H. G., Ahmadi, M., Quian Quiroga, R. Single trial analysis of field potentials in perception, learning and memory. *Curr. Op. Neurobiol.*, 2015, 31, 148–155.
35. Donchin, E. A multivariate approach to the analysis of average evoked potentials. *IEEE Trans. Biomed. Eng.*, 1966, 3, 131–139.
36. John, E.R., Ruchkin, D.S., Vilegas, J. Experimental background: signal analysis and behavioral correlates of evoked potential configurations in cats. *Ann. N.Y. Acad. Sci.*, 1964, 112, 362–420.
37. Chapman, R.M., McCrary, J.W. EP component identification and measurement by principal component analysis. *Brain Cognit.*, 1995, 27, 288–310.
38. Lagerlund, T.D., Sharbrough, F.W., Busacker, N.E. Spatial filtering of multichannel electroencephalographic recordings through principal component analysis by singular value decomposition. *J. Clin. Neurophysiol.*, 1997, 14(1), 73–82.
39. Kayser, J., Tenke, C.E. Trusting in or breaking with convention: towards a renaissance of principal components analysis in electrophysiology. *Clin. Neurophysiol.*, 2005, 116(8), 1747–1753.
40. Dien, J. Evaluating two-step PCA of ERP data with Geomin, Infomax, Oblimin, Promax, and Varimax rotations. *Psychophysiology*, 2010, 47, 170–183.
41. Picton, T.W. *Human Auditory Evoked Potentials*. 1st ed. San Diego, CA: Plural Publ., 2010.
42. Koles, Z.J. The quantitative extraction and topographic mapping of the abnormal components in the clinical EEG. *Electroencephalogr. Clin. Neurophysiol.*, 1991, 79, 440–447.
43. Koles, Z.J., Soong, A. EEG source localization: implementing the spatio-temporal decomposition approach. *Electroencephalogr. Clin. Neurophysiol.* 1998, 107, 343–352.
44. Fukunaga K. *Statistical Pattern Recognition*. 2nd ed. New York: Academic Press, 1990.
45. Ramoser, H., Muller-Gerking, J., Pfurtscheller, G. Optimal spatial filtering of single trial EEG during imagined hand movement. *IEEE Trans. Rehab. Eng.*, 2000, 8(4), 441–446.
46. Rivet, B., Souloumiac, A., Attina, V., Gibert, G. xDAWN algorithm to enhance evoked potentials: application to brain-computer interface. *IEEE Trans. Biomed. Eng.*, 2009, 56(8), 2035–2043.
47. Souloumiac, A., Rivet, B. Improved estimation of EEG evoked potentials by jitter compensation and enhancing spatial filters. *Proceedings of the ICASSP*, Vancouver, Canada, 2013, 1222–1226.
48. Yu, K., Shen, K., Shao, S., Ng, W.C., Li, X., Bilinear common spatial pattern for single-trial ERP-based rapid serial visual presentation triage. *J. Neural Eng.*, 2012, 9(4), 046013.
49. Congedo, M., Korczowski, L., Delorme, A., Lopes da Silva, F. Spatio-temporal common pattern: A companion method for ERP analysis in the time domain. *J. Neurosci. Meth.*, 2016, 267, 74–88.
50. Parra, L.C., Spence, C.D., Gerson, A.D., Sajda, P. Recipes for the linear analysis of EEG. *Neuroimage*, 2005, 28, 326–341.
51. Blankertz, B., Lemm, S., Treder, M., Haufe, S., Müller, K-R. Single-trial analysis and classification of ERP components—a tutorial. *Neuroimage*, 2011, 56, 814–825.
52. Jung, T.P., Makeig, S., McKeown, M.J., et al. Imaging brain dynamics using independent component analysis. *Proc. IEEE*, 2001, 89(7), 1107–1122.
53. Makeig, S., Jung, T.P., Bell, A.J., et al. Blind separation of auditory event-related brain responses into independent components. *Proc. Natl. Acad. Sci. USA*, 1997, 94(20), 10979–10984.
54. Jung, T.P., Makeig, S., Humphries, C., et al. Removing electroencephalographic artifacts by blind source separation, *Psychophysiology*, 2000, 37(02), 163–178.
55. Makeig, S., Debener, S., Onton, J., Delorme, A. Mining event-related brain dynamics. *Trends Cogn. Sci.*, 2004, 8(5), 204–210.
56. Congedo, M. *EEG Source Analysis*. HDR thesis presented at Doctoral School EDISCE, University of Grenoble Alpes, 2013.
57. Ruchkin, D.S. An analysis of average response computations based upon aperiodic stimuli. *IEEE Trans. Biomed. Eng.*, 1965, 12(2), 87–94.
58. Woldorff, M. Distortion of ERP averages due to overlap from temporally adjacent ERPs: analysis and correction. *Psychophysiology*, 1993, 30(1), 98–119.
59. Wolpaw, J., Wolpaw, E.W., eds. *Brain-Computer Interfaces. Principles and Practice*. London: Oxford University Press, 2012.
60. Sereno, S.C., Rayner, K. Measuring word recognition in reading: eye-movements and event-related potentials. *Trends Cogn. Sci.*, 2003, 7(11), 489–493.
61. Smith, N.J., Kutas, M. Regression-based estimation of ERP waveforms: II. Nonlinear effects, overlap correction, and practical considerations. *Psychophysiology*, 2015, 52(2), 169–181.
62. Woody, C.D. Characterization of an adaptive filter for the analysis of variable latency neuroelectric signals. *Med. Biol. Eng.*, 1967, 5(6), 539–554.
63. Jaśkowski, P., Verleger, R. Amplitudes and latencies of single-trial ERPs estimated by a maximum-likelihood method. *IEEE Trans. Biomed. Eng.*, 1999, 46(8), 987–993.
64. Cabasson, A., Meste, O. Time delay estimation: a new insight into the Woody's method. *IEEE Signal Process. Lett.*, 2008, 15, 573–576.
65. Leonowicz, Z., Karvanen, J., Shishkin, S.L. Trimmed estimators for robust averaging of event-related potentials. *J. Neurosci. Meth.*, 2005, 142(1), 17–26.
66. Hosking, L.R.M. L-moments: analysis and estimation of distributions using linear combinations of order statistics, *J.R. Statist. Soc. B*, 1990, 52(1), 105–124.

67. Möcks, J., Gasser, T., Köhler, W., de Weerd, J.P.C. Does filtering and smoothing of average potentials really pay? A statistical comparison. *Electroencephalogr. Clin. Neurophysiol.*, 1986, 64, 469–480.

68. Raij, T., Ahveninen, J., Lin, F.H., et al. Onset timing of cross-sensory activations and multisensory interactions in auditory and visual sensory cortices. *Eur. J. Neurosci.*, 2010, 31(10), 1772–1782.

69. Letham, B., Raij, T. Statistically robust measurement of evoked onset latencies. *J. Neurosci. Meth.*, 2011, 194, 374–379.

70. Spekreijse, H., Reits, D. Sequential analysis of the visual evoked potential system in man: nonlinear analysis of a sandwich system. *Ann. NY Acad. Sci.*, 1982, 388, 72–97.

71. Regan, D. Some early uses of evoked brain responses in investigations of human visual function. *Vision Res.*, 2009, 49, 882–897.

72. Vialatte, F.B., Maurice, M., Dauwels, J., Cichocki, A. Steady-state visually evoked potentials: focus on essential paradigms and future perspectives. *Progr. Neurobiol.*, 2010, 90, 418–438.

73. Picton, T.W., Skinner, C.R., Champagne, S.C., et al. Potentials evoked by the sinusoidal modulation of the amplitude or frequency of a tone. *J. Acoust. Soc. Am.*, 1987, 82(1), 165–178.

74. Picton, T.W., Bentin, S., Berg, P., et al. Guidelines for using human event-related potentials to study cognition: recording standards and publication criteria. *Psychophysiology*, 2000, 37(2), 127–152.

75. Picton, T.W., John, M.S., Purcell, D.W., et al. Human auditory steady-state responses: the effects of recording technique and state of arousal. *Anesth. Analg.*, 2003, 97(5), 1396–1402.

76. Lehmann, D., Skrandies, W. Spatial analysis of evoked potentials in man—a review. *Prog. Neurobiol.*, 1984, 23, 227–250.

77. Murray, M.M., Brunet, D., Michel, C.M. Topographic ERP analyses: a step-by-step tutorial review. *Brain Topogr.*, 2008, 20(4), 249–64.

78. Hochberg, Y., Tamhane, A.C. *Multiple Comparison Procedures.* New York: John Wiley & Sons, 1987.

79. Lehmann, E.L., Romano, J.P. Generalizations of the family error rate. *Ann. Stat.*, 2005, 33(3), 1138–1154.

80. Shaffer, J.P. Multiple hypothesis testing. *Ann. Rev. Psychol.*, 1995, 46, 561–584.

81. Fisher, R. A. *Design of Experiments.* Edinburgh: Oliver and Boyd, 1935.

82. Petersson, K.M., Nichols, T.E., Poline, J-B., Holmes, A.P. Statistical limitations in functional neuroimaging II. Signal detection and statistical inference. *Philos. Trans. Royal Soc. London*, 1999, 354, 1261–1281.

83. Pesarin, F. *Multivariate Permutation Tests.* New York: John Wiley & Sons, 2001.

84. Westfall, P.H., Young, S.S., *Resampling-Based Multiple Testing. Examples and Methods for p-Values Adjustment.* New York: John Wiley & Sons, 1993.

85. Benjamini, Y., Hochberg, Y. Controlling the false discovery rate: a practical and powerful approach to multiple testing. *J. Royal Stat. Soc. B*, 1995, 57(1), 289–300.

86. Benjamini, Y., Yekutieli, D. The control of the false discovery rate in multiple testing under dependency? *Ann. Stat.*, 2001, 29(4), 1165–1188.

87. Yekutieli, D. Hierarchical false discovery rate-controlling methodology. *J. Am. Stat. Assoc.*, 2008, 103(481), 309–316.

88. Oostenveld, R., Fries, P., Maris, E., Schoffelen, J.M. FieldTrip: open source software for advanced analysis of MEG, EEG, and invasive electrophysiological data. *Comput. Intell. Neurosci.*, 2011, 156869.

89. Maris, E., Oostenveld, R. Nonparametric statistical testing of EEG- and MEG-data. *J Neurosci Meth.*, 2007, 164(1), 177–190.

90. Holmes, A.P., Blair, R.C., Watson, J.D.G., Ford, I. Nonparametric analysis of statistic images from functional mapping experiments. *J. Cerebr. Blood Flow Metab.*, 1996, 16(1), 7–22.

91. Donchin, E. Discriminant analysis in average evoked response studies: the study of single trial data. *Electroencephalogr. Clin. Neurophysiol.*, 1969, 27, 311–314.

92. Farwell, L.A., Donchin, E. Talking off the top of your head: toward a mental prosthesis utilizing event-related brain potentials. *Electroencephalogr. Clin. Neurophysiol.*, 1988, 70, 510–523.

93. Krusienski, D.J., Sellers, E.W., Cabestaing, F., et al. A comparison of classification techniques for the P300 Speller. *J. Neural Eng.*, 2006, 3(4), 299–305.

94. Mak, J.N., Arbel, Y., Minett, J.W., et al. Optimizing the P300-based brain-computer interface: current status, limitations and future directions. *J. Neural Eng.*, 2011, 8(2), 025003.

95. Jrad, N., Congedo, M., Phlypo, R., et al. A sw-SVM: sensor weighting support vector machines for EEG-based brain-computer interfaces. *J. Neural Eng.*, 2011, 8(5), 056004.

96. Barachant, A., Bonnet, S., Congedo, M., Jutten, C. Multi-class brain-computer interface classification by Riemannian geometry. *IEEE Trans. Biomed. Eng.*, 2012, 59(4), 920–928.

97. Barachant, A., Bonnet, S., Congedo, M., Jutten, C. Classification of covariance matrices using a Riemannian-based kernel for BCI applications. *Neurocomputing*, 2013, 112, 172–178.

40 | EEG EVENT-RELATED DESYNCHRONIZATION AND EVENT-RELATED SYNCHRONIZATION

GERT PFURTSCHELLER, PHD AND FERNANDO H. LOPES DA SILVA, MD, PHD

ABSTRACT: Event-related desynchronization (ERD) reflects a decrease of oscillatory activity related to internally or externally paced events. The increase of rhythmic activity is called event-related synchronization (ERS). They represent dynamical states of thalamocortical networks associated with cortical information-processing changes. This chapter discusses differences between ERD/ERS and evoked response potentials and methodologies for quantifying ERD/ERS and selecting frequency bands. It covers the interpretation of ERD/ERS in the alpha and beta bands and theta ERS and alpha ERD in behavioral tasks. ERD/ERS in scalp and subdural recordings, in various frequency bands, is discussed. Also presented is the modulation of alpha and beta rhythms by 0.1-Hz oscillations in the resting state and phase-coupling of the latter with slow changes of prefrontal hemodynamic signals (HbO$_2$), blood pressure oscillations, and heart rate interval variations in the resting state and in relation to behavioral motor tasks. Potential uses of ERD-based strategies in stroke patients are discussed.

KEYWORDS: event-related desynchronization, ERD, event-related synchronization, ERS, stroke

PRINCIPAL REFERENCES

1. Pfurtscheller, G., Lopes da Silva, F.H. Event-related EEG/MEG synchronization and desynchronization: basic principles. *Clin. Neurophysiol.* 1999;110:1842–1857.
2. Crone, N.E., Miglioretti, D.L., Gordon, B., et al. Functional mapping of human sensorimotor cortex with electrocorticographic spectral analysis. I. Alpha and beta event-related desynchronization. *Brain* 1998;121: 2271–2299.
3. Crone, N.E., Miglioretti, D.L., Gordon, B., et al. Functional mapping of human sensorimotor cortex with electrocorticographic spectral analysis. II. Event-related synchronization in the gamma band. *Brain* 1998;121:2301–2315.
4. Klimesch, W. EEG alpha and theta oscillations reflect cognitive and memory performance: A review and analysis. *Brain Res. Rev.* 1999;29:169–195.
5. Neuper, C., Pfurtscheller, G. Event-related dynamics of cortical rhythms: frequency-specific features and functional correlates. *Int. J. Psychophysiol.* 2001;43:41–58.
6. Neuper, C., Klimesch, W., eds. *Event-Related Dynamics of Brain Oscillations.* Progress in Brain Research. Vol. 158. Amsterdam: Elsevier, 2006.
7. Takemi, M., Masakado, Y., Liu, M., Ushiba, J. Event-related desynchronization reflects downregulation of intracortical inhibition in human primary motor cortex. *J. Neurophysiol.* 2013;110:1158–1166.
8. Lopes da Silva, F.H. EEG and MEG: relevance to neuroscience. *Neuron* 2013;80(5):1112–1128.

1. INTRODUCTION

Electroencephalographic (EEG) desynchronization or blocking of alpha band rhythms associated with sensory processing or motor behavior was first reported by Berger (1). This desynchronization reflects a decrease of oscillatory activity related to an internally or externally paced event and is known as *event-related desynchronization* (ERD) (2). The opposite, namely the increase of rhythmic activity, is termed *event-related synchronization* (ERS). ERD and ERS are characterized by their fairly localized topography, phasic behavior, and frequency specificity (3). Both phenomena can be studied as functions of time and space (ERD/ERS maps). There is general agreement that EEG alpha ERD and ERS represent different dynamical states of the activity of thalamocortical networks associated with changes in cortical information processing, as discussed in detail in Chapter 2.

2. EVENT-RELATED POTENTIALS VERSUS EEG INDUCED REACTIVITY

Two types of changes in the electrical activity of the cortex may occur upon sensory stimulation: (1) the so-called evoked responses, which are time-locked and phase-locked to a stimulus and can be extracted from the ongoing activity by simple linear methods such as averaging; and (2) the induced responses, that are elicited by changes in the dynamical state of on-going EEG oscillations and are time-locked but not phase-locked and can only be extracted through methods such as envelope detection or power spectral analysis. Which mechanisms underlie these types of responses? The time- and phase-locked response can easily be understood in terms of the response of a quasi-stationary system to an external stimulus that can be accounted for, in a first approximation, by a process of addition of the evoked response to the ongoing activity of the neural networks, although the latter may undergo some degree of reorganization as well. Whether or not this occurs is a matter of debate (see discussion in Chapter 39).

The induced changes can be understood as resulting from changes in the dynamical state of neural networks leading to increases, or decreases, in the degree of synchrony of cortical neuronal populations. These changes can be due to a variety of factors; in particular, they may depend on modulating influences arising from subcortical systems, leading to changes in the strength of synaptic interactions and/or affecting intrinsic membrane properties of the local neurons.

3. QUANTIFICATION OF EEG REACTIVITY

The ERD/ERS can be quantified in time and space domains. For the quantification, a number of event-triggered EEG trials

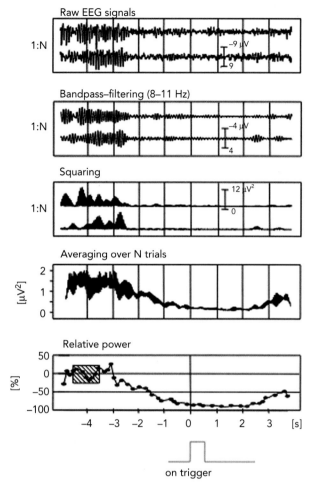

Raw EEG signals

1:N

Bandpass–filtering (8–11 Hz)

1:N

Squaring

1:N

Averaging over N trials

Relative power

on trigger

Figure 40.1. Schema of the classic ERD processing method, showing an example of movement-related mu ERD. The raw EEG signals (0.5–50 Hz) are first bandpass-filtered (8–12 Hz), and thereafter all samples are squared and averaged over all N trials. After averaging over consecutive power samples (compression) and specifying a reference interval (e.g., –3.5 to –4.5), the relative band power values are displayed. Power decrease corresponds to ERD.

are necessary, including some seconds before and some seconds after the event. The event can be externally paced (e.g., by acoustical, visual, or somatosensory stimulation) or internally paced (e.g., triggered by a voluntary finger movement). The classic procedure of processing (Fig. 40.1) once the frequency band has been selected comprises the following steps:

1. Bandpass filtering of each event-related trial

2. Squaring of each amplitude sample to obtain power samples

3. Averaging over all trials

4. Averaging over a small number of consecutive power samples to reduce the variance

An alternative method is based on the calculation of the intertrial variance (4,5). Absolute band power is converted into percentage power by setting the power within a reference interval as 100%. By convention, a power decrease corresponds to an ERD and a power increase to an ERS (3). ERD/ERS time

courses can also be calculated using the Hilbert transform and determining the envelope of a bandpass-filtered signal (6). Hilbert-based ERD calculation yields very similar results as the method of bandpass filtering (7).

4. SELECTION OF EEG FREQUENCY BANDS

One way of defining the EEG frequency bands of interest is to search for the most reactive frequency components. Classically this search involves comparing power spectra calculated during a reference period (i.e., during rest) with that of two subsequent periods, one *before* and one *after* the relevant event, in order to identify frequency bands showing statistically significant differences. For example, in this way pre-movement alpha ERD and post-movement beta ERS can be displayed (Fig. 40.2). A frequency band with a significant power decrease is selected for ERD calculation (e.g., 8–12 Hz in Fig. 40.2), while a band with a significant power increase (e.g., 12–19 Hz in Fig. 40.2) is defined for ERS calculation (8–10). Theoretically, the frequency band can be defined for each derivation. In practice, a few derivations overlying the areas of interest—depending on the specific study being performed—are used to determine the frequency bands of interest in a given case; for example, temporal and parietal electrodes are selected in a memory task and central electrodes in a movement study. Another method of frequency band selection can be applied specifically subdividing the alpha band into sub-bands, as proposed by Klimesch et al. (11). Indeed, the functional specificity particularly of alpha frequency bands can better be put in evidence if frequency boundaries are adjusted to the peak of individual alpha frequency of a given subject, and if rather narrow bands are used (a detailed description of methods is given in 12,13). The dominant alpha peak in the power spectrum calculated for the whole trial is first detected. The upper alpha band is then defined as consisting of the frequencies between this alpha peak frequency and the upper edge of the classically defined alpha band, while the lower alpha band is defined as those frequencies between the alpha peak frequency and the lower edge of the alpha band.

To obtain a dynamic representation of changing activity within a broad frequency range, the calculation of time-frequency maps using bandpass filtering (14) (Fig. 40.3) and wavelet transformation is recommended (3,15). A method with high time-frequency resolution is the matching pursuit with stochastic Gabor dictionaries as estimator for the signal's energy density (16).

5. ERD AND ERS IN ALPHA AND BETA FREQUENCY BANDS

The alpha band rhythm displays a relatively widespread desynchronization (ERD) in verbal judgments and perceptual and memory tasks (17,18). An increase of task complexity or of attention demand results in an increased magnitude of ERD (19,20). Moreover, it has been shown that there is a relationship

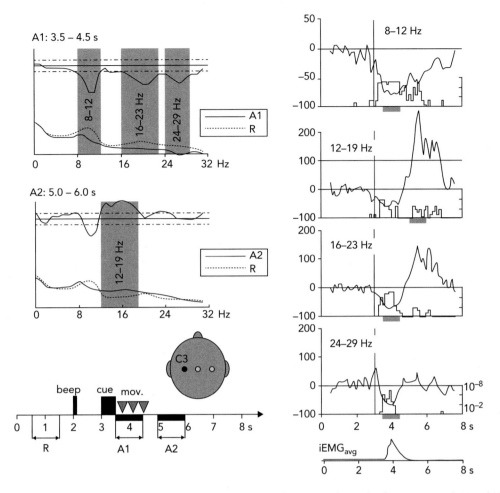

Figure 40.2. Left side: Superimposed logarithmic 1-sec power spectra calculated in the reference period (R) and in the activity periods A1 and A2 in a cue-paced right finger movement experiment. A1 and A2 correspond to two 1-sec time intervals; one is selected during the cue-triggered finger movement (A1) and the other after termination of the movement (A2), as shown in the lower left. In addition, the differences between the two superimposed spectra are displayed with 95% confidence intervals (indicated by the dotted lines). The frequency ranges displaying significant power decrease or increase are marked. Right side: Band power time course calculated for the frequency bands indicated in the spectra on the left. Data are triggered according to cue onset (vertical line). The integrated and averaged EMG shows the beginning and end of the movements. The step function indicates the significance level (sign test p from 10^{-2} to 10^{-8}) for the respective power changes. The horizontal line marks the band power in the reference period. Downward deflection indicates power decrease or ERD; upward deflection indicates power increase or ERS. Modified from Neuper and Pfurtscheller (8).

between the P300 event-related potential and ERD of alpha band activity (21,22). It has to be kept in mind, however, that the ERD is measured as a percentage of power relative to the reference interval, and therefore it depends on the amount of rhythmic activity in this interval. To make a reliable estimate of the power at the resting level (reference epoch), the intervals between consecutive events (e.g., cues, self-paced movements) should be randomized and should not be shorter than ~10 sec.

It is important to note that alpha desynchronization is not a unitary phenomenon. If different frequency bands within the range of the extended alpha band are distinguished, two distinct patterns of desynchronization can be observed. Lower alpha desynchronization (in the range of about 8–10 Hz) is obtained in response to almost any type of task. It is topographically widespread over the entire scalp and probably reflects general task demands and attentional processes. Upper alpha desynchronization (in the range of about 10–12 Hz), in contrast, is topographically restricted and is rather related to task-specific aspects (23,24). ERD and ERS are quite often not uniformly distributed over the scalp but show spatial

specificities such that even simultaneously occurring ERD and ERS can occur over different cortical areas.

It is of interest to note that blocking of alpha band rhythms occurs not only in response to a specific stimulation, but also in anticipation of a stimulus. Modality-specific ERD patterns, for instance, have been demonstrated during anticipatory attention to a feedback stimulus presented in different modalities. Examples are the occipitally maximal ERD preceding visual stimuli and the temporally maximal ERD (in magnetoencephalographic [MEG] data) prior to an auditory feedback stimulus (25). The functional relevance of ERD and ERS in memory tasks is discussed in a subsequent section.

In addition to sensory and cognitive processing, *voluntary movement* also results in a circumscribed ERD in the upper alpha and lower beta bands, localized over sensorimotor areas (2,8,26–30). The ERD starts over the contralateral rolandic region and becomes bilateral symmetric with execution of movement. It is of interest that the time course of the contralateral mu ERD is almost identical in case of brisk and slow finger movements, and it starts more than 2 sec prior

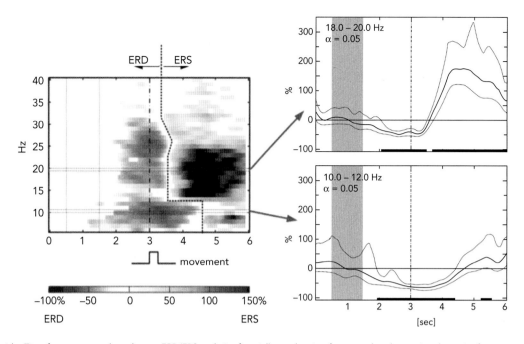

Figure 40.3. *Left side: Time-frequency map based on an ERD/ERS analysis of partially overlapping frequency bands covering the entire frequency range of interest (e.g., 5–40 Hz). This ERD/ERS map is a matrix, the rows of which correspond to ERD/ERS calculations for specific frequency bands. In this example, the ERD/ERS map was constructed from ERD/ERS curves with a bandwidth of 2 Hz and an overlap of 1 Hz. The trigger time point is marked by a dashed-dotted vertical line. The reference interval is indicated by two dotted vertical lines. Right side: Examples of corresponding ERD/ERS time curves for two selected frequency bands (10–12 Hz, 18–20 Hz).*

to movement onset (31). Finger movement of the dominant hand is accompanied by a pronounced ERD in the contralateral hemisphere and by a very low ERD in the ipsilateral side, whereas movement of the nondominant finger is preceded by a less lateralized ERD (32). Different reactivity patterns have been observed with mu rhythms in the lower and upper alpha frequency band (33).

In addition to motor preparation and movement execution, *motor imagery* can produce replicable EEG patterns over primary sensory and motor areas (e.g., 34–36). This is in accordance with the concept that motor imagery is realized via the same brain systems as those involved in programming and preparing movements (37,38). For example, imagination of right and left hand movements results in ERD of mu and beta rhythms over the contralateral hand area, very similar in topography to planning and execution of real movements (39) (Fig. 40.4). Besides movement execution and imagination, the *observation of movement* has an impact on sensorimotor rhythms and results in alpha and beta ERD: a clear correlation was found between the velocity profile of the observed movements and the beta ERD (40).

During repeated training sessions with a motor imagery task, the pattern of contralateral ERD of alpha band components becomes even more pronounced, and a concomitant power increase (ERS) over the ipsilateral side can develop. These findings strongly indicate the existence of activity in primary motor cortex during mental simulation of movement. Hence, we can assume that the pre-movement ERD and the ERD during motor imagery reflect a similar type of readiness, or presetting, of neural networks in sensorimotor areas. Involvement of the primary sensorimotor cortex in motor imagery was further supported by functional brain imaging

(e.g., 41–43) and by transcranial magnetic stimulation (TMS) studies that showed an increase of motor responses to TMS during mental imagination of movements (44).

The observation that, in parallel with the contralateral ERD, imagining a movement also triggers a significant ipsilateral ERS supports the concept of antagonistic behavior of

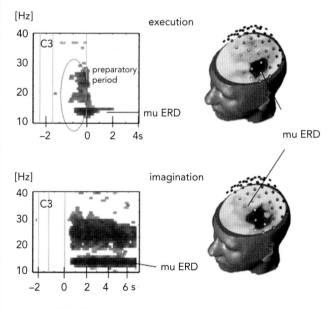

Figure 40.4. *ERD/ERS time-frequency maps (left side) and topographical maps of mu ERD (right side) of a representative subject during execution (upper panel) versus imagination of a right-hand movement (lower panel). Time-frequency maps are recorded from electrode position C3; time point 0 indicates movement onset and the onset of cue presentation in the execution and imagination task, respectively.*

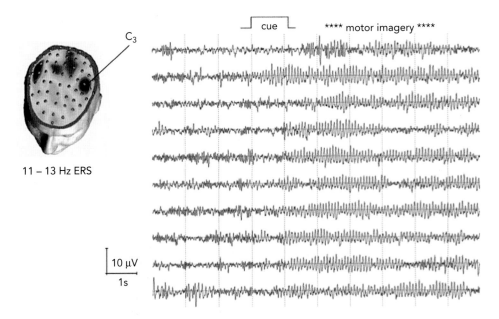

Figure 40.5. Left side: Topographic map indicating the localized 10-Hz ERS on electrode positions C3 and C4 during foot motor imagery. Right side: Examples of single EEG trials, recorded from electrode position C3, in a cue-based motor imagery experiment. Note the enhancement of mu rhythm at C3 (corresponding to the cortical are representing the hand) during the imagination of foot movements.

neural networks ("focal ERD/surround ERS," 45) described in the next section. A comparable effect, induced ERS alpha oscillations in the hand area during foot movement, is demonstrated in Figure 40.5. It is of interest to note that the antagonistic behavior of alpha components (ERD/ERS) is a dominant feature of the upper alpha band and is not seen with lower-frequency components.

6. INTERPRETATION OF ERD AND ERS IN THE ALPHA BAND

Changes in thalamocortical systems result in a low-amplitude desynchronized EEG (see for details Chapter 2). ERD can be interpreted as an electrophysiological correlate of activated cortical areas involved in the processing of sensory or cognitive information or the production of motor behavior (46). The fact that sensorimotor cortex excitability is correlated with ERD was elegantly demonstrated by Takemi et al. (47). Using TMS, these authors showed that ERD during wrist motor imagery is associated with enhanced excitability in primary motor cortex; indeed, the response to TMS applied to this cortical area elicited a larger motor potential and a reduced short-interval intracortical inhibition during ERD compared with a control condition. An increased and/or more widespread ERD can be the result of the involvement of a larger neural network or of more cell assemblies in information processing. Factors contributing to such an enhancement of the ERD are increased task complexity, more efficient task performance (19,20,48,49), and more effort and attention that may be needed in the case of some subjects, such as elderly people or those with a low IQ (27,50,51).

Explicit learning of a movement sequence (e.g., key pressing with different fingers) is accompanied by an enhancement of ERD over the contralateral central regions. Once the movement sequence has been learned and the movements are performed more automatically, the ERD is reduced. These ERD findings strongly suggest that the activity in primary sensorimotor areas increases in association with learning a new motor task and decreases after the task has been learned (52). The involvement of the primary motor area in learning motor sequences was also suggested by Pascual-Leone et al. (53), who studied motor output maps using TMS.

The opposite phenomenon to desynchronization (ERD) is synchronization (ERS); in this case the amplitude enhancement is likely mediated by the cooperative or synchronized behavior of a large number of neurons. When the summed synaptic events become sufficiently large, the field potentials can be recorded with macroelectrodes not only within the cortex but also over the scalp. To be recorded at the scalp, cortical activity must be coherent over an appreciable surface of cortical tissue (54–56; see also Chapter 2). When patches of neurons display coherent activity in the alpha band, a depressed state of processing of information in the underlying cortical neuronal populations can be assumed to exist.

It is of interest to note that ~85% of cortical neurons are excitatory, with the other 15% being inhibitory (57). Inhibition in neural networks, however, is very important, not only to optimize energy demands but also to limit and control excitatory processes. Klimesch (58) suggested that synchronized alpha band rhythms may produce powerful inhibitory effects, which could act to block a memory search from entering irrelevant parts of neural networks. Adrian and Matthews (59) described a system that is neither receiving nor processing sensory information as an "idling system." This concept is, however, outdated. We noted above that synchronized alpha band rhythms may produce powerful inhibitory effects (58) and thus cannot be considered idle; rather, they are actively involved in inhibitory control, associated with attentional processes (56). Accordingly, the state of alpha activity modulates the threshold for perception, as shown experimentally (30,60,61). Furthermore, the phase of alpha oscillations can predict subsequent detection of visual stimuli (62). Thus, we may propose that alpha oscillations constitute a form of "pulsed inhibition" of cortical excitability. Along the same line, Haegens et al. (63), recording alpha oscillations and spike firing in monkey cortex, showed that as alpha oscillations decreased, the spike firing frequency increased. This implies that alpha oscillations exert an inhibitory modulating influence in the cortex and are far from representing an idling state.

7. SPATIAL DISTRIBUTIONS OF ERD AND ERS PHENOMENA: OPPOSITE FEATURES

As mentioned above, an important feature of ERD and ERS is that changes in opposite directions can occur in different brain areas at the same time, the so-called focal ERD/surround ERS phenomenon that is described in detail in (45). This aspect, however, was often overlooked in many early studies and may cause misinterpretations of what ERD or ERS may represent if the corresponding spatial distribution is not clearly indicated. In this context a paradigmatic observation is that mu ERD over sensorimotor cortex associated with the hand movements is not a generalized phenomenon but is accompanied by mu ERS over central cortical areas, as illustrated in Figure 40.6 (see also 36, 64). A similar antagonistic

behavior with ERD of central mu rhythm and ERS of parieto-occipital alpha rhythms during repetitive brief finger movement was reported in (65). The opposite phenomenon, the enhancement of central mu rhythm and blocking of occipital alpha rhythm during visual stimulation, was reported in (66, 67). Jones et al. (68), using MEG recordings, found ERD of mu rhythm over the contralateral cortical area when subjects had their attention cued to one hand; however, when subjects directed their attention to the foot, mu ERS was seen over the hand area. Furthermore, Popov et al. (69), also using MEG, found that the perception of faces expressing emotions was associated with ERD in the frequency band 10 to 15 Hz over the visual cortical areas, whereas ERS of the same frequency band was seen over sensorimotor areas.

The focal mu ERD in the upper alpha band (~10–13 Hz) may reflect a mechanism responsible for selective attention focused to a motor subsystem. This effect of focal attention may be accentuated when other cortical areas, not directly involved in the specific motor task, display ERS (i.e., are "inhibited"). The interplay between thalamocortical modules and the corresponding reticular nucleus neurons may play an important role in this process, as shown by the model simulations (45).

Support for the phenomenon of "focal ERD/surround ERS" also comes from regional cerebral blood flow and functional magnetic resonance imaging (fMRI) studies. A decrease of cerebral blood flow was reported in the somatosensory cortical representation area of one body part whenever attention

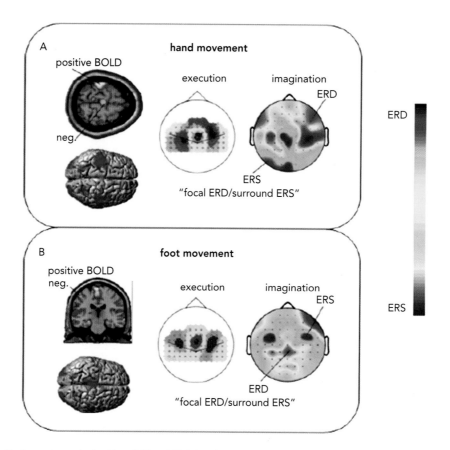

Figure 40.6. Examples of activation patterns obtained from fMRI and EEG data during execution and imagination of hand (**A**) and foot movements (**B**), respectively. Note the correspondence between the focus of the positive BOLD signal and ERD on the one side and between negative BOLD signal and ERS on the other side.

was directed to a distant body part (70). An increase of the BOLD signal in the foot area and a decrease of the BOLD signal (negative BOLD) in the hand area was observed when the subject imagined or executed movements of the toes (43; see also examples in Fig. 40.6). Hemodynamic BOLD (fMRI) and cortical alpha power are, in general, inversely correlated. Indeed, several groups (71–74) have shown that temporal variations of alpha power are negatively correlated to the BOLD signal in several cortical regions (visual cortex, pre-and postcentral gyrus) but positively correlated with the thalamic BOLD signal. Taking these observations together, we may conclude that this indicates that enhanced alpha rhythm corresponds to a relatively low average spiking rate level in the cortex. Of interest in this context is also an fMRI study during execution of a learned complex finger movement sequence and inhibition of the same sequence (inhibition condition); overt movement was accompanied by a positive BOLD signal and a focal, broad-banded mu ERD in the hand area, while movement inhibition resulted in a negative BOLD signal and a narrow-banded (11–13 Hz) mu ERS in the same area (75,76).

The phenomenon of focal ERD/surround ERS emerges also in cortical areas outside the sensorimotor areas. This has been shown in the visual cortex, where it was found that retinotopic ERD/ERS can be elicited by visual stimulation of specific retinal sectors: while alpha ERD is seen over the cortical area corresponding to the retinal sector being stimulated, contralateral cortical areas exhibit ERS (77,78). Furthermore, when attention is directed to one visual hemi-field, there is alpha ERD over the contralateral parieto-occipital areas and ERS ipsilaterally (30,79,80). This ERD–ERS opposition in the space domain has also been found between cortical areas processing different sensory modalities. Anderson and Ding (81) demonstrated that lateralized spatial attention elicits mu-rhythm ERD in the corresponding somatotopic somatosensory cortex, while alpha ERS occurs over the visual cortex This is in line with the MEG findings reported in (82), where a cross-modal attention task was used in which subjects had to discriminate between a visual and an auditory stimulus. Preparation for visual versus auditory discrimination resulted in alpha (9–11Hz) ERD in occipital cortex, while alpha and beta (14–16 Hz) power increased in the supramarginal gyrus. These examples illustrate the existence of *cross-modal ERD–ERS effects*.

8. FUNCTIONAL MEANING OF ERD AND ERS IN MEMORY PROCESSES

A number of studies have addressed the question of whether alpha frequency ERS and ERD were associated with memory processing. Pesonen et al. (83), studying EEG in an auditory Sternberg memory task, reported ERS of both low-frequency components (~1–6 Hz) and alpha (~7–12 Hz) during the *encoding phase* of a memory set, more conspicuous in the parietal, right temporal, and occipital areas; as the number of items to be encoded increased, the alpha ERS became stronger. These changes were accompanied by beta (~18–28 Hz) ERD in left temporal and frontal electrodes. During the *recognition phase*, similarly low frequency (≈1–6 Hz) ERS and beta (≈15–30 Hz)

ERD were also recorded, but alpha (~8–12 Hz) now showed ERD; the ERD/ERS responses evolved at different phases of the memory task. These studies, however, do not make a detailed spatial analysis since only a limited number of electrodes were available. Interestingly, during investigations of ERD/ERS in similar memory tasks but using letters presented visually, Jensen et al. (84) also showed alpha (7–12 Hz) ERS during the encoding of a set of letters to be memorized, an effect that became more pronounced as the number of items to be held in memory increased. This is described in more detail below.

The differential behavior of different frequency bands in memory tasks can be put in evidence in tasks where items to be remembered are presented visually. In a study by Sauseng et al. (85), a cue (pointing to the left or to the right hemi-field) was used to indicate whether visual items in the left or right hemi-field had to be remembered. The findings showed that during the retention interval, the lateralized increase in alpha ERS over the ipsilateral hemisphere was correlated with the subject's individual memory capacity. This result suggests that alpha ERS mediates the inhibition of task-irrelevant and distracting information (in the not-cued hemi-field), which is an important factor for keeping the relevant information in mind. In addition, a selective, lateralized phase coupling of theta and gamma was observed over the contralateral hemisphere and appeared to be correlated with memory capacity.

A growing number of studies of EEG and MEG activities associated with memory processing have appeared in the last years, but they go beyond the scope of this chapter's focus on ERD/ERS phenomena. The reader is referred to Chapter 46 for a more general account of the relationships between such phenomena and neurocognitive processes.

9. BETA BAND ERS/ERD

Termination of movement, motor imagery, and somatosensory stimulation are accompanied by a short-lasting beta burst known as beta rebound or post-movement beta ERS. One characteristic feature of this beta ERS is its strict somatotopical organization reported in MEG (86) and EEG recordings (3,87). Another feature is its frequency specificity, with a slightly lower frequency over the lateralized sensorimotor areas than the midcentral area (88). Frequency bands in the range of 16 to 20 Hz were reported for the hand representation area and of 20 to 24 Hz for the midcentral area close to the vertex. The observation that a self-paced finger movement can activate neuronal networks in the hand and foot representation areas with different frequency in both areas (Fig. 40.7; see also 89) provides further support for the notion that the frequency of these oscillations may be characteristic for the underlying neural circuitry.

The post-movement beta synchronization is found after both active and passive movements (26). This indicates that proprioceptive afferents play an important role in the desynchronization of the central beta rhythm and the subsequent beta rebound. However, electrical nerve stimulation (88), mechanical finger stimulation (90), motor imagery (39,91), and even observing another person's movements (92) also can

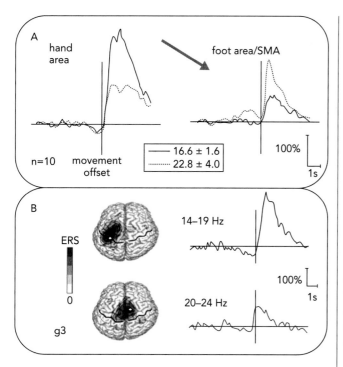

Figure 40.7. A: Grand average time courses of the relative beta band power calculated for subject-specific frequency bands. Average hand-area specific frequency was 16.6 Hz ± 1.6 (full line curves) and foot-area specific frequency was 22.8 Hz ± 4.0 (stippled line curves). Data are triggered at movement offset (indicated by the vertical line). Note the large band power increase (beta ERS, indicated by upward deflection) over the hand area, with the lower-frequency component, and the larger power increase over the foot area, with the high-frequency components. The horizontal line marks the average band power in the 1-sec reference interval that started 4 sec before the trigger. B: ERS distributions of one representative subject calculated in the bands 14–19 Hz and 20–24 Hz shown over the cortical surface (left side). A light disk marks the location of the maximal beta ERS. Each map corresponds to a time interval of 125 msec. ERS results over the cortical surface were computed based on the linear estimation method. A realistically shaped head model (brain-skull-scalp compartments) was constructed from 200 transversal T1-weighted MR images. For the indicated positions of maximal beta ERS, the corresponding ERD/ERS time courses are shown (right side). The horizontal line indicates the band power in the reference interval, the vertical line the time of movement offset. Modified from Pfurtscheller et al. (89).

induce a beta ERD followed by a short-lasting beta ERS or beta rebound. A general explanation for the induced beta bursts in the motor cortex *after* movement, somatosensory stimulation, motor imagery, and movement observation is that parts of the beta-generating network shift from a highly activated state during movement activation to a deactivated or inhibited state immediately after cessation of the motor task, whether real, imagined, or observed.

By applying TMS during self-paced movement or median nerve stimulation, it was shown that the excitability of motor cortex neurons was significantly reduced in the first second after termination of movement or of stimulation, respectively (93,94). This gives support to the interpretation that the beta rebound might represent a deactivated or inhibited cortical state. This is also in line with the finding of the suppression of the beta rebound during continuous sensory motor cortex activation in MEG (95) and EEG (96) (Fig. 40.8). Such a continuous activation, as for example during manipulation of a cube with one

hand, is accompanied not only by an intense outflow from the motor cortex to the hand muscles but also by an afferent flow from mechanoreceptors and proprioceptors to the somatosensory cortex. This strong activation of the sensorimotor cortex could be responsible for the suppression of the beta rebound. At movement arrest the networks of the motor area may be reset, which would be reflected in the beta rebound or beta bursts in the sensorimotor area. The latter could be interpreted as representing a "resetting of functions" in contrast to a "binding function" that may be related to some types of gamma oscillations.

The sensorimotor beta rhythm can be used to study the underlying neuronal mechanisms of response preparation, decision making, and response inhibition. Recordings in monkey during a go/no-go task (97) showed that during motor preparation, signaled by a visual cue, there is a frontal beta ERD regardless of the subsequent response, whether go or no go. Alegre et al. (98) recorded scalp EEG in healthy subjects using two different go/no-go protocols to dissociate EEG changes related to motor preparation/execution from those related to decision making. These authors found that in the phase of decision making a conspicuous frontal beta ERS was manifest.

Interestingly, Pfurtscheller et al. (99) reported in a cue-paced movement imagination task, also using a go/no-go paradigm (motor imagery or withholding of motor imagery), a beta ERD localized to the central area occurring during imagery followed by post-imagery beta ERS (rebound), akin to the observations by Alegre et al. (98) (Fig. 40.9). The subjects, however, can also show, in the case of withholding motor imagery, a beta ERD without this being followed by beta ERS. In agreement with these observations, Solis-Escalante et al. (100) showed that ERS beta rebound is stronger after termination and withholding of real movements than during withholding of imaginary movements. It is remarkable that beta ERD, associated with motor imagery in the Go condition (see Fig. 40.9), is accompanied by a short-lasting heart rate deceleration. These concomitant responses in cerebral and cardiovascular systems give support to the existence of a strong mutual interaction between the central and autonomic nervous systems (101), reflecting processes operating automatically and unconsciously as part of the orienting reflex (102,103).

10. GAMMA BAND ERD/ERS

In the tasks involving sensorimotor activities, at least three different types of oscillations can be found at the same scalp electrode locations during brisk finger lifting, as documented in Figure 40.10. Besides a mu ERD (10–12 Hz) and a post-movement rebound beta ERS (14–18 Hz), induced gamma oscillations (36–40 Hz) are also present. These 36- to 40-Hz oscillations reach a maximum ERS shortly before movement onset, whereas the beta ERS has its maximum after movement offset (104).

Gamma oscillations in the frequency range from 60 to 90 Hz associated with movement were studied also in subdural recordings (electrocorticography [ECoG] 105, 106). In contrast to the alpha band rhythms, the gamma oscillations reflect a stage of active information processing. A prerequisite for

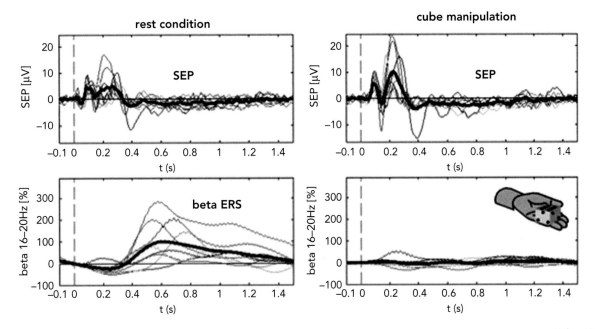

Figure 40.8. *Superimposed individual sensory evoked potentials (upper panels, referential recording, Cpz) and the individual beta ERS curves (middle and lower panels, bipolar, channel C3, frequency range 16–20 Hz and 20–24 Hz) for six subjects. The left part of the figure represents condition A (resting), and the right part indicates condition B (cube manipulation). The mean curve of each panel is displayed with a thick line. Modified from Pfurtscheller et al. (96).*

the development of gamma bursts may be the desynchronization of alpha band rhythms. The examples in Figure 40.11 show that induced gamma and beta oscillations are embedded in desynchronized alpha band activity. Opposite changes in the alpha and gamma power have been found in several other studies. Siegel et al. (107), using MEG during a spatially cued motion discrimination task, reported that attention was associated with ERD of alpha-beta oscillations in the hemisphere

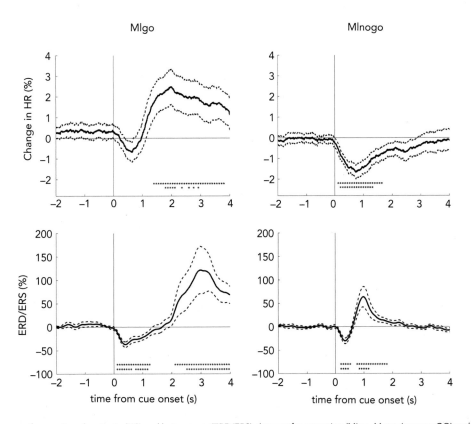

Figure 40.9. *Grand averages of percentage heart rate (HR) and beta power (ERD/ERS) changes for execution (MIgo, Motor Imagery GO) and withholding (MInogo) of foot motor imagery (MI). In addition to the mean and the standard error (stippled lines), the significant changes (bootstrap) are displayed (one asterisk vertically indicates significance at p < .05, and two asterisks at p < .01). Data from 16 subjects. Note the significant HR decrease in the no-go condition and the significant early beta ERD in both the go and no-go conditions. Modified from Pfurtscheller et al. (99).*

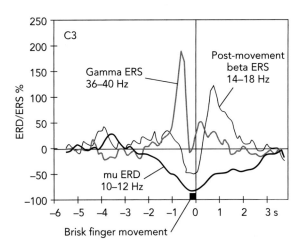

Figure 40.10. Superposition of different band power versus time courses triggered with respect to brisk finger movement offset. The duration of the index finger extension and flexion was 0.2 sec. Note the relatively long-lasting mu rhythm (10–12 Hz) desynchronization starting ~2 sec prior to movement onset, the post-movement beta (14–18 Hz) ERS following a beta ERD, and the short-lasting increase of gamma power ~40 Hz prior to movement onset.

representing the attended hemi-field and was followed by gamma ERS. A number of studies along the same line (108) led to a better understanding of how gamma and alpha oscillations interact in order to temporally organize neuronal coding in the visual system (109).

Another interesting finding is that separate foci of synchronized gamma activities occurring in cortical regions that are widely separated—often even in different lobes— can display high correlation or coherence during the performance of cognitive or motor tasks.

These results are also in line with the animal studies by Bressler et al. (110), who reported task-related increases of coherence in high-frequency activities in the monkey neocortex during the performance of a pattern-discrimination task: gamma band activities in the striate and motor cortex were briefly correlated when a motor response occurred and were uncorrelated when no response occurred. Andrew and Pfurtscheller (111) reported a phasic increase in 40-Hz event-related coherence between the contralateral sensorimotor and the supplementary motor areas during the performance of unilateral finger movements. In contrast, the 40-Hz coherence between the left and right sensorimotor areas showed no changes in coherence during the movement and remained low throughout. These findings suggest that increases in gamma band coherence are functionally related to the task being performed. Possibly, the coherence between the gamma oscillations in these distant regions is facilitated by specific cortico-cortical connections between the corresponding neural masses sustaining the gamma oscillations.

11. EEG OSCILLATORY ACTIVITIES: RELATIONSHIPS WITH HEMODYNAMIC VARIABLES

The modulation of the amplitude of EEG rhythmic activities is not only associated with sensory stimulation or motor behavior during cognitive processing, but it can also be put in evidence in the resting state in connection with processes operating automatically and unconsciously, as we alluded to above with respect to heart rate changes and beta ERD. Slow oscillations modulating the power of high gamma, theta, and theta/high gamma, with dominant frequencies ~0.1 Hz in human posteromedial cortex, have been described in the resting state (112). Furthermore, the modulation of beta power by oscillations at frequencies ~0.1 Hz in sensorimotor areas was reported (113). These slow fluctuations of beta power displayed not only a temporary phase coupling with slow changes of prefrontal hemodynamic signals (HbO$_2$) but were also associated with the Mayer waves of blood pressure (periodicity of 10 sec) and with the variability of heart rate intervals (113).

The close relationship between beta ERD/ERS and BOLD phenomena can also be put in evidence in simple button press experiments. A button press is always accompanied by a pre- and peri-movement ERD and a post-movement beta ERS (3). Stancak et al. (114) investigated the effect of external load opposing brisk voluntary extension of the right index finger, and found that the pre-movement ERD of beta rhythms (18–25 Hz) over the contralateral sensorimotor area was greater with larger loads; similarly, the post-movement beta ERS was longer under the heaviest loads. It is interesting to consider these findings in relation to what has been observed with respect to BOLD signals. Fox et al. (115) found spontaneous BOLD signals with significantly different magnitudes 2 to 3 sec after button press for soft compared with hard pressing; this relationship between BOLD and button press force was named the BOLD-behavior effect (115). This may be considered the counterpart of the ERD-behavior effect in the EEG domain described above. In addition, the example in Figure 40.12 documents such a short-lasting phase coupling between prefrontal hemodynamic (oxyhemoglobin) and central beta power oscillations with a dominant frequency at 0.1 Hz in the resting state (113).

12. ERD/ERS PATTERNS IN INTRACRANIAL AND SUBDURAL RECORDINGS IN HUMANS

Different types of movement-related ERD patterns have been observed in subdural (30,106,116,117) and intracerebral recordings (118,119). Stereo-electroencephalographic (SEEG) studies with intracerebral depth electrodes in pre- and postcentral gyri and the frontal medial cortex in epileptic patients, during self-paced hand movement, revealed a relative widespread mu and beta ERD followed by a more focused beta ERS in primary sensorimotor areas and supplementary motor area (SMA) proper (119). In general, the spatial distribution of gamma ERS is discrete and somatotopically more specific than power changes in lower-frequency bands (alpha–mu or beta) (120; see also Chapter 33). In a similar SEEG study on one epileptic surgery candidate, Sochurkova and Rektor (118) reported a mu and beta ERD recorded by means of depth electrodes located in the basal ganglia (putamen) in a "self-paced" motor task. The post-movement beta ERS was in this case most prominent in the 28- to 32-Hz band.

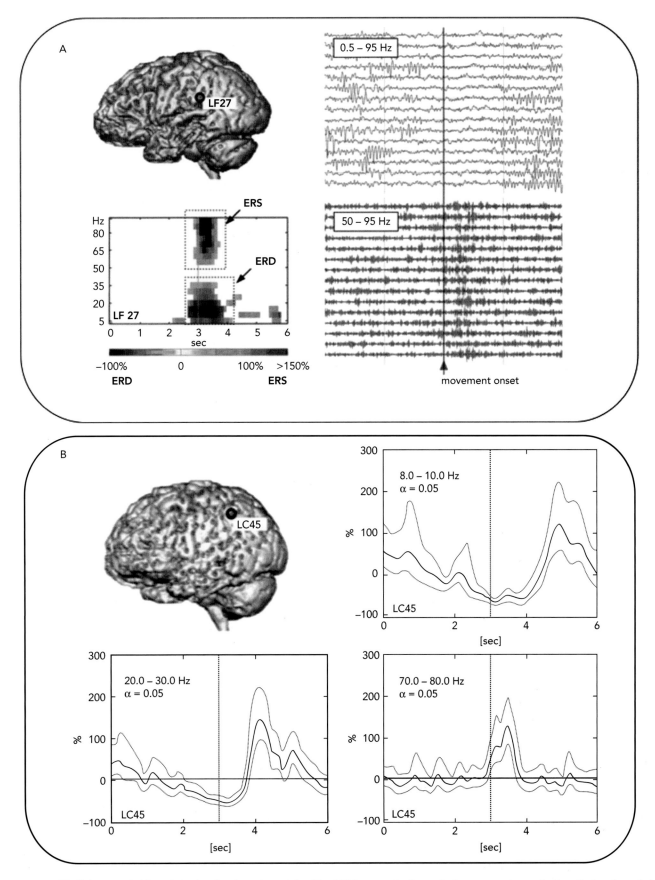

Figure 40.11. ECoG data recorded from electrodes placed over temporal and frontal lobe neocortex for monitoring purposes in an epileptic patient, and sampled at 200 Hz. The subject performed self-paced movement tasks such as index finger movement and palmar pinch with a minimum of 4 sec between repetitions. ERD/ERS was quantified from ~40 trials at movement onset and with a statistical significance of p = .05. **A:** Raw ECoG trials of two different frequency bands (0.5–95 Hz and 50–95 Hz) for channel LF27 of subject C16 performing palmar pinch (right side). Corresponding ERD/ERS time-frequency map spanning a frequency range of 5 to 90 Hz with a frequency resolution of 5 Hz and frequency bands of 10 Hz (left side). **B:** ERD/ERS curves with 95% confidence intervals for channel LC45 of subject C17 performing index finger movement. In both cases (**A** and **B**) gamma activity (gamma ERS) ~70 to 80 Hz, which is embedded in alpha and beta ERD, is clearly visible.

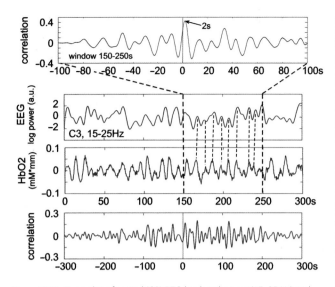

Figure 40.12. *Examples of central (C3) EEG log band power (15–25 Hz) and prefrontal oxyhemoglobin (HbO₂) time courses of a representative subject during 300 sec of rest. Cross-correlations of both signals are shown: in the top trace for a selected 100-sec interval (r = .49, p < .01) and in the bottom trace for the whole 300-sec interval (r = .2, non-significant). Note the short-lasting significant phase coupling between EEG and hemodynamic (HbO₂) signals. Modified from Pfurtscheller et al. (113).*

Gamma activity (>30 Hz) can also be associated with cortical activation during auditory perception. Auditory stimuli induced a broad-band gamma activity (40 Hz, as well as 80–100 Hz) in ECoG of greater amplitude during presentation of phonemes than to tones.

13. EEG REACTIVITY AND NEUROLOGICAL DISORDERS

Although movement-related ERD/ERS were identified in patients with cerebrovascular disorders, these have not been systematically applied in diagnosis. Nonetheless, ERD/ERS analysis had been of interest not only to monitor recovery after stroke but also to provide online measurements of ERD and ERS during motor imagery and execution for biofeedback, with the objective of enhancing recovery after stroke (121). This is a new field of research supported by brain–computer interface (BCI) technology (see more details in Chapter 47). Recently it was shown that BCI-based ERD evaluation with somatosensory feedback can improve functional recovery from severe hemiplegia after stroke (122,123).

Early studies in Parkinson's disease (124–126) revealed that the pre-movement ERD is less lateralized over the contralateral sensorimotor area and is delayed compared to control subjects. In Parkinson's patients with unilateral predominant clinical signals, Labyt et al. (127) made an interesting comparison of the ERD/ERS in mu and beta frequency bands elicited by movements (finger extension or visually guided targeted movement) of the less akinetic and the more akinetic hand. They found that the simple finger extension made with the less akinetic limb elicited a pre-movement mu ERD focused over the contralateral central region, while the visually guided movement induced additional mu ERD over the contralateral

parietal region as well as an earlier ipsilateral mu ERD. When the same movements, however, were performed with the more affected hand, the contralateral ERD was delayed and the ERD induced by the visually guided movement occurred earlier, while the contralateral parietal ERD was absent. Furthermore, there was a clear post-movement beta ERS focused on the contralateral central area for the less affected hand, but this was remarkably attenuated for the more akinetic hand.

Treatment with L-dopa in patients with idiopathic Parkinson's disease can significantly reduce the delayed ERD onset (126). Further, it was reported that stimulation of the internal globus pallidus in Parkinson's patients can enhance the mu ERD before and during self-paced wrist movement (128). Interestingly, recordings in Parkinson's patients of local field potentials in subcortico-cortical loops linked to movement (125) showed ERD and ERS of mu, beta, and gamma rhythms. A study of the reaction of normal subjects and patients with Parkinson's disease to a postural perturbation, cued by a visual warning stimulus, showed that beta ERD exhibited differences between the two groups of subjects: Parkinson's patients displayed greater beta ERD than the normal subjects at the central electrode sites (CZ), and the increased beta ERD was associated with decreased adaptability of postural responses (129). These findings indicate that ERD/ERS studies can give interesting information regarding the pathophysiology of the dynamics of sensorimotor integration in Parkinson's patients.

REFERENCES

1. Berger, H. Uber das Elektrenkephalogramm des Menschen II. *J. Psychol. Neurol.* 1930;40:160–179.
2. Pfurtscheller, G., Aranibar, A. Evaluation of event-related desynchronization (ERD) preceding and following voluntary self-paced movements. *Electroencephalogr. Clin. Neurophysiol.* 1979;46:138–146.
3. Pfurtscheller, G., Lopes da Silva, F.H. Event-related EEG/MEG synchronization and desynchronization : basic principles. *Electroencephalogr. Clin. Neurophysiol* 1999;110:1842–1857.
4. Kalcher, J., Pfurtscheller, G. Discrimination between phase-locked and non-phase-locked event-related EEG activity. *Electroencephalogr. Clin. Neurophysiol.* 1995;94:381–483.
5. Kaufman, L., Schwartz, B., Salustri, C., et al. Modulation of spontaneous brain activity during mental imagery. *J. Cogn. Neurosci.* 1989;2:124–132
6. Clochon, P., Fontbonne, J.M., Lebrun, N., et al. A new method for quantifying EEG event-related desynchronization: amplitude envelope analysis. *Electroencephalogr. Clin. Neurophysiol.* 1996;98(2):126–129.
7. Knosche, T.R., Bastiaansen, M.C. On the time resolution of event-related desynchronization: a simulation study. *Clin. Neurophysiol.* 2002;113(5):754–763.
8. Neuper, C., Pfurtscheller, G. Event-related dynamics of cortical rhythms: frequency-specific features and functional correlates. *Int. J. Psychophysiol.* 2001;43:41–58.
9. Pfurtscheller, G., Stancak A. Jr. , Neuper, C. Post-movement beta synchronization. A correlate of an idling motor area? *Electroencephalogr. Clin. Neurophysiol.* 1996;98:281–293.
10. Pfurtscheller, G., Stancak A. Jr. , Edlinger, G. On the existence of different types of central beta rhythms below 30 Hz. *Electroencephalogr. Clin. Neurophysiol.* 1997;102:316–325.
11. Klimesch, W., Schimke, H., Schwaiger, J. Episodic and semantic memory: an analysis in the EEG theta and alpha band. *Electroencephalogr. Clin. Neurophysiol.* 1994;91:428–441.
12. Doppelmayr, M., Klimesch, W., Pachinger, T., et al. Individual differences in brain dynamics: important implications for the calculation of event-related band power measures. *Biol. Cybernet.* 1998;79:49–57.
13. Klimesch, W., Schimke, H., Doppelmayr, M., et al. Event–related desynchronization (ERD) and the Dm-effect: Does alpha desynchronization

during encoding predict later recall performance? *Int. J. Psychophysiol.* 1996;24:47–60.

14. Graimann, B., Huggins, J.E., Levine S.P., et al. Visualization of significant ERD/ERS patterns in multichannel EEG and ECoG data. *Clin. Neurophysiol.* 2002;113(1):43–47.

15. Alegre, M., Gurtubay, I.G., Labarga, A., et al. Alpha and beta oscillatory changes during stimulus-induced movement paradigms: effect of stimulus predictability. *Neuroreport* 2003;14(3):381–385.

16. Durka, P.J., Ircha, D., Neuper, C., et al. Time-frequency microstructure of electroencephalogram desynchronization and synchronization. *Med. Biol. Eng. Comput.* 2001;39(3):315–321.

17. Pfurtscheller, G., Klimesch, W. Functional topography during a visuo-verbal judgement task studied with event-related desynchronization mapping. *J. Clin. Neurophysiol.* 1992;9:120–131.

18. Van Winsum, W., Sergeant, J., Gueze, R. The functional significance of event-related desynchronization of alpha rhythms in attentional and activating tasks. *Electroencephalogr. Clin. Neurophysiol.* 1984;58:469–524.

19. Boiten, F., Sergeant, J., Geuze, R. Event-related desynchronization: the effects of energetic and computational demands. *Electroencephalogr. Clin. Neurophysiol.* 1992;82:302–309.

20. Dujardin, K., Derambure, P., Defebvre, L., et al. Evaluation of event-related desynchronization (ERD) during a recognition task: effect of attention. *Electroencephalogr. Clin. Neurophysiol.* 1993;86:353–356.

21. Sergeant, J., Geuze, R., Van Winsum, W. Event-related desynchronization and P300. *Psychophysiology* 1987;24:272–277.

22. Yordanova, J., Kolev, V., Polich, J. P300 and alpha event-related desynchronization (ERD). *Psychophysiology* 2001;38(1):143–152.

23. Klimesch, W. EEG alpha and theta oscillations reflect cognitive and memory performance: A review and analysis. *Brain Res. Rev.* 1999;29:169–195.

24. Klimesch, W., Pfurtscheller, G., Schimke, H. Pre- and poststimulus processes in category judgment tasks as measured by event-related desynchronization (ERD). *J. Psychophysiol.* 1992;6:186–203.

25. Bastiaansen, M.C.M., Böcker, K.B.E., Brunia, C.H.M., et al. Event-related desynchronization during anticipatory attention for an upcoming stimulus: a comparative EEG/EMG study. *Clin. Neurophysiol.* 2001;112:393–403.

26. Cassim, F., Monaca, C., Szurhaj, W., et al. Does post-movement beta synchronization reflect an idling motor cortex? *Neuroreport* 2001;12(17):3859–3863.

27. Derambure, P., Defebvre, L., Dujardin, K., et al. Effect of aging on the spatio-temporal pattern of event-related desynchronization during a voluntary movement. *Electroencephalogr. Clin. Neurophysiol.* 1993;89:197–203.

28. Pfurtscheller, G., Berghold, A. Patterns of cortical activation during planning of voluntary movement. *Electroencephalogr. Clin. Neurophysiol.* 1989;72:250–258.

29. Stancak A. Jr., Pfurtscheller, G. Event-related desynchronization of central beta rhythms in brisk and slow self-paced finger movements of dominant and non-dominant hand. *Cogn. Brain Res.* 1996;4:171–184.

30. Toro, C., Deuschl, G., Thatcher, R., et al. Event-related desynchronization and movement-related cortical potentials on the ECoG and EEG. *Electroencephalogr. Clin. Neurophysiol.* 1994;93:380–389.

31. Stancak A. Jr., Pfurtscheller, G. Mu-rhythm changes in brisk and slow self-paced finger movements. *Neuroreport* 1996;7:1161–1164.

32. Stancak A. Jr., Pfurtscheller, G. The effects of handedness and type of movement on the contralateral preponderance of mu-rhythm desynchronization. *Electroencephalogr. Clin. Neurophysiol.* 1996;99:174–182.

33. Pfurtscheller, G., Neuper, C., Krausz, G. Functional dissociation of lower and upper frequency mu rhythms in relation to voluntary limb movement. *Clin. Neurophysiol* 2000;111:1873–1879.

34. Beisteiner, R., Höllinger, P., Lindinger, G., et al. Mental representations of movements. Brain potentials associated with imagination of hand movements. *Electroencephalogr. Clin. Neurophysiol.* 1995;96:83–193.

35. Leocani, L., Magnani, G., Comi, G. Event-related desynchronization during execution, imagination and withholding of movement. In: Pfurtscheller, G., Lopes da Silva, F.H., eds. *Event-Related Desynchronization. Handbook of Electroencephalography and Clinical Neurophysiology*, revised ed. Amsterdam: Elsevier, 1999: vol. 6, 291–301.

36. Pfurtscheller, G., Neuper C. Motor imagery activates primary sensorimotor area in humans. *Neurosci. Lett.* 1997;239:65–68.

37. Decety, J. The neurophysiological basis of motor imagery. *Behav. Brain Res.* 1996;77:45–52.

38. Jeannerod, M. Mental imagery in the motor context. *Neuropsychologia* 1995;33(11):1419–1432.

39. Neuper, C., Pfurtscheller, G. Motor imagery and ERD. In: Pfurtscheller, G., Lopes da Silva, F.H., eds. *Event-Related Desynchronization. Handbook of Electroencephalography and Clinical Neurophysiology*, revised ed. Amsterdam: Elsevier, 1999; vol. 6, 303–325.

40. Avanzini, G., Fabbri-Destro, M., Volta, R.D. et al. The dynamics of sensorimotor oscillations during observation of hand movements: An EEG study. *PLoS ONE* 2012;7(5):e37534.

41. Porro, C.A., Francescato, M.P., Cettolo, V., et al. Primary motor and sensory cortex activation during motor performance and motor imagery: a functional magnetic resonance imaging study. *J. Neurosci.* 1996;16:7688–7698.

42. Roth, M., Decety, J., Raybaudi, M., et al. Possible involvement of primary motor cortex in mentally simulated movement: a functional magnetic resonance imaging study. *Neuroreport.* 1996;7:1280–1284.

43. Ehrsson, H.H., Geyer, S., Naito, E. Imagery of voluntary movement of fingers, toes and tongues activates corresponding body-part specific motor representations. *J. Neurophysiol.* 2003;90:3304–3316.

44. Rossi, S., Pasqualetti, P., Tecchio, F., et al. Corticospinal excitability modulation during mental simulation of wrist movements in human subjects. *Neurosci. Lett.* 1998;243:147–151.

45. Suffczynski, P., Kalitzin, S, Pfurtscheller, G., Lopes da Silva, F.H. Computational model of thalamo-cortical networks: dynamical control of alpha rhythms in relation to focal attention. *Int. J. Psychophysiol.* 2001;43:25–40.

46. Pfurtscheller, G. Event-related synchronization (ERS): an electrophysiological correlate of cortical areas at rest. *Electroencephalogr. Clin. Neurophysiol.* 1992;83:62–69.

47. Takemi, M., Masakado, Y., Liu, M., Ushiba, J. Event-related desynchronization reflects downregulation of intracortical inhibition in human primary motor cortex. *J. Neurophysiol.* 2013;110:1158–1166.

48. Klimesch, W., Doppelmayr, M., Russegger, H., et al. Theta band power in the human scalp EEG and the encoding of new information. *NeuroReport* 1996;7:1235–1240.

49. Sterman, M.B., Kaiser, D.A., Veigel, B. Spectral analysis of event-related EEG responses during short-term memory performance. *Brain Topogr.* 1996;9(1):21–30.

50. Defebvre, L., Bourriez, J.L., Destee, A., et al. Movement-related desynchronization pattern preceding voluntary movement in untreated Parkinson's disease. *J. Neurol. Neurosurg. Psychiatry* 1996;60:307–312.

51. Labyt, E., Szurhaj, W., Bourriez, J.L., et al. Influence of aging on cortical activity associated with a visuo-motor task. *Neurobiol. Aging* 2004;25(6):817–827.

52. Zhuang, P., Toro, C., Grafman, J., et al. Event-related desynchronization (ERD) in the alpha frequency during development of implicit and explicit learning. *Electroencephalogr. Clin. Neurophysiol.* 1997;102:374–381.

53. Pascual-Leone, A., Dang, N., Cohen, L.G., et al. Modulation of muscle responses evoked by transcranial magnetic stimulation during the acquisition of new fine motor skills. *J. Neurophysiol.* 1995;74:1037–1045.

54. Cooper, R., Winter, A.L., Crow, H.J., et al. Comparison of subcortical, cortical and scalp activity using chronically indwelling electrodes in man. *Electroencephalogr. Clin. Neurophysiol.* 1965;18:217–228.

55. Lopes da Silva, F.H. Neural mechanisms underlying brain waves: from neural membranes to networks. *Electroencephalogr. Clin. Neurophysiol.* 1991;79:81–93.

56. Lopes da Silva, F.H. EEG and MEG: relevance to neuroscience. *Neuron* 2013;80(5):1112–1128.

57. Braitenberg, V., Schuz, A. *Anatomy of the Cortex.* New York: Springer, 1991.

58. Klimesch, W. Memory processes, brain oscillations and EEG synchronization. *J. Psychophysiol.* 1996;24:61–100.

59. Adrian, E.D., Matthews, B.H. The Berger rhythm: potential changes from the occipital lobes in man. *Brain* 1934;57:355–385.

60. Ergenoglu, T., Demiralp, T., Bayraktaroglu, Z., et al. Alpha rhythm of the EEG modulates visual detection performance in humans. *Brain Res. Cogn. Brain Res.* 2004;20:376–383.

61. Hanslmayr, S., Asian, A., Staudigl, T., et al. Prestimulus oscillations predict visual perception performance between and within subjects. *Neuroimage* 2007;37:1465–1473.

62. Mathewson, K.E., Gratton, G., Fabiani, M., Beck, D.M., Ro, T. To see or not to see: prestimulus alpha phase predicts visual awareness. *J. Neurosci.* 2009;29:2725–2732.

63. Haegens, S., Nacher, V., Luna, R., Romo, R., Jensen, O. Alpha-oscillations in the monkey sensorimotor network influence discrimination performance by rhythmical inhibition of neuronal spiking. *Proc. Natl. Acad. Sci. USA* 2011;108:19377–19382.

64. Pfurtscheller, G., Neuper, C. Event-related synchronization of mu rhythm in the EEG over the cortical hand area in man. *Neurosci. Lett.* 1994;174:93–96.

65. Gerloff, C., Hadley, J., Richard, J., et al. Functional coupling and regional activation of human cortical motor areas during simple, internally paced and externally paced finger movements. *Brain* 1998;121:1463–1531.

66. Koshino, Y., Niedermeyer, E. Enhancement of rolandic mu-rhythm by pattern vision. *Electroencephalogr. Clin. Neurophysiol.* 1975;38:535–538.

67. Kreitmann, N., Shaw, J.C. Experimental enhancement of alpha activity. *Electroencephalogr. Clin. Neurophysiol.* 1965;18:147–155.
68. Jones, S.R., Kerr, C.E., Wan, Q., Pritchett, D.L., Hämäläinen, M., Moore, C.I. Cued spatial attention drives functionally relevant modulation of the mu rhythm in primary somatosensory cortex. *J. Neurosci.* 2010;30:13760–13765.
69. Popov, T., Steffen, A., Weisz, N., Miller, G.A., Rockstroh, B. Cross-frequency dynamics of neuromagnetic oscillatory activity: two mechanisms of emotion regulation. *Psychophysiology* 2012;49:1545–1557.
70. Drevets, W., Burton, H., Videen, T., Snyder, A., Simpson, J., Raichle, M. Blood flow changes in human somatosensory cortex during anticipated stimulation. *Nature* 1995;373(6511):198–199.
71. Goldman, R.I., Stern, J.M., Engel, J., Cohen, M. Simultaneous EEG and fMRI of the alpha rhythm. *NeuroReport* 2002;13(18):2487–2492.
72. Laufs, H., Krakow, K., Sterzer, P., et al. Electroencephalographic signatures of attentional and cognitive default modes in spontaneous brain fluctuations at rest. *Proc. Natl. Acad. Sci. USA* 2003;100(19):11053–11058.
73. Moosmann, M., Ritter, P., Krastel, I., et al. Correlates of alpha rhythm in functional magnetic resonance imaging and near infrared spectroscopy. *Neuroimage* 2003;20:145–158.
74. De Munck, J.C., Gonçalves, S.I., Mammoliti, R., Heethaar, R.M., Lopes da Silva, F. Interactions between different EEG frequency bands and their effect on alpha-fMRI correlations. *Neuroimage* 2009;47:69–76.
75. Hummel, F., Andres, F., Altenmuller, E., Dichgans J., Gerloff, C. Inhibitory control of acquired motor programmes in the human brain. *Brain* 2002;125:404–420.
76. Hummel, F.C., Gerloff, C. Interregional long-range and short-range synchrony: a basis for complex sensorimotor processing. *Prog. Brain Res.* 2006;159:223–236.
77. Kelly, S.P., Lalor, E.C., Reilly, R.B., Foxe, J.J. Increases in alpha oscillatory power reflect an active retinotopic mechanism for distracter suppression during sustained visuospatial attention. *J. Neurophysiol.* 2006;95:3844–3851.
78. Rihs, T.A., Michel, C.M., Thut, G. Mechanisms of selective inhibition in visual spatial attention are indexed by alpha-band EEG synchronization. *Eur. J. Neurosci.* 2007;25:603–610
79. Worden, M.S., Foxe, J.J., Wang, N., Simpson, G.V. Anticipatory biasing of visuospatial attention indexed by retinotopically specific alpha band electroencephalography increases over occipital cortex. *J. Neurosci.* 2000;20:RC63.
80. Medendorp, W.P., Kramer, G.F., Jensen, O., et al. Oscillatory activity in human parietal and occipital cortex shows hemispheric lateralization and memory effects in a delayed double-step saccade task. *Cereb. Cortex* 2007;17:2364–2374.
81. Anderson, K.L., Ding, M. Attentional modulation of the somatosensory mu rhythm. *Neuroscience* 2011;180:165–180.
82. Mazaheri, A., van Schouwenberg, M.R., Dimitrijevic, A., et al. Region-specific modulations in oscillatory alpha activity serve to facilitate processing in the visual and auditory modalities. *Neuroimage* 2014;87:356–362.
83. Pesonen, M., Haarala Björnberg, C., Hämäläinen, H., Krause, C.M. Brain oscillatory 1–30 Hz EEG ERD/ERS responses during the different stages of an auditory memory search task. *Neurosci. Lett.* 2006;309:45–50.
84. Jensen, O., Gelfand, J., Kounios, J., Lisman, J.E. Oscillations in the alpha band (9–12Hz) increase with memory load during retention in a short-term memory task. *Cereb. Cortex* 2002;12:887–882.
85. Sauseng,P., Klimesch, W., Gerloff, C., Hummel, F.C. Spontaneous locally restricted EEG alpha activity determines cortical excitability in the motor cortex. *Neuropsychologia* 2009;47:284–288.
86. Salmelin, R., Hamalainen, M., Kajola, M., et al. Functional segregation of movement-related rhythmic activity in the human brain. *Neuroimage* 1995;2:237–243.
87. Neuper, C., Pfurtscheller, G. Post-movement synchronization of beta rhythms in the EEG over the cortical foot area in man. *Neurosci. Lett.* 1996;216:17–20.
88. Neuper, C., Pfurtscheller, G. Evidence for distinct beta resonance frequencies related to specific sensorimotor cortical areas. *Clin. Neurophysiol.* 2001;112(11):2084–2097.
89. Pfurtscheller, G., Neuper, C., Pichler-Zalaudek, K., et al. Do brain oscillations of different frequencies indicate interaction between cortical areas in humans? *Neurosci. Lett.* 2000;286:66–68.
90. Pfurtscheller, G., Krausz, G., Neuper, C. Mechanical stimulation of the fingertip can induce bursts of beta oscillations in sensorimotor areas. *J. Clin. Neurophysiol.* 2001;18(6):559–564.
91. Pfurtscheller, G., Solis-Escalante, T. Could the beta rebound in the EEG be suitable to realize a "brain switch"? *Clin. Neurophysiol.* 2009;120:24–29.
92. Hari, R. Action-perception connection and the cortical mu rhythm. *Prog. Brain Res.* 2006;159:253–260.
93. Chen, R., Yassen, Z., Cohen, L.G., et al. The time course of corticospinal excitability in reaction time and self-paced movements. *Ann. Neurol.* 1998;44:317–325.
94. Chen, R., Corwell, B., Hallett M. Modulation of motor cortex excitability by median nerve and digit stimulation. *Exp. Brain Res.* 1999;129:77–86.
95. Schnitzler, A., Salenius, S., Salmelin, R., et al. Involvement of primary motor cortex in motor imagery: a neuromagnetic study. *Neuroimage* 1997;6(3):201–208.
96. Pfurtscheller, G., Woertz, M., Müller, G., et al. Contrasting behavior of beta event-related synchronization and somatosensory evoked potential after median nerve stimulation during finger manipulation in man. *Neurosci. Lett.* 2002;323:113–116.
97. Zhang, Y., Chen, Y., Bressler, S.L., Ding, M. Response preparation and inhibition: The role of the cortical sensorimotor beta rhythm. *Neuroscience* 2008;156:238–246
98. Alegre, M., Gurtubay, I.G., Labarga, A., et al. Frontal and central oscillatory changes related to different aspects of the motor process: a study in go/no-go paradigms. *Exp. Brain Res.*, 2004;159:14–22
99. Pfurtscheller, G., Solis-Escalante, T., Barry, R.J., et al. Brisk heart rate and EEG changes during execution and withholding of cue-paced foot motor imagery. *Front. Hum. Neurosci.* 2013;7: 379.
100. Solis-Escalante, T., Müller-Putz, G., Pfurtscheller, G., Neuper, C. Cue-induced beta rebound during withholding of overt and covert foot movement. *Clin. Neurophysiol.* 2012;123:1182–1190.
101. Thayer, J.F., Lane, R.D. Claude Bernard and the heart-brain connection: Further elaboration of a model of neurovisceral integration. *Neurosci. Biobehav. Rev.* 2009;33(2):81–88.
102. Haggard, P. Conscious intention and motor cognition. *Trends Cogn. Sci.* 2005;9(6):290–295.
103. Barry, B. Promise versus reality in relation to the unitary orienting reflex: A case study examining the role of theory in psychophysiology. *Int. J. Psychophysiol.* 2006;62:353–366.
104. Pfurtscheller, G., Neuper, C.,Kalcher, J. 40-Hz oscillations during motor behavior in man. *Neurosci. Lett.* 1993;162(1–2):179–182.
105. Crone, N.E., Miglioretti, D.L., Gordon, B., et al. Functional mapping of human sensorimotor cortex with electrocorticographic spectral analysis. II. Event-related synchronization in the gamma band. *Brain* 1998;121:2301–2315.
106. Pfurtscheller, G., Graimann, B., Huggins, J.E., et al. Spatiotemporal patterns of beta desynchronization and gamma synchronization in corticographic data during self-paced movement. *Clin. Neurophysiol.* 2003;114:1226–1236.
107. Siegel, M., Donner, T.H., Oostenveld, R., Fries, P., Engel, A.K. Neural synchronisation along the dorsal visual pathway reflects the focus of spatial attention. *Neuron* 2008;60(4):709–719.
108. Van Kerkoerle, T., Self, M.W., Dagnino, B., et al. Alpha and gamma oscillations characterize feedback and feedforward processing in monkey visual cortex. *Proc. Natl. Acad. Sci. USA* 2014;111(40):14332–14341.
109. Jensen, O., Bonnefond, M., Marshall, T.R., Tiesinga, P. Oscillatory mechanisms of feedforward and feedback visual processing. *Trends Neurosci.* 2015;38(4):192–194.
110. Bressler, S.L., Coppola, R., Nakamura, R. Episodic multi-regional cortical coherence at multiple frequencies during visual task performance. *Nature* 1993;366:153–156.
111. Andrew, C., Pfurtscheller, G. Event-related coherence as a tool for studying dynamic interaction of brain regions. *Electroencephalogr. Clin. Neurophysiol.* 1996;98:144–148.
112. Foster, B.L., Parvizi, J. Resting oscillations and cross-frequency coupling in the human posteromedial cortex. *Neuroimage.* 2012;60(1):384–391.
113. Pfurtscheller, G., Daly, I., Bauernfeind, G., Müller-Putz, G.R. Coupling between intrinsic prefrontal Hbo2 and central EEG beta power oscillations in the resting brain. *PLoS ONE.* 2012;7(8):1–9.
114. Stancak, A. Jr., Riml, A., Pfurtscheller, G. Effects of external load on movement-related changes of sensorimotor EEG rhythms. *Electroencephalogr. Clin. Neurophysiol.* 1997;102:495–504.
115. Fox, M.D., Snyder, A.Z., Vincent, J.L., Raichle, M.E. Intrinsic fluctuations within cortical systems account for intertrial variability in human behavior. *Neuron* 2007;56(1):171–184.
116. Crone, N.E., Miglioretti, D.L., Gordon, B., et al. Functional mapping of human sensorimotor cortex with electrocorticographic spectral analysis. I. Alpha and beta event-related desynchronization. *Brain* 1998;121:2271–2299.
117. Ohara, S., Ikeda, A., Kunieda, T., et al. Movement-related change of electrocorticographic activity in human supplementary motor area proper. *Brain* 2000;123:1203–1215.
118. Sochurkova, D., Rektor, I. Event-related desynchronization/synchronization in the putamen. An SEEG case study. *Exp. Brain Res.* 2003;149(3):401–404.

119. Szurhaj, W., Derambure, P., Labyt, E., et al. Basic mechanisms of central rhythms reactivity to preparation and execution of voluntary movement: a stereoencephalographic study. *Clin. Neurophysiol.* 2003;114(1):107–119.

120. Crone, N.E., Boatman, D., Gordon, B., et al. Induced electrocorticographic gamma activity during auditory perception. *Clin. Neurophysiol.* 2001;112:565–582.

121. Kaiser, V., Daly, I., Pichiurri, F., et al. Relationship between electrical brain responses to motor imagery and motor impairment in stroke. *Stroke* 2012;43(10):2735–2740.

122. Ramos-Manguialday, A., Broetz, D., Rea, M., et al. Brain-machine interface in chronic stroke rehabilitation: A controlled study. *Ann. Neurol.* 2013;74:100–108.

123. Ono, T., Shindo, K., Kawashima, K., et al. Brain-computer interface with somatosensory feedback improves functional recovery from severe hemiplegia due to chronic stroke. *Front. Neuroeng.* 2001;19:1–18.

124. Defebvre, L., Bourriez, J.L., Dujardin, K., et al. Spatiotemporal study of Bereitschaftspotential and event-related desynchronization during voluntary movement in Parkinson's disease. *Brain Topogr.* 1994;6:237–244.

125. Devos, D. Defebvre, L. Effect of deep brain stimulation and L-Dopa on electrocortical rhythms related to movement in Parkinson's disease. *Prog. Brain Res.* 2006;159:331–349.

126. Magnani, G., Cursi, M., Leocani, L., et al. Acute effects of L-dopa on event-related desynchronization in Parkinson's disease. *Neurol. Sci.* 2002;23(3):91–97.

127. Labyt, E., Devos, D., Bourriez, J.L., et al. Motor preparation is more impaired in Parkinson's disease when sensorimotor integration is involved. *Clin. Neurophysiol.* 2003;114(12):2423–2433.

128. Devos, D., Derambure, P., Bourriez, J.L., et al. Influence of internal globus pallidus stimulation on motor cortex activation pattern in Parkinson's disease. *Clin. Neurophysiol.* 2002;113:1110–1120.

129. Smith, B.A., Jacobs, J.V., Horak, F.B. Effect of magnitude and magnitude predictability of postural perturbations on preparatory cortical activity in older adults with and without Parkinson's disease. *Exp. Brain Res.* 2012;222(4): 455–470.

41 | VISUAL EVOKED POTENTIALS AND ELECTRORETINOGRAMS

GASTONE G. CELESIA, MD AND NEAL S. PEACHEY, PHD

ABSTRACT: Electrophysiological testing of vision permits the objective assessment of the function of the retina, visual pathways, and cortices. This chapter covers visual evoked potentials (VEPs) and electroretinography (ERG). Flash ERG is useful in evaluating the outer retinal function and specifically helping in the diagnosis of retinal degeneration, monitoring the progress of retinal diseases, monitoring the retinal toxicity of drugs, and understanding the pathophysiology of retinal disorders. VEPs to various stimuli are useful in evaluating macular disorders, diagnosing optic neuropathies, detecting silent pathologies in the absence of other clinical signs of visual impairment, and evaluating disturbances of visual processing in degenerative diseases of the central nervous system. Simultaneous recording of pattern ERG and pattern VEP permits the differentiation between maculopathies and optic neuropathy.

KEYWORDS: vision, visual evoked potentials, retina, electroretinogram, VEP, ERG, retinal degeneration, macular, optic neuropathy

PRINCIPAL REFERENCES

1. Celesia GG. *Disorders of visual processing.* Amsterdam: Elsevier, 2005.
2. Heckenlively JR, Arden GB. *Principles and practice of clinical electrophysiology of vision.* Cambridge, MA: MIT, 2006.
3. Hubel DH. *Eye, brain, and vision.* New York: Scientific American Library, 1995.
4. Kaas J, Collins CE. *The primate visual system.* Boca Raton: CRC Press, 2004.
5. Regan D. *Human brain electrophysiology. Evoked potentials and evoked magnetic fields in science and medicine.* New York: Elsevier, 1989.
6. Zeki S. *A vision of the brain.* Oxford: Blackwell, 1993.

1. INTRODUCTION

The visual system can be studied noninvasively by recording field potentials from the surface of the cornea or the scalp overlying the visual cortex. Retinal potentials recorded at the cornea constitute the electroretinogram (ERG) and reflect the initial processes of phototransduction and retinal transmission. Cortical potentials constitute the visual evoked potential (VEP) and reflect the output features of the entire visual pathways. ERGs were first recorded directly from the eye by Holmgren in 1865 (1). However, the routine use of ERGs in clinical practice did not occur until the development of reliable differential amplifiers and safe contact lenses in the 1950s. ERGs evoked by bright flashes can reach amplitudes of several hundred microvolts (uV) and reflect the activity of retinal photoreceptors and the early retinal pathways (2). Utilization of chromatic stimuli under scotopic (dark-adapted) and photopic (light-adapted) conditions allows, respectively, the rod and cone pathways to be examined separately (1–3).

VEPs were initially recorded in animals directly from the striate cortex; they could not be recorded from the scalp due to their small amplitude. VEP recording from the scalp became feasible with the introduction of summation and computer averaging techniques. The functional integrity of the visual pathways can be evaluated by VEPs (4,5). Furthermore, manipulation of visual stimuli permits the preferential evaluation of the various segments of the visual pathways (5). The clinician applying these technologies to the study of the visual system must be aware that, as Floyd Ratliff (6) stated, "There is no 'best method' of stimulus control or of data analysis in the study of visual evoked potentials"; rather, recordings and stimulation must be tailored to the clinical problem to be studied. Evaluation of peripheral retinal function, for example, can be achieved best by flash ERG techniques, whereas optic nerve function may be assessed by pattern-reversal VEPs. In this chapter, evaluations of retinal function, anterior visual pathways, and retrochiasmal pathway function are discussed separately.

2. RETINA

2.1. Retinal Anatomy and Function

The eye is an optical device. The pupil controls the amount of light that enters the eye, and its diameter is controlled by the iris, a diaphragm that can be contracted or dilated by the ciliary muscles. Light entering the eye must pass through normally transparent media (the cornea, the aqueous humor, the lens, and the vitreous humor) to reach the retina. A prerequisite for normal retinal function is an intact optic system, and in the evaluation of visual function, one must always be aware of the optical status of the eye. Thus, while visual neurons may be intact, a cataract will impair transmittance of a pattern stimulus from reaching the retina and will result in abnormal retinal and/or visual cortical function.

The retina is a neuronal membrane lining the back of the eye chamber (7,8). The retina contains five types of neurons: photoreceptors, horizontal cells, bipolar cells, amacrine cells, and ganglion cells. These and other non-neuronal cells are organized into eight cellular and synaptic layers (Fig. 41.1) and two limiting membranes, which, from outer to inner, are referred to as follows:

1. The retinal pigmented epithelium made up of cells containing melatonin

2. The Pigmented layer (PL), housing retinal pigment epithelial cells

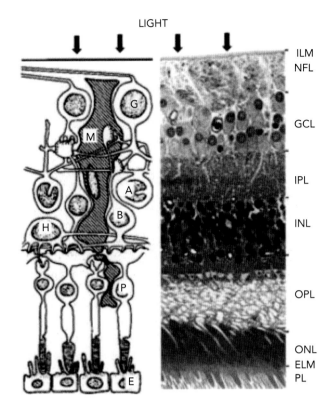

LIGHT

ILM
NFL

GCL

IPL

INL

OPL

ONL
ELM
PL

Figure 41.1. Left: *Diagram of the cellular components of the retina. G, ganglion cells; M, glial Müller cells; A, amacrine cells; B, bipolar cells; H, horizontal cells; E, pigmented epithelium; P, photoreceptors. Right: Photomicrograph of a radial section of the human parafoveal retina illustrating its laminar organization. The layers are PL, photoreceptor layer; ELM, external limiting membrane; ONL, outer nuclear layer; OPL, outer plexiform layer; INL, inner nuclear layer; IPL, inner plexiform layer; GCL, ganglion cell layer; NFL, nerve fiber layer; and ILM, internal limiting membrane. Modified from Brown (10) and Dacheu (11).*

3. External limiting membrane (ELM) formed by the endfeet of retinal Müller glial cells

4. Outer nuclear layer (ONL) containing fibers and bodies of photoreceptors

5. Outer plexiform layer (OPL) containing photoreceptors horizontal and bipolar cells

6. Inner nuclear layer (INL) containing the bodies of horizontal, bipolar amacrine, interplexiform and Müller cells

7. Inner plexiform layer (IPL) containing dendrites of bipolar, amacrine and ganglion synapsing with each other cells

8. Ganglion cell layer (GCL) (9–12) containing the bodies of ganglion cells, displaced amacrine cells ant the feet of Müller cells.

9. Nerve fiber layer (NFL) containing ganglion cell axons

10. The inner limiting membrane (ILM) consists of the basal lamina between the foot processes of ther Müller cells and the vitreous body.

Neuronal connections are made primarily in two synaptic layers: the OPL and the IPL. Retinal neurons are organized

within the ONL (rod and cone photoreceptors), INL (horizontal, bipolar, amacrine and Müller glial cells), and GCL (retinal ganglion and displaced amacrine cells). The OPL contains the synaptic connections between photoreceptors and their second-order neurons (horizontal and bipolar cells) while the IPL contains synapses between bipolar, amacrine, and ganglion cells. Detailed reviews of retinal anatomy have been published (11–14).

The outer surface of the retina is delimited by the retinal pigment epithelium (RPE). The RPE is critically involved in many activities required for normal retinal function, including the flow of nutrients and waste products between the photoreceptor and the choroidal circulation, the visual cycle by which light-sensitive photopigments are regenerated, and the phagocytosis of outer-segment disks, which are shed on a daily basis (15,16).

In the retina, there are two classes of photoreceptors: cones and rods. The human retina is rod-dominated, containing only about 5% cones (15). Photoreceptors have three highly specialized compartments: (1) the outer segment contains the light-sensitive photopigments along with the phototransduction machinery, which are organized into a series of bilipid membrane disks; (2) the inner segment houses the nucleus and cellular organelles, including mitochondria; and (3) the photoreceptor terminal contains synapses where glutamate is released to communicate with second-order neurons. All rods contain the same photopigment, rhodopsin. In the human retina, there are three types of cones differentiated by the photopigment contained in the outer segment: short-wavelength (420 mm or blue), medium-wavelength (531 mm or green), and long-wavelength (558 mm or red) cones (8–13). Visual pigments are activated by light and initiate a phototransduction cascade that culminates in the closure of ion channels along the outer segment membrane, membrane hyperpolarization, and a consequent reduction in the rate of neurotransmitter release at the synaptic terminal (16). In the human eye, the amplification gained from the phototransduction cascade is such that a visual sensation can result from one quantal absorption in only three rod photoreceptors (17). Rods are responsible for high-sensitivity vision in darkness, whereas the activity of spectrally different cones is processed in the inner retina to extract wavelength information.

The central transmission of rod and cone activity differs in other ways. For example, information from rods is carried by one primary pathway, from rods to rod depolarizing bipolar cells (DBCs), to rod amacrine cells, and then to on- and off-center ganglion cells via an excitatory synapse to cone DBCs and an inhibitory signal to cone hyperpolarizing bipolar cells (HBCs) (18–21). Cone activity is carried through DBCs and also HBCs, and then to the on- and off-center ganglion cells. Information from medium-wavelength and long-wavelength cones are segregated at the bipolar cell level into ON and OFF retino-geniculo-cortical pathways (22,23). Short-wavelength cones convey their signals through DBCs, but a short-wavelength-cone HBC is absent in the primate retina. Lateral inhibitory connections, mediated by horizontal and amacrine cells, form the basis for the development of antagonistic receptive fields, which are instrumental in the coding of spatial patterns and contrast (24). Chromatic information is derived from circuits comparing the responses of the different types of cone photoreceptors. The net result is that the output of the photoreceptors is extensively processed by the time that corresponding signal exits the retina via ganglion cell axons that form the optic nerve and project to the lateral geniculate nucleus (LGN) and from there to the visual cortex.

Different regions of the retina are specialized for different functions. These are mirrored by changes in the organization of the retinal architecture (24–27). For example (Fig. 41.2), the best acuity is achieved by the central part of the fovea, the foveola. This region contains only cones in a highly ordered packing. Moreover, each foveal cone makes contact with only a single bipolar and ganglion cell of each class (28,29). As a result, the response of each foveal cone is transmitted with high fidelity through the retina. Across the retina, Frisen and Frisen (28) have shown that the decrease in visual acuity that

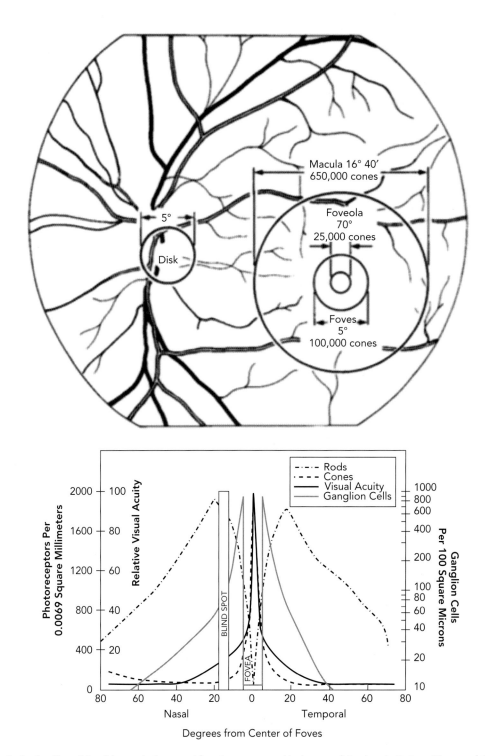

Figure 41.2. Top: *Ocular fundus. Sizes of the disk, macula, fovea, and foveola are expressed in degrees of visual angle.* Bottom: *Diagram of the distribution of photoreceptors (rods and cones) and ganglion cells and their relationship to visual acuity. Data on visual acuity from Jones and Higgins (24), distribution of rods and cones from Osterberg (25), distribution of ganglion cells from Van Buren (26) and Oppel (27). Note the logarithmic scale for the ganglion cell distribution.*

occurs at more peripheral locations is highly correlated with the decrease in ganglion cell density. In comparison, the retinal region with the best sensitivity to light is located some 20 to 30 degrees away. This sensitivity increase reflects the increased concentration of rods in the periphery (see Fig. 41.2) and the increased degree of synaptic convergence that is achieved at more peripheral locations.

Ganglion cells transmit information to the LGN via action potentials. Each ganglion cell responds to light stimulation only in a certain retinal area called the receptive field. If stimulation of the center of the receptive field induces on-discharges, stimulation of the periphery produces off-discharges (28). This center-surround opponent arrangement (29,30) represents a key initial coding step of the central visual system (Fig. 41.3). There are three major classes of ganglion cells: midget cells represent 80% of the ganglion cell population and make up the parvocellular (P) pathway; parasol cells represent 5% to 8% of ganglion cells and constitute the magnocellular (M) pathway; and bistratified ganglion cells represent 5% to 10% of cells and constitute the koniocellular (K) pathways. Consistent with their small size, parvocellular cells have a small receptive field, are slow-conducting, have a

color opponency mechanism (i.e., red center, green surround spectral opponency), and have a fine spectral discrimination. The magnocellular cells have high conduction velocity and a center-surround opponent mechanism and provide analysis of movement. The koniocellular cells have no center-surround mechanisms. The function of the koniocellular pathway is less clear; it processes blue-ON information from the S-cone retinal input and may also be involved in processing moving stimuli (31–33). The reader is referred to the literature for a more extensive review of the electrophysiology of the retina (8,12,13).

To summarize, rods are responsible for achromatic scotopic (night) vision, while cones are activated by color. There are three types of cones: short-wavelength (blue), medium-wavelength (green), and long-wavelength (red) cones. Photoreceptors via visual pigments transduce light into electrical signals that activate the neuronal retina. The retina starts the initial steps of visual processing and contains four types of neurons: horizontal, bipolar, amacrine, and ganglion cells. Ganglion cells transmit information to the lateral geniculate body via action potentials. Three functional pathways originate in the retina: the parvocellular, magnocellular, and koniocellular pathways.

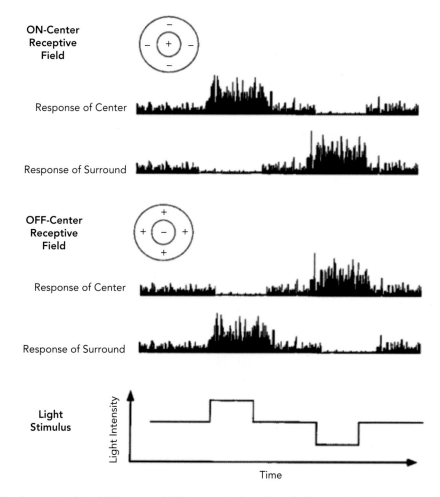

Figure 41.3. *Receptive profiles for receptive field of ON-center and OFF-center retinal ganglion cells. The receptive fields shown represent an area of the retina that, when stimulated by an increment or decrement of light, affects the response of the cell. The cell's response will depend on whether the central or annular region is stimulated in the receptive field. The response elicited from stimulation of each region, represented as the cumulative sum of action potentials over time, is shown on the right. Note how responses from the center and surround are always complementary to each other. Modified from Celesia and De Marco (30).*

2.2. Clinical Applications

Many aspects of retinal function can be studied by ERG. Manipulation of visual stimuli permits evaluation of the functional integrity of photoreceptors and retina neuronal circuitry. Three general ERG protocols have been used in clinical practice: flash ERGs, multifocal ERGs, and pattern ERGs.

In response to the short-duration (1 msec) stimuli typically used in clinical settings, the ERG is composed of two major components, the "a wave" and the "b wave," as well as a series of higher-frequency oscillatory potentials (OPs) (2,3). The source of these underlying components has been investigated by intracellular and intraretinal recordings as well as by using pharmacologic agents that selectively interfere with different aspects of retinal function (12,13,18,20,28–30,34,35). The cornea-negative a wave reflects in large measure the massed response of the rod or cone photoreceptors, although postreceptoral contributions are clearly present (36–39).

In comparison, the cells that contribute to the cornea-positive b wave change depending on whether stimulus conditions elicit rod- or cone-mediated potentials. Under dark-adapted conditions, which isolate rod-mediated responses, the b wave reflects the activity of the rod DBCs. Under stimulus conditions that isolate cone-mediated activity, the b wave reflects the combined activity of both DBCs and HBCs (34–41). OPs are generated in the IPL; while not completely understood, they likely reflect the activity of amacrine and interplexiform neuronal cells (2,40).

The International Society for Clinical Electrophysiology of Vision (ISCEV) has defined a standard ERG testing protocol for clinical purposes (42). The standard incorporates a series of stimulus conditions designed to isolate rod-mediated responses by presenting stimuli to the dark-adapted eye and cone-mediated responses by rapid flicker and light adaptation. The ISCEV standard for clinical ERGs specifies six response including the background adaptation and the flash strength (Fig. 41.4):

1. Dark-adapted 0.01 ERG (rod ERG)

2. Dark-adapted 3.0 ERG (combined rod and cone standard flash ERG)

3. Dark-adapted 10 ERG (strong flash ERG)

4. Dark-adapted 3 oscillatory potentials

5. Light-adapted 3 ERG (standard flash "cone" ERG)

6. Light-adapted 30 Hz flicker ERG (42)

The ISCEV guidelines are meant to define the minimal stimulus and recording conditions for a meaningful clinical ERG, and it is important to recognize that ISCEV "encourages the use of additional ERG protocols for testing beyond this minimum standard" for research studies and for clinical evaluation (42). In our laboratory we routinely use blue and red flashes under scotopic conditions as well as yellow-red and blue-green flashes in light-adapted conditions (Fig. 41.5). In addition, the standard addresses other important issues such as electrodes, amplifier settings, stimulus calibration, and the establishment of normative data.

Flash ERGs have important applications:

1. To evaluate outer retinal function, which is of particular relevance to the diagnosis of hereditary and acquired retinal degenerations

2. To monitor the progress of retinal disease within an individual patient

3. To monitor the potential retinal toxicity of drugs

4. To understand the pathophysiology of retinal disorders

The flash ERG is particularly useful in the diagnosis of retinal pigmentary degeneration (Fig. 41.6). The ERG is reduced in amplitude or absent in retinitis pigmentosa (RP) (43–45). RP is an inherited retinal dystrophy involving multiple genes (retnet.org). The initial stages of RP affect predominantly the rods; cones are affected only at advanced stages. In the early

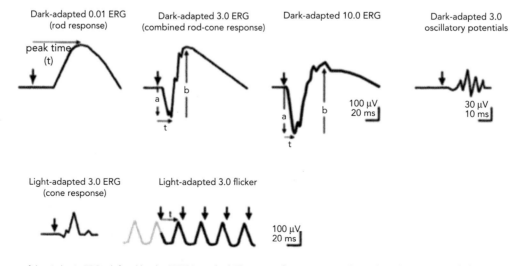

Figure 41.4. Diagram of the six basic ERGs defined by the ISCEV standard. These waveforms are exemplary only and are not intended to indicate minimum, maximum, or typical values. Bold arrowheads indicate the stimulus flash; solid arrows illustrate a-wave and b-wave amplitude; horizontal arrows exemplify how to measure time to peak (t implicit time or latency). Reproduced with permission from McCulloch, Marmor, Brigell, et al. (42).

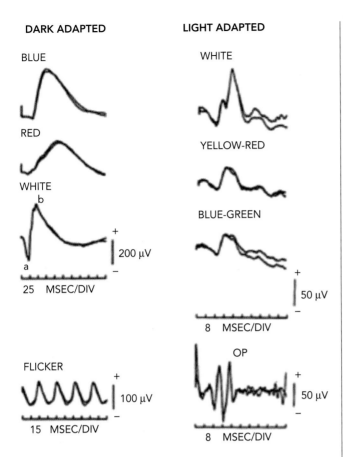

DARK ADAPTED   LIGHT ADAPTED

BLUE

RED

WHITE
b

a

+

−

200 µV

25   MSEC/DIV

FLICKER

+

−

100 µV

15   MSEC/DIV

WHITE

YELLOW-RED

BLUE-GREEN

+

−

50 µV

8   MSEC/DIV

OP

+

−

50 µV

8   MSEC/DIV

Figure 41.5. Flash ERGs in a normal 32-year-old man. Two ERGs tracings are superimposed to demonstrate reproducibility. The left column represents ERGs to dim suprathresold and scotopically matched blue and red flashes, to white flashes, and to 32-Hz flicker in the absence of background light. The right column represents ERGs to white and photopically matched yellow-red and blue-green flashes in the presence of background light. OP refers to oscillatory potentials obtained by selected filtering at 100–500 Hz. Note the different time and amplitude calibration for the various ERGs.

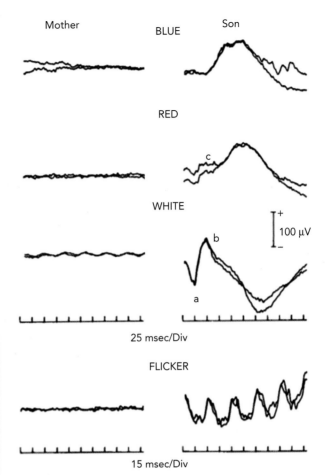

Mother   BLUE   Son

RED
c

WHITE
b

a

+

−

100 µV

25 msec/Div

FLICKER

15 msec/Div

Figure 41.6. Full-field flash ERG in two members of a family. The mother (left) suffers from retinitis pigmentosa; her central vision is spared, although her peripheral vision is severely affected. She has nyctalopia. Note the absence of any recognizable ERG. The son (right), age 15, has normal fundus and normal visual acuity. The dark-adapted ERGs show small-amplitude b wave, particularly to red and white light, suggesting early rod dysfunction. The flicker ERG is normal, indicating normal cone function. a = a wave; b = b wave; c = cone response. Modified from Celesia (182).

stages RP patients have involvement limited to the dark-adapted rod ERG response, accompanied by impaired night vision (nyctalopia). As the disease progresses, they show evidence of impaired cone vision, including reduced amplitude of light-adapted ERG responses. In RP patients, a reduced dark-adapted b-wave amplitude with normal b-wave latency (often referred to as implicit time) indicates a focal disease that leaves segments of the retina normal and able to respond to light with normal latency (46). A general rule of flash ERG is that conditions that preserve latency in the presence of decreased amplitude are focal or patchy retinal disorders. In comparison, ERGs of prolonged latency indicate diffuse retinal disease, as most retinal cells respond abnormally to the stimulus. Early reduction in amplitude and prolongation of latency of dark-adapted rod responses have been found, even before classic funduscopic changes appear, in subjects with dominantly inherited RP. Reduced amplitude and prolonged latencies in the dark-adapted rod responses were also found in female carriers of X-linked RP (47,48). Therefore, the ERG is a useful adjunct to genetic counseling for carriers and young subjects (see Fig. 41.6) in families with a history of retinal pigmentary degeneration.

Other inherited retinal diseases demonstrate a more selective involvement of rod or cone systems. Congenital stationary night blindness is characterized by impaired night vision, normal daylight vision, and normal fundi. In these patients the ERG (49) shows normal cone amplitude with abnormal rod function with absent or severe reduction of the dark-adapted/scotopic b wave (Fig. 41.7). Oguchi disease, another form of night blindness, is characterized by diffuse graying of the fundus and specific ERG changes (50). The dark-adapted/scotopic ERG shows low-amplitude or absent b waves similar to the ERG of congenital nyctalopes. However, if the eye is allowed to adapt to darkness for an extended period (more than 12 hours), a normal b wave can be obtained. Congenital achromatopsia (rod monochromatism) affects the cone system selectively. It is characterized by absent color vision and impaired visual acuity. The ERG (see Fig. 41.7) shows normal b waves in the dark-adapted state but no cone responses (49,50).

The ERG is also useful in evaluating paraneoplastic retinopathies. Cancer-associated retinopathy (CAR) involves photoreceptor degeneration, with an attendant decline in overall

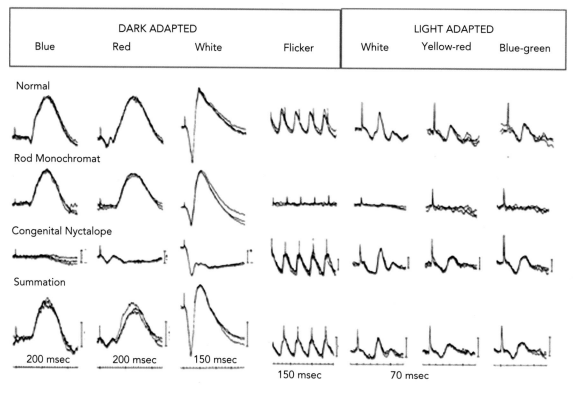

DARK ADAPTED				LIGHT ADAPTED		
Blue	Red	White	Flicker	White	Yellow-red	Blue-green

Normal

Rod Monochromat

Congenital Nyctalope

Summation

200 msec   200 msec   150 msec

150 msec   70 msec

Figure 41.7. Left: *Under the dark-adapted column are three superimposed single-trace ERGs elicited by standard, dim, full-field, scotopically matched, blue, red, white flashes and 30-Hz white flicker stimulus in the absence of background light in a normal subject, a rod monochromat, and a congenital nyctalope. Waveforms under "Summation" were obtained by algebraic summation of individual traces from rod monochromat and congenital nyctalope respectively.* Right: *Under the light-adapted column are ERGs evoked by standard single white, photopically matched yellow-red and blue-green flashes in the presence of white background light. Note the different time calibration for dark adapted and light adapted situations Modified from Chatrian et al. (49).*

ERG amplitude (51–53). Melanoma-associated retinopathy (MAR) impairs DBC signal transduction and presents as a selective reduction in the ERG b wave (54,55).

In central retinal occlusion (CRO), only the retinal circulation supplying the inner retina including DBCs is impaired; the choroidal circulation remains intact. Sparing of the choroidal circulation supports photoreceptor function, so the ERG, therefore, is characterized by a prominent a-wave but one depressed or absent b-wave (56,57).

ERGs can also help assess degrees of retinal ischemia (58,59). Sabates et al. (59) have shown in central retinal venous occlusion (CRVO) that the b-wave amplitude varies with the amount of retinal ischemia, the presence of which often precedes the development of neurovascular glaucoma. Johnson and Hood (60) showed that ERG changes arise at the photoreceptor level. ERG can be used to select CRVO patients requiring photocoagulation to prevent neurovascular glaucoma (61,62).

Other potentially damaging conditions, particularly those that affect the retina diffusely, may be associated with reduced ERG amplitude (Fig. 41.8). Damage of the retinal periphery will affect ERG rod components more severely than it will cone components. Flash ERG testing, therefore, can be utilized in assessing retinal damage and has been shown to be abnormal in many disorders, including diabetic (63,64) and sickle cell retinopathies (65), retinoschisis (66), cone and rod degenerations (2,43,45,49), as well as other disorders (56).

ERGs can also be used to monitor the health of the retina in an attempt to detect early changes before they are clinically detectable with the hope of preventing further damage (64,67–71). ERG changes have been reported in diabetes before the presence of a clinically detectable retinopathy (64,68). Similarly, the ERG can be "a proxy for visual function to monitor for retinal toxicity" (69), and it has been utilized to monitor chemotherapy toxicity in cancer and epilepsy treatment (69–71).

Superimposed on the ascending slope of the flash ERG b-wave are a series of four to six wavelets, the OPs. The OPs are a high-frequency response component in the region of 100 to 160 Hz and can be easily isolated from slower ERG components by selective filtering using an amplifier bandpass of 100 to 500 or 1,000 Hz (72,73). OPs can be utilized as selective probes of the functional integrity of the neuronal circuitry of the proximal retina. Clinically, they have been shown to be abnormal in diabetic and ischemic retinopathies (Fig. 41.9) independently and often before abnormalities of the b-wave have been detected (64,73–75).

2.2.1. MULTIFOCAL ERG

While the flash ERG provides a useful index of overall retinal function, many retinal disorders impair only the macular region. Macular disorders are particularly disabling because they affect the high-acuity fovea. Flash ERGs in such patients are typically normal. Multifocal ERG is a technique

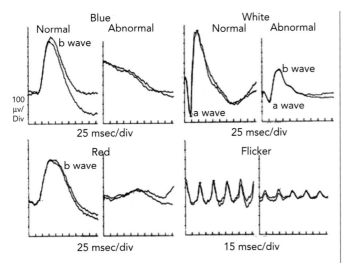

Figure 41.8. ERGs in in a 54-year-old man with diabetic retinopathy. He reported impaired night vision and dimmed vision. Visual acuity was 20/25. Left: ERGs in the dark-adapted state to dim blue and red flashes in a normal subject (left column) and in the diabetic patient (right column). Right: ERGs to white flashes obtained in the dark-adapted state and to 32-Hz white flicker in a normal subject and the diabetic patient. Note that the b wave is almost absent to blue flashes and very small to red flashes, indicating severe impairment of the rod system. Both a and b waves to a white flash have a small amplitude. The latency of the b wave to flicker is delayed at 43.2 msec (boundary of normality, 36.0). These findings indicate the presence of a diffuse retinopathy. Note the different time calibration for dark adapted and light adapted situations. Modified from Celesia (96).

that provides a focal analysis of retinal function by isolating responses to a large number of retinal areas simultaneously, generating a map of retinal function that defines local outer

retinal involvement in cases of visual loss (76–80). As stated by Creel, "Small scotomas in retina can be mapped and degree of retinal dysfunction quantified" (56). Standards for clinical multifocal ERG have been suggested by ISCEV (79) and should be adhered to. Multifocal ERGs are effective for early detection and assessment of a wide range of conditions that involve the retina in focal areas, such as macular disease (Fig. 41.10), diabetes, vascular disease, and inflammatory disorders.

2.2.2. PATTERN ERG

Pattern ERGs (P-ERGs) were first obtained by pattern-reversal stimuli, in which patterns alternate but mean luminance is kept constant (81). The spatial frequency amplitude function of the P-ERG shows a band-passing tuning behavior (82–84) with attenuation at low and high spatial frequencies. Attenuation at low spatial frequencies indicates that the P-ERG originates in cells with lateral inhibition and center-surround receptive field organization. Bipolar and ganglion cells both have center-surround receptive field organization. Transection of the optic nerve in cats and monkeys results in retrograde degeneration of the ganglion cells and abolition of steady-state and transient P-ERGs (82,84–86). Zrenner and Nelson (87) recorded the membrane depolarizing potentials of amacrine cells and showed their remarkable similarity to the transient P-ERG. They suggested that P-ERGs may be a mixture of ganglion and amacrine cell responses. Holder (88) suggests that the N95 component of P-ERGs arises in the spiking activity of the retinal ganglion cells. Steady-state P-ERG reflects mainly spike-related ON pathway ganglion cell activity (89). It is now generally agreed that the P-ERG is *predominantly a foveal response* that originates in the

CENTRAL RETINAL VEIN OCCLUSION

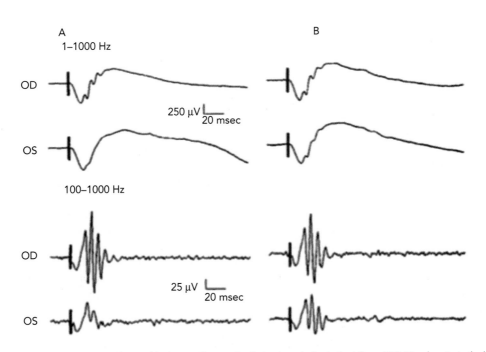

Figure 41.9. ERG under scotopic conditions in a 32-year-old woman with central retinal vein occlusion in the left eye (OS). Visual acuity in the left eye was 20/200. ERGs were recorded (A) at the onset of the disorder and (B) 6 months later, when the patient's vision had recovered to 20/30. The upper half of the illustration shows the oscillatory potential (OP) riding on the ascending slope of the b wave. The lower half shows the simultaneously recorded OP with the low bandpass at 100 Hz to eliminate the a and b waves. The OPs are then easily recognizable. Note normal responses from the right eye (OD) and the small OPs from the left eye. The a and b waves were normal from both eyes. From N.S. Peachey, unpublished data, 1991.

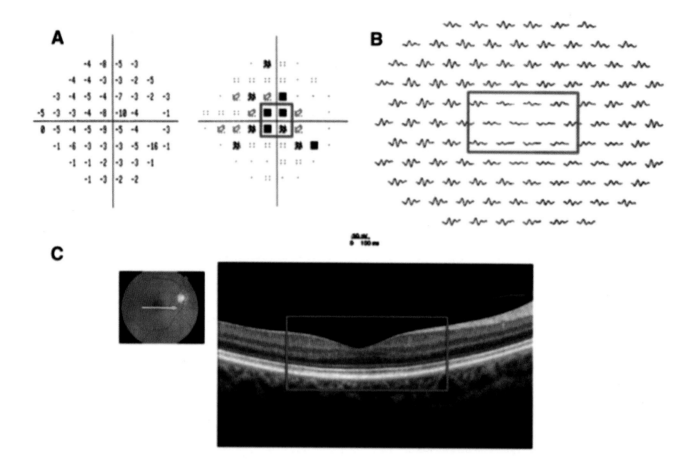

Figure 41.10. *A 57-year-old woman presented with a complaint of a "dark spot" in her central vision. A: Standard automated perimetry (SAP) demonstrates a central scotoma in the right eye (red box). B: Multifocal ERG with reduced amplitude in the right eye in the retinal region corresponding to the SAP defect (red box). C: Frequency domain optical coherence tomography (OCT) demonstrates a normal-appearing retina in the region corresponding to the visual field and multifocal ERG abnormalities (red box). Reproduced with permission from Talamini et al. (78).*

proximal retina. The size of the spatial features of stimuli used to evoke the P-ERG is an important variable that may influence response amplitude (85,90–92).

P-ERGs to high- and medium-spatial-frequency stimuli (i.e., with small stimulus elements) are dependent on the integrity of ganglion cells, with a contribution from amacrine cells (85,90,92–94). However, the pattern reversal to low-spatial-frequency stimuli is a mixed response containing a second harmonic response to luminance (85,90).

ISCEV has also published a standard for P-ERG testing (91). We will adhere to ISCEV's proposed nomenclature in this chapter. P-ERGs to transient stimuli consist of a series of negative-positive waves: a negative N35, a positive P50, followed by another negative wave N95 (Fig. 41.11). The amplitude and latency of P-ERG waves are shown in Table 41.1.

If the P-ERG reflects post-receptor retinal activity and possibly ganglion cell activity, it can be used as a marker to determine retinocortical transient time (RCT), provided VEPs are recorded simultaneously. RCT will then reflect activity outside the retina in the visual pathways (5,92,93,95). RCT is defined as the difference in milliseconds between VEP and ERG wave latencies. Two RCTs have been calculated: RCT1 (P50-N70) equals the latency of N70 minus P50 latency and RCT2 (P50-P100) equals the latency of P100 minus P50 latency.

P-ERGs to steady-state stimulation consist of quasi-sinusoidal deflections as shown in Figure 41.11. In retinal lesions affecting the macula preferentially, Celesia and Kaufman (5) described abnormal transient P-ERGs in 89% of cases with checks of 15 minutes (15′)and in 67% of patients with checks of 31 minutes (31′). Small or absent P-ERG has also been noted in age-related macular degeneration (Fig. 41.12). In cases of early macular degeneration, P-ERG was present but delayed (5,95,96). Similar absent or greatly depressed P-ERGs in macular diseases were described by Holder (88,97) and Sherman (98).

Robson et al. (99) report that P50 abnormalities "may reveal macular dysfunction in the absence of significant ophthalmoscopic changes." In 20 cases of central serous retinopathy, Goyal (100) reported that P50 was reduced, indicating functional disturbance of the macular photoreceptors (Fig. 41.13). In these cases a normal flash ERG indicates that pathology is "electrophysiologically localised to macula without affecting general retina" (100).

P-ERG abnormalities are not limited to maculopathies; they are also present in any optic nerve lesions with associated retrograde ganglion cell degeneration (5,82,84,86,89,94,101–104). The implications of P-ERG abnormalities in optic nerve dysfunction are discussed in more detail in the section on anterior visual pathway function.

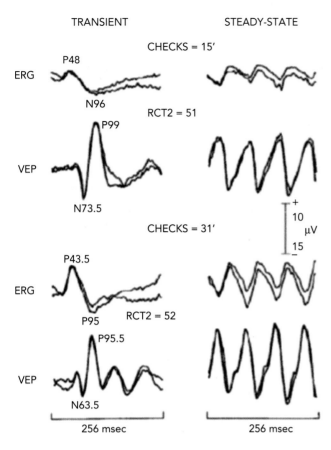

TRANSIENT — STEADY-STATE

CHECKS = 15'

ERG P48 N96

RCT2 = 51

VEP P99 N73.5

CHECKS = 31'

+
10
μV
15
−

ERG P43.5 P95

RCT2 = 52

VEP P95.5 N63.5

256 msec — 256 msec

Figure 41.11. Normal P-ERG and VEP to transient and steady-state pattern stimulation in a 36-year-old woman. Positive is upward for both P-ERG and VEP. In the calibration, 10 refers to P-ERG amplitude and 15' to VEP amplitude. Two responses are superimposed to verify reproducibility of the data. The upper half of the figure shows the responses to 15' checks, the lower half to 31' checks. RCT2, retinocortical transmission time in milliseconds from the ERG P50 to the P100 deflection. Steady-state VEPs were obtained at the reversal rate of 8 Hz.

A delayed P-ERG occurs only in macular diseases; absent or markedly depressed P-ERGs are present in either maculopathies or severe optic nerve diseases associated with axonal involvement and retrograde ganglion cell degeneration. In a study of glaucoma patents Bach (104) used P-ERG to identify "incipient" damage before visual field changes occurred. He concluded that P-ERG is "a sensitive biomarker for retinal ganglion cell function."

It should be emphasized that in macular lesions flash ERGs are normal. Thus, P-ERGs are useful in the assessment of macular function and retinal ganglion cell function. Holder (88, 97) suggests that the P-ERG P50 can be used as an index of macular function. Reduction in P-ERG N95 with preservation of P50 may indicate dysfunction at the level of the retinal ganglion cells (97). These data support the principle of selective activation: different structures of the retina can be preferentially, if not exclusively, activated by varying the type of stimulation (5). Flashes selectively activate retinal luminance and color detectors, whereas small pattern stimuli preferentially activate contrast and edge detectors.

In summary, the flash ERG a-wave reflects the massed response of rod or cone photoreceptors; the b-wave reflects the activity of bipolar cells. Oscillatory potentials are generated by amacrine and interplexiform cells. Flash ERGs are useful in (1) evaluating the outer retinal function and specifically helping in the diagnosis of retinal degenerations; (2) monitoring the progress of retinal diseases; (3) monitoring retinal toxicity of drugs; and (4) understanding the pathophysiology of retinal disorders. Multifocal ERG is a technique that extends simultaneously focal analysis of retinal function to a large number of retinal areas. P-ERG is generated in the ganglion cells with a contribution from amacrine cells and is predominantly a foveal response. It is abnormal in macular dysfunctions and in optic nerve atrophy.

TABLE 41.1. Pattern ERGs and VEPS: Normative Data

PARAMETER	15' CHECKS		31' CHECKS	
	RANGE	(MEAN ± SD)	RANGE	(MEAN ± SD)
ERG				
N35 latency	20.5–37.0	28.3± 3.0	20.0–36.0	27.1 ± 2.6
P50 latency	38.0–55.5	47.3 ± 2.7	39.0–54.0	46.1 ± 2.5
P50 amplitude	0.4–5.1	1.8 ± 0.8	0.5–7.1	2.3 ± 1.1
VEP				
P60 latency	50.0–75.0	60.9 ± 4.2	44.5–67.0	56.1 ± 3.5
N70 latency	63.5–87.5	75.5 ± 4.1	60.0–87.5	70.8 ± 3.7
N70 amplitude	1.0–18.2	5.1 ± 3.1	0.7–14.5	3.9 ± 2.2
P100 latency	83.5–107.5	98.1 ± 4.4	81.5–107.0	94.7 ± 5.0
P100 amplitude	1.1–38.1	9.9 ± 5.9	1.9–29.9	8.7 ± 4.7
Retinocortical time				
RCT1 (P50-N70)	17.0–40.5	28.3 ± 3.9	13.5–38.5	24.8 ± 3.3
RCT2 (P50-P100)	39.0–63.0	50.8 ± 4.0	36.5–60.5	48.7 ± 4.4

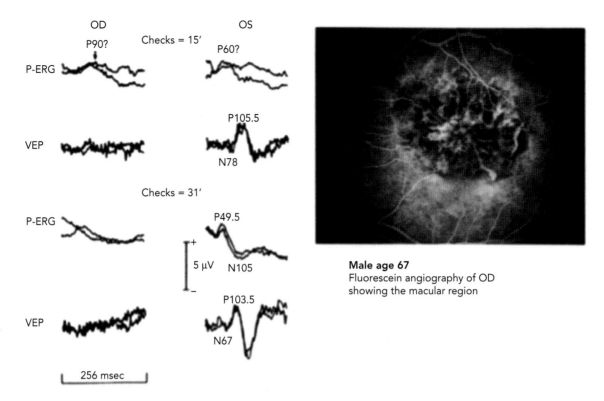

Male age 67
Fluorescein angiography of OD
showing the macular region

Figure 41.12. Male age 67 with age-related macular degeneration of the right eye (OD). Left: Stimulation of OD shows absent or greatly diminished P-ERG and absent VEP. Stimulation of the left eye (OS) shows very small P-ERG to 15′ checks but normal P-ERG to 31′ checks and normal VEPs to both 15′ and 31′ checks. Right: Fluorescein angiography of OD demonstrates dilated capillary and extravasation of fluorescein in the macular region. Fluorescein angiography of OS was normal (not shown).

3. VISUAL PATHWAYS AND VISUAL CORTICES

3.1. Anatomy and Physiology

The optic nerve comprises nerve fibers originating in the ganglion cells. The optic nerve spans approximately 50 mm long from the eye to the chiasm. Nerve fibers originating from ganglion cells in the macula constitute the papillomacular bundle that occupies the entire temporal side of the optic disk. This bundle of fibers then moves toward the center of the optic disk as it approaches the chiasma. Fibers from peripheral ganglion cells occupy less central positions in the optic disk and optic nerve (105,106). The optic nerve fibers are small myelinated fibers; 92% of the axons are 2 μm or less in diameter, 6% have a diameter around 4 μm, and only 2% have a large axon (>4 μm) (107). Calculated conduction velocities range from 1.3 to 20 meters/sec (108,109).

The human retina projects to both ipsilateral and contralateral sides of the cortex. Fibers from the nasal retina cross in the chiasma; crossed and uncrossed fibers begin to separate at the termination of the optic nerve. Macular fibers also are subdivided into crossed and uncrossed fibers; the macular fibers from the nasal portion of the macula cross in the chiasma into the contralateral optic tract, whereas the macular temporal fibers travel into the ipsilateral optic tract. Information from the contralateral hemifield travels in the optic tract and, after synaptic transfer to LGN neurons, continues into the striate area 17 (also named V1) via the geniculocalcarine tract.

Two major visual pathways or systems have been described (110–114): the magnocellular (M) and the parvocellular (P) visual systems (Fig. 41.14). The magnocellular pathway originates in large ganglion cells in the retina and projects to layers 1 and 2 of the LGN. The magnocellular ganglion cells receive input mainly from rods. The parvocellular pathway receives input mainly from the cones via the parvocellular ganglion cells and projects to layers 3 through 6 of the LGN, which projects directly to striate area V1. A third system representing approximately 5% to 10% of the ganglion cells is the koniocellular pathway. It originates in the bistratified ganglion cells and projects to the LGN. The function of this pathway is unclear, although it may contribute to spatial and temporal processing. The two major pathways (magnocellular and parvocellular) remain anatomically separate (113).

Both in the LGN and in striate cortex (V1), the information from the right and left eyes remains distinct. V1 has a modular organization, with a sequence of ocular dominance columns (receiving input from only one eye), blobs (involved in color processing), and orientation columns (consisting of neurons that respond to specific orientation visual stimuli). This sequence is repeated precisely over the entire surface of V1. The two pathways (Fig. 41.15) project to different cortical areas. The magnocellular pathway travels to V2 and continues to the middle temporal area (also called V5) and other parietal cortical areas, including area 7A. The magnocellular pathway projects to the dorsal parietal region; thus, it is also called the dorsal pathway. The magnocellular pathway

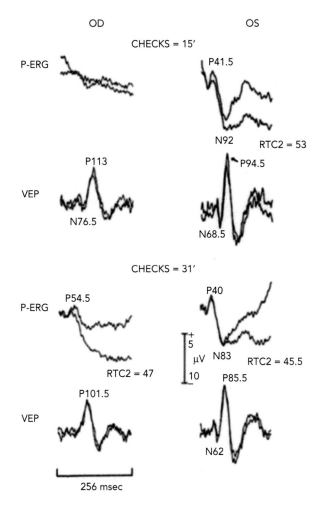

OD   OS

CHECKS = 15'

P-ERG   P41.5

N92   RTC2 = 53

P113   P94.5

VEP

N76.5   N68.5

CHECKS = 31'

P54.5   P40

P-ERG

+
5
μV   N83   RTC2 = 45.5
RTC2 = 47
10   P85.5

P101.5

VEP

N62

256 msec

Figure 41.13. Male age 35 with central serous chorioretinitis of the right eye (OD). P-ERG and VEP are normal for the left eye (OS). In OD P-ERG is absent and VEP slightly delayed to 15' checks; P-ERG is decreased in amplitude but VEP is normal to 31' checks. Flash ERG was normal for both eyes. These findings suggest that the functional disturbance was localized to the macular region.

processes motion, dynamic form, and spatial relationships among objects, and it is involved in the control of visually guided movements representing the "where system." The parvocellular pathway continues via V2 to area V4 and the inferior temporal cortex. Because the system processes form and color and is most active in the recognition of objects, it is also called the "what system" or, due to its anatomical location, the ventral system (110–112). This dichotomy is not absolute: there are many interconnecting pathways between the two systems and many visual cortical areas have more than one function. Anatomical studies in primates have demonstrated 305 interconnecting pathways among the various visual areas (115,116). In the primate brain, 35 visual cortical areas have been identified (115,116). Many of these areas have a full retinotopic representation of the visual field. V1 contains the retinotopic representation of the entire contralateral visual field. The representation of the fovea, however, is larger than the peripheral field: this phenomenon is named the *cortical magnification*. The magnification factor or *M-factor* indicates that the visual cortex is biased for processing information from the central portion of the visual field (117–121). The M-factor is also present in V2, V3, V4, and other visual areas (122). Kaas (123) proposed that multiple cortical representations are the most efficient way to increase information processing in the phylogenetic scale as mammals require more sophisticated and selective information of the visual environment.

Approximately one-third of the human brain is involved in visual processing. Although it is not yet possible to subdivide the human visual cortex with the same detail as has been achieved in non-human primates, more than 10 cortical areas have been identified in humans by a combination of anatomical, functional (functional magnetic resonance imaging, positron emission tomography), and behavioral studies (115,120,125,126). Although certain areas have specific

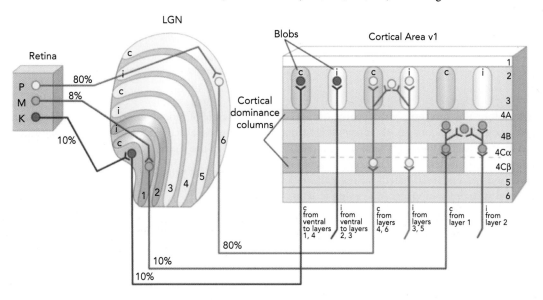

Figure 41.14. Schematic representation of retino-geniculate-striate pathways. Note that the output from the retina is subdivided into three pathways: the parvocellular (P; yellow) pathway originating from midget ganglion cells, the magnocellular (M; green) pathway originating from parasol ganglion cells; and the koniocellular (K; blue) pathway originating from bistratified ganglion cells. The three pathways remain segregated in the LGN striate cortex V1. Input from the contralateral (C) and ipsilateral (I) eye remains separated throughout the system until it is processed in the visual cortex. Reprinted with permission from Celesia, 2005.

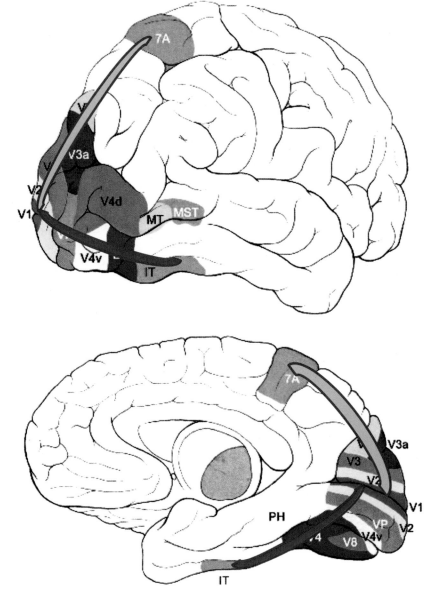

Figure 41.15. *Schematic representation of the multiple visual cortical areas and the magnocellular (M) dorsal "where" and the parvocellular (P) ventral "what" pathways. The magnocellular pathway (green arrow) travels to parietal areas, whereas the P pathway (red arrow) travels to ventral temporal areas.*

functions (V4, color; V5, motion), visual perception (i.e., the capacity to recognize and consciously interpret information processed by the visual system) is the result of a parallel activity of many interconnected areas. The complexity of the visual system cannot be underestimated; however, there are some fundamental principles of visual processing that must be considered in any study of vision. These principles are as follows:

- Principle of parallel processing: Visual information is processed simultaneously via multiple parallel pathways or channels (124–126).

- Principle of modular design: The visual system is composed of a collection of small modules partially independent from one another (127,128).

- Principle of functional specialization: Different attributes of the visual scene are processed in anatomically separate parts of the visual cortex (125,126).

- Principle of primacy: Attributes separately processed in the cerebral cortex are those that have primacy in vision— color, form, and motion (129,130).

- Principle of hierarchical organization: The multiple visual modules are organized in a hierarchical fashion (116,124).

- Principle of distributed network: The multiple visual modules are operating via a distributed network (131–135) with crucial nodal points. The distributed network is involved in object and space recognition, binding, spatial attention, and memory.

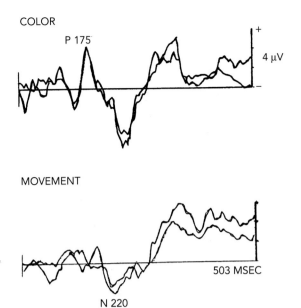

COLOR

P 175

4 μV

+

−

MOVEMENT

503 MSEC

N 220

Figure 41.16. Top: The "color" VEPS were elicited by equiluminant chromatic field alternating between yellow and green color low frequencies aimed at stimulating the parvocellular pathways. Bottom: The "motion" VEPS were elicited by white dots moving on a dark background aimed at stimulating the magnocellular pathways. The responses were obtained in the same subject.

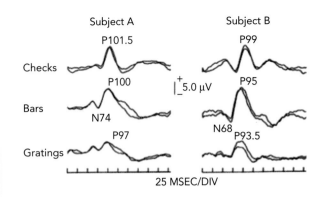

Subject A   Subject B

P101.5   P99

Checks

P100   P95

+ 5.0 μV

Bars   −

N74   N68 P93.5

P97

Gratings

25 MSEC/DIV

Figure 41.17. VEP to three varieties of stimuli from two normal volunteers. All stimuli subtended 30' of visual angle and were equiluminant. Note that the morphology, latency, and amplitude differ depending on the type of stimulus.

These principles can be effectively applied in obtaining VEPs. Thus, because changes in color, luminance, and motion are processed separately, these different attributes of the visual scene can be isolated and studied by utilizing visual stimuli that preferentially activate one of the parallel channels. VEPs elicited from equiluminant chromatic (color) stimuli and VEPs elicited from moving dots have a different morphology (Fig. 41.16) and are distributed over the scalp in separate but overlapping topographical regions. VEPs to chromatic stimuli have a maximum distribution over temporal areas, whereas VEPs to movement are distributed maximally over the parietal area (136–138).

In summary, two major visual pathways are the magnocellular and the parvocellular. These visual pathways remain partially separated from the retina to the LGN and to the striate cortex (V1). The magnocellular pathway travels to V2 and continues to the middle temporal (MT) area and other parietal cortical areas; it processes motion, dynamic form, and spatial relationships among objects. The parvocellular pathway continues via V2 to area V4 and the inferior temporal cortex; it processes form and color and the recognition of objects. Approximately one-third of the human brain is involved in visual processing. More than 10 areas have been described in humans. Many visual cortical areas have a retinotopic representation of the entire contralateral visual field. The representation of the fovea is larger than the peripheral field; this phenomenon is named cortical magnification. The magnification factor indicates that the visual cortex is biased for processing information from the central portion of the visual field.

3.2. Clinical Applications

The functional integrity of the visual pathways, once they enter the optic nerve, can be assessed using VEPs recorded from the occipital scalp region. It is presumed that these potentials are near-field potentials from the visual cortices (139–141). VEPs can be elicited by a variety of visual stimuli, including flashes, light-emitting diodes (LEDs), bars, and gratings. Empirically, it has been shown that full-field stimulation with patterned stimuli (Fig. 41.17) is best suited to evaluating visual pathway function (4,5,96,142–144). Clinically the preferred stimulus is checkerboard pattern reversal because it evokes reproducible and relatively large potentials (123,152) and can be readily standardized across labs. Checkerboard-patterned stimuli consist of series of black and white checks reversing at a set reversal rate. Check sizes and contrast are important variables in the use of patterned stimuli.

Pattern stimuli with individual checks, bars, or gratings smaller than 30 minutes of visual angle (min) stimulate predominantly contrast and spatial frequency detectors, whereas patterns of lower spatial frequency (checks larger than 40 min) inevitably stimulate luminance channels (103). Checks equal to or smaller than 15 min not only stimulate contrast and spatial frequency channels but also preferentially stimulate the fovea (Fig. 41.18) (119,145,146).

Field and check sizes may have to be changed relative to the region of the visual pathways to be studied. To detect small demyelinating lesions affecting optic nerve fibers originating in ganglion cells subserving the fovea (the papillomacular bundle), checks equal to or smaller than 30 min with a small total field should be used. On the other hand, to stimulate areas outside the fovea to detect chiasmal or retrochiasmal lesions, large fields with check sizes greater than 60 min may be preferable. VEPs are critically dependent on many parameters: stimulus brightness or luminance, contrast level, type of photic stimulus (patterned or unpatterned), type and size of patterned stimuli, total field size, and method and presentation rate (147). We recommend that clinicians consult the guidelines set by ISCEV (148) and the International Federation of Clinical Neurophysiology (149).

3.2.1. Transient Full-Field Pattern VEPs: Normative Data

The typical transient full-field pattern VEP (P-VEP) consists of a series of positive–negative deflections that are designated by capital letters indicating polarity followed by a number

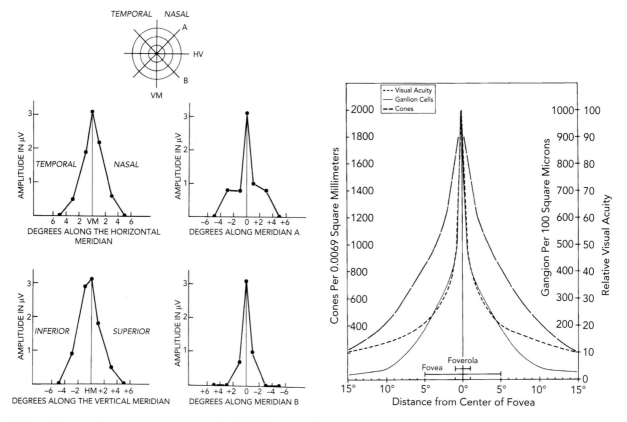

Figure 41.18. Left: *Relationship between the amplitude of the VEP P100 and retinal eccentricity. Each point represents the mean amplitude of wave P100 of eight volunteers. The stimulus was a field of 2 degrees with checks of 34'. Right: Visual acuity, ganglion cells density, and cones density along the retina horizontal meridian. Note that VEPs correlate well with cones, ganglion cells density, and visual acuity in the foveal region. Data from Meredith & Celesia (119), Jones & Higgins (24), Osterberg (25), Van Buren (26), and Oppel (27).*

indicating the average latency. The two most frequent waves (Fig. 41.19) are designated N70 (negative wave occurring at about 70 msec) and P100 (positive wave occurring at around 100 msec). Sometimes, a positive wave around 50 msec (P50) precedes N70.

Normative data values for responses to 15 min and 31 min checks are shown in Table 41.1. Normative data were obtained with bandpass filters of 5 to 250 Hz. If the recording is noisy, digital filtering and/or waveform smoothing (151,152) can be applied to eliminate some of the noise in

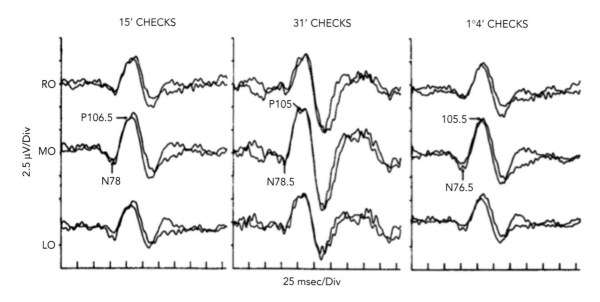

Figure 41.19. *Normal P-VEPs to stimulation of the right eye with three different size checks in a 71-year-old man. The two major waves, N70 and P100, have been labeled. Positive waves have an upward deflection. RO, right occipital; MO, mid-occipital; LO, left occipital; All responses were from the roght eye. Modified from Celesia & Cone (150).*

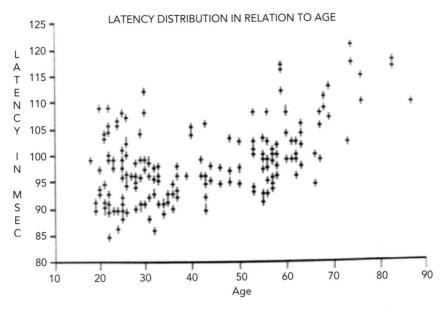

LATENCY DISTRIBUTION IN RELATION TO AGE

Figure 41.20. VEPs P100 latency to checks of 31' in relation to age. Each cross point represents a data point from a normal volunteer.

the tracing without introducing any latency shift. N70 and P100 latencies change with age (143,153–158). An increased latency is most evident after 45 years (Fig. 41.20) and is probably caused by a combination of age-related phenomena: decreased conduction velocity in the optic nerve and optic pathways due to defective myelin regeneration (159) or axonal dystrophy (160), corpora amylacea in the optic nerve and chiasm (161), degeneration of retinal ganglion cells (162,163), changes in neurotransmitter function and increased synaptic delay (164,165), and/or neuronal loss in the LGN and striate cortex (166). Gender also affects response latency, with females displaying slightly shorter latencies (143,167). It is suggested that the small differences in latencies between sexes can be accounted for by differences in brain size and the related smaller and shorter pathways in females (143,167).

VEPs to checkerboard reversal and to other patterned stimuli must be interpreted with caution. Refractive errors may affect both latency and amplitude. Delayed latency and decreased amplitude have been reported with as little as two diopters of refractive error, which will impact especially stimuli composed of small checks with low contrast (168,169). Pupil size is another variable (Fig. 41.21) that influences the amplitude and latency of P-VEP. Tobimatsu et al. (170) showed that the increase in P100 latency associated with decreased pupillary diameter is caused by decreased retinal illuminance. They estimated that P100 latency will increase by 10 to 15 msec/log unit of decreased retinal illuminance. *It is of paramount importance to avoid misinterpretation of VEP abnormalities due to refractory errors, pupillary changes, or lens opacities.*

We recommend the following precautions:

1. Measure the visual acuity and pupil diameter of each eye.

2. Use corrective lenses to compensate for refractory errors.

3. In cases of refractive errors greater than 20/100, determine whether the acuity can be corrected with a "pinhole."

4. Pupils should not be dilated with mydriatics.

5. Use monocular stimulation.

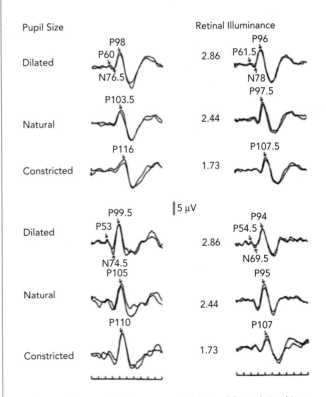

Figure 41.21. VEPs recorded from a normal subject and their relationship to pupil diameter (left) and retinal illuminance (right). Two trials are superimposed to demonstrate the reproducibility of the potentials. Note the increased latency as the pupil diameter decreased and similarly as the retinal illuminance decreased. The upper half of the illustration represents responses to 15' checks, the lower half to 31' checks. Calibration bar = 5 microvolts; time bar = 25 msec/division. Retinal illuminance is expressed in log trolands.

3.2.2. Transient Full-Field Pattern VEPs: Abnormalities

In the interpretation of P-VEP it is important to answer two questions: Are the VEPs abnormal? And if so, what is their significance? Abnormalities in VEPs are defined either as absent responses (case E in Fig. 41.22) or potentials with prolonged P100 latencies. Because N70 is sometimes absent in normal subjects it cannot be used as a reliable indicator of visual abnormalities. As shown in Figure 41.22, there are considerable varieties of morphological changes in abnormal responses. Prolonged P100 may have normal amplitude (case A in Fig. 41.22) or the amplitude may be smaller while preserving a normal morphology (case B in Fig. 41.22). Alternatively, P100 may be wider and smaller with prolonged latency (cases C and D in Fig. 41.22).

VEP abnormalities are nonspecific and thus must be interpreted in the context of the clinical features and ophthalmological complaints of each patient. The significance of a particular set of electrophysiological abnormalities may depend on the associated ophthalmological findings. An algorithm for clinical use in subjects with complaints of visual dysfunction is shown in Figure 41.23.

This algorithm is modified from Brigell and Celesia (171) and will answer the following questions:

1. Can vision loss be accounted for by media opacities (e.g., cataract, corneal abnormalities)?

2. Does the patient suffer from a rod or cone dysfunction?

3. Is the visual defect (usually a central visual field defect) related to a maculopathy or an optic neuropathy?

If flash ERG, P-ERG, and P-VEP are all normal and the patient still complains of visual dysfunction, one should not necessarily conclude that the complaints are psychogenic without first excluding dysfunction related to cortical visual disorders (see later discussion on retrochiasmatic disorders).

ABNORMAL TYPES of VEPs

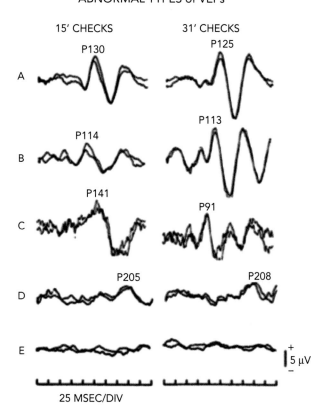

Figure 41.22. Different varieties of abnormal VEPs. Each subject (A to E) was tested with 15' and 31' checks. Note that case C had a small and prolonged P100 with checks but a normal P100 latency with 31' checks.

Another approach to determine the significance of a delayed P-VEP was proposed by Holder (172) and is shown in Figure 41.24. Here again it is emphasized that the true meaning of an abnormal VEP requires additional electrophysiological testing. Abnormal P-VEPs have been reported in many retinal diseases

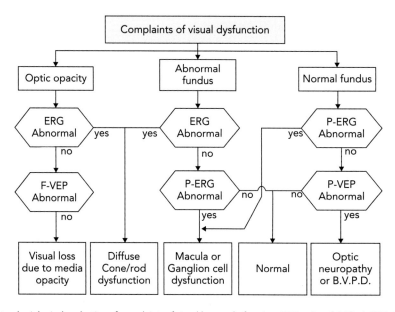

Figure 41.23. Flow chart for electrophysiological evaluation of complaints of visual loss or dysfunction. ERG = Ganzfeld flash ERG; P-ERG = pattern ERG; F-VEP = flash VEP; P-VEP = pattern VEP; B.V.P.D. = bilateral visual pathways dysfunction.

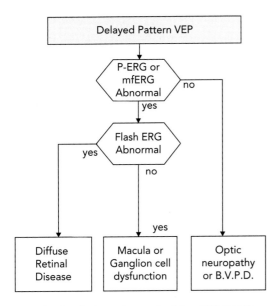

Figure 41.24. *Flow chart for the evaluation of a delayed VEP (P-VEP). mfERG = multifocal ERG; B.V.P.D. = bilateral visual pathways dysfunction.*

(see Figs. 41.12 and 41.13) and in disorders affecting the optic nerve, including retrobulbar neuritis, papillitis, ischemic optic neuropathy, toxic and metabolic optic neuropathy, optic nerve compression, and optic atrophy (4,5,92,93,95,98,144,169,173–178). P-VEPs are quite useful in helping to establish the diagnosis of multiple sclerosis (MS). The presence of delayed (Fig. 41.25) or absent P-VEPs (Fig. 41.26) in the absence of retinal pathology suggests the presence of an optic nerve lesion. A normal P-ERG with prolonged VEPs and RCT suggests the

presence of an optic neuropathy or with bilateral optic radiation lesions (174–176,179). The demonstration of an optic nerve lesion in a subject with evidence of a central nervous system disorder may establish the presence of multiple lesions, the hallmark of MS. In the authors' laboratory, P-VEPs were delayed or absent in 70% of patients with MS (Fig. 41.27). More important is the great sensitivity of VEPs to subclinical optic nerve lesions. Indeed, VEPs can reveal silent pathologies in the absence of other clinical signs of visual impairment: 50% of MS patients without visual dysfunction and with a normal neuro-ophthalmological examination had delayed VEPs (4,5,93,144,176,178,180,181)., The visual system process spatial, temporal, luminance and chromatic aspects of objects, via multiple parallel channels, it is therefore possible that a given disease may affect only one of these channels. Thus the use of multimodal stimuli (e.g., chromatic or moving stimuli and patterns of different frequency or spatial orientation) may more accurately detect abnormalities (182,183). For instance, patients with suspected MS have been found to have delayed VEPs only when the stimulus pattern was presented in a specific orientation or with a specific spatial frequency (184,185). Similarly, Tobimatsu and Kato (183) found in MS patients that while VEPs to pattern stimulation were normal, VEPs to chromatic or motion stimuli showed delayed responses, suggesting that in some cases the dysfunction was limited to selective visual pathways.

With the advent of MRI, optical coherence tomography (OCT), and other visual evaluation techniques, an important issue is the usefulness of VEPs in the neurologist's armamentarium. Although there are few studies comparing these new modalities, the available data show a good correlation between

FR♂ AGE 38 OD
MULTIPLE SCLEROSIS

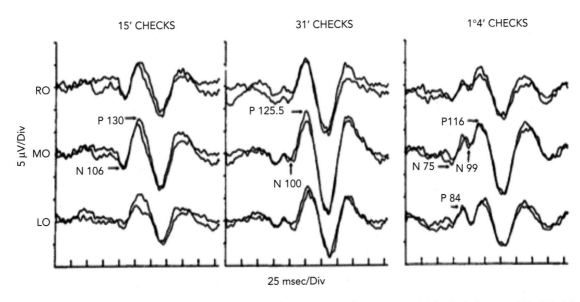

Figure 41.25. *P-VEPs in a patient with the diagnosis of definite MS but no evidence of visual dysfunction. Upward deflection indicates positivity. RO, right occipital; MO, mid-occipital: LO, left occipital; OD, right eye. Pattern reversal with checks of three different sizes were used. Note that the latency prolongation of wave N70 and P100 is more severe for smaller checks than for larger ones. The major positive wave of the VEPs to 1°4' stimuli is dispersed into two waves. Pattern ERG (not shown) was normal. Modified from Celesia & Cone (150).*

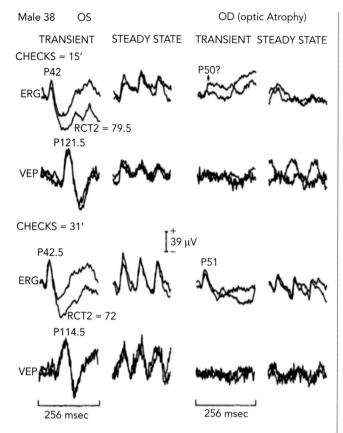

Male 38   OS   OD (optic Atrophy)

TRANSIENT   STEADY STATE   TRANSIENT   STEADY STATE
CHECKS = 15'
P42   P50?
ERG
RCT2 = 79.5
P121.5
VEP

CHECKS = 31'
                    +
                   39 µV
                    −
P42.5   P51
ERG
RCT2 = 72
P114.5
VEP

256 msec   256 msec

Figure 41.26. Optic atrophy in a 38-year-old woman with retrobulbar neuritis due to MS. Note the probable absence of transient P-ERG at 15' checks stimulation, but its presence at 31' checks in the affected eye (OD). Steady-state P-ERG to 15' checks is also absent. Larger checks of 31' produce a small P-ERG, probably related to stimulation of the perimacular area. There is a total block of nerve conduction through the optic nerve manifested by absence of VEPs to both 15' and 31' checks. Stimulation of the normal left eye (OS) shows normal P-ERGs but prolonged P100 and RCT to stimulation with 15' and 31' checks.

reduced retinal fiber layer thickness as measured by OCT and reduced VEP amplitude/delayed latency (186,187). MRI scans showing demyelinating lesions of the optic nerve correlate well with abnormal VEP (187). Other studies found OCT to be

VEPs ABNORMALITIES in MS

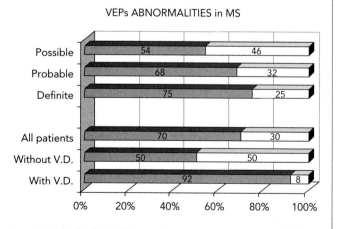

Possible	54	46
Probable	68	32
Definite	75	25
All patients	70	30
Without V.D.	50	50
With V.D.	92	8

0%   20%   40%   60%   80%   100%

Figure 41.27. P-VEP abnormalities in 180 patients with a diagnosis of MS. Note that 50% of patients without any complaints or findings of visual dysfunction had abnormal VEP indicating a subclinical lesion in the optic nerve. Similarly, 54% of patients with a suspicion of MS (possible MS) had abnormal VEP. V.D. = visual disturbance.

less sensitive than VEP in MS (180,188). There will always be cases in which one test will be more sensitive than the other (186,188,189); VEP, MRI, and OCT should be viewed as complementary tests that provide information about the integrity of the visual pathways (187).

P-VEPs can also detect chiasmic compression (174,190). In a study of 83 patients with pituitary tumors Gott et al. (190) found that "Each of the patients who had suprasellar extension of the tumor sufficient to produce a visual field abnormality also had an abnormal VER. In addition, some patients with suprasellar extension had normal visual fields but abnormal visual evoked responses." Absent or prolonged P-VEPs to full-field pattern stimulation indicate direct optic nerve compression or compromise by vascular impairment. Detection of chiasmatic lesions in the absence of optic nerve involvement requires the use of hemifield stimulation. Absence or prominent amplitude depression of responses to stimulation of both temporal or both nasal hemifields is unequivocal evidence of chiasmatic impairment.

3.3.3. Steady-State VEPs

Steady-state potentials are electrical events evoked by rapid repetitive sensory stimulation. Continuous rapid stimulation evokes responses of constant amplitude and frequency. The different potentials overlap so that no individual response can be related to any particular stimulus cycle (191–193). Steady-state potentials have the advantage that they can be studied by conventional averaging methods (see Figs. 41.11 and 41.26) and also by Fourier analysis. Steady-state VEPs (SSVEPs) to flashes, pattern-reversal checks, or gratings consist of sinusoidal deflections at frequencies that are multiples of the stimulus frequency. For pattern-reversal stimuli, the most prominent response is at double the frequency of the reversal cycle. Thus, an 8-Hz pattern-reversal rate evokes 16 responses/sec (see Fig. 41.11). The rapid stimulation rates possible in steady-state studies permit considerable time savings and therefore a more complete analysis of visual system physiology and pathophysiology (192–196). Spatial and temporal frequency tuning in the human retina and cortex, contrast modulation threshold, and visual working memory were evaluated with steady-state responses (194–198). Clinically, steady-state responses to grating have been successfully used to establish the contrast sensitivity of infants (199) and to demonstrate contrast sensitivity loss in MS (200).

SSVEPs to flashes determine the critical frequency of photic driving (CFPD), which is defined as the highest frequency at which a response is detectable, measured in flashes per second (143,191,201). CFPD represents the objective counterpart of critical flicker fusion. CFPD was abnormal in 42% of a group of 104 MS patients (Fig. 41.28); although it was less sensitive than P-VEPs, it was the sole abnormality in two patients. Patients with optic opacities cannot be tested with P-VEPs, but CFPD measurement permits evaluation of the function of the retinal cone system as well as the functional integrity of the visual pathways that process luminance. Fourier analysis has been used to study SSVEPs to various visual stimuli. The utilization of fast Fourier analysis with interfaced computer-generated visual stimulation permits the rapid evaluation of

43 | SOMATOSENSORY AND PAIN EVOKED POTENTIALS: NORMAL RESPONSES, ABNORMAL WAVEFORMS, AND CLINICAL APPLICATIONS IN NEUROLOGICAL DISEASES

FRANÇOIS MAUGUIÈRE, MD, PHD AND LUIS GARCIA-LARREA, MD, PHD

ABSTRACT: This chapter discusses the use of somatosensory evoked potentials (SEPs) and pain evoked potentials for diagnostic purposes. The generators of SEPs following upper limb stimulation have been identified through intracranial recordings, permitting the analysis of somatosensory disorders caused by neurological diseases. Laser activation of fibers involved in thermal and pain sensation has extended the applications of evoked potentials to neuropathic pain disorders. Knowledge of the effects of motor programming, paired stimulations, and simultaneous stimulation of adjacent somatic territories has broadened SEP use in movement disorders. The recording of high-frequency cortical oscillations evoked by peripheral nerve stimulation gives access to the functioning of SI area neuronal circuitry. SEPs complement electro-neuro-myography in patients with neuropathies and radiculopathies, spinal cord and hemispheric lesions, and coma. Neuroimaging has overtaken SEPs in detecting and localizing central nervous system lesions, but SEPs still permit assessment of somatosensory and pain disorders that remain unexplained by anatomical investigations.

KEYWORDS: stimulation, evoked potentials, somatosensory, SEPs, pain, neuropathies, radiculopathies, spinal cord lesions, movement disorders, coma

PRINCIPAL REFERENCES

1. Desmedt JE, Cheron G. Central somatosensory conduction in man: Neural generators and interpeak latencies of the far-field components recorded from neck and right or left scalp or earlobes. Electroencephalogr Clin Neurophysiol. 1980;50:382–403.
2. Cruccu G, Aminoff MJ, Curio G, et al. Recommendations for the clinical use of somatosensory-evoked potentials. Clin Neurophysiol. 2008;119:1705–1719.
3. Cheron G, Dan B, Borenstein S. Sensory and motor interfering influences on somatosensory evoked potentials. J Clin Neurophysiol. 2000;17:280–294.
4. Frot M, Mauguière F. Dual representation of pain in the operculo-insular cortex in humans. Brain. 2003;126:438–450.
5. Garcia-Larrea L, Perchet C, Creac'h C, et al. Operculo-insular pain (parasylvian pain): a distinct central pain syndrome. Brain. 2010;133:2528–2539.
6. Mauguière F, Desmedt JE, Courjon J. Astereognosis and dissociated loss of frontal or parietal components of somatosensory evoked potentials in hemispheric lesions. Brain. 1983;106:271–311.
7. Ozaki I, Hashimoto I. Exploring the physiology and function of high-frequency oscillations (HFOs) from the somatosensory cortex. Clin Neurophysiol. 2011;122:1908–1923.
8. Restuccia D. Anatomic origin of P13 and P14 scalp far-field potentials. J Clin Neurophysiol. 2000;17:246–257.
9. Sonoo M. Anatomic origin and clinical application of the widespread N18 potential in median nerve somatosensory evoked potentials. J Clin Neurophysiol. 2000;17:258–268.
10. Treede RD, Lorenz J, Baumgartner U. Clinical usefulness of laser-evoked potentials. Neurophysiol Clin. 2003;33:303–314.

1. INTRODUCTION

The modern history of clinical somatosensory evoked potential (SEP) testing began over 60 years ago with George Dawson's (1) recordings, in patients with myoclonus, of what is known today as giant somatosensory cortical responses. Because of their relatively large amplitude and low frequency, compatible with a slow sampling rate of analog–digital conversion, the cortical SEPs were the first studied in both healthy subjects and patients. In the 1970s and early 1980s the spinal potentials and subcortical far-field potentials were identified and correlations among abnormal waveforms, lesion sites, and clinical findings were established. Recent advances stem from the development of multichannel recordings of SEPs and somatosensory evoked magnetic fields (SEFs) coupled with MRI source imaging in the brain volume. While electroclinical correlations had tended toward the identification of a single generator for each SEP component, source modeling suggested that the field distribution of cortical SEPs at a given moment often results from activities of multiple distributed sources that overlap in time, thus reflecting the parallel activations and the feedback controls that characterize the processing of somatosensory inputs at the cortical level. Lastly, the development of laser evoked potentials (LEPs) and of high-frequency oscillations (HFOs) evoked by somatosensory stimuli now allow access to the clinical physiology of the spinothalamic pathways and intracortical synaptic networks, respectively.

2. STIMULATION PROCEDURES

Only the essential technical requirements for recording SEPs and pain EPs will be given here. Technical details concerning electrodes, recording montages, filters, sampling rates, and safety can be found elsewhere in this book as well as in guidelines published by the International Federation of Clinical Neurophysiology (2).

2.1. Stimulus Types

2.1.1. ELECTRICAL STIMULI

Brevity and strict control in the time of stimulus onset and cutoff, and thus of the averaging trigger, are the major advantages of electrical stimulation over any other types of stimulus. SEPs are usually evoked by bipolar transcutaneous electrical stimulation applied on the skin over the trajectory of peripheral nerves at motor threshold for mixed nerves and three times sensation threshold for pure sensory nerves. Dermatomal electrical stimulation can also be used to explore root lesions (see below). Monophasic electrical pulses of 100 to 300 μsec depolarize nerve fibers directly by generating a potential difference in the medium adjacent to the nerve trunk and thus across the nerve fiber membrane, causing a depolarization close to the site of the cathode. Electrical stimuli thus bypass the peripheral encoding of natural stimuli (pressure, vibration, joint movement) by the receptors. The different categories of fibers that subserve the different types of sensations can be individualized on the basis of their diameter and the thickness of their myelin sheets. There is an inverse relation between the fiber diameter on the one hand and its threshold to electrical stimulation and conduction velocity on the other hand. In most clinical applications of SEPs electrical stimuli are delivered at intensities equivalent to three to four times the sensory threshold; these produce a twitch in the muscles innervated by the stimulated nerve when it contains a contingent of motor fibers. At this stimulus intensity the rapidly conducting large myelinated fibers, including fibers subserving touch and joint sensation but also muscle afferents, are activated. The contribution of muscle afferents to cortical SEPs after stimulation of upper limb mixed nerves has long been considered negligible. However, selective intrafascicular stimulation of hand muscle afferents at the wrist and motor-point stimulation were shown to produce short-latency cortical SEPs with the same waveforms (3) and sources (4) as those obtained by stimulating the trunk of a mixed nerve. These cortical responses are relatively small compared to the potentials evoked from the whole mixed nerve or digital nerves because only relatively few afferents are activated. Their first cortical component peaks later than for median nerve stimulation at the wrist and at approximately the same latency as for stimulation of the digital nerves (5). Therefore, the possibility remains that, when stimulating a mixed nerve of the upper limb, the cortical response to muscle afferents inputs could be gated by the response to cutaneous and joint inputs. In short, the contribution of muscle afferents to median nerve cortical SEPs can be considered weak compared to that of cutaneous afferents.

The situation is quite different after electric stimulation of lower limb sensorimotor nerves such as the tibial nerve, for which muscle afferents have been shown to have a major contribution to cortical SEPs (6). The latency of the earliest cortical response is shorter after stimulation of the abductor hallucis muscle fascicle than after stimulation of the tibial nerve, and its amplitude is approximately half that of the tibial nerve response. It has been shown that, after stimulation of the tibial nerve, inputs conveyed by muscle afferents, which have the fastest conduction velocity, are able to occlude the response to cutaneous inputs (7). Because of this gating, the cutaneous afferent volley may make little or no contribution to the cerebral potential evoked by electric stimulation of lower limb mixed nerves. Electric simulation of pure sensory nerves, such as digital nerves for the upper limb and the sural nerve for the

lower limb, activates exclusively skin and joint peripheral and dorsal column fibers. It is advisable to use this type of stimulus in any attempt to correlate the quality of perception with SEP data in normal subjects as well as in patients with impaired sensation. At the upper limb, stimulation of the fingertip (8) or distal phalanx of the fingers (9) activates selectively skin fibers, while stimulation of digital nerves at the level of the first or second phalanx concerns both joint and skin afferents.

Paired electric stimuli delivered to the same nerve at various interstimulus intervals can be used to characterize distinct components of a given response according to their refractoriness after the response to the first stimulus of the pair (conditioning stimulus), and also to combine SEP testing with psychophysical evaluation of time discrimination performances in detecting the second stimulus of the pair (10). The voltage of the response to the second stimulus of the pair is evaluated by subtracting the response to the test stimulus delivered alone in a separate session.

The effect on SEPs of spatial interference between two electric stimuli delivered simultaneously but at two distinct sites was first described by Burke et al. (7) and Gandevia et al. (11). These authors showed that after simultaneous stimulation of both index and middle fingers of the same hand, the size of the early component of the cerebral potential is less than predicted by simple addition of the potentials produced by stimulation of the fingers individually. The interfering influences of sensory and motor events on electrically evoked SEPs have been widely used in the context of gating paradigms (see reference 12 for a review). In particular, models of centrifugal and centripetal SEP gating during movement programming or execution are based on the results from these studies (see below).

2.1.2. NATURAL STIMULI

Physiological stimuli have a higher selectivity than that of electrical stimulation of sensory nerves. SEPs and SEFs can be obtained in response to a brief mechanical impact on the fingertip or air puffs (see the seminal studies by Debecker and Desmedt (13) and Schieppati and Ducati (14)). Due to the small population of excited fibers, these mechanical stimuli produce low-voltage responses and are not used routinely in the clinical setting despite their potential advantage over conventional electrical stimuli. Dedicated devices have been developed to activate selectively finger joint afferents (8) or muscle afferents (15). Despite close similarities between stimulation paradigms and evoked responses in these two studies, the authors diverge about the nature of afferent peripheral fibers involved in cortical response genesis: joint afferents for Desmedt and Osaki (8) versus spindle afferents of finger extensor muscles for Mima et al. (15).

2.1.3. PAIN STIMULI

Nociceptive afferents can be excited by a variety of techniques, but only few of them are specific. The three most widely used techniques are electrical, contact heat, and laser pulsed stimulation. Electrical stimuli used routinely in clinical neurophysiology laboratories excite large-diameter afferents that have a lower electrical threshold than nociceptive fibers; consequently, they do not explore the small myelinated Aδ or unmyelinated C afferents to spinothalamic tracts subserving temperature and pain sensation. Although increasing the intensity of electrical stimulation can induce a pain response, nociceptive afferents are excited simultaneously with non-nociceptive fibers, hence precluding the recording of specifically "nociceptive" EPs. By stimulating simultaneously large and thin peripheral afferents, electrical stimuli set out interactions between noxious and non-noxious inputs all along the ascending pathways: the large-afferent input inhibits nociceptive signals at spinal and supraspinal levels, and therefore the specific nociceptive response is diminished when large and small afferents are simultaneously stimulated. Attempts to render electrical stimuli "nociceptive-specific" have been based on stimulating regions innervated exclusively by small-diameter fibers, such as the tooth pulp (16), and more recently by using small electrodes delivering very superficial currents, which limits current spread to the intra-epidermal level (17). Although promising and useful for research, this latter attempt has not yet gained access to clinical practice.

Thermal stimulation without skin contact permits selective activation of thermo-nociceptive receptors. However, conventional heat sources such as lightbulbs or xenon lamps cannot ensure their synchronous activation and are hardly useful for recording neurophysiological responses. Furthermore, they mainly emit in the visible spectral range, where skin energy absorption is poor and widely affected by changes in skin pigmentation, thus making the control of heat transfer virtually impossible (18). These problems are avoided by using monochromatic high-intensity light sources such as those provided by laser stimulators, of which CO_2 and solid-state (YAG/YAP) laser stimulators are the most commonly used. Infrared laser pulses increase the local skin temperature very rapidly, allowing synchronized activation of free nerve endings of Aδ and C-fibers without concomitant activation of A-beta fibers. The corresponding cortical responses are called laser evoked potentials (LEPs) (19,20). LEPs are currently the most reliable neurophysiological tool to investigate patients with neuropathic pain (2).

Nociceptive activation can also be achieved using fast-acting contact heat thermodes, which evoke a pinprick sensation and cortical responses attributed to A-δ fiber stimulation (21). Contact heat-evoked potentials (CHEP) are less ample and delayed by 200 to 300 msec relative to laser EPs due to the low slope of the heating ramp (~50–70°C/s), which desynchronizes the afferent volley and makes the precise moment of afferent fiber activation hard to establish (22). With further refinements, however, the CHEP technique may become a useful tool to study pain-related responses (23).

3. NORMAL RESPONSES

3.1. Short-Latency SEPs to Upper Limb Stimulation (Electrical Stimulation of Median, Ulnar, Radial, or Finger Nerves)

The main early SEP components will be described as they appear on recordings using a non-cephalic reference electrode placed at the shoulder on the non-stimulated side after

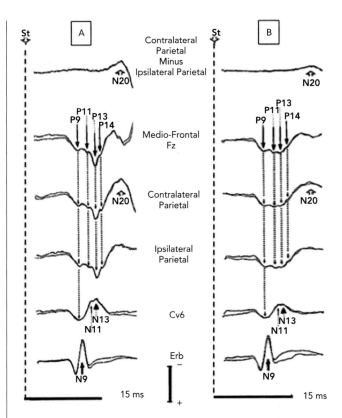

Figure 43.1. Early median nerve SEPs (non-cephalic reference recording). This figure illustrates the Erb's point N9, spinal N11, N13, far-field P9, P11, P13, P14, and cortical N20 components (A) and the effect of vibrations applied to the stimulated hand (B). The far-field potentials are picked up at all cephalic recording sites. Only the potentials reflecting the moving action potentials in peripheral (N9, P9) and central segments (N11, P11) of the first-order neuron are unaffected by the interfering vibrations. Conversely, all potentials reflecting activities generated after the first synapse in the cord dorsal horn (N13), brainstem (P13, P14), and SI cortex (N20) are reduced by the interfering stimulus. In this normal subject the N11 spinal potential, reflecting the ascending volley in dorsal column fibers, is discernible in the ascending slope of the postsynaptic dorsal horn N13 potential. Note that the P9 far-field potential is recorded at all recording sites above Erb's point. Calibration: 10 µV for Erb's point trace and 5 µV for all other traces. From Ibañez, Deiber, and Mauguière (24) (modified, with permission of authors).

stimulation of the median nerve at the wrist (Fig. 43.1) (24). When necessary we will discuss the modifications of waveform and latency related to the use of other reference electrode sites.

3.1.1. PERIPHERAL N9 COMPONENT

Stimulation of a mixed nerve such as the median nerve elicits a compound action potential (CAP) reflecting the peripheral ascending volley that can be recorded at different levels of forearm and arm. In most routine SEP recordings carried out in patients with lesions of the central nervous system (CNS), the peripheral ascending volley is recorded only at Erb's point in the supraclavicular fossa. The CAP appears as a triphasic positive-negative-positive waveform with a negative peak culminating at about 9 msec (N9) for a body height of 170 cm. If necessary, a CAP with a shape similar to that of the N9 potential peaking at an earlier latency can also be recorded more distally over the trajectory of the nerve. Mixed nerve CAPs are a mixture of motor antidromic and sensory orthodromic responses and thus are qualitatively different from SEPs generated in central somatosensory pathways. Because of their large amplitude (5–10 μV at Erb's point) they are easily obtained using runs of 500 stimuli. The amplitude of peripheral CAPs is unaffected by interfering stimuli applied on the stimulated hand (see Fig. 43.1) or when the stimulus rate is increased up to 50 Hz (24).

3.1.2. Spinal Segmental N13 Component

Electrical stimulation of large-diameter myelinated fibers of peripheral nerves produces a dorsal horn potential with a posterior-negative and anterior-positive dipolar field perpendicular to the cord axis (Fig. 43.2). The cervical N13 potential is recorded at the posterior neck, with a maximum voltage at the level of C5–C7 spinous processes and decreases in amplitude at more rostral or caudal electrode positions. N13 does not show any latency shift between C6 and C2 recordings in normal subjects (25). When recorded anterior to the cord by an electrode placed at the anterior aspect of the neck. the cervical dorsal horn response is recorded as a spinal P13 positivity (26). This polarity reversal has been demonstrated with esophageal (27), epidural (28), and direct recordings from the surface of the cervical cord (29) (Fig. 43.3).

Both N13 and P13 spinal components are reduced in amplitude when the stimulation rate is over 10/sec (24), both persist in brain death or in cervicomedullary lesions (26, 30), and both are selectively reduced or abolished in lesions of the cervical cord gray matter sparing the spinal somatosensory tracts (31). Thus the most likely generator of the N13/P13 cervical potentials is the compound segmental postsynaptic potential triggered in the dorsal horn gray matter by the afferent volley in fast-conducting myelinated fibers. A cervical transverse derivation between two electrodes located respectively over the C6 spinal process and above the laryngeal cartilage is

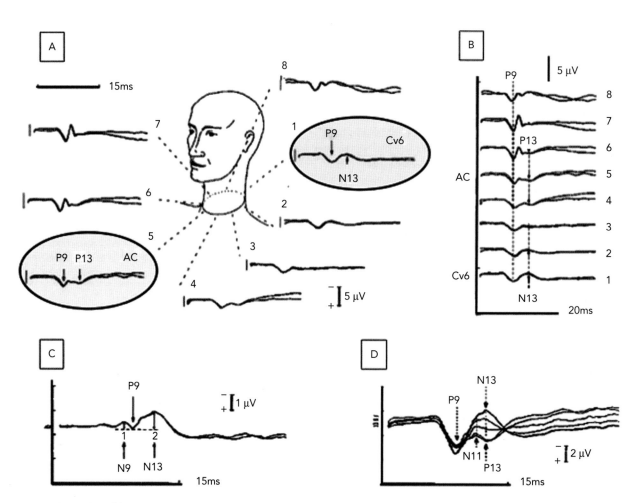

Figure 43.2. Neck recording of the N13/P13 segmental potential. Normal distribution of the N13/P13 recorded using an array of electrodes placed around the neck and a reference electrode at the shoulder contralateral to the stimulated right median nerve (A). The triphasic root activity is picked up at lateral neck electrodes on the stimulated side (6,7) and its initial positivity is synchronous with that of the P9 potentials picked up at all other recording sites (B). The trace obtained using a derivation between the posterior Cv6 and anterior cervical (AC) electrodes illustrated in C shows the N9/P9 reflecting the incoming volley in dorsal roots followed by the N13 potential reflecting the postsynaptic response of dorsal horn neurons. The dipolar source of N13 is oriented perpendicular to the cord axis and the segmental N13 is picked up with a maximal voltage by a CV6-AC derivation. The N11 potential is not clearly visible in this subject as compared with that illustrated in Figure 43.1; it appears as a notch on the initial phase of the segmental N13/P13 potential and does not reverse its polarity at anterior neck recording sites (D), suggesting that it is generated by the ascending volley of action potentials in the dorsal columns of the cervical spinal cord. N11 is often difficult to differentiate from the following N13 component. This seriously hampers the use of N11 in clinical practice, which is limited to cervical cord lesions that selectively obliterate the N13 potential. In direct recordings on the cervical cord surface during surgery, N11 appears as a fast polyphasic component that overlaps in time with the slower N13 segmental postsynaptic potential (Fig. 43.3).

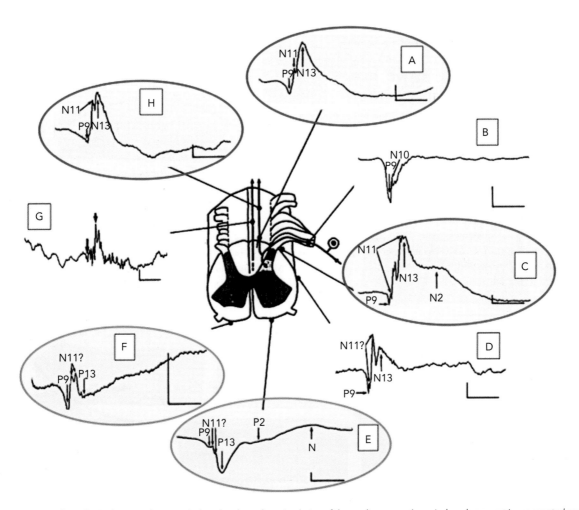

Figure 43.3. *Direct recording of spinal potentials on cervical cord surface after stimulation of the median nerve. A cervical cord segment is represented containing one axon from a cervical dorsal root ganglion cell on the stimulated side. The dorsal recordings (A and C) show the P9, N11, N13, and later N2 wave. The anterior recordings (E and F) show the polarity reversal of the dorsal horn N13 response (P13). Recording at the root spinal entry zone shows the P9 and N10 dorsal root potentials (B). The ascending action potentials in dorsal columns corresponding to the surface N11 potential are illustrated in G; these fast action potentials also visible in A, C, and H on the ascending phase of the N13 potential. The origin of fast N11 activities recorded at lateral and anterior electrode sites (D–F) is not firmly assessed (presynaptic afferents in the dorsal horn, spinocerebellar pathways). Calibration: horizontal bars 10 msec, vertical bars 10 μV except in G, where it represents 1 μV. Modified from Jeanmonod, Sindou, and Mauguière (29).*

the most adapted for recording the spinal N13/P13 segmental response (see Fig. 43.2). The segmental N13 potential often shows amplitude reduction, rather than latency prolongation, when the dorsal afferent volley is time dispersed, or when the number of responding dorsal horn neurons is reduced. For clinical purposes, the amplitude ratio between the N13 and its preceding positive wave (P9) generated in proximal dorsal roots has been proposed as a reliable procedure to assess the amplitude of dorsal horn potentials in the clinics.

An "upper cervical N13" has been described, supposedly generated by the presynaptic volley in the dorsal column fibers close to the cuneate nucleus (32,33). The difficulty of separating it from the dorsal horn N13 lessens its reliability in routine clinical recordings (see reference 34 for a review).

3.1.3. CONDUCTED CERVICAL N11 COMPONENT

The nuchal N11 potential is recorded all along the posterior aspect of the neck, where it usually appears to encroach upon the ascending slope of N13. In direct recordings on the cervical cord surface N11 appears as a fast polyphasic component that overlaps in time with the slower N13 segmental postsynaptic potential (see Fig. 43.3). In non-cephalic reference recordings the N11 onset latency increases from C6 to C1 spinal processes by 0.9 ± 0.15 msec (25,35), suggesting that it reflects the ascending volley in dorsal columns at the cervical cord level.

3.1.4. FAR-FIELD SCALP POSITIVITIES (P9, P11, P13, P14)

On scalp non-cephalic reference recordings three or four stationary positivities are consistently observed with a wide distribution and a mediofrontal predominance. In normal adults these potentials peak with mean latencies of 9, 11, 13, and 14 msec and are labeled P9, P11, P13, and P14 (36), respectively, according to the polarity-latency nomenclature (Figs. 43.1 and 43.4A). Contrary to that of the dorsal horn N13, the amplitude of these far-field positive potentials is not affected when the stimulation rate is increased up to 50 Hz (24).

The P9 potential is picked up at the neck as well as on the scalp. It reflects the afferent volley in the trunks of the brachial plexus in the axilla and supraclavicular fossa (37).

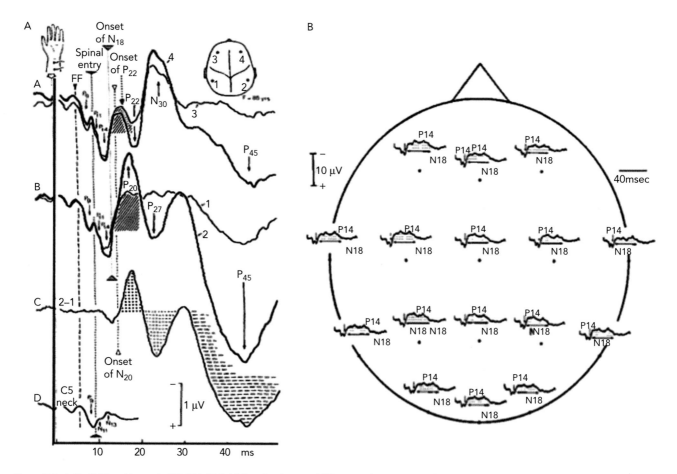

Figure 43.4. **A:** Far-field positive peaks (P9, P11, P14), N18, and early cortical SEPs to median nerve stimulation recorded with a non-cephalic reference electrode. The P9, P11, and P14 far-field potentials are picked up on all scalp derivations: contralateral (2, parietal; 4, frontal) and ipsilateral (1, parietal; 3, frontal) to stimulation. The N18 potential is identifiable only in the parietal region ipsilateral to the stimulation where no cortical response is present. The hatched area indicates the N18 onset and ascending phase, but note that N18 takes end only after the 35-msec post stimulus (trace 1). By subtracting the ipsilateral parietal response from the contralateral, the genuine early cortical parietal SEPs can be isolated. **B:** Scalp topography of the P14 and N18 potentials. In this patient with a large left centro-parietal lobe lesion eliminating all cortical SEPs, the N18 is recorded on the whole surface of the scalp, preceded by the P9 and P14 potentials (non-cephalic reference recording). Note that the amplitude of the P14 potential is maximal in the frontal region, whereas that of the P9 potential is similar at all recording sites. **A**, from Desmedt and Cheron (36) (modified, with permission of authors).

The P11 potential reflects the ascending volley in the fibers of dorsal columns at the cervical level; it is not recorded in about 20% of normal controls and thus the clinical significance of its absence in patients is questionable. Conversely, its persistence when later scalp components are abnormal is a reliable indicator of preserved dorsal column function in patients with lesions located in the medulla oblongata or at the cervicomedullary junction.

The P13-P14 far-field potentials are consistently recorded in normal subjects (see reference 38 for a review). Both may be of similar amplitude, or either of them may be the larger of the two. P14, but not P13, peaks later than the cervical segmental N13 potential. The P9 potential is smaller than the P14 potential when recorded with a broad bandpass, which allows quantifying the P14 amplitude decrease using a P9/P14 amplitude ratio (39). The P13–P14 complex, but not the earlier far-fields, can be recorded with a scalp–earlobe montage. Patients with thalamic lesions usually show a normal P14, suggesting that this component originates at the subthalamic level (40,41). Conversely, in cervicomedullary lesions (26) or in brain-dead patients (30), the P14 potential is absent. These

findings suggest that the generator of P14 is situated above the level of the foramen magnum. Recordings in patients having undergone hemispherectomy (42) or in brain death support the hypothesis that P13 and P14 potentials are generated at different levels along the medial lemniscus (see the section below on brain death).

3.1.5. N18 Scalp Negativity

This potential, identified by Desmedt and Cheron (36), is a long-lasting scalp negative shift that immediately follows P14 (see Fig. 43.4A). In normal conditions N18 can be identified only in the posterior parietal region ipsilateral to the stimulation, where there is no or minimal interference with cortical potentials. If low frequencies are cut off by excessive filtering the N18 can become a "peak" falsely interpreted as an ipsilateral cortical N20. When all cortical responses are eliminated by deafferentation due to a lesion of the ventroposterolateral thalamic nucleus (43) or by direct lesion of the centroparietal cortex (44), N18 can be recorded on the whole surface of the scalp (see Fig. 43.4B). After hemispherectomy, which entails retrograde degeneration of the thalamocortical neurons, the

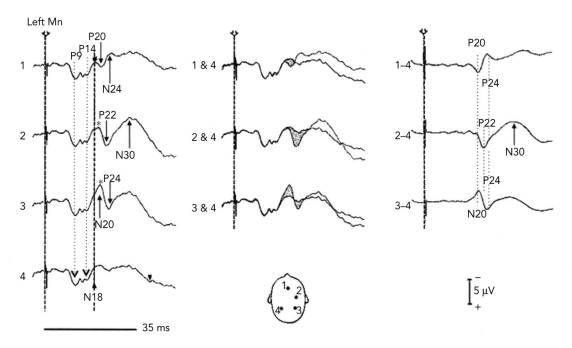

Figure 43.5. Identification of early cortical N20/P20, P22, P24/N24, and N30 potentials (left median nerve stimulation, non-cephalic reference recording). Since the subcortical far-field positivities and N18 potentials are recorded uncontaminated by cortical potentials in the parietal region ipsilateral to stimulation (trace 4, left column), responses obtained in this region can be used as a baseline to assess cortical responses, either by superimposition to (middle column) or subtraction from (right column) the contralateral responses. This shows that the N20/P20, P22, and P24 potentials have distinct peak latencies. Moreover, the negativities (asterisks) recorded in the contralateral central (2) and midfrontal region (1) disappear in difference waveforms. They correspond to interruption of the widespread N18 (Fig. 43.4) by the cortical positive responses P20 and P22. Due to the restricted filter bandpass used for this recording, the P14 amplitude is less than that of the P9 potential.

N18 potential is most often preserved (45). These observations rule out the possibility that N18 could reflect a cortical or a thalamic response to ascending inputs. N18 has been considered a postsynaptic response of the brainstem nuclei connected with the dorsal column nuclei, because intracerebral human SEP recordings show a stationary negativity between the upper pons and the midbrain, peaking at the same latency as the scalp N18 (46). Other authors, however, have suggested an origin in the nucleus cuneatus itself, based on nasopharyngeal recordings and similarity with responses evoked in cats (47,48). Cortical SEPs in the range of 20 to 40 msec are superimposed on the widespread N18 plateau, which entails some problems when estimating their true amplitude. Since most of the N18 is also picked up at the earlobe, the use of the earlobe or parietal electrode ipsilateral to stimulation as a reference point eliminates the N18 negative shift in the resulting waveforms, hence allowing easy estimation of cortical potentials amplitude (Figs. 43.4B and 43.5).

3.1.6. EARLY CORTICAL SEPs

These cortical SEPs peak in the 18- to 35-msec latency range and are all obtained with optimal voltage in response to stimuli delivered at a slow rate (<2/sec). They are recorded on the scalp in the parietal region contralateral to stimulation and in a large frontocentral area, mostly contralateral to stimulation.

3.1.7. N20-P20 AND P22 POTENTIALS

Two sets of early cortical potentials are consistently recorded in normal subjects on the scalp contralateral to stimulation.

The first is made of a parietal N20 and frontal P20 dipolar field (N20-P20); the second is composed of a central P22 positivity (see Fig. 43.5). These components are also present after finger stimulation with a latency delay of 2 to 3 msec, as compared with median nerve SEPs, because of finger-to-wrist conduction time.

The parietal N20 and frontal P20 reflect the activity of a dipolar generator in Brodmann's area 3b situated in the posterior bank of the rolandic fissure (49) and represent the earliest cortical potential elicited by median nerve stimulation. All source modeling studies of electrical and magnetic fields, as well as direct cortical recordings, converge on the conclusion that the N20-P20 field is produced by a dipolar source tangential to the scalp surface reflecting the response of area 3b to cutaneous inputs.

On scalp (see Fig. 43.5) and direct cortical recordings a P22 wave recorded over the central region was found to peak 1 to 2 msec later than the N20-P20 potentials (50–52). Spatial maps have shown that the N20-P20 dipolar field is followed by a positive P22 field with little or no negative counterpart on the scalp (53,54), suggesting that its source is radial to the scalp surface. Most studies of SEFs failed to confirm such a radial source in the central region, possibly because magnetic recordings are blind to magnetic fields produced by dipolar sources radial to the scalp surface (55–57). The question of whether the radial source of the central P22 is located behind the central sulcus, in primary somatosensory area (SI), or in front of it, in in primary motor area (MI), is not easy to address by scalp recordings, even when assisted by source imaging (58–60). In favor of a precentral origin, the P22 may be selectively lost in patients with hemispheric lesions who have normal sensations but signs of upper motor neuron dysfunction, and selectively preserved in patients with hemianesthesia or astereognosis and no motor deficit (61–64, see Fig. 43.15 later in the chapter). Some direct cortical recordings in monkeys and humans failed to identify a P22 in the precentral cortex (65,66) but individualized a surface positive potential, labeled as P25, with a source radial to the scalp surface and located at the posterior edge of the rolandic fissure in Brodmann's area 1. However, more recent simultaneous intracortical recordings of median nerve SEPs in SI and MI areas showed that a genuine early response is generated in M1 (51,52). Lastly, Nicholson-Peterson et al. (67), recording median nerve SEPs in the cortex of monkeys, showed that the earliest cortical responses to upper limb stimulation are likely to result from the approximately coincident activation of three dipolar sources in areas 3b, 4, and 1 with orientations opposing and orthogonal to each other. Sources in area 3b and 4 have opposite orientations tangential to the scalp surface, while the source located in area 1, at the crown of the postcentral gyrus, is oriented radial to the scalp surface. Dipole source analysis of either magnetoencephalography (MEG) or subdural electroencephalographic (EEG) recordings in humans located the P22 slightly posterior and superficial to the N20 generator, and suggested an origin in the crown of the postcentral gyrus (BA1) (54,68).

3.1.8. PARIETAL P24 AND P27 POTENTIALS

These potentials are recorded in the parietal region contralateral to stimulation; their peaking latencies show large interindividual variations, between 24 and 27 msec. In some subjects two distinct P24 and P27 potentials can be identified, while only one of the two peaks is observed in others. This explains why, according to the polarity-latency nomenclature, the first parietal positive potential following N20 has received various labels in the literature (P24, P25, or P27). These variations reflect the fact that the activities of several parietal sources overlap in time in this latency range. The P27 potential was found to be abnormal in patients with focal lesions of the parietal cortex, presenting with astereognosis and preserved N30 frontal responses (62). A P27 source in the primary somatosensory area (Brodmann's area 1), radial to the scalp surface, would accord with these findings. The P24 potential on its own is associated with a frontal N24 potential (see below). The dipolar source of the P24-N24 field is tangential to the scalp surface (69) and thus presumed to be located in the posterior bank of the rolandic fissure (Figs. 43.4, 43.5, and 43.6).

3.1.9. FRONTAL N24-N30 WAVEFORM

The frontal potential peaking at 30 msec after stimulus, labeled as N30 in most clinical studies, has warranted much attention in the SEPs literature because it shows some abnormality in patients with various types of motor disorders. It is picked up in the frontal region contralateral to stimulation; however, it often spreads to the midfrontal region and to the frontal region ipsilateral to stimulus. Early hypotheses of a single N30-P30 dipolar field, frontal negative and parietal positive, generated by a single source in area 3b were challenged by data showing

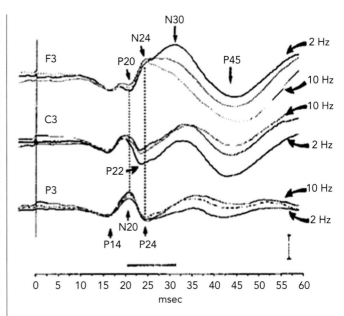

Figure 43.6. Identification of the P24-N24 dipolar field and frontal N30 responses. Responses to right median nerve stimulation have been recorded in the left parietal (P3), central (C3), and frontal (F3) regions at stimulus rates of 2 (thick traces), 5, and 10 Hz. The dipolar P24-N24 response is unaffected, while the frontal N30 is dramatically depressed, by increasing the stimulus rates. Calibration: 2 μV. From Garcia-Larrea, Bastuji, and Mauguière (69) (with permission of authors).

that this potential was composed of a first response (N24-P24 or N27-P27) of clearly dipolar field distribution (69), followed by a more widespread radial component, or "genuine" (N30). While the early N24-P24 remains unaffected if the stimulus frequency is increased up to 10 Hz, the later N30 decreases at stimulus rates higher than 1/sec and is virtually absent at 10/sec (69,70) (see Fig. 43.6). The administration of tiagabine, which enhances aminobutyric acid (GABA) inhibition, increases selectively the voltage of the N24-P24 dipolar field, suggesting that it could reflect hyperpolarization of deep spiny cells that follows their initial depolarization and is strongly influenced by inhibitory inputs from layer IV GABAergic cells. Interestingly, the firing properties of the cell population generating high-frequency SEPs were unaffected by the increase of GABAergic inhibition (71).

While the existence of any N30 potential generated in the precentral cortex has been questioned (65,66) on the basis of direct cortical recordings in monkeys and humans, several observations support the existence of an N30 generator distinct from early parietal components:

1. N30 amplitude decreases with aging while that of P27 increases (50).

2. N30 can be selectively absent, or decreased, with preserved parietal P27, in patients with focal lesions of the frontal lobe (62) presenting with motor symptoms and normal sensation.

3. N30 was found to be selectively reduced in Parkinson's disease with a decrease of the N30/P27 amplitude ratio (see below).

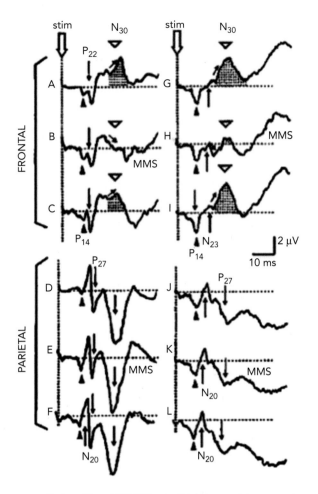

Figure 43.7. *Gating of frontal SEP N30 potential during mental movement simulation (MMS). These responses were obtained in two distinct normal subjects (right and left traces) before (A, D, G, J), during (B, E, H, K), and after (C, F, I, L) MMS. The dotted areas indicate the N30 potential surface above the baseline. Note that parietal responses are not affected by MMS. From Cheron and Borenstein (72) (with permission of authors).*

4. The most convincing evidence that the N30 potential may have a frontal origin stems from its relation with motor programming (see reference 12 for a review). Voluntary movements of the fingers on the stimulated side exert a gating effect on frontal SEPs by reducing selectively the amplitude of N30, with no effect on parietal potentials. The gating of N30 does not require that the intended movement be executed and is also observed when the subject mentally simulates a complex sequence of finger movements on the stimulated side (Fig. 43.7) (72,73). When the mental movement simulation (MMS) concerns the nonstimulated hand, or when the subject performs a mental task other than motor simulation, this gating effect does not occur. N30 gating during MMS has been considered as indirect evidence that the supplementary motor area (SMA) might be the generator of the N30 potential. Lastly, the N30 potential, as well as the homolog M30 magnetic field, is enhanced when subject observes repetitive grasping movements or complex sequences of finger movements performed by an examiner during stimulation. This effect is independent of the complexity of the observed movements; it has been interpreted as reflecting storage of the subject's somatosensory information connected with the observed movements (74).

While there is little doubt that the N30 amplitude is linked to motor programming, its origin in SMA is challenged by data from direct cortical recordings, which favor a N30 dipolar source radial to the scalp surface, located in Brodmann's area 1 of the SI cortex (49) and do not show a N30 potential in SMA (75). Moreover, after subtraction of the N24-P24 field, the maximum of the remaining scalp N30 field has the same location as that of the P22 potential in the central region, suggesting an origin close to the central sulcus and not in the premotor cortex (76,77).

3.1.10. Ipsilateral Short-Latency Cortical Potentials

No early cortical potential is observed on the scalp ipsilateral to electrical stimulation of the median nerve in normal subjects as well as in the majority of direct cortical recordings. However, a few median nerve SEP recordings with subdural electrodes placed over the central cortical area have shown an early ipsilateral median nerve potential with an amplitude 4 to 16 times smaller than that of the contralateral response, which can be maximal anterior to the rolandic fissure (78). The functional significance of these ipsilateral responses and the nature of their afferent pathways remain speculative.

3.2. Middle- and Long-Latency SEPs to Upper Limb Stimulation

These responses have been identified either by scalp and cortical SEP recordings or through modeling of magnetic SEFs. They have, however, not proved their clinical utility, and most of them are modulated by cognitive factors.

3.2.1. P45 and N60 Potentials

Both P45 and N60 potentials are recorded contralaterally to the stimulation in the central and frontal regions. It is still debated whether they reflect the activation of associative cortical areas, via cortico-cortical connections, or cortical responses to inputs transmitted directly from the thalamus. SEP studies in patients with focal lesions have shown that P45 is always preserved in patients with isolated loss of pain and temperature sensations (79) and may persist in patients with lesion of the parietal cortex causing astereognosis and abnormal N20 or P27 over the damaged hemisphere (62). This latter finding has been interpreted as suggesting a possible P45 origin from parallel ascending inputs rather than through cortico-cortical fibers from the generators of the N20-P27 potentials. However, the higher amplitude and broader scalp distribution of P45 relative to earlier cortical responses, its higher attenuation by repetition of stimuli at rapid stimulation rates (80), and its sensitivity to attentional modulation (81,82) rather suggest that P45 generation may indeed depend on cortico-cortical projections from SI 3a-3b to the crown of the postcentral gyrus and/or associative parietal areas.

Little is known about the N60 potential. Recordings coupled with source modeling of scalp responses suggest that three distinct sources contribute to the N60; one is located in the frontocentral cortex contralateral to stimulation, and the two others are located in the suprasylvian cortex (somatosensory area SII) on both sides (83). In scalp recordings two distinct components can also be identified on the basis of their latencies and scalp distributions, namely a frontocentral N60 contralateral to stimulation and a bilateral N70 in the temporal regions.

3.2.2. RESPONSES OF THE SECOND SOMATOSENSORY AREA (SII)

The most precise available descriptions of the human SII area have long been those by Penfield and Rasmussen (84) and Woolsey et al. (85), based, respectively, on electrical stimulation and intracortical recordings of SEPs. Both electric SEPs and magnetic SEFs in the latency range of 90 to 120 msec have scalp topography and estimated generators compatible with sources located in the suprasylvian parietal operculum of both hemispheres (86,87). Opercular SEPs/SEFs show somatotopic organization, higher inter-individual variability than SI responses, and exquisite sensitivity to the interstimulus interval (ISI) (80,88,89).

Early corticographic recordings on the surface of the suprasylvian cortex also showed responses, interpreted as originating in SII, peaking in the 100- to 120-msec latency range, ipsilateral and contralateral to the stimulus and sensitive to the ISI and task condition (see reference 90 for a review). Direct intracortical recordings using electrodes stereotactically implanted in the upper bank of the sylvian fissure have shown a robust N60-P90 response to median nerve stimulation (Fig. 43.8) (91), which, contrary to SI responses, continues to increase up to and above pain threshold (92). Ipsilateral SII responses are consistently recorded 10 to 12 msec later than contralateral ones, a delay compatible with a transcallosal

transmission. The difference between corticography and depth intracortical SII responses remains unclear. It is probable that the first N60 potential of depth recordings contributes to the scalp N60 potential (see above) while the second response may be reflected by scalp/corticographic N120.

At a latency of about 140 msec a scalp negativity distributed over both central regions and the vertex is of maximal amplitude when the subject's attention is drawn to the stimulus and he or she is instructed to mentally count the stimuli (93). This response is modulated by attention and shows the same behavior as the endogenous processing negativity originally described in response to auditory tones (see reference 94 for a review). Bilateral activation of SII areas and the midcingulate gyrus could contribute to the generation of this N140 negativity.

The existence of SII SEPs peaking earlier than 40 msec after median nerve stimulus remains a debated issue. Lüders et al. (95), using subdural electrodes in a single epileptic patient, recorded responses in the inferior frontal gyrus, peaking only 2.4 msec later than SI evoked responses, which they considered as originating in the SII area. Stereotactic recordings in the suprasylvian cortex have also shown early bilateral responses peaking at about 30 msec in area SII (96). Using MEG, Karhu and Tesche (97) found, in roughly half of the recordings, neuromagnetic activity localized in the SII area starting at the same time as the first activation in SI. Major thalamic input to SII comes from the ventroposterior inferior nucleus, which has been shown to receive input via the dorsal column system in cats and might be responsible for these somewhat inconsistent early SII responses.

3.2.3. LONG-LATENCY RESPONSES OF POSTERIOR PARIETAL, MESIAL, AND FRONTAL CORTEX

SEF sources have been modeled in the posterior parietal (98) and mesial cortex (99) contralateral to stimulation and in both frontal lobes (100,101), which are all active in the latency range of 70 to 160 msec, in response to stimuli delivered at

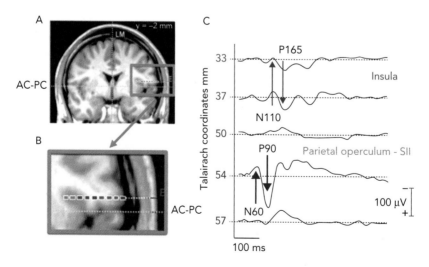

Figure 43.8. Intracortical median nerve SEPs recorded in the parietal operculum and insula contralateral to stimulation. SEPs were recorded through intracortical multi-contact electrodes implanted perpendicular to the midsagittal plane (**A**) referred to a distant electrode placed in cranial bone thickness. The external contacts in blue are located in the suprasylvian parietal opercular SII area; the internal contacts in red are located in the cortex of the dorsal insula (**B**). In **C** the trace recorded at 54 mm from the midsagittal plane shows the N60-P90 SII response; the trace recorded more deeply, at 37 mm from the midsagittal plane, shows the N110-P165 insular response. Note the delay of 50 msec between the opercular SII (N60, P90) and insular (N110, P165) SEPs. AC-AP: anterior commissure–posterior commissure horizontal plane in the Talairach's stereotaxic system of coordinates.

long interstimulus intervals, in particular when mentally counted by the subject. Thus the magnetic field distribution at these latencies reflects simultaneous activation of multiple and largely distributed sources.

3.3. Short-Latency SEPs to Lower Limb Stimulation

Most authors use electrical stimulation of the tibial nerve at the ankle to test the sensory pathways of the lower limb. However, the electrical stimulation can also be applied to the sural nerve at the ankle, or to the peroneal nerve at the knee, without major changes in the general waveform of the spinal or scalp responses. Compared with tibial nerve SEPs, only the peaking latencies are modified; they are delayed by ~3 msec, or shortened by ~5 to 6 msec, respectively, for sural and peroneal nerve stimulation. In what follows, tibial nerve SEPs are taken as the reference for describing the normal waveforms (Fig. 43.9).

3.3.1. Peripheral Nerve and Dorsal Root Responses
A compound action potential corresponding to the activation of tibial nerve fibers is recorded at the posterior aspect of the knee using a bipolar montage. The negativity of this near-field potential peaks at a latency of ~7 to 8 msec in adults. This N7 potential reflects a mixed response of motor and sensory fibers, which is clinically useful to assess the function of the

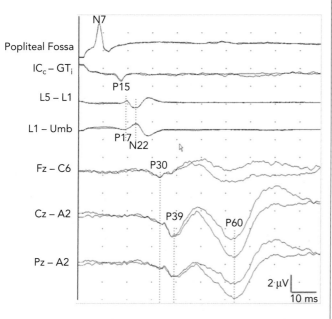

Figure 43.9. Short-latency tibial nerve SEPs. The N7 potential recorded in the popliteal fossa reflects the afferent volley of action potentials in the tibial nerve. The P15 potential recorded between the iliac crest contralateral to stimulus (ICc) and greater trochanter ipsilateral to stimulus (GTi) is generated at the entry of the sciatic nerve in the pelvis at the level of the greater sciatic foramen. The P17 and N22 potentials recorded with a transverse derivation between the spinous process of the L1 vertebra and the supra-umbilical region (Umb) reflect the afferent volley in the cauda equina and the postsynaptic response of dorsal horn neurons, respectively. The P30 potential recorded in the medio-frontal scalp region (Fz) referred to an electrode placed over the spinous process of C6 vertebra (C6) is generated at the cervicomedullary junction. On the scalp midline derivations between the central (Cz) and parietal (Pz) sites and the earlobe ipsilateral to the stimulus (A2) pick up the first cortical P39 potential.

peripheral segment of the pathway. Using a contralateral iliac crest (ICc)—ipsilateral greater trochanter (GTi) derivation, a P15 potential is recorded, which is a junctional potential generated at the entry of the sciatic nerve in the pelvis at the level of the greater sciatic foramen (102). The afferent volley in cauda equina roots can be recorded as an N17 potential using bipolar leads between adjacent skin electrodes placed at the spinous processes of the L2 to L5 vertebrae (103), or as a P17 when the activity is derived between lumbar electrodes and a distant reference site (104,105).

3.3.2. Spinal Potentials
A derivation between the spinal process of the T12 or L1 vertebrae and a distant reference electrode records a spinal negative potential peaking at 21 to 24 msec in normal subjects. According to different authors, this segmental response has been labeled N20, N21 N22 N23, or N24. These differences in nomenclature are mostly due to differences in the mean body height of the subjects sampled for normative studies. In what follows this response is labeled N22. After tibial nerve stimulation the lumbar N22 originates mostly from the spinal segment receiving fibers from the S1 root (104).

Like all segmental dorsal horn responses (see reference 106 for a review), the N22 demonstrates a polarity reversal when recorded anterior to the cord, a field distribution consistent with a horizontal dipolar source reflecting the postsynaptic response of dorsal horn neurons to incoming inputs. The N22 amplitude is maximal close to the entry zone of the S1 root in cord surface recordings and decreases steeply without any latency shift at more rostral or caudal electrode sites (29). In intraoperative direct recording of the cord, several fast negativities are superimposed on the ascending slope of the N22; they reflect the action potentials ascending in the dorsal columns. In most skin surface recordings these negativities cannot be individualized.

3.3.3. Scalp Far-Field P30 Potential
With non-cephalic reference montages widespread far-field positivities can be recorded on the scalp that peak before the onset of the earliest cortical potential in the latency range of 25 to 32 msec (104,105). Only the latest of these positivities, identified by Yamada et al. (104) as the P31 potential, is consistently recorded in healthy subjects after tibial nerve stimulation at the ankle. This potential was labeled as P28, P30, or P31. Its latency varies according to body height; it is labeled P30 in this chapter, according to our normative data.

The P30 potential is widely distributed on the scalp with a predominance in the frontal region (107) and therefore is drastically reduced in scalp-reference recordings. When recorded with electrodes located in the fourth ventricle during surgery, this potential shows the same intracranial spatiotemporal distribution as the P14 component of median nerve SEPs (108). Therefore, the P30 potential is likely to be generated in the lower brainstem (104,105) and can be viewed as the homolog, for the lower limb, of the far-field P14 recorded on the scalp after median nerve stimulation.

Recording of P30 is made easier if the scalp electrode is placed in the midfrontal region at Fz or Fpz, with a reference electrode at the spinous process of the sixth cervical vertebra (109). Since no segmental response is evoked by lower limb stimulation at the cervical cord level, the neck can be considered as virtually inactive at the peaking latency of P30. In some normal subjects a scalp far-field P27 potential distinct from P30 is recordable in the frontal region, which reflects the ascending volley in the cervical cord (104,105).

3.3.4. N33 Scalp Potential

In non-cephalic or earlobe reference recordings a small N33 negativity (107) may precede the P39 potential. This negativity is widely distributed over the scalp; part of it is also picked up at the earlobe so that it is reduced in earlobe reference recordings (110). N33 is considered as the homolog of the N18 upper limb SEPs and is likely to have a similar origin in the lower brainstem (see above).

3.3.5. Cortical Potentials

The earliest cortical potential elicited by the stimulation of tibial nerve at the ankle is a positive potential usually labeled P37, P39, or P40 because it peaks at a mean latency of 37 to 40 msec in normal subjects (see reference 111 for a review). In what follows this potential is labeled P39. This potential peaks 6 to 7 msec earlier after stimulation of the tibial nerve at the popliteal fossa, and ~3 msec later after stimulation of the sural nerve at the ankle. In normal subjects P39 can be recorded on the vertex and can be reliably obtained midway between Pz and Cz using a scalp-to-earlobe montage. Frequently the maximum of P39, although close to the midline, is slightly shifted on the side of the scalp ipsilateral to the stimulation. The most likely reason for this paradoxical lateralization is that the somatotopic representation of the lower limb in the somatosensory SI, and in particular that of the foot, is situated at the inner aspect of the hemisphere. SEP mapping in normals often shows a dipolar field distribution for P39, with a maximum of positivity ipsilateral to the stimulation in the parietal region and a maximum of negativity (N39) in the contralateral frontocentral region (107,112). The negative N39 maximum of this dipolar field is not consistently obtained, probably because of intersubject differences in the orientation of the leg area in SI with respect to the scalp surface.

The question is still debated whether all of these potentials reflect the activity of the lower limb area in SI, or whether some could be generated in other cortical areas. Another question is to determine whether the P39-N39 dipolar field has only a single source in SI tangential to the scalp or several. The following observations support the latter hypothesis:

1. N39 and P39 can show some latency differences, the former peaking earlier than the latter (113).

2. P39 is reduced at high stimulation rates (114), while the frontal N39 amplitude remains unaffected at stimulus rates up to 7.5 Hz (112).

3. Source modeling studies of scalp responses and direct intracerebral recordings have suggested that two sources located in the central region are quasi-simultaneously involved in the generation of the N39-P39 field on the

scalp surface (115,116). One is tangential to the scalp surface and responsible for a dipolar field with a positive maximum in the centroparietal region ipsilateral to stimulus, and a negative maximum in the frontotemporal region contralateral to stimulus. The other is perpendicular to the scalp surface and responsible for part of the vertex P39 potential.

4. Studies of the effects of movement on cortical tibial SEPs have shown that P39, but not N39, is gated during voluntary movement of the stimulated foot (117,118).

P39 is followed by N50 and P60 components, these three waves forming the "W" profile (P39-N50-P60) of the cortical response recorded in the centroparietal region. This waveform has been reported in all studies on tibial nerve SEPs (see reference 110 for a review). The N50 and P60 potentials culminate at the vertex (Cz) and do not show the same clear dipolar distribution as the P39-N39 response on the scalp, thus suggesting that the W-shaped P39-N50-P60 waveform could be generated by several sources with distinct orientations (107). N50 and P60 show the same attenuation as P39 during active movement (117).

3.4. Scalp SEPs Evoked by Stimulation of the L5 and S1 Dermatomes

Electrical stimulation of the L5 and S1 dermatomes, applied at the medial side of the first metatarsophalangeal joint and at the lateral side of the fifth metatarsophalangeal joint, respectively, yields consistent W-shaped evoked potentials on the scalp (119). The first scalp positive potential peaks at mean latencies of about 48.5 and 50 msec, respectively, for stimulation of the L5 and S1 dermatomes.

3.5. Short-Latency SEPs to Pudendal Nerve Stimulation

Stimulation of the dorsal nerves of the penis or the clitoris elicits spinal and scalp responses with a waveform very similar to that of SEPs obtained by stimulation of the posterior tibial nerve. A spinal negative N15 potential equivalent to the tibial nerve N22 potential can be recorded on the skin surface of the lumbar region after stimulation of the penis or clitoris (120). On direct cord recordings the N15 potential shows a polarity reversal on the anterior aspect of the cord and is preceded by a P10 potential that has the same origin as the tibial nerve P17 potential (121). Electrical stimulation of the dorsal nerve of the penis (or clitoris) also yields consistent, W-shaped, EPs on the scalp (122). The earliest positivity of this response culminates at 40 msec after stimulation. Direct cortical recordings have located the genitalia somatotopic area anterior to the foot area on the mesial aspect of SI (123).

3.6. SEPs to Trigeminal Nerve Stimulation

A P19 scalp component can be evoked by electrical stimulation of the lips (124). Other authors using various methods of stimulation described similar cortical SEP components. The scalp response to stimulation of trigeminal afferents recorded by means of surface electrodes can be contaminated by muscular artifacts. To detect, but also to locate, the trigeminal nerve dysfunction, it has been proposed to stimulate the infraorbital nerve through needle electrodes inserted into the infraorbital foramen (125). With this type of stimulation three far-field positive waves can be recorded that reflect the compound action potential at the entry of the maxillary nerve into the gasserian ganglion (W1), at the entry zone of the trigeminal root into the pons (W2), and in the presynaptic portion of the trigeminal spinal tract (W3) (for a discussion of trigeminal SEPs see reference 2).

3.7. Measurement of the Central Conduction Time

One of the advantages of SEP recording in clinical routine is to permit an evaluation of the transit time of the ascending volley in the central segments of the somatosensory pathways. In most studies this transit time is referred to as the central conduction time (CCT).

3.7.1. CCT in Upper Limb SEPs

Various montages and procedures have been proposed for measuring the CCT depending on whether the aim is merely to detect a conduction slowing and to follow up CCT values during the evolution of a disease in the same individual, or to locate accurately the site where conduction velocity is slowed down. Conduction in the proximal segment of brachial plexus roots can be evaluated by measuring the interval between the peaks of the supraclavicular N9 (or far-field P9) and of the spinal N13 potentials. Since its early description (126) the interpeak interval between the cervical N13 and the parietal N20 potentials has been the most widely used method for assessing CCT from cervical spinal cord to cortex. However, this procedure evaluates the CCT from the peak of a postsynaptic dorsal horn potential (N13), which is produced in parallel to the ascending volley in the dorsal columns. In intramedullary cervical cord lesions, for instance, a normal conduction in the dorsal columns may coexist with a clearly abnormal, or even absent, N13 potential (127). Moreover, the N13-N20 interval does not allow a separate assessment of conduction times in the intraspinal and intracranial segments of the somatosensory pathways (Fig. 43.10).

The N13-N20 CCT is usually measured from the peak of the cervical negativity recorded at C6 to the peak of the contralateral parietal N20 using mediofrontal (Fz) reference montages. The use of a frontal reference may introduce some uncertainty in the identification of the N13 and N20 potentials because the brainstem P14 and cortical P22 potentials recorded by the scalp Fz reference are injected as negative N14 and N22 potentials in the C6-Fz and parietal-Fz traces, respectively, so that their peaks can be confused with those of the genuine cervical N13 and parietal N20 potentials.

In non-cephalic reference recordings three transit times can be calculated to assess central conduction (see Fig. 43.10 (128)). Conduction from the brachial plexus roots to the brainstem and from the brainstem to the parietal cortex can be

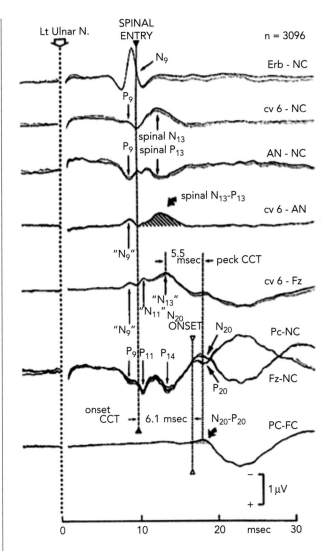

Figure 43.10. CCT measurements: ulnar nerve SEPs. The entry time of the afferent volley in the spinal cord corresponds to the onset latency of the N11 potential at C6 or anterior neck (AC) recorded with a non-cephalic (NC) or Fz reference, and to the P11 recorded in the parietal region contralateral to stimulation (Pc) or mid-frontal region (Fz) with an NC reference. The N20 onset latency can be measured either after superimposition of contralateral parietal and frontal traces, or by subtraction of these two responses (PC-FC). In this normal subject the peak CCT between N13 and N20 is 5.5 msec, while the onset CCT measured from the entry time of the afferent volley in the cord and the onset of the cortical N20 is 6.1 msec. From Ozaki, Takada, Shimamura, Baba, and Matsunaga (128) (with permission of authors).

explored, respectively, by calculating the P9-P14 and the P14-N20 intervals. The global CCT can be evaluated by measuring the intervals either between peaks of N13 and N20 potentials (peak CCT) or between the onsets of N11 and N13 potentials (onset CCT). Only the interval between the onsets of N11 and of N20 that actually assesses the transit time from the spinal entry to the cortex, shows that the ulnar nerve CCT is longer than the median nerve CCT, and correlates with body height in normal subjects (128).

3.7.2. CCT in Lower Limb SEPs

In most clinical applications of tibial nerve SEPs the CCT from the lumbosacral spinal cord to the cortex is evaluated by the interval between the peak of the lumbar N22 negativity and the peak of the cortical P39 potential. As for upper limb SEPs, one can argue (1) that the N22 potential reflects a postsynaptic dorsal horn response, which can be abnormal in patients with lesions of the lumbosacral spinal cord whose CCT is preserved and (2) that only the onset of N22 reflects the spinal entry time of the afferent volley. However, only N22-P39 interpeak CCT has been validated in clinical studies. The peaking latencies of N22 and P39 correlate with body height in normal subjects, while authors' opinions diverge concerning the correlation between N22-P39 interpeak interval and height. Several attempts have been made to evaluate separately the intraspinal and intracranial CCT using lower limb SEPs. Recordings of a dorsal column CAP, the latency of which increases from caudal to rostral levels of the spine, have been reported by several authors (104,105)). However, due to the time dispersion of the ascending volley at the cervical level, as evidenced by direct recordings of the cord (121), the amplitude of the spinal CAP drops dramatically from T12 to T6 and cervical responses recorded with skin electrodes are small (104,129) or even nonrecordable at C6 or C2 in shoulder reference recordings. It has been shown that measuring the N22-P30 and P30-P39 interpeak intervals provides a reliable evaluation of the intraspinal and intracranial CCTs in normal subjects and patients with focal cervical cord, brainstem, and hemispheric lesions (109,130).

3.8. Cortical High Frequency Oscillations (HFOs) Evoked by Somatosensory Stimuli

In the1980s digital bandpass filtering between 300 and 2,500 Hz revealed that several wavelets with a frequency of ~600 Hz are synchronous with the ascending and descending slopes of the N20-P20 potential (131). Several of these HFOs were shown to be markedly attenuated in non–rapid-eye-movement (NREM) sleep while the voltage of the N20-P20 "slow wave" was preserved (132) and magnetic recordings showed that HFOs and N20 sources are co-localized in the posterior bank of the central sulcus (area 3b) (133). Since these early studies somatosensory evoked cortical HFOs have been extensively explored in humans and animal models as potential markers of cortex sensitivity to thalamocortical afferent inputs. Ozaki and Hashimoto (134) recently reviewed these numerous studies. Five to eight HFO peaks underlying the parietal N20 and frontal P20 show a phase reversal between parietal and frontal traces, while a few HFO peaks synchronous with the central P22 show a phase alignment across the central fissure, thus suggesting that dipolar sources of these two sets of HFOs are differently oriented, respectively tangential and radial to the scalp surface (135) (Fig. 43.11). A distinction was proposed between HFOs occurring before (early HFOs) and after (late HFOs) the N20 peak because responsiveness to various modulations differs between early and late HFOs. As observed for N20 potential, late HFOs are strongly depressed when stimuli frequency is >12 Hz, favoring the view that both reflect postsynaptic activities, while early HFOs, as action potentials in afferent thalamocortical fibers, are relatively unaffected at high-frequency stimulation rates. The amplitudes and durations of both late HFOs and N20 are increased in children and aged subjects compared to young adults. Conversely, reciprocal changes have been

observed for late HFOs and N20 in other conditions: (1) late HFOs, but not early HFOs, decrease during hyperventilation while the N20 increases and (2) tactile stimulation of the stimulated hand also has opposite effects on magnetic N20 and HFO amplitudes. The mechanisms of HFOs at a cellular level are still matter of controversy; if there is a consensus that early HFOs reflect activity of thalamocortical axon terminals in layer IV of area 3b, it remains open whether late HFOs reflect excitatory postsynaptic activities of pyramidal cells or are produced by the activity of inhibitory interneurons (see reference 134 for a review, and Chapters 2 and 33 in this book) (see Fig. 43.11).

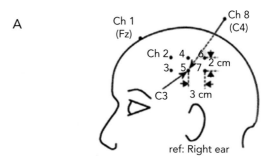

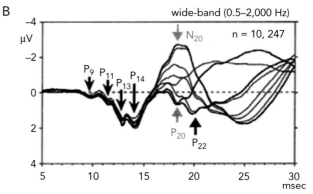

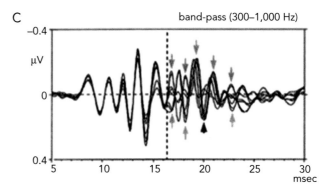

Figure 43.11. *HFOs evoked by median nerve stimulation.* **A:** *Positions of the eight electrodes over the scalp.* **B:** *Superimposition of all traces recorded with a wide-band filter (0.5–2,000 Hz).* **C:** *The digitally high pass-filtered traces extracted from B. Following the high-frequency components embedded in P9-P14, cortical HFOs start at the onset of the N20-P20 response about 16 msec, and their phase reversal is clearly discerned between the frontal and parietal regions (gray arrows). In addition, at around 20 msec, when the central P22 culminates in wide-band recordings, a single HFO is in phase (black arrow), suggesting a radial current source. From Ozaki, Suzuki, Yaegashi, Baba, Matsunaga, and Hashimoto (135) (reprinted and modified with permission of authors).*

3.9. Potentials Evoked by Nociceptive Stimulation

The easiest and most robust way to activate selectively the small Aδ and C fibers responding to painful stimuli are brief heat pulses delivered by infrared laser beams (136). Cortical responses to laser stimuli (LEPs) depend on inputs conveyed in the spinothalamic tracts and are clinically useful in patients with suspected impairment of pain and temperature sensation (reviewed in references 137 and 138). LEPs are particularly useful in patients with neuropathic pain, which is mainly associated with lesions of pain and temperature pathways (139,140). The involvement of the large fibers-dorsal-column-lemniscal system is, on the contrary, not crucial for most cases of neuropathic pain.

Due to the small number of fibers stimulated by laser beams, and the temporal dispersion of afferent volleys in small-diameter axons, segmental responses of the dorsal horn are not elicited on skin recordings, and LEPs inform exclusively about cortical potentials. As shown in Figure 43.12 the earliest cortical potential evoked by laser stimulation of the hand has a dipolar N1-P1 distribution on the scalp with a negative maximum peaking at ~160 msec in the temporal region contralateral to stimulation, and a positive maximum in the midfrontal region (141). It is followed by a negative-positive "vertex complex" commonly labeled N2-P2, peaking respectively at 200 to 250 msec and 300 to 350 msec (reviewed in references 2, 20, and 142).

Both source modeling and intracranial recordings have permitted the determination of the main cortical origin of LEPs recorded within the first 500 msec following Aδ laser

stimulation. The earliest responses (scalp N1-P1) reflect activation of the operculo-insular cortex (SII and posterior insula) (143) in the suprasylvian region, with a simultaneous and weak contribution of the primary somatosensory areas (S1). The vertex "N2-P2" complex reflects the combined activation of bilateral posterior insular and midcingulate cortex (20, 142). In addition, intracranial recordings have shown a sequential activation of other brain regions, including the amygdala, anterior insular cortex, hippocampus, perigenual and posterior cingulate cortices, and frontoparietal regions (144), but their contribution to scalp-recorded potentials has not been demonstrated yet.

The vertex complex, and in particular its late positive component (P2), is subject to cognitive influences, the amplitude of which may vary widely with attention, vigilance, and other cognitive factors (145–147). The P2 wave, despite its modulation by attention, is different from the later P3 wave peaking at ~600 msec after laser stimulation. This late P3 appears when the subject is detecting actively the stimulus applied on a target hand (148). For clinical purposes it is advisable to rely, whenever possible, on the early responses N1 and N2, which are less subject to cognitive modulation.

Although laser stimuli excite simultaneously Aδ and C receptors (136), the cortical responses most often reflect Aδ activation exclusively (149). To obtain evoked potentials specific of C-fiber stimulation, the Aδ component of the afferent volley must be suppressed, either by pressure block of A-fibers or by a number of easier procedures, the most reliable of which are the "microspot" technique (stimulation of tiny skin areas 0.15–0.30 mm²) and the stimulation of large skin areas at low intensities (2,18,20). All these manipulations yield the so-called ultra-late LEPs, occurring 700 to 1,000 msec after a hand stimulus and depending exclusively on C-fiber activation.

LEPs are not contingent on the stimulation of nerve trunks and can be applied to explore the function of Aδ fibers in any body region (excluding mucosae). It is therefore strongly advised in clinical practice to always stimulate the territory where pain and/or sensory abnormalities are present, whatever its location, rather than sticking to some "standard" body region. C-fiber–specific LEPs are difficult to obtain from the distal lower limbs but can be recorded easily from the trigeminal areas and in more than 60% of cases from the trunk and upper limbs.

4. NONLESIONAL FACTORS OF VARIATION

4.1. Maturation

The development of somatosensory pathways from birth to adult life is dominated by two coexisting phenomena, which have opposite effects on SEPs: myelinogenesis causes a progressive increase in conduction velocities and synchronization of potentials with age, while body growth increases latencies and desynchronization. Differences in recording procedures make it difficult to compare latency and amplitude values reported in the available studies of SEP maturation. The largest series of SEP normative data in children was published by Taylor and Boor et al. (150–153). During the first 4 to 5 years of life SEP

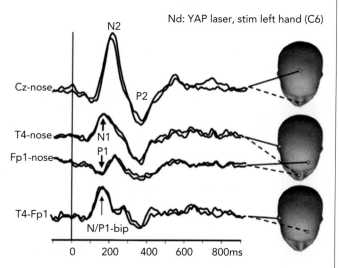

NORMAL LEPs

Nd: YAP laser, stim left hand (C6)

Figure 43.12. Normal LEPs after stimulation of the superficial radial territory (C6) on the left hand (C6) with a solid-state laser (Nd:YAP; λ = 1.34 μm). The vertex complex (N2-P2, upper traces) is best recorded over the midline, with a nose reference (Cz-nose). An earlier negative wave (opercular N1) generated in the suprasylvian operculum can be recorded over the temporal region (top of the middle traces, T4-nose); this component inverts polarity across the midline and is recorded as a positive wave (opercular P1) from frontal or frontopolar electrodes ipsilateral to the stimulus (bottom of the middle traces, Fp1-nose). Taking advantage of such phase reversal, a bipolar montage linking the contralateral temporal to the ipsilateral frontopolar electrodes maximizes the amplitude of the opercular N1/P1 response (bottom trace, T4-Fp1).

maturation is marked by a progressive synchronization and a latency reduction of all potentials. Conduction velocities are known to reach adult values before the age of 3 years in the peripheral nervous system, but this acceleration is slower in the central somatosensory pathways (154,155). Spinal cord conduction in lower limb fibers reaches adult values at the age of 5 to 6 years (154). Later on, changes in conduction velocity related to fiber maturation interact with those of body growth and the peaking latencies progressively increase so that adult values are reached at the age of 15 to 17 years.

When divided by arm's length or body height, the latencies of all central SEPs decrease from birth to the age of 10 years and stabilize thereafter. The rising time between onsets and peaks of the cortical N20 and P39 evoked respectively by median and tibial nerve stimulations decreases steadily from birth to the age of 16 years (156). In children aged 7 to 14 years the voltage of the cervical N13 median nerve SEPs recorded with an anterior cervical electrode tends to be higher than in adults, while the P14 component tends to be lower, with a greater P9/P14 amplitude ratio.

4.2. Aging

The effects of age on SEP latencies mainly reflect conduction slowing in the peripheral nerves, evidenced by the increase of the N9 component after median nerve stimulation. The CCT between the spinal N13 and the parietal N20 was reported as unaffected (50) or increased (157) during normal aging. Uncertainties as to the measurement of the spinal N13 peaking latency on traces obtained using a cervical to Fz montage (see above) may account for these diverging results. The amplitude of the frontal N30 tends to decrease with age, and this component can be virtually absent on both sides in healthy octogenarians, whereas the parietal N20 tends to increase (50).

Aging reduces the amplitude of LEPs after stimulation of any territory and correlates positively with the latencies of all components (158,159). The effects on latencies may reflect a distal loss of peripheral inputs and a length-dependent desynchronization of the ascending nociceptive volley.

4.3. Body Height in Adults

The absolute latencies of SEPs vary according to the distance between the stimulated site and the SEP sources. This effect is naturally more pronounced for lower than for upper limb SEPs. This variability is less for the interpeak intervals used for calculating CCT than for absolute latencies. It is usually not considered when estimating norms of CCT values for upper limb SEPs. Absolute latencies of N22, P30, and P39 potentials evoked by lower limb stimulation are correlated with body height (109). The upper normal values of the N22-P39 interval vary between 18 and 20 msec for body heights of 1.50 and 1.90 m, respectively (160).

4.4. Skin and Core Temperature

Peripheral nerve conduction velocities are affected by changes in limb temperature. A marked decrease in body temperature,

as observed during drug-induced hypothermia, increases the absolute and interpeak latencies of both the early cortical N20 and the positive far-field positive potentials. Moreover, the curves of amplitude decrease versus body temperature during hypothermia are not the same for peripheral, spinal, brainstem, and cortical SEPs (161). The N20 potential disappears at temperatures ranging from 17° to 25°C, the P14 at 17° to 20°C. The peripheral N9 and spinal N13 potentials remains identifiable down to a body temperature of 17°C. SEP changes related to hypothermia warrant special attention in comatose patients, in whom they can combine with those induced by CNS depressant drugs. These effects are described below (see the sections on coma and brain death).

4.5. Attention

It has been assumed for years that the cortical SEPs peaking before 50 msec following stimulation of the upper limb are not significantly affected by cognitive processes. However, Desmedt et al. (81), in an odd-ball detection task of somatosensory stimuli, described an enhancement of the positive waves P27-P45, which they labeled "P40," in response to target stimuli, suggesting that attention-related processes could affect the early cortical SEPs. This positive enhancement can also be identified in response to non-target stimuli during "lie" experiments in which the subject is instructed to detect rare deviant target stimuli that are never delivered (162). A similar positive shift enhancing the amplitude of the P45 is observed in response to non-target electrical stimuli when the attention of the subject is drawn toward the stimulated area (82). These attention-related changes of early cortical SEPs are not likely to affect the amplitude of the P27, N30, and P45 potentials as recorded in routine conditions—that is, using runs of 500 stimuli or more with no instruction given to the subject.

4.6. Sleep and Vigilance

Some changes in the amplitude, waveform, and latency of the parietal N20 have been reported during natural sleep in normal subjects (132). The main change consisted of a prolongation of N20 latency of ~0.4 msec between the awake state and sleep stage II and in a reduction of N20 latency of ~0.3 msec between stage II and REM sleep. The disappearance of sharp inflections superimposed over the rising phase of N20 in non-REM sleep reflects the attenuation of HFOs (see above). The latency changes observed during sleep are not likely to affect the interpretation of the SEP waveform in patients. However, a maximal prolongation of 0.9 msec of the N9-N20 interval have been reported between wake and sleep (163), suggesting that the patient state should be monitored using EEG in patients with a fluctuating state of vigilance.

4.7. Drugs

Significant group differences in CCT were reported between controls and ambulatory epileptic patients treated with phenobarbital or phenytoin (164), whereas primidone, and valproic acid seem to have no demonstrable effect. Similarly,

Mavroudakis et al. (165) have reported a latency increase of N13 and N20 potentials after a single intravenous injection of phenytoin with blood levels of the drug between 19 and 25 mg/L. When drug sedation is necessary, low oral anxiolytic doses of benzodiazepines can be used and have not been reported to provoke false SEP abnormalities. A prospective study of median nerve SEPs showed that vigabatrin, as an add-on therapy in patients with refractory partial seizures, did not cause any significant prolongation of CCT over a follow-up period of 2 years (166). Only serious overdoses of CNS depressant drugs are associated with abnormally prolonged N13-N20 CCT in comatose patients. These effects are clinically relevant for the interpretation of SEPs in coma and brain death (see below).

5. ABNORMAL WAVEFORMS AND CLINICAL APPLICATIONS

5.1. Peripheral Lesions

SEPs can be useful for the evaluation of peripheral pathology in three circumstances: (1) to measure peripheral conduction velocities when sensory nerve action potentials (SNAPs) cannot be obtained at the periphery because of the neuropathic process; (2) to explore proximal lesions of the peripheral sensory pathways that are not accessible to EMG studies; and (3) to study the whole pathway up to the cortex in pathologies combining peripheral and central lesions.

5.1.1. NEUROPATHIES

Early in the history of SEPs it was demonstrated that the N20 potential to stimulation of median, ulnar, or digital nerves could be recorded in neuropathies when SNAPs cannot be obtained from recording the nerve itself. The difference between the latencies of the N20 potentials obtained by stimulation of the same nerve at two different levels permits estimation of the conduction velocity in the segment between the two stimulated points. The utility of this method for assessing peripheral conduction velocity has been validated in chronic acquired demyelinating neuropathies (167). Because muscle afferents contribute to the cortical response after stimulation of mixed nerves, the sensory conduction velocities measured by SEPs may not be equivalent to those obtained by direct recording of SNAPs after selective stimulation of cutaneous afferents. In pure sensory neuropathies with conduction abnormalities in the proximal segment of peripheral sensory fibers, distal conduction velocities, as assessed by conventional EMG testing, can be normal. SEPs are useful in this condition to assess conduction in the damaged segment of sensory fibers (168,169). Nociceptive cortical EPs can also be useful to explore sensory neuropathies affecting preferentially the Aδ myelinated fibers, and reduced responses parallel the impairment of pain and temperature sensation as well as the decreased density of small-diameter fibers, as assessed by histological examination of skin biopsy (170,171).

5.1.2. BRACHIAL AND LUMBOSACRAL PLEXUS LESIONS

In traumatic lesions of the brachial plexus the persistence of a normal Erb's point potential (N9) and far-field P9 at the neck and on the scalp with abolition of all subsequent components indicates a root avulsion proximal to the ganglia with a very poor prognosis for recovery (172). The reliability of SEP recording can be increased by stimulating several nerves and/or dermatomes to study selectively different trunks or roots of the brachial plexus; to this aim, stimulation of musculocutaneous, radial, median, and ulnar nerves has been proposed. Upper limb SEPs are normal in most patients with thoracic outlet syndrome. The value of SEPs in this syndrome is limited to patients in whom another pathology is suspected.

In lumbosacral plexopathies the persistence of a reproducible P39 cortical potential, even if delayed or reduced, indicates that some ascending inputs are reaching the CNS. Conversely, side-to-side asymmetries of N22 with reduced or absent N22 on the affected side can be viewed as a sign of spinal deafferentation. SEPs to femorocutaneous nerve stimulation medial to the anterior iliac crest can be useful in meralgia paresthetica. In retroperitoneal compressive lesions of the femoral nerve scalp, SEPs to saphenous nerve stimulation at the lateral aspect of the knee can be absent or delayed.

5.1.3. GUILLAIN-BARRÉ SYNDROME AND CHRONIC INFLAMMATORY DEMYELINATING POLYRADICULOPATHIES

These pathologies predominantly affect roots and proximal nerve segments, hence peripheral conduction velocities are often normal in the early stages of the disease. Moreover, F-wave recording assesses motor conduction in proximal nerve segments and ventral roots, but not in dorsal roots. Upper limb SEPs show absent, delayed, or dispersed N9 potential with a reduced or absent N13 and increased N9-N13 interval (when measurable). If lesions are confined to the proximal segments of dorsal roots, N9 may be normal. Lower limb SEPs are more frequently abnormal than upper limb SEPs in Guillain-Barré syndrome, showing a normal or delayed peripheral response at the popliteal fossa with a reduced or absent lumbar N22 potential (173). In chronic inflammatory demyelinating polyradiculopathies (CIDP), the electrodiagnostic criteria based on motor nerve conduction studies and F-wave recording may be missing either because of secondary axonal degeneration or in pure sensory forms of the disease. In this circumstance the recording of preserved peripheral SEPs, combined with delayed and/or reduced N13 or N22 spinal potentials, may reveal abnormal conduction in proximal segments of sensory fibers or dorsal roots (174). Such abnormalities were recently reported in 85% of patients with CIDP and no other electrodiagnostic sign of peripheral demyelination (175).

5.1.4. FOCAL MONORADICULOPATHIES OR POLYRADICULOPATHIES

SEPs to stimulation of mixed nerves are seldom useful in radiculopathies since they explore multiple roots, so a monoradiculopathy may be masked by normal responses mediated through unaffected roots. Selective nerve stimulation using saphenous, superficial peroneal, and sural nerves is more appropriate for exploring radiculopathies. Despite dermatomal overlapping between roots and interindividual variations, these techniques proved to be useful for exploring radiculopathies, especially those that present only with pain or sensory symptoms (119). The recording of compound nerve action potentials at the periphery and of scalp N20 or P39, respectively, for upper and lower limb stimulations, provides enough information for detecting conduction abnormalities but does not provide information as to the exact site where conduction is impaired. For upper limb stimulation, it is possible to obtain reliable N13 and P14 potentials after digital stimulation, but for lower limb studies the reliability of lumbar N22 and far-field P30 to dermatomal stimulation has not been validated in patients.

5.1.5. COMBINED INVOLVEMENT OF PERIPHERAL AND CENTRAL SOMATOSENSORY PATHWAYS IN HEREDITARY ATAXIAS

In Friedreich's ataxia sensory nerve conduction velocity is only moderately decreased, whereas sensory nerve action potentials are reduced or absent. In most patients with a history of more than 10 years of clinical symptoms, no SEPs can be obtained after stimulation of upper or lower limbs. When a parietal N20 persists after median nerve stimulation, it peaks with a delayed latency and its amplitude is reduced (176). Even when severely reduced, the N9 and P9 potentials may have latencies within normal limits. When P14 persists, the N9-P14 (or P9-P14) transit time is usually normal; conversely, the P14-N20 interval is often prolonged. The cervical N13, when recorded with a non-cephalic reference, cannot be identified in most cases. In hereditary ataxias other than Friedreich's, SEPs proved to be of potential value for the classification of subtypes in this group of diseases (177). In familial spastic paraplegia and hereditary cerebellar ataxia, the incidence of abnormal responses is smaller than in Friedreich's, and peripheral N9-P9 components are normal in most cases (178). Most patients with progressive early-onset hereditary ataxias have a normal N9; P9 and P14 potentials are present but N20 is delayed or absent. SEPs in clinically unaffected members of families with hereditary spastic paraplegia may be used to detect asymptomatic heterozygotes.

5.2. Spinal Cord Lesions

5.2.1. SPINAL CORD TRAUMA

In most cases of complete functional transection of the spinal cord, scalp, cortical SEPs are absent after stimulation of nerves whose roots enter the spinal cord below the lesion, while spinal segmental responses recorded caudal to the lesion are unaffected. At the early stage the persistence of SEPs on the scalp may suggest some residual spinal cord function when clinical examination would lead to more pessimistic conclusions. In the chronic stage of functionally incomplete lesions, abnormalities correlate well with clinical somatosensory signs, in particular discriminative skin and joint sensation. In the acute stage SEPs may antedate clinical improvement.

5.2.2. TUMORS OF THE SPINAL CORD

Abnormalities of CCT and of segmental spinal N13 and N22 SEPs can be observed in >75% of spinal cord tumors (179). In cervical intramedullary tumors, median nerve SEPs show unilateral or bilateral abnormalities of P14, N13, and N22-P39 CCT, respectively, in 75%, 86%, and 78% of cases. These abnormalities are clinically silent (i.e., not associated with sensory deficit or abnormal reflexes in the explored territory) in more than one third of cases. The highest rate of clinically silent SEP abnormality in cervical intramedullary tumors is that of the N13 potential, which exceeds 50%. There is no large series of thoracic intramedullary tumors investigated using SEPs in the literature; in our series a prolonged N22-P39 interval or an absent P39 potential was observed, at least on one side, in 75% of cases and was clinically silent in only 10%. There is no simple relation between the size of the lesion as assessed by MRI and the severity of SEP abnormalities in intramedullary spinal cord tumors; thus, SEPs are useful for preoperative evaluation of the cord dysfunction. Extrinsic compression of the cord by an extramedullary tumor affects more central conduction than spinal segmental responses. Normalization of CCTs can be observed after surgical decompression and return to normal sensation.

5.2.3. SYRINGOMYELIA

SEPs can be normal when the syrinx does not involve the dorsal horn and when the dorsal columns are not constricted by herniation of cerebellar tonsils through the foramen magnum (Arnold-Chiari malformation). However, this eventuality is exceptional (31). The most frequent upper limb SEP abnormality is the amplitude reduction or absence of the segmental N13 potential, associated with normal P14 and N20 potential (Fig. 43.13). N13 abnormalities are correlated with abnormal tendon reflexes and with pain and temperature hypesthesia in the upper limbs. Since the N13 potential does not reflect the response of dorsal horn spinothalamic cells to $A\delta$ and C fibers, afferent volley N13 reduction reflects a global dysfunction of the cord dorsal horn in syringomyelia. Cortical responses to painful stimuli delivered via CO_2 laser peaking in the latency range of 200 to 350 msec are abnormal in all patients with cervical syringomyelia showing reduced or absent N13 potential (180).

5.2.4. CERVICAL SPONDYLOTIC MYELOPATHY

Cervical spondylotic myelopathy is the most frequent type of myelopathy seen in general hospitals. Numerous studies have emphasized the diagnostic utility of SEP recording in cervical spondylotic myelopathy (181). Globally these first reports demonstrated abnormalities of median and/or tibial nerve SEPs in ~50% of patients with cervical myelopathy. Lower limb stimulation is more effective than upper limb stimulation for disclosing abnormalities of central somatosensory conduction in such patients. The recording of the segmental N13 spinal potential, using an anterior cervical reference electrode, increases the sensitivity of upper limb SEPs for detecting dorsal horn dysfunction in cervical spondylotic myelopathy. Restuccia et al. (182) reported an incidence of 84%, 93%, and 65% of N13 abnormality in median, radial, and ulnar nerves SEPs, respectively (Fig. 43.14). Neither narrowing of the cord diameter nor increased intramedullary T2 signal is necessarily associated with SEP signs of cervical cord dysfunction. However, prolonged CCT after stimulation of the lower limbs is observed in more than two thirds of these patients, so by combining median and tibial nerve stimulation most of the patients with such severe MRI abnormalities have abnormal SEPs. The practical utility of median and tibial nerve SEP recording is definitely more obvious in patients without MRI evidence of a cervical cord lesion due to compression.

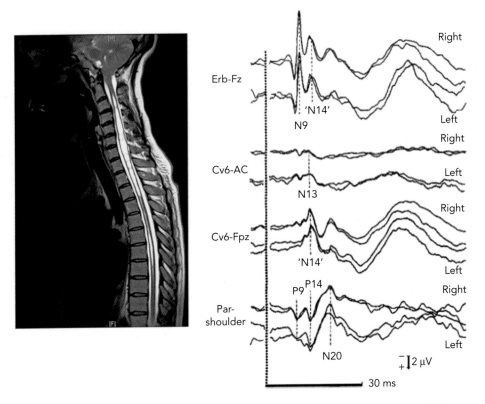

Figure 43.13. *Absence of the segmental cervical N13 potential with preserved cervical cord conduction in a case of syringomyelia. This figure illustrates that when the P14 and N20 upper limb SEPs are preserved in intramedullary lesions, as shown by traces recorded in the scalp parietal region contralateral to stimulus referred to the shoulder contralateral to stimulus (Par-shoulder), the absence of the segmental N13, which is evident in cervical transverse derivation Cv6-AC, is masked in Cv6-Fz recordings due to contamination of the waveform by the injection of the scalp P14 potential as an N14 negativity in traces recorded with a reference electrode placed on the scalp frontal region (Erb-Fz and Cv6-Fpz). Note that conduction is preserved in dorsal columns despite the large cervical syrinx.*

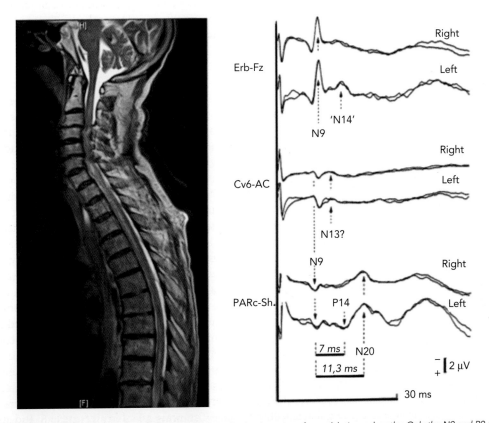

Figure 43.14. *Absence of the segmental N13 with impaired cervical cord conduction in a case of spondylotic myelopathy. Only the N9 and P9 potentials are normal. The N13 potential is absent after stimulation of both median nerves. The P14 is absent after stimulation of the left median nerve and the P9-P14 interval is prolonged after stimulation of the right median nerve (upper normal value 6 msec).*

5.2.5. LESIONS OF THE CERVICOMEDULLARY JUNCTION

When the volley of impulses ascending in the cervical dorsal columns is blocked or dispersed at the cervicomedullary junction, the segmental N13 potential to upper limb stimulation is normal, whereas far-field P14 and later components are absent or abnormal (183). The lower limb P39 SEP is most often abnormal but can be preserved in association with severe upper limb SEP abnormalities (26); this occurs when the lesion compresses only the outer dorsal column fibers. When the P39 potential is abnormal, an absent or delayed P30 is consistently observed (109).

5.3. Amyotrophic Lateral Sclerosis and Hirayama Disease

5.3.1. AMYOTROPHIC LATERAL SCLEROSIS

SEPs are not indicated as a routine diagnostic procedure in amyotrophic lateral sclerosis (ALS). However, several authors have reported central SEP abnormalities in ALS, including abnormal central conduction and/or amplitude reduction of cortical SEPs (113,184). These findings were not confirmed by others (160). Abnormal SEPs in a patient with clinical signs of motor neuron disease are expected in various diseases that may mimic ALS, where peripheral or central somatosensory pathways can be affected, such as spondylotic myelopathy, lymphoma, AIDS, paraneoplastic syndromes, and monoclonal paraproteinemia. Abnormal central conduction SEPs are more surprising in the idiopathic form of ALS where the dorsal columns, somatosensory thalamic relays, and SI granular cell layers are spared. Reduced cortical response to tibial nerve stimulation is the most consistent SEP abnormality reported in ALS. Zanette et al. (113) observed it in 22 of 29 ALS patients, whereas tibial nerve SEPS were unaffected in 10 patients with progressive muscular atrophy.

Reduced cortical tibial nerve SEPs could be related to axonal loss in muscle afferent fibers. However, this explanation does not hold for lower limb SEP abnormalities in response to stimulation of cutaneous nerves such as sural, saphenous internus, and medial plantar nerves (185). Other proposed explanations for tibial nerve SEP abnormalities are a neuronal loss in the somatosensory cortex that may selectively affect the generators of the cortical SEPs to lower limb stimulation, or a perturbation of the control exerted by the motor cortex over the subcortical sensory relays and somatosensory cortex. At the upper limb some authors reported a selective loss or abnormality of the central P22 potential to median nerve stimulation, suggesting that this abnormality might reflect the loss of pyramidal cells in the motor area (113). This view was reinforced by some correlation between SEP abnormalities and the severity of or the stage in the evolution of the disease, but this is not unanimously accepted.

5.3.2. HIRAYAMA DISEASE

Hirayama disease is a sporadic lateralized spinal amyotrophy of distal upper limb muscles affecting young males that was described for the first time in Japan. It has been considered either as a focal form of ALS (or of progressive spinal amyotrophy) or due to a compression of the lower cervical cord during neck flexion producing ischemia of motor neurons in the spinal cord ventral horn. N9 and spinal N13 were reported as reduced after median and ulnar nerve stimulation in association with preserved CCTs (186). These SEP abnormalities are bilateral and infra-clinical since sensation is normal in the affected limb. An N13 reduction has been reported during neck flexion by some authors (187), but this was not confirmed by others (188).

5.4. Brainstem Lesions

Upper limb P14 and N18 potentials and lower limb P30 are generated close to the dorsal columns nuclei in the medulla oblongata. Therefore, these components are clearly reduced, delayed, or absent in lesions of the medulla oblongata affecting somatosensory input transmission at this level. When not completely canceled, the P14 potential is delayed and the P9/P14 amplitude ratio is abnormally high in such patients. This pattern combining normal spinal N13 potential with absent or clearly abnormal P14 and cortical SEPs is similar to that observed in upper cervical cord lesions. It can be observed in any destructive or compressive lesion of this region as well as in brain-dead patients. Conversely, interruption of the spinothalamic tract in medulla oblongata (Wallenberg's syndrome) does not modify early SEPs (79). The behavior of the P30 potential evoked by lower limb stimulation is the same as that of the median nerve P14 in brainstem lesions (109,130).

5.5. Thalamic, Capsulo-Thalamic, and Cortical Lesions

SEPs to median nerve stimulation are abnormal in >70% of capsulo-thalamic and in nearly 90% of posterior thalamic lesions (44). After stimulation of the affected side, amplitude reduction or loss of both parietal N20-P27 and frontal P22-N30 potentials with preserved scalp far-field positivities, including P14, represents the most frequent SEP abnormality in thalamic or capsular lesions interrupting the somatosensory pathways (189). The N18 potential persists in this condition in non-cephalic reference recordings (43). There is no simple relation between thalamic pain and deafferentation of area S1 as evidenced by loss of the primary cortical components of SEPs (41). Early cortical SEPs, including the N20, P22, P27, N30, and P45 potentials, are consistently absent or abnormal in posterolateral infarctions of the geniculo-thalamic artery territory with loss of touch and position sense. Conversely, they are normal in infarctions in other thalamic arterial territories. In capsular infarcts in the territory of the anterior choroid artery or in thalamo-capsular hematomas, there is no clear correlation between neuroimaging data and SEP findings. In these patients the degree of hemispheric somatosensory deafferentation cannot be accurately predicted from computed tomography or MRI. Selective loss of frontal or parietal SEPs is infrequently observed in capsulo-thalamic lesions (61).

In large cortical lesions involving the central and parietal areas, SEP abnormalities are very similar to those encountered in posterior thalamic lesions deafferenting the hemisphere, showing a loss of all cortical SEPs with preserved P14 and N18 potentials. In lesions outside the centroparietal area, early cortical SEPs are normal. Less than 10% of patients with

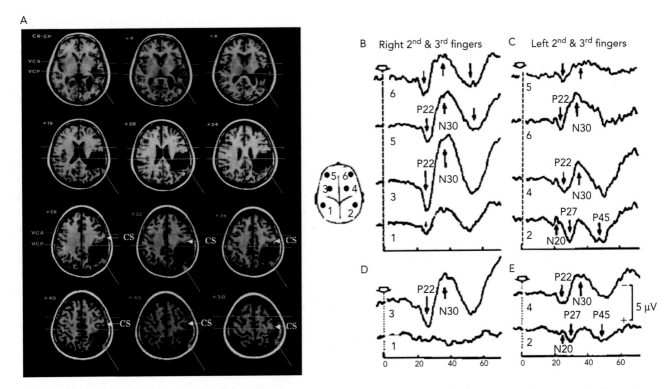

Figure 43.15. The paradigmatic case of dissociated loss of parietal SEPs. These traces are those of case 10 published in Brain by Mauguière et al. (62), recorded 5 years after a complete ischemic lesion of the left parietal lobe (**A**). These responses were obtained after stimulation of the second and third fingers at an intensity of three times the sensory threshold in **B** and **C**, and at the sensory threshold intensity of the normal side in **D** and **E**. Parietal N20, P27, and P45 potentials are definitely absent, and frontal P22 and N30 clearly preserved, over the damaged side. Seven years after this recording a brain MRI of this patient was performed. MRI slices parallel to the anterior commissure–posterior commissure (AC-AP) stereotactic planes (**A**) show that the left parietal cortex behind the central sulcus (CS) is entirely damaged (the left side is represented on the right in MRI slices). Furthermore, the lesion extended in the posterior white matter of the internal capsula and corona radiata. Therefore, there is no doubt that in this particular patient the SEPs recorded in the frontal region of the damaged left hemisphere cannot be generated in the left parietal lobe. This case remains unique because the parietal branches of the left middle cerebral artery had been selectively, and accidentally, obstructed during intracarotid embolization of a malformation of the occipital branch of the left external carotid artery, producing a lesion that is almost never encountered in spontaneous infarctions. Despite the large ischemic area, this patient was not hemiplegic but presented with a complete anesthesia of her right side. On verbal instruction she was also able to locate approximately tactile stimulations applied on her right anesthetic side ("blind-touch" phenomenon). The existence of large prerolandic responses in this patient can result from synaptic reorganization of the cortical circuitry long after the stroke and does not necessarily imply that short-latency responses are generated in the prerolandic cortex of normal subjects.

focal hemispheric lesions present with dissociated abnormalities of frontal and parietal early cortical SEPs, showing either reduced or absent N20P27 with preserved P22-N30, or the reverse (Fig. 43.15). When elementary touch and joint sensation is preserved, astereognosis of the hand opposite to the cortical lesion is consistently associated with abnormal N20 and/or P27 abnormality; conversely, precentral lesions eliminating specifically the P22 component are usually associated with central hemiparesis (44,62).

5.6. Multiple Sclerosis

Historically SEPs have been the first evoked responses tested in patients with multiple sclerosis (MS) (190). The main effect of central demyelination is to slow down the conduction and thus to increase the time dispersion of impulses in the dorsal columns, medial lemniscus, and thalamocortical fibers. Abnormal SEPs can be observed in the absence of any sensory symptoms. By providing a quantitative index of central conduction that can be periodically reassessed, SEPs, like all other types of EPs, are useful in all situations where a functional follow-up of the disease is requested, including long-term therapeutic trials of new pharmacological agents.

5.6.1. Types of SEP Abnormalities in MS
The most frequent SEP abnormality in MS is the latency increase or absence of the P39 component evoked by tibial nerve stimulation followed by delayed or absent P14 and N20 potentials to median nerve stimulation. Latency abnormalities are associated with prolonged CCT, while peripheral SEPs are normal (see references 160 and 191 for reviews). Delayed or reduced N13 is infrequent. Amplitude reduction of the scalp P14 potential, as evaluated by measuring the P9/P14 amplitude ratio in scalp to shoulder traces, is observed in >90% of MS patients with abnormal SEPs (39). The frequency of abnormal SEPs is maximal when the four limbs are tested and increases by <10% by testing the upper limb when tibial SEPs are normal.

5.6.2. Diagnostic Indications of SEPs in MS
SEPs are less profitable than visual evoked potentials when searching for silent demyelination in MS. At present the

diagnosis of MS is based on MRI and the consensus is that SEPs are no longer considered as useful for diagnosis. The introduction of MRI has thus dramatically modified the role of SEP testing at the early stage of the disease, which is now done more to assess the organicity of subjective symptoms and to follow up the course of the disease than to detect lesion dissemination. SEPs remain useful in screening the many patients consulting the neurologist for poorly reliable or unspecific "soft" symptoms, such as paresthesias or sensation of numbness in one limb, compatible with CNS dysfunction, in whom the clinical examination is uninformative or unconvincing.

5.7. Adrenoleukodystrophy

Adrenoleukodystrophy is a peroxisomal disorder caused by an abnormal gene localized in the Xq28 area, which shows variable clinical features, from severe cerebral symptoms in childhood to progressive peripheral and spinal symptoms in adults (adrenomyeloneuropathy). SEPs have proved their usefulness in detecting subclinical abnormalities of the segmental N13 cervical potential or of CCT in adrenoleukodystrophy carriers (192).

5.8. Coma

Interpretation of SEPs in deeply comatose patients must take into account the combined effects of hypothermia and CNS depressant drugs. Hypothermia increases CCT, with a linear relation between the two parameters between 35° and 40°C and an exponential relation below 35°C (161). The use of CNS depressant drugs has considerably increased for the past 20 years in intensive care units (ICUs), in particular that of intravenous barbiturate perfusion, which depresses the EEG activity and brainstem reflexes. Fortunately, short-latency SEPs are rather resistant to barbiturate anesthesia and remain within normal limits in this condition. However, transient SEP latency increases can be observed after injection of barbiturates, which should not be misinterpreted as signs of neurological deterioration when observed in the course of continuous SEP monitoring.

Most SEP studies in coma and brain death have been limited to short-latency potentials peaking before 30 msec after stimulation of the median nerve. The absence of all early N20-P24 cortical responses to median nerve stimulation on both sides with preserved peripheral N9 and cervical N13 potentials carries a prognosis of death or permanent vegetative state (PVS) in almost 100% of post-anoxic comas (193,194). Conversely, the prognostic value of this SEP pattern is less unfavorable when the coma is caused by a primary brainstem lesion, which can interrupt ascending somatosensory pathways, or in non-comatose patients presenting with a locked-in syndrome caused by a lesion of the tegmentum pontis. If the percentage of deaths or PVS is high when the cortical N20 is lost on both sides in head-injured or vascular brain-damaged comatose patients, moderate disability or good recovery, according to the Glasgow Outcome Scale, has been reported in patients with no recordable early cortical SEPs (195).

Furthermore, in the interpretation of absent cortical SEPs in a comatose patient whose past medical history is unknown, the possibility should not be overlooked of preexisting pathologies such as MS, heredo-degenerative diseases, and Arnold-Chiari malformation, which may themselves lead to absence of N20, and eventually of P14. Logi et al. (196) reviewed the literature data published since 1984 on the prognostic value of SEPs in 1,818 patients. Since neither SEP methodology nor criteria for estimation of clinical outcome are uniform across studies from different authors, the overall results presented are to be taken as a general indication. However, all studies converge to a 100% specificity of bilateral N20 absence in predicting poor outcome in post-anoxic comatose adult patients.

The loss of early cortical SEPs on one side only, with preserved P14 potential, does not provide by itself clear information concerning the vital prognosis in comatose patients with hemispheric traumatic or vascular lesions. Conversely, this pattern is associated with a high incidence of severe sensorimotor lateralized disability in case of survival. Increased CCT has been considered as predictive of severe coma outcome in the early SEP studies (195,197). However, 42% of head-injured comatose patients in whom a single SEP recording shows prolonged CCT completely recover or have a moderate disability. This suggests that, contrary to the complete loss of early cortical SEPs, a prolonged CCT may be a reversible phenomenon.

The recording of normal N20 and early cortical responses in the acute phase of a coma does not provide any certitude of good recovery since only two thirds of these patients will have a good recovery, either complete or with minimal disability. This reflects the fact that contingent events during the course of the coma may worsen the final outcome. The recording of normal middle- and long-latency cortical SEPs increases to ~85% the chances of complete recovery (198). One drawback is that these components are much more sensitive to CNS depressant drugs than early cortical responses.

5.9. Brain Death

Our concepts on the assessment of brain death have considerably evolved from the early clinical description of the "coma dépassé" (coma beyond coma), where the recording of an isoelectric EEG played a key role, toward the idea that the brain is dead when brainstem functions are irreversibly lost (see reference 199 for a review). Neuroimaging techniques now offer the possibility of assessing, in comatose patients kept alive by respiratory assistance, whether a focal brainstem or supratentorial lesion can be considered responsible for this critical clinical condition. In a patient whose comatose state is directly related to an identified brain lesion, the absence of segmental brainstem reflexes tested by two experienced neurologists would be theoretically sufficient to ascertain brainstem death after eliminating any interference from depressant drug treatment (199). Such an ideal situation is not met in all instances, and objective proof of brain death has been steadily sought, since the very beginning of the intensive care history, to avoid the unacceptable risk of a false diagnosis of brain death based exclusively on a clinical report. Therefore, the pending question, which is more pragmatic than conceptual, is to identify the neurophysiological tests that are reliable enough to state that no activity persists in the CNS rostral to the foramen magnum, in all conditions where the diagnosis of brain death is at stake. In many ICUs the EEG and multimodal EPs, including SEPs, are routinely recorded for monitoring cerebral functions in deeply comatose patients, and the eventuality that brain death could be diagnosed without the help of confirmatory electrophysiological techniques is not envisaged (Fig. 43.16).

In this clinical context the loss of cortical and brainstem SEPs is clinically relevant only after peripheral or spinal damage has been eliminated by the recording of normal peripheral N9 and spinal N13 potentials and appropriate neuroimaging investigations. The disappearance of the P14 and N18 potentials in comatose patients, whose N20 potentials are absent on both sides, indicates a dysfunction of the lower brainstem. Conversely, the segmental spinal N13 can persist long after the P14 potential has disappeared in brainstem death (see Fig. 43.16) (30). Therefore, the median nerve SEP pattern of brainstem death consists of the persistence of the spinal N13 at the neck and of far-field P9 and P11 on the scalp, with absent P14, N18, and cortical responses (40). When interpreting SEPs in the context of brain death diagnosis, the possibility of a lesion at the cervicomedullary junction must be eliminated, since it can reproduce the SEP pattern observed in brain death (see above).

The P14 potential recorded between the scalp (Fz) and a nasopharyngeal electrode was shown to disappear in brain

death, while it persists in non–brain-dead comatose patients (200). It was thus proposed to consider the loss of this rostral P14 as an indicator of brainstem death even in patients whose scalp SEPs recorded with a non-cephalic reference show a persisting positivity peaking at 13 to 14 msec. Scalp-to-nasopharynx recordings of the rostral SEPs in brainstem death diagnosis might thus be useful in this condition.

The recording of the EEG, SEPs, and brainstem auditory evoked potentials (BAEPs) is recommended as a confirmatory test of cerebral death in many countries; however, it has been questioned whether electrophysiological explorations are indispensable for the diagnosis of brain death on the following three arguments: (1) the brain is dead when the brainstem is dead; (2) "electro-cerebral silence" on EEG recordings does not demonstrate brainstem death, while clinical examination of brainstem reflexes does; and (3) the recording of SEPs and BAEPs is technically more demanding than the use of the EEG. The reservation that a peripheral, cervical cord, or brainstem pathology predating that causing the coma can hamper the use of EPs also applies to the clinical testing of brainstem reflexes, which also have the disadvantage of being less resistant to anesthetic drugs than brainstem and early cortical SEPs. Any neurologist aware of the pitfalls of brainstem reflexes testing is able to interpret correctly SEP and BAEP abnormalities and will be helped in that by neuroimaging techniques. Therefore, the question is not whether EPs could replace clinical testing, but rather whether adding SEP and BAEP recording to the list of maneuvers used to assess brainstem function would increase the reliability of brainstem death diagnosis in the hands of an experienced practitioner. The answer to this question, based on 20 years of routine use of EPs in intensive care patients, is definitely positive.

5.10. Myoclonus

Since the first description by Dawson in 1947 (1), it has been known that giant SEPs can occur in association with the cortical reflex myoclonus observed in progressive myoclonic epilepsy (PME) and with focal motor seizures in lesions of the perirolandic area. The giant SEPs in PME were first described as a P25-N33 complex by Shibasaki and Kuroiwa (201), the amplitude of which, when measured from peak to peak, can reach 50 μV or more and is usually >15 μV (Fig. 43.17). Most PME patients with cortical myoclonus show a parietal positive and frontal negative dipolar field peaking at ~25 msec contralateral to median nerve stimulation. Jerk-locked back-averaging the EEG prior to the myoclonus shows that spontaneous myoclonus can be associated with an abnormal cortical spike in some patients with cortical myoclonus.

When identifiable, the parietal N20 potential to median nerve stimulation has normal latency and amplitude in most patients with cortical myoclonus (202). Similarly, P14 is normal in such patients. The normal size of the N20 component indicates that both the sensory input into the cortex and the primary cortical response itself are not grossly abnormal. It has been suggested on the basis of waveform decomposition and computerized modeling that the giant SEPs result from an abnormal enhancement of certain components of the normal SEPs (203). This has been confirmed by dipole modeling

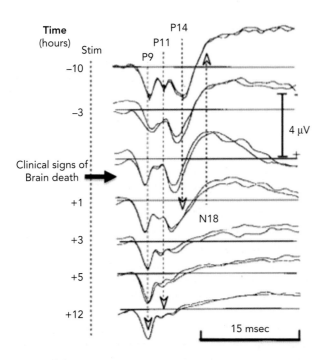

Figure 43.16. Rostrocaudal deterioration of median nerve SEPs in brain death. This figure shows that 1 hour after clinical diagnosis of brain death (time +1) a P14 potential persists, with a shorter peaking latency than that of the P14 recorded before brain death (time –10). This potential disappears by time +3. The amplitude of the subcortical N18 potential decreases in parallel with that of the P14 potential. Three hours after clinical diagnosis of brain death, only the P9 (brachial plexus) and P11 (cervical cord) are recordable on the scalp. Modified from Buchner, Ferbert, and Hacke (30) (with permission of authors).

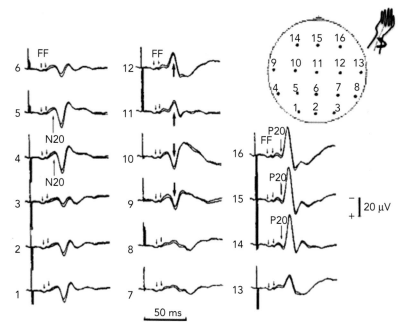

Figure 43.17. Scalp topography of giant SEPs in a case of progressive myoclonic epilepsy. The giant response (bold arrows) has a clear dipolar field distribution and shows a phase reversal in the central region contralateral to stimulation with a voltage gradient of >50 μV between the two extremes. Note that the far-field P9 and P14 and the N20 parietal potentials have normal amplitudes.

showing that the scalp distribution of both normal and giant SEPs can be explained by the same cortical sources and suggesting that giant SEPs mostly reflect an enhanced response of the N24-P24 generator in area 3b (204). An enhanced cortical response to proprioceptive inputs can be observed in some of the PME patients with giant median nerve SEPs, in association with an exaggerated EMG response to passive movements (205). Thus, cortical hyperresponses either to cutaneous inputs alone or to both cutaneous and proprioceptive inputs can occur in PME with cortical reflex myoclonus.

Giant SEPs can be recorded in the absence of myoclonus-related spikes and vice versa. Thus, patients who apparently have similar clinical symptoms can show different SEP abnormalities. Complete electrophysiological investigation of patients with myoclonus includes jerk-locked EEG averaging (201), conventional SEP recordings to median nerve and finger stimulation, and the recording of the long-latency myogenic reflex activity (C reflex) to median nerve stimulation, which reflects the myoclonus itself. Shibasaki et al. (202) proposed classifying myoclonus into four subtypes according to electrophysiological data:

Type I is the above-described pyramidal myoclonus.

In type II giant SEPs are absent and myoclonus-related spike is present, suggesting that myoclonus is not triggered by a hyperresponse of the SI cortex to afferent inputs.

In type III only giant SEPs are present, possibly because the epileptic discharge causing the myoclonic jerk is generated in deep cortical layers and has no recordable scalp correlates.

In type IV both giant SEPs and jerk-locked spikes are absent, and the efferent impulses generating myoclonus in response to afferent inputs might be generated in subcortical reticular structures; this type could correspond to the reticular reflex myoclonus (206).

Not all of the patients with myoclonus have giant SEPs. In particular, enhanced SEPs are usually not observed in benign forms of juvenile myoclonic epilepsies and in essential nonprogressive isolated myoclonus. They are inconstant in Creutzfeldt-Jakob disease and post-hypoxic myoclonus. In the two latter conditions the existence of giant SEPs probably depends on the stage of the disease. Conversely, giant SEPs are an almost constant feature in the various forms of PME.

Giant SEPs can also be observed over the damaged hemisphere in patients with supratentorial tumors, in patients with posttraumatic cortical atrophies, or long after an ischemic or hemorrhagic stroke. In these patients the enhancement of the cortical response is often less than that observed in PME patients with cortical reflex myoclonus. Loss of inhibitory control and postlesional collateral sprouting of cortical afferents could be responsible for such SEP abnormalities. In focal lesions, giant SEPs are often observed in the absence of myoclonus triggered by somatosensory stimuli, but the occurrence of focal motor seizures is frequent in the history of such patients.

In some children aged 3 to 13 years with normal neurological status, vertex and parietal EEG spikes, corresponding to high-voltage SEPs (up to 400 μV), can be evoked by a single tactile stimulation; the presence of these "extreme SEPs" might forecast the possible occurrence of partial motor seizures with benign outcome (207). "Extreme SEPs" culminate after the first 60 msec following median nerve stimulation, reach their maximum for low stimulation frequencies of 0.2 to 0.5 Hz, and have the same scalp topography and modeled source as spontaneous rolandic spikes in children with benign rolandic epilepsy (208).

5.11. Parkinson's Disease and Movement Disorders

5.11.1. PARKINSON'S DISEASE

Rossini et al. (209) were the first to report a reduction of the frontal N30 median nerve SEPs in patients with Parkinson's disease (PD), in association with parietal SEPs of normal amplitude. These authors hypothesized that the rigidity or akinesia of PD patients could be related to this SEP abnormality. Analysis of SEP topography showed that differences in temporal and power spectrum distributions of SEPs between normal subjects and PD patients are confined to frontal scalp areas (210). Moreover, the amplitude of the N30 potential was found to be inversely correlated with that of the second component (latency range 50–60 msec) of the long-latency reflexes evoked by electrical stimulation of the median nerve (211), which are commonly increased in PD. It has also been shown (212) that, though reduced, the N30 potential in PD shows the same amplitude decrease as in normal subjects during voluntary finger movements (see reference 12 for a review) There are, however, conflicting reports concerning attenuation of the frontal N30 potential in patients with PD. A reduced N30 was observed in only 32.5% of PD patients by Onofrj et al. (213), with no clear relation between N30 amplitude and motor performances, and several authors failed to confirm this N30 reduction, either when comparing PD patients with normal subjects matched for age, or when comparing the SEPs to stimulation of the more affected side with those to stimulation of the less affected side in patients with hemi-parkinsonism (214–216). SEPs to median nerve stimulation have also been reported as normal in multiple system atrophy (217).

Another open question is whether the amplitude of the N30 potential actually correlates with motor performances in PD and could be used as an objective marker of the stage of the disease. The effects of subcutaneous apomorphine injection on the amplitude of the frontal N30 have been studied with controversial results. Some authors (212,218) reported a clear-cut and selective amplitude increase of N30 in association with clinical improvement, while other authors did not observe this effect on frontal SEPs, despite a clear improvement of motor performance (216). In line with this latter negative result, acute or chronic administration of L-dopa and bromocriptine did not modify the frontal SEP amplitude in PD patients, despite positive clinical effects (213). Differences in the severity of the disease between the patient cohorts included in these studies may account for such divergences. Pierantozzi et al. (219) provided some evidence in favor of a link between N30 amplitude and motor performances in PD patients treated with deep brain stimulation of the internal globus pallidus or of the nucleus subthalamicus. These authors reported that during stimulation the N30 amplitude increase correlated with the positive effects on motor abilities; conversely, after interruption of stimulation the N30 enhancement faded nearly in parallel with the clinical effects. HFOs to median nerve and tibial nerve stimulation were reported as enhanced in patients with PD or multiple system atrophy (220,221), but other authors (222) failed to replicate this finding in a group of PD patients with an akinetic rigid form of the disease.

5.11.2. DYSTONIA

Abnormal central integration of afferent somatosensory inputs is, among others, a possible causative mechanism of dystonia. The first report on SEPs in patients with focal or generalized dystonia was that by Reilly et al. (223), who described a selective increase of the N30 potential, which could reflect hyperactivity of the striatocortical loops. However, in this study, N30 abnormalities were similar after stimulation of either the affected or unaffected side in patients with unilateral dystonia. Kanovsky et al. (224) replicated this finding in patients with spasmodic torticollis, and Ng and Jones (225) found that an increased "N35" potential recorded in C3' and C4' referred to Fz showed a sensitivity of 65% and a specificity of 78% in dystonia. Tinazzi et al. (226) reported an increase of tibial nerve P39 and N50 potentials that was unrelated to the severity of the disease and was present on both sides in patients with unilateral dystonia. These findings can be interpreted as reflecting an abnormal central processing of somatosensory inputs related to increased excitability of the motor cortex and are coherent with the early findings by Reilly et al. (223). HFOs to median nerve stimulation were found decreased in patients with writer's cramp (227), suggesting that cortical excitability might be associated with a disorganization of inputs to the somatosensory cortex in this condition.

Responses to paired interfering stimuli have been studied by comparing the amplitudes of SEPs to simultaneous stimulation of the median and ulnar nerves on the same side with that of the sum of SEP amplitudes after stimulation of each nerve individually. In normal subjects the former are smaller than the latter for N13, P14, N20, P27, and N30 potentials, while this does not occur for the peripheral N9 potential. This gating phenomenon, which can be interpreted as reflecting a central surround inhibition of incoming volleys from neighboring territories, was found to be less efficient in dystonic patients than in normal subjects (228). Moreover, Frasson et al. (229) reported an abnormal SEP recovery cycle in response to paired stimulation (i.e., less in-field inhibition) in patients with generalized dystonia. Recently, MEG responses to high-rate and novel stimuli in S2 and parietal ventral somatosensory areas were reported increased in patients with task-specific hand dystonia (230). Thus, a sensory overflow could play a role in the distortion of sensory and motor cortical maps of dystonic patients and explain why the temporal discrimination threshold, which is the shortest time interval at which two electrical tactile stimuli are perceived as separate, is higher in patients with generalized and focal dystonia than in normal subjects in affected but also in unaffected body regions (see reference 228 for a review).

Abnormal movement-related gating of SEPs has been carefully investigated in patients with writer's cramp using a reaction time paradigm (231). The main finding was that pre-movement gating of N24 and N30 frontal SEPs, usually observed in normal subjects with this paradigm, is lacking or reduced in patients with writer's cramp. This abnormality was identical in dystonic as well as in simple writer's cramp. Conversely, there was no difference in SEP gating during voluntary movements between patients and normal subjects. During movement preparation, changes in SEPs might be due mainly to changes in central sensory transmission produced by the intention to move. Thus, dystonia could be related to some defect in a premotor subroutine, which includes the specification of motor commands for a forthcoming action, as well as the specific setting of cortical responsiveness to afferent somatosensory inputs.

5.12. Huntington's Disease

Since the first study by Oepen et al. (232), early cortical N20-P27 potentials have been known to be depressed in patients with Huntington's disease. Amplitude decrease of both N20 and N30 SEPs was reported in Huntington's disease that correlated with functional decline over a two-year period (233). Moreover, abnormal SEPs have been reported in clinically asymptomatic subjects at risk for the disease (234), and reduction of early parietal and frontal SEPs is correlated with the CAG repeat length on chromosome 4 (235).

5.13. Trigeminal Neuralgia

Arterial compression of the trigeminal roots in the cerebellopontine angle has been recognized as a frequent etiology of the so-called idiopathic trigeminal neuralgia; pain relief in these cases can be achieved by decompressive microsurgery. Several attempts have been made to detect conduction slowing reflecting trigeminal compression using trigeminal SEPs. However, the routine use of trigeminal SEPs remained limited for three main reasons: (1) the clinical presentation of trigeminal neuralgia is in most cases so typical that ancillary techniques are not needed to make the diagnosis; (2) imaging studies (computed tomography or MRI and/or angiography) are usually performed routinely whenever an extrinsic compressive lesion is suspected and/or neurosurgical treatment is envisaged; and (3) some uncertainties remain as to the most adequate recording method and identification of normal components of the evoked response (see the section above on SEPs to trigeminal nerve stimulation). The P19 scalp component evoked by electrical stimulation of the lips was reported as delayed in 40% of patients with trigeminal neuralgia (124). Leandri et al. (125) used the early potentials evoked by stimulation of the infraorbital nerve in these patients. Nine patients out of the 38 of their series with clinically idiopathic trigeminal neuralgia showed abnormal responses on the affected side. The most frequent abnormality was an increase of the interpeak interval between waves W1 and W3, supposed to take origin respectively at the entry of the maxillary nerve into the gasserian ganglion and in the presynaptic portion of the trigeminal spinal tract. The latency of wave W2, thought to originate at the entry zone of the trigeminal root into the pons, was normal in eight of the nine patients with abnormal responses. These authors reported similar abnormalities in tumors of the cerebellopontine angle, while both waves W2 and W3 were delayed in patients with trigeminal neuralgia or hypesthesia symptomatic of a parasellar tumor.

5.14. Pain Syndromes

Two major categories of chronic pain have been recognized on clinical grounds. One is referred to as *somatic pain* and is thought to be due to prolonged activation of nociceptors; chronic pain in malignant disease, for example, is usually included in this category. The second type of pain, often referred to as *neuropathic pain*, results from direct injury or disease of the somatosensory systems. A third category is being progressively added to this classification, termed *dysfunctional pain*, which refers to chronic pain syndromes such as fibromyalgia, myofascial pain, irritable bowel or painful bladder syndromes, vulvodynia, or primary dysmenorrhea, which do not show evidence of primary alteration of somatosensory transmission but do show indices of central sensitization and deficits in descending pain control systems (236,237).

EPs are useful mainly for investigating chronic neuropathic and dysfunctional pain syndromes. The most direct approach is to record responses evoked by nociceptive stimuli, since neuropathic pain is usually associated with lesions of pain and temperature pathways (see above). LEPs have demonstrated their ability to detect lesions in peripheral and central pain pathways, including small-fiber neuropathies (170,140), spinal cord lesions (180, 238), brainstem infarcts affecting the spinothalamic system (239, 240), and focal cortical lesions affecting the spinothalamic projections (241) (Fig. 43.18).

While early studies mostly attempted to identify lesions of the nociceptive system, more recent work uses LEPs as tools for the diagnosis of neuropathic pain (reviewed in reference 138). Recent clinical reports using contact-heat evoked potentials (CHEPs) suggest that this technique might soon become a useful adjunct to LEPs in the neurophysiological assessment of pain syndromes (242).

Abnormal somatosensory responses to stimulation of a painful territory substantiate the neuropathic origin of the pain. Providing objective evidence of conduction abnormalities in somatosensory pathways defines the pain as neuropathic. Study of thermo-algesic pathways using LEPs is a crucial step for the diagnosis of neuropathic pain, since the results of standard exams such as nerve conduction velocity or SEPs will be normal in a substantial proportion of patients with neuropathic pain. Significant abnormality of LEPs to stimulation of a painful territory should be considered as an electrophysiological signature of neuropathic pain and can be commonly observed in small-fiber neuropathy, central spinal lesions (syringomyelia), and brainstem, thalamic, or cortical stroke. The exquisite sensitivity of LEPs to spinothalamic impairment allows the detection of minute lesions and gives LEPs medicolegal value in a number of countries.

The type of SEP/LEP abnormality depends on the lesion site and the pathophysiology of the pain. Ischemic necrosis interrupting transmission where the spinothalamic tract occupies a small volume (e.g., brainstem lesions) will entail profound LEP abnormalities, to a greater extent than slowly

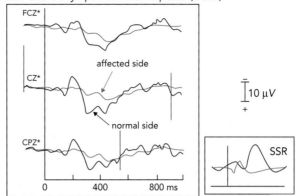

Abnormal nocieptive laser evoked potentials (LEPs)
and laser-evoked sympathetic skin response (L-SSR)

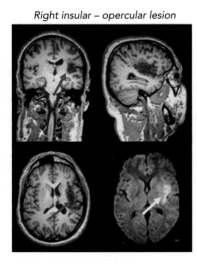

Right insular – opercular lesion

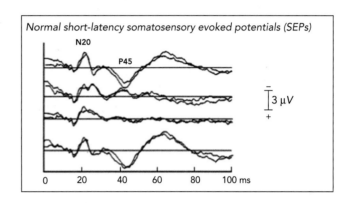

Normal short-latency somatosensory evoked potentials (SEPs)

Figure 43.18. SEPs and LEPs in operculo-insular pain syndrome. Anatomical lesion and electrophysiological tests after an ischemic lesion covering two thirds of the right insula, with extension to the inner operculum. There was left-sided neuropathic pain and left hemi-hypesthesia for pain and temperature but preserved lemniscal sensory modes. LEPs were significantly attenuated to the stimulation of the painful left hand (red traces, upper right), as were vegetative responses after stimulation to the affected hand (framed responses, skin sympathetic response, red traces). In contrast, short-latency SEPs to non-noxious electric shocks were normal and symmetrical (bottom right).

progressive lesions that tend to distort structures without much axonal loss (e.g., syringomyelia). Focal thalamic lesions may produce alterations of both SEPs and LEPs, but only the latter are related to the development of central pain (243). Focal cortical lesions in the posterior operculo-insular cortex, where the spinothalamic system mainly projects, may cause profound alteration of LEPs but total sparing of SEPs (240).

Partial preservation and desynchronization of LEPs in neuropathic pain increase the probability of hyperalgesia and allodynia. Although this conclusion would benefit from further validation, it has been supported by a number of independent studies so far, in both peripheral and central pain. A study on 54 patients reported that the prevalence of allodynia or hyperalgesia increased significantly when LEP alteration was only partial, and in particular when LEPs appeared desynchronized or included late abnormal components (253). The notion that partial preservation of thermo-algesic pathways is associated with hyperalgesia has been supported by studies in patients with peripheral, spinal and supraspinal neuropathic pain, in whom LEPs and/or thermal thresholds were more severely affected in patients with exclusively ongoing pain than in those with superimposed allodynia/hyperalgesia (140).

Normal or enhanced SEPs/LEPs to stimulation of a painful territory suggest functional integrity of somatosensory pathways and do not support a diagnosis of neuropathic pain.

Demonstration of unaltered somatosensory transmission at peripheral and central levels after stimulation of a territory alleged as painful tends to exclude the diagnosis of neuropathic pain, or at least raises a reasonable doubt. In case of normal LEPs, it is however important to ascertain that normal responses are also obtained to the selective stimulation of C-fibers, as the latter may prove to be selectively abnormal while Aδ LEPs remain within normal limits (138). Association of chronic pain with normal or enhanced LEPs is the rule in fibromyalgia, chronic myofascial pain, chronic fatigue syndrome, tension headache, and migraine, which underlines the pathophysiological differences between these conditions and neuropathic pain. In some of these diseases, notably migraine and fibromyalgia, a deficit of LEP habituation to repeated series of stimuli has been described (244), consistent with failure of mechanisms of descending pain control rather than a primary dysfunction of nociceptive transmission (236). Also, normal or enhanced LEPs in patients with nonorganic pain syndromes or *sine materia* pain anesthesia are useful to document the psychogenic participation in the syndrome.

EP interpretation benefits from concomitant recording of psychophysical measures and vegetative responses. The interpretation of nociceptive EPs greatly benefits from the simultaneous analysis of reaction times, sensory and nociceptive thresholds, subjective intensity reports, and vegetative skin responses. Thresholds should be obtained preferably before initiating the electrophysiological exam, for which they serve as a useful guide. The clinical somatosensory exam will indicate the territory to be stimulated and the stimulation modalities. Stimulation should always concern the affected territory, and results should be compared whenever possible with its contralateral homolog. Normal responses obtained to stimulation of an unaffected region have *no clinical value*. Simultaneous with LEPs, the motor reaction times and sympathetic skin responses can be recorded using a single bipolar montage between the palm and the dorsum of the hand. Reaction time latencies commonly are in the same range as those of vertex potentials, while sympathetic skin responses develop 3 to 8 seconds following the laser stimulus, and therefore need long interstimulus intervals. Sympathetic skin response is a peripheral manifestation of stimulus-related arousal and in healthy subjects correlates with both subjective intensity ratings and the amplitude of cortical responses (245,246). Dissociation between these variables therefore has diagnostic relevance, in particular in patients in whom conversion disorder or malingering is suspected.

Nociceptive EP abnormalities reflect abnormalities in thermo-algesic transmission but do not reflect pain itself. SEPs and LEPs provide objective information on the functional status of somatosensory pathways, the lesion of which is the crucial element of the so-called neuropathic pain paradox: the association of a negative symptom (hypesthesia) and a positive symptom (pain) in the same territory. While this is important for diagnosis, it is also important to remember that we can detect the lesion, but the pain itself. Neither electrophysiology nor functional imaging has so far been able to devise clinical routine tests detecting neuronal activities directly and unequivocally associated with the subjective sensation of pain, and cortical activities subtending the pain experience remain transparent to classical EP techniques. More sophisticated approaches such as time frequency wavelet decomposition (see Chapters 36 and 44) might be able in the future to address in a more direct way the detection of the neuropathic abnormal sensation, of which the lesion of nociceptive pathways is just the *primum movens*.

5.15. Migraine

Most SEP studies reported normal amplitudes and latencies of early cortical responses to median nerve stimulation in migraine (247) and normal LEPs to trigeminal and extra-trigeminal stimulations. Recent SEP studies in migraine patients focused on HFOs triggered by somatosensory stimulation and SEP habituation, which have been recently reviewed (248). Somatosensory evoked HFOs, especially the early HFOs, were found to be smaller in migraine patients than in matched normal controls between attacks, particularly in those whose attack frequency had worsened over the 6 months before the recording. Furthermore, they tended to be larger in patients who had improved during the same period and to return to normal during migraine attacks (249). Interictal decrease with ictal normalization of early HFOs may thus reflect a fluctuating dysfunction of thalamocortical afferents in migraine patients.

In a MEG study the equivalent current dipole strength of N20m was found enhanced in migraine patients compared to controls, but no N20m habituation was observed at various stimulus frequencies in any of the two groups (250). Conversely, deficient habituation of N20 on six consecutive runs of 500 median nerve stimulations has been reported in migraine patients between attacks while early HFOs, which were reduced in patients, showed no habituation in both patients and control subjects (251). Between attacks, a reduced habituation of LEPs to repeated runs of painful trigeminal and extra-trigeminal stimulations repetitive stimulation has also been reported in migraine patients (244).

5.16. Dysfunctional Pain

Patients with dysfunctional pain (see the pain syndromes section above) present without an obvious cause on physical examination, imaging studies, or laboratory tests. The pathophysiology of such conditions is thought to be a dysfunctional sensory processing (rather than lesion or disease) within the CNS. The most commonly adduced mechanism is central sensitization, which refers to CNS mechanisms leading to increased sensitivity to somatic signals (i.e., somatosensory amplification), either through increased facilitation or a decrease in central inhibition (252). The similar pattern of clinical presentation and the frequent comorbidity among these pain syndromes may reflect a commonality of central sensitization mechanisms, for which a possible genetic propensity remains to be determined.

The main use of SEPs/LEPs in dysfunctional pain is in its differential diagnosis versus neuropathic pain syndromes. While depressed SEPs/LEPs are signatures of neuropathic pain, normal or enhanced cortical responses after stimulation of painful areas are typical of dysfunctional pains. The flagship condition of these are fibromyalgia and myofascial-related disorders, which affect ~2% of the general population in Western countries, with a much stronger prevalence in women. In these patients, standard SEPs are normal. Also consistent with the lack of neuropathic alteration in sensory transmission, nociceptive LEPs to stimulation of painful territories in fibromyalgia patients were normal or even significantly enhanced in most studies (e.g., 253,254,255). Habituation to paired stimuli or to repeated trains is decreased in fibromyalgia and related syndromes (256), in a similar fashion as in migraine (see above). All these data strongly support the existence of central sensitization mechanisms entailing somatosensory amplification; this hypothesis is also substantiated by the failure of descending pain control systems in these conditions (236).

Loss of intraepidermal fibers suggesting small-fiber pathology has recently been described in subgroups of fibromyalgia patients (257), sometimes associated with depressed LEPs (256). These notions are difficult to reconcile with the above data, and considering fibromyalgia as the result of peripheral neuropathy is at odds with the bulk of clinical, therapeutic, and epidemiological results on dysfunctional pain (237). Loss of peripheral thin fibers is prevalent in a number of central conditions entailing chronic loss of physical mobility, from critical illness to Parkinson's disease or central post-stroke pain. Chronic loss of physical activity in fibromyalgia might contribute to the observed peripheral changes. The fact that exercise-based therapy is considered one of the most efficient treatments in these patients abounds in this view.

5.17. Factitious Sensory Loss

The finding of normal early somatosensory responses to stimulation of a territory that is alleged to be anesthetic provides a firm basis for the diagnosis of fictitious sensory loss. The use of SEP components with longer latency, originating in high-level association areas, may allow distinguishing genuine conversion (i.e., unconsciously driven anesthesia) from conscious simulation (i.e., malingering). Patients with genuine conversion symptoms have normal early SEPs but a reduction in the P300 potential (258), reflecting a lack of conscious processing of sensory stimuli (259), whereas P300 responses remain normal or even enhanced when hypesthesia is consciously faked (138,258). The concomitant recording of late SEPs/LEPs and sympathetic skin responses assessing vegetative arousal has been recently suggested to contribute further to the objective distinction between malingering and conversion (138).

REFERENCES

1. Dawson GD. Investigations on a patient subject to myoclonic seizures after sensory stimulation. J Neurol Neurosurg Psychiatry 1947;10:141–162.
2. Cruccu G, Aminoff MJ, Curio G, et al. Recommendations for the clinical use of somatosensory-evoked potentials. Clin Neurophysiol. 2008;119:1705–1719.
3. Gandevia SC, Burke D. Projection to the cerebral cortex from proximal and distal muscles in the human upper limb. Brain. 1988;111:389–403.
4. Restuccia D, Valeriani M, Insola A. et al. Modality-related scalp responses after selective electrical stimulation of cutaneous and muscular upper limb afferents in humans: specific and unspecific components. Muscle Nerve. 2002;26:44–54.
5. Gandevia SC, Burke D. Projection of thenar muscle afferents to frontal and parietal cortex of human subjects. Eleectroencephalogr Clin Neurophysiol. 1990;77:353–361.
6. Macefield G, Burke D, Gandevia SC. The cortical distribution of muscle and cutaneous afferent projections from the human foot. Electroencephalogr Clin Neurophysiol. 1989;72:518–528.
7. Burke D, Gandevia SC, McKeon B, Skuse NF. Interactions between cutaneous and muscle afferent projections to cerebral cortex in man. Electroencephalogr Clin Neurophysiol. 1982;53:349–360.
8. Desmedt JE, Osaki I. SEPs to finger joint input lack the N20-P20 response that is evoked by tactile inputs: contrast between cortical generators in areas 3b and 2 in humans: Electroencephalogr Clin Neurophysiol. 1991;80:513–521.
9. Restuccia D, Valeriani M, Barba C, Le Pera D, Tonali P, Mauguière F. Different contribution of joint and cutaneous inputs to early scalp somatosensory evoked potentials. Muscle Nerve. 1999;22:910–919.
10. El Kharoussi M, Ibañez V, Ben Jelloun W, Hugon M, Mauguière F. Potentiels évoqués somesthésiques: Interférences et masquage perceptif des afférences cutanées chez l'homme. Neurophysiol Clin. 1996;26:85–101.
11. Gandevia SC, Burke D, McKeon BB. Convergence in the somatosensory pathway between cutaneous afferents from the index and middle fingers in man. Exp Brain Res. 1983;50:415–425.
12. Cheron G, Dan B, Borenstein S. Sensory and motor interfering influences on somatosensory evoked potentials. J Clin Neurophysiol. 2000;17:280–294.
13. Debecker J, Desmedt JE. Les potentiels évoqués cérébraux et les potentiels de nerf sensible chez l'homme. Acta Neurol Belg. 1964;64:1212–1248.
14. Schieppati M, Ducati A. Short latency cortical potentials evoked by tactile air-jet stimulation of body and face in man. Electroencephalogr Clin Neurophysiol. 1984;58:418–425.
15. Mima T, Terada K, Maekawa M, Nagamine T, Ikeda A, Shibasaki H. Somatosensory evoked potentials following proprioceptive stimulation of fingers in man. Exp Brain Res. 1996;29:440–443.
16. Harkins SW, Chapman CR. Cerebral evoked potentials to noxious dental stimulation: relationship to subjective pain report. Psychophysiology. 1978;15:248–252.
17. Inui K, Tran TD, Hoshiyama M, Kakigi R. Preferential stimulation of A-delta fibers by intra-epidermal needle electrode in humans. Pain. 2002;96:247–252.
18. Plaghki L, Mouraux A. How do we selectively activate skin nociceptors with a high power infrared laser? Physiology and biophysics of laser stimulation. Neurophysiol Clin. 2003;33:269–277.
19. Bromm B, Treede RD. Human cerebral potentials evoked by CO2-laser stimuli causing pain. Exp Brain Res. 1987;67:153–162.
20. Kakigi R, Inui K, Tamura Y. Electrophysiological studies on human pain perception. Clin Neurophysiol. 2005;116:743–763.
21. Chen AC, Niddam DM, Arendt-Nielsen L. Contact heat evoked potentials as a valid means to study nociceptive pathways in human subjects. Neurosci Lett. 2001;316:79–82.
22. Baumgärtner U, Greffrath W, Treede RD. Contact heat and cold, mechanical, electrical and chemical stimuli to elicit small fiber-evoked potentials: merits and limitations for basic science and clinical use. Neurophysiol Clin/ 2012;42:267–280.
23. Truini A, Galeotti F, Pennisi E, Casa F, Biasiotta A, Cruccu G. Trigeminal small-fibre function assessed with contact heat evoked potentials in humans. Pain. 2007;132:102–107.
24. Ibañez V, Deiber MP, Mauguière F. Interference of vibrations with input transmission in dorsal horn and cuneate nucleus in man: a study of somatosensory evoked potentials (SEPs) to electrical stimulation of median nerve and fingers. Exp Brain Res. 1989;75:599–610.
25. Desmedt JE, Cheron G. Central somatosensory conduction in man: Neural generators and interpeak latencies of the far-field components recorded from neck and right or left scalp or earlobes. Electroencephalogr Clin Neurophysiol. 1980;50:382–403.
26. Mauguière F, Ibañez V. The dissociation of early SEP components in lesions of the cervico-medullary junction: a cue for routine interpretation of abnormal cervical responses to median nerve stimulation. Electroencephalogr Clin Neurophysiol. 1985;62:406–420.
27. Desmedt JE, Cheron G. Prevertebral (oesophageal) recording of subcortical somatosensory evoked potentials in man: the spinal P13 component and the dual nature of the spinal generators. Electroencephalogr Clin Neurophysiol. 1981;52:257–275.
28. Cioni B, Meglio M. Epidural recordings of electrical events produced in the spinal cord by segmental, ascending and descending volleys. Appl Neurophysiol. 1986;49:315–326.
29. Jeanmonod D, Sindou M, Mauguière F. The human cervical and lumbo-sacral evoked electrospinogram. Data from intra-operative spinal cord surface recordings. Electroencephalogr Clin Neurophysiol. 1991;80:477–489.
30. Buchner H, Ferbert A, Hacke W. Serial recording of median nerve stimulated subcortical somatosensory evoked potentials (SEPs) in developing brain death. Electroencephalogr Clin Neurophysiol. 1988;69:14–23.
31. Restuccia D, Mauguière F. The contribution of median nerve SEPs in the functional assessment of the cervical spinal cord in syringomyelia. A study of 24 patients. Brain. 1991;114:361–379.
32. Morioka T, Shima F, Kato M, Fukui M. Direct recordings of the somatosensory evoked potentials in the vicinity of the dorsal column nuclei in man: their mechanisms and contribution to the scalp far-field potentials. Electroencephalogr Clin Neurophysiol. 1991;80:215–220.
33. Zanette G, Tinazzi M, Manganotti P, Bonato C, Polo A. Two distinct cervical N13 potentials are evoked by ulnar nerve stimulation. Electroencephalogr Clin Neurophysiol. 1995;96:114–120.
34. Mauguière F. Anatomical origin of the cervical N13 potential evoked by upper extremity stimulation. J Clin Neurophysiol. 2000;17:236–245.
35. Mauguière F. Les potentiels évoqués somesthésiques cervicaux chez le sujet normal. Analyse des aspects obtenus selon le siège de l'électrode de référence. Rev EEG Neurophysiol. 1983;13:259–272.
36. Desmedt JE, Cheron G. Non-cephalic reference recording of early somatosensory potentials to finger stimulation in adult or aging man: differentiation of widespread N18 and contralateral N20 from the prerolandic P22 and N30 components. Electroencephalogr Clin Neurophysiol. 1981;52:553–570.
37. Cracco RQ, Cracco JB. Somatosensory evoked potential in man: Far-field potentials. Electroencephalogr Clin Neurophysiol. 1976;41:460–466.
38. Restuccia D. Anatomic origin of P13 and P14 scalp far-field potentials. J Clin Neurophysiol. 2000;17:246–257.
39. Garcia-Larrea L, Mauguière F. Latency and amplitude abnormalities of the scalp far-field P14 to median nerve stimulation in multiple sclerosis. Electroencephalogr Clin Neurophysiol. 1988;71:180–186.

40. Anziska A, Cracco RQ. Short-latency somatosensory evoked potentials: studies in patients with focal neurological disease. Electroencephalogr Clin Neurophysiol. 1980;49:227–239.

41. Mauguière F, Desmedt JE. Thalamic pain syndrome of Dejerine-Roussy. Differentiation of four subtypes assisted by somatosensory evoked potentials data. Arch Neurol. 1988;45:1312–1320.

42. Restuccia D, Di Lazzaro V, Valeriani M, et al. Brainstem somatosensory dysfunction in a case of long-standing left hemispherectomy with removal of the left thalamus thalamus: a nasopharyngeal and scalp SEP study. Electroencephalogr Clin Neurophysiol. 1996;100:184–188.

43. Mauguière F, Desmedt JE, Courjon J. Neural generators of N18 and P14 far-field somatosensory evoked potentials studied in patients with lesions of thalamus or thalamo-cortical radiations. Electroencephalogr Clin Neurophysiol. 1983;56:283–292.

44. Mauguière F. Short-latency somatosensory evoked potentials to upper limb stimulation in lesions of brainstem, thalamus and cortex. In Ellingson RJ, Murray NMF, Halliday AM, eds. The London Symposia. Electroencephalogr Clin Neurophysiol. 1987(Suppl 39):302–309.

45. Mauguière F, Desmedt JE. Bilateral somatosensory evoked potentials in four patients with long-standing surgical hemispherectomy. Ann Neurol.1989;26:724–731.

46. Urasaki E, Wada S, Kadoya C, Yokota A, Matsuoka S, Shima F. Origin of scalp far-field N18 of SSEPs in response to median nerve stimulation. Electroencephalogr Clin Neurophysiol. 1990;77:39–51.

47. Tomberg C, Desmedt JE, Ozaki I, Noël P. Nasopharyngeal recordings of somatosensory evoked potentials document the medullary origin of the N18 far-field. Electroencephalogr Clin Neurophysiol. 1991;80:496–503.

48. Sonoo M. Anatomic origin and clinical application of the widespread N18 potential in median nerve somatosensory evoked potentials. J Clin Neurophysiol. 2000;17:258–268.

49. Allison T, McCarthy G, Wood CC, Darcey TM, Spencer DD, Williamson PD. Human cortical potentials evoked by stimulation of the median nerve. I. Cytoarchitectonic areas generating short-latency potentials. J Neurophysiol. 1989;62:694–710.

50. Desmedt JE, Cheron G. Somatosensory evoked potentials to finger stimulation in healthy octogenarians and in young adults: waveforms, scalp topography and transit times of parietal and frontal components. Electroencephalogr Clin Neurophysiol. 1980;50:404–425.

51. Balzamo E, Marquis P, Chauvel P, Régis J. Short-latency components of evoked potentials to median nerve stimulation recorded by intracerebral electrodes in the human pre- and postcentral areas. Clin Neurophysiol. 2004;115:1616–1623.

52. Frot M, Magnin M, Mauguière F, Garcia-Larrea L. Cortical representation of pain in primary sensory-motor areas (S1/M1): a study using intracortical recordings in humans. Hum Brain Mapp. 2013;34:2655–2668.

53. Deiber MP, Giard MH, Mauguière F. Separate generators with distinct orientations for N20 and P22 somatosensory evoked potentials to finger stimulation. Electroencephalogr Clin Neurophysiol. 1986;65:321–334.

54. Baumgärtner U, Vogel H, Ohara S, Treede RD, Lenz FA. Dipole source analyses of early median nerve SEP components obtained from subdural grid recordings. J Neurophysiol. 2010;104:3029–3041.

55. Brenner D, Lipton J, Kaufman L, Williamson SJ. Somatically evoked magnetic fields of the human brain. Science. 1978;199:81–83.

56. Okada YC, Tanenbaum R, Williamson SJ, Kaufman L. Somatotopic organization of the human somatosensory cortex revealed by neuromagnetic measurements. Exp Brain Res. 1984;56:197–205.

57. Wood CC, Cohen D, Cuffin BN, Yarita M, Allison T. Electrical sources in human somatosensory cortex: identification by combined magnetic and potential recordings. Science. 1985;227:1051–1053.

58. Buchner H, Adams L, Müller A, et al. Somatotopy of human hand somatosensory cortex revealed by dipole source analysis of early somatosensory evoked potentials and 3D-NMR tomography. Electroencephalogr Clin Neurophysiol. 1995;96:121–134.

59. Buchner H, Waberski TD, Fuchs M, Drenckhahn R, Wagner M, Wischmann HA. Postcentral origin of P22: evidence from source reconstruction in a realistically shaped head model and from a patient with a post-central lesion. Electroencephalogr Clin Neurophysiol. 1996;100:332–342.

60. Franssen H, Stegeman DF, Molemen J, Schoobaar RP. Dipole modelling of median nerve SEPs in normal subjects and patients with small subcortical infarcts. Electroencephalogr Clin Neurophysiol. 1992;84:401–417.

61. Mauguière F, Desmedt JE. Focal capsular vascular lesions can selectively deafferent the prerolandic or the parietal cortex: Somatosensory evoked potentials evidence. Ann Neurol. 1991;30:71–75.

62. Mauguière F, Desmedt JE, Courjon J. Astereognosis and dissociated loss of frontal or parietal components of somatosensory evoked potentials in hemispheric lesions. Brain. 1983;106:271–311.

63. Slimp JC, Tamas LB, Stolov WC, Wyler AR. Somatosensory evoked potentials after removal of somatosensory cortex in man. Electroencephalogr Clin Neurophysiol. 1986;65:111–117.

64. Tsuji S, Muray Y, Kadoya C. Topography of somatosensory evoked potentials to median nerve stimulation in patients with cerebral lesions. Electroencephalogr Clin Neurophysiol. 1988;71:280–288.

65. Allison T, McCarthy G, Wood CC, Jones SJ. Potentials evoked in human and monkey cerebral cortex by stimulation of the median nerve: a review of scalp and intracranial recordings. Brain. 1991;114:2465–2503.

66. McCarthy G, Wood CC, Allison T. Cortical somatosensory evoked potentials: I. Recordings in the monkey Macaca fascicularis. J Neurophysiol. 1991;66:53–63.

67. Nicholson-Peterson N, Schroeder CE, Arezzo JC. Neural generators of the early cortical somatosensory evoked potentials in the awake monkey. Electroencephalogr Clin Neurophysiol. 1995;96:248–260.

68. Papadelis C, Eickhoff SB, Zilles K, Ioannides AA. BA3b and BA1 activate in a serial fashion after median nerve stimulation: direct evidence from combining source analysis of evoked fields and cytoarchitectonic probabilistic maps. Neuroimage. 2011;54:60–73.

69. Garcia-Larrea L, Bastuji H, Mauguière F. Unmasking of cortical SEP components by changes in stimulus rate a topographic study. Electroencephalogr Clin Neurophysiol. 1992;84:71–83.

70. Delberghe X, Mavroudakis N, Zegers de Beyl D, Brunko E. The effect of stimulus frequency on post- and precentral short latency somatosensory evoked potentials (SEPs). Electroencephalogr Clin Neurophysiol. 1990;77:86–92.

71. Restuccia D, Valeriani M, Grassi E, et al. Contribution of GABAergic circuitry in shaping scalp somatosensory evokes responses in humans: specific changes after single-dose administration of tiagabine. Clin Neurophysiol. 2002;113:656–671.

72. Cheron G, Borenstein S. Mental movement stimulation affects the N30 frontal component of the somatosensory evoked potential. Electroencephalogr Clin Neurophysiol. 1992;84:288–292.

73. Rossini PM, Caramia D, Bassetti MA, Pasqualetti P, Tecchio F, Bernardi G. Somatosensory evoked potentials during the ideation and execution of individual finger movements. Muscle Nerve. 1996;19:191–202.

74. Rossi S, Tecchio F, Pasqualetti P, et al. Somatosensory processing during movement observation in humans. Clin Neurophysiol. 2002;113:16–24.

75. Barba C, Frot M, Guénot M, Mauguière F. Stereotactic recordings of median nerve SEPs in the human supplementary motor area. Eur J Neurosci. 2001;13:347–356.

76. Waberski TD, Buchner H, Perkuhn M, et al. N30 and the effect of explorative finger movements: a model of the contribution of the motor cortex to early somatosensory potentials. Clin Neurophysiol. 1999;110:1589–1600.

77. Valeriani M, Restuccia D, Barba C, Tonali P, Mauguière F. Central scalp projection of the N30 SEP source activity after median nerve stimulation. Muscle Nerve. 2000;23:353–360.

78. Noachtar S, Lüders HO, Dinner DS, Klem G. Ipsilateral median somatosensory evoked potentials recorded from human somatosensory cortex. Electroencephalogr Clin Neurophysiol. 1997;104:189–198.

79. Halliday AM, Wakefield GS. Cerebral evoked potentials in patients with dissociated sensory loss. J Neurol Neurosurg Psychiatry. 1963;26:211–219.

80. Bradley C, Joyce N, Garcia-Larrea L. Adaptation in human somatosensory cortex as a model of sensory memory construction: a study using high-density EEG. Brain Struct Funct. 2016;221:421–431.

81. Desmedt JE, Nguyen TH, Bourguet M. The cognitive P40, N60, P100 components of somatosensory evoked potentials and the earliest signs of sensory processing in man. Electroencephalogr Clin Neurophysiol. 1983;56:272–282.

82. Garcia-Larrea L, Bastuji H, Mauguière F. Mapping study of somatosensory evoked potentials during selective spatial attention. Electroencephalogr Clin Neurophysiol. 1991;80:201–214.

83. Barba C, Frot M, Valeriani M, Tonali P, Mauguière F. Distinct fronto-central N60 and suprasylvian N70 middle-latency components of the median nerve SEPs as assessed by scalp topographic analysis, dipolar source modelling and depth recordings. Clin Neurophysiol. 2002;113:981–992.

84. Penfield W, Rasmussen T. The Cerebral Cortex of Man: A Clinical Study of Localization. New York: Macmillan, 1957.

85. Woolsey CN, Erickson TC, Gilson WE. Localization in somatic sensory and motor areas of human cerebral cortex as determined by direct recording of evoked potentials and electrical stimulation. J Neurosurg. 1979;51:476–506.

86. Hari R, Hämäläinen M, Kaukoranta E, Reinikainen K, Tezner D. Neuromagnetic responses from the second somatosensory cortex in man. Acta Neurol Scand. 1983;68:207–212.

87. Hari R, Reinikainen K, Kaukoranta E, et al. Somatosensory evoked cerebral magnetic fields from SI and SII in man. Electroencephalogr Clin Neurophysiol. 1984;57:254–263.

88. Hari R, Hämäläinen H, Hämäläinen M, Kekoni J, Sams M, Tiihonen J. Separate finger representations at the human second somatosensory cortex. Neuroscience. 1990;37:245–249.

89. Hari R, Karhu J, Hämäläinen M, et al. Functional organization of the human first and second somatosensory cortices: a neuromagnetic study. Eur J Neurosci. 1993;5:724–734.

90. Allison T, McCarthy G, Wood CC. The relationship between human long-latency somatosensory evoked potentials recorded from the cortical surface and from the scalp. Electroencephalogr Clin Neurophysiol. 1992;84:301–314.

91. Frot M, Mauguière F. Timing and spatial distribution of somatosensory responses recorded in the upper bank of the sylvian fissure (SII area) in humans. Cerebral Cortex. 1999;9:854–863.

92. Frot M, Garcia-Larrea L, Guénot M, Mauguière F. Responses of the supra-sylvian (SII) cortex in humans to painful and innocuous stimuli. A study using intra-cerebral recordings. Pain. 2001;94:65–73.

93. Garcia-Larrea L, Lukaszewicz AC, Mauguière F. Somatosensory responses during selective spatial attention: the N120 to N140 transition. Psychophysiology. 1995;32:526–537.

94. Näätänen R. The role of attention in auditory information processing as revealed by event-related potentials and other brain measures of cognitive function. Behav Brain Sci. 1990;13:201–288.

95. Lüders H, Lesser RP, Dinner DS, Hahn JF, Salanga V, Morris HH. The second somatosensory area in humans: Evoked potentials and electrical stimulation studies. Ann Neurol. 1985;17:177–184.

96. Barba C, Frot M, Mauguière F. Early secondary somatosensory area (SII) SEPs. Data from intracerebral recordings in humans. Clin Neurophysiol. 2002;113:1778–1786.

97. Karhu J, Tesche CD. Simultaneous early processing of sensory input in human primary (SI) and secondary (SII) somatosensory cortices. J Neurophysiol. 1999;81:2017–2025.

98. Forss N, Hari R, Salmelin R, et al. Activation of the human posterior parietal cortex by median nerve stimulation. Exp Brain Res. 1994;99:309–315.

99. Forss N, Merlet I, Vanni S, Hämäläinen M, Mauguière F, Hari R. Activation of human mesial cortex during somatosensory attention task. Brain Res. 1996;734:229–235.

100. Mauguière F, Merlet I, Forss N, et al. Activation of a distributed cortical network in the human brain. A dipole modelling study of magnetic fields evoked by median nerve stimulation. Part I: Location and activation timing of SEF sources. Electroencephalogr Clin Neurophysiol. 1997;104:281–289.

101. Mauguière F, Merlet I, Forss N, et al. Activation of a distributed cortical network in the human brain. A dipole modelling study of magnetic fields evoked by median nerve stimulation. Part II: Effects of stimulus rate attention and stimulus detection. Electroencephalogr Clin Neurophysiol. 1997;104:290–295.

102. Sonoo M, Genba K, Iwatsubo T, Mannen T. P15 in tibial nerve SEPs as an example of the junctional potential. Electroencephalogr Clin Neurophysiol. 1992;84:486–491.

103. Miura T, Sonoo M, Shimizu T. Establishment of standard values for the latency, interval an amplitude parameters of tibial nerve somatosensory evoked potentials (SEPs). Clin Neurophysiol. 2003;114:1367–1378.

104. Desmedt JE, Cheron G. Spinal and far-field components of human somatosensory evoked potentials to posterior tibial nerve stimulation analysed with oesophageal derivations and non-cephalic reference recording. Electroencephalogr Clin Neurophysiol. 1983;56:635–651.

105. Yamada T, Machida M, Kimura J. Far-field somatosensory evoked potentials after stimulation of the tibial nerve. Neurology. 1982;32: 1151–1158.

106. Dimitrijevic MR, Halter JA, eds. Atlas of Human Cord Evoked Potentials. Boston: Butterworth-Heinemann, 1995.

107. Desmedt JE, Bourguet M. Color imaging of parietal and frontal somatosensory potential fields evoked by stimulation of median or posterior tibial nerve in man. Electroencephalogr Clin Neurophysiol. 1985;62:1–17.

108. Urasaki E, Tokimura T, Yasukouchi H, Wada S, Yokota A. P30 and N33 of posterior tibial nerve SSEPs are analogous to P14 and N18 of median nerve SSEPs. Electroencephalogr Clin Neurophysiol. 1993;88:525–529.

109. Tinazzi M, Mauguière F. Assessment of intraspinal and intracranial conduction by P30 and P39 tibial nerve somatosensory evoked potentials in cervical cord and hemispheric lesions. J Clin Neurophysiol. 1995;12:237–253.

110. Tinazzi M, Zanette G, Manganotti B, et al. Amplitude changes of tibial nerve cortical SEPs when using ipsilateral or contralateral ear as reference. J Clin Neurophysiol. 1997;14:217–225.

111. Yamada T. Neuroanatomic substrates of lower extremity somatosensory evoked potentials. J Clin Neurophysiol. 2000;17:269–279.

112. Tinazzi M, Zanette G, Fiaschi A, Mauguière F. Effects of stimulus rate on the cortical posterior tibial nerve SEPs: a topographic study. Electroencephalogr Clin Neurophysiol. 1996;100:210–219.

113. Zanette G, Tinazzi M, Polo A, Rizzuto N. Motor neuron disease with pyramidal tract dysfunction involves the cortical generators of the early somatosensory evoked potential to tibial nerve stimulation. Neurology. 1996;47:932–938.

114. Chiappa KH, Ropper AH. Evoked potentials in clinical medicine. N Engl J Med. 1982;306:1205–1211.

115. Valeriani M, Insola A, Restuccia D, et al. Source generators of the early somatosensory evoked potentials to tibial nerve stimulation: an intracerebral and scalp recording study. Clin Neurophysiol. 2001;112:1999–2006.

116. Baumgärtner V, Vogel H, Ellrich J, Gawehn J, Stoeter P, Treede RD. Brain electrical source analysis of primary cortical components of the tibial nerve somatosensory evoked potential using regional sources. Electroencephalogr Clin Neurophysiol. 1998;108:588–599.

117. Tinazzi M, Zanette G, La Porta F, et al. Selective gating of lower limb cortical somatosensory evoked potentials (SEPs) during passive and active foot movements. Electroencephalogr Clin Neurophysiol. 1997;104:312–321.

118. Valeriani M, Restuccia D, Di Lazzaro V, Barba C, Le Pera D, Tonali P. Dissociation induced by voluntary movement between two different components of the centro-parietal P40 SEP to tibial nerve stimulation. Electroencephalogr Clin Neurophysiol. 1998;108:190–198.

119. Katifi HA, Sedgwick EM. Somatosensory evoked potentials from posterior tibial nerve and lumbosacral dermatomes. Electroencephalogr Clin Neurophysiol. 1986;65:249–259.

120. Opsomer RJ, Caramia MD, Zarola F, Pesce F, Rossini PM. Neurophysiological evaluation of central-peripheral sensory and motor pudendal fibres. Electroencephalogr Clin Neurophysiol. 1989;74:260–270.

121. Turano G, Sindou M, Mauguière F. Spinal cord evoked potentials monitoring during spinal surgery for pain and spasticity. In Dimitrijevic MR, Halter JA, eds. Atlas of Human Cord Evoked Potentials. Boston: Butterworth-Heinemann, 1995:107–122.

122. Guérit JM, Opsomer RJ. Bit-mapped imaging of somatosensory evoked potentials after stimulation of the posterior tibial nerves and dorsal nerve of the penis/clitoris. Electroencephalogr Clin Neurophysiol. 1991;80:228–237.

123. Allison T, McCarthy G, Luby M, Puce A, Spencer DD. Localization of functional regions of human mesial cortex by somatosensory evoked potential recording and by cortical stimulation. Electroencephalogr Clin Neurophysiol. 1996;100:126–140.

124. Stöhr M, Petruch F, Scheglman K. Somatosensory evoked potentials following trigeminal nerve stimulation in trigeminal neuralgia. Ann Neurol.1981;9:63–66.

125. Leandri M, Parodi CI, Favale E. Early trigeminal evoked potentials in tumours of the base of the skull and trigeminal neuralgia. Electroencephalogr Clin Neurophysiol. 1988;71:114–124.

126. Hume AL, Cant BR. Conduction time in central somatosensory pathways in man. Electroencephalogr Clin Neurophysiol. 1978;45:361–375.

127. Mauguière F, Restuccia D. Inadequacy of the forehead reference montage for detecting spinal N13 potential abnormalities in patients with cervical cord lesion and preserved dorsal column function. Electroencephalogr Clin Neurophysiol. 1991;79:448–456.

128. Ozaki I, Takada H, Shimamura H, Baba M, Matsunaga M. Central conduction in somatosensory evoked potentials. Comparison of ulnar and median data evaluation of onset versus peak methods. Neurology. 1996;47:1299–1304.

129. Tsuji S, Lüders H, Lesser RP, Dinner DS, Klem G. Subcortical and cortical somatosensory potentials evoked by posterior tibial nerve stimulation: normative values. Electroencephalogr Clin Neurophysiol. 1984;59:214–228.

130. Tinazzi M, Zanette G, Bonato C, et al. Neural generators of tibial nerve P30 somatosensory evoked potential studied in patients with a focal lesion of the cervico-medullary junction. Muscle Nerve. 1996;19:1538–1548.

131. Eisen A, Roberts K, Low M, Hoirch M, Lawrence P. Questions regarding the sequential neural generator theory of the somatosensory evoked potentials raised by digital filtering. Electroencephalogr Clin Neurophysiol. 1984;59:388–395

132. Yamada T, Kameyama S, Fuchigami Y, Nakasumi Y, Dickins QS, Kimura J. Changes of short latency somatosensory evoked potential in sleep. Electroencephalogr Clin Neurophysiol. 1988;70:126–136.

133. Curio G, Mackert BM, Burghoff M, Koetitz R, Abraham-Fuchs K, Härer W. Localization of evoked neuromagnetic 600Hz activity in the cerebral somatosensory system. Electroencephalogr Clin Neurophysiol. 1994;91:483–487.

134. Ozaki I, Hashimoto I. Exploring the physiology and function of high-frequency oscillations (HFOs) from the somatosensory cortex. Clin Neurophysiol. 2011;122: 1908–1923.

135. Ozaki I, Suzuki C, Yaegashi Y, Baba M, Matsunaga M, Hashimoto I. High-frequency oscillations in early cortical somatosensory evoked potentials. Electroencephalogr Clin Neurophysiol. 1998;108:536–542.
136. Bromm B, Treede RD. Nerve fibre discharge, cerebral potentials and sensations induced by CO2 laser stimulation. Hum Neurobiol. 1984;3:33–40.
137. Treede RD, Lorenz J, Baumgartner U. Clinical usefulness of laser-evoked potentials. Neurophysiol Clin. 2003;33:303–314.
138. Garcia-Larrea L. Objective pain diagnostics: clinical neurophysiology. Clin Neurophysiol. 2012;42:187–197.
139. Boivie J, Leijon G, Johansson I. Central post-stroke pain: a study of the mechanisms through analyses of the sensory abnormalities. Pain. 1989;37:173–185.
140. Truini A, Biasiotta A, La Cesa S, et al. Mechanisms of pain in distal symmetric polyneuropathy: a combined clinical and neurophysiological study. Pain. 2010;150:516–521.
141. Valeriani M, Rambaud L, Mauguière F. Scalp topography and dipolar source modelling of potentials evoked by CO2 laser stimulation of the hand. Electroencephalogr Clin Neurophysiol. 1996;100:343–352.
142. Garcia-Larrea L, Frot M, Valeriani M. Brain generators of laser-evoked potentials: from dipoles to functional significance. Neurophysiol Clin. 2003;33:279–292.
143. Frot M, Mauguière F. Dual representation of pain in the operculo-insular cortex in humans. Brain. 2003;126:438–450.
144. Bastuji H, Frot M, Perchet C, Magnin M, Garcia-Larrea L. Pain networks from the inside: Spatiotemporal analysis of brain responses leading from nociception to conscious perception. Hum Brain Mapp. 2016, 37: 4301–4315.
145. Legrain V, Guérit J, Bruyer R, Plaghki L. Attentional modulation of the nociceptive processing into the human brain: selective spatial attention, probability of stimulus occurrence, and target detection effects on laser evoked potentials. Pain. 2002;99:21–39.
146. Lorenz J, Garcia-Larrea L. Contribution of attentional and cognitive factors to laser evoked brain potentials. Neurophysiol Clin. 2003;33:293–301.
147. Bastuji H, Perchet C, Legrain V, Montes C, Garcia-Larrea L. Laser-evoked responses to painful stimulation persist during sleep and predict subsequent arousals. Pain. 2008;137:589–599.
148. Siedenberg R, Treede D. Laser-evoked potentials: Exogenous and endogenous components. Electroencephalogr Clin Neurophysiol. 1996;100:240–249.
149. Garcia-Larrea L. Somatosensory volleys and cortical evoked potentials: "first come, first served"? Pain. 2004;112:5–7.
150. Taylor MJ, Fagan ER. SEPs to median nerve stimulation: normative data for paediatrics. Electroencephalogr Clin Neurophysiol. 1988;71:323–330.
151. George SR, Taylor MJ. Somatosensory evoked potentials in neonates and infants: developmental and normative data. Electroencephalogr Clin Neurophysiol. 1991;80:94–102.
152. Boor R, Goebel B, Taylor MJ. Subcortical somatosensory evoked potentials after median nerve stimulation in children. Eur J Paediatr Neurol. 1998;2:137–143.
153. Boor R, Goebel B, Doepp M, Taylor MJ. Somatosensory evoked potentials after posterior tibial nerve stimulation. Normative data in children. Eur J Paediatr Neurol. 1998;2:145–152.
154. Cracco JB, Cracco RQ, Stolove R. Spinal evoked potentials in man: A maturational study. Electroencephalogr Clin Neurophysiol. 1979;46:58–64.
155. Desmedt JE, Brunko J, Debecker J. Maturation of the somatosensory evoked potential in normal infants and children, with special reference to the early N1 component. Electroencephalogr Clin Neurophysiol. 1976;40:43–58.
156. Zhu Y, Geogesco M, Cadilhac J. Normal latency values of early cortical somatosensory evoked potentials in children. Electroencephalogr Clin Neurophysiol. 1987;68:471–474.
157. Hume AL, Cant BR, Shaw NA, Cowan JC. Central somatosensory conduction time from 10 to 79 years. Electroencephalogr Clin Neurophysiol. 1982;54:49–54.
158. Truini A, Galeotti F, Romaniello A, Virtuoso M, Ianetti GD, Cruccu G. Laser-evoked potentials: normative values. Clin Neurophysiol. 2005;116: 821–826.
159. Creac'h C, Bertholon A, Convers P, Garcia-Larrea L, Peyron R. Effects of aging on laser evoked potentials. Muscle Nerve. 2015;51:736–742.
160. Chiappa KH. Evoked Potentials in Clinical Medicine, 2nd ed. New York: Raven Press, 1990.
161. Guérit JM, Soveges L, Baele P, Dion R. Median nerve evoked potentials in profound hypothermia for ascending aorta repair. Electroencephalogr Clin Neurophysiol. 1990;77:163–173.
162. Desmedt JE, Tomberg C. Mapping early somatosensory evoked potentials in selective attention: critical evaluation of control conditions used for titrating by difference the cognitive P30, P40, P100 and N140. Electroencephalogr Clin Neurophysiol. 1989;74:321–346.

163. Emerson RG, Sgro JA, Pedley TA, Hauser WA. State-dependent changes in the N20 component of the median nerve somatosensory evoked potentials. Neurology. 1988;38:64–68.
164. Green JB, Walcoff MR, Lucke JF. Comparison of phenytoin and phenobarbital effects on far-field auditory and somatosensory evoked potentials interpeak latencies. Epilepsia. 1982;23:417–421.
165. Mavroudakis N, Brunko E, Nogueira MC, Zegers de Beyl D. Acute effects of diphenylhydantoin on peripheral and central somatosensory conduction. Electroencephalogr Clin Neurophysiol. 1991;78:263–266.
166. Mauguière F, Chauvel P, Dewailly J, Dousse N. No effect of long-term vigabatrin treatment on central nervous system conduction in patients with refractory epilepsy: results of a multicenter study of somatosensory and visual evoked potentials. Epilepsia. 1997;38:301–308.
167. Parry GJ, Aminoff MJ. Somatosensory evoked potentials in chronic acquired demyelinating peripheral neuropathy. Neurology. 1987;37: 313–316.
168. Petiot P, Vial C, Mauguière F. Proximal sensory neuropathy with preserved distal conduction and SEPs. Muscle Nerve. 1999;22:650–652.
169. Yiannikas C, Vusik S. Utility of somatosensory evoked potentials in chronic acquired demyelinating neuropathy. Muscle Nerve. 2008;38:1447–1454.
170. Kakigi R, Shibasaki H, Tanaka K. CO2 laser induced pain-related somatosensory evoked potentials in peripheral neuropathies: correlation between electrophysiological and histopathological findings. Muscle Nerve. 1991;14:441–450.
171. Casanova-Molla J, Grau-Junyent JM, Morales M, Valls-Solé J. On the relationship between nociceptive evoked potentials and intraepidermal nerve fiber density in painful sensory polyneuropathies. Pain. 2011;152:410–418.
172. Jones SJ, Wynn Parry CB, Landi A. Diagnosis of brachial plexus traction lesions by sensory nerve action potentials and somatosensory evoked potentials. Injury. 1981;12:376–382.
173. Ropper AH, Chiappa KH. Evoked potentials in Guillain-Barré syndrome. Neurology. 1986;36:587–590.
174. Tsukamoto H, Sonoo M, Shimizu T. Segmental evaluation of the peripheral nerve using tibial nerve SEPs for the diagnosis of CIDP. Clin Neurophysiol. 2010;121:77–84.
175. Devic P, Petiot P, Mauguière F. Diagnostic utility of somatosensory evoked potentials in chronic polyradiculopathy without electrodiagnostic signs of peripheral demyelination. Muscle Nerve. 2016;53:78–83.
176. Nuwer MR, Perlman SL, Packwood JW, Kark RA. Evoked potential abnormalities in the various inherited ataxias. Ann Neurol. 1983;13:20–27.
177. Vanasse M, Garcia-Larrea L, Neuschwander L, Trouillas P, Mauguière F. Evoked potentials studies in Friedreich's ataxia and progressive early onset cerebellar ataxia. Can J Neurol Sci. 1988;15:292–298.
178. Pedersen L, Trojaborg W. Visual, auditory and somatosensory pathway involvement in hereditary cerebellar ataxia, Friedreich's ataxia and familial spastic paraplegia. Electroencephalogr Clin Neurophysiol. 1981;52:283–297.
179. Ibañez V, Fischer G, Mauguière F. Dorsal horn and dorsal column dysfunction in intramedullary cervical cord tumours: a SEP study. Brain. 1992;115:1209–1234.
180. Kakigi R, Shibasaki H, Kuroda Y, et al. Pain-related somatosensory evoked potentials in syringomyelia. Brain. 1991;114:1871–1889.
181. Yu YL, Jones SJ. Somatosensory evoked potentials in cervical spondylosis. Correlation of median, ulnar and posterior tibial nerve re- sponses with clinical and radiological findings. Brain. 1985;108:273–300.
182. Restuccia D, Valeriani M, Di Lazzaro V, Tonali P, Mauguière F. Somatosensory evoked potentials after multisegmental upper limb stimulation in the diagnosis of cervical spondylotic myelopathy. J Neurol Neurosurg Psychiatry. 1994;57:301–308.
183. Mauguière F, Schott B, Courjon J. Dissociation of early SEP components in unilateral traumatic section of the lower medulla. Ann Neurol. 1983;13:309–313.
184. Anziska A, Cracco RW. Short-latency somatosensory evoked potentials to median nerve stimulation in patients with diffuse neurologic disease. Neurology. 1983;33:989–993.
185. Georgesco M, Salerno A, Camu W. Somatosensory evoked potentials elicited by stimulation of lower-limb nerves in amyotrophic lateral sclerosis. Electroencephalogr Clin Neurophysiol. 1997;104:333–342.
186. Polo A, Curro-Dossi M, Fiaschi A, Zanette GP, Rizzuto N. Peripheral and segmental spinal abnormalities of median and ulnar somatosensory evoked potentials in Hirayama's disease. J Neurol Neurosurg Psychiatry. 2003;74:627–632.
187. Restuccia D, Rubino M, Valeriani M, Mirabella M, Sabatelli M, Tonali P. Cervical cord dysfunction during neck flexion in Hirayama's disease. Neurology. 2003;60:1980–1983.

188. Misra UK, Kalita J, Mishra VN, Phadke RV, Hadique A. Effect of neck flexion on F wave, somatosensory evoked potentials, and magnetic resonance imaging in Hirayama disease. J Neurol Neurosurg Psychiatry. 2006;77:695–698.

189. Graff-Radford NR, Damasio H, Yamada T, Eslinger PJ, Damasio AR. Nonhaemorrhagic thalamic infarction: clinical, neuropsychological and electrophysiological findings in four anatomical groups defined by computerized tomography. Brain. 1985;108:485–516.

190. Namerow NS. Somatosensory evoked responses in multiple sclerosis patients with varying sensory loss. Neurology. 1968;18:1197–1204.

191. Halliday AM. Evoked Potentials in Clinical Testing. Edinburgh: Churchill Livingstone, 1993.

192. Restuccia D, Di Lazzaro M, Valeriani M, et al. Neurophysiological abnormalities in adrenoleukodystrophy carriers. Evidence of different degrees of central nervous system involvement. Brain. 1997;120:1139–1148.

193. Robinson LR, Micklesen PJ, Tirschwell DL, Lew HL. Predictive value of somatosensory evoked potentials for awakening from coma. Crit Care Med. 2003;31:960–967.

194. Fischer C, Luaute J, Nemoz C, Morlet D, Kirkorian G, Mauguière F. Improved prediction of awakening or nonawakening from severe anoxic coma using tree-based classification analysis. Crit Care Med. 2006;34:1520–1524.

195. Rumpl E, Prugger M, Gerstenbrand F, Hackl JM, Pallua A. Central somatosensory conduction time and short-latency somatosensory evoked potentials in posttraumatic coma. Electroencephalogr Clin Neurophysiol. 1983;56:583–596.

196. Logi F, Fischer C, Murri L, Mauguière F. The prognostic value of evoked responses from primary somatosensory and auditory cortex in comatose patients. Clin Neurophysiol. 2003;114:1615–1627.

197. Hume AL, Cant BR, Shaw NA. Central somatosensory conduction time in comatose patients. Ann Neurol. 1979;5:379–384.

198. Greenberg RP, Newlon PG, Becker DP. The somatosensory evoked potentials in patients with severe head injury: outcome prediction and monitoring of brain function. Ann New York Acad Sci. 1982;388:683–688.

199. Pallis C. Brainstem death. In Braakman RD, ed. Handbook of Clinical Neurology, vol. 13, Head Injury. Amsterdam: Elsevier, 1990:441–496.

200. Wagner W. Scalp, earlobe and nasopharyngeal recordings of the median nerve somatosensory evoked P14 potential in coma and brain death. Brain. 1996;119:1507–1521.

201. Shibasaki H, Kuroiwa Y. Electroencephalographic correlates of myoclonus. Electroencephalogr Clin Neurophysiol. 1975;39:455–463.

202. Shibasaki H, Yamashita Y, Neshige R, Tobimatsu S, Fukui R. Pathogenesis of giant somatosensory evoked potentials in progressive myoclonic epilepsy. Brain. 1985;108:225–240.

203. Shibasaki H, Nakamura M, Nishida S, Kakigi R, Ikeda A. Waveform decomposition of "giant SEP" and its computer model for scalp topography. Electroencephalogr Clin Neurophysiol. 1990;77:286–294.

204. Valeriani M, Restuccia D, Di Lazzaro V, Le Pera D, Tonali P. The pathophysiology of giant SEPs in cortical myoclonus: a scalp topography and dipolar source modelling study. Electroencephalogr Clin Neurophysiol. 1997;104:122–131.

205. Mima T, Terada K, Ikeda H, et al. Afferent myoclonus studied by proprioception-related SEPs. Electroencephalogr Clin Neurophysiol.1997;104:51–59.

206. Hallett M, Chadwick D, Adam J, Marsden CD. Reticular reflex myoclonus; a physiological type of human post-hypoxic myoclonus. J Neurol Neurosurg Psychiatry. 1977;40:253–264.

207. De Marco P, Tassinari CA. Extreme somatosensory evoked potential (ESEP): an EEG sign forecasting a possible occurrence of seizures in children. Epilepsia. 1981;22:569–575.

208. Manganotti P, Miniussi C, Santorum E, et al. Scalp topography and source analysis of interictal spontaneous spikes and evoked spikes by digital stimulation in benign rolandic epilepsy. Electroencephalogr Clin Neurophysiol. 1998;107:18–26.

209. Rossini PM, Babiloni F, Bernardi G, et al. Abnormalities of short-latency somatosensory evoked potentials in parkinsonian patients. Electroencephalogr Clin Neurophysiol. 1989;74:277–289.

210. Babiloni F, Babiloni C, Cecchi L, Onorati P, Salinari S, Urbano A. Statistical analysis of topographic maps of short-latency somatosensory evoked potentials in normal and parkinsonian subjects. IEEE Trans Biomed Eng. 1994;41:617–624.

211. Rossini PM, Paradiso C, Zarola F, et al. Brain excitability and long-latency muscular arm responses: non-invasive evaluation in healthy and parkinsonian subjects. Electroencephalogr Clin Neurophysiol. 1991;81:454–465.

212. Cheron G, Piette T, Thiriaux A, Jacquy J, Godaux E. Somatosensory evoked potentials at rest and during movement in Parkinson's disease: evidence for a specific apomorphine effect on the frontal N30 wave. Electroencephalogr Clin Neurophysiol. 1994;92:491–501.

213. Onofrj M, Fulgente T, Malatesta G, et al. The abnormality of N30 somatosensory evoked potential in idiopathic Parkinson's disease is unrelated to disease stage or clinical scores and insensitive to dopamine manipulations. Mov Disord. 1995;10:71–80.

214. Garcia PA, Aminoff MJ, Goodin DS. The frontal N30 component of the median-derived SEP in patients with predominantly unilateral Parkinson's disease. Neurology. 1995;45:989–992.

215. Huttunen J, Teravainen H. Pre- and post–central cortical somatosensory evoked potentials in hemiparkinsonism. Mov Disord. 1993;8:430–436.

216. Mauguière F, Broussolle E, Isnard J. Apomorphine induced relief of the akinetic-rigid syndrome and early median nerve somatosensory evoked potentials in Parkinson's disease. Electroencephalogr Clin Neurophysiol. 1993;88:243–254.

217. Abbruzzese G, Marchese R, Trompetto C. Sensory and motor evoked potentials in multiple system atrophy: a comparative study with Parkinson's disease. Mov Disord. 1997;12:315–321.

218. Rossini PM, Traversa R, Boccasena P, et al. Parkinson's disease and somatosensory evoked potentials: apomorphine-induced transient potentiation of frontal components. Neurology. 1993;43:2495–2500.

219. Pierantozzi M, Mazzone P, Bassi A, et al. The effect of deep brain stimulation on the frontal N30 component of somatosensory evoked potentials in advanced Parkinson's disease patients. Clin Neurophysiol. 1999;110:1700–1707.

220. Mochizuki H, Ugawa Y, Machii K, et al. Somatosensory evoked high-frequency oscillation in Parkinson's disease and myoclonus epilepsy. Clin Neurophysiol. 1999;110:185–191.

221. Inoue K, Hashimoto I, Nakamura S. High-frequency oscillations in human posterior tibial somatosensory evoked potentials are enhanced in patients with Parkinson's disease and multiple system atrophy. Neurosci Lett. 2001;297:89–92.

222. Gobbelé R, Thyerlei D, Kawohl W, Buchner H, Waberski TD. Evaluation of thalamo-cortical impulse propagation in the akinetic rigid type of Parkinson's disease using high-frequency (600Hz) SEP oscillations. J Clin Neurophysiol. 2008;25: 274–280.

223. Reilly JA, Hallett M, Cohen LG, Tarkka IM, Dang M. The N30 component of somatosensory evoked potentials in patients with dystonia. Electroencephalogr Clin Neurophysiol. 1992;84:243–247.

224. Kanovsky P, Streitova H, Dufek J, Rektor I. Lateralization of the P22/N30 component of somatosensory evoked potentials of the median nerve in patients with cervical dystonia. Mov Disord. 1997;12:553–560.

225. Ng K, Jones S. The "enhanced N35" somatosensory evoked potential: its associations and potential utility in the clinical evaluation of dystonia and myoclonus. J Neurol. 2007;254:46–52.

226. Tinazzi M, Frasson E, Polo A. Evidence for an abnormal cortical sensory processing in dystonia: selective enhancement of lower limb P37-N50 somatosensory evoked potential. Mov Disord. 1999;14:473–480.

227. Cimatti Z, Schwartz DP, Bourdain F, et al. Time-frequency analysis reveals decreased high-frequency oscillations in writer's cramp. Brain. 2007;130:198–205.

228. Tinazzi M, Priori A, Bertolasi L, Frasson E, Mauguière F, Fiaschi A. Abnormal central integration of a dual somatosensory input in dystonia: evidence for sensory overflow. Brain. 2000;123:42–50.

229. Frasson E, Priori A, Bertolasi L, Mauguière F, Fiaschi A, Tinazzi M. Somatosensory disinhibition in dystonia. Mov Disord. 2001;16:674–682.

230. Dolberg R, Hinkley LB, Honma S. Amplitude and timing of somatosensory cortex activity in task-specific focal hand dystonia. Clin Neurophysiol. 2011;122:2441–2445.

231. Murase N, Kaji R, Shimazu H, et al. Abnormal premovement gating of somatosensory input in writer's cramp. Brain. 2000;123:1813–1829.

232. Oepen G, Doerr M, Thoden U. Visual (VEP) and somatosensory (SSEP) evoked potentials in Huntington's chorea. Electroencephalogr Clin Neurophysiol. 1981;51:666–670.

233. Lefaucheur JP, Ménard-Lefaucheur I, Maison P, et al. Electrophysiological deterioration over time in patients with Huntington's disease. Mov Disord. 2006;21:1350–1354.

234. Yamada T, Rodnitzky RL, Kameyama S, Matsuoka H, Kimura J. Alteration of SEP topography in Huntington's patients and their relatives at risk. Electroencephalogr Clin Neurophysiol. 1991;80:251–261.

235. Beniczky S, Kéri S, Antal A, et al. Somatosensory evoked potentials correlate with genetics in Huntington's disease. Neuroreport. 2002;13: 2295–2298.

236. Julien N, Goffaux P, Arsenault P, Marchand S. Widespread pain in fibromyalgia is related to a deficit of endogenous pain inhibition. Pain. 2005;114:295–302.

237. Hoffman D. Central and peripheral pain generators in women with chronic pelvic pain: patient centered assessment and treatment. Curr Rheumatol Rev. 2015;11:146–166.

238. Treede RD, Lankers J, Frieling A, et al. Cerebral potentials evoked by painful laser stimuli in patients with syringomyelia. Brain. 1991;114:1595–1607.

239. Bromm B, Frieling A, Lankers J. Laser evoked potentials in patients with dissociated loss of pain and temperature sensibility. Electroencephalogr Clin Neurophysiol. 1991;100:342–353.

240. Kanda M, Mima T, Xu X, et al. Pain-related somatosensory evoked potentials can quantitatively evaluate hypalgesia in Wallenberg's syndrome. Acta Neurol Scand. 1996;94:131–136.

241. Garcia-Larrea L, Perchet C, Creach'h C, et al. Operculo-insular pain (parasylvian pain): a distinct central pain syndrome. Brain. 2010;133:2528–2539.

242. Ulrich A, Haefeli J, Blum J, Mink K, Curt A. Improved diagnosis of spinal cord disorders with contact heat evoked potentials. Neurology. 2013;80:1393–1399.

243. Vartiainen N, Perchet C, Magnin M, et al. Thalamic pain anatomical and physiological indices of prediction. Brain. 2016;139:708–722.

244. Valeriani M, de Tommaso M, Restuccia D, et al. Reduced habituation to experimental pain in migraine patients: a CO2 laser evoked potential study. Pain. 2003;105:57–64.

245. Schestatsky P, Valls-Solé J, Costa J, Leon J, Veciana M, Chaves ML. Skin autonomic reactivity to thermoalgesic stimuli. Clin Auton Res. 2007;17:349–355.

246. Veciana M, Valls-Solé J, Schestatsky P, et al. Abnormal sudomotor skin responses to temperature and pain stimuli in syringomyelia. J Neurol. 2007;254: 638–645.

247. Schoenen J, Ambrosini A, Sandor PS, Maertens de Noordhout A. Evoked potentials and transcranial magnetic stimulation in migraine: Published data and viewpoint on their pathophysiologic significance. Clin Neurophysiol. 2003;114:955–972.

248. Demarquay G, Mauguière F. Central nervous system underpinnings of sensory hypersensitivity in migraine: Insights from neuroimaging and electrophysiological studies. Headache. 2015 Sep 9 [Epub ahead of print].

249. Coppola G, Vandenheede M, Di Clemente L, et al. Somatosensory evoked high-frequency oscil ations reflecting thalamo-cortical activity are decreased in migraine patients between attacks. Brain. 2005;128:98–103.

250. Lang E, Kaltenhäuser M, Neundörfer B, Seider S. Hyperexcitability of the primary somatosensory cortex in migraine: a magnetoencephalographic study. Brain. 2004;127:2459–2469.

251. Restuccia D, Vollono C, Virdis D, et al. Patterns of habituation and clinical fluctuations in migraine. Cephalalgia. 2014;34:201–210.

252. Woolf C. Central sensitization: Implications for the diagnosis and treatment of pain. Pain. 2011;152: S2–S15.

253. Garcia-Larrea L, Convers P, Magnin M, et al. Laser-evoked potential abnormalities in central pain patients: the influence of spontaneous and provoked pain. Brain. 2002;125:2776–2781.

254. Lorenz J, Grasedyck K, Bromm B. Middle and long latency somatosensory evoked potentials after painful laser stimulation in patients with fibromyalgia syndrome. Electroencephalogr Clin Neurophysiol. 1996;100:165–168.

255. Truini A, Gerardi MC, Di Stefano G, et al. Hyperexcitability in pain matrices in patients with fibromyalgia. Clin Exp Rheumatol. 2015;33:S68–72.

256. de Tommaso M, Nolano M, Iannone F, et al. Update on laser-evoked potential findings in fibromyalgia patients in light of clinical and skin biopsy features. J Neurol. 2014;261:461–472.

257. Üçeyler N, Zeller D, Kahn AK, et al. Small fibre pathology in patients with fibromyalgia syndrome. Brain. 2013;136:1857–1867.

258. Lorenz J, Kunze K, Bromm B. Differentiation of conversive sensory loss and malingering by P300 in a modified oddball task. Neuroreport. 1998;9:187–191.

259. Harvey SB, Stanton BR, David AS. Conversion disorder: towards a neurobiological understanding. Neuropsychiatr Dis Treat. 2006;2:13–220.

PART VII | NEW FRONTIERS IN CLINICAL NEUROPHYSIOLOGY/EEG

44 | EEG ANALYSIS: THEORY AND PRACTICE

**FABRICE WENDLING, ENG, PHD, MARCO CONGEDO, PHD
AND FERNANDO H. LOPES DA SILVA, MD, PHD**

ABSTRACT: This chapter addresses the analysis and quantification of electroencephalographic (EEG) and magnetoencephalographic (MEG) signals. Topics include characteristics of these signals and practical issues such as sampling, filtering, and artifact rejection. Basic concepts of analysis in time and frequency domains are presented, with attention to non-stationary signals focusing on time-frequency signal decomposition, analytic signal and Hilbert transform, wavelet transform, matching pursuit, blind source separation and independent component analysis, canonical correlation analysis, and empirical model decomposition. The behavior of these methods in denoising EEG signals is illustrated. Concepts of functional and effective connectivity are developed with emphasis on methods to estimate causality and phase and time delays using linear and nonlinear methods. Attention is given to Granger causality and methods inspired by this concept. A concrete example is provided to show how information processing methods can be combined in the detection and classification of transient events in EEG/MEG signals.

KEYWORDS: EEG, MEG, electroencephalography, magnetoencephalographic, filtering, artifact rejection, denoising, Granger causality

PRINCIPAL REFERENCES

1. Blinowska KJ, Kaminski M, Brzezicka A, Kaminski J. Application of directed transfer function and network formalism for the assessment of functional connectivity in working memory task. Philos Trans A Math Phys Eng Sci. 2013;371(1997):20110614.
2. Colombet B, Woodman M, Badier JM, Benar CG. AnyWave: a cross-platform and modular software for visualizing and processing electrophysiological signals. J Neurosci Meth. 2015;242:118–126.
3. Delorme A, Makeig S. EEGLAB: an open source toolbox for analysis of single-trial EEG dynamics including independent component analysis. J Neurosci Meth. 2004;134(1):9–21.
4. Durka P, Ircha D, Blinowska K. Stochastic time-frequency dictionaries for matching pursuit. IEEE Trans Signal Proc. 2001;49(3):507–510.
5. Kalitzin SN, Parra J, Velis DN, Lopes da Silva FH. Quantification of unidirectional nonlinear associations between multidimensional signals. IEEE Trans Biomed Eng. 2007;54(3):454–461.
6. Lachaux JP, Rodriguez E, Martinerie J, Varela FJ. Measuring phase synchrony in brain signals. Hum Brain Map. 1999;8(4):194–208.
7. Pascual-Marqui RD, Biscay RJ, Bosch-Bayard J, et al. Assessing direct paths of intracortical causal information flow of oscillatory activity with the isolated effective coherence (iCoh). Front Human Neurosci. 2014;8:448.
8. Wendling F, Bartolomei F, Bellanger JJ, Chauvel P. Interpretation of interdependencies in epileptic signals using a macroscopic physiological model of the EEG. Clin Neurophysiol. 2001;112(7):1201–1218.
9. Friston K, Moran R, Seth AK. Analysing connectivity with Granger causality and dynamic causal modelling. Curr Opin Neurobiol. 2013;23(2):172–178.
10. Oostenveld R, Fries P, Maris E, Schoffelen JM. FieldTrip: Open source software for advanced analysis of MEG, EEG, and invasive electrophysiological data. Comput Intell Neurosci. 2011;2011:156869.
11. Blinowska K, Zygierewicz J. Practical Biomedical Signal Analysis Using MATLAB. New York: CRC Press, 2012.

1. INTRODUCTION

1.1. The Need to Quantify

Analysis of electroencephalographic (EEG) signals always involves quantification; the determination of the precise value of the dominant frequency, or the estimation of the degree of similarity between two signals recorded from symmetric derivations at the same time, are examples of questions that imply quantification of EEG signals. Without quantification, EEG appraisal remains subjective and can hardly lead to logical systematization.

The primary aim of EEG analysis is to support EEG-ers' evaluations with objective data in numerical or graphic form. EEG analysis, however, can go further, actually extending EEG-ers' capabilities by giving them new tools with which they can perform such difficult tasks as quantitative analysis of long-duration EEG in epileptic patients, or sleep and psychopharmacologic studies.

The choice of an analytic method should be determined mainly by the goal of the application, although budget limitations must also be taken into consideration. The development of an appropriate strategy rests on such practical facts as whether analysis results must be available in real time and online or may be presented offline. In the past, the former requirement would pose considerable problems, solvable only by adopting rather simple forms of analysis; the development of new computer technology has provided a wide range of solutions. Another practical consideration is the number of derivations to be analyzed and whether the corresponding topographic relations have to be determined or the analysis of a couple of derivations is enough; the latter may suffice during anesthesia monitoring or in simple sleep monitoring. Whether the analysis of a relatively short EEG epoch is sufficient or must involve very long records (e.g., up to 24 hours) is another important factor.

In short, the method of analysis must be suited to the purpose of the analysis. In this chapter we address these kind of questions from both a theoretical and a practical viewpoint.

1.2. The Evolution of EEG Signal Processing Since the Middle of the Last Century

The need for "quantified EEG" was felt since the early days of EEG studies (for a historical discussion see (1), but it became more visible in the early 1960s with the development of

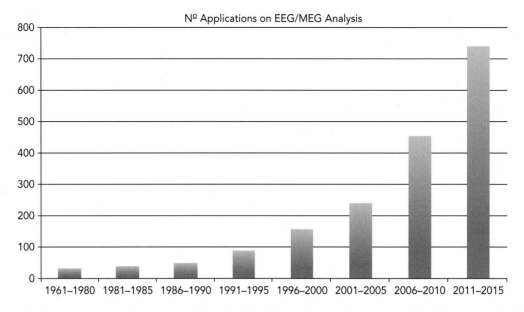

Figure 44.1. Number of publications in the past 50 years retrieved from the Web of Science (Thomson Reuters) using keyword "applications for EEG analysis."

computers. In the past half century a spectacular development of digital signal processing methods took place, due, in particular, to the growing use of digitized video-EEG monitoring systems in clinical practice. Nowadays, the panel of available methods is very wide. Proposed methods mainly depend on well-defined objectives that can be either clinical (diagnostic aid in neurological, psychiatric, or sleep disorders) or related to cognitive research (assessment of brain activity during resting state or during specific cognitive and motor tasks) (Fig. 44.1).

The growth of these applications is exponential, as can be seen in Figure 44.1, where the number of applications in the course of the last 50 years are displayed, retrieved from the Web of Science (Thomson Reuters) under the keywords "applications for EEG analysis," which cover the field, although not perfectly. The increase in the last five years is spectacular. Several software packages are being used worldwide. In Section 6.2 we mention some of the most popular ones, most of which belong to the category of open-source software.

2. GENERAL CHARACTERISTICS OF EEG SIGNALS

2.1. EEG Signal as the Realization of a Random Process

The exact characteristics of EEG signals are, in general terms, unpredictable. This means that one cannot foresee precisely the amplitude of an EEG grapho-element or the duration of an EEG wave. Therefore, it can be said that an EEG signal is a realization of a random or stochastic process. Indeed, it is possible to determine some statistical measures of EEG signals that show considerable regularity, such as an average amplitude or an average frequency. This is a general feature of random processes, which are characterized by probability distributions and their moments (e.g., mean, variance, skewness, and kurtosis) or by frequency power spectra or correlation functions. Such

a description of an EEG signal as a realization of a random process implies a mathematical, but not a biophysical, model.

It should be stressed that the neurophysiological and biophysical processes underlying EEG generation are not necessarily random in nature, but may have such a high degree of complexity that only a description in statistical terms is justified. Gasser (2) has also emphasized this point; even in the case of signals that are deterministic (e.g., sinusoids) but very complex (e.g., made of many components), a stochastic approach may be the most adequate.

2.2. Sampling: The Nyquist-Shannon Theorem

To make quantitative analysis of EEG signals, the latter must be digitized so that they can be processed by a digital computer. This means that the EEG signal must be processed in such a way that the random variable, electric potential difference as a function of time, will have only one set of discrete values at a set of discrete time instances. In technical terms, the process of analog-to-digital conversion involves sampling combined with the operation of quantizing. According to definitions commonly used, sampling is the "process of obtaining a sequence of instantaneous values of a wave at regular or intermittent intervals" and quantization is the "process in which the continuous range of amplitude values of an input signal is divided into non-overlapping sub-ranges and to each sub-range a discrete value of the output is uniquely assigned."

EEG signal sampling must be performed without changing the statistical properties of the continuous signal. Generally, one samples an EEG signal at T equidistant times t ($t = 1, \ldots, T$) where T_s denotes the sampling period. This sampling process-thus transforms the continuous signal into a set of impulses with different heights separated by intervals T_s. An important question is the choice of the sampling frequency F_s—that is, the inverse of the sampling period T_s. This choice is based on Shannon's sampling theorem that provides a condition on

F_s: no information is lost when a signal is reconstructed from its samples if the sampling frequency F_s is at least equal to two times the highest frequency F_{max} of the frequencies contained in the sampled signal spectrum:

$$F_s = \frac{1}{T_s} \geq 2F_{max}.$$

The consequence is that on an acquisition system that samples EEG signals at F_s, information is lost for all frequencies beyond $F_s/2$. This limit, in practice, is often taken as $F_s/3$.

2.3. Filtering and Artifact Rejection

2.3.1. FILTERING
Filtering refers to a process that enhances some components of interest in EEG signals or, on the contrary, it may attenuate or suppress unwanted components. See (3) for didactic and practical information about filtering methods of digital signals.

Classically, EEG reviewing systems include low-pass, high-pass, bandpass, and notch linear time-invariant filters as preprocessing methods of raw EEG. Typically, a low-pass filter with a low cutoff frequency (<0.5 Hz, for instance) will enhance delta oscillations. Technically, linear time-invariant filters may be implemented in various different ways, in either the time or the frequency domain, depending on the desired filter characteristics and the desired performance. Two classical implementations are based on (1) the convolution product (digital filters) and (2) the Fourier transform and inverse transform after alteration of the frequency components to be filtered. Note that both implementations are theoretically equivalent since the convolution product in the time domain is equivalent to a simple product in the frequency domain. Any linear filter is characterized by an impulse response that contains all information about the filter. By definition, this impulse response is the filter output to a Dirac impulse input. Once this impulse response is specified, the frequency response can be calculated. Therefore, a straightforward implementation of digital filters is performed by convolving EEG signals with an impulse response corresponding to the desired filter characteristics. In this case, the filter is referred to as a finite impulse response (FIR) filter.

Another way to build a digital filter is by recursion. Recursive filters are also based on a convolution of the input signal, but with a very long filter kernel. This is why they are referred to as infinite impulse response (IIR) filters. As only few coefficients are necessary to design an IIR filter, they execute very rapidly; they have, however, less flexibility than FIR filters. Unlike FIR filters, in which phase response is linear, IIR filters have a nonlinear phase response. This might be important as filtering is often used as a preprocessing step before more sophisticated analysis. For instance, due to the phase linearity, a FIR filter would be preferred to an IIR filter in methods aimed at measuring time delays among EEG signals. It is worth mentioning that forward-backward digital filtering has no phase distorsion. However it can only be applied off-line.

Similarly, when bandpass filters are being used to reveal specific EEG oscillations, one should not make a confusion between the "true" oscillations actually present in the EEG signals to be analyzed and the "false" oscillations induced by the filter response to sharp transients that often contaminate the raw time series (see Section 6.1.3.2 for examples of the pitfalls of bandpass filtering in the detection of fast ripples). A remarkable example of such a pitfall was put in evidence by the study by Yuval-Greenberg et al. (4), who demonstrated that spike potentials associated with microsaccades, especially in recordings where the subject scans visual images, can often contaminate EEG recordings. Due to filtering of these spiky signals, the power of the gamma frequency band (30–100 Hz) can be appreciably enhanced; this may be misinterpreted as genuine EEG gamma oscillations, which led to an open controversy (4–6).

2.3.2. ARTIFACT REJECTION
In practice, EEG signals are often contaminated by noise and by various types of artifacts with physiological (i.e., subject-related) or extra-physiological (acquisition system-related) origin. Table 44.1 lists artifacts commonly encountered during EEG recording.

Artifact removal from EEG signals is still a matter of intensive research. More particularly, the online detection and correction of both physiological and non-physiological artifacts is currently one of the great challenges of EEG research for areas such as the development of brain–computer interfaces (BCI) and for neurofeedback research. Unfortunately, there exists no unique method that can deal with all the above-listed artifacts. This is why a number of methods were proposed, each accounting for the artifact specificity as well as for technical

TABLE 44.1. List of Artifacts Frequently Encountered in EEG Recordings

SUBJECT-RELATED ARTIFACTS (PHYSIOLOGICAL)	ACQUISITION SYSTEM-RELATED ARTIFACTS (EXTRA-PHYSIOLOGICAL)	STIMULATION-RELATED ARTIFACTS (BOTH PHYSIOLOGICAL AND EXTRA-PHYSIOLOGICAL)
- Eye (saccades, movements, blinks; electro-oculogram = EOG) - Muscles (subject movements and muscular tension; electromyogram = EMG) - Heart (electrocardiogram = EKG, ECG) - Respiration (can be monitored using a resistive belt) - Tongue (glossokinetic) artifact	- Cable movements - Power-line (alternating current: 50 or 60 Hz, depending on the country) - Ground instability - Electromagnetic interferences with nearby electric/ electronic devices - Movement of other persons around the patient - Ballistocardiogram (functional magnetic resonance imaging)	Stimulation techniques like transcranial Direct Current Stimulation (tDCS) or Transcranial Magnetic Stimulation (TMS) generally induce prominent artifacts on the EEG

features like the capability of achieving (pseudo) real-time processing (here "pseudo" means that a small delay introduced by the artifact removal method is acceptable).

2.3.3. ADAPTIVE-FILTER–BASED METHODS

Generally speaking, an adaptive filter is a filter that self-adjusts its coefficients in order to adapt its performance based on the input signal. The main advantage of adaptive filtering methods is that they are generally simple enough to allow online processing. The disadvantage is that they usually require strong a priori information about the signal to be filtered. Regarding eye-related artifacts (e.g., movements, blinks. electro-oculogram [EOG]), these methods proved to be relatively efficient, given that both horizontal and vertical EOGs can be recorded simultaneously with the EEG. An example of implementation is provided in (7) and illustrated in Figure 44.2A.

This method produces an output signal, $e(n)$ in the figure (clean EEG), that is as close to the input EEG ($x(n)$ in the figure) as possible, by continuously adjusting the coefficients of two filters $h_h(m)$ and $h_v(m)$ of order M, the input of which is the EOG (signals HEOG and VEOG, respectively). The algorithm used to optimize the transfer function of both filters is a recursive least square (RLS). Authors claim that the method is fast enough (order M is small) to allow for online implementation

and that performances are excellent (see Fig. 44.2B). For a comparison of other EEG denoising methods, see Section 4.2.

2.4. EEG Signals Depend on Space; the Inverse Problem

The fact that EEG signals have different characteristics depending on the site over the head where they are recorded is essential to all EEG recordings. Therefore, in any method of EEG analysis, not only the evolution in time but also the spatial characteristics must be taken into account. This means that one should choose EEG montages carefully depending on the objectives of the analysis.

A common pitfall in EEG analysis is to interpret EEG signals as representing unequivocally the activity of brain areas lying under the scalp area where the recordings were made. Two main aspects undermine such a simplistic interpretation. The first is that EEG signals are always potential differences, and thus a given signal depends not only on the so-called active electrode but also on the position of the reference electrode. The second is that the transfer of electrical fields from the cortex to the scalp is a complex process such as electric cortical fields are attenuated and deformed by the tissues of the head. The inverse problem (i.e., the estimation of the brain sources from a given EEG scalp distribution) has no unique solution,

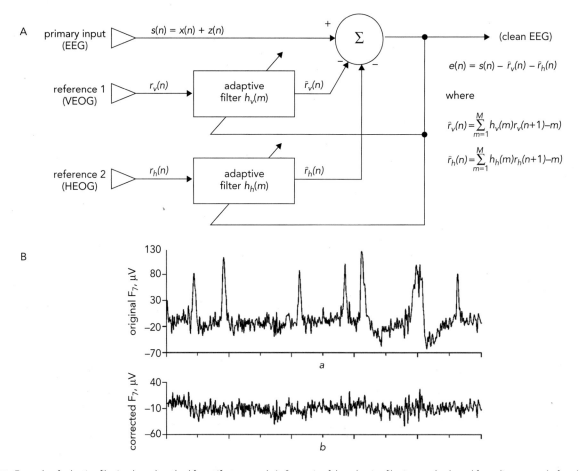

Figure 44.2. Example of adaptive filtering-based method for artifact removal. A: Synopsis of the adaptive filtering method used for online removal of ocular artifacts from EEG signals. B: Original EEG contaminated by eye movements (top) and corrected EEG after online processing (bottom). Adapted with permission from He, Wilson, and Russell (7).

as Helmholtz demonstrated in the 19th century. A solution to the inverse problem may be estimated, however, assuming a number of constraints—that is, by making a specific model of the head volume conductor based on reasonable assumptions. The situation is somewhat simpler with magnetoencephalography (MEG; see also Chapter 35) than EEG, since MEG is less affected by the inhomogeneity of the head tissues than EEG. These issues are discussed in detail in Chapter 45 and the underlying biophysics are discussed in Chapter 4.

2.5. EEG Signals and Stationarity

An important general issue in EEG analysis (which, however, receives less attention than it merits) is the concept of stationarity. Indeed. with respect to any EEG analysis, a basic precaution is whether the signal is stationary or not. Strictly speaking, the signal $x(t)$ is stationary if its statistical moments and joint moments do not depend on time. In other words, the distribution of a stationary process is not affected by a shift in time: $x(t)$ and $x(t + k)$ have the same distribution for any k.

Usually one may relax those requirements and consider the signal as weak stationary if simply the mean value and the autocorrelation do not depend on time (8). McEwen and Anderson (9) introduced the concept of wide-sense stationarity in EEG analysis; they proposed a procedure for determining whether a set of EEG signals can be considered to belong to a wide-sense stationarity process. Their procedure consisted of calculating the amplitude distributions and power spectra of sample subsets; if the latter did not differ significantly using the Kolmogorov-Smirnov statistic, then the EEG signals could be accepted as weakly stationary. From this study it was concluded that for EEG epochs (awake condition or during anesthesia) with a duration of <32 sec, the assumption of wide-sense stationarity was valid >50% of the time. On the basis of this type of empirical observation, it is generally assumed that relatively short EEG epochs (~10 sec) recorded under constant behavioral conditions are quasi-stationary.

A basis for this assumption is the classic findings of Isaksson and Wennberg (10). These authors found that given that the subject's behavioral state is kept almost constant, as in the resting state, ~90% of EEG signals displayed time-invariant properties during ~20 sec, whereas <75% remained time-invariable after 60 sec. Empirical observations indicate that EEG records obtained under equivalent behavioral conditions show highly stable characteristics. For example, Dumermuth et al. (11) showed that variations in mean peak (beta activity) of only 0.8 Hz were obtained in a series of 11 EEGs over a long period of 29 weeks.

3. STATIONARY SIGNALS

3.1. Analysis in Time Domain (Probability Functions, Autocorrelation)

3.1.1. PROBABILITY FUNCTIONS
The digitized EEG signal values $x(t)$ can be considered realizations of one stochastic variable $\underline{X}(t)$; when in an interval $0 > t > T$

there are n_a sample points in the interval $a \pm 1/2\Delta$ (where the partitioning variable Δ defines the interval width around a), n_a/N is called the relative frequency of occurrence of the value a, where N is the total number of samples available (Δ: arbitrarily defined). One can define the relative frequencies of all other values similarly. When N becomes infinitely large and Δ infinitely small, n_a/N will tend to a limit value $p(x(t) = a)$, called the probability of occurrence of $x(t)=a$. The set of values of $p(x(t))$ is called the signal probability distribution, characterized by a mean and a number of moments. Considering that the discrete random variable x can take any of a set of values from 1 to Q, the mean or average of the sample functions is given as follows (E is the symbol for expectation):

$$E\left[\underline{X}(t)\right] = \sum_{a=1}^{Q}\left[a \cdot p(x(t) = a)\right].$$

Also definable is a class of statistical functions characteristic of the random process:

$m_i = E\left[\underline{X}(t)\right]$ with $i = 1, 2, 3, \ldots$; these functions are called the ith moments of the discrete random variable $\underline{X}(t)$. The implicit assumption here and in the following discussion is that the signal is stationary—in other words, the statistical properties of the signal do not change in the interval T. Therefore, the moments are independent of time t.

The first moment $E\left[\underline{X}(t)\right]$ that we have just described is called the mean of $\underline{X}(t)$. It is often useful to consider the central moments (i.e., the moments around the mean); the second central moment is then:

$$E\left[\left(\underline{X}(t) - E[\underline{X}(t)]\right)^2\right] = m_2$$

or σ^2 or variance of $\underline{X}(t)$.

Similarly, the third central moment $E[(\underline{X}(t) - E[\underline{X}(t)])^3] = m_3$ can be defined; from this can be derived the *skewness factor* $\beta_1 = m_3/(m_2)^{3/2}$.

The fourth central moment is $E[(\underline{X}(t) - E[\underline{X}(t)])^4] = m_4$, from which can be derived the *kurtosis excess*: $\beta_2 = m_4/(m_2)^2$. In case of a symmetric amplitude we have $\beta_1 = 0$; all odd moments are equal to zero. For a Gaussian distribution the even moments have specific values (e.g., $\beta_2 = 3$); deviations from this value indicate the peakedness ($\beta_2 > 3$) or flatness ($\beta_2 < 3$) of the distribution.

3.1.2. AUTOCORRELATION FUNCTION
In general terms, successive values of a signal, such as an EEG, which result from a stochastic process, are not necessarily independent. On the contrary, it is often found that successive discrete values of an EEG signal have a certain degree of interdependence. To describe this interdependence, one may compute the signal joint probability distribution. As an example, consider the definition of the joint probability applied to a pair of values at two discrete times, $\underline{X}(t_1)$ and $\underline{X}(t_2)$; assume that one disposes of N realizations of the signal and let the number of times that at time t_1 a value v and at time t_2 a value u

are encountered be equal to n_{12}. Thus, the joint probability of $\underline{X}(t_1) = v$ and $\underline{X}(t_2) = u$ may be defined as follows:

$$p\left(\underline{X}(t_1) = v, \underline{X}(t_2) = u\right) = \lim_{x \to \infty} \frac{n_{12}}{N}$$

A complete description of the properties of the signal generated by a random process can be achieved by specifying the *joint probability density function*:

$$\rho\left(\underline{X}(t_1), \underline{X}(t_2), \ldots, \underline{X}(t_N)\right)$$

for every choice of the discrete time samples $t_1, t_2, \ldots, t_N$ and for every finite value of N. The computation of this function, however, is rather complex. A simpler alternative to this form of description is to compute a number of average characteristics of the signals, such as their covariance, correlations, and spectra. These averages do not necessarily describe stochastic signals completely, but they may be very useful for a general description of signals such as EEG.

The covariance between a random variable at two time samples $\underline{X}(t_1)$ and $\underline{X}(t_2)$ is given by the following expectation:

$$E\left[\left(\underline{X}(t_1) - E\left[\underline{X}(t_1)\right]\right)\left(\underline{X}(t_2) - E\left[\underline{X}(t_2)\right]\right)\right].$$

Estimating the covariance between any two $\underline{X}(t_1)$ and $\underline{X}(t_2)$ requires averaging over a number of realizations of an ensemble. Another way to estimate the covariance, provided that the signal is stationary and ergodic (for a discussion of these concepts see (12)), is by computing a time average of the product of the signal and a replica of itself shifted by a certain time τ_k along the time axis, for one realization of the signal. This time average is called the *autocorrelation function*:

$$\Phi_{XX}(\tau_k) = \left\langle \underline{X}(t_1) \cdot \underline{X}(t_1 + \tau_k) \right\rangle = \frac{1}{N} \sum_{i=1}^{N} x(t_1) \cdot x(t_1 + \tau_k),$$

where $\tau_K = K.\Delta t$.

3.1.3. Entropy and Information Measures

A measure that is often used to characterize statistical properties of EEG signals is the *information content* of a signal, or its *entropy*. In the case of an EEG signal, the *entropy* can be derived from the amplitude distribution. The amplitude range of the signal is subdivided in a number of quanta Q for a number of intervals $i = 1, \ldots, K$. This constitutes the process of *quantization*. Given an EEG signal constituted by N samples, the probability distribution of samples N_i falling within a given amplitude interval Q_i is:

$$p_i = N_i / N.$$

The corresponding information I is, according to Shannon's theorem, $I_i = -\log p_i$.

The entropy is defined as the expected value of the information I:

$$Entropy = -\sum p_i \log p_i.$$

It is a measure of uncertainty. The largest value of entropy corresponds to the case where all probabilities are equal. In the EEG field a number of measures related to, or derived from, the definition of entropy have been used, particularly in the analysis of the effects of anesthetics on the EEG, as a measure of signal unpredictability or complexity. We may simply state that an EEG signal with a regular pattern such as during slow-wave sleep or deep anesthesia has a low entropy value, whereas the EEG of an awake subject, usually a more complex signal, has a high entropy. Several authors (13,14) reported studies where measures derived from the concept of entropy were applied to EEG signals in order to assess the state of vigilance of subjects under anesthesia, or of those who are in a vegetative/unresponsive wakefulness state.

3.2. Analysis in the Frequency Domain (Fourier Spectrum, 1/F Power Law)

3.2.1. Fourier Analysis and Spectral Estimates

The fundamental mathematical tool for frequency analysis is the discrete Fourier transform (DFT). The DFT decomposes a finite signal in a finite sum of sinusoids with different *frequency, amplitude*, and *phase*. It can be computed efficiently by means of the celebrated fast Fourier transform (FFT) algorithm (15,16). The application of DFT to a signal in a time window results in a complex number $z(f) = a(f) + ib(f)$ for each discrete Fourier frequency f; the real numbers $a(f)$ and $b(f)$ are named the FFT coefficients, and i is the imaginary unit defined as $- i = \sqrt{-1}$. The measures of interest are the *amplitude* and *phase* at frequency f, given by the *modulus* of $z(f)$, $r(f) = |z(f)| = \sqrt{(a(f)^2 + b(f)^2)}$ and by its *argument* $\varphi(f) = Arg(z(f)) = ArcTan(b(f)/a(f))$, respectively. The amplitude and phase are real quantities and have a straightforward geometrical interpretation in the complex plane (Box 44.1); for each frequency f, $r(f)$ is the amplitude of the decomposed sinusoid and $\varphi(f)$ is its position in time (lag). The values $r(f)^2$ and $\varphi(f)$ along all discrete frequencies, appropriately averaged and smoothed, provide then the *power spectrum* and *phase spectrum*, respectively. The square root of the power spectrum provides the *amplitude spectrum*.

Note that the estimate of the spectral value at one frequency point of a power spectrum has a chi-square distribution with only two degrees of freedom. To obtain reliable estimates the number of degrees of freedom must be increased, for example up to 60, and the estimated variance reduced, either by averaging of a number of equivalent epochs or by smoothing over adjacent frequency components. Technical details can be found in many standard books, for example that by Jenkins and Watts (12) (see Box 44.1).

3.2.2. EEG Power Law (1/F) and Criticality

In the EEG field most attention is dedicated to studying rhythmic activities of different frequency bands. Notwithstanding this long tradition, more recently some researchers put in evidence the arrhythmic behavior of EEG signals, stimulated by the concept of scaling laws imported from physics. Indeed, EEG spectral power $C(f)$ estimates may obey scaling laws—in other words, power may be a function of frequency, raised to a power: $C(f) \approx f^{-\beta}$. Taking the log at both sides of the expression

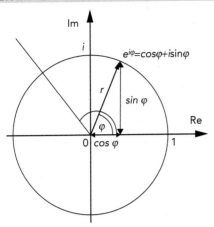

In the complex plane the abscissa is the real line and the ordinate is the imaginary line endowed with the imaginary unit i, which is defined as $I = \sqrt{-1}$. A complex number z can be represented in Cartesian coordinates as $\Re(z) + i\Im(z)$, where $\Re(z)$ is the real coordinate and $\Im(z)$ the imaginary coordinate. It can also be represented by a position vector (that is, the vector joining the origin and the point, with length r and angle φ, the angle being defined with respect to the real axis). r and φ are known as the polar coordinates of a complex number. In trigonometric form the coordinates are $r\cos\varphi$ and $ir\sin\varphi$; therefore, using Euler's formula $ei\varphi = \cos\varphi + i\sin\varphi$, we can also express any complex number as $rei\varphi$. This reduces to $ei\varphi$ if the point is on the unit circle (i.e., wherever $r = 1$), which is the case of the thick vector in the figure. In the frequency domain (see Section 3.2.1) we obtain a complex number for each frequency. In the time-frequency domain (see Section 4.1) we obtain a complex number for each time-frequency point. Regardless of the representation, the amplitude r is expressed in μV units, while the phase φ, which is a circular quantity, is usually reported in the radians interval $(-\pi, \ldots, \pi]$ or $(0, \ldots, 2\pi]$.

yields a straight line with slope β. Thus we can state that if $\beta = 1$, $C(f)$ displays $1/f$ scaling.

The estimation of the power-law exponent of a given EEG spectrum is not trivial. To realize this, He et al. (17) used the method of Yamamoto and Hughson (18), which permits separating the oscillatory frequency components from the scale-free components, the so-called coarse-graining spectral analysis. It is sometimes assumed that $1/f^\beta$ power laws are considered a footprint of self-organized criticality, in variety of phenomena, as in the distribution of earthquakes, econometric series, and resistor noise, and also in global aspects of EEG signals. Applied to neuronal systems, criticality means that neuronal networks operate between premature termination and runaway excitation (19–22). However, $1/f^\beta$ spectra are not necessarily associated with critical states (23). Bédard et al. (24) investigated whether $1/f^\beta$ power scaling can be demonstrated in local field potentials (LFPs) in vivo (in cat). They concluded that to obtain a $1/f$ scaling of LFPs, it is sufficient to take into account the biophysical fact that the extracellular

current underlying the LFPs has, on its own, a classic $1/f$ scaling property; this property confers the $1/f$ spectral characteristic to the LFPs. These conclusions do not support the hypothesis that $1/f$ scaling of EEG signals power spectra is evidence for the existence of neuronal critical states; rather, they point out the importance of taking into account straightforward biophysical properties when interpreting LFPs and EEG signals.

Furthermore, Pettersen et al. (24a), using a simplified compartmental model of the soma-dendritic membrane of a neuron, demonstrated analytically, solving the cable equation and assuming ion channel noise sources evenly distributed along the neuronal membrane, that the power spectral density of subthreshold membrane potentials follows a $1/f^\beta$ power law. Channel noise sources have been known since Verveen et al. (24b) showed that the spectrum of membrane noise follows a $1/f$ power law; the source of this noise was identified as due to the passage of potassium ions through ionic channels.

Notwithstanding the fact that the power-law property appears ubiquitous and omnipresent in many natural phenomena, and also in some EEG signals, a general or universal explanation for the underlying process is lacking. It is likely that specific natural phenomena, although displaying power-law scaling, do not share a common physical underlying mechanism, and that no universal encompassing explanation can fit all such phenomena.

3.2.3. PARAMETRIC MODELS

It is reasonable to argue that EEG signals may be analyzed by any suitable method regardless of precise knowledge of their biophysical origins. It may be asked, however, whether more appropriate methods of EEG analysis might be developed, if more precise models of the biophysical processes underlying the generation of EEG phenomena (e.g., alpha rhythms, delta waves, spike and wave complexes) were available. In the particular case of alpha-rhythm generation, there are biophysical models that can help in formulating an answer. These alpha-rhythm models have indicated that an EEG with a dominant rhythmic component in the alpha frequency range can be described by a filter network with parameters related to physiologically acceptable variables submitted to a noise input. This filter network can be analyzed in a first approximation as a linear processor. This processor can be realized in terms of a mathematical model. A special case of this model is the mixed autoregressive model as described by Zetterberg (25) and the autoregressive model used by Gersch (26). Such methods are called parametric, because in such cases the EEG signals are described in terms of a mathematical model characterized by a set of parameters.

A few examples of the application of autoregressive models in the field of EEG analysis are the following: in the detection of EEG transient nonstationary events such as epileptiform spikes and sharp waves (27), in subdividing the EEG into quasistationary segments (28), in providing EEG features to apply in BCI (29), in estimating functional connectivity by means of directed transfer function and partial directed coherence (reviewed in (30)), in estimating partial coherence between EEG signals using a multivariate autoregressive model (31), in investigating interactions between EEG signals by means of Granger causality (see Section 5.2.2.1) using vector autoregressive processes (32), and in estimating the epileptic seizure onset zone (33).

Parametric methods allow considerable EEG data reduction and have more robust statistical properties than FFT estimates. For instance, using an autoregressive model, it is possible to describe an EEG signal using a few coefficients; by following the values of these coefficients, the time-varying properties of the signal can be traced.

In general, according to this approach, the EEG signal, given as a set of samples $x(t)$, results from a filter operation on an input noise signal $e(t)$ with zero mean. The filter, corresponding to the *autoregressive moving average (ARMA) model*, is described by a linear difference equation of the following form:

$$a_0 x(t) + a_1 x(t-1) + \cdots + a_p x(t-p) = b_0 e(t) + b_1 e(t-1)$$
$$+ \cdots + b_q e(t-q),$$

where $q \leq p$. The relation between $x(t)$ and $e(t)$ is given by the sets of coefficients $a_1, \ldots, a_p$ and $b_1, \ldots, b_q$ with $a_0 = 1$. In case $b_0 = 1$ and $b_i = 0$ for $i = 1, \ldots, q$, we are left with the so-called *autoregressive (AR) model*:

$$x(t) + a_1 x(t-1) + \cdots + a_p x(t-p) = e(t)$$

The computation problem, therefore, is to estimate the parameters of the model. The optimal order p is chosen to optimize a given criterion. Schneider and Neumaier published a MATLAB package for this purpose (34).

Using Durbin's algorithm, it was found in a group of EEG recordings of epileptic patients that the minimal order of the model was, in ~70% of the cases, equal to or less than 5 (35). However, when one wishes a faithful reproduction of the power spectral density, many coefficients may be needed (36). In most applications it is sufficient to compute the AR model of the EEG signal, so this section need not consider the special problems regarding ARMA model computation.

4. NONSTATIONARY SIGNALS

4.1. Time-Frequency Signal Decomposition

In the case of nonstationary signals the concept of Fourier spectra characterized by amplitude, frequency, and phase is a rough abstraction, since these quantities vary in time. To deal with this feature the concept of time-frequency analysis has been introduced to determine the instantaneous amplitude and frequency. From the conceptual point of view, a time-frequency analysis consists of representing a signal $x(t)$ by means of a linear combination of elementary functions with a specific form as a function of both time and frequency. With DFT (see Section 3.2.1) an accurate localization of the basis functions is obtained in the frequency domain, but DFT provides no information about the times at which a given frequency component occurs. To overcome this problem, short-term Fourier transform can be implemented to obtain a time-frequency distribution of the analyzed signal. Current practice entails the use of more advanced tools such as the analytic signal obtained by the Hilbert transform and wavelets.

In practice, the result of a time-frequency analysis is usually displayed as a color-coded image (see example in Fig. 44.4C) in which the horizontal axis represents time and the vertical axes represents frequency (analytic signal) or scale (wavelets) and where the color encodes the signal energy. Algorithms for computing the Hilbert transform and wavelets are implemented, for example, in the MATLAB signal processing toolbox.

4.1.1. Analytic Signal and the Hilbert Transform

The analytic signal representation of time-series $x(t)$ has the form $z(t) = x(t) + iy(t)$, where $y(t)$ is the Hilbert transform of $x(t)$. $z(t)$ is a complex signal in the time domain with the same sampling rate as the original signal. By applying a filter bank to the input signal—that is, a series of bandpass filters centered at successive frequencies f (e.g., centered at 1Hz, 2Hz, ...)—and by computing the Hilbert transform for each filtered signal, we obtain the *analytic signal* in the time-frequency domain—that is, for all points $z(t, f) = x(t, f) + iy(t, f)$ in the time-frequency plane. Since this is a complex quantity, we can express it in polar coordinates as $z(t,f) = r(t,f)e^{i\varphi(t,f)}$, where $r(t,f)$ is the instantaneous amplitude (or envelope) and $\varphi(t,f)$ is the instantaneous phase, as a functions of time (see Box 44.1). The physical interpretation of the instantaneous amplitude and phase in case of simple sinusoidal signals is illustrated in Figure 44.3. The analytic signal is efficiently computed by means of the FFT algorithm, as described concisely by Marple (36a).

4.1.2. Wavelet Transform

Due to the inverse relationship that exists between time and frequency resolution, the short-term Fourier transform cannot provide homogenous resolution over the two domains. The wavelet transform (WT) solves this issue by introducing the convolution between signal $x(t)$ and a set of basis functions, the so-called wavelet functions $\psi_{a,b}(t)$ that have special properties: $W\psi X(a, b) = <x(t) \mid \psi_{a,b}(t)>$. $\psi_{a,b}(t)$ is the basis wavelet function, which may be dilated or contracted, and shifted in time according to two essential parameters, a that controls scaling, and b that controls translation along the time axis: $\psi_{a,b} = \mid a \mid^{-1/2} \psi(t-b/a)$. If $0 < a < 1$, $\psi_{a,b}$ is contracted along the time axis and if $a > 1$, $\psi_{a,b}$ is stretched. Intuitively, we can see that the WT provides a decomposition of $x(t)$ over "analyzing waveforms" obtained from the different values of a. Wavelet coefficients represent the similarity between the wavelet $\psi_{a,b}$ and signal $x(t)$ at different scaling and translation parameters. They tend to be maximum at those scale and time locations where the wavelet best resembles the signal.

The WT can be implemented by using either arbitrary scales and almost arbitrary wavelets (continuous wavelet transform [CWT]) or wavelet scales and translations obeying some defined mathematical rules (discrete wavelet transform [DWT]). Typically, in the DWT, the signal content is analyzed using mutually orthogonal wavelets. This transform can be seen as a reversible multiresolution analysis (or filter bank) where signal $x(t)$ is decomposed into a discrete set of orthogonal details from which the original signal can be reconstructed exactly (37).

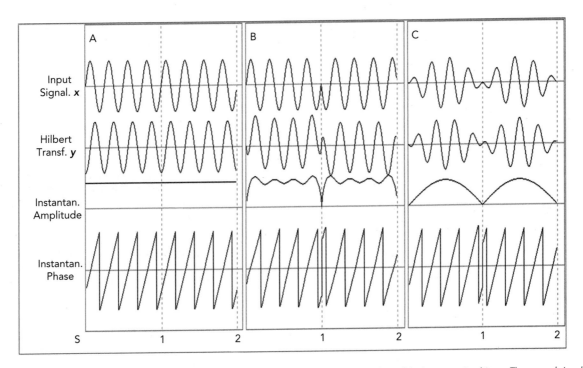

Figure 44.3. *Three 2-sec signals are shown as the top traces (x). Time is on the abscissa. The vertical scaling of the last traces is arbitrary. The second signal (y) is the Hilbert transform of the input signal x. The next two traces are the instantaneous amplitude (envelope) and instantaneous phase. A: The input signal is a sine wave at 4 Hz. The amplitude is constant in the whole epoch. The phase oscillates regularly in between its bounds at 4 Hz. B: As before, but the sine wave features a phase reversal at 1 sec. As expected, the phase features an abrupt change at 1 sec. C: The input signal is a sine wave at 4 Hz as in A, but it is multiplied by a sine wave at 0.5 Hz with the same amplitude. The result input signal is a sine wave at 4 Hz, the amplitude of which is modulated by the sine wave at 0.5 Hz. The phase features an abrupt change at 1 sec also in this case, and the change happens to be similar to the abrupt change observed in B. This simple example demonstrates that caution should be applied when interpreting the instantaneous phase.*

4.1.3. Example of Time-Frequency Analysis

This brief theoretical introduction on time-frequency analysis is complemented by a practical example, namely the problem of detection of interictal epileptic events in scalp EEG signals. The example illustrates the use of wavelets. Interictal epileptiform spikes (IESs) are "brief" events and occur in EEG signals as singularities well localized in time. In this context, time-scale approaches like wavelets offer a sound framework for automatic detection. As illustrated in Figure 44.4A, one can notice the presence of IESs on the left (see derivations C3, P3, and O1, Fig. 44.4B). The CWT applied to selected EEG signals allows interictal events to be enhanced over particular scales, as illustrated in Figure 44.4C, where a clear difference appears between selected left derivations and contralateral ones. This enhancement of the sharp component of epileptic events (white arrows) shows that CWT could serve as a first stage in an automated detection method. This approach was followed by Senhadji et al. (38), who proposed the first EEG interictal event detector using CWT. For more information, see the review in (39).

4.1.4. Matching Pursuit

To represent nonstationary EEG signals, a wide repertoire of basis functions is desirable, since these signals present a very large number of distinct features. With the aim of analyzing nonstationary signals, the method called matching pursuit (MP) was developed by Mallat and Zhang (40). This method was intensively applied to the detection of various kinds of features in EEG/MEG signals by Durka, Ircha, and Blinowska

(41) as an extension of the wavelet transform approach. The MP algorithm is iterative; at each step a basis function is found that better matches the signal. The corresponding waveform $g_{\gamma i}$ is called an element, or an "atom," taken from a dictionary of waveforms D. The latter consists of a vast collection of basic functions including Gabor functions, sinusoids, Dirac deltas (a detailed description is given in (8) and also in http://eeg.pl/mp). According to this approach the signal $x(t)$ to be analyzed is called the "null residue" (symbolically $R^0 x = x$). A succession of iterations is then performed as follows:

$$R^n x = < R^n x, g_{\gamma n} > g_{\gamma n} + R^{n+1} x,$$

$$g_{\gamma n} = \arg\max_{g_{\gamma i} \in D} |< R^n x, g_{\gamma i} >|,$$

where $\arg\max_{g_{\gamma i} \in D}$ represents the "atom $g_{\gamma i}$" that gives the highest inner product with the current residue $R^n x$. The signal $x(t)$ is then given finally by the expression:

$$x = \sum_{n=0}^{M-1} < R^n x, g_n > g_n,$$

where M represents the number of iterations. The iterative procedure is stopped as the set of waveforms obtained by the application of the MP algorithm is able to explain a given amount of the signal's variance. The corresponding results can be visualized by means of the so-called Wigner maps, an

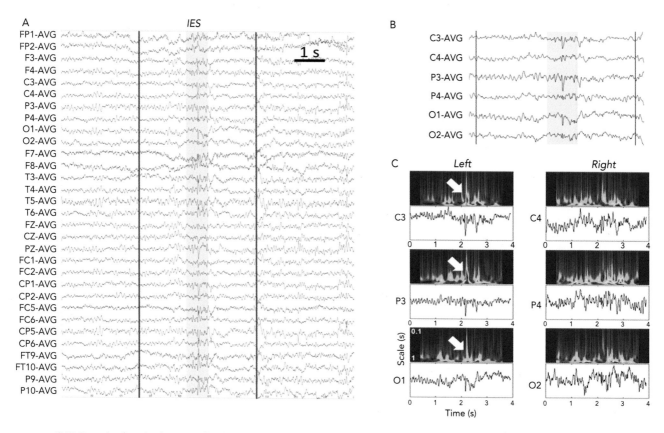

Figure 44.4. *CWT. Example of use for detection of epileptic interictal spikes (IESs) in scalp EEG.* **A:** *A 10-sec segment of EEG recorded in a patient with partial epilepsy. A relatively extended IES is denoted by the light blue rectangle.* **B:** *Selection and magnification of EEG signals (4 sec) recorded at the level of C, P, and O electrodes (left and right hemispheres). Note the presence of the IES on the left (C3, P3, and O1).* **C:** *CWT computed on selected signals. Note the enhancement of the epileptic events on the left electrodes (white arrows) over the considered range of scaling analysis, showing that this method is relevant for elaboration of an automatic detector.*

example of which is given in Figure 44.5, for the analysis of an epoch of sleep EEG where the detection of different types of sleep spindles is put in evidence. A comprehensive MP algorithm with multivariate extensions has been implemented in a software program using an interface, as described in the review by Kus et al. (42), which also illustrates the variety of applications in EEG (e.g., effects of drugs, sleep monitoring, evolution of epileptic seizures, gamma oscillations).

4.1.5. BLIND SOURCE SEPARATION AND INDEPENDENT COMPONENT ANALYSIS

Scalp EEG recording can be reasonably assumed to be a mixture of various activities generated by statistically independent sources. As far as physiological sources that can be captured by scalp electrodes are concerned, these are located not only in the brain but also in the eyes, heart, and muscles. Regarding the source–electrode relationship, two assumptions can be made: (1) the summation of potentials arising from the different parts of the brain and the body is linear at the electrodes (superposition principle) and (2) diffusion delays from the sources to the electrodes are negligible (instantaneous diffusion due to volume conduction).

Typically we face a situation where a tool like blind source separation (BSS) can be favorably applied in order to separate by linear decomposition the various contributions of sources (EEG, EMG-EOG, ECG) to the mixed signal collected at the level of scalp electrodes. The term "blind"

refers to the fact that the separation relies only on statistical assumptions on the source process, whereas no information or hypothesis is required about the biophysical or physiological aspects of the sources and volume conductor. The superposition principle and instantaneous diffusion allows us to relate linearly the source process $s(t)$ to the sensor measurement $x(t)$, such as

$$x(t) = As(t) + e(t)$$

where A is named the *mixing matrix* and $e(t)$ is an error ("noise") term. The problem to be solved is to determine both A and $s(t)$, knowing only $x(t)$ (42a).

A popular member of the BSS family is independent component analysis (ICA). In the case of ICA, the only assumption is that the sources are statistically independent. As a consequence, at most one of them may be Gaussian, which is the main limitation of this method. The application of ICA-based methods in the EEG field has been extensively developed over the past decade. Readers may refer to James and Hesse (43) for a review on ICA applied to biosignals. As illustrated in Figure 44.6, the measured observations are multiplied by the pseudo-inverse (Moore-Penrose matrix inverse) of the estimated mixing matrix, namely the "un-mixing" matrix B, in order to identify the source processes as

$$\hat{s}(t) = Bx(t).$$

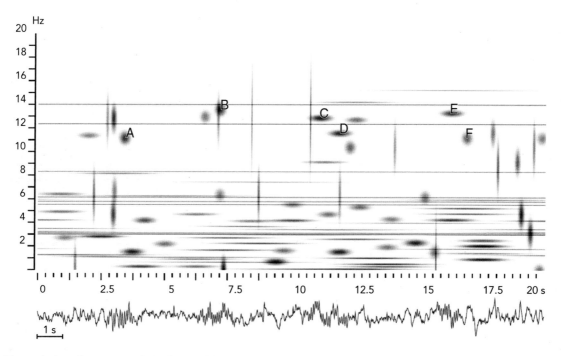

Figure 44.5. Wigner plot (time-frequency energy distribution) of the analysis of an EEG epoch of 20 sec during light sleep using an MP algorithm. The main objective of the analysis was to detect and characterize sleep spindles automatically and to compare the results with the evaluation of experts by visual inspection. The sleep spindles automatically detected are indicated by the letters A to F. Spindles A, B, C, D, and E were also detected by the experts as single spindles; F, however, was not. Adapted with permission from Durka PJ. From wavelets to adaptive approximations: time-frequency parametrization of EEG. BioMedical Engineering OnLine. 2003;2:1. DOI: 10.1186/1475-925X-2-1 (Fig. 9).

For instance, EOG and EMG components may be removed, zeroing the corresponding components of $\check{s}(t)$ to reconstruct the signal without those artifacts. A member of the BSS family particularly adapted to EEG data releases the assumption of independence and non-Gaussianity; instead, in this approach it is assumed that the sources are uncorrelated (hence it does not matter if they are Gaussian or not) and that they have a unique power spectrum or unique pattern of energy changes over time (43a). A comparison of the performance of different algorithms (JADE, CoM2, Infomax, SOBI, and FastICA) proposed to solve the BSS problem can be found in Delorme et al. (44).

4.1.6. CANONICAL CORRELATION ANALYSIS

The canonical correlation analysis (CCA) method originally proposed by Hotelling (45) seeks a linear transformation of

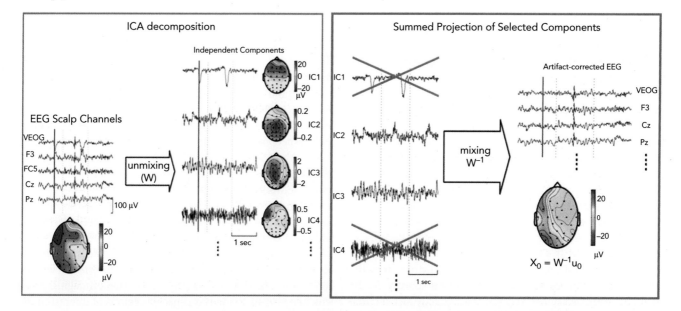

Figure 44.6. Basic principles of ICA methods applied to removal of artifacts from scalp EEG signals. Adapted from Jung et al. (http://sccn.ucsd.edu/~jung/artifact.html).

two sets of variables maximizing their correlation. CCA can be effectively used to improve the signal-to-noise ratio of EEG events, namely with respect to event-related potentials, by constructing spatial filters that achieve a very good classification accuracy. A systematic comparison with other methods is presented in Spueler et al. (46).

4.1.7. EMPIRICAL MODE DECOMPOSITION

Originally proposed by Huang et al. (47), empirical mode decomposition (EMD) aims at sequentially decomposing a given signal into a sum of amplitude- and frequency-modulated zero-mean oscillatory signals called intrinsic mode functions, plus a non-zero mean low-degree polynomial reminder. Thus EMD is an iterative algorithm by means of which the highest-frequency component is removed from the data at each iteration until only a very slow trend remains. This method of decomposition yields components for which instantaneous phase may be identified, and thus it provides a convenient way to assess phase synchrony or phase locking between EEG signals, and is particularly robust in cases of nonstationary signals. Sweeney-Reed and Nasato (48) present a comprehensive comparative analysis of this approach in comparison with other methods (Fourier analysis, bandpass filtering, wavelet analysis) in order to estimate synchrony measures of EEG signals.

4.2. EEG Denoising: An Illustrative Example

The four approaches described above (ICA, CCA, EMD, DWT) were evaluated in a simulation context where artifactual EMG activity (s_{ART}) contaminates EEG signals displaying normal background activity (s_{BCG}) and where epileptiform events (s_{AOI}) can randomly occur (49). The behavior of the four approaches was evaluated on simulated signals generated using a physiologically based mean field model (50) wherein the sources were represented as a dipole layer distributed over the cortical surface. In this mean field model (see also Chapter 3), adjustable parameters control the generation of either epileptiform (epileptic spikes) or background activity. A realistic head model representing the brain, the skull, and the scalp was used to generate EEG signals observed at surface electrodes (51). Regarding muscle artifacts, real segments exhibiting prominent EMG activity (caused by jaw clenching) were extracted from 32-channel EEG recordings. This model offers two advantages. First, the sources of cortical (s_{AOI}) and muscle (s_{ART}) activity, along with corresponding time series, are completely determined. Second, the signal-to-noise ratio can be adjusted.

Results are reported in Figure 44.7. The activity to be recovered (simulated EEG with epileptic spikes) is shown on the left. A signal mixture results from contaminating this activity with real muscular artifacts for two different values of SNR (top: −25 dB, bottom: −15 dB). Finally, four denoising methods based on ICA, CCA, EMD, and DWT are used to extract from the mixture the signals generated by the cortical sources. In the ideal case, extracted signals (right) should exactly match initial ones (left). As depicted in this figure, the CCA and Contrast Maximization 2 algorithm (CoM2) for ICA methods offer good

to quasi-optimal performance even at low signal-to-noise levels, while the performances of DWT and 2T-EMD to a lesser extent are affected by the contamination with muscle artifact.

This simple example illustrates that advanced signal processing techniques based on source separation can recover signals of interest when the source signal statistical independence assumption is met. Although in the four studied cases EEG signals could be extracted from the mixture, this example shows that final results may strongly depend on the method used to implement the denoising technique.

Finally, a conclusion of the study was that other criteria may also be considered in the performance comparison, such as numerical complexity (CCA, DWT preferred) or configuration of epileptic sources (2T-EMD and CoM2 preferred in the multifocal case).

5. ASSESSING FUNCTIONAL AND EFFECTIVE CONNECTIVITY WITH EEG/MEG

In the assessment of brain functions using EEG or MEG signals, in general an important aspect is the determination of the statistical relationships between different EEG/MEG signals. Multivariate analytic methods provide the basic tools to estimate functional relationships of brain signals. It should be stressed that *functional connectivity* measures address statistical dependencies between brain signals that are *instantaneous or undirected,* as pointed out by Friston et al. (52). The distinction made by these authors between *functional connectivity* and *effective connectivity* is useful to clarify the different dimensions of the relationships between brain systems. In the next section we deal with approaches dedicated to assess *effective connectivity*—that is, the *directed or causal* influence of one system upon another one. The basic concepts on which statistical functional analysis are based can be found in several comprehensive textbooks and reviews (53).

5.1. Linear and Nonlinear Analytic Measures

Cross-power and phase spectra and the derived coherence function (Box 44.2) have been used in a wide variety of research and clinical investigations of EEG/MEG signals for decades. In the case of scalp derivations, there are a number of hurdles that make the interpretation of these functions with respect to functional connectivity difficult or ambiguous, namely the reference electrode (this is not the case for MEG), the volume conductor effect, and noise of different sources, mainly EMG and eye movements. Therefore, whenever computing indices of functional connectivity, it is recommended to use EEG bipolar derivations with closely spaced electrodes, without a common electrode, and it is even preferable to use Laplacian derivations or to compute these indices at the level of brain sources. In Chapter 45 methods to remove volume conductor effects by solving the EEG source imaging problem, allowing us to focus on specific regions of interest in the brain, are further presented and discussed. The estimation of cross-correlation and coherence functions can be considered

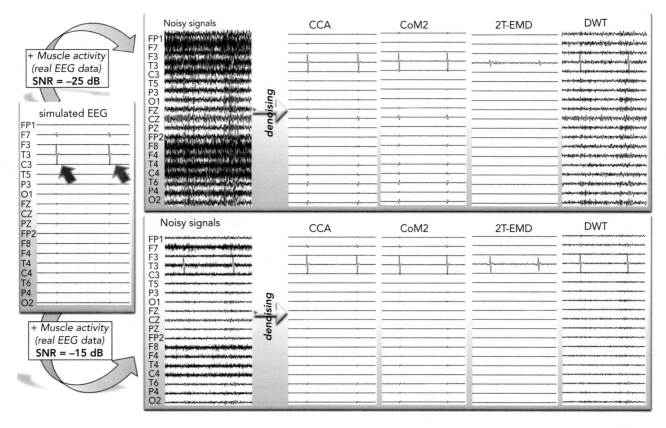

Figure 44.7. Performance of EEG denoising techniques evaluated on simulated data. Left: Example of the noise-free simulation of EEG data with interictal spikes (blue arrows). These EEG signals were obtained by solving the EEG forward problem in a realistic head model in which epileptic spikes arise from activation of a single patch (5 cm²) located in the superior temporal gyrus. Resulting spikes at scalp EEG level culminated at electrode T3 (facing the cortical patch). Right, top: Simulated signals contaminated with real muscle activity (signal-to-noise ratio −25 dB) are displayed along with the result of denoising using, respectively, the CCA, CoM2, 2T-EMD, and DWT algorithms. Right, bottom: The same noise-free simulation is now displayed after the injection of a lower amount of real muscle activity (signal-to-noise ratio −15 dB). The result of denoising for these data is also illustrated. Note that the original EEG signals could be extracted from the mixture in the four studied cases, but CCA and CoM2 methods offer the best results (see text). Adapted with permission from Safieddine et al. (49).

the forerunner of modern recent analytic tools developed to realize EEG *functional connectivity analysis.* A variety of analytic approaches are being applied in this field. The ultimate purpose of these tools is to estimate functional relationships, or more specifically the causality, among neural activities recorded from different brain areas. We cannot describe here the basic mathematical concepts underlying all these analytic methods. It is preferable to make a review of the most used methods in a way that may satisfy the perspective of the potential clinical neurophysiologist user, who is mainly interested in understanding the relative value of the different methods available but may be overwhelmed by the plethora of sophisticated theoretical concepts, which very often leave the user wondering which method to choose for a particular practical application.

Comprehensive critical assessments of the advantages and disadvantages of the most commonly used analytic methods have been published, and these can help the user to better understand the issues at stake. A difficulty in assessing the value of different methods is that the descriptions published are usually based on a particular set of data from a specific environment, very often from the author's own laboratories, and this precludes an unbiased comparison of specific methods. Indeed, several studies do not include a comparison with a general standardized dataset.

In the scope of this discussion we will distinguish three studies in which straightforward comparisons of different methods were carried out. The first study, by Quian Quiroga et al. (54), applied various measures of synchronicity to rat EEG (nonlinear interdependencies, phase synchronization, mutual information, cross-correlation, and coherence function) and concluded that all are valuable measures. The second study, by David et al. (55), used a neural mass model to generate different kinds of simulated EEG signals and applied several measures of synchronicity (generalized synchronization, phase synchronization, mutual information) to the same set of simulated signals. An important conclusion that we may derive from these two qualitative comparative studies is that none of the methods tested is perfect, and that it is recommendable to apply a battery of tests that are sensitive to different aspects of synchronization, depending on whether the interaction involves broadband frequency range or is restricted to a narrow band, and whether the nature of the interaction is linear or nonlinear.

A third study, by Wendling et al. (56), used a quantitative approach, also model-based, as illustrated in Figure 44.8. The

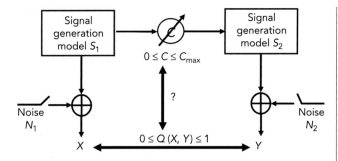

Figure 44.8. Model constructed to simulate EEG signals S_1 and S_2, with unidirectional coupling, the strength of which is tuned using parameter C, which varies from 0 to a maximum; Q is the estimated coupling value obtained by applying a given analytic method to the signals X and Y, obtained from S_1 and S_2 after the addition of noise sources N_1 and N_2. Adapted with permission from Wendling et al. (56).

methods analyzed in this study and the corresponding basic concepts are presented here in abridged form:

1. Regression methods: linear (Pearson correlation R^2, coherence function) and nonlinear (h^2)

2. Phase synchronization: Hilbert phase entropy; Hilbert mean phase coherence; wavelet phase entropy; wavelet mean phase coherence

3. Generalized synchronization: similarity indices, synchronization likelihood.

These researchers quantified and statistically evaluated the results obtained using different methods on the same data. For simplicity we focus here only on major findings:

1. With respect to broadband background simulated EEG signals, regression methods (linear and nonlinear) exhibited better sensitivity than coherence and phase synchrony methods, which may be interpreted as indicating that interdependence between signals is not entirely determined by a phase relationship.

2. Regarding narrow-band signals sharing a phase relationship, phase synchronization methods performed better, but R^2 and h^2 regression methods also yielded correct results. However, this was not the case for coherence functions and generalized synchronization methods.

3. In the case of simulated EEG signals with spikes, most methods, except the coherence function and wavelet entropy, could detect the increase of the coupling parameter in the model, but R^2, Hilbert entropy, and wavelet mean phase coherence displayed smaller variance of the estimates of the coupling factor.

A general conclusion of this comparative study is that none of the tested methods can be considered ideal. Further, the authors recommended (1) applying regression methods, linear and nonlinear, before using other ones, and (2) applying different methods to the same data to compare results, since different methods have different sensitivity to distinct properties of the signals.

The concept of *functional connectivity* and the methods to measure phase synchronization imply relationships between EEG signals that are instantaneous and undirected. The question is which mechanism can account for synchronization of phase, assuming that the latter is constant within a given frequency band. A trivial case is when two EEG signals have a 180-degree phase shift, since this occurs if the two signals are recorded from two opposite sides of the same dipolar source. This is what happens with signals recorded from different cortical layers, where the signal source has a dipolar configuration between deep and superficial layers, as has been shown for the alpha rhythm (see Chapter 2). Depending on the relative orientation of the dipolar source and the position of the recording electrodes, values of phase different from 180 degrees may be obtained. But how can an instantaneous phase around 0 degrees arise?

Experimentally, a case of global instantaneous synchronization, or "synchronization without substantial time lag," was reported by Roelfsema et al. (57). In this case signals from different cortical areas were recorded in cats, as the animals focused their attention on a prominent visual stimulus. This was interpreted as possibly due to the influence of a third system, an attention-related process, probably mediated by nonspecific thalamocortical projections (58). The model study of Sompolinsky et al. (59) gives an alternative explanation for this phenomenon. These authors demonstrated that synchronized states of neuronal populations with zero phase shifts are stable if the time delay τ_d (subscript "d" stands for delay) associated with neural propagation between two oscillating neuronal clusters obeys the relation: $0 < \tau_d < \pi/2\omega$ where ω is the angular frequency. In the case that the neuronal clusters oscillate at the gamma frequency of 40 Hz, as in the experimental case of (57), this means that instantaneous synchronization is not disrupted for values of time delay $\tau_d < 6$ msec, which corresponds to a propagation delay of neural activity between clusters separated by ~5 mm, which may be realistic. This means that it is not necessary to invoke a third system to account for instantaneous phase synchronization as found in experimental data where oscillations in the gamma frequency range are dominant, although it does not exclude the possibility of a third modulating system influencing the instantaneous synchronization of coupled systems.

In the next section we consider more specifically the issue of causality that goes beyond simple synchronization.

5.2. Assessing "Effective Connectivity": Estimates of Causality

The discussion about functional connectivity is dominated by the concept of instantaneous phase synchronization. The relationship between two neurophysiological signals, however, goes beyond the notion of phase locking. This leads to the question of how to assess *effective connectivity*, as introduced above. We consider, first, methods based on the concepts of phase and time delay, and next methods based on the Granger causality concept, which was developed initially in the realm of the analysis of econometric time series (60).

5.2.1. METHODS BASED ON THE CONCEPTS OF PHASE AND TIME DELAY

5.2.1.1. LINEAR METHODS

As stated above, we have to take into consideration the fact that neural activity reflected in a local field potential and in an EEG signal in a certain brain area A most often is transmitted to another brain site B and thus may be recorded at the latter site after a certain delay time Δt (in seconds). This delay is naturally caused by the finite velocity of the signal along the axons and the time needed for synaptic transmission. In such a simple case the activity at the first site, A, *causes* the activity at the second site, B. If these activities have oscillatory components there will be a phase difference $\Delta\varphi_d$ (subscript "d" for difference) between the two signals. In the simplest case $\Delta\varphi_d$ is linearly related with frequency, within a given range Δf (in Hz); in this case, the following relationship is valid:

$$\Delta t = \Delta\varphi_d / 360°.\Delta f$$

This means that from the slope of the relation between phase shift $\Delta\varphi_d$ and frequency Δf, a time delay Δt can be deduced indicating the direction and the time involved in the propagation of the neural activity. It should be emphasized, however, that phase is determined modulo 2π, which may lead to ambiguous interpretations concerning the direction of propagation. Indeed, knowledge of the neurophysiological system responsible for the generation of the signals can help in determining the direction of causality. Therefore, time delays may be interpreted in terms of propagation delays unambiguously only if Δt is estimated from the linear slope of a linear phase-frequency relation over a stable coherent frequency range. If the coherence between the two signals is significant only over a very narrow frequency band (e.g., around a peak), it may be impossible to define a best line fit to the phase function. In such a case, the result may be impossible to interpret definitively in terms of time delay. Further, instead of using the simple phase function, it may be recommended to use a weighted phase function, as proposed by (61), in the type of problems just discussed.

However, this model may be too simple. The transmission of the neural activity can involve a transformation of the signal being transmitted due to the frequency characteristics of the system involved, most likely due to some form of filtering. For example, if the neural activity, consisting of a time series of action potentials generated at site A, arrives at synapses in the dendrites of the receiving neuronal population at site B, the cable properties of the dendrites exert a filtering effect, such that high-frequency components are more attenuated with distance along the dendrite-soma membrane than lower frequencies (62). This means that, although the signal at site B follows that of site A, the frequency content of the former can differ from that of the latter. Moreover, in analyzing neurophysiological signals, one encounters quite often nonlinear relations, for which methods based on linear assumptions, such as coherence and cross-correlation, are not appropriate.

5.2.1.2. NONLINEAR METHODS

To estimate the degree of association between two signals and the corresponding time delay in a more general way, the nonlinear correlation coefficient h^2 as a function of time shift between two signals $x(t)$ and $y(t)$ (see Box 44.2) has been introduced by Pijn et al. (63). The time delay Δt is given by the time shift for which h^2 reaches the maximal value.

This method has also been shown to give reliable measures for the degree and direction of functional coupling between intracerebral EEG signals both in an animal model of epilepsy (64) and in human epileptic patients (65,66). Note that the value of h^2 is asymmetric ($h^2_{xy} \neq h^2_{yx}$). The asymmetry information and the time-delay information were combined in a single quantity named "direction index" (67) for a given relation between signals $x(t)$ and $y(t)$:

$$D = \frac{1}{2}\left[sign(\Delta h^2) + sign(\Delta t) \right]$$

where $sign(\Delta h^2)$ is the sign of the difference between the values of h^2_{xy} and h^2_{yx} and $sign(\Delta t)$ is the sign of the estimated delay; D = +1 (respectively −1) denotes that Y (respectively X) is dependent on, and delayed with respect to, X (respectively Y). An algorithm for the estimation of h^2 was incorporated in a modular software program for processing neurophysiological signals (68).

The computation of h^2 can give indications about causality with respect to whether signal x is caused by signal y, or vice versa, or whether it is impossible to decide on the basis of the available signals. It can also be related to causality as the delayed activity is more likely *caused by* rather than *causing* the preceding activity. Thus, bidirectional associations reflect the invertibility of the nonlinear mapping while highly asymmetric, unidirectional associations indicate noninvertible mapping. This implies that high asymmetric association values may indicate essentially nonlinearity. Kalitzin et al. (69) presented a general definition of the nonlinear association index h^2, demonstrating rigorously that the index measures the best dynamical range of any nonlinear map between signals.

A further refinement of the nonlinear association analysis is the so-called partialization of the association measure between two signals. Indeed, in cases where a nonlinear association index h^2 between two signals may be caused by a third one, acting as a common source, the influence of the third one can be removed and the residual signals' correlations may be computed to determine whether the association between them depends on the third signal or not (69).

An example of results obtained with nonlinear regression analysis in temporal lobe epilepsy is illustrated in Figure 44.9. Analyzed EEG signals were recorded from intracerebral electrodes (SEEG) positioned in nine distinct brain structures (see Fig. 44.9A) during the transition from pre-ictal to seizure activity. h^2 values were computed pairwise and averaged over six periods of 10 sec each (see Fig. 44.9B). These values were then represented in two complementary manners: matrices of color-coded nonlinear correlation values (see Fig. 44.9C) and undirected graphs (see Fig. 44.9D) in which the nodes denote the explored brain structures and in which the links are proportional to h^2 values (the greater the h^2 value, the thicker the line). As depicted, remarkable changes in h^2 values (interpreted as functional couplings among the local SEEG signals)

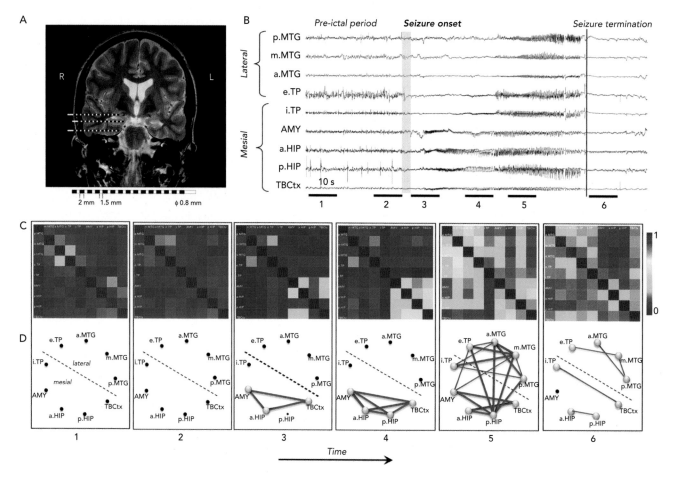

Figure 44.9. Signal processing method based on nonlinear regression analysis and aimed at characterizing brain connectivity during the transition from ongoing to seizure activity. **A, B:** In this example, stereo-EEG recordings were performed in a patient with mesial temporal lobe epilepsy as part of the presurgical investigation. **C:** Color-coded nonlinear correlation matrices obtained from the pairwise computation of nonlinear correlation coefficient h^2 over six 10-sec intervals chosen during the pre-ictal period (1 and 2), the ictal period (3, 4, and 5), and after seizure termination (6). **D:** Graphical representation of the correlation matrices as graphs in which edges indicate significantly high couplings (based on a statistical test) among considered brain structures (graph nodes). Line thickness is proportional to h^2 values. Note the increase of couplings in mesial structures at seizure onset (3) and the extended synchronization of ictal activity as the seizure develops (5). Adapted with permission from Wendling et al. (70).

occur during the transition from ongoing background activity to seizure activity. Typically, a dramatic increase of h^2 values is observed at seizure onset, characterized by the appearance of fast oscillations in the limbic system (see Fig. 44.9D, period #3). As the seizure develops (see Fig. 44.9D, periods #4 and #5) and the ictal activity is spreading, coupling values significantly increase, not only among depth-EEG signals recorded from the limbic system but also between signals generated by the limbic system and by lateral neocortical structures. Detailed inspection of adjacency matrices also reveals a strong asymmetry in nonlinear correlation values, suggesting a possible propagation of the seizure from the external temporal pole to the posterior middle temporal gyrus, which is plausible from an anatomic-functional viewpoint.

This example illustrates the usefulness of methods aimed at characterizing functional and effective connectivity among brain structures explored by depth-electrodes, before and during seizures. In this context, nonlinear regression analysis was shown to provide relevant results (70) with the unique advantage that it does not require strong assumptions regarding the relationship between analyzed EEG signals (Box 44.2).

5.2.2. FURTHER ESTIMATION OF EFFECTIVE CONNECTIVITY: TESTING FOR CAUSALITY

In this section, we describe general methods that can provide information about the direct or indirect *causal* influence that a brain neuronal system may exert on another one. We use the term "testing for causality" (60), to paraphrase the title of the influential work of Granger, who introduced the concept in 1969, inspired by a hint from Wiener (79). This type of causal relationships fits in the general concept of *effective connectivity* (52).

5.2.2.1. GRANGER CAUSALITY

Granger causality analysis is a signal processing method that provides a quantitative measure of the causal association (and by extension of the effective connectivity) between timeseries. Besides in econometrics, the approach has been applied in various fields including neurophysiology, namely in the analysis of local field potentials form the cat visual system (80), and it has also inspired applications of related methods in EEG analysis (*directed transfer function* (81) and *partial directed coherence* (82)). Since these early years many studies have appeared

BOX 44.2. ASSESSING FUNCTIONAL CONNECTIVITY WITH EEG/MEG

A. Regression Methods

First, we consider the *linear case* (71): for two signals $x(t)$ and $y(t)$ (i.e., stochastic variables with mean zero), the cross-correlation function between the two signals is given by the following expression, where E denotes expectancy or average:

$$\Phi_{xy}(\tau) = E[x(t)\,y(t+\tau)].$$

This expression can be converted to the frequency domain by taking the Fourier transform (FT) of $\Phi_{xy}(\tau)$; this operation yields the cross-power frequency spectrum of the two signals:

$$S_{xy}(f) = FT\,[\Phi_{xy}(\tau)].$$

To obtain an estimate of $S_{xy}(f)$ this quantity has to be smoothed by a window function $W(f)$ with duration of $(2p+1)$ sample points. This yields the smoothed cross-power spectrum:

$$C_{xy}(f_i) = \Sigma\, W(f_k)\; S_{xy}(f_{i+k}),$$

where the summation Σ ranges from $k = -p$ to p. $C_{xy}(f)$ is a complex quantity and therefore can be expressed in term of magnitude and phase, as we saw in Box 44.1. The cross-spectrum normalized with respect to the power spectra of both signals Cxx and Cyy defines the *coherence function*, as follows:

$$Coh_{xy}(f) = \left|C_{xy}(f)\right|^2 / C_{xx}(f)C_{yy}(f)$$

Second, we consider the more general case of *nonlinear regression* between two signals $x(t)$ and $y(t)$ ((69,72)). The nonlinear correlation ratio h^2 expresses the reduction of variance of $y(t)$ that can be obtained by predicting the $x(t)$ values according to the regression curve, as follows:

$$h^2_{xy}(\tau) = 1 - \mathrm{var}\,[y(t+\tau)\,/\,x(t)]\,/\,\mathrm{var}[y(t+\tau)],$$

where h^2 is a nonlinear fitting curve that is obtained, in practice, from the piece-wise linear approximation between the samples of the two time series. The estimated time delay between the two signals corresponds to the value of Δt for which h^2 is maximum.

B. Phase Synchronization Methods

These methods are based on the concept of instantaneous phase. Two alternative methods have been developed, one based on the analytic signal and the Hilbert transform (Section 4.1.1) and the other based on wavelets (Section 4.1.2). Differences between the performances of the two methods are minor (73). Basically, the instantaneous phases of two signals $x(t)$ and $y(t)$, φ_x and φ_y, estimated by one of these methods, are compared and statistically evaluated; phase synchrony (74) or phase locking means that the difference $\varphi_d = |n\varphi_x - m\varphi_y| = $ constant (modulo 2π), where n and m are integers that indicate the ratios of possible frequency locking. This difference is determined within a limited time window, in general with a duration of a few hundreds of milliseconds. The phases of the two signals φ_x and φ_y are extracted from the

coefficients of the corresponding wavelet (or Hilbert) transform at the desired frequency f, centered at time τ; the index is the phase-locking value (PLV(t, f)), estimated by averaging over a number of trials N, given as:

$$PLV(t,f) = \left| \frac{1}{N} \sum_{n=1}^{N} e^{i(\varphi_{x,n}(t,f) - \varphi_{y,n}(t,f))} \right|$$

The estimation of phase synchronization can be affected by the same hurdles that condition the interpretation of EEG signals in general, particularly recorded from the scalp: the reference electrode, the volume conductor effects, and noise sources. This led several researchers to develop variants of the phase synchronization methodology, namely methods based on the imaginary component of the cross-spectrum, such as that proposed by Nolte et al. (75), the so-called phase-lag index (PLI) of Stam et al. (76), and the weighted phase lag index (77).

C. Generalized Synchronization

This quantity derives from the theory of nonlinear dynamical systems (78). According to this concept, synchronization between two dynamical systems X (the driver) and Y (the response) exists when the state of the response system Y is a function of the state of the driving system, X: $Y\, F(X)$. Thus, if two points on the attractor of X, x_i and x_j, are close to each other, the corresponding points on attractor Y, y_i and y_j, will also be close. The probability that embedded vectors are closer to each other than a certain small critical distance is estimated for each discrete time pair (i, j). This is done for each signal, or channel k of a set of M channels.

and very comprehensive evaluative comparisons of different methodological approaches were published. Among these we may especially note that of Kaminski et al. (83), who proposed that the *directed transfer function* can be interpreted within the framework of Granger causality and introduced a method for evaluating the significance of causality measures; that of Hesse et al. (84), who presented an adaptive time-variant Granger causality approach allowing the estimation of causal relations within time intervals of <100 msec; and that of Friston et al. (52), who combined the estimation of directed connectivity using Granger causality with dynamic neural causal modeling; and also the MATLAB toolbox for Granger causal connectivity analysis of Seth (85).

Granger formulated a general axiom on which his methodology is based—"The past and present may cause the future, but the future cannot cause the past"—and a general definition of the statement that Y_t is said to cause X_{t+1} if:

$$\mathrm{Pr}\,ob\left(X_{t+1} \in A\,|\,\Omega_t\right) \neq \mathrm{Pr}\,ob\left(X_{t+1} \in A\,|\,\Omega_t - Y_t\right) \quad \text{for some } A.$$

This means that Y_t has unique information about what value X_{t+1} will take in the immediate future; in other words, the knowledge of Y_t affects the conditional distribution of X_{t+1} (see Box 44.3). In his original paper (1980), Granger pointed out

BOX 44.3. MATHEMATICAL FORMULATION OF LINEAR GRANGER CAUSALITY

The mathematical formulation of Granger causality is based on linear regression modeling of stochastic processes. For illustration in the bivariate case, let X and Y be two zero-mean time series with observation times denoted by $x(t)$ and $y(t)$, with $t = 1, \ldots, T$. Let us also assume that both X and Y can be represented by a univariate autoregressive model of order p (i.e., maximum number of lagged observations included in the model):

$$x(t) = \sum_{k=1}^{p} a_1(k) x(t-k) + e_1(t),$$

$$y(t) = \sum_{k=1}^{p} a_2(k) y(t-k) + e_2(t),$$

where e_1 and e_2 denote the prediction error that depends only on the past of respective time series. In this case, the model to be considered to analyze Granger causality assumes that $x(t)$ and $y(t)$ are suitably represented by the following bivariate coupled autoregressive model (also called ARX model):

$$x(t) = \sum_{k=1}^{p} A_{11}(k) x(t-k) + \sum_{k=1}^{p} A_{12}(k) y(t-k) + E_1(t),$$

$$y(t) = \sum_{k=1}^{p} A_{21}(k) y(t-k) + \sum_{k=1}^{p} A_{22}(k) x(t-k) + E_2(t),$$

which is equivalent to:

$$\begin{bmatrix} x(t) \\ y(t) \end{bmatrix} = \sum_{k=1}^{p} A_k \begin{bmatrix} x(t-k) \\ y(t-k) \end{bmatrix} + \begin{bmatrix} E_1(t) \\ E_2(t) \end{bmatrix} \quad \text{with } A_k = \begin{bmatrix} A_{11} & A_{12} \\ A_{21} & A_{22} \end{bmatrix}$$

and where p is the model order, E_1 and E_2 are residual prediction errors for the respective time series, and where the A matrix contains the coefficients of the model (i.e., the contributions of each lagged observation to the predicted values of $x(t)$ and $y(t)$).

From the above equation, one can notice that the inclusion of y (respectively x) terms in the first (resp. second) equation can have an impact on the variance of the residual E_1 (resp. E_2). If this variance is reduced, then X (resp. Y) is said to Granger-cause Y (resp. X). In other words, X causes Y if the p coefficients in A_{22} are significantly different from zero. Similarly, Y causes X if the A_{12} coefficients are significantly different from zero. An F-test of the null hypothesis ($A_{12} = 0$ or $A_{22} = 0$) can be performed to assess the statistical significance of A_{12} or A_{22} coefficients being jointly different from zero. Some criteria (like the Akaike information criterion (86)) can be used to determine the appropriate model order p.

It is worth noting that the above-described model does not account for latent confounding effects like X and Y processes being unrelated directly but caused by a common third process, nor does it account for instantaneous and non-linear causal relationships. Finally, this model can be readily extended to the multivariate case.

some difficulties that should be discussed since they may affect the application of this methodology. One major difficulty is caused by inadequacy of the data, specifically by an insufficient sampling rate. In this case the relationship may appear "instantaneous," but this is a weak proposition since it is not possible to differentiate between whether X is caused by Y or viceversa, or due to feedback between X and Y. Another difficulty is due to the so-called missing variables. These difficulties presented by Granger constitute an important warning for neurophysiologist, since they may easily occur in applications of Granger methodology in assessing causal relationships between neuronal brain activities based on incomplete sets of EEG/MEG signals.

5.2.2.2. Directed Transfer Function and Related Approaches in EEG/MEG Analysis

Methods akin to Granger causality have been introduced and applied in recent decades, namely directed transfer function (DTF), direct directed transfer function (dDTF), and partial directed coherence (PDC). All these methods are based on a multivariate autoregressive model (MVAR)—that is, an extension to an arbitrary number of signals of the univariate autoregressive model (AR) described in Section 3.2.3. The basics of these measures are described in several publications indicated in this chapter and in several books on EEG signal analysis; a comprehensive overview is provided by Blinowska and Zygierewicz (8). Here we will only sketch the main properties of the methods mentioned above. Further, we will comment on a comparative evaluation of the performance of these methods in some practical applications.

DTF (83) is based on the properties of the MVAR of a group of k EEG signals that contains spectral and phase information with respect to the relations between all the signals in the format of a matrix. In this way the information of the inflow from channel i to channel j relative to all inflows to channel i are estimated. Formally a vector $x(t)$, in other words, the data vector at time t can be expressed as:

$$x(t) = \sum_{i=1}^{p} A(i) x(t-i) + e(t),$$

where $A(i)$ are the MVAR coefficients, $e(t)$ is the vector constituted by white noise, and p is the model order.

Transforming the above equation into the frequency domain, we obtain:

$$x(f) - A^{-1}(f) e(f) = H(f) e(f),$$

where $H(f)$ is the transfer matrix and f is the frequency. From $H(f)$ the power spectra can be calculated. The normalized DTF is given by:

$$\Upsilon^2_{ij}(f) = |H_{ij}(f)|^2 / \sum_{m=1}^{k} |H_{im}(f)|^2,$$

where $H_{ij}(f)$ represents the causal influence from channel j to channel i, and $H_{im}(f)$ that from all channels m to channel i. The quantity $\Upsilon^2_{ij}(f)$ is a measure of the ratio between the influence of channel j to channel i (i.e., the outgoing flow of transferred information from $j \to i$) and the joint influences from all the other channels to channel i; it has a value from 0 to 1. The transmission from $j \to i$ is given by Υ^2_{ij}; this is a measure of the transmitted outflow of information; values close to 1 represent that most of the signal in i comes from channel j, whereas a value of 0 means that there is no flow from j to i at the frequency f (83). These authors further show that it is possible to interpret the multivariate DTF in terms of Granger causality.

This method was modified in order to separate direct from indirect flows and led to the development by Korzeniewska et al. (87) of dDTF. This modification entails taking into account the partialization of the coherence. In that paper a number of further variants of the DTF were introduced. In practice it is important to note the possibility of calculating DTF for short EEG epochs (SDTF) in order to be able to follow the dynamics of fast-occurring cognitive processes (88), similar to the short-time Fourier spectra (see Section 4.1.1). An example of the results obtained using SDTF during a working memory task is shown in Figure 44.10, where the outflow of information from a number of sites on the scalp is shown as a function of time elapsed as the subject performed a memory task.

Among variants of these methods, partial directed coherence (PDC), which separates direct from indirect connections, can estimate the strength and direction of direct interactions between EEG signals (88a, 88b). Interestingly, Plomp et al. (88c) evaluated the performance of several variants of time-varying PDC and DTF experimentally in a study of somatosensory evoked potentials in rat cortex and were able to validate the estimates of effective connectivity obtained with these methods in this well-characterized physiological preparation.

In conclusion, Granger causality yields measures in the time domain, whereas PDC and DTF operate in the frequency domain, which may be preferable since brain rhythmic activities play an important role in information processing and

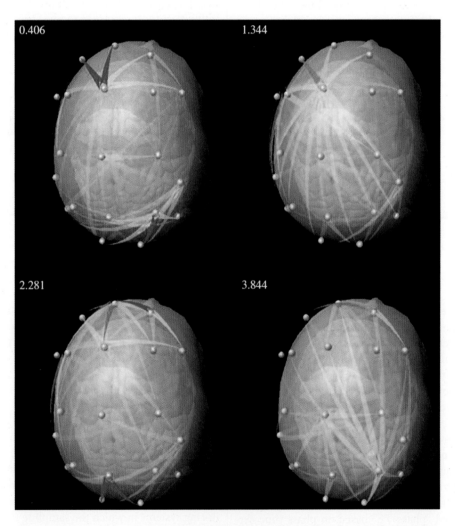

Figure 44.10. Four snapshots from a movie showing the time-varying pattern of the most significant outflows from specific electrode sites on the scalp. The color of the arrows indicates the intensity of outgoing flows (red is the strongest, followed by bright and pale yellow). The numbers on the left upper corner indicate the times after stimulus presentation. The latter was a memory task; the data analyzed correspond to the phase where the subjects integrated incoming information to be memorized. EEG was recorded by 64 electrodes using the 10-20 System, with linked mastoids as reference. For DTF analysis 20 electrode sites were chosen. The estimates of SDTF were obtained using a short sliding time window; ensemble averaging of a number of repetitions was applied. Statistical evaluation was performed by randomization of the original datasets. Note the initial strong outflow of information from a frontal site to more posterior sites, what the authors call an active frontal module, that in about 2 sec is followed by a strong posterior parietal active module. Adapted with permission from Blinowska et al. (126).

modulation in the brain. The physiological interpretation of these measures of effective connectivity, particularly at the level of EEG scalp recordings, however, has to be performed with reservation, taking always in account that scalp recordings give, in general, distorted images of the relationships between cortical areas, and may be influenced by volume conduction effects. Therefore, direct interpretations, based on these or equivalent measures, with respect to interacting cortical sources should always be corroborated by additional and independent information.

5.2.2.3. Mutual Information and Transfer Entropy; Applications to EEG Signals

The concept of mutual information was defined in the field of Shannon's information theory (89). Gel'fand and Yaglom (90) generalized and operationalized the corresponding calculation. This approach was applied to EEG signals recorded during epileptic seizures and allowed estimations to be made of the evolution of time delays in the course of epileptic seizures in animals and humans (91,92). This method, however, in its original form has not been widely applied in clinical cases, most likely because it is heavy from a computational point of view.

A method also based on the concept of mutual information that is becoming widely applied is transfer entropy (TE). This method (detailed in Box 44.4) was introduced by Schreiber (93). TE can be defined in synthetic form as follows:

$$TE(X \rightarrow Y, u) = I(Y_t; X_{t-u} | Y_{t-1})$$

where X and Y are two random signals and u is the delay from X to Y. The mutual information (I) between the past of the source (X_{t-u}) and the current value of the target process (Y_t) is conditional on the past state of the target (Y_{t-1}); further, the interaction conduction delay is given by:

$$\Delta t = \arg\max_u \left(TE \cdot (X \rightarrow Y, u) \right)$$

A detailed overview of the literature on entropy and mutual information and on methods for computing TE is presented by Hlavackova-Schindler et al. (94). Vicente et al. (95) give a comprehensive and general account of applications of TE in neuroscience. Wibral et al. (96) extended TE to include time-delayed source-target interactions applied to numerically simulated signals and also to local field potentials.

Most interesting, Roux et al. (97), based on MEG data, used TE analysis to analyze the coupling between gamma and alpha oscillations in cortical and thalamic sources and estimated time delays between thalamic and cortical sources that are compatible with independent neurophysiological findings obtained in animals. Lobier et al. (98) proposed a variant of TE that they called "phase TE" based on phase time series extracted from neuronal signals. An unbiased comparative analysis of the different variants of methods to estimate causality and time delays in this field is necessary in order to gain insight concerning the strong and weak points of different approaches. In any case, Barnett et al. (99) showed analytically that Granger causality and TE are, for Gaussian variables, strictly equivalent (see Box 44.4).

5.3. Cross-Frequency Phase Coupling

There is experimental evidence that oscillatory processes encoding cognitive functions often involve a combination of different types of EEG oscillations (74,101). With the aim of investigating quantitatively these combined oscillations, we can resort to cross-frequency methods of analysis. The latter can reveal phase and amplitude cross-frequency coupling between EEG channels, as proposed by Canolty et al. (102). This is also clearly put in evidence in the study by He et al. (17), who investigated systematically nested-frequency patterns in different intracerebral EEG recordings in humans. These authors sorted the lower-frequency phase into a series of bins, along with the corresponding higher-frequency amplitude; these plots were then tested statistically, using shuffled data, against a uniform distribution. In this way significant nested oscillations could be identified even beyond the range of rhythmic frequency components. Although the significance of these nested arrhythmic components, in general, is not clear yet, in some specific cases nested rhythmic activities appear to have functional significance. This is the case of the observation by Jensen et al. (103) of gamma oscillations phase-locked to alpha oscillations in the visual cortex. This led these authors to hypothesize that gamma oscillations phase-locked to alpha oscillations would serve processing of visual information by segmenting visual representations in time.

6. SPECIFIC APPLICATIONS

6.1. Detection and Classification of Transient Events in EEG Signals

In this section we will provide an example showing an integrated method involving multiple processing steps often required to solve a specific problem in EEG analysis. The chosen example is that of the detection and classification of epileptiform transient events (a few tens or hundreds of msec) in EEG signals, typically interictal epileptic spikes (IESs) and high-frequency oscillations (HFOs).

6.1.1. Interictal Epileptic Spikes and High-Frequency Oscillations

IESs have long been a topic of great interest in epilepsy research, although the exact relationship between networks generating IESs on the one hand and seizures on the other hand is a recurrent question in epileptology. The detection of IESs has long been—and is still—the subject of new methodological developments. More recently, and due to the wider use of EEG monitoring systems in which the sampling frequency can be set to high frequencies (1 or 2 kHz), a number of studies reported that interictal HFOs (30–600 Hz) are also potential biomarkers of the epileptogenic zone (104). In humans, HFOs can be easily observed in intracerebral EEG signals recorded with multicontact depth electrodes. HFOs are non-stationary oscillations of low amplitude with various frequencies, morphologies, and

BOX 44.4. THE CONCEPT OF TRANSFER ENTROPY

Shannon entropy quantifies the expected value of the information contained in a message. If a discrete variable I can take one of i values with a probability $p(i)$, the definition of Shannon's entropy is:

$$H_I = -\Sigma_i \int p(i) \log p(i)$$

where the Σ extends over all states i that the process may display.

Assuming two processes I and J with joint probability $p_{ij}(i, j)$, the corresponding mutual information (MI) is given by:

$$M(i, j) = \Sigma p(i, j) \log \frac{p(i.j)}{p(i)p(j)}$$

MI is symmetric—that is, one can exchange i and j without affecting the result. To give it a directional sense it is necessary to introduce a time lag in one of the variables, as proposed by Mars and van Arragon (100), who introduced the concept of average amount of mutual information (AAMI) as a function of time delay.

Schreiber (93) extended the concept of MI in order to incorporate dynamical structure in a more fundamental way, by introducing transitional instead of static probabilities. In simplified terms, Schreiber assumed two processes (I, J), where J has influence on the transition probabilities of system I, and he used the generalized notion of Markov processes—that is, processes where the conditional probability of the process being in a given state, say I_{n+1} at time $n+1$, is independent of the state i_{n-k}; in this case k is the order of Markov process i, and l that of another related process j. Under these assumptions, the transfer entropy (TE) is defined as:

$$TE_{J \rightarrow I} = p\left(i_{n+1}, i_n^{(k)}, j_n^{(l)}\right) \log \frac{p(i_{n+1} \mid i_n^{(k)}, j_n^{(l)})}{p(i_{n+1} \mid i_n^{(k)})}$$

Thus TE is nonsymmetric; this quantity is a measure of dependency of I on J, but not vice versa. Schreiber proposed an algorithm to implement TE and presented a number of examples of applications, among them a physiological bivariate time series. However, the coupling between both signals might be due to a common, unknown, source (the missing variable in Granger's nomenclature).

Statistical measures of a detector performance are based on the comparison between the detector output ("an event is detected at time t") and the ground truth ("an event is actually present at time t").

DETECTOR OUTPUT	GROUND TRUTH	
	"An event is actually present"	*"There is no event"*
Positive	*True positive* (correct detection)	*False positive* (false alarm)
Negative	*False negative* (wrong rejection)	*True negative* (correct rejection)

The detector sensitivity is the proportion of correctly identified positives (true-positive rate):

$$\text{Sensitivity} = \frac{\#\text{correct detections}}{\#\text{correct detections} + \#\text{wrong rejections}} = \frac{\#\text{correct detections}}{\text{Total} \# \text{events}}$$

The detector specificity is the proportion of correctly identified negatives (true-negative rate):

$$\text{Specificity} = \frac{\#\text{correct rejections}}{\#\text{correct rejections} + \#\text{false alarms}} = \frac{\#\text{correct rejections}}{\text{Total} \# \text{rejections}}$$

The above definitions are classically used in the case of a binary test. However, in some detection problems, the determination of "correct rejections" may not be possible. This is typically the case where events must be detected in the background activity. To cope with this difficulty the false discovery rate (FDR) might be preferred. FDR provides the number of wrongly detected events normalized by the total number of detected events. It is defined as:

$$FDR = \frac{\#\text{false alarms}}{\#\text{false alarms} + \#\text{correct detection}}.$$

---

underlying pathophysiological mechanisms that can have clinical significance. Compared with IESs, the resection of brain structures generating interictal HFOs was shown to be correlated with a favorable surgical outcome and to provide essential complementary information to ictal pattern analysis (104).

See Chapter 33 for more detailed information about the clinical value of IESs and HFOs.

6.1.2. AUTOMATIC DETECTION OF TRANSIENT EVENTS IN EEG: A TOUGH PROBLEM

It is generally agreed that the automatic detection of IESs is a nontrivial problem. It has been—and is still—the topic of a large number of publications in the field of EEG analysis. Many algorithms have been proposed based on Fourier or wavelet transforms, on mimetic and rule-based approaches, on neural networks, on adaptive filtering (template matching), and on principal or independent component analysis. See (39,105,106) for partial reviews. As shown in many studies (107), the ideal spike detector does not exist, as the false-alarm and non-detection rates remain difficult to control in a context where human experts themselves have difficulty assessing the presence of spikes in EEG signals.

The automatic detection of HFOs (30–600 Hz) is also recognized as a challenging problem because of (1) the poor signal-to-noise ratio, (2) the contamination of signals by transient broadband events (e.g., spikes or artifacts) causing pitfalls in classical filtering techniques (108), and (3) the wide diversity of oscillations, ranging from gamma (30–80 Hz), high gamma (80–120 Hz), ripple (120–250 Hz) and up to the fast ripple (250–600 Hz) frequency band. Automated detection methods were first proposed in the time domain (109–111), but more recent methods make use of algorithms in the time-frequency domain (112,113). However, a universal HFO detector (i.e., one that would offer high performance in all situations) has not been proposed yet. This is partly due to the absence of a "ground truth" (i.e., the exact knowledge of the type and instants of occurrence of the events to be detected). Indeed, the visual inspection of HFOs is time-consuming, quite subjective, and marginally consistent among experts.

6.1.3. FROM RAW EEG SIGNALS TO DETECTED AND LABELED EVENTS: A CHAIN OF INFORMATION PROCESSING

Whatever the type of event to be automatically detected and classified, the general approach proceeds according to a number of processing steps, as illustrated in Figure 44.11. These processing steps, detailed below, are (1) pre-processing of raw data, (2) detection of events of interest in pre-processed signals, (3) characterization of detected events, and finally (4) classification steps that ultimately lead to labeling the detected events.

6.1.3.1. PRE-PROCESSING OF RAW EEG SIGNALS

In most cases, raw EEG signals are contaminated by various types of artifacts that can be removed prior to detection of events of interest. Several methods for artifact removal were presented in Section 2.3. Along the same line, various sources of noise (e.g., equipment, muscle activity) can also alter the quality of EEG signals. Again, denoising techniques (see Section 4.2) can be used as a pre-processing step in order to improve the performance of detection techniques. In the particular case of epileptiform events, high-pass filtering is often used as pre-processing. Indeed, IESs are usually characterized by a sharp component (spike) that corresponds to the presence of energy at high frequencies (typically beyond 20 Hz). Similarly, and by definition, HFOs are events occurring in a frequency band starting from ~80 Hz.

Interestingly, and as emphasized in the study by Benar et al. (108), the detection of interictal HFOs cannot be based only on high-pass filtering of raw EEG signals. Indeed, as mentioned in Section 2.3.1, a filter is entirely characterized by its impulse response. Consequently, when sharp transient events are used as input to a high-pass filter, the output signal is close to the impulse response of the filter, which is typically a short-duration oscillation that can be confounded with an actual oscillation present in the signal (see also discussion in Section 2.3.1, and Yuval-Greenberg et al. (4)). For instance, and as illustrated in Figure 44.12, some sharp transient events such as IESs, after filtering, can result in "false" ripples that resemble genuine "fast" ripples: both types of events correspond to a fast oscillatory activity in the frequency band defined by the filter.

6.1.3.2. DETECTION OF EVENTS OF INTEREST

Formally, in signal theory, the term "detection" refers to the ability to discern between information-bearing patterns (i.e., signals) and random patterns that distract from the information (i.e., noise). In our case, "detection" is defined as the ability to identify specific events of interest (typically IESs or HFOs) in EEG data. Technically, the general approach consists, first in building a new signal, referred to as a "statistics," from pre-processed raw EEG signals. This "statistics" must be relevant with respect to events to be detected—that is, it must exhibit changes whenever an event of interest is present in the EEG signal. An example is provided in Figure 44.13. In this case based on intracerebral EEG signals containing both IESs and HFOs (ripples), and for simplicity, the statistics w was chosen to be the EEG signal energy in a frequency band ranging from 30 to 600 Hz. As depicted, the mean of w significantly increases whenever an HFO or an IES is present as compared with the background activity (outside events of interest). The approach then consists in "analyzing" the "statistics" w—in other words, finding the time instants at which significant changes occur due to the presence of events of interest. The simplest method to achieve this is by comparing w to a threshold value λ, which is critical for the detection performance as it determines both the sensitivity and specificity of the detector (see Box 44.4). As illustrated in the didactical example of Figure 44.13, the λ value was set to automatically detect HFOs but not IESs. This simple

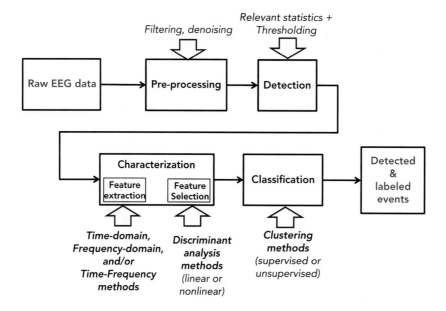

Figure 44.11. Processing steps usually implemented to solve the problem of detection/classification of events of interest from raw EEG data.

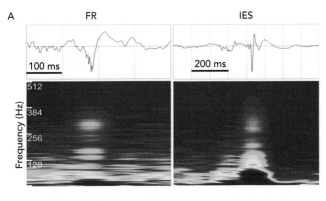

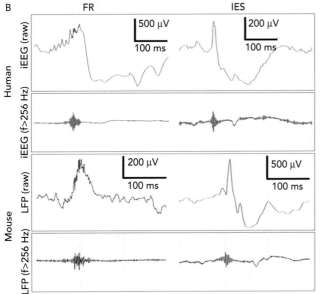

Figure 44.12. Typical fast ripples (FRs) and IESs recorded from hippocampus in human Temporal Lobe Epilepsy (TLE) and in an animal model of epilepsy (mouse, kainate model). **A:** Human FRs and IESs (depth-EEG signals) with corresponding spectrograms. Note that both events of interest (the FR and the IES) exhibit energy in the range of 250 to 600 Hz. **B:** FRs and IESs recorded from hippocampus using macro-electrodes (human: depth-EEG, mouse: LFPs). Upper plots: raw signals. Lower plots: filtered signals (high-pass cutoff frequency = 256 Hz). Note that the two types of epileptic events can hardly be discriminated using a simple high-pass filtering procedure. Adapted with permission from Birot et al. (112).

example shows how crucial the threshold value is. If λ were set to a lower value, then the method would also detect IESs; if it were set to a higher value, some HFOs would be missed.

A standard procedure to assess the detector performance as a function of λ is to analyze its receiver operating characteristic (ROC). The ROC curve is a plot of the true-positive rate (sensitivity) versus the false-positive rate (λ – specificity) for different values of the threshold parameter λ. The ideal detector has a ROC curve passing through the upper left corner (false-positive rate = 0, true-positive rate = 1). Therefore, the closer the ROC curve is to the upper left corner, the higher the detection performance.

6.1.3.3. CHARACTERIZATION OF DETECTED EVENTS AND CONSTRUCTION OF A FEATURE VECTOR

This step aims at defining a number of features that best describe the spectral and/or morphological content of events

detected in raw EEG signals. Many of the methods presented in this chapter, operating either in the time, frequency, or time-frequency domain, can be used for this purpose, depending on the type of events to be characterized. For instance, spike-and-waves are, by definition, characterized by a sharp component ("spike") generally followed by a slower component of the same or opposite polarity ("wave"). In the case of HFOs, a typical feature is the presence of low-amplitude fast oscillations superimposed on a large-amplitude slow wave. These non-stationary properties can be typically captured by time-frequency methods like wavelets (see Section 4.1.2) or MP (see Section 4.1.4. Matching Pursuit). In both cases, a feature vector can be built from the "atoms" obtained from the decomposition of the raw EEG signal. It is noteworthy that this feature extraction/selection step usually leads to a dimensionality reduction as the dimension of the retained feature vector is usually lower than that of the signal. An illustrative example (114) based on MP is provided in Figure 44.14.

6.1.3.4. CLASSIFICATION OF DETECTED EVENTS

In general, the term "classification" refers to the categorization of objects or items presenting with similar features. In signal processing, this step naturally follows the characterization step in which feature vectors are defined to quantify the time and/or frequency content of signals under analysis. A large number of classification algorithms are available, which can be used to cluster and label signal events detected in raw EEG, after feature extraction and selection. The aim of this section is to provide a brief overview of classification techniques and associated classifiers. See detailed reviews on signal classification (115), some of which are specifically related to well-known problems in EEG like the recognition of brain activity patterns in BCI (116).

A first dichotomy is to distinguish supervised classification methods from unsupervised methods. According to the supervised approach, a training dataset containing reference signals (i.e., already grouped into classes that are known a priori) is used to "optimize" the classifier (i.e., to produce clusters as close as possible to reference classes). Unsupervised methods proceed from the data itself without prior information about classes. The aim is to automatically group items of similar type into clusters so that a model representing the structure of the data can be obtained. In (116), a survey of classification algorithms used in BCI research is proposed. Classifiers are divided into five categories:

1. Linear classifiers (based on linear discriminant analysis or support vector machine) that make use of hyperplanes to separate the different classes

2. Neural networks, which allow for producing nonlinear decision boundaries based on the interconnected artificial neurons

3. Nonlinear Bayesian classifiers, which assign classes to feature vectors under the constraint of highest probability

4. Nearest neighbor classifiers, which group items based on their distance in the feature space

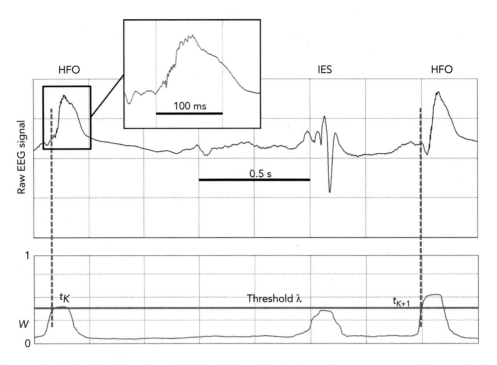

Figure 44.13. Detection step. A statistics w is built from the raw EEG signal. This statistics is relevant with respect to events of interest to be detected. In this case, w was chosen to be the EEG signal energy in a frequency band ranging from 30 to 600 Hz. As depicted, the mean of w significantly increases whenever an HFO or an IES occurs, as compared with the mean during background activity (outside events of interest). The detection step then consists in determining the occurrence times t_k of events of interest. The simplest way to achieve this is by comparing w to a threshold value λ.

5. "Combined classifiers," in which a strategy (boosting, voting, stacking) is used to aggregate the results obtained from several classifiers known to increase performance and to decrease variance.

6.2. Software Packages

At present, several of the methods described in this chapter are available in the form of software packages that can easily be downloaded. The reader may encounter useful general information and practical tools in these packages. We mention here some of the most popular ones, most of which belong to the category of open-source software.

EEGLAB is a toolbox for analyzing EEG dynamics including independent component analysis (117) that was extended with new EEG processing tools, including the ability to perform statistical analyses, a forward head modeling toolbox, a toolbox to model effective connectivity between cortical areas, a toolbox for building online BCI, and an experimental real-time control and analysis environment (118).

Fieldtrip (119) is a general software package for analysis of EEG/MEG and invasive electrophysiological data. It includes algorithms for time-frequency analysis, source reconstruction using dipolar models, as well as distributed sources and beamformers, connectivity analysis tools, and nonparametric permutation tests.

A number of other software packages have more specific aims. We distinguish here a number of widely known systems that cover most applications in the domain of EEG/MEG analysis in practice:

LORETA (low-resolution electromagnetic tomography) is dedicated to estimating brain electrical activity based on multichannel surface EEG recordings and thus to construct the smoothest possible three-dimensional current distribution that corresponds to a given distribution of EEG at the scalp (120,121).

Brainstorm is dedicated to EEG/MEG data visualization, analysis, and processing, with emphasis on the estimation of cortical sources and their integration in MRI (122).

CARTOOL is a software package aiming at the analysis of spatial properties of multichannel EEG signals, in particular topographic analysis and source imaging (123).

SPM8 (EEG/MEG data analysis in statistical parameter mapping) is a system that, besides standard EEG/MEG pre-processing, provides tools for the statistical analysis of scalp maps, time-frequency, Bayesian source reconstruction images, and dynamic causal modeling. It is integrated with the Fieldtrip toolbox, described above.

EEGNET is a software pipeline particularly dedicated to the reconstruction of cortical sources of EEG/MEG signals, the identification of functional brain networks from EEG/MEG signals, and the visualization of brain networks at the scalp (two-dimensional) and at the cortex (three-dimensional) levels (124).

eConnectome (http://econnectome.umn.edu) is an open-source MATLAB software package for imaging brain functional connectivity from electrophysiological signals developed by Dai et al. (125). It provides interactive

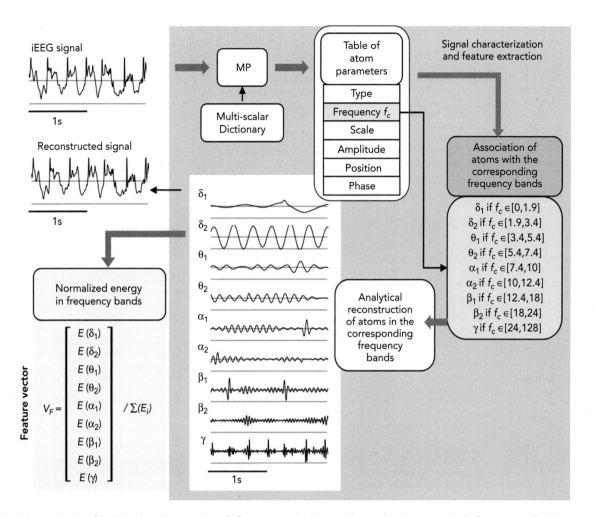

Figure 44.14. *Characterization of EEG signals and construction of a feature vector. In this example, the objective was to build a feature vector for short segments of intracranial EEG signals. The approach made use of the MP algorithm (with a dictionary of Gabor, Fourier, and Dirac atoms). Parameters of detected atoms (atom type, central frequency fc, scale, phase, amplitude, and position) were extracted by MP applied on intracranial EEG signals. Detected atoms were then associated with frequency bands ($\delta1$ to γ) depending on their proper central frequency. Sub-band ($\delta1$ to γ) signals were reconstructed from the sum of corresponding atoms. The normalized energy vector $[E(\delta1) \ldots E(\gamma)]/(E(\delta1) + \ldots + E(\gamma))$ was chosen as the feature vector. Note that the sum of identified atoms leads to a reconstructed signal that is (almost) identical to the original intracranial EEG signal. Adapted with permission from Mina et al. (114).*

graphical interfaces for EEG/ECoG/MEG pre-processing, source estimation, connectivity analysis, and visualization.

Epilab (http://www.epilepsiae.eu/project_outputs/epilab_software) was developed by a consortium of European laboratories and is dedicated to the analysis of EEG in epilepsy.

IFT (http://sccn.ucsd.edu/wiki/SIFT) is a software package for analysis and visualization of multivariate causality and information flow between EEG/ECoG/MEG sources, maintained by T. Mullen. (Information source, (88).)

The Svarog package is a signal viewer, analyzer and recorder on GPL (http://braintech.pl/svarog). (Information source, (42).)

REFERENCES

1. Vogel T, Grey Walter W. Discussion sur les bases mathématiques de l'analyse de fréquence. Electroenceph Clin Neurophysiol. 1951;40(3):435–442.

2. Gasser T. General characteristics of the EEG as a signal. In: Remond A, ed. EEG Informatics. A Didactic Review of Methods and Applications of EEG Data Processing. Amsterdam: Elsevier. 1977.

3. Smith SW. The Scientist and Engineer's Guide to Digital Signal Processing. San Diego: California Technical Publishing, 2002.

4. Yuval-Greenberg S, Tomer O, Keren AS, Nelken I, Deouell LY. Transient induced gamma-band response in EEG as a manifestation of miniature saccades. Neuron. 2008;58(3):429–441.

5. Fries P, Scheeringa R, Oostenveld R. Finding gamma. Neuron. 2008;58(3):303–305.

6. Melloni L, Schwiedrzik CM, Wibral M, Rodriguez E, Singer W. Response to Yuval-Greenberg et al. Neuron. 2009;62(1):8–10.

7. He P, Wilson G, Russell C. Removal of ocular artifacts from electro-encephalogram by adaptive filtering. Med Biol Eng Comput. 2004;42(3):407–412.

8. Blinowska K, Zygierewicz J. Practical Biomedical Signal Analysis Using MATLAB. New York: CRC Press, 2012.

9. McEwen JA, Anderson GB. Modeling the stationarity and Gaussianity of spontaneous electroencephalographic activity. IEEE Trans Biomed Eng. 1975;22(5):361–369.

10. Isaksson A, Wennberg A. Spectral properties of nonstationary EEG signals, evaluated by means of Kalman filtering: application examples from a vigilance test. In: Kellaway P, Petersén I, eds. Quantitative Analytic Studies in Epilepsy. New York: Raven, 1976.

11. Dumermuth G, Gasser T, Hecker A. Exploration of EEG components in the beta frequency range. In: Kellaway P, Petersén I, eds. Quantitative Analytic Studies in Epilepsy. New York: Raven, 1976.

12. Jenkins G, Watts D. Spectral Analysis and Its Applications. San Francisco: Holden Day, 1968.

13. Bruhn J, Ropcke H, Rehberg B, Bouillon T, Hoeft A. Electroencephalogram approximate entropy correctly classifies the occurrence of burst suppression pattern as increasing anesthetic drug effect. Anesthesiology. 2000;93(4):981–985.

14. Gosseries O, Schnakers C, Ledoux D, et al. Automated EEG entropy measurements in coma, vegetative state/unresponsive wakefulness syndrome and minimally conscious state. Funct Neurol. 2011;26(1):25–30.

15. Cooley J, Tukey J. An algorithm for the machine calculation of complex Fourier series. Math Comp. 1965;19:297–301.

16. Frigo M, Johnson S. The design and implementation of FFTW3. Proc IEEE. 2005;93(2):216–231.

17. He BJ, Zempel JM, Snyder AZ, Raichle ME. The temporal structures and functional significance of scale-free brain activity. Neuron. 2010;66(3):353–369.

18. Yamamoto Y, Hughson RL. Coarse-graining spectral analysis: new method for studying heart rate variability. J Appl Physiol (1985). 1991;71(3):1143–1150.

19. Beggs JM, Plenz D. Neuronal avalanches in neocortical circuits. J Neurosci. 2003;23(35):11167–11177.

20. Gireesh ED, Plenz D. Neuronal avalanches organize as nested theta- and beta/gamma-oscillations during development of cortical layer 2/3. Proc Nat Acad Sci USA. 2008;105(21):7576–7581.

21. Petermann T, Thiagarajan TC, Lebedev MA, Nicolelis MA, Chialvo DR, Plenz D. Spontaneous cortical activity in awake monkeys composed of neuronal avalanches. Proc Nat Acad Sci USA. 2009;106(37):15921–15926.

22. Shriki O, Alstott J, Carver F, et al. Neuronal avalanches in the resting MEG of the human brain. J Neurosci. 2013;33(16):7079–7090.

23. De Los Rios P, Zhang Y-C. Universal 1/f noise from dissipative self-organized criticality models. Phys Rev Lett. 1999;82(3):472–475.

24. Bedard C, Kroger H, Destexhe A. Does the 1/f frequency scaling of brain signals reflect self-organized critical states? Phys Rev Lett. 2006;97(11):118102.

24a. Pettersen KH, Lindén H, Tetzlaff T, Einevoll GT. Power Laws from Linear Neuronal Cable Theory: Power Spectral Densities of the Soma Potential, Soma Membrane Curent and Single-Neuron Contribution to the EEG. PLoS Comput Biol. 2014;10(11):e1003928. doi:10.1371/journal.pcbi.1003928

24b. Verveen AA, DeFelice LJ. Membrane Noise. Progress in Biophysics and Molecular Biology. 1974;28:189–234.

25. Zetterberg L. Estimation of parameters for a linear difference equation with application to EEG analysis. Math Biosci. 1969;5:227–275.

26. Gersch W. Spectral analysis of EEGs by autoregressive decomposition of time series. Math Biosci. 1970;7:205–222.

27. Lopes da Silva F, Dijk A, Smits H. Detection of nonstationarities in EEGs using the autoregressive model. An application to EEGs of epileptics. In: Dolce G, Künkel H, eds. CEAN-Computerized EEG Analysis. Stuttgart: Fischer, 1975.

28. Praetorius HM, Bodenstein G, Creutzfeldt OD. Adaptive segmentation of EEG records: a new approach to automatic EEG analysis. Electroencephalogr Clin Neurophysiol. 1977;42(1):84–94.

29. McFarland DJ, Wolpaw JR. Sensorimotor rhythm-based brain-computer interface (BCI): model order selection for autoregressive spectral analysis. J Neural Eng. 2008;5(2):155–162.

30. Blinowska KJ. Review of the methods of determination of directed connectivity from multichannel data. Med Biol Eng Comput. 2011;49(5):521–529.

31. Pascual-Marqui RD, Biscay RJ, Bosch-Bayard J, et al. Assessing direct paths of intracortical causal information flow of oscillatory activity with the isolated effective coherence (iCoh). Front Hum Neurosci. 2014;8:448.

32. Sommerlade L, Thiel M, Mader M, et al. Assessing the strength of directed influences among neural signals: an approach to noisy data. J Neurosci Meth. 2015;239:47–64.

33. Geertsema EE, Visser GH, Velis DN, Claus SP, Zijlmans M, Kalitzin SN. Automated seizure onset zone approximation based on nonharmonic high-frequency oscillations in human interictal intracranial EEGs. Int J Neural Syst. 2015;25(5):1550015.

34. Schneider T, Neumaier A. ARfit—A Matlab package for the estimation of parameters and eigenmodes of multivariate autoregressive models. ACM Trans Math Software. 2001;27(1):58–65.

35. Lopes Da Silva FH. Analysis of EEG non-stationarities. Electroencephalogr Clin Neurophysiol Suppl. 1978;34:163–179.

36. Zetterberg L. Means and methods for processing of physiological signals with emphasis on EEG analysis. In: Lawrence JH, ed. Advances in Biology and Medical Physics. New York: Academic Press, 1977.

36a. Marple SL. Computing the discrete-time "analytic" signal via FFT. IEEE Trans Signal Processing. 1999;47(9):2600–2603.

37. Mallat SG. A theory of multiresolution signal decomposition: the wavelet representation. IEEE Trans Patt Anal Mach Intell. 1989;31:674–693.

38. Senhadji L, Dillenseger JL, Wendling F, Rocha C, Kinie A. Wavelet analysis of EEG for three-dimensional mapping of epileptic events. Ann Biomed Eng. 1995;23(5):543–552.

39. Senhadji L, Wendling F. Epileptic transient detection: wavelets and time-frequency approaches. Clin Neurophysiol. 2002;32(3):175–192.

40. Mallat S, Zhang Z. Matching pursuits with time-frequency dictionaries. IEEE Trans Signal Proc. 1993;12:3397–3415.

41. Durka P, Ircha D, Blinowska K. Stochastic time-frequency dictionaries for matching pursuit. IEEE Trans Signal Proc. 2001;49(3):507–510.

42. Kus R, Rozanski PT, Durka PJ. Multivariate matching pursuit in optimal Gabor dictionaries: theory and software with interface for EEG/MEG via Svarog. Biomed Eng Online. 2013;12:94.

42a. Comon P, Jutten C. (Eds). Handbook of Blind Source Separation: Independent Component Analysis and Applications. Academic Press/Elsevier, Amsterdam, 2010.

43. James CJ, Hesse CW. Independent component analysis for biomedical signals. Physiol Measure. 2005;26(1):R15–39.

43a. Congedo M, Gouy-Pailler C, Jutten C. On the Blind Source Separation of Human Electroencephalogram by approximate joint diagonalization of second order statistics. Clin Neurpohysiol. 2008;119(12):2677–2686.

44. Delorme A, Palmer J, Oostenveld R, Onton J, Makeig S. Comparing results of algorithms implementing blind source separation of EEG data. Unpublished 2007 manuscript, available at http://sccnucsdedu/~arno/mypapers/delorme_unpubpdf.

45. Hotelling H. Relations between two sets of variates. Biometrika. 1936;28:321–377.

46. Spueler M, Walter A, Rosenstiel W, Bogdan M. Spatial filtering based on canonical correlation analysis for classification of evoked or event-related potentials in EEG data. IEEE Trans Neural Systems Rehab Eng. 2014;22(6):1097–1103.

47. Huang N, Shen Z, Long S, et al. The empirical mode decomposition and the Hilbert spectrum for nonlinear and non-stationary time series analysis. Proc R Soc Lond A. 1998;454:903–995.

48. Sweeney-Reed CM, Nasuto SJ. A novel approach to the detection of synchronisation in EEG based on empirical mode decomposition. J Comp Neurosci. 2007;23(1):79–111.

49. Safieddine D, Kachenoura A, Albera L, et al. Removal of muscle artifact from EEG data: comparison between stochastic (ICA and CCA) and deterministic (EMD and wavelet-based) approaches. EURASIP, J Ad SigPro. 2012:1–15.

50. Cosandier-Rimele D, Merlet I, Bartolomei F, Badier JM, Wendling F. Computational modeling of epileptic activity: from cortical sources to EEG signals. J Clin Neurophysiol. 2010;27(6):465–470.

51. Goncalves SI, de Munck JC, Verbunt JP, Bijma F, Heethaar RM, Lopes da Silva F. In vivo measurement of the brain and skull resistivities using an EIT-based method and realistic models for the head. IEEE Trans Biomed Eng. 2003;50(6):754–767.

52. Friston K, Moran R, Seth AK. Analysing connectivity with Granger causality and dynamic causal modelling. Curr Op Neurobiol. 2013;23(2):172–178.

53. Sanei S, Chambers J. EEG Signal Processing. Chichester, UK: John Wiley & Sons, 2007.

54. Quian Quiroga R, Kraskov A, Kreuz T, Grassberger P. Performance of different synchronization measures in real data: a case study on electroencephalographic signals. Phys Rev E. 2002;65(4 Pt 1):041903.

55. David O, Cosmelli D, Friston KJ. Evaluation of different measures of functional connectivity using a neural mass model. NeuroImage. 2004;21(2):659–673.

56. Wendling F, Ansari-Asl K, Bartolomei F, Senhadji L. From EEG signals to brain connectivity: a model-based evaluation of interdependence measures. J Neurosci Meth. 2009;183(1):9–18.

57. Roelfsema PR, Engel AK, Konig P, Singer W. Visuomotor integration is associated with zero time-lag synchronization among cortical areas. Nature. 1997;385(6612):157–161.

58. Singer W. Neuronal synchrony: a versatile code for the definition of relations? Neuron. 1999;24(1):49–65, 111–125.

59. Sompolinsky H, Golomb D, Kleinfeld D. Cooperative dynamics in visual processing. Phys Rev A. 1991;43(12):6990–7011.

60. Granger CWJ. Investigating causal relations by econometric models and cross-spectral methods. Econometrica. 1969;37:424–438.

61. Carter G. Time Delay Estimation. New London, CT: Naval Underwater Systems Center. Report TR5335, 1976.

62. Buzsaki G, Anastassiou CA, Koch C. The origin of extracellular fields and currents--EEG, ECoG, LFP and spikes. Nature Rev Neurosci. 2012;13(6):407–420.

63. Pijn JP, Vijn PC, Lopes da Silva FH, Van Ende Boas W, Blanes W. Localization of epileptogenic foci using a new signal analytical approach. Clin Neurophysiol. 1990;20(1):1–11.

64. Meeren HK, Pijn JP, Van Luijtelaar EL, Coenen AM, Lopes da Silva FH. Cortical focus drives widespread corticothalamic networks during spontaneous absence seizures in rats. J Neurosci. 2002;22(4):1480–1495.

65. Wendling F, Bellanger JJ, Bartolomei F, Chauvel P. Relevance of nonlinear lumped-parameter models in the analysis of depth-EEG epileptic signals. Biol Cybernet. 2000;83(4):367–378.

66. Uva L, Librizzi L, Wendling F, de Curtis M. Propagation dynamics of epileptiform activity acutely induced by bicuculline in the hippocampal-parahippocampal region of the isolated guinea pig brain. Epilepsia. 2005;46(12):1914–1925.

67. Wendling F, Bartolomei F, Bellanger JJ, Chauvel P. Interpretation of interdependencies in epileptic signals using a macroscopic physiological model of the EEG. Clin Neurophysiol. 2001;112(7):1201–1218.

68. Colombet B, Woodman M, Badier JM, Benar CG. AnyWave: a cross-platform and modular software for visualizing and processing electrophysiological signals. J Neurosci Meth. 2015;242:118–126.

69. Kalitzin SN, Parra J, Velis DN, Lopes da Silva FH. Quantification of unidirectional nonlinear associations between multidimensional signals. IEEE Trans Biomed Eng. 2007;54(3):454–461.

70. Wendling F, Bartolomei F, Senhadji L. Spatial analysis of intracerebral electroencephalographic signals in the time and frequency domain: identification of epileptogenic networks in partial epilepsy. Phil Trans A. 2009;367(1887):297–316.

71. Bendat J, Piersol A. Random Data: Analysis and Measurement Procedures. Hoboken, NJ: John Wiley & Sons, 1971.

72. Pijn JP, Velis DN, Lopes da Silva FH. Measurement of interhemispheric time differences in generalised spike-and-wave. Electroencephalogr Clin Neurophysiol. 1992;83(2):169–171.

73. Le Van Quyen M, Foucher J, Lachaux J, et al. Comparison of Hilbert transform and wavelet methods for the analysis of neuronal synchrony. J Neurosci Meth. 2001;111(2):83–98.

74. Lachaux JP, Rodriguez E, Martinerie J, Varela FJ. Measuring phase synchrony in brain signals. Hum Brain Map. 1999;8(4):194–208.

75. Nolte G, Bai O, Wheaton L, Mari Z, Vorbach S, Hallett M. Identifying true brain interaction from EEG data using the imaginary part of coherency. Clin Neurophysiol. 2004;115(10):2292–2307.

76. Stam CJ, Nolte G, Daffertshofer A. Phase lag index: assessment of functional connectivity from multichannel EEG and MEG with diminished bias from common sources. Hum Brain Map. 2007;28(11):1178–1193.

77. Vinck M, Oostenveld R, van Wingerden M, Battaglia F, Pennartz CM. An improved index of phase-synchronization for electrophysiological data in the presence of volume-conduction, noise and sample-size bias. NeuroImage. 2011;55(4):1548–1565.

78. Rulkov N, Sushchik M, Tsimring L. Generalized synchronization of chaos in directionally coupled chaotic systems. Phys Rev E. 1995;51(2):980–994.

79. Wiener N. The theory of prediction. In: EF Bec, ed. Modern Mathematics for Engineers, Series 1, Chapter 8. New York: McGraw-Hill, 1958.

80. Bernasconi C, Konig P. On the directionality of cortical interactions studied by structural analysis of electrophysiological recordings. Biol Cybernet. 1999;81(3):199–210.

81. Kaminski MJ, Blinowska KJ. A new method of the description of the information flow in the brain structures. Biol Cybernet. 1991;65(3):203–210.

82. Baccala LA, Sameshima K. Partial directed coherence: a new concept in neural structure determination. Biol Cybernet. 2001;84(6):463–474.

83. Kaminski M, Ding M, Truccolo WA, Bressler SL. Evaluating causal relations in neural systems: Granger causality, directed transfer function and statistical assessment of significance. Biol Cybernet. 2001;85(2):145–157.

84. Hesse W, Moller E, Arnold M, Schack B. The use of time-variant EEG Granger causality for inspecting directed interdependencies of neural assemblies. J Neurosci Meth. 2003;124(1):27–44.

85. Seth AK. A MATLAB toolbox for Granger causal connectivity analysis. J Neurosci Meth. 2010;186(2):262–273.

86. Akaike H. A new look at the statistical model identification. IEEE Trans Automatic Control. 1974;19(6):716–723.

87. Korzeniewska A, Manczak M, Kaminski M, Blinowska KJ, Kasicki S. Determination of information flow direction among brain structures by a modified directed transfer function (dDTF) method. J Neurosci Meth. 2003;125(1-2):195–207.

88. Kaminski M, Blinowska K. Directed transfer function is not influenced by volume conduction—inexperient pre-processing should be avoided. Front Comput Neurosci. 2014;8(art 61):1–3.

88a. Baccalá LA, Sameshima K. Partial coherence: a new concept in neural structure determination. Biol Cybernetics. 2001;84(6):463–474.

88b. Astolfi L, Cincotti F, Mattia D, et al. Comparison of different cortical connectivity estimators for high-resolution EEG recordings. Human Brain Mapp. 2007;28(2):143–157.

88c. Plomp G, Quairiaux C, Michel CM, Astolfi L. The physiological plausicility of time-varying Granger-causal modeling: Normalization and weighting by spectral power. Neuroimage. 2014;97:206–216.

89. Shannon CE, Weaver W. The Mathematical Theory of Communication. Chicago: University of Illinois Press, 1948.

90. Gel'fand IM, Yaglom AM. Calculation of the amount of information about a random function contained in another such function. Am Math Sac Transl. 1959;12:199–246.

91. Mars NJ, Lopes da Silva FH. Propagation of seizure activity in kindled dogs. Electroencephalogr Clin Neurophysiol. 1983;56(2):194–209.

92. Mars NJ, Thompson PM, Wilkus RJ. Spread of epileptic seizure activity in humans. Epilepsia. 1985;26(1):85–94.

93. Schreiber T. Measuring information transfer. Phys Rev Lett. 2000;85(2):461–464.

94. Hlaváčková-Schindler K, Palus M, Vejmelka M, Bhattachyria J. Causality detection based on information-theoretic approaches in time series analysis. Physics Reports. 2007;441:1–46.

95. Vicente R, Wibral M, Lindner M, Pipa G. Transfer entropy—a model-free measure of effective connectivity for the neurosciences. J Comp Neurosci. 2011;30(1):45–67.

96. Wibral M, Pampu N, Priesemann V, et al. Measuring information-transfer delays. PLoS One. 2013;8(2):e55809.

97. Roux F, Wibral M, Singer W, Aru J, Uhlhaas PJ. The phase of thalamic alpha activity modulates cortical gamma-band activity: evidence from resting-state MEG recordings. J Neurosci. 2013;33(45):17827–17835.

98. Lobier M, Siebenhuhner F, Palva S, Palva JM. Phase transfer entropy: a novel phase-based measure for directed connectivity in networks coupled by oscillatory interactions. NeuroImage. 2014;85(Pt 2):853–872.

99. Barnett L, Barrett AB, Seth AK. Granger causality and transfer entropy are equivalent for Gaussian variables. Phys Rev Lett. 2009;103(23):238701.

100. Mars NIJ, van Arragon GW. Time delay estimation in non-linear systems using average amount of mutual information analysis. Signal Processing. 1982;4:139–153.

101. Palva JM, Palva S, Kaila K. Phase synchrony among neuronal oscillations in the human cortex. J Neurosci. 2005;25(15):3962–3972.

102. Canolty RT, Cadieu CF, Koepsell K, Knight RT, Carmena JM. Multivariate phase-amplitude cross-frequency coupling in neurophysiological signals. IEEE Trans Biomed Eng. 2012;59(1):8–11.

103. Jensen O, Gips B, Bergmann TO, Bonnefond M. Temporal coding organized by coupled alpha and gamma oscillations prioritize visual processing. Trends Neurosci. 2014;37(7):357–369.

104. Jacobs J, Zijlmans M, Zelmann R, et al. High-frequency electroencephalographic oscillations correlate with outcome of epilepsy surgery. Ann Neurol. 2010;67(2):209–220.

105. Gotman J. Automatic detection of seizures and spikes. J Clin Neurophysiol. 1999;16(2):130–140.

106. Tzallas AT, Oikonomou VP, Fotiadis DI. Epileptic spike detection using a Kalman filter-based approach. Conf Proc IEEE Eng Med Biol Soc. 2006;1:501–504.

107. Brown MW, 3rd, Porter BE, Dlugos DJ, et al. Comparison of novel computer detectors and human performance for spike detection in intracranial EEG. Clin Neurophysiol. 2007;118(8):1744–1752.

108. Benar CG, Chauviere L, Bartolomei F, Wendling F. Pitfalls of high-pass filtering for detecting epileptic oscillations: a technical note on "false" ripples. Clin Neurophysiol. 2010;121(3):301–310.

109. Staba RJ, Wilson CL, Bragin A, Fried I, Engel J, Jr. Quantitative analysis of high-frequency oscillations (80–500 Hz) recorded in human epileptic hippocampus and entorhinal cortex. J Neurophysiol. 2002;88(4):1743–1752.

110. Gardner AB, Worrell GA, Marsh E, Dlugos D, Litt B. Human and automated detection of high-frequency oscillations in clinical intracranial EEG recordings. Clin Neurophysiol. 2007;118(5):1134–1143.

111. Crepon B, Navarro V, Hasboun D, et al. Mapping interictal oscillations greater than 200 Hz recorded with intracranial macroelectrodes in human epilepsy. Brain. 2010;133(Pt 1):33–45.

112. Birot G, Kachenoura A, Albera L, Benar C, Wendling F. Automatic detection of fast ripples. J Neurosci Meth. 2013;213(2):236–249.

113. Burnos S, Hilfiker P, Surucu O, et al. Human intracranial high frequency oscillations (HFOs) detected by automatic time-frequency analysis. PLoS One. 2014;9(4):e94381.

114. Mina F, Benquet P, Pasnicu A, Biraben A, Wendling F. Modulation of epileptic activity by deep brain stimulation: a model-based study of frequency-dependent effects. Front Comp Neurosci. 2013;7:94.

115. Schürmann J. Pattern Classification: A Unified View of Statistical and Neural Approaches. New York: John Wiley & Sons, Inc, 1996.

116. Lotte F, Congedo M, Lecuyer A, Lamarche F, Arnaldi B. A review of classification algorithms for EEG-based brain-computer interfaces. J Neural Eng. 2007;4(2):R1–R13.

117. Delorme A, Makeig S. EEGLAB: an open source toolbox for analysis of single-trial EEG dynamics including independent component analysis. J Neurosci Meth. 2004;134(1):9–21.

118. Delorme A, Mullen T, Kothe C, et al. EEGLAB, SIFT, NFT, BCILAB, and ERICA: new tools for advanced EEG processing. Comp Intell Neurosci. 2011;2011:130714.

119. Oostenveld R, Fries P, Maris E, Schoffelen JM. FieldTrip: Open source software for advanced analysis of MEG, EEG, and invasive electrophysiological data. Comp Intell Neurosci. 2011;2011:156869.

120. Pascual-Marqui RD, Michel CM, Lehmann D. Low-resolution electromagnetic tomography: a new method for localizing electrical activity in the brain. Int J Psychophysiol. 1994;18(1):49–65.

121. Pascual-Marqui RD, Esslen M, Kochi K, Lehmann D. Functional imaging with low-resolution brain electromagnetic tomography (LORETA): a review. Methods Findings Exp Clin Pharmacol. 2002;24(Suppl C):91–95.

122. Tadel F, Baillet S, Mosher JC, Pantazis D, Leahy RM. Brainstorm: a user-friendly application for MEG/EEG analysis. Comp Intell Neurosci. 2011;2011:879716.

123. Brunet D, Murray MM, Michel CM. Spatiotemporal analysis of multichannel EEG: CARTOOL. Comp Intell Neurosci. 2011;2011:813870.

124. Hassan M, Shamas M, Khalil M, El Falou W, Wendling F. EEGNET: An open source tool for analyzing and visualizing M/EEG Connectome. PLoS One. 2015;10(9):e0138297.

125. Dai Y, Zhang W, Dickens DL, He B. Source connectivity analysis from MEG and its application to epilepsy source localization. Brain Topography. 2012;25(2):157–166.

126. Blinowska KJ, Kaminski M, Brzezicka A, Kaminski J. Application of directed transfer function and network formalism for the assessment of functional connectivity in working memory task. Philosoph Trans A. 2013;371(1997):20110614.

45 | EEG MAPPING AND SOURCE IMAGING

CHRISTOPH M. MICHEL, PHD AND BIN HE, PHD

ABSTRACT: This chapter describes methods to analyze the scalp electric field recorded with multichannel electroencephalography (EEG). With advances in high-density EEG, systems now allow fast and easy recording from 64 to 256 channels simultaneously. Pattern-recognition algorithms can characterize the topography of scalp electric fields and detect changes in topography over time and between experimental or clinical conditions. Methods for estimating the sources underlying the recorded scalp potential maps have increased the spatial resolution of EEG. The use of anatomical information in EEG source reconstruction has increased the precision of EEG source localization. Algorithms of functional connectivity applied to the source space allow determination of communication between large-scale brain networks in certain frequencies and identification of the directionality of this information flow and detection of crucial drivers in these networks. These methods have boosted the use of EEG as a functional neuroimaging method in experimental and clinical applications.

KEYWORDS: EEG, electroencephalography, source localization, high-density EEG, functional connectivity, algorithm, topography

PRINCIPAL REFERENCES

1. Michel CM, Murray MM, Lantz G, Gonzalez S, Spinelli L, Grave de Peralta R. EEG source imaging. Clin Neurophysiol. 2004;115(10):2195–222.
2. David O, Kiebel SJ, Harrison LM, Mattout J, Kilner JM, Friston KJ. Dynamic causal modeling of evoked responses in EEG and MEG. Neuroimage. 2006;30(4):1255–1272.
3. Vulliemoz S, Lemieux L, Daunizeau J, Michel CM, Duncan JS. The combination of EEG source imaging and EEG-correlated functional MRI to map epileptic networks. Epilepsia. 2010;51(4):491–505.
4. He B, Yang L, Wilke C, Yuan H. Electrophysiological imaging of brain activity and connectivity-challenges and opportunities. IEEE Trans Biomed Eng. 2011;58(7):1918–1931.
5. Michel CM, Murray MM. Towards the utilization of EEG as a brain imaging tool. Neuroimage. 2012;61(2):371–385.
6. Babiloni F, Cincotti F, Babiloni C, Carducci F, Mattia D, Astolfi L, et al. Estimation of the cortical functional connectivity with the multimodal integration of high-resolution EEG and fMRI data by directed transfer function. Neuroimage. 2005;24(1):118–131.
7. Brodbeck V, Spinelli L, Lascano AM, Wissmeier M, Vargas MI, Vulliemoz S, et al. Electroencephalographic source imaging: a prospective study of 152 operated epileptic patients. Brain. 2011;134(Pt 10):2887–2897.
8. van de Ville D, Britz J, Michel CM. EEG microstate sequences in healthy humans at rest reveal scale-free dynamics. Proc Natl Acad Sci USA. 2010;107:18179–18184.
9. Michel CM, Koenig T, Brandeis D, Gianotti LRR, Wackermann J, eds. Electrical Neuroimaging. Cambridge: Cambridge University Press, 2009.
10. He B, Ding L. Electrophysiological neuroimaging. In: He B, ed. Neural Engineering. New York: Springer, 2013:499–544.

1. INTRODUCTION

Neuronal activities in the brain generate current flows in the head volume conductor, reflected as electric potentials over the scalp, where they give rise to a specific topographical map. Proper recording and analysis of these maps are precursors for source localization and imaging. A great deal of spatial information can be derived from these maps, but their incorrect interpretation can also lead to a misleading conclusion about the putative source generators. The first part of this chapter will deal with the recording of the scalp potential fields and the characterization, description, and statistical comparison of scalp potential maps. It will also summarize analysis methods that are based on spatio-temporal characteristics of potential maps, thereby leading to data reduction and a priori constraints for subsequent source localization and imaging.

The propagation of the electric potential in the brain that is generated by the active neuronal populations is modulated by the electric conductivity properties of the different tissues and by the shape of the head. If these parameters are known the electric potentials that a given current source in the brain produces on the surface electrodes can be calculated. This so-called forward solution is the basis, albeit well studied, of every source localization method (see Chapter 4 for the biophysical basis of these processes). The second part of the chapter will discuss the electroencephalographic (EEG) forward problem and the different source and head models.

EEG source localization has evolved from equivalent dipole searching methods to distributed source estimation procedures without constraint to a few sources. However, solving the underdetermined inverse problem requires a priori assumptions based on information other than the number of sources, preferentially incorporating physiological or biophysical knowledge. The correctness of these assumptions determines the correctness of the source estimation. The third section will discuss the different source reconstruction algorithms that are currently used and show examples of applications and validations.

The spatial resolution of high-density EEG with sophisticated source localization methods in realistic geometry head models has become impressive and the images that are produced are as tempting as pictures from other functional imaging methods, particularly because they show direct neuronal signaling rather than indirect metabolic changes. But EEG has a second important attraction: the high temporal resolution. This temporal resolution combined with electrophysiological neuroimaging leads to the possibility of elucidating the temporal dynamics of neuronal signaling in large-scale neuronal networks and directly estimating network connectivity. The last section will discuss such functional connectivity methods based on EEG.

The power of EEG as a functional neuroimaging method is largely underestimated, and many impressive experimental and clinical studies using these tools have not received the attention they merit. The reasons are manifold. First, functional magnetic resonance imaging has received a unique status of being able to reduce brain activity to the underlying brain activation unambiguously. Second, misinterpretations of EEG and evoked potential waveforms due to a lack of understanding of the properties of electromagnetic fields, of the role of the reference electrode, and of the influence of non-neuronal signals such as myogenic or oculomotor sources, resulted in a number of claims that later proved to be unsubstantiated or simply wrong. Third, the EEG is somehow harmed by history. The term *EEG* is still often related to the cryptic interpretation of grapho-elements by some skilled neurophysiologists. The magnetoencephalogram (MEG), which basically measures the same neuronal activity, does not suffer from this history and is easily considered as a neuroimaging method. With this chapter we would like to diminish this incorrect historical view and show that the EEG has considerably matured and can now be considered as a powerful, flexible, and affordable imaging technology (1,2).

2. MAPPING OF THE SCALP ELECTRIC FIELD

Electrophysiological neuroimaging is based on the recording of the electric potential from a multitude of electrodes distributed over the surface of the head. From these simultaneous recordings a potential map can be constructed for any single moment in time, depicting the momentary configuration of the potential field on the scalp (11). The idea of analyzing these topographies instead of waveform morphologies was formulated decades ago (12) and has been called EEG topographical mapping. EEG mapping is a precursor to source imaging, and the proper analysis and interpretation of EEG maps can give a great deal of information about the putative sources in the brain. Most importantly, by physical laws, different map topographies must have been produced by different source configurations in the brain (13). Thus, statistical methods that allow the determination of significantly different map topographies over time or between conditions, or subjects, provide important a priori insights about whether and when differences in the source localization algorithms can be expected. Analysis of topographic maps is therefore an important step in electric source imaging (3).

In the following we discuss some practical issues related to the recording and construction of topographic maps. This concerns the number of electrodes that are needed to provide an adequate spatial sampling of the potential field. It also concerns the parametric description of the map configuration and the comparison of map topographies in a global and reference-independent way. Finally, methods to decompose maps in space and in time are discussed. Such methods allow reducing the large amount of data to the most relevant components. Further details can be found in (10).

2.1. Spatial Sampling

It is clear that proper sampling of the electromagnetic field over the whole scalp needs a large number of sensors. The MEG community has consequently quickly moved from low- to high-resolution systems, and most of the MEG laboratories are nowadays recording from over 200 channels. Until recently, this was a severe limitation for the EEG, because application of a large number of electrodes was time-consuming, uncomfortable, and expensive. However, this is no longer a limiting factor. EEG systems of up to 256 electrodes are commercially available and are easily and quickly applied, even in clinical settings (14) (Fig. 45.1).

The question of how many electrodes are needed for proper EEG mapping and source imaging is not completely answered. It depends on the spatial frequency of the scalp potential field, which is limited by the blurring caused by volume conductor effects, particularly induced by the low conductivity of the skull (15). The maximal spatial frequency has to be correctly sampled to avoid aliasing, which appears when the frequency of the measured signal is higher than the sampling frequency. In the case of discrete sampling of time-varying signals, a sampling frequency that is twice as high as the highest frequency in the signal is required to avoid aliasing (Nyquist rate). Similar rules apply to sampling in space, since the potential distribution is only sampled at discrete measurement points (electrodes) (16). Spatial frequencies of the potential field that are higher than the spatial sampling frequency (i.e., the distance between electrodes) will distort the map topography (17) and will lead to misinterpretation of maps and consequently to potential mislocalization of the sources.

Many years ago, researchers tried to estimate the maximal spatial frequency of the scalp electric field based on theoretical considerations and modeling. These works suggested that inter-electrode distances of ~2 to 3 cm are preferable (18) for proper sampling of the field, which would lead to ~100 required electrodes. Several studies performed simulations using dipole forward modeling to calculate the dipole localization error of different source localization algorithms when different numbers of electrodes were used (3,19). These studies showed that the localization precision increases with increasing number of electrodes up to ~100 electrodes for fully distributed inverse solution algorithms. In addition, these simulations also showed that increasing the number of electrodes could remedy the localization error of deep sources.

Several experimental studies used subsampling techniques to establish the number of electrodes that are needed to correctly reconstruct potential maps and localize the sources. Michel et al. (3) demonstrated incorrect lateralization of the source estimated for the P100 component of the visual evoked potential when down-sampling from 46 to 19 electrodes and showed that an incomplete coverage of the scalp surface can lead to complete misplacement of the sources. Luu et al. (20) and Lantz et al. (21) used the down-sampling method in clinical data to evaluate the correctness of localization of pathological activity. Luu et al. (20) studied patients with acute focal ischemic stroke recorded with 128 electrodes and down-sampled to 64, 32, and 19 channels. Visual comparison of the EEG maps with radiographic images led to the conclusion that more than 64 electrodes were desirable to avoid mislocalizations of the affected region. Lantz et al. (21) used the down-sampling approach on 123-electrode recordings from patients

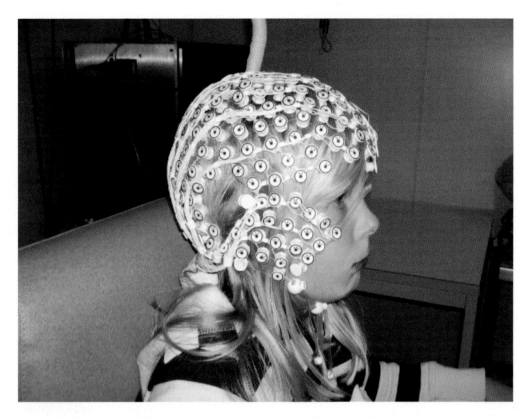

Figure 45.1. High-resolution EEG. *Example of an EEG system that allows fast application of 256 electrodes. The electrodes are connected by thin rubber bands and each contains a small sponge that touches the subject's head directly (180). The nets are soaked in saline before being put on the subject's head. The entire net is applied at once and needs no skin abrasion or electrode paste. (HydroCel Geodesic Sensor Net, Electrical Geodesics Inc., Eugene, OR, USA)*

with partial epilepsy. Fourteen patients with different focus localization were recorded before successful surgery; thus, the location of the epileptic focus was retrospectively known. Several interictal spikes were manually identified and then down-sampled to 63 and 31 electrodes. Source localization was applied to each single spike and the distance of the source maximum to the resected area was determined and statistically compared between the different electrode sets. Significant smaller localization error was found when using 63 versus 31 electrodes. Accuracy still systematically increased from 63 to 123 electrodes, but less significantly (Fig. 45.2A). The study by Sohrabpour et al. (19) used the same method in a pediatric population of epileptic patients and evaluated the localization error by comparing the source localization with the seizure onset zone defined by intracranial recordings. A continuous increase in localization precision was again demonstrated when the number of electrodes was increased up to 128, with significant improvement observed when using 64 versus 32 electrodes (see Fig. 45.2B).

The above-described experimental studies estimate that ~64 to 128 electrodes are desirable for accurate spatial sampling and reconstruction of the scalp potential field. However, as shown by Ryynänen et al. (17,22) in computer simulation studies, these estimations were made when we assume a conductivity ratio of ~1:80 between skull and brain, as proposed by Rush and Driscoll (23). These traditional values were used in most of the above explained simulation and down-sampling studies, but they are most probably misestimated (24–26). If the conductivity of the skull is higher, the spatial blurring is smaller and the

spatial frequency is higher. He and colleagues (27) measured the scalp and subdural potentials simultaneously during cortical current injection and used them to estimate the brain-to-skull conductivity ratio. These measurements suggested that the averaged brain-to-skull conductivity ratio is ~1:25 when using the three-sphere head model (26) and ~1:20 when using the realistic geometry finite element head model (27). In newborns the skull thickness is approximately seven to eight times lower than in adults, leading to a ratio of ~1:14 (28). Ryynänen et al. (17) showed that with this ratio, spatial resolution still increases with 256 versus 128 electrodes. Grieve et al. (28) also suggested that a 256-electrode array is needed in infants to obtain a spatial sampling error of <10%. However, larger electrode arrays are also more influenced by measurement noise, which affects the spatial resolution. As suggested by Ryynänen et al. (17,22), the measurement noise is a critical limiting factor for the spatial resolution of high-density EEG systems. Thus there is an important interplay between the number of electrodes, measurement noise, and conductivity values of the different compartments of the head.

Given that the spatial frequency of the EEG is higher than previously assumed, the general assumption that ~6 to 10 cm^2 of cortex has to be active in order to be detected, as distinct electrophysiological events on the scalp surface (29,30) can be questioned. In Chapter 2, the factors that determine the size of a cortical area responsible for producing a measurable EEG/MEG signal are discussed. Density of active neurons, correlation among them, and the decay of the amplitude with distance are important factors. In the study by Zelmann et al. (31) simultaneous scalp and intracranial recordings provided evidence that

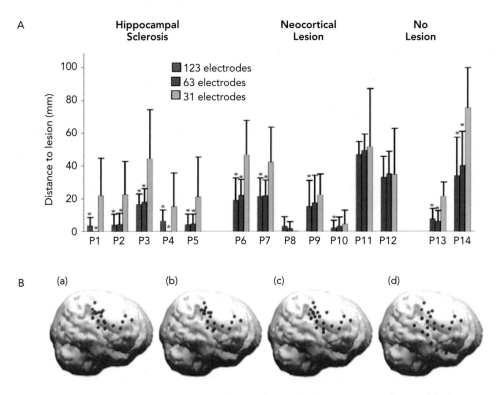

A
Hippocampal Sclerosis | Neocortical Lesion | No Lesion

Figure 45.2. Influence of number of electrodes on source localization. *A: Evaluation of source localization precision of interictal discharges in 14 epileptic patients, recorded with 123 electrodes. Single spikes were localized with the LORETA linear inverse solution in the individual brain and the distance of the source maximum to the resected area was measured. Mean ± standard deviation (across spikes) of the distance was compared between the original high-resolution recording and with down-sampling of the same data to fewer channels (but still equally distributed). The bar graph shows the mean distance to the lesion. Stars indicate significant differences between the different number of electrodes. A clear and significant amelioration of the localization precision was observed when the number of recording channels was increased. B: Source location of interictal spikes in a pediatric patient obtained using (a) 128, (b) 96, (c) 64, and (d) 32 electrodes. The blue dot represents the location of maximum of the sLORETA inverse solution. The red dot represents the ECoG electrodes marked as seizure onset zone electrodes. A: From (181), modified after (182). B: From (19).*

high-frequency oscillations (HFOs; frequency range 80–500 Hz) can be recorded on the scalp despite their low amplitude and their very focal generators. Lu et al. (32) further demonstrated that focal HFO sources can be not only detected with EEG but also correctly localized with source imaging methods. The explanation for the detection of such focal events is that there is no specific increased attenuation of high frequencies by the skull, as sometimes stated in textbooks. The conductivity of the skull remains the same from 1 Hz to 10 kHz (24,33). Since the noise level in the range of HFOs is smaller than at the typical EEG frequencies, they can be detected on the scalp despite the low amplitude (31). These studies clearly again demonstrated the effect of spatial under-sampling: electrophysiological events of such small spatial extent can only be detected by proper sampling of the electric field. To illustrate this fact, Zelmann et al. (31) simulated distributed sources of ~1 cm² in size. They showed that only 14% of these small sources were visible on the scalp with the 10-20 system, 38% with the 10-10 system, and 71% with 256 electrodes.

Nevertheless, these results do not necessarily mean that imperfect spatial sampling precludes source localization and imaging. Some data did suggest that even with a low number of electrodes, we can gain important insight about the underlying brain electric sources by applying source localization algorithms (34,35), particularly when the precision request remains on the level of larger regions of interest.

2.2. Topographic Analysis

The traditional analysis of EEG and evoked potentials relies on waveforms. Parameters of interest are thereby changes in amplitude or frequency, or peaks at certain latencies time-locked to stimulus presentation. These measures are ambiguous because the EEG is by definition a bipolar signal. Changes of the location of one of the two electrodes will change the values of the above parameters. This ambiguity is well known and led to a large discussion in the 1990s on the reference dependency of the EEG and the question of the correct recording reference for a certain experimental or clinical condition (36,37).

This reference problem of the EEG is less of an issue when topographic analysis methods are applied and is completely resolved for source localization and imaging. The potential map topography does not depend on the reference. The reference changes only the zero level (DC shift), but the topographic features of the map remain unaffected (38). Elimination of the DC shift can be achieved by calculating the so-called common average reference at each moment in time, which removes the potential common to all electrodes (12). However, topographic analysis of EEG data in the frequency domain is *not* reference-free (39,40). This is also a problem for connectivity analysis on the sensor level (41,41a). In such applications, the choice of the EEG reference is a critical issue since reference-free potential measures are not possible. One offline re-referencing method that shows optimal properties is the so-called infinity reference (42): the reference electrode standardization technique (REST) proposes to solve the generalized linear minimum norm solution with a given head-model and a given recording reference. Since the source is not affected by the reference, a forward solution can then be calculated for an infinity reference potential, at the expense of solving the EEG inverse problem. These reconstructed standardized potentials have been suggested to improve mapping of frequency power (43), evoked potentials (44), and coherency (41).

One way to sharpen the spatial details of the scalp potential maps is to calculate the scalp current source density, or the surface Laplacian of the potential (45,46). The surface Laplacian of the scalp potential is the second spatial derivative of the potential field in the local curvature in $\mu V/cm^2$. The surface Laplacian has been mainly derived from unipolar potential recordings on the scalp, using algorithms such as the finite difference algorithm (47), spherical spline algorithm (48), or realistic geometry spline algorithm (49). The surface Laplacian has been widely used in applications when one wishes to enhance the sensitivity to local activity. It can be interpreted as an estimation of the current density entering or exiting the scalp. It emphasizes superficial sources because deeper sources produce smaller potentials and much smaller surface Laplacian on the surface. Like the other topographic measures that will be described below, the surface Laplacian estimates are independent of the position of the recording reference, because (as with the common average reference) the potential common to all electrodes is automatically removed (50).

Scalp potential maps can be characterized by their strength and their topography. A reference-independent measure of map strength is the global field power (GFP) (51)). GFP is the standard deviation of the potentials at all electrodes of an average-reference map. It is defined as:

$$GFP = \sqrt{\sum_{i=1}^{N} (u_i - \bar{u})^2 \bigg/ N} \tag{1}$$

where u_i is the voltage of the map u at the electrode i, $\bar{u}$ is the average voltage of all electrodes of the map u (the average reference), and N is the number of electrodes of the map u. Scalp potential fields with pronounced peaks and troughs and steep gradients (i.e., very "hilly" maps) will result in high GFP, while GFP is low in maps that have a "flat" appearance with shallow gradients. GFP is a one-number measure of the map at each moment in time. Displaying this measure over time allows us to identify moments of high signal-to-noise ratio, corresponding to moments of high global neuronal synchronization (52).

A reference-independent measure of topographic differences of scalp potential maps is the so-called global map dissimilarity measure (GMD) (51), defined as:

$$GMD = \sqrt{\frac{1}{N} \sum_{i=1}^{N} \left\{ \frac{u_i - \bar{u}}{\sqrt{\sum_{i=1}^{N} \frac{(u_i - \bar{u})^2}{N}}} - \frac{v_i - \bar{v}}{\sqrt{\sum_{i=1}^{N} \frac{(v_i - \bar{v})^2}{N}}} \right\}^2} \tag{2}$$

where u_i is the voltage of map u at the electrode i, v_i is the voltage of map v at the electrode i, $\bar{u}$ is the average voltage of all electrodes of map u, $\bar{v}$ is the average voltage of all electrodes of map v, and N is the total number of electrodes. To ensure that only topographic differences are taken into account, the two maps that are compared are first normalized by dividing the potential values at each electrode of a given map by its GFP.

The GMD is 0 when two maps are equal and maximally reaches 2 when two maps have the same topography with reversed polarity. It can be shown that the GMD is equivalent to the spatial Pearson's product-moment correlation coefficient between the potentials of the two maps to be compared (53).

If two maps differ in topography independent of their strength, this directly indicates that the two maps were generated by a different configuration of sources in the brain (3,54). However, the inverse is not necessarily true: an infinite number of source configurations may produce the same scalp potential topography (13). The GMD calculation is therefore considered as a first step in defining whether different sources were involved in the two processes being compared. When comparing subsequent maps in time using the GMD, periods where source configuration changes appeared can be defined. It is interesting to note that the GMD inversely correlates with the GFP: GMD is high when GFP is low. In other words, maps tend to be stable during high GFP and change the configuration when GFP is low (Fig. 45.3). The GMD is itself not a statistical measure. However, if two groups of maps are compared, a statistical statement of the significance of the topographic differences can be made. This is achieved by performing non-parametric randomization tests based on the GMD values (55). Koenig et al. (56) extended the use of randomization test on map topographies to detect reliable events (e.g., event-related potential [ERP] components) across single trials or across subjects.

2.3. Spatio-Temporal Decomposition

Source localization procedures can be applied to multichannel EEG and ERP data at any instant in time. With the high sampling rate of modern EEG systems, easily exceeding 1,000 Hz, this leads to a large amount of data from which the relevant information must be extracted. Consequently, experimenters typically pre-determine relevant events within a continuous time series of data to which source analysis will be applied. This particularly concerns ERP research, where peaks in certain time windows at certain electrodes are identified and spatially analyzed (57). This traditional approach is, however, less tenable with high-density EEG and ERP recordings because (1) different scalp sites have different peak latencies and (2) the waveforms (and thus the peaks) at certain electrodes change when the position of the reference electrode is changed.

An alternative to the traditional pre-selection of relevant events based on ERP waveforms is to define components on the basis of the topography of the potential field (58). Most commonly, some kinds of spatial factor analysis methods are used for this purpose (see also Chapter 36 for examples). These methods produce a series of factors that represent a weighted sum of all recorded channels across time. The aim of this factor analysis

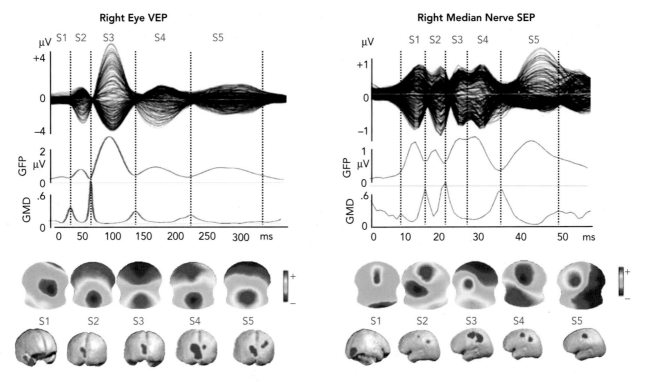

Right Eye VEP

Right Median Nerve SEP

Figure 45.3. Spatial analysis of evoked potentials. *Example of 256 channel visual (VEP) and somatosensory (SEP) evoked potentials. VEP from full-field checkerboard reversal presented to the right eye only (left eye covered). SEP from electrical stimulation of the right median nerve. Data represent the grand mean of >20 subjects. Top row: overlaid traces of all 256 channels against the average reference. Second row: Global field power curve as a measure of field strength indicates five dominant peaks in both EPs. Third row: Global map dissimilarity curve measuring topography differences between successive time points. It shows low values during extended periods and sharp peaks at moments of low GFP. Fourth row: Potential maps (seen from top, nose up, left ear left) that were derived from a k-means cluster analysis of the whole datasets. In both EPs, five maps best explained the data. Each one dominated a given period as determined by spatial correlation analysis. Vertical dashed lines mark these periods. Last row: Distributed linear inverse solution applied to each of the five maps, revealing activation and propagation of visual and sensory-motor cortex, respectively. Note that the first period represents extra-cortical activity in both cases (activity in the right retina for the VEP and in the brainstem for the SEP). Both areas were not included in the solution space, leading to incorrect localization in the source estimation. (For more details see (92)).*

approach is to find a limited number of optimal factors that best represent a given dataset. The load for each of these factors (i.e., the goodness of fit) then varies in time. Each factor represents a certain potential topography—that is, a prototypical map. Source localization applied to these maps results in a limited number of putative sources in the brain that explain a full time series of multichannel EEG data with time-varying strength.

A commonly used variant of spatial factor analyses is the principal component analysis (PCA) (59)). The first factor of the PCA solution accounts for the maximum possible amount of data variance, and each next orthogonal factor accounts for the maximum possible residual variance. Since factors that contribute little to the explained variance can be neglected, the PCA is a powerful exploratory tool to reduce complex multi-channel EEG data in space and time. It has been repeatedly applied to ERP studies with the aim of extracting ERP components whose variance is related to a given experimental condition. It can provide useful information on how a given experimental manipulation affects ERP components without any a priori assumption about the shape or number of components in the dataset (60,61).

The PCA does not allow for cross-correlations between activities corresponding to separate factors and thus excludes linear dependencies between the factor maps. However, it does not exclude dependencies based on higher-order correlations.

The factor analysis method that also removes these higher-order relations is called independent component analysis (ICA) (62; see also Chapter 45). The objective of the ICA is sometimes illustrated by the so-called cocktail party problem, where the ICA allows decomposing a sound record from a party into the independent contributions of the individual persons. Like the PCA, the ICA produces a weight coefficient for each factor. Each factor is supposed to represent a temporally independent component.

The ICA can be very useful for detecting and removing artifacts such as eye-blinks (63), or artifacts produced by brain-independent sources such as the ballistocardiogram artifact of the EEG recorded in a magnetic resonance imaging (MRI) scanner (64,65), although negative results have been reported as well (66). The ICA has also been used for decomposing the brain activity into a number of maps that can then be used to determine the sources of these statistically independent brain processes (62,67). Recent source localization studies indicated the excellent performance and applicability of ICA to EEG source imaging, such as localizing seizure sources from recorded ictal EEG (68).

An alternative to the above-described component analysis approaches is the so-called microstate segmentation method (69). It is based on the highly reproducible observation that the topography of the EEG or ERP potential maps remains stable for several tens of milliseconds and then abruptly switches to a new configuration in which it remains stable again. This can easily be seen in the ERP examples in Figure 45.3 by the stable low global dissimilarity over extended time periods separated by sharp dissimilarity peaks indicating periods of topographic change. The same observation holds for spontaneous EEG, if polarity inversion caused by the intrinsic oscillatory activity of the generator processes is ignored (70,71) (Fig. 45.4). This fundamental observation led to the proposal to apply cluster analysis to the dataset to identify a set of topographies that explain a maximum amount of the variance of the data (72). The difference from the above-described factor analysis approach is that the microstate model allows only one single topography to occur at one moment in time. Evidently, each topography can represent multiple simultaneously active sources, but they are active together for a certain time period, forming a large-scale neuronal network configuration that is expressed as unique stable map topography. During the period of stable topography, the strength of the field varies, indicating different levels of synchronization of the simultaneously active areas. In contrast to the ICA-based models of independent brain processes that overlap in time, the microstate model proposes one global brain state per time period, consisting of an interdependent and synchronized network (73). This corresponds well to the neuronal workspace model, which suggests that episodes of coherent activity last a certain amount of time (~100 msec) and are separated by sharp transitions (74,75), as well as to the proposal that neurocognitive networks evolve through a sequence of quasi-stable coordinated states rather than a continuous flow of neuronal activity (76,77). Cross-validation methods following cluster analysis have shown that a very limited number of map topographies are needed to explain extended periods of spontaneous EEG, and that these few configurations follow each other according to certain rules. Several studies over the last 20 years (for reviews see (73,78,79)) have shown that the temporal properties of the microstates are selectively modulated by different states of consciousness such as hypnosis (80), meditation (81), and sleep (82), and are altered in diseases such as schizophrenia (83–85) and dementia (86). In normal subjects, the duration and the frequency of appearance of the four most dominant microstate configurations vary with age (71). It has been shown that subjects can actively modulate microstate presence using neurofeedback (87). Simultaneous EEG and functional MRI (fMRI) recordings showed close relations between the resting-state networks defined by correlated BOLD activity in the fMRI and the EEG microstates (88,89). This relation, despite the different time scales in which fMRI BOLD signals and EEG microstates fluctuate, is partly explained by the fact that microstate time series show scale-free monofractal behavior over six dyadic scales that cover the time scales between 256 msec and 16 sec (i.e., the temporal scales at which microstate changes and BOLD oscillations can be observed, respectively) (9,90).

Concerning ERPs, the cluster analysis is an efficient way to determine different ERP components on the basis of their topography (91). The statistical specificity of these component maps for different experimental conditions can then be assessed by spatial fitting procedures using the global dissimilarity value as metric (55). Such methods can be used for an objective analysis of clinical evoked potentials, for example in multiple sclerosis (92). It has been used in numerous experimental ERP studies on sensory and cognitive information processing and has allowed the creation of a microstate dictionary for different brain functions (93,94). Source localization applied to these microstate maps has proven to be an efficient way to describe those brain areas that are crucially implicated in the processing of stimuli and that differ depending on the task demands (91,95) (see Fig. 45.3).

3. EEG FORWARD PROBLEM

In this section, we introduce methods for solving the so-called EEG forward problem, which deals with how to model (1) the neuronal sources within the brain volume and (2) the head volume conduction process in order to quantitatively link neuronal electrical sources with the electric potentials over the scalp. Solving the EEG forward problem can help us understand the relationship between neuronal sources and the recorded EEG signals, and is also an integrative part of the EEG source localization—the inverse problem, which will be discussed in Section 4.

3.1. Source Models

The primary sources of EEG are considered to be the post-synaptic currents flowing through the apical dendritic trees of cortical pyramidal cells. Such neuronal currents, when viewed from a location on the scalp surface that is relatively remote from where the neuronal excitation takes place (far-field), can be modeled as an electrical current dipole composed of a pair of current source and sink with an infinitely small inter-distance (relative to the distance from the dipole to scalp electrodes). When the brain electrical activity is confined to a few focal regions, each of these focal areas of neuronal excitation may be modeled as an equivalent current dipole (ECD) based on the far-field theory (for the biophysical concepts see Chapters 2 and 4). While the ECD is a simplified model and higher-order equivalent source models such as the quadrupole have also been studied to represent the neural electric sources (96), the dipole model has so far been the most commonly used brain electric source model and is the basis for dipole fitting methods as well as for distributed current density source localization and imaging methods.

The initially utilized equivalent current dipole source model has been largely replaced by distributed current source models (97,98). The essence of the distributed current source modeling is to model the neuronal activities over a small region by a current dipole located at each region. The brain activity with any distribution of neuronal currents can be approximately represented by a source model consisting of a distribution of current dipoles that are evenly placed within the entire brain volume. At each location, three orthogonal dipoles can be used in that the weighted combination of them is capable of representing an averaged current flow with an arbitrary direction in the region. Such source model is usually called the volume

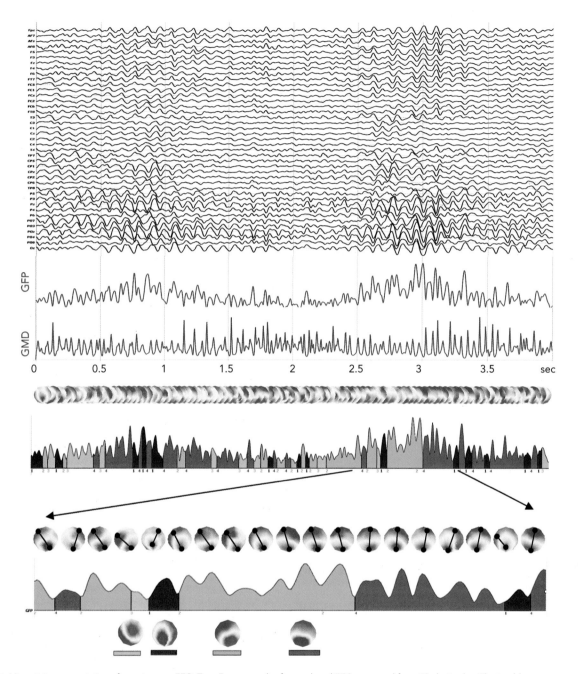

Figure 45.4. Microstate segmentation of spontaneous EEG. *Top: Four seconds of eyes-closed EEG measured from 42 electrodes. The two blue curves represent the global field power (GFP) and the global map dissimilarity, respectively. A series of potential maps illustrate the data that have been submitted to a k-means cluster analysis with ignoring strength and polarity. Four maps best explained the whole 4 sec of data. Examples of the four prototypical microstate maps across subjects are illustrated on the bottom (taken from (88)). On the GFP curve below the map series, the time periods during which each map was dominant are marked in different colors. A shorter period is zoomed in and all maps during this period are shown. Marking and connecting the extreme potentials illustrates the stability of topography during each period. From (181).*

current density model (97). The brain anatomical information can also be used to constrain the current source space to the cortical gray matter due to the dominant presence of large pyramidal cells. Such anatomical constraints can be obtained from existing structural neuroimaging modalities, particularly T1-weighted MRI. The current source orientations can be further constrained to be perpendicular to the cortical surface, because the columnar organization of neurons within the cortical gray matter constrains the regional current flow in either outward or inward normal direction with respect to the local cortical patch (99), and the gray matter thickness (~2–4 mm)

is much smaller relative to the "source-to-sensor" distance (50). Under such cortical constraints, the source model is usually called the cortical current density model, in which current dipoles distribute over a surface in parallel to the epicortical surface.

All of the above current source models are often referred to as distributed current density models. Physically, any bioelectric source activity can be represented by a continuous distribution of primary current density. Mathematically, the current density and current dipole share the identical form of equations for computing the extracellular potential, supporting the use of distributed current dipoles to approximate the continuous current density distribution. The dipole distribution may be viewed as a discretized version of the continuous current density distribution in the space domain. Each of these current dipoles represents the regional neuronal activity, and its amplitude represents the amount of synchronized neuronal activity in the local region.

In addition to current dipole-based source models, the current monopole model (100) was also proposed to equivalently represent brain electric activity. Mathematically, the current monopole model can also represent the source activities in a sense that it produces almost the same electric potentials on the scalp electrodes. As discussed in detail in Chapter 2, current monopoles can contribute to EEG signals but do not contribute to MEG signals, which may explain the differences that have been described between MEG and EEG in simultaneous recordings.

3.2. Volume Conductor Models

When the source model is determined, the EEG forward problem consists of obtaining the distribution of electric potential ϕ on the scalp surface, given any known distribution of current density $\bar{j}$ inside the brain as well as conductivity values throughout the head volume. Such solution is usually called the EEG forward solution for a given head volume conductor model. The head volume conductor model refers to our assumption about the shape and conductivity properties of the tissues of head. Head volume conductor models include the infinite homogeneous model, single-sphere model, three-concentric-spheres model, four-concentric-spheres model, adaptive local spherical model, realistic geometry homogenous head model, realistic geometry multicompartment head model, and realistic geometry inhomogeneous head model (1,2).

The simplest EEG forward solution is that in the infinite homogeneous model, where the entire space is assumed to be occupied by a homogeneous conductive medium (98,101). The electric potential over the scalp electrodes can then be given as:

$$\Phi = \frac{1}{4\pi\sigma}\int_V \nabla\left(\frac{1}{r}\right)\cdot\bar{j}^i\, dv \qquad (3)$$

where the source element $\bar{j}^i\, dv$ behaves like a dipole source, with a field that varies as $1/r^2$, and ∇ represents the gradient operator. The impressed current density $\bar{j}^i$, representing neuronal currents, may be interpreted as an equivalent dipole source density, which behaves as a fundamental driving force establishing the electric potentials within the head volume conductor with an electrical conductivity σ. Eq. (3) can be transformed into another representation that illustrates the monopole source model:

$$\Phi = \frac{1}{4\pi\sigma}\int_V \left(\frac{1}{r}\right)\nabla\cdot\bar{j}^i\, dv \qquad (4)$$

where the divergence of impressed current density $\nabla\cdot\bar{j}^i$ can be interpreted as volume current density, a scalar quantity that may be considered as current monopole in the brain.

A more reasonable representation of the head is a series of spherical models, including a single-sphere model (102), three-concentric-spheres model (23,103), and four-concentric-spheres model (104). In these spherical models, the shape of the head is approximated by spherical surfaces, including the scalp, the skull surface, the brain surface, and so forth. In such cases, the electric potentials over the scalp surface (the outer sphere) due to a current dipole can be derived analytically for the single-sphere model, or by use of special function for the multiple-spheres models. Since the low-conductivity layer of the skull smears significantly the electric potential, the three-spheres model (brain, skull, and scalp), in which the skull layer is incorporated, has been used widely and found to be a good approximation to head volume conductor when the head shape is ignored. Further, the cerebrospinal fluid layer can also be incorporated as in the four-spheres model (104), although there is no converging agreement that it must be incorporated when modeling the head volume conductor.

We should note that the influence of the inhomogeneities of the tissues of the head as volume conductor affect the EEG and the MEG differently, since the brain and surrounding tissues behave as a medium with constant magnetic permeability. Therefore, the magnetic field, in contrast to the electric field, is not directly influenced by those layers for a given current source. On the other hand, head electrical conductivity inhomogeneities will result in secondary currents that generate external magnetic fields in addition to the primary neuronal currents. The effect of head conductivity inhomogeneity to the MEG is reflected through the secondary currents.

A major disadvantage of the spherical head models is that they do not make any distinction between areas that generate electrical activity (gray matter) and those that do not (white matter and ventricles). Constraining the source space to the gray matter of the individual brain is an important anatomical constraint that improves the accuracy of the EEG forward solution. A simple straightforward way is to map the individual segmented MRI to a sphere and use the analytic multi-shell spherical model described above, but with the solution space constrained to the individual gray matter (105) (Fig. 45.5A). This spherical model with anatomical constraints (SMAC) can be improved by an adaptive local spherical model (LSMAC) where the lead field is calculated iteratively using a spherical model with a different radius for each electrode position (106).

More advanced EEG forward solutions have used numerical techniques to take into consideration both the conductivity inhomogeneity and the geometry of the head. The most popular EEG forward solution is based on the boundary element method (BEM) (107,108). He et al. (107) first reported the use of BEM in solving the EEG forward and inverse problem using a realistic geometry homogeneous head model. The skull's low-conductivity layer was incorporated later by (108) and others. In particular, the numerical treatment of the low-conductivity skull layer developed by Hämäläinen and Sarvas (108) made the BEM forward solution widely used for EEG as well as MEG studies. An example of the three-shell BEM head model is illustrated in Figure 45.5B, as derived from structural MRI of a human subject.

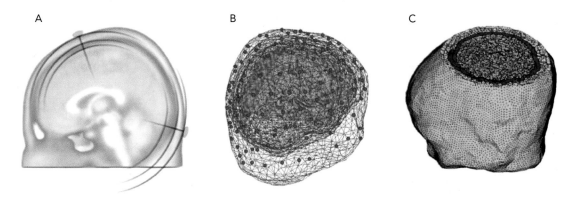

Figure 45.5. Head models. **A:** *Illustration of the LSMAC head model: local radiuses of the scalp and skull are calculated, under each electrode position, to generate different sets of three shell spherical models (from (106)).* **B:** *A realistic geometry multi-shell boundary element head model as derived from structural MRI of a human subject (136). The scalp, skull, and brain surfaces are represented by a number of surface triangles. Brown and blue surfaces refer to the right and left cortical surfaces. Pink circles refer to the scalp electrodes.* **C:** *A realistic geometry inhomogeneous finite element head model as derived from structural MRI and CT of a human subject (183). Green, gray, blue, and yellow regions refer to the scalp, skull, cerebrospinal fluid, and brain. Red refers to the subdural pad of the ECoG electrode array, which has low electrical conductivity. The red layer is not displayed continuously in this figure due to the angle of view.*

In addition to the boundary element method, which provides forward solutions when the head can be modeled by the multicompartment model with homogeneous conductivity profiles within each compartment, the finite element method (FEM) has been further used to handle the inhomogeneous conductivity distribution within the head (109) (see Fig. 45.5C). The FEM modeling allows proper handling of the inhomogeneity of head tissues, including those caused by surgical alterations such as the very-low-conductivity subdural pad of electrocorticography (ECoG) electrodes (183). The FEM forward solutions enable the incorporation of the realistic geometries and inhomogeneous conductivities of the head, even allowing inclusion of the anisotropic conductivity distribution of the white matter (110). The challenge of using FEM to solve the EEG forward problem is not the FEM algorithm, which has been fairly well developed, but the need to build an FEM mesh model of the head from MRI or computed tomography (CT) images. It remains a laborious effort to build FEM head models from a subject's MRI. Alternative efforts, such as the finite difference method, have been reported to solve the EEG forward problem in which the finite difference grids can be reasonably easily built from the MRI of a subject. However, it is still not a straightforward procedure to automatically segment and classify head tissues into the finite difference model. For a review of image segmentation for the purpose of solving the EEG forward problem, see (111). All of these numerical techniques must use the anatomical information provided by other structural imaging modalities, particularly T1- and proton-density-weighted MRI, in order to segment different brain tissues (i.e., the gray matter and the white matter) and head structures (i.e., cerebrospinal fluid, skull, and scalp).

Birot et al. (112) directly compared the BEM, the FEM, and the simpler LSMAC model in 38 epileptic patients who were recorded with high-density (128–256 channels) EEG. The source localization maximum of a distributed inverse solution (see below) was evaluated with respect to intracranial recordings in the same patient and to the distance to the surgical resection. The study suggested that in this specific clinical application (epilepsy) and for the source localization algorithm used, the use of the more complex and difficult-to-implement head models is not a crucial factor for an accurate source localization: for all three head models, at least 74% of the source maxima were within the resection in patients having a positive postoperative outcome. The median distance from the source maximum to the nearest intracranial electrode showing interictal discharges was 13.2, 15.6, and 15.6 mm for LSMAC, BEM, and FEM, respectively.

Diffusion tensor magnetic resonance imaging (DT-MRI) provides a means to estimate the anisotropic conductivity of the cerebral white matter (109), which may further improve the accuracy of the EEG forward solution. The white matter anisotropy is caused by the bundled axon fibers, which restrict the direction of ionic movements (109). While a computer simulation study (109) suggested that the white matter conductivity anisotropy may affect the EEG forward and inverse solutions, a recent experimental study suggested otherwise. Lee et al. (110) conducted a human study to localize the sources in primary visual cortex using the single dipole solution and compared the results with the fMRI activation under the same visual stimuli in the same subjects. Their results indicated that use of the anisotropic white matter model did not return significantly different solutions from that using the isotropic white matter model. Further experimental investigation is needed to examine the effects of white matter anisotropy in other brain regions.

4. EEG INVERSE PROBLEM—SOURCE IMAGING

The EEG inverse problem refers to the reconstruction of brain electric sources from scalp-recorded EEG signals. In experimental and clinical studies, it is desirable to image

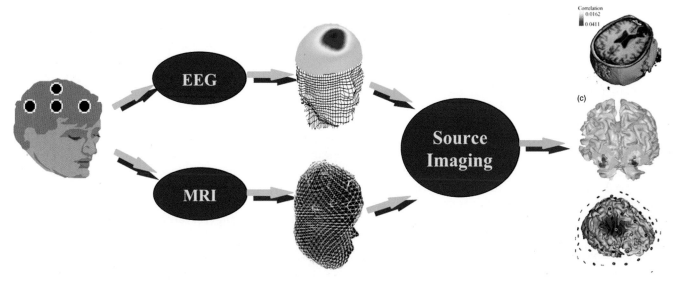

Figure 45.6. Schematic diagram of EEG source imaging. Adapted from (2).

the neuronal activity that generates recordable scalp EEG signals. When the neuronal activity is assumed to be localized in a few focal regions, the problem is usually referred to as the source localization problem. Source localization methods have been found to be particularly useful in localizing epileptogenic foci in epilepsy patients. On the other hand, when the brain activity is not localized in a few focal areas, one needs to image the distribution of neural electrical sources within the brain. This problem becomes the so-called source imaging problem, which will include source localization since focal sources are special cases of distributed sources. Figure 45.6 illustrates the EEG source imaging approach from noninvasive multichannel scalp EEG recordings to three-dimensional brain source distributions with the aid of anatomical information that is readily available via T1-weighted MRI.

4.1. Dipole Source Localization

The most classic solution to the EEG inverse problem is the so-called dipole source localization (DSL). This approach is applicable when the primary generators of scalp-recorded EEG signals are localized in one or a few small regions within the brain. Given a specific dipole source model, DSL can yield solutions to the EEG inverse problem by using a non-linear multidimensional optimization procedure to estimate the dipole parameters that can best explain the observed scalp potential measurements in a least-square sense (107,113). Further improvement of the DSL has been shown by combining EEG with MEG data, which may increase information content and improve the overall signal-to-noise ratio (114) (see also Chapter 35), or integrated with fMRI (see Section 4.5 and Chapter 46 for details).

The EEG dipole source localization can be solved for single "snapshots" of the measured scalp EEG (115) or for a time series of EEG measurements, which is sometimes termed spatiotemporal source localization (113).

All equivalent dipole localization algorithms need a priori knowledge of the number and class of the underlying dipole sources. If the number of dipoles is underestimated for a given model, then the DSL inverse solution is biased by the missing dipoles. On the other hand, if too many dipoles are specified, then spurious dipoles may be introduced.

The EEG DSL solution can be further improved when prior information is available with regard to the possible solution space. If the observed EEG signals are known to be mainly produced by cortical sources, then the solution space can be restricted to the cortex while excluding subcortical source locations. In particular situations when a priori information is known with respect to the possible source region (e.g., the sensory evoked potentials data, or based on preliminary diagnosis of the epilepsy), the solution space can be restricted to only half of the brain or even a certain lobe.

The EEG dipole source localization was an effective tool in detection of epileptic foci (116), presurgical localization of sensorimotor cortex, and some other applications. However, recent development in distributed brain source imaging has offered more exciting options to image and localize brain sources from scalp EEG signals. These methods do not make a priori assumption as to the number of dipoles and dipolar nature of sources, and will be discussed below.

4.2. Distributed Source Imaging

In the EEG research community the dipole source localization has been largely replaced by distributed source imaging methods. Such distributed imaging approaches are motivated by the need to image brain electric activity that may not be limited to a few focal sources, and to minimize the error due to misspecification of the number of dipole sources.

Unlike the point dipole source models, the distributed source models do not make any ad hoc assumption as to the number or configuration of brain electric sources. Instead, the equivalent sources are distributed over the source space.

For example, the distributed source model may consist of a large number of current dipoles (e.g., 5,000–7,000) placed over the three-dimensional brain volume (97) or over the gray matter of cortex (99,105). Regardless of the current source models being used, the current dipoles (or monopoles) are fixed at preset locations so they are not movable. The parameters to be estimated are the dipole moments (or monopole strength), which are estimated by minimizing the difference between the measurements and source model predicted scalp potentials.

Assuming quasi-static condition and the linear properties of the head volume conductor, the brain electric sources and the scalp EEG could be mathematically described by the following linear matrix equation:

$$\bar{\varphi} = A\bar{X} + \bar{n} \qquad (5)$$

where $\bar{\varphi}$ refers to scalp EEG measurements, $\bar{X}$ is the source distribution, $\bar{n}$ refers to measurement noise, and A is the transfer matrix from brain sources to the scalp EEG. So the distributed source imaging is to estimate the source distribution $\bar{X}$ from the noninvasive scalp EEG measurements $\bar{\varphi}$. Mathematically, this is equivalent to designing an inverse filter B, which can project the measured data into the solution space:

$$\bar{X} = B\bar{\varphi} \qquad (6)$$

Eq. (6) indicates that the distributed source imaging can be a linear inverse problem, which avoids the difficulty of a nonlinear multidimensional optimization problem as in the dipole source localization approach. However, the EEG linear inverse approach is underdetermined because the number of unknown distributed sources is larger than the limited number of scalp EEG electrodes. Additional constraints have to be imposed in order to obtain unique and well-posed linear inverse solutions. A well-studied solution to this linear inverse problem is the so-called general inverse, which is also termed the minimum norm least-squares (MNLS) inverse, minimizing the least-square error of the estimated inverse solution $\bar{X}$ under the constraint $\bar{\varphi} = A\bar{X}$ in the absence of noise (117). Variations of the MNLS include the lead-field normalized weighted minimum norm (WMN) (118), low-resolution brain electromagnetic tomography (LORETA) (97), local autoregressive average (LAURA) (119), and others. LORETA is basically a WMN solution where the weighting is a discrete Laplacian operator. The solution's second spatial derivative is minimized so the estimation is smooth. Further, by normalizing the source estimates with respect to the corresponding noise sensitivity, one can assess the statistical significance of the inverse solution and obtain a map of source estimate statistics. Along this line, Dale et al. and Pascual-Marqui et al. have developed two statistical functional mapping techniques, known as dynamic statistical parametric mapping (dSPM) (120) and standardized LORETA (sLORETA) (121), based on the MNLS and LORETA algorithms respectively (122).

The EEG linear inverse solutions enjoy the merits of solving a linear inverse problem but sometimes end up with limited resolution images of current density or its statistics. One way to improve its spatial resolution is to generate images with focal source distribution by iteratively repeating the linear inverse computation (123). For each step during the iteration, the linearly computed inverse solution from the previous step is used as the weighting factor to constrain the linear source estimates in the current step. As such a reiterative process continues until convergence, the estimated source distribution tends to shrink to be more focalized. Other than L2 norm estimates, which are to minimize the signal energy, L1 norm estimates, which are to minimize the signal magnitude (or Lp norm), have also been explored (124–127). The selective minimum norm method (128), minimum current estimate, and sparse source imaging (127) are some of these methods. These methods basically use L1 norms in the regularization term and seek to minimize the L1 norm of the solution. The study by Ding and He (127) demonstrates the merits of L1 norm-based distributed current density imaging in imaging and localizing focal sources in human as induced by somatosensory stimulation (Fig. 45.7).

A recent advancement in EEG source imaging is the development of oscillatory source imaging with the aid of the ICA (68). He and colleagues (68,129) decomposed oscillatory brain activity into multiple independent components, performed source estimation on selected independent components, and then recombined the estimated source distributions. This approach enabled imaging of seizure activity from seizure EEG instead of interictal EEG in partial epilepsy patients, and returned results on the seizure onset zone in adult (68) and pediatric (129) patients that are in accordance with intracranial EEG recordings and successful surgical resection results. Figure 45.8 illustrates an example of EEG source imaging of seizure sources from 76 scalp electrodes and its comparison with successful surgical resection in two adult patients.

4.3. Validation and Clinical Yield of EEG Source Imaging

The increasing availability of high-density EEG, together with the development of individual realistic geometry head models and powerful inverse solution algorithms, led to an increased use of EEG source imaging in the presurgical evaluation of patients with pharmacoresistant epilepsy, in whom surgical resection of the epileptic zone is a therapeutic option. The introduction of EEG source imaging has the aim of (1) better determining the epileptogenic focus noninvasively and (2) guiding the location of intracranial electrodes if deemed necessary. Studies that evaluated the accuracy of EEG source imaging compared the location of the source maximum to the location of either the subsequently resected zone or the intracranial electrodes that recorded interictal discharges or seizures (8,68,129,130). These studies showed very good localization precision, in the range of 70% to 80%, with respect to the resected area (8) and on average a distance of ~15 mm to the seizure onset zone determined by intracranial EEG (130). The study by Brodbeck et al. (8) included 152 patients, all of whom

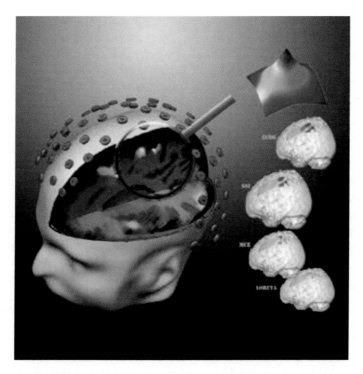

Figure 45.7. *Sparse source imaging (SSI) and its validation using ECoG in a patient. The left panel shows SSI imaging results of SEP. The right lower part of the illustration shows that the new SSI is evaluated using somatosensory evoked potential data with subdural ECoG recordings in a human subject, and compared with other algorithms. Cover image of* Human Brain Mapping, *September 2008 issue (127).*

underwent surgery. This allowed calculation of the sensitivity and specificity of electric source imaging. The study showed a sensitivity of 84% and a specificity of 88% of electrical source imaging, values higher than those of the conventional noninvasive imaging methods (MRI, positron emission tomography [PET], and single-photon-emission computed tomography [SPECT]). However, these high values were reached only with high-density (>128 channels) EEG allied with the use of the individual MRI for the head model. The values dropped significantly when only the routine clinical EEG of 20 to 32 channels was used and were even worse when a generic head model derived from a single MRI was used. A follow-up study by Lascano et al. (131) specifically evaluated the additional clinical yield of EEG source imaging with respect to the routine imaging methods. They evaluated a database of 190 patients recorded with high-density EEG and who underwent surgery.

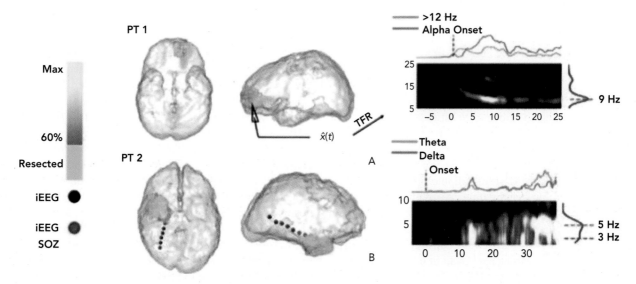

Figure 45.8. *Seizure onset zones (SOZs) estimated from a typical seizure in each of the patients. A, B: The estimated SOZ (yellow to orange color bar) is co-localized with surgically resected zones (shown in green) in patients. Intracranial electrodes were implanted in patient 2 (dots). Yellow color displays estimated source distributions; green color refers to surgically resected regions quantified by postoperative MRI. TFR= Time Frequency Representation. From (68).*

They showed that of all methods, only MRI and high-density EEG source imaging (HD-ESI) were favorable outcome predictors and that patients with concordant structural MRI and HD-ESI results had a 92.3% (24/26) probability of favorable outcome. An independent study on 43 temporal lobe epilepsy patients recorded with 256-channel EEG confirmed the findings of these studies (132); the researchers reported a sensitivity of 91.4% and a specificity of 75% on the sub-lobule level.

In a review that appeared in 2008, Plummer et al. (133) concluded that electric source imaging deserves a place in the routine workup of patients with localization-related epilepsy. However, they noted that prospective validation studies conducted on larger patient groups are still required. The studies cited above with large patient cohorts published after this review article filled this gap.

4.4. Multimodal Integration of EEG with fMRI

Integrating electrophysiological source imaging with hemodynamic imaging modalities has drawn great attention during the past decade (6,134) (see Chapter 46 for detailed reviews). The motivation for integrating EEG/MEG source imaging with fMRI is based on the different strengths and limitations of these two modalities, which are complementary. In other words, EEG/MEG has high temporal resolution but limited spatial resolution, and fMRI has high spatial resolution but poor temporal resolution. The fundamental assumption of the multimodal integration approach is that regions in the brain that show increased metabolic activity are also on average more electrically active over time. Due to the current inability of simultaneous MEG and fMRI recordings, the integration of EEG with fMRI that can be recorded simultaneously has shown great promise and will be the focus of discussion in this section.

The earliest efforts in EEG–fMRI integrated imaging used fMRI statistical parametric maps to obtain a priori information on where brain electric sources are likely to be located. The spatial information derived from fMRI has been used to constrain the locations of multiple current dipoles in the independently recorded EEG or MEG (135) or to constrain the distributed source distribution (7,136–138). When neural activity is confined to a few small regions, fMRI activation mapping should yield several hotspots, which can be used to constrain the equivalent dipole locations or to estimate initial locations in the dipole source localization. Once the dipole locations are reconstructed from the EEG data, the time course of dipole moments represents the temporal dynamics of the regional neural activity. This fMRI-seeded dipole fitting technique is usually applied to retrieve the time course of the brain activity at identified fMRI activation foci instead of imaging brain activity. On the other hand, the fMRI-constrained distributed source imaging (i.e., fMRI is used as a constraint in the distributed source imaging) can be applied to brain sources that are either focal or extended. The fMRI-constrained current density imaging has been explored in the framework of the Wiener filter (99,139) or weighted minimum norm frameworks (140). The major technical limitations of these approaches are primarily due to the fundamental mismatches between fMRI and EEG (or MEG) owing to the different temporal scales in which fMRI and EEG (or MEG) temporal dynamics are generated and collected. The fMRI–EEG/MEG mismatches include fMRI extra sources, fMRI invisible sources, and the fMRI displacement (138), and it is problematic to constrain the temporally variable current source estimates to "time-invariant" fMRI spatial priors, which may result in fMRI false positives or false negatives.

Efforts have been made to tackle this challenge caused by the different time scales of BOLD fMRI signals and EEG signals by means of data-driven approaches. For example, the fMRI weighting factor may be selected from data by means of the expectation maximization (EM) algorithm (137,141) or by using an adaptive Wiener filter framework for fMRI–EEG/MEG integrated neuroimaging as proposed in (136). In this approach, the system assumes a common neuronal source (i.e., synaptic activity), from which fMRI and EEG signals are generated via a temporal low-pass filter and a spatial low-pass filter, respectively. The EEG inverse problems essentially deal with the spatial deconvolution—the process of reversing the head volume conductor contribution. The EEG inverse solution retains the temporal source evolution even though it may fail to reconstruct the spatial source distribution. In other words, at every source location, the source waveform estimated from EEG is much less distorted than its absolute magnitude, since the filtering applies to the spatial domain instead of the time domain. This feature is opposed to the temporal regression of fMRI data, which theoretically ends up with high-resolution spatial maps of brain activations but with little temporal information. To integrate the EEG and BOLD signals, the BOLD effect size estimated from the fMRI signal in each voxel is set to be proportional to the time integral of the local source power underlying the ERP signals (136). The source estimates are further fitted to the EEG data by means of an adaptive Wiener filter (136).

Figure 45.9 shows an experimental example in a human subject exploring the cortical pathway specialized in processing unilateral visual stimuli (136). The experiment included two separate sessions with the identical visual stimuli for the EEG and fMRI data collection. The visual stimulation was a rectangular checkerboard within the lower left quadrant of the visual field; the checkerboard pattern was reversed at 2 Hz. The dynamically integrated EEG–fMRI imaging algorithm (136) revealed a pathway sequentially activating V1/V2, V3/V3a, V5/V7, and intraparietal sulcus, in general agreement with the hierarchical organization of the visual system (142). This pathway was also observed in the source images reconstructed from the visual evoked potentials alone. In contrast, an fMRI-weighted source imaging algorithm (120) showed a false-positive source region in and around V1/V2 at the latency of 212 msec, whereas a more likely high-tier EEG source around V5, as observed from the EEG data, was missed. This experimental result indicates the potential of dynamic neuroimaging by integrating fMRI with EEG using the model-based adaptive Wiener filter (143).

New EEG recording systems, together with advanced artifact correction algorithms (66,144), allow recovery of the EEG signal that is acquired in the scanner. This opens new

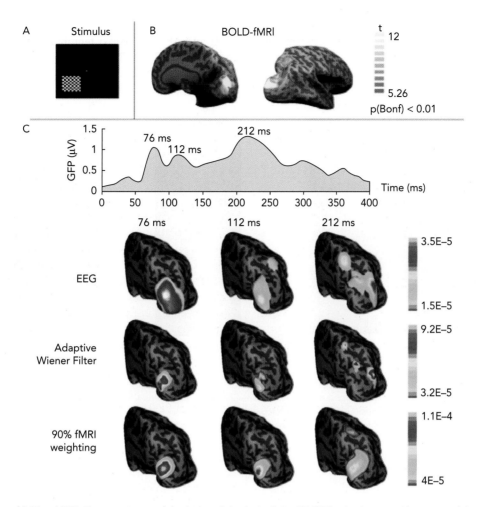

Figure 45.9. Integration of fMRI and EEG. *The pattern-reversal checkerboard visual stimulation (A), fMRI activation map with a corrected threshold (p < .01) (B), and (C) the global field power of VEP and the dynamic cortical source distribution at three VEP latencies (76, 112, and 212 msec after the visual onset) imaged from EEG alone (first row), or fMRI–EEG integration using our proposed adaptive Wiener filter (second row) and the conventional 90% fMRI weighted algorithm (third row). Both the source images and the fMRI activation map are visualized on an inflated representation of cortical surface. Note the excellent spatio-temporal resolution by adaptively integrating the BOLD with EEG signals. From (136).*

possibilities not only to study the relation between hemodynamic and electrical activity, but also to directly combine the temporal resolution of the EEG and the spatial resolution of the fMRI during the same brain state. Several recent studies have used this technique to study the relation between different brain rhythms and the BOLD response (145) and the relation between the so-called brain resting state and specific oscillatory activity recorded with the EEG (146). With the use of high-density EEG in the scanner, source imaging of this EEG has also become possible. This is particularly interesting in epilepsy, where the spike-related fMRI activity can be compared with the source imaging result of the very same spikes (5,134,147). Such studies have demonstrated the capability of the EEG source imaging to temporally disentangle the different activated regions seen in the spike-triggered fMRI, as illustrated in Figure 45.10 (148,149). This figure also shows that EEG source imaging is possible in patients with large brain lesions, indicating that conductivity changes due to such lesions are not as important as one might believe. This has been demonstrated in a systematic study in a series of epileptic patients with large brain lesions (150).

5. CONNECTIVITY ANALYSIS

Static images indicating brain regions responsible for the execution of particular tasks do not convey sufficient information with respect to how these regions communicate with each other. The concept of brain connectivity now plays an important role in neuroscience as a way to understand the organized behavior of brain regions (151). Previously, some investigators have computed cortical connectivity patterns based on hemodynamic or metabolic measurements such as fMRI (152, 153), whereas the sluggishness of the hemodynamic process confounds its interpretation in terms of neuronal interaction (154). The use of EEG data to examine the functional connectivity has a long and rich history (155). A variety of techniques have been used to evaluate the relationship between pairs of scalp electrodes or sensors (156). Wendling et al. (157) distinguished three main families of methods: regression methods (158), phase synchrony, and general synchronization (159). They tested the performance of 10 different methods belonging to these three families on simulated data. The results showed that none of the methods performed best

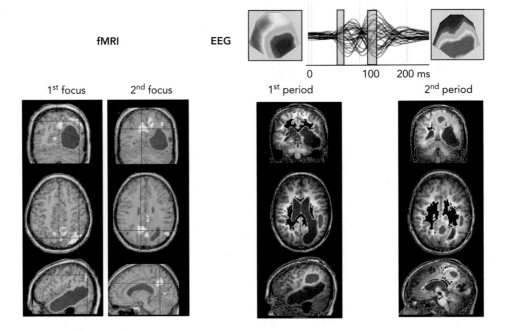

Figure 45.10. Combined EEG source imaging and fMRI in epilepsy. *A patient with focal epilepsy was recorded using 32-channel EEG in a 1.5T MR scanner. Spikes were marked and the significant BOLD responses related to these spikes were determined. Two foci were found around the large lesion: one right lateral parietal, the other mesial parietal. The same spikes recorded in the scanner were cleaned and subjected to EEG source imaging using a distributed linear inverse solution (LAURA) constrained to the gray matter determined from the patient's MRI. A temporal propagation of the activity was found, with the initial activity in the right parietal lobe, followed by activation in mesial parietal areas. Thus the foci found in the fMRI were confirmed and temporally resolved. The patient was seizure-free after surgical resection of the right lateral parietal focus. Data collected by M. Siniatchkin, University Hospital of Pediatric Neurology, Kiel, Germany. For details and more examples see (148).*

in all stimulations. Frequency properties of the signals as well as coupling parameters influenced the results. The authors concluded that "it is recommended to compare the results obtained from different connectivity methods to get more reliable interpretation of measured quantities with respect to underlying coupling" (157).

The functional connectivity methods evaluated in this study give information about the amount but not the direction of coupling between the different sites. Various time-varying methods exist that estimate directed interactions between brain areas using effective connectivity measures in the framework of Wiener-Granger causality or dynamic causal modeling (4,160–164). Tools based on graph theory from the study of complex networks have also been developed to describe directed connectivity of large-scale networks (165). In the study by Plomp et al. (166), multichannel scalp EEG recordings from rats were used as a benchmark to test different directed, time-varying connectivity methods. They used unilateral whisker stimulation as a test paradigm as the spatio-temporal activation patterns are very well known (167). The results showed clear differences between methods in terms of physiological plausibility, effect size, and temporal resolution, while row-normalized partial directed coherence weighted by the spectral power density gave the most plausible solutions.

A major problem when applying connectivity analysis on EEG or MEG signals measured on the scalp is the influence of volume conduction. Electromagnetic signals disperse from the cortex to the sensors, and thus each sensor measures a mixture

of all active sources, leading to spurious connectivities. Methods that ignore zero-phase lag between channels have been applied when working on the sensor level (168). Still, the reference problem in the case of scalp EEG time series makes the results ambiguous and interpretation of the results difficult (41a).

An important development over the past decade has been to perform connectivity analysis in the source domain after solving the EEG inverse problem (6,168–170). In this approach, the head volume conductor effect is first removed by solving the EEG source imaging, allowing one to focus on specific regions of interest in the brain. Functional connectivity analysis is then performed to estimate the connectivity or causality among the regions of interest, including structural equation modeling (SEM) (171), the directed transfer function (DTF) (7), adaptive DTF (172), partial directed coherence (170,173), and graph theory (174). Figure 45.11 shows an example of functional connectivity patterns as estimated by DTF from EEG and fMRI of a human subject during a motor task (7). It shows connectivity among several regions of interest involved in the motor task. A eConnectome MATLAB toolbox (175) (freely available to the public at http://econnectome.umn.edu/) has been developed that provides the capability to process the EEG data, including scalp topography mapping, cortical current density source imaging, and functional connectivity analysis using DTF or adaptive DTF algorithms.

DTF-based connectivity analysis methods in the inverse space have shown promise in localizing epileptogenic foci from seizures (184). Ding et al. (184) conducted a study in a group of

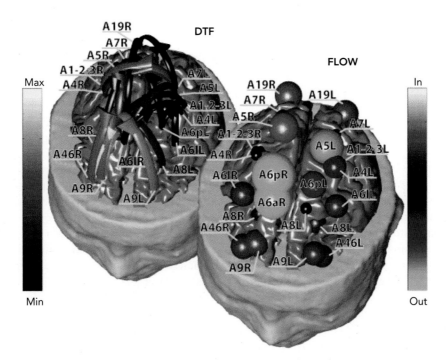

Figure 45.11. Connectivity estimation. Left panel: *Functional connectivity patterns estimated in a subject during the performance of finger-tapping movement, after the EMG onset. Each pattern is represented with arrows moving from one cortical area toward another. The color and size of the arrows code the level of strength of the functional connectivity observed between regions of interest (ROIs). The labels indicate the names of the ROIs employed. Right panel: Outflow patterns in all the ROIs obtained for the same connectivity pattern depicted in top left. The figure summarizes in red hues the behavior of an ROI in terms of reception of information flow from other ROIs by adding all the values of the links arriving on the particular ROI from all the others. The information is represented by the size and the color of a sphere, centered on the particular ROI analyzed. The larger the sphere, the higher the value of inflow or outflow for any given ROI. The blue hues code the outflow of information from a single ROI toward all the others. DTF = Direct Transfer Function. From (7).*

epilepsy patients, estimating brain sources from scalp EEG and then performing DTF analysis in the source domain. Statistical analysis of DTF estimates revealed a robust estimation of primary seizure sources versus propagated activities, as judged by other clinical information. Coito et al. (173) used partial directed coherence in the inverse space to study patients with right and left temporal lobe epilepsy. The results revealed clear differences between the two groups: the right temporal lobe epilepsy patients showed strong bilateral connectivity patterns while the connectivity network was more limited to the left temporal lobe in patients with left temporal lobe epilepsy (Fig. 45.12). Interestingly, the right temporal lobe patients also had more neuropsychological dysfunctions related to the contralateral hemisphere than the left temporal lobe patients. While this study applied connectivity measures to interictal spikes, a subsequent study showed that the same epileptic networks were active during rest in the absence of spikes in these two patient groups (177).

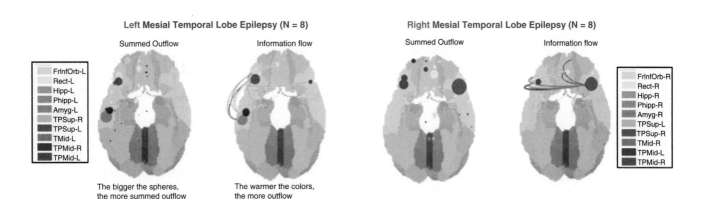

Figure 45.12. Effective connectivity analysis of epileptic spikes. *Sixteen patients with right or left temporal lobe epilepsy were analyzed. Electrical source activity of individual spikes was estimated in 82 cortical regions of interest (ROIs) using an individual head model and a distributed linear inverse solution. A multivariate, time-varying and frequency-resolved Granger causality analysis (partial directed coherence) was then applied to the activities in these ROIs. The figure shows the summed outflow for each ROI at the beginning of the spike and the main information flow during the whole spike, separately for the left and the right temporal lobe patients. For the summed outflow only the regions in which at least half of the patients show a statistically significance are displayed. The bigger the sphere, the more summed outflow that region has. For the information flow, the warmer the color, the stronger the connection. Adapted from (173).*

In summary, a plethora of methods for estimating functional connectivity is currently available, and they have been applied to EEG, MEG, and ECoG data. Since they are based on different assumptions, their suitability for the data at hand must be carefully evaluated. Further validation studies such as the ones described above (157,166,168,178,179) are still needed using simulated and benchmark data.

6. CONCLUSION

This chapter focused on modern analytic techniques that convert the EEG to a functional neuroimaging modality. This translation from waveforms to images includes several processing steps that need to be understood and performed properly. It starts with the appropriate spatial sampling of the scalp potential field and ends with proper statistical evaluation of the reconstructed time series of electrical activity in the brain.

Concerning spatial sampling, the recent literature strongly suggests that the use of a high number of recording channels is desirable to avoid under-sampling of the spatial frequency of the EEG. With modern technology this is no longer a limiting issue, and 64 to 128 channels of EEG are recorded in many labs. At present EEG can easily be sampled from 200 or more electrodes, with electrode nets that allow fast application even in a clinical setting.

Reconstruction and visualization of the scalp potential maps are important steps in EEG source imaging. On the one hand, this serves to detect map distortions due to artifacts that are invisible on the EEG traces. On the other hand, EEG mapping allows one to statistically assess time points where map topographies changed over time or between experimental conditions. By physical laws, different map topographies indicate a different configuration of the active sources in the brain. Analytic strategies that are based on the topography of the potential field also have the important advantage of being reference-free, which is not the case for the analysis of peaks and troughs of EEG or ERP waveforms, and also not for the analysis of coherence or correlations between different electrode sites.

Two main models are involved in EEG source imaging: the head model and the source model. In this chapter we not only described the historical evolution of these models but also made clear that a distinction between simple source localization and comprehensive source imaging should be made. The once-popular single equivalent dipole fitting approach in a simple spherical head model has been largely replaced by imaging of distributed sources in a realistic geometry head model defined by structural MRI. A rapidly growing number of experimental and clinical studies have appeared, demonstrating the promising capability of these new techniques. Most impressive are the results in epilepsy, where EEG source imaging is used to localize the epileptogenic zone. The fact that the very same methods also allow one to localize eloquent cortex with impressive precision renders electrical neuroimaging one of the most promising methods in the presurgical evaluation of patients with functional and structural brain lesions.

The high temporal resolution is the key advantage of EEG. However, it also increases the complexity and demands additional analytic steps for electrical neuroimaging compared to the other (static) imaging procedures. We have described different methods to deal with the temporal dynamics of brain electrical activity. One of them is based on spatio-temporal decomposition of the topographic maps. This allows one to define the most dominant scalp topographies during given time periods and thus permits a reduction of the complex data in time and space. Source imaging procedures can then be applied to this reduced dataset. Since the potential maps represent the real recordings and do not yet rely on models, pre-processing of the data based on the maps might be more prudent than directly converting the raw data to source images and then performing all analysis in the source space. Nevertheless, several interesting studies have appeared recently that showed the possibilities of analysis of the source waveforms. Most interesting are the applications of functional connectivity analysis techniques to these source waveforms. They allow one to study the causal interactions between different sources in the brain.

In summary, this chapter illustrated that the temporal resolution of the EEG, together with the capability and reliability of modern source imaging algorithms, has converted EEG to a fully fledged functional neuroimaging method that is not secondary to, but instead is a perfect companion to, fMRI and other neuroimaging methods (3).

ACKNOWLEDGMENTS

C.M. is supported by the Swiss National Science Foundation (Grant No. 320030_159705) and by the Swiss National Center of Competence in Research; "Synapsy: the Synaptic Basis of Mental Diseases" financed by the Swiss National Science Foundation (Grant no.51AU40_125759). B.H. is supported in part by NIH R01NS096761, R01EB021027, RF1MH114233, and U01HL117664.

REFERENCES

1. Michel CM, Murray MM. Towards the utilization of EEG as a brain imaging tool. Neuroimage. 2012;61(2):371–385.
2. He B, Ding L. Electrophysiological neuroimaging. In: He B, ed. Neural Engineering. New York: Springer; 2013:499–544.
3. Michel CM, Murray MM, Lantz G, Gonzalez S, Spinelli L, Grave de Peralta R. EEG source imaging. Clin Neurophysiol. 2004;115(10):2195–2222.
4. David O, Kiebel SJ, Harrison LM, Mattout J, Kilner JM, Friston KJ. Dynamic causal modeling of evoked responses in EEG and MEG. Neuroimage. 2006;30(4):1255–1272.
5. Vulliemoz S, Lemieux L, Daunizeau J, Michel CM, Duncan JS. The combination of EEG source imaging and EEG-correlated functional MRI to map epileptic networks. Epilepsia. 2010;51(4):491–505.
6. He B, Yang L, Wilke C, Yuan H. Electrophysiological imaging of brain activity and connectivity-challenges and opportunities. IEEE Trans Biomed Eng. 2011;58(7):1918–1931.
7. Babiloni F, Cincotti F, Babiloni C, Carducci F, Mattia D, Astolfi L, et al. Estimation of the cortical functional connectivity with the multimodal integration of high-resolution EEG and fMRI data by directed transfer function. Neuroimage. 2005;24(1):118–131.
8. Brodbeck V, Spinelli L, Lascano AM, Wissmeier M, Vargas MI, Vulliemoz S, et al. Electroencephalographic source imaging: a prospective study of 152 operated epileptic patients. Brain. 2011;134(Pt 10):2887–2897.

9. van de Ville D, Britz J, Michel CM. EEG microstate sequences in healthy humans at rest reveal scale-free dynamics. Proc Natl Acad Sci USA. 2010;107:18179–18184.
10. Michel CM, Koenig T, Brandeis D, Gianotti LRR, Wackermann J, eds. Electrical Neuroimaging. Cambridge: Cambridge University Press, 2009.
11. Lehmann D. Multichannel topography of human alpha EEG fields. Electroencephalogr Clin Neurophysiol. 1971;31:439–449.
12. Lehmann D, Skrandies W. Spatial analysis of evoked potentials in man—a review. Prog Neurobiol. 1984;23(3):227–250.
13. Helmholtz HLP. Ueber einige gesetze der vertheilung elektrischer ströme in körperlichen leitern mit anwendung aud die thierisch-elektrischen versuche. Ann Physik und Chemie. 1853;9:211–233.
14. Michel CM, Lantz G, Spinelli L, De Peralta RG, Landis T, Seeck M. 128-channel EEG source imaging in epilepsy: clinical yield and localization precision. J Clin Neurophysiol. 2004;21(2):71–83.
15. Malmivuo JA, Suihko VE. Effect of skull resistivity on the spatial resolutions of EEG and MEG. IEEE Trans Biomed Eng. 2004;51(7):1276–1280.
16. Li T-H, North G. Aliasing effects and sampling theorems of SRFs when sampled on a finite grid. Ann Inst Stat Math. 1996;49(2):341–354.
17. Ryynanen OR, Hyttinen JA, Malmivuo JA. Effect of measurement noise and electrode density on the spatial resolution of cortical potential distribution with different resistivity values for the skull. IEEE Trans Biomed Eng. 2006;53(9):1851–1858.
18. Gevins A, Brickett P, Costales B, Le J, Reutter B. Beyond topographic mapping: towards functional-anatomical imaging with 124-channel EEGs and 3-D MRIs. Brain Topogr. 1990;3(1):53–64.
19. Sohrabpour A, Lu Y, Kankirawatana P, Blount J, Kim H, He B. Effect of EEG electrode number on epileptic source localization in pediatric patients. Clin Neurophysiol. 2015;126(3):472–480.
20. Luu P, Tucker DM, Englander R, Lockfeld A, Lutsep H, Oken B. Localizing acute stroke-related EEG changes: assessing the effects of spatial undersampling. J Clin Neurophysiol. 2001;18(4):302–317.
21. Lantz G, Grave de Peralta R, Spinelli L, Seeck M, Michel CM. Epileptic source localization with high density EEG: how many electrodes are needed? Clin Neurophysiol. 2003;114(1):63–69.
22. Ryynanen OR, Hyttinen JA, Laarne PH, Malmivuo JA. Effect of electrode density and measurement noise on the spatial resolution of cortical potential distribution. IEEE Trans Biomed Eng. 2004;51(9):1547–1554.
23. Rush S, Driscoll DA. EEG electrode sensitivity—an application of reciprocity. IEEE Trans Biomed Eng. 1969;16(1):15–22.
24. Oostendorp TF, Delbeke J, Stegeman DF. The conductivity of the human skull: results of in vivo and in vitro measurements. IEEE Trans Biomed Eng. 2000;47(11):1487–1492.
25. Hoekema R, Wieneke GH, Leijten FS, van Veelen CW, van Rijen PC, Huiskamp GJ, et al. Measurement of the conductivity of skull, temporarily removed during epilepsy surgery. Brain Topogr. 2003;16:29–38.
26. Lai Y, van Drongelen W, Ding L, Hecox KE, Towle VL, Frim DM, et al. Estimation of in vivo human brain-to-skull conductivity ratio from simultaneous extra- and intra-cranial electrical potential recordings. Clin Neurophysiol. 2005;116(2):456–465.
27. Zhang Y, van Drongelen W, He B. Estimation of in vivo brain-to-skull conductivity ratio in humans. Appl Phys Lett. 2006;89(22):223903–2239033.
28. Grieve PG, Emerson RG, Isler JR, Stark RI. Quantitative analysis of spatial sampling error in the infant and adult electroencephalogram. Neuroimage. 2004;21(4):1260–1274.
29. Tao JX, Baldwin M, Hawes-Ebersole S, Ebersole JS. Cortical substrates of scalp EEG epileptiform discharges. J Clin Neurophysiol. 2007;24(2):96–100.
30. Cosandier-Rimele D, Merlet I, Badier JM, Chauvel P, Wendling F. The neuronal sources of EEG: modeling of simultaneous scalp and intracerebral recordings in epilepsy. Neuroimage. 2008;42(1):135–146.
31. Zelmann R, Lina JM, Schulze-Bonhage A, Gotman J, Jacobs J. Scalp EEG is not a blur: it can see high frequency oscillations although their generators are small. Brain Topogr. 2014;27(5):683–704.
32. Lu Y, Worrell GA, Zhang HC, Yang L, Brinkmann B, Nelson C, et al. Noninvasive imaging of the high frequency brain activity in focal epilepsy patients. IEEE Trans Biomed Eng. 2014;61(6):1660–1667.
33. Tang C, You F, Cheng G, Gao D, Fu F, Yang G, et al. Correlation between structure and resistivity variations of the live human skull. IEEE Trans Biomed Eng. 2008;55(9):2286–2292.
34. Ding L, Worrell GA, Lagerlund TD, He B. Ictal source analysis: localization and imaging of causal interactions in humans. Neuroimage. 2007;34(2):575–586.
35. Sperli F, Spinelli L, Seeck M, Kurian M, Michel CM, Lantz G. EEG source imaging in pediatric epilepsy surgery: a new perspective in presurgical workup. Epilepsia. 2006;47(6):981–990.
36. Desmedt JE, Tomberg C, Noel P, Ozaki I. Beware of the average reference in brain mapping. Electroencephalogr Clin Neurophysiol Suppl. 1990;41:22–27.
37. Pascual-Marqui RD, Lehmann D. Comparison of topographic maps and the reference electrode: comments on two papers by Desmedt and collaborators. Electroencephalogr Clin Neurophysiol. 1993;88(6):530–536.
38. Geselowitz DB. The zero of potential. IEEE Eng Med Biol Mag. 1998;17:128–132.
39. Lehmann D, Michel CM. Intracerebral dipole source localization for FFT power maps. Electroencephalogr Clin Neurophysiol. 1990;76:271–276.
40. Lehmann D, Ozaki H, Pal I. Averaging of spectral power and phase via vector diagram best fits without reference electrode or reference channel. Electroencephalogr Clin Neurophysiol. 1986;64(4):350–363.
41. Marzetti L, Nolte G, Perrucci MG, Romani GL, Del Gratta C. The use of standardized infinity reference in EEG coherency studies. Neuroimage. 2007;36(1):48–63.
41a. Chella F, Pizzella V, Zappasodi F, Marzetti L. Impact of the reference choice on scalp EEG connectivity estimation. J Neural Eng. 2016 Jun;13(3):036016.
42. Yao D, Wang L, Oostenveld R, Nielsen KD, Arendt-Nielsen L, Chen AC. A comparative study of different references for EEG spectral mapping: the issue of the neutral reference and the use of the infinity reference. Physiol Meas. 2005;26(3):173–184.
43. Qin Y, Xu P, Yao D. A comparative study of different references for EEG default mode network: the use of the infinity reference. Clin Neurophysiol. 2010;121(12):1981–1991.
44. Tian Y, Yao D. Why do we need to use a zero reference? Reference influences on the ERPs of audiovisual effects. Psychophysiology. 2013;50(12):1282–1290.
45. Perrin F, Pernier J, Bertrand O, Giard MH, Echallier JF. Mapping of scalp potentials by surface spline interpolation. Electroencephalogr Clin Neurophysiol. 1987;66(1):75–81.
46. Srinivasan R, Nunez PL, Tucker DM, Silberstein RB, Cadusch PJ. Spatial sampling and filtering of EEG with spline Laplacians to estimate cortical potentials. Brain Topogr. 1996;8:355–366.
47. Hjorth B. An on-line transformation of EEG scalp potentials into orthogonal source derivations. Electroencephalogr Clin Neurophysiol. 1975;39(5):526–530.
48. Perrin F, Bertrand O, Pernier J. Scalp current density mapping: value and estimation from potential data. IEEE Trans Biomed Eng. 1987;34(4):283–288.
49. He B, Lian J, Li G. High-resolution EEG: a new realistic geometry spline Laplacian estimation technique. Clin Neurophysiol. 2001;112(5):845–852.
50. Nunez PL, Srinivasan R. Electric Fields of the Brain: The Neurophysics of EEG, 2nd ed. New York: Oxford University Press, 2006.
51. Lehmann D, Skrandies W. Reference-free identification of components of checkerboard-evoked multichannel potential fields. Electroencephalogr Clin Neurophysiol. 1980;48:609–621.
52. Skrandies W. The effect of stimulation frequency and retinal stimulus location on visual evoked potential topography. Brain Topogr. 2007;20(1):15–20.
53. Brandeis D, Naylor H, Halliday R, Callaway E, Yano L. Scopolamine effects on visual information processing, attention, and event-related potential map latencies. Psychophysiology. 1992;29(3):315–336.
54. Fender DH. Source localization of brain electrical activity. In: Gevins AS, Remont A, eds. Methods of Analysis of Brain Electrical and Magnetic Signals. Amsterdam: Elsevier, 1987:335–403.
55. Murray MM, Brunet D, Michel CM. Topographic ERP analyses: a step-by-step tutorial review. Brain Topogr. 2008;20(4):249–264.
56. Koenig T, Melie-Garcia L. A method to determine the presence of averaged event-related fields using randomization tests. Brain Topogr. 2010;23(3):233–242.
57. Picton TW, Bentin S, Berg P, Donchin E, Hillyard SA, Johnson R, Jr., et al. Guidelines for using human event-related potentials to study cognition: recording standards and publication criteria. Psychophysiology. 2000;37(2):127–152.
58. Brandeis D, Lehmann D. Event-related potentials of the brain and cognitive processes: approaches and applications. Neuropsychologia. 1986;24(1):151–168.
59. Skrandies W. Data reduction of multichannel fields: global field power and principal component analysis. Brain Topogr. 1989;2(1-2):73–80.
60. Pourtois G, Delplanque S, Michel C, Vuilleumier P. Beyond the conventional event-related brain potential (ERP): exploring the time-course of visual emotion processing using topographic and principal component analyses. Brain Topogr. 2008;20(4):265–277.

61. Kayser J, Tenke CE. Trusting in or breaking with convention: towards a renaissance of principal components analysis in electrophysiology. Clin Neurophysiol. 2005;116(8):1747–1753.
62. Makeig S, Jung TP, Bell AJ, Ghahremani D, Sejnowski TJ. Blind separation of auditory event-related brain responses into independent components. Proc Natl Acad Sci USA. 1997;94(20):10979–10984.
63. Jung TP, Makeig S, Humphries C, Lee TW, McKeown MJ, Iragui V, et al. Removing electroencephalographic artifacts by blind source separation. Psychophysiology. 2000;37(2):163–178.
64. Benar C, Aghakhani Y, Wang Y, Izenberg A, Al-Asmi A, Dubeau F, et al. Quality of EEG in simultaneous EEG-fMRI for epilepsy. Clin Neurophysiol. 2003;114(3):569–580.
65. Mantini D, Perrucci MG, Cugini S, Ferretti A, Romani GL, Del Gratta C. Complete artifact removal for EEG recorded during continuous fMRI using independent component analysis. Neuroimage. 2007;34(2):598–607.
66. Debener S, Mullinger KJ, Niazy RK, Bowtell RW. Properties of the ballistocardiogram artefact as revealed by EEG recordings at 1.5, 3 and 7 T static magnetic field strength. Int J Psychophysiol. 2008;67(3):189–199.
67. Makeig S, Westerfield M, Townsend J, Jung TP, Courchesne E, Sejnowski TJ. Functionally independent components of early event-related potentials in a visual spatial attention task. Philos Trans R Soc Lond B Biol Sci. 1999;354(1387):1135–1144.
68. Yang L, Wilke C, Brinkmann B, Worrell GA, He B. Dynamic imaging of ictal oscillations using non-invasive high-resolution EEG. Neuroimage. 2011;56(4):1908–1917.
69. Lehmann D, Ozaki H, Pal I. EEG alpha map series: brain micro-states by space-oriented adaptive segmentation. Electroencephalogr Clin Neurophysiol. 1987;67:271–288.
70. Lehmann D. Brain electric fields and brain functional states. In: Friedrich R, Wunderlin A, eds. Evolution of Dynamical Structures in Complex Systems. Berlin: Springer, 1992:235–248.
71. Koenig T, Prichep L, Lehmann D, Sosa PV, Braeker E, Kleinlogel H, et al. Millisecond by millisecond, year by year: normative EEG microstates and developmental stages. Neuroimage. 2002;16:41–48.
72. Pascual-Marqui RD, Michel CM, Lehmann D. Segmentation of brain electrical activity into microstates: model estimation and validation. IEEE Trans Biomed Eng. 1995;42:658–665.
73. Lehmann D, Pascual-Marqui R, Michel CM. EEG microstates. Scholarpedia. 2009;4(3):7632.
74. Baars BJ. The conscious access hypothesis: origins and recent evidence. Trends Cogn Sci. 2002;6(1):47–52.
75. Dehaene S, Sergent C, Changeux JP. A neuronal network model linking subjective reports and objective physiological data during conscious perception. Proc Natl Acad Sci USA. 2003;100(14):8520–8525.
76. Bressler SL, Tognoli E. Operational principles of neurocognitive networks. Int J Psychophysiol. 2006;60(2):139–148.
77. Grossberg S. The complementary brain: unifying brain dynamics and modularity. Trends Cogn Sci. 2000;4(6):233–246.
78. Lehmann D, Michel CM. EEG-defined functional microstates as basic building blocks of mental processes. Clin Neurophysiol. 2011;122(6):1073–1074.
79. Khanna A, Pascual-Leone A, Michel CM, Farzan F. Microstates in resting-state EEG: current status and future directions. Neurosci Biobehav Rev. 2015;49:105–113.
80. Katayama H, Gianotti LR, Isotani T, Faber PL, Sasada K, Kinoshita T, et al. Classes of multichannel EEG microstates in light and deep hypnotic conditions. Brain Topogr. 2007;20(1):7–14.
81. Kopal J, Vysata O, Burian J, Schatz M, Prochazka A, Valis M. Complex continuous wavelet coherence for EEG microstates detection in insight and calm meditation. Conscious Cogn. 2014;30C:13–23.
82. Brodbeck V, Kuhn A, von Wegner F, Morzelewski A, Tagliazucchi E, Borisov S, et al. EEG microstates of wakefulness and NREM sleep. Neuroimage. 2012;62(3):2129–2139.
83. Lehmann D, Faber PL, Galderisi S, Herrmann WM, Kinoshita T, Koukkou M, et al. EEG microstate duration and syntax in acute, medication-naive, first-episode schizophrenia: a multi-center study. Psychiatry Res. 2005;138(2):141–156.
84. Strelets V, Faber PL, Golikova J, Novototsky-Vlasov V, Koenig T, Gianotti LR, et al. Chronic schizophrenics with positive symptomatology have shortened EEG microstate durations. Clin Neurophysiol. 2003;114(11):2043–2051.
85. Tomescu MI, Rihs TA, Becker R, Britz J, Custo A, Grouiller F, et al. Deviant dynamics of EEG resting state pattern in 22q11.2 deletion syndrome adolescents: A vulnerability marker of schizophrenia? Schizophr Res. 2014;157(1-3):175–181.
86. Nishida K, Morishima Y, Yoshimura M, Isotani T, Irisawa S, Jann K, et al. EEG microstates associated with salience and frontoparietal networks in

87. Diaz Hernandez L, Rieger K, Baenninger A, Brandeis D, Koenig T. Towards using microstate-neurofeedback for the treatment of psychotic symptoms in schizophrenia. A feasibility study in healthy participants. Brain Topogr. 2016;29(2):308–321.
88. Britz J, Van De Ville D, Michel CM. BOLD correlates of EEG topography reveal rapid resting-state network dynamics. Neuroimage. 2010;52(4):1162–1170.
89. Musso F, Brinkmeyer J, Mobascher A, Warbrick T, Winterer G. Spontaneous brain activity and EEG microstates. A novel EEG/fMRI analysis approach to explore resting state networks. Neuroimage. 2010;52(4):1149–1161.
90. Van de Ville D, Britz J, Michel CM. EEG microstate sequences in healthy humans at rest reveal scale-free dynamics. Proc Natl Acad Sci USA. 2010;107(42):18179–18184.
91. Michel CM, Thut G, Morand S, Khateb A, Pegna AJ, Grave de Peralta R, et al. Electric source imaging of human brain functions. Brain Res Brain Res Rev. 2001;36(2-3):108–118.
92. Lascano AM, Brodbeck V, Lalive PH, Chofflon M, Seeck M, Michel CM. Increasing the diagnostic value of evoked potentials in multiple sclerosis by quantitative topographic analysis of multichannel recordings. J Clin Neurophysiol. 2009;26(5):316–325.
93. Spierer L, Murray MM, Tardif E, Clarke S. The path to success in auditory spatial discrimination: electrical neuroimaging responses within the supratemporal plane predict performance outcome. Neuroimage. 2008;41(2):493–503.
94. Thierry G, Martin CD, Downing P, Pegna AJ. Controlling for interstimulus perceptual variance abolishes N170 face selectivity. Nat Neurosci. 2007;10(4):505–511.
95. Schnider A, Mohr C, Morand S, Michel CM. Early cortical response to behaviorally relevant absence of anticipated outcomes: a human event-related potential study. Neuroimage. 2007;35(3):1348–1355.
96. Jerbi K, Baillet S, Mosher JC, Nolte G, Garnero L, Leahy RM. Localization of realistic cortical activity in MEG using current multipoles. Neuroimage. 2004;22(2):779–793.
97. Pascual-Marqui RD, Michel CM, Lehmann D. Low resolution electromagnetic tomography: a new method for localizing electrical activity in the brain. Int J Psychophysiol. 1994;18:49–65.
98. He B, Lian J. Electrophysiological neuroimaging: solving the EEG inverse problem. In: He B, ed. Neural Engineering. Norwell, MA: Kluwer Academic Publishers, 2005:221–261.
99. Dale AM, Sereno MI. Improved localization of cortical activity by combining EEG and MEG with MRI cortical surface reconstruction: a linear approach. J Cogn Neurosci. 1993;5(2):162–176.
100. He B, Yao D, Lian J, Wu D. An equivalent current source model and Laplacian weighted minimum norm current estimates of brain electrical activity. IEEE Trans Biomed Eng. 2002;49(4):277–288.
101. Plonsey R. Bioelectric Phenomena. New York: McGraw-Hill, 1969.
102. Wilson FN, Bayley RH. The electric field of an eccentric dipole in a homogeneous spherical conducting medium. Circulation. 1950;1(1):84–92.
103. Wang Y, He B. A computer simulation study of cortical imaging from scalp potentials. IEEE Trans Biomed Eng. 1998;45(6):724–735.
104. Cuffin BN, Cohen D. Comparison of the magnetoencephalogram and electroencephalogram. Electroencephalogr Clin Neurophysiol. 1979;47(2):132–146.
105. Spinelli L, Andino SG, Lantz G, Seeck M, Michel CM. Electromagnetic inverse solutions in anatomically constrained spherical head models. Brain Topogr. 2000;13(2):115–125.
106. Brunet D, Murray MM, Michel CM. Spatiotemporal analysis of multichannel EEG: CARTOOL. Comput Intell Neurosci. 2011;2011:813870.
107. He B, Musha T, Okamoto Y, Homma S, Nakajima Y, Sato T. Electric dipole tracing in the brain by means of the boundary element method and its accuracy. IEEE Trans Biomed Eng. 1987;34(6):406–414.
108. Hämäläinen M, Sarvas J. Realistic conductor geometry model of the human head for interpretation of neuromagnetic data. IEEE Trans Biomed Eng. 1989;36:165–171.
109. Wolters CH, Anwander A, Tricoche X, Weinstein D, Koch MA, MacLeod RS. Influence of tissue conductivity anisotropy on EEG/MEG field and return current computation in a realistic head model: a simulation and visualization study using high-resolution finite element modeling. Neuroimage. 2006;30(3):813–826.
110. Lee WH, Liu Z, Mueller BA, Lim K, He B. Influence of white matter anisotropic conductivity on EEG source localization: Comparison to fMRI in human primary visual cortex. Clin Neurophysiol. 2009;120:2071–2081.
111. Withey DJ, Koles ZJ. A review of medical image segmentation: methods and available software. Int J Bioelectromagnetism. 2008;10:125–148.

frontotemporal dementia, schizophrenia and Alzheimer's disease. Clin Neurophysiol. 2013;124(6):1106–1114.

112. Birot G, Spinelli L, Vulliemoz S, Megevand P, Brunet D, Seeck M, et al. Head model and electrical source imaging: A study of 38 epileptic patients. Neuroimage Clin. 2014;5:77–83.

113. Scherg M, von Cramon D. A new interpretation of the generators of BAEP waves I-V: results of a spatio-temporal dipole model. Electroencephalogr Clin Neurophysiol. 1985;62(4):290–299.

114. Fuchs M, Wagner M, Wischmann HA, Kohler T, Theissen A, Drenckhahn R, et al. Improving source reconstructions by combining bioelectric and biomagnetic data. Electroencephalogr Clin Neurophysiol. 1998;107(2):93–111.

115. Cuffin BN. A method for localizing EEG sources in realistic head models. IEEE Trans Biomed Eng. 1995;42(1):68–71.

116. Lantz G, Holub M, Ryding E, Rosen I. Simultaneous intracranial and extracranial recording of interictal epileptiform activity in patients with drug resistant partial epilepsy: patterns of conduction and results from dipole reconstructions. Electroencephalogr Clinl Neurophysiol. 1996;99(1):69–78.

117. Hämäläinen MS, Ilmoniemi RJ. Interpreting Measured Magnetic Fields of the Brain: Estimation of Current Distributions. Technical Report. Helsinki: Helsinki University of Technology, 1984. Report No.: TKK-F-A559.

118. Wang JZ, Williamson SJ, Kaufman L. Magnetic source images determined by a lead-field analysis: the unique minimum-norm least-squares estimation. IEEE Trans Biomed Eng. 1992;39:665–675.

119. Grave de Peralta Menendez R, Murray MM, Michel CM, Martuzzi R, Gonzalez Andino SL. Electrical neuroimaging based on biophysical constraints. Neuroimage. 2004;21(2):527–539.

120. Dale AM, Liu AK, Fischl BR, Buckner RL, Belliveau JW, Lewine JD, et al. Dynamic statistical parametric mapping: combining fMRI and MEG for high-resolution imaging of cortical activity. Neuron. 2000;26(1):55–67.

121. Pascual-Marqui RD. Standardized low-resolution brain electromagnetic tomography (sLORETA): technical details. Methods Find Exp Clin Pharmacol 2002;24:5–12.

122. Pascual Marqui RD, Sekihara K, Brandeis D, Michel CM. Imaging the electrical neuronal generators of EEG/MEG. In: Michel CM, Koenig T, Brandeis D, Gianotti LRR, Wackermann J, eds. Electrical Neuroimaging. Cambridge: Cambridge University Press, 2009.

123. Gorodnitsky IF, George JS, Rao BD. Neuromagnetic source imaging with FOCUSS: a recursive weighted minimum norm algorithm. Electroencephalogr Clin Neurophysiol. 1995;95:231–251.

124. Uutela K, Hamalainen M, Somersalo E. Visualization of magnetoencephalographic data using minimum current estimates. Neuroimage. 1999;10(2):173–180.

125. Huang MX, Dale AM, Song T, Halgren E, Harrington DL, Podgorny I, et al. Vector-based spatial-temporal minimum L1-norm solution for MEG. Neuroimage. 2006;31(3):1025–1037.

126. Bai X, Towle VL, He EJ, He B: Evaluation of cortical current density imaging methods using intracranial electrocorticograms and functional MRI, Neuroimage. 2007;35:598–608.

127. Ding L, He B. Sparse source imaging in electroencephalography with accurate field modeling. Hum Brain Mapp. 2008;29(9):1053–1067.

128. Matsuura K, Okabe Y. Selective minimum-norm solution of the biomagnetic inverse problem. IEEE Trans Biomed Eng. 1995;42(6):608–615.

129. Lu Y, Yang L, Worrell GA, Brinkmann B, Nelson C, He B. Dynamic imaging of seizure activity in pediatric epilepsy patients. Clin Neurophysiol. 2012;123(11):2122–2129.

130. Megevand P, Spinelli L, Genetti M, Brodbeck V, Momjian S, Schaller K, et al. Electric source imaging of interictal activity accurately localises the seizure onset zone. J Neurol Neurosurg Psychiatry. 2014;85(1):38–43.

131. Lascano AM, Perneger T, Vulliemoz S, Spinelli L, Garibotto V, Korff CM, et al. Yield of MRI, high-density electric source imaging (HD-ESI), SPECT and PET in epilepsy surgery candidates. Clin Neurophysiol. 2015;125:150–155.

132. Feng R, Hu J, Pan L, Wu J, Lang L, Jiang S, et al. Application of 256-channel dense array electroencephalographic source imaging in presurgical workup of temporal lobe epilepsy. Clin Neurophysiol. 2015;127(1):108–116.

133. Plummer C, Harvey AS, Cook M. EEG source localization in focal epilepsy: where are we now? Epilepsia. 2008;49(2):201–218.

134. Pittau F, Grouiller F, Spinelli L, Seeck M, Michel CM, Vulliemoz S. The role of functional neuroimaging in pre-surgical epilepsy evaluation. Front Neurol. 2014;5:31.

135. Ahlfors SP, Simpson GV, Dale AM, Belliveau JW, Liu AK, Korvenoja A, et al. Spatiotemporal activity of a cortical network for processing visual motion revealed by MEG and fMRI. J Neurophysiol. 1999;82(5):2545–2555.

136. Liu Z, He B. FMRI-EEG integrated cortical source imaging by use of time-variant spatial constraints. Neuroimage. 2008;39(3):1198–1214.

137. Phillips C, Mattout J, Rugg MD, Maquet P, Friston KJ. An empirical Bayesian solution to the source reconstruction problem in EEG. Neuroimage. 2005;24(4):997–1011.

138. Liu Z, Ding L, He B. Integration of EEG/MEG with MRI and fMRI. IEEE Eng Med Biol Mag. 2006;25(4):46–53.

139. Liu AK, Belliveau JW, Dale AM. Spatiotemporal imaging of human brain activity using functional MRI constrained magnetoencephalography data: Monte Carlo simulations. Proc Natl Acad Sci USA. 1998;95(15):8945–8950.

140. Wagner M, Fuchs M, Kastner J. fMRI-constrained dipole fits and current density reconstructions. Proceedings of the 12th Intl Conf Biomag. 2000:785–788.

141. Mattout J, Phillips C, Penny WD, Rugg MD, Friston KJ. MEG source localization under multiple constraints: an extended Bayesian framework. Neuroimage. 2006;30(3):753–767.

142. Felleman DJ, Van Essen DC. Distributed hierarchical processing in the primate cerebral cortex. Cereb Cortex. 1991;1(1):1–47.

143. He B, Liu Z. Multimodal functional neuroimaging: integrating functional MRI and EEG/MEG. IEEE Rev Biomed Eng. 2008(1):23–40.

144. Iannotti GR, Pittau F, Michel CM, Vulliemoz S, Grouiller F. Pulse artifact detection in simultaneous EEG-fMRI recording based on EEG map topography. Brain Topogr. 2015;28(1):21–32.

145. Tyvaert L, Levan P, Grova C, Dubeau F, Gotman J. Effects of fluctuating physiological rhythms during prolonged EEG-fMRI studies. Clin Neurophysiol. 2008;119(12):2762–2774.

146. Laufs H, Hamandi K, Salek-Haddadi A, Kleinschmidt AK, Duncan JS, Lemieux L. Temporal lobe interictal epileptic discharges affect cerebral activity in "default mode" brain regions. Hum Brain Mapp. 2007;28(10):1023–1032.

147. Vulliemoz S, Carmichael DW, Rosenkranz K, Diehl B, Rodionov R, Walker MC, et al. Simultaneous intracranial EEG and fMRI of interictal epileptic discharges in humans. Neuroimage. 2010;54(1):182–190.

148. Groening K, Brodbeck V, Moeller F, Wolff S, van Baalen A, Michel CM, et al. Combination of EEG-fMRI and EEG source analysis improves interpretation of spike-associated activation networks in paediatric pharmacoresistent focal epilepsies. Neuroimage. 2009;46(3):827–833.

149. Vulliemoz S, Thornton R, Rodionov R, Carmichael DW, Guye M, Lhatoo SA, et al. The spatio-temporal mapping of epileptic networks: Combination of EEG-fMRI and EEG Source Imaging. Neuroimage. 2009;46(3):834–843.

150. Brodbeck V, Lascano AM, Spinelli L, Seeck M, Michel CM. Accuracy of EEG source imaging of epileptic spikes in patients with large brain lesions. Clin Neurophysiol. 2009;120(4):679–685.

151. Ioannides AA. Dynamic functional connectivity. Curr Opin Neurobiol. 2007;17(2):161–170.

152. Arthurs OJ, Donovan T, Spiegelhalter DJ, Pickard JD, Boniface SJ. Intracortically distributed neurovascular coupling relationships within and between human somatosensory cortices. Cereb Cortex. 2007;17(3):661–668.

153. McIntosh AR, Gonzalez-Lima F. Structural equation modeling and its application to network analysis in functional brain imaging. Hum Brain Mapp. 1994;2:2–22.

154. Otte A, Halsband U. Brain imaging tools in neurosciences. J Physiol Paris. 2006;99(4–6):281–292.

155. Gevins AS, Cutillo BA, Bressler SL, Morgan NH, White RM, Illes J, et al. Event-related covariances during a bimanual visuomotor task. II. Preparation and feedback. Electroencephalogr Clin Neurophysiol. 1989;74(2):147–160.

156. Lachaux JP, Rodriguez E, Martinerie J, Varela FJ. Measuring phase synchrony in brain signals. Hum Brain Mapp. 1999;8(4):194–208.

157. Wendling F, Ansari-Asl K, Bartolomei F, Senhadji L. From EEG signals to brain connectivity: a model-based evaluation of interdependence measures. J Neurosci Methods. 2009;183(1):9–18.

158. Lopes da Silva F, Pijn JP, Boeijinga P. Interdependence of EEG signals: linear vs. nonlinear associations and the significance of time delays and phase shifts. Brain Topogr. 1989;2(1-2):9–18.

159. Stam CJ, van Dijk BW. Synchronization likelihood: an unbiased measure of generalized synchronization in multivariate data sets. Physica D: Nonlin Phenom. 2002;163(3-4):236–251.

160. Lin FH, Hara K, Solo V, Vangel M, Belliveau JW, Stufflebeam SM, et al. Dynamic Granger-Geweke causality modeling with application to interictal spike propagation. Hum Brain Mapp. 2009;30(6):1877–1886.

161. Porcaro C, Coppola G, Pierelli F, Seri S, Di Lorenzo G, Tomasevic L, et al. Multiple frequency functional connectivity in the hand somatosensory network: an EEG study. Clin Neurophysiol. 2013;124(6):1216–1224.

162. Martino J, Honma SM, Findlay AM, Guggisberg AG, Owen JP, Kirsch HE, et al. Resting functional connectivity in patients with brain tumors in eloquent areas. Ann Neurol. 2011;69(3):521–532.

163. Brovelli A, Ding M, Ledberg A, Chen Y, Nakamura R, Bressler SL. Beta oscillations in a large-scale sensorimotor cortical network: directional influences revealed by Granger causality. Proc Natl Acad Sci USA. 2004;101(26):9849–9854.

164. Urbano A, Babiloni C, Onorati P, Babiloni F. Dynamic functional coupling of high resolution EEG potentials related to unilateral internally triggered one-digit movements. Electroencephalogr Clin Neurophysiol. 1998;106(6):477–487.

165. Strogatz SH. Exploring complex networks. Nature. 2001;410(6825):268–276.

166. Plomp G, Quairiaux C, Michel CM, Astolfi L. The physiological plausibility of time-varying Granger-causal modeling: normalization and weighting by spectral power. Neuroimage. 2014;97:206–216.

167. Quairiaux C, Megevand P, Kiss JZ, Michel CM. Functional development of large-scale sensorimotor cortical networks in the brain. J Neurosci. 2011;31(26):9574–9584.

168. Haufe S, Nikulin VV, Muller KR, Nolte G. A critical assessment of connectivity measures for EEG data: a simulation study. Neuroimage. 2013;64:120–133.

169. Schoffelen JM, Gross J. Source connectivity analysis with MEG and EEG. Hum Brain Mapp. 2009;30(6):1857–1865.

170. Plomp G, Hervais-Adelman A, Astolfi L, Michel CM. Early recurrence and ongoing parietal driving during elementary visual processing. Sci Rep. 2015;5:18733.

171. Astolfi L, Cincotti F, Mattia D, Salinari S, Babiloni C, Basilisco A, et al. Estimation of the effective and functional human cortical connectivity with structural equation modeling and directed transfer function applied to high-resolution EEG. Magn Reson Imaging. 2004;22(10):1457–1470.

172. Wilke C, van Drongelen W, Kohrman M, He B: "Identification of epileptogenic foci from causal analysis of ECoG interictal spike activity," Clinical Neurophysiology. 2010;120(8):1449–1456.

173. Coito A, Plomp G, Genetti M, Abela E, Wiest R, Seeck M, et al. Dynamic directed interictal connectivity in left and right temporal lobe epilepsy. Epilepsia. 2015;56(2):207–217.

174. Astolfi L, Cincotti F, Mattia D, De Vico Fallani F, Colosimo A, Salinari S, et al. Time-varying cortical connectivity by adaptive multivariate estimators applied to a combined foot-lips movement. Conference Proceedings, IEEE Eng Med Biol Soc. 2007;2007:4402–4405.

175. He B, Dai Y, Astolfi L, Babiloni F, Yuan H, Yang L. eConnectome: A MATLAB toolbox for mapping and imaging of brain functional connectivity. J Neurosci Meth. 2011;195(2):261–269.

176. Wilke C, Worrell G, He B. Graph analysis of epileptogenic networks. Epilepsia. 2011;52(1):84–93.

177. Coito A, Genetti M, Pittau F, Iannotti G, Thomschewski A, Höller Y, et al. Altered directed connectivity in temporal lobe epilepsy in the absence of interictal spikes: a high density EEG study. Epilepsia. 2016;57(3):402–411.

178. Astolfi L, Cincotti F, Mattia D, Marciani MG, Baccala LA, de Vico Fallani F, et al. Comparison of different cortical connectivity estimators for high-resolution EEG recordings. Hum Brain Mapp. 2007;28(2):143–157.

179. David O, Cosmelli D, Friston KJ. Evaluation of different measures of functional connectivity using a neural mass model. Neuroimage. 2004;21(2):659–673.

180. Tucker DM. Spatial sampling of head electrical fields: the geodesic sensor net. Electroencephalogr Clin Neurophysiol. 1993;87:154–163.

181. Michel CM, Brandeis D. Data acquisition and pre-processing standards for electrical neuroimaging. In: Michel CM, Koenig T, Brandeis D, Gianotti LRR, Wackermann J, eds. Electrical Neuroimaging. Cambridge: Cambridge University Press, 2009.

182. Lantz G, Spinelli L, Seeck M, Grave de Peralta Menendez R, Sottas C, Michel C. Propagation of interictal epileptiform activity can lead to erroneous source localizations: A 128 channel EEG mapping study. J Clin Neurophysiol. 2003;20(5):311–319.

183. Zhang Y, van Drongelen W, Kohrman M, He B. Three-dimensional brain current source reconstruction from intra-cranial ECoG recordings. Neuroimage. 2008;42(2):683–695.

184. Ding L, Worrell GA, Lagerlund TD, He B: "Ictal Source Analysis: Localization and Imaging of Causal Interactions in Humans," Neuroimage. 2007;34(2):575–586.

46 | COMBINATION OF BRAIN FUNCTIONAL IMAGING TECHNIQUES: EEG/MEG, FMRI, PET, SPECT—CLINICAL APPLICATIONS IN NEUROLOGY

MARGITTA SEECK, MD, LAURENT SPINELLI, PHD, JEAN GOTMAN, PHD, AND FERNANDO H. LOPES DA SILVA, MD, PHD

ABSTRACT: Several tools are available to map brain electrical activity. Clinical applications focus on epileptic activity, although electric source imaging (ESI) and electroencephalography-coupled functional magnetic resonance imaging (EEG–fMRI) are also used to investigate non-epileptic processes in healthy subjects. While positron-emission tomography (PET) reflects glucose metabolism, strongly linked with synaptic activity, and single-photon-emission computed tomography (SPECT) reflects blood flow, fMRI (BOLD) signals have a hemodynamic component that is a surrogate signal of neuronal (synaptic) activity. The exact interpretation of BOLD signals is not completely understood; even in unifocal epilepsy, more than one region of positive or negative BOLD is often observed. Co-registration of medical images is essential to answer clinical questions, particularly for presurgical epilepsy evaluations. Multimodal imaging can yield information about epileptic foci and underlying networks. Co-registering MRI, PET, SPECT, fMRI, and ESI (or magnetic source imaging) provides information to estimate the epileptogenic zone and can help optimize surgical results.

KEYWORDS: EEG, positron-emission tomography, PET, single-photon-emission computed tomography, SPECT, functional magnetic resonance imaging, fMRI, co-registration, epilepsy

PRINCIPAL REFERENCES

1. Chassoux F, Landré E, Mellerio C, et al. Type II focal cortical dysplasia: electroclinical phenotype and surgical outcome related to imaging. Epilepsia. 2012;53(2):349–358.
2. Lascano AM, Perneger T, Vulliemoz S et al. Yield of MRI, high-density electric source imaging (HD-ESI), SPECT and PET in epilepsy surgery candidates. Clin Neurophysiol. 2016;127:150–155.
3. Carne RP, O'Brien TJ, Kilpatrick CJ, et al. MRI-negative PET-positive temporal lobe epilepsy: a distinct surgically remediable syndrome. Brain. 2004;127:2276–2285
4. Gotman J, Kobayashi E, Bagshaw AP, Bénar CG, Dubeau F. Combining EEG and fMRI: a multimodal tool for epilepsy research. J Magn Reson Imaging. 2006;23(6):906–920.
5. Ives JR, Warach S, Schmitt F, Edelman RR, Schomer DL. Monitoring the patient's EEG during echo planar MRI. Electroencephogr Clin Neurophysiol. 1993;87:417–420.
6. Mégevand P, Spinelli L, Genetti M, et al. Electric source imaging of interictal activity accurately localises the seizure onset zone. J Neurol Neurosurg Psychiatry. 2004;85(1):38–43.
7. Klein A, Andersson J, Ardekani BA, et al. Evaluation of 14 nonlinear deformation algorithms applied to human brain MRI registration. Neuroimage. 2014;46:786–802.

1. INTRODUCTION

Why combine electroencephalography (EEG) and other brain functional modalities? The fundamental reason is to better understand the dynamical neural substrates of brain functions, with the ultimate goal of improving the diagnosis of brain disorders. The fundamental problem in studying these processes is that it is difficult to obtain precise information about the underlying neural mechanisms from outside the brain. The brain has a complicated structure, intricate connectivity, and manifold functions. Furthermore, it is enclosed in a space surrounded by three connective tissue layers (meninges) with cerebrospinal fluid, the skull, and the scalp. All these features make brain processes difficult to unravel from the scalp. Nonetheless, relevant information about such processes can be obtained using several kinds of techniques, in particular EEG, magnetoencephalography (MEG), and functional magnetic resonance imaging (fMRI), as well as positron emission tomography (PET) and single-photon-emission computed tomography (SPECT). Every one of these techniques has strong and weak features. Thus, EEG (the recording of electric fields) and MEG (the recording of magnetic fields) have the advantage of yielding signals of neuronal processes that evolve at the millisecond time scale. These signals can play an important role in providing measures of functional and effective connectivity in the brain, but they have intrinsically limited spatial resolution and low sensitivity to deep brain structures. Further, the inverse transfer from EEG/MEG signals measured at the scalp to the sources in the brain is an ill-posed problem and has no unique solution. The fMRI blood-oxygen-level-dependent (BOLD) signal has the strong feature of being able to reflect changes of activity throughout the entire brain with a high spatial resolution, but it has the drawback that its time resolution is much lower than what is required to catch the dynamics of most neural processes. Neural activity can be also assessed by measuring other physiological signals, namely cerebral regional blood flow or brain tissue metabolism, as estimated by PET, SPECT, or fMRI (1–5). How the information gathered by means of these different methods can be integrated with EEG/MEG, with the objective of enhancing our understanding of brain functions, constitutes the core of this chapter.

Neuronal metabolic activity can be estimated using PET by means of tracers such as $C^{15}O_2$ and $H_2^{15}O$ and using the ^{18}Fluoro-2-deoxy-D-glucose (FDG) isotope. Also by means of fMRI, changes in regional cerebral flow may be estimated either by using paramagnetic tracers or, more commonly, by making use of the deoxyhemoglobin/oxyhemoglobin ratio, the so-called BOLD signal. For both PET and fMRI the estimation of the activity of brain regions is based on comparisons between task/pathological conditions and control conditions, or on the correlation between the evolution in time of the signals with the performance of a behavioral task. Regarding fMRI, the BOLD signal reflects that, associated with neural activity, there is an increase in oxygen consumption by the cells, followed by a larger increase in blood flow and blood volume, which results in a net decrease of the concentration of the local deoxyhemoglobin.

In this respect, two important questions are as follows:

1. What are the precise relationships between changes in electrical neural activity and changes in BOLD signals, cerebral blood flow (CBF), venous cerebral blood volume (CBV_v), and cerebral metabolic rate of oxygen consumption ($CMRO_2$)?

2. What kinds of neural activity are relevant with respect to BOLD signals: (a) neural firing, (b) excitatory and/or inhibitory synaptic activity, (c) glial activity?

With respect to the first question, it is not easy to disentangle the relative contributions of CBF, $CMRO_2$, and CBV_v to the BOLD signal related to the onset of a neural dynamic response (6). The experimental and modeling study of these authors showed that the BOLD response can be explained by a close coupling between CBF and $CMRO_2$, while the CBV_v is a much slower process. In interpreting BOLD signals with respect to behavioral and cognitive processes, one must take into account that it is still difficult to assess precisely the contributions of these different physiological components of the BOLD signal to a given dynamical BOLD response.

Regarding the second question, it is well known that there is much more glucose consumption at the level of axon terminals and perisynaptic region than in the neuronal soma, since oxidative metabolism occurs in mitochondria, and these are highly concentrated in presynaptic terminals. In a number of classic experiments, where glucose utilization was compared between orthodromic and antidromic stimulation of nerve fibers, it was found that the glucose utilization was significantly increased only in the presynaptic terminal (1). Furthermore, experiments where the sodium pump was blocked showed that the critical event coupling glucose utilization and neuronal activity is the activation of the sodium pump (7). Therefore, (a) neural firing is strongly coupled to energy consumption. In light of the previous observation that the neural firing of presynaptic terminals is the critical event in this process, it may be assumed that (b) both excitatory and inhibitory processes would contribute to the enhancement of energy consumption. Regarding (c) the contribution of glial activation to energy consumption, experimental data are not abundant, but only about 15% of oxidative cerebral glucose utilization appears to be accounted for by glial activity (1). The physiological observations described above imply that

neural activity is associated with an increase of $CMRO_2$ since it is necessary, for the normal functioning of the nervous system, that ion gradients and the stores of neurotransmitters are restored, and also with an increase in CBF; the latter may be, at least partially, the consequence of the release of glutamate and other neurotransmitters (2). This overview emphasizes that BOLD effects should be interpreted primarily as reflecting changes in neural signaling, whereas CBF changes should be considered as resulting from processes operating in parallel. Further, neural activity mediated by a diversity of neurotransmitter systems, such as cholinergic, dopaminergic, noradrenergic, and serotoninergic, can contribute to BOLD signals directly as well as associated with blood flow changes in the cortex, diffusely or locally.

Summarizing these various physiological observations, we should emphasize that the BOLD response is a combination of a *hemodynamic response,* related to changes in blood flow and venous blood volume, and a *metabolic response* related to oxygen metabolism (6).

SPECT requires, similarly to PET, the delivery of a gamma-emitting radioisotope (radionuclide) to a subject, usually through injection into the bloodstream. Therefore, it provides a snapshot of activated areas in the brain, and, if injected early in a seizure, can visualize the seizure onset zone. SPECT is also easier to obtain than PET because it uses radioisotopes with a long half-life, which do not require a cyclotron in the hospital and allow scanning to be performed one or two hours after injection. However, in contrast to PET, in SPECT the gamma radiation is measured directly, whereas PET tracers emit positrons that collide with electrons within the tissue, resulting in positron annihilation and the simultaneous emission of energy in the form of two photons, or γ-rays, that travel in opposite directions. The latter can be detected by multiple detectors arranged in rings around the head such that a pair of detectors, lying opposite to each other, is able to identify the position of the annihilation event inside the head. Given that the direction of the photons is almost 180 degrees to each other, it is possible with PET to obtain quantitative information on the metabolism if arterial blood is sampled, allowing one to calculate precisely the pharmacokinetic function of uptake in an individual patient. Since this is usually not possible in a clinical setting, semi-quantitative measurements using body weight or body surface area and/or measures relative to reference regions at later, steady-state time points are used to obtain an approximation of local or whole-body concentration of the injected radioactivity. Using tomographic techniques analogous to those used in CT scans, images of the distribution of the radioactivity within the brain tissue can thus be obtained. In this way these events can be localized more precisely in PET than in SPECT; however, this can be overcome with other localization algorithms discussed below.

With respect to the use of combinations between EEG and MEG and between the latter and fMRI/PET, see Chapter 35 on MEG. In short, the use of multimodal methodologies to study the brain can yield relevant information and insights depending on a deep understanding of the biophysical processes that underlie the signals of different modalities, including

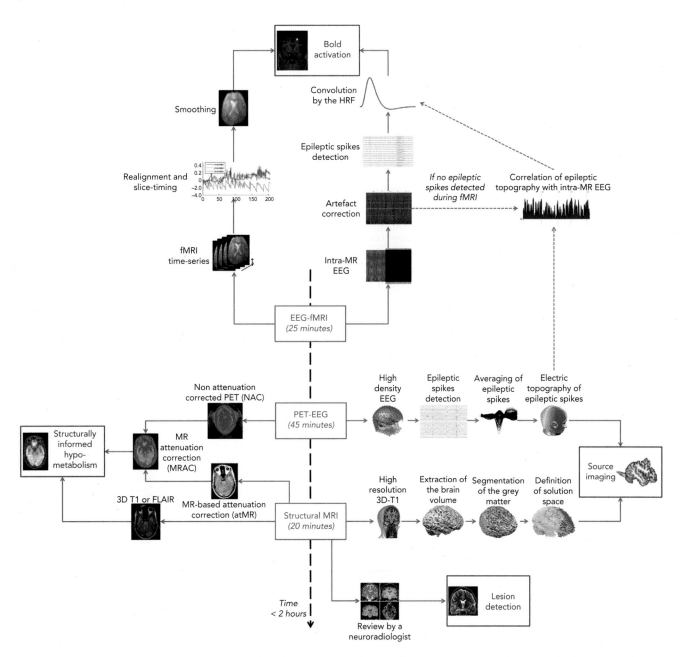

Figure 46.1. *Multimodal integration procedure: acquisition of EEG-fMRI, PET-EEG, and structural MRI in one session to analyze interictal epileptic activity if surgery for epilepsy is being considered. Adapted with permission from Grouiller F, Delattre BMA, Pittau F, Heizer S, Lazeyras F, Spinelli L, et al. All-in-one interictal presurgical imaging in patients with epilepsy: single-session EEG/PET/(f)MRI. Eur J Nucl Med Mol Imaging. 2015;42:1133–1143.*

biochemical, electrophysiological, and hemodynamic dimensions. In the University Hospital in Geneva structural MRI, PET, EEG (electric source imaging [ESI]) and EEG–fMRI are routinely performed for interictal presurgical imaging in patients with epilepsy (8), according to the scheme shown in Figure 46.1. In the following, we pay special attention to the combinations EEG and fMRI, EEG and PET, and EEG and SPECT, ending with a brief analysis of the technical aspects of medical image registration.

2. EEG–FMRI

Given that fMRI has excellent spatial but poor temporal resolution, and for EEG the reverse is true, the idea that the combination of both techniques might overcome the weaknesses of each one has gained momentum in recent times. Moreover, fMRI is sensitive to all parts of the brain, including deep cortex and deep nuclei, which are not visible on EEG (although sensitivity can be reduced for some parts of the inferior temporal and frontal lobe, near air cavities). This idea may be exciting, but a basic problem is that it is not clear if the signals recorded using both techniques correspond to the same neural processes. Indeed, BOLD signals, having a hemodynamic component by nature, are neural surrogate signals, reflecting activities of relatively large masses of brain tissue including vascular components. Although the measurement of BOLD signals is the most popular MRI method used in the study of the brain, MRI can offer other kinds of relevant information related to neural activities, such as estimates of tissue perfusion (arterial spin labeling), and may even yield information about activated neural tissue by means of diffusion MRI.

In contrast, it has been argued that changes in hemodynamic signals may be observed in situations where neuronal firing is absent. This issue, however, is controversial, as illustrated by the discussion between Viswanathan and Freeman (9) on the one hand and Nir, Dinstein, Malach, and Heeger (10) on the other. The former devised an experimental situation where a visual stimulus elicited synaptic activity without associated spike discharges in cat primary visual cortex showing a strong coupling between local field potentials and changes in tissue oxygen concentration in the absence of spikes. From these results the authors concluded that the BOLD signal is more closely coupled to synaptic activity, reflected in local field potentials, than to spike firing. Nir et al. (10), however, pointed out that in the experimental setup of Viswanathan and Freeman (9) it is difficult to convincingly make the decoupling between synaptic and spiking activity. On the contrary, they concluded that these experiments show that 80% to 90% of the local vascular response is coupled to local spiking activity. Nonetheless, Logothetis (5) noted that a series of experiments using various techniques show evidence for the claim that hemodynamic responses may occur in situations where neuronal firing is apparently absent. There are also situations where the sources of neuronal activity form closed fields that are not reflected in electrophysiological signals at a distance but may nevertheless cause measurable hemodynamic signals. Despite these special circumstances, the BOLD signal reflects most often the intensity of neuronal activity, as both synaptic activity and action potentials contribute to the metabolic activity measured by BOLD. The relationship between BOLD and neuronal activity is most often linear (11).

Another controversial issue regards the meaning of *decreases of BOLD signals* (i.e., negative BOLD signals), associated with neuronal activity. In general, a negative BOLD response (a BOLD value lower than the baseline) is most likely to reflect a decrease in neuronal activity compared to baseline; as indicated above, the BOLD signal largely reflects neuronal activity. In exceptional circumstances, when a negative BOLD signal is observed at the same time as an expected increase in neuronal activity, it has been proposed that a vascular blood steal phenomenon could take place: a local decrease in blood flow could compensate for an increase in other more active brain regions and thus would not have a neural origin, but mainly a hemodynamic one (12). A study in the visual cortex of anesthetized macaque monkeys shed light on this question. Shmuel et al. (4) demonstrated that negative BOLD responses were indeed found beyond the stimulated regions of the visual cortex, coupled to decreases in neuronal activity below baseline level. This does not imply, however, that a vascular component might not also contribute to the negative BOLD signal by the phenomenon of "vascular steal," as indicated above. A negative BOLD could be caused, also exceptionally, by an increase in deoxyhemoglobin associated with an increase in neuronal activity and oxygen consumption without a significant change in CBF.

Logothetis (5) also warned that "the impulse response function of fMRI is strongly site- and structure dependent." It has

been demonstrated in healthy and epileptic humans that there is inter-individual and inter-regional variability in hemodynamic responses, although the responses have many common characteristics (13–15). Thus one must keep in mind this dependency of BOLD responses on brain area when interpreting fMRI data.

Another form of dependency of BOLD responses that has emerged from combined studies of fMRI and EEG is the fact that EEG frequency bands are not reflected uniformly in the amplitude of BOLD signals (16). Thus, modulations of BOLD signals were found to follow closely modulations of EEG gamma power (40–100 Hz). The amplitude of BOLD signals may depend on the ratio between low and high EEG frequency components because the latter appear to correspond to stronger spiking activity. Indeed, several groups (17–22) have shown that temporal variations of alpha power are negatively correlated to the BOLD signal in several cortical regions, namely the visual cortex and the pre- and post-central gyrus, but positively correlated with the thalamic BOLD and also with the insula according to Goldman et al. (17). We may speculate (18) that this indicates that enhanced power of alpha rhythm corresponds to a relatively low average spiking rate level in the cortex, but not in the thalamus, where probably a high level of neural spiking of the reticular neurons may be dominant during alpha activity. These EEG–BOLD correlations were further refined by Sadaghiani et al. (23). They found (i) positive correlations of global upper alpha band (10–12 Hz) and a wide beta band (17–24 Hz) power with BOLD signals in a cingulo-insula–prefrontal cortex–thalamic network, a network identified as the tonic alertness system maintaining vigilance but (ii) negative correlations between BOLD and lower alpha (7–10 Hz) and a narrow beta band (15–18 Hz) power in the dorsal attention system including visual cortex, in areas that are associated with selective attention. Thus, sub-bands of alpha may show different signs of correlations with BOLD signals. Further, not only the frequency (sub) band of alpha or beta activity but also the corresponding spectral bandwidth may be important. The latter is often not specifically mentioned in most papers. This is a shortcoming since this information should be always taken into account.

This discussion illustrates the statement that we need to have a model of the relationship between neural processes and hemodynamic variables in order to draw valid conclusions from these relationships. The above examples show that when a model is available, the combination of EEG and fMRI allows us to draw conclusions that would be impossible to obtain in humans with any other noninvasive technique, as it measures metabolic activity simultaneously in cortex and subcortical structures at the time of specific EEG activity. It has thus been possible to study the role of different thalamic nuclei during epileptic discharges (24).

Above, we mentioned that by means of diffusion fMRI (DfMRI) (20), we may also obtain information about activated neural tissue. This is still a technique in development. In essence, it consists of detecting changes in water diffusion associated with cell swelling that may take place as neurons are activated. Changes of DfMRI elicited by neural activation take place much faster than BOLD responses and display temporal precedence with respect to the latter. The increase in DfMRI signal corresponds to a decrease of the apparent diffusion coefficient (ADC) of water molecules in the cortex. The underlying mechanism of this process is still a matter of debate. Nonetheless, Le Bihan (25) formulated the hypothesis that this decreased ADC could result from variations in cell shape and size, such as neural and/or glial cell swelling associated with neuronal activation, which is supported by experimental observations in hippocampal slices in vitro (26).

Next we consider *practical applications* of EEG–fMRI data integration in two main fields of paramount importance: epilepsy and neurocognitive functional studies.

In epilepsy applications, we have to distinguish *interictal* and *ictal* activities. *Interictal* analyses consist primarily in finding BOLD correlates of interictal epileptiform discharges (IEDs), as shown in Figure 46.2, and more recently of high-frequency oscillations.

The estimation of the spatial localization of IEDs was pioneered by Ives et al. (27), and since then many papers have been published describing interesting applications with clinically relevant results. A comprehensive review of early studies

is that by Gotman et al. (28); besides describing the methodology used for recording interictal EEG continuous signals inside the MRI scanner, including artifact removal (gradient and pulse artifacts), and different approaches to data statistical analyses, this review also discusses pertinent questions with respect to the interpretation of BOLD changes associated with the occurrence of IEDs. From this review we may extract a number of general conclusions: finding significant relationships between EEG and IEDs and BOLD signals depends on the signal-to-noise ratio and thus on the strength of the electric or magnetic field, on the number of IEDs analyzed (bursts of spikes being, in most cases, easier to detect than isolated spikes), and on the kind of hemodynamic response function (HRF) applied. Indeed, using multiple HRFs yields relatively more IED datasets with fMRI activations than using just the standard HRF peaking 5.4 sec after the IED (29). A caveat regarding the specificity of the spatial extent of the brain area estimated to be responsible for the generation of a given IED is that BOLD signals may have important contributions from venous cerebral blood volume changes, which may be detected

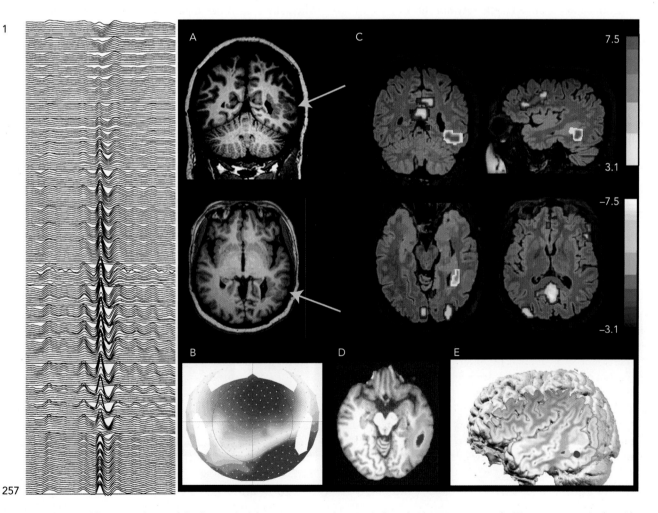

*Figure 46.2. A 20-year-old patient with cortical dysplasia at the left temporo-occipital junction indicated with a green arrow in the T1 sequences acquired outside the EEG-fMRI (**A**). Left: Marked events inside the EEG-fMRI session: spikes and slow waves with maximum at TP7 (257 channels EEG, reference: Fz). **B**: The voltage topographic map of the event has maximal negativity at TP7. **C**: The positive BOLD response showed a focal activation in the left posterior cortex (p < .001, 20 voxels extent cluster, for visualization; color code indicates t-values). Note also negative BOLD responses, outside the focus and in this case, corresponding to the default network. **D**: Electric source localization in the right posterior region. **E**: Both ESI and maximal positive BOLD response co-registered with the patient's MRI, both very close to each other and corresponding to the lesion. Right hemisphere is on the left of the image. Courtesy of Dr. Francesca Pittau.*

at some distance from the sites of IED generation. It is estimated that most BOLD responses occur 3 to 4 mm from the corresponding neuronal activity, but in some circumstances (very high responses) this distance can reach 1 cm (30,31). This effect depends on magnet strength, but not in a straightforward fashion (32).

Recent studies have demonstrated the clinical potential of EEG–fMRI in providing localizing information in epileptic patients (33) and in helping to predict surgical outcome (34,35). Although the studies in patients with focal epilepsy often point to several regions of BOLD response, these studies have shown that the peak response is often a good predictor of the epileptogenic zone. Distinguishing the sites of IED generation and propagation regions is a question that deserves further investigation, as reviewed by Murta et al. (36), where several recent approaches are described. In this respect it is pertinent to take into account the information based on IED-related BOLD signals recorded using intracerebral electrodes. In selected epileptic patients significant changes in IED-related BOLD signals were detected not only localized at the most active EEG sites, but also spread to remote regions, leading to the identification of an "epileptic network" (37).

Another limitation in the investigation of BOLD correlates with interictal epileptiform events is the limited time resolution of the usually employed echo-planar imaging technique (EPI), on the order of ~2 to 3 sec. New approaches have decreased this value to about 100 msec; one of these sequences, called fast magnetic resonance EEG (MREG), was introduced by Zahneisen et al. (38). Jacobs et al. (39) carried out a comparative investigation of EPI and MREG in epileptic patients

with infrequent interictal spikes. They found both positive and negative BOLD effects, more frequently using MREG than EPI (Fig. 46.3). The conclusion of this investigation is that simultaneous EEG and MREG can yield a higher sensitivity with respect to the localization of spike-related BOLD findings than EEG–EPI. To test this kind of conclusion in a systematic way, Safi-Harb et al. (40) performed a simulation study focusing on the advantages and disadvantages of this fast sequence with respect to the identification of BOLD correlates of interictal spikes. In general, MREG yielded more significant results but at the cost of more false positives. Clearly there is much to be studied concerning this new EEG–fMRI sequence.

Studies of *ictal* events based on EEG–fMRI are less abundant than interictal studies, mainly because it is not easy to investigate seizures while video-EEG and BOLD signals are being recorded. Chaudhary et al. (41) reported a review of such studies particularly regarding epileptic seizures with *focal onset*. Based on this review, we may put forward a number of general points. A first-line approach in studying seizure-related EEG–fMRI signal changes is to use the EEG-based general linear model (GLM). However, one must choose an appropriate HRF, since the latter may be specific for a particular type of epileptic condition. Further, since seizures are dynamical processes that evolve through different stages, taking a seizure as a single block, as in the GLM approach, does not represent a seizure adequately. To overcome this limitation Thornton et al. (42) subdivided the seizure event into phases—(i) an early phase characterized by ictal EEG changes, (ii) a clinical seizure onset phase, and (iii) a late ictal EEG phase—and determined EEG–fMRI correlations. Tyvaert et al. (43) applied a sliding

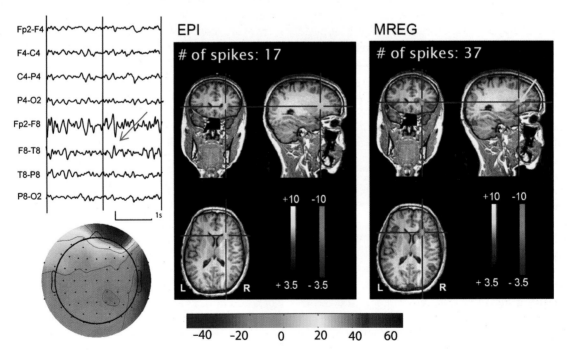

Figure 46.3. A 28-year-old patient with unclear epilepsy and spikes over the right frontal areas. The anatomical MRI showed volume reduction in this area of unclear etiology. The echo-planar imaging (EPI) measurement did not show any significant BOLD changes, while the MREG measurement revealed a strong BOLD effect in agreement with the epileptic spike topography. The yellow arrow indicates the area with the strongest BOLD response. Note that off-resonance artifacts are present in the inferior frontal areas, causing some distortion of the activation pattern in fast magnetic resonance EEG (MREG). In the left upper corner a typical epileptic spike is visible in the EEG trace over the right posterior frontal area (F8) as well as a voltage map derived from this spike. Adapted with permission from Jacobs J, Stich J, Zahneisen B, et al. Fast fMRI provides high statistical power in the analysis of epileptic networks. Neuroimage. 2014;88:282–294.

window approach to the analysis of EEG–fMRI by which the evolution of a seizure with 2-sec time resolution and 5-mm spatial resolution can be obtained. In this way dynamical images of the onset and the propagation of epileptic seizures of the whole human brain were made noninvasively, yielding information on regions with increased or decreased metabolism associated with the evolution of seizures. This form of analysis of seizures of 10 focal epileptic patients showed that the first activation was likely to reflect the region of seizure onset with a limited extent, whereas a more extended and complex network was observed during seizure propagation.

A practical method for assessing the ictal hemodynamic evolution is the application of independent component analysis (ICA) to the fMRI data, even when scalp EEG does not reflect appropriately the seizure evolution. In the dataset of these authors, ICA yielded spatially independent components that could identify the seizure onset zone in all cases studied by this group (33). Notwithstanding these good results, seizures are essentially non-stationary signals, whereas ICA methodology assumes stationarity. Nonetheless, a series of criteria have been explored to estimate cluster of voxels with the most robust association between BOLD and EEG changes (32). Improvements of these combined studies may be expected from more investigations where intracranial EEG is combined with BOLD recordings (28).

With respect to *idiopathic generalized epilepsies*, several studies (44–48) revealed some common patterns of BOLD changes associated with generalized spike-and-wave discharges (GSWDs). There were BOLD decreases in frontal and parietal cortices, posterior cingulate, precuneus, and caudate, which largely reflect the default mode network, while there were increases in the thalamus, mesial frontal region, and insulae. The time relation between the onset of GSWDs and BOLD changes, both in cortex and thalamus, has been investigated, but with variable results, likely due to insufficient time resolution of the BOLD signal. To overcome this limitation, Moeller et al. (49) used sequences of short blocks to represent the time evolution of GSWDs in GLM (Fig. 46.4); in this way these authors were able to determine that BOLD increases in the cortex preceded those in the thalamus, in general agreement with the experimental findings obtained in genetic animal models of absence seizures (50). The dynamical changes found in this animal model during GSWD take place quickly (in a fraction of a second) and propagate to the thalamus, several cortical areas, striatum, and other brain systems very rapidly, at a pace that is difficult to follow with hemodynamic variables.

This is nicely illustrated in an EEG–fMRI study in a similar rat animal model by David et al. (51), where the neuronal driver of spike–wave discharges (SWDs) was found in the primary somatosensory cortex based on both intracerebral EEG and fMRI, using a dynamic causal model and Granger causality after deconvolution of hemodynamic effects. More complex, however, are the observations by Bai et al. (52), who found, in children with absence seizures, BOLD increases in the orbital/medial frontal and medial/lateral parietal cortex preceding by >5 sec the apparent onset of the seizures, followed by BOLD decreases that could be followed for >20 sec after seizure termination, while the thalamus showed delayed BOLD increases after seizure onset. These findings need

still confirmation, and deep scrutiny from a physiological viewpoint.

In short, this multiplicity of studies, taken together, allow us to draw the conclusion that BOLD signal changes complement EEG findings in identifying neuronal systems responsible for GSWDs, particularly by showing the involvement of a diversity of brain systems in the evolution of absence seizures, although not being able to follow the quick evolution in time of GSWDs.

3. EEG–PET

3.1. PET Tracers Used in Epilepsy

In the mid-1970s, PET was introduced as a tool to visualize gamma rays emitted by a positron-emitting radiotracer injected into the human body (53,54). The most commonly used tracer is fluorodeoxyglucose (FDG) (i.e., labeled glucose). In epileptic patients PET provides images of interictal brain glucose metabolism (Fig. 46.5). The observation of hypometabolism in epileptogenic cortex revealed by PET is a finding of great interest, but the underlying mechanisms are still being discussed. It appears that FDG PET distribution reflects synaptic activity rather than cellular loss (55). Then why do we see hypometabolism in PET and positive BOLD in the epileptogenic zone? fMRI takes into account the spikes and relates to these events, where between-spikes metabolism may be depressed, and there are many more periods between spikes than spike periods.

Reduction of glucose metabolism is correlated with the duration of epilepsy and inherently with the severity of the disease (56)—in other words, with longer disease and overall more spike counts (albeit not necessarily during the PET exam). There are also more interictal periods with severe metabolic dysfunction. It has been hypothesized that repeated seizures or dysfunctional cortex (like dysplasia or tubers) may induce a protective inhibitory effect through synaptic plasticity (57). In addition, the use of antiepileptic drugs can affect metabolism. Patients taking GABAergic drugs (e.g., benzodiazepines, barbiturates) often exhibit a diffuse hypometabolism that may hinder the identification of discrete areas of hypometabolic epileptogenic tissue (58). This study, as well as the absence of correlation of neuronal density with PET hypometabolism in epilepsy patients, supports the notion that PET reflects mainly synaptic activity and not neuronal loss (59).

Tracers other than FDG are less commonly used. Only a few centers have the necessary facilities and dedicated research programs to create new tracers. Most of the latter use radio-labeled carbon, whose production and use are more difficult than FDG. These tracers are either ligands of specific receptors or neurotransmitter precursors or transporters, specific for the main neurotransmitter systems: GABA, glutamate, serotonin, adenosine, acetylcholine, and the opioid system. Alpha-methyltryptophan (AMT)-PET showed promising results in patients with tuberous sclerosis, since an increased uptake of the epileptogenic tuber, among the other non-epileptogenic tubers, could be identified in most cases (60). Other developmental malformations might also benefit from AMT-PET imaging, such as dysplasia type IIb with balloon cells (61) or periventricular

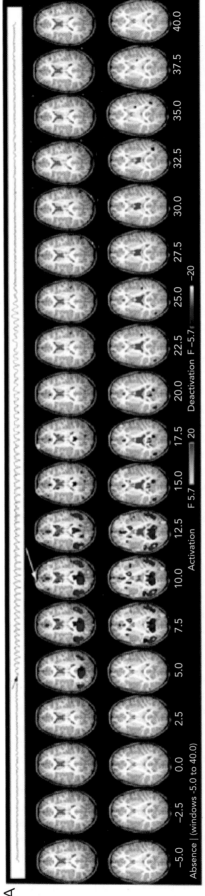

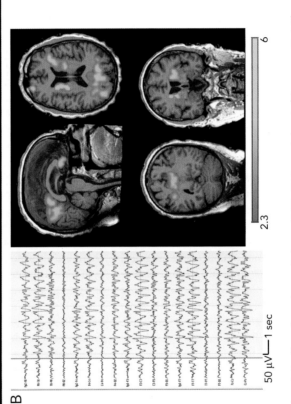

Figure 46.4. **A:** Sliding window fMRI analysis of two absences characterized by spike-and-wave discharges (SWDs; EEG record above) of the same patient. These windows (from 0 to 52.5 sec) overlapped by 5 sec, providing a statistical F-value every 2.5 sec. Windows before the onset and after the end of typical absence seizures with 3 Hz spike-wave pattern were observed. Each row shows the evolution of the BOLD signal for one typical absence characterized by SWDs. First activation consistent for both absences was found in the right inferior frontal cortex (white arrows). In the first absence this activation started 2.5 sec after the EEG onset; for the second absence it coincided with the EEG onset. The thalamic activation and deactivation in default mode areas and caudate nucleus started between 5 and 7.5 sec after onset. BOLD signal changes in the thalamus and default mode areas exceeded the duration of the absence by several windows. **B:** A 51-year-old patient with probable left cingulate seizures, characterized by bilateral 2- to 3-Hz spike–waves pattern. Deactivation of default mode areas are similar to the previous example (A), except that the thalamus is not affected. In fact, during these discharges the patient could execute orders and did not lose consciousness. Thalamic activation or deactivation of the fMRI might be a biomarker to discriminate idiopathic generalized epilepsy from focal epilepsy syndrome. **A:** Adapted with permission from (49).

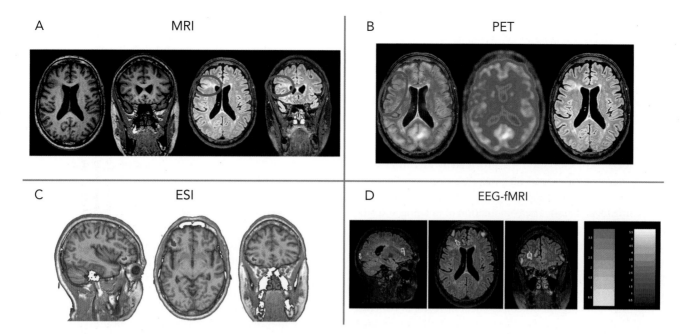

Figure 46.5. *Multimodal imaging in a patient with lesional right frontal epilepsy. A: Right frontal transmantle cortical dysplasia is apparent on the structural MRI (left T1; right FLAIR; lesion is highlighted by the red circles). B: Extended zone of hypometabolism, encompassing the lesion, in the right frontal lobe on interictal PET images (hypometabolism is highlighted by the red circle). C: EEG source imaging (ESI). D: Topography-related fMRI activation located in right prefrontal cortex (fMRI activation in red, deactivation in blue) in close proximity to the lesion. Right hemisphere is on the left of the image. Adapted with permission from Grouiller F, Delattre BMA, Pittau F, Heizer S, Lazeyras F, Spinelli L, et al. All-in-one interictal presurgical imaging in patients with epilepsy: single-session EEG/PET/(f)MRI. Eur J Nucl Med Mol Imaging. 2015;42:1133–1143, Fig. 2.*

heterotopia, although these studies are still limited and uptake is not always noted (62). The GABA antagonist flumazenil (FMZ) has been studied mainly in temporal lobe epilepsy and appears to be more sensitive than FDG for lateralizing the focus in this form of epilepsy (63,64). Its use in extratemporal lobe epilepsy has been less often studied, and signs of both hyperactivity and hypoactivity were identified, making FMZ-PET less useful in non-lesional extratemporal lobe epilepsy (65). Increased periventricular [11C] (FMZ) binding, perhaps reflecting the presence of heterotopic neurons, has been associated with the lack of postoperative seizure freedom in patients with temporal lobe epilepsy and hippocampal sclerosis (66,67).

3.2. Clinical Use and Relation to EEG Findings

PET studies showed a good correlation with scalp EEG findings in patients with focal abnormalities. They can even provide better localization than scalp EEG in some patients. The expectation in the early years was that the arrival of PET would obviate the need for intracranial evaluation (57,68), but this view turned out to be too optimistic. Later studies found a good localization/lateralization value of FDG-PET in temporal lobe epilepsy (TLE), less so in extratemporal lobe epilepsy, especially if the focus is deeply buried in brain tissue, due to nonlinear signal decrease with depth of dysfunctional tissue.

In patients with TLE and hippocampal sclerosis, FDG-PET often showed ipsilateral temporal hypometabolism of the mesial and to a variable degree lateral temporal structures, but also beyond the lesions/foci and the final resected volume. Thus, in these patients, PET tends to overestimate the epileptogenic zone (although it estimates the dysfunctional zone well) and therefore is not helpful for determining the exact limits of the epileptogenic zone. It probably reflects not only the ictal focal area but also the areas involved by the initial ictal spread (69). Nonetheless, it has also been shown that larger resections of the hypometabolic region are related to better outcome of the surgery (70). However, "more equals better" is true for any surgical procedure of this kind, since it increases the likelihood that the totality of abnormal tissue will be removed; of course, this must be weighed against the possible cognitive and physical deficits. Patients with resection limited to the anterior and mesial temporal lobe (i.e., smaller than the abnormal zone) often have excellent outcome.

PET turned out to be very useful in non-lesional TLE. In several studies on surgical candidates with unilateral temporal lobe epilepsy, unilateral hypometabolism helped to confirm TLE. The surgical results were as good as in patients with TLE and hippocampal sclerosis (~80% seizure-free), and PET is now an established tool to identify epileptogenic lesions, even subtle ones, in the temporal lobe of patients with chronic epilepsy (71–73). Patients with PET hypometabolism concordant with EEG findings benefit from surgery as much as patients with hippocampal sclerosis or other lesions identified on MRI. ~80% of them were seizure-free at >1 year follow-up.

The role of PET in extratemporal lobe epilepsy is less clear. A recent retrospective study of 194 patients with nonfocal or normal MRI showed unifocal hypometabolism in only 50.5%. PET findings were more often useful regarding the decision for or against surgery in TLE patients (63%) versus patients with frontal (38%) or other extratemporal lobe epilepsy (50%) (74). In another study, interictal discharges were localized using EEG–fMRI and compared with FDG-PET (75). The relationship appears to be complex, and several BOLD changes and several areas of hypometabolism were found. Most BOLD changes were at the margin or outside the hypometabolic zone(s), despite the presence of unifocal dysplasia, indicating that both techniques can identify the underlying epileptogenic network but may also provide potentially ambiguous results. In a study of 62 patients with type II focal cortical dysplasia (76), consisting of patients with MRI-positive (n = 37) and MRI-negative epilepsy (n = 25), no differences in the electroclinical pattern (stereo-EEG) between both groups were found. A correct localization was provided by PET in 21 of the 25 MRI-negative cases, and PET was also positive in 28 of the 37 MRI-positive patients, although in 4 of these PET yielded a misleading localization. The combination of imaging and EEG data allowed these authors to perform restricted resections, limited to a single gyrus in more than half of the cases.

In a retrospective study of 23 patients with MRI-negative focal cortical dysplasia, the metabolic data obtained with PET were compared with the epileptogenic zone determined by stereo-EEG and surgical outcome. Focal or regional concordant PET abnormalities were detected either by visual analysis alone or by PET/MRI co-registration (77). Twenty of 23 patients were seizure-free at 4 years after a limited resection that included the PET hypometabolic zone, showing the value of PET in localizing the epileptogenic zone in patients with MRI-negative findings.

Another study of 14 patients with similar clinical characteristics showed that the complete resection of the dysplastic cortex, localized by FDG-PET, subtraction ictal SPECT co-registered to MRI (SISCOM), or intracranial EEG, is a reliable predictor of favorable postoperative outcome (78). Therefore, PET is probably best used as a guide for focusing the review of MRI in the search for subtle overlooked cortical dysplasia. In addition, it is useful to guide the placement of intracranial electrodes.

Several studies in patients with anteromesial TLE have shown that hypometabolism can be found not only in the affected area but also, to a lesser extent, ipsilaterally in the frontal, parietal, insular cortex, thalamus, and basal ganglia (79), suggesting the existence of an epileptic network as described also for EEG–fMRI (see above). In unilateral mesial temporal lobe epilepsy, bilateral temporal lobe hypometabolism can often be detected, causing ambiguity with respect to lateralizing the epileptogenic zone. Having had a recent seizure is the major factor related to this situation: this can be avoided by performing the PET scan >2 days after the last seizure and/or with EEG-monitoring during and 30 min after tracer injection (80).

3.3. Visual Versus Statistical Analysis

In most clinical studies, and also in clinical practice, visual analysis is deemed to be sufficient. However, this appears not to be the case, since in this way discrete abnormal hypometabolic regions can be overlooked. A systematic comparison between the performance of visual analysis and automated quantified analysis of FDG-PET images in detecting the epileptogenic area, which was defined by a combination of clinical semiology, ictal and interictal EEG, SPECT, MRI, and FMZ-PET, showed similar sensitivity in patients with TLE but not in patients with extratemporal lobe epilepsy. Automated voxel-based analysis improved the yield of FDG-PET in patients with extratemporal lobe epilepsy, and the sensitivity rose from 19-38% to 67% (81).

4. SPECT

Nuclear medicine imaging techniques are widely used in the investigation of patients with pharmacoresistant epilepsy (82–84). SPECT allows in vivo estimates of cerebral perfusion changes on a fine time scale. Because cerebral blood flow is closely linked to neuronal activity and is maximal during a seizure, the distribution of perfusion changes is presumed to reflect neuronal activity levels in different areas of the brain. While PET "summarizes" the activity over 30 minutes or so, SPECT reflects activity in the second range (10–30 sec). Radiotracers cross promptly the blood–brain barrier and distribute over the brain. The distribution obtained over the first minutes after injection is stable for a few hours. Consequently, the acquired images reveal the perfusion at the time of injection, providing an "ictal snapshot" when the radiotracer is injected at the moment a seizure occurs (85). SPECT images provide information about the relative variation of brain perfusion between regions but do not yield quantitative values as regards regions of interest (86).

A lipophilic, pH-neutral radiopharmaceutical tracer is generally used, most commonly ^{99m}Tc-hexamethylpropyleneamine oxime (HMPAO) or ^{99m}Tc-ethylene cysteine diethylester (Tc-ECD) (87). Previously iodine-123-labeled N-isopropyl-p-iodoamphetamine (I-123-IMP) was also used, but it does not allow ictal imaging (88). A case report of three interictal I-123-IMP-SPECTs in a patient with frontal lobe epilepsy provided highly variable results (between right frontal hyperperfusion and normal) that could not be explained by seizure occurrence (89). ^{99m}Tc-ECD offers the advantage that it is stable for a long time (6–8 hours) and does not have to be reconstituted during the day when ictal SPECTs can be performed. ECD uptake is supposedly rather linear with regard to rCBF, although this may be less relevant in epilepsy. Comparisons between HMPAO and ECD are inconclusive: one study found higher sensitivity and specificity with regard to focus localization by ECD (89), but the other favored HMPAO, in particular for neocortical epilepsy (mostly neocortical temporal and frontal) (90).

SPECT can help to identify the seizure onset zone noninvasively if it is carried out at the correct time with respect to the development of the seizure. Performing SPECT during an epileptic event enables visualization of the perfusion changes occurring during these events; however, similar to fMRI, (ictal) SPECT often shows more than one hyperperfused region. Thus, there is growing evidence that epilepsy implies the activation of a network rather than a single focus (91,92), which is readily picked up by techniques measuring blood flow. It has been shown that SPECT/SISCOM hyperperfusions coincide with the areas of BOLD changes revealed by the EEG–fMRI in most of the patients (93). The best-established technique is SISCOM (89) (see below).

In most studies, radiotracer injection is done manually at bedside. To reveal perfusion patterns related to the seizure5 the tracer should be injected as soon as possible (94) after the seizure onset. This implies that a nurse or a physician should continuously and carefully watch both the patient and the EEG. Thus, performing ictal SPECT requires significant staffing and logistics. During the evolution of temporal lobe seizures, hyperperfusion switches to isoperfusion and then to hypoperfusion. Thus, if the injection is performed too late, focus localization is not obtained. To the best of our knowledge, no systematic studies on postictal perfusion changes have been carried out on extratemporal seizures. Nonetheless, the yield in extratemporal lobe epilepsy is as high as in TLE, albeit it is more difficult to achieve due the brevity of some extratemporal seizures (95).

In the case of a seizure with motor components, safety considerations can arise to protect the medical staff against radiotracer projection. A few centers have reported the use of automatic or remote pump systems. Feichtinger et al. (96) proposed a setup that allowed injections to be started remotely by the nurse. The efficacy of remote-controlled injection is demonstrated in terms of SPECT image quality compared to manual injection. Lee et al. (97) decreased the delay of injection from seizure onset from 40 (± 26) to 12 sec (± 12) using an attachable automated injector.

SPECT image review should be interpreted in the light of the simultaneous ongoing EEG and clinical observations at the time of injection. Therefore, the time of injection with respect to seizure onset should be carefully documented and marked on the tracing. Comparison between ictal and interictal SPECT is mandatory to extract the exact localization of the focus; interictal images alone are useless. Visual inspection of both images is limited due to low spatial resolution and difficulties in appreciating subtle changes with just a black-and-white or color scale. Thus, several statistical approaches have been proposed to increase the yield of this exam in term of epileptic foci localization.

Applying SISCOM, once the ictal and interictal images have been co-registered, both images are normalized and then subtracted (Fig. 46.6). The subtraction image is thresholded to display only values greater than two standard deviations of the subtraction pixel distribution. The computed image is then displayed over the anatomical image and interpreted. The SISCOM algorithm is implemented, for example, in the Analyze software (AnalyzeDirect, Overland Park, KS).

Several more methods of SPECT image analysis are available. Statistical parametric mapping (SPM) is used for a variety of imaging sets and has been also used to evaluate differences between pairs of ictal and interictal images and SPECT images of healthy controls (98). Significant increases or decreases of perfusion are computed (99). The method is referred as ictal–interictal SPECT analysis by SPM (ISAS). The method is available through SPM scripts or BioImage suite software programs. STATISCOM (statistical ictal SPECT co-registered to MRI) is similar. As for the ISAS approach, the ictal–interictal difference image is compared to a normal control set; however, images are obtained twice within a subject to compensate for possible perfusion

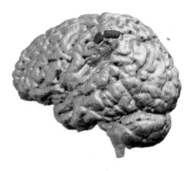

Figure 46.6. *Three-dimensional co-registration of multimodal information, including also eloquent cortex localization. Electric source imaging (ESI) related to scalp EEG spikes (green), SISCOM maximum (blue), localization of the somatosensory area of the right hand by high-density somatosensory evoked potentials (pink), motor area of the right hand localized by fMRI (yellow). All activation has been projected orthogonally to the surface using option "depth shifting" of Cartool. Note the proximity of epileptogenic cortex (green, blue) and vital cortex (pink, yellow), which was confirmed by electrocorticography and subdural EEG recordings. Focus resection, sparing as much as possible hand area cortex, led to postoperative distal hand paresis, which improved to almost normal preoperative levels over the next months.*

changes between two time points (100). HERMES BRASS software (Brain Registration & Analysis Software Suite) offers the possibility of comparing individual SPECT images to a database of healthy subjects. Processing includes comparisons between individuals as much as comparison with the template derived from control subjects. This technique is also used for FDG-PET. On a voxel-by-voxel analysis, deviations from the control group can be localized, using for example the Talairach atlas (101,102).

Sulc et al. (103) compared the performance of each technique to localize correctly epileptic foci in a cohort of 49 patients, 21 with TLE and 28 with extratemporal epilepsy, all having an unrevealing MRI (MRI-negative). Only patients were included who had undergone surgery and had a follow-up of >1 year. For ISAS and STATISCOM, two SPECT scans from 30 normal subjects served as control. For both non-lesional TLE and extratemporal epilepsy groups, SPM-based analysis techniques (ISAS and STATISCOM) often showed concordance of the focal ictal hyperperfusion to the resection site, particularly for TLE patients (STATISCOM 71% correct, ISAS 67%, SISCOM 38%). If the area of hyperperfusion as identified by ISAS or STATISCOM was included in the resection, the likelihood of the patient being seizure-free after surgery was significantly higher compared to SISCOM. This relationship was not obtained for non-lesional extratemporal epilepsy; however, ISAS and STATISCOM tend to provide correctly localizing results more often than SISCOM (57%, 53%, and 36%, respectively).

5. ELECTRIC SOURCE IMAGING

Apart from PET and SPECT imaging, the role of EEG in the presurgical workup of epileptic patients who are candidates for a surgical resection is essential, especially if the EEG is recorded with a large number of electrodes (128–256 channels [i.e., high-density EEG, or HD-EEG]) in order to

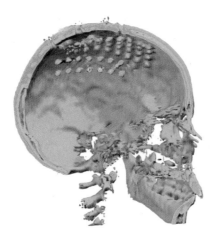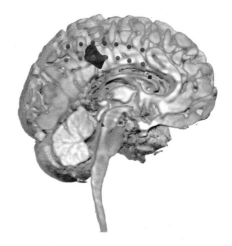

Figure 46.7. *Three-year-old patient with left mesial parietal epilepsy, requiring intracranial monitoring with subdural electrodes. Left: Postoperative CT shows artifacts produced by subdural electrodes, which can be used to reconstruct their position. Right: After co-registration with the preoperative MRI, intra-hemispheric subdural electrodes are shown with a three-dimensional rendering of the brain. The lesion (red) was detected by morphometric analysis. Co-registration of subdural electrodes, MRI, and morphometric data allowed verification that subdural electrodes cover the suspicious area. The patient underwent surgery and has been seizure-free for 4 years.*

perform *high-density electric source imaging* (HD-ESI) (104), as described in Chapter 45 (see also Fig. 46.2). Lascano et al. (105) published a prospective study of 190 patients, 58 of whom underwent all four noninvasive techniques (HD-ESI, MRI, PET, and SPECT). In this patient group MRI and HD-ESI showed the highest predictive value of surgical outcome (both at a significant level of $p < .004$). Patients with concordant MRI and HD-ESI had a 92.3% probability of favourable outcome, while the probability was 0% when the results of these two methodologies were not taken into account and/or did not provide localizing results. These results indicate clearly the importance of including HD-ESI in the workup of candidates for epilepsy surgery. With new systems allowing long-term recording with 64 to 256 channels, ictal HD-ESI is technically also possible and has been done in a few small studies (106). However, the search for optimal algorithms for analysis is ongoing (e.g., frequency-based, global field power maxima, repetitive spikes) (106a). It is also noteworthy that HD-EEG can be used to localize eloquent cortex (107).

An alternative neurophysiological tool is MEG, which has shown its usefulness in the context of presurgical evaluation (108). Due to the more complex setup, ictal recordings are less easily obtained. For detailed discussion on this technique and the neuronal substrates, see Chapter 35.

6. ELECTRODE LOCALIZATION

To evaluate the performance of ESI in identifying an epileptogenic zone, co-registration is mandatory; in this way the distance between ESI maxima and the seizure onset zone defined by intracranial electrodes can be estimated (109,110). Visualization of intra-cerebral electrodes can be achieved either using CT scan or MRI (111). The latter has the advantage of being radiation-free, although the detection and the individualization of intra-cerebral electrodes on CT scan provide more reliable results and less ambiguous artifacts

(112,113). Localization of the electrodes with respect to the anatomy requires co-registration of the postoperative images with the preoperative ones (114) (Fig. 46.7). As both datasets are from the same patient, one might think that the rigid body co-registration would be sufficient to perform good anatomical matching of the electrodes. However, introducing external material inside the skull can produce bleeding, which may accumulate between the brain and the skull, or edema, and consequently shifts in brain position. Without taking into account this deformation, a rigid co-registration can lead to the wrong anatomical correlation for the implanted electrodes. In Stieglitz et al. (115), elastic matching was introduced to co-register pre and post datasets. Pieters et al. (116) presented a survey of different ways to label correctly the subdural electrodes with respect to brain anatomy. The use of intraoperative high-resolution digital photos may be helpful, even though sometimes not all the electrodes are visible and co-registration of two- and three-dimensional images is not obvious (117).

7. TECHNICAL ASPECTS OF MEDICAL IMAGE REGISTRATION

Medical images are used intensively in health care, bringing together different levels of information. Images are major tools in diagnosis and are also important in planning interventions, which may be surgical or radiotherapeutic. Usually a variety of images have to be combined to obtain insight into pathological processes. This implies that image registration must bring all images into the same frame of reference and with the same resolution (118). Registration, co-registration, alignment, and matching are different terms that refer to the same process of bringing two or more images within the same frame of view. The registration process can be divided into sub-processes. First, one has to define the features (distinctive objects, points, contours, corners, surface) that will be used for matching. This is the question of "what to register."

The salient objects can be detected automatically or manually. These objects are divided in two categories: intrinsic and extrinsic. Then the question of "how to register" has to be answered. Depending on the distance between the two images to be registered (different orientation, intra- vs. inter-subject, intra- vs. inter-modality), rigid body, affine, or elastic matching should be used to achieve a good alignment. Registration parameters are then estimated or computed. Finally the transformation parameters are applied to deform the images using interpolation algorithms (119).

Image registration is used for a large number of applications in the medical domain (120). In the context of this chapter we focus on applications in patients with epilepsy. This means bringing together MRI sequences (T1, T2, FLAIR, fMRI) nuclear imaging techniques (PET, SPECT) and three-dimensional ESI to enhance the quality of the diagnosis and to guide more accurately the neurologist and the neurosurgeon in planning a surgical intervention. This approach refers to the intra-subject co-registration. Further, intra-subject co-registration is also used to co-register images, whether two- or three-dimensional, from the same modality when the data were acquired in different clinical conditions or at different times. For example, this allows monitoring the evolution of a tumor over time, or comparing different exams obtained during the ictal and the interictal phase in the case of epilepsy.

Co-registration involves a number of technical steps; here we refer to only a few main procedures that have to be considered. Alignment of images of the same modality is usually performed using rigid body algorithms. For a formal description and the implementation of rigid-body transformations, see http://www.fil.ion.ucl.ac.uk/spm/doc/books/hbf2/pdfs/Ch2.pdf from John Ashburner and Karl J. Friston (121). Applications using this approach are numerous and widely present in the clinical environment. Further, the same reference deals with registration methods between different modalities such as PET and MRI. In this case rigid body co-registration cannot perform adequate alignment of the images. Elastic matching is then rquired to make the alignment between two different objects precise and accurate. This is also the case when inter-subject registration is required (122). Ardekani et al. (123) presented a review of three different software programs that perform elastic matching. Klein et al. (124) evaluated and discussed up to 14 nonlinear algorithms. Using a brain parcellation atlas, the authors computed the quality of each algorithm in terms of volume and surface overlap, similarity and distance measures, over 45,000 registrations. This paper has the merit of presenting an independent analysis of the tested software.

Even though accuracy is the main factor that should be taken into account when choosing an algorithm, robustness and reliability are equally important. The algorithm's robustness, or stability (125), is defined as its ability to give stable results in the presence of noise. Different noise sources can affect the result of the computation. The images themselves can be noisy, for example due to movement during the scan (126). High-field MRI scanners present more important gradient non-uniformity-inducing geometric distortion in MR images and therefore are more prone to error; distortion algorithms were very effective with 1.5T and 3T machines in reducing positional errors but still need to be validated in 7T imaging (127).

Finally, we have to take into account the availability of several techniques for MRI segmentation of the human brain (128–131). Different approaches were evaluated (132), in particular volume-based and surface-based brain imaging registration methods (133). The major challenge of all methods is that they allow the detection of small dysfunctional structures, the detection of abnormalities in only a subset of sequences or processed images (e.g., junction image) and in the individual patient.

ACKNOWLEDGMENTS

M.S. was supported by SNSF 140332, 127608, 146633. J.G. was supported by the Canadian Institutes of Health Research grant FDN 143208.

REFERENCES

1. Jueptner M, Weiller C. Review: does measurement of regional cerebral blood flow reflect synaptic activity? Implications for PET and fMRI. Neuroimage. 1995;2:148–156.
2. Attwell D, Iadecola C. The neural basis of functional brain imaging signals. Trends Neurosci. 2002;25:621–625.
3. Arthurs OJ, Boniface S. How well do we understand the neural origins of the fMRI BOLD signal? Trends Neurosci. 2002;25:27–31.
4. Shmuel A, Augath M, Oeltermann A, Logothetis NK. Negative functional MRI response correlates with decreases in neuronal activity in monkey visual area V1. Nat Neurosci. 2006;9:569–577.
5. Logothetis NK. Intracortical recordings and fMRI: an attempt to study operational modules and networks simultaneously. Neuroimage. 2012;62:962–969.
6. Simon AB, Buxton RB. Understanding the dynamic relationship between vertebral blood flow and the BOLD signal: implications for quantitative functional MRI. Neuroimage. 2015;116:158–167.
7. Mata M, Fink DJ, Gainer H, et al. Activity-dependent energy metabolism in rat posterior pituitary primarily reflects sodium pump activity. 1980. J Neurochem. 1980;34:213–215.
8. Grouiller F, Delattre BMA, Pittau F, et al. All-in-one interictal presurgical imaging in patients with epilepsy: single-session EEG/PET/(f)MRI. Eur J Nucl Med Mol Imaging. 2015;42:1133–1143.
9. Viswanathan A, Freeman RD. Neurometabolic coupling in cerebral cortex reflects synaptic more than spiking activity. Nat Neurosci. 2007;10:1308–1312
10. Nir Y, Dinstein I, Malach R, Heeger DJ. BOLD and spiking activity. Nat Neurosci. 2008;11: 523–524.
11. Shmuel A, Maier A. Neurophysiological basis of functional MRI. In: Ugurbil K, Uludag K, Berliner LJ, eds. fMRI: From Nuclear Spins to Brain Function. Biological Magnetic Resonance, Vol. 30. New York: Springer Science and Business Media, 2015.
12. Harel N, Lee SP, Nagaoka T, et al. Origin of negative blood oxygenation level-dependent fMRI signals. J Cereb Blood Flow Metab. 2002;22:908–917.
13. Bénar CG, Gross DW, Wang Y, et al. The BOLD response to interictal epileptiform discharges. Neuroimage. 2002;17:1182–1192.
14. Handwerker DA, Ollinger JM, D'Esposito M. Variation of BOLD hemodynamic responses across subjects and brain regions and their effects on statistical analyses. Neuroimage. 2004;21:1639–1651.
15. Proulx S, Safi-Harb M, LeVan P, et al. Increased sensitivity of fast BOLD fMRI with a subject-specific hemodynamic response function and application to epilepsy. Neuroimage. 2014;93:59–73.
16. Magri C, Schridde U, Murayama Y, et al. The amplitude and timing of the BOLD signal reflects the relationship between local field potential power at different frequencies. J Neurosci. 2012;32:1395–1407.
17. Goldman RI, Stern JM, Engel J, Cohen M. Simultaneous EEG and fMRI of the alpha rhythm. Neuroreport. 2002;13:2487–2492.

18. Laufs H, Krakow K, Sterzer P, et al. Electroencephalographic signatures of attentional and cognitive default modes in spontaneous brain fluctuations at rest. Proc Natl Acad Sci USA. 2003;100:11053–11058.
19. Laufs H, Holt JL, Elfont R, et al. Where the BOLD signal goes when alpha EEG leaves. Neuroimage. 2006;31:1408–1418.
20. Moosmann M, Ritter P, Krastel I, et al. Correlates of alpha rhythm in functional magnetic resonance imaging and near infrared spectroscopy. Neuroimage. 2003;20:145–158.
21. Gonçalves SI, de Munck, JC, Pouwels PJW, et al. Correlating the alpha rhythm to BOLD using simultaneous EEG/fMRI: inter-subject variability. Neuroimage. 2006;30:203–213.
22. De Munck JC, Gonçalves SI, Mammoliti R, et al. Interactions between different EEG frequency bands and their effect on alpha-fMRI correlations. Neuroimage 2009;47:69–76.
23. Sadaghiani S, Scheeringa R, Lehongre K, et al. Intrinsic connectivity networks, alpha oscillations, and tonic alertness: a simultaneous electroencephalography/functional magnetic resonance imaging study. J Neurosci. 2010;30(30):10243–10250.
24. Tyvaert L, Chassagnon S, Sadikot A, et al. Thalamic nuclei activity in idiopathic generalized epilepsy: an EEG-fMRI study. Neurology. 2009;73:2018–2022.
25. Le Bihan D. The "wet mind": water and functional neuroimaging. Phys Med Biol. 2007;52(7):R57–90.
26. Flint J, Hansen B, Vestergaard-Poulsen P, Blackband SJ. Diffusion-weighted magnetic resonance imaging of neuronal activity in the hippocampal slice model. Neuroimage. 2009;46:411–418.
27. Ives JR, Warach S, Schmitt F, et al. Monitoring the patients's EEG during echo planar MRI. Electroencephogr Clin Neurophysiol. 1993;87:417–420.
28. Gotman J, Kobayashi E, Bagshaw AP, et al. Combining EEG and fMRI: a multimodal tool for epilepsy research. J Magn Reson Imaging. 2006;23:906–920.
29. Bagshaw AP, Aghakhani Y, Bénar C-G, et al. EEG-fMRI of focal epileptic spikes: analysis with multiple haemodynamic functions and comparison with gadolinium-enhanced MR angiograms. Hum Brain Mapp. 2004;22:179–192.
30. Turner R. How much cortex can a vein drain? Downstream dilution of activation-related cerebral blood oxygen changes. Neuroimage. 2002;16:1062–1067.
31. Parkes LM, Schwarzbach JV, Bouts AA, et al. Quantifying the spatial resolution of the gradient echo and spin echo BOLD response at 3 Tesla. Magn Reson Med. 2005;54:1465–1472.
32. Nencka AS, Rowe DB. Reducing the unwanted draining vein BOLD contribution in fMRI with statistical post-processing methods. Neuroimage. 2007;37:177–188.
33. Pittau F, Grova C, Moeller F, et al. Patterns of altered functional connectivity in mesial temporal lobe epilepsy. Epilepsia. 2012;53:1013–1023.
34. Thornton R, Vulliemoz S, Rodionov R, et al. Epileptic networks in focal cortical dysplasia revealed using electroencephalography-functional magnetic resonance imaging. Ann Neurol. 2011;70:822–837.
35. An D, Fahoum F, Hall J, et al. Electroencephalography/functional magnetic resonance imaging responses help predict surgical outcome in focal epilepsy. Epilepsia. 2013;54:2184–2194.
36. Murta T, Leite M, Carmichael DW, et al. Electrophysiological correlates of the BOLD signal for EEG-informed fMRI. Hum Brain Mapp. 2015;36:391–414.
37. Vulliemoz S, Rodionov R, Carmichael DW, et al. Continuous EEG source imaging enhances analysis of EEG-fMRI in focal epilepsy. Neuroimage. 2010;49:3219–3229.
38. Zahneisen B, Grotz T, Lee KJ, et al. Three-dimensional MR-encephalography: fast volumetric brain imaging using rosette trajectories. Magn Reson Med. 2011;65:1260–1268.
39. Jacobs J, Menzel A, Ramantani G, et al. Negative BOLD in default-mode structures measured with EEG-MREG is larger in temporal than extra-temporal epileptic spikes. Front Neurosci. 2014;8:335.
40. Safi-Harb M, Proulx S, von Ellenrieder N, Gotman J. Advantages and disadvantages of a fast fMRI sequence in the context of EEG-fMRI investigation of epilepsy patients: A realistic simulation study. Neuroimage. 2015;119:20–32.
41. Chaudhary UJ, Duncan JS, Lemieux L. Mapping hemodynamic correlates of seizures using fMRI: a review. Hum Brain Mapp. 2013;34:447–466.
42. Thornton RC, Rodionov R, Laufs H, et al. Imaging haemodynamic changes related to seizures: comparison of EEG-based general linear model, independent component analysis of fMRI and intracranial EEG. 2010. Neuroimage. 2010;53:196–205.
43. Tyvaert L, LeVan P, Dubeau F, Gotman J. Non-invasive dynamic imaging of seizures in epileptic patients. Hum Brain Mapp. 2009;30:3993–4011.
44. Salek-Haddadi A, Lemieux L, Merschhemke M, et al. Functional magnetic resonance imaging of human absence seizures. Ann Neurol. 2003;53:663–667.
45. Aghakhani Y, Bagshaw AP, Bénar, C-G, et al. fMRI activation during spike and wave discharges in idiopathic generalized epilepsy. Brain. 2004;127:1127–1144.
46. Gotman J, Grova C, Bagshaw A, et al. Generalized epileptic discharges show thalamocortical activation and suspension of the default state of the brain. Proc Natl Acad Sci USA. 2005;102:15236–15240.
47. Hamandi K, Laufs H, Nöth U, et al. Bold and perfusion changes during epileptic generalized spike wave activity. Neuroimage. 2008; 9:608–618.
48. Laufs H, Langler U, Hamandi K, et al. Linking generalized spike-and-wave discharges and resting state brain activity by using EEG/fMRI in a patient with absence seizures. Epilepsia. 2006;47:444–448.
49. Moeller F, Levan P, Muhle H, et al. Absence seizures: individual patterns revealed by EEG-fMRI. Epilepsia. 2010;51:2000–2010.
50. Meeren HK, Pijn JP, van Luijtelaar EL, et al. Cortical focus drives widespread corticothalamic networks during spontaneous absence seizures in rats. J Neurosci. 2002;22:1480–1495.
51. David O, Guillemin I, Saillet S, et al. Identifying neural drivers with functional MRI: an electrophysiological validation. PLoS Biol. 2008;6(12).
52. Bai X, Vestal M, Berman R, et al. Dynamic time course of typical childhood absence seizures: EEG, behavior, and functional magnetic resonance imaging. J Neurosci. 2010;30:5884–5893.
53. Ter-Pogossian MM, Phelps ME, Hoffman EJ, Mullani NA. A positron-emission transaxial tomograph for nuclear imaging (PET). Radiology. 1975;114:89–98.
54. Phelps ME, Hoffman EJ, Mullani NA, Ter-Pogossian MM. Application of annihilation coincidence detection to transaxial reconstruction tomography. J Nucl Med. 1975;16:210–224.
55. Magistretti PJ. Cellular bases of functional brain imaging: insights from neuron-glia metabolic coupling. Brain Res. 2000;886:108–112.
56. Theodore WH, Fishbein D, Dubinsky R. Patterns of cerebral glucose metabolism in patients with partial seizures. Neurology. 1998;38:1201–1206.
57. Kumar A, Semah F, Chugani HT, Theodore WH. Epilepsy diagnosis: positron emission tomography. Handb Clin Neurol. 2012;107:409–424.
58. Varrone A, Sjöholm N, Eriksson L, et al. Advancement in PET quantification using 3D-OP-OSEM point spread function reconstruction with the HRRT. Eur J Nucl Med Mol Imaging. 2009;36:1639–1650.
59. Foldvary N, Lee N, Hanson MW, et al. Correlation of hippocampal neuronal density and FDG-PET in mesial temporal lobe epilepsy. Epilepsia. 1999;40:26–29.
60. Kagawa K, Chugani DC, Asano E, et al. Epilepsy surgery outcome in children with tuberous sclerosis complex evaluated with alpha-[11C] methyl-L-tryptophan positron emission tomography (PET). J Child Neurol. 2005;20:429–438.
61. Chugani HT, Kumar A, Kupsky W, et al. Clinical and histopathological correlates of 11C-alpha-methyl-L-tryptophan (AMT) PET abnormalities in children with intractable epilepsy. Epilepsia. 2011;52:1692–1698.
62. Natsume J, Bernasconi N, Aghakhani Y, et al. Alpha-[11C]methyl-L-tryptophan uptake in patients with periventricular nodular heterotopia and epilepsy. Epilepsia. 2008;49:826–831.
63. Koepp MJ, Richardson MP, Brooks DJ, et al. Central benzodiazepine/gamma-aminobutyric acid A receptors in idiopathic generalized epilepsy: an [11C]flumazenil positron emission tomography study. Epilepsia. 1997;38:1089–1097.
64. Vivash L, Gregoire MC, Lau EW, et al. 18F-flumazenil: a γ-aminobutyric acid A specific PET radiotracer for the localization of drug-resistant temporal lobe epilepsy. J Nucl Med. 2013;54:1270–1277.
65. Richardson MP, Koepp MJ, Brooks DJ, Duncan JS. 11C-flumazenil PET in neocortical epilepsy. Neurology. 1998;51:485–492.
66. Hammers A, Koepp MJ, Brooks DJ, Duncan JS. Periventricular white matter flumazenil binding and postoperative outcome in hippocampal sclerosis. Epilepsia. 2005;46:944–948.
67. Yankam Njiwa J, Bouvard S, Catenoix H, et al. Periventricular [C]flumazenil binding for predicting postoperative outcome in individual patients with temporal lobe epilepsy and hippocampal sclerosis. Neuroimage Clin. 2013;3:242–248.
68. Theodore WH, Brooks R, Sato S, et al. The role of positron emission tomography in the evaluation of seizure disorders. Ann Neurol. 1984;15 Suppl:176–179.
69. Nelissen N, Van Paesschen W, Baete, K, et al. Correlations of interictal FDG-PET metabolism and ictal SPECT perfusion changes in human temporal lobe epilepsy with hippocampal sclerosis. Neuroimage. 2006;32:684–695.
70. Vinton AB, Carne R, Hicks RJ, et al. The extent of resection of FDG-PET hypometabolism relates to outcome of temporal lobectomy. Brain. 2007;130:548–560.
71. Carne RP, O'Brien TJ, Kilpatrick CJ, et al. MRI-negative PET-positive temporal lobe epilepsy: a distinct surgically remediable syndrome. Brain. 2004;127:2276–2285.

72. Gok B, Jallo G, Hayeri R. The evaluation of FDG-PET imaging for epileptogenic focus localization in patients with MRI positive and MRI negative temporal lobe epilepsy. Neuroradiology. 2013;55:541–550.

73. LoPinto-Khoury C, Sperling M, Skidmore C. Surgical outcome in PET-positive, MRI negative patients with temporal lobe epilepsy. Epilepsia. 2012;53:342–348.

74. Rathore C, Dickson JC, Teotónio R, et al. The utility of 18F-fluorodeoxyglucose PET (FDG PET) in epilepsy surgery. Epilepsy Res. 2014;108:1306–1314.

75. Donaire A, Capdevila A, Carreño M, et al. Identifying the cortical substrates of interictal epileptiform activity in patients with extratemporal epilepsy: An EEG-fMRI sequential analysis and FDG-PET study. Epilepsia. 2013;54:678–690.

76. Chassoux F, Landré E, Mellerio C, et al. Type II focal cortical dysplasia: electroclinical phenotype and surgical outcome related to imaging. Epilepsia. 2012;53:349–358.

77. Chassoux F, Rodrigo S, Semah F, et al. FDG-PET improves surgical outcome in negative MRI Taylor-type focal cortical dysplasias. Neurology. 2010;75:2168–2175.

78. Kudr M, Krsek P, Maton B, et al. Predictive factors of ictal SPECT findings in paediatric patients with focal cortical dysplasia. Epileptic Disord. 2013;15:383–391.

79. Nelissen N, Van Paesschen W, Baete K, et al. Correlations of interictal FDG-PET metabolism and ictal SPECT perfusion changes in human temporal lobe epilepsy with hippocampal sclerosis. Neuroimage. 2006;32:684–695.

80. Tepmongkol S, Srikijvilaikul T, Vasavid P. Factors affecting bilateral temporal lobe hypometabolism on 18F-FDG PET brain scan in unilateral medial temporal lobe epilepsy. Epilepsy Behav. 2013;29:386–389.

81. Drzezga A, Arnold S, Minoshima S, et al. 18F-FDG PET studies in patients with extratemporal and temporal epilepsy: evaluation of an observer-independent analysis. J Nucl Med. 1999;40:737–746.

82. Kumar A, Chugani HT. The role of radionuclide imaging in epilepsy, part 2: epilepsy syndromes. J Nucl Med. 2013;54:1924–1930.

83. Fernández S, Donaire A, Serès E, et al. PET/MRI and PET/MRI/SISCOM coregistration in the presurgical evaluation of refractory focal epilepsy. Epilepsy Res. 2015;111:1–9.

84. Joo EY, Seo DW, Hong SC, Hong SB. Functional neuroimaging findings in patients with lateral and mesio-lateral temporal lobe epilepsy; FDG-PET and ictal SPECT studies. J Neurol. 2015;262:1120–1129.

85. So EL, O'Brien TJ. Peri-ictal single-photon emission computed tomography: principles and applications in epilepsy evaluation. Handb Clin Neurol. 2012;107:425–436.

86. Kapucu OL, Nobili F, Varrone A, et al. EANM procedure guideline for brain perfusion SPECT using 99mTc-labelled radiopharmaceuticals, version 2. Eur J Nucl Med Mol Imaging. 2009;36:2093–2102.

87. Juni JE, Waxman AD, Devous MD, et al. Procedure guideline for brain perfusion SPECT using 99mTc radiopharmaceuticals 3.0*. J Nucl Med Technol 2009;37:191–195.

88. Jibiki I, Yamaguchi N, Matsuda H, Hisada K. Fluctuations of interictal brain imaging in repeated 123I-IMP SPECT scans in an epileptic patient. J Neurol. 1990;237:372–375.

89. O'Brien TJ, Brinkmann BH, Mullan BP, et al. Comparative study of 99mTc-ECD and 99mTc-HMPAO for peri-ictal SPECT: qualitative and quantitative analysis. J Neurol Neurosurg Psychiatry. 1999;66:331–339.

90. Lee DS, Lee SK, Kim YK, et al. Superiority of HMPAO ictal SPECT to ECD ictal SPECT in localizing the epileptogenic zone. Epilepsia. 2002;43:263–269.

91. Pittau F, Vulliemoz S. Functional brain networks in epilepsy: recent, advances in noninvasive imaging. Curr Opinion Neurol. 2015;28:338–343.

92. Cleeren E, Casteels C, Goffin K, et al. Ictal perfusion changes associated with seizure progression in the amygdala kindling model in the rhesus monkey. Epilepsia. 2015;56:1366–1375.

93. Tousseyn S, Dupont P, Goffin K, et al. Correspondence between large-scale ictal and interictal epileptic networks revealed by single photon emission computed tomography (SPECT) and electroencephalography (EEG)–functional magnetic resonance imaging (fMRI). Epilepsia. 2015;56:382–392.

94. Rowe CC, Berkovic SF, Austin MC, et al. Patterns of postictal cerebral blood flow in temporal lobe epilepsy: qualitative and quantitative analysis. Neurology. 1991;41:1096–1103.

95. Newton MR, Berkovic SF, Austin MC, et al. SPECT in the localisation of extratemporal and temporal seizure foci. J Neurol Neurosurg Psychiatry. 1995;59:26–30.

96. Feichtinger M, Eder H, Holl A, et al. Automatic and remote controlled ictal SPECT injection for seizure focus localization by use of a commercial contrast agent application pump. Epilepsia. 2007;48:1409–1413.

97. Lee JJ, Lee SK, Choi JW, et al. Ictal SPECT using an attachable automated injector: clinical usefulness in the prediction of ictal onset zone. Acta Radiol. 2009;50:1160–1168.

98. Friston KJ, Ashburner J, Kiebel SJ, et al., eds. Statistical Parametric Mapping: The Analysis of Functional Brain Images. Academic Press, 2007.

99. McNally KA, Paige AL, Varghese G, et al. Localizing value of ictal-interictal SPECT analyzed by SPM (ISAS). Epilepsia. 2005;46:1450–1464.

100. Kazemi NJ, Worrell GA, Stead SM, et al. Ictal SPECT statistical parametric mapping in temporal lobe epilepsy surgery. Neurology. 2010;74:70–76.

101. Koch W, Radau PE, Hamann C, Tatsch K. Clinical testing of an optimized software solution for an automated, observer-independent evaluation of dopamine transporter SPECT studies. J Nucl Med. 2005;46:1109–1118.

102. Pencharz DR, Hanlon P, Chakravartty R, et al. Automated quantification with BRASS reduces quivocal reporting of DaTSCAN (123I-FP-CIT) SPECT studies. Nucl Med Rev Cent East Eur. 2014;17:65–69.

103. Sulc V, Stykel S, Hanson DP, et al. Statistical SPECT processing in MRI-negative epilepsy surgery. Neurology. 2014;82:932–939.

104. Brodbeck V, Spinelli L, Lascano AM, et al. Electroencephalographic source imaging: a prospective study of 152 operated epileptic patients. Brain. 2011;134:2887–2897.

105. Lascano AM, Perneger T, Vulliemoz S, et al. Yield of MRI, high-density electric source imaging (HD-ESI), SPECT and PET in epilepsy surgery candidates. Clin Neurophysiol. 2016;127:150–155.

106. Holmes MD, Tucker DM, Quiring JM, et al. Comparing noninvasive dense array and intracranial electroencephalography for localization of seizures. Neurosurgery. 2010;66:354–362.

106a. Nemtsas P, Birot G, Pittau F, et al. Source localization of ictal epileptic activity based on high-density scalp EEG data. *Epilepsia.* 2017 Jun;58(6):1027–1036.

107. Lascano AM, Grouiller F, Genetti M, et al. Surgically relevant localization of the central sulcus with high-density somatosensory-evoked potentials compared with functional magnetic resonance imaging. Neurosurgery. 2015;74:517–526.

108. Kharkar S, Knowlton R. Magnetoencephalography in the presurgical evaluation of epilepsy. Epilepsy Behav. 2015;46:19–26.

109. Rikir E, Koessler L, Gavaret M, et al. Electrical source imaging in cortical malformation–related epilepsy: A prospective EEG-SEEG concordance study. Epilepsia. 2014;55:918–932.

110. Mégevand P, Spinelli L, Genetti M, et al. Electric source imaging of interictal activity accurately localises the seizure onset zone. J Neurol Neurosurg Psychiatry. 2014;85:38–43.

111. Yang AI, Wang X, Doyle WK, et al. Localization of dense intracranial electrode arrays using magnetic resonance imaging. Neuroimage. 2012;63:157–165.

112. Darcey TM, Roberts DW. Technique for the localization of intracranially implanted electrodes. J Neurosurg. 2010;113:1182–1185.

113. Azarion AA, Wu J, Pearce A, et al. An open-source automated platform for three-dimensional visualization of subdural electrodes using CT-MRI coregistration. Epilepsia. 2014;55:2028–2037.

114. Mirzadeh Z, Chapple K, Lambert M, et al. Validation of CT-MRI fusion for intraoperative assessment of stereotactic accuracy in DBS surgery. Mov Disord. 2014;29:1788–1795.

115. Stieglitz LH, Ayer C, Schindler K, et al. Improved localization of implanted subdural electrode contacts on magnetic resonance imaging with an elastic image fusion algorithm in an invasive electroencephalography recording. Neurosurgery. 2014;10:506–513.

116. Pieters TA, Conner CR, Tandon N. Recursive grid partitioning on a cortical surface model: an optimized technique for the localization of implanted subdural electrodes. J Neurosurg. 2013;118:1086–1097.

117. Mahvash M, König R, Wellmer J, et al. Coregistration of digital photography of the human cortex and cranial magnetic resonance imaging for visualization of subdural electrodes in epilepsy surgery. Neurosurgery. 2007;61(5 Suppl 2):340–344.

118. Hill DLG, Batchelor PG, Holden M, Hawkes DJ. Medical image registration. Phys Med Biol. 2001;46:1–45.

119. Van den Elsen PA, Pol EJD, Viergever MA. Medical image matching: A review with classification. IEEE Eng Med Biol. 1993:26–30.

120. Maintz JB, Viergever MA. A survey of medical image registration. Med Image Anal. 1998;2:1–36.

121. Ashburner J, Friston KJ. Rigid body registration. In: Frackowiak RSJ, Friston KJ, Frith C, et al., eds. Human Brain Function, 2nd ed. Academic Press, 2003.

122. Liu P, Eberhardt B, Wybranski C, et al. Nonrigid 3D medical image registration and fusion based on deformable models. Comput Math Methods Med. 2013;2013:902470.

123. Ardekani BA, Guckemus S, Bachman A, et al. Quantitative comparison of algorithms for inter-subject registration of 3D volumetric brain MRI scans. J Neurosci Methods. 2005;142:67–76.

124. Klein A, Andersson J, Ardekani BA, et al. Evaluation of 14 nonlinear deformation algorithms applied to human brain MRI registration. Neuroimage. 2014;46:786–802.
125. Sotiras A, Davatzikos C, Paragios N. Deformable medical image registration: A survey. IEEE Trans Med Imaging. 2013;32:1153–1190.
126. Schulz J, Siegert T, Bazin P-L, et al. Prospective slice-by-slice motion correction reduces false positive activations in fMRI with task-correlated motion. Neuroimage. 2014;84:124–132.
127. Neumann JO, Giese H, Biller A, et al. Spatial distortion in MRI-guided stereotactic procedures: Evaluation in 1.5-, 3- and 7-Tesla MRI scanners. Stereotact Funct Neurosurg. 2015;93:380–386.
128. Aljabar P, Heckemann RA, Hammers A, et al. Multi-atlas based segmentation of brain images: Atlas selection and its effect on accuracy. Neuroimage. 2009;46:726–738

129. Cabezas M, Oliver A, Lladóa X, et al. A review of atlas-based segmentation for magnetic resonance brain images. 2011. Comput Methods Programs Biomed. 2011;104:158–177.
130. Tohka J. Partial volume effect modeling for segmentation and tissue classification of brain magnetic resonance images: A review. World J Radiol. 2014;6:855–864.
131. Despotovic I, Goossens B, Philips W. MRI segmentation of the human brain: Challenges, methods, and applications. Comput Math Methods Med. 2015;2015:450341.
132. Pluim JPW, Maintz JBA, Viergever MA. Mutual-information-based registration of medical images: A survey. IEEE Trans Med Imaging. 2003;22:986–1004.
133. Klein A, Ghosh SS, Avants B, et al. Evaluation of volume-based and surface-based brain image registration methods. Neuroimage. 2010;51:214–220.

47 | EEG-BASED BRAIN–COMPUTER INTERFACES

GERT PFURTSCHELLER, PHD, CLEMENS BRUNNER, PHD, AND CHRISTA NEUPER, PHD

ABSTRACT: A brain–computer interface (BCI) offers an alternative to natural communication and control by recording brain activity, processing it online, and producing control signals that reflect the user's intent or the current user state. Therefore, a BCI provides a non-muscular communication channel that can be used to convey messages and commands without any muscle activity. This chapter presents information on the use of different electroencephalographic (EEG) features such as steady-state visual evoked potentials, P300 components, event-related desynchronization, or a combination of different EEG features and other physiological signals for EEG-based BCIs. This chapter also reviews motor imagery as a control strategy, discusses various training paradigms, and highlights the importance of feedback. It also discusses important clinical applications such as spelling systems, neuroprostheses, and rehabilitation after stroke. The chapter concludes with a discussion on different perspectives for the future of BCIs.

KEYWORDS: brain–computer interface, BCI, electroencephalogram, EEG, feedback, stroke, rehabilitation, spelling systems, neuroprostheses

PRINCIPAL REFERENCES

1. Wolpaw JR, Birbaumer N, McFarland DJ, et al. Brain–computer interfaces for communication and control. Clin Neurophysiol. 2002;113:767–791.
2. Wolpaw JR, Wolpaw EW. Brain–computer interfaces: something new under the sun. In: Wolpaw JR, Wolpaw EW, eds. Brain–Computer Interfaces: Principles and Practice. New York: Oxford University Press, 2012:3–12.
3. Brunner C, Birbaumer N, Blankertz B, et al. BNCI Horizon 2020: towards a roadmap for the BCI community. BCI Journal. 2015;2.
4. Lemm S, Blankertz B, Dickhaus T, Müller K-R. Introduction to machine learning for brain imaging. Neuroimage. 2011;56:387–399.
5. Blankertz B, Lemm S, Treder M, et al. Single-trial analysis and classification of ERP components—a tutorial. Neuroimage. 2011;56:814–825.
6. Pfurtscheller G, Allison BZ, Bauernfeind G, et al. The hybrid BCI. Front Neurosci. 2010;4:30.
7. Graimann B, Allison BZ, Pfurtscheller G, eds. Brain–Computer Interfaces—Revolutionizing Human–Computer Interaction. Heidelberg, London, New York: Springer, 2010.

1. INTRODUCTION AND BASIC PRINCIPLES

Over the last decades, the field of brain-computer interfaces (BCIs) has grown exponentially from a futuristic concept in applied neurophysiology (1) to a full-fledged research field with hundreds of active researchers worldwide. Initially, BCIs targeted mainly patients with highly compromised motor functions such as tetraplegic patients, but nowadays applications for healthy people are becoming increasingly feasible (2).

Essentially, a BCI provides a non-muscular communication channel that can be used to convey messages and commands without any muscle activity (3). According to a widely adopted definition, any BCI must meet the following four requirements:

1. Signals must be recorded directly from the brain. If a device records signals after they pass through peripheral nerves or muscles, it is not a BCI.

2. Users must intentionally modulate the recorded brain signals used by the BCI.

3. Signal processing must be performed online.

4. Users must obtain feedback about the success or failure of their efforts to communicate or control.

In a more recent definition, the requirement that a BCI must rely on intentional modulations of brain patterns was dropped (4), which broadened the scope of the BCI definition to include so-called passive BCIs (5). Such BCIs can rely on covert aspects of ongoing brain activity, and therefore operate without requiring the user to produce intentional control commands. More specifically, a BCI can be defined according to its intended use as follows: "A BCI is a system that measures central nervous system (CNS) activity and converts it into artificial output that replaces, restores, enhances, supplements, or improves natural CNS output and thereby changes the ongoing interactions between the CNS and its external or internal environment" (4).

Therefore, BCIs can be used to replace, restore, enhance, supplement, and improve natural CNS output. In addition, BCIs can also be used as a research tool to study CNS functions in clinical and non-clinical research settings (6). Examples for these six application scenarios include communication through a spelling system (replace), functional electrical stimulation of muscles in a paralyzed person (restore), detecting lapses of attention during a demanding task (enhance), providing a third robotic arm (supplement), improving motor function in stroke rehabilitation (improve), and studying brain patterns on a single-trial basis (research tool).

It follows from these definitions that a BCI is a closed-loop system with two adaptive controllers: the user's brain, which produces the signals and provides the input to the BCI, and the BCI itself, which analyzes the brain signals and transforms them into control signals (Fig. 47.1).

In general, a BCI extracts features from the recorded brain signals and translates these into control signals. The feature

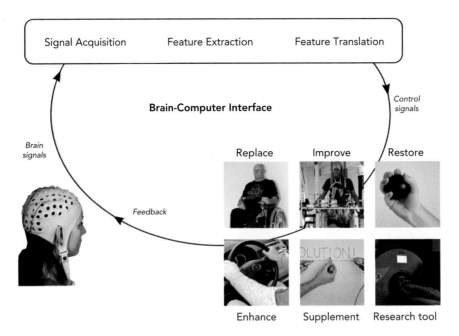

Replace   Improve   Restore

Enhance   Supplement   Research tool

Figure 47.1. *Principle of a BCI system with internal processing blocks signal acquisition, feature extraction, and feature translation. Feedback to the user is essential and creates a closed-loop system. Modified from (6).*

extraction stage finds a suitable representation of the recorded signals to simplify subsequent classification or detection of specific patterns of brain activity. That is, good signal features should encode the commands sent by the user, but should also attenuate noise and other signal components that can impede the classification process. A multitude of feature extraction methods are used in current BCI systems. A non-exhaustive list of these methods includes amplitude and band power measures, Hjorth parameters, autoregressive parameters, and wavelet coefficients. A comprehensive review of commonly used features can be found in (7).

The feature translation stage assigns the signal features to a given category of brain patterns. Essentially, this corresponds to a classification problem, but a regression approach can also be used if there are no discrete categories. In its most basic form, a simple threshold is sufficient to detect specific brain patterns (8). However, a great variety of machine learning algorithms (including shrinkage linear discriminant analysis, support vector machines, and ensemble classifiers) may be used to improve classification performance (9,10).

The classifier output, which can be a simple discrete signal or a signal that encodes the probabilities for different classes, is transformed into a signal that can be used to control a variety of devices. For most current BCI systems, the output device is a computer screen and the desired output consists of the selection of certain targets such as in a spelling system (11). Other applications include control of prostheses (12) and multimedia applications, including gaming (13).

Feedback of performance is usually obtained by visualizing the classifier output on a computer screen or by providing auditory, tactile, or other visual feedback signals. Feedback is an integral part of a BCI system, because users directly observe the actions of the BCI (such as selected letters or specific movements) as a result of their brain patterns.

2. EEG PATTERNS USED AS INPUT FOR A BCI

BCIs based on the electroencephalogram (EEG) are particularly widely used because they can be realized with inexpensive and portable recording devices and offer a high time resolution. Two types of signals can be extracted from the ongoing EEG:

1. Event-related (evoked) potentials (ERPs) are time-locked and phase-locked changes in response to an external or internal event. Evoked signals include slow cortical potentials (SCPs), P300 components, and steady-state evoked potentials (SSEPs) (14).

2. Event-related (induced) changes in ongoing EEG activity in specific frequency bands are time-locked but not phase-locked to an external or internal event. Event-related desynchronization (ERD) is associated with power decrease of a rhythmic component, whereas event-related synchronization (ERS) is characterized by power increase (15).

Depending on the analyzed and classified phenomena, a number of widely used EEG-based BCI systems can be differentiated.

2.1. The Slow Cortical Potential BCI

Beginning in 1979, Birbaumer et al. published a series of experiments demonstrating operant control of slow cortical potential (SCP) shifts (16). Operant conditioning is a learning process with the goal to self-regulate brain potentials (such as SCPs) or brain waves (such as sensorimotor rhythms) using suitable feedback. This approach does not require continuous feedback, but a reward for achieving the desired brain potential (wave) change is necessary. Operant conditioning was successfully used in communication systems for completely paralyzed (locked-in) patients (17).

2.2. The P300 BCI

The P300 (or P3) is a positive component of the evoked potential that develops around 300 msec after a stimulus is perceived (18). In a widely used BCI application, the user focuses on a particular item on a computer screen while ignoring all other stimuli. Whenever the target stimulus flashes, it produces a larger P300 than the other possible choices. P300 BCIs are typically used to spell texts (19–22) but have been validated with other tasks such as controlling a mobile robot (23).

2.3. The Steady-State Visual Evoked Potential BCI

Steady-state (visual) evoked potentials (SSVEPs) occur when sensory stimuli are repetitively delivered fast enough that the relevant neuronal structures do not return to their resting states. In a common BCI application, the user focuses on one of several simultaneously presented visual stimuli, each of which flickers at a different rate and/or phase (24). Gao et al. described a BCI with 48 flickering lights and a high information transfer rate of 68 bits/min (25). Like P300 BCIs, SSVEP BCIs require no training and facilitate rapid communication (26,27). SSVEP BCIs have also recently expanded to tasks beyond spelling, such as controlling an avatar in a computer game (28–30) or controlling an orthosis (31). Some BCI researchers argued that SSVEP BCIs can only be used for communication when users have some conscious control of eye muscles and are therefore not applicable for patients in the late stages of amyotrophic lateral sclerosis (ALS) (3). Later work showed that this assumption is not entirely correct: in some cases, SSVEP BCIs can function even when users do not shift their gaze, but performance is significantly higher in paradigms that allow shifts in gaze direction (32–35).

2.4. The Event-Related Desynchronization BCI

Brain rhythms can exhibit ERD (power decrease) or ERS (power increase) (15). An ERD BCI is a BCI system that detects these power changes in sensorimotor (mu and central beta rhythms) and/or other brain oscillations such as short-lasting post-imagery beta bursts (beta ERS, beta rebound) (36–38).

The first reports on online classification of ERD/ERS patterns quantified via band power measures were published in (39) and (40). Many current BCIs use ERD/ERS as features for single-trial EEG classification, including the Wadsworth BCI (3,41), the Berlin BCI (42,43), the Graz BCI (44), the EPFL BCI (45), the Würzburg BCI (46), and the Tübingen BCI (47). The reported bit rates are between 2 and 17 bits/min (48,49) and can be up to 35 bits/min (42).

The ERD BCI can be operated in two different modes, which defines when the user performs a mental task and thus intends to transmit a message. The first mode is called externally paced (cue-based, computer-driven, synchronous BCI),

and the second mode is referred to as internally paced (user-driven, asynchronous BCI) (50). In a synchronous BCI, a fixed predefined time window is used. After a visual or auditory cue, the user produces a specific brain pattern. Most BCI systems still operate in such a cue-based mode (3,51). An asynchronous protocol entails a continuous analysis and classification of the recorded brain signals, which allows the user to produce control signals at any time. Thus, such BCIs are generally more demanding and more complex than BCIs operating with a fixed timing scheme.

2.5. The Hybrid BCI

To overcome the limitations of traditional BCIs such as long training periods, slow information throughput, and a limited number of classes, so-called hybrid BCIs have been increasingly used in practical applications (52). These devices combine a BCI with another input device (including another BCI) (53). Examples include two-dimensional cursor control by combining ERD and SSVEP BCIs (54) or SSVEP and P300 BCIs (55,56), control of a hand orthosis (31), and a BCI based on both EEG and near infrared spectroscopy (NIRS) (57). Hybrid BCIs also include systems consisting of several input devices, including at least one BCI, which is constantly available but which may or may not be used during operation of the system (58).

3. MOTOR IMAGERY AS CONTROL STRATEGY

Several EEG studies demonstrated that primary sensorimotor areas are activated when subjects imagine the execution of a hand movement. Klass and Bickford (59) and Chatrian et al. (60) observed blocking or desynchronization of the central mu rhythm with motor imagery. By quantifying spatio-temporal ERD patterns, it was clearly shown that one-sided hand motor imagery can result in a lateralized activation of sensorimotor areas, similarly to that found in the preparatory phase of a self-paced hand movement (61). Furthermore, measurements of slow potential shifts (62) have demonstrated that similar changes over the contralateral hand area can be observed during execution and imagination of movement. In addition, multichannel neuromagnetic measurements provided further evidence of the effect of motor imagery on brain oscillations generated in primary motor areas (63).

Figure 47.2 shows example band power time courses of 11 to 13 Hz EEG activity. The ERD/ERS curves show different reactivity patterns during right and left motor imagery, displaying a significant band power decrease (ERD) over the contralateral hand area. ERD is present at sites contralateral and ERS is present at sites ipsilateral to the side of motor imagery. Furthermore, feedback enhances the difference between both patterns, and therefore also improves classification accuracy (64).

The enhancement of oscillatory EEG activity (ERS) during motor imagery is a very important aspect in BCI research. For example, foot motor imagery can induce long-lasting beta

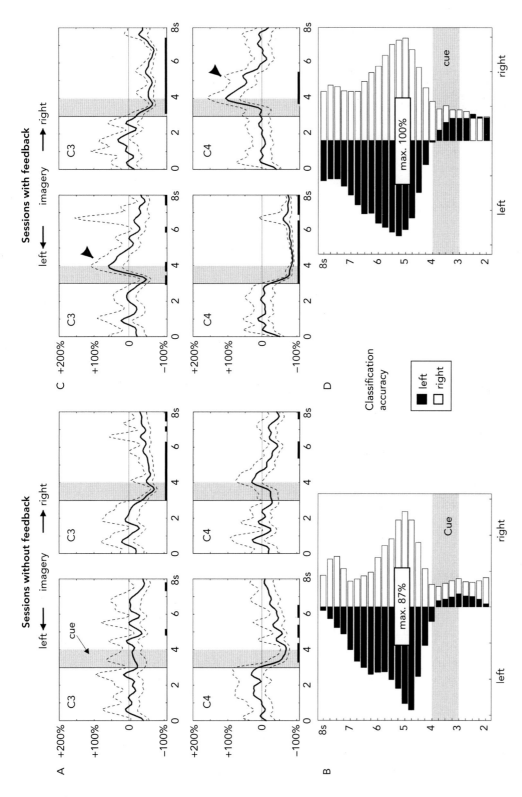

Figure 47.2. Event-related desynchronization (ERD) and event-related synchronization (ERS) time courses in the frequency range 11 to 13 Hz (solid lines; 95% confidence intervals indicated by dashed lines). A representative BCI user performed imagined movements of the left versus right hand in sessions without feedback (**A**) and in sessions with continuous feedback (**C**). Data were recorded from sites over the sensorimotor cortex (C3, C4). Cues were presented from second 3 to 4 (gray vertical bars). Examples of classification results of single trials (based on linear discriminant analysis [LDA]) of two selected sessions are shown, one without (**B**) and one with feedback (**D**), respectively. The x-axis denotes the average size of the distance function (resulting from LDA) for all left and right trials of one session. For details, see (64). In the session with feedback, the average distance corresponds to the average length of the feedback bar presented on the screen. Black bars indicate bar movements to the left side of the screen, whereas white bars indicate bar movements to the right side. The y-axis displays the time points used for classification. The best classification accuracy for each session is indicated.

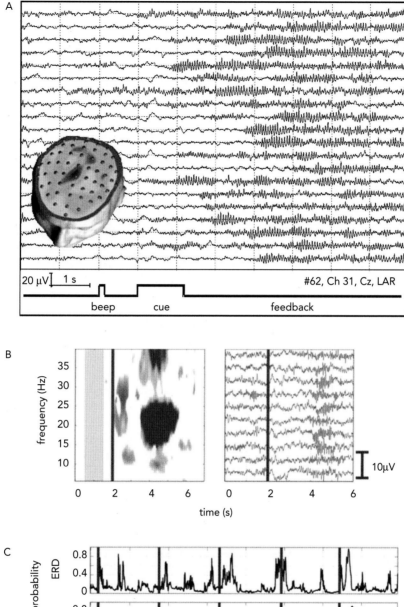

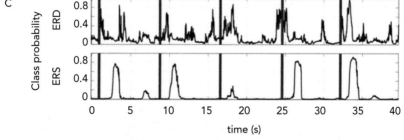

Figure 47.3. *A: Examples of a series of single EEG trials showing peri-imagery beta ERS recorded at electrode position Cz with topographic map indicating the localized 10-Hz ERS. **B:** Examples of EEG trials during cue-based brisk foot motor imagery with post-imagery beta ERS recorded at Cz (right panel) and time-frequency map displaying peri-imagery ERD and post-imagery ERS at Cz (left panel). **C:** Single-trial classification of peri-imagery ERD and post-imagery ERS with indicated true positives.*

oscillations during imagery (peri-imagery ERS) (Fig. 47.3A) and/or short-lasting beta bursts after the end of the imagery process (post-imagery ERS) (see Fig. 47.3B) over the foot representation area close to the vertex (38,65). The post-imagery ERS is dominant in the beta band with a maximum approximately 2.5 sec after brisk cue-based imagery, which can be detected with high accuracy (see Fig. 47.3C) in the ongoing EEG. This so-called beta rebound is therefore a good candidate to realize a single-channel EEG-based BCI (38,65,66).

In summary, motor imagery can modify sensorimotor rhythms in a similar way to that observed in the preparatory phase of an executed movement. Since motor imagery results in a somatotopically organized activation pattern, mental imagination of different movements (e.g., left vs. right hand or hand vs. foot) can be an efficient strategy to operate a BCI based on oscillatory EEG activity. The challenge is to detect these imagery-related changes in ongoing EEG recordings.

4. TRAINING PARADIGM

In general, BCIs are set up by training the user (67), the system (43), or both (co-adaptive training) (68–70). Lotte et al. (71) give a comprehensive overview of existing training protocols, point out weaknesses, and suggest promising alternatives.

In the first approach, users participate in a training (calibration) session before using the BCI. This allows them to obtain some control of their brain signals, which in turn optimizes classification performance of different brain states. Prior to starting online feedback sessions with a specific user, the individual brain patterns (related to, e.g., different types of motor imagery) must be known. To this end, the training session of an imagery-based BCI protocol requires users to repeatedly imagine different kinds of movements (e.g., hand, feet, or tongue movement) in a cue-based mode while their EEG is being recorded (Fig. 47.4A). Optimally, this training session provides high-density EEG recordings, which are subjected to a fine-grained topographical time-frequency analysis of ERD/ERS patterns, and subsequent classification of different imagery conditions. By applying suitable algorithms to the training data, features and electrode locations that best discriminate between different imagery tasks can be identified for each participant, as well as the classification accuracy (see Fig. 47.4B). After setting up the initial classifier, subsequent training sessions can start where the user receives online feedback of motor imagery-related changes in the EEG (see Fig. 47.4C). Depending on the classification accuracy, an update of the classifier and further feedback experiments may be recommended (see Fig. 47.4D). This adaptation process between brain and computer can last for many days or weeks, especially in patients.

In co-adaptive approaches, the BCI continuously updates the classifier and/or relevant features based on online data. Therefore, feedback can be provided from the very beginning of the calibration process, which might be beneficial for naïve users or people who cannot achieve control with conventional training paradigms (69,70,72).

5. FEEDBACK

To keep the training period as short as possible, a well-designed training protocol and helpful feedback signals are essential. Feedback provides the user with information about the efficiency of his/her strategy and supports learning. In this context, two aspects are crucial: (1) the exact manner of how brain signals are translated into the feedback signal (i.e., information content of the feedback) and (2) the type of feedback presentation. In any case, the influence of the feedback on the capacity for attention, concentration, and motivation of the user (aspects that are closely related to the learning process) should be considered; see also (73).

One example of an efficient feedback strategy is the so-called basket game. In this paradigm, the user has to mentally move a falling ball into the correct goal (basket) marked on the screen (Fig. 47.5A). If the ball hits the correct basket, it becomes highlighted and points are earned. The horizontal position of the ball is controlled with the BCI output signal and the vertical velocity can be adjusted by the investigator. The speed of the ball can be increased run by run until the person considers it too fast. This approach can find the optimal speed for a maximum information transfer rate (ITR). Experiments with two bipolar EEG channels and two motor imagery tasks performed by volunteers with spinal cord injuries (SCIs) revealed a maximum ITR of 17 bits/min with a trial length (falling time of the ball) of 2.5 sec (49) (see Fig. 47.5B).

BCI studies can use different feedback modalities. Using the auditory modality, SCP amplitude shifts could be encoded in ascending and descending pitches on a major tone scale (74,75). A BCI using only auditory (rather than visual) stimuli is relevant for providing communication for severely paralyzed patients with visual impairment (76,77). Although these studies could show that BCI communication using only auditory stimuli is possible, visual feedback turned out to be superior to auditory feedback. Chatterjee et al. (78) presented an ERD BCI using a motor imagery paradigm and haptic feedback provided by vibrotactile stimuli to the upper limb. Although further work will be needed to determine how neural correlates of vibrotactile feedback modulate the mu rhythm, haptic information may become a critical component of BCIs, especially if they are designed to control an advanced neuroprosthetic device (79).

Despite successful approaches in developing non-visual BCI systems, visual presentation of stimuli remains the most frequently used feedback modality in BCI research (3). Typical visual feedback stimuli comprise cursor movement (42,80),

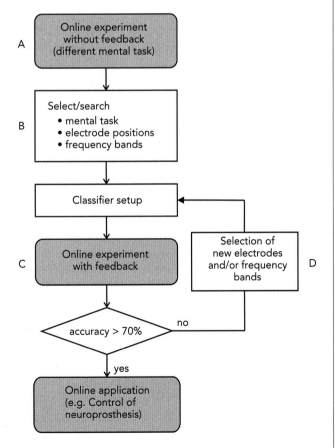

Figure 47.4. Workflow for an imagery-based BCI.

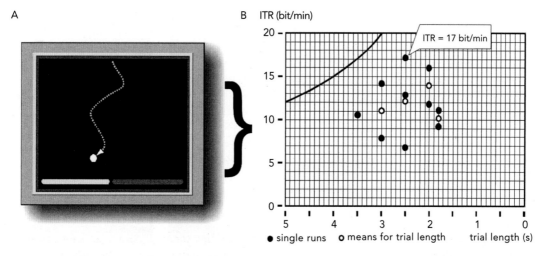

Figure 47.5. **A:** *Graphical display of the "basket paradigm." The user has to direct the ball to the indicated goal (basket). The trial length varies across runs.* **B:** *Information transfer rate (ITR) for one subject in relation to trial length. The black line represents the maximum possible ITR for an error-free classification. Modified from (49).*

a moving bar of varying size (64,78), and the trajectory of a moving object (42,49). Other interesting variants include color coding (81) and complex virtual reality environments (82–84).

There is evidence that rich visual feedback (e.g., a three-dimensional video game or virtual reality environment) may enhance the learning process in a BCI task (73,85,83). For example, multimodal feedback can enhance performance and motivation in a motor imagery BCI task (86). Combining BCI and virtual reality technologies could lead to highly realistic and immersive feedback scenarios. As an important step in this direction, it was demonstrated that EEG recording and single-trial processing with sufficiently high classification results are possible in an immersive multi-projection and head-tracked virtual reality system, and that the obtained signals are even suitable to control events within a virtual environment in real time (83).

6. SOME EEG-BASED BCI APPLICATIONS

Currently, the most important applications of BCIs include communication for locked-in patients and control of neuroprostheses for paralyzed patients (3,87,88). In addition, BCIs can be used to provide neurofeedback for people with stroke (89–91), SCI (92), and cerebral palsy (93). Daly and Wolpaw (94) provide a general review on BCIs in neurorehabilitation. Currently, the plurality of BCI applications is expanding and new fields are emerging. One promising opportunity is to use BCIs to control multimedia applications (13), while another is to use BCIs for user authentication (51,95). Some applications are explained in more detail below and are illustrated in Figure 47.6.

6.1. Control of Spelling Systems in Severely Paralyzed Patients

Spelling systems are communication aids that allow users to express themselves by selecting letters and other characters to write words and sentences. The simplest case involves a binary control signal requiring two distinctive mental activities. Patients with ALS can learn to control their slow cortical potentials (SCP BCI) and to operate a BCI-based spelling device (87,96). By using such a dichotomous selection strategy, an ALS patient and a patient with severe cerebral palsy learned to operate a virtual keyboard spelling application (97). The spelling rates in these studies varied from 0.15 to approximately 1.0 letters per minute. An example for such a spelling system with an ERD BCI is displayed in Figure 47.6B.

Other examples include the Wadsworth speller, based on mu and beta activity, which divides the alphabet into four parts (98). Millán et al. (99) reported an average spelling rate of three letters per minute using a three-class BCI. A novel spelling concept using an asynchronous protocol was introduced by Scherer et al. (100). Another efficient selection strategy was introduced by Müller and Blankertz (101). The Hex-O-Spell application combines asynchronous two-class ERD BCI control and divides the alphabet into six parts. This improved the average spelling rate to about six letters per minute. Furdea et al. created an auditory oddball speller relying on the P300 (102), which might be particularly relevant for patients who cannot control their eye movements. Leeb et al. (103) successfully evaluated various online applications, including a spelling system, in a group of 24 patients.

6.2. Control of Neuroprosthesis to Restore Grasp Function

In general, systems for functional electrical stimulation (FES)—so-called neuroprostheses—are able to restore lost motor functions after SCI. Typically, the control signal generated by the BCI switches the FES on and off. In a project with a tetraplegic patient, FES resulting in hand grasp was controlled by ongoing EEG activity based on an asynchronous BCI. The patient participated in a large number of BCI training sessions with varying types of motor imagery over a period of several months (104). At the end, he was able to induce trains of

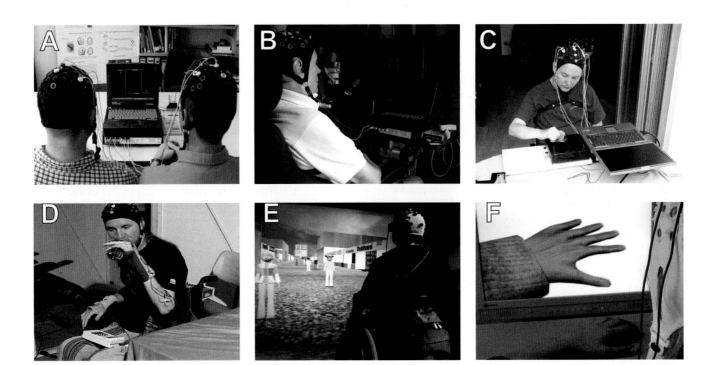

Figure 47.6. **A:** *Two people playing virtual table tennis.* **B:** *ALS patient operating a spelling system at home.* **C:** *Motor imagery-based control of a neuroprosthesis through implanted functional electrical stimulation (FES) of hand muscles.* **D:** *Motor imagery-based control of a neuroprosthesis through FES of hand muscles using surface electrodes.* **E:** *Wheelchair control in a virtual environment.* **F:** *Control of virtual hand movement.*

17-Hz beta oscillations focused on the electrode position near the vertex (Cz) by foot motor imagery. These mentally induced 17-Hz oscillations were used as a simple asynchronous brain switch to generate a control signal for the operation of the FES using surface electrodes (see Fig. 47.6D). With this method, the patient was able to voluntarily grasp a glass of water; for a detailed description of the procedure, see (105). Müller-Putz et al. (12) reported on an implantable neuroprosthesis (106) coupled with an ERD BCI, which was used in a tetraplegic patient to perform a grasp sequence (see Fig. 47.6C). A review of applications of noninvasive hybrid BCI-controlled upper extremity neuroprostheses in individuals with high SCIs is available in (107).

6.3. Rehabilitation After Stroke

Typically, physical therapy aimed at post-stroke motor recovery focuses on active movement training. However, some patients cannot engage in movement without assistance. Novel protocols based on motor imagery represent an intriguing backdoor approach to access the motor system, because they can induce activation of sensorimotor networks affected by the lesions (108,109).

It is well established that unilateral hand motor imagery can result in contralateral ERD and simultaneously in ipsilateral ERS after some training sessions (61). Hence, an ERD BCI based on motor imagery can provide some measure of attempted activity in the motor regions and reinforce a patient's sensorimotor experience during post-stroke motor recovery. Feedback from the BCI can be solely visual, as in the movement of a virtual hand (see Fig. 47.6F), or it can occur

through a prosthetic device like an orthotic hand attached to the patient's own hand (88). In both cases, not only can positive feedback reinforce the motor imagery process, but the act of observing the hand movement can itself activate sensorimotor areas.

Two fundamental questions must be addressed in this context: (1) how can synaptic connections be recovered after a lesion caused by a stroke, and (2) how may BCIs improve this recovery of motor functions?

First, neurophysiological animal experiments showed how synaptic potentiation may occur in motor cortex. Fetz et al. (110,111) demonstrated that synaptic connections between artificially synchronized neuronal populations could be potentiated. They conclude that natural stimulation under volitional control could provide a way of strengthening neural pathways in the course of a rehabilitation protocol.

Second, synaptic plasticity is strongly modulated by the dynamical state of the involved neuronal population. Haegens et al. (112) investigated local field potentials and spike firing in monkeys performing a vibrotactile discrimination task. They found that spikes tended to occur at the trough of an alpha cycle rather than at the peak. A decrease of alpha power was also associated with an increase in firing rate, supporting the notion that alpha oscillations exert an inhibitory modulating influence. In addition, a decrease of alpha oscillations (ERD) facilitates performance of a tactile stimulus discrimination task and reflects downregulation of intracortical inhibition. Takemi et al. (113) directly showed increased motor potential amplitudes with transcranial magnetic stimulation (TMS) applied when ERD exceeded a predefined threshold during motor imagery.

Therefore, combining mu ERD with appropriate stimulation of cortical neurons can facilitate motor learning at the cortical level, which may promote recovery of motor functions in stroke patients. Using BCIs for the purpose of stroke rehabilitation, a disinhibitory state can be achieved by simply imagining a hand movement, which induces ERD over the corresponding brain areas. Stimulating specific neuronal populations can be achieved by two strategies. First, proprioceptive sensory feedback can be elicited by passive movement of the paretic hand via a hand orthosis (114–116). Second, ERD can be used to trigger functional electrical stimulation of the paralyzed hand muscles (117).

7. PERSPECTIVES FOR THE FUTURE

BCI technology is a rapidly growing research field with the potential to improve the quality of life of severely disabled people. To date, several BCI prototypes exist, but most of them have been tested only in a laboratory environment. Before BCIs can be used for reliable communication and control at home or work, several problems have to be solved, such as (i) making BCIs easy and comfortable to use (e.g., with dry electrodes), (ii) making BCIs affordable, (iii) automatically selecting optimal electrode positions and frequency components in a motor imagery task, (iv) minimizing the number of recording electrodes, (v) minimizing training time through game-like feedback, and (vi) automatically detecting and/or correcting artifacts. To close the translational and reliability gaps BCIs are currently facing, these issues should be addressed by studies that investigate BCI use at home (118).

A clear challenge is to develop more effective BCI control paradigms, offering, for instance, three-dimensional neuroprosthesis control or fast and reliable operation of a spelling device. Such an improvement of speed and accuracy is possible by analyzing cortical potential changes recorded with electrocorticographic (ECoG) electrode strips or grids or the detection of firing patterns in intracortical recordings. The advantage of ECoG (as compared to EEG) is its better signal-to-noise ratio, which affords easier detection of gamma activity. Bursts of gamma activity between 60 and 90 Hz during self-paced limb and tongue movements were reported in ECoG recordings (119,120). These gamma bursts are short-lasting, display high somatotopic specificity, and are embedded in the alpha and beta ERD lasting for some seconds. Patient-oriented work with subdural electrodes and ECoG single-trial classification have shown first promising results (121,122).

Studies in monkeys have shown that three-dimensional control is possible when multiunit activity is recorded in cortical areas. Between 32 and 96 microwires were implanted in different cortical motor areas. After a training period with distinct motor tasks, the monkeys were able to control the movement of a robotic device by real-time transformation of neuronal multiunit neuronal activity (123). The feasibility of a prosthetic device control in a tetraplegic patient based on recording of neural ensemble activity through a 96-microelectrode array has been reported (124). These preliminary results suggest that recording of intracortical neuronal multiunit activity could

provide a new neurotechnology to restore independence for humans with paralysis.

The beta rebound is a relatively stable EEG phenomenon (36) that can be detected in single-trial EEG during foot motor imagery to realize a brain switch (38,66). One desirable feature of such a brain switch is a low number of unintended activations in the output signal; that is, the false-positive rate should be zero or close to zero. An imagery-based brain switch can be used, for instance, to turn the flickering lights of an SSVEP-controlled hand orthosis on or off (31). This type of BCI, composed of two sequentially operating BCIs, is an example of a hybrid BCI (53).

Stroke rehabilitation based on BCIs is a promising area of research. Using noninvasive measures of brain activity, BCIs could improve existing therapy by promoting recovery of motor functions at the cortical level.

It can be expected that making BCIs useful to a wider group of users will open up new fields of (non-medical) applications such as entertainment in the next several years. Applications for healthy users include gaming and entertainment as well as monitoring and decoding of covert user states such as attention, performance, and workload (2,6). Most of these applications do not entail intentional control but fall in the category of passive BCIs. These systems continuously monitor brain activity and react to changes in specific brain patterns. For example, BCIs have been proposed to detect emergency braking intentions (125), lapses of attention (126), and workload monitoring (127) during driving a car; control computer games and multimedia applications (128,129); enhance image classification in a rapid serial visual presentation (RSVP) paradigm (130); and provide authentication without passwords (131,132).

Finally, there is growing evidence that cortical excitability displays ongoing intrinsic fluctuations with a dominant frequency at ~0.1 Hz (133–135). These slow fluctuations reflect excitability dynamics of cortical networks and are correlated with human psychophysical performance (136). It is worth noting that there exists an intimate coupling between the brain and the heart through vagal nerve activation (137). Whether these slow oscillations in cortical excitability and heart rate can be used to optimize the training procedure of an ERD BCI (e.g., cue presentation controlled by spontaneous activity) is still a topic of ongoing research.

ACKNOWLEDGMENTS

We would like to thank Josef Faller for reviewing the text and for providing helpful comments.

REFERENCES

1. Vidal JJ. Toward direct brain-computer communication. Annu Rev Biophys Bioeng. 1973;2:157–180.
2. Blankertz B, Tangermann M, Vidaurre C, et al. The Berlin brain-computer interface: non-medical uses of BCI technology. Front Neurosci. 2010;4:00198.
3. Wolpaw JR, Birbaumer N, McFarland DJ, et al. Brain-computer interfaces for communication and control. Clin Neurophysiol. 2002;113:767–791.

4. Wolpaw JR, Wolpaw EW. Brain–computer interfaces: something new under the sun. In: Wolpaw JR, Wolpaw EW, eds. Brain–Computer Interfaces: Principles and Practice. New York: Oxford University Press, 2012:3–12.
5. Zander TO, Kothe C. Towards passive brain–computer interfaces: applying brain-computer interface technology to human–machine systems in general. J Neural Eng. 2011;8:025005.
6. Brunner C, Birbaumer N, Blankertz B, et al. BNCI Horizon 2020: towards a roadmap for the BCI community. BCI Journal. 2015;2.
7. Bashashati A, Fatourechi M, Ward RK, Birch GE. A survey of signal processing algorithms in brain–computer interfaces based on electrical brain signals. J Neural Eng. 2007;4:R32.
8. Schalk G, Wolpaw JR, McFarland DJ, Pfurtscheller G. EEG-based communication: presence of an error potential. Clin Neurophysiol. 2000;111:2138–2144.
9. Lotte F, Congedo M, Lécuyer A, Lamarche F, Arnaldi B. A review of classification algorithms for EEG-based brain-computer interfaces. J Neural Eng. 2007;4:R1.
10. Lemm S, Blankertz B, Dickhaus T, Müller K-R. Introduction to machine learning for brain imaging. Neuroimage. 2011;56:387–399.
11. Cecotti H. Spelling with non-invasive brain–computer interfaces—current and future trends. J Physiol Paris. 2011;105:106–114.
12. Müller-Putz GR, Scherer R, Pfurtscheller G, Rupp R. EEG-based neuroprosthesis control: a step into clinical practice. Neurosci Lett. 2005;382:169–174.
13. Gürkök H, Nijholt A. Brain–computer interfaces for multimodal interaction: a survey and principles. Int J Hum-Comput Int. 2012;28:292–307.
14. Luck SJ. An Introduction to the Event-Related Potential Technique. Cambridge, MA: MIT Press, 2014.
15. Pfurtscheller G, Lopes da Silva FH. Event-related EEG/MEG synchronization and desynchronization: basic principles. Clin Neurophysiol. 1999;110:1842–1857.
16. Birbaumer N, Elbert T, Canavan AG, Rockstroh B. Slow potentials of the cerebral cortex and behavior. Physiol Rev. 1990;70:1–41.
17. Birbaumer N, Gallegos-Ayala G, Wildgruber M, et al. Direct brain control and communication in paralysis. Brain Topogr. 2014;27:4–11.
18. Polich J. Updating P300: an integrative theory of P3a and P3b. Clin Neurophysiol. 2007;118:2128–2148.
19. Farwell LA, Donchin E. Talking off the top of your head: toward a mental prosthesis utilizing event-related brain potentials. Electroencephalogr Clin Neurophysiol. 1988;70:510–523.
20. Donchin E, Spencer KM, Wijesinghe R. The mental prosthesis: assessing the speed of a P300-based brain-computer interface. IEEE Trans Rehabil Eng. 2000;8:174–179.
21. Allison BA, Pineda JA. Effects of SOA and flash pattern manipulations on ERPs, performance, and preference: implications for a BCI system. Int J Psychophysiol. 2006;59:127–140.
22. Blankertz B, Lemm S, Treder M, et al. Single-trial analysis and classification of ERP components—a tutorial. Neuroimage. 2011;56:814–825.
23. Bell CJ, Shenoy P, Chalodhorn R, Rao RP. Control of a humanoid robot by a non-invasive brain-computer interface in humans. J Neural Eng. 2008;5:214.
24. Vialatte F-B, Maurice M, Dauwels J, Cichocki A. Steady-state visually evoked potentials: focus on essential paradigms and future perspectives. Prog Neurobiol. 2010;90:418–438.
25. Gao X, Xu D, Cheng M, Gao S. A BCI-based environmental controller for the motion-disabled. IEEE Trans Neural Syst Rehabil Eng. 2003;11:137–140.
26. Krusienski DJ, Sellers EW, Cabestaing F, et al. A comparison of classification techniques for the P300 Speller. J Neural Eng. 2006;3:299–305.
27. Allison BZ, McFarland DJ, Schalk G, et al. Towards an independent brain–computer interface using steady-state visual evoked potentials. Clin Neurophysiol. 2008;119:399–408.
28. Lalor E, Kelly SP, Finucane C, et al. Steady-state VEP-based brain-computer interface control in an immersive 3D gaming environment. EURASIP J Adv Signal Process. 2005;2005:706904.
29. Martinez P, Bakardjian H, Cichocki A. Fully online multicommand brain-computer interface with visual neurofeedback using SSVEP paradigm. Comput Intell Neurosci. 2007;94561.
30. Faller J, Müller-Putz GR, Schmalstieg D, Pfurtscheller G. An application framework for controlling an avatar in a desktop based virtual environment via a software SSVEP brain-computer interface. Presence-Teleop Virt. 2010;19:25–34.
31. Pfurtscheller G, Solis-Escalante T, Ortner R, et al. Self-paced operation of an SSVEP-based orthosis with and without an imagery-based "brain switch": a feasibility study towards a hybrid BCI. IEEE Trans Neural Syst Rehabil Eng. 2010;18:409–414.
32. Kelly SP, Lalor EC, Reilly RB, Foxe JJ. Visual spatial attention tracking using high-density SSVEP data for independent brain-computer communication. IEEE Trans Neural Syst Rehabil Eng. 2005;13:172–178.
33. Allison BZ, McFarland DJ, Schalk G, et al. Towards an independent brain-computer interface using steady-state visual evoked potentials. Clin Neurophysiol. 2008;119:399–408.
34. Brunner P, Joshi S, Briskin S, et al. Does the 'P300' speller depend on eye gaze? J Neural Eng. 2010;7:056013.
35. Treder MS, Blankertz B. (C)overt attention and visual speller design in an ERP-based brain–computer interface. Behav Brain Funct. 2010;6:28.
36. Pfurtscheller G, Neuper C, Brunner C, Lopes da Silva FH. Beta rebound after different types of motor imagery in man. Neurosci Lett. 2005;378:156–159.
37. Pfurtscheller G, Brunner C, Schlögl A, Lopes da Silva FH. Mu rhythm (de)synchronization and EEG single-trial classification of different motor imagery tasks. Neuroimage. 2006;31:153–159.
38. Pfurtscheller G, Solis-Escalante T. Could the beta rebound in the EEG be suitable to realize a "brain switch"? Clin Neurophysiol. 2009;120:24–29.
39. Pfurtscheller G, Kalcher J, Flotzinger D. A new communication device for handicapped persons: the brain–computer interface. In: Ballabio E, Placencia-Porrero I, Puig de la Bellacasa R, eds. Rehabilitation Technology. Amsterdam: IOS Press, 1993:123–127.
40. Kalcher J, Flotzinger D, Neuper C, et al. Graz brain–computer interface II: towards communication between humans and computers based on online classification of three different EEG patterns. Med Biol Eng Comput. 1996;34:382–388.
41. Vaughan TM, McFarland DJ, Schalk G, et al. The Wadsworth BCI Research and Development Program: at home with BCI. IEEE Neural Syst Rehabil Eng. 2006;14:229–233.
42. Blankertz B, Dornhege G, Krauledat M, et al. The non-invasive Berlin Brain–Computer Interface: fast acquisition of effective performance in untrained subjects. Neuroimage. 2007;37:539–550.
43. Blankertz B, Losch F, Krauledat M, et al. The Berlin Brain–Computer Interface: accurate performance from first-sessions in BCI-naïve subjects. IEEE Trans Biomed Eng. 2008;55:2452–2462.
44. Pfurtscheller G, Müller-Putz GR, Schlögl A, et al. 15 years of BCI research at Graz University of Technology: current projects. IEEE Trans Neural Syst Rehabil Eng. 2006;14:205–210.
45. Carlson T, Millán JR. Brain-controlled wheelchairs: a robotic architecture. IEEE Robot Autom Mag. 2013;20:65–73.
46. Kübler A, Holz EM, Riccio A, et al. The user-centered design as novel perspective for evaluating the usability of BCI-controlled applications. PLoS ONE. 2014;9:e112392.
47. Hinterberger T, Nijboer F, Kübler A, et al. Brain–computer interfaces for communication in paralysis: a clinical-experimental approach. In: Dornhege G, Millán JR, Hinterberger T, et al., eds. Toward Brain-Computer Interfacing. Cambridge, MA: MIT Press, 2007:43–64.
48. McFarland DJ, Sarnacki WA, Wolpaw JR. Brain–computer interface (BCI) operation: optimizing information transfer rates. Biol Psychol. 2003;63:237–251.
49. Krausz G, Scherer R, Korisek G, Pfurtscheller G. Critical decision-speed and information transfer in the "Graz Brain–Computer Interface." Appl Psychophysiol Biofeedback. 2003;28:233–240.
50. Mason SG, Bashashati A, Fatourechi M, et al. A comprehensive survey of brain interface technology designs. Ann Biomed Eng. 2007;35:137–169.
51. Pfurtscheller G, Neuper C. Future prospects of ERD/ERS in the context of brain–computer interface (BCI) developments. In: Neuper C, Klimesch W, eds. Event-Related Dynamics of Brain Oscillations, Progress in Brain Research. Amsterdam: Elsevier, 159:19–27.
52. Amiri S, Fazel-Rezai R, Asadpour V. A review of hybrid brain–computer interface systems. Advances in Human–Computer Interaction. 2013;2013:187024.
53. Pfurtscheller G, Allison BZ, Bauernfeind G, et al. The hybrid BCI. Front Neurosci. 2010;4:30.
54. Allison BZ, Brunner C, Altstätter C, et al. A hybrid ERD/SSVEP BCI for continuous simultaneous two dimensional cursor control. J Neurosci Methods. 2012;209:299–307.
55. Li YQ, Pan J, Wang F, Yu Z. A hybrid BCI system combining P300 and SSVEP and its application to wheelchair control. IEEE Trans Biomed Eng. 2013;60:3156–3166.
56. Wang M, Daly I, Allison BZ, et al. A new hybrid BCI paradigm based on P300 and SSVEP. J Neurosci Methods. 2015;244:16–25.
57. Fazli S, Mehnert J, Steinbrink J, et al. Enhanced performance by a hybrid NIRS-EEG brain computer interface. Neuroimage. 2011;59:519–529.
58. Müller-Putz GR, Breitwieser C, Cincotti F, et al. Tools for brain–computer interaction: a general concept for a hybrid BCI. Front Neuroinform. 2011;5:30.

59. Klass DW, Bickford RG. Observations on the rolandic arceau rhythm. Electroencephalogr Clin Neurophysiol. 1957;9:570.

60. Chatrian GE, Petersen MC, Lazarte JE. The blocking of the rolandic wicket rhythm and some central changes related to movement. Electroencephalogr Clin Neurophysiol. 1959;11:497–510.

61. Pfurtscheller G, Neuper C. Motor imagery activates primary sensorimotor area in humans. Neurosci Lett. 1997;239:65–68.

62. Beisteiner R, Höllinger P, Lindinger G, et al. Mental representations of movements. Brain potentials associated with imagination of hand movements. Electroencephalogr Clin Neurophysiol. 1995;96:183–193.

63. Schnitzler A, Salenius S, Salmelin R, et al. Involvement of primary motor cortex in motor imagery: a neuromagnetic study. Neuroimage. 1997;6:201–208.

64. Neuper C, Schlögl A, Pfurtscheller G. Enhancement of left-right sensorimotor EEG differences during feedback-regulated motor imagery. J Clin Neurophysiol. 1999;16:373–382.

65. Solis-Escalante T, Müller-Putz GR, Pfurtscheller G. Overt foot movement detection in one single Laplacian EEG derivation. J Neurosci Methods. 2008;175:148–153.

66. Solis-Escalante T, Müller-Putz GR, Brunner C, et al. Analysis of sensorimotor rhythms for the implementation of a brain switch for healthy subjects. Biomed Signal Process Control. 2010;5:15–20.

67. Neuper C, Scherer R, Wriessnegger S, Pfurtscheller G. Motor imagery and action observation: modulation of sensorimotor brain rhythms during mental control of a brain-computer interface. Clin Neurophysiol. 2009;120:239–247.

68. Vidaurre C, Schlögl A, Cabeza R, et al. A fully on-line adaptive BCI. IEEE Trans Biomed Eng. 2006;54:550–556.

69. Vidaurre C, Sannelli C, Müller K-R, Blankertz B. Machine-learning-based coadaptive calibration for brain-computer interfaces. Neural Comput. 2011;23:791–816.

70. Vidaurre C, Sannelli C, Müller K-R, Blankertz B. Co-adaptive calibration to improve BCI efficiency. J Neural Eng. 2011;8:025002.

71. Lotte F, Larrue F, Mühl C. Flaws in current human training protocols for spontaneous brain–computer interfaces: lessons learned from instructional design. Front Hum Neurosci. 2013;7:568.

72. Faller J, Scherer R, Costa U, et al. A co-adaptive brain–computer interface for end users with severe motor impairment. PLoS ONE. 2014;9:e101168.

73. Pineda JA, Silverman DS, Vankov A, Hestenes J. Learning to control brain rhythms: making a brain-computer interface possible. IEEE Trans Neural Syst Rehabil Eng. 2003;11:181–184.

74. Hinterberger T, Schmidt S, Neumann N, et al. Brain–computer communication and slow cortical potentials. IEEE Trans Biomed Eng. 2004;51:1011–1018.

75. Pham M, Hinterberger T, Neumann N, et al. An auditory brain–computer interface based on the self-regulation of slow cortical potentials. Neurorehabil Neural Repair. 2005;19:206–218.

76. Riccio A, Mattia D, Simione L, et al. Eye-gaze independent EEG-based brain-computer interfaces for communication. J Neural Eng. 2012;9:045001.

77. Gao S, Wang Y, Gao X, Hong B. Visual and auditory brain–computer interfaces. IEEE Trans Biomed Eng. 2014;61:1436–1447.

78. Chatterjee A, Aggarwal V, Ramos A, et al. A brain–computer interface with vibrotactile biofeedback for haptic information. J Neuroeng Rehabil. 2007;4:40.

79. Lebedev MA, Nicolelis MAL. Brain–machine interfaces: past, present and future. Trends Neurosci. 2006;29:536–546.

80. McFarland DJ, McCane LM, Wolpaw JR. EEG-based communication and control: short-term role of feedback. IEEE Trans Rehabil Eng. 1998;6:7–11.

81. Kaplan AY, Byeon J-G, Lim J-J, et al. Unconscious operant conditioning in the paradigm of brain–computer interface based on color perception. Int J Neurosci. 2005;115:781–802.

82. Leeb R, Friedman D, Müller-Putz GR, et al. Self-paced (asynchronous) BCI control of a wheelchair in virtual environments: a case study with a tetraplegic. Comput Intell Neurosci. 2007;2007:79642.

83. Pfurtscheller G, Leeb R, Keinrath C, et al. Walking from thought. Brain Res. 2006;1071:145–152.

84. Graimann B, Allison BZ, Pfurtscheller G, eds. Brain–Computer Interfaces—Revolutionizing Human–Computer Interaction. Heidelberg, London, New York: Springer, 2010.

85. Ron-Angevin R, Díaz-Estrella A. Brain-computer interface: changes in performance using virtual reality techniques. Neurosci Lett. 2009;449:123–127.

86. Sollfrank T, Ramsay A, Perdikis S, et al. The effect of multimodal and enriched feedback on SMR-BCI performance. Clin Neurophysiol. 2015;127:490–498.

87. Birbaumer N, Ghanayim N, Hinterberger T, et al. A spelling device for the paralysed. Nature. 1999;398:297–298.

88. Birbaumer N, Cohen LG. Brain–computer interfaces: communication and restoration of movement in paralysis. J Physiol. 2007;579:621–636.

89. Grosse-Wentrup M, Mattia D, Oweiss K. Using brain–computer interfaces to induce neural plasticity and restore function. J Neural Eng. 2011;8:025004.

90. Belda-Lois J-M, Mena-del Horno S, Bermejo-Bosch I, et al. Rehabilitation of gait after stroke: a review towards a top-down approach. J Neuroeng Rehabil. 2011;8:66.

91. Silvoni S, Ramos-Murguialday A, Cavinato M, et al. Brain–computer interface in stroke: a review of progress. Clin EEG Neurosci. 2011;42:245–252.

92. Cramer SC, Orr ELR, Cohen MJ, Lacourse MG. Effects of motor imagery training after chronic, complete spinal cord injury. Exp Brain Res. 2007;177:233–242.

93. Steenbergen B, Crajé C, Nilsen DM, Gordon AM. Motor imagery training in hemiplegic cerebral palsy: a potentially useful therapeutic tool for rehabilitation. Dev Med Child Neurol. 2009;51:690–696.

94. Daly JJ, Wolpaw JR. Brain–computer interfaces in neurological rehabilitation. Lancet Neurol. 2008;7:1032–1043.

95. Marcel S, Millán JR. Person authentication using brainwaves (EEG) and maximum a posteriori model adaption. IEEE Trans Pattern Anal Mach Intell. 2007;29:743–748.

96. Kübler A, Kotchoubey B, Hinterberger T, et al. The thought translation device: a neurophysiological approach to communication in total motor paralysis. Exp Brain Res. 1999;124:223–232.

97. Obermaier B, Müller GR, Pfurtscheller G. "Virtual keyboard" controlled by spontaneous EEG activity. IEEE Trans Neural Syst Rehabil Eng. 2003;11:422–426.

98. Wolpaw JR, McFarland DJ, Vaughan TM, Schalk G. The Wadsworth Center brain–computer interface (BCI) research and development program. IEEE Trans Neural Syst Rehabil Eng. 2003;11:204–207.

99. Millán J, Mouriño J. Asynchronous BCI and local neural classifiers: an overview of the Adaptive Brain Interface project. IEEE Trans Neural Syst Rehabil Eng. 2003;11:159–161.

100. Scherer R, Müller GR, Neuper C, et al. An asynchronously controlled EEG-based virtual keyboard: improvement of the spelling rate. IEEE Trans Biomed Eng. 2004;51:979–984.

101. Müller K-R, Blankertz B. Toward noninvasive brain computer interfaces. IEEE Signal Process Mag. 2006;23:125–128.

102. Furdea A, Halder S, Krusienski DJ, et al. An auditory oddball (P300) spelling system for brain–computer interfaces. Psychophysiology. 2009;46:617–625.

103. Leeb R, Perdikis S, Tonin L, et al. Transferring brain–computer interfaces beyond the laboratory: successful application control for motor-disabled users. Artif Intell Med. 2013;59:121–132.

104. Pfurtscheller G, Guger C, Müller GR, et al. Brain oscillations control hand orthosis in a tetraplegic. Neurosci Lett. 2000;292:211–214.

105. Pfurtscheller G, Müller GR, Pfurtscheller J, et al. 'Thought'-control of functional electrical stimulation to restore hand grasp in a patient with tetraplegia. Neurosci Lett. 2003;351:33–36.

106. Keith MW, Peckham PH, Thrope GB, et al. Implantable functional neuromuscular stimulation in the tetraplegic hand. J Hand Surg Am. 1989;14:524–530.

107. Rupp R, Schneiders M, Kreilinger A, Müller-Putz GR. Functional rehabilitation of the paralyzed upper extremity after spinal cord injury by noninvasive hybrid neuroprostheses. Proc IEEE. 2015;103:954–968.

108. Sharma N, Pomeroy VM, Baron JC. Motor imagery: a backdoor to the motor system after stroke? Stroke. 2006;37:1941–1952.

109. Dimyan MA, Cohen LG. Neuroplasticity in the context of motor rehabilitation after stroke. Nature Rev Neurol. 2011;7:76–85.

110. Jackson A, Mavoori J, Fetz EE. Long-term motor cortex plasticity induced by an electronic neural implant. Nature. 2006;444:56–60.

111. Fetz EE. Volitional control of neural activity: implications for brain–computer interfaces. J Physiol. 2007;579:571–579.

112. Haegens S, Nácher V, Luna R, et al. α-oscillations in the monkey sensorimotor network influence discrimination performance by rhythmical inhibition of neuronal spiking. Proc Nat Acad Sci USA. 2011;108:19377–19382.

113. Takemi M, Masakado Y, Liu M, Ushiba J. Event-related desynchronization reflects downregulation of intracortical inhibition in human primary motor cortex. J Neurophysiol. 2013;110:1158–1166.

114. Buch E, Weber C, Cohen LG, et al. Think to move: a neuromagnetic brain-computer interface (BCI) system for chronic stroke. Stroke. 2008;39:910–917.

115. Ramos-Murguialday A, Broetz D, Rea M, et al. Brain–machine interface in chronic stroke rehabilitation: a controlled study. Ann Neurol. 2013;74:100–108.

116. Gharabaghi A, Kraus 1, Leão MT, et al. Coupling brain–machine interfaces with cortical stimulation for brain-state dependent stimulation: enhancing motor cortex excitability for neurorehabilitation. Front Human Neurosci. 2014;8:122.

117. Mukaino M, Ono T, Shindo K, et al. Efficacy of brain–computer interface-driven neuromuscular electrical stimulation for chronic paresis after stroke. J Rehabil Med. 2014;46:3780382.

118. Kübler A, Holz E, Kaufmann T, Zickler C. A user-centred approach for bringing BCI controlled applications to end-users. In: Fazel-Rezai R, ed. Brain–Computer Interface Systems—Recent Progress and Future Prospects. InTech Open, 2013.

119. Crone NE, Miglioretti DL, Gordon B, et al. Functional mapping of human sensorimotor cortex with electrocorticographic spectral analysis. I. Alpha and beta event-related desynchronization. Brain. 1998;121:2271–2299.

120. Pfurtscheller G, Graimann B, Huggins JE, et al. Spatiotemporal patterns of beta desynchronization and gamma synchronization in corticographic data during self-paced movement. Clin Neurophysiol. 2003;114:1226–1236.

121. Graimann B, Huggins JE, Schlögl A, et al. Detection of movement-related desynchronization patterns in ongoing single-channel electrocorticogram. IEEE Trans Neural Syst Rehabil Eng. 2003;11:276–281.

122. Schalk G, Miller KJ, Anderson NR, et al. Two-dimensional movement control using electrocorticographic signals in humans. J Neural Eng. 2008;5:75.

123. Wessberg J, Stambaugh CR, Kralik JD, et al. Real-time prediction of hand trajectory by ensembles of cortical neurons in primates. Nature. 2000;408:361–365.

124. Hochberg LR, Serruya MD, Friehs GM, et al. Neuronal ensemble control of prosthetic devices by a human with tetraplegia. Nature. 2006;442:164–171.

125. Haufe S, Kim JW, Kim IH, et al. Electrophysiology-based detection of emergency braking intention in real-world driving. J Neural Eng. 2014;11:056011.

126. Wang Y-T, Huang K-C, Wei C-S, et al. Developing an EEG-based online closed-loop lapse detection and mitigation system. Front Neurosci. 2014;8:321.

127. Kohlmorgen J, Dornhege G, Braun M, et al. Improving human performance in a real operating environment through real-time mental workload detection. In: Dornhege G, Millán JR, Hinterberger T, et al., eds. Toward Brain–Computer Interfacing. Cambridge, MA: MIT Press, 2007:409–422.

128. Lécuyer A, Lotte F, Reilly RB, et al. Brain–computer interfaces, virtual reality, and videogames. Computer. 2008;41:66–72.

129. van de Laar B, Gürkök H, Plass-Oude Bos D, et al. Experiencing BCI control in a popular computer game. IEEE Trans Comput Intell AI in Games. 2013;5:176–184.

130. Bigdely-Shamlo N, Vankov A, Ramirez RR, Makeig S. Brain activity-based image classification from rapid serial visual presentation. IEEE Trans Neural Syst Rehabil Eng. 2008;16:432–441.

131. Thorpe J, van Oorschot PC, Somayaji A. Pass-thoughts: authenticating with our minds. Proc New Security Paradigms Workshop. 2005;45–56.

132. Chuang J, Nguyen H, Wang C, Johnson B. I think, therefore I am: usability and security of authentication using brainwaves. Lect Notes Comput Sci. 2013;7862:1–16.

133. Vanhatalo S, Palva JM, Miller JW, et al. Infraslow oscillations modulate excitability and interictal epileptic activity in the human cortex during sleep. Proc Natl Acad Sci USA. 2004;101:5053–5057.

134. Foster BL, Parvizi J. Resting oscillations and cross-frequency coupling in human posteromedial cortex. Neuroimage. 2012;60:384–391.

135. Pfurtscheller G, Daly I, Bauernfeind G, Müller-Putz GR. Coupling between intrinsic prefrontal HbO2 and central EEG beta power oscillations in the resting brain. PloS ONE. 2012;7:e43640.

136. Monto S, Palva S, Voipio J, Palva JM. Very slow EEG fluctuations predict the dynamics of stimulus detection and oscillation amplitudes in humans. J Neurosci. 2008;28:8268–8272.

137. Thayer JF, Lane RD. Claude Bernard and the heart brain connection: further elaboration of a model of neurovisceral integration. Neurosci Biobehav Rev. 2009;33:81–88.

48 | NEUROCOGNITIVE PROCESSES

FERNANDO H. LOPES DA SILVA, MD PHD AND ERIC HALGREN, PHD

ABSTRACT: Transmembrane neuronal currents that embody cognition in the cortex produce magnetoencephalographic and electroencephalographic signals. Frequency-domain analysis reveals standard rhythms with consistent topography, frequency, and cognitive correlates. Time-domain analysis reveals average event-related potentials and field (ERP/ERF) components with consistent topography, latency, and cognitive correlates. Standard rhythms and ERP/ERF components underlie perceiving stimuli; evaluating whether stimuli match predictions, and taking appropriate action when they do not; encoding stimuli to permit semantic processing and then accessing lexical representations and assigning syntactic roles; maintaining information in primary memory; preparing to take an action; and closing processing of an event–response sequence. Sustained mental processes are associated with theta and gamma. Consolidating memories appears to occur mainly during replay of specific firing patterns during sleep spindles and slow oscillations. Biophysical, neuroanatomical, and neurophysiological factors interact to render cognitive rhythms and components particularly sensitive to the large-scale modulatory processes that sequence and integrate higher cortical processing.

KEYWORDS: cognition, rhythms, perception, memory, stimulus, electroencephalography

PRINCIPAL REFERENCES

1. Kutas M, Van Petten C. Psycholinguistics electrified: Event-related brain potential investigations. In: Gernsbacher M, ed. Handbook of Psycholinguistics. New York: Academic, 1994:83–143.
2. Luck SJ, Kappenman ES. The Oxford Handbook of Event-Related Potential Components. New York: Oxford University Press, 2011.
3. Buzsaki G. Rhythms of the Brain. New York: Oxford University Press, 2012.
4. Donchin E, Coles MG. Is the P300 component a manifestation of context updating? Behav Brain Sci. 1988;11(3):357–427.
5. Gray CM, König P, Engel AK, Singer W. Oscillatory responses in cat visual cortex exhibit inter columnar synchronization which reflects global stimulus properties. Nature. 1989;338(6213):334–337.
6. Halgren E, Kaestner E, Marinkovic K, et al. Laminar profile of spontaneous and evoked theta: Rhythmic modulation of cortical processing during word integration. Neuropsychologia. 2015;76:108–124.
7. Kahana MJ. The cognitive correlates of human brain oscillations. J Neurosci. 2006;26(6):1669–1672.
8. Klimesch W, Sauseng P, Hanslmayr S. EEG alpha oscillations: the inhibition-timing hypothesis. Brain Res Rev. 2007;53(1):63–88.
9. Lopes da Silva FH. EEG and MEG: relevance to neuroscience. Neuron. 2013;80:1112–1128.
10. Picton TW, Stuss DT. The component structure of the human event-related potentials. Progress Brain Res. 1980;54:17–49.

1. INTRODUCTION

The interest in using electroencephalographic (EEG) signals to understand cognitive processes has existed since Berger recorded EEG signals for the first time. According to Niedermeyer (1), Berger's driving force "was the quest for the nature of the all-powerful force of mental energy (Psychische Energie)." Subsequently, many researchers pursued this question and tried to use EEG signals to understand the material basis of cognitive processes. The strategy followed by most researchers in this field has been essentially correlative. Many EEG studies in the field of neurocognition involve averaged evoked or event-related potentials or magnetic fields (ERPs or ERFs); in parallel, investigations of ongoing EEG/magnetoencephalographic (MEG) signals associated with cognitive events have also been actively pursued, mainly in the last few decades. In the first part of this chapter we focus on the latter; in the second part we focus on studies concerning ERPs in the same context.

2. MAIN EEG/MEG NEUROCOGNITIVE CORRELATES

In most studies the subject performs a specific task, usually according to a standard psychological paradigm, while EEG or MEG signals are recorded. The researchers extract some properties of these signals and use statistical approaches to find significant associations between cognitive and EEG features. These investigations are based on a number of assumptions that span the microscopic level of neuronal firing and synaptic activities, the mesosocopic level of local field potentials (LFPs), up to the macroscopic level of EEG/MEG signals. The basic assumptions are the following:

1. Sensory processing, motor programming, and specific cognitive functions (perception, attention, memory, decision making) depend on patterns of neuronal spike firing.

2. Neuronal spike firing is reflected, at least partially, in LFPs according to biophysical rules that account for the transfer of soma–dendritic membrane processes to field electrical potentials and magnetic fields.

3. LFPs are the basic building blocks of EEG/MEG signals (and also of functional magnetic resonance imaging signals (fMRI), as discussed in Chapter 46; the basic neurophysiology is presented and discussed in Chapters 2, 3, and 4).

These assumptions, however, have a number of limitations and some caveats are needed. A fundamental one is that EEG/MEG signals, recorded at the scalp or even intracranially, are not capable of reflecting all neuronal activities that take place in the brain in the context of cognitive processes. It is not possible to sample brain space in a satisfactory way in order to detect the complete set of neuronal activities underlying a given cognitive process, in spite of outstanding advances in high-density whole-head electrophysiological and MEG technologies, or intracranial multiple electrode recordings.

Palva et al. (2) attempted to sample brain space and constructed a global picture of the distribution of different interrelated brain activities based on a combination of EEG and MEG signals using estimates of phase coherence according to the methodology proposed by Womelsdorf et al. (3). This was done within the framework of an investigation of brain signals associated with a working memory task. In this way these authors mapped all recordable interactions of those signals distributed over the whole scalp, and they concluded that phase synchrony in the alpha, beta, and gamma frequency bands, among fronto-parietal and visual regions, was "sustained and stable during the memory task retention period." The authors assumed that the inter-areal phase interactions correspond to "communication pathways," but no explicit information about causality or time delays was given. Thus these studies need further validation.

This limitation in spatial sampling can to some extent be compensated by simultaneous recordings of EEG and hemodynamic signals (fMRI, blood oxygen level dependent [BOLD]), but the latter are too slow to catch the quick dynamics of most cognitive processes, as discussed further in Chapter 46.

2.1. EEG/MEG Signals Reflect the Dynamics of Neuronal Assemblies

A common assumption in neuroscience is that neurons do not work in isolation; rather, they form dynamical assemblies that work in synchrony to realize determined functions. This assumption stems from the classic concept of Hebb (4), who postulated that neuronal assemblies are dynamical systems with plastic properties that underlie learning and memory. These assemblies may vary in dimension and in degree of synchrony. A multitude of neuronal assemblies are usually simultaneously active in the brain, such that we may state that the brain constitutes a complex system where parallel processing, under normal conditions, is constantly going on. These neuronal assemblies may occupy different cortical areas that are not necessarily anatomically contiguous. Therefore, the brain must integrate the operations of multiple neuronal units and neuronal assemblies. In other words, the brain has to integrate distributed sets of neuronal activities spread over multiple cortical and subcortical systems in order to achieve a coherent representation of events and to effectuate coordinated actions. The experimental observations of Vaadia et al. (6), who recorded populations of single units (6–10) in the cortex of cats and monkeys during several behavioral conditions, support the concepts put forward above. A salient finding was that information processing in the cortex is represented by *co-activation* of sets of neurons rather than by independent modulation of single-unit firing rates. The strength of the co-activation among adjacent neurons is modulated by sensory stimulation and by arousal. This co-activation between neurons is reflected in the properties of LFPs.

2.2. Do Neuronal Oscillations Have Functional Significance?

An essential note that deserves emphasis concerns the notion of *oscillation* in the EEG/MEG field. EEG/MEG signals are noisy and thus may be conceived as being made of a very large number of sinusoidal components with different frequency, amplitude, and phase. This is, in short, the essence of the decomposition of a signal in a Fourier series, as the sum of simple oscillating functions (sines and cosines), constituting the Fourier spectrum (see also Chapter 44 for a general discussion of EEG/MEG spectra, 1/f law, etc.). In the EEG /MEG field most attention, however, is dedicated to studying rhythmic activities within specific frequency bands. These rhythmic activities can be put in evidence as peaks in the Fourier spectrum; these peaks are characterized by the corresponding frequency, bandwidth, and power (or squared amplitude). The bandwidth may be narrow or broad. In general terms, in EEG/MEG signals the narrow-band activities correspond to neuronal natural oscillations, taking into account, however, that the signal has been filtered appropriately (i.e., in a frequency band appreciably wider than the spectral peak bandwidth of interest). We should note that broad-band EEG/MEG activities do not correspond to a simple oscillation, and should not be named as such, but simply as "activity in a given frequency band." By using narrow-bandwidth filters, however, one may artificially create what may appear as a narrow-band oscillation reflected in a peak in the Fourier spectrum. This should not be confused with a neuronal natural oscillation. In interpreting descriptions of EEG/MEG activities, it is important to keep this in mind.

There are many instances of oscillations in nervous systems, from the simpler organisms to the more complex. A comprehensive review of oscillations in nervous systems, from the level of very simple neural networks in invertebrate ganglia, to the more complex level of the mammalian brain, can be found in the book edited by Levine et al. (6), at the molecular, cellular, synaptic, and network levels. A characteristic property of these neuronal assemblies is that they display nonlinear dynamical oscillations. Thus we should be aware that neuronal oscillations constitute a biological property that has been conserved in the course of evolution. Rhythm-generating circuits can be very flexible in responding to external stimuli. Indeed, rhythmic activities can become manifest in the form of oscillations of LFPs at various scales. Some of these are very local, but some are manifest as mass field potentials, ultimately contributing to the electrocorticogram (ECoG), EEG, or MEG.

EEG/MEG oscillations occur at different frequencies, from the infraslow, say 0.1 Hz, to the very fast, reaching values of several hundreds of Hz. We may advance that different kinds of oscillations correspond to different sorts of operations in brain systems. Thus oscillations at the lower end of the frequency spectrum tend to engage large spatial domains, while those at higher frequencies are usually localized in restricted cortical areas. With the risk of oversimplifying, we may state that the slow oscillations can modulate the excitability of extensive neuronal populations, as occurs in the case of the "up and down states" of infraslow waves (7). Oscillations at intermediate frequencies, such as in the theta and alpha/mu ranges, are optimal to modulate, or to gate, the transfer of information within and between neuronal populations, such as those of the hippocampal formation and associated cortical areas in the case of theta (8) and of thalamocortical systems in the case of alpha/mu (see Chapter 2). Interestingly, this process of modulation may be realized by means of phase-amplitude cross-frequency coupling, where a low-frequency oscillation, such as theta or alpha, acts as the modulating signal, and a high-frequency signal, such as gamma activity, is the modulated signal. Oscillations at the higher frequencies, in the beta and gamma range, are especially adequate in promoting the transfer of packets of specific information (9) between neuronal systems. In short, specific oscillations have different kinds of functional connotations.

2.3. Neuronal Oscillations: A Role of LFPs in Promoting Synchrony and Oscillations in Neural Assemblies

A specific role for LFP oscillations emerges from the findings of Murthy and Fetz (10), who observed in the motor cortex that cortical neurons can become transiently synchronized, particularly during LFP oscillations, even if their spikes are uncorrelated during non-oscillatory periods, showing that oscillatory behavior can play a role in promoting synchrony of neuronal units. Also in the visual system, Fries et al. (11) suggested that the adjustment of spike timing by oscillations in the gamma frequency band is not an epiphenomenon but a fundamental mechanism in cortical information processing. A number of similar correlates that reinforce the statements presented here can be found, among others, in the review by Mazzoni et al. (12). Thus we may conclude, based on these experimental findings, that LFPs are neurophysiological phenomena that permit the establishment of bridges between the level of neuronal activity and the level of cognitive processes.

2.4. Contribution of EEG/MEG Analysis to Neurocognitive Studies: Skepticism and Realism

There may be reasons for some skepticism regarding the value of neuronal network oscillations and EEG/MEG rhythmic activities for neurocognitive studies. In particular, many simplistic claims of correlates between gross EEG/MEG features and cognitive processes may give rise to controversies. Nonetheless, the evidence built up in recent decades provides a realistic basis to propose that it is worthy to analyze the neuronal activities underlying cognitive processes to advance our understanding of how cognitive functions arise as emerging properties of dynamical brain systems. We discuss here experimental evidence that justifies the statement that EEG/MEG features can provide useful windows into cortical functional states underlying relevant cognitive processes (13).

In this first part of the chapter we discuss the role of the main EEG/MEG frequency bands according to what is common practice in the literature. It is important to emphasize, however, that different frequency bands are *not* independent variables, and the same cognitive process may be associated with changes of EEG/MEG signals at different frequencies. Indeed, there are interesting concatenations between frequency components that are relevant correlates of cognitive phenomena. In this respect it is pertinent to mention that different kinds of neuronal oscillations, at a variety of frequencies, can show consistent phase relations that may differ for different cortical areas. The importance of these phase relations is discussed in general terms by Maris et al. (14). An abridged overview of these phenomena is presented in the following.

3. LOW-FREQUENCY EEG/MEG ACTIVITIES, MEMORY PROCESSES, AND EXCITABILITY CYCLES

In the last decades considerable advances were made regarding the neurophysiological basis of EEG low-frequency activities (e.g., 0–4 Hz), the basic properties of which are discussed in Chapters 2 and 32. Definitions based exclusively on specific frequency bands may conceal underlying mechanisms. Thus the EEG low-frequency band that is traditionally called *the delta frequency band* may comprise different electrophysiological processes, such as ultra-slow components, with distinct basic mechanisms. Basic ionic currents and intrinsic membrane phenomena underlying slow waves and oscillations are described in Chapter 2. The first reason why it is interesting to discuss EEG slow-wave activity in the context of the topic of this chapter—*EEG phenomena and cognitive processes*—is that while these EEG slow rhythms are distinctive of slow-wave sleep (SWS), sleep plays a role in memory processes. The second reason is that it appears that infraslow oscillations may modulate behavioral variables also in the awake state. First we consider the association between slow oscillations, sleep, and memory processes, since these are well documented. Later we describe briefly the modulation of behavioral variables with infraslow oscillations in the awake state.

There is ample evidence showing that sleep plays a critical role in memory consolidation (reviewed in Walker and Stickgold (15)), where consolidation means the post-learning stabilization process that strengthens new memory traces. This was shown for procedural memory tasks (16) and for declarative memory (17). Even an ultra-short period of sleep (a diurnal nap) is sufficient to enhance declarative memory processing (18). Payne et al. (19) showed that sleep preferentially enhances memories with emotional charge, particularly if this has a negative connotation.

Following the analysis by Diekelmann and Born (20), the associations between the two stages of sleep and memory processes can be summarized according to two main features. First, SWS comprises characteristic features—slow oscillations, spindles, and ripples. Spindle activity and ripples increase during the "up-state" and become suppressed during the "down-state" of the slow oscillation. A current hypothesis is that during the "up-state" the ripples and spindles would provide a mechanism by which information would be transferred from the hippocampal formation to the neocortex, where the information would be stored. Second, rapid eye movement (REM sleep), which is characterized by a cortical desynchronized EEG and ponto-geniculate-occipital waves concomitant with a regular theta rhythm in the hippocampal formation and associated structures, is associated with a high level of cholinergic activity and a local increase in the expression of plasticity-related genes. This neuronal state would facilitate the subsequent synaptic stabilization of memories in the cortex.

This role of the sleep state in optimizing memory consolidation has been mainly put in evidence for hippocampus-dependent memories but may be extended to other types of memories (21). A central question is whether the EEG pattern characteristic of SWS is directly relevant for memory functions or whether it is the duration of sleep, as such, that is the important variable. van der Werf et al. (22) showed that a disruption of sleep that suppressed slow-wave activity (SWa) while inducing shallow sleep, although not reducing total sleep time, was sufficient to affect subsequent memory performance in healthy human subjects. These observations are in line with the experimental findings of Marshall et al., (23) who showed that slow oscillations induced in humans by transcranial magnetic stimulation (TMS) during non-REM sleep at low frequency (0.75 Hz) were able to improve the retention of hippocampus-dependent memory, but stimulation at higher frequencies (5 Hz) did not; the low-frequency stimulation, however, was not effective in improving procedural (hippocampus-independent) memory. This suggests a causal role of cortical SWa (≈0.75 Hz) in those kinds of memory processes. A similar conclusion regarding the role of ripples can be drawn from the findings of Ego-Stengel and Wilson (24), who showed that selectively disrupting neuronal activity during ripple events in the hippocampus, by stimulating hippocampal afferents at the rat, impairs spatial learning.

Taken together, these various experimental findings lead to the conclusion that SWS promotes memory consolidation and the distribution of memory traces in the brain, which is complemented in the local synaptic consolidation stage during REM. Based on this and other experimental evidence that we cannot discuss here in detail (see for a comprehensive recent review Stickgold and Walker (25)), it may be concluded that sleep physiological phenomena, sleep spindles and SWa, actively promote memory improvement.

Do infraslow oscillations also modulate cognitive functions in the awake state? In this respect the study by Monto et al. (26) is interesting (see also Chapter 32). These authors investigated whether the 0.01- to 0.1-Hz infraslow oscillations may influence slow fluctuations in human psychophysical performance. To this purpose they used an uncued somatosensory detection task; they applied weak electrical pulses to the right index finger while simultaneously recording DC coupled full-band EEG. The subjects were asked to report a detected stimulus by twitching the right thumb while keeping their eyes closed. Statistical analyses showed that behavioral performance was correlated with the phase of infra-slow EEG oscillations (both phase and amplitude) recorded at Fpz and Cz. These findings allow us to draw the conclusion that EEG infraslow oscillations are associated with fluctuations of the excitability of cortical networks also in the awake state.

In conclusion, EEG slow oscillations can modulate cognitive processes, particularly memory formation, but also cognitive performance.

4. SPATIAL COGNITION AND MEMORY PROCESSES: THE ROLE OF THETA RHYTHMS AS SUCH AND IN COMBINATION WITH HIGHER-FREQUENCY OSCILLATIONS

Most of the knowledge about the neurophysiology of theta rhythms at the cellular level and at neuronal network levels pertains to the activities recorded in the hippocampal formation and associated limbic structures, including the cingulate cortex, in rodents and other animals (see Chapter 2). The relations between theta, sensory, and motor events is well documented, particularly regarding spatial orientation. Further, the modulation of theta frequency with levels of motor actions (locomotion, orientation, vestibular stimulation) is also well established in animals. In the case of human theta rhythms a series of experimental findings, as reviewed by Kahana (27), provide good arguments to support a similar role in humans, as in other mammals.

4.1. Are Theta Oscillations Associated with Movement and Spatial Navigation?

A good deal of the human studies that yield insight in the relations between theta rhythms and cognitive processes were obtained using indwelling electrodes, either implanted intracerebrally or incorporated in subdural grids. These recordings permitted the direct exploration of the hippocampal formation in humans during the performance of behavioral tasks and showed that hippocampal low-frequency theta, also in humans, is modulated by overt movement in a situation with a working memory component (28).

Epileptic patients were investigated during a task where the subjects had to navigate through a virtual maze by Kahana (29). The hippocampal EEG recordings showed periods of theta rhythmic activity as the subjects learned to navigate virtual mazes, and the occurrence of these periods co-varied with the degree of difficulty of the task, suggesting an association between the occurrence of theta oscillations and spatial navigation. These experimental findings were elaborated by Caplan et al. (30), who showed, in a virtual taxi driver task, that theta oscillations appeared more frequently during virtual movement than during periods of voluntary stillness. These effects were widespread throughout many recording sites, including, bilaterally, the peri-rolandic region and the temporal lobes. Cornwell et al. (31), also using whole-head MEG, reported hippocampal and parahippocampal theta, centered around 5 Hz, during an ingenious spatial navigation task (virtual reality Morris water maze). They showed larger theta activity in the left anterior hippocampus especially during the early stages of training, indicating that this region plays a role in early learning.

A conclusion that can be drawn from these studies is that theta activity is preeminent during learning of associations between sensory stimuli and motor behavior that are essential for the performance of spatial navigation.

4.2. Are Theta Oscillations Associated with Memory Processes?

This question was tackled by Raghavachari et al. (32), who investigated whether theta occurs during a non-spatial task, namely as subjects performed the Sternberg working memory task (Fig. 48.1). They found that the amplitude of theta rhythmic activity in the range from 4 to 9 Hz, but predominantly between 6 and 8 Hz, increased from the start of a Sternberg task, persisted during the delay period, and decreased only at the end. In this study the electrode sites where increases of theta oscillations were found were distributed over many cortical areas. A conclusion is that theta oscillations can mediate the organization of working memory, incorporating multiple items of information.

Sederberg et al. (33) investigated EEG changes in epileptic patients using intracranial cortical and subcortical electrodes during the encoding stage in a basic memory task. A relationship was observed between increased theta activity in right frontal and temporal regions during encoding. In the human hippocampus EEG intracranial recordings revealed phase-coupling between a frequency band, which the authors called slow theta (2.5–5 Hz), and a broad gamma band activity (34–130 Hz) during the formation of new episodic memories; it was greater in the case of successful encoding compared with unsuccessful trials (34).

Theta rhythmic activity has been also shown to be strongly associated with language processing mainly in the anteroventral temporal lobe, but also in other cortical areas, as reviewed by Halgren et al. (35). The role of theta in this context is discussed in more detail in the second part of this chapter, particularly in relation with ERPs, in a variety of cognitive tasks, mainly involving language processing and word memory formation ((36), see further in this chapter).

In scalp EEG there is also evidence in healthy human subjects that theta oscillations are related to memory processes such as successful encoding of new information (37). An important aspect that is considered only in some studies is how theta oscillations recorded from different areas are interrelated and which are the corresponding sources in the brain. In this respect Sarnthein et al. (38) found increased 4- to 7-Hz coherence between frontal and posterior association cortex during retention periods involved in a verbal and a visuo-spatial working memory task. Schack et al. (39), investigating subjects using a modified Sternberg paradigm, reported maximal theta power at Fz and Cz during retention periods, and noted strong phase-coupling, estimated using cross-bicoherence, between theta (3–7 Hz) recorded at Fz and gamma oscillations (30–33 Hz) at frontal areas (F3 and Fp1) as the subjects memorized number words.

Several studies using MEG also revealed associations between theta activity and memory functions, although focusing on different frequency bands. Tesche and Karhu (40) showed a relation between the duration of episodes of theta increased activity (4–8 Hz) and memory demands in a working memory task, based on an analysis of MEG signals likely recorded from the hippocampal formation. Jensen and Tesche (41) recorded whole-head MEG signals while subjects were performing a Sternberg memory task. These authors found that

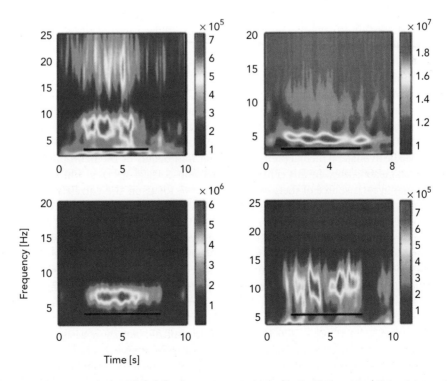

Time [s]

Figure 48.1. Theta is gated during the Sternberg task. Averaged time-frequency power shows sustained theta activity in four subjects: right frontal site in subject 1 (top left); left temporal site in subject 2 (top right); right frontal site in subject 3 (bottom left); depth electrode in left temporal lobe in subject 4 (bottom right). The color scale represents power in square microvolts. Adapted with permission from Raghavachari et al., 2001 (32).

oscillations in the band around 8 Hz (called theta by them), particularly in frontal areas, increased with the number of items retained in working memory. Also using MEG recordings de Araújo et al. (42) found an oscillation with a peak at ~3.7 Hz that increased during a task where subjects had to navigate through a computer-generated virtual reality town. Using a single-dipole model they localized this source to near the superior temporal gyrus and the deeper temporal structures. Guderian and Düzel (43) also used whole-head MEG to find out whether MEG phenomena associated with recognition memory judgments could be put in evidence. They showed pictures of human faces to the subjects, some of which had been seen previously and some not. Theta oscillations, both high (7–8 Hz) and low (4.5 Hz), had a larger amplitude for those trials where the subjects had good recollection of the pictures versus trials where accurate memory was poor. This analysis led to the conclusion that recollection of the memorized information is associated with a distributed network characterized by theta oscillations that includes the prefrontal, mediotemporal, and occipital areas.

We note that there is a considerable variability among several of these studies with respect to the frequency of theta oscillations that were studied. In several of these investigations the frequency observed is relatively high (≈8 Hz) to be assigned with certainty to the hippocampal formation and associated limbic cortex, since the electrical activity recorded locally from electrodes implanted in the human hippocampus (28) is usually much lower (≈4 Hz), which is close to that reported by de Araújo et al. (42) using MEG.

4.3. What Are the Correlates of Frontal Midline Theta?

An EEG phenomenon in the theta frequency range that has been investigated intensively in relation to cognitive functions is the so-called frontal midline theta (Fmθ) that can be recorded from the scalp (44). An Fmθ rhythm at 6 to 7 Hz, particularly evident during mental arithmetic calculations appearing in relatively short bursts, was recorded in MEG recordings combined with EEG, and during tasks engaging focused attention such as mental calculation and musical imagining (45). Later Ishii et al. (46), using an adaptive beamforming method, estimated that the sources of FMθ lie in bilateral medial prefrontal cortices, including anterior cingulate cortex. In this context it is also appropriate to note that in rat a source of theta rhythmic activity was found in the cingulate cortex by Leung and Borst (47); the latter, if also present in human, may contribute to FMθ. In line with this finding, Onton et al. (48), investigating EEG activities associated with the performance of a form of Sternberg verbal memory task, focused on FMθ 6-Hz oscillatory activity and estimated the major source of FMθ as being a "field activity in and/or above the dorsal anterior cingulate cortex." The strength of the FMθ was related to memory load. In addition to this midline theta, a beta1 oscillation (12–15 Hz) was identified as a significant correlate, the spectral power of which was enhanced while encoding an internal representation of the stimulus. These authors point out an important aspect, which is that theta and beta1 frequency oscillations of frontal midline sources may sometimes reflect periodic non-sinusoidal wave sequences that are decomposed by time/frequency analysis into two or more harmonic frequencies.

Based on data obtained directly from the human hippocampus and from scalp EEG, the hypothesis has been put forward that the cortical theta rhythm reflects dynamic interactions between the hippocampal system and the neocortex (49). According to this hypothesis the study of scalp EEG theta may provide relevant information about hippocampal theta activities that, as we saw above, are associated with memory processes.

In short, we may conclude that similar to what has been seen in other species, the human theta may represent a dynamic state of neuronal networks engaged in memory processing that may be instrumental in facilitating the formation of these dynamic neural assemblies in an extensive brain workspace.

5. ALPHA RHYTHMS, "MODULATING GATE FUNCTION" AND ATTENTION MODULATION

It is important to emphasize, from the start, that a unique and homogenous alpha rhythm does not exist. Three independent alpha rhythms must be distinguished, depending on the brain system where they are dominant:

1. The occipito-parietal alpha associated with the visual system

2. The central alpha, also called mu rhythm, associated with the somatomotor system

3. The temporal alpha, also called tau rhythm. This one is difficult to detect on scalp EEG but can be detected more readily in the MEG (see Chapter 35) and with intracranial electrodes (50).

5.1. Neuronal Mechanisms Underlying the Generation of Alpha Oscillations

To understand the role of alpha rhythms in cognitive processes it is important to consider basic mechanisms of the generation of alpha oscillations at the neuronal level. Without getting into details of the neurophysiology of alpha rhythms in thalamo-cortical systems, which was discussed in Chapter 2, here we focus on the correlation between alpha oscillations and neuronal firing at the level of the cortex. Bollimunta et al. (51) recorded LFPs and current source density (CSD) profiles and multi-unit activity (MUA) in monkey visual cortical areas V2 and V4. They found that neuronal firing in the granular (layer 4) and infra-granular layers was modulated by local alpha oscillations; firing was higher during the local sinks, corresponding to local neuronal depolarization, and it was low during the local sources, but, in contrast, the supra-granular multi-unit did not show a significant modulation. Using an experimental approach similar to Bollimunta's (51) and also in the awake monkey, the relationship between alpha oscillations and neuronal firing (MUA) was more recently investigated in more detail by van Kerkoerle et al. (52) and by Haegens et al. (53). Applying estimates of Granger causality, van Kerkoele et al. reported that alpha waves are initiated mainly in infragranular layer 5, but also in supragranular layers 1 and 2; alpha activity both from layer 5 and from layers 1 and 2 showed phase advance with respect to activity in layer 4, as illustrated in Chapter 2, Figure 2.16. The study by Haegens et al. (53), also using CSD and MUA, described alpha current generators in the supragranular, granular, and infragranular layers. These findings were not exclusive to the visual cortex and were also encountered in the somatomotor and auditory cortices.

The picture that arises from these more advanced experimental studies, however, is complex. Although it confirms that the main neuronal generators of alpha are situated in deep cortical layers (layer 5), it shows that alpha field generators can be found in all layers, and that alpha can modulate neuronal excitability and the firing rate of cortical neurons. Accordingly, alpha modulation may be involved both in cortical feedback and feed-forward processes.

5.2. The Alpha Rhythm Is Not Monolithic: The Existence of a Variety of Alpha Oscillations

Even within the visual cortex there are many sources of alpha rhythms. This has been put in evidence in dog, where cortical "epicenters" of alpha rhythms were described that are interconnected via dense cortico-cortical connections (54), but also more recently in monkey (51–53). This shows that we have to be careful in generalizing about "the" alpha rhythm because there are several alpha rhythms generated in different cortical areas and with different cortical laminar organization. The degree of synchronization between the diverse alpha rhythms may vary depending on local inputs either from subcortical structures or from other cortical areas.

A large body of evidence revealed that both visual alpha and somatomotor mu rhythms may show enhancement or attenuation, simultaneously or successively, at different sites on the scalp or on the ECoG (55) depending on cognitive tasks. This can be explained taking into consideration the interaction between different thalamocortical modules, as explained in Chapter 40 (ERD/ERS phenomena). In this respect, the experimental findings by Rihs et al. (57), showing enhancement of occipital alpha associated with active suppression of unattended positions in the visual field during a visual spatial orienting task, provides further evidence for the *facilitatory role* of alpha-power decreases (event-related alpha desynchronization [ERD]) versus the *inhibitory role* of alpha-power enhancement (event-related alpha synchronization [ERS]), with respect to attentional processes (see below for a more detailed description).

Regarding associations between alpha rhythms and cognitive events, one must always take into consideration not only the frequency and reactivity of the rhythmic activity but also the spatial distribution over the scalp.

5.3. Misconceptions Around the Concept of an "Idling Alpha Rhythm"; Alpha as a "Modulating Gate" for Information Flow

Long ago Adrian and Matthews (57) named a system that is neither receiving nor processing sensory information as an "idling system"; subsequently, occipital alpha rhythms were considered as idling rhythms of the visual areas and mu rhythms as idling rhythms of sensorimotor areas (58). Nonetheless, the "idling concept" does not account for the real neuronal processes going on as alpha oscillations are present. As described above basic neurophysiological data show clearly that during alpha oscillations the main feature is that the thalamo-cortical relay neurons are in a dynamic state of phasic inhibition (see also Chapter 2). This state does not imply that these neuronal populations are idling; on the contrary, they can play an active inhibiting role in gating the transfer of information in certain neuronal pathways. In short, the alpha rhythm state may fulfill, in itself, a relevant functional role, namely a "modulating gate function" (54).

This neurophysiological interpretation is compatible with the theoretical considerations of Klimesch et al. (59), who stated that alpha ERS plays an active role in the inhibitory control and timing of cortical processing, whereas ERD reflects the gradual release of inhibition associated with the emergence of activation processes.

The experimental evidence obtained in many studies that a state of enhanced focalized attention on a given stimulus that is being processed is associated with a decrease of alpha power, whereas alpha power increases simultaneously in other cortical areas not involved in the task, appears to corroborate the notion that an enhanced alpha "shuts off" distracting inputs. We proposed that in this condition alpha rhythm fulfills a "modulating gate function." We mean by this term "modulating gate" a process that controls, or filters, the flow of information and its timing—in other words, that information flow would be phased according to the periodicity of the alpha waves.

5.4. Experimental Evidence for a Modulator Inhibiting Role of Alpha Oscillations in Perceptual Processes

Several studies showed that perception performance is reduced in the cases where stimuli are presented while the power in the alpha band is large compared to the opposite condition. Hanslmayr et al. (60) found (Fig. 48.2) that not only do strong oscillations in the alpha frequency band inhibit the perception of visual stimuli, but also increases of synchrony in higher frequency ranges (>20 Hz) enhance visual perception. Further, Mathewson et al. (61) revealed not only that the power of the alpha oscillations is important with respect to perception, but also that the phase of EEG alpha rhythm recorded from posterior brain regions can reliably predict detection of visual stimuli.

These studies, taken together, support the concept that an increase of alpha oscillations in cortical areas directly involved in information processing functions as a "modulating gate" that inhibits and/or modulates temporarily the information flow necessary for visual perception.

5.5. Experimental Evidence that Alpha Oscillations Exert Phased Inhibition on Information Flow

The idea that the *phase* of alpha oscillations represents oscillations in cortical excitability has been alive in the field of

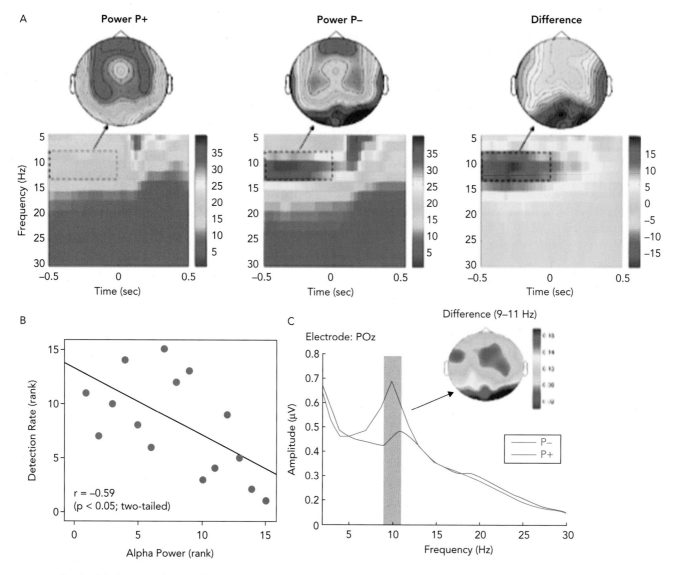

Figure 48.2. Results of the between-subjects analysis: perceivers (P+) vs. non-perceivers (P−) and the difference between both are shown. *A:* Time–frequency plot of power is shown for the electrode O2. Stimulus is presented at time 0. Differences between perceivers and non-perceivers are most evident in the alpha frequency range (8–12 Hz) in the time window of 500 msec prior to stimulus presentation. The scalp maps indicate that alpha power was strongest at parieto-occipital electrode leads. The square indicates the time window that was used for statistical comparison. *B:* The scatterplot between rank transformed alpha power (x-axis) and perception performance (y-axis) is shown. Alpha power was collapsed for parieto-occipital electrode sites. *C:* Power spectrum of the resting condition with eyes open is plotted for electrode POz. The resting condition was recorded prior to the start of the experiment. Perceivers showed significantly lower alpha amplitudes than non-perceivers. The gray bar indicates the frequency window that was used for statistics (9–11 Hz). Power spectra were calculated using a fast Fourier transformation. Adapted with permission from Hanslmayr et al., 2007 (60).

EEG for a long time. A possible role of alpha oscillations in phased inhibition has been addressed in a number of more recent studies, such as that by Matthewson et al. (61) referred above. Another one is that by Busch et al. (62). In this investigation the authors presented brief flashes of light to subjects near the subject's threshold so that they detected approximately only half of the flashes (hits) and missed the other half (misses) while the EEG was recorded. Stimuli that were presented when the EEG displayed large power in (theta) alpha band (6–12 Hz) were significantly less likely to be detected. More relevant regarding the question formulated above is that the visual detection threshold fluctuated over time with the phase of the ongoing EEG activity. Curiously, the major effect, however, was seen at 7 Hz (as the authors note, at "the intersection between theta and alpha frequency bands"), and it had a fronto-central topography, which could correspond to a source in fronto-central midline structures assumed to be associated with sources of theta rhythms, as described above. Nonetheless, this study presents interesting evidence for the fact that during EEG oscillations there are cyclic variations of neuronal excitability that may filter the flow of incoming stimuli within successive discrete time windows.

Mathewson et al. (61) called the functional state associated with alpha rhythm a form of "pulsed inhibition." This interpretation is in line with the "inhibition-timing hypothesis," proposed by Klimesch et al. (59), and the "modulating gate hypothesis," proposed by us (54), as described above.

5.6. Is There Complementary Evidence Supporting the Modulating Inhibiting Role of Alpha Oscillations in Perception?

Interesting support for this concept has been given by the investigation (63) of the effects of TMS applied to the visual cortex under different conditions of alpha oscillations. TMS induces illusory visual percepts, the so-called phosphenes. These authors report a remarkable result: whether TMS stimuli evoked such a percept or not depended on pre-stimulus alpha power. While TMS applied during low pre-stimulus alpha power resulted in phosphenes, the same TMS stimulus applied during the condition of large pre-stimulus alpha power failed to evoke phosphenes. These findings give support to the concept that during the state characterized by strong alpha power the excitability of the local cortex is markedly decreased.

Another, although indirect, contribution to the concept that alpha rhythms may exert a modulating role in perception is given by the observation that alpha activity in subjects with attention-deficit/hyperactivity disorder (ADHD) displays, in a visuo-spatial covert attention task, a different reactivity than in healthy subjects. Whereas healthy subjects display a decrease of alpha (8–12 Hz) in the contralateral hemisphere, in contrast with an increase in the ipsilateral hemisphere, in the ADHD subjects this lateralized reactivity is not apparent (64). This effect may be interpreted in the light of the concept that alpha oscillations play a role in the dorsal fronto-parietal network for top-down control of visual attention, but much more information is needed to better understand these phenomena.

5.7. Alpha Rhythm Reactivity: Top-Down Inhibitory Attentional Processes

The most common correlate of alpha rhythm can be summarized in the concept proposed by Klimesch et al. (59): the functional state where alpha oscillations are dominant (alpha ERS) reflects a "top-down inhibitory control process" (i.e., a state of reduced information processing). As a consequence, the reverse situation (i.e., the decrease of alpha power [alpha ERD]) corresponds to a situation where attentional processes are facilitated. One can envisage the alpha rhythm state as a functional state where some brain systems are protected from the influence of disturbing stimuli, as it may occur as a subject is keeping information to be encoded and refrains from responding before a given command, as shown in several experimental situations (59). This concept was further refined by Klimesch (65) by adding the qualification "timing" to the "inhibiting role of alpha activity" in light of the hypothesis that entrainment of alpha phase, associated with the inhibitory phase, is responsible for the attentional blink (AB) phenomenon. This is also supported by the findings of Zauner et al. (66), who demonstrated that the failure to detect a second stimulus (T2) in an AB trial (i.e., the reduced ability to report a second target after identifying a first one in a serial presentation of visual stimuli at approximately 10 items per second) is associated with the phase of the alpha oscillation.

One of these situations merits special mention since it exemplifies the dynamical interaction between different neuronal systems during the performance of a cognitive task. Jensen et al. (67) showed that alpha power (9–12 Hz) increases with memory load during retention of a short-term memory task. These authors formulated two alternative explanations: "the increase in alpha band activity with memory load appears either to be a consequence of active inhibition of alpha producing brain areas, or it is explained by a mechanism in which alpha band oscillations are directly involved in memory maintenance." In light of what we presented above about alpha power increase as exerting a "modulating gate function" (54) or the alpha as representing a mechanism underlying a "top-down control inhibitory process" (59), our interpretation is that the first alternative suggested by Jensen et al. (67) is the more likely. Indeed, an increase in alpha power under these conditions represents a condition where interfering inputs that may disturb memory processing are actively inhibited or filtered out. It does not mean, however, that alpha activity as such operates directly on the process of memory. In the section on gamma oscillations we will discuss further the fact that an alpha power decrease very often goes together with an increase in gamma oscillations.

In short, there is solid evidence to conclude that modulations of alpha power correspond to modulations of attentional processes.

6. BETA RHYTHMS, FOCUSED ATTENTION AND MOTOR PROGRAMMING

A variety of cortical beta rhythms exist, with different spatial distribution and reactivity. In classic EEG literature it is common to distinguish, within the beta frequency range, two sub-bands (beta1, 14–20 Hz, and beta2, 20–30 Hz), while the gamma band is reserved for frequency components beyond 30 Hz (in some cases even three beta bands are distinguished). In general, we may state that beta oscillations are associated with cortical output from pyramidal neurons of deep layers (V). The neural mechanisms underlying the generation of beta oscillations are discussed in Chapters 2 and 3. Beta oscillations are recorded over most cortical areas, in particular areas involved in motor functions (supplementary motor, premotor, somato-motor), but are widespread over neocortex, limbic and olfactory cortex, and basal ganglia, in animal and man. A number of classic animal studies demonstrated the presence of 14- to 30-Hz waves (beta1 and beta2) in various cortical areas, during different conditions of increased alertness. Since the limits between the different sub-bands of beta and gamma are somewhat arbitrary, it is always preferable to state the specific frequency band of a particular EEG or LFP activity that one is dealing with.

Fast rhythmic activities in the frequency range from 35 to 85 Hz dominate the LFPs of olfactory areas of the forebrain (68) but are also recorded from the temporal cortex, namely the entorhinal cortex (16–20 and 35–40 Hz) (69) and the hippocampus (20–60 Hz), typically during behavioral active states and accompanied by theta rhythm (6–9 Hz) (70), and also in the fronto-parietal cortex during focused attention on a specific target (35–45 Hz) (71); in the visual cortex during behavioral immobility associated with an enhanced level of vigilance of a dog expecting a conditioned visual stimulus, what was called beta-frequency cortical selectivity peaking at 28 Hz (72); and in the visual cortex of a monkey during accurate performance of a conditioned response (20–40 Hz) (73). In many cases fast oscillations, however, are associated with overt movement, such as during tasks requiring fine finger movements and focused attention.

6.1. Some Beta Oscillations Are Harmonically Coupled to Lower-Frequency Spectral Components: Bispectral Analysis

An interesting feature of EEG signals in the beta frequency range is that some components within this frequency band are harmonically related to alpha frequencies due to the fact that alpha rhythms result from the activity of nonlinear neuronal processes and thus display second harmonic (~20 Hz) and even third harmonic (~30 Hz) components (74). This is particularly evident in the case of rhythmic activity recorded from the central region, the so-called mu rhythm that has a "comb-like "appearance (75). Using bispectral analysis, one can check whether different EEG frequency components are harmonically related: if a significant bispectrum between any pair of frequency components exists these are, of course, not independent.

6.2. Beta Oscillations, Attention, Motor Programming, Execution and Relaxation

An important feature of human beta rhythms is that there is a variety of activities within the same frequency range that differ in frequency, spatial localization, and behavioral correlates. This diversity is probably a factor that contributes to the notion that the EEG beta band "seems to be the least well understood in terms of its functional significance," according to Engel and Fries (76). Nonetheless, a good number of experimental observations in primates and in humans, in particular studies of beta oscillations in relation to motor activities, demonstrate the functional significance of some types of beta oscillations.

Murthy and Fetz (77) showed that bursts of 20- to 40-Hz oscillations can be recorded in monkey motor cortical cells. These bursts become synchronized over a large cortical area during exploratory forelimb movements. Further, they concluded that the burst of beta oscillations had no reliable relation to particular components of the movement but likely constituted a neural correlate of attention during demanding sensorimotor behaviors. In awake monkey Baker et al. (78) obtained experimental evidence that supports this conclusion. They recorded LFPs (local EEG) from the primary motor cortex as well as pyramidal tract neuronal discharges. The former showed bursts of oscillations in the beta2 frequency range (20–30 Hz) that were coherent with the rectified electromyogram (EMG) of hand and forearm muscles active during the hold phase of a precision grip task. In humans, Salenius et al. (79) recorded whole-scalp MEG signals simultaneously with the surface EMG from upper and lower limb muscles

during voluntary isometric contractions and found a significant coherence between MEG signals in the beta1 and beta2 frequency bands (15–33 Hz) recorded from the primary motor cortex, with motor unit firing for all muscles (Fig. 48.3). The cortical signals preceded motor unit firing by 12 to 53 msec. These results indicate that these beta cortical rhythms are intimately associated with the pattern of motor neuronal activity necessary to realize the motor cortex output during isometric contractions.

A prominent example of the relation between beta oscillations and motor functions is the phenomenon of post-movement event-related beta synchronization (ERS) or beta rebound that is induced by simple voluntary movements (75). These beta oscillations are somatotopically organized in the cortex, but the frequency differs depending on whether the movement is of the hand or the foot, being in the range of 16 to 20 Hz in the former and 20–24 Hz in the latter. The application of TMS during these beta bursts showed that at this time there is a reduction of the motor cortex excitability, which indicates that these beta bursts correspond to a state of cortical deactivation. These phenomena are covered in more detail in Chapter 28.

Interestingly, modulations of alpha/mu (10–12 Hz) and beta (18–30 Hz) EEG oscillations were investigated with respect to human upright robot-assisted walking (80). Both frequency spectral components decreased (ERD) in the central sensorimotor areas corresponding to the somatotopic cortical location of the legs during active walking in comparison with upright standing, reflecting an active state of the sensorimotor cortex during walking. In addition, the amplitude of gamma oscillations was modulated, predominantly in the frequency range of 28 to 36 Hz, in relation to the gait phase, with the maximum located in central sensorimotor areas. Although there was a partial overlap between the beta frequency range showing ERD and the low gamma frequency range displaying amplitude modulation, these two phenomena could be shown to be distinct. The gait phase modulation of gamma oscillations likely corresponds to synchronization of the neuronal populations involved in sensorimotor integration of walking.

A particular aspect of beta rhythms around 20 Hz recorded using MEG over the primary motor cortex is their occurrence during the observation of movement realized by another person, which has been interpreted as reflecting the activity of the human mirroring system (81). This phenomenon is described and discussed in Chapter 32. Babiloni et al. (82) compared EEG (≈20 Hz) rhythmic reactivity to movement observation and execution and noted a similar topographical distribution for central beta ERD/ERS for both conditions, but this needs more detailed experimental analysis.

In conclusion, four main aspects regarding beta oscillations are as follows:

1. Mental states in which subjects program a voluntary motor act are represented at the EEG level by an enhancement of beta2 rhythms with specific spatial distribution.

2. There are different kinds of EEG beta rhythms, with diverse dynamics and localizations.

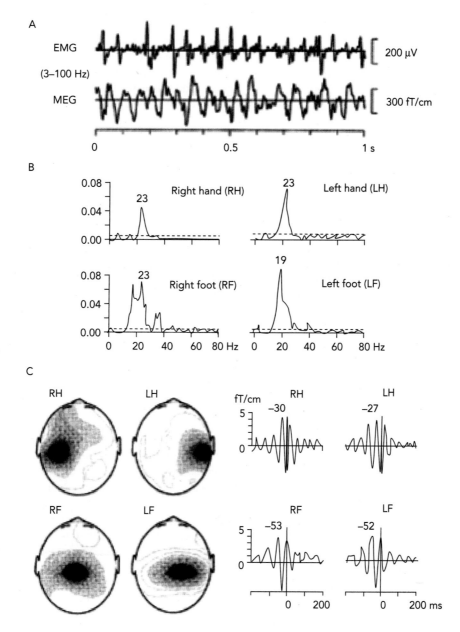

Figure 48.3. *A: EMG from contracting left flexor hallucis brevis muscle, and coincident MEG signal over right foot area. B: Coherence spectra between MEG and EMG for isometric contraction of left and right interosseus (hand) and flexor hallucis brevis (foot) muscles. Dashed lines, 1% significance level. C: Spatial distributions of strongest peaks of coherence spectra. Head is viewed from above. D: Time domain MEG signals, averaged with respect to onset of motor unit potentials in EMG. Adapted with permission from Salenius et al., 1997 (79).*

3. Beta rhythmic oscillations can promote synchrony of neuronal elements in different cortical systems, associated with diverse motoric and cognitive functions.

4. The boundary between beta2 and gamma is not precisely defined.

7. GAMMA OSCILLATIONS, BINDING HYPOTHESIS, PERCEPTION AND MEMORY

Several studies have put in evidence EEG gamma oscillations, typically in the range of 30 to 100 Hz, associated with conscious perception. We mention here only a few that are particularly relevant to the discussion with respect to the relation between gamma oscillations and cognitive functions such as attention and perception.

7.1. Gamma Oscillations, Binding and Synchronization

Since the reports by Eckhorn et al. (83), Gray and Singer (84), and Gray et al. (85) that the firing probability of neurons of the visual cortex of the cat, in response to the presentation of appropriate visual stimuli, can display oscillations in the gamma frequency range, predominantly around 40 Hz, these cortical gamma oscillations are considered to form the mechanism by which various features of a visual scene may be bound together ("binding hypothesis"). Beyond this observation it was also shown that gamma oscillations may operate as a general mechanism that is capable of binding together, by a process of phase synchronization, not only the firing of neurons at the local level but also neural activities of spatially separate cortical areas (86). Thus, phase synchronization may operate whenever neural dynamic processes involving spatially separate brain regions are integrated (87). In general, we may state that synchronization of neuronal networks by way of common oscillations in the gamma frequency range may enable fast routing of information in the cortex with respect to processing of cognitive information (11).

The association between gamma oscillations (30–100 Hz) and attention processes has been clearly demonstrated in several studies in experimental animals and also in humans. Experiments by Fries et al. (88) in behaving monkeys showed that focusing attention to a behaviorally relevant stimulus is associated with the enhancement of gamma frequency rhythmicity (35–90 Hz) in visual area V4, while low-frequency oscillations were reduced. These changes in gamma synchronization may facilitate the efficacy of the output of these neurons to activate downstream targets, since gamma frequency synchronization recruits spikes to cluster within ~10 msec and in this way may enhance their effect on postsynaptic neurons.

These experimental findings show that visual cortical neurons that are activated by an attended stimulus display much stronger synchronized firing, reflected in LFP, than do neurons that are activated by a distracters. How gamma oscillations, which can display a wide range of frequencies, can bind together neuronal populations that are spatially distributed is a question that requires reflection. This has been approached in detailed studies of gamma oscillations in the hippocampus of rodents. This model allows detailed physiological analysis and thus can be optimal to investigate the detailed neurophysiological mechanism of brain oscillations. Colgin (89) and Colgin et al. (90) showed that in CA1 area gamma oscillations split into fast (65–140 Hz) and slow (25–50 Hz) components; the former are coupled to similar oscillations in the entorhinal cortex, a system that encodes information about the spatial position of an animal, while the latter are coupled to CA3, a system that plays an important role in memory. Interestingly, the two types of gamma oscillations occurred at different phases of the local CA1 theta rhythm. These experimental findings are important in order to better understand how gamma oscillations coupled to theta oscillations may operate as a mechanism for rerouting information in a brain system.

7.2. Gamma Oscillations and Visuo-Motor Integration

It may be expected that only if relatively large populations of neurons are synchronously active the corresponding oscillations may be reflected in measurable fields at the level of the EEG or MEG. It can be shown that the occurrence of gamma oscillations is associated with an enhanced efficiency of a behavioral response. This can be illustrated in the case of a visuo-motor reaction-time task (91). These authors investigated whether there was a relationship between behavioral efficiency, reflected in a shorter reaction time, and the properties of the EEG signals at the moment that the subjects received a warning cue. They found that the larger the power of the gamma frequency band (>30 Hz) in a fronto-parietal network, measured before stimulus onset, the shorter the reaction time. These findings are especially interesting because they indicate that the brain state characterized by gamma activity can enhance the efficiency of visuo-motor tasks and may function as a top-down attentional control mechanism.

EEG/MEG gamma band signals also play an important role in establishing synchronization between different cortical areas, and thus these synchronized oscillations may mediate the formation of a dynamic workspace in the brain, which is necessary for the realization of specific cognitive processes. In this context the findings by Roelfsema et al. (86), who recorded LFPs of the cerebral cortex of cats performing a visual guided motor response (described above) are a good illustration. In humans, stimulus-locked neural coupling within the EEG gamma band (30–40 Hz) across hemispheres in visual cortex was also encountered during processing of visual stimuli with spatially distributed features (92).

7.3. Gamma Oscillations and Conscious Perception

The studies by Rodriguez et al. (93) and Trujillo et al. (94) are particularly relevant in this respect because they enable us to pinpoint a few aspects that are important for the interpretation of correlates between EEG signals and cognitive processes in general. Rodriguez et al. (93) reported results that they interpreted as demonstrating a specific role of EEG gamma activity in human visual perception. They showed that gamma synchrony (20–60 Hz), estimated by an index of phase synchrony, was significantly more likely to occur when observers perceived a face than when they did not, because the face presented was inverted, what was called the "non-face" condition. Trujillo et al. (94) confirmed these observations, showing that larger gamma spectral power and greater phase synchrony occurs when upright faces are presented compared to the "non-face" condition, but noted that in all conditions studied—presentation of upright faces, inverted faces, or scrambled faces—widespread gamma synchrony was observed in all perceptual conditions but at different gamma frequencies, roughly within the range of 38 to 49 Hz.

7.4. Opposite Changes of Gamma and Alpha Oscillations

In a number of studies a remarkable interplay between decreases of alpha and increases of gamma has been put in evidence. Spaak et al. (95) observed what may be called "nested oscillations" in the monkey visual cortex, where there is a layer-specific phase-coupling between the phase of alpha oscillations and gamma power (in two bands, 30–70 and 100–200 Hz), where the phase of alpha oscillation of the deeper cortical layers modulates the amplitude of the gamma oscillation of the superficial layers. These findings support the concept proposed by Jensen et al. (96) that "gamma and alpha oscillations interact in order to temporally organize neuronal coding in the visual system." For a detailed discussion see Jensen et al. (97). Thus we may conclude that neural synchrony revealed by gamma frequency synchronization is associated with the perception of a stimulus, regardless of its precise form, and that this synchrony can be expressed in LFPs, and also at the level of the EEG/MEG, at least in some cases.

7.5. Gamma Oscillations and Attentional Processing

Debener et al. (98) attempted to differentiate bottom-up aspects of attention, which are directly associated with the presentation of a stimulus, and top-down related attentional demands. They noted that gamma band activity, detected using a 40-Hz centered wavelet, was enhanced when auditory targets were presented, but not by novel stimuli, which they interpreted as indicating that the gamma response cannot be accounted for simply by arousal associated with stimulus presentation. They concluded that the enhancement of gamma oscillations accompanies top-down attentional processing.

7.6. Gamma Oscillations and Memory Processes

It is important to consider how gamma oscillations, often jointly with oscillations in other frequency bands, are associated with object representation in short- and long-term memory. Sederberg et al. (99), using intracranial EEG recordings, found that gamma oscillations (44–64 Hz) in the hippocampus and the left temporal and frontal (left inferior prefrontal cortex) cortices predicted successful encoding of new verbal memories for nouns. These were the same brain structures that were activated during similar investigations using fMRI. These authors made a very detailed analysis of the time course of the different EEG changes and noted that the increase in gamma activity in the left inferior prefrontal cortex began at stimulus onset and lasted throughout the encoding interval, which may signal a state of increased attention, while the increases in gamma in the hippocampus, which differentiated successful from unsuccessful encoding, began 500 msec following stimulus onset, and may be interpreted as being more directly related to episodic memory encoding. This task involves semantic processing, which is reflected in an increase in hippocampal gamma oscillations 1500 msec after the word presentation. This second process is probably related to associative encoding, which occurs after the initial processing of a verbal item.

Also using EEG recordings obtained using implanted electrodes in epileptic patients, Fell et al. (100) found that successful memory formation for words is accompanied within 1 sec by a transient enhancement and later by a decrease of phase synchronization in the gamma range (32–48 Hz) between rhinal cortex and hippocampus, as well as enhanced coupling in the sub-gamma range. This effect, however, depended on the task, namely on whether the words presented were common or uncommon words.

In another experimental setting Tallon-Baudry et al. (101) investigated subjects during a delayed-matching-to-sample task, using visual stimuli, while recording the EEG. During the delay period when the subjects had to keep the information in short-time memory for further action, the gamma band (24–60 Hz) was conspicuous, but this was not the case when no memorization was required. These enhanced gamma-band activities were localized at both occipito-temporal and frontal sites. This topographic distribution suggest that during the period of holding the visual information in short-term memory there is an enhancement of synchronized gamma activity that may mediate the establishment of a distributed brain workspace that includes the ventral visual areas and the frontal cortex.

These effects have been demonstrated not only for visual information but also for other kinds of sensory information. Kaiser et al. (102) investigated an auditory spatial delayed-matching-to-sample short-term memory task in normal subjects. Subjects received an auditory stimulus, consisting of a burst of 200-msec noise at a given lateralization angle, and were required, after a 800-msec delay period, to compare this stimulus to test stimuli, which could be presented at the same or at a more medial or lateral angle. They found enhanced gamma oscillations (55–70 Hz, but also 75–100 Hz in another set of experiments) peaking during the middle 200 to 500 msec of the delay phase, over parieto-occipital cortex contralateral to the side of stimulation. These findings suggest that the observed gamma oscillations may reflect the engagement of neuronal networks, tuned to spatial sound features, while keeping the information relevant to the task in short-term memory.

Further, gamma oscillations have been shown to be associated with retrieval from memory. Gruber et al. (103) investigated this issue using EEG recordings and found induced gamma oscillations (spectral peak ≈ 54 Hz) occurring during encoding for items that were afterwards recognized in contrast to forgotten items. They also found that retrieval of items that were recognized was associated with higher gamma oscillations than new items. Thus gamma oscillations may be associated not only with memory encoding but also with retrieval. These results suggest that gamma-induced oscillations may represent cortical mechanisms involved in episodic memory encoding.

Findings along the same line were reported by Osipova et al. (104), who approached this issue in a wider way, looking also to other frequency bands besides gamma (Fig. 48.4). They used pictorial stimuli to investigate declarative memory processing while recording the MEG of normal subjects. They found that oscillatory activity in two frequency bands, gamma (60–90 Hz) and theta (4.5–8.5 Hz), was much stronger for the later-remembered compared with the later-forgotten items. Further, during retrieval, theta and gamma oscillations were stronger for recognized items compared with correctly rejected new items. The gamma activity was also stronger for recognized compared with forgotten old items. The effects in the theta band were observed over right parieto-temporal areas, whereas the sources of the effects in the gamma band were attributed to Brodmann's area 18/19.

These data corroborate the conclusion that theta oscillations are directly engaged in mnemonic operations, as presented above in the section on theta rhythms. With respect to gamma oscillations it appears that the increase of gamma oscillations over the occipital areas with respect to a task involving pictorial items to be memorized indicates that these oscillations may facilitate both memory encoding and

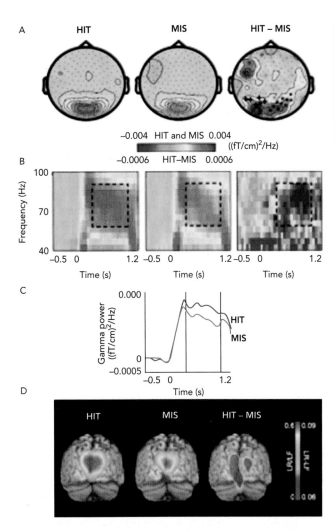

A HIT MIS HIT − MIS

−0.004 HIT and MIS 0.004
((fT/cm)²/Hz)
−0.0006 HIT−MIS 0.0006

B

Frequency (Hz)

100

70

40

−0.5 0 1.2 −0.5 0 1.2 −0.5 0 1.2
Time (s) Time (s) Time (s)

C

Gamma power ((fT/cm)²/Hz)

0.000

0

−0.0005

HIT

MIS

−0.5 0 1.2
Time (s)

D HIT MIS HIT − MIS

Figure 48.4. MEG recorded gamma activity associated with a memory task showing the results of the recognition effect. A: The grand average of the topography of gamma power for hits (HIT) and missed (MIS) items and their difference (HIT-MIS). Two adjacent clusters of occipital sensors showed significant increase in gamma power (*p < .01; p < .05). B: Grand-averaged time–frequency representations of power from one significant sensor associated with hits versus missed items and the subtraction of two conditions. C: Grand-averaged gamma power averaged between 60 and 90 Hz for both conditions for the same sensor as in B. D: Source reconstruction of gamma activity, averaged over subjects and overlaid on the Montreal Neurological Institute standard brain. The sources for HIT and MIS conditions were located bilaterally in Brodmann's area 18/19. The difference in power (HIT-MIS) revealed sources in Brodmann's area 18/19 as well. The power of the source representations was thresholded at half-maximum. Adapted with permission from Osipova et al., 2006 (104).

retrieval. These findings are in line with the hypothesis that representations of objects (in whatever modality or combination of modalities) are mediated by the synchronization in distributed neural assemblies, which is reflected, at least partially, in gamma oscillations at the level of LFPs, and also at the scalp level of EEG/MEG signals.

7.7. Neural Mechanisms Underlying Gamma Oscillations

The basic physiology of gamma oscillations is discussed in detail in Chapters 2 and 3.

8. EEG NEUROCOGNITIVE CORRELATES BEYOND CLASSIC FREQUENCY BANDS: AMPLITUDE AND PHASE MODULATION AND NESTED FREQUENCY OSCILLATIONS

At several points in this chapter we noted that different neuronal oscillations may be phase-coupled, as for example the sensorimotor mu rhythm in the alpha frequency range (~10 Hz) and the beta rhythm (~20 Hz) in the same region. There exist, however, other forms by which neuronal oscillations at different frequencies may be coupled. This is the case of the modulation of gamma rhythms by the "up-state" of the slow oscillation that we discussed in the section on slow rhythms. Similarly, many other cases occur where oscillations at different frequencies are apparently amplitude-modulated by other frequency components, such as theta and gamma rhythms in the hippocampus (105). In the auditory neocortex Lakatos et al. (106) showed an interesting interaction of different EEG frequency components where delta (1–4 Hz) phase modulates theta (4–10 Hz) amplitude and theta phase modulates gamma (30–50 Hz) amplitude. These authors proposed that this hierarchy of frequency components would operate to enable the auditory cortex to optimize the processing of rhythmic inputs. They found that for each frequency, there are both ideal and less optimal phases during which stimulus responsiveness is respectively enhanced or suppressed.

Another case where cross-frequency coupling occurs is in the study of memory tasks based on EEG recordings made in epileptic patients with implanted electrodes in the hippocampus. Axmacher et al. (107) found that maintenance of an increasing number of items in working memory is associated with modulation of beta/gamma (modulated frequency at 14–50 Hz) amplitude by theta/alpha band (modulating frequency at 6–10 Hz) oscillation. It appears that cross-frequency phase-coupling can predict individual working memory performance. In this context it is important to refer to the findings of Canolty et al. (108), who investigated ECoGs obtained using subdural electrodes and reported that the phase of the low-frequency theta (4–8 Hz) rhythm can modulate the power of the high gamma (80–150 Hz) EEG band and different patterns of theta/high gamma coupling occur depending on behavioral state. The interaction between neuronal oscillations at different frequencies emerges also from the work of Doesburg et al. (109), who studied perceptual switching during binocular rivalry. In their task subjects viewed rivaling visual images and pressed buttons to indicate which stimulus was being perceived at that moment. These authors found increases of gamma-band activity (38–42 Hz) that recurred at a theta (5.7–7.3 Hz) rate, time-locked to the moment of button press indicating the emergence of a new percept. The main sources of the burst of gamma activity were estimated, using beamformer analysis, to be located preferentially in prefrontal and parietal cortical areas. The authors computed phase-locking values to assess interregional relationships and reported gamma phase synchronization among several cortical areas. The results are suggestive but need further critical validation not only due to the complexity of this kind of EEG scalp data, but also due to the risk of mixing real EEG and artifactual signals. These are very interesting results but they pose some complex challenges, for example:

How are cross-frequency relationships established?

What regulates the phase relations between gamma and theta oscillations within and between areas?

Where are the theta oscillations generated?

What are the phase and time relations between gamma oscillations at the different cortical areas?

9. CAVEATS AND PITFALLS CONCERNING SCALP EEG RECORDINGS OF BETA, GAMMA, AND HIGHER FREQUENCIES

To end this section, it is appropriate, in general terms, to add the caveat that EEG activities in the high frequency bands (i.e., beta, gamma, and higher frequencies) at the level of the human scalp are liable to suffer contamination by several kinds of artifacts, not only EMG, especially in cases where subjects are required to make movements in the context of a behavioral task, but also strongly filtered (as in the study referred to above between 38 and 42 Hz) physiological transients. In particular, those caused by spike potentials associated with eye microsaccades have been shown to contribute to the power within the gamma (30–100 Hz) frequency band by Yuval-Greenberg et al. (110). This may result in what appears to be an intrinsic oscillation but is just the ringing of the filter used. Therefore it is important to control for these artifacts, particularly in awake subjects performing visual tasks; complementary eye-tracking recordings may be considered in specific cases using an infrared camera. Recordings of beta, gamma, and higher frequency phenomena in MEG are less prone to these kinds of pitfalls (see also Chapter 32).

10. EVENT-RELATED POTENTIALS

10.1. Components: Ambiguous but Powerful

Averaged ERP and ERFs have been recorded for several decades across a wide variety of time-locked cognitive tasks. Regular constellations of latency, topography, and response to task manipulations have been reified as named "components" (for reviews see 111–115). No single characteristic is absolutely defining, so there is always some degree of circularity in ERP/ERF studies. Ultimately, we would like a component to be linked to a particular brain process, but noninvasive EEG and MEG are inadequate for this task. Here we describe the most commonly studied cognitive ERP/ERF components and consider what they may represent within the brain.

10.2. Orienting, Predicting, and Correcting

We minimally process most sensory input so that we can concentrate on that which may be important. We cannot know if input is important until we evaluate it. Sometimes a cursory evaluation is adequate but sometimes it needs to be more in depth, so this evaluation and the ERPs that embody it unfold in time, with later components reflecting progressively more complex evaluations. Stimuli are selected for evaluation because they are not predicted or expected. One assumption guiding expectations is that repeating stimuli will continue to repeat. Indeed, many ERPs decrease when a stimulus is repeated (termed "stimulus specific adaptation" or "habituation") and then recover when the stimulus changes ("dishabituation") (116). However, tone sequences may be complex and still generate an expectation, and a corresponding reaction when that expectation is violated, leading to the inference that there is a "sensory memory" that is continuously compared to incoming stimuli. In one view, this comparison could be implemented as dishabituation, but of neurons that respond to correspondingly complex patterns. In another view, expectation is an active process termed "predictive coding." This mechanism is needed to explain the typical mismatch ERPs evoked by the omission of a stimulus from a regular stream (117). In short, violation of expectation evokes further activity that may reflect processing, dishabituation, prediction, and/or consequent processing, including orienting and memory updating.

Variations in the auditory environment evoke a characteristic set of ERPs at the scalp. Small deviations from a constant stream of tones evoke pre-attentively a "mismatch negativity" (MMN) (118). When the stimulus change is sufficient to demand attention, then additional processes embodied in the ERP component termed "P3a" are invoked (119), as a larval form of the orienting response (120). When the auditory stream is explicitly attended and a behavioral target is identified, the supramodal "N2b-P3b" is emitted (112), which will be discussed in the next section. Figure 48.5 and Table 48.1 summarize the distinctions between P3a and P3b.

A variety of methods have been used to identify the neural substrates of these ERP components. Imaging of hemodynamic increases with positron emission tomography (PET) or fMRI has identified a circuit that is involved in auditory pattern processing; it is centered in the posterior superior temporal plane (pSTP) but interacts with prefrontal cortex for ongoing context (121). Hemodynamic studies also suggest that an extended cortical network is activated by deviant auditory stimuli (122). However, the sequence of involvement of these structures, and their relation to different scalp ERP components (e.g., MMN vs. P3a vs. P3b), cannot be determined with hemodynamic measures because of their lack of temporal resolution, and because hemodynamic activation reflects a different neural substrate than ERPs (Fig. 48.6). Cognitive processes necessarily involve a network of structures, not all of which evoke electromagnetic fields that can be measured outside the skull (i.e., "propagating generators") (Fig. 48.7).

10.3. Mismatch Negativity

The field patterns of the MMN and its MEG counterpart, the MMF, correspond well to that expected for a generator in the pSTP (116,123). However, the same scalp topography can result from different intracranial generators. Unambiguous

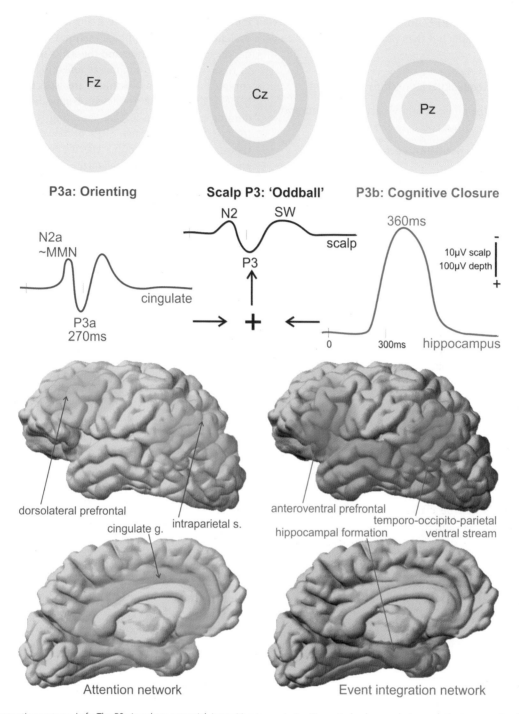

Figure 48.5. *P3 generating systems. Left: The P3a is a sharp potential, insensitive to overt attention or task relevance but responsive to unusual and unexpected events that involuntarily grab attention. Diffusely generated, it is largest and most reliable in supramarginal gyrus and area 46, as well as the limbic lobe, including cingulate, subgenual, retrosplenial, and parahippocampal regions. Right: In contrast to the P3a, the P3b is broad, late, and large, and requires overt attention. Diffusely generated, it is largest in the hippocampus proper, but also prominent in other convergence zones in the anterior parietal and ventrolateral prefrontal regions. Top middle: The scalp P3 usually reflects both systems, but when isolated, the scalp P3a is earlier and more frontal, whereas the scalp P3b is later and more parietal, relative to the composite potential.*

evidence for local generation of the MMN in the pSTP has been provided by intracranial recordings in humans (124–126), monkeys (127), and cats (128). Unit responses to deviant auditory stimuli are found from brainstem to cortex (129).

In addition to the classical MMN reflecting the local shift from the immediately preceding tone, a "deviance related negativity" can be evoked by shifts in the global pattern of the prior several tones. This negativity has been interpreted as a

MMN, based on its scalp topography and its latency of 125 to 210 msec (130). Although this pattern-shift MMN and MMF occurs even when the tone sequence is ignored, it is strongly modulated by attention. MMN-like potentials have previously been recorded from medioventral and polar temporal cortices, but not until about 200 msec after stimulus onset (131, 132). Furthermore, hippocampal lesions do not affect the MMN (133), but they do influence the related P3a to novel

TABLE 48.1. P3 Components Identified in Depth Recordings

TYPE OF P3	COGNITIVE CORRELATE	REQUIRES ATTENTION?	MODALITY SELECTIVITY	LATENCY RELATIVE TO SCALP P3	DURATION	ASSOCIATED WAVES	ANTECEDENT GENERATOR	OCCULT GENERATOR	PROPAGATING GENERATOR
P3a	Orienting response	No	Auditory>visual	~50 msec earlier	~60 msec	Middle of triphasic complex	Prefrontal, para-hippocampal?	Nucleus reticularis thalami?	Anterior/posterior cingulate, dorsolateral prefrontal, intraparietal sulcus, parahippocampal gyrus
P3b	Cognitive closure	Yes	Auditory=visual	~50 msec later	~400 msec	Usually monophasic	Parietal, hippocampus, prefrontal in different tasks	Hippocampus	Ventrolateral prefrontal, anteroventral temporal, parietal

stimuli (134). Also, the hippocampal formation receives direct input from auditory association cortex, and human hippocampal units may show strongly habituating responses to simple auditory stimuli with a latency of ~100 msec (135). Thus, it is possible that the anteroventromedial temporal region works with the superior temporal cortex in detecting mismatches. Predictive coding models suggest that a memory trace of the repeated regularity is stored in superficial layers, which is compared against the incoming evidence in layer 4 (136).

10.4. P3a: Orienting

The classical MMN can be evoked by stimuli that are neither attended, task-relevant, nor noticed. Infrequent stimulus changes that *are* noticed (regardless of task relevance) evoke a P3a, maximal at Fz (137). The P3a overlaps with the P3b, which peaks later at Pz, as discussed below. In intracranial recordings, such stimuli evoke a triphasic waveform with sharp negative, positive, and negative peaks at ~215, 270 and 390 msec, respectively (124,138,139). The largest amplitudes were near the inferior frontal sulcus and supramarginal gyrus, with clear polarity inversions in the anterior cingulate and subgenual cortices (139,140). Depth-P3a's have also been recorded in the posterior cingulate (124) and its continuation in retrosplenial and parahippocampal cortices (131,141). In lateral-to-medial penetrations by depth electrodes with multiple recording points, N2a/P3a/SWa amplitudes often change only slowly with distance, suggesting additional diffuse cortical generation. The dorsolateral prefrontal, inferior parietal, and cingulate cortices are highly interconnected anatomically, and lesions in these sites are associated with neglect and other attentional deficits. Novel stimuli may evoke BOLD activation in similar areas (122).

Among these areas, the prefrontal cortex may perform an essential antecedent role (in the terminology of Fig. 48.7), inasmuch as the scalp P3a can be eliminated by prefrontal lesions

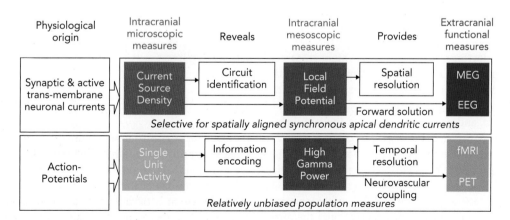

Figure 48.6. Measurements used to localize and understand ERPs and ERFs. Upper row: EEG and MEG are generated by synaptic and active transmembrane currents, but because of summation and cancellation at multiple scales, they are highly selective for spatially and temporally aligned currents in apical dendrites. CSD can measure these net transmembrane currents intracortically, which are reflected in the LFP (measured with stereoencephalography or ECoG) and ultimately MEG and EEG. Lower row: Hemodynamic activation measured with fMRI or PET is well correlated with overall neuronal firing, without cancellation between neuron and sensor. Firing can be measured intracranially with different levels of spatial precision with unit recordings and high gamma (HG), both of which provide temporal resolution lacking in fMRI and PET. Due to cancellation and to their origin in different aspects of neuronal activity, MEG/EEG and fMRI/PET often provide different localization in the same task contrasts.

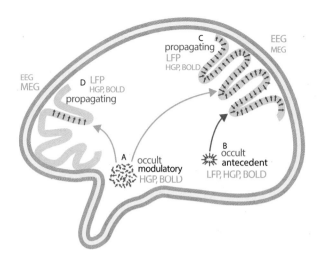

Figure 48.7. Visible and invisible neural systems underlying ERPs and ERFs. Cognitive ERPs/ERFs are often very widespread and may reflect currents evoked by modulatory structures (A) such as the locus coeruleus. Because of their lack of lamination and distance from the scalp, such structures are unlikely to contribute directly to the EEG or MEG (i.e., they are occult generators), but they may show HG activation in stereoencephalography (SEEG) and hemodynamic activation in fMRI or PET. Other occult generators may perform essential antecedent calculations necessary for a particular ERP component but not generate activity that propagates to the scalp, for example because of mesoscopic cancellation such as sometimes occurs in the hippocampus (B). Such structures would generate LFP and HG in SEEG recordings, and possibly BOLD responses. Lesions of these areas may abolish the component in all locations even though it is generated mainly, or entirely, elsewhere. Finally, propagating generators (C, D) contain the equivalent current dipoles (ECDs) that are recorded by EEG and MEG sensors. Note that highly distributed generators would tend to produce relatively large EEG signals (C) due to ECDs with consistent orientations close to the scalp in the gyral crowns, whereas much smaller generators in a single bank of a sulcus would tend to produce relatively large MEG signals (D), which would cancel mesoscopically in the more distributed case. Both propagating generators would necessarily have to produce LFP signals, and thus could be localized with SEEG, but they may or may not produce HG or BOLD signals.

(142,143). The earliest locally generated P3a peaks occur in prefrontal cortex (139), and this decrease is correlated across patients with apathy and lack of interest in novel stimuli (144). Apparently the P3a antecedent system also includes some part of the medial temporal lobe, as lesions in that location also produce a general decrease in the P3a (134). Knight (134) suggests that the hippocampus maintains a continuous store of the recent past, and that when a current event does not match that template, a novelty signal is emitted. Locally, this encourages memory formation, and globally, it results in the P3a. While the broad outlines of this hypothesis may be correct, intracranial recordings suggest that the parahippocampal rather than the hippocampal portion of the medial temporal lobe may play the critical role. The hippocampus itself does not generate P3a activity (131,141). Further, the onset of differential hippocampal activity to novel tones is ~200 msec (141), and the onset of differential activity to novel words or faces is ~270 to 300 msec (145). These latencies are considerably longer than the ~140-msec onset latency of the N2a/P3a/SWa complex (139), so it is unlikely that the hippocampus is making the antecedent calculations necessary for their appearance. However, as noted above, the immediately adjacent parahippocampal region

anchors one end of the limbic lobe, including also the retrosplenial, cingulate, and subgenual regions. All parts of this limbic lobe generate P3a's, and it could link the essential medial temporal and prefrontal contributions to its occurrence. Furthermore, unit studies in monkeys as well as humans suggest that detection of novelty relies on parahippocampal areas, whereas the hippocampus itself may be more concerned with recall of complex integrative memories.

The N2a/P3a/SWa thus is evoked by stimuli that demand processing because of their potential biological significance. It prominently engages areas that can localize in space the evoking stimuli, as well as those that can help prepare the organism to make a rapid response. The additional less prominent diffuse activation observed during the N2a/P3a/SWa may represent the widespread polling of cortical areas to arrive at a rapid evaluation of the stimulus. Stimuli that automatically attract attention due to their potential biological importance also evoke the orienting response, typically measured as various autonomic phenomena that prepare the organism to respond (146). The most reliable autonomic index of orienting is the skin conductance response, which has a complicated relationship to different N2 and P3 components (147). However, across individual trials, the skin conductance response and the P3a to rare distracting sounds may be highly correlated (120), supporting interpretation of the P3a as a cortical manifestation of the orienting response (120).

10.5. Error-Related Negativity

In a variety of situations, errors are accompanied by a sharp negativity at fronto-central sites beginning at about the same time as the motor response (148). It also occurs when observing others commit errors (149). The scalp topography of this error-related negativity (ERN) is consistent with generation in the anterior cingulate, where error-related activity can be recorded with intracranial electrodes (150). Recent intracranial recordings indicate that the primary location driving the ERN is the supplementary motor cortex (151). Lesion studies suggest that the medial frontal and lateral frontal areas both participate in its elaboration (148). Scalp recordings are consistent with the ERN reflecting phase-reset of ongoing theta activity (152).

11. PROCESSING AND RESPONDING

In a generic cognitive task, a stimulus is briefly exposed and a rapid response is required. The processing is synchronized across individual trials embodied in a typical sequence of ERPs (after the sensory peaks). Numerous components have been distinguished at ~100 msec, which are generically termed the N1. Lesions suggest generators in the superior-posterior temporal lobe (for reviews see (142,143)), consistent with MEG and human intracranial data, which also suggest prefrontal sources in multiple modalities (153). Superimposed on the N1-P2 are processing negativities (variously termed Nd, NA, N200, and N2pc) that are strongly affected by attention and task demands and that decline rapidly with repetition

(113,115,154–157). Aspects of stimuli that can be rapidly detected (such as location in space) tend to be associated with the shorter latency negativities. The NA is related to perceptual processing of a stimulus regardless of its rarity (115). The N2b is most easily evoked by attended events of any modality that are rare within the context of the task (113,115). The longest latency processing negativity, the N4, will be discussed below. These negativities are usually followed by a positivity associated with cognitive closure, termed the P3, P300, or LPC ("late positive component") (112,113,154,155,158).

11.1. P3b: Cognitive Closure

Cognitive correlates of the P3 (or P300) have been reviewed many times (112,154). The P3 is evoked by simple or complex attended stimuli in the auditory, visual, or somatosensory modalities. If the stimuli are simple and if they are occurring at a rapid rate, then the P3 will occur at the time when a stimulus was expected but did not occur. If the stimuli are complex and well known, or if they are simple but occurring at a slow rate (< .3/sec), then a P3 will occur to every stimulus. However, if the stimuli are simple, are rapidly presented, and belong to two task-relevant categories, then stimuli belonging to the less frequently occurring category (termed "rare") will evoke a much bigger P3 than the stimuli belonging to the other category. Most of this effect is due to sequence: to a first approximation, a rare tone will evoke a large P3 if and only if it is preceded by a series of frequent tones. Although the P3 is evoked in a large variety of tasks, the "auditory oddball" task has become a de facto standard because its simplicity and reliability make it useful for clinical and developmental studies as well as for psychological analysis. The relation of the P3 to rarity within context, in the auditory oddball and related tasks, has led to hypothesized correlations of the P3 with "context-updating" (112) and "context-closure" (159).

In the context-updating hypothesis, the P3 represents the updating of internal models of the external environment (112). This hypothesis has been extended in the "trace-formation hypothesis," which posits that the amplitude of the P3 evoked by a stimulus reflects the strength of the memory trace formed at that time. Indeed, words that are subsequently recalled (160) or recognized (161) may evoke a larger-amplitude P3 on their initial input presentation than do words that are not subsequently remembered. This effect during memory input complements the finding that at memory output, the P3b is associated with successful conscious retrieval, but only if the left anterior temporal lobe is intact (162).

The largest potentials evoked by rare target events are found in the human hippocampus. These responses, up to ~300 μV, have been reported by at least eight independent laboratories (131,141,163–168). This potential occurs to auditory, visual, and somatosensory rare stimuli (141, 166), and it is eliminated if the subject is instructed to ignore the tones (131,141). It is evoked not only by oddball target tones but also by the absence of expected tones and by non-target distractors (131). The latency of this response is ~380 msec, between the scalp P3 and scalp slow wave. However, the hippocampus (HC) potential behaves more like the scalp P3 to the omissions of tones from a rapidly repeated constant stream, or to a series of identical tones at long irregular intervals (141), so it is referred to here as the HC-P3b. The P3b in simple oddball tasks has similar but not identical generators to the LPC occurring at ~620 msec in more complex tasks involving, for example, semantic processing of words (145,169,170).

The HC-P3b can be accompanied by changes in unit activity. Since unit activity must be local, there must be local synaptic activity, and this makes accompanying field potentials more likely (163). Another important piece of evidence for local generation is that the HC-P3b is large within the hippocampus and declines dramatically on all sides, lateral, medial, above, below, in front, and behind (131,165). Further evidence that the HC-P3b is locally generated is that its amplitude is decreased in the presence of ipsilateral hippocampal sclerosis (164,167).

Despite the proven local hippocampal generation of the P3b, no significant effect on the scalp P3b is found after unilateral anterior temporal lobectomy removing the hippocampus unilaterally (171,172) or after bilateral hippocampal lesions in amnesia (173,174). In contrast, left anterior temporal lobectomy (162) or bilateral hippocampal lesions (175,176) do abolish the P3b to repeated words, even when they are recognized as repeated. Thus, the hippocampus functions as an *occult* rather than *propagating* generator of the P3b; it is also a necessary *antecedent* structure for the P3b in declarative memory (see Fig. 48.7 and Table 48.1).

With rare exceptions (177), BOLD recordings fail to detect the HC-P3b (178). MEG may be more successful, with medial temporal P3b sources estimated to auditory (123,179,180) and visual stimuli (181,182). Confirmation of local generation was obtained when the hippocampal source was lost ipsilaterally after unilateral anterior temporal lobectomy (183). However, it is also possible that the MEG signal is actually arising in medioventral temporal structures outside the hippocampus (131,141,163).

Some previous MEG studies have estimated P3b generators to the thalamus rather than the medial temporal lobe (184,185). A similar localization was reported for the P3b-like activity identified using independent component analysis applied to high-density EEG (186). These studies failed to identify the parietal, temporal, and prefrontal generators demonstrated with intracranial recordings. Intracranial studies have also found potentials with the latency and task correlates of the P3 in the thalamus (187–192) and putamen (193). In published examples, these potentials are typically small and do not exhibit steep complex gradients or inversions. Such potentials may reflect passive volume conduction from the cortex rather than local generation; if locally generated, their size and distance from the scalp make it unlikely that they are the source of the scalp P3.

In addition to the hippocampus, the depth P3b can be recorded in several neocortical structures with evidence for local generation, including large amplitude, steep voltage gradients, and frequent polarity inversions. These areas include a limited region of the superior temporal sulcus, the ventrolateral prefrontal cortex, and the intraparietal sulcus (124,131,139,163). Although the P3b can be commonly recorded in the amygdala, it is presumed to be volume conducted from the underlying anteroventral temporal cortex (141). These regions roughly correspond to those most commonly activated by rare target events in BOLD recordings (for review see (122)).

Neocortical P3b sources modeled in MEG studies include the inferior parietal lobule (180), superior temporal plane (179,180), superior temporal sulcus (123,182), left superior parietal lobule, and posteromedial frontal cortex (194). Interestingly, the large ventral temporal and ventral prefrontal generators demonstrated with intracranial recordings were detected in only one study (123). Overall, noninvasive electric, magnetic, and hemodynamic measures have provided poor localization of the P3b (compared to gold-standard intracranial recordings).

A complex but reliable pattern of effects on the scalp P3 is also seen after cortical lesions (for reviews see (142,143)). Temporo-parietal lesions attenuate the P3a and P3b to auditory (142,143) and visual (195) attended target oddball stimuli, as recorded on the posterior scalp. A P3 decrement also is observed in the somatosensory modality where the P3 to contralateral stimulation is entirely abolished (suggesting that this location provides an essential antecedent calculation), whereas the decrement to ipsilateral stimulation is only over the lesion (142,143), suggesting that this cortex is now functioning as a propagating generator (196). Thus, temporo-parietal, prefrontal, and hippocampal areas all function as an essential antecedent structure in different tasks, as well as occult or propagating generators across tasks (see Fig. 48.7). Although lesion-induced ERP decrements are often interpreted as removing generators, often they act on prior processing pathways.

The widespread prefrontal, parieto-temporal, and limbic system underlying the P3b corresponds to the supramodal event integration network encoding stimuli within the current cognitive context and associations derived from declarative, semantic, and primary memories (197). As noted above, the cognitive correlates of the scalp P3b indicate that it reflects the closure of the controlled processing of an event (112). For example, the P3b is present if, and only if, independent behavioral data show that the stimulus has reached awareness and been subjected to controlled processing. P3b onset occurs at about the same latency as the specification of the subject's response, suggesting that the P3b begins when event-encoding activities are substantially complete and the brain is ready to move on to its next task (158,198,199). Presumably, this entails updating the contents and instructions in the mental workspace, as well as entering the conclusions of the event-encoding process into working and declarative memories (159). In summary, the task correlates, latency, topography, and generators of the depth P3b suggest that it embodies updating of working memory and the closure of the cognitive event-encoding cycle (see Fig. 48.5).

Because the P3a and P3b have distinctive waveforms and generating structures, intracranial recordings can clarify the relationship of the P3a and P3b in a manner that is not possible at the scalp, where they strongly overlap (see Fig. 48.5 and Table 48.1). Intracranial recordings show that the P3a and P3b systems are often evoked by the same task stimuli, especially auditory stimuli that are sufficiently salient. Compared to what

would have been recorded at the scalp during the P3 if only the P3b were active, the superposition of the P3a causes the scalp P3 to be earlier, with a latency between the P3a (~265 msec) and P3b (~360 msec). In addition, the SWa following the P3a may superimpose on the P3b to bring the scalp P3 waveform back to baseline, prior to the termination of the depth P3b.

The co-occurrence of P3a and P3b may occur to either targets or distractors, with the relative contributions of the P3a or P3b to the scalp P3 varying between these conditions as expected. Conversely, if a target stimulus is not intrinsically salient (as is often the case with complex visual targets), then only the P3b may be evoked, or if the stimulus is salient but unattended, then only the P3a may be evoked (as is often the case for auditory stimuli). Thus, the P3a and P3b are neither mutually exclusive (as they often occur on the same trials) nor necessarily sequential (as the P3b can occur without a preceding P3a).

Some theories emphasize a sequential linkage from P3a to P3b reflecting a passage from novelty to memory formation (119). However, the P3a and P3b have distinct generators, waveforms, and behavioral correlates. The P3a can be abolished by lesions without affecting the P3b. Although they can be evoked together by rare attended target stimuli, they can also be evoked independently. Indeed, their temporal overlap when they are evoked together is actually more consistent with them representing separate and independent processes. Obviously, the involuntary orientation of attention can interact with the intentional encoding and retrieval of memory, but perhaps they are best viewed as good examples of independent systems rather than a single integrated sequential system.

In summary, the scalp P3 to attended rare auditory stimuli reflects contributions from three separate generating systems. Two of these systems, P3a and P3b, simultaneously engage multiple structures in frontal, parietal, and temporal lobes, one concerned with orienting attention toward a possibly significant stimulus and the other for the transition between mental events, including possibly cognitive closure and memory updating.

11.2. Readiness Potential

As might be expected, the movement potentials begin diffuse and related to psychological variables (i.e., cognitive), become progressively more focal and specific as the movement approaches, and then become more diffuse and more associated with cognitive processes with increasing time after the movement (200,201). The readiness potential (RP = "Bereitschaftspotential") is a widespread negativity beginning about 1 sec before the movement (202,203). The later RP is larger over the hemisphere contralateral to the pressing hand, and in central recording sites. This has led to the subdivision of the RP into two components:

An RP proper beginning 1 to 3 sec prior to the movement

A negative slope (NS) superimposed on the RP and signaled by an inflection in the RP slope occurring ~500 to 700 msec prior to movement (200, 204).

This asymmetry can be leveraged to focus analysis on the contralateral-minus-ipsilateral difference wave, termed the "lateralized readiness potential" (205).

Intracranial recordings in monkeys (206) and humans (207) indicate that most of the peri-movement potentials arise in rolandic cortex, with earlier activity generated more broadly in contralateral parietal postcentral, precentral, and frontal cortex (208). Primate studies indicate that in simple tasks the main generator of the RP may be deep pyramids in contralateral precentral cortex (206). Especially in more complex tasks, widespread areas are also engaged, including subcortical (thalamus, basal ganglia, and hippocampus), premotor, supplementary motor, prefrontal, and parietal cortices (208–210). In humans, lesions often greatly reduce the RP without producing the pyramidal signs that would be expected were the precentral cortex involved (211).

Even with simple movements, it has been found that the RP varies substantially with cognitive factors. For example, the amplitude of the NS (like subsequent components) increases with increased force of contractions, whereas an RP of maximum amplitude can be observed to the voluntary contraction of a single motor unit. Similarly, the RP is much larger prior to movements that are self-initiated than to those that are triggered by a sensory stimulus. RPs to self-initiated movements are larger if instructions emphasize spontaneity over planning. When the subject expects the consequence of his or her movement to be more rewarding, or risky, or interesting, a larger RP may be seen. Sustained RPs with distinct topographies have been reported during writing as compared to visual tracking. The temporal relationship of RP to volition is controversial (212).

11.3. Contingent Negative Variation

The continent negative variation (CNV) is a large scalp negativity during the interval between two stimuli, when the first stimulus (S1) conditions the reaction to the second (S2) (202). The early CNV resembles the slow wave that can also be observed following isolated significant stimuli, and the late CNV resembles the RP seen before isolated movements—thus, the CNV may be largely noncontingent (213). When the S1–S2 interval exceeds 4 sec, the early CNV has a modality-specific distribution, being maximal frontocentrally to auditory, and centro-parieto-occipital to visual stimuli, and corresponds to what is termed "SW," "SNW1," or "O wave" in other contexts, peaking ~400 to 800 msec after S1 (115). CNVs are evoked in paradigms that evoke quite varied behavioral activity required during the S1–S2 interval, including (i) holding a motor response in readiness; (ii) preparing for a perceptual judgment; (iii) anticipating a positive or negative reinforcer; (iv) preparing to make a cognitive decision regarding S2, taking into account S1; or (v) waiting to receive feedback (202,204). CNV amplitude and topography are quite consistent for a given subject, task, and conditions but are highly variable across many task and individual factors. For example, the CNV has been reported to be larger when S2 is noxious, is near threshold, or requires a larger muscular response, if the occurrence of S2 is uncertain, or if the subject is moderately aroused. The CNV may have some relationship to the "infraslow potentials" (see also Chapter 32) and may be difficult to differentiate from electrodermal changes or sustained eye movements (204).

Widespread field potentials are observed inside the human brain simultaneous with the scalp CNV (214–216). Cortical surface recordings are negative parietally, centrally, and frontally (209,217). These cortical CNVs are similar in distribution to the P3 and RP but not identical. In particular, the CNV is relatively more anterior than the P3 in most tasks. Subcortically, the CNV is positive in gray matter anterior to the thalamus, negative posterior to the thalamus, and small in the white matter. Within the thalamus itself, negative CNVs are recorded in the midline nuclei, whereas only transient potentials are present in motor nuclei.

In monkeys, cortical CNVs are found frontally, occipitally, and centrally. Subcortically, many structures anterior to the thalamus (e.g., caudate, preoptic, amygdala) are positive, whereas many posterior (e.g., posterior hypothalamus, mesencephalic reticular formation) are negative (218). Within the monkey thalamus, midline nuclei are negative, whereas other nuclei (e.g., the pulvinar) show little response.

In general, negative slow potentials are accompanied by increases in local unit firing rates (219). The behavioral correlates of prefrontal unit firing have been studied during the CNV in S1-S2-R paradigms when the task is to compare S1 and S2 (delayed-match-to-sample) or to delay the response to S1 until S2 appears (delayed response) (220). In a given area, different cells will fire during the original (cue) stimulus, the delay, the second (imperative) stimulus, and the post-response reinforcement. During the delay, some cells will fire differentially according to different aspects of the cue and others according to different aspects of the intended response (220). Similar firing patterns are seen in widespread frontal, temporal, parietal, and hippocampal regions, suggesting a coherent network maintained by recurrent excitation (216).

Widespread neural generation of the CNV is further supported by the effects of lesions. Localized or even widespread cortical lesions in humans usually decrease the CNV recorded at the overlying scalp but not grossly over normal cortex, although widespread effects on the early CNV (possibly equivalent to the slow wave) have been reported after frontal lesions (221). In contrast, widespread effects on the CNV may occur after small diencephalic lesions (222). Moderate decreases in CNV amplitude are seen after lesions of the centromedian but not the ventralis lateralis nucleus (223). Conversely, the CNV is affected by stimulation of midline, but not motor, thalamic nuclei. Further evidence for a widespread generator activated by a diffuse system originating in the brainstem is the observation of bilateral CNVs after a unilateral warning cue in split-brain patients (224).

Skinner (219) proposed that the CNV is generated in the cortex due to sustained excitatory influences from their specific nuclei (e.g., from dorsalis medialis to the prefrontal cortex). These specific thalamic nuclei are inhibited by nucleus reticularis thalami, which in turn is inhibited (they propose) by the mesencephalic reticular formation (MRF) (see Chapter 2). MRF activation thus leads to cortical CNV by releasing their afferent thalamic nuclei from inhibition by nucleus reticularis thalami. Prefrontal control over the nucleus reticularis is thus hypothesized to direct attention by activating the relevant thalamocortical circuits (as reflected in the CNV and sustained cellular firing) (158,219). They further suggest that the P3 results when this MRF drive is released when cognitive processing on a given topic is completed and the focus of attention is shifted—that is, at the time of cognitive closure. However, situations where P3 occurs without a preceding CNV, and where CNVs occur without a subsequent P3, have been described (225). Alternatively, inferior thalamic lesions may have abolished the CNV by injuring the cholinergic neurons in the nucleus basalis (226). Unilateral lesions of these cells produce a large decrease in the ipsilateral CNV, these cells respond differentially during the CNV, and blockade of their effects at the cortex (with subdural atropine) decreases the ipsilateral CNV. It appears most likely that the CNV reflects a gross summation of neural activation within the neocortex. The timing, task and individual correlates, and apparent frontal location of the CNV have led to it being assigned various roles, including expectancy, motivation, volition, conation, and arousal (202).

12. UNDERSTANDING AND COMMUNICATING

The ERPs evoked by words are found in the context of the responses described in the previous section but have been the subject of vigorous investigation in search of insights into the neural dynamics of language (227). Special responses are found to written word forms (N170), to the meaning of words (N400), and to syntactic integration (P600) (Fig. 44.8). While each of these ERP components show some specificity for language, similar or perhaps even identical components can be evoked by non-linguistic semantic stimuli such as faces and namable objects. What these stimuli have in common is that they each point beyond their surface form to many layers and dimensions of associated characteristics, categories, and implications.

12.1. N170: Word Encoding

Neuroimaging studies have identified a "visual word-form area" (VWFA) showing increased hemodynamic activation to words compared to sensory controls and centered in the left posterior fusiform gyrus (lpFg; for review see (228)). Critically, activation in this area to letter-strings increases with their similarity to actual words, especially in more anterior VWFA, suggesting that it actually comprises a succession of detectors responding to progressively more abstract lexico-semantic aspects of the letter-strings. A word-selective response can also be recorded with EEG, peaking over the left occipital scalp at ~140 to 220 msec. This response has been localized to lpFg with MEG (229,230) and intracranial LFPs (231–233).

The N170 in the VWFA is part of a posterior-to-anterior sweep of activity. Earlier and posterior to the VWFA-N170, converging fMRI, MEG (see also Chapter 35), and intracranial

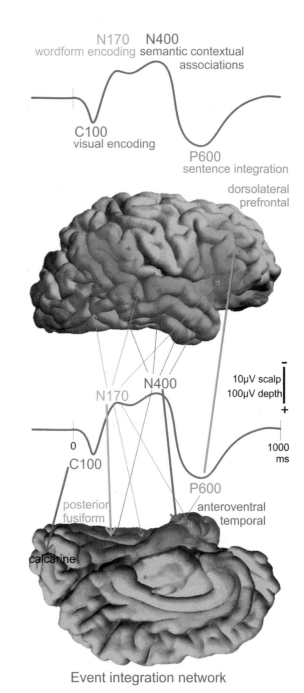

Figure 48.8. ERP components evoked by words. The connection of written words to their meaning within context is tracked by a series of ERP/ERF components. Contextual letter frequency effects may occur shortly after the main early visual component (C100), but the first component dominated by lexical effects peaks at ~170 msec in the visual wordform area in the posterior fusiform gyrus (N170). Feed-forward activation begins earlier and more posteriorly with letterform effects and continues later along the ventral visual processing stream with increasingly semantic correlates, even extending to the ventrolateral prefrontal cortex by ~200 msec, where it feeds into syntactic processing. Pronounceable letter-strings access their meaning within the current cognitive context from ~240 msec, peaking at ~400 msec (N400), in widespread areas, most prominently in anterobasal temporal cortex. Closure of the sentence or other word context results in a P600, especially prominent when initial associative activation is inadequate. Responses are bilateral but larger in the dominant hemisphere. Auditory words evoke a similar N400 but preceded by phoneme encoding peaking at ~100 msec in the posterior superior temporal gyrus. Faces also evoke a similar series of ERP components, peaking at ~170 msec in the fusiform face area, in the posterior fusiform gyrus, mainly nondominant, and again followed by an N400 with similar task correlates.

evidence shows selectivity for letters versus false fonts, but not to words versus consonant-strings typical of VWFA-N170 (234). Increasingly semantic responses are revealed in more anterior locations in humans with MEG (235,236), consistent with the general posterior-to-anterior gradient in the complexity of visual stimulus processing in the ventral stream demonstrated in humans with fMRI, and in monkeys with unit recordings. The N170 eventually arrives in Broca's area, according to MEG (235) and intracranial recordings (170,233,237). In the anteroventral temporal lobe (AVTL), the N170 distinguishes between words referring to animals versus objects (238). N170 amplitude also varies with word frequency, both at the scalp (239) and intracranially (237). Thus, lexical access must begin during the N170 (239), although it is clearly elaborated and integrated with the cognitive context during the N400 (see below).

The synaptic circuitry generating the N170 has been inferred using CSD estimated using "laminar electrodes" in AVTL (240). Laminar electrodes are linear arrays of microelectrodes sampling LFP in different layers of a cortical column. CSD estimates the currents across neuronal membranes, which can be produced by excitatory and inhibitory synaptic activity or voltage-gated channels (see Chapter 2 and Fig 2.3). Laminar recordings show that the N170 is generated by a current sink in layer IV associated with sharply increased firing (240). An initial excitatory layer IV sink is the typical pattern produced by feed-forward input from lower (i.e., more sensory) to higher cortical areas. Thus, the N170 is generated by first-pass bottom-up activation.

In the auditory modality, ERFs are evoked by phonemes as compared to noise-vocoded control sounds, beginning at ~60 msec and peaking at ~100 msec (241). Inverse modeling and correlated LFP and high gamma (HG) localize the generators to the posterior superior temporal gyrus (241), consistent with hemodynamic studies (242).

Faces also selectively generate a scalp ERP with a similar latency (243). Intracranial (169,170,244), fMRI (245), and MEG (246) recordings show that these arise in the right hemisphere area homologous to the VWFA, termed the "fusiform face area" (228), with possible contributions from the nearby "occipital face area" (243).

12.2. N400: Semantic Contextual Associations

In the initial studies, the N400 was observed to the terminal word of sentences, when that word was not expected given the preceding words in the sentence. The N400 was not evoked if the terminal word was syntactically or orthographically incongruent with those preceding it. Conversely, an N400 was evoked by words that formed a meaningful ending, as long as they were unexpected (i.e., in Garden Path Sentences; for reviews see (247,248)). This gave rise to the hypothesis that the N400 is actually evoked by "semantic incongruity," a special case of the hypothesized cognitive correlate of the N2-P3 with incongruity in general (112). However, subsequent studies have found that the N400 is evoked in many situations that do not appear to involve incongruity with the established context. The evoking stimulus can be individually presented

words, printed, spoken, or signed. Effective tasks include reading, recognizing, naming, categorizing, and rhyming. A negativity with the same latency, similar topography, and (when possible to test) identical task correlates is evoked by drawings of meaningful objects and by photographs of faces (249). It is apparently necessary that the stimulus be intrinsically meaningful within a complex associative cognitive system: complex abstract sounds and pictures have not been found to evoke an N400. In some cases, the N400 is not evoked by words if the discrimination required by the task depends solely upon the physical features of the stimulus. Thus, it appears that the N400 is evoked by any stimulus capable of activating a widespread cerebral associative network, within any task that requires or permits such activation (for reviews see (247,248)). Although slight topographical differences exist between the N4s evoked by various stimuli and circumstances, limited intracranial data suggest that their generators are highly overlapping (145).

The N400 is exquisitely sensitive to the ease with which the stimulus is integrated into the current cognitive context. "Ease" is greater if a memory trace (remote, recent, or immediate) for that stimulus-contextual gestalt already exists. It appears that the N400 is emitted after an initial evaluation indicates that the stimulus belongs to a meaningful class (e.g., words, objects, or people), and then it terminates when that stimulus is integrated with the current context, or when the attempt at integration fails. The existence of this pre-N400 screening for potential meaningfulness is suggested both by the N4's latency and by the special circumstances under which an N400 can be evoked by meaningless stimuli (250). Letter-strings that cannot be pronounced evoked no N400, but pronounceable non-word letter-strings do, as do the faces of unknown people. The latency at which words and non-pronounceable letter-strings diverge, ~250 msec, marks the beginning of the N400. Thus, the wordform analysis during the N170 discussed above provides an initial evaluation that the stimulus *may* be meaningful, thus triggering an N400, where the meaning of the word is accessed within the current cognitive context (Fig. 48.9).

Intracranial studies also found that the AVTL N400 and the associated LFP oscillations in the high gamma (HG) frequency band respond differentially to words referring to animals versus objects, with different recording sites showing preferences for one or the other semantic word category (238). Microelectrode recordings found that neurons in the medial temporal lobe may fire to particular words during the N400 (251). Further, both spoken and written words were found to activate the same sites with the same semantic preferences, supporting the proposal that the AVTL comprises a supramodal semantic hub for word understanding (252).

In its purest form, the influence of remote lexical memory is apparent in the smaller N400 evoked by commonly used English words, as compared to uncommon words (250). Remote semantic memory also influences the N400; if the terminal word in a sentence makes that sentence false, then a larger N400 will be evoked than if the sentence were true (253). The N400 to semantically incongruous words at the ends of sentences is another example of this effect. The N400 to a target word is also decreased if it is preceded by words of the same category or by a synonym. These experiments illustrate the

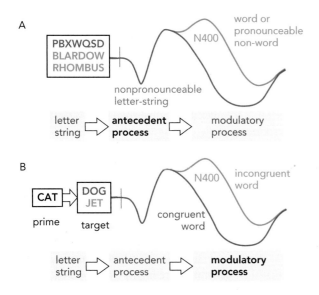

Figure 48.9. N400 task correlates reflect both (**A**) antecedent and (**B**) modulatory processes. **A:** Feed-forward first-pass processing determines if the stimulus fulfills the minimal requirements to be a word. Thus, antecedent processing accepts pronounceable non-words as potential words and an N400 is evoked (green line), whereas antecedent processing rejects non-pronounceable letter-strings as potential words, and no N400 is evoked (purple line). **B:** After the antecedent requirement has been met, continued processing integrates the word's meaning within the current cognitive context. This processing is maximal if the word is presented without context (green line) and is abbreviated if the word has been primed by a word in the same or another modality or language, or by a nonverbal sound or picture (purple line). The prime could be in working, recent episodic, or remote semantic memory; it could consist of a repetition, an association, or a semantic inference. Thus, the N400 is conceived as being evoked by potential words and modulated by ease of integration. N400 would be decreased if (**A**) the stimulus can be rejected in early processing as not word-like or (**B**) integration of the stimulus is facilitated by a congruent cognitive context.

effects of the current context (primary memory). The strongest modulatory effects on the N400 are induced by contextual repetition in recent memory. Repetition of a word or face induces a large decrease of the N400, even if the repetition is not relevant to the task.

N400 context effects have also been observed for nonverbal but meaningful stimuli, albeit with somewhat different scalp distributions than for words. When line drawings are preceded by either printed sentences or other line drawings, the difference between semantically related and unrelated drawings is similar to the linguistic N400 in waveshape and latency, but it is somewhat larger at anterior scalp sites. Interpretable environmental sounds (e.g., glass breaking, horse hooves on pavement) also elicit N400-like potentials that are modulated by semantic context, but the context effect for these nonspeech sounds has a different hemispheric asymmetry than that observed for words (254). In contrast to these results from various sorts of stimuli that convey a meaning (or could possibly convey a meaning, as in the case of pronounceable non-words), stimuli that cannot be mapped onto existing semantic knowledge (e.g., novel geometric shapes, unpronounceable non-words) do not elicit N400s (250, 255). The differing scalp distributions of the family of N400 potentials elicited by words versus nonverbal stimuli suggest the engagement of different

(although likely overlapping) populations of neurons in processing their meanings. Overall, N400-like potentials seem to be triggered by stimuli whose physical forms can be used to access other knowledge about the referent of the stimulus (256) (see Fig. 48.9).

Even for the N400 elicited by words, little progress has been made in inferring the underlying brain generators from the EEG scalp distribution of the component. The word-elicited N400 is largest at midline centro-parietal scalp sites, and larger at lateral sites over the right hemisphere as compared to the left (257). This right-greater-than-left scalp asymmetry is a clear indication of the difficulty of mapping scalp distribution onto cortical regions, as studies of both split-brain patients and patients with unilateral damage have suggested that the N400 context effect is critically dependent on an intact left hemisphere (257–259), as is the N400 repetition effect (162). High-density EEG recordings were unable to identify topographic features of the N400 using Laplacian estimates of radial current density (260). Similarly, minimum-norm and minimum-current distributed solutions constrained to lie on the cortical surface reconstructed from MRI produced no findings that were consistent across individuals (261).

In contrast to the lack of clear localization from scalp EEG, MEG has provided good localization. Initially, an equivalent current dipole for the N400m was localized to the left postero-superior temporal lobe (262,263). A noise-normalized cortically constrained minimum norm solution ("dSPM") suggested additional sources in the anteroventral temporal, orbitofrontal, and posteroventral prefrontal cortices in the left hemisphere, as well as orbitofrontal and (weakly) anterior temporal cortices in the right hemisphere. Similar N400m's have been identified to sentence-terminal incongruous words; to content (vs. function) words, especially if they are early (rather than late) in the sentence (264); and to isolated words or wordstems in a variety of tasks (265,266). As for the N400, the N400m is evoked by words in any modality and by signs (235,267). Remarkably, an N400m with typical localization and latency is evoked by words that do not match a preceding picture in 14-month-old infants, indicating that this lexico-semantic integration mechanism is present during word acquisition (268). However, there appears to be a critical period for N400 acquisition, because it is absent in children who do not learn their first language until adolescence (267).

The distributed locations estimated by MEG to generate the N400 match those that have been demonstrated to generate potentials at this latency in the same or similar paradigms using intracranial recordings. These include comparisons between congruous and incongruous sentence completions (269), related and unrelated word pairs (270), high- and low-frequency words (271), content and function words (270), and repeated versus initial presentations of isolated words (145,169,170,271–275). Many of these studies have converged to suggest an N400 generator in the anterior medial temporal lobe. In addition to the anterior medial temporal lobe, intracranial recordings have demonstrated prominent N400 generators in the posteroventral prefrontal cortex (169,276,277), lateral temporal lobe in the vicinity of the superior temporal sulcus (170,273,278), and posterior parietal sites (170,276).

Intracranially, HG LFP activity above 70 Hz generally increases during the local N400, with similar task correlates, indicating that it reflects neuronal excitation (238,279) and thus should be correlated with increased BOLD response (fMRI) or metabolism (PET). This correlation has indeed been observed in several studies (235,266,279,280), with the proviso that AVTL responses prominent in MEG and intracranial recordings are not always captured with fMRI due to signal loss.

As noted above, the initial response to words in AVTL is a sink in layer IV with increased unit firing associated with the N170 (240). The initial layer IV sink occurs to words occurring for the first time in a task ("new") and to those that have been repeated many times ("old"). However, the layer IV sink to old words quickly returns to baseline while the response to new words continues. The timing and task correlates of this divergence are similar to that of the scalp N400, implying that the N400 is an extended feed-forward sink in layer IV (240).

While the AVTL N400 occasionally polarity-inverts locally within the AVTL, it is largest, most reliable, and invariably negative in locations dorsal to the ventral surface of the anterior temporal lobe (145,169). In contrast, when recorded in a similar task by intracranial subdural strips immediately below this surface, the corresponding potential is positive (269). This mesoscopic surface-positive/depth-negative field distribution inferred from intracranial recordings is consistent with the layer IV sink and layer II/III source in the ventral surface of the temporal lobe, which would produce an equivalent current dipole in the temporal lobe with intracellular positive current flowing toward the neck, as was observed with MEG (264).

12.3. Early Left Anterior Negativity and P600: Syntax

Syntax refers to modifications, selection, or ordering of words to enable them to convey meaning beyond that inherent in their base lexical referent. The early left anterior negativity peaks ~100 to 300 msec after the onset of a grammatically incorrect stimulus such as phrase structure violations (e.g., "the chair was in the painted" rather than "the chair was painted") (281–283). More complex syntactic violations (such as subject–verb violations) evoke a P600 (284), beginning ~500 msec after the word producing the violation begins, and lasting ~300 msec. Commonly, it is assumed that the P600 embodies syntactic revision/reanalysis/repair (285,286). However, others have found that even correct sentences can evoke a P600, provided that they are syntactically (287) or semantically (288) complex, and thus may embody more general construction of sentence representations. Still others, noting that grammatical errors are rare, suggest that the P600 may be a variety of P3b. Little data exist localizing either the early left anterior negativity or P600. Generation of the appropriate morphosyntactic verb or noun forms given a brief sentence context is associated with an intracranially recorded LFP peaking at ~320 msec in Broca's area (237). MEG recordings suggest that the P600 may be generated in either posterior temporal (289) or right prefrontal (290) areas; laminar recordings suggest that the late P3b to words corresponds to the upper-layer sink, which follows the middle-layer sink associated with the N400 (240).

Since associative and feedback connections terminate in superficial layers (291), this implies that the arrival of a word focuses processing in middle layers (N170, N400), which rises to upper layers as processing involves larger cortical domains (P600). This is consistent with studies in macaques, where the latencies and durations of unit responses in ventral visual stream areas imply their sequential then simultaneous activation. This basic pattern of an initial layer IV sink followed by a sink in more superficial cortical layers has been repeatedly observed in response to visual, somatosensory, and auditory input in animals, suggesting engagement of a canonical cortical circuit (292,293). Laminar analysis of single trials shows that the AVTL N400-P600 are actually due to the phase-resetting of an ongoing slow theta oscillation between middle and upper layers. Source estimation of theta recorded with EEG and MEG during working memory and executive control tasks indicate prominent generators in the anterior cingulate and dorsolateral prefrontal cortices (see also the earlier section on the correlates of frontal midline theta and Fig. 48.1).

Theta in the rodent hippocampus is generated by the interplay of active currents, local interneurons, and synchronizing inputs from the medial septum and other structures (see Chapter 2 for details of the basic neurophysiology of theta activity). Neocortical theta generation is less well understood, but it may involve similar mechanisms, with modulation from the basal forebrain. The role of these mechanisms in generating the human slow theta, and by extension the N400/LPC, is unknown. The cellular-synaptic level of analysis is particularly relevant to the late cognitive ERPs, which modulate many structures simultaneously. Thus, more important than knowing where these ERPs are located is finding out what they are doing there.

13. CONCLUDING REMARKS

Oscillatory mechanisms involve always local populations of neurons interconnected by loops where different kinds of neurons (main cells or interneurons) participate. Although it is not well known, as yet, how synchronous activity of different neuronal populations results in specific neuronal operations, some hypotheses can be put forward. It appears that memory formation and its distribution throughout the cortex may be facilitated during SWS. Similarly, inhibition of inputs that may disturb perception, or memory encoding, may be accomplished by oscillations in the alpha frequency range, and the decrease of alpha, as a mechanism subserving attention, may enable, or facilitate, perception. On the other hand, theta, beta2, and gamma rhythms appear to mediate processes that recruit neuronal populations into joint action, such as in motor programming, and in binding neuronal assemblies to enable the formation of a conscious percept. Especially with respect to high-frequency oscillations (beta2 and gamma), an important property is that during these oscillations the repetitive firing of groups of neurons can provide a periodic barrage of impulses that can modulate the synaptic strength of postsynaptic targets. Tight phasing of neuronal firing reflected in an evident oscillation at the LFP level can induce synaptic plasticity and an increase in synaptic transfer of information. Neuronal synchronization and the corresponding oscillatory LFPs should not be considered epiphenomena; rather, these phenomena can constitute the foundation of the neuronal processes underlying cognitive functions.

We only have one brain, so the same neural currents must generate ERPs and ERFs; the difference is in analysis methods and historical framework. Rhythms provide sensitivity to single trials, but temporal accuracy is inevitably limited, especially for lower frequencies. ERP/ERFs provide temporal accuracy limited only by the sampling rate and bandpass, and sensitivity to sub-microvolt changes, but at the cost of requiring hundreds or thousands of trials. Rhythms are compared across subjects, tasks, and recording modalities by referring to their topography, frequency, and cognitive characteristics. Such standard rhythms (e.g., visual alpha, frontal midline theta) correspond to ERP/ERF components, which are also defined by their topography, latency, and cognitive characteristics. Because extracranial EEG/MEG studies are irretrievably ambiguous regarding generators, definition of both standard rhythms and ERP/ERF components from extracranial measures are always circular. Indeed, source localization is particularly challenged by the distributed generators producing standard rhythms and long-latency cognitive components, so the results of inverse solutions must be validated against intracranial recordings.

Our cortices contain about as many pyramidal cells as there are people on earth, and each pyramidal cell is a complex computational unit, exchanging information with tens of thousands of other cells, using highly modifiable links. Each cell is not a passive capacitor, collecting excitation and discharging occasionally, but is rather a highly active participant, with thousands of synaptic spines, and dozens of dendritic domains and active channels, which are co-equal participants with synaptic input in shaping the neuron's activity. Yet, these billions of complex semi-independent entities are somehow organized to act as a unit while at the same time retaining their essential ability to make unique contributions. When something unpredicted happens, we quickly focus our attention and processing resources. When a word arrives, we access a broad network of associations, integrate with the ongoing sentence and pragmatic contexts, as well as primary, recent, and remote memories, and create a single interpretation of its meaning. We do one volitional movement at a time.

Due to a lucky convergence of cortical anatomy, physiology, and biophysics, standard rhythms and ERP/ERF components are exquisitely tuned to detect the modulatory processes used by the brain to organize its activity into a coherent whole. At the microscopic level, significant equivalent current dipoles will only occur in pyramidal cells due to global inputs on different laminae of their dendritic domains; laminar selectivity reflects the basic parameters of cortico-cortical connectivity (feed-forward vs. feedback/associational) and thalamo-cortical connectivity (matrix vs. core). At the mesoscopic level, only spatially and temporally aligned microscopic sources will summate to produce EEG/MEG that rises above the noise. Thus, EEG and MEG provide uniquely powerful insights into the mechanisms underlying the unity of our cortical function and subjective experience.

REFERENCES

1. Niedermeyer E. Historical aspects. In: Niedermeyer E, Lopes da Silva FH, eds. Electroencephalography: Basic Principles, Clinical Applications and Related Fields. Philadelphia: Lippincott, Williams and Wilkins, 2005.
2. Palva JM, Monto S, Kulashekhar S, Palva S. Neuronal synchrony reveals working memory networks and predicts individual memory capacity. Proc Nat Acad Sci USA. 2010;107:7580–7585.
3. Womelsdorf T, Fries P. The role of neuronal synchronization in selective attention. Curr Opin Neurobiol. 2007;17:154–160.
4. Hebb DO. The Organization of Behavior. New York: Wiley, 1949.
5. Vaadia E, Bergman H, Abelcs M. Neuronal activities related to higher brain functions—theoretical and experimental implications. IEEE Trans Biomed Eng. 198936(1):25–35.
6. Levine DS, Brown V, Shirey VT, eds. Oscillations in Neural Systems. Mahwah, NJ: Lawrence Erlbaum Assoc., 2009.
7. Steriade M. Grouping of brain rhythms in corticothalamic systems. Neuroscience. 2006;137:1087–1106.
8. Mizuseki K, Sirota A, Pastalkova E, Buzsáki G. Theta oscillations provide temporal windows for local circuit computation in the entorhinal-hippocampal loop. Neuron. 2006;64:267–280.
9. Freeman WJ. The wave packet: an action potential for the 21st century. J Integr Neurosci. 2003;2:3–30.
10. Murthy VN, Fetz EE. Synchronization of neurons during local field potential oscillations in sensorimotor cortex of awake monkeys. J Neurophysiol. 1996;76(6):3968–3982.
11. Fries P, Nikolić D, Singer W. The gamma cycle. Trends Neurosci. 2007;30(7):309–316.
12. Mazzoni A, Panzeri S, Logothetis NK, Brunel N. Encoding of naturalistic stimuli by local field potential spectra in networks of excitatory and inhibitory neurons. PLoS Comput Biol. 2008;4(12):e1000239.
13. Lopes da Silva FH. EEG and MEG: relevance to neuroscience. Neuron. 2013;80:1112–1128.
14. Maris E, Fries P, van Ende F. Diverse phase relations among neuronal rhythms and their potential function. Trends Neurosci. 2016;39(2):86–99.
15. Walker MP, Stickgold R. Sleep, memory, and plasticity. Annu Rev Psychol. 2006;57:139–166.
16. Walker MP, Stickgold R. Sleep-dependent learning and memory consolidation. Neuron. 2004;44:121–133.
17. Gais S, Albouy G, Boly M, et al. Sleep transforms the cerebral trace of declarative memories. Proc Natl Acad Sci USA. 2007;104(47):18778–18783.
18. Lahl O, Wispel C, Willigens B, Pietrowsky R. An ultra-short episode of sleep is sufficient to promote declarative memory performance. J Sleep Res. 2008;17(1):3–10.
19. Payne JD, Stickgold R, Swanberg K, Kensinger EA. Sleep preferentially enhances memory for emotional components of scenes. Psychol Sci. 2008;19(8):781–788.
20. Diekelmann S, Born J. The memory function of sleep. Nat Rev Neurosci. 2010;11(2):114–126.
21. Bjorn R, Born J. About sleep's role in memory. Physiol Revs. 2013;93(2):681–766.
22. Van Der Werf YD, Altena E, Schoonheim MM, et al. Sleep benefits subsequent hippocampal functioning. Nat Neurosci. 2009(2):122–123.
23. Marshall L, Helgadottir H, Molle M, Born J. Boosting slow oscillations during sleep potentiates memory. Nature. 2006;444:610–613.
24. Ego-Stengel V, Wilson MA. Disruption of ripple-associated hippocampal activity during rest impairs spatial learning in the rat. Hippocampus. 2010;20(1):1–10.
25. Stickgold R, Walker MP. Sleep-dependent memory triage: evolving generalization through selective processing. Nature Neurosci. 2013;16(2):139–145.
26. Monto S, Palva S, Voipio J, Palva JM. Very slow EEG fluctuations predict the dynamics of stimulus detection and oscillation amplitudes in humans. J Neurosci. 2008;28(33):8268–8272.
27. Kahana MJ. The cognitive correlates of human brain oscillations. J Neurosci. 2006;26(6):1669–1672.
28. Arnolds DE, Lopes da Silva FH, Aitink JW, et al. The spectral properties of hippocampal EEG related to behaviour in man. Electroencephalogr Clin Neurophysiol. 1980;50(3-4):324–328.
29. Kahana MJ, Seelig D, Madsen JR. Theta returns. Curr Opin Neurobiol. 2001;11:739–744.
30. Caplan JB, Madsen JR, Schulze-Bonhage A, et al. Human theta oscillations related to sensorimotor integration and spatial learning. J Neurosci. 2003;23(11):4726–4736.
31. Cornwell BR, Johnson LL, Holroyd T, et al. Human hippocampal and parahippocampal theta during goal-directed

spatial navigation predicts performance on a virtual Morris water maze. J Neurosci. 2008;28(23):5983–5990.

32. Raghavachari S, Kahana MJ, Rizzuto DS, et al. Gating of human theta oscillations by a working memory task. J Neurosci. 2001;121(9):3175–3183.

33. Sederberg PB, Kahana MJ, Howard MW, et al. Theta and gamma oscillations during encoding predict subsequent recall. J Neurosci. 2003;23(34):10809–10814.

34. Lega B, Burke J, Jacobs J, Kahana MJ. Slow-theta-gamma phase-amplitude coupling in human hippocampus supports the formation of new episodic memories. Cerebral Cortex. 2016;26(1):268–278.

35. Halgren E, Kaestner E, Marinkovic K, et al. Laminar profile of spontaneous and evoked theta: Rhythmic modulation of cortical processing during word integration. Neuropsychologia. 2015;76:108–124.

36. Halgren E, Boujon C, Clarke J, et al. Rapid distributed fronto-parieto-occipital processing stages during working memory in humans. Cerebral Cortex. 2002;12:710–728.

37. Klimesch W. Memory processes, brain oscillations and EEG synchronization. Int J Psychophysiol. 1996;24(1-2):61–100.

38. Sarnthein J, Petsche H, Rappelsberger P, et al. Synchronization between prefrontal and posterior association cortex during human working memory. Proc Natl Acad Sci USA. 1998;95:7092–7096.

39. Schack B, Vath N, Petsche H, et al. Phase-coupling of theta-gamma EEG rhythms during short-term memory processing. Int J Psychophysiol. 2002;449(2):143–163.

40. Tesche CD, Karhu J. Theta oscillations index human hippocampal activation during a working memory task. Proc Nat Acad Sci USA. 2000;97:919–924.

41. Jensen O, Tesche CD. Frontal theta activity in humans increase with memory load in a working memory task. Eur J Neurosci. 2002;15:1395–1399.

42. de Araújo DB, Baffa O, Wakai RT. Theta oscillations and human navigation: a magnetoencephalography study. J Cogn Neurosci. 2002;14(1):70–78.

43. Guderian S, Düzel E. Induced theta oscillations mediate large-scale synchrony with mediotemporal areas during recollection in humans. Hippocampus. 2005;15(7):901–912.

44. Mitchell DJ, McNaughton N, Flanagan D, Kirk IJ. Frontal-midline theta from the perspective of hippocampal "theta." Progr Neurobiol. 2008;86:156–185.

45. Sasaki K, Tsujimoto T, Nishikawa S, Nishitani N, Ishihara T. Frontal mental theta wave recorded simultaneously with magnetoencephalography and electroencephalography. Neuroscience Res. 1996;26(1):79–81.

46. Ishii R, Shinosaki K, Ukai S, et al. Medial prefrontal cortex generates frontal midline theta rhythm. Neuroreport. 1999;10:675–679.

47. Leung LS, Borst JG. Electrical activity in the cingulated cortex of the rat. I. Generating mechanisms and relations to behavior. Brain Res. 1987;407:68–80.

48. Onton J, Delorme A, Makeig S. Frontal midline EEG dynamics during working memory. Neuroimage. 2005;27(2):341–356.

49. Bastiaansen M, Hagoort P. Event-induced theta responses as a window on the dynamics of memory. Cortex. 2003;39(4-5):967–992.

50. Niedermeyer E. Alpha like rhythmical activity of the temporal lobe. Clin Electroencephalogr. 1990;21:210–224.

51. Bollimunta A, Chen Y, Schroeder CE, Ding M. Neuronal mechanisms of cortical alpha oscillations in awake-behaving macaques. J Neurosci. 2008;28(40):9976–9988.

52. Van Kerkoerle T, Self MW, Dagnino B, et al. Alpha and gamma oscillations characterize feedback and feedforward processing in monkey visual cortex. Proc Nat Acad Sci USA. 2014; 111940:14332–14341.

53. Haegens S, Barczak A, Musacchia G, et al. Laminar profile and physiology of alpha rhythm in primary visual, auditory and somatosensory regions of neocortex. J Neurosci, 2015;35(42):14341–14352.

54. Lopes da Silva FH. Neural mechanisms underlying brain waves: from neural membranes to networks. Electroencephalogr Clin Neurophysiol. 1991;79:81–93.

55. Crone NE, Miglioretti DL, Gordon B, et al. Functional mapping of human sensorimotor cortex with electrocorticographic spectral analysis. I. Alpha and beta event-related desynchronization. Brain. 1998;121:2271–2299.

56. Rihs TA, Michel CM, Thut G. Mechanisms of selective inhibition in visual spatial attention are indexed by alpha-band EEG synchronization. Eur J Neurosci. 2007;25(2):603–610.

57. Adrian ED, Matthews BH. The interpretation of potential waves in the cortex. J Physiol. 1934;81(4):440–471.

58. Chatrian GE, Petersen MC, Lazarte JA. The blocking of the rolandic wicket rhythm and some central changes related to movement. Electroencephalogr Clin Neurophysiol. 1959;11(3):497–510.

59. Klimesch W, Sauseng P, Hanslmayr S. EEG alpha oscillations: the inhibition-timing hypothesis. Brain Res Rev. 2007;53(1):63–88.

60. Hanslmayr S, Aslan A, Staudigl T, et al. Prestimulus oscillations predict visual perception performance between and within subjects. Neuroimage. 2007;37(4):1465–1473.

61. Mathewson KE, Gratton G, Fabiani M, et al. To see or not to see: prestimulus alpha phase predicts visual awareness. J Neurosci. 2009;29(9):2725–2732.

62. Busch NA, Dubois J, van Rullen R. The phase of ongoing EEG oscillations predicts visual perception. J Neurosci. 2009;29(24):7869–7876.

63. Romei V, Brodbeck V, Michel C, et al. Spontaneous fluctuations in posterior alpha-band EEG activity reflect variability in excitability of human visual areas. Cereb Cortex. 2008;18(9):2010–2018.

64. Vollebregt MA, Zumer JM, ter Huurne N, et al. Posterior alpha oscillations reflect attentional problems in boys with attention deficit hyperactive disorder. Clin Neurophysiol. 2016;127:2182–2191.

65. Klimesch W. Alpha-band oscillations, attention, and controlled access to stored information. Trends Cogn Sci. 2012;16(12):606–617.

66. Zauner A, Fellinger R, Gross J, et al. Alpha entrainment is responsible for the attentional blink phenomenon. Neuroimage. 2012;63:674–686.

67. Jensen O, Gelfand J, Kounios J, Lisman JE. Oscillations in the alpha band (9–12 Hz) increase with memory load during retention in a short-term memory task. Cereb Cortex. 2002;12(8):877–882.

68. Bressler SL, Freeman WJ. Frequency analysis of olfactory system EEG in cat, rabbit, and rat. Electroencephalogr Clin Neurophysiol. 1980;50(1-2):19–24.

69. Boeijinga PH, Lopes da Silva FH. Modulations of EEG activity in the entorhinal cortex and forebrain olfactory areas during odour sampling. Brain Res. 1989;478(2):257–268.

70. Leung LS. Generation of theta and gamma rhythms in the hippocampus. Neurosci Biobehav Rev. 1998;22(2):275–290.

71. Bouyer JJ, Montaron MF, Vahnée JM, et al. Anatomical localization of cortical beta rhythms in cat. Neuroscience. 1987;22(3):863–869.

72. Lopes da Silva FH, van Rotterdam A, Storm van Leeuwen W, Tielen AM. Dynamic characteristics of visual evoked potentials in the dog. II. Beta frequency selectivity in evoked potentials and background activity. Electroencephal Clin Neurophysiol. 1970;29:260–268.

73. Freeman WJ, van Dijk BW. Spatial patterns of visual cortical fast EEG during conditioned reflex in a rhesus monkey. Brain Res. 1987;422(2):267–276.

74. Stam CJ, Pijn JPM, Suffczynski P, Lopes da Silva FH. Dynamics of the human alpha rhythm: evidence for non-linearity? Clinical Neurophysiol. 1999;110(10):1801–1813.

75. Pfurtscheller G, Lopes da Silva FH. Event-related EEG/MEG synchronization and desynchronization: basic principles. Clin Neurophysiol. 1999;110(11):1842–1857.

76. Engel AK, Fries P. Beta-band oscillations—signaling the status quo? Curr Opin Neurobiol. 2010;20:156–165.

77. Murthy VN, Fetz EE. Oscillatory activity in sensorimotor cortex of awake monkeys: synchronization of local field potentials and relation to behavior. J Neurophysiol. 1996;76(6):3949–3967.

78. Baker SN, Olivier E, Lemon RN. Coherent oscillations in monkey motor cortex and hand muscle EMG show task-dependent modulation. J Physiol. 1997;501(Pt 1):225–241.

79. Salenius S, Portin K, Kajola M, et al. Cortical control of human motoneuron firing during isometric contraction. J Neurophysiol. 1997;77(6):3401–3405.

80. Seeber M, Scherer R, Wagner J, et al. EEG beta suppression and low gamma modulation are different elements of human upright walking. Front Hum Neurosci. 2014;8(art 485):1–9.

81. Caetano G, Jousmäki V, Hari R. Actor's and observer's primary motor cortices stabilize similarly after seen or heard motor actions. Proc Natl Acad Sci USA. 2007;104:9058–9062.

82. Babiloni C, Babiloni F, Carducci F, et al. Human cortical electroencephalography (EEG) rhythms during the observation of simple aimless movements: a high-resolution EEG study. Neuroimage. 2002;17:559–572.

83. Eckhorn R, Bauer R, Jordan W, et al. Coherent oscillations: a mechanism of feature linking in the visual cortex? Multiple electrode and correlation analyses in the cat. Biol Cybern. 1988;60(2):121–130.

84. Gray CM, Singer W. Stimulus-specific neuronal oscillations in orientation columns of cat visual cortex. Proc Natl Acad Sci USA. 1989;86(5):1698–16702.

85. Gray CM, König P, Engel AK, Singer W. Oscillatory responses in cat visual cortex exhibit inter-columnar synchronization which reflects global stimulus properties. Nature. 1989;338(6213):334–337.

86. Roelfsema PR, Engel AK, König P, Singer W. Visuomotor integration is associated with zero time-lag synchronization among cortical areas. Nature. 1997;385(6612):157–161.

87. Varela F, et al. The brainweb: phase synchronization and largescale integration. Nat Rev Neurosci. 2001;2:229–239.

88. Fries P, Reynolds JH, Rorie AE, Desimone R. Modulation of oscillatory neuronal synchronization by selective visual attention. Science. 2001;291:1560–1563.

89. Colgin LL. Rhythms of the hippocampal network. Nature Rev Neurosci. 2016;17:239–249.

90. Colgin LL, Denninger T, Fyhn M, et al. Frequency of gamma oscillations routes flow of information in the hippocampus. Nature. 2009;462:353–358.

91. Gonzalez Andino SL, Michel CM, Thut G, et al. Prediction of response speed by anticipatory high-frequency (gamma band) oscillations in the human brain. Hum Brain Mapp. 2005;24(1):50–58.

92. Rose M, Sommer T, Buchel C. Integration of local features to a global percept by neural coupling. Cerebral Cortex. 2006;16:1522–1528.

93. Rodriguez E, George N, Lachaux JP, et al. Perception's shadow: long-distance synchronization of human brain activity. Nature. 1999;397(6718):430–433.

94. Trujillo LT, Peterson MA, Kaszniak AW, Allen JJ. EEG phase synchrony differences across visual perception conditions may depend on recording and analysis methods. Clin Neurophysiol. 2005;116(1):172–189.

95. Spaak E, Bonnefond M. Maier A, et al. Layer-specific entrainment of gamma-band neural activity by alpha rhythm in monkey visual cortex. Curr Biol. 2012;22: 2313–2318.

96. Jensen O, Gips B, Bergmann TO, Bonnefond M. Temporal coding organized by coupled alpha and gamma oscillations prioritize visual processing. Trends Neurosci. 2014;37(7):358–369.

97. Jensen O, Bonnefond M, Marshall TR, Tiesenga P. Oscillatory mechanisms of feedforward and feedback visual processing. Trends Neurosci. 2015;38(4):192–194.

98. Debener S, Herrmann CS, Kranczioch C, et al. Top-down attentional processing enhances auditory evoked gamma band activity. Neuroreport. 2003;14(5):683–686.

99. Sederberg PB, Schulze-Bonhage A, Madsen JR, et al. Hippocampal and neocortical gamma oscillations predict memory formation in humans. Cereb Cortex. 2007;17(5):1190–1196.

100. Fell J, Fernández G, Klaver P, et al. Rhinal-hippocampal coupling during declarative memory formation: dependence on item characteristics. Neurosci Lett. 2006;407(1):37–41.

101. Tallon-Baudry C, Bertrand O, Peronnet F, Pernier J. Induced gamma activity and visual short-term memory. J Neurosci. 1998;18(11):4244–4254.

102. Kaiser J, Heidegge T, Wibral M, et al. Distinct gamma-band components reflect the short-term memory maintenance of different sound lateralization angles. Cereb Cortex. 2008;18:2286–2295.

103. Gruber T, Tsivilis D, Montaldi D, Müller MM. Induced gamma band responses: an early marker of memory encoding and retrieval. Neuroreport. 2004;15(11):1837–1841.

104. Osipova D, Takashima A, Oostenveld R, et al. Theta and gamma oscillations predict encoding and retrieval of declarative memory. J Neurosci. 2006;26(28):7523–7531.

105. Buzsaki G. Rhythms of the Brain. New York: Oxford University Press, 2006.

106. Lakatos P, Shah AS, Knuth KH, et al. An oscillatory hierarchy controlling neuronal excitability and stimulus processing in the auditory cortex. J Neurophysiol. 2005;94:1904–1911.

107. Axmacher N, Henseler MM, Jensen O, et al. Cross-frequency coupling supports multi-item working memory in the human hippocampus. Proc Natl Acad Sci USA. 2010;107(7):3228–3233.

108. Canolty RT, Edwards E, Dalal SS, et al. High gamma power is phase-locked to theta oscillations in human neocortex. Science. 2006;313(5793):1626–1628.

109. Doesburg SM, Green JJ, McDonald JJ, Ward LM. Rhythms of consciousness: binocular rivalry reveals large-scale oscillatory network dynamics mediating visual perception. PLoS One. 2009;4(7):e6142.

110. Yuval-Greenberg S, Tomer O, Keren AS, et al. Transient induced gamma-band response in EEG as a manifestation of miniature saccades. Neuron. 2008;58(3):429–441.

111. Donchin E, Ritter W, McCallum WC. Cognitive psychophysiology: the endogenous components of the ERP. In: Callaway E, Tueting P, Koslow S, eds. Brain and Information: Event-Related Potentials. New York: New York Academy of Science, 1978:349–411.

112. Donchin E, Coles MG. Is the P300 component a manifestation of context updating? Behav Brain Sci. 1988;11(3):357–427.

113. Picton TW, Stuss DT. The component structure of the human event-related potentials. Progress Brain Res. 1980;54:17–49.

114. Luck SJ, Kappenman ES. The Oxford Handbook of Event-Related Potential Components. New York: Oxford University Press, 2012.

115. Ritter W, Ford JM, Gaillard AWK, et al. Cognition and event-related potentials. I. The relation of negative potentials and cognitive processes. Ann NY Acad Sci. 1984;425:24–38.

116. Jaaskelainen IP, Ahveninen J, Bonmassar G, et al. Human posterior auditory cortex gates novel sounds to consciousness. Proc Natl Acad Sci USA. 2004;101(17):6809–6814.

117. Renault B. The visual emitted potentials: Clues for information processing. In: Gaillard AWK, Ritter W, eds. Tutorials in event-related potential research: Endogenous components. Amsterdam: North-Holland, 1983:159–175.

118. Naatanen R, Kreegipuu K. The mismatch negativity (MMN). In: Luck SJ, Kappenman ES, eds. The Oxford Handbook of Event-Related Potential Components. Oxford: Oxford University Press, 2012:143–157.

119. Polich J. Updating P300: an integrative theory of P3a and P3b. Clin Neurophysiol. 2007;118(10):2128–2148.

120. Marinkovic K, Halgren E, Maltzman I. Arousal-related P3a to novel auditory stimuli is abolished by a moderately low alcohol dose. Alcohol Alcoholism. 2001;36(6):529–539.

121. Zatorre RJ. Neural specializations for tonal processing. Ann NY Acad Sci. 2001;930:193–210.

122. Linden DEJ. The P300: Where in the brain is it produced and what does it tell us? Neuroscientist. 2005;11:563–576.

123. Halgren E, Sherfey J, Irimia A, et al. Sequential temporo-fronto-temporal activation during monitoring of the auditory environment for temporal patterns. Hum Brain Mapp. 2011;32(8):1260–1276.

124. Halgren E, Baudena P, Clarke JM, et al. Intracerebral potentials to rare target and distractor auditory and visual stimuli. I. Superior temporal plane and parietal lobe. Electroencephalogr Clin Neurophysiol. 1995;94(3):191–220.

125. Kropotov JD, Alho K, Naatanen R, et al. Human auditory-cortex mechanisms of preattentive sound discrimination. Neurosci Lett. 2000;280(2):87–90.

126. Rosburg T, Trautner P, Dietl T, et al. Subdural recordings of the mismatch negativity (MMN) in patients with focal epilepsy. Brain. 2005;128(Pt 4):819–828.

127. Javitt DC, Steinschneider M, Schroeder CE, et al. Detection of stimulus deviance within primate primary auditory cortex: intracortical mechanisms of mismatch negativity (MMN) generation. Brain Res. 1994;667(2):192–200.

128. Pincze Z, Lakatos P, Rajkai C, et al. Effect of deviant probability and interstimulus/interdeviant interval on the auditory N1 and mismatch negativity in the cat auditory cortex. Brain Res Cogn Brain Res. 2002;13(2):249–253.

129. Escera C, Malmierca MS. The auditory novelty system: an attempt to integrate human and animal research. Psychophysiology. 2014;51(2):111–123.

130. Horvath J, Czigler I, Sussman E, Winkler I. Simultaneously active preattentive representations of local and global rules for sound sequences in the human brain. Brain Res Cogn Brain Res. 2001;12(1):131–144.

131. Halgren E, Baudena P, Clarke JM, et al. Intracerebral potentials to rare target and distractor auditory and visual stimuli: 2. Medial, lateral and posterior temporal lobe. Electroencephalogr Clin Neurophysiol. 1995;94(4):229–250.

132. Rosburg T, Trautner P, Ludowig E, et al. Hippocampal event-related potentials to tone duration deviance in a passive oddball paradigm in humans. Neuroimage. 2007;37(1):274–281.

133. Alain C, Woods DL, Knight RT. A distributed cortical network for auditory sensory memory in humans. Brain Res. 1998;812(1-2):23–37.

134. Knight RT, Nakada T. Cortico-limbic circuits and novelty: a review of EEG and blood flow data. Rev Neurosci. 1998;9(1):57–70.

135. Wilson CL, Babb TL, Halgren E, et al. Habituation of human limbic neuronal response to sensory stimulation. Exp Neurol. 1984;84(1):74–97.

136. Kanai R, Komura Y, Shipp S, Friston K. Cerebral hierarchies: predictive processing, precision and the pulvinar. Philos Trans R Soc B Biol Sci. 2015;370(1668):20140169.

137. Polich J. Neuropsychology of P300. In: Luck SJ, Kappenman ES, eds. The Oxford Handbook of Event-Related Potential Components. Oxford: Oxford University Press, 2012:159–188.

138. Alain C, Richer F, Achim A, Saint-Hilaire JM. Human intracerebral potentials associated with target, novel and omitted auditory stimuli. Brain Topogr. 1989;1:237–245.

139. Baudena P, Halgren E, Heit G, Clarke JM. Intracerebral potentials to rare target and distractor auditory and visual stimuli. III. Frontal cortex. Electroencephalogr Clin Neurophysiol. 1995;94(4):251–264.

140. Halgren E, Marinkovic K. Neurophysiological networks integrating human emotions. In: Gazzaniga M, ed. The Cognitive Neurosciences. Cambridge, MA: MIT Press, 1995:1137–1151.

141. Stapleton JM, Halgren E. Endogenous potentials evoked in simple cognitive tasks: Depth components and task correlates. Electroencephalogr Clin Neurophysiol. 1987;67:44–52.

142. Knight R. Neural mechanisms of event-related potentials: Evidence from human lesion studies. In: Rohrbaugh JW, Parasuraman R, Johnson R, eds. Event-Related Brain Potentials: Basic Issues and Applications. New York: Oxford University Press, 1990:3–18.

143. Soltani M, Knight RT. Neural origins of the P300. Crit Rev Neurobiol. 2000;14(3-4):199–224.

144. Daffner KR, Mesulam MM, Scinto LF, et al. The central role of the prefrontal cortex in directing attention to novel events. Brain. 2000;123(Pt 5):927–939.

145. Smith ME, Stapleton JM, Halgren E. Human medial temporal lobe potentials evoked in memory and language tasks. Electroencephalogr Clin Neurophysiol. 1986;63:145–159.

146. Sokolov EN. The orienting response, and future directions of its development. Pavlovian J Biol Sci. 1990;25:142–150.

147. Näätänen R, Gaillard AWK. The orienting reflex and the N2 deflection of the ERP. In: Gaillard AWK, Ritter W, eds. Tutorials in Event Related Potential Research: Endogenous Components. Amsterdam: Elsevier, 1983:119–141.

148. Gehring WJ, Liu Y, Orr JM, Carp J. The error-related negativity (ERN/Ne). In: Luck SJ, Kappenman ES, eds. The Oxford Handbook of Event-Related Potential Components. Oxford: Oxford University Press, 2012:231–291.

149. Van Schie HT, Mars RB, Coles MG, Bekkering H. Modulation of activity in medial frontal and motor cortices during error observation. Nature Neurosci. 2004;7(5):549–554.

150. Wang C, Ulbert I, Schomer DL, et al. Responses of human anterior cingulate cortex microdomains to error detection, conflict monitoring, stimulus-response mapping, familiarity, and orienting. J Neurosci. 2005;25(3):604–613.

151. Bonini F, Burle B, Liegeois-Chauvel C, et al. Action monitoring and medial frontal cortex: leading role of supplementary motor area. Science. 2014;343(6173):888–891.

152. Cavanagh JF, Zambrano-Vazquez L, Allen JJ. Theta lingua franca: a common mid-frontal substrate for action monitoring processes. Psychophysiology. 2012;49(2):220–238.

153. Quinn BT, Carlson C, Doyle W, et al. Intracranial cortical responses during visual-tactile integration in humans. J Neurosci. 2014;34(1):171–181.

154. Rosler F, Sutton S, Johnson R, Jr., et al. Endogenous ERP components and cognitive components: A review. In: McCallum WC, Zappoli R, Denoth F, eds. Cerebral Psychophysiology Studies in Event-Related Potentials (EEG Supplement 38). Amsterdam: Elsevier, 1986:51–92.

155. Hillyard SA, Picton TW. Electrophysiology of cognition. In: Plum F, ed. Handbook of Physiology—The Nervous System V. Bethesda, MD: American Physiological Society, 1988:519–584.

156. Luck SJ, Kappenman ES. ERP components and selective attention. In: Luck SJ, Kappenman ES, eds. The Oxford Handbook of Event-Related Potential Components. Oxford: Oxford University Press, 2012:295–327.

157. Luck SJ. Electrophysiological correlates of the focusing of attention within complex visual scenes: N2pc and related ERP components. In: Luck SJ, Kappenman ES, eds. The Oxford Handbook of Event-Related Potential Components. Oxford: Oxford University Press, 2012:329–360.

158. Desmedt JE. Scalp-recorded cerebral event-related potentials in man as point of entry into the analysis of cognitive processing. In: Schmitt FO, Worden FG, Edelmann G, Dennis SD, eds. The Organization of the Cerebral Cortex. Cambridge, MA: MIT, 1981:441–473.

159. Verleger R. Event-related potentials and cognition: A critique of the context updating hypothesis and an alternative interpretation of P3. Behav Brain Sci. 1988;11(3):343–356.

160. Paller KA, McCarthy G, Wood CC. ERPs predictive of subsequent recall and recognition performance. Biol Psychol. 1988;26(1-3):269–276.

161. Neville HJ, Kutas M, Chesney G, Schmidt AC. Event-related brain potentials during initial encoding and recognition memory of congruous and incongruous words. J Memory Language. 1986;25:75–92.

162. Smith ME, Halgren E. Dissociation of recognition memory components following temporal lobe lesions. J Exp Psychol Learning Memory Cognition. 1989;15:50–60.

163. Halgren E, Squires NK, Wilson CL, et al. Endogenous potentials generated in the human hippocampal formation and amygdala by infrequent events. Science. 1980;210(4471):803–805.

164. Puce A, Kalnins RM, Berkovic SF, et al. Limbic P3 potentials, seizure localization, and surgical pathology in temporal lobe epilepsy. Ann Neurol. 1989;26:377–385.

165. McCarthy G, Wood CC, Williamson PD, Spencer DD. Task-dependent field potentials in human hippocampal formation. J Neurosci. 1989;9:4253–4268.

166. Brazdil M, Roman R, Daniel P, Rektor I. Intracerebral somatosensory event-related potentials: effect of response type (button pressing versus mental counting) on P3-like potentials within the human brain. Clin Neurophysiol. 2003;114(8):1489–1496.

167. Grunwald T, Beck H, Lehnertz K, et al. Limbic P300s in temporal lobe epilepsy with and without Ammon's horn sclerosis. Eur J Neurosci. 1999;11(6):1899–1906.

168. Watanabe N, Hirai N, Maehara T, et al. The relationship between the visually evoked P300 event-related potential and gamma band oscillation in the human medial and basal temporal lobes: an electrocorticographic study. Neurosci Res. 2002;44(4):421–427.

169. Halgren E, Baudena P, Heit G, et al. Spatio-temporal stages in face and word processing. 1. Depth-recorded potentials in the human occipital, temporal and parietal lobes. J Physiol Paris. 1994;88:1–50.

170. Halgren E, Baudena P, Heit G, et al. Spatio-temporal stages in face and word processing. 2. Depth-recorded potentials in the human frontal and Rolandic cortices. J Physiol Paris. 1994;88:51–80.

171. Stapleton JM, Halgren E, Moreno KA. Endogenous potentials after anterior temporal lobectomy. Neuropsychologia. 1987;25:549–557.

172. Johnson R, Jr. Scalp-recorded P300 activity in patients following unilateral temporal lobectomy. Brain. 1988;111(Pt 6)(3):1517–1529.

173. Polich J, Squire LR. P300 from amnesic patients with bilateral hippocampal lesions. Electroencephalogr Clin Neurophysiol. 1993;86:408–417.

174. Onofrj M, Fulgente T, Nobilio D, et al. P3 recordings in patients with bilateral temporal lobe lesions. Neurology. 1992;42(9):1762–1767.

175. Duzel E, Vargha-Khadem F, Heinze HJ, Mishkin M. Brain activity evidence for recognition without recollection after early hippocampal damage. Proc Natl Acad Sci USA. 2001;98(14):8101–8106.

176. Olichney JM, Van Petten C, Paller KA, et al. Word repetition in amnesia. Electrophysiological measures of impaired and spared memory. Brain. 2000;123(Pt 9):1948–1963.

177. Kiehl KA, Laurens KR, Duty TL, et al. Neural sources involved in auditory target detection and novelty processing: an event-related fMRI study. Psychophysiology. 2001;38(1):133–142.

178. Halgren E. Considerations in source estimation of the P3. In: Ikeda A, Inoue Y, eds. Event-Related Potentials in Patients with Epilepsy. Paris: John Libbey Eurotext, 2008.

179. Tarkka IM, Stokic DS, Basile LF, Papanicolaou AC. Electric source localization of the auditory P300 agrees with magnetic source localization. Electroencephalogr Clin Neurophysiol. 1995;96(6):538–545.

180. Nishitani N, Nagamine T, Fujiwara N, et al. Cortical-hippocampal auditory processing identified by magnetoencephalography. J Cogn Neurosci. 1998;10(2):231–247.

181. Okada YC, Kaufman L, Williamson SJ. The hippocampal formation as a source of the slow endogenous potentials. Electroencephalogr Clin Neurophysiol. 1983;55(4):417–426.

182. Basile LF, Rogers RL, Simos PG, Papanicolaou AC. Magnetoencephalographic evidence for common sources of long latency fields to rare target and rare novel visual stimuli. Int J Psychophysiol. 1997;25(2):123–137.

183. Nishitani N, Ikeda A, Nagamine T, et al. The role of the hippocampus in auditory processing studied by event-related electric potentials and magnetic fields in epilepsy patients before and after temporal lobectomy. Brain. 1999;122(Pt 4):687–707.

184. Rogers RL, Baumann SB, Papanicolaou AC, et al. Localization of the P3 sources using magnetoencephalography and magnetic resonance imaging. Electroencephalogr Clin Neurophysiol. 1991;79(4):308–321.

185. Mecklinger A, Maess B, Opitz B, et al. A MEG analysis of the P300 in visual discrimination tasks. Electroencephalogr Clin Neurophysiol. 1998;108(1):45–56.

186. Makeig S, Delorme A, Westerfield M, et al. Electroencephalographic brain dynamics following manually responded visual targets. PLoS Biol. 2004;2(6):747–762.

187. Yingling CD, Hosobuchi Y. A subcortical correlate of P300 in man. Electroencephalogr Clin Neurophysiol. 1984;59:72–76.

188. Katayama Y, Tsukiyama T, Tsubokawa T. Thalamic negativity associated with the endogenous late positive component of cerebral evoked potentials (P300): Recordings using discriminative aversive conditioning in humans and cats. Brain Res Bull. 1985;14:223–226.

189. Velasco M, Velasco F, Velasco AL. Intracranial studies on potential generators of some vertex auditory evoked potentials in man. Stereotact Funct Neurosurg. 1989;53(1):49–73.

190. Kropotov JD, Ponomarev VA. Subcortical neuronal correlates of component P300 in man. Electroencephalogr Clin Neurophysiol. 1991;78(1):40–49.

191. Rektor I, Kanovsky P, Bares M, et al. Event-related potentials, CNV, readiness potential, and movement accompanying potential recorded from posterior thalamus in human subjects. A SEEG study. Neurophysiol Clin. 2001;31(4):253–261.

192. Klostermann F, Wahl M, Marzinzik F, et al. Mental chronometry of target detection: human thalamus leads cortex. Brain. 2006;129(Pt 4):923–931.

193. Rektor I, Bares M, Kanovsky P, et al. Cognitive potentials in the basal ganglia-frontocortical circuits. An intracerebral recording study. Exp Brain Res. 2004;158(3):289–301.

194. He B, Lian J, Spencer KM, et al. A cortical potential imaging analysis of the P300 and novelty P3 components. Hum Brain Mapp. 2001;12(2):120–130.

195. Verleger R, Heide W, Butt C, Koempf D. Reduction of P3-sub(b) in patients with temporo-parietal lesions. Cogn Brain Res. 1994;2(2):103–116.

196. Yamaguchi S, Knight RT. Anterior and posterior association cortex contributions to the somatosensory P300. J Neurosci. 1991;11(7):2039–2054.

197. Mesulam M. Large-scale neurocognitive networks and distributed processing for attention, language, and memory. Ann Neurol. 1990;28(5):597–613.

198. Kutas M, McCarthy G, Donchin E. Augmenting mental chronometry: the P300 as a measure of stimulus evaluation time. Science. 1977;197:792–795.

199. McCarthy G, Donchin E. A metric for thought: a comparison of P300 latency and reaction time. Science. 1981;211:77–80.

200. Shibasaki H, Barrett G, Halliday E, Halliday AM. Components of the movement-related cortical potential and their scalp topography. Electroencephalogr Clin Neurophysiol. 1980;49:213–226.

201. Vaughan HG, Jr. The motor potentials. Handbook of Electroencephalography and Clinical Neurophysiology, Vol. 8A. Amsterdam: Elsevier, 1975:86–92.

202. Brunia CHM, van Broxel GJM, Bocker KBE. Negative slow waves as indices of anticipation: The Bereitschaftspotential, the contingent negative variation, and the stimulus-preceding negativity. In: Luck SJ, Kappenman ES, eds. The Oxford Handbook of Event-Related Potential Components. Oxford: Oxford University Press, 2012:189–207.

203. Jahanshahi M, Hallet M. Bereitschaftspotential Movement-Related Cortical Potentials. New York: Kluwer Academic/Plenum, 2003.

204. Hillyard SA. The CNV and human behavior: A review. In: McCallum WC, Knott JR, eds. Event-Related Slow Potentials of the Brain. Amsterdam: Elsevier, 1973:161–171.

205. Smulders FTY, Miller JO. The lateralized readiness potential. In: Luck SJ, Kappenman ES, eds. The Oxford Handbook of Event-Related Potential Components. Oxford: Oxford University Press, 2012:209–229.

206. Arezzo JC, Vaughan HG, Kraut MA, et al. Intracranial generators of event-related potentials in the monkey. In: Cracco R, Bodis-Wollner I, eds. Evoked Potentials. New York: Liss, 1986:141–154.

207. Lee BI, Luders H, Lesser RP, et al. Cortical potentials related to voluntary and passive finger movements recorded from subdural electrodes in humans. Ann Neurol. 1986;20(1):32–37.

208. Pieper CF, Goldring S, Jenny AB, McMahon JP. Comparative study of cerebral evoked potentials associated with voluntary movements in monkey and man. Electroencephalogr Clin Neurophysiol. 1980;48:266–292.

209. Groll-Knapp E, Ganglberger JA, Haider M, Schmid H. Stereoelectroencephalographic studies on event-related slow potentials in the human brain. In: Lechner H, Aranibar A, eds. Electroencephalography and Clinical Neurophysiology. Amsterdam: Excepta Medica, 1980:746–760.

210. Tanji J. The neuronal activity in the supplementary motor area of primates. Trends Neurosci. 1984;7:282–285.

211. Shibasaki H. Movement-associated cortical potentials in unilateral cerebral lesions. J Neurol. 1975;209:189–198.

212. Libet B, Gleason CA, Wright EW, Jr., Pearl DK. Time of conscious intention to act in relation to onset of cerebral activities (readiness-potential): the unconscious initiation of a freely voluntary act. Brain. 1983;106:623–642.

213. Rohrbaugh JW, Syndulko K, Sanquist TF, Lindsley DB. Synthesis of the contingent negative variation brain potential from noncontingent stimulus and motor elements. Science. 1980;208:1165–1168.

214. McSherry JW. Multiple-contact probes for intracortical CNV research. In: McCallum WC, Knott JR, eds. Event-Related Slow Potentials of the Brain: Their Relations to Behavior (EEG Suppl. 33). Amsterdam: Elsevier, 1973:25–27.

215. Rebert CS. Elements of a general cerebral system related to CNV genesis. In: McCallum WC, Knott JR, eds. Event-Related Slow Potentials of the Brain: Their Relations to Behavior (EEG Suppl. 33). Amsterdam: Elsevier, 1973:63–67.

216. Rockstroh B, Elbert T, Birbaumer N, Lutzenberger W. Slow Brain Potentials and Behavior. Baltimore, MD: Urban and Schwartzenberg, 1982.

217. Papakostopoulos D, Crow HJ. Electrocorticographic studies of the contingent negative variation and "P300" in man. In: McCallum WC, Knot JR, ed. The Responsive Brain. Bristol, UK: Wright, 1976:205–210.

218. Rebert CS. Neurobehavioral aspects of brain slow potentials. In: Kornhuber HH, Deecke L, eds. Motivation, Motor and Sensory Processes of the Brain. Amsterdam: North-Holland Biomedical Press, Elsevier, 1980:381–402.

219. Skinner JE, Yingling CD. Central gating mechanisms that regulate event-related potentials and behavior. A neural model for attention. In: Desmedt JE, ed. Attention, Voluntary Contraction and Event-Related Cerebral Potentials. Progress in Clinical Neurophysiology, Vol. 1. Basel: Karger, 1977:30–69.

220. Fuster JM. The Prefrontal Cortex: Anatomy, Physiology and Neuropsychology of the Frontal Lobe. New York: Raven Press, 1980.

221. Lutzenberger W, Birbaumer N, Elbert T, et al. Self-regulation of slow cortical potentials in normal subjects and patients with frontal lobe lesions. Prog Brain Res. 1980;54:427–430.

222. Low MD. Event-related potentials and the electroencephalogram in patients with proven brain lesions. In: Desmedt JE, ed. Cognitive Components in Cerebral Event-Related-Potentials and Selective Attention. Basel: Karger, 1979:258–264.

223. Tsubokawa T, Moriyasu N. Motivational slow negative potential shift (CNV) related to thalamotomy. Appl Neurophysiol. 1978;41:202–208.

224. Gazzaniga MS, Hillyard SA. Attention mechanisms following brain bisection. In: Kornblum S, ed. Attention and Performance, Vol. 4. New York: Academic, 1973:221–238.

225. Ruchkin DS, Sutton S. CNV and P300 relationships for emitted and for evoked cerebral potentials. In: Desmedt JE, ed. Cognitive Components in Cerebral Event-Related-Potentials and Selective Attention. Basel: Karger, 1979:119–131.

226. Pirch JH, Corbus MJ, Rigdon GC, Lynes WH. Generation of cortical event-related slow potentials in the rat involves nucleus basalis cholinergic innervation. Electroencephalogr Clinical Neurophysiol. 1986;63:464–465.

227. Swaab TY, Ledoux K, Camblin CC, Boudewyn MA. Language-related ERP components. In: Luck SJ, Kappenman ES, eds. The Oxford Handbook of Event-Related Potential Components. OxfordY: Oxford University Press; 2012:397–439.

228. Dehaene S, Cohen L. The unique role of the visual word form area in reading. Trends Cogn Sci. 2011;15(6):254–262.

229. Tarkiainen A, Helenius P, Hansen PC, et al. Dynamics of letter string perception in the human occipitotemporal cortex. Brain. 1999;122(Pt 11):2119–2132.

230. Leonard MK, Brown TT, Travis KE, et al. Spatiotemporal dynamics of bilingual word processing. Neuroimage. 2010;49(4):3286–3294.

231. Allison T, McCarthy G, Nobre A, et al. Human extrastriate visual cortex and the perception of faces, words, numbers, and colors. Cerebr Cortex. 1994;4:544–554.

232. Gaillard R, Naccache L, Pinel P, et al. Direct intracranial, FMRI, and lesion evidence for the causal role of left inferotemporal cortex in reading. Neuron. 2006;50(2):191–204.

233. Mainy N, Jung J, Baciu M, et al. Cortical dynamics of word recognition. Hum Brain Mapp. 2008;29(11):1215–1230.

234. Thesen T, McDonald CR, Carlson C, et al. Sequential then interactive processing of letters and words in the left fusiform gyrus. Nature Communications. 2012;3: 1284.

235. Marinkovic K, Dhond RP, Dale AM, et al. Spatiotemporal dynamics of modality-specific and supramodal word processing. Neuron. 2003;38(3):487–497.

236. Solomyak O, Marantz A. Evidence for early morphological decomposition in visual word recognition. J Cogn Neurosci. 2010;22(9):2042–2057.

237. Sahin NT, Pinker S, Cash SS, et al. Sequential processing of lexical, grammatical, and phonological information within Broca's area. Science. 2009;326(5951):445–449.

238. Chan AM, Baker JM, Eskandar E, et al. First-pass selectivity for semantic categories in human anteroventral temporal lobe. J Neurosci. 2011;31(49):18119–18129.

239. Hauk O, Davis MH, Ford M, et al. The time course of visual word recognition as revealed by linear regression analysis of ERP data. Neuroimage. 2006;30(4):1383–1400.

240. Halgren E, Wang C, Schomer DL, et al. Processing stages underlying word recognition in the anteroventral temporal lobe. Neuroimage. 2006;30(4):1401–1413.

241. Travis KE, Leonard MK, Chan AM, et al. Independence of early speech processing from word meaning. Cereb Cortex. 2013;23(10):2370–2379.

242. Hickok G, Poeppel D. The cortical organization of speech processing. Nat Rev Neurosci. 2007;8(5):393–402.

243. Rossion B, Jacques C. The N170: Understanding the time course of face perception in the human brain. In: Luck SJ, Kappenman ES, eds. The Oxford Handbook of Event-Related Potential Components. Oxford: Oxford University Press, 2012:115–141.

244. Klopp J, Marinkovic K, Chauvel P, et al. Early widespread cortical distribution of coherent fusiform face activity. Hum Brain Mapp. 2000;11(4):286–293.

245. Halgren E, Dale AM, Sereno MI, et al. Location of human face-selective cortex with respect to retinotopic areas. Hum Brain Mapp. 1999;7(1):29–37.

246. Halgren E, Raij T, Marinkovic K, et al. Cognitive response profile of the human fusiform face area as determined by MEG. Cereb Cortex. 2000;10(1):69–81.

247. Kutas M, Federmeier KD. Electrophysiology reveals semantic memory use in language comprehension. Trends Cogn Sci. 2000;4(12):463–470.

248. Kutas M, Van Petten C. Psycholingusistics electrified: Event-related brain potential investigations. In: Gernsbacher M, ed. Handbook of Psycholinguistics. New York: Academic, 1994:83–143.

249. Smith ME, Halgren E. Event-related potentials elicited by familiar and unfamiliar faces. Electroencephalogr Clin Neurophysiol Suppl. 1987;40:422–426.

250. Smith ME, Halgren E. Event-related potentials during lexical decision: effects of repetition, word frequency, pronounceability, and concreteness. Electroencephalogr Clin Neurophysiol Suppl. 1987;40:417–421.

251. Heit G, Smith ME, Halgren E. Neural encoding of individual words and faces by the human hippocampus and amygdala. Nature. 1988;333(6175):773–775.

252. Patterson K, Nestor PJ, Rogers TT. Where do you know what you know? The representation of semantic knowledge in the human brain. Nat Rev Neurosci. 2007;8(12):976–987.

253. Fischler I, Bloom PA, Childers DG, et al. Brain potentials during sentence verification: late negativity and long-term memory strength. Neuropsychologia. 1984;22:559–568.

254. Van Petten C, Rheinfelder H. Conceptual relationships between spoken words and environmental sounds: event-related brain potential measures. Neuropsychologia. 1995;33(4):485–508.

255. Van Petten C, Senkfor AJ. Memory for words and novel visual patterns: repetition, recognition, and encoding effects in the event-related brain potential. Psychophysiology. 1996;33(5):491–506.

256. Halgren E. Insights from evoked potentials into the neuropsychological mechanisms of reading. In: Scheibel A, Weschsler A, eds. Neurobiology of Cognition. New York: Guilford, 1990:103–150.

257. Kutas M, Hillyard SA, Gazzaniga MS. Processing of semantic anomaly by right and left hemispheres of commissurotomy patients. Evidence from event-related brain potentials. Brain. 1988;111:553–576.

258. Friederici AD, Hahne A, von Cramon DY. First-pass versus second-pass parsing processes in a Wernicke's and a Broca's aphasic: electrophysiological evidence for a double dissociation. Brain Lang. 1998;62(3):311–341.

259. Hagoort P, Brown CM, Swaab TY. Lexical-semantic event-related potential effects in patients with left hemisphere lesions and aphasia, and patients with right hemisphere lesions without aphasia. Brain. 1996;119(Pt 2):627–649.

260. Curran T, Tucker DM, Kutas M, Posner MI. Topography of the N400: brain electrical activity reflecting semantic expectancy. Electroencephalogr Clin Neurophysiol. 1993;88:188–209.

261. Haan H, Streb J, Bien S, Rosler F. Individual cortical current density reconstructions of the semantic N400 effect: using a generalized minimum norm model with different constraints (L1 and L2 norm). Hum Brain Mapp. 2000;11(3):178–192.

262. Simos PG, Basile LF, Papanicolaou AC. Source localization of the N400 response in a sentence-reading paradigm using evoked magnetic fields and magnetic resonance imaging. Brain Res. 1997;762(1-2):29–39.

263. Helenius P, Salmelin R, Service E, Connolly JF. Semantic cortical activation in dyslexic readers. J Cogn Neurosci. 1999;11(5):535–550.

264. Halgren E, Dhond RP, Christensen N, et al. N400-like magnetoencephalography responses modulated by semantic context, word frequency, and lexical class in sentences. Neuroimage. 2002;17(3):1101–1116.

265. Dhond RP, Buckner RL, Dale AM, et al. Spatiotemporal maps of brain activity underlying word generation and their modification during repetition priming. J Neurosci. 2001;21(10):3564–3571.

266. Dale AM, Liu AK, Fischl BR, et al. Dynamic statistical parametric mapping: combining fMRI and MEG for high-resolution imaging of cortical activity. Neuron. 2000;26(1):55–67.

267. Ferjan Ramirez N, Leonard MK, Torres C, et al. Neural language processing in adolescent first-language learners. Cereb Cortex. 2014;24:2772–2783.

268. Travis KE, Leonard MK, Brown TT, et al. Spatiotemporal neural dynamics of word understanding in 12- to 18-month-old-infants. Cereb Cortex. 2011;21(8):1832–1839.

269. McCarthy G, Nobre AC, Bentin S, Spencer DD. Language-related field potentials in the anterior-medial temporal lobe: I. Intracranial distribution and neural generators. J Neurosci. 1995;15(2):1080–1089.

270. Nobre AC, McCarthy G. Language-related field potentials in the anterior-medial temporal lobe: II. Effects of word type and semantic priming. J Neurosci. 1995;15(2):1090–1098.

271. Fernandez G, Weyerts H, Tendolkar I, et al. Event-related potentials of verbal encoding into episodic memory: dissociation between the effects of subsequent memory performance and distinctiveness. Psychophysiology. 1998;35(6):709–720.

272. Grunwald T, Lehnertz K, Helmstaedter C, et al. Limbic ERPs predict verbal memory after left-sided hippocampectomy. Neuroreport. 1998;9(15):3375–3378.

273. Elger CE, Grunwald T, Lehnertz K, et al. Human temporal lobe potentials in verbal learning and memory processes. Neuropsychologia. 1997;35(5):657–667.

274. Puce A, Andrewes DG, Berkovic SF, Bladin PF. Visual recognition memory. Neurophysiological evidence for the role of temporal white matter in man. Brain. 1991;114(Pt 4):1647–1666.

275. Helmstaedter C, Grunwald T, Lehnertz K, et al. Differential involvement of left temporolateral and temporomesial structures in verbal declarative learning and memory: evidence from temporal lobe epilepsy. Brain Cogn. 1997;35(1):110–131.

276. Guillem F, Rougier A, Claverie B. Short- and long-delay intracranial ERP repetition effects dissociate memory systems in the human brain. J Cogn Neurosci. 1999;11(4):437–458.

277. Marinkovic K, Trebon P, Chauvel P, Halgren E. Localized face-processing by the human prefrontal cortex: 2. Face-selective intracerebral potentials and post-lesion deficits. Cogn Neuropsychol. 2000;17:187–199.

278. Guillem F, N'Kaoua B, Rougier A, Claverie B. Intracranial topography of event-related potentials (N400/P600) elicited during a continuous recognition memory task. Psychophysiology. 1995;32:382–392.

279. McDonald CR, Thesen T, Carlson C, et al. Multimodal imaging of repetition priming: Using fMRI, MEG, and intracranial EEG to reveal spatiotemporal profiles of word processing. Neuroimage. 2010;53(2):707–717.

280. Nenov VI, Halgren E, Smith ME, et al. Localized brain metabolic response correlated with potentials evoked by words. Behav Brain Res. 1991;44(1):101–104.

281. Frisch S, Hahne A, Friederici AD. Word category and verb—argument structure information in the dynamics of parsing. Cognition. 2004;91(3):191–219.

282. Pulvermuller F, Shtyrov Y, Hasting AS, Carlyon RP. Syntax as a reflex: neurophysiological evidence for early automaticity of grammatical processing. Brain Lang. 2008;104(3):244–253.

283. Steinhauer K, Drury JE. On the early left-anterior negativity (ELAN) in syntax studies. Brain Lang. 2012;120(2):135–162.

284. Osterhout L, Holcomb PJ. Event-related brain potentials elicited by syntactic anomaly. J Memory Language. 1992;31:785–806.

285. Friederici AD. Towards a neural basis of auditory sentence processing. Trends Cogn Sci. 2002;6(2):78–84.

286. Kaan E, Swaab TY. Repair, revision, and complexity in syntactic analysis: an electrophysiological differentiation. J Cogn Neurosci. 2003;15(1):98–110.

287. Hagoort P. Interplay between syntax and semantics during sentence comprehension: ERP effects of combining syntactic and semantic violations. J Cogn Neurosci. 2003;15(6):883–899.

288. Kuperberg GR. Neural mechanisms of language comprehension: challenges to syntax. Brain Res. 2007;1146:23–49.

289. Service E, Helenius P, Maury S, Salmelin R. Localization of syntactic and semantic brain responses using magnetoencephalography. J Cogn Neurosci. 2007;19(7):1193–1205.

290. Marinkovic K, Baldwin S, Courtney MG, et al. Right hemisphere has the last laugh: neural dynamics of joke appreciation. Cogn Affect Behav Neurosci. 2011;11(1):113–130.

291. Felleman DJ, VanEssen DC. Distributed hierarchical processing in the primate cerebral cortex. Cerebr Cortex. 1991;1:1–47.

292. Schroeder CE, Mehta AD, Givre SJ. A spatiotemporal profile of visual system activation revealed by current source density analysis in the awake macaque. Cereb Cortex. 1998;8(7):575–592.

293. Barth DS, Di S. Three-dimensional analysis of auditory-evoked potentials in rat neocortex. J Neurophysiol. 1990;64(5):1527–1536.

INDEX

Tables, figures, and boxes are indicated by an italic t, f, and b following the page/paragraph number.